Rosen's Emergency Medicine

Volume 3

ROSEN'S EMERGENCY MEDICINE

Concepts and Clinical Practice

sixth edition

Editor-in-Chief

John A. Marx, MD, FAAEM, FACEP
Chair and Chief
Department of Emergency Medicine
Carolinas Medical Center
Charlotte, North Carolina
Adjunct Professor
Department of Emergency Medicine
University of North Carolina School of Medicine
Chapel Hill, North Carolina

Senior Editors

Robert S. Hockberger, MD, FACEP, FAAEM
Chair
Department of Emergency Medicine
Harbor–UCLA Medical Center
Torrance, California
Professor of Clinical Medicine
David Geffen School of Medicine at UCLA
Westwood, Los Angeles, California

Ron M. Walls, MD, FAAEM, FACEP, FRCPC
Chair
Department of Emergency Medicine
Brigham and Women's Hospital
Associate Professor of Medicine (Emergency Medicine)
Harvard Medical School
Boston, Massachusetts

Editors

James G. Adams, MD, FACP, FACEP
Chair
Department of Emergency Medicine
Northwestern Memorial Hospital
Professor of Medicine
Northwestern University Feinberg School of Medicine
Chicago, Illinois

William G. Barsan, MD
Professor and Chair
Department of Emergency Medicine
University of Michigan Medical School
Ann Arbor, Michigan

Michelle H. Biros, MD, MS, FAAEM, FACEP
Research Director and Faculty Physician
Department of Emergency Medicine
Hennepin County Medical Center
Professor of Emergency Medicine
University of Minnesota Medical School
Minneapolis, Minnesota

Daniel F. Danzl, MD
Professor and Chair
Department of Emergency Medicine
University of Louisville School of Medicine
Louisville, Kentucky

Marianne Gausche-Hill, MD, FACEP, FAAP
Professor of Medicine
David Geffen School of Medicine at UCLA
Director of EMS and Pediatric Emergency Medicine Fellowship
Department of Emergency Medicine
Harbor–UCLA Medical Center
Torrance, California

Glenn C. Hamilton, MD, MSM
Professor and Chair
Department of Emergency Medicine
Wright State University School of Medicine
Dayton, Ohio

Louis J. Ling, MD, FACEP, FACMT
Professor of Emergency Medicine and Pharmacy
Associate Dean for Graduate Medical Education
University of Minnesota Medical School
Associate Medicine Director for Medical Education
Hennepin County Medical Center
Senior Associate Medical Director
Hennepin Regional Poison Center
Minneapolis, Minnesota

Edward J. Newton, MD, FACEP
Chair
Department of Emergency Medicine
Los Angeles County and University of Southern California Medical Center
Professor of Clinical Emergency Medicine
University of Southern California Keck School of Medicine
Los Angeles, California

MOSBY
ELSEVIER

MOSBY
ELSEVIER

1600 John F. Kennedy Boulevard, Suite 1800
Philadelphia, PA 19103-2899

ROSEN'S EMERGENCY MEDICINE: Concepts and Clinical Practice, 6th Edition
Three-Volume Set 0–323–02845–4
Online Edition 0–323–03686–4
E-dition 0–323–04302–X

Notice

Knowledge and best practice in this field are constantly changing. As new research and experience broaden our knowledge, changes in practice, treatment, and drug therapy may become necessary or appropriate. Readers are advised to check the most current information provided (i) on procedures featured or (ii) by the manufacturer of each product to be administered, to verify the recommended dose or formula, the method and duration of administration, and contraindications. It is the responsibility of the practitioner, relying on their own experience and knowledge of the patient, to make diagnoses, to determine dosages and the best treatment for each individual patient, and to take all appropriate safety precautions. To the fullest extent of the law, neither the Publisher nor the Editors and Authors assume any liability for any injury and/or damage to persons or property arising out of or related to any use of the material contained in this book.

Library of Congress Cataloging-in-Publication Data

Rosen's emergency medicine : concepts and clinical practice.—6th ed. / editor-in-chief, John A. Marx ; senior editors, Robert S. Hockberger, Ron M. Walls ; editors, James Adams . . . [et al.]
p. ; cm.
Includes bibliographical references and index.
ISBN 0-323-02845-4
1. Emergency medicine. I. Title: Emergency medicine. II. Marx, John A. III. Hockberger, Robert S. IV. Walls, Ron M. V. Adams, James. VI. Rosen, Peter Emergency medicine.
[DNLM: 1. Emergencies. 2. Emergency Medicine. WB 105 E555 2006]
RC86.7.E5784 2006
616.02′5—dc22 2005041694

Acquisitions Editor: Todd Hummel
Developmental Editor: Kimberly Cox
Publishing Services Manager: Frank Polizzano
Project Manager: Robin E. Hayward
Cover Design Direction: Steven Stave
Text Designer: Jayne Jones
Marketing Manager: Dana Butler

Printed in China

Last digit is the print number: 9 8 7 6 5 4 3 2 1

Contents

Volume 1

PART ONE
Fundamental Clinical Concepts

Section I
Critical Management Principles **2**

Chapter 1
Airway **2**
Ron M. Walls

Chapter 2
Mechanical Ventilation and Noninvasive Ventilatory Support **26**
Charles V. Pollack, Jr.

Chapter 3
Monitoring the Emergency Patient **35**
Michael F. Murphy and Timothy A. D. Graham

Chapter 4
Shock... **41**
Alan E. Jones and Jeffrey A. Kline

Chapter 5
Blood and Blood Components **56**
Gwendolyn L. Hoffman

Chapter 6
Brain Resuscitation **62**
Robert Silbergleit and Norman S. Abramson

Chapter 7
Adult Resuscitation **75**
Robert W. Neumar and Kevin R. Ward

Chapter 8
Pediatric Resuscitation **97**
Brian P. Gilligan and Robert C. Luten

Chapter 9
Neonatal Resuscitation **118**
Eileen Klein and Linda Quan

Section II
Cardinal Presentations **125**

Chapter 10
Clinical Decision Making **125**
Dane M. Chapman, Douglas M. Char, and Chandra D. Aubin

Chapter 11
Fever in the Adult Patient **134**
Frederick C. Blum

Chapter 12
Weakness **138**
Robert C. Reiser

Chapter 13
Dizziness and Vertigo **142**
Jonathan S. Olshaker

Chapter 14
Confusion **150**
J. Stephen Huff and William J. Brady

Chapter 15
Coma and Depressed Level of Consciousness **156**
Richard E. Wolfe and David F. M. Brown

Chapter 16
Seizures **164**
Charles V. Pollack, Jr.

Chapter 17
Headache **169**
Gregory L. Henry and Christopher S. Russi

Chapter 18
Dyspnea **175**
Sabina Braithwaite and Debra Perina

Chapter 19
Chest Pain **183**
James E. Brown and Glenn C. Hamilton

Chapter 20
Syncope **193**
Robert A. De Lorenzo

Chapter 21
Nausea and Vomiting **200**
Leslie S. Zun and Amardeep Singh

Chapter 22
Abdominal Pain **209**
Kelly E. King and John M. Wightman

Chapter 23
Gastrointestinal Bleeding **220**
Philip L. Henneman

Chapter 24
Diarrhea 227
John E. Gough and Phillip A. Clement

Chapter 25
Constipation 237
Natalie Cullen

Chapter 26
Jaundice 243
Katherine L. Heilpern and Tammie E. Quest

Chapter 27
Acute Pelvic Pain 248
Robert Dart

Chapter 28
Vaginal Bleeding 254
John C. Bradford and Christ G. Kyriakedes

Chapter 29
Back Pain 260
Kevin G. Rodgers and James B. Jones

Chapter 30
Cyanosis 268
Jennifer Bocock and Joan Kolodzik

Chapter 31
Sore Throat 274
Jonathan I. Singer and Mark E. Gebhart

Chapter 32
Hemoptysis 279
Brian Springer and Timothy G. Janz

Chapter 33
Red and Painful Eye 283
John M. Wightman and Glenn C. Hamilton

PART TWO
Trauma

Section I
General Concepts 300

Chapter 34
Multiple Trauma 300
Susan L. Gin-Shaw and Robert C. Jorden

Chapter 35
Trauma in Pregnancy 316
John D. G. Neufeld

Chapter 36
Pediatric Trauma 328
Richard M. Cantor

Chapter 37
Geriatric Trauma 344
Diane M. Birnbaumer

Section II
System Injuries 349

Chapter 38
Head 349
William G. Heegaard and Michelle H. Biros

Chapter 39
Facial Trauma 382
Mary Pat McKay

Chapter 40
Spinal Injuries 398
Robert S. Hockberger, Amy H. Kaji,
and Edward J. Newton

Chapter 41
Neck 441
Kim Newton

Chapter 42
Thoracic Trauma 453
Marc Eckstein and Sean Henderson

Chapter 43
Abdominal Trauma 489
John A. Marx and Jennifer Isenhour

Chapter 44
Genitourinary System 514
Robert E. Schneider

Chapter 45
Peripheral Vascular Injury 536
Edward J. Newton

Section III
Orthopedic Lesions 549

Chapter 46
General Principles of Orthopedic
Injuries 549
Joel M. Geiderman

Chapter 47
Hand 576
Everett Lyn and Robert E. Antosia

Chapter 48
Wrist and Forearm 622
Karen G. H. Woolfrey and Mary A. Eisenhauer

Chapter 49
Humerus and Elbow 647
Joel M. Geiderman

Chapter 50
Shoulder 670
Mohamud Daya

Chapter 51
Musculoskeletal Back Pain 701
Michelle Lin

Chapter 52
Pelvis 717
A. Adam Cwinn

Chapter 53
Femur and Hip 735
Michael A. Gibbs, Edward J. Newton, and James F. Fiechtl

Chapter 54
Knee and Lower Leg 770
Everett Lyn, Daniel Pallin, and Robert E. Antosia

Chapter 55
Ankle and Foot 808
Kendall Ho and Riyad B. Abu-Laban

Section IV
Soft Tissue Injuries 842

Chapter 56
Wound Management Principles 842
Barry Simon and H. Gene Hern, Jr.

Chapter 57
Foreign Bodies 859
Stephen H. Thomas and David F. M. Brown

Chapter 58
Mammalian Bites 882
Ellon J. Wobor

Chapter 59
Venomous Animal Injuries 894
Edward J. Otten

Chapter 60
Thermal Burns 913
Richard F. Edlich, Marcus L. Martin, and William B. Long III

Chapter 61
Chemical Injuries 929
Richard F. Edlich, Marcus L. Martin, and William B. Long III

Section V
Violence and Abuse 940

Chapter 62
Injury Prevention and Control 940
Stephen W. Hargarten and Jeffrey W. Runge

Chapter 63
Forensic Emergency Medicine 952
William S. Smock

Chapter 64
Child Maltreatment 968
Carol D. Berkowitz

Chapter 65
Sexual Assault 977
Laura Slaughter

Chapter 66
Intimate Partner Violence and Abuse 994
Patricia R. Salber

Chapter 67
Elder Abuse and Neglect 1008
Deirdre Anglin and Diana C. Schneider

Chapter 68
Youth, Gangs, and Violence 1017
H. Range Hutson

Index i

Volume 2

PART THREE
Medicine and Surgery

Section I
Head and Neck Disorders 1026

Chapter 69
Oral Medicine 1026
James T. Amsterdam

Chapter 70
Ophthalmology 1044
Douglas D. Brunette

Chapter 71
Otolaryngology 1066
James A. Pfaff and Gregory P. Moore

Section II
Pulmonary System 1078

Chapter 72
Asthma 1078
Richard M. Nowak and Glenn Tokarski

Chapter 73
Chronic Obstructive Pulmonary Disease 1097
Stuart P. Swadron and Diku P. Mandavia

Chapter 74
Upper Respiratory Tract Infections 1109
Frantz R. Melio

Chapter 75
Pneumonia 1128
Gregory J. Moran and David A. Talan

Chapter 76
Pleural Disease 1143
Joshua M. Kosowsky

Section III
Cardiac System 1154

Chapter 77
Acute Coronary Syndromes 1154
William J. Brady, Richard A. Harrigan, and Theodore Chan

Chapter 78
Dysrhythmias **1199**
Donald M. Yealy and Theodore R. Delbridge

Chapter 79
Implantable Cardiac Devices................. **1246**
James T. Niemann

Chapter 80
Heart Failure **1258**
John F. O'Brien and Jay L. Falk

Chapter 81
Pericardial and Myocardial Disease **1280**
Nicholas J. Jouriles

Chapter 82
Infective Endocarditis and Valvular Heart Disease **1300**
Susan M. Dunmire

Section IV
Vascular System............................... 1310

Chapter 83
Hypertension **1310**
Richard O. Gray

Chapter 84
Aortic Dissection **1324**
Felix Ankel

Chapter 85
Abdominal Aortic Aneurysm **1330**
Howard A. Bessen

Chapter 86
Peripheral Arteriovascular Disease **1342**
Tom P. Aufderheide

Chapter 87
Pulmonary Embolism and Deep Venous Thrombosis **1368**
Jeffrey A. Kline and Michael S. Runyon

Section V
Gastrointestinal System 1382

Chapter 88
Esophagus, Stomach, and Duodenum **1382**
Mark J. Lowell

Chapter 89
Liver and Biliary Tract **1402**
David A. Guss

Chapter 90
Pancreas **1426**
Sally A. Santen and Robin R. Hemphill

Chapter 91
Disorders of the Small Intestine **1440**
Susan P. Torrey and Philip L. Henneman

Chapter 92
Acute Appendicitis **1451**
Jeannette M. Wolfe and Philip L. Henneman

Chapter 93
Acute Gastroenteritis **1460**
Robert A. Bitterman and David K. Zich

Chapter 94
Large Intestine **1490**
Michael A. Peterson

Chapter 95
Anorectum **1507**
Wendy C. Coates

Section VI
Genitourinary System 1524

Chapter 96
Renal Failure **1524**
Allan B. Wolfson

Chapter 97
Sexually Transmitted Diseases **1556**
Diane M. Birnbaumer and Christine Anderegg

Chapter 98
Selected Urologic Problems **1572**
John Kahler and Ann L. Harwood-Nuss

Section VII
Neurology...................................... 1606

Chapter 99
Stroke **1606**
Rashmi U. Kothari, Todd J. Crocco, and William G. Barsan

Chapter 100
Seizures... **1619**
Charles V. Pollack, Jr.

Chapter 101
Headache **1631**
Thomas Kwiatkowski and Kumar Alagappan

Chapter 102
Delirium and Demetia **1645**
Jeffrey Smith and Jennifer Seirafi

Chapter 103
Brain and Cranial Nerve Disorders **1664**
Brian Stettler and Arthur M. Pancioli

Chapter 104
Spinal Cord Disorders **1675**
Andrew D. Perron and J. Stephen Huff

Chapter 105
Peripheral Nerve Disorders **1687**
E. John Gallagher

Chapter 106
Neuromuscular Disorders **1702**
Peter Shearer and Andrew Jagoda

Chapter 107
Central Nervous System Infections **1710**
Frank W. Lavoie and John R. Saucier

Section VIII
Psychiatric and Behavioral Disorders **1726**

Chapter 108
Thought Disorders **1726**
Robert S. Hockberger and John R. Richards

Chapter 109
Mood Disorders **1734**
Douglas A. Rund and Marshall G. Vary

Chapter 110
Anxiety Disorders **1744**
Eugene E. Kercher and Joshua L. Tobias

Chapter 111
Somatoform Disorders **1753**
Thomas B. Purcell

Chapter 112
Factitious Disorders and Malingering **1761**
Thomas B. Purcell

Chapter 113
Suicide **1766**
Stephen A. Colucciello

Section IX
Immunologic and Inflammatory **1776**

Chapter 114
Arthritis **1776**
Douglas W. Lowery III

Chapter 115
Tendinopathy and Bursitis **1794**
Ted Koutouzis and Stephen L. Adams

Chapter 116
Systemic Lupus Erythematosus and the Vasculitides **1805**
Clare T. Sercombe

Chapter 117
Allergy, Hypersensitivity, and Anaphylaxis **1818**
T. Paul Tran and Robert L. Muelleman

Chapter 118
Dermatologic Presentations **1838**
Rita K. Cydulka and Mary Hancock

Section X
Hematology and Oncology **1867**

Chapter 119
Anemia, Polycythemia, and White Blood Cell Disorders **1867**
Glenn C. Hamilton and Timothy G. Janz

Chapter 120
Disorders of Hemostasis **1892**
Timothy G. Janz and Glenn C. Hamilton

Chapter 121
Selected Oncologic Emergencies **1907**
Nnamdi Nkwuo, Neil Schamban, and Marc Borenstein

Section XI
Metabolism and Endocrinology **1922**

Chapter 122
Acid-Base Disorders **1922**
Jamie L. Collings

Chapter 123
Electrolyte Disturbances **1933**
Michael A. Gibbs and Vivek S. Tayal

Chapter 124
Diabetes Mellitus and Disorders of Glucose Homeostasis **1955**
Rita K. Cydulka and Jeffrey Pennington

Chapter 125
Rhabdomyolysis **1975**
Laura J. Bontempo

Chapter 126
Thyroid and Adrenal Disorders **1985**
Jeffrey Sternlicht and John M. Wogan

Section XII
Infectious Disease **2001**

Chapter 127
Bacteria **2001**
Madonna Fernández-Frackelton

Chapter 128
Viruses **2033**
Michael Alan Polis and Tenagne Haile-Mariam

Chapter 129
Rabies **2061**
Ellen J. Weber

Chapter 130
AIDS and HIV 2071
Richard E. Rothman, Catherine A. Marco, Samuel Yang, and Gabor D. Kelen

Chapter 131
Parasites 2096
Bruce M. Becker and John D. Cahill

Chapter 132
Tick-Borne Illnesses 2116
Edward B. Bolgiano and Joseph Sexton

Chapter 133
Tuberculosis 2145
Peter E. Sokolove and Dennis Chan

Chapter 134
Bone and Joint Infections 2174
Brian J. Zink

Chapter 135
Soft Tissue Infections 2195
Harvey W. Meislin and John A. Guisto

Chapter 136
Sepsis Syndromes 2211
Nathan I. Shapiro, Gary D. Zimmer, and Adam Z. Barkin

Index i

Volume 3

PART FOUR
Environment and Toxicology

Section I
Environment 2228

Chapter 137
Frostbite 2228
Daniel F. Danzl

Chapter 138
Accidental Hypothermia 2236
Daniel F. Danzl

Chapter 139
Heat Illness 2254
Salvator Vicario

Chapter 140
Electrical and Lightning Injuries 2267
Timothy G. Price and Mary Ann Cooper

Chapter 141
Scuba Diving and Dysbarism 2279
Lee W. Shockley

Chapter 142
High-Altitude Medicine 2296
Michael Yaron and Benjamin Honigman

Chapter 143
Submersion 2311
Andrew L. Knaut and Kim M. Feldhaus

Chapter 144
Radiation Injuries 2316
Vincent Markovchick

Section II
Toxicology 2325

Chapter 145
General Approach to the Poisoned Patient 2325
Ken Kulig

Chapter 146
Acetaminophen 2331
Kenneth E. Bizovi and Robert Hendrickson

Chapter 147
Aspirin and Nonsteroidal Agents 2339
Donna L. Seger and Lindsay Murray

Chapter 148
Anticholinergics 2345
Wilfredo Rivera and Larissa I. Velez

Chapter 149
Antidepressants 2352
Elisabeth F. Bilden and Frank G. Walter

Chapter 150
Cardiovascular Drugs 2368
David J. Roberts

Chapter 151
Caustics 2380
Paul M. Wax and Sandra M. Schneider

Chapter 152
Cocaine and Other Sympathomimetics 2386
Rama B. Rao and Robert S. Hoffman

Chapter 153
Toxic Alchohols 2395
Suzanne R. White and Joseph Kosnik

Chapter 154
Hallucinogens 2406
Binh T. Ly, Richard F. Clark, and Saralyn R. Williams

Chapter 155
Heavy Metals 2418
Larissa I. Velez and Kathleen A. Delaney

Chapter 156
Hydrocarbons 2428
David C. Lee

Chapter 157
Inhaled Toxins 2432
Lewis S: Nelson and Robert S. Hoffman

Chapter 158
Lithium 2442
Keith K. Burkhart

Chapter 159
Antipsychotics 2445
Mary A. Wittler and Eric J. Lavonas

Chapter 160
Opioids 2451
Christina E. Hantsch

Chapter 161
Pesticides 2457
Cynthia K. Aaron

Chapter 162
Plants, Mushrooms, and Herbal Medications 2471
Richard D. Shih

Chapter 163
Sedative Hypnotics 2481
Leon Gussow and Andrea Carlson

PART FIVE
Special Populations

Section I
The Pediatric Patient 2494

Chapter 164
General Approach to the Pediatric Patient 2494
Robert A. Wiebe

Chapter 165
Fever 2505
Roger M. Barkin and D. Demetrios Zukin

Chapter 166
Pediatric Respiratory Emergencies: Upper Airway Obstruction and Infections 2519
Mariann Manno

Chapter 167
Pediatric Respiratory Emergencies: Lower Airway Obstruction 2532
Christine D. Darr

Chapter 168
Pediatric Respiratory Emergencies: Disease of the Lungs 2554
Susan Kirelik and Brian Alverson

Chapter 169
Cardiac Disorders 2567
Alson S. Inaba

Chapter 170
Gastrointestinal Disorders 2601
Mark A. Hostetler

Chapter 171
Infectious Diarrheal Disease and Dehydration 2623
Roger M. Barkin and David G. Ward

Chapter 172
Renal and Genitourinary Tract Disorders 2635
Maureen McCollough and Ghazala Sharieff

Chapter 173
Neurologic Disorders 2657
David H. Rubin, Dina Halpern Kornblau, Edward E. Conway, Jr., and Stuart M. Caplen

Chapter 174
Musculoskeletal Disorders.................... 2689
Kemedy K. McQuillen

Chapter 175
Sudden Infant Death Syndrome and Apparent Life-Threatening Events 2713
Marianne Gausche-Hill

Section II
The Pregnant Patient 2722

Chapter 176
General Approach to the Pregnant Patient 2722
Laurie J. Morrison

Chapter 177
Acute Complications of Pregnancy 2739
Debra E. Houry and Jean T. Abbott

Chapter 178
Chronic Medical Illness During Pregnancy....................................... 2761
Edward J. Newton and Kirsten K. Calder

Chapter 179
Drug Therapy and Substance Abuse 2779
Rania Habal and Diane Sauter

Chapter 180
Labor and Delivery and Their Complications 2797
Sean Henderson and William K. Mallon

Section III
The Geriatric Patient 2824

Chapter 181
The Elder Patient............................... 2824
Diane M. Birnbaumer

Section IV
The Patient with Compromised Immune Function 2831

Chapter 182
The Immunocompromised Patient 2831
Michael J. Burns and Mark I. Langdorf

Section V
The Patient with an Organ Transplant...................................... 2846

Chapter 183
The Solid-Organ Transplant Patient 2846
Matthew T. Keadey and Douglas W. Lowery III

Section VI
The Alcoholic or Substance Abuse Patient.. 2858

Chapter 184
Alcohol-Related Disease 2858
David B. McMicken and John T. Finnell

Chapter 185
Substance Abuse 2882
Stephen A. Colucciello and Christian Tomaszewski

Section VII
The Developmentally or Physically Disabled Patient 2898

Chapter 186
Evaluation of the Developmentally and Physically Disabled Patient 2898
Maria Stephan

Section VIII
The Patient in Pain 2913

Chapter 187
Pain Management 2913
Paul M. Paris and Donald M. Yealy

Chapter 188
Procedural Sedation and Analgesia 2938
Carl R. Chudnofsky and Marie M. Lozon

Section IX
The Problem Patient 2956

Chapter 189
The Combative Patient 2956
Gregory P. Moore and Louise Kao

Chapter 190
The Difficult Patient............................ 2972
David W. Harrison and Robert J. Vissers

PART SIX
Emergency Medical Services

Chapter 191
Emergency Medical Service: Overview and Ground Transport 2984
Thomas H. Blackwell

Chapter 192
Air Medical Transport.......................... 2994
Howard Rodenberg and Ira J. Blumen

Chapter 193
Tactical Emergency Medical Support and Urban Search and Rescue 3000
Richard Schwartz, John G. McManus, and Jeffrey Orledge

Chapter 194
Disaster Preparedness 3010
Carl H. Schultz, Kristi L. Koenig, and Eric K. Noji

Chapter 195
Weapons of Mass Destruction 3021
Carl H. Schultz and Kristi L. Koenig

PART SEVEN
The Practice of Emergency Medicine

Section I
Clinical Practice and Administration 3034

Chapter 196
Guidelines in Emergency Medicine 3034
J. Stephen Bohan

Chapter 197
Medical Literature and Evidence-Based Medicine 3046
Kelly D. Young and Roger J. Lewis

Chapter 198
Observation Medicine and Clinical Decision Units 3062
Malcolm Mahadevan and Louis Graff

Chapter 199
Occupational Medicine and Occupational Health in the Emergency Department 3076
Andrew R. Barnosky, Daniel K. Chapman, and Victor S. Roth

Chapter 200
Hyperbaric Medicine 3088
Enoch T. Huang and Stephen R. Thom

Chapter 201
The Social Role of Emergency Medicine 3092
James A. Gordon

Chapter 202
Information Technology in Emergency Medicine **3097**
Jonathan M. Teich and William H. Cordell

Chapter 203
Multiculturalism and Care Delivery **3107**
Edward Bernstein, Judith Bernstein, and Thea James

Chapter 204
Process Improvement and Patient Safety in the Emergency Department **3119**
Pat Croskerry, Marc J. Shapiro, Shawna J. Perry, and Robert L. Wears

Section II
Philosophical Issues of Practice **3127**

Chapter 205
Bioethics **3127**
Kenneth V. Iserson

Chapter 206
End of Life **3139**
Jean T. Abbott and Susan Stone

Chapter 207
Medicolegal and Risk Management **3156**
Robert A. Bitterman

Chapter 208
Wellness, Stress, and the Impaired Physician **3174**
Richard Goldberg

Index .... **i**

PART FOUR

Environment and Toxicology

CHAPTER 137

Frostbite

Daniel F. Danzl

PERSPECTIVE

Peripheral cold injuries occur primarily in humans. The highest homeostatic priority is to maintain the body's core temperature. This is accomplished through vasoconstriction and shunting, which prevents adequate heat distribution to the extremities. Therefore, unlike cold-adapted animals, the peripheral tissue temperatures of humans can drop below freezing. As a result, failure to achieve adequate protection from the environment results in injuries that are usually preventable.[1-3]

Peripheral cold injuries include both freezing and nonfreezing syndromes, which may occur independently or in conjunction with systemic hypothermia. Frostbite is the most common freezing injury. Trench foot and immersion foot are nonfreezing injuries that result from exposure to wet cold. Nonfreezing injury that occurs after exposure to dry cold is termed *chilblains* (pernio).

The incidence and severity of frostbite correlate with the predisposing factors associated with the cold stress. Most cases of civilian frostbite result from routine exposure to cold by individuals who have not given due consideration to risk factors for cold injury.[4] Well-equipped treks up the world's highest peaks have been completed without cold injury when appropriate steps are taken to address these factors.[5] Current trends show an increase in outdoor recreational activities that produce exposure to unanticipated drastic climatic changes.[6] Unsheltered and homeless people are no longer the most likely group at risk.

Military history is replete with accounts of the effects of cold injury on combat troops. Amputations and time lost to local cold injuries in both World Wars and the Korean conflict were extensive. Trench foot was particularly common among the Royal Marines in the Falkland Islands and United States troops in the Vietnam War.

Napoleon's surgeon general, Baron de Larrey, first recorded the disastrous effects of the freeze-thaw-refreeze cycle.[7] During the 1812 to 1813 Russian invasion and retreat, soldiers would acutely thaw frozen extremities directly over open fires. The subsequent refreeze further increased tissue destruction. Unfortunately, the resultant gangrene was misattributed to this rapid thawing of frostbite and trench foot injuries. Therefore, gradual thawing, often including friction massage with snow, remained the standard treatment regimen until the 1950s.[8,9]

In addition to dry radiant heat rewarming and massage, another misdirected rewarming modality was immersion thawing in icy water. In 1961, Mills ultimately popularized rapid warm immersion rewarming after extensive experience with severe Alaskan frostbite cases.[9,10]

PRINCIPLES OF DISEASE

Physiology

Human cold stress should produce adaptive behavioral reactions such as an attempt to find heat or shelter. In addition, complex endocrinologic and cardiovascular physiologic responses are engaged. Peripheral cooling of the blood activates the pre-optic anterior hypothalamus. This central thermostat orchestrates temperature regulation. This dynamic process encompasses catecholamine release, thyroid stimulation, shivering thermogenesis, and peripheral vasoconstriction.

Cutaneous circulation is one of the keys to maintaining thermoneutrality. Baseline cutaneous circulation greatly exceeds the nutritional requirements. This reflects the skin's "radiator" function to maintain thermostability. Cutaneous blood flow in the euthermic 70 kg human averages 200 to 250 mL/min. Heat stress causes vasodilation that can increase this amount to 7000 mL/min. In contrast, extreme cold-induced vasoconstriction reduces flow 10-fold to less than 50 mL/min.

During cold stress, peripheral vasoconstriction limits radiant heat loss. Acral skin structures (fingers, toes, ears, nose) contain a plethora of arteriovenous anastomoses. These facilitate shunting and subsequent drastic reductions in blood flow to these areas. This "life-vs.-limb" mechanism reflects the homeostatic attempt to prevent systemic hypothermia.

In contrast to heat exposure, humans do not appear to display significant physiologic adaptation to the cold. Exposing extremities to cold temperatures down to 15° C results in maximal peripheral vasoconstriction with minimal blood flow. Continued exposure to progressively colder temperatures down to 10° C produces the "hunting response," which is termed *cold-induced vasodilation*. These periods of vasodilation, recurring in 5-minute to 10-minute cycles, interrupt vasoconstriction and serve to protect the extremity. Eskimos, as well as Lapps and others of Nordic extraction, are capable of stronger cold-induced vasodilation responses than individuals from tropical regions.[11]

BOX 137-1. Freezing Injury Cascade

Prefreeze Phase
Superficial tissue "cooling"
Increased viscosity of vascular contents
Microvascular constriction
Endothelial plasma leakage

Freeze-Thaw Phase
*Extra*cellular fluid ice-crystal formation*
Water diapedesis across cell membrane
*Intra*cellular dehydration and hyperosmolality
Cell membrane denaturation or disruption
Cell shrinkage and collapse

Vascular Stasis and Progressive Ischemia
Vasospasticity and stasis coagulation
Arteriovenous shunting
Vascular endothelial cell damage or prostanoid release
Interstitial leakage or tissue hypertension
Necrosis, demarcation, mummification, or slough

*Extremely rapid cooling produces more initial intracellular than extracellular ice crystallization.

Pathophysiology

The pathologic phases that occur with local cold injury often overlap and vary with the extent and rapidity of the cold response (Box 137-1). Frostbite occurs when the tissue temperature drops to less than 0° C. There are two putative mechanisms of tissue injury: architectural cellular damage from ice-crystal formation and microvascular thrombosis and stasis.

In the *prefreeze* phase, tissue temperatures drop below 10° C and cutaneous sensation is lost. Before ice-crystal formation, microvascular vasoconstriction occurs along with endothelial leakage of plasma into the interstitium. Radiation and conduction of heat from deeper tissues prevent crystallization until the skin temperature drops well below 0° C.

In the *freeze-thaw* phase, the timing, location, and rate of ice-crystal formation depend on the exposure circumstances. In addition to ambient temperatures, wind and moisture increase the freezing rate. Skin must cool below 0° C to freeze because of the underlying radiation of heat.[11]

During usual exposure conditions, ice-crystal formation initially occurs extracellularly. This results in diapedesis of water exiting the cell to maintain osmotic equilibrium. Cellular dehydration increases the intracellular osmolarity and electrolyte concentrations. When approximately one third of the cellular volume is lost, cellular collapse and death result. This may occur with or without direct architectural damage from the crystals. Extracellular crystallization also increases the tissue pressure on cell membranes and surrounding vascular structures.

Sludging, stasis, and cessation of flow are initiated at the capillary level. The third phase, progressive microvascular collapse, first affects venules and then arterioles. Red blood cells sludge and form microthrombi during the first few hours after the tissues are thawed. Factors adversely affecting flow include hypoxic vasospasm, hyperviscosity, and direct endothelial cell damage. Anaerobic metabolism subsequently extends the surrounding injury. Tissues are deprived of nutrients and oxygen. Ultimately, plasma leakage and arteriovenous shunting result in thrombosis, increased tissue pressure, ischemia, and necrosis.

Some direct skin injury is reversible. For example, frozen skin grafted to a normal site can survive. Zones immediately surrounding injured areas are potentially salvageable. The histopathology of frostbite suggests that some changes in the epidermis are primary and some reflect damage to the endothelial cells. During initiation of rewarming, these tissues are revitalized.

An additional insult, progressive dermal ischemia, is partially mediated by thromboxane.[12] Fluid analysis of clear vesicles suggests that prostaglandins are involved. When subdermal vascular plexi are injured, hemorrhagic blisters develop that also contain these prostanoids. The arachidonic acid breakdown products released from underlying damaged tissue into the blister fluid include both prostaglandins and thromboxane. These mediators produce platelet aggregation, vasoconstriction, and leukocyte immobilization.[13]

The ultimate determinant of progressive tissue damage appears to be injury to the microvasculature. Endothelial cells are the tissue most susceptible to freezing injury.[14] After thawing, the vasculature is patent only temporarily. Platelet and erythrocyte aggregates promptly clog and distort the vasculature. Intense vasoconstriction coupled with arteriovenous shunting occurs at the interface between normal and damaged tissue. The injured viable vasculature remains distorted. Local arteritis, medial degeneration, and intimal proliferative thickening are seen.

Nerve and muscle tissues are more susceptible to cold injury than connective tissue. For example, nonviable hands and feet can be moved after thawing if the tendons are intact.

Edema progresses for 48 to 72 hours after tissue has been thawed. Leukocyte infiltration, thrombosis, and early necrosis become apparent as this edema resolves. The dry gangrene carapace of frostbite is superficial in comparison to arteriosclerotic-induced, full-thickness gangrene. Final demarcation between viable and nonviable tissue can require more than 60 to 90 days, hence the historical surgical aphorism, "Frostbite in January, amputate in July."[10]

Predisposing Factors

The extent of peripheral cold injury is determined by the type and duration of cold contact with the skin (Box 137-2).

Any conditions affecting judgment can jeopardize the physiologically tropical human. In urban settings, cold injuries are often attributed to overt or covert psychiatric impairment or ingestion of intoxicants.[15] Ethanol also produces peripheral vasodilation, which increases heat loss. Whenever self-protective instincts are blunted, appropriate adaptive maneuvers may not be undertaken.

BOX 137-2. Predisposing Factors

Physiologic
Genetic
Core temperature
Previous cold injury
± Acclimatization
Dehydration
Overexertion
Trauma: multisystem, extremity
Dermatologic diseases
Physical conditioning
Diaphoresis, hyperhidrosis
Hypoxia

Mechanical
Constricting or wet clothing
Tight boots
Vapor barrier, alveolite liners
Inadequate insulation
Immobility or cramped positioning

Psychological
Mental status
Fear, panic
Attitude
Peer pressure
Fatigue
Intense concentration on tasks
Hunger, malnutrition
Intoxicants

Environmental
Ambient temperature
Humidity
Duration of exposure
Wind chill factor
Altitude ± associated conditions
Quantity of exposed surface area
Heat loss: conductive, evaporative`
Aerosol propellants

Cardiovascular
Hypotension
Atherosclerosis
Arteritis
Raynaud's syndrome
Cold-induced vasodilation
Anemia
Sickle cell disease
Diabetes
Hypovolemia, shock
Vasoconstrictors, vasodilators

Direct skin contact with good thermal conductors such as metal, water, and volatile liquids affects the extent and rapidity of tissue destruction.[11] Commercial aerosol spray propellants such as propane and butane are potentially hazardous. Clinicians will see more frostbite from these agents as they replace chlorohydrofluorocarbons. One passenger on a commercial airline flight suffered a full-thickness lumbar injury from a "cold pack" provided by the stewardess that contained dry ice.[16] Overenthusiastic application of standard ice packs while treating soft tissue injuries can also result in tissue loss. Although air alone is a poor thermal conductor, associated cold and wind (windchill index) markedly increase heat loss.

CLINICAL FEATURES

Symptoms and Signs

The symptoms of frostbite usually reflect the severity of the exposure. The most common presenting symptom is numbness, present in more than 75% of patients. All patients have some initial sensory deficiency in light touch, pain, or temperature. Anesthesia is produced by intense vasoconstrictive ischemia and neurapraxia. Acral areas and distal extremities are the usual insensate sites. The distal extremities—the nose, ears, and penis—are specific locations at risk.[11,17]

Patients often complain of clumsiness and report a "chunk of wood" sensation in the extremity. The history of complete acute anesthesia in a painful cold digit suggests a severe injury.

"Frostnip" is a superficial cold insult manifested by transient numbness and tingling that resolves after rewarming. This does not represent true frostbite, because no tissue destruction occurs.

Significant pain usually accompanies reestablishment of perfusion. With partial tissue destruction, intermittent pain may be noticed during ongoing exposure. The dull continuous ache evolves into a throbbing sensation in 48 to 72 hours. This often persists until tissue demarcation several weeks to months later.

Chilblains (pernio) is a mild form of dry-cold injury that often follows repetitive exposure. These "cold sores" appear less than 24 hours after exposure and usually affect facial areas, the dorsa of the hands and feet, and the pretibial areas. Young women with a history of Raynaud's phenomenon are especially at risk. Persistent vasospasm and vasculitis result in pruritus, erythema, and mild edema. Plaques, blue nodules, and ulcerations can develop.

Management of the chilblain syndrome is usually supportive. Nifedipine (20-60 mg daily) may be an effective treatment for refractory perniosis.[18] Topical or systemic corticosteroids have also been useful. Other options include oral pentoxifylline or limaprost, a prostaglandin E_1 analogue.

The other common nonfreezing cold injury is trench foot (immersion foot). This remains a significant threat during recreational activities and expeditions in cold, wet climates.[19] Trench foot is produced by prolonged exposure to wet cold at temperatures above freezing. It usually develops slowly over several days and results in neurovascular damage in the absence of ice-crystal formation. Immersion foot commonly develops while a person is wearing sweat-dampened or neoprene socks, vapor-barrier boots, or constrictive gaiters.[20]

The clinical presentation varies. Most patients' symptoms include cool, pale feet that are numb or tingle. Later the feet appear cyanotic, cold, and edematous. Often, numbness and leg cramping are present. The clinical hallmark is that, after rewarming, the skin remains erythematous, dry, and very painful to touch. Rubor on dependency and pallor on elevation are caused by vasomotor paralysis.

Bullae that are indistinguishable from those seen with frostbite commonly develop. Vesiculation proceeds to ulceration and liquefaction gangrene in severe cases.[11] Protracted symptoms of pain during weight bearing, cold sensitivity, and hyperhidrosis often last for years. Prevention of trench foot often simply requires continual drying of socks.

Classically, the initial presentation of frostbite is deceptively benign. Most patients do not arrive in the emergency department with frozen, insensate tissue. Frozen tissues often appear mottled or violaceous-white, waxy, or pale yellow. In severe cases, the examiner will not be able to roll the dermis over bony prominences. Rapid rewarming results in an initial hyperemia, even in severe cases. After thawing, partial return of sensation should be expected until blebs form.[10]

Favorable initial symptoms include normal sensation, warmth, and color. Soft, pliable subcutaneous tissue suggests a superficial injury. A residual violaceous hue after rewarming is ominous. Early formation of clear large blebs that extend to the tips of the digits are more favorable than delayed appearance of small hemorrhagic blebs. These dark vesicles are produced by damage to the subdermal vascular plexi. Vesicles and large bullae eventually form in 6 to 24 hours.

Lack of edema formation suggests significant tissue damage. Post-thaw edema usually develops in less than 3 hours. In severe cases, frostbitten skin forms an early black, dry eschar until mummification and apparent demarcation.

Historically, frostbite, like burns, has been classified into degrees of injury. Anesthesia and erythema are characteristic of first-degree frostbite. Superficial vesiculation surrounded by edema and erythema is considered second-degree. Third-degree frostbite produces deeper hemorrhagic vesicles. Fourth-degree injuries extend into subcuticular, osseous, and muscle tissues.

Classification by degrees is often incorrect in relation to the actual severity of the frostbite and thus therapeutically misleading. Mills suggests two simple classifications.[9,10] Superficial or mild frostbite does not entail eventual tissue loss, whereas deep or severe frostbite does result in tissue loss. These frostbite classifications, however, are based on retrospective analysis. As a result, it is not feasible to predict, on presentation, the eventual tissue loss. A new classification attempts to establish severity based on clinical features coupled with early bone scan results.[21]

DIAGNOSTIC STRATEGIES

Many ancillary diagnostic imaging techniques have been used in an attempt to diagnose the severity of injury. Unfortunately, none consistently and accurately predict tissue loss at the time of initial examination.

Routine baseline radiographs should be obtained, and at follow-up radiographs will begin to demonstrate specific frostbite abnormalities 4 to 10 weeks after injury. Intravenous isotope studies have mixed success experimentally and clinically.[22,23] In one study, triple-phase bone scans performed 2 days after cold injury demonstrate ischemic tissue at risk.[24] Delayed bone scans in 7 to 10 days can image deep tissue and bone infarction. The absence of radionuclide uptake even after 10 days, however, does not reliably predict the eventual need for amputation. The patient should be advised that accurate prediction of eventual tissue loss is not possible. As an ancillary tool, scintigraphy may predict the eventual demarcation line better than thermography.[25-27] Scintigraphy as early as day 2 may predict tissue loss and monitor the efficacy of treatment.[28]

Large-vessel angiography is useful weeks after the injury unless vasodilators have been injected. This does not assess the microvasculature at presentation because of vasospasm. Transitory vascular instability often lasts 2 to 3 weeks. Angiography does facilitate evaluation of associated traumatic or chronic vascular abnormalities. Doppler ultrasonography and digital plethysmography are insensitive but may help determine the need for sympathetic blockade.

In clinical practice, magnetic resonance imaging and magnetic resonance angiography may be superior to technetium bone scanning. In one study, the clear-cut line of demarcation was noted before clinical demarcation.[29]

MANAGEMENT

Field rewarming of frozen tissue is rarely practical. If possible, constricting or wet clothing should be removed and affected areas insulated and immobilized. Friction massage is not efficacious and increases tissue loss. Frozen parts should be kept away from dry heat sources in the transport vehicle to prevent a gradual partial thaw.

A direct relationship exists between the length of time that tissue is frozen and the ultimate extent of cellular damage. Rewarming should not be initiated in the field, however, if there is any potential for interrupted or incomplete thawing. Tissue refreezing is disastrous, and it is preferable to ambulate to safety on frozen extremities if rescue will be delayed.

When evacuation is not possible, rapid field rewarming, preferably in water at 40° C to 42° C, may be the only option. Logistic considerations that affect this medical decision include risks to the party, the availability of shelter and necessary equipment, and the anticipated mode of eventual transportation.

Emergency Department

Prethaw

In the emergency department, pertinent history regarding the ambient temperature, wind velocity, and duration of exposure should be obtained. The type of apparel worn, the circumstances surrounding rescue, and the presence of preexisting cardiovascular or neurologic diseases that could affect tissue loss should be noted.

After stabilizing the core temperature and addressing associated conditions, rapid thawing should be initiated. Treatment should not be delayed while awaiting the results of laboratory and radiographic studies. Most patients have some degree of dehydration and benefit from crystalloid administration. Poor oral intake and hypothermia-induced cold diuresis further increase blood viscosity and sludging.[11]

Thaw

Frozen or partially thawed tissue should be rapidly and actively rewarmed by immersion in gently circulating water that is carefully maintained at a temperature of 40° C to 42° C by thermometer measurement.[9] Marginal tissue can be thermally injured when the water temperature exceeds 42° C. Although a circulating tank is ideal for the extremities, a large container suffices for the hands or feet. In some cases, 35° C to 40° C water is better tolerated and less painful.

Incomplete thawing and increased tissue loss are hazards when lower water temperatures are used. Rewarming should be continued until the part feels pliable and distal erythema is noted. This usually requires 10 to 30 minutes of submersion. Active gentle motion of the part by the patient during rewarming should be encouraged, but direct tissue massage should be avoided.

Parenteral analgesia is often indicated during rewarming of deep frostbite. Reperfusion is intensely painful.[30] It produces throbbing, burning pain, and tenderness. A common error is premature termination of rewarming, which results in a partial thaw. Sensation is often diminished after thawing until it disappears with bleb formation.

Patients with completely frozen extremities are invariably hypothermic and at risk for significant fluid and electrolyte fluxes during rewarming. The acute thawing of large amounts of distal musculature extinguishes peripheral vasoconstriction. This results in the sudden return of cold, hyperkalemic, acidotic blood to the central circulation. This produces "core temperature after-drop," which is dysrhythmogenic. In the most severe cases, extracorporeal rewarming should be considered to manage these massive metabolic and electrolyte derangements (Box 137-3).

BOX 137-3. Emergency Department Rewarming Protocol

Prethaw
- Protect part—no friction massage
- Stabilize core temperature
- Address medical and surgical conditions
- Rehydrate patient
- Prevent partial thaw and refreeze

Thaw
- Provide parenteral ketorolac and analgesia
- Administer ibuprofen 400 mg q 8 hours PO
- Immerse part in circulating water that is thermometer-monitored at 37° C to 40° C
- Encourage gentle motion of part

Post-thaw
- Dry and elevate part
- Aspirate clear vesicles
- Debride broken vesicles and apply topical antibiotic or sterile aloe vera ointment every 6 hours
- Leave hemorrhagic vesicles intact
- Consider tetanus and streptococcal prophylaxis
- Provide hydrotherapy at 37° C tid
- Consider Dibenzyline in severe cases

Post-thaw

The injured extremities should be kept elevated to minimize edema formation. Sterile dressings should be applied and involved areas handled gently. Persistent cyanosis in the extremities after a complete thaw may reflect increased fascial compartment pressure. Because of the cold-induced anesthesia, this and other occult soft tissue injuries are often not appreciated by the patient or physician. Tissue pressures should be monitored carefully, although decompressing escharotomies are usually not necessary during the initial treatment rendered in the emergency department.

The clinical role of thromboxane inhibition in frostbite is limited. Thromboxane inhibition does not appear to result in additional clinically significant tissue salvage. In one experimental model, methimazole did not improve tissue survival even when therapy was initiated immediately.[31] Progressive secondary dermal ischemia is addressed by attempts to limit the accumulation of the products of arachidonic acid breakdown. Topical aloe vera (Dermaide) every 6 hours is a specific thromboxane inhibitor when applied directly to frostbitten areas,[13] but has not definitively been proven to salvage tissue. Other alternatives include topical antibiotic ointment or limaprost 20 µg tid. Systemically, ibuprofen appears preferable to salicylates. The dose is 12 mg/kg per day in divided doses. Although both agents inhibit this cascade, ibuprofen also produces fibrinolysis. Parenteral ketorolac should also be considered.

Frostbite blister management varies widely. Earlier recommended options for large clear blisters included leaving them intact, debridement, or aspiration (Figure 137-1). Although all authors debride broken blisters, many prefer to aspirate intact clear blisters rather than leaving them intact. In contrast, if hemorrhagic blisters are debrided, secondary desiccation of deep dermal layers appears to extend the injury (Figure 137-2). In this case, aspiration is preferable to debridement.

In severe cases, parenteral penicillin is indicated for streptococcal prophylaxis. Cultures and Gram stains of areas adjacent to the damaged tissue should be performed. Common organisms include staphylococci, streptococci, and *Pseudomonas* species. Broad-spectrum prophylaxis should be considered if excessive heat was used to thaw tissue, since liquefaction and infection are inevitable. Tetanus can also occur after frostbite.

Adjunctive Treatment

Numerous ancillary modalities have been suggested. The only treatment consensus is removal from the cold and rapid complete thawing in a 40° C to 42° C bath.

Capillary flow ceases early after cold injury, whereas thrombosis proceeds.[11,32] This observation has led to

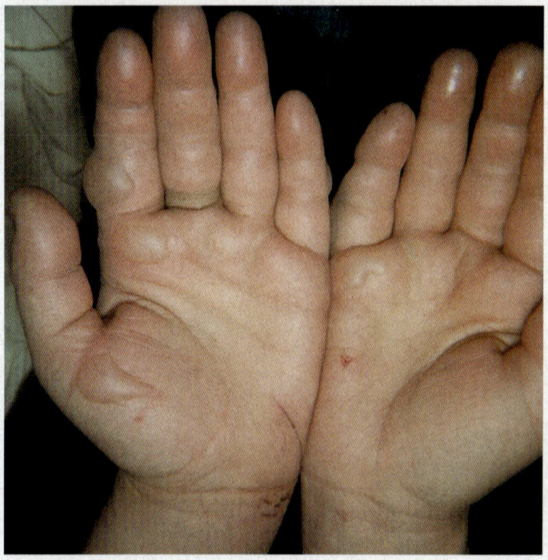

Figure 137-1. Frostbite with clear vesiculations.

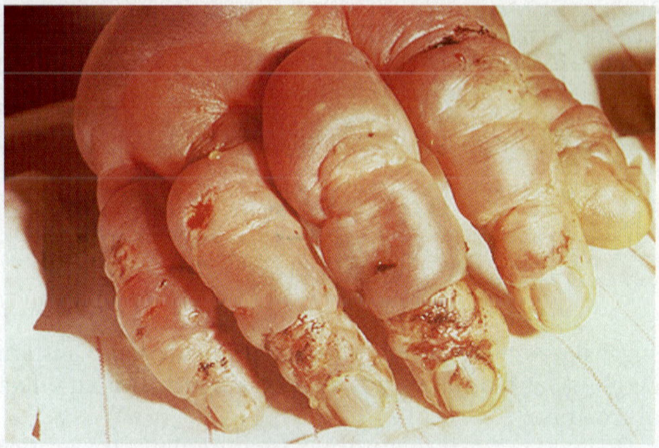

Figure 137-2. Severe frostbite with early hemorrhagic vesicles. (Courtesy of Bill Mills, MD.)

multiple experimental antithrombotic and vasodilation treatment regimens. Most of these studies were conducted before the elucidation of some of the pathophysiologic consequences of frostbite. As demonstrated in a pilot study on triple-phase bone scans, thrombolytic agents may restore some flow to severely frostbitten limbs.[33] The fibrinolytic agent urokinase can also conserve slowly thawed tissue.[34]

Low-molecular-weight dextran may inhibit intravascular cellular aggregation. Clinical observations suggest that low-molecular-weight dextran is not harmful. Therapeutic anticoagulation with heparin fails to enhance tissue salvage. Tissue edema may be increased. Pentoxifylline may decrease blood viscosity and increase tissue oxygenation.[35] Its ability to increase red blood cell flexibility facilities revascularization and may enhance tissue survival. Although still considered a research modality in frostbite, the suggested dosage is 400 mg three times daily for 2 to 6 weeks.[36]

Various anti-inflammatory drugs and other agents have not been conclusively evaluated. These include steroids, nonsteroidal anti-inflammatory drugs, dipyridamole, dimethyl sulfoxide, nonionic detergents, and calcium channel blockers. A long-acting α-blocker, phenoxybenzamine, may decrease vasospasm while increasing peripheral blood flow. The dosage starts with 10 mg/day to a maximum of 60 mg/day. With this agent, adequate hydration is necessary to prevent orthostatic hypotension.

The role of hyperbaric oxygen therapy is unclear. It produces vasoconstriction and subsequently reduces cutaneous blood flow. A small number of patients have reported a temporary flush and increased limb motion, but this appears to depend on the elapsed time interval after injury. Hyperbaric oxygen could accelerate demarcation. Insufficient data on severe frostbite exist to assess the potential value of hyperbaric oxygen therapy for tissue salvage.[37,38]

Sympathectomy

The theoretical benefits of sympathectomy include relief of painful vasospasm, decreased edema, and tissue salvage. Long-term vasodilation could protect against repeated cold injury and some of the degenerative sequelae of frostbite. The value of these benefits is highly debatable.[39] Epidural spinal cord stimulation combined with conventional treatment may reduce pain and conserve tissue.

A "medical" sympathectomy results from direct injection of an agent such as reserpine into an artery. Common injection sites include the radial, brachial, and femoral arteries. This injection produces local depletion of arterial wall norepinephrine for 2 to 4 weeks. No significant systemic effects are appreciated with the recommended dose of 0.5 mg. This can be repeated in 2 to 3 days. Parenteral reserpine is not commercially available in the United States. Guanethidine is also recommended for this purpose.

There is angiographic documentation of temporary improvement in perfusion and vasospasm after medical sympathectomy. When tissue is rapidly thawed, experimental attempts to demonstrate further enhancement of tissue salvage have failed. Intra-arterial reserpine may prove most useful in patients with residual pain after gradual thawing.

Early results with surgical sympathectomy were encouraging. Decreased pain, edema, and residual autonomic dysfunction were reported. Tissue demarcation also appeared to accelerate. Bouwman and colleagues[40] performed unilateral surgical sympathectomy on 10 patients with bilateral matched frostbite injuries. Delayed protection against reinjury was one direct benefit. Ultimately, however, there was no increased tissue salvage. Mills observes that surgical sympathectomy produces a smoother initial clinical course but no long-term benefits, with the possible exception of decreased causalgia.[9,10]

DISPOSITION

Except in minor cases, all patients should be hospitalized for 24 to 48 hours to determine the extent of injury. Superficial injuries to facial structures may be followed on an outpatient basis. In preparation for hospitaliza-

BOX 137-4. Sequelae of Frostbite

Neuropathic

Pain

Phantom
Causalgia
"Tabes" burning
Chronic

Sensation

Hypesthesia
Dysesthesia
Paresthesia
Anesthesia

Thermal Sensitivity

Heat
Cold

Autonomic Dysfunction

Hyperhidrosis
Raynaud's syndrome

Musculoskeletal

Atrophy
Compartment syndrome
Rhabdomyolysis
Tenosynovitis
Stricture
Epiphyseal fusion
Osteoarthritis
Osteolytic lesions
Necrosis
Amputation

Dermatologic

Edema
Lymphedema
Chronic or recurrent ulcers
Epidermoid or squamous cell carcinoma
Hair or nail deformities

Miscellaneous

Core temperature afterdrop
Acute tubular necrosis
Electrolyte fluxes
Psychological stress
Gangrene
Sepsis

tion, damaged tissues are best protected with loose sterile sheets and towels rather than compressive dressings. Feet must be kept elevated under a protective cradle. Sterile cotton pledgets should be placed between the toes, and the hands may rest elevated on the chest.

Whirlpool hydrotherapy with the antiseptic Hibiclens should be performed two to three times daily for 20 to 30 minutes. Range-of-motion exercises should be encouraged during immersion. Severe cases may require position-of-function splinting. Hydrotherapy is continued as the eschar sloughs. At this point, sterile precautions may be discontinued. During hospitalization, all vasoconstrictive agents, including nicotine, should be avoided.

SEQUELAE

Direct neuronal damage and residual abnormalities in sympathetic tone are responsible for most of the common symptomatic sequelae of frostbite.[41] In a series of military patients with documented frostbite, 65% had long-term residual symptoms.[42] Vasospasm with secondary cold intolerance is the other major sequela.[43]

Intermittent paresthesias resulting from ischemic neuritis are reported after the first week. The severity of this symptom often reflects the extent of tissue damage. Symptoms may persist for many months. Burning electric-shock sensations are worse at night, after heat exposure, and on first returning to ambulation. Thermal perception is also altered. Hyperhidrosis suggests an abnormal sympathetic nervous system response and often serves as both a cause and an effect of frostbite.

Delayed cutaneous findings include nail deformities and pigmentation changes. Squamous and epidermoid cell carcinoma can occur. Osseous reabsorption and subchondral lytic defects develop months after the cold insult. In pediatric patients, concerns include premature fusion, destruction, and fragmentation of epiphyses.[44] Shortening of the distal phalanges is common.[40] Frostbite arthritis also occurs.[45] In severe cases involving extremity muscle compartments, rhabdomyolysis and subsequent renal failure are a concern. Continuous monitoring of serum muscle enzymes and urinalyses is warranted.

Surgical decisions regarding amputation are complex.[46-48] The amount of tissue eventually salvaged often exceeds even optimistic initial estimates. Historically, the natural progression of demarcation, mummification, and eventual sloughing was allowed to occur. Necrotic tissue was classically debrided at least 1 to 2 months after injury when the line of demarcation is clear.[49] Exceptions include refractory pain, sepsis, and supervening gangrene. Recent advances in radiologic assessment of tissue viability are facilitating earlier surgical intervention. Most grafts and amputations now occur at 3 to 4 weeks after injury. Free flap tissue transfer to salvage function after earlier debridement of soft tissues should be a consideration.[46,47]

Various neuropathic, musculoskeletal, and dermatologic sequelae of frostbite are listed in Box 137-4.[50]

KEY CONCEPTS

- The initial presentation of frostbite can be deceptively benign. Rapid rewarming in 40° C to 42° C water should begin promptly.
- Premature termination of thawing is a common error. Reperfusion of completely frozen tissue is very painful and often requires parenteral analgesia.
- The early formation of clear blebs is more favorable than delayed hemorrhagic blebs, since the latter reflect damage to the subdermal vascular plexi.
- The patient should be advised that accurate prediction of eventual tissue loss is not possible at presentation.

REFERENCES

1. Berg A, Aas P, Lund T: Frostbite injuries. *Tidsskr Nor Laegeforen* 119:382, 1999.
2. Hamlet MP: Prevention and treatment of cold injury. *Int J Circumpolar Health* 59:108, 2000.
3. Rintamaki H: Predisposing factors and prevention of frostbite. *Int J Circumpolar Health* 59:114, 2000.
4. Hassi J, Makinen TM: Frostbite: Occurrence, risk factors and consequences. *Int J Circumpolar Health* 59:92, 2000.
5. Hashmi MA, et al: Frostbite: Epidemiology at high altitude in the Karakoram mountains. *Ann R Coll Surg Engl* 80:91, 1998.
6. Nissen ER, Melchert PJ, Lewis EJ: A case of bullous frostbite following recreational snowmobiling. *Cutis* 63:21, 1999.
7. Paton BC: "From Larrey to Mills": The road to rapid rewarming—a commentary. *Wilderness Environ Med* 9:223, 1998.
8. Paton BC: A history of frostbite treatment. *Int J Circumpolar Health* 59:99, 2000.
9. Mills WJ Jr, Whaley R, Fish W: Frostbite: Experience with rapid rewarming and ultrasonic therapy: Part III, 1961. *Alaska Med* 35:19, 1993.
10. Mills WJ Jr: Summary of treatment of the cold injured patient, 1980. *Alaska Med* 35:50, 1993.
11. Purdue GF, Hunt JL: Cold injury: A collective review. *J Burn Care Rehabil* 7:331, 1986.
12. Ozyazgan I, et al: Eicosanoids and inflammatory cells in frostbitten tissue: Prostacyclin, thromboxane, polymorphonuclear leukocytes, and mast cells. *Plast Reconstr Surg* 101:1881, 1998.
13. Heggers JP, et al: Frostbite: Experimental and clinical evaluations of treatment. *J Wilderness Med* 1:27, 1990.
14. Marzella L, et al: Morphologic characterization of acute injury to vascular endothelium of skin after frostbite. *Plast Reconstr Surg* 83:67, 1989.
15. Pinzur MS, Weaver FM: Is urban frostbite a psychiatric disorder? *Orthopedics* 20:43, 1997.
16. Gamble WB, Bonnecarre ER: Coffee, tea, or frostbite? A case report of inflight freezing hazard from dry ice. *Aviat Space Environ Med* 67:880, 1996.
17. Svartling N, et al: Life-threatening airway obstruction from nitrous oxide induced frostbite of the oral cavity. *Anaesth Intens Care* 24:717, 1996.
18. Rustin MH, et al: The treatment of chilblains with nifedipine: The results of a pilot study, a double-blind placebo-controlled randomized study and a long-term open trial. *Br J Dermatol* 120:267, 1989.
19. Tek D, Mackey S: Non-freezing cold injury in a Marine infantry battalion. *J Wilderness Med* 4:353, 1993.
20. Burr RE: Trench foot. *J Wilderness Med* 4:348, 1993.
21. Cauchy E, et al: Retrospective study of 70 cases of severe frostbite lesions: A proposed new classification scheme. *Wilderness Environ Med* 12:248, 2001.
22. Kenney A III, Vyas P: Frostbite injury: Appearance on three-phase bone scan. *Clin Nucl Med* 23:188, 1998.
23. Greenwald D, Cooper B, Gottlieb L: An algorithm for early aggressive treatment of frostbite with limb salvage directed by triple-phase scanning. *Plast Reconstr Surg* 102:1069, 1998.
24. Mehta RC, Wilson MA: Frostbite injury: Prediction of tissue viability with triple-phase bone scanning. *Radiology* 170:511, 1989.
25. Bhatnagar A, et al: Diagnosis, characterization and evaluation of treatment response of frostbite using pertechnetate scintigraphy: A prospective study. *Eur J Nuc Med* 29:170, 2002.
26. Junila J, Kaarela O, Waris T: The formation of the demarcation line at experimental frostbite. *Int J Circumpolar Health* 58:44, 1999.
27. Aygit AC, Sarikaya A: Imaging of frostbite injury by technetium-99m-sestamibi scintigraphy: A case report. *Foot Ankle Intern* 23:56, 2002.
28. Cauchy E, et al: The value of technetium 99 scintigraphy in the prognosis of amputation in severe frostbite injuries of the extremities: A retrospective study of 92 severe frostbite injuries. *J Hand Surg* 25:969, 2000.
29. Barker JR, et al: Magnetic resonance imaging of severe frostbite injuries. *Ann Plast Surg* 38:275, 1997.
30. Punja K, Graham M, Cartotto R: Continuous infusion of epidural morphine in frostbite. *J Burn Care Rehabil* 19:142, 1998.
31. Goldberg BD, Robinson WA, Watson WA: Impact of delayed presentation on the efficacy of thromboxane inhibition in the treatment of frostbite. *J Wilderness Med* 5:325, 1994.
32. Zook N, et al. Microcirculatory studies of frostbite injury: Discussion. *Ann Plast Surg* 40:254, 1998.
33. Skolnick AA: Early data suggest clot-dissolving drug may help save frostbitten limbs from amputation. *JAMA* 267: 2008, 1992.
34. Zdeblick TA, Field GA, Shaffer JW: Treatment of experimental frostbite with urokinase. *J Hand Surg [Am]* 13:948, 1988.
35. Miller MB, Koltai PJ: Treatment of experimental frostbite with pentoxifylline and aloe vera cream. *Arch Otolaryngol Head Neck Surg* 121:678, 1995.
36. Hayes DW Jr, et al: Pentoxifylline: Adjunctive therapy in the treatment of pedal frostbite. *Clin Podia Med Surg* 17: 715, 2000.
37. Finderle Z, Cankar K: Delayed treatment of frostbite injury with hyperbaric oxygen therapy: A case report. *Aviat Space Environ Med* 73:392, 2002.
38. von Heimburg D, et al: Hyperbaric oxygen treatment in deep frostbite of both hands in a boy. *Burns* 27:404, 2001.
39. Porter JM, et al: Intra-arterial sympathetic blockade in the treatment of clinical frostbite. *Am J Surg* 132:625, 1976.
40. Bouwman DL, et al: Early sympathetic blockade for frostbite: Is it of value? *J Trauma* 20:744, 1980.
41. Arvesen A, Wilson J, Rosen L: Nerve conduction velocity in human limbs with late sequelae after local cold injury. *Eur J Clin Invest* 26:443, 1996.
42. Taylor MS, Kulungowski MA, Hamelink JK: Frostbite injuries during winter maneuvers: A long-term disability. *Mil Med* 154:411, 1989.
43. Ervasti O, et al: Sequelae of moderate finger frostbite as assessed by subjective sensations, clinical signs, and thermophysiological responses. *Int J Circumpolar Health* 59:137, 2000.
44. Reed MH: Growth disturbances in the hands following thermal injuries in children, 2. frostbite. *Can Assoc Radiol J* 39:95, 1988.

45. Saxena A: Achilles peritendinosis: An unusual case due to frostbite in an elite athlete. *J Foot Ankle Surg* 33:87, 1994.
46. Leonard LG, et al: Salvage of a vascular bone from frostbite with free tissue transfer. *Ann Plast Surg* 46:431, 2001.
47. Classen DA: Free flap coverage of bilateral frostbite of the feet. *Plast Reconstr Surg* 106:1316, 2000.
48. Su CW, Lohman R, Gottlieb LJ: Frostbite of the upper extremity. *Hand Clin* 16:235, 2000.
49. McAdams TR, Swenson DR, Miller AR: Frostbite: An orthopedic perspective. *Am J Orthop* 28:21, 1999.
50. Oumlish OY, Parish LC: Marching in the army: Common cutaneous disorders of the feet. *Clin Dermatol* 20:445, 2002.

CHAPTER 138

Accidental Hypothermia

Daniel F. Danzl

PERSPECTIVE

The amazing "reanimations" of profoundly cold victims in prolonged cardiac arrest help to explain the contemporary allure of hypothermia. A physician recently presented her own case report at an international conference. She was successfully resuscitated from accidental hypothermia at 13.7° C after 9 hours, which included cardiopulmonary resuscitation (CPR) initiated at the scene and 179 minutes of cardiopulmonary bypass.[1] Although used for medical purposes for millennia, cold modalities were not scientifically evaluated until the 18th century. The hemostatic, analgesic, and therapeutic effects of cold on a wide variety of conditions were well known. Although fever remained the most common disorder of thermoregulation, accidental hypothermia was also common and its treatment controversial. Biblical references cite truncal rewarming of King David by a damsel, and various remedies, including rubbing the extremities with hot oil, were mentioned by Hippocrates, Aristotle, and Galen.

Cold weather has had a major impact on military history.[2] Hannibal lost nearly half of his army of 46,000 while traversing the Pyrenees Alps in 218 BC. Baron Larrey, Napoleon's chief surgeon, reported that only 350 of the 12,000 men in the 12th division survived the cold during their retreat from Russia in 1812. He also observed that those soldiers who were rapidly rewarmed closest to the campfire died.

The winter of 1777 to 1778 took its toll on Washington's troops at Valley Forge. The French subsequently suffered heavy losses to the cold in the Crimean War (1845-1855). These Crimean lessons were relearned during both world wars. Many pilots and U-boat crews perished from the cold water temperature in the North Atlantic. Approximately 10% of the United States casualties in Korea were cold related.

Innumerable cold-related tragedies affect both military personnel and civilians, in particular hunters, sailors, skiers, climbers, boaters, and swimmers. Widespread participation in outdoor winter sports has also increased the number of patients who develop hypothermia.[3]

Hypothermia is geographically and seasonally pervasive.[4-6] Most cases occur in urban settings. "Primary" hypothermia fatalities are classified as accidental, homicidal, or suicidal; however, death certificate data under-report secondary hypothermia deaths, in which cold complicates many systemic diseases. The effect of cold on mortality from cardiovascular and neurologic disorders is greatly underestimated.[7]

Hypothermia is defined as a core temperature less than 35° C. Many variables contribute to the development of accidental hypothermia. Exposure, age, health, nutrition, medication, and intoxicants can decrease heat production, increase heat loss, or interfere with thermostability. The healthy individual's compensatory responses to heat loss through conduction, convection, radiation, and evaporation are often overwhelmed by exposure. Medications can also interfere with thermoregulation, and central nervous system (CNS) processes commonly decrease the efficiency of thermoregulation.[8]

PRINCIPLES OF DISEASE

Physiology of Temperature Regulation

In humans, basal heat production generates approximately 40 to 60 kcal/m^2 of body surface area per hour. This increases with food ingestion, muscular activity, fever, and acute cold exposure. Cold stress increases preshivering muscle tone, and heat production can double. Maximal heat production lasts only a few hours because of fatigue and glycogen depletion.

Shivering thermogenesis increases the basal metabolic rate two to five times. This shivering, which markedly increases oxygen consumption, is modulated by the posterior hypothalamus and the spinal cord.

The preoptic anterior hypothalamus orchestrates nonshivering heat conservation and dissipation. Serotonergic and dopaminergic neurons are pivotal. They exert immediate control through the autonomic

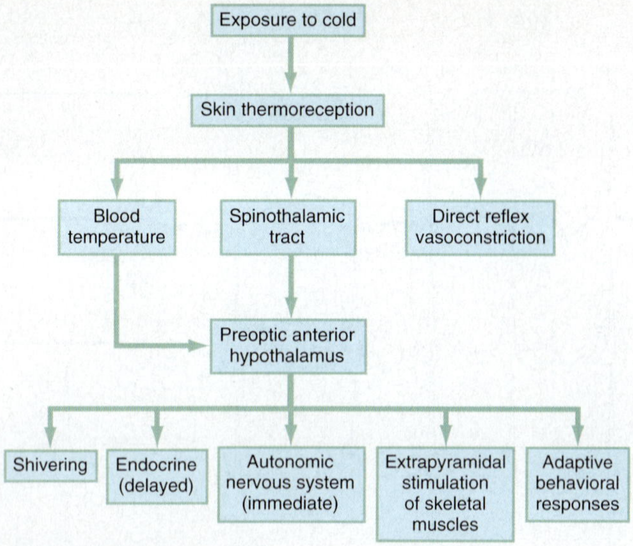

Figure 138-1. Physiology of cold exposure.

nervous system and delayed control through the endocrine system. Thermal suppression or activation of the sympathetic nervous system with cold-induced release of norepinephrine also occurs. Cold also stimulates the hypothalamus to release thyrotropin-releasing hormone. This activates the anterior pituitary gland, which releases thyroid-stimulating hormone, and results in the release of thyroxine (T_4) from the thyroid gland.[9]

The discomfort of cold can be reduced after long periods of exposure. No evidence exists, however, that there is any significant physiologic adaptation to the cold (Figure 138-1).

Normal heat loss occurs through five mechanisms. Assuming an average basal metabolic rate, 55% to 65% of this loss is through radiation. Heat loss by radiation is greatest when one is spread nude and least when curled and insulated. Radiative heat loss depends on the temperature gradient between the environment and the exposed body surface area. Conduction normally accounts for only approximately 2% to 3% of the heat loss, but this may increase up to five times in wet clothing and up to 25 times in cold water.

Close correlation exists between subcutaneous fat thickness and cooling rates. Individuals with greater insulation lose heat more slowly. Conduction and convection normally account for about 15% of the body's heat loss, but convective losses increase with shivering. Respiration and evaporation account for the remainder of the loss, with 2% to 9% lost in heating inspired air and 20% to 27% lost to insensible evaporation from the skin and lungs.

Cutaneous and respiratory heat loss is markedly influenced by the ambient temperature, air motion, and relative humidity. Greater losses occur in a cool, dry, windy environment (windchill index). When the body is not perspiring, most heat loss is through radiation and convection. Conductive losses become significant in immersion-induced hypothermia. Children cool faster than adults because of the elevated ratios of surface area to mass.

When the temperature is between 37° C and 32° C, vasoconstriction, shivering, and nonshivering basal and endocrinologic thermogenesis generate heat. From 32° C to 24° C, a progressive depression of the basal metabolic rate occurs without shivering thermogenesis. At temperatures less than 24° C, autonomic and endocrinologic mechanisms for heat conservation become inactive.

Pathophysiology

Cardiovascular

After an initial tachycardia, a progressive bradycardia develops. The pulse usually decreases by 50% at 28° C. If an observed tachycardia is inconsistent with a patient's temperature, associated conditions such as hypoglycemia, drug ingestion, or hypovolemia should be considered.

The bradycardia of hypothermia results from decreased spontaneous depolarization of the pacemaker cells. As a result, the bradydysrhythmia is refractory to atropine. Hypothermia also decreases the mean arterial pressure and the cardiac index.

The electrocardiographic features of hypothermia are unique.[10] Initially described by Tomaszewkski in 1938, the Osborn (J) wave is seen at the junction of the QRS complex and ST segment (Figure 138-2). J waves are potentially diagnostic but not prognostic. They may appear at any temperature less than 32° C. The size of the J wave is not related to arterial pH but does increase with temperature depression.

J waves are normally upright in aVL, aVF, and the left precordial leads. The J deflection may be a result of hypothermic ion flux alterations, with delayed depolarization or early repolarization of the left ventricular wall. It can also be seen during local cardiac ischemia, with sepsis or CNS lesions, and occasionally in young normothermic patients.

Some J waveform abnormalities can simulate a myocardial injury current. Hypothermic electrocardiographic changes are not easily computer programmable. Reliance on computer interpretations can result in mistaken admissions to coronary care units. Thrombolytic therapy in patients with hypothermia is unstudied but would be expected to exacerbate preexistent coagulopathies.[11]

All atrial and ventricular dysrhythmias are common in cases of moderate to severe hypothermia. Reentrant dysrhythmias result from decreased conduction velocity with increased myocardial conduction time and a decreased absolute refractory period. Independent electrical foci also precipitate dysrhythmias.

Because the conduction system is more sensitive to the cold than the myocardium, cardiac cycle prolongation occurs. Fluctuations of available oxygen, pH, electrolytes, and nutrients also alter conduction. As hypothermia worsens, the PR interval, then the QRS interval, and finally (and most characteristically) the QT interval become prolonged. In the absence of obvious shivering, thermal muscular tone may obscure P waves or produce artifacts.

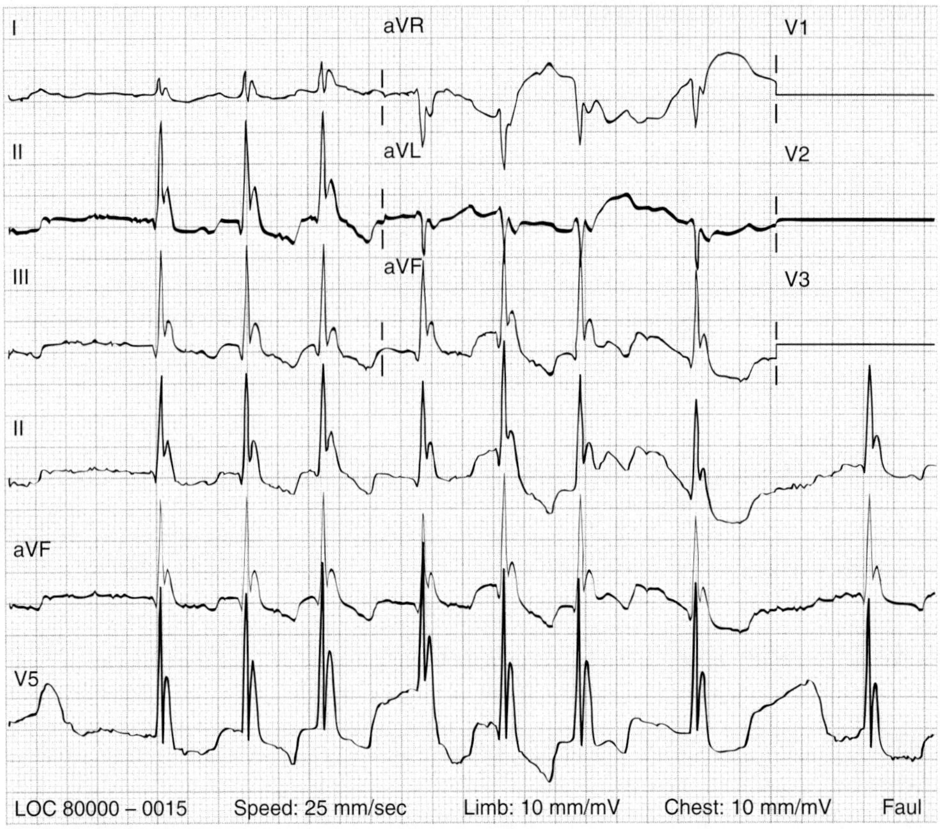

Figure 138-2. Hypothermic J waves.

Atrial fibrillation is common when the core temperature is less than 32° C. Other rhythms are sinus, atrial, or junctional. Atrial fibrillation usually converts spontaneously during rewarming, and mesenteric embolization is a hazard.

The development of ventricular fibrillation (VF) or asystole in hypothermia is multifactorial. Putative explanations include tissue hypoxia, physical jostling, electrophysiologic or acid-base disturbances, and autonomic dysfunction. Asystole and VF can occur spontaneously when the core temperature falls below 25° C.[12] Hypothermia causes a decrease in transmembrane resting potential, which, in turn, decreases the threshold for ventricular dysrhythmias. VF can also result from an independent focus or a reentrant phenomenon. When the heart is cold, a large dispersion of repolarization exists, which facilitates the development of a conduction delay. The action potential is also prolonged, and this increases the temporal dispersion of the recovery of excitability.

The term *core temperature afterdrop* refers to a further decline in an individual's core temperature after removal from the cold. The two processes that contribute to afterdrop are simple temperature equilibration across a gradient and circulatory changes. Countercurrent cooling of the blood, which is perfusing cold tissues, results in a temperature decline until the gradient is eliminated.[13]

Active external rewarming of the extremities obliterates peripheral vasoconstriction and reverses arteriovenous shunting. This was most vividly demonstrated by Hayward, who measured his own esophageal, rectal, tympanic, and cardiac temperatures (using a flotation tip catheter) after cooling in 10° C water on 3 different days.[14] Warm bath immersion rewarming caused a 30% fall in mean arterial pressure, coupled with a 50% decline in peripheral vascular resistance.

Core temperature afterdrop is a clinically relevant consideration when treating patients with a large temperature gradient between the core and the periphery. This is common in dehydrated patients after chronic exposure. Major afterdrops also occur in severely hypothermic patients if frostbitten extremities are thawed before thermal stabilization.

Central Nervous System

Hypothermia progressively depresses the CNS.[15] Significant alteration of the brain's electrical activity begins below 33.5° C, and the electroencephalogram goes silent at 19° C to 20° C.

Cerebral autoregulation is maintained with an increase in vascular resistance until 25° C. In cases of severe hypothermia, there is a disproportionately higher redistribution of blood flow to the brain. Visually evoked potentials are an objective measure of cerebral function and depend on cerebral blood flow. The potentials become smaller as the temperature decreases. Like the heart, the brain has a critical period of tolerance to hypothermia. There are temperature-dependent neural enzyme systems that are unable to function at temperatures that are well tolerated by the kidney.

Table 138-1. Physiologic Characteristics of the Four Zones of Hypothermia

State	Core temperature ° C (°F)	Characteristics
Mild	35 (95)	Urine temperature 34.8° C; maximum shivering thermogenesis; increase in metabolic rate
	34 (93.2)	Amnesia and dysarthria develop; normal blood pressure; maximum respiratory stimulation
	33 (91.4)	Ataxia and apathy develop
Moderate	32 (89.6)	Stupor; 25% decrease in oxygen consumption
	31 (87.8)	Extinguished shivering thermogenesis
	30 (86)	Atrial fibrillation and other dysrhythmias; poikilothermia; pulse and cardiac output two thirds normal; insulin ineffective
	29 (85.2)	Progressive decrease in level of consciousness, pulse, and respiration; pupils dilated
Severe	28 (82.4)	Ventricular fibrillation susceptibility; 50% decrease in oxygen consumption and pulse
	27 (80.6)	Losing reflexes and voluntary motion
	26 (78.8)	Major acid-base disturbances; no reflexes or response to pain
	25 (77)	Cerebral blood flow one third normal; cardiac output 45% normal; pulmonary edema may develop
	24 (75.2)	Significant hypotension
	23 (73.4)	No corneal or oculocephalic reflexes
	22 (71.6)	Maximum risk of ventricular fibrillation; 75% decrease in oxygen consumption
Profound	20 (68)	Lowest resumption of cardiac electromechanical activity; pulse 20% of normal
	19 (66.2)	Flat electroencephalogram
	18 (64.4)	Asystole develops
	14.2 (57.6)	Lowest accidental hypothermia survival in an infant[93]
	13.7 (56.7)	Lowest accidental hypothermia survival in an adult[1]
	9 (48.2)	Lowest therapeutic hypothermia survival[88]

Renal System

Simple exposure to cold induces a diuresis regardless of an individual's state of hydration. Hypothermia depresses renal blood flow, reducing it by 50% at 27° C to 30° C. The kidneys then excrete a large amount of dilute urine, termed the *cold diuresis.* Cold diuresis is essentially glomerular filtrate, which does not clear nitrogenous waste products. Severe hypothermia causes an initial relative central hypervolemia as a consequence of peripheral vasoconstriction. Cold diuresis may act as a volume regulator to diminish the vasoconstriction-induced capacitance vessel overload. Cold water immersion can further increase urinary output by 3.5 times, and ethanol doubles that increase.[16]

Respiratory System

Hypothermia initially stimulates respiration. This is followed by a progressive decrease in the respiratory minute volume, which is proportional to the decreasing metabolism. Carbon dioxide production decreases 50% with an 8° C fall in temperature. The normal stimuli for respiratory control are altered in severe hypothermia, and carbon dioxide retention with respiratory acidosis can occur.

Numerous other pathophysiologic factors adversely affect the respiratory system (Table 138-1). These include viscous bronchorrhea, decreased ciliary motility, and noncardiogenic pulmonary edema.

Predisposing Factors

Predisposing factors that contribute to the pathophysiologic changes accompanying core temperature depression can be categorized as those that decrease heat production, increase heat loss, or impair thermoregulation (Box 138-1).

Decreased Heat Production

Decreased thermogenesis is often secondary to an endocrinologic failure such as hypopituitarism, hypoadrenalism, or myxedema. Myxedema coma is several times more common in women, and up to 80% of these persons are hypothermic. Hypothyroidism is often occult in this setting. There is usually no available history of lassitude, dry skin, arthralgias, or cold intolerance.

Hypoglycemia with central neuroglycopenia also predisposes to hypothermia. Another cause of decreased heat production is malnutrition, which corresponds to a decrease in subcutaneous fat. Severe malnutrition, as with marasmus, contributes to heat loss. Kwashiorkor is less commonly associated with hypothermia because of the insulating effect of the hypoproteinemic edema.[9]

The young and the old are commonly at risk. The neonate has a large surface area-to-mass ratio, a relatively deficient subcutaneous tissue layer, and an inefficient shivering mechanism. Since neonates lack behavioral defense mechanisms, they are more likely to develop hypothermia.

Acute neonatal hypothermia is common after emergency deliveries or resuscitations. Many neonates are lethargic, fail to thrive, and have a weak cry. Half have deceptively rosy cheeks. Late-onset hypothermia, which occurs after 72 hours of life, is commonly a result of septicemia. Hypothermia can occur in the shaken baby syndrome and may be a factor in some cases of sudden infant death syndrome.

Homeostatic capability progressively decreases with aging. Thermal perception is altered, and elderly people manipulate the indoor ambient temperature less precisely. Most elderly patients are capable of normal thermoregulation but are prone to conditions, includ-

Box 138-1. Factors Predisposing to Hypothermia

Decreased Heat Production
Endocrinologic failure
- Hypopituitarism
- Hypoadrenalism
- Hypothyroidism
- Diabetes

Insufficient fuel
- Hypoglycemia
- Malnutrition
- Marasmus
- Kwashiorkor
- Extreme exertion

Neuromuscular inefficiency
- Age extremes
- Impaired shivering
- Inactivity
- Lack of adaptation

Increased Heat Loss
Environmental
- Immersion
- Nonimmersion

Induced vasodilation
- Pharmacologic
- Toxicologic

Erythrodermas
- Burns
- Psoriasis
- Ichthyosis
- Exfoliative dermatitis

Iatrogenic
- Emergency deliveries
- Cold infusions
- Heat stroke treatment

Impaired Thermoregulation
Peripheral failure
- Neuropathies
- Acute spinal cord transection
- Diabetes

Central failure/neurologic
- CNS trauma
- Cerebrovascular accident
- Toxicologic
- Metabolic
- Subarachnoid hemorrhage
- Pharmacologic
- Hypothalamic dysfunction
- Parkinson's disease
- Anorexia nervosa
- Cerebellar lesion
- Neoplasm
- Congenital intracranial anomalies
- Multiple sclerosis

Miscellaneous Associated Clinical States
Recurrent hypothermia
Episodic hypothermia
Sepsis
Pancreatitis
Carcinomatosis
Cardiopulmonary disease
- Vascular insufficiency

Uremia
Paget's disease
Giant cell arteritis
Sarcoidosis
Shaken baby syndrome
Multisystem trauma
Shapiro's syndrome
Wernicke-Korsakoff syndrome
Hodgkin's disease

ing immobility and systemic diseases, that interfere with heat production and conservation. Evidence exists that normal aging factors can predispose to hypothermia. Inability to sense cold, abnormal adaptive behavioral responses, and decreased peripheral blood flow reflect autonomic dysfunction.[17-19]

Increased Heat Loss

Unacclimated individuals often conserve heat poorly during exposure to the cold. Patients with erythrodermas, including psoriasis, exfoliative dermatitis, ichthyosis, eczema, and burns, can have increased peripheral blood flow.

Iatrogenic causes of heat loss include exposure during resuscitations, massive cold infusions, overcooling of patients with heat stroke, and overzealous burn treatment.

Ethanol is metabolized at a slower rate in hypothermic individuals and interacts with every putative thermoregulatory neurotransmitter. It may directly damage the posterior hypothalamus and the mammillary bodies. Cutaneous heat loss increases through vasodilation, and shivering thermogenesis is decreased.

Ethanol is the most common cause of heat loss in urban settings.[6,12] Patients often lack protective adaptive behavior to avoid the cold. "Paradoxical undressing," which is the removal of clothing in response to a cold stress, is common.[20] Aging is associated with an increased sensitivity to the hypothermic actions of ethanol. Hypothermic alcoholic ketoacidosis also occurs. The incidence of hypothermia in patients with Wernicke's encephalopathy is common. Hypothermia can mask the usual clinical triad of ophthalmoplegia, confusion, and truncal ataxia. Intravenous thiamine can be both diagnostic and therapeutic.

Impaired Thermoregulation

Thermoregulation can be impaired centrally, peripherally, or metabolically. Skull fractures, particularly basilar fractures, and chronic subdural hematomas, are implicated. Other causes include cerebrovascular accidents, neoplasms, anorexia nervosa, and Hodgkin's and Parkinson's diseases. The final common pathway in these disorders may be centrally mediated vasodilation. Cerebellar lesions produce choreiform, less efficient shivering.

In therapeutic or toxic doses, benzodiazepines, phenothiazines, cyclic antidepressants, barbiturates, and general anesthetics interfere with thermoregulation by impairing centrally mediated vasoconstriction. Overdosage of these medications and others (e.g., the organophosphates, heroin, glutethimide, and carbon monoxide) predisposes to hypothermia. Core temperature reduction can be a prodrome of lithium toxicity. Clonidine, fluphenazine, acetaminophen, cannabis, bethanechol, and atropine are also implicated.

Peripheral thermoregulatory failure classically occurs after acute spinal cord transections. The interruption of the autonomic nervous system eliminates vasoconstrictive control and the patient effectively becomes poikilothermic. Neuropathies and diabetes are additional peripheral causes of heat loss. An abnormal plasma osmolality may be the mechanism of hypothalamic interference in cases of uremia, lactic acidosis, diabetic ketoacidosis, and hypoglycemia.[21]

Miscellaneous Causes

Hypothermia occurs in conjunction with several infections, most commonly overwhelming gram-negative sepsis, pneumonia, meningitis, and encephalitis. Other associated infections include bacterial endocarditis, brucellosis, malaria, syphilis, typhoid, miliary tuberculosis, and trypanosomiasis.

Medical conditions associated with hypothermia include carcinoma, pancreatitis without secondary infection, peritonitis from any cause, and severe cerebrovascular disease. Low cardiac output resulting from a myocardial infarction can induce hypothermia. Fetal and maternal bradycardia and hypothermia may result from magnesium sulfate infusion during preterm labor. Delayed recovery from neuromuscular blockade may also result from unrecognized hypothermia.

Traumatic Factors

Trauma victims often suffer from hypothermia.[22] Hypotension and hypovolemia jeopardize thermostability. In patients with major injuries, a fall in core and skin temperature with no compensatory shivering thermogenesis occurs. Thermoregulation is impaired, and heat production decreases.

Hypothermia may exacerbate blood loss by inducing a coagulopathy via three mechanisms: the coagulation cascade of enzymatic reactions is impaired, plasma fibrinolytic activity is enhanced, and platelets are sequestered and poorly functional.[23]

Traumatic injuries may be overlooked if hypotension or neurologic findings such as areflexia or paralysis are misattributed to hypothermia. Major risk factors for hypothermia in trauma patients include age; type of injury; level of intoxicants; transfusion requirements; and elapsed time spent in the field, emergency department, and operating room.

Hypothermia does protect the brain from ischemia, but it seems to be protective only when it is induced before shock develops. This reduces adenosine triphosphate (ATP) use while the ATP stores are near normal. In traumatized patients, the ATP stores are already depleted. The target core temperature when rewarming a patient with an isolated head injury should balance neuroprotection against the adverse hematologic consequences of hypothermia.[24]

CLINICAL FEATURES

When exposure is obvious, the diagnosis is simple. Appreciation of more subtle presentations helps facilitate the early diagnosis of mild to moderate hypothermia. Vague symptoms include hunger, nausea, confusion, dizziness, chills, pruritus, or dyspnea (Box 138-2). During an expedition, individuals may simply become uncooperative, uncoordinated, moody, or apathetic. Indoors, elderly patients may exhibit confusion or simply become less communicative and display lassitude or a peculiar "flat" affect. Subtle progression of mental deterioration or motor skill impairment may mimic senility. Symptoms such as slurred speech and ataxia may resemble symptoms of a cerebrovascular accident.[21]

Some elderly people have a decreased ability to sense cold and thus fail to take appropriate adaptive action. The maladaptive phenomenon of *paradoxical undressing* is not uncommon. The last preterminal effort of the victim may be related to the peripheral vasoconstrictive changes of profound hypothermia. The patient can be mistaken for a victim of sexual assault.

In urban settings, hypothermia is most commonly associated with ethanol ingestion or underlying illness. Other common presentations include strokes, overdoses, psychiatric emergencies, or coexistent major trauma.[12]

Neurologic manifestations vary widely. A progressive decrease in the level of consciousness is usually proportional to the degree of hypothermia. Some patients, however, continue to be verbally responsive and display intact reflexes at 27° C to 25° C.

Eye movement abnormalities and extensor plantar responses do not correlate directly with the degree of hypothermia. Cranial nerve signs may be seen with bulbar damage from central pontine myelinolysis. Above 22° C, it should be assumed that nonreactive dilated pupils reflect inadequate tissue perfusion and not hypothermia per se.

The rest of the neuromuscular examination may suggest the diagnosis. The patient's posture ranges from stiff to pseudo-rigor mortis to opisthotonos. Reflexes are usually hyperactive down to 32° C, then become hypoactive until they disappear around 26° C. Cremasteric reflexes are expectedly absent with testicular retraction. The plantar response usually remains flexor until 26° C. The knee jerk, when intact, is the last reflex to disappear and the first to reappear with rewarming. The diagnosis of an antecedent CNS disorder, including cord lesions, may be obscured by hypothermia.

Between 30° C and 26° C, both contraction and relaxation phases of the reflexes are equally prolonged. If intact, the ankle jerk is helpful in diagnosing hypothermic myxedema. Myxedema prolongs the relaxation phase more than the contraction phase.

Box 138-2. Presenting Signs of Hypothermia

Head, Eye, Ear, Nose, Throat
Mydriasis
Decreased corneal reflexes
Extraocular muscle abnormalities
Erythropsia
Flushing
Facial edema
Epistaxis
Rhinorrhea
Strabismus

Cardiovascular
Initial tachycardia
Subsequent bradycardia
Dysrhythmias
Decreased heart tones
Hepatojugular reflux
Jugular venous distention
Hypotension

Respiratory
Initial tachypnea
Adventitious sounds
Bronchorrhea
Progressive hypoventilation
Apnea

Gastrointestinal
Ileus
Constipation
Abdominal distention or rigidity
Poor rectal tone
Gastric dilation in neonates or in adults with myxedema

Genitourinary
Anuria
Oliguria
Polyuria
Testicular torsion

Neurologic
Depressed level of consciousness
Ataxia
Hypesthesia
Dysarthria
Anti-nociception
Amnesia
Initial hyperreflexia
Anesthesia
Hyporeflexia
Areflexia
Central pontine myelinolysis

Psychiatric
Impaired judgment
Perseveration
Mood changes
Peculiar flat affect
Altered mental status
Paradoxical undressing
Neuroses
Psychoses
Suicide
Organic brain syndrome

Musculoskeletal
Increased muscle tone
Shivering
Rigidity or pseudo–rigor mortis
Paravertebral spasm
Opisthotonus
Compartment syndrome

Dermatologic
Erythema
Pernio
Pallor
Frostnip
Cyanosis
Frostbite
Icterus
Popsicle panniculitis
Sclerema
Cold urticaria
Ecchymosis
Necrosis
Edema
Gangrene

No psychiatric disorder improves when the patient is cold. Mental status alterations include anxiety, perseveration, neurosis, and psychosis. Many individuals who are functional in temperate climates decompensate in colder weather. Hypothermic-induced psychiatric presentations and suicide attempts are commonly misdiagnosed.[9]

DIAGNOSTIC STRATEGIES

Laboratory Evaluations

Acid-Base Balance

Blood gas analyzers warm blood to 37° C, which increases the partial pressure of dissolved gases. This results in an arterial blood gas (ABG) report showing higher oxygen and carbon dioxide levels and a lower pH than the patient's actual values. Optimal ABG levels in the setting of hypothermia dictate that correction of ABGs for temperature is unnecessary as a guide to therapy.[25-28] In fact, attempting to maintain a corrected pH at 7.4 and P_{CO_2} at 40 mm Hg during hypothermia depresses cerebral and coronary blood flow and cardiac output and increases the incidence of ventricular fibrillation.[29] Although the ideal acid-base strategy continues to be debated, the ectothermic alpha-stat approach appears preferable.[8] The goal is an uncorrected pH at 7.4 and Pa_{CO_2} at 40 mm Hg.

Cold blood buffers poorly. In normothermia, when the P_{CO_2} increases 10 mm Hg, the pH decreases 0.08 units. At 28° C, the decrease in pH doubles. Because the neutral point of water at 37° C is a pH of 6.8, the normal 0.6 unit pH offset between blood and intracellular water should be maintained at all temperatures. Just as the neutral pH rises with cooling, so should actual blood pH (Figure 138-3).

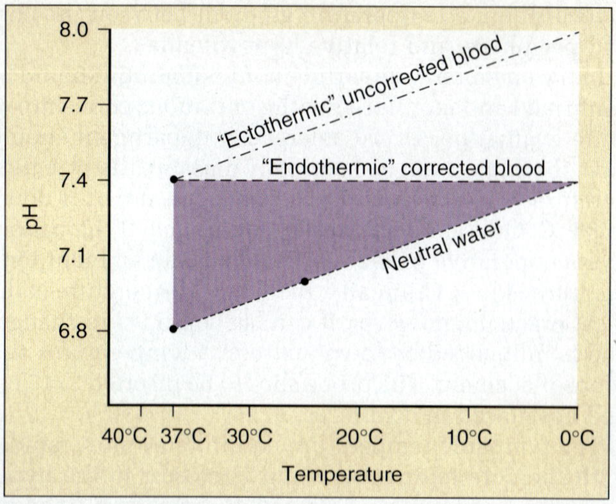

Figure 138-3. Neutrality reflects the pH of water at any given temperature. The pH of water is 6.8 at 37° C and 7.0 at 25° C. The physiologically ideal intracellular-to-extracellular 0.6 pH unit offset will be maintained if the arterial pH is kept uncorrected for temperature at 7.42.

Intracellular electrochemical neutrality ensures optimal enzymatic function at all temperatures.[26] Relative alkalinity affords myocardial protection and improves the heart's electrical stability.[29] Carbogen could prove valuable in the treatment of accidental hypothermia because it flattens and shifts the oxyhemoglobin dissociation curve to the right.

Hematologic Evaluation

A patient's hematocrit can be deceptively high as the result of a decreased plasma volume. As a rule of thumb, the hematocrit level should increase 2% for every 1° C fall in temperature. A normal hematocrit level in a moderate to severely hypothermic patient should raise suspicion for acute blood loss or suggest the possibility of a preexisting anemia.

A normal white blood cell count does not exclude infection, especially if the patient is debilitated, alcoholic, myxedematous, or at either age extreme. Splenic, hepatic, and splanchnic sequestration in hypothermia decreases leukocyte and platelet counts.

Frequent evaluation of serum electrolytes during rewarming is essential. There appears to be no safe predictor of their values or trends.[12] Changes occur in both membrane permeability and in the sodium-potassium (K^+-Na^+) pump. The patient's preexisting physiologic status, the severity and chronicity of hypothermia, and the method of rewarming alter the serum electrolyte values.

The plasma potassium level is independent of the primary hypothermic process. Hyperkalemia is often associated with metabolic acidosis, rhabdomyolysis, or renal failure. An important caveat is that hypothermia enhances the cardiac toxicity and obscures the premonitory electrocardiographic changes associated with hyperkalemia.

Hypokalemia is most common with chronic hypothermia. It results from potassium entering muscle, not a kaliuresis. A discrepant decline in serum potassium level despite a decreasing serum pH is caused by intracellular pH fluxes greater than extracellular pH fluxes.

Conditions associated with hypokalemia include preexisting diabetic ketoacidosis, hypopituitarism, inappropriate secretion of antidiuretic hormone, previous diuretic therapy, and alcoholism. If the potassium level is less than 3 mEq/L, the addition of 20 to 30 mEq K^+/L of crystalloid fluid may be necessary for treatment of gastrointestinal ileus or congestive heart failure during rewarming.

The blood urea nitrogen (BUN) and creatinine levels are elevated with preexisting renal disease or decreased clearance. Because of hypothermic fluid shifts, the hematocrit and BUN levels are poor indicators of a patient's actual fluid status.

The blood sugar level may also provide a subtle clue to the type of hypothermia. Acute hypothermia initially elevates blood sugar levels through catecholamine-induced glycogenolysis, diminished insulin release, and inhibition of cellular membrane glucose carrier systems. On the other hand, subacute and chronic hypothermia produce glycogen depletion, leading to hypoglycemia. Symptoms of hypoglycemia can be masked by hypothermia. A cold-induced renal glycosuria does not imply hyperglycemia.[21]

When hyperglycemia persists during rewarming, one should suspect hemorrhagic pancreatitis or diabetic ketoacidosis. Patients with the latter must be actively rewarmed past 30° C because insulin is ineffective below that temperature. Correction of hypoglycemia only corrects the level of consciousness to that of the corresponding level of hypothermia.

Severe hypothermia causes serum enzyme elevation because of the ultrastructural cellular damage. Rhabdomyolysis is commonly associated with cold exposure.

The relationship between hypothermia and hyperamylasemia is poorly defined. The extent of hyperamylasemia can correlate with mortality. Ischemic pancreatitis may result from the microcirculatory shock of hypothermia. The decreased pancreatic blood flow then activates proteolytic enzymes.[6]

Hypothermic Coagulation

A physiologic increase in coagulation occurs with hypothermia, and a disseminated intravascular coagulation type of syndrome occurs. The cause may be catecholamine or steroid release, simple circulatory collapse, or release of tissue thromboplastin from cold, ischemic tissue.[23,30]

Hypothermic patients also develop coagulopathies because the enzymatic nature of the activated clotting factors is depressed by the cold. The clotting prolongation is proportional to the number of steps in the cascade. Because the kinetic tests of coagulation are performed in the laboratory at 37° C, the physician will see a disparity between the in vivo clinically evident coagulopathy and the deceptively "normal" prothrombin time or partial thromboplastin time reported by the laboratory.[31] The only effective treatment is rewarming, not administration of clotting factors.[32]

The leukopenia and thrombocytopenia usually reverse with rewarming. Clinically significant coagulopathies occur, particularly in association with trauma. Cold-induced thrombocytopenia is observed with induced hypothermia. The mechanism may be either direct bone marrow suppression or splenic and hepatic sequestration. Platelet thromboxane B_2 production is also temperature dependent. Thrombocytopenia is more common at both age extremes.

The elevated viscosity seen with hypothermia may be exacerbated in patients with cryoglobulinemia or cryofibrinogenemia, both of which are more common in elderly patients. Cryofibrinogen, which is a cold-precipitated fibrinogen, is associated with the collagen vascular diseases, carcinomas, and coliform sepsis. The pathophysiology of cold hemagglutination results from cold agglutinins that produce either hemolysis or agglutination with thrombosis. This could explain the increase in coronary and cerebral thromboses in winter.

In summary, except in mild cases, the immediate laboratory evaluations should include glucose; ABGs uncorrected for temperature; complete blood cell count; a comprehensive medical panel including serum calcium, serum magnesium, and serum amylase/lipase levels; and coagulation studies. Baseline serum BUN and creatinine tests are indicated because renal failure may occur after rewarming in patients with chronic hypothermia.

A toxicologic screen is necessary when the depression of the level of consciousness is inconsistent with the degree of hypothermia. Thyroid function studies, cardiac markers, and serum cortisol levels have selective utility.

The indications for radiography should be liberalized from those followed for normothermic patients. If the patient is not alert, spinal radiographs should be obtained. Abdominal radiographs or computed tomography films show pancreatic calcifications, unsuspected pneumoperitoneum, small bowel dilation from hypothermia-induced mesenteric vascular occlusion, or colonic dilation associated with myxedema coma.[21]

MANAGEMENT

Patients who are cold, stiff, and cyanotic, with fixed pupils and inaudible heart tones, without visible thoracic excursions continue to be successfully resuscitated. Some patients still recover completely in the morgue.

An adequate history includes available pertinent information regarding preexisting cardiac, pulmonary, neurologic, or endocrinologic disease. The duration of exposure, circumstances of discovery, associated injuries, and predisposing conditions should be documented. Initial management should emphasize the prevention of further heat loss.[33] The goals of prehospital care are to rescue, examine, insulate, and rapidly transport.[34,35]

If the patient is unresponsive and not shivering, the hypothermia should be presumed to be severe. At temperatures below 32° C, one should expect an irritable myocardium, a temperature gradient between the core and periphery, and relative hypovolemia.

In the emergency department, hypothermia should be confirmed and monitored with continuous core temperature evaluation. Every emergency department should have the equipment to accurately measure the core temperature. Standard oral thermometers record only down to 35° C. Oral temperatures are unreliable if the patient is uncooperative or tachypneic, or if the ambient temperature is low. Clinically, the rectal temperature is the most practical; however, it can lag behind core changes and is influenced by lower extremity temperatures and probe placement. The probe should be inserted to 15 cm and not placed in cold feces.

The tympanic temperature equilibrates most rapidly with the core temperature and is closest to the hypothalamic temperature. Infrared thermography should not be used alone in the setting of suspected hypothermia because the reliability of commercially available devices remains uncertain. If the patient is tracheally intubated, an esophageal probe reads falsely high with heated inhalation.

A Doppler measuring device may be necessary to establish the presence of a spontaneous pulse or blood pressure. The accuracy of pulse oximetry during conditions of poor perfusion and hypothermia is uncertain. Similarly, end-tidal carbon dioxide measurements accurately assess tissue perfusion and tracheal tube placement only at normal temperatures. Commercially available devices do not function with humidified air used for airway rewarming.

Endotracheal intubation is necessary unless the patient is alert with intact protective airway reflexes.[5,12] Cold depression of ciliary activity allows secretory accumulation, with the production of frothy sputum and chest congestion. Failure to differentiate between this bronchorrhea and pulmonary edema may explain the conflicting reports of the association of hypothermia with pulmonary edema. Blind nasotracheal intubation may be the simplest option when cold-induced trismus is present, unless there is a significant coagulopathy.

In a multicenter survey, endotracheal intubation was performed on 117 patients by multiple operators in various settings.[12] No induced dysrhythmias were recognized, which is consistent with several other reports. Factors commonly precipitating dysrhythmias include failure to preoxygenate, mechanical jostling, acid-base changes, and electrolyte fluctuations.

A nasogastric tube is indicated in patients with moderate and severe hypothermia after endotracheal intubation. Decreased gastric motility and gastric dilation occur commonly. Physical examination of the abdomen is unreliable because the cold can induce rectus muscle rigidity. A large percentage of moderate and severely hypothermic patients have decreased or absent bowel sounds. Because physical examination of the abdomen is unreliable, it is important to evaluate the patient carefully for an associated ileus, pancreatitis, or occult trauma.

In cases of moderate and severe hypothermia, indwelling bladder catheters with urine meter bags are essential to monitor urinary output and to help determine the severity of vascular fluid shifts.

Cardiac monitoring should be continued, and peripheral or central intravenous catheters inserted as necessary. Inserting a central venous pressure catheter tip into the heart can precipitate dysrhythmias and should be avoided. Arterial catheters for continuous monitoring of intra-arterial blood pressure may be necessary in selected profoundly hypothermic patients. Placement of pulmonary artery catheters, although they are potentially useful, risks perforation of the cold, stiff pulmonary artery.[36]

Volume Resuscitation

Patients with moderate or severe hypothermia are usually dehydrated, and they are also prone to thromboembolism resulting from the increased viscosity. During rewarming, a relatively high total plasma volume and low circulatory plasma volume are often present. As hypothermia develops, other effects include an increased peripheral vascular resistance with a decreased circulatory volume.[37]

Rapid volume expansion is critical. In hypothermic neonates, the mortality risk is dramatically lessened. Adult patients with moderate or severe hypothermia should initially receive a 250 to 500 mL fluid challenge of heated 5% dextrose in normal saline solution until laboratory values are available. Lactated Ringer's solution should in theory be avoided because the cold liver inefficiently metabolizes lactate.

Fluids administered intravenously should be heated to 40° C to 42° C. This is done primarily to avoid worsening hypothermia, because the amount of heat provided only becomes significant with large-volume resuscitations.[38,39] One heating option is to microwave intravenous fluids in plastic containers. A 1 L bag of crystalloid requires an average of 2 minutes on high power. The fluid should be shaken before administration to avoid hot spots. Rapid central venous administration, which may produce myocardial thermal gradients, should also be avoided.

There can be significant conductive heat loss through intravenous tubing. Long lengths of this tubing increase heat loss, especially at slow flow rates. There are various methods to achieve and maintain ideal delivery temperature of intravenous and lavage fluids in hypothermia. On option is to preheat the fluid to 60° C when using long segments of tubing, and 40° C with short segments. Another option is to administer fluid in intermittent boluses at higher flow rates rather than continuously.[40] Countercurrent heat exchangers such as the Level I Fluid Warmer (Life Systems, Southfield, Mich) effectively heat crystalloids and blood from 10° C to 35° C. Various other blood-warming devices are also available.

Normally, hypothermia induces an increased natriuresis. Preexisting gastrointestinal losses or previous diuretic treatment can also contribute to sodium loss. Patients with normal sodium and osmolality values may have preexisting sodium overload as a result of cirrhosis, nephrosis, or congestive heart failure; however, most patients will be free-water depleted, which elevates their sodium and osmolality values.

Hemoconcentration resulting from decreased plasma volume, fluid shifts, and increased vascular permeability usually is present. Hemodilution can occur from parenteral crystalloid administration, but a low hematocrit can also result from acute hemorrhage or preexisting anemia.

During rewarming, the patient should be monitored for clinical signs of fluid overload. In severe cases with persistent cardiovascular instability, central venous pressure catheters provide useful information but should be inserted carefully to avoid irritating the right atrium. Generally, it is wise to defer pulmonary wedge pressure measurements until after rewarming.[36]

Advanced Life Support

Blood flow during CPR in patients with hypothermia differs from that during normothermia, when some flow results from phasic alterations in the intrathoracic pressure, not necessarily from direct cardiac compression.[41] During hypothermic cardiac arrest in swine, the cardiac output and cerebral and myocardial blood flows average 50%, 55%, and 31%, respectively, of those achieved during normothermic closed-chest compressions.[42]

In hypothermia, the "thoracic pump" concept with the heart as a passive conduit contributes to blood flow. The phasic alterations in the intrathoracic pressure are exerted equally on all cardiac chambers. The mitral valve remains patent during systole, and blood continues to circulate through the left side of the heart. This could explain the observation of Althaus and associates,[43] who note that in one of three survivors at thoracotomy, "the heart was found to be hard as stone and it is hardly conceivable how effective external cardiac massage could have been." There are many neurologically intact survivors after prolonged closed-chest compressions.[44,45]

Chest wall elasticity and pulmonary compliance are decreased with cold. Therefore, more force is needed to depress the chest wall sufficiently to generate intrathoracic pressure gradients. Pneumatic-powered thoracic compression devices may be useful during prolonged resuscitations pending decisions regarding extracorporeal rewarming. Other perfusion enhancers could include abdominal binding to inhibit paradoxical diaphragmatic motion and simultaneous compression ventilation.

Tissue decomposition, apparent rigor mortis, dependent lividity, and fixed dilated pupils are not always reliable criteria for withholding CPR in the hypothermic patient. Because intermittent flow may provide adequate support during evacuation, CPR should not be withheld just because continuous compressions cannot be ensured.

In a multicenter survey of 428 cases, 9 of the 27 patients receiving CPR initiated in the field survived, as did 6 of 14 patients with CPR initiated in the emergency department.[12] The rescuer should initiate CPR in cases of accidental hypothermia unless do-not-resuscitate status is documented and verified, obviously lethal injuries are present, chest wall depression is impossible, signs of life are present, or rescuers are endangered by evacuation delays or altered triage conditions.

PHARMACOLOGY

The efficacy of most drugs is temperature dependent. Protein binding increases during hypothermia, and liver metabolism is decreased. Overmedication could be required to achieve a therapeutic response, and subsequent toxic levels would develop with rewarming. No medication should be given orally because of decreased gastrointestinal motility; none should be given intramuscularly because of poor absorption from vasoconstricted sites.

Cardiovascular

The effects of hypothermia on the autonomic nervous system vary. In primate studies, the sympathetic nervous system responds rapidly to cooling from 37° C to 31° C. It then switches off around 29° C, which suggests that some catecholamine support might be useful below that temperature.[46]

In general, pharmacologic manipulation of the pulse and blood pressure should be avoided. Vasoconstrictors may be dysrhythmogenic while having a minimal effect on the maximally constricted peripheral vasculature. Epinephrine and other vasoconstrictors should be avoided.

Inotropes usually are not necessary to support the blood pressure. Low-dose (2-5 μg/min) dopamine infusions should be considered in disproportionately hypotensive patients who do not maintain a mean arterial pressure of 60 in response to crystalloids, colloids, and rewarming. To facilitate perfusion of a vasoconstricted cardiovascular system while on dopamine, some investigators add an infusion of low-dose nitroglycerin.

Dysrhythmia Treatment

Preexisting chronic premature ventricular contractions can be suppressed during hypothermia and recur during rewarming. Most hypothermia-induced dysrhythmias convert spontaneously during rewarming. Asystole that develops during rewarming is *not* a more ominous rhythm than VF. VF should be defibrillated at 2 W sec/kg up to 200 W sec. A successful reestablishment of electromechanical activity has been reported at 20° C.[47] If the defibrillation attempt is unsuccessful, active rewarming should be initiated with available equipment while CPR is continued. Defibrillation attempts are usually unsuccessful until the core temperature is well above 28° C to 30° C. Nevertheless, at any temperature, three defibrillation attempts should be initiated. If unsuccessful, the core temperature should be raised to 30° C before further reattempts.

Virtually all atrial dysrhythmias are common below 32° C and are associated with a slow ventricular response. Atrial fibrillation is common and considered innocent. It usually converts spontaneously during rewarming. Digitalization and calcium channel blockade are not warranted. Mesenteric embolization may occur when the rhythm converts.

The ideal approach to the prevention and treatment of ventricular dysrhythmias is unresolved. Lidocaine and propranolol have minimal hemodynamic effects during hypothermia. Their efficacy in treating ventricular dysrhythmias appears limited.

Although no longer available, bretylium tosylate was extremely effective in several animal studies before invasive maneuvers performed *after* induction of hypothermia. Several clinical chemical defibrillations with bretylium in cases of severe hypothermia are reported.[21] The prophylactic value of bretylium or lidocaine during hypothermia has not been evaluated. In a canine model of severe hypothermic VF, neither amiodarone nor bretylium was effective.[48]

In cases of normothermia, group I ventricular antidysrhythmics directly decrease conduction velocity and possess indirect anticholinergic activity. In cases of hypothermia, at least one agent in this group, procainamide, reportedly increases the incidence of VF. Another drug in the group, quinidine, has prevented VF during induced profound hypothermia and during cardiac manipulation at 25° C to 30° C.

Transvenous intracardiac pacing is extremely hazardous for hypothermia-induced bradydysrhythmias. External noninvasive pacing by means of large low-resistance electrodes is a successful alternative to emergency transvenous pacing and is preferable in cases of hypothermia.[49]

Miscellaneous

Cold exposure normally induces adrenal unresponsiveness to adrenocorticotropic hormone. A false diagnosis of decreased adrenal reserve in hypothermia is possible. The increase in adrenocorticotropic hormone level seen in hypothermic individuals may be a neurogenic or emotional response to the cold.

Acute cold stress initially stimulates cortisol secretion. The patient may already have a very high level as a result of an underlying stress. In clinical series, serum cortisol levels are commonly elevated. The percentage of cortisol bound to protein is increased with hypothermia, and therefore the active free fraction is decreased.

If a patient fails to rewarm, a history should be taken for evidence of adrenocortical insufficiency or steroid dependence. At that juncture, administration of 30 mg/kg methylprednisolone sodium succinate or 250 mg hydrocortisone IV should be considered.

Empirical treatment with thyroxine should be reserved for patients thought to be myxedematous. Thyroid hormone replacement is recommended if a history of hypothyroidism is present, a suggestive neck scar is present, or a failure to rewarm occurs. After thyroid function study samples are drawn, 250 to 500 μg of levothyroxine should be administered cautiously intravenously over several minutes. Daily injections of 50 to 100 μg are necessary for 5 to 7 days.

Hydrocortisone (100-200 mg) should be added to the first several liters of crystalloid fluid.

The absorption of levothyroxine is variable when it is administered orally or intramuscularly. Administration intravenously results in a smooth effect after the onset of action at 6 to 12 hours. This is evidenced by improvement in the vital signs and the rewarming rate. Half the dose is converted by the peripheral tissues into 1-triiodothyronine (T_3). If there is no improvement, 25 µg T_3 should also be given every 6 hours through a nasogastric tube.[21]

Septicemia

Hypothermia compromises host defenses and predisposes to infection. The usual signs of infection, including fever, are absent. Shaking chills from sepsis may be mistaken for shivering. If a patient's mental status remains altered despite rewarming, CNS injury or infection should be suspected.

Diminished bone marrow release and circulation of neutrophils, along with impaired neutrophil migration and bacterial phagocytosis, are factors contributing to infection. In children younger than 3 months, prophylactic antibiotics after culturing are indicated. No reliable clinical or laboratory indicators of infection exist, but bradycardia, anemia, uremia, and serum glucose levels, as well as leukocyte abnormalities, are common clues.

The role of antibiotic prophylaxis in adults is less clear. Although gram-negative septicemia may be the cause of hypothermia, coexistent infections from gram-positive cocci, enterobacteriaceae, and oral anaerobes are common.

Elderly patients with thermoregulatory failure have a high risk of mortality and should be considered septic until proven otherwise. Routine antibiotic prophylaxis in hypothermic adults, unlike in elderly patients and in children, does not appear warranted. Antibiotics should be administered if the clinical picture is consistent with septic shock, if there is failure to rewarm, or if aspiration has occurred. Cellulitis, myositis, bacteriuria, or infiltrates present on chest radiographs all warrant immediate antimicrobial therapy.[9]

REWARMING

No controlled studies compare rewarming methods in cases of moderate and severe hypothermia, and rigid treatment protocols are not advisable.[34,50] The treatment choice must be based on clinical reports, animal experiments, and experiments on mildly hypothermic humans.[51] The advantages, disadvantages, indications, contraindications, and specific guidelines for the various reported techniques of rewarming patients with accidental hypothermia are given here.

Passive External Rewarming

Spontaneous passive external rewarming is noninvasive, and it is the treatment of choice for most patients with mild hypothermia. During passive external rewarming, the patient must be able to metabolically generate sufficient heat to maintain an acceptable rate of spontaneous rewarming.

The normal processes of heat dissipation are minimized by passive external rewarming. Cessation of evaporization and convection are coupled with insulation against further radiation of heat. This technique simply involves covering the patient with an insulating material in a favorable atmospheric condition. The ambient temperature should exceed 21° C. When the air is stationary, less heat is lost to conduction, convection, and radiation. If the air is of high humidity, less heat is lost in the respiratory process of heating and humidification.

Below 30° C, humans are functionally poikilothermic. No shivering thermogenesis occurs. Shivering is the thermoregulatory neuromuscular response to cold that increases heat production from 250 to 1000 kcal/hr. Without it, the endogenously generated metabolic heat is insufficient to raise the core temperature. For example, the basal metabolic rate is less than 50% of normal below 28° C. When the core temperature exceeds 32° C, the major source of heat production is shivering thermogenesis, unless complete glycogen depletion occurs. Sufficient body insulation is more critical than muscle glycogen levels in passive rewarming.

Recommended rewarming rates vary between 0.5° C and 2.0° C/hr. In a multicenter survey, the first three hourly rewarming rates exceeded 0.5° C with no increase in mortality.[12] The rewarming rate should be rapid enough to avoid prolonged exposure to dysrhythmias. Elderly patients are commonly glycogen depleted, centrally hypovolemic, and not capable of normal cardiovascular or metabolic homeostasis.

Active Rewarming

Active rewarming is the direct transfer of exogenous heat to the patient. It can be accomplished by either external or internal techniques.

Cardiovascular instability and decompensation require rapid elevation of the core temperature (Box 138-3). Defibrillation is rarely successful at temperatures below 28° C to 30° C. Active rewarming is indicated in patients with cerebrovascular accidents and other conditions that impair CNS control of thermoregulation. Active rewarming is also indicated in patients when endogenous thermogenesis is insufficient or when glycogen depletion is present. These diseases are usually endocrinologic and include hypo-

Box 138-3. Indications for Active Rewarming

1. Cardiovascular instability
2. Moderate or severe hypothermia (<32.2° C)
3. Inadequate rate or failure to rewarm
4. Endocrinologic insufficiency
5. Traumatic or toxicologic peripheral vasodilation
6. Secondary hypothermia impairing thermoregulation

pituitarism, adrenal insufficiency, hypothyroidism, and Wernicke's encephalopathy. Active rewarming is also indicated if diabetic ketoacidosis is present because the core temperature must be elevated well above 30° C before insulin becomes effective.[52]

Pharmacologically induced peripheral vasodilation or acute spinal cord transection makes a patient incapable of sufficient thermogenesis, and such patients should be actively rewarmed. Active rewarming in patients with moderate or severe hypothermia is also indicated because of the potential for cardiovascular decompensation or ventricular irritability. Patients with severe hypothermia and a sustained perfusing rhythm do not necessarily require invasive extracorporeal rewarming techniques.[53]

Aggressive treatment of hypothermia in infants is indicated. Rapid rewarming may be advantageous because it minimizes energy expenditures.[54] Vigorous monitoring for infectious, respiratory, hematologic, and metabolic complications is needed.

Active External Rewarming

Early concern with active external rewarming (AER) was voiced by Duguid and collagues[55] in 1961 when 20 of their 23 patients died. Retrospective analysis of numerous clinical series notes widely varying mortality rates with AER.[5,12,52] Interpretation of these clinical series is affected by risk factors and patient selection.

Various methods are available to conduct heat directly to the skin. Immersion in a bath of 40° C is one option. Disadvantages of this approach include the inability to monitor or resuscitate the patient in water and the difficulty of performing CPR on a floating body.

Other rewarming options include plumbed garments that recirculate warm fluids, hot water bottles, heating pads, forced-air warming systems, and radiant sources. Thermal injury to vasoconstricted hypoperfused skin is a common hazard with local heat application.[56]

Forced air warming systems efficiently transfer heat.[57-60] The Bair Hugger uses hot forced air circulated through a blanket. The air exits apertures on the patient side of the cover, which allows a convective transfer of heat. In one study in which accidental hypothermia victims were rewarmed in the emergency department, rewarming shock and core temperature afterdrop were not noted.[61] Both groups of patients were also treated with heated inhalation and warmed intravenous fluids. The use of forced-air warming systems is currently most practical in the emergency department.[61,62] Although these devices decrease shivering thermogenesis, afterdrop is minimized and heat transfer can be significant.

Arteriovenous anastomoses rewarming is another noninvasive AER technique that was first described by Vangaard in 1979.[63] Exogenous heat is provided by immersion of the lower parts of the extremities (hands, forearms, feet, calves) in 44° C to 45° C water. The heat opens the arteriovenous anastomoses (AVAs). These organs are 1 mm below the epidermal surface in the digits.[64] As a result, there is an increased flow of warmed venous subcutaneous blood returning directly to the heart. Countercurrent heat loss is minimized because the superficial veins are not close to the arterial tree.

A permutation of AVA rewarming is negative pressure rewarming. Under hypothermic conditions, the AVAs remain closed during peripheral vasoconstriction. In combination with localized heat application, the application of subatmospheric pressure theoretically distends the venous rete and increases flow through the AVAs.

To initiate negative pressure rewarming, the forearm is inserted through an acrylic tubing sleeve device fitted with a neoprene collar. This allows an airtight seal to form around the forearm. After a −40 mm Hg vacuum pressure is created, heat is applied over the dilated AVAs.[65] The clinical efficacy and safety of AVA rewarming in cases of accidental hypothermia remains to be determined.

Optimal candidates for AER are previously healthy patients with acute hypothermia. In these patients, minimal pathophysiologic circulatory changes have occurred.[66] If AER is chosen and the extremities are vasoconstricted, the heat source should generally be applied only to the thorax. Application of heat to the extremities increases the cardiovascular load by increasing the metabolic requirements of the peripheral musculature. The depressed cardiovascular system may not be able to meet the demands, and cardiovascular collapse can occur.

Combining truncal AER with core rewarming is also successful. Some authors believe that providing heated humidified oxygen and warmed intravenous fluids in addition to AER may anticipate and avert hypoxia, metabolic acidosis, core temperature afterdrop, and hypotension. If AER is chosen as the method of treatment for moderate or severe hypothermia, it should be combined with one of the active core rewarming techniques.

Active Core Rewarming

Numerous alternatives have been explored to achieve active rewarming of the core. These techniques minimize rewarming collapse in patients with temperatures below 32° C.

Airway Rewarming

Airway rewarming as an adjunctive active core rewarming technique has been explored in research laboratories and clinically since first suggested by Lloyd.[16] This simple technique is indicated in all cases of moderate or severe hypothermia.[67]

Advantages of heated humidified oxygen include noninvasiveness, cost, simplicity, assurance of adequate oxygenation, and avoidance of afterdrop. Additional benefits are the stimulation of pulmonary cilia, a decrease in pulmonary secretion viscosity, and a reduction of cold-induced bronchorrhea. Pulmonic absorption occurs without adverse affects on surfactant or increased pulmonary congestion.

Table 138-2. Oxygenation Considerations During Hypothermia

Detrimental Factors	Protective Factors
Oxygen consumption increases ×3/10° C rise in temperature; caution if rapid rewarming; shivering increases demand	Reduction of oxygen consumption 50% at 28° C; 75% at 22° C, 92% at 10° C
Clinical evidence of increased muscle enzymes with decreased Pa_{O_2}	Increased oxygen solubility in plasma
Decreased temperature shifts oxyhemoglobin dissociation curve to left	Decreased pH, increased Pa_{CO_2}, shift oxyhemoglobin dissociation curve to right
Ventilation-perfusion mismatch, atelectasis, decreased respiratory minute volume, bronchorrhea, decreased protective airway reflexes	
Decreased tissue perfusion from vasoconstriction, increased viscosity	
"Functional hemoglobin" concept—capacity of hemoglobin to unload oxygen is low	

The respiratory tract is a limited site for heat exchange.[38] Nevertheless, both the oxygen content and the temperature in the pulmonary vasculature rise. The myocardium is perfused by warmer oxygenated blood, stabilizing against intermittent temperature gradients.

A sufficient respiratory minute volume and complete humidification are necessary for maximal heat delivery. Because of the low thermal conductivity of dry air, ventilation with warm dry air provides negligible heat. Depending on the technique used (endotracheal tube more than mask), one should expect a rewarming rate between 1° C and 2.5° C/hr.[5,12]

Heated mask ventilation is of interest. A thermal countercurrent heat exchanger is in the cerebrovascular bed of humans. This system, known as the rete mirabile, could preferentially rewarm the brainstem. Another option is heated inhalation through face mask continuous positive airway pressure.

Maintenance of sufficient oxygenation is critical in moderate and severe cases. Fisher considered the effects of hypothermia, pH, Pa_{CO_2}, and the level of 2,3-diphosphoglycerate on the shift of the oxyhemoglobin dissociation curve. In patients on cardiopulmonary bypass cooled to 28° C to 30° C, the capacity of hemoglobin to unload oxygen to the tissue is less than half that found in normothermic patients.[68] Despite lower metabolic requirements, this decrease in "functional" hemoglobin, combined with a depressed respiratory minute volume, results in minimum oxygen reserves (Table 138-2).

Some patients maintain a level of spontaneous respiration appropriate to the depressed carbon dioxide production. This is not the case in patients with coexisting toxicologic or metabolic depression of their respiratory centers. During spontaneous or assisted ventilation with heated ventilation, there is the flexibility to alter the Fi_{O_2}, monitor airway pressure, and deliver continuous positive airway pressure or positive end-expiratory pressure.

The technique for patients with spontaneous respirations requires a heated cascade nebulizer. An immersion heater can be connected to a hose with a warming wire. Because patients with a depressed level of consciousness do not complain of pain, it is essential to frequently check the temperature of the inspired air with an in-line temperature probe. The gas temperature should be maintained at 42° C to 45° C. Most heater modules require modification to allow the temperature to reach 42° C to 45° C and should be so labeled to avoid routine use.

Most humidifiers are manufactured in accordance with the International Standards regulations. The humidifier does not exceed 41° C close to the patient outlet with a 6-foot tubing length.

Strategies to circumvent the 41° C ceiling include reduction of tubing length, adding more heat sources, disabling the humidifier safety system, and placing the temperature probe outside the patient circuit.[69] Due to the modest clinical benefit in stable patients, circumventing the 41° C ceiling may not be worth the effort. The only report of thermal airway injury is in a patient ventilated via endotracheal tube for 11 hours with 80° C inhalant. A volume ventilator with a heated cascade humidifier can also deliver continuous positive airway pressure or positive end-expiratory pressure if needed during rewarming.

Complete airway protection averts aspiration. Hypothermia is associated with ileus, bronchorrhea, and depressed protective airway reflexes. Although the airway rewarming technique provides less heat than other forms of active core rewarming, it is safe, noninvasive, and practical.

Peritoneal Dialysis

Peritoneal dialysis delivers heated dialysate at 40° C to 45° C to the peritoneal cavity. Heat is conducted directly to the intraperitoneal structures. Heat is also conducted through the posterior parietal peritoneum to the solid viscera and through the hemidiaphragms to the heart and lungs.

A double-catheter system can be used to increase the rate of rewarming with suction at the outflow. The usual clinically attainable rate is 6 L/hr. Two liters are infused, retained for 20 to 30 minutes, and then aspirated. Rewarming rates average 1° C to 3° C/hr, depending on flow rates and dwell times.

An additional benefit of this invasive technique is hepatic rewarming, which reactivates depressed detoxification and conversion enzymes. Peritoneal dialysis can exacerbate preexistent hypokalemia; therefore, serum electrolytes should be carefully monitored. Peritoneal lavage rewarming should not be routinely selected for stable patients. It should be considered for use in severe cases and in combination with all available rewarming techniques for patients without spontaneous perfusion.[21]

Heated Irrigation

Heat transfer from irrigation fluids is usually very limited because the surface area available for heat exchange is minimal. Gastric or colonic irrigation can cause fluid and electrolyte fluxes. Exceeding 200 to 300 mL aliquots may force fluid into the duodenum; therefore, frequent fluid removal via gravity drainage minimizes "lost" fluid. A log of input and output is essential. A double-lumen esophageal tube has been investigated, as have other modified Sengstaken tubes.[70]

Clinical experience with closed thoracic lavage in accidental hypothermia is expanding.[71] Two large-bore thoracostomy tubes are inserted into one or both hemithoraces. One is placed anteriorly in the second or third intercostal space at the midclavicular line. The other is placed in the posterior axillary line at the fifth to sixth intercostal space. Normal saline solution is heated to 40° C to 42° C and sterilely infused and drained.[72]

The efficiency of heat transfer varies with the flow rate and dwell times. Pleural adhesions prevent adequate infusion rates. Adequate drainage must be ensured to prevent intrathoracic hypertension.

Thoracic lavage should be reserved for severely hypothermic patients who do not respond to standard techniques. It should be combined with all other available rewarming modalities in potentially salvageable cardiac arrest patients.[45,73,74]

Mediastinal irrigation and direct myocardial lavage should only be considered in patients without spontaneous perfusion. The procedure begins with a standard left lateral thoracotomy incision. The pericardium is not opened unless an effusion or tamponade is present. The heart is bathed in 1 to 2 L of an isotonic solution heated to 40° C for several minutes. The fluid is then removed and the lavage repeated. Internal defibrillation is attempted at 1° C to 2° C intervals after the myocardial temperature exceeds 26° C to 28° C. When a perfusing rhythm is achieved, lavage is continued until the myocardial temperature exceeds 32° C. A median sternotomy approach allows ventricular decompression in addition to direct defibrillation. Open cardiac massage of a cold, rigid, and contracted heart may not generate flow.[41,43]

Diathermy

Diathermy involves the conversion of energy waves into heat. Large amounts of heat can be delivered to deep tissues with ultrasonic and low-frequency microwave radiation. Frostbite, burns, significant edema, and the presence of all types of metallic implants and pacemakers contraindicate diathermy.

Regional heating of hypothermic dogs after immersion does not damage tissue at 4 to 6 W/kg and rapidly elevates the core temperature. Zhong and associates[54] rewarmed 16 piglets with microwave irradiation "until they squealed and suckled." In a subsequent experiment, 20 of 28 human infants were rewarmed with microwave irradiation at 90 to 100 W and survived.

Table 138-3. Extracorporeal Blood Rewarming Options

Options	Considerations
Venovenous rewarming	Circuit: CU catheter to CV or peripheral catheter No oxygenator/circulatory support Flow rates 150-400 mL/min ROR 2-3° C/hr
Hemodialysis	Circuit: single or dual vessel cannulation Stabilizes electrolyte or toxicologic abnormalities Exchange cycle volumes 200-500 mL/min ROR 2-3° C/hr
CAVR	Circuit: percutaneous 8.5 Fr femoral catheters Requires blood pressure of 60 mmHg No perfusionist/pump/anticoagulation Flow rates 225-375 mL/min ROR 3-4° C/hr
CPB	Circuit: full circulatory support with the pump and oxygenator Perfusate: temperature gradient (5-10° C) Flow rates 2-7 mL/min (average, 3-4) ROR up to 9.5° C/hr

CAVR, continuous arteriovenous rewarming; CPB, cardiopulmonary bypass; CV, central venous; ROR, rate of rewarming.
From Danzl DF: Hypothermia and frostbite. In: Kasper DL, et al (eds): *Harrison's Principles of Internal Medicine*, 16th ed. New York, McGraw-Hill Professional, 2005.

Extracorporeal Blood Rewarming

The four common techniques to rewarm blood are cardiopulmonary bypass (CPB), continuous arteriovenous rewarming, venovenous rewarming, and hemodialysis (Table 138-3).[75-78]

Cardiopulmonary bypass utilizes the standard femoral-femoral circuit and includes arterial and venous catheters, a mechanical pump, a membrane or bubble oxygenator, and a heat exchanger.[79] A 16 to 30 French venous cannula is inserted via the femoral vein to the right atrium/inferior vena cava junction. The tip of the shorter 16 to 20 French arterial cannula is inserted 5 cm or just proximal to the aortic bifurcation. Transesophageal echocardiography can help evaluate ventricular load and valve function.

There are techniques to decrease the need for intravenous anticoagulation that previously limited clinical applicability. Heparin-coated perfusion equipment and the use of nonthrombogenic pumps can be coupled with the enhanced physiologic fibrinolysis seen in the first hour of CPB.[80,81]

Heated, oxygenated blood is returned via the femoral artery. Femoral flow rates of 2 to 3 L/min can elevate the core temperature 1° C to 2° C every 3 to 5 minutes. In Splittgerber's review the mean CPB temperature increase was 9.5° C/hr.[82] Most pumps can generate full flow rates up to 7 L/min.

The optimal temperature gradient and bypass rewarming rates are unknown. An excessive temperature gradient between brain tissue and circulant can adversely affect electroencephalographic regeneration. The other concern is the possibility of increased bubbling if high perfusate temperature gradients are used. Most investigators use 5° C to 10° C gradients.[83]

The major advantage of CPB in perfusing patients is the preservation of flow if mechanical cardiac activity is lost during rewarming. Other candidates for CPB are patients who do not respond to less invasive rewarming techniques, those with completely frozen extremities, and those with rhabdomyolysis accompanied by major electrolyte disturbances.

Continuous arteriovenous rewarming is another option if the blood pressure is at least 60 mm Hg. As described by Gentilello, continuous arteriovenous rewarming involves the use of percutaneously inserted femoral arterial and contralateral femoral venous catheters.[22,84] The Seldinger technique is used to insert the 8.5 French catheters. Heparin-bonded tubing circuits obviate the need for systemic anticoagulation. Continuous arteriovenous rewarming has principally been performed on traumatized patients.

The blood pressure of spontaneously perfusing traumatized hypothermic patients creates a functional arteriovenous fistula by diverting part of the cardiac output out the femoral artery through a countercurrent heat exchanger (e.g., Level 1; Flo Temp-IIe). The heated blood is then returned with admixed heated crystalloids via the femoral vein.

Continuous arteriovenous rewarming does not require the specialized equipment and perfusionist necessary for CPB. The average flow rates are 225 to 375 mL/min, resulting in a rate of rewarming of 3° C to 4° C/hr. Since the catheters are 8.5 French, the patient must weigh at least 40 kg.

Extracorporeal venovenous rewarming is another option for warming and recirculating the blood. With this technique, blood is removed, usually from a central venous catheter, heated to 40° C, and returned via a second central or large peripheral venous catheter. Flow rates of 150 to 400 mL/min have been achieved.[85,86]

The circuit is not complex and is more efficient than many other non-bypass modalities. There is no oxygenator, and, since the method does not provide full circulatory support, volume infusion is the only option to augment inadequate cardiac output.[87]

Standard hemodialysis is a widely available and practical rewarming technique. It is portable and efficient, and it should be considered in patients with electrolyte abnormalities, renal failure, or intoxication with a dialyzable substance. Two-way flow catheters allow cannulation of a single vessel. A Drake-Willock single-needle dialysis catheter can be used with a portable hemodialysis machine and external warmer. After central venous cannulation, exchange cycle volumes of 200 to 250 mL/min are possible.

Although heat exchange is less than with standard two-vessel hemodialysis, the ease of percutaneous subclavian vein placement is a major advantage. Hemodialysis via two separate single-lumen catheters placed in the femoral vein can achieve continuous blood flow at 450 to 500 mL/min.

Of note, rapid acceleration of the rate of rewarming does not necessarily improve survival rates. Complications of rapid rewarming in severe hypothermia include disseminated intravascular coagulation, pulmonary edema, hemolysis, and acute tubular necrosis.

Extracorporeal blood rewarming should be attempted in hypothermic cardiac arrest patients when no contraindications to CPR exist. A realistic assessment of the risk-to-benefit ratio for debilitated patients with secondary hypothermia should be made. The lowest temperature in a survivor of induced hypothermia was 9° C.[88] Extracorporeal blood rewarming is unlikely to succeed below 5° C.[89] Resuscitation should be discontinued if frozen or clotted intravascular contents are identified.

DISPOSITION

Otherwise healthy patients who have mild primary accidental hypothermia (35° C to 32.2° C) usually rewarm easily in the emergency department. They can be safely discharged if a warm environment is available.

Patients with more severe hypothermia (< 32.2° C) almost always require admission. These patients should be evaluated for the presence of underlying medical disorders (see Box 138-1). Cardiac monitoring should be considered in patients with persistent toxicologic or metabolic abnormalities. This is essential for those patients displaying cardiovascular instability or an inadequate rate of rewarming. Transferring patients to tertiary care centers is generally not necessary; however, some severely hypothermic patients are best managed in facilities with CPB capabilities.

OUTCOME

In the past, the treatment dictum was that "no one is dead until they are warm and dead." Some patients are cold and dead, and it would be useful and humane if they could be safely identified. Because of the variability of human physiologic responses, outcome is difficult to predict.[89-92] The type and severity of the underlying or precipitating disease process are the major determinants.[93] Patient age is not an independent predictor of mortality.

Trauma, infection, and toxin ingestions also affect survival unpredictably.[24] Outcome prediction based on the Glasgow Coma Scale score is unreliable. A hypothermia outcome score developed from a large database may enable multiple observers at different sites to assess treatment modalities and outcome predictors.[94] Significant predictors of outcome include asphyxia, prehospital cardiac arrest, a low or absent blood pressure, elevated BUN level, and the need for either endotracheal or nasogastric intubation in the emergency department.[78]

The search for a valid triage marker of death continues.[95-97] Grave prognostic indicators include evidence of intravascular thrombosis (fibrinogen less than 50 mg/dL), cell lysis (hyperkalemia more than 10 mEq/L), and ammonia levels greater than 250 mmol/L.[98] These indicators have not been prospectively validated.

KEY CONCEPTS

- The emergency physician must decide rapidly whether passive rewarming will suffice or whether the patient should be actively rewarmed.
- Indications for active rewarming include cardiovascular instability, temperature below 32° C, poor rate of rewarming, endocrinologic insufficiency, and vasodilation.
- Consider hypoglycemia, hypovolemia, or an overdose if there is a tachycardia disproportionate to the temperature.
- The efficacy of most medications is temperature dependent. Overmedication to achieve an effect when the patient is cold could cause toxicity during rewarming.
- Kinetic laboratory tests of coagulation are performed at 37° C. Despite a clinically obvious coagulopathy, the values will be deceptively "normal."
- There are no safe predictors of serum electrolytes. Hypothermia enhances the cardiac toxicity of hyperkalemia and obscures premonitory electrocardiographic changes.

REFERENCES

1. Gilbert M, et al: Resuscitation from accidental hypothermia of 13.7° C with circulatory arrest. *Lancet* 355:375, 2000.
2. Moran DS, et al: Hypothermia and local injuries in combat and non-combat situations: The Israeli experience. *Aviat Space Environ Med* 74:281, 2003.
3. Marsigny B: Medical mountain rescue in the Mont-Blanc massif. *Wilder Environ Med* 10:152, 1999.
4. Danzl DF, Pozos RS: Accidental hypothermia. *N Engl J Med* 331:1756, 1994.
5. Miller JW, Danzl DF, Thomas DM: Urban accidental hypothermia: 135 cases. *Ann Emerg Med* 9:456, 1980.
6. White JD: Hypothermia: The Bellevue experience. *Ann Emerg Med* 11:417, 1982.
7. Centers for Disease Control and Prevention: Hypothermia related deaths: Philadelphia, 2001, and United States, 1999. 52:86, 2003.
8. Kempainen RR, Brunette DD: The evaluation and management of accidental hypothermia. *Resp Care* 49:192, 2004.
9. Giesbrecht GG: Cold stress, near drowning and accidental hypothermia: A review. *Aviat Space Environ Med* 71:733, 2000.
10. Vassallo SU, et al: A prospective evaluation of the electrocardiographic manifestations of hypothermia. *Acad Emerg Med* 6:1121, 1999.
11. Danzl DF, O'Brien DJ: The ECG computer program: Mort de froid. *J Wilderness Med* 3:328, 1992.
12. Danzl DF, et al: Multicenter hypothermia survey. *Ann Emerg Med* 16:1042, 1987.
13. Giesbrecht GG, Johnston CE, Bristow GK: The convective afterdrop component during hypothermic exercise decreased with delayed exercise onset. *Aviat Space Environ Med* 69:17, 1998.
14. Hayward JS, Eckerson JD, Kemna D: Thermal and cardiovascular changes during three methods of resuscitation from mild hypothermia. *Resuscitation* 11:21, 1984.
15. Irwin BR: A case report of hypothermia in the wilderness. *Wilder Environ Med* 13:125, 2002.
16. Lloyd EL: Accidental hypothermia. *Resuscitation* 32:111, 1996.
17. Pedley DK, Paterson B, Morrison W: Hypothermia in elderly patients presenting to accident and emergency during the onset of winter. *Scott Med J* 47:10, 2002.
18. Mallet ML: Pathophysiology of accidental hypothermia. *QJM* 95:775, 2002.
19. Ranhoff AH: Accidental hypothermia in the elderly. *Int J Circumpolar Health* 59:255, 2000.
20. Kibayashi K, Shojo H: Accidental fatal hypothermia in elderly people with Alzheimer's Disease. *Med Sci Law* 43:127, 2003.
21. Danzl DF: Hypothermia. *Semin Respir Crit Care Med* 23:57, 2002.
22. Gentilello LM, et al: Is hypothermia in the victim of major trauma protective or harmful? A randomized, prospective study. *Ann Surg* 226:439, 1997.
23. Cosgriff N, et al: Predicting life-threatening coagulopathy in the massively transfused trauma patient: Hypothermia and acidoses revisited. *J Trauma* 42:857, 1997.
24. Walpoth BH, et al: Outcome of survivors of accidental deep hypothermia and circulatory arrest treated with extracorporeal blood warming. *N Engl J Med* 337:1500, 1997.
25. White FN: Reassuring acid-base balance in hypothermia: A comparative point of view. *West J Med* 138:255, 1983.
26. Baraka AS, et al: Effect of alpha-stat versus pH-stat strategy on oxyhemoglobin dissociation and whole body oxygen consumption during hypothermia cardiopulmonary bypass. *Anesth Analg* 74:32, 1992.
27. Delaney KA, et al: Assessment of acid-base disturbances and their physiologic consequences. *Ann Emerg Med* 18:72, 1989.
28. McInerney JJ, et al: Accidental hypothermia and active rewarming: The metabolic and inflammatory changes observed above and below 32 degrees C. *Emerg Med J* 19:219, 2002.
29. Kroncke GM, et al: Ectothermic philosophy of acid-base balance to prevent fibrillation during hypothermia. *Arch Surg* 121:303, 1986.
30. Eddy VA, Morris JA Jr, Cullinane DC: Hypothermia, coagulopathy and acidosis. *Surg Clin North Am* 80:845, 2000.
31. Rohrer MJ, Natale AM: Effect of hypothermia on the coagulation cascade. *Crit Care Med* 20:1402, 1992.
32. Watts DD, et al: Hypothermic coagulopathy in trauma: Effect of varying levels of hypothermia on enzyme speed, platelet function and fibrinolytic activity. *J Trauma* 44:846, 1998.
33. Mills WJ Jr: Field care of the hypothermic patient. *Int J Sports Med* 1:S199, 1992.
34. Samuelson T: Experience with standardized protocols in hypothermia, boom or bane? The Alaska experience. *Arctic Med Res* 50:28, 1991.
35. Grief R, et al: Resistive heating is more effective than metallic foil insulation in an experimental model of accidental hypothermia: A randomized controlled trail. *Ann Emerg Med* 35:337, 2000.
36. Cohen JA, et al: Increased pulmonary artery perforating potential of pulmonary artery catheters during hypothermia. *J Cardiothorac Vasc Anesth* 5:235, 1991.
37. Lazar HL: The treatment of hypothermia. *N Engl J Med* 337:1545, 1997.
38. Myers RA, Britten JS, Cowley RA: Hypothermia: Quantitative aspects of therapy. *JACEP* 8:523, 1979.
39. Silbergleit R, et al: Hypothermia from realistic fluid resuscitation in a model of hemorrhagic shock. *Ann Emerg Med* 31:339, 1998.
40. Handrigan MT, et al: Factors and methodology in achieving ideal delivery temperatures for intravenous and lavage fluid in hypothermia. *Am J Emerg Med* 15:350, 1997.
41. Danzl DF: Blood flow during closed chest compressions in hypothermic humans. *Wilder Med* 7:12, 1991.
42. Maningas PA, et al: Regional blood flow during hypothermic arrest. *Ann Emerg Med* 15:390, 1986.
43. Althaus U, Aeberhard P, Schupbach P: Management of profound accidental hypothermia with cardiorespiratory arrest. *Ann Surg* 195:492, 1982.

44. Lexow K: Severe accidental hypothermia: Survival after 6 hours 30 minutes of cardiopulmonary resuscitation. *Arctic Med Res* 50:112, 1991.
45. Brunette DD, et al: Internal cardiac massage and mediastinal irrigation in hypothermic cardiac arrest. *Am J Emerg Med* 10:32, 1992.
46. Weiss SJ, et al: The physiological response to norepinephrine during hypothermia and rewarming. *Resuscitation* 39:189, 1998.
47. DaVee TS, Reineberg EJ: Extreme hypothermia and ventricular fibrillation. *Ann Emerg Med* 9:100, 1980.
48. Stoner J, et al: Amiodarone and bretylium in the treatment of hypothermic ventricular fibrillation in a canine model. *Acad Emerg Med* 10:187, 2003.
49. Dixon RG, et al: Transcutaneous pacing in a hypothermic dog model. *Ann Emerg Med* 29:602, 1997.
50. Rogers I: Which rewarming therapy in hypothermia? A review of the randomized trials. *Emerg Med* 9:213, 1997.
51. Shields CP, Sixsmith DM: Treatment of moderate-to-severe hypothermia in an urban setting. *Ann Emerg Med* 19:1093, 1990.
52. Gregory RT, Doolittle WH: Accidental hypothermia. II. Clinical implications of experimental studies. *Alaska Med* 15:48, 1973.
53. Roggla M, et al: Severe accidental hypothermia with or without hemodynamic instability: Rewarming without the use of extracorporeal circulation. *Wien Klin Wochen* 114:315, 2002.
54. Zhong H, Qinyi S, Mingjlang S: Rewarming with microwave irradiation in severe cold injury syndrome. *Chin Med J* 93:19, 1980.
55. Duguid H, Simpson RG, Stowers JM: Accidental hypothermia. *Lancet* 2:1213, 1961.
56. Hamilton RS, Paton BC: The diagnosis and treatment of hypothermia by mountain rescue teams: A survey. *Wilderness Environ Med* 7:37, 1996.
57. Giesbrecht GG, Bristow GK: Recent advances in hypothermia research. *Ann N Y Acad Sci* 813:676, 1997.
58. Goheen MSL, et al: Efficacy of forced-air and inhalation rewarming using a human model for severe hypothermia. *J Appl Physiol* 83:1635, 1997.
59. Kornberger E: Forced air surface rewarming in patients with severe accidental hypothermia. *Resuscitation* 41:105, 1999.
60. Taguchi A: Negative pressure rewarming vs. forced air warming in hypothermia postanesthetic volunteers. *Anesth Analg* 92:261, 2001.
61. Steele MT, et al: Forced air speeds rewarming in accidental hypothermia. *Ann Emerg Med* 27:479, 1996.
62. Koller R, Schnider TW, Neidhart P: Deep accidental hypothermia and cardiac arrest rewarming with forced air. *Acta Anaesthesiol Scand* 41:1359, 1997.
63. Vangaard L, et al: Arteriovenous anastomoses (AVA) rewarming in 45° C water is effective in moderately hypothermic subjects. *FASEB J* 12:A90, 1998.
64. Ducharme MG, et al: Forced-air rewarming in −20° C simulated field conditions. *Ann N Y Acad Sci* 813:676, 1997.
65. Soreide E, et al: A non-invasive means to effectively restore normothermia in cold stressed individuals: A preliminary report. *J Emerg Med* 17:725, 1999.
66. Ereth MH, Lennon RL, Sessler DL: Limited heat transfer between thermal compartments during rewarming in vasoconstricted patients. *Aviat Space Environ Med* 63:1065, 1992.
67. Weinberg AD: The role of inhalation rewarming in the early management of hypothermia. *Resuscitation* 36:101, 1998.
68. Fisher A, et al: Oxygen availability during hypothermic cardiopulmonary bypass. *Crit Care Med* 5:154, 1977.
69. Wallace W: Does it make sense to heat gases higher than body temperature for the treatment of cold water near-drowning or hypothermia? A point of view paper. *Alaska Med* 39:75, 1997.
70. Levitt MA, et al: A comparative rewarming trial of gastric versus peritoneal lavage in a hypothermic model. *Am J Emerg Med* 8:285, 1990.
71. Winegard C: Successful treatment of severe hypothermia and prolonged cardiac arrest with closed thoracic cavity lavage. *J Emerg Med* 15:629, 1997.
72. Hall KN, Syverud SA: Closed thoracic cavity lavage in the treatment of severe hypothermia in human beings. *Ann Emerg Med* 19:204, 1990.
73. Brunette DD, et al: Comparison of gastric and closed thoracic lavage in the treatment of severe hypothermia in dogs. *Ann Emerg Med* 16:1222, 1987.
74. Iverson RJ, et al: Successful CPR in a severely hypothermic patient using continuous thoracostomy lavage. *Ann Emerg Med* 19:1335, 1990.
75. Kjaergaard B, et al: A mobile system for the treatment of accidental hypothermia with extracorporeal circulation. *Perfusion* 16:453, 2001.
76. Gregory JS, et al: Comparison of three methods of rewarming from hypothermia: Advances of extracorporeal blood rewarming. *J Trauma* 31:1247, 1991.
77. Long WB: Cardiopulmonary bypass for rewarming profound hypothermia patients: Critical decisions in hypothermia. Presented at the Annual International Forum, Portland, Oregon, February 28, 1992.
78. Farsted M, et al: Rewarming from accidental hypothermia by extracorporeal circulation: A retrospective study. *Eur J Cardiothorac Surg* 20:58, 2001.
79. Walpoth BH, et al: Accidental deep hypothermia with cardiopulmonary arrest: Extracorporeal blood rewarming in 11 patients. *Eur J Cardiothorac Surg* 4:390, 1990.
80. von Segesser LK, et al: Reduction and elimination of systemic heparinization during cardiopulmonary bypass. *J Thorac Cardiovasc Surg* 103:790, 1992.
81. Kirkpatrick AW, et al: Use of a centrifugal vortex blood pump and heparin-bonded circuit for extra corporeal rewarming of severe hypothermia in acutely injured and coagulopathic patients. *J Trauma* 55:407, 2003.
82. Splittgerber FH, et al: Partial cardiopulmonary bypass for core rewarming in profound accidental hypothermia. *Am Surg* 52:407, 1986.
83. Bolgiano E, Sykes L, Barish RA: Accidental hypothermia with cardiac arrest: Recovery following rewarming by cardiopulmonary bypass. *J Emerg Med* 10:427, 1992.
84. Gentilello LM, et al: Continuous arteriovenous rewarming: Experimental results and thermodynamic model simulation of treatment for hypothermia. *J Trauma* 30:1436, 1990.
85. Gregory JS, et al: Incidence and timing of hypothermia in trauma patients undergoing operations. *J Trauma* 31:795, 1991.
86. Heise D, Rathgeber J, Burchardi H: Severe, accidental hypothermia: Active rewarming with a simple extracorporeal veno-venous warming-circuit. *Anaesthesist* 45:1093, 1996.
87. Brauer A, et al: Severe accidental hypothermia: Rewarming strategy using a venovenous bypass system and a convective air warmer. *Intensive Care Med* 25:520, 1999.
88. Niazi SA, Lewis FJ: Profound hypothermia in man: Report of a case. *Ann Surg* 147:264, 1958.
89. Danzl DF, Lloyd EL: Treatment of accidental hypothermia. In Pandolk KB, Burr RE, Wenger CB, Pozos RS (eds): *Medical Aspects of Harsh Environment*, vol 1.
90. Vassal T, et al: Severe accidental hypothermia treated in an ICU: Prognosis and outcome. *Chest* 120:1998, 2001.
91. Wittmers LE: Pathophysicology of cold exposure. *Minn Med* 84: 30, 2001.
92. Megarbane B, et al: Hypothermia with indoor occurrence is associated with a worse outcome. *Intensive Care Med* 25:1943, 2000.

93. Dobson JAR, Burgess JJ: Resuscitation of severe hypothermia by extracorporeal rewarming in a child. *J Trauma* 40:483, 1996.
94. Danzl DF, et al: Hypothermia outcome score: Development and implications. *Crit Care Med* 17:227, 1989.
95. Locher T, et al: Accidental hypothermia in Switzerland (1980-1987): Case reports and prognostic factors. *Schweiz Med Wochenschr* 121:1020, 1991.
96. Pillgram-Larsen J, et al: Accidental hypothermia: Risk factors in 29 patients with body temperature of 30° C and below. *Tidsskr Nor Laegeforen* 111:180, 1991.
97. Schaller MD, Fischer AP, Perret CH: Hyperkalemia: A prognostic factor during acute severe hypothermia. *JAMA* 264:1842, 1990.
98. Hauty MG, et al: Prognostic factors in severe accidental hypothermia: Experience from the Mt. Hood tragedy. *J Trauma* 27:1107, 1987.

CHAPTER 139 Heat Illness

Salvator Vicario

PERSPECTIVE

Whereas humans must use their intellect to seek heat and insulation to survive in cold environments, heat stress is generally tolerated well, even without air conditioning or special clothing. Nevertheless, humans have been plagued by heat illness throughout recorded history. The Bible describes a young man's death after laboring in hot fields during harvest (II Kings 4:18-20). The ancient Greeks named a disease that resembled heatstroke *siriasis* after the dog star Sirius, which accompanies the summer sun.

Many military campaigns have been lost because of the lack of heat acclimatization and subsequent heat illness. King Edward and his metal-armored crusaders allegedly lost the final battle of the Holy Land against the well-adapted and well-ventilated Arab horsemen because of heat illness.[1] Modern military organizations continue to encounter heat illness because of the requirement to train unacclimatized troops with forced heavy physical exercise. The U.S. Army reported at least 125 deaths from heatstroke during basic training in the years 1941 to 1944.[2] In 1999 there were 51 reported cases of heat stress among military trainees at Lackland Air Force base, including 5 cases of heatstroke.[3] Athletes are also prone to heat illness. Between 1961 and 1971, 46 American football players died of heatstroke. Heatstroke was once third only to head and spinal cord injuries and cardiac arrest as a cause of death among American athletes.[4]

When environmental heat stress is maximal, strenuous exercise is not required to produce heat illness. The elderly and poor, often lacking adequate air conditioning and nutrition, and those with preexisting disease are prone to heat illness during environmental extremes. In heat wave years in the United States, about 10 times as many deaths are reported as during non-heat wave years. It is also estimated that at least 10 times as many heat-aggravated illnesses occur because of myocardial infarction, cerebrovascular accident, and other causes. Despite advances in prevention and treatment, more than 700 excess deaths were caused by the heat during the 1995 heat wave in Chicago.[5,6] Cincinnati and Dayton, Ohio, also reported 21 and 7 heat-related deaths per million, respectively, during a 1999 heat wave.[7] The heat wave during the summer of 2003 is estimated to have caused 14,802 deaths in France.[8]

PRINCIPLES OF DISEASE

Physiology of Heat

Heat Production

Humans can be considered biochemical "furnaces" that burn food to fuel a complex array of metabolic functions. These chemical reactions consume substrate, generate usable energy, and produce byproducts that must be eliminated for continued operation of the system. Water and carbon dioxide are produced and eliminated in large quantities, as are urea, sulfates, phosphates, and other chemical products. All of these reactions are exothermic and combine to produce a basal metabolic rate that amounts to approximately 100 kcal for a 70-kg person. In the absence of cooling mechanisms, this baseline metabolic activity would result in a 1.1° C hourly rise in body temperature.

Heat production can be increased up to 20-fold by strenuous exertion. Rectal temperatures as high as 42° C are recorded without ill effects in trained marathon runners. Metabolic factors, such as hyperthyroidism or sympathomimetic drug ingestion, can dramatically increase heat production. Environmental heat not only adds to the heat load, it also interferes with heat dissipation. The physics of heat transfer as it relates to human physiology involves four mechanisms: conduction, convection, radiation, and evaporation.[9]

Conduction

Conduction is the transfer of heat energy from warmer to cooler objects by direct physical contact. Air is a good insulator; therefore, only approximately 2% of the body heat loss is by conduction. In contrast, the thermal conductivity of water is at least 25 times that of air.

Convection

Heat loss to air and water vapor molecules circulating around the body is termed *convection*. As ambient temperature rises, the amount of heat dissipated by convection becomes minimal, and once air temperature exceeds the mean skin temperature, heat is gained by the body. Convective heat loss varies directly with wind velocity. Loose-fitting clothing maximizes convective (and also evaporative) heat loss.

Radiation

Radiation is heat transfer by electromagnetic waves. Although radiation accounts for approximately 65% of heat loss in cool environments, it is a major source of heat gain in hot climates. Up to 300 kcal/hr can be gained from radiation when a person is directly exposed to the hot summer sun.[10]

Evaporation

Evaporation is the conversion of a liquid to the gaseous phase. Evaporation of 1 mL of sweat from the skin cools the body by 0.58 kcal. As ambient temperature rises, evaporation becomes the dominant mechanism of heat loss. Panting mammals such as dogs have an oropharyngeal countercurrent flow mechanism (carotid rete mirabile) that results in selective cooling of the brain. In humans, respiratory and countercurrent mechanisms are minimal sources of heat loss, and the dominant mode of cooling in hot conditions is evaporation of sweat from the skin.

Heat Regulation

The regulation of body temperature involves three distinct functions: thermosensors, a central integrative area, and thermoregulatory effectors.

Thermosensors

Temperature-sensitive structures are located both peripherally in the skin and centrally in the body. Skin temperature changes, however, correlate poorly with changes in the rate of heat loss.[11] Thermosensitive neurons are in the preoptic area of the anterior hypothalamus. They are activated when the temperature of the blood circulating through that area exceeds a certain "set point."

The skin temperature affects heat loss, since a person resting in a warm environment initiates sweating, even though the core temperature remains constant. In contrast, changes in core temperature are more potent in producing heat-dissipating responses than skin temperature changes.[12]

Central Integrative Area

The central nervous system (CNS) interprets information received from the thermosensors to properly instruct thermoregulatory effectors. The concept of a central thermostat by which an alteration shifts effector thresholds in the same direction fits a variety of clinical situations. For example, fever, the circadian rhythm of temperature variation, and the 0.5° C difference in rectal temperature after ovulation can be explained by variation of a thermal set-point.

Thermoregulatory Effectors

Sweating and peripheral vasodilation are the major mechanisms by which heat loss can be accelerated. In a warm environment, evaporation of sweat from the skin is the most important mechanism of heat dissipation. Heat loss from the skin by convection and radiation is maximized by increased skin blood flow to facilitate sweating.

Humans possess apocrine and eccrine sweat glands. Apocrine glands are concentrated in the axillae and produce milky sweat rich in carbohydrate and protein. They are adrenergically innervated and respond to emotional stress as well as to heat. Most glands producing "thermal sweat" are eccrine glands. These are cholinergically innervated and distributed over the entire body, with the largest number on the palms and soles. Eccrine sweat is colorless, odorless, and devoid of protein. Individuals exercising in hot environments commonly lose 1 to 2 L/hr of sweat; loss of 4 L/hr for short periods is possible.

Cooling is best achieved by evaporation from the body surface; sweat that drips from the skin does not cool the body, and sweat evaporated from clothing is considerably less efficient. Each liter of completely evaporated sweat consumes 580 kcal of heat. The ability of the environment to evaporate sweat is termed *atmospheric cooling power* and varies primarily with humidity, but also with wind velocity. As humidity approaches 100%, evaporative heat loss ceases.

The vascular response to heat stress is cutaneous vasodilation and compensatory vasoconstriction of splanchnic and renal beds. These vascular changes are under neurogenic control and allow heat to be dissipated quickly and efficiently, but they place a tremendous burden on the heart.[13] To maintain blood pressure, cardiac output must increase dramatically. For this reason, saunas and hot tubs may be dangerous for patients with cardiac disease. Cardiovascular and baroreceptor reflexes also affect skin blood flow. Reduced forearm sweating and vasodilation are observed in severely dehydrated subjects exercising in a warm environment.[14]

Acclimatization

Acclimatization is defined as "a constellation of physiologic adaptations that appear in a normal person as the result of repeated exposures to heat stress." Daily exposure to work and heat for 100 min/day results in near-maximal acclimatization in 7 to 14 days. This is characterized by an earlier onset of sweating (at a lower core temperature), increased sweat volume, and lowered sweat electrolyte concentration. Acclimatization is hastened by modest salt deprivation and delayed by high dietary salt intake.[15] As acclimatization proceeds, the sweat sodium concentration drops while the volume increases.

The cardiovascular system plays a major role in both acclimatization and endurance training, largely resulting from an expansion of plasma volume.[16] Heart rate is lower and associated with a higher stroke volume. Other physiologic changes include earlier release of aldosterone, although acclimatized individuals generate lower plasma levels of aldosterone during exercise heat stress. Total body potassium depletion of up to 20% (500 mEq) by the second week of acclimatization can occur as a result of sweat and urine losses coupled with inadequate repletion.[16]

Although many similarities exist between thermoregulatory responses to heat and exercise, the well-conditioned athlete is not necessarily heat acclimatized. To maintain heat and exercise-induced adaptive responses, heat exposure needs to continue intermittently at least on 4-day intervals. Plasma volume decreases considerably within 1 week in the absence of heat stress.[16]

PATHOPHYSIOLOGY

Predisposing Factors for Heat Illness

Elderly patients or those with chronic diseases who are taking medications predisposing to heat illness are prone to classic heatstroke during periods of high ambient heat and humidity. Adequate fluid intake is essential. Elderly patients sometimes dress inappropriately for hot weather; heat loss is maximized by light, loose-fitting garments.

Exertional heatstroke is most likely to occur in young, healthy people involved in strenuous physical activity, especially if they have not acclimatized to environmental factors that overwhelm heat-dissipating mechanisms. Fluid intake is the most critical variable. Dehydration can be minimized by education on work-rest cycles and fluid consumption and through provision of cool, pleasantly flavored fluids.

The goal is to maximize voluntary fluid intake and gastric emptying so that fluid can rapidly enter the small intestine, where it is absorbed. Gastric emptying is accelerated to 25 mL/min by large fluid volumes (500-600 mL) and cool temperatures (10° C to 15.8° C). Soldiers under conditions of heat stress provided with cool, flavored water consume significantly more fluid than those given warm tap water.[17] High osmolality inhibits gastric emptying; osmolality of less than 200 mOsm/L is optimal. Most commercially available electrolyte solutions contain excessive sugar. Hydration can be monitored by measuring body weight before and after training or athletic competition. An athlete with a loss of 2% to 3% body weight (1.5-2 L in a 70-kg man) should drink extra fluid and be permitted to compete only when within 0.5 to 1 kg (1-2 pounds) of the starting weight on the previous day. A weight loss of 5% to 6% represents a moderately severe deficit and usually is associated with intense thirst, scanty urine, tachycardia, and an increase in rectal temperature of about 2° C. Such athletes should be restricted to light workouts after hydration to their normal weight. A loss of 7% or more of body weight represents severe water depletion; the athlete should not participate in sports until examined by a physician. Wrestlers frequently fast, restrict food and fluid intake, and exercise vigorously wearing vapor-impermeable clothing to lose weight quickly so that they can compete in a lower weight class.[18]

The administration of salt tablets during strenuous exercise can cause delayed gastric emptying, osmotic fluid shifts into the gut, gastric mucosal damage, and hypernatremic dehydration. A 6-g sodium diet is sufficient for successful adaptation for work in the heat, with sweat losses averaging 7 L/day. Excessively high salt intake in relation to salt losses in sweat during initial heat exposure can impair acclimatization because of inhibition of aldosterone secretion. Excessive salt ingestion can also exacerbate potassium depletion.

Evaporative cooling can be lost when clothing inhibits air convection and evaporation. Loose-fitting clothing or ventilated fishnet jerseys allow efficient evaporation. Light-colored clothing reflects rather than absorbs light. Water evaporated from clothing is much less efficient for body cooling than is water evaporated from the skin.[19]

The body's heat dissipation mechanisms are analogous to the cooling system of an automobile (Figure 139-1). Coolant (blood) is circulated by a pump (heart) from the hot inner core to a radiator (skin surface cooled by the evaporation of sweat). Temperature is sensed by a thermostat (CNS), which alters coolant flow by a system of pipes, valves, and reservoirs (vasculature). Failure of any of these components can result in overheating.

Effective circulation requires both an intact pump and adequate coolant levels. Individuals with cardiac disease or those taking β-adrenergic blocking agents may be unable to increase their cardiac output sufficiently to produce the necessary peripheral vasodilation to dissipate heat. Dehydration caused by gastroenteritis, diuretics, or inadequate fluid intake predisposes to heat illness. Individuals working in the heat seldom voluntarily drink as much fluids as they lose and replace only approximately two thirds of net water loss ("voluntary dehydration"). Dehydration alone increases body temperature at rest by increasing the work of the sodium–potassium adenosine triphosphatase (ATPase) pump, which accounts for 25% to 45% of basal metabolic rate.[20] This is particularly true in cases of hypernatremic dehydration. The pipes and valves of the coolant system may be abnormal in diabetic or elderly patients with extensive atherosclerosis.

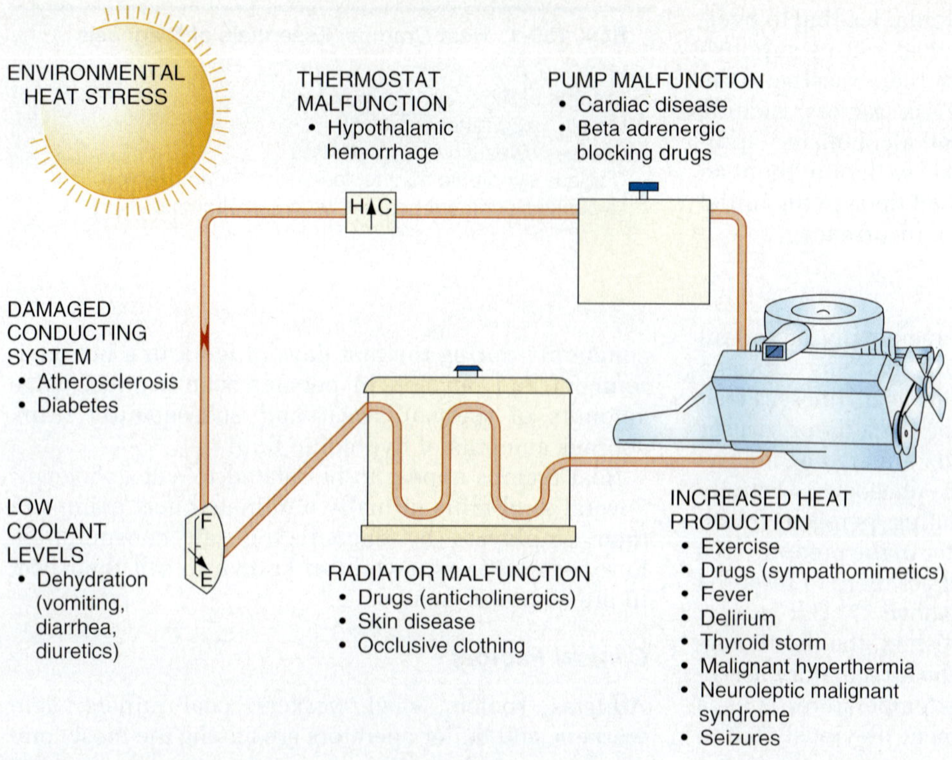

Figure 139-1. Predisposing factors for heat illness: an automotive analogy.

Radiator function depends on the skin and sweat glands. Occlusive, vapor-impermeable clothing hinders evaporative and convective cooling. Anticholinergic drugs, including atropine, Jimson weed, phenothiazines, benztropine mesylate, tricyclic antidepressants, and antihistamines, interfere with sweating and produce heat illness.[21] Various skin diseases, including miliaria (prickly heat rash), extensive burns, scleroderma, ectodermal dysplasia, and cystic fibrosis, are all risk factors. Anhidrosis can be secondary to either central or peripheral nervous system disorders as well.

Increased heat production causing heat illness most often accompanies exercise in hot, humid environments. Athletes and military recruits are commonly affected. When heat and humidity are extreme, exertion is not necessary to produce heat-related problems. The Wet Bulb Globe Thermometer index is an excellent measure of environmental heat stress. It includes the effects of temperature, humidity, and wind speed. When climatic conditions exceed 25° C wet bulb, even healthy people are at high risk if they choose to exercise. Above 28° C, exercise and strenuous work should be avoided or limited to extremely short periods.[22]

Before the advent of air conditioning, mortality increased threefold to fivefold in nursing homes and threefold in the general population during heat waves. Mortality in geriatric patients correlates with average weekly peak air temperature. Most deaths in the 2003 European heat wave occurred in elderly patients.[8] Microclimates conducive to heat illness are produced in the interiors of automobiles, tanks, and tents in the sun, as well as engine rooms, hot tubs, and saunas. Children are more susceptible to heat stressors because the higher surface area-to-mass ratios allow increased absorption of heat. They also have lower sweat rates per gland.[23]

Endogenous factors such as hyperthyroidism or pheochromocytoma can also drastically increase heat production. An overdose of sympathomimetics (e.g., amphetamines or cocaine) can cause fatal hyperpyrexia. High ambient temperature is associated with a significant increase in mortality from cocaine overdose. Many younger patients dying of hyperthermia test positive for cocaine.[24] Heatstroke also can occur with delirium resulting from alcohol withdrawal.[25] Phencyclidine also causes heatstroke. There are also reports of heatstroke occurring in well-trained military soldiers who ingest dietary supplements containing ephedrine.[26]

Certain patients undergoing general anesthesia rapidly experience severe hyperthermia, muscular rigidity, and acidosis. This syndrome, termed *malignant hyperthermia*, is the result of a genetically determined instability of skeletal muscle sarcoplasmic reticulum that allows inappropriate intracellular calcium release. Dantrolene, which lowers myoplasmic calcium, is effective in the prevention and treatment of this syndrome.[27]

Malignant hyperthermia is rarely seen in outpatient settings, but a clinically similar entity, *neuroleptic malignant syndrome*, is often encountered. This syndrome is induced by antipsychotic medications and is characterized by muscular rigidity, severe dyskinesia or akinesia, hyperthermia, tachycardia, dyspnea, dysphagia, and urinary incontinence. Although the rigidity and hyperthermia are reminiscent of malignant hyperthermia, the putative mechanism is different. Dopamine receptor blockade in the corpus striatum caused by haloperidol and similar drugs produces severe muscle spasticity and dystonia, leading to overproduction of heat. Haloperidol also causes suppression of thirst recognition, which further exacerbates the problem. Other miscellaneous risk factors include obesity,[28] fatigue, lack of sleep, and alcoholism.[29] Individuals with a history of heatstroke, with or without an inherent aberration that predisposed them to the initial episode, are at increased risk for a recurrence.

Fever versus Hyperthermia

It is both diagnostically and therapeutically important to understand fever and to identify patients suffering from a febrile response rather than heat illness. Fever is caused by pyrogens released by bacteria or viruses (exogenous pyrogens) or from cells undergoing autolysis after having participated in phagocytic activity (endogenous pyrogens).[30] Circulating pyrogens reach the thermoregulatory control center in the preoptic area of the anterior hypothalamus and act there to reset the thermal set point at a new level above 37° C.[31]

Once this temperature is established, the thermoregulatory center uses all available heat-regulatory servomechanisms to maintain the new temperature. Thus, a patient with fever in an environment previously felt to be thermally comfortable begins to feel cold and chooses a warmer environment. This behavioral drive is coordinated with the autonomic mechanisms such as shivering to increase body temperature to the new set point. Under most circumstances, temperature elevation is not a significant problem, and therapy is directed at the underlying disease state. Fever does not cause primary pathologic or physiologic damage to humans and does not require primary emphasis in the therapeutic regimen, which is directed at the underlying disease state.[30] If temperature-related physiologic changes such as febrile seizures or tachycardia in a patient with marginal cardiac reserve compromise the individual, however, temperature must be artificially regulated.

Since fever is the product of a molecular interaction that establishes a new physiologic thermal set point, therapeutic attempts to lower temperature are opposed by body mechanisms that attempt to maintain the new set point. Thus, attempts at whole-body cooling produce violent shivering and discomfort.[32] The use of agents to block the causative molecular interaction is the most clinically effective approach. Aspirin and other antipyretics block the action of the pyrogen at hypothalamic receptor sites through inhibition of prostaglandin synthesis.[31] These antipyretics are not effective against and should not be used to control environmental hyperthermia.

MINOR HEAT ILLNESS

Heat Cramps

Physiology

Heat cramps are brief, intermittent, and often severe muscular cramps occurring typically in muscles that are fatigued by heavy work. Heat cramps occur most commonly during the first days of work in a hot environment and develop in persons who produce large amounts of thermal sweat and subsequently drink copious amounts of hypotonic fluid.[33]

Heat cramps appear to be related to salt deficiency. Several steel mills virtually eliminated heat cramps in their employees by encouraging salt consumption. European laborers have been known to salt their beer to prevent heat cramps.

BOX 139-1. Heat Cramps: Essentials of Diagnosis

- Cramps of most worked muscles
- Usually occur after exertion
- Copious sweating during exertion
- Copious hypotonic fluid replacement during exertion
- Hyperventilation not present in cool environment

Clinical Factors

Athletes, roofers, steel workers, coal miners, field workers, and boiler operators are among the most commonly reported victims of heat cramps. Heat cramps tend to occur after exercise when the victim has stopped working and is relaxing (Box 139-1). In this respect, they differ from the cramps experienced by athletes during exercise, which tend to last for several minutes, are relieved by massage, and resolve spontaneously.

Heat cramps are occasionally confused with hyperventilation tetany, which can occur during heat exhaustion. The latter syndrome can be distinguished by the presence of carpopedal spasm and paresthesias in the distal extremities and perioral area. If accompanied by systemic symptoms, heat cramps may be part of salt-depletion heat exhaustion. Heat cramp victims exhibit hyponatremia, hypochloremia, and low serum sodium and chloride levels. Rhabdomyolysis or resultant renal damage is not present with isolated heat cramps.

Management

Heat cramps are usually rapidly relieved by salt solutions. Commercially available flavored electrolyte solutions are commonly ingested. Mild cases without concurrent dehydration may be treated orally with 0.1% to 0.2% salt solution (two to four 10-grain salt tablets [56 to 112 mEq] or ¼ to ½ teaspoon table salt dissolved in a quart of water), which is the general limit of palatability. Severe cases respond rapidly to intravenous isotonic solution (0.9% NaCl). Salt tablets are gastric irritants and are not recommended.[34]

Heat Edema

Physiology and Clinical Features

Swollen feet and ankles are often reported by nonacclimatized individuals, especially the elderly, who encounter climatic stresses of tropical and semitropical areas. Such individuals often have no underlying cardiac, hepatic, venous, or lymphatic disease. They commonly have assumed rigorous schedules with long periods of sitting or standing. The edema is usually minimal, not accompanied by any significant impairment in function, and often resolves after several days of acclimatization.

It is presumed that hydrostatic pressure and vasodilation of cutaneous vessels, combined with some degree of orthostatic pooling, lead to vascular leak and accumulation of interstitial fluid in the lower extremities. Simultaneously, aldosterone increases in response to the heat stress and perceived central volume deficit.

Awareness of this clinical presentation prevents overly vigorous diagnostic and therapeutic intervention. Brief diagnostic evaluation to rule out thrombophlebitis, lymphedema, or congestive heart failure is appropriate, but invasive diagnostic techniques or vigorous pharmacologic therapy is not indicated.

Management

No evidence exists that diuretic therapy is effective. Rather, simple leg elevation or thigh-high support hose should be used. In most individuals, the problem resolves either through adequate acclimatization or with the individual's return to a home climate.

Heat Syncope

Physiology and Clinical Features

Heat syncope is a perplexing disorder in which a host of serious and an even larger number of nonserious underlying mechanisms can also result in temporary loss of consciousness. The elderly have a special predilection for this disorder. Individuals adapt to a hot, humid environment by dilation of cutaneous vessels to deliver heat to the body surface. Thus, an increased portion of the intravascular pool is located in the periphery at any given time. Increasing blood flow to compliant cutaneous veins raises skin vascular volume at the expense of thoracic blood volume. Individuals who stand for protracted periods tend to pool blood in the lower extremities. Combined with volume loss and peripheral vasodilation, this pooling can result in inadequate central venous return, a concomitant drop in cardiac output, and a cerebral perfusion inadequate to maintain consciousness.

Management

The disorder is self-limited, because assumption of a horizontal position is the cure. Individuals at risk for heat syncope should be warned to move often, flex leg muscles repeatedly when standing stationary, avoid protracted standing in hot environments, and assume a sitting or horizontal position when prodromal warning signs or symptoms occur. These include scintillating scotomata, tunnel vision, vertigo, nausea, diaphoresis, and weakness. Adequate education prevents many serious injuries.

Prickly Heat

Physiology and Clinical Features

Prickly heat, also known as miliaria rubra, lichen tropicus, and heat rash, is an acute inflammatory disorder of the skin that occurs in tropical climates. It is the result of blockage of sweat gland pores by macerated stratum corneum and secondary staphylococcal infection. The acute phase is characterized by vesicles in the malpighian layer of the skin caused by dilation and rupture of the obstructed sweat gland ducts.

Clinically, this initially produces intensely pruritic vesicles on an erythematous base. The rash is confined to clothed areas, and the affected area is often completely anhidrotic. Over the next week or so, a keratin plug arises and fills these vesicles, causing a deeper obstruction of the sweat gland duct. The obstructed duct then ruptures a second time, producing a deeper vesicle within the dermis. This is known as the profunda stage, and it can persist for weeks. Profunda vesicles are not pruritic and closely resemble the white papules of piloerection; chronic dermatitis is a common complication.

Management

Chlorhexidine in a light cream or lotion is the antibacterial treatment of choice during the acute phase. Salicylic acid, 1%, can be applied three times daily to localized, affected areas to assist in desquamation, but it should not be used over large areas because of possible salicylate intoxication. For diffuse or pustular rashes, erythromycin can be helpful.

Prickly heat can be prevented by wearing light, loose-fitting, clean clothing and avoiding situations that produce continuous sweating. Routine use of talcum or baby powder should be avoided. Spending 8 to 12 hours a day in an air-conditioned environment is helpful.

HEAT EXHAUSTION

Physiology

Heat exhaustion (heat prostration) is a clinical syndrome characterized by volume depletion that occurs under conditions of heat stress. Two types of heat exhaustion are classically described: water depletion and salt depletion. *Water depletion* heat exhaustion results from inadequate fluid replacement by individuals working in a hot environment, usually laborers, athletes, military personnel, or invalids without free access to water. People working in the heat seldom drink as much as they lose and replace only approximately two thirds of net water loss. This "voluntary dehydration" results in progressive hypovolemia. Left untreated, water depletion heat exhaustion will progress to heatstroke.

Salt depletion heat exhaustion takes longer to develop than the water depletion form. It occurs when large volumes of thermal sweat are replaced by water with too little salt. It differs from heat cramps in that

BOX 139-2. Heat Exhaustion: Diagnosis

Vague malaise, fatigue, headache
Core temperature often normal; if elevated, less than 40° C (104° F)
Mental function essentially intact; no coma or seizures
Tachycardia, orthostatic hypotension, clinical dehydration (may occur)
Other major illness ruled out
If in doubt, treat as heat stroke

BOX 139-3. Heat Exhaustion: Treatment

Rest
Cool environment
Assess volume status (orthostatic changes, BUN, hematocrit, serum sodium)
Fluid replacement: normal saline to replete volume if patient orthostatic, replace free water deficits slowly to avoid cerebral edema.
Healthy young patients usually treated as outpatients; consider admission if patient is elderly, has significant electrolyte abnormalities, or would be at risk for recurrence if discharged.

BUN, blood urea nitrogen.

systemic symptoms occur. This syndrome is characterized by hyponatremia, hypochloremia, and low urinary sodium and chloride concentrations. Symptoms are similar to those seen in water-depletion heat exhaustion; body temperature usually remains near normal.

Clinical Features

The symptoms and signs associated with both types of heat exhaustion are variable and nonspecific and include weakness, fatigue, frontal headache, impaired judgment, vertigo, nausea and vomiting, and occasionally muscle cramps (Box 139-2). Orthostatic dizziness and syncope can occur. Sweating persists and may be profuse. The core temperature is only moderately elevated, usually less than 40° C, and signs of severe CNS dysfunction are not present.

Mild heat exhaustion and full-blown heatstroke represent extremes of the spectrum of heat illness, and intermediate cases may prove difficult to differentiate. Nevertheless, heat exhaustion should not be diagnosed in the presence of major CNS dysfunction (seizures, coma) or severe hyperthermia (greater than 40.5° C). If uncertainty exists, measurement of hepatic transaminases may prove helpful. Elevations to several thousand units can be seen in patients with heat exhaustion or healthy runners after a marathon, whereas in patients with heatstroke, such levels are usually in the tens of thousands after 24 hours.[35,36]

Management

Pure forms of either type of heat exhaustion are rare, and most cases of heat exhaustion involve mixed salt and water depletion. Heat exhaustion is primarily a volume depletion problem, and rapid recovery generally follows fluid administration. Decisions regarding the type of fluid and electrolyte replacements should be based on serum electrolyte measurements and the estimation of hydration status by clinical and laboratory parameters.

In mild cases, rest in a cool environment and an oral electrolyte solution, such as 0.1% saline, may suffice. Patients with significant volume depletion or electrolyte abnormalities generally require intravenous fluids. If the patient is orthostatic, normal saline should be administered until the patient is hemodynamically stable.

Free water deficits should be replaced slowly over 48 hours so as not to decrease serum osmolality more than 2 mOsm/hr. Overly rapid correction of hypernatremia is associated with seizures caused by cerebral edema.

Disposition

Young, otherwise healthy patients who do not have significant laboratory abnormalities and who respond rapidly to treatment do not require hospitalization. These patients can be discharged with instructions to drink plenty of fluids and avoid heat stress for 24 to 48 hours. Older patients, particularly those with cardiovascular disease or other predisposing factors described in Figure 139-1, require more cautious fluid and electrolyte replacement and frequent reassessment. They are best managed as inpatients (Box 139-3).

HEATSTROKE

In the previously discussed forms of heat illness, although the body temperature rises, homeostatic thermoregulatory mechanisms remain intact. Heatstroke is the catastrophic life-threatening emergency that occurs when these mechanisms fail. This failure results in elevation of body temperature to extreme levels, usually greater than 40.5° C (105° F), producing multisystem tissue damage and organ dysfunction.

Physiology

As heatstroke develops, energy will be insufficient to sustain thermoregulatory mechanisms, resulting in dramatic increases in core temperature and the clinical manifestations of heatstroke.[37] An exact temperature at which cellular damage begins to occur in an individual patient varies. Credible reports exist of full recovery despite rectal temperatures of 44.4° C to 46.5° C.[38] Damage is a function not only of temperature but also of the exposure time.[39] The resultant damage to tissues is a function of a complex interaction of body temperature, exposure time, work load, tissue perfusion, and individual factors, which vary markedly.

Neurologic dysfunction is a hallmark of heatstroke, and cerebral edema is common. Other pathologic changes include petechiae in the walls of the third and fourth ventricles and marked cerebellar Purkinje cell damage.[40] Interestingly, the hypothalamus, the predominant site of central thermoregulatory control, is usually not damaged.

Heat stress creates tremendous demands on the cardiovascular system, and patients who succumb to heatstroke show signs of circulatory failure. Although such pathologic changes are common, cardiac damage alone is not lethal.

Prolonged heat stress produces impressive increases in skin blood flow (peripheral vasodilation) and a reduction of the thermal gradient between the core and the skin. Functional hypovolemia is avoided by compensatory vasoconstriction of the splanchnic and renal vasculature. The resulting splanchnic and renal ischemia may explain the nausea, vomiting, and diarrhea observed in postmarathon runners. Hepatic damage is such a consistent feature of heatstroke that its absence should cast doubt on the diagnosis. This is manifested pathologically by centrilobular necrosis with extensive cholestasis.

If severe heat stress continues, compensatory splanchnic vasoconstriction will eventually fail. Failure to perfuse the skin with heated blood from the core results in a dramatically increased rate of heat storage. This produces elevated intracranial pressure, which, in combination with a reduction in mean arterial pressure caused by failure of compensatory splanchnic vasoconstriction, conspires to produce a fall in cerebral blood flow; this results in the major CNS dysfunction characteristic of heatstroke.

BOX 139-4. Heat Stroke: Diagnosis

Exposure to heat stress, endogenous or exogenous
Signs of severe CNS dysfunction (coma, seizures, delirium)
Core temperature usually above 40.5° C (105° F), but may be lower
Dry, hot skin common, but sweating may persist
Marked elevation of hepatic transaminases

CNS, central nervous system.

Table 139-1. Usual Characteristics of Heat Stroke

Exertional	Classic
Healthy	Predisposing factors/medications
Younger	Older
Exercise	Sedentary
Sporadic	Heat wave occurrence
Diaphoresis	Anhidrosis
Hypoglycemia	Normoglycemia
DIC	Mild coagulopathy
Rhabdomyolysis	Mild CPK elevation
Acute renal failure	Oliguria
Marked lactic acidosis	Mild acidosis
Hypocalcemia	Normocalcemia

CPK, creatinine phosphokinase; DIC, disseminated intravascular coagulation.

Clinical Features

Heatstroke versus Heat Exhaustion

The onset of heatstroke is sudden and the patient's level of consciousness is altered.[40] Prodromal symptoms lasting minutes to hours occur in approximately 20% of cases. These are nonspecific and may include weakness, dizziness, nausea, vomiting, anorexia, frontal headache, confusion, drowsiness, disorientation, muscle twitching, ataxia and signs of cerebellar dysfunction, and psychiatric symptoms ranging from anxiety and irritability to psychosis.[41,42]

These prodromal symptoms are reminiscent of the description of heat exhaustion. Heat exhaustion, particularly the water depletion variety, can progress to heatstroke if untreated. These two syndromes should be considered extremes on a spectrum of responses to heat stress. Heatstroke occurs when the thermoregulatory responses are overwhelmed and fail. If the patient is evaluated as this is occurring, differentiation between heat exhaustion and heatstroke is very difficult. If heatstroke cannot be excluded, efforts to cool the patient should begin immediately.

The usual manifestations of heatstroke include hyperpyrexia above 40.5° C, profound CNS dysfunction, and hot, dry skin (Box 139-4). Persistent sweating can be observed in patients with rectal temperatures of 41.5° C to 42.4° C with heatstroke. In one large series of exertional heatstroke victims, sweating persisted in 50% of cases.[43] Therefore, the cessation of sweating is not the cause of heatstroke, and continued sweating does not preclude the diagnosis.

Although in heatstroke the core temperature is elevated above 40.5° C, significant cooling may occur in the prehospital phase, and the first temperature obtained in the emergency department may not represent the original maximum. An oral or axillary temperature does not represent central or hypothalamic temperatures.

Classic Heatstroke versus Exertional Heatstroke

The two forms of heatstroke have significantly different presentations and manifestations: classic (epidemic) heatstroke (CHS) and exertional heatstroke (EHS) (Table 139-1).

Classic heatstroke occurs during periods of sustained high ambient temperatures and humidity, as during summer heat waves. Victims are often elderly and poor and live in underventilated dwellings without air conditioning. Debilitated patients who have limited access to oral fluids may develop water-depletion heat exhaustion, which progresses to heatstroke if untreated. Victims of CHS commonly suffer from chronic diseases, alcoholism, or schizophrenia, which predispose to heat illness. Such patients are often prescribed medications (e.g., diuretics, antihypertensives, neuroleptics, and anticholinergics) that impair the ability to tolerate heat stress. Sweating is totally absent in the majority of CHS patients. Factors such as advanced age, hypotension, altered coagulation status, and the necessity for endo-

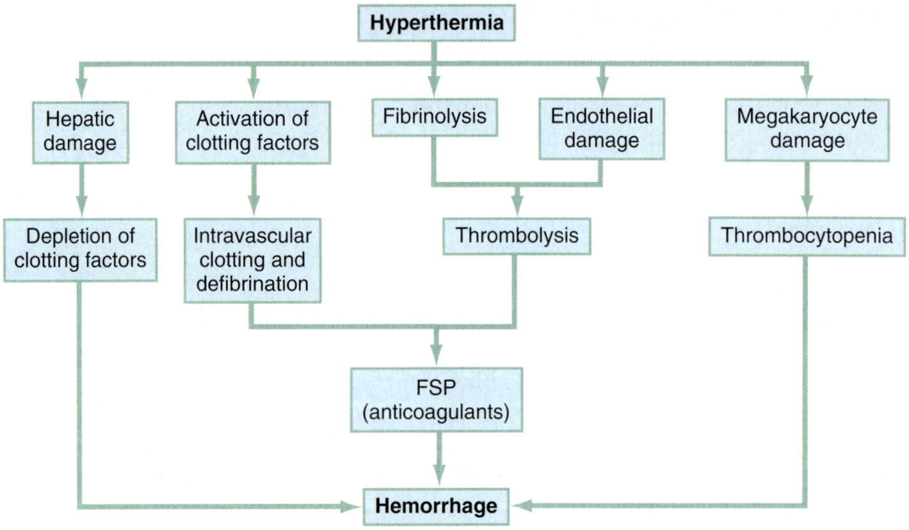

Figure 139-2. Pathogenesis of hemorrhage. FSP, fibrin split products.

tracheal intubation on arrival at the emergency department dictated a poor outcome despite successful cooling measures.[44]

In contrast, patients with EHS are usually young and healthy individuals whose heat-dispelling mechanisms are overwhelmed by endogenous heat production. Athletes and military recruits are typical victims.[45-47] Rhabdomyolysis and acute renal failure, rarely seen in patients with CHS, are common in patients with EHS.[48] Sweating is present in half the cases of EHS. Hypoglycemia may occur as the result of increased glucose metabolism and hepatic damage resulting in impaired gluconeogenesis. Coagulopathy is common. Hyponatremia with serum sodium levels less than 130 mmol/L has been detected in summer hikers in the Grand Canyon; many present with neurologic symptoms or seizures.[46]

Signs of profound CNS dysfunction dominate the early course of heatstroke. Delirium or coma is characteristic, but virtually any neurologic abnormality, including bizarre behavior, opisthotonus, hallucinations, decerebrate rigidity, oculogyric crisis, and cerebellar dysfunction, can be seen.[43] Convulsions occur in up to 75% of patients and can be precipitated by therapeutic maneuvers (such as ice water immersion). Profound muscle rigidity with tonic contractions, coarse tremor, and dystonic movements can mimic seizures. Pupils may be fixed and dilated, and the electroencephalogram may be isoelectric. All these changes are potentially reversible, although permanent damage, including cerebellar deficits, hemiplegia, dementia, and personality changes, is common in severe cases. Patients with heatstroke usually have hyperdynamic cardiovascular systems with low peripheral vascular resistance, tachycardia (up to 180 beats/min), and an elevated cardiac index. These changes are expected because skin blood vessels dilate to dissipate heat; however, this low peripheral vascular resistance has persisted in patients treated with ice water immersion and reduction of body temperature to near normal.

The central venous pressure (CVP) is usually elevated. The combination of elevated CVP with right-sided cardiac dilation suggests right-sided cardiac failure, which is also seen after shock or sepsis.[49] Nevertheless, crystalloid resuscitation is essential. Respiratory alkalosis is a physiologic response to active or passive heating and may be severe enough to produce tetany. Although most patients with CHS have respiratory alkalosis, those with EHS usually have a relatively pure lactic acidosis. Lactic acidosis is associated with a poor prognosis in cases of CHS but not necessarily in cases of EHS.

Aberrations in coagulation are common in patients with severe heatstroke, and their presence is a poor prognostic sign (Figure 139-2). Abnormal hemostasis is manifested clinically by purpura, conjunctival hemorrhage, melena, bloody diarrhea, hemoptysis, hematuria, myocardial bleeding, or hemorrhage into the CNS.[50]

Hepatic damage is so consistently featured in heatstroke that its absence should cast doubt on the diagnosis. Hepatic injury is evidenced by markedly elevated levels of hepatic aminotransferases (serum aspartate transaminase and alanine transaminase). Jaundice typically appears 24 to 72 hours after the onset of severe heatstroke and gradually recedes if the victim survives. Survivors generally have no permanent impairment of liver function. Hypoglycemia with a serum glucose level less than 65 mg/dL is common in cases of exertional heatstroke.[51]

Renal damage is common. The initial urine specimen, usually obtained by catheterization, is a scanty, brownish, turbid fluid resembling machine oil. Microscopic examination reveals proteinuria with abundant granular casts and red blood cells. Acute oliguric renal failure complicates 25% to 30% of EHS cases and 5% of CHS cases. Glomerular filtration rate, renal plasma flow, urine flow, and sodium excretion diminish markedly during exercise. Heavy physical exertion in hot climates produces acidic and maximally concentrated urine, which can result in acute oliguric renal failure when combined with hypotension and myoglobinuria.[33] Cocaine use is also associated with rhabdomyolysis and hyperthermia.[52]

BOX 139-5. Differential Diagnosis of Heatstroke

CNS hemorrhage
Toxins/drugs
Seizures
Malignant hyperthermia
Neuroleptic malignant syndrome
Serotonin syndrome
Thyroid storm
High fever/sepsis
Encephalitis/meningitis

CNS, central nervous system.

Diarrhea, probably caused by intense splanchnic vasoconstriction, is commonly seen. Cooling aggravates the diarrhea, creating an unpleasant treatment problem. Pancreatitis is described with elevated serum amylase and lipase levels.

Diagnostic Strategies

Thermometry

Unfortunately, most standard measurements of body temperature vary significantly from the actual core temperature. Oral thermometry is affected by mouth breathing and is a poor approximation of the core. Rectal thermometry is less variable but responds to changes in core temperature slowly. Thermistors that are inserted 15 cm into the rectum offer continuous monitoring of temperature and less variability. Although slower to respond to changes in core temperature than tympanic temperature readings, rectal measurements are not biased by head skin temperature. An esophageal thermistor positioned adjacent to the heart is another option.

Placement of a tympanic temperature sensor directly on the tympanic membrane may be difficult and is not used clinically. Commercially available infrared thermometers do not physically contact the tympanic membrane and are unreliable in detecting hyperthermia.[53] If a patient is being monitored with a catheter, pulmonary arterial temperature can be measured precisely with a thermistor catheter.

Only after the initial assessment and cooling have begun is the differential diagnosis relevant. When a history of collapse under conditions of heat stress is present, rapid improvement in mental status and blood pressure with cooling eliminates alternative diagnoses. If, however, the temperature does not respond and the patient does not recover neurologically, other causes of fever and coma must be considered (Box 139-5).

The history may be helpful; shaking chills suggest fever with an altered hypothalamic set point rather than heat illness. Meningitis and encephalitis can masquerade as heatstroke. In patients with heatstroke, the spinal fluid should be crystal clear, with occasional lymphocytic pleocytosis and elevated protein levels. Cerebral falciparum malaria, which presents a clinical picture of high fever and encephalitis, is seen in tropical areas where heat illness can also occur.

In patients with thyroid storm, the clinical symptoms resemble those of heatstroke. It should be suspected if the thyroid gland is enlarged or nodular, but a normal thyroid gland does not exclude the diagnosis. Thyroid function test results are elevated, but these are not available on an emergency basis. Fortunately, thyroid storm is rare, and some critical aspects of treatment, such as rapid cooling, coincide with those for heatstroke.

Drug-induced heat illness is an important consideration, particularly anticholinergic poisoning. Differentiation may be difficult because both heatstroke and anticholinergic poisoning produce hyperpyrexia, hot and dry skin, tachycardia, and abnormal mental status. Constricted pupils are present in many heatstroke patients.[54] Mydriasis should be present in patients with anticholinergic poisoning, and its absence argues strongly against this diagnosis. Typhoid fever, typhus, delirium tremens, and hypothalamic hemorrhage all produce symptom complexes similar to that of heatstroke.

Hepatic transaminase elevations may be diagnostically helpful. In most febrile states that include altered mental status or coma, these enzymes will be normal or minimally elevated, although they are usually dramatically elevated early in the course of heatstroke.

Malignant hyperthermia and neuroleptic malignant syndrome are characterized by "lead pipe" rigidity. The serotonin syndrome can mimic heatstroke because of the elevated body temperature tremors and CNS alterations that occur. Recent exposure to illicit or therapeutic medication is important.

MANAGEMENT

It does not take long either to boil an egg or to cook neurons.

D. Hamilton[55]

Cooling

Immediate cooling is the cornerstone of treatment. Cooling must be initiated as soon as possible, in conjunction with the initiation of stabilizing treatment. Mortality increases significantly when cooling is delayed.[56,57] Cooling efforts take precedence over any time-consuming search for the cause. In the prehospital setting, cooling should be initiated by removing the patient from the hot environment and fanning. When the patient arrives at the hospital, clothes should be removed, a thermistor probe should be inserted, and the temperature should be continuously monitored.

The ideal method of evaporative cooling uses a body cooling unit on which the patient lies suspended on a net surface while being sprayed with atomized 15° C water from above and below.[58] Air warmed to 45° C to 48° C is blown over the skin surface at 3 m/min. The unit, not widely available, maximizes evaporative cooling by maintaining cutaneous vasodilation and avoiding heat generation caused by shivering.

BOX 139-6. Cooling Modalities to Lower Body Temperature in Heat Stroke

Preferred

Evaporative cooling using large circulating fans and skin wetting

Ice water immersion

Adjuncts

Ice packs to axillae and groin

Cooling blanket

Peritoneal lavage (unproven efficacy in humans)

Rectal lavage

Gastric lavage

Cardiopulmonary bypass

Less complex equipment can also be used to maximize evaporative cooling. Evaporative cooling is the most widely used cooling method. The combination of atomized tepid water at 40° C from a spray bottle and standing fans cool at rates comparable to both body cooling unit and immersion.[59] Other evaporative techniques, including the use of downdraft from a helicopter, can be applied successfully.[60]

Immersion in ice water results in a rapid reduction of core temperature to less than 39° C within 10 to 40 minutes[56] but complicates the resuscitation. Vigorous skin massage to maintain cutaneous circulation has been advocated but no objective evidence exists that this is efficacious. When the body temperature reaches 39° C, cooling measures should be discontinued to avoid hypothermic overshoot. Continuous monitoring is necessary to maintain the core temperature at 37° C to 38° C.[57]

Cooling modalities other than evaporation and immersion should be considered adjunctive treatments (Box 139-6). Application of ice packs to high heat transfer areas (neck, groin, axillae) is commonly used. Cooling blankets may be a useful adjunct but will not produce rapid cooling if used exclusively. Cardiopulmonary bypass with a heat exchanger has been successful in the treatment of malignant hyperthermia.[61] Peritoneal dialysis with cold fluids, although successful in a canine model, remains untested in humans. Cold-irrigant gastric or rectal lavage will not provide significant heat exchange if used as the primary cooling modality.

Military studies of EHS patients treated with ice water immersion report no fatalities or permanent sequelae.[45] A mortality rate of 14% is reported in a study of 28 patients with CHS treated by immersion.[54] Immersion is technically difficult in the emergency department. Vasoconstriction from ice water immersion may be beneficial to hypotensive patients and may be better than evaporative cooling for victims in shock who have poor peripheral circulation.

Resuscitation

Aspiration and seizures are common in patients with heatstroke, and airway control is essential.[62] Hypoxemia may occur because of aspiration, pneumonitis and pulmonary infarction, hemorrhage, or edema. Metabolic demands are high, and normal pulmonary ventilation may be inadequate in this setting.

Circulatory fluid requirements are modest in some cases, averaging 1200 mL of isotonic crystalloid solution in the first 4 hours. Pulmonary edema occurs in patients with heatstroke and can be exacerbated by overzealous fluid administration. The use of a CVP catheter to monitor fluid resuscitation may be deceptive. Most patients have a hyperdynamic circulation with high cardiac index, low peripheral vascular resistance, and elevated CVP as a result of right-sided heart failure. These patients may require only modest intravenous fluids because cooling produces vasoconstriction and increases blood pressure.[63]

Hypotension is common in patients with heatstroke and is usually caused by peripheral vasodilation resulting in high-output cardiac failure, in addition to dehydration. Blood pressure usually rises with cooling. Hypothermia attenuates circulatory shock and cerebral ischemia in an experimental model of heatstroke.[64] If this does not occur, or if the patient monitored invasively has a low central venous or pulmonary capillary wedge pressure, a fluid challenge of 250 to 500 mL of 0.9% saline should be given rapidly while blood pressure, pulse, and urine output are monitored. If the blood pressure rises, further fluids are given with careful monitoring of the CVP. Aggressive fluid replacement is continued until the blood pressure reaches 90/60 mm Hg or the CVP exceeds 12 mL H_2O. Occasionally, patients exhibit hypodynamic responses with low cardiac index, elevated CVP, and hypotension. These patients may be cyanotic, whereas patients with hyperdynamic circulation are initially pink. This clinical observation can be helpful in identifying patients who may respond to catecholamines (Figure 139-3).

A variety of tachyarrhythmias commonly occur during heatstroke. These usually resolve with cooling, and electrical cardioversion should be avoided until the myocardium is cooled. The use of α-adrenergic agents such as norepinephrine is not recommended because they promote vasoconstriction without improving cardiac output or perfusion, decrease cutaneous heat exchange, and may enhance ischemic renal and hepatic damage. Atropine and other anticholinergic drugs that inhibit sweating should be avoided.

Because the pathophysiologies of heatstroke and fever differ, antipyretics such as aspirin and acetaminophen are not indicated and may be harmful. Salicylates, particularly in large doses, can worsen hyperthermia by uncoupling oxidative phosphorylation and aggravate coagulopathies. Large doses of acetaminophen can result in further hepatic damage. The efficacy of dantrolene is not established.[64]

After volume repletion, administration of mannitol in an initial intravenous dose of 12.5 g, followed by 12.5 g mannitol per liter of intravenous fluid increases renal blood flow and minimizes damage from myoglobinuria secondary to rhabdomyolysis. If myoglobinuria is documented, maintenance of urine output of at least 50 mL/hr and urinary alkalinization are indicated. Dextran is contraindicated because of its propensity to

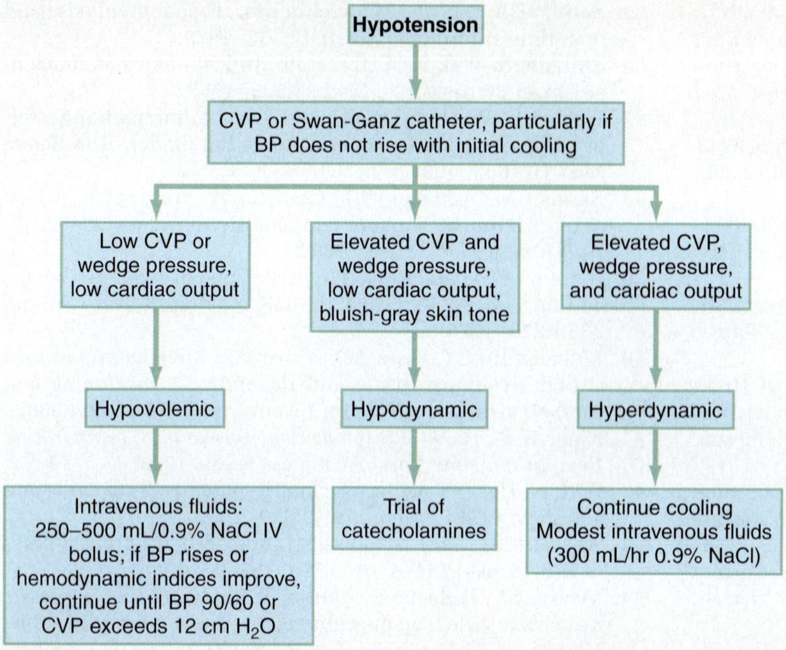

Figure 139-3. Treatment of hypotension in heat stroke. BP, blood pressure; CVP, central venous pressure. (Modified from Auerbach PS, Geehr EC: *Management of Wilderness and Environmental Emergencies*, 2nd ed. St. Louis, Mosby, 1989.)

coat platelets and impair coagulation. Persistent anuria, uremia, or hyperkalemia is an indication for consideration of hemodialysis.

Hematologic evaluation should include arterial blood gas determination, complete blood cell count and platelet counts; electrolytes, blood urea nitrogen, glucose, creatinine, aspartate aminotransferase, alanine aminotransferase, lactate dehydrogenase, creatine phosphokinase, uric and lactic acid, and calcium levels; prothrombin and partial thromboplastin times; international normalized ratio; and fibrin degradation products and hepatic enzymes. Acidosis is common, especially in patients with exertional heatstroke. Lactate levels are usually elevated; this may persist or even worsen with improved extremity perfusion.

Cooling modalities that drastically lower skin temperature may induce violent shivering; this increases metabolic heat production and may impede cooling. In this situation, chlorpromazine (25 mg IV) can be efficacious. Chlorpromazine has anticholinergic properties that can interfere with sweating and cause hypotension or, rarely, precipitate seizures. Therefore, its use should be reserved for instances when cooling is not adequate because of vigorous shivering.

Many patients are agitated during the initial cooling period. Short-acting benzodiazepines can be used for sedation and to control seizures.[65] Barbiturates are less desirable for treatment of seizures, since metabolism is altered by hepatic dysfunction.

Coagulopathies can occur during the first day of illness but are more common on the second and third days. Initial treatment should include replacement therapy with fresh frozen plasma and platelets.[1] The clinician should monitor the laboratory signs of disseminated intravascular coagulation (hypofibrinogenemia, elevated fibrin split products, prolonged prothrombin time, and thrombocytopenia).[50] The bleeding diathesis in patients with heatstroke may be the result of fibrinolysis. Although ε-amino caproic acid can impede fibrinolysis, administration of this compound is associated with rhabdomyolysis and its use is not recommended in patients with heatstroke.

KEY CONCEPTS

- Antipyretics are ineffective and should not be used to control environmental hyperthermia.
- The symptoms and signs of heat exhaustion often mimic those of viral illnesses.
- Patients with exertional heatstroke are commonly diaphoretic.
- Rapid (convective) cooling of the potential heatstroke patient should be initiated before the diagnosis is firmly established.
- Heatstroke can cause right-sided cardiac dilation and elevated CVP, clinically resemble pulmonary edema, and yet require vigorous crystalloid resuscitation.

REFERENCES

1. Shibolet S, Lancaster MC, Danon Y: Heat stroke: A review. *Aviat Space Environ Med* 47:280, 1976.
2. Dickenson JG: Heat illness in the services. *J R Army Med Corps* 140:7, 1994.
3. Smalley B, Janke RM, Cole D: Exertional heat illness in Air Force basic military trainees. *Mil Med* 168:298, 2003.
4. Knochel JP: Dog days and siriasis: How to kill a football player. *JAMA* 233:513, 1975.
5. Heat-related mortality—United States, 1997. *MMWR Morb Mortal Wkly Rep* 47:473, 1998.
6. Dematte JE, et al: Near-fatal heat stroke during the 1995 heat wave in Chicago. *Ann Intern Med* 129:173, 1998.
7. Heat-related illnesses, deaths, and risk factors—Cincinnati and Dayton, Ohio 1999 and United States 1979-1997. *MMWR Morb Mortal Wkly Rep* 49:470, 2000.

8. Vanhems P, Gambotti L: Excess rate of in-hospital death in Lyons, France, during the August 2003 heat wave. *N Engl J Med* 349:2007, 2003.
9. Bouchama A, Knochel JP: Heat stroke. *N Engl J Med* 346:1978, 2002.
10. Gisolfi CV, Wenger CB: Temperature regulation during exercise: Old concepts, new ideas. *Exerc Sport Sci Rev* 12:339, 1984.
11. Charkoudian N: Skin blood flow in adult human thermoregulation: How it works, when it does not, and why. *Mayo Clin Proc* 78:603, 2003.
12. Rowell LB: General principles in vascular control. In *Human Circulation: Regulation during Physical Stress.* New York, Oxford University Press, 1986.
13. Rowell LB: Cardiovascular adjustments to thermal stress (Section 2: the cardiovascular system). In Shepherd JT, Aboud PM (eds): *Handbook of Physiology,* vol 3. Bethesda, Md, American Physiological Society, 1983.
14. Nadel ER, Fortney SM, Wenger CB: Effect of hydration state of circulatory and thermal regulations. *J Appl Physiol Respir Environ Exerc Physiol* 49:715, 1980.
15. Knochel J: Heat illness. In Callaham ML (ed): *Current Therapy in Emergency Medicine.* Toronto, BC Decker, 1987.
16. Appenzeller O: Physical training, heat acclimatization and diet. In *Heat Stroke.* New York, Academic Press, 1983.
17. Hubbard RW, et al: Voluntary dehydration and allesthesia for water. *J Appl Physiol* 57:868, 1984.
18. Hyperthermia and dehydration-related deaths associated with intentional rapid weight loss in three collegiate wrestlers—North Carolina, Wisconsin, and Michigan, November-December 1997. *MMWR Morb Mortal Wkly Rep* 47:105, 1998.
19. Pascoe DD, Bellingar TA, McCluskey BS: Clothing and exercise: II. Influence of clothing during exercise/work in environmental extremes. *Sports Med* 18:94, 1994.
20. Edelman IS, Ismail-Beigi F: Thyroid thermogenesis and active sodium transport. *Recent Prog Horm Res* 30:235, 1974.
21. Greenblatt DJ, Shader RJ: Anticholinergics. *N Engl J Med* 288:1217, 1978.
22. Olshaker JS, Tek D: Environmental emergencies. *Emerg Med Clin North Am* 10:299, 1992.
23. Falk B: Effect of thermal stress during rest and exercise in the pediatric population. *Sports Med* 25:221, 1998.
24. Marzuk PM, et al: Ambient temperature and mortality from unintentional cocaine overdose. *JAMA* 279:1795, 1998.
25. Martinez M, Devenport L, Saussy J, Martinez J: Drug-associated heat stroke. *So Med J* 95:799, 2002.
26. Oh RC, Henning JS: Exertional heatstroke in an infantry soldier taking ephedra-containing dietary supplements. *Mil Med* 168:129, 2003.
27. Ester EA, Harrison J, Stasiewicz ED, Wang D: Malignant hyperthermia in an adult trauma patient. *Am Surg* 68:883, 2002.
28. Chung NK, Pin CH: Obesity and the occurrence of heat disorders. *Mil Med* 161:739, 1996.
29. Kilbourne EM, et al: Risk factors for heat stroke. *JAMA* 247:3332, 1982.
30. Stitt JT: Fever versus hyperthermia. *Fed Proc* 38:39, 1979.
31. Saper CB, Breder CD: Endogenous pyrogens in the CNS: Role in the febrile response. *Prog Brain Res* 93:419, 1992.
32. Kashmeery AMS: Physiological studies on heat exhaustion victims among Mecca Pilgrims: Response to relevant hormones, and effect of cold IV infusion on recovery. *Acta Med Austr* 22:16, 1995.
33. Noakes TD: Fluid and electrolyte disturbance in heat illness. *Int J Sports Med* 2:5146, 1998.
34. Brake DJ, Bates GP: Fluid losses and hydration status of industrial workers under thermal stress working extended shifts. *J Occup Environ Med* 60:90, 2003.
35. Schiff HB, et al: Myoglobinuria, rhabdomyolysis and marathon running. *Q J Med* 47:463, 1978.
36. Shibolet S, et al: Heat stroke: Its clinical picture and mechanism in 36 cases. *Q J Med* 36:525, 1967.
37. Hubbard RW, et al: Novel approaches to the pathophysiology of heatstroke: The energy depletion model. *Ann Emerg Med* 16:1066, 1987.
38. Slovis CM, Anderson GF, Casolaro A: Survival in a heat stroke victim with a core temperature in excess of 46.5° C. *Ann Emerg Med* 11:269, 1982.
39. Bynum GD, et al: Induced hyperthermia in sedated humans and the concept of critical thermal maximum. *Am J Physiol* 235:R228, 1978.
40. McLaughlin CT, Kane AG, Auber AE: MR imaging of heat stroke, external capsule and thalamic T1 shortening and cerebellar injury. *AJNR Am J Neuroradiol* 24:1372, 2003.
41. Khogali M, Hales JRS (eds): *Heat Stroke and Temperature Regulation.* New York, Academic Press, 1983.
42. Bark N: Heat stroke in psychiatric patients: Two cases and a review. *J Clin Psychiatry* 43:377, 1982.
43. Austin MG, Berry JW: Observations on one hundred cases of heat stroke. *JAMA* 161:1525, 1956.
44. Vicario SJ, Okabajue R, Haltom T: Rapid cooling in classic heatstroke: Effect on mortality rates. *Am J Emerg Med* 4:394, 1986.
45. Beller GA, Boyd AE III: Heat stroke: A report of 13 consecutive cases without mortality despite severe hyperpyrexia and neurologic dysfunction. *Mil Med* 140:464, 1975.
46. Backer HD, et al: Exertional heat illness and hyponatremia in hikers. *Am J Emerg Med* 17:532, 1999.
47. Porter AM: Collapse from exertional heat illness: Implications and subsequent decisions. *Mil Med* 168:76, 2003.
48. Phillips RA: The relationship between proinflammatory mediators and heat stress induced rhabdomyolysis in exercising marines. *Crit Care Nurs Clin North Am* 15:163, 2003.
49. Shahid MS, et al: Echocardiographic and Doppler study of patients with heatstroke and heat exhaustion. *Int J Cardiac Imag* 15:279, 1999.
50. al-Mashhadani SA, et al: The coagulopathy of heat stroke: Alterations in coagulation and fibrinolysis in heat stroke patients during the pilgrimage (Haj) to Makkah. *Blood Coagul Fibrinol* 5:731, 1994.
51. Gumma K, et al: The metabolic status of heat stroke patients. In Khogali M, Hales JRS (eds): *Heat Stroke and Temperature Regulation.* New York, Academic Press, 1983, pp 157-170.
52. Roth D: Acute rhabdomyolysis associated with cocaine intoxication. *N Engl J Med* 319:673, 1988.
53. Hansen RD, et al: Infrared thermometry in the diagnosis and treatment of heat exhaustion. *Int J Sports Med* 17:66, 1996.
54. Hart GR, et al: Epidemic heat stroke: Clinical characteristics and course of 28 patients. *Medicine (Baltimore)* 61:189, 1982.
55. Hamilton D: The immediate treatment of heatstroke. *Anaesthesia* 31:270, 1976.
56. Costrini A: Emergency treatment of exertional heatstroke and comparison of whole body cooling techniques. *Med Sci Sports Exerc* 22:15, 1990.
57. Olson KR, Benowitz NL: Environmental and drug-induced hyperthermia: Pathophysiology, recognition, and management. *Emerg Med Clin North Am* 2:459, 1984.
58. Weiner JS, Khogali M: A physiological body-cooling unit for treatment of heat stroke. *Lancet* 1:507, 1980.
59. Graham BS, et al: Nonexertional heat stroke: Physiologic management and cooling in 14 patients. *Arch Intern Med* 146:87, 1986.
60. Poulton TJ, Walker RA: Helicopter cooling of heatstroke victims. *Aviat Space Environ Med* 58:358, 1987.

61. Ryan JF, et al: Cardiopulmonary bypass in the treatment of malignant hyperthermia. *N Engl J Med* 290:1121, 1974.
62. Al-Khawashki MJ, et al: Clinical presentation of 172 heat stroke cases seen at Mina and Arafat—September 1982. In Khogali M, Hales JRS (eds): *Heat Stroke and Temperature Regulation.* New York, Academic Press, 1983, pp 99-108.
63. Atar S, Royner E, Rosenfeld T: Transient cardiac dysfunction and pulmonary edema in exertional heat stroke. *Mil Med* 168:671, 2003.
64. Channa AB, et al: Is dantrolene effective in heat stroke patients? *Crit Care Med* 18:290, 1990.
65. Eichner ER: Treatment of suspected heat illness. *Int J Sports Med* 19:S150, 1998.

CHAPTER 140

Electrical and Lightning Injuries

Timothy G. Price and Mary Ann Cooper

PERSPECTIVE

Electrical Injury

The first recorded death caused by electrical current from an artificial source was reported in 1879, when a carpenter in Lyons, France, inadvertently contacted a 250-V AC generator.[1] The first U.S. fatality occurred in 1881, when an inebriated man passed out on a similar generator in front of a crowd in Buffalo, New York. The apparent painlessness of his death impressed the crowd, and electrocution became considered a "humane" mode of execution. In 1890, Kemmeler was the first person executed in New York State's electric chair.[2]

Electrical burns account for 4% to 6.5% of all admissions to burn units in the United States and for approximately 1000 fatalities per year in the United States.[3] Most electrical fatalities and adult admissions to burn centers from electrical injury are occupationally related. Children have a predisposition to injuries from low-voltage sources, such as electric cords, because of their limited mobility within a relatively confined environment. During adolescence, a more active exploration of the environment leads to more severe high-voltage injuries or death. At the time of presentation, documentation of injuries is important not only for the immediate resuscitation of the victim, but also for medicolegal reasons. Many cases of electrical injuries eventually involve litigation for negligence, product liability, or worker compensation.

Lightning Injury

Because no agency requires the reporting of lightning injuries, and because some victims do not seek treatment at the time of their injury, the incidence of injury and death from lightning is unknown. In the United States, 3239 deaths were reported in a 35-year period ending in 1994.[4] Currently, it is estimated that lightning is fatal in 1 of 10 lightning strike victims.[5] In typical years, lightning kills more people in the United States than any other natural disaster except floods and is consistently among the top four weather-related killers (Figure 140-1).

Participants in sports and recreational activities are common victims; mountain activities, golf, ball field games, and water activities account for the largest numbers of fatalities and injuries.[5] Outdoor workers also are vulnerable. Lightning incidents often involve more than one victim when the current "splashes" to other individuals or as ground current spreads the electrical power throughout the area where a group may be sheltered in a storm. The largest number of victims reported to be injured from a single lightning strike is 35 (28 people and 7 dogs). Four children and four dogs were fatally injured. All of the victims were sleeping in a large tent.[6]

Certain snowy conditions also can result in lightning and put skiers at risk for lightning injury. The formation of sleet and *graupel,* a type of frozen precipitation sometimes referred to as *snow pellets* or *soft hail,* may indicate the presence of large differences in electrical potential in the atmosphere. Winter sports enthusiasts should learn to recognize the appearance of graupel and appreciate the associated lightning risks.[7]

PRINCIPLES OF DISEASE

Physics of Injury

The exact pathophysiology of electrical injury is not well understood because of the numerous variables that cannot be measured or controlled when an electrical current passes through tissue. With high voltage, most of the injury seems to be thermal, and histologic studies reveal coagulation necrosis consistent with thermal injury.[8,9] The theory of *electroporation* is that electrical charges insufficient to produce thermal damage cause protein configuration changes that threaten cell wall integrity and cellular function.[10]

The nature and severity of electrical burn injury are directly proportional to the current strength, resistance,

Figure 140-1. Global frequency and distribution of lightning as observed from space by the Optical Transient Detector. (From Christian HJ, et al: Global frequency and distribution of lightning as observed from space by the Optical Transient Detector. *J Geophys Res* 108[D1]:4005, 2003.)

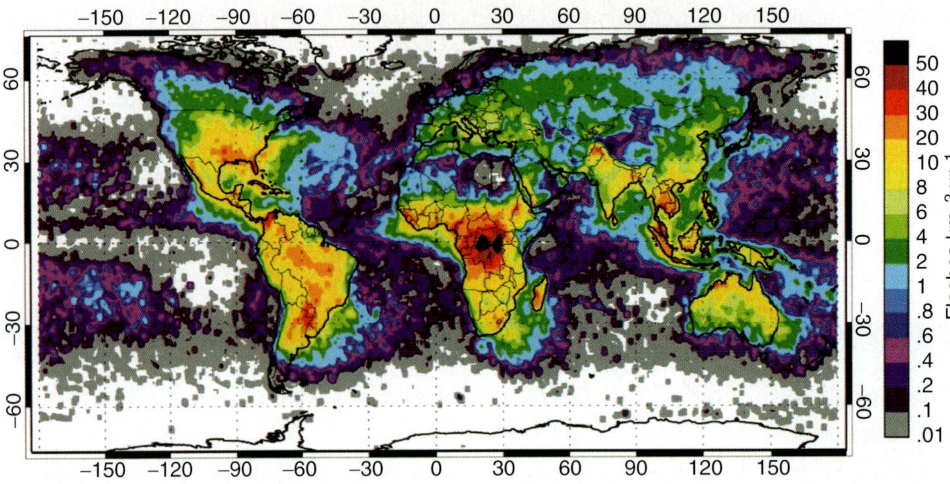

BOX 140-1. Electrothermal Heating Formulas

$P = I^2Rt$

and

$I = V/R$

where:
P = thermal power (heat), in joules
I = current, in amperes
R = resistance, in ohms
t = time, in seconds
V = potential, in volts

BOX 140-2. Factors Determining Electrical Injury

- Type of circuit
- Duration
- Resistance of tissues
- Voltage
- Amperage
- Pathway of current

and duration of current flow (Box 140-1). *Current strength* is expressed in amperes and is a measure of the amount of energy flowing through an object. Current is determined by the voltage and resistance.[11] Resistance is determined by the current's pathway through the body. The factors determining the severity of burn injury are summarized in Box 140-2.

Type of Circuit

One of the factors affecting the nature and severity of electrical injury is the type of circuit involved, either direct current (DC) or alternating current (AC). High-voltage DC contact tends to cause a single muscle spasm, often throwing the victim from the source; this results in a shorter duration of exposure, but increases the likelihood of traumatic blunt injury. Brief contact with a DC source also can result in disturbances in cardiac rhythm, depending on the phase of the cardiac cycle affected.

AC exposure to the same voltage tends to be *three* times more dangerous than DC. Continuous muscle contraction, or tetany, can occur when the muscle fibers are stimulated at between 40 and 110 times per second. The standard frequency of electrical transmission in the United States is 60 Hz (cycles per second), which is near the lowest frequency at which an incandescent light appears to be continuously lit.

The terms *entry* and *exit* are commonly used to describe electrical injuries. The terms *source contact point* and *ground contact point* are more appropriate, however, when referring to AC injuries. The hand is the most common site of contact via a tool that is in contact with an AC electrical source. Because the flexors of the hand and forearm are much stronger than the extensors, contraction of the flexors at the wrist, elbow, and shoulder occurs, causing the hand grasping the current source to pull the source even closer to the body. Currents greater than the "let-go threshold" (6 to 9 mA) can prevent the victim from releasing the current source, which prolongs the duration of exposure to the electrical current.

Resistance

Resistance is the tendency of a material to resist the flow of electrical current; it is specific for a given tissue, depending on its moisture content, temperature, and other physical properties. The higher the resistance of a tissue to the flow of current, the greater the potential for transformation of electrical energy to thermal energy. Nerves, designed to carry electrical signals, and muscle and blood vessels, because of their high electrolyte and water content, have a low resistance and are good conductors. Bone, tendon, and fat, which all contain a large amount of inert matrix, have a high resistance and tend to heat and coagulate rather than transmit current. The other tissues of the body are intermediate in resistance (Box 140-3).[12]

Skin is the primary resistor to the flow of current into the body. Skin on the inside of the arm or back of the hand has a resistance of about 30,000 Ω/cm^2. Deeply

BOX 140-3. Resistance of Body Tissues

Least
Nerves
Blood
Mucous membranes
Muscle

Intermediate
Dry skin

Most
Tendon
Fat
Bone

Table 140-1. Skin Resistance (Ω/cm²)

Tissue	Resistance (Ω/cm²)
Mucous membranes	100
Vascular areas	
Volar arm, inner thigh	300-10,000
Wet skin	
Bathtub	1200-1500
Sweat	2500
Other skin	10,000-40,000
Sole of foot	100,000-200,000
Heavily calloused palm	1-2 million

calloused skin can have 20 to 70 times greater resistance (Table 140-1).[9] This high resistance may result in a significant amount of energy being expended at the skin surface as the current burns its way through deep callus, resulting in greater thermal injury to the skin but less internal damage than would be expected if the current were delivered undiminished to the deep tissues. As the duration of contact increases, however, the skin begins to blister and offer decreased resistance. A surge of current internally can cause extensive deep tissue destruction. Moisture also lowers resistance. Sweating can decrease the skin's resistance to 2500 to 3000 Ω/cm², and immersion in water causes a further reduction to 1200 to 1500 Ω/cm².

Amperage

Current, expressed in amperes, is a measure of the amount of energy that flows through an object. As defined by Joule's law, the heat generated is proportional to the amperage squared.[11] Amperage depends on the source voltage and the resistance of the conductor and normally must be estimated in human electric exposures. Although the voltage of the source is often known, the resistance varies according to the involved tissues. Additionally, as tissue changes occur secondary to the energy of the current flow, resistance may change markedly, rendering predictions of amperage difficult for any given electrical injury.

The physical effects vary with different amperages at 50 to 60 Hz, which is the AC frequency used in European countries and the United States (Table 140-2). A narrow range exists between the threshold of perception of current (0.2 to 0.4 mA) and *let-go current* (6 to 9 mA). The let-go current is the level above which muscular tetany prevents release of the current source. Thoracic tetany also can occur at levels just above this *let-go current* and result in respiratory arrest. Ventricular fibrillation occurs at an amperage of 60 to 120 mA. Dry skin in contact with a 120-V household source results in significantly lower current than the same voltage across skin submerged in water. This wet skin may result in current sufficient to cause electrocution with cardiac arrest but no surface burns.

Table 140-2. Physical Effects of Different Amperage Levels at 50 to 60 Hz

Physical Effect	Current (mA)
Tingling sensation	1-4
Let-go current	
Children	4
Women	7
Men	9
Freezing to circuit	10-20
Respiratory arrest from thoracic muscle tetany	20-50
Ventricular fibrillation	60-120

Duration of Contact

In general, the longer the duration of contact with high-voltage current, the greater the electrothermal heating and degree of tissue destruction. When carbonization of tissue occurs, the resistance to current flow increases. The physics are different with lightning. The extremely short duration and extraordinarily high voltage and amperage of lightning result in a short flow of current internally, with little, if any, skin damage and almost immediate flashover of current around the body.

Voltage

Voltage is a measure of the difference in electrical potential between two points and is determined by the electrical source. Electrical injuries conventionally are divided into high or low voltage, with 1000 V being the most commonly used dividing line.[13] Although high and low voltage can cause significant morbidity and mortality, high voltage results in greater current flow and has a greater potential for tissue destruction, leading to major amputations and tissue loss.

No fatalities are recorded from contact with the low voltages associated with long distance communications lines (24 V) or telephone lines (65 V). Fatalities are reported, however, with exposure to 110 V household current, especially in special environmental circumstances, such as bathtub-related electrocutions.

Pathway

The pathway of high, low, or lightning voltages determines the tissues at risk, the type of injury, and the degree of conversion of electrical energy to heat.

Current passing through the heart or thorax can cause dysrhythmias and direct myocardial damage. Cerebral current can result in respiratory arrest, seizures, and paralysis. Current with ocular proximity can cause cataracts.

Truncal current causes less damage than current that passes through a single digit. As current density increases, its tendency to flow through the less resistant tissues is overcome. Eventually it flows through tissues indiscriminately, as if the body were a volume conductor, with the potential to destroy all tissues in the current's path. Because the current often is concentrated at the source and ground contact points, the greatest degree of damage is often observed there. Nevertheless, extensive deep destruction of the tissues may exist between these sites with high-voltage injuries, and the surface damage is often only "the tip of the iceberg." Damage to the internal structures of the body may be noncontiguous, with areas of normal-appearing tissue adjacent to burned tissue and with damage to structures at sites distant from the apparent contact points.

The pathway between contact points is a major determinant of the electrical field strength, which is the voltage per unit of length. For a given current, the shorter the distance between contact points, the greater the electrical field strength. Current from a 20,000-V power line passing from head to toe (approximately 2 m) results in an electrical field strength of 10,000 V/m. Approximately the same electrical field strength is created when 120-V household current passes between two close contact points on the mouth of a child chewing on a power cord (120 V/0.01 m). While the electrical field strengths are similar, there is a tremendous difference in the amount of at-risk tissue in the respective pathways.[13,14]

Although lightning is governed by the same physical laws as artificial electricity, the rapid rise and decay of the energy complicates predictions of the extent of lightning injury more than artificial electrical injury. The most important difference between lightning and high-voltage electrical injuries is the duration of exposure to the current.

Lightning is neither a direct current nor an alternating current, but rather a unidirectional massive current impulse. Lightning is classed as a *current,* rather than a *voltage,* phenomenon. The cloud-to-ground lightning impulse results from the breakdown of a large electrical field between a cloud and the ground that is measured in millions of volts. When connection is made with the ground, this voltage difference between the cloud and ground disappears, and a large current flows impulsively for a short time. The study of these massive discharges of such short duration on the human body is not well advanced.

Mathematical modeling of a lightning strike to the human body is substantiated on animal models.[15] After lightning meets the body, current initially is transmitted internally, after which skin breaks down, and ultimately external "flashover" occurs. Experimental evidence suggests that a fast flashover appreciably diminishes the energy dissipation within the body and results in survival.[16]

BOX 140-4. Types of Electrical Burns

Direct contact
- Electrothermal heating

Indirect contact
- Arc
- Flame
- Flash

Although lightning current may flow internally for an instant and short-circuit electrical systems, it seldom causes significant burns or tissue destruction. Burns and myoglobinuric renal failure are not a common injury pattern from lightning. More common manifestations include cardiac and respiratory arrest, vascular spasm, neurologic damage, and autonomic instability.

Lightning tends to cause asystole rather than ventricular fibrillation. Although cardiac automaticity may re-establish a rhythm, the duration of the respiratory arrest may cause secondary deterioration of the rhythm to refractory ventricular fibrillation and asystole.[2,4,17] This secondary arrest occurs experimentally in sheep. Other injuries caused by blunt trauma or ischemia from vascular spasms, such as myocardial infarction or spinal artery syndromes, also occur.[18-20]

Mechanisms of Injury

Electrical Injury

The primary electrical injury is the burn. Secondary blunt trauma results from falls or being thrown from the electrical source by an intense muscular contraction or the explosive force that may occur with electric flashes from circuit box or transformer accidents. Electrical burns are classified into four different types (Box 140-4).[21]

Heating of tissues secondary to current causes electrothermal burns. Usually, these burns are a result of a low-voltage shock with a limited affected area. Severe electrothermal burns can occur, however, if a person grips a high-voltage conductor. The prolonged flow of current can result in significant burns anywhere along the current path. Typically, the skin lesions of electrothermal burns are well-demarcated, deep, partial-thickness to full-thickness burns.

The most destructive indirect injury occurs when a victim becomes part of an electrical arc. An electrical arc is a current spark formed between two objects of differing potential that are not in contact with each other, usually a highly charged source and a ground. Because the temperature of an electrical arc is approximately 2500° C, it causes deep thermal burns at the point where it contacts the skin.[12] With electrical arcs, burns may be caused by the heat of the arc itself, electrothermal heating due to current flow, or flames that result from the ignition of clothing. Instead of a discrete arc, current may jump the gap by splashing across the entire body. These splash burns may cover a large portion of the body, but are generally only partial thickness.[21]

At the time of presentation, it is often difficult to determine the mechanism of injury that caused an electrically injured patient's burns. Electrothermal heating is the main cause of muscle damage and is seen almost exclusively in high-voltage accidents with prolonged (seconds) contact and current flow.[21]

The histologic change in muscle injury that results from direct contact with an electrical source is coagulation necrosis with shortening of the sarcomere.[9,12] Muscle damage can be erratic, so areas of viable and nonviable muscle often are found in the same muscle group. Periosteal muscle damage may occur even though overlying muscle appears to be normal. Similar to the muscle damage, serious vascular damage usually occurs only after a high-voltage accident.

Vascular damage is greatest in the media; this can lead to delayed hemorrhage when the vessel eventually ruptures.[2,12] Intimal damage may result in either immediate or delayed thrombosis and vascular occlusion as edema and clots form on the damaged internal surface of the vessel over a period of days. The injury is usually most severe in the small muscle branches, where blood flow is slower.[22] This damage to small muscle arteries, combined with mixed muscle viability that is not visible to gross inspection, creates the illusion of "progressive" tissue necrosis.

Immediate arterial thrombosis results in the absence of a pulse on initial examination. The absence of a pulse also can be due to transient vascular spasm. Pulselessness resulting from vascular spasm should resolve within a few hours. If pulselessness persists after this time, serious vascular injury is likely.

Damage to neural tissue also may occur via several mechanisms. A nerve may show an immediate decrease in conductivity as it undergoes coagulation necrosis similar to that observed in muscle. In addition, it may suffer indirect damage as its vascular supply or myelin sheath is injured or as progressive edema results in a compartment syndrome. The signs of neural damage may develop immediately or be delayed hours to days. The skull is a common contact point. Histologic studies of the brain reveal focal petechial hemorrhages in the brainstem, cerebral edema, and widespread chromatolysis (the disintegration of chromophil bodies of neurons).[12]

Lightning Injury

Lightning injury may occur by electrical mechanisms (Box 140-5) and by secondary blunt trauma.[23] With a direct strike, the mechanism of injury is self-evident. It has been substantiated experimentally in sheep that lightning strikes near the head may enter orifices such as the eyes, ears, and mouth to flow internally. This study may help explain the myriad eye and ear symptoms and signs reported with lightning injury.

Injury from contact occurs when the person is touching an object that is part of the pathway of lightning current, such as a tree or tent pole. Side flash or splash occurs as lightning jumps from its primary strike object to a nearby person on its way to the ground.[18,24,25] Step voltage, a difference in electrical potential between a person's feet, may occur as lightning current spreads radially through the ground. A person is a far better conductor of electricity than the earth. A person who has one foot closer than the other to the strike point has a potential difference between the feet so that the lightning current preferentially flows through the legs and body rather than the ground. This ground current is a common killer of large livestock such as cattle and horses because of the distance between their hind legs and forelegs.

BOX 140-5. Mechanisms of Lightning Injury

Direct strike
  Orifice entry
Contact
Side flash, "splash"
Ground current or step voltage
Blunt trauma

A proposed fifth electrical mechanism is from low-current upward streamers. Cloud-to-ground lightning approaches the earth as charged downward leaders. As the leaders approach, the large electrical field induces a build-up of ground charges that surge upward as upward streamers. This upward surge can travel through objects, including people. If the upward streamer connects with a downward leader, a completed lightning strike occurs. Not all upward streamers connect. Individuals in the path of an upward streamer may be injured even in the absence of a completed lightning strike.

Blunt injury from lightning can occur from two mechanisms. First, the person may be thrown a considerable distance by the sudden, massive contraction caused by current passing through the body. Second, an explosive or implosive force occurs as the lightning pathway is instantaneously superheated then rapidly cooled after the passage of the lightning. The heating is seldom long enough to cause severe burns, but it does cause rapid expansion of air followed by rapid implosion of the cooled air as it rushes back into the void.[4]

CLINICAL FEATURES

Patients with high-voltage injury commonly present with devastating burns. Patients with lightning injury and low-voltage injury may have little evidence of injury or, alternatively, may be in cardiopulmonary arrest. After the initial resuscitation of patients lightning and low-voltage injuries, other conditions may be identified. These patients may have significant residual morbidity from pain syndromes or cerebral damage.

Head and Neck

Electrical Injury

The head is a common point of contact for high-voltage injuries, and the patient may exhibit burns and neurologic damage. Cataracts develop in approximately 6% of patients with high-voltage injuries, especially whenever electrical injury occurs in the vicinity of the head.[26] Although cataracts may be present initially or develop shortly after the accident, they more typically appear months after the injury. Visual acuity and funduscopic examination should be performed at presentation.

Lightning Injury

Lightning strikes may cause skull fractures and cervical spine injury from associated blunt trauma.[18,19,27] Tympanic membrane rupture commonly is found in lightning victims and may be secondary to the shock wave, a direct burn, or a basilar skull fracture.[4,17,28] Although most patients recover without serious sequelae, disruption of the ossicles and mastoid, otorrhea, hemotympanum, and permanent deafness may occur.[17,28]

Ocular injuries include corneal lesions, uveitis, iridocyclitis, hyphema, vitreous hemorrhage, optic atrophy, retinal detachment, and choroidoretinitis. As a result, dilated, unreactive pupils are not a reliable indicator of death. As with electrical injuries, cataracts may develop later in some patients.[4,17,29]

Cardiovascular System

Electrical Injury

Cardiac arrest, either from asystole or from ventricular fibrillation, is a common presenting condition in electrical accidents. Other electrocardiographic findings include sinus tachycardia, transient ST segment elevation, reversible Q-T segment prolongation, premature ventricular contractions, atrial fibrillation, and bundle branch block.[2] Acute myocardial infarction is relatively rare. Damage to skeletal muscles may produce an increase in the creatine kinase (CK)–MB fraction, leading to a spurious diagnosis of myocardial infarction.

Lightning Injury

In lightning injury, cardiac arrest may be caused by the electrical shock or induced vascular spasm.[30] Numerous dysrhythmias are reported in the absence of cardiac arrest.[4,14] Nonspecific ST–T wave segment changes and prolongation of the Q-T interval may occur, and serum levels of cardiac enzymes are often elevated.[4,31,32] Hypertension is commonly present after lightning injury but usually resolves without treatment within a few hours.

Skin

Electrical Injury

Other than cardiac arrest, the most devastating injuries are burns, which are most severe at the source and ground contact points. The most common sites of contact with the source include the hands and the skull. The most common areas of ground contact are the heels. A patient may have multiple source and ground contact points. Burns in severe electrical accidents often appear as painless, depressed, yellow-gray, punctate areas with central necrosis, or the areas may be mummified.[12] High-voltage current often flows internally and can create massive muscle damage. If contact is brief, however, minimal flow may have occurred, and the visible skin damage may represent nearly all of the damage. Prediction of the amount of underlying tissue damage from the amount of cutaneous involvement is not possible.

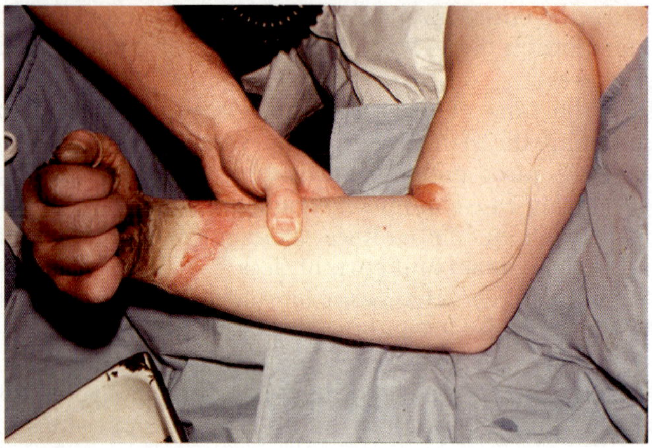

Figure 140-2. Kissing burn. (Courtesy of Mary Ann Cooper, MD.)

A peculiar type of burn associated with electrical injury is the "kissing burn," which occurs at the flexor creases (Figure 140-2).[12] As the current causes flexion of the extremity, the skin of the flexor surfaces at the joints touches. Combined with the moist environment that often occurs at the flexor areas, the electrical current may arc across the flexor crease, causing arc burns on both flexor surfaces and extensive underlying tissue damage.

Electrical flash burns are usually superficial partial-thickness burns, similar to other flash burns. Isolated thermal burns also may be seen when clothing ignites. The total body surface area affected by burns in electrical injury averages 10% to 25%. Severe burns to the skull and occasionally to the dura may occur.

The most common electrical injury seen in children younger than 4 years old is the mouth burn that occurs from sucking on a household electrical extension cord. These burns usually represent local arc burns, may involve the orbicularis oris muscle, and are especially worrisome when the commissure is involved because of the likelihood of cosmetic deformity. A significant risk of delayed bleeding from the labial artery exists when the eschar separates. Damage to developing dentition is reported, and referral to an oral surgeon familiar with electrical injuries is recommended.[33]

Lightning Injury

Deep burns occur in fewer than 5% of lightning injuries.[17,34] Patients may exhibit one or more of the fol-

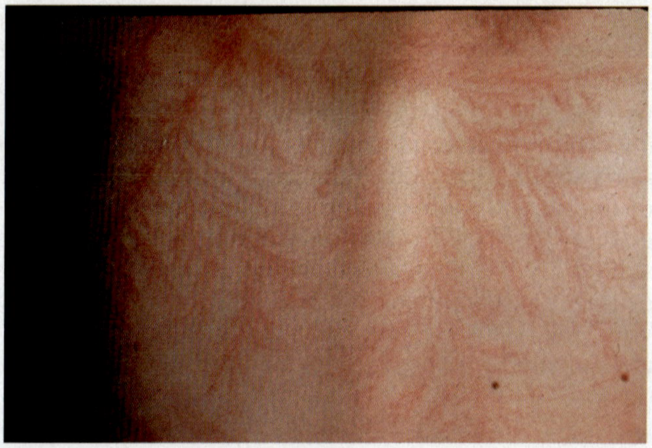

Figure 140-3. Feathering burn. (Courtesy of Mary Ann Cooper, MD.)

lowing four types of superficial burns or skin changes: linear, punctate, feathering, or thermal burns.[4,10,17,34] *Linear burns* tend to occur in areas where sweat or water accumulate, such as under the arms or down the chest. These are superficial burns that appear to be caused by steam production from the flashover phenomenon. *Punctate burns* appear as multiple, small cigarette-like burns, often with a heavier central concentration in a rosette-like pattern. They range from a few millimeters to 1 cm in diameter and seldom require grafting. *Feathering burns* are not true burns because there is no damage to the skin itself.[34] They seem to be caused by electron showers induced by the lightning, which make a fern pattern on the skin.[34] These transient lesions are pathognomonic for lightning injury and require no therapy (Figure 140-3).[35] *Thermal burns* occur if the clothing is ignited or may be caused by metal that the person is wearing or carrying during the flashover.[21]

Extremities

Electrical Injury

In high-voltage injuries, muscle necrosis can extend to sites distant from the observed skin injury, and compartment syndromes occur as a result of vascular ischemia and muscle edema. Decompression fasciotomy or amputation is often necessary.[36] Massive release of myoglobin from the damaged muscle may lead to myoglobinuric renal failure.

Joint areas may exhibit more severe injury than the muscle along the long bone portions of an extremity for several reasons. Burn injury becomes concentrated at joints because there is less cross-sectional area of muscle to conduct the energy than at long bone portions. There is also a much lower proportion of muscle to more poorly conductive tendons as they cross a joint surface. In addition, as the energy is concentrated in these areas, it may cause skin surface burns, particularly where skin surfaces touch, such as the antecubital fossae.

Vascular damage from the electrical energy may become evident at any time.[22] Neurovascular checks should be reassessed continually in all extremities. Because the arteries are a high-flow system, heat may be dissipated and cause little initial apparent damage but result in subsequent deterioration. In contrast, the veins are a low-flow system, allowing the heat energy to heat blood rapidly, with resulting thrombosis. Consequently, an extremity may appear edematous initially. With severe injuries, the entire extremity may appear mummified when all tissue elements, including the arteries, experience coagulation necrosis.

Damage to the vessel wall at the time of injury also may result in delayed thrombosis and hemorrhage, especially in the small arteries to muscle.[22] This ongoing vascular damage can cause a partial-thickness burn to progress into a full-thickness burn as the vascular supply diminishes to the area. Progressive loss of muscle because of vascular ischemia downstream from damaged vessels may mandate repeated deep debridements.[22]

Lightning Injury

Lightning injury may cause transient vasospasm so severe that the extremities appear cold, blue, mottled, and pulseless. This condition usually resolves within a few hours and rarely requires vascular imaging or surgical intervention.[17]

Skeletal System

As with electrical injury, numerous types of fractures and dislocations are reported with lightning injury.[4] Fractures of the long bones are possible secondary to the trauma associated with electrical injury. Posterior and anterior shoulder dislocations caused by tetanic spasm of the rotator cuff muscles and spinal fractures occur.

Nervous System

Electrical Injury

In high-voltage injuries, loss of consciousness is usually transient, unless there is a significant concomitant head injury. Prolonged coma with eventual recovery also occurs. Patients may exhibit confusion, flat affect, and difficulty with short-term memory and concentration. Electrical injury to the central nervous system may cause a seizure, either as an isolated event or as part of a new-onset seizure disorder. Other possible causes of seizures, such as hypoxia and traumatic central nervous system injury, should be considered. Neurologic symptoms may improve, but long-term disability is common. Lower extremity weakness is commonly undiagnosed until ambulation is attempted.[37]

In high-voltage exposures, spinal cord injury may result from fractures or ligamentous disruption of the cervical, thoracic, or lumbar spine.[37,38] Neurologic damage in patients without evidence of spinal injury can be immediate or delayed. Patients with immediate damage have symptoms of weakness, and paresthesias develop within hours of the insult. Lower extremity findings are more common than upper extremity findings. These patients have a good prognosis for partial or complete recovery. Delayed neurologic damage may present days to years after the insult. There are three clinical presentations: ascending paralysis, amyotrophic lateral sclerosis, or transverse myelitis.[38] Motor findings predominate. Sensory findings also are common, but they may be patchy and may not match the motor levels. Although recovery is reported, the prognosis is usually poor.[37]

Lightning Injury

On initial presentation, two thirds of seriously injured lightning patients have *keraunoparalysis,* which is a unique temporary paralysis secondary to lightning strike. It is characterized by lower and sometimes upper extremities that are blue, mottled, cold, and pulseless. These findings are secondary to vascular spasm and sympathetic nervous system instability.[39] Generally, this condition clears within a few hours, although some patients may be left with permanent paresis or paresthesias.

Paraplegia, intracranial hemorrhages, cardiac enzyme elevations, seizures, and electroencephalographic changes are reported after lightning injuries.[31,32,39-42] Loss of consciousness for varying periods is common, and confusion and anterograde amnesia are almost universal findings. Peripheral nerve damage is common, and recovery is usually poor.[43,44] A syndrome of delayed muscle atrophy caused by electrical injury of the nerves is described, even in the absence of cutaneous burns.[45]

Other Viscera

Electrical Injury

Injury to the lungs may occur because of associated blunt trauma but is rare from electrical current, perhaps because air is a poor conductor. Injury to visceral organs also is rare, but damage to the pancreas, liver, small intestine, large intestine, bladder, and gallbladder is reported.[46]

Lightning Injury

Pulmonary contusion and hemorrhage are seen with lightning injury.[19,47] Blunt abdominal injuries occur rarely. None of the other intra-abdominal catastrophes commonly associated with high-voltage electrical injury, such as gallbladder necrosis or mesenteric thrombosis, are seen with lightning injury.

Other Low-Voltage Injuries

An accurate history is essential to ensure that an apparent low-voltage injury was not caused by the discharge from a capacitor (as in the repair of a television, microwave oven, or computer monitor) or other high-voltage source. Although burns from low-voltage sources are usually less severe than burns from high-voltage sources, patients still may complain of paresthesias for an extended period, experience cardiac dysrhythmias, or have cataracts develop if the shock occurs close to the face or head.

As law enforcement use of electromechanical disruption devices (stun guns [Tasers]) increases, more subjects exposed to the associated electrical current will be evaluated in emergency departments. These devices deliver brief pulses of electrical energy that incapacitate the target subject. There have been no deaths directly attributable to the electrical discharge of these devices. Evaluation and treatment of persons subdued with such devices should focus on wounds caused by the probes, secondary injuries associated with the induced fall, and the organic or psychiatric conditions prompting the officers' use of the device.[48]

Complications

Electrical Injury

Cardiac arrest generally occurs only at the initial presentation or as a final event after a long and complicated hospital course. Many of the complications are similar to complications of thermal burns and crush injuries, including infection, clostridial myositis, and myoglobinuria. The incidence of acute myoglobinuric renal failure has decreased since the widespread adoption of aggressive alkalinized fluid resuscitation. Fasciotomies or carpal tunnel release may be necessary for treatment of compartment syndromes.[36] Tissue loss and major amputations are common with severe high-voltage injuries and result in the need for extensive rehabilitation.

Neurologic complications, such as loss of consciousness, peripheral nerve damage, and delayed spinal cord syndromes, may occur.[37,38,44] Damage to the brain may result in a permanent seizure disorder.[27] Long-term neuropsychiatric complications include depression, anxiety, inability to continue in the same profession, aggressive behavior, and suicide. Stress ulcers are the most common gastrointestinal complication after burn ileus. Abdominal injuries from ischemia, vascular damage, burns, or associated blunt trauma may be overlooked initially.[12,46]

Lightning Injury

Complications of lightning injury fall into three categories: (1) complications that could be reasonably predicted from the presenting signs, such as hearing loss from tympanic membrane rupture or paresthesias and paresis from neurologic damage; (2) long-term neurologic deficits similar to deficits associated with blunt head injury and chronic pain syndromes; and (3) iatrogenic complications, which are secondary to overaggressive management. In the past, patients with lightning injuries often were treated similarly to patients with high-voltage electrical injuries. These injuries are distinctly different, however. The treatment of lightning victims seldom requires massive fluid resuscitation, fasciotomies for compartment syndromes, mannitol and furosemide diuretics, alkalinization of the urine, amputations, or large repeated debridements.[17,31]

DIFFERENTIAL CONSIDERATIONS

Electrical Injury

Electrical injuries are usually self-evident from historical factors except in the case of bathtub accidents, instances when no burns occur, or instances of foul play. The mechanism of burn injury is relevant; flash burns have a much better prognosis than arc or conductive burns. Alterations in consciousness or seizures can be caused by the electrical injury or result from an associated traumatic brain injury.

Lightning Injury

The differential diagnosis of lightning injury is more complex, often because the incident is unobserved. It includes many of the causes of unconsciousness, paralysis, or disorientation of unclear etiology [4] Evidence of a thunderstorm or a witness to the lightning strike may not be available, particularly when victims are alone when injured. The presence of typical burn patterns, such as feathering, may be helpful.

MANAGEMENT

Prehospital

Securing the Scene

When first reaching the scene, prehospital personnel should secure the area so that bystanders and rescuers do not sustain other injuries. For high-voltage incidents, the power source must be turned off. Although many approaches to achieving this goal are recommended, the safest approach is to involve the local power company in high-voltage accidents. Accidents involving discrete electrical sources that are disconnected easily through a circuit box or switch are easier to manage, although rescuers still should ensure that the power is off before approaching the victim. The use of electrical gloves by emergency medical service personnel is dangerous. A microscopic hole in a glove can result in an explosive injury to the hand inside it, as thousands of volts from the circuit concentrate there to enter the glove.

Although a line may be on the ground and appear to be de-energized, it may have substantial current flowing from it to the ground, making the surrounding area dangerous. This ground current spreads out in a circle along and just below the surface of the ground. De-energized lines may be re-energized by automatic circuit reclosers resulting in surges of current.[49] During lightning incidents, prehospital personnel must be vigilant because lightning *can* strike the same place twice.

Triage Considerations

Field evaluation of patients may involve triage of multiple victims. Traditional rules of mass casualty triage do not apply to lightning victims. The major cause of death in lightning injuries is cardiorespiratory arrest.[17] In the absence of cardiopulmonary arrest, victims are highly unlikely to die in the field. Triage of lightning victims should concentrate on victims who appear to be in cardiorespiratory arrest. When multiple victims are involved, the evaluation of victims who are breathing may be delayed because they are likely to survive the incident. Although intrinsic cardiac automaticity may ensue, the respiratory arrest caused by central nervous system injury often prevails. If the victim is adequately ventilated during the interval, perfusion may be maintained.

Initial Prehospital Resuscitation

Electrical injury victims may require a combination of cardiac and trauma care because they often have blunt injuries and burns and possible cardiac damage. Spinal immobilization is indicated whenever associated spinal trauma is suspected. Fractures and dislocations should be splinted, and burns should be covered with clean, dry dressings.

All patients with conductive injury should have at least one large-bore intravenous line established. Hypotensive patients initially should receive a bolus of 20 mL/kg of isotonic fluid, and subsequent fluid management should be based on the patient's vital signs and clinical status.

Emergency Department

Assessment

The history obtained from bystanders and the prehospital personnel regarding the type of electrical source, duration of contact, or environmental factors is helpful. An electrical injury should be treated similarly to a crush injury, rather than a thermal burn, because of the large amount of tissue damage that is often present under normal-appearing skin. As a result, none of the formulas for intravenous fluids based on percentage of burned body surface area are reliable. Standard crystalloid resuscitation in anticipation of myoglobinuria should be maintained. Cardiac monitoring is indicated for severely injured patients and for patients who have the indications listed in Box 140-6.[50] All patients with high-voltage injury and patients with low-voltage injury and cardiorespiratory complaints should have an electrocardiogram (ECG) and cardiac isoenzyme determinations. Although electrocardiographic changes and dysrhythmias are common with electrical injuries, anesthesia and surgical procedures performed in the first 48 hours of care can be accomplished without cardiac complications.[50,51] The patient's clinical status should guide the use of invasive monitoring with central venous pressure catheters, intracranial pressure monitors, or Swan-Ganz catheters.

Victims of electrical injury with altered mentation should have a computed tomography (CT) scan performed. Most lightning victims behave as though they have had electroconvulsive therapy, with confusion

BOX 140-6. Indications for Electrocardiogram Monitoring

- Cardiac arrest
- Documented loss of consciousness
- Abnormal ECG
- Dysrhythmia observed in prehospital or emergency department setting
- History of cardiac disease
- Presence of significant risk factors for cardiac disease
- Concomitant injury severe enough to warrant admission
- Suspicion of conductive injury
- Hypoxia
- Chest pain

and anterograde amnesia for several days. If any neurologic deterioration occurs after an electrical injury, a CT scan is indicated to assess for intracranial hemorrhage.[17,42]

Lightning victims who do not experience cardiopulmonary arrest at the time of the strike generally do well with supportive therapy. Patients who have cardiopulmonary arrest may have a poor prognosis, particularly if there is hypoxic brain damage.[4,50]

Ancillary Tests

Electrical Injury

Patients sustaining an electrical injury should receive cardiac monitoring in the emergency department and an ECG despite the source voltage. The following laboratory tests may be performed in patients with evidence of conductive injury or significant surface burns: complete blood count, electrolyte levels, serum myoglobin, blood urea nitrogen, serum creatinine, and urinalysis. Patients with severe electrical injury or suspected intra-abdominal injury also should have pancreatic and hepatic enzymes measured and a coagulation profile obtained. If major debridements may be necessary, the emergency physician may consider ordering a type and crossmatch. Arterial blood gas analysis is indicated if the patient needs ventilatory intervention or alkalinization therapy. Patients should be evaluated for myoglobinuria, a common complication of high-voltage electrical injury. If the urine is pigmented or the dipstick examination of the urine is positive for blood, and no red blood cells (RBCs) are seen on microscopic analysis, the patient should be assumed to have myoglobinuria.

CK levels and isoenzyme analysis should be performed. Peak CK levels predict muscle injury, risk of amputation, and length of hospitalization; the clinical value of a single level in the acute setting is not established. Cardiac enzyme levels should be interpreted with care when diagnosing myocardial infarction in the setting of electrical injury. The peak CK level is not indicative of myocardial damage in electrical injury because of the large amount of injured skeletal muscle cells, which can contain a 20% to 25% CK-MB fraction. CK-MB fractions, electrocardiographic changes, thallium studies, angiography, and echocardiography correlate poorly in acute myocardial infarction after electrical injury. Other cardiac enzymes (e.g., troponin) are not well studied in electrical injury but may prove useful in determining myocardial injury.

Radiographs of the spine should be obtained if spinal injury is clinically suspected or in cases in which patients cannot be assessed adequately because of altered mentation or the presence of other painful injuries. Radiographs also should be obtained to assess for fractures in other areas in which the patient complains of pain or has an apparent deformity. Angiography is not shown to be useful in the planning of debridements or amputations and is not routinely indicated.[22] Technetium pyrophosphate scanning to detect areas of clinically unsuspected myonecrosis can be useful.[30,36] "Hot spots" may reflect 20% to 80% viable muscle and should be followed clinically.[36,52,53] CT or magnetic resonance imaging may be useful in the evaluation of associated trauma and is essential for evaluation of possible intracranial injuries.

Lightning Injury

In patients injured by lightning, an ECG should be obtained. Serum markers for cardiac injury are indicated in patients with chest pain, abnormal ECGs, or altered mentation. The severity or nature of the injuries may require other laboratory studies. Radiographic studies, particularly cranial CT evaluation, may be indicated, depending on the patient's level of consciousness at presentation and throughout the evaluation and treatment.

Specific Therapies

Rhabdomyolysis

Victims of electrical injury who have heme pigment in the urine usually have myoglobinuria. Alkalinization of the urine increases the solubility of myoglobin in the urine, increasing the rate of clearance. Urine output should be maintained at 1 to 1.5 mL/kg/hr until all traces of myoglobin have cleared from the urine, while the blood is maintained at a pH of at least 7.45 using sodium bicarbonate. Furosemide or mannitol may be used to cause further diuresis. In contrast to high-voltage injuries, in lightning injuries, rhabdomyolysis is rare.

Burn Wound Care

Cutaneous burns should be dressed with antibiotic dressings, such as sulfadiazine silver (Silvadene). Mafenide acetate (Sulfamylon) occasionally is used for selected burns; however, its use may result in electrolyte abnormalities because of its carbonic anhydrase inhibitory activity.

Electrical burns are especially prone to tetanus, and patients should receive tetanus toxoid and tetanus immune globulin on the basis of their immunization history. Clostridial myositis is common, but prophylactic administration of high-dose penicillin to prevent clostridial myonecrosis is controversial.

Extremity Injuries

Management of electrical injuries of the extremities entails surgical management, including early fasciotomy, carpal tunnel release, or amputation of an obviously nonviable extremity. Extremities should be splinted in a functional position to minimize edema and contracture formation. The hand should be splinted in 35- to 45-degree extension at the wrist, 80- to 90-degree flexion at the metacarpophalangeal joints, and almost full extension at the proximal and distal interphalangeal joints.

DISPOSITION

Electrical Injuries

Admission

Indications for admission for electrocardiographic monitoring are listed in Box 140-6. In general, when corporeal conduction is suspected, the patient should be admitted for 12 to 24 hours of cardiac monitoring. Most patients with significant electrical burns should be stabilized and transferred to a regional burn center for burn care and extensive occupational and physical rehabilitation.

Outpatient Management

Asymptomatic patients with a normal physical examination after low-voltage exposure can be reassured and discharged without performing any ancillary tests.[54] Patients with cutaneous burns or mild persistent symptoms can be discharged if they have a normal ECG and no urinary heme pigment. Outpatient referral is provided in the event that current symptoms persist or new symptoms (delayed cataracts, weakness, or paresthesias) develop.

Electrical injury during pregnancy from low-voltage sources may result in fetal demise. A prospective cohort study of electric shock in pregnancy suggests that electric shock usually does not pose a major fetal risk.[55] Nevertheless, obstetric consultation or referral is advisable for all pregnant patients reporting electrical injury, regardless of symptoms at the time of presentation. Placental abruption, the most common cause of fetal death after blunt trauma, may result from even minor trauma, such as may be associated with electrical injuries. Patients in the latter half of pregnancy should receive fetal monitoring if there has been even minor blunt trauma and be considered high-risk patients for the remainder of their pregnancy.[14] First-trimester patients should be informed of the remote risk of spontaneous abortion and, if no other indications for admission exist, may be discharged with instructions for threatened miscarriage and close obstetric follow-up evaluation. The prognosis for fetal survival after lightning strike varies with the mother's injuries.

Pediatric patients with oral burns generally may be discharged safely if close adult care is ensured. There is no evidence that an isolated oral burn correlates with cardiac injury or myoglobinuria. In general, these patients require surgical and dental consultation for oral splinting, eventual debridement, and occasionally reconstructive surgery. After appropriate consultation, if hospitalization is not deemed necessary, the child's parents should be warned about the possibility of delayed hemorrhage and receive instructions to apply direct pressure by pinching the bleeding site and to return immediately to the emergency department.

Lightning Injuries

Many of the signs of lightning injuries, such as lower extremity paralysis and mottling, confusion, and amnesia, resolve with time. After spinal cord and intracranial processes are excluded, observation is the mainstay of treatment.

Consultation with other specialists may be indicated for otic and ophthalmic damage. More severely injured patients require trauma surgeon and cardiologist consultations, although with lightning injuries medical pathology predominates. If there is a history of a loss of consciousness or if the patient exhibits confusion, hospital admission and observation are suggested. After evaluation, if the ECG is normal, asymptomatic patients (including patients with feathering burns) may be discharged home with referral for follow-up from an ophthalmologist and other specialists as indicated.

KEY CONCEPTS

- High-voltage electrical injury causes significant tissue and organ damage along the path between the entrance and exit wounds. As a result, victims are often more severely injured than they initially appear. Injury assessment must be detailed, fluid requirements during resuscitation are much greater than one would calculate from the surface burns alone, and extensive tissue debridement is often necessary.
- Victims of lightning injury may appear to have significant injuries, but symptoms (extremities that are cold and pulseless, mottled skin, paralysis, and confusion) usually resolve with time. After spinal cord and intracranial injuries are excluded, observation is the mainstay of treatment.
- Patients with low-voltage electrical injury who have only minor cutaneous burns or persistent minor symptoms may be discharged safely if they have a normal ECG and no urinary heme pigment.

REFERENCES

1. Jex-Blake AJ: The Gulstonian lectures on death from electricity in the late nineteenth century. *Med Instrum* 9:267, 1975.
2. Kobernick M: Electrical injuries: Pathophysiology and emergency management. *Ann Emerg Med* 11:633, 1982.
3. Lee RC: Injury by electrical forces: Pathophysiology, manifestations, and management. *Curr Probl Surg* 34:684, 1997.
4. Cooper MA, Andrews CJ: Lightning injuries. In Auerbach P (ed): *Wilderness Medicine: Management of Wilderness and Environmental Emergencies,* 3rd ed. St. Louis, Mosby, 1995.
5. Cherington M: Lightning injuries in sports. *Sports Med* 31:301, 2001.

6. Carte AE, et al: A large group of children struck by lightning. *Ann Emerg Med* 39:665, 2002.
7. Cherington M, et al: Lightning injuries during snowy conditions. *Sports Med* 32:333, 1998.
8. Childbert M, et al: Measure of tissue resistivity in experimental electric burns. *J Trauma* 25:209, 1985.
9. Puschel K, Brinkman B, Lieske K: Ultrastructural alteration of skeletal muscles after electrical shock. *Am J Forensic Med Pathol* 6:246, 1985.
10. Lee RC, et al: Role of cell membrane rupture in the pathogenesis of electrical trauma. *J Surg Res* 44:709, 1988.
11. Jain S, Bandi V: Electrical and lightning injuries. *Crit Care Clin* 15:319, 1999.
12. Jaffe RH: Electropathology: A review of the pathologic changes produced by electric currents. *Arch Pathol* 5:839, 1928.
13. Capelli-Schellpfeffin M, et al: Advances in the evaluation and treatment of electrical and thermal injury emergencies. *IEEE Trans Industry Applications* 31:1147, 1995.
14. Fish RM: Electric injury: Part III. Cardiac monitoring indications, the pregnant patient, and lightning. *J Emerg Med* 18:181, 2000.
15. Ishikawa T, et al: Experimental study on the lethal threshold value of multiple successive voltage impulses to rabbits simulating multi-stroke lightning flash. *Int J Biometeor* 29:157, 1986.
16. Ohashi M, Kitagawa N, Ishikawa T: Lightning injury caused by discharges accompanying flashover: A clinical and experimental study of death and survival. *Burns* 12:496, 1986.
17. Cooper MA: Lightning injuries: Prognostic signs for death. *Ann Emerg Med* 9:134, 1980.
18. Woods J: Spinal atrophic paralysis following lightning stroke. *S Afr Med J* 26:92, 1952.
19. Buechner HA, Rothbaum JC: Lightning stroke injury: A report of multiple casualties from a single lightning bolt. *Milit Med* 126:775, 1961.
20. Leys K: Spinal atrophic paralysis case following lightning stroke. *Edinburgh Med J* 49:657, 1942.
21. ten Duis HJ: Acute electrical burns. *Semin Neurol* 15:381, 1995.
22. Hunt JL, et al: Vascular lesions in acute electrical injuries. *J Trauma* 14:461, 1974.
23. Cooper MA: A fifth mechanism of lightning injury. *Acad Emerg Med* 9:172, 2002.
24. Jaffe R: Electropathology: Review of the pathological changes produced by electric current. *Arch Pathol* 5:839, 1928.
25. Arden GP, et al: Lightning accident at Ascot. *BMJ* 1:1453, 1956.
26. Saffle JR, Crandall A, Warden GD: Cataracts: A long-term complication of electrical injury. *J Trauma* 25:17, 1985.
27. Critchley M: Neurological effects of lightning and electricity. *Lancet* 1:68, 1934.
28. Bergstrom L, et al: The lightning-damaged ear. *Arch Otolaryngol* 100:117, 1974.
29. Fish RM: Electric injury: Part I. Treatment priorities, subtle diagnostic factors, and burns. *J Emerg Med* 17:977, 1999.
30. Romero B, et al: Myocardial necrosis by electrocution: Evaluation of noninvasive methods. *J Nucl Med* 38:250, 1997.
31. Yost JW, Holmes FF: Myoglobinuria following lightning stroke. *JAMA* 228:1147, 1974.
32. Andrews CJ, Colquhoun DM, Darveniza M: The QT interval in lightning injury with implications for the "cessation of metabolism" hypothesis. *J Wilderness Med* 4:155, 1993.
33. Alexander WN: Composite dysplasia of a single tooth as a result of electrical burn damage: Report of a case. *J Am Dent Assoc* 69:589, 1961.
34. Barthlome CW, Jacoby WD, Ramchand SC: Cutaneous manifestations of lightning injury. *Arch Dermatol* 111:1466, 1975.
35. Wetli CV: Keraunopathology. *Am J Forens Med Pathol* 17:89, 1996.
36. Holliman CJ, et al: Early surgical decompression in the management of electrical injuries. *Am J Surg* 144:133, 1982.
37. Varghese G, Mani MM, Redford JB: Spinal cord injuries following electrical accidents. *Paraplegia* 24:159, 1986.
38. Levine NS, et al: Spinal cord injury following electrical accidents: Case reports. *J Trauma* 15:459, 1975.
39. Duis HJ, Klasen HJ: Keraunoparalysis, a "specific" lightning injury. *Burns* 12:54, 1985.
40. Baker R: Paraplegia as a result of lightning injury. *BMJ* 4:1464, 1978.
41. Cherington M, Yarnell P, Hallmark D: MRI in lightning encephalopathy. *Neurology* 43:1437, 1993.
42. Cherington M, Yarnell P, Lammereste D: Lightning strikes: Nature of neurological damage in patients evaluated in hospital emergency departments. *Ann Emerg Med* 21:575, 1992.
43. Shantha TR: Causalgia induced by telephone-mediated lightning electrical injury and treated by interpleural block. *Anesth Analg* 73:507, 1991.
44. Mankani MH, et al: Detection of peripheral nerve injury in electrical shock patients. *Ann N Y Acad Sci* 720:206, 1994.
45. Francis DA, Heron JR: Progressive muscular atrophy and posterior dislocation of the humerus following electrical shock. *Postgrad Med J* 60:143, 1984.
46. Newsome TW, Curreri PW, Eurenius K: Visceral injuries: An unusual complication of an electrical burn. *Arch Surg* 105:494, 1972.
47. Solterman B, Frutiger A, Kuhn M: Lightning injury with lung bleeding in a tracheotomized patient. *Chest* 99:240, 1991.
48. Heck JJ: Stun guns: The medical implications. *Emerg Med Serv* 32:96, 2003.
49. Bernstein T: Electrical injury: Electrical engineer's perspective and an historical review. *Ann N Y Acad Sci* 720:1, 1994.
50. Andrews CJ, et al: The pathology of electrical and lightning injuries. In Wecht CJ (ed): *Forensic Sciences*. New York, Matthew Bender, 1995.
51. Purdue GF, Hunt JL: Electrocardiographic monitoring after electrical injury: Necessity or luxury? *J Trauma* 26:166, 1986.
52. Karczmar GS, et al: Prospects for assessment of the effects of electrical injury by magnetic resonance. *Ann N Y Acad Sci* 720:176, 1994.
53. Chen CT, et al: Radionuclide probes for tissue damage. *Ann N Y Acad Sci* 720:181, 1994.
54. Garcia CT, et al: Electrical injuries in a pediatric emergency department. *Ann Emerg Med* 26:604, 1995.
55. Einarson A, et al: Accidental electric shock in pregnancy: A prospective cohort study. *Am J Obstet Gynecol* 176:678, 1997.

CHAPTER

141 Scuba Diving and Dysbarism

Lee W. Shockley

PERSPECTIVE

Underwater free diving (breath holding) to salvage wrecks and to harvest seafood, sponges, coral, and mother-of-pearl has been practiced for more than 5000 years.[1] Historic records indicate that the Persian King Xerxes employed a diver to recover sunken treasure in the fifth century BC.[1] Alexander the Great used divers to remove obstacles in the harbor of the city of Tyre in 332 BC.[1] Navies since the time of Alexander have used divers to construct defenses, sabotage enemy ships and harbor defenses, and salvage wrecks.

The earliest divers were limited by the depths that they could achieve and by the duration that they could remain submerged. To extend the duration of time underwater, some divers have used breathing tubes, such as hollow reeds. These tubes, however, become nearly impossible to use at depths greater than 3 feet because of the underwater pressure restricting inspiration. Breathing bags (animal skins inflated with air) have been tried but make submersion impossible because of their buoyancy.

Shakespeare's description of Clarence's dream in King Richard III* (~1597) may have been influenced by reports of the first diving bell (1531). Subsequent inventions, including diving dresses, from the 16th to the 19th centuries allowed divers to remain underwater for prolonged periods at depths of up to 12 fathoms (72 feet).[2] The first diving dress (1715) was a reinforced, leather-covered barrel with watertight arm holes and a viewing porthole.[2]

Colonel William Pasley, the officer in charge of a unit of the British Royal Engineers salvaging the sunken warship HMS *Royal George* in 1840, probably observed symptoms of "the bends" (decompression sickness, type I) in his divers: "of the seasoned divers, not a man escaped the repeated attacks of rheumatism and cold," after working up to 7 hours a day at depths of 60 to 70 feet.[3] At about the same time, similar symptoms and even fatalities were observed among caisson workers.†

*Clarence: "Methought I saw a thousand fearful wracks; a thousand men that fishes gnawed upon; wedges of gold, great anchors, heaps of pearl, inestimable stones, unvalued jewels, all scattered in the bottom of the sea. Some lay in dead men's skulls; and in the holes where eyes did once inhabit there were crept, as t'were in scorn of eyes, reflecting gems, that woo'd the slimy bottom of the deep, and mocked the dead bones that lay scatter'd by."
The Keeper: "Had you such leisure in the time of depth to gaze upon these secrets of the deep?"

†Caissons are construction chambers filled with pressurized air that permit working in a dry environment. They have been used in the construction of bridge footings and tunnels in places that would otherwise have been underwater.

The disease became known as Caisson's disease, but the construction workers on the Brooklyn Bridge (built from 1870 to 1883) attached the name the bends characterizing the symptoms that often caused the victim to bend forward in pain.[3]

The first clinical description of Caisson's disease was by Paul Bert in 1878.[3] He correctly attributed the disease to nitrogen gas coming out of solution in the tissues during decompression. This led to the recommendation of slow ascents for pressurized workers and the development of the first recompression chambers. Heavy diving helmets with their surface-supplied air dominated underwater diving operations until the development of the *s*elf-*c*ontained *u*nderwater *b*reathing *a*pparatus (scuba). Scuba requires a demand regulator and high-pressure air tanks that allow the delivery of an air supply at an appropriate pressure for the depth of the diver. The significant breakthrough in making scuba possible was the invention of the Aqua-Lung, by Jacques-Yves Cousteau and Emile Gagnan in 1943.[2] The lighter and less expensive scuba equipment did not require a surface supply of air and the support personnel that are necessary for helmet diving.

The sport of scuba diving has become increasingly popular. Since 1967, more than 10 million people have been certified as scuba divers. Worldwide, more than 500,000 new diver certifications are issued annually. The sport is relatively safe, with an estimated risk of an accident during a dive of 1 in 250,000.[4] The vast majority of amateur divers use compressed air, open-circuit scuba equipment at depths less than 130 feet of seawater (fsw).

Mixed gas scuba open-circuit systems using nitrogen and oxygen mixtures are becoming more popular with sport divers. More than a dozen mixtures of enriched air Nitrox (EAN) or oxygen-enriched air have been developed. The two most commonly cited are NOAA Nitrox I (32% oxygen, 68% nitrogen) and Nitrox II (36% oxygen, 64% nitrogen). Only Nitrox I, however, has been approved for recreational dive use. The benefits of EAN include reduced decompression risk, risk of nitrogen narcosis, residual nitrogen time, decompression times, and surface intervals between diving and flying. Further, EAN may extend bottom times up to twice as long as with compressed air scuba for bottom depths between 50 and 130 fsw. Specific decompression tables for the standard EAN mixtures minimize the risks of decompression sickness (DCS) and acute oxygen toxicity.[5] EAN does not eliminate the risk of DCS, however, and requires special training, equipment and computers. There is also a potential fire hazard in working with EAN. Long-duration EAN dives may increase the risk of pulmonary and central nervous system (CNS) oxygen toxicity.[3]

Heliox diving involves a gas mixture of helium and oxygen. The inert helium is used to replace the nitrogen and part of the oxygen that would be in compressed air. Helium is not associated with narcosis and can, therefore, be used for commercial deep diving (greater than 130 fsw). Tri-Mix diving involves a gas mixture of helium, nitrogen, and oxygen. The concentration mixture formulated is varied for the depth profile. The depths at which Tri-Mix can be used effectively exceed 190 fsw. At extreme depths, a different "travel gas" may be required for the diver during the descent and ascent. Because of its inherent difficulties, expense, and limited applications, most Tri-Mix is used for military and specialized commercial applications.

There is some civilian experience with oxygen-enriched Tri-Mix. A mixture of 26% oxygen, 17% helium, and 57% nitrogen (TX 26/17) has been used for depths as deep as 150 fsw. For decompression after using TX 26/17, Nitrox I has been used or, during ascent, the diver may switch to 100% oxygen at a 20 fsw decompression stop. Oxygen-enriched Tri-Mix remains controversial because several deaths have been associated with using the equipment.

Closed-circuit and semiclosed-circuit diving apparatus ("rebreathers") use calcium hydroxide, $Ca(OH)_2$, to absorb expired carbon dioxide. Oxygen is then added to the decarboxylated gas prior to rebreathing. The four types of rebreathers are closed-circuit oxygen rebreathers, closed-circuit mixed-gas rebreathers, semiclosed-circuit rebreathers using premixed gases, and semiclosed-circuit rebreathers that mix gases on board. The advantages of rebreathers over compressed air scuba are that they are more efficient (less gas used for a given time), allow deeper dives, allow longer bottom times, and generate few, if any, bubbles.

PRINCIPLES OF DISEASE

Medical emergencies encountered by scuba divers include those common to environmental exposures (e.g., hypothermia, sunburn, and physical trauma), those common to aquatic activities (e.g., submersion accidents, motion sickness, and marine envenomations), and dysbarisms (problems unique to the sport of diving). *Dysbarisms* are illnesses that result directly or indirectly from exposure to increased ambient pressure. The pathophysiology of these conditions primarily results from volume-pressure changes within the air-filled cavities of the body and from increased dissolution of gases, particularly nitrogen, in body tissues.

To understand the pathophysiology of dysbarisms, one should be familiar with several of the laws of physics that define the behavior of liquids and gases. Atmospheric pressure varies with altitude and weather patterns, but 760 mm Hg, or 14.7 lb/in^2 (psi), is the standard used at sea level. The pressure exerted on the human body at sea level is 1 atmosphere. A scuba diver's depth gauge reads pressure in addition to the pressure at sea level. Therefore, at sea level, a pressure gauge reads zero. The absolute pressure, or *atmospheres absolute* (ATA), is the total pressure on a diver, which is the sum of gauge pressure and atmospheric pressure. It is most useful to speak in terms of ATA. Water is far denser than air and, as a diver descends, each foot of seawater exerts an additional pressure of 23 mm Hg or 0.445 psi on the diver. Although a mountain climber would need to ascend to 18,000 feet to reduce atmospheric pressure by 50%, a diver needs to descend only 33 feet in seawater (34 feet in freshwater) to double atmospheric pressure.

Pressure changes are perceived only as they affect the air-filled spaces in the body. The human body is composed mostly of water and behaves as a liquid subject to Pascal's law, which states that a pressure applied to any part of a liquid is transmitted equally throughout. Pascal's law is the reason that toothpaste comes out of the tube when you squeeze the other end. Pressure changes, however, do alter the volume within the air-filled spaces of the body, including the lungs, bowel, sinuses, and middle ear. These spaces compress on descent and expand on ascent according to Boyle's law, which states that at constant temperature, the absolute pressure and the volume of gas are inversely proportional ($PV = k$). As pressure increases, the gas volume is reduced; as the pressure is reduced, the gas volume increases (Figure 141-1).

When working with Boyle's law, the temperature of the gas is a constant value. Temperature, however, affects the pressure and volume of a gas. Charles' law describes the relationships of temperature, volume, and pressure; at a constant pressure, the volume of a gas is directly proportional to the change in the absolute temperature ($V_1/T_1 = V_2/T_2$).

The general gas law combines the laws to predict the behavior of a given quantity of gas when any of the factors change. The formula expressing the general gas law is

$$P_1 * V_1 / T_1 = P_2 * V_2 / T_2$$

where:

P_1 = initial pressure (absolute)
V_1 = initial volume
T_1 = initial temperature (absolute)
P_2 = final pressure (absolute)
V_2 = final volume
T_2 = final temperature (absolute)

Dalton's law states that the total pressure exerted by a mixture of gases is equal to the sum of the pressures (partial pressures) of the individual gases making up the mixture, with each gas acting as if it alone was present and occupied the total volume ($P_{total} = P_1 + P_2 + P_3 + \ldots + P_n$). Henry's law states that the amount of any gas that dissolves in a liquid at a given temperature is directly proportional to the partial pressure of that gas. At higher ambient pressures, the concentration of each component of air in solution with blood and tissues increases until a new steady-state concentration is achieved. Nitrogen accumulates in tissues and blood in

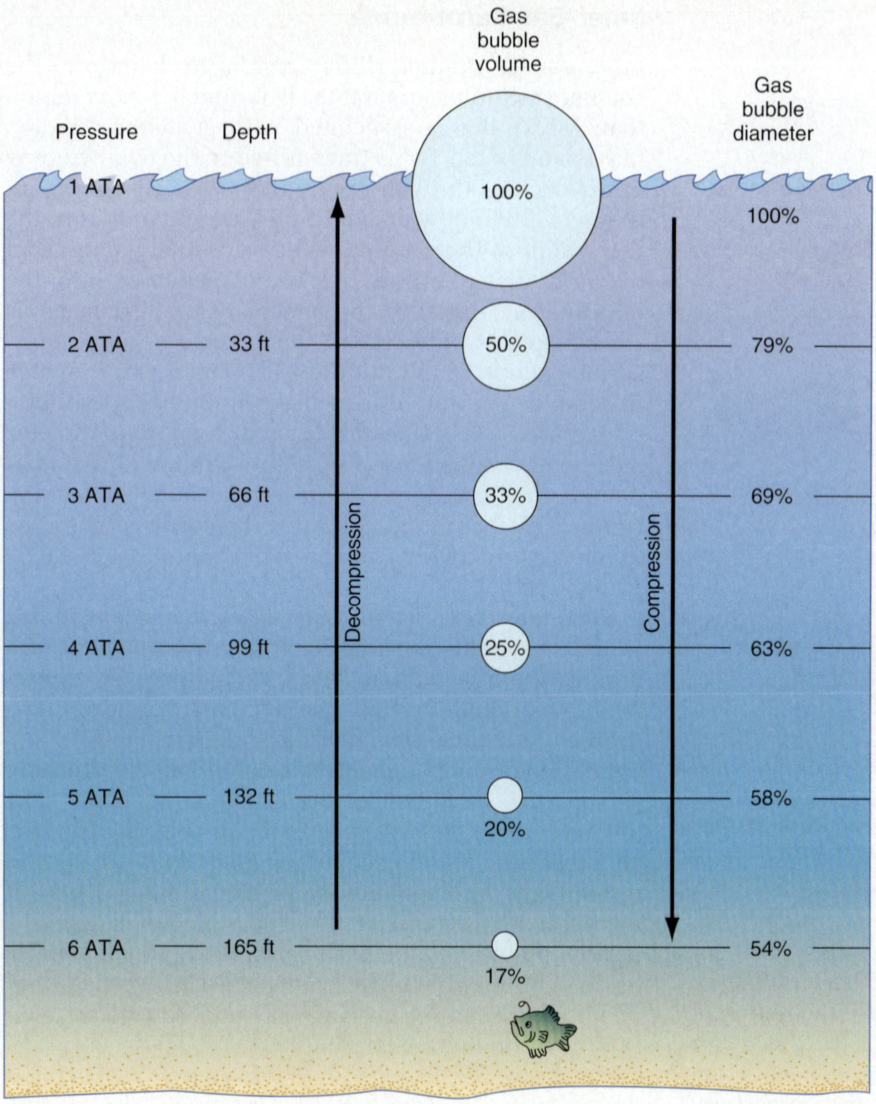

Figure 141-1. Boyle's law. The volume of a given quantity of gas at constant temperature varies inversely with pressure: $P_1V_1 = P_2V_2$. (From Kizer KW: Diving medicine. In Auerbach PS [ed]: *Wilderness Medicine*, 4th ed. St. Louis, Mosby, 2001, p 1375.)

proportion to the depth and length of a dive. If a diver ascends too rapidly to the surface, nitrogen comes out of solution, forming gas bubbles in the tissues and blood. A familiar example is the opening of a bottle of soda, which allows bubbles of carbon dioxide to come out of solution rapidly.

The solubility of gases is affected by temperature; the lower the temperature, the higher the solubility. As the temperature of a solution increases, some of the dissolved gas leaves the solution. The gases in a diver's breathing mixture are dissolved into the body in proportion to the partial pressure of each gas in the mixture. Because of the varied solubility of different gases, the quantity of a particular gas that becomes dissolved is also governed by the length of time the diver is breathing the gas at the increased pressure. The dissolved gas in a diver's body, regardless of quantity, depth, or pressure, remains in solution as long as the pressure is maintained. As the diver ascends, however, more and more of the dissolved gas comes out of solution and may form microbubbles in the circulation. If the ascent rate is controlled (i.e., through the use of the safe decompression tables or submersible dive computers), the gas is carried to the lung vascular bed and is exhaled before it accumulates to form significantly large or numerous bubbles in the tissues. If, however, the ascent occurs suddenly and the pressure is reduced at a rate higher than the body can accommodate, the nitrogen bubbles may accumulate and disrupt body tissues and systems to produce DCS.

Barotrauma, or injury caused by pressure changes, results when a diver is unable to equalize the pressure within air-filled structures to the ambient pressure of the environment during ascent or descent. Proportionally, changes in volume are greater as a diver approaches the surface. Thus, the greatest risk for barotrauma is in shallow water.

CLINICAL FEATURES

Middle Ear Barotrauma

Middle ear barotrauma (MEBT), also known as barotitis or "ear squeeze," is the most common complaint of scuba divers. It is experienced by 30% of novice scuba divers and 10% of experienced divers.[6] The middle ear

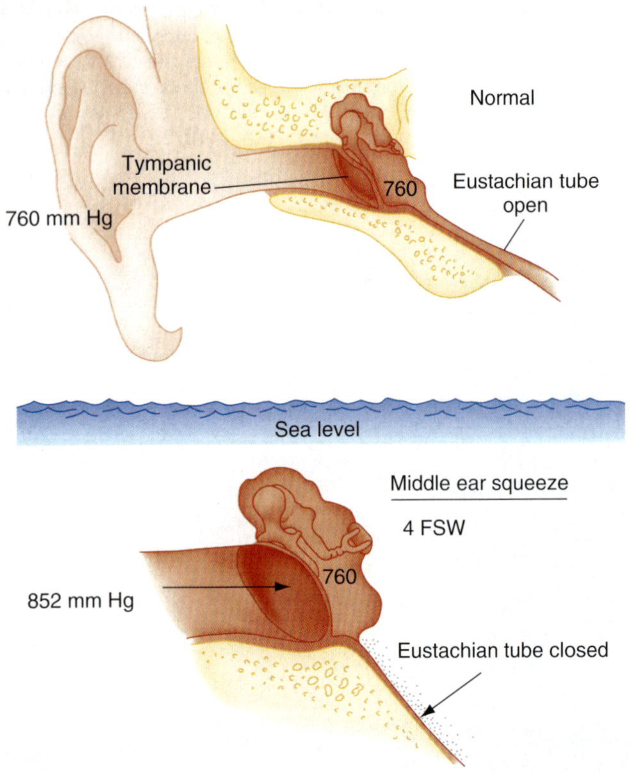

Figure 141-2. Anatomy of the ear and middle ear trauma. FSW, feet of seawater. (From Kizer KW: Diving medicine. In Auerbach PS [ed]: *Wilderness Medicine*, 4th ed. St. Louis, Mosby, 2001, p 1376.)

is an air-filled space with solid bony walls except for the tympanic membrane (Figure 141-2). The eustachian tube is the only anatomic passage to the external environment.

As the diver descends, each foot of water exerts an additional 23 mm Hg pressure against the intact tympanic membrane (TM). Under normal circumstances, the diver performs maneuvers to force passage of additional air into the middle ear through the eustachian tubes, maintaining an equal pressure across the TM. Ear squeeze occurs when a negative differential pressure is created within the middle ear because the diver could not equalize to ambient pressure. If equilibration of middle ear pressure does not occur, the floppy medial third of the eustachian tube collapses shut, making any further attempts at equalization futile. Further pressure increases can cause the TM to rupture. The pain may or may not resolve as the TM ruptures. The ruptured TM, however, exposes the middle ear to cold water, inducing a caloric nystagmus and vertigo. A seventh nerve facial palsy may also occur together with MEBT.

External Ear Barotrauma

External ear barotrauma is less common than MEBT and results from the outward bulging of the TM during descent. Normally, the external auditory canal is filled with water during descent. If air becomes trapped because of obstruction from cerumen, stenosis, earplugs, or a tight-fitting wet suit hood, a relative negative pressure develops in the external canal.

Inner Ear Barotrauma

Inner ear barotrauma (IEBT) results in damage to the cochleovestibular apparatus. It is much less common than MEBT but is associated with greater morbidity. Movement of the TM is transmitted to the oval window of the cochlea through the ossicles. Inward movement of the oval window creates a pressure wave within the perilymph of the cochlea, which eventually causes an outward distention of the round window into the middle ear. Initially, the mechanism of damage is similar to that of MEBT in that a large negative pressure develops in the middle ear if the diver is unable to equalize pressure during descent. Sudden equilibration of pressure in the middle ear or a vigorous Valsalva maneuver may rupture the round window. Two other pathologic changes may not be associated with frank rupture of the round window: hemorrhage into the inner ear and tearing of the labyrinthine (Reissner's) membrane.

Symptoms associated with IEBT include variable hearing loss, severe vertigo, nausea, tinnitus, and fullness in the affected ear. Signs include severe nystagmus, positional vertigo, ataxia, and vomiting. The degree of sensorineural hearing loss is variable.

The history and physical examination are probably as sensitive as operative confirmation of IEBT.[7] The (Hennebert) fistula test may help. To perform this test, an insufflator and otoscope are used to compress and decompress air sequentially in the auditory canal. If nystagmus or vertigo is induced, the test suggests a perilymphatic fistula. Audiogram and tympanometric testing can provide objective data regarding the severity of sensorineural hearing loss and can detect concomitant conductive hearing loss.

Barosinusitis

The air-filled maxillary, frontal, and ethmoidal sinuses are all susceptible to volume-pressure changes. Equilibration of pressure within the paranasal sinuses requires patent nasal passages. Obstruction by mucosal thickening, polyps, pus, or a deviated septum predisposes to sinus barotrauma. Pain is felt over the ethmoid, frontal, or maxillary sinuses during descent or ascent. Epistaxis may also occur.

Facial Barotrauma

Facial barotrauma results from negative pressure generation within the "artificial" airspace created by a dive mask over the eyes and nose. As water pressure increases during descent, a negative pressure develops within the mask, which must be equalized by forced exhalation through the nose. When this is not adequately performed, the large negative pressure produces facial and conjunctival edema, diffuse petechial hemorrhages on the face, and subconjunctival hemorrhages. Rarely, optic nerve damage can result from severe facial barotrauma.

Temporomandibular Joint Dysfunction

Temporomandibular joint dysfunction can be seen in divers who experience teeth clenching and poor occlusion because of a poorly fitting regulator mouthpiece. The pain associated with this condition is typically felt in the region of the ear and can be mistaken for MEBT. Customized mouthpieces are available to relieve the problem.

Nitrogen Narcosis

Nitrogen narcosis, known as "rapture of the deep," results from the intoxicating effects of increased tissue nitrogen concentration at depth. Symptoms include euphoria, a false feeling of well-being, confusion, loss of judgment or skill, disorientation, inappropriate laughter, diminished motor control, and tingling and vague numbness of the lips, gums, and legs.[3] Symptoms typically begin to occur around 100 feet but often become profound at depths greater than 150 fsw.[3] There is a large degree of individual variability in susceptibility to nitrogen narcosis. Although the effects of nitrogen narcosis resolve with ascent to shallower depths, the diver may drown because of poor judgment or seriously impaired motor skills in the presence of a dive emergency. Because of the dangers of breathing nitrogen at increased partial pressures, the use of compressed air is not recommended for sport diving to depths greater than 120 feet.

Oxygen Toxicity

At elevated partial pressures for extended periods of time, oxygen can be toxic to the CNS or lungs. Oxygen becomes toxic to the CNS when its partial pressure exceeds 1.6 ATA.* Oxygen partial pressures less than 1.4 ATA are unlikely to produce CNS toxicity. Symptoms of CNS oxygen toxicity may be remembered by the mnemonic VENTIDC[3]:

V: Visual symptoms (tunnel vision or blurred vision)
E: Ear symptoms (tinnitus)
N: Nausea or spasmodic vomiting
T: Twitching and tingling symptoms (small facial muscles, lips, or muscles of the extremities)
I: Irritability, confusion, agitation, and anxiety
D: Dizziness, clumsiness, incoordination, and unusual fatigue
C: Convulsions

Deep divers prevent oxygen toxicity by breathing mixed gases with a decreased oxygen content. Breathing EAN or oxygen-enriched air at depth makes a diver more susceptible to oxygen toxicity.

Pulmonary oxygen toxicity (low-pressure oxygen poisoning) can occur after 24 hours of exposure to partial pressures of oxygen in excess of 0.6 ATA.† The symptoms of pulmonary oxygen toxicity include a burning sensation or pain on inspiration and coughing. Pulmonary function gradually becomes normal after the exposure is terminated, but pneumonitis and permanent fibrosis are possible.

Contaminated Air

Rarely, other gases, such as carbon monoxide and carbon dioxide, can contaminate the air that is compressed into a tank. This can happen, for example, if the compressor intake is placed too close to the compressor's engine exhaust. As in the case of oxygen and nitrogen, the partial pressure of these contaminants in the tissues increases dramatically with depth, potentiating their clinical effects. The symptoms of hypercarbia or carbon monoxide poisoning are more severe at elevated partial pressures. Hypercarbia increases a diver's susceptibility to CNS oxygen toxicity.[3]

Rebreathers release microscopic calcium hydroxide or "soda lime" dust particles into the apparatus.[8] The smallest of these particles are less than 1 μm in diameter and have geometric characteristics that allow them to be deposited in the alveoli of the diver. When soda lime comes into contact with water, it forms a caustic liquid. In the event of a hose rupture allowing seawater contamination of the circuit, caustic burns to the mouth, throat, and airways may result. Chronic exposure to soda lime dust may contribute to long-term effects on respiratory function.

Decompression Sickness

The term *decompression sickness* refers to a spectrum of clinical illnesses that result from the formation of small bubbles of nitrogen gas in the blood and tissues.[9,10] The clinical expression of DCS depends on the location, destination, and degree of nitrogen bubble formation in blood and tissues. Small, asymptomatic venous gas emboli are common in the ascending diver and are filtered by the lungs without apparent permanent damage.[11-13] Persistent intravascular bubbles, however, elicit inflammatory cascades, cytokines, the complement system, platelet aggregation, and thrombosis.[14] Further, the bubbles can cause mechanical obstruction, ischemia, and tissue hypoxia. Nitrogen is highly fat soluble, and the heavily myelinized white matter of the CNS is at particular risk for DCS.

The incidence of DCS is estimated to be 1 case per 5000 to 10,000 dives.[15] The potential for development of DCS increases with the length and depth of a dive. Other risk factors include age, obesity, fatigue, heavy exertion, dehydration, fever, cold ambient temperatures after diving, diving at high altitude, and flying

*A diver breathing compressed air would attain a partial pressure of 1.6 ATA of oxygen at a depth of 218 feet of seawater. This far exceeds the depth to which sport divers would go. Treatment in a hyperbaric chamber with 100% oxygen attains this partial pressure at only 20 feet of seawater. Therefore, hyperbaric treatment combines alternating periods of delivering 100% oxygen and air.

†A diver breathing compressed air would attain a partial pressure of 0.6 ATA of oxygen at a depth of 60 feet of seawater. It is extremely unlikely that a sport diver would ever be exposed for the duration that is required to produce toxicity; however, long exposures to higher levels of oxygen, such as administered according to Recompression Treatment Tables 4, 7, and 8, may lead to pulmonary oxygen toxicity.

after diving. Tobacco and alcohol use may also increase susceptibility to DCS. The risk of DCS is 2.6 times greater for men than women.[16] This difference is possibly due to risk-taking behaviors. There appears to be no increase in DCS in women who are taking oral contraceptive agents or menstruating during diving.

A patent foramen ovale (PFO) may be a risk factor for increased susceptibility to DCS. Sixty-five percent of divers who present with serious DCS have a PFO.[17] Ruel and colleagues[18] reported an increased prevalence of brain lesions in 27% of the sport divers studied. This percentage is roughly the same as the prevalence of PFO or other right-to-left shunts in the general population. These multiple brain lesions may be caused by bubbles in the venous circulation that are not filtered by the vasculature of the lungs but enter the arterial circulation, even in the absence of DCS symptoms.[19] Most sport divers do not undergo screening for PFO with echocardiographic bubble studies, and there is reason to believe that some PFOs may open only at increased ambient pressures, so that bubble studies are negative if conducted at 1 ATA.[20]

The U.S. Navy dive tables estimate the amount of nitrogen that accumulates in the body during a dive to a particular depth for a specific duration.[3] The tables calculate a maximal dive time, called the no-decompression limit, which represents the amount of time a diver may spend at a maximum depth and return to the surface without sufficiently exceeding the solubility of nitrogen at sea level to produce DCS. The diver still must ascend in a slow, controlled manner to allow the gradual release of nitrogen. Off-gassing continues after the diver has surfaced; it takes up to 12 hours at the surface for nitrogen stores to return to normal sea level values. Repetitive dives within several hours result in accumulation of tissue nitrogen and shorter no-decompression limits. Because dive tables are based on several assumptions regarding N_2 elimination, even strict adherence to these tables does not ensure that DCS will not occur.[3]

If the no-decompression limits are exceeded, underwater decompression stops are recommended. The depth and duration of these stops can be derived from the U.S. Navy Standard Air Decompression Dive Tables.[3]

Submersible dive computers are being used more often by sport scuba divers to calculate maximum dive times. These computers use mathematical algorithms to model nitrogen saturation in human tissues. Although they remove human calculation errors, such computers also tend to extend no-decompression times to their maximum limits.

The clinical manifestations of DCS are divided into two categories, type I and type II. Type I DCS affects the musculoskeletal system, skin, and lymphatic vessels. Type II DCS involves any other organ system. Type II DCS is more commonly reported and more serious than type I.

Type I DCS is also called the bends. It is experienced as variable and periarticular pain in the arms and legs. The elbow and shoulder joints are most commonly affected. Local tenderness and erythema are uncommon. Classically, the placement and inflation of a blood pressure cuff to 150 to 200 mm Hg on an affected joint produces relief of pain and helps confirm the diagnosis; however, the sensitivity of this maneuver was as low as 61% in one study.[21] Skin manifestations of type I DCS may include pruritus, erythema, and marbling. Pruritus without other signs, however, usually occurs only during decompression in hyperbaric chamber workers as a result of nitrogen diffusing through the skin; it is not considered a true form of DCS and is rare in scuba divers. Skin marbling, known as cutis marmorata (patchy cyanotic marbling of the skin), is a true form of DCS and results from venous stasis. It may begin as severe pruritus and progress into an erythematous rash and then to skin mottling. Cutis marmorata does not follow a dermatomal distribution and commonly involves the trunk and torso. Lymphatic obstruction by air bubbles can also occur, causing extremity edema.

Type II DCS includes symptoms beyond those described for type I DCS. These symptoms can involve the CNS, the inner ear, and the lungs. The CNS is particularly susceptible to decompression illness because of its high lipid content. The spinal cord, especially the upper lumbar area, is more often involved than cerebral tissue. Symptoms of spinal DCS include limb weakness or paralysis, paresthesias, numbness, and low back and abdominal pain. Limb symptoms often begin as a distal prickly sensation that advances proximally, followed by progressive sensory or motor loss. A dermatome sensory level occurs in some spinal DCS patients, often at the T12 to L1 dermatomes. Bladder symptoms, fecal incontinence, and priapism may occur.

Spinal DCS can occur alone or in combination with cerebral, inner ear, or pulmonary symptoms. Cerebral symptoms include mild to moderate headache, blurred vision, diplopia, dysarthria, unusual fatigue, inappropriate behavior, and a sense of detachment. Loss of consciousness in CNS DCS is rare (in marked contrast to the presentation in arterial gas embolism [AGE]).[22] Magnetic resonance imaging, computed tomography (CT), and single photon emission CT using technetium 99m–labeled hexamethylpropyleneamine can identify the bubbles of CNS DCS.

Inner ear DCS is commonly called "the staggers." The symptoms of inner ear DCS are the same as those of IEBT and include nausea, dizziness, vertigo, and nystagmus.

Pulmonary DCS is called "the chokes." All divers are exposed to some degree of microbubble emboli to the lungs on ascent. The progression to symptoms probably depends on the number and volume of bubbles. The deposition of venous gas emboli in the pulmonary arterial circulation produces progressive dyspnea, cough, and chest pain. The cough may progress to paroxysmal fits with worsening pain.

The physical examination in patients suffering from pulmonary DCS may reveal cyanosis and hypotension in association with increased central venous pressure and pulmonary arterial pressure, right-sided strain on an electrocardiogram, and a decreased end-tidal CO_2 level. The condition may progress to respiratory arrest.

DCS may be particularly dangerous to a developing fetus in the womb of a scuba diving mother because the majority of the fetal circulation bypasses the pulmonary bed through the foramen ovale and the ductus arteriosus. This bypass prevents the lungs from acting as a filter for microbubbles. In addition, venous gas emboli may appear in the fetal circulation before they are apparent in the maternal circulation.[23,24] Human data on the effects of diving on pregnant women suggest a higher incidence of low-birth-weight infants, prematurity, congenital malformations, stillbirths, and spontaneous abortions.[25-27] There are no safe-diving tables that would protect a fetus from DCS, and therefore pregnant women should be advised to refrain from scuba diving. Ancillary tests for pulmonary DCS not only are insensitive but also lead to unnecessary delays in treatment. Although microbubbles in the venous circulation can be routinely detected by M-mode ultrasonography even after ascent from very shallow saturation dives, their presence does not necessarily correlate with symptoms.[28-31]

Pulmonary Barotrauma

Without continuously expiring on ascent, a scuba diver who takes a full breath at 33 fsw has twice the lung volume at the surface. Because the volume expansion of the alveoli is limited, the increase in pressure either forces gas bubbles across the alveolar-capillary membrane or causes the wall of the alveoli to rupture. A differential pressure of only 80 mm Hg between the alveoli and chest wall, corresponding to a change in depth of 3 to 4 feet, is all that is required to force air bubbles across the alveolar-capillary membrane.[32] The greatest risk for pulmonary barotrauma occurs in less than 10 feet of water. Pulmonary barotrauma can result in five conditions: AGE, pneumothorax, pneumomediastinum, subcutaneous emphysema, and alveolar hemorrhage.

Risk factors sought from the dive and medical history may suggest the diagnosis of pulmonary barotrauma. In most cases, fast ascent, panic, problems regulating buoyancy, or running out of air is noted.

Scuba divers who suffer from asthma probably have a twofold increased risk for a dive accident compared with the general diver population.[4] There are six mechanisms by which asthmatics are at higher risk for pulmonary barotrauma:

1. Bronchospasm and mucus plugging predispose local regions of lung to injury.[33]
2. When air is compressed it becomes more dense (Boyle's law). This may contribute to greater turbulent flow through narrow airways.
3. During scuba diving there is a reduction in breathing capacity related to the effects of immersion. At 33 feet underwater, the maximum breathing capacity of a normal scuba diver is only 70% of the surface value. At 100 feet underwater, the reduction is approximately 50%.
4. When compressed air (from the scuba tank) expands in the regulator before delivery to the lungs, it cools (Charles' law). Breathing chilled air may trigger bronchospasm in asthmatics who have a cold-induced component of their disease.
5. Scuba diving takes some effort, and asthmatics who have an exercise-induced component of their disease may experience bronchospasm.
6. Compressed air may be contaminated by pollen and other allergens.

Traditionally, asthmatics are advised not to dive. A consensus of experts at a 1995 Undersea and Hyperbaric Medical Society workshop proposed more liberal guidelines. The risk of diving is probably acceptable if the diving candidate with some asthmatic history demonstrates normal pulmonary function at rest (forced vital capacity [FVC], midexpiratory flow, forced expiratory volume in 1 second, and forced expiratory flow between 25% and 75% of FVC) and after strenuous exercise. Asthma severity can wax and wane. Because symptoms may worsen for 4 to 6 weeks after an upper respiratory infection or during certain seasons, an asthmatic should refrain from diving until completely free of symptoms despite the pulmonary function criteria.[34]

Arterial Gas Embolism

The most severe form of pulmonary barotrauma is AGE. AGE is the second leading cause of mortality of sport divers after drowning, accounting for approximately 30% of diving-related deaths.[35] Typically, it results when air bubbles are forced across the alveolar-capillary membrane, escape into the pulmonary venous circulation, and proceed through the left atrium and ventricle into the arterial circulation. Clinical symptoms and signs are in part the result of mechanical obstruction by gas bubbles. AGE can also result from a right-to-left shunt of venous bubbles, such as in a diver with a PFO.

Although air bubbles may embolize to any organ, the coronary and cerebral arteries are associated with the most serious consequences. Emboli to the coronary arteries may cause cardiac ischemia, myocardial infarction, dysrhythmias, or cardiac arrest. Dysrhythmias are also indirectly caused by centrally mediated autonomic dysfunction from cerebral emboli.[36,37] Mechanical occlusion of the cerebral vasculature from emboli, most commonly to the anterior and middle cerebral arteries, causes a variety of symptoms and signs similar in appearance to an acute stroke.

The clinical manifestations of AGE may be sudden, dramatic, and life threatening. Divers who have supposedly "drowned" may actually have lost consciousness during ascent as a result of cerebral gas emboli. Any diver who has breathed compressed air at any depth underwater and who surfaces unconscious or who loses consciousness within 10 minutes of reaching the surface should be assumed to be suffering from AGE. The most commonly reported presentation of AGE includes a global alteration of consciousness, headache, dizziness, convulsions, and visual changes. Other common presenting symptoms and signs include cranial nerve symptoms, unilateral weakness, unilateral or bilateral sensory loss, ataxia, and speech changes.[35] Pulmonary symptoms, including dyspnea, pleuritic chest pain, and hemoptysis, occur in 25% to 50% of cases.[38]

Pneumothorax

When the air that escapes from alveoli as a result of pulmonary barotrauma crosses the visceral pleura, it may result in a pneumothorax. A tension pneumothorax is a rare complication. The symptoms and signs of a pulmonary barotrauma–related pneumothorax are typical for a pneumothorax of any cause. Pulmonary barotrauma can also cause alveolar hemorrhage. Hemoptysis is coincident with chest pain and dyspnea.

Pneumomediastinum and Subcutaneous Emphysema

Pneumomediastinum results when air crosses the alveolar endothelium and dissects into the pulmonary interstitium. Most commonly, the air then travels into the neck, mediastinum, or pericardium. The manifestations of pneumomediastinum may include fullness in the neck, palpable subcutaneous crepitance, and a change in voice quality or timbre. Unless evidence of either hemodynamic instability or airway compromise exists, interstitial air or subcutaneous emphysema is not a life-threatening condition.

Alternobaric Vertigo

Alternobaric vertigo (ABV) results from an inability to equalize pressure within the middle ear during ascent. Although equalization during descent requires active maneuvers to maintain eustachian tube patency, air normally exits the middle ear without difficulty during ascent because the pressure within the middle ear exceeds ambient pressure. In the setting of mucosal edema or thickening within the eustachian tube, however, the passage of air may be impeded. The problem is typically unilateral. When the pressure gradient within the middle ear reaches 60 cm H_2O, increased labyrinthine discharge produces nystagmus, with the fast phase toward the affected ear. Clinically, the patient experiences a profound but transient sense of vertigo during ascent that may be associated with nausea and vomiting. Unlike those of IEBT, the symptoms are self-limited.

Barodontalgia

Occasionally, air that is trapped beneath a poorly filled dental cavity expands on ascent, leading to dental pain. This condition is relatively benign and self-limited.

Gastrointestinal Barotrauma

Serious gastrointestinal barotrauma is a rare condition in scuba divers. It results from the expansion of bowel gas in the small intestine and colon on ascent after diving. Predisposing factors include consumption of carbonated beverages, large meals, or gas-producing foods before diving as well as performing the Valsalva maneuver in the head-down position. Symptoms include eructation, flatulence, bloating, and crampy abdominal pain. In divers with inguinal or other hernias, the potential for expansion of trapped gas within the hernia exists, and expansion may result in incarceration or strangulation.[39] Gastric rupture is a rare complication.[40] Although gastrointestinal barotrauma is a rare entity, it must be suspected in the diver-patient with a provocative history and abdominal pain.

Avascular Osteonecrosis

Dysbaric avascular osteonecrosis may occur months to decades after hyperbaric exposure. This condition can lead to joint degeneration, medullary infarcts, and malignancy and require orthopedic intervention.[41]

Pulmonary Edema

Pulmonary edema while scuba diving was first reported in 1981.[42] An increase in afterload (from vascular hyper-reactivity, possibly triggered by cold) combined with an increase in preload (from the hyperbaric underwater environment) may be the cause.

DIAGNOSTIC STRATEGIES

Focused questions concerning the dive profile, including the depth and length of the dive and a careful assessment of when the symptoms first occurred, may provide important diagnostic clues (Box 141-1).

A physician unfamiliar with the specifics of scuba diving may rely on the assessment of members of the dive group in determining whether maximum dive limits were approached. When making the diagnosis of a dive injury, it is helpful to think of the injuries in terms of occurring during descent, while at depth, or during ascent (Figure 141-3).

The diagnosis of MEBT can be established by history and physical examination alone (Table 141-1). Symp-

BOX 141-1. Focused Dive History

- When was the first onset of symptoms?
- What type of equipment was used? Compressed air, mixed gas, enriched air, rebreather? What was the source of the gas?
- Did the dive approach or exceed decompression limits? Was a dive computer used?
- What were the number, depth, bottom time, total time, and surface intervals for all dives in the 72 hours preceding symptoms (the dive "profiles")?
- Were decompression stops used? Was in-water decompression attempted?
- What was the time delay from the last dive to air travel?
- Did the diver experience difficulty with ear or sinus equilibration? Did the pain occur on descent or ascent?
- Was the diver intoxicated? Dehydrated? Working strenuously?
- How long after the dive did symptoms present? Were they present at surfacing? Delayed? Progressive?
- Is a medical history of ear or sinus infections or abnormalities present? Emphysema or asthma? Coronary artery disease? Patent foramen ovale? Neurologic illness?

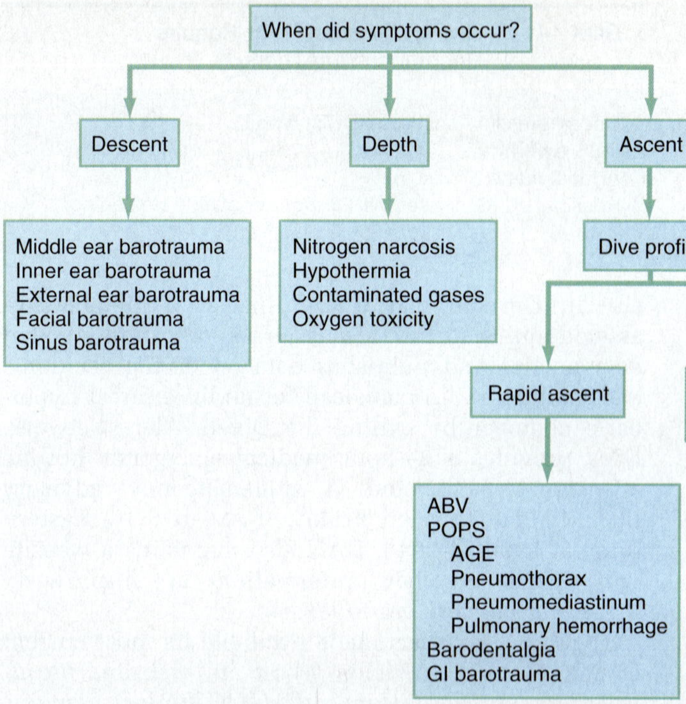

Figure 141-3. The approach to the injured diver. ABV, alternobaric vertigo; AGE, arterial gas embolism; DCS, decompression sickness; GI, gastrointestinal; POPS, pulmonary overpressure syndrome.

Table 141-1. Middle Ear Barotrauma, Inner Ear Barotrauma, and Alternobaric Vertigo

	MEBT	IEBT	ABV
Symptoms	Ear pain during descent Hearing loss Possible transient vertigo	Ear pain during descent Hearing loss Severe vertigo and nausea	Ear pain during ascent Transient hearing loss Nausea
Signs	Conductive hearing loss TM injury Unilateral face paralysis	Nystagmus Emesis Ataxia Romberg's sign Neural hearing loss	Nystagmus Emesis TM injury

ABV, alternobaric vertigo; IEBT, inner ear barotraumas; MEBT, middle ear barotraumas; TM, tympanic membrane

toms include ear pain during descent, transient vertigo, and hearing loss. A grading system for MEBT based on symptoms and signs is useful in selecting treatment regimens (Table 141-2).[43,44] Other signs may include conductive hearing loss and occasional unilateral facial paralysis.

DIFFERENTIAL CONSIDERATIONS

Most diving injuries have limited differential diagnoses that include medical disorders and trauma unrelated to dysbarism. The differential diagnosis of IEBT includes inner ear DCS, ABV, and isolated MEBT with a rupture of the TM. It is relatively easy to distinguish IEBT from MEBT and ABV because the vestibular symptoms associated with the latter two entities are transient and self-limited. When IEBT occurs simultaneously with MEBT, the presence of both may be documented by an audiogram, which demonstrates both a conductive and a sensorineural hearing loss.

The differentiation of IEBT from inner ear neurologic DCS is crucial, particularly because the treatments

Table 141-2. Grading of Middle Ear Barotrauma

Grade	Findings	Treatment
Type 1	Postdive symptoms with normal examination	Avoid diving until symptoms clear; systemic or topical decongestants
Type 2	Symptoms plus otoscopic findings without perforation	Avoid further diving until complete resolution; systemic or topical decongestants; non-narcotic analgesics
Type 3	Symptoms plus otoscopic findings with perforation	Avoid further diving until complete resolution and healing; systemic and topical decongestants; consider prophylactic antibiotics, analgesics

Modified from Farmer JC: Ear and sinus problems in diving. In Bove AA, Davis JC (eds): *Diving Medicine,* 2nd ed. Philadelphia, WB Saunders, 1990.

Table 141-3. Decompression Sickness versus Arterial Gas Embolism

Decompression Sickness	Arterial Gas Embolism
Dive History	
Depth and length dependent	Independent of dive profile
Decompression limits approached	Rapid ascent
Flying after diving	Inexperience
Diving at altitude	Out of air
Risk Factors	
Fatigue	Obstructive lung disease
Dehydration	Emphysema
Fever, hypothermia	Mucous plugging
Obesity	Patent foramen ovale
Strenuous activity	
Signs and Symptoms	
Progressive onset	Rapid onset
Spinal symptoms predominate	Cerebral symptoms predominate
Headache	Headache
Unusual fatigue	Loss of consciousness
Limb weakness or paralysis	Confusion
Paresthesias	Convulsions
Abdominal pain	Motor or sensory loss
Urinary retention	Cardiac dysrhythmias or arrest
Fecal incontinence	
Periarticular joint pain	
Skin marbling	
Vertigo or nystagmus	
Treatment	
Recompression	Recompression

differ. A careful history is the most important tool in diagnosis. An IEBT is more likely when symptoms began during descent or the diver relates a history of difficulty equilibrating or performing a vigorous Valsalva maneuver. If the dive profile is examined and the no-decompression limits are approached or exceeded and symptoms began soon after surfacing, inner ear DCS is more likely.[45]

The differentiation of inner ear DCS from barotrauma is based on the history, particularly the time of onset of symptoms. A history of difficulty equalizing the ears on descent, or the onset of symptoms early in the dive, suggests barotrauma. A history of a dive that approaches decompression limits, or the onset of symptoms during or shortly after ascent, and the presence of other neurologic findings suggest DCS. A trial of recompression therapy is indicated if concern about DCS exists.

The differential diagnosis of pulmonary DCS includes AGE (Table 141-3). Although the treatment of both requires recompression therapy, attempts should be made to distinguish the two forms of injury. Almost all cases of AGE present within the first 10 minutes of surfacing, whereas DCS presents more typically after 10 minutes: 42% of pulmonary DCS symptoms begin within 1 hour of surfacing, 60% within 3 hours, 83% within 8 hours, and 98% within 24 hours.[3]

MANAGEMENT

There are several invaluable resources available for advice in the management of diving accidents. The Divers Alert Network (DAN), located at Duke University in Durham, North Carolina, is a membership association that provides courses on diving-related emergencies and publishes data on diving accidents and fatalities. Clinicians can locate the nearest hyperbaric chamber by calling the Divers Alert Network. DAN provides a 24-hour medical emergency hotline at 919-684-8111 and a nonemergency advisory line Monday through Friday, 9 AM to 5 PM Eastern time, at 919-684-2948. DAN also maintains a website with links to key information at *http://www.diversalertnetwork.org/index.asp.*

BOX 141-2. Diving Disorders That Require Recompression Therapy

Decompression sickness (DCS) type I
DCS type II
Arterial gas embolism
Possibly contaminated air (carbon monoxide poisoning)

The U.S. Navy has made available its most current Diving Manual (revision 4) at its website, *http://www.vnh.org/DivingManual/DMTOC.html.* It contains a wealth of information about diving principles, equipment, and operations. It also has extensive information on diving medicine and recompression chamber operations.

Diving Disorders Requiring Recompression Therapy (Box 141-2)

Recompression is the only definitive treatment for DCS (types I and II) and AGE. Immediate treatment should include the administration of 100% oxygen. This reduces the bubble size by increasing the differential pressure for nitrogen diffusion out of the bubbles and speeds the washout of nitrogen from the tissues.[46] Treatment of DCS or AGE should not be withheld even if a significant time delay in transfer to a hyperbaric chamber is unavoidable. In-water recompression is risky, demanding, time consuming, and not typically recommended.

Hyperbaric therapy for AGE should be initiated as soon as possible for optimal results, but there was a case of improvement of symptoms in a patient with a suspected AGE treated with recompression therapy 27 days after the incident dive.[47] Patients with AGE who are recompressed within 5 minutes of surfacing have a mortality rate of 5%, with an extremely low risk of morbidity among the survivors.[48] If recompression is delayed by 5 hours or more, the mortality rate climbs to 10% with 50% morbidity.[48] Although spontaneous resolution of symptoms may occur in patients with AGE, all patients should be recompressed. One rationale for this approach is that although microbubbles may clear from the cerebral circulation, secondary capillary edema and swelling may result in a delayed recurrence of symptoms. Furthermore, more subtle symptoms may be appreciated only after the resolution of more prominent ones. Finally, minor symptoms may progress, and the relapse rate is high in untreated cases.

Similarly, the prognosis for DCS when treated with recompression is generally good but depends on the

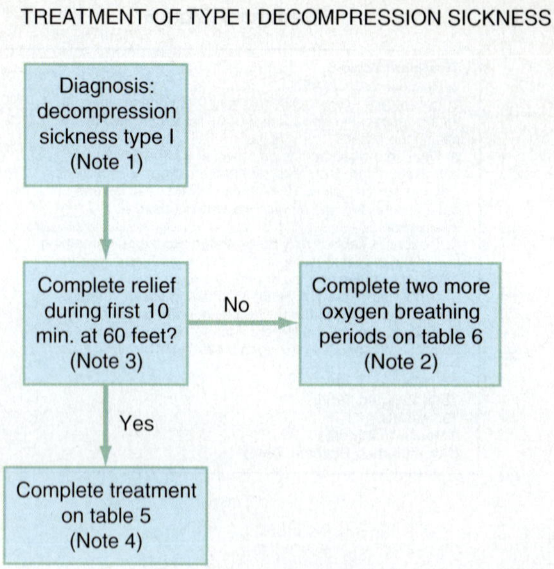

NOTES

1. If a complete neurological exam was not completed before recompression, treat as a Type II symptom.
2. Treatment Table 6 may be extended up to four additional oxygen-breathing periods, two at 30 feet and/or two at 60 feet.
3. May elect to treat on Treatment Table 6.
4. Treatment Table 5 may be extended two oxygen-breathing periods at 30 fsw.

Figure 141-4. Decompression sickness treatment from diving or altitude exposures. (Modified from Figure 21-4 from Naval Sea Systems Command: *U.S. Navy Diving Manual*, revision 4. Published by direction of Commander of Naval Sea Systems, United States Navy, January 1999: Decompression Sickness Treatment from Diving or Altitude Exposures.)

severity of symptoms at onset and the delay to recompression. A delay to definitive recompression treatment is associated with a worse outcome in cases of severe DCS. Patients can obtain some benefit from recompression, however, even if treatment is initiated more than 24 hours after the dive. Recompression therapy for DCS may be initiated as late as 10 to 14 days after exposure if necessary.[49]

Monoplace hyperbaric chambers are compact, lightweight, and more widely available than multiplace chambers. Unfortunately, because of their design, most cannot be pressurized beyond 3 ATA or deliver air-oxygen mixtures. The 3 ATA limit renders U.S. Navy Treatment Tables 2A, 3, 4, 6A, and 8 unsuitable for monoplace chambers. The U.S. Navy Treatment Tables 5, 6, 7, and 9 can be used in either a monoplace or multiplace chamber. The small size of a monoplace chamber prevents the unstable patient from receiving attendance within the chamber. The decision to bypass a monoplace chamber for a potentially more distant multiplace hyperbaric chamber must be weighed carefully. The DAN hotline may be helpful in locating the closest suitable chamber.

Ground transport to a hyperbaric facility is preferred over air transportation, if feasible, because an increase in altitude lowers the ambient pressure and allows microbubbles to expand. If air transportation must be used, it is important to maintain cabin pressure at less than 1000 feet. Commercial aircraft are typically pressurized to a cabin altitude of 5000 to 8000 feet in cruise flight. Most of these aircraft are capable of near-sea-level cabin pressures if flying no higher than 20,000 to 25,000 feet. The transferring physician can also consider transportation of the patient in a portable, monoplace chamber, if one is available.

The goals of recompression therapy are to reduce the mechanical obstruction of air bubbles, to facilitate the washout of nitrogen by increasing the tissue-blood nitrogen gradient, and to increase oxygen delivery to ischemic tissue. It is generally accepted that hyperbaric oxygen treatment is superior to hyperbaric air treatment for DCS or AGE. The selection of a treatment protocol for a particular patient, however, is best made by a qualified hyperbaricist. The U.S. Navy Treatment Tables are one of several widely accepted sets of treatment protocols. Patients suffering from DCS type I should be treated with recompression and the clinician should search for symptoms of the more severe manifestations of DCS.

The recompression treatment of DCS type I (except for cutis marmorata) with no neurologic abnormalities, as recommended by the U.S. Navy, begins with compression to 60 fsw (Figure 141-4).[3] If the patient has complete relief of symptoms at this depth within the first 10 minutes, treatment is continued according to Treatment Table 5 (Figure 141-5A).[3] Treatment Table 5 is also used for asymptomatic omitted decompression of shallow surfacing (20 fsw or less), asymptomatic omitted decompression of rapid ascent (from deeper than 20 fsw) if the missed decompression time is less than 30 minutes, and follow-up treatments for residual symptoms. If the patient with DCS type I does not have complete relief of symptoms at 60 fsw within the first 10 minutes, treatment is continued according to Treatment Table 6 (Figure 141-5B).[3]

The treatment of AGE and DCS type II, as recommended by the U.S. Navy, depends on the patient's stability (Figure 141-6).[3] If the patient has no pulse and if advanced cardiac life support (ACLS) capabilities are available within 20 minutes, the patient is treated with ACLS protocols and Treatment Table 6 (see Figure 141-5B).[3] If the patient has a pulse or if ACLS capabilities are not available within 20 minutes, the patient is compressed to 60 fsw while receiving 100% oxygen. If the patient's symptoms improve, treatment according to Treatment Table 6 is continued. If the symptoms worsen or do not improve at this depth, the patient is given air and compressed to a depth of complete or significant relief (not to exceed 165 fsw). After 30 minutes at this new depth breathing air, the patient is treated with Treatment Table 6A (Figure 141-5C).[3]

If the patient requires additional recompression time after the 30 minutes on air at the depth of complete or significant relief, Treatment Tables 4 or 7 can be used.[3] Treatment Table 4 is typically used for non–life-threatening symptoms and can be used with or without oxygen, depending on the facilities available (Figure 141-5D).[3] The length and complexity of Treatment Table 4 may limit its usefulness.

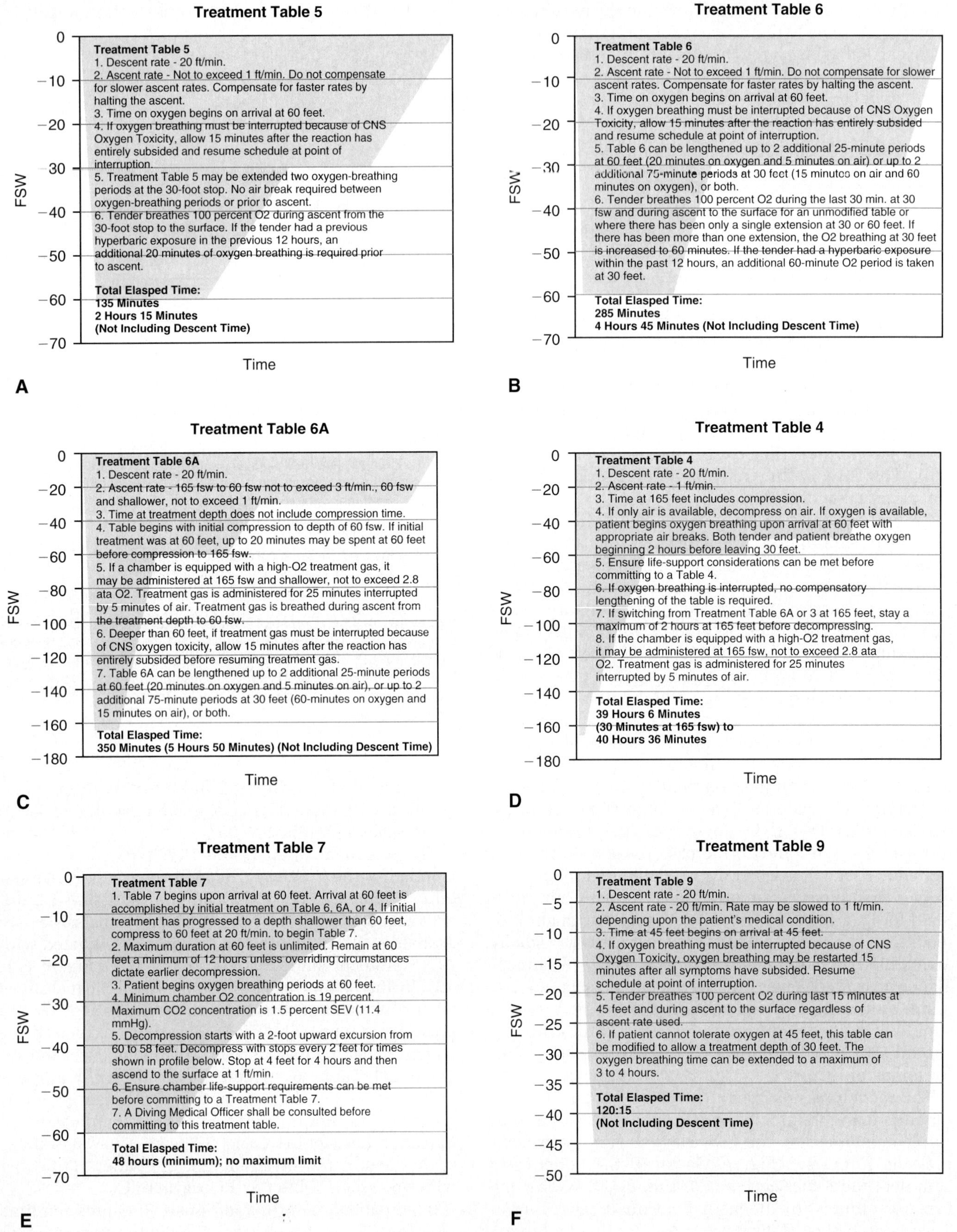

Figure 141-5. Treatment tables. (Modified from the Naval Sea Systems Command: *U.S. Navy Diving Manual*, revision 4. Published by direction of Commander of Naval Sea Systems, United States Navy, January 1999. **A,** From Figure 21-7: Treatment Table 5; **B,** from Figure 21-8: Treatment Table 6; **C,** from Figure 21-9: Treatment Table 6A; **D,** from Figure 21-10: Treatment Table 4; **E,** from Figure 21-11: Treatment Table 7; **F,** from Figure 21-13: Treatment Table 9. The clinician is strongly advised to obtain a copy of the Naval Sea Systems Command: *U.S. Navy Diving Manual*, revision 4. Published by direction of Commander of Naval Sea Systems, United States Navy, January 1999, if any attempt to use these tables in practice is to be made. The manual may be downloaded from the Internet at http://www.vnh.org/DivingManual/DMTOC.html.)

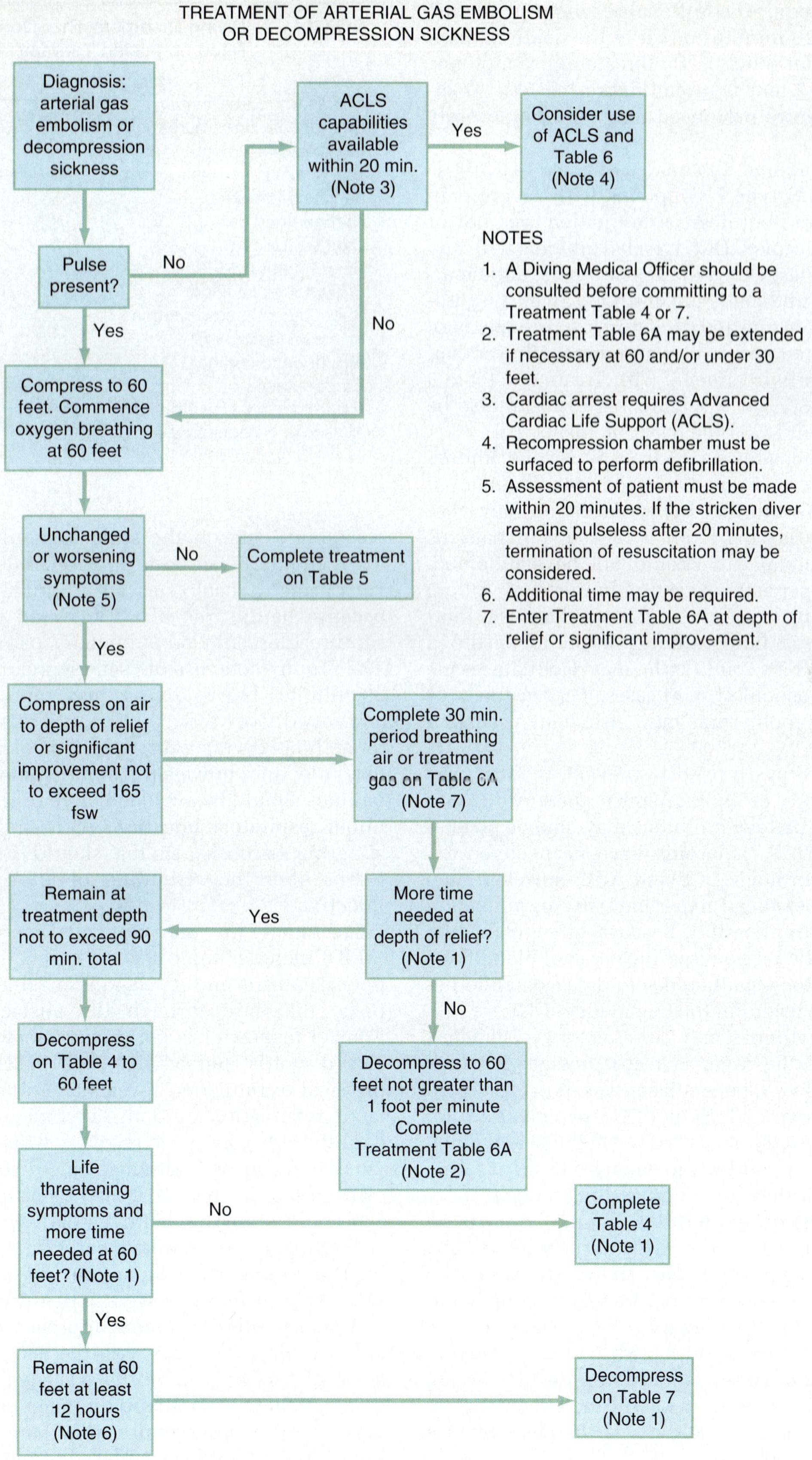

Figure 141-6. Treatment of arterial gas embolism or decompression sickness. (Modified from Figure 21-5 from Naval Sea Systems Command: *U.S. Navy Diving Manual*, revision 4. Published by direction of Commander of Naval Sea Systems, United States Navy, January 1999: Treatment of Arterial Gas Embolism or Decompression Sickness.)

If the patient requires additional recompression time after the initial 30 minutes on air at the depth of complete or significant relief of life-threatening symptoms, Treatment Table 7 may be used (Figure 141-5E).[3] Treatment Table 7 allows prolonged treatment for severely ill patients.

U.S. Navy Treatment Table 6 (see Figure 141-5B)[3] is also used for DCS type I symptoms with severe pain when a complete neurologic examination was not or could not be performed, DCS type I symptoms with any neurologic findings, DCS type II symptoms, cutis marmorata, AGE, symptomatic uncontrolled ascent, asymptomatic divers with omitted decompression greater than 30 minutes, or a recurrence of symptoms shallower than 60 fsw. Twice-daily treatments with Treatment Table 5 (see Figure 141-5A)[3] or 9 (Figure 141-5F)[3] can also be used for persistent DCS type II symptoms.

In addition to recompression therapy, several adjunctive treatments have been advocated in the treatment of DCS and AGE. Controlled hyperventilation may very transiently decrease intracranial pressure in patients with CNS symptoms but should not be maintained. One hundred percent oxygen administered before recompression may facilitate the washout of inert gases. Intravenous fluid administration to ensure a urine output of 1 to 2 mL/kg/hr may facilitate tissue perfusion and washout of inert gases. The treatment or prevention of hypothermia may also help perfusion and off-gassing.

There are no drugs proved to prevent or lessen the symptoms of DCS or AGE. Aspirin therapy (325 to 650 mg) or other platelet inhibitors may impede platelet aggregation in DCS.[50] Steroids have been advocated clinically for neurologic DCS and AGE; however, they have not been beneficial experimentally in animals.[51] Lidocaine therapy, possibly because of reducing the cerebral metabolic rate, preserving cerebral blood flow, or reducing leukocyte adherence to damaged endothelium, may prove useful in the treatment of DCS.[3,52]

Cardiac dysrhythmias may be refractory to standard treatments until the diver is recompressed. Seizures may be managed with benzodiazepines; however, mannitol should be avoided. Spinal DCS patients develop urinary retention. Of note, endotracheal tube and Foley catheter balloons should be inflated with water or saline (not air) before initiating recompression therapy.

Transport of the patient with AGE in the supine position is recommended to maximize arterial-venous flow. The Trendelenburg position, once thought to reduce the degree of cerebral embolization, increases intracranial pressure and facilitates coronary gas embolization.[53]

There is limited experience with carbon monoxide poisoning from contaminated air supplies in a diving environment. This condition should be treated immediately with normobaric 100% oxygen and may require hyperbaric oxygen therapy.

Diving Disorders Not Requiring Recompression Therapy (Box 141-3)

Prevention of MEBT requires that the diver equalize the pressure in both middle ears. Any diver who cannot clear both ears on the surface should not dive. The diver should never perform a forceful Valsalva maneuver during descent or ascent in order to clear the ears because of the risk of ABV, round or oval window rupture (descent), or pulmonary barotrauma (ascent). The prophylactic use of pseudoephedrine, 60 mg taken 30 minutes before diving, may reduce the incidence and severity of MEBT.[54] The use of this drug as a means to facilitate diving with symptoms of an upper respiratory infection, however, is not recommended. Antihistamines should be avoided before diving. Sinusitis and upper respiratory infections increase the likelihood of suffering barotitis. Diving should be avoided for 2 weeks after the resolution of an upper respiratory infection.[55]

BOX 141-3. Diving Disorders That Do Not Require Recompression Therapy

- Middle ear barotrauma
- External ear barotrauma
- Inner ear barotrauma
- Barosinusitis
- Facial barotrauma
- Nitrogen narcosis
- Oxygen toxicity
- Pneumothorax
- Pneumomediastinum
- Subcutaneous emphysema
- Alveolar hemorrhage
- Alternobaric vertigo
- Barodentalgia
- Gastrointestinal barotrauma
- Avascular osteonecrosis

Treatment for uncomplicated serous otitis from MEBT includes topical nasal vasoconstrictors such as phenylephrine and repeated Frenzel maneuvers to displace the fluid through the eustachian tube. The Frenzel maneuver is performed by swallowing with a closed glottis, pursed lips, and pinched nose. If the physical examination reveals a ruptured TM, prophylactic treatment should also include an oral antibiotic. Oral steroids may speed recovery when a seventh nerve palsy is diagnosed, although this disorder is typically self-limited. Diving must also be suspended until the TM is healed to prevent calorically induced vertigo.

Treatment of external ear barotrauma includes cleaning the external canal and removing foreign bodies. Ear plugs should never be worn when diving.

A conservative treatment approach to IEBT includes bed rest for 5 to 7 days with the head elevated, avoidance of straining and the Valsalva maneuver, and decongestants to facilitate drainage of the middle ear. Early surgical intervention may benefit patients with total or near-total hearing loss but not divers with isolated high-frequency hearing loss. All patients with IEBT should be provided referral to an otolaryngologist because IEBT suggests significant injury to the cochleovestibular system.

Treatment of barosinusitis is typically conservative, including the use of decongestants and, occasionally, antibiotics. If symptoms persist, referral for antrostomy should be considered, particularly to prevent future recurrences. The patient should be advised not to dive until any underlying respiratory infection or acute inflammatory process has resolved completely.

The victim of facial barotrauma may have a dramatic appearance, but the condition is usually benign and requires no specific treatment. The patient should be advised not to resume diving until facial edema has resolved.[56]

Nitrogen narcosis symptoms should resolve on surfacing when the partial pressure of nitrogen drops. Seemingly persistent symptoms should prompt a search for other etiologies, such as DCS, cerebral AGE, contaminated air, and near drowning.

With the exception of AGE, none of the pulmonary barotrauma disorders (pneumothorax, pneumomediastinum, subcutaneous emphysema, and alveolar hemorrhage) requires recompression therapy. Treatment with 100% oxygen may aid in the resolution of the disorders. Although tube thoracostomy may not be required for the treatment of a small pneumothorax, such a tube should be placed if the diver is to undergo recompression therapy for concomitant AGE or DCS to prevent a tension pneumothorax. Catheter aspiration of the pneumothorax is an acceptable alternative to tube thoracostomy if the patient will not receive positive-pressure ventilation.

Treatment of pneumomediastinum consists of bed rest. One hundred percent oxygen therapy may hasten the resolution of symptoms. In the case of respiratory compromise, tracheal intubation may be required. Most important, the presence of interstitial pulmonary emphysema should alert the physician to the possible coexistence of more severe forms of pulmonary barotrauma. The need for a surgical decompressive treatment of subcutaneous emphysema alone is extremely unlikely. Supportive therapy to correct hypoxia is indicated in the treatment of alveolar hemorrhage.[57]

Careful equalization during a slow ascent can prevent the occurrence of ABV. Oral and topical decongestants may be indicated if symptoms persist. Occasionally, myringotomy is required.[58]

DISPOSITION

Decompression tables are based on the premise that the diver returns to an ambient pressure of 1 atmosphere on surfacing; however, a further reduction in ambient pressure occurs either when ascending in altitude after diving or when diving at altitude. Commercial airliners may be pressurized to a cabin altitude of 5000 to 8000 feet in cruise flight. Many cases of DCS have a delay in the onset of symptoms in divers who fly after diving without symptoms before departure. Divers who experience DCS symptoms before departure but nevertheless fly are more likely to have type II DCS, less likely to achieve complete relief after recompression, and more likely to have residual symptoms for at least 3 months.

The recommended postdive preflight surface interval (PFSI) before ascending to higher altitudes (or flying) depends on the diver's repetitive group designator (residual nitrogen time). The relative risk of developing DCS increases with greater residual nitrogen times and shorter PRSI (Figure 141-7).[59] For example, the risk of developing DCS is seven times greater for PFSIs of 12 hours after a dive to 130 fsw than for PFSIs of 24 hours after a dive to 60 fsw.[59] Long PFSIs (up to 48 hours) may be necessary to reduce the risk of DCS after deep, multiday repetitive diving, particularly if the dives required decompression stops (exceeding the no-decompression limits).[60] Some dive computers calculate time-to-flight intervals, which tend to be somewhat shorter than most guidelines based on residual nitrogen timetables. Flying should be delayed for at least 12 hours after diving if less than 2 hours of total dive time was accumulated in the preceding 48 hours. For multiple-day, unlimited diving, flying should be delayed for at least 24 hours. The diver should be advised not to fly for 3 to 7 days after treatment for DCS

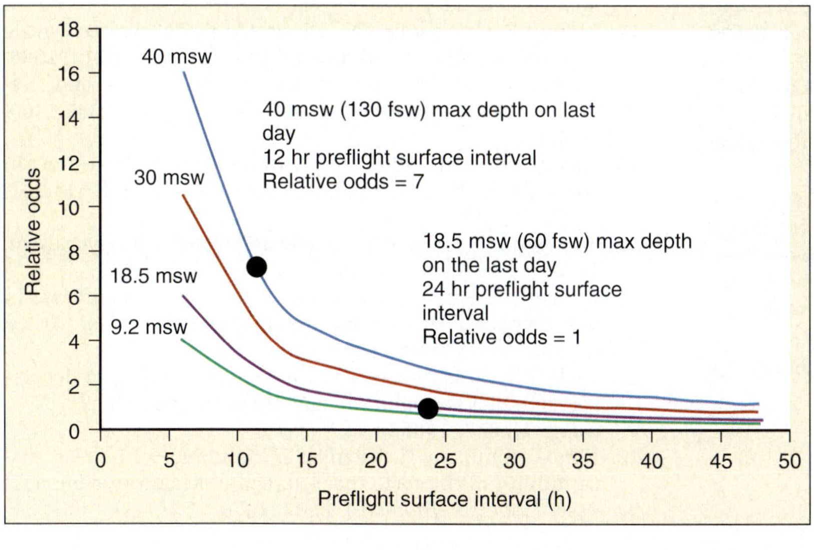

Figure 141-7. The risk of decompression sickness relative to flying. fsw, feet of seawater; msw, meters of seawater. (From Freiberger JJ, et al: The relative risk of decompression sickness during and after air travel following diving. *Aviat Space Environ Med* 73:983, 2002.)

type I and for 4 weeks after recompression therapy for DCS type II.

Patients treated according to Treatment Table 5 should remain in the hyperbaric facility for at least 2 hours. After recompression for DCS II symptoms according to Treatment Table 6, the diver should be observed for at least 6 hours. It is prudent to admit all recompressed patients or to advise them to remain within 60 minutes of the hyperbaric facility for 24 hours. Patients recompressed after DCS or AGE should not fly for 72 hours.

The U.S. Navy's guidelines recommend that the patient not return to diving for 7 days after recompression for type I DCS and for 4 weeks after type II DCS.[3] The sport diver who experiences DCS type II symptoms or AGE should probably never dive again.

After recompression therapy according to Treatment Table 5, a patient should not dive again for at least 7 days. After recompression according to Treatment Table 6, the diver should not dive again for at least 4 weeks and only after the recommendation of a hyperbaricist.

After treatment for pulmonary barotrauma, it is advisable to evaluate the diver with a spiral volumetric chest CT scan to determine whether there are any preexisting pathologic conditions (e.g., bullae) that could put the diver at risk for recurrence before further diving.[61] Chest CT is not recommended in routine medical screening before participating in scuba diving without a history of pulmonary barotrauma.

KEY CONCEPTS

- There is a large population of sport scuba divers at risk for diving injuries. The land-locked emergency physician may be confronted with these problems.
- The Trendelenburg position, once thought to reduce cerebral embolization, increases intracranial pressure and facilitates coronary gas embolization.
- The majority of dive injuries are diagnosed on the basis of the focused dive history and physical examination alone and are best differentiated into disorders of descent, disorders of depth, and disorders of ascent. The U.S. Navy Dive Manual and the Divers Alert Network (DAN) are valuable resources for the clinician presented with a diving emergency. The nonemergency advisory line Monday through Friday, 9 AM to 5 PM Eastern time, is 919-684-2948. The 24-hour medical emergency hotline is 919-684-8111. Emergency physicians should be familiar with their local hyperbaric capabilities.
- With the exception of decompression sickness (DCS), arterial gas embolism (AGE), and, possibly, carbon monoxide poisoning from contaminated air, most dive-related disorders can be treated without recompression therapy. Recompression treatment is always recommended for victims of DCS and AGE.
- After multiple-day unlimited diving, flying should be delayed for at least 24hours.

REFERENCES

1. Brylske A: A brief history of diving: Free divers, bells, and helmets (part 1). *Dive Training* Aug 4:20, 1994.
2. Brylske A: A brief history of diving: Evolution of the self-contained diver (part 2). *Dive Training* Sep 4:20, 1994.
3. Naval Sea Systems Command: *U.S. Navy Diving Manual,* revision 4. Published by direction of Commander of Naval Sea Systems, United States Navy, January 1999 (http://www.vnh.org/DivingManual/DMTOC.html).
4. Neuman TS, et al: Asthma and diving. *Ann Asthma* 73:344, 1994.
5. Joiner JT (ed): *NOAA Diving Manual: Diving for Science and Technology*, 4th ed. Flagstaff, Best Publishing, 2001.
6. Green SM, Rothrock SG, Green EA: Tympanometric evaluation of middle ear barotrauma during recreational scuba diving. *Int J Sports Med* 14:411, 1993.
7. Kohut RI: Perilymph fistulas: Clinical criteria. *Arch Otolaryngol Head Neck Surg* 118:687, 1992.
8. Neubauer B, Mutzbauer TS, Tetzlaff K: Exposure to soda-lime dust in closed and semi-closed diving apparatus. *Aviat Space Environ Med* 71:1248, 2000.
9. Baj Z, Olszanski R, Majewska E, Konarski M: The effect of air and nitrox divings on platelet activation tested by flow cytometry. *Aviat Space Environ Med* 71:925, 2000.
10. Masurel G: The value of ultrasonic detection of circulating bubbles in animal and man. The contribution to physiopathogenesis of a decompression accident. *Schweiz Z Sportmed* 37:41, 1989.
11. Pilmanis AA: Intravenous gas emboli in man after selected open air scuba dives [abstract 5.1]. Undersea Medical Society Annual Scientific Meeting, May 10-12, 1997, Miami.
12. Spencer MP, Clarke JF: Precordial monitoring of pulmonary gas embolism and decompression bubbles. *Aerospace Med* 43:762, 1972.
13. Butler BD, Hills BA: The lung as a filter for microbubbles. *J Appl Physiol* 47:537, 1979.
14. Francis TJR, Gorman DF: The pathogenesis of the decompression disorders. In Bennet PB, Elliot DH (eds): *The Physiology and Medicine of Diving,* 4th ed. Philadelphia, WB Saunders, 1993, p 463.
15. Divers Alert Network: *Report on Decompression Illness and Diving Fatalities: DAN's Annual Review of Recreational Scuba Diving Injuries and Fatalities Based on 1998 Data.* Durham, NC, Divers Alert Network, 2000.
16. St. Leger Dowse M, Bryson P, Gunby A, Fife W: Comparative data from 2250 male and female sports divers: Diving patterns and decompression sickness. *Aviat Space Environ Med* 73:743, 2002.
17. Moon RE, Camporesi EM, Kisslo JA: Patent foramen ovale and decompression sickness in divers. *Lancet* 1:513, 1989.
18. Ruel J, et al: Central nervous system lesions and cervical disc herniations in amateur divers. *Lancet* 345:1403, 1995.
19. Knauth M, et al: Cohort study of multiple brain lesions in sport divers: Role of a patent foramen ovale. *BMJ* 314:701, 1997.
20. Tomassoni A: Cardiac problems associated with dysbarism. *Cardiol Clin* 13:266, 1995.
21. Rudge FW, Stone JA: The use of the pressure cuff test in the diagnosis of decompression sickness. *Aviat Space Environ Med* 62:266, 1991.
22. Dick APK, Massey EW: Neurologic presentation of decompression sickness and air embolism in sport divers. *Neurology* 35:667, 1985.
23. Fife W, Simmang C, Kitzman J: Preliminary study on susceptibility of the fetal sheep to acute decompression sickness. *Undersea Biomed J* 5:287, 1978.

24. Stock MK, et al: Responses of fetal sheep to simulated no-decompression dives. *J Appl Physiol* 48:776, 1980.
25. Bolton M: Scuba diving and fetal well-being: A survey of 208 women. *Undersea Biomed Res* 7:183, 1989.
26. Bangasser SA: Medical profile of the woman scuba diver. Proceedings of the 10th International Conference on Underwater Education. NAUI PO Box 14650, Montclair, Calif, 91763-1150, 10:31-40, 1978.
27. Turner G, Unsworth I: Intrauterine bends? *Lancet* 1:905, 1982.
28. Eckenhoff RG, Olstad CS, Carrod G: Human dose-response relationship for decompression and endogenous bubble formation. *J Appl Physiol* 69:914, 1990.
29. Ikeda T, et al: M-mode ultrasonic detection of microbubbles following saturation diving: A case report and proposal for a new grading system. *Aviat Space Environ Med* 60:166, 1989.
30. Bayne CG, et al: Doppler bubble detection and decompression sickness: A prospective clinical trial. *Undersea Biomed Res* 12:327, 1985.
31. Ikeda T, Okamoto Y, Hashimoto A: Bubble formation and decompression sickness on direct ascent from shallow air saturation diving. *Aviat Space Environ Med* 64:121, 1993.
32. Kizer KW: Diving medicine. In Auerbach PS (ed): *Wilderness Medicine*, 4th ed. St. Louis, Mosby, 2001, p 1380.
33. Møllem H, Emhjellen S, Horgen O: Pulmonary barotrauma and arterial gas embolism caused by an emphysematous bulla in a scuba diver. *Aviat Space Environ Med* 61:559, 1990.
34. Elliott DH: Are asthmatics fit to dive? Presented at the Undersea and Hyperbaric Medical Society (UHMS) Annual Scientific Meeting, Denver, June 21, 1995.
35. Kizer KW: Dysbaric cerebral air embolism in Hawaii. *Ann Emerg Med* 16:535, 1987.
36. Cales RH, et al: Cardiac arrest from gas embolism in scuba diving. *Ann Emerg Med* 10:589, 1981.
37. Evans DE, et al: Cardiovascular effects of cerebral air embolism. *Stroke* 12:338, 1981.
38. Ball R: Effect of severity, time to recompression with oxygen, and re-treatment on outcome in forty-nine cases of spinal cord decompression sickness. *Undersea Hyperb Med* 20:133, 1993.
39. Landon CW: Gastrointestinal barotrauma in scuba divers. *West J Med* 135:242, 1981.
40. Cramer FS, Heimbach RD: Stomach rupture as a result of gastrointestinal barotrauma in a scuba diver. *J Trauma* 22:238, 1982.
41. Wilmshurst P, Ross P: Dysbaric osteonecrosis of the shoulder in a sport scuba diver. *Br J Sports Med* 32:344, 1998.
42. Wilmshurst PT, et al: Forearm vascular responses in subjects who develop recurrent pulmonary edema when scuba-diving: A new syndrome. *Br Heart J* 45:349, 1981.
43. Hunter SE, Farmer JC: Ear and sinus problems in diving. In Bove AA (ed): *Bove and Davis' Diving Medicine,* 4th ed. Philadelphia, WB Saunders, 1993, pp 442-443.
44. Clenney TL, Lassen LF: Recreational scuba diving injuries. *Am Fam Physician* 53:1761, 1996.
45. Adkisson GH, Meredith AP: Inner ear decompression sickness combined with a fistula of the round window: Case report. *Ann Otol Rhinol Laryngol* 99:733, 1990.
46. Strauss MB, Borer RC: Diving medicine: Contemporary topics and their controversies. *Am J Emerg Med* 19:232, 2001.
47. Tirpitz D, Schipke JD: Delayed recompression after scuba diving-induced barotrauma: A case report. *Aviat Space Environ Med* 67:266, 1996.
48. Tomassoni AJ: Cardiac problems associated with dysbarism. *Cardiol Clin* 13:266, 1995.
49. Myers RA, Bray P: Delayed treatment of serious decompression sickness. *Ann Emerg Med* 14:254, 1985.
50. Kizer KW: Diving medicine. In Auerbach PS (ed): *Wilderness Medicine*, 4th ed. St. Louis, Mosby, 2001, p 1391.
51. Francis TJR, Dutka AJ: Methylprednisolone in the treatment of acute spinal cord decompression sickness. *Undersea Biomed Res* 16:165, 1989.
52. Drewry A, Gorman DF: Lidocaine as an adjunct to hyperbaric therapy in decompression illness: A case report. *Undersea Biomed Res* 19:187, 1992.
53. Butler BD, et al: Effect of the Trendelenburg position on the distribution of arterial air emboli in dogs. *Ann Thorac Surg* 45:198, 1988.
54. Brown M, Jones J, Krohmer J: Pseudoephedrine for the prevention of barotitis media: A controlled clinical trial in underwater divers. *Ann Emerg Med* 21:849, 1992.
55. Parell GJ, Becker GD: Conservative management of inner ear barotrauma resulting from scuba diving. *Otolaryngol Head Neck Surg* 93:393, 1985.
56. Rudge FW: Ocular barotrauma caused by mask squeeze during a scuba dive. *South Med J* 87:749, 1994.
57. Balk M, Goldman JM: Alveolar hemorrhage as a manifestation of pulmonary barotrauma after scuba diving. *Ann Emerg Med* 19:930, 1990.
58. Becker GD: Recurrent alternobaric facial paralysis resulting from scuba diving. *Laryngoscope* 93:596, 1983.
59. Freiberger JJ, et al: The relative risk of decompression sickness during and after air travel following diving. *Aviat Space Environ Med* 73:980, 2002.
60. Sheffield PJ: Flying after diving guidelines: A review. *Aviat Space Environ Med* 61:1130, 1990.
61. Tetzlaff K, Neubauer B, Reuter M, Waringhoff V: Pulmonary barotrauma of a diver using an oxygen rebreathing diving apparatus. *Aviat Space Environ Med* 67:1198, 1996.

CHAPTER

142 High-Altitude Medicine

Michael Yaron and Benjamin Honigman

EPIDEMIOLOGY

High-altitude illness represents a spectrum of clinical entities that have hampered the activities of mountaineers, merchants, military forces, aviators, and explorers throughout time. This illness is seen clinically in one of several forms that overlap and share a common pathophysiology. Acute mountain sickness (AMS) is the relatively benign and self-limited presentation, whereas high-altitude pulmonary edema (HAPE) and high-altitude cerebral edema (HACE) represent the potentially life-threatening manifestations of high-altitude illness.

Worldwide, it is estimated that approximately 40 million individuals live above 8000 feet, and 25 million live above 10,000 feet.[1] Rather than these high-altitude residents, the groups at risk for altitude illnesses are those who ascend into mountainous regions. Mountain sports activities and tourism are attracting increasing numbers of participants each year. This, combined with the rapid ascent made possible by air transportation, results in more unacclimatized individuals at risk for high-altitude illness. More than 1 million visitors travel annually to the remote high mountain ranges of Asia, Africa, and South America.[1] Approximately 35 million visitors travel annually to high-altitude recreation areas in the western United States.[1]

The incidence of high-altitude illness depends on many variables. The rate of ascent, sleeping altitude, final altitude reached, duration of stay at any altitude, and individual susceptibility are the most important factors. AMS is very common (67% incidence) among mountain climbers on Mt. Rainier who ascend quickly (1 to 2 days) to 14,410 feet.[2] Trekkers who fly into the Khumbu region to explore the Mt. Everest area have a higher incidence of AMS (47%) compared with those who walk (23%).[3] Skiers who visit resorts in the western United States from sea level generally fly or drive to the region but sleep at relatively lower altitudes than the other groups mentioned. Among this population, AMS occurs in approximately 25%.[4] Given the large number (approximately 2 million) of visitors skiing in Colorado each year, this is not a trivial matter. The incidence of HAPE varies from 0.01% to 2% in most studies but has reached 15.5% among soldiers flown directly to 14,500 feet without a chance to acclimatize at a lower altitude.[3,5] The incidence of HACE is lower, and although it usually occurs with HAPE, it can be seen as an isolated entity. Both HAPE and HACE are more common with a longer duration of visit and higher sleeping altitude.

Age appears to be a relative risk factor. Children probably have the same incidence of AMS as adults.[6-8] Younger individuals (younger than 20 years old) are more likely to develop HAPE, although HAPE is extremely rare in children younger than 2 years of age. Gender does not affect the incidence of AMS; however, women may have less risk of developing HAPE.[3,4]

The number of elderly persons visiting mountain resorts is increasing. Many of these individuals have underlying health problems, including lung disease (10%), heart disease (25%), and hypertension (30%). Despite these conditions, the risk for AMS development in this subset of older adults is less than that in other age groups.[9] Nevertheless, clues exist that elderly persons may not react well to acute high-altitude exposure. Pulmonary vital capacity decreases almost one third in elderly persons ascending from sea level to 14,000 feet for 1 week, producing a large fall in both oxygen saturation and maximal oxygen uptake during exercise. For elderly persons residing at moderate elevations, oxygen saturation is approximately 92% at rest.[9]

DEFINITIONS

Moderate altitude is between 8000 and 10,000 feet of elevation. Although most people do not experience significant arterial oxygen desaturation until they reach higher altitudes, high-altitude illness is common with rapid ascent above 8200 feet. Individuals with underlying medical problems may be predisposed to developing altitude illness at these lower levels.

High altitude is between 10,000 and 18,000 feet. Most serious altitude illness occurs at these levels. The pathophysiologic effects of high altitude begin when the oxygen saturation of the arterial blood begins to fall below the 90% level. The sigmoidal shape of the oxyhemoglobin dissociation curve prevents a significant fall of arterial oxygen saturation (SaO_2) in most individuals until an altitude of approximately 12,000 feet. At this altitude, the steep portion of the curve is encountered, and rapid desaturation begins, with relatively small increases in altitude (Figure 142-1). Some predisposed individuals may desaturate to less than 90% at altitudes as low as 8000 feet.

Extreme altitude is above 18,000 feet. At this height, complete acclimatization generally is not possible and long visits above this level result in progressive deterioration.

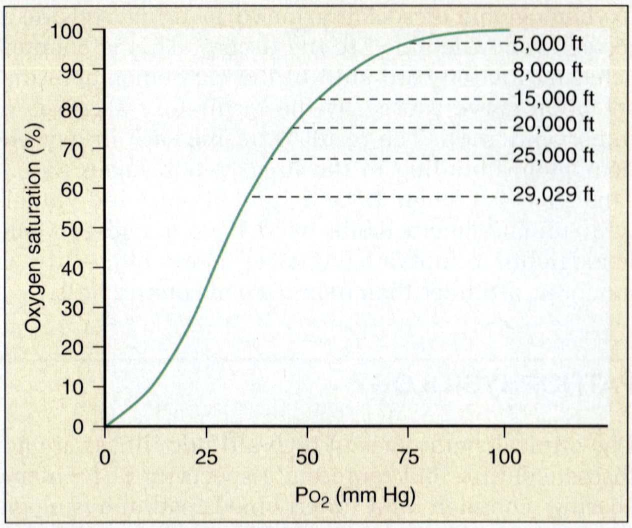

Figure 142-1. Oxygen-hemoglobin dissociation curve. Approximate oxygen saturations are marked for several altitudes. PO_2, partial pressure of oxygen. (Data for 15,000 to 29,029 feet from Sutton JR, et al: Operation Everest II: Oxygen transport during exercise at extreme simulated altitude. *J Appl Physiol* 64:1309, 1988.)

ENVIRONMENTAL CONSIDERATIONS

Barometric pressure decreases logarithmically as the altitude rises. The partial pressure of oxygen (PO_2) in the atmosphere also decreases as altitude rises, but it remains a constant 20.93% of the barometric pressure. The shape of the earth is slightly flat at the poles and bulging at the equator. The atmospheric envelope that surrounds the earth has a similar shape; therefore, the barometric pressure is lower at higher latitudes than it is at the equator. For example, it has been calculated that it would be impossible for a climber to reach the summit of Mt. Everest without supplemental oxygen if the mountain happened to be in a more northern latitude.

The atmospheric envelope also undergoes a seasonal tide that causes a variation in its local thickness. This results in barometric pressures that are lower and "relative altitudes" that are higher during the winter season. Local weather can also have a significant effect on barometric pressure from day to day. A low-pressure front can reduce the barometric pressure 12 to 40 mm Hg (500 to 2500 feet) and result in a significant temporary increase in relative altitude.

ACCLIMATIZATION

The term *acclimatization* refers to the series of integrated adaptations that take place at high altitudes, which tend to restore the oxygen pressures within the tissues toward normal sea level values despite the lowered PO_2 of the atmosphere. These processes occur gradually and involve multiple respiratory, cardiovascular, and hematologic adjustments. Gradual ascents made by mountaineers over several weeks have allowed the successful ascent of many of the world's highest summits, including Mt. Everest (29,029 feet), without supplemental oxygen and without the serious manifestations of altitude illness. If rapid exposure to extreme altitudes is attempted, acclimatization is impossible, and the individual loses consciousness and may die in a matter of minutes.

BOX 142-1. Alveolar Gas Equation

$PaO_2 = piO_2 - (PaCO_2/R)$
PaO_2 = Partial pressure of oxygen in alveolus
PiO_2 = Partial pressure of oxygen in inspired air
$PaCO_2$ = Partial pressure of oxygen in carbon dioxide in alveolus
R = Respiratory quotient

Acclimatization begins at the altitude that causes the oxygen saturation of arterial blood to fall below sea level values. The altitude at which this occurs depends on the rate of ascent, the duration of exposure, and individual physiology. People with preexisting conditions that reduce oxygen saturation or content will have a decreased altitude tolerance. Of particular importance are both acute and chronic cardiac and respiratory illnesses. Most healthy, unacclimatized visitors to high altitude will not desaturate significantly (to less than 90%) until they reach elevations higher than 8000 feet.[1]

The risk of high-altitude illness also depends on an individual's inherent ability to acclimatize. Some people acclimatize easily without any clinical symptoms developing, whereas others may have AMS develop transiently during acclimatization. This variability may involve the genetic mediation of oxygen transport capabilities between individuals. Previous, successful acclimatization may be predictive of future responses in similar conditions.

The most important physiologic change that occurs during acclimatization is an increase in minute ventilation, causing a decrease in the partial pressure of carbon dioxide in arterial gas ($PaCO_2$). The alveolar gas equation states that, as the $PaCO_2$ decreases, a corresponding increase in PaO_2 occurs, thereby increasing arterial oxygenation (Box 142-1). Thus, the level of ventilation determines alveolar oxygen for a given inspired oxygen tension.

When a person arrives at high altitude, the peripheral chemosensors in the carotid bodies respond to a decrease in PaO_2 and signal the respiratory control center in the medulla to increase ventilation. This increase in ventilation is known as the hypoxic ventilatory response (HVR) and can be inhibited or stimulated by numerous factors, including alcohol, sleep medications, caffeine, cocoa, prochlorperazine, and progesterone. The magnitude of the HVR varies among individuals and may be genetically predetermined.

As ventilation increases, a respiratory alkalosis occurs that acts as a negative feedback system on the central respiratory center, limiting any further increase in ventilation. The kidneys, within 24 to 48 hours of ascent, begin to excrete bicarbonate in an effort to compensate for the alkalosis. As the pH normalizes, ventilation continues to rise slowly, reaching a maximum after 6 to 8 days. The ability to achieve an adequate HVR varies among individuals and is related to the ability to acclimatize; thus, a poor HVR makes an individual more likely to fail acclimatization and suffer from AMS. For the majority of people with intermediate hypoxic ventilatory response values, ventilatory drive probably has no predictive value for AMS development.[10] A low HVR and relative hypoventilation have been implicated in the pathogenesis of both AMS and HAPE.[11]

The release of catecholamines on ascent stimulates the circulatory system to increase cardiac output; this is manifested by an elevation in heart rate, blood pressure, and venous tone. Except at extreme altitudes, acclimatization results in the resting heart rate gradually returning to near sea level values. A resting heart rate that remains high is evidence of poor acclimatization. As the altitude increases, a decrease in maximal heart rate capacity occurs and, at the limits of acclimatization, maximal and resting heart rates converge.

Another component of the acclimatization process is the hematopoietic response to high altitude, consisting of an increase in both hemoglobin and number of red blood cells. An early increase of up to 15% occurs in hemoglobin concentration after rapid ascent to high altitude. This is primarily a result of a fluid shift into the extravascular space. Long-term acclimatization leads to an increase in plasma volume and, therefore, to an increase in total blood volume. Erythropoietin is secreted in response to hypoxemia, which in turn stimulates the production of red blood cells, leading to new circulatory red blood cells in 4 to 5 days. Over the next 2 months, red blood cell mass increases in proportion to the degree of hypoxemia (Figure 142-2).[12]

Hypoxemia also results in an increase in 2,3-diphosphoglycerate, resulting in a rightward shift of the oxyhemoglobin dissociation curve, favoring a release of oxygen from the blood to the tissues. This is counteracted by the leftward shift of the oxyhemoglobin dissociation curve caused by the respiratory alkalosis of hyperventilation. The result is an increase in oxygen-hemoglobin binding in the lung, which raises SaO_2.[13] This effect is thought to be helpful because individuals with mutant hemoglobins who have a high oxygen-hemoglobin affinity acclimatize more efficiently at moderate altitudes than their normal counterparts.

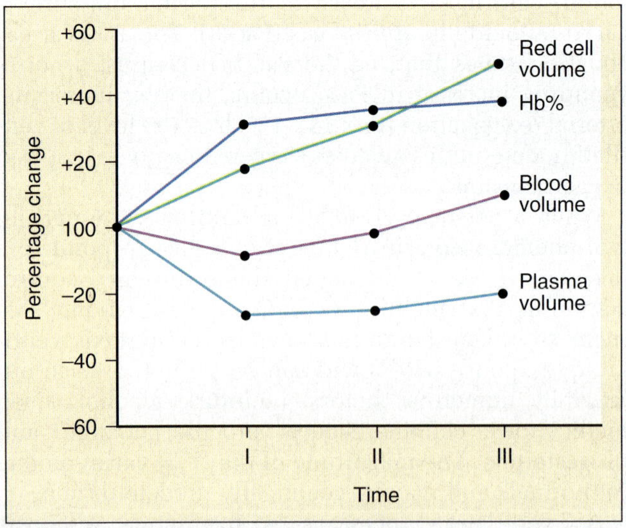

Figure 142-2. Acclimatization: Hematopoietic and volume adaptation. Point I, altitude 4000 to 5800 m, 18 weeks after arrival; point II, altitude 5800 m, 21 to 24 weeks after arrival; point III, altitude above 5800 m, 30 to 38 weeks after arrival. (Redrawn from Pugh LG: High altitudes. In Edholm AG, Bacharach AL (eds): *The Physiology of Human Survival*. London, Academic Press, 1965, p 138.)

PATHOPHYSIOLOGY

The clinical syndromes of high-altitude illness are not discrete entities but represent a spectrum of problems sharing common and intertwined pathophysiologic mechanisms. AMS and HACE represent differing manifestations of altitude illness on the same continuum, although HAPE appears to have an independent pathophysiology.

The symptoms of AMS develop several hours after arrival at high altitude, whereas the development of HAPE and HACE generally requires several days of altitude exposure. Because hypobaric hypoxemia occurs within minutes of arrival, it cannot be the direct cause of high-altitude illness. Instead, it appears to be the initiating factor for a complex pathologic process that leads to the development of the various clinical syndromes. The proposed mechanisms for the development of AMS, HAPE, and HACE are represented schematically in Figure 142-3.

A poor HVR resulting in relative hypoventilation may result from either the individual's genetic predisposition or extrinsic factors, such as medications, that decrease the ventilatory drive. Whenever the HVR is decreased, the protective effects of hyperventilation are lost and the hypoxemia of high-altitude exposure is exacerbated.

The periodic breathing associated with high-altitude exposure may result in periods of apnea during sleep, causing severe arterial oxygen desaturation, which further exacerbates hypoxemia.[14] Significant hypoxemia initiates multiple systemic responses that involve the circulatory, pulmonary, endocrine, and central nervous systems.

Hypoxemia alters fluid homeostasis, resulting in a generalized fluid retention followed by the shift of fluid into the intracellular spaces. This is manifested by peripheral edema, decreased urinary output, and increased body weight in patients with AMS. Several different mechanisms may account for these fluid shifts. Antidiuretic hormone levels are elevated in many patients with AMS and HAPE,[15] and this release of antidiuretic hormone may be centrally mediated.[16] Aldosterone, plasma renin, and atrial natriuretic levels are higher in persons with AMS.[17,18]

The hypoxemia that results from high-altitude exposure causes pulmonary artery hypertension and elevated capillary pressures that play the cardinal role in the development of HAPE. Exercise and cold stress at altitude may increase hypoxemia and exacer-

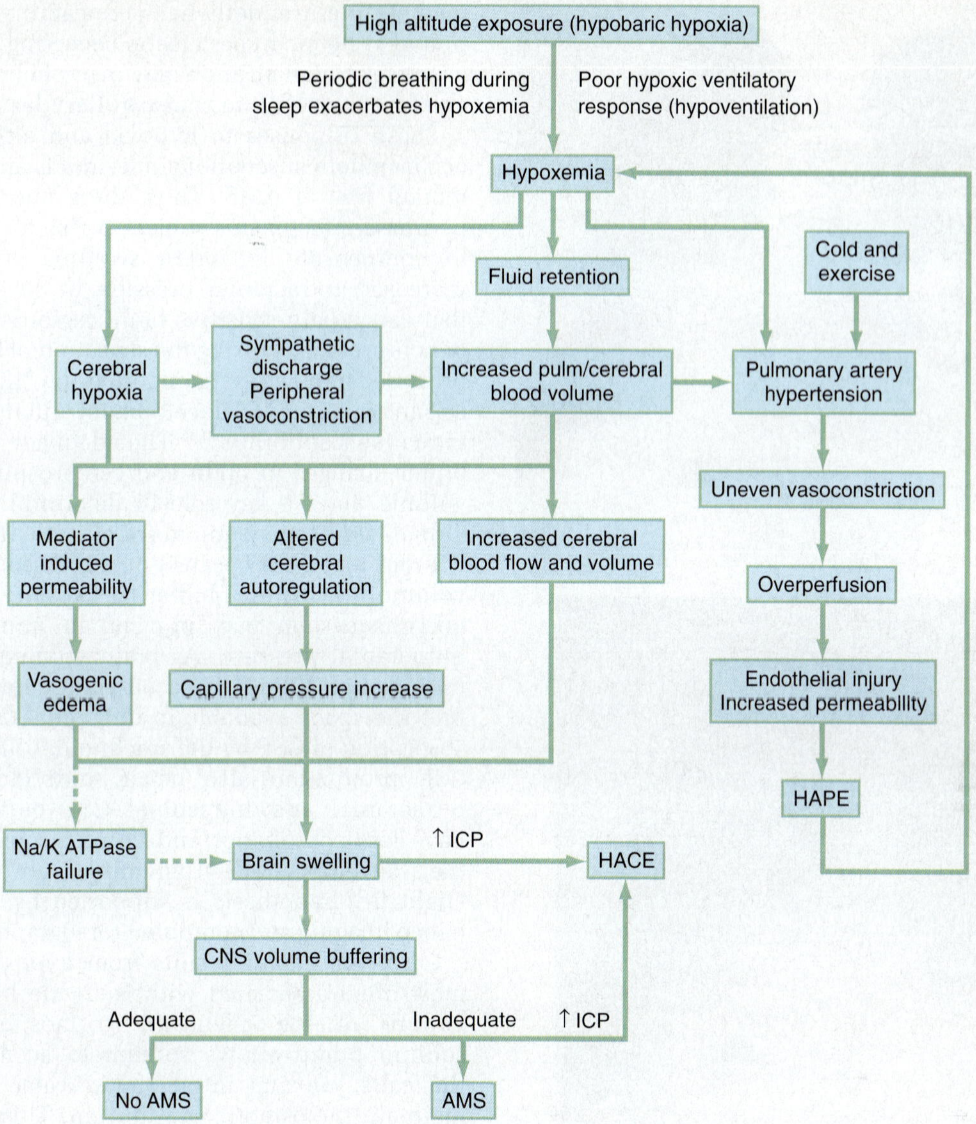

Figure 142-3. Proposed mechanisms for the development of acute mountain sickness (AMS), high-altitude pulmonary edema (HAPE), and high-altitude cerebral edema (HACE). CNS, central nervous system; ICP, intracranial pressure.

bate pulmonary hypertension.[19,20] Pulmonary blood volumes and pulmonary hypertension are increased by sympathetic nervous system stimulation and catecholamine release.[21,22] In HAPE-susceptible individuals, pulmonary hypertension becomes severe and an uneven distribution of pulmonary vasoconstriction results in overperfusion, increased capillary pressures, distention, and leakage in the remaining vessels.[23,24] This explains the patchy nature of the infiltrate seen on a chest radiograph with HAPE (Figure 142-4). Overperfusion of a restricted vascular bed as the pathogenesis of HAPE is supported by the observation that people born with congenital unilateral absence of a pulmonary artery are very susceptible to HAPE.[25] These individuals deliver their entire cardiac output to one lung, predisposing them to overperfusion injury.

The nature of the pulmonary vascular leak is unclear. Overperfusion and the resultant mechanical shear forces that lead to endothelial damage and changes in membrane permeability appear to be the primary mechanism.[26] Inflammatory mediators now appear to be a secondary response to the mechanical injury caused by overperfusion.[24,27] Once the vascular leak occurs and alveolar fluid accumulates, HAPE may develop due to a defect in transepithelial sodium transport that impairs the clearance of alveolar fluid.[28]

Preexisting inflammation, however, may also be a risk factor for HAPE. A preexisting respiratory infection during ascent to high altitude increases susceptibility to HAPE, particularly in children.[29] Inflammation may therefore "sensitize" the pulmonary endothelium to mechanical injury and increase susceptibility to HAPE during ascent.

The clinical manifestations of AMS/HACE are the result of central nervous system dysfunction. Vasogenic edema resulting from increased permeability of brain capillary endothelial cells appears to be the primary mechanism responsible for the development of HACE.[30] Magnetic resonance imaging in patients with HACE reveals white matter changes consistent with

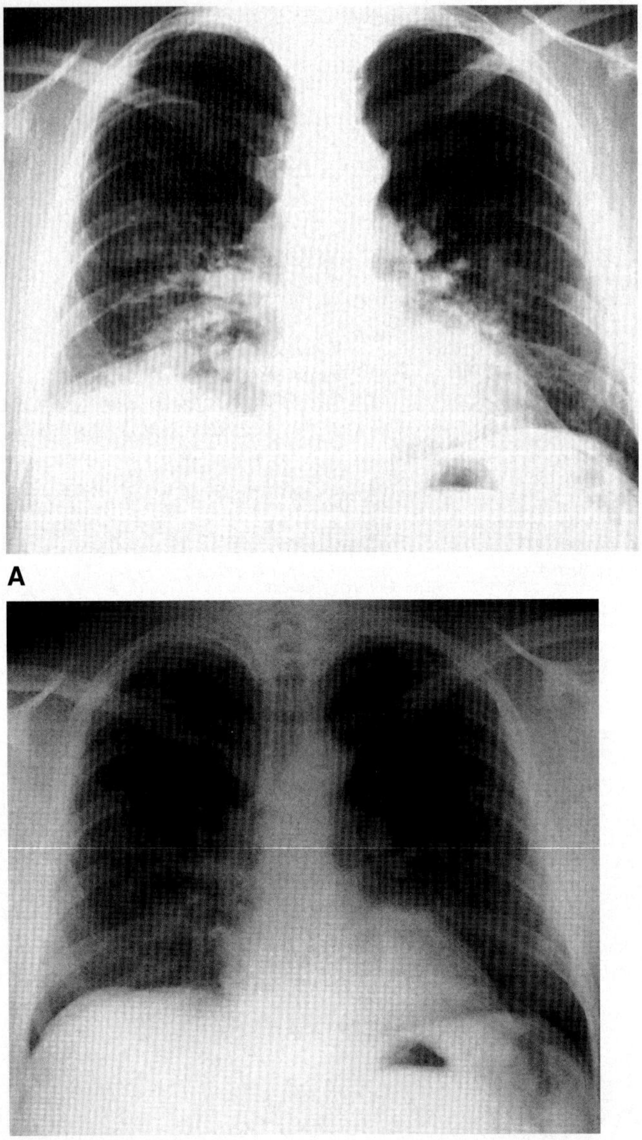

A

B

Figure 142-4. Chest radiograph of a patient with high-altitude pulmonary edema. **A,** Before treatment. **B,** After treatment. (Courtesy of Richard Nicholas, MD, Snake River Health Clinic, Keystone, Colo.)

vasogenic edema[31] (see Figure 142-6). Vasogenic edema is also implicated in the origin of AMS. This breakdown of the blood-brain barrier is most likely the result of both mechanical factors and biochemical mediation of permeability.

The vasodilatory response to hypoxemia causes an increase of cerebral blood flow and cerebral blood volume.[30,32] In susceptible individuals, this vasodilation may be responsible for the headache in patients with mild AMS.[33] Hypoxemia can also result in impaired vascular autoregulation,[34] causing increased pressure transmission to the brain's capillary beds, resulting in vasogenic edema.[16] Additional circumstances, however, may be necessary for the development of vasogenic edema. Biochemical inflammatory mediators may contribute to vasogenic edema formation. Vascular endothelial growth factor, the inducible form of nitric oxide synthase, and bradykinin may mediate brain endothelial permeability.[35-37] The addition of systemic hypertension occurring with strenuous exercise at high altitude may overwhelm the brain vasculature, resulting in transcapillary leakage.

These responses to hypoxia and altitude exposure occur in both susceptible individuals and in those who remain free of AMS. Thus, there must be an overall permissive factor in a subject at risk for AMS that fails to compensate for brain swelling. This results in increased intracranial pressure or structural changes that cause pain-sensitive brain regions to be stretched or compressed, causing the sensation of headache. Ross proposed and Hackett supported the "tight fit" hypothesis to explain AMS development and its inherent individual susceptibility.[30,38] The adequacy of the space to buffer changes in brain and cerebrospinal fluid (CSF) volume plays a key role in determining which individuals develop symptoms of altitude illness. As brain volume increases because of increased cerebral blood volume, the volume-buffering capacity of the central nervous system may prevent an immediate rise of intracranial pressure. As brain volume increases, the intracranial CSF is displaced via the foramen magnum into the space available in the spinal canal. Increased absorption of CSF by the arachnoid villi and decreased CSF production also occur. Individuals with less intracranial and intraspinal CSF buffering capacity have less compliance and become more symptomatic (i.e., develop AMS) from mild brain swelling. This "tight fit" hypothesis is supported by magnetic resonance imaging and computed tomography studies.[30,38,39]

Cytotoxic edema results from hypoxic cell damage most often associated with ischemic hypoxic insults. Failure of the adenosine triphosphate–dependent sodium pump allows sodium to accumulate within the cells, causing intracellular water to increase to maintain the osmotic equilibrium. This mechanism of pathologic intracellular water accumulation is not likely to be a primary mechanism for the development of HACE but rather the result of the increased cell ischemia caused initially by vasogenic edema[31]; thus, cytotoxic edema may develop as HACE progresses but cannot explain the pathophysiology of AMS or early HACE.

Hypobaria appears to play a role in the development of AMS. Sea level experiments that expose subjects to hypoxia alone do not result in AMS; however, when hypoxia is combined with hypobaria, AMS does occur.[40] Although microbubble formation may be a mechanism, the exact role of hypobaria regarding altitude pathophysiology remains unclear.

ACUTE MOUNTAIN SICKNESS

The syndrome of high-altitude illness represents a spectrum of clinical conditions that range in severity from mild AMS with an unpleasant yet not severe constellation of symptoms to the life-threatening conditions of HAPE and HACE. AMS, however, may be the benign presentation of a process that can rapidly progress to life-threatening HAPE or HACE.

BOX 142-2. Acute Mountain Sickness

Incidence	12% to 67%, varies with rate of ascent; rare below 8000 feet, most common with rapid ascent to altitudes greater than 10,000 feet
Signs and symptoms	Headache, anorexia, nausea, fatigue, dizziness, difficulty sleeping
Treatment	Mild cases are usually self-limited and do not require treatment; discontinue ascent, rest; for moderate case, administer acetazolamide, aspirin, or acetaminophen for headache; prochlorperazine for nausea; supplemental oxygen if available; descend if persistent or severe; add dexamethasone in severe cases
Prevention	Gradual ascent to allow acclimatization; high-carbohydrate diet, avoidance of alcohol or smoking; acetazolamide if ascent is rapid or know history of recurrent acute mountain sickness

Clinical Presentation

The symptoms of mild AMS are very similar to those of a viral syndrome, an ethanol "hangover," or simple physical exhaustion. The vague nature of this presentation results in many misdiagnoses. In the setting of recent high-altitude exposure, symptoms suggestive of AMS should be considered as being caused by high altitude until proven otherwise.

To diagnose AMS, a patient must be in the setting of a recent gain in altitude, be at the new altitude for at least several hours, and report a headache *plus* at least one of the following symptoms: gastrointestinal upset (anorexia, nausea, or vomiting), general weakness or fatigue, dizziness or light-headedness, or difficulty sleeping (Box 142-2).[41] The headache may vary from mild to severe, is generally bitemporal and throbbing in nature, and is worse during the night and on awakening or suddenly becoming upright. Anorexia and nausea, with or without vomiting, are common, and the other symptoms described can range in severity from mild to incapacitating. The disturbance of sleep caused by periodic breathing is common in all visitors to high altitudes but is exacerbated in the setting of AMS. The symptoms of AMS develop within a few hours after arrival at high altitude and generally reach maximum severity between 24 and 48 hours, followed by a gradual resolution. Most individuals become symptom free by the third or fourth day.

Among infants and very young children, AMS is manifested by increased fussiness, decreased playfulness, decreased appetite, and sleep disturbance.[7] In most cases of AMS in very young children, all of these symptoms are present. Many of the symptoms manifested by AMS can also result from the disruption of normal routine. A change in environment, sleeping accommodation, or eating habits can result in a fussy, unhappy child. Additionally, the occurrence of an acute illness can also mimic AMS in young children. If occult bacteremia or another serious illness is suspected in a young child, descent to lower altitude is recommended to eliminate the confounding variable of altitude illness.

There are no diagnostic physical findings in cases of mild AMS. Although dyspnea on exertion is universal at high altitudes, dyspnea at rest is an early indication of HAPE, and a careful examination for pulmonary edema is indicated. Similarly, any evidence of cerebellar dysfunction, such as mild ataxia or alteration in mentation, mandates descent because of early evidence of HACE.

Management

The proper management of AMS must include adherence to the principle that, *after the symptoms of altitude illness occur, further ascent to a higher sleeping altitude is contraindicated.* Halting ascent or activity to allow further acclimatization may reverse the symptoms; however, continuing the ascent exacerbates the underlying pathologic processes and may lead to disastrous results.

The presence of neurologic abnormalities (e.g., ataxia or altered mentation) or evidence of severe pulmonary edema mandates immediate descent because these signs indicate a progression of AMS to the more dangerous forms of altitude illness. AMS that becomes worse or does not respond to maintenance of altitude, rest, and pharmacologic intervention also constitutes an indication for descent. A descent of 1500 to 3000 feet effectively reverses high-altitude illness in most cases. Descent should be continued until improvement is seen, and efforts to minimize exertion should be instituted during the descent.

Treatment of AMS with acetazolamide speeds the process of acclimatization and, if given early in the development of the illness, leads to a more rapid resolution of symptoms. A dose of 250 mg of acetazolamide given at the onset of symptoms and repeated twice daily is effective therapy for AMS.[42] The treatment of AMS in children is not studied but there is no reason to believe that their response would be any different from that of adults. The dose for children is 2.5 mg/kg/dose to a maximum of 250 mg given twice daily.

Acetazolamide is a carbonic anhydrase inhibitor that induces a renal bicarbonate diuresis, causing a metabolic acidosis and thereby increasing ventilation and arterial oxygenation. This respiratory stimulation improves sleep when the severe hypoxemia caused by periodic breathing is eradicated by acetazolamide. The diuretic effects may be of benefit for the fluid retention common in patients with AMS. This drug also lowers CSF volume and pressure, which may play an additional role in its therapeutic and prophylactic use.

The most common adverse reactions to acetazolamide include paresthesias and polyuria. Less common reactions include nausea, drowsiness, tinnitus, and transient myopia. Carbonic anhydrase inhibition at the tongue causes dysgeusia, altering the flavor of carbonated beverages. This drug should be avoided in patients with a sulfa allergy, breast-feeding mothers, and pregnant women.

Supplemental oxygen administration addresses the primary insult of high-altitude exposure. In most cases, oxygen relieves the headache that is common in victims of AMS. Oxygen is also effective for AMS when given in small amounts (1-2 L/min) during sleep. In the wilderness, oxygen tanks are heavy and are usually unavailable in adequate amounts; therefore, oxygen therapy is usually reserved for the more serious manifestations of high-altitude illness. In resort settings, oxygen may be easily available for use in the hotel or condominium.

Treatment of headache, nausea, and insomnia can be beneficial during the course of mild AMS. Aspirin, ibuprofen, and acetaminophen are useful for the treatment of headache; however, narcotic analgesics should be avoided because they depress the HVR and the respiratory drive during sleep. Nausea and vomiting can be treated with prochlorperazine, which, unlike other antiemetics, stimulates the HVR.

Insomnia generally results from periodic breathing, experienced by most visitors to altitude. This is best treated with the respiratory stimulant acetazolamide.[43] Doses of acetazolamide as low as 62.5 to 125 mg at bedtime may prevent periodic breathing and eradicate insomnia. Benzodiazepines and other sedative-hypnotics should be avoided because of their tendency to decrease ventilation during sleep. Some climbers experience unusual reactions to diazepam at high altitudes, including agitation, hallucinations, and disorientation. These reactions occur in individuals who had previously used diazepam at lower altitudes without any difficulties. Zolpidem does not depress ventilation and may prove useful in cases of AMS-related insomnia.[44]

Dexamethasone is an effective treatment for AMS. A dose of 8 mg is given initially, followed by 4 mg every 6 hours.[45] No significant adverse reactions are reported; however, symptoms can recur when the treatment is withdrawn. The reduction of symptoms while using dexamethasone may be the result of its euphoric effects. Although dexamethasone can resolve the symptoms of AMS, it does not play a role in acclimatization. Dexamethasone should be reserved for use in the setting of acetazolamide intolerance, or in more advanced cases of AMS, especially to help facilitate descent.

Prevention

Most of the symptoms of mild AMS are benign in nature, and many individuals tolerate them without difficulty. These symptoms, however, can be unpleasant and debilitating to the point that travel, business, or vacation plans must be interrupted. Up to 50% of individuals with AMS report a decrease in activity.[4]

Slow ascent, allowing adequate time for acclimatization, is the best method of prevention; however, often the time constraints of most vacationers make slow ascent unrealistic. The major concern lies in the sleeping altitude during any individual ascent. Ideally, the first night should not be spent at an altitude higher than 8000 feet, with a subsequent increase of not more than 2000 feet each night. One extra night of acclimatization should be added for every 3000 to 4000 feet of altitude gain above 10,000 feet. If the journey begins at an altitude above 10,000 feet, then three nights should be spent acclimatizing before any further increase in sleeping altitude. Excursions during the day to higher altitudes with a return to a lower sleeping altitude are acceptable and aid in acclimatization.

Mild to moderate exercise is thought to aid in acclimatization; however, overexertion can contribute to the development of AMS. Intake of a high-carbohydrate diet and maintenance of adequate hydration are also recommended. Normal urine output and relatively clear (unconcentrated) urine are good guidelines for adequate hydration. Recommendations for hyperhydration are frequently recommended in the lay literature, yet no scientific evidence to support this advice exists. Drinking excessive amounts of free water may lead to hyponatremia and possibly complicate altitude illness.

In some cases, such as arrival at a high-altitude airport or the immediate dispatch of rescue personnel to high altitude, a slow ascent is impossible. Mountain climbers commonly ascend at rates that are higher than recommended, and some individuals continue to suffer AMS symptoms despite gradual ascent. Individuals who have a known susceptibility to the development of AMS and those for whom slow ascent is impractical may consider pharmacologic prophylactic intervention.

Numerous studies have demonstrated the effectiveness of acetazolamide in preventing AMS in adults, and many dosage protocols have proven successful.[2,3,46] Lower dosages provide similar prophylaxis with fewer adverse reactions than higher dosages. The recommended dosage is 125 mg twice daily starting 24 hours before ascent and continuing for the first 2 days at high altitude. Although unstudied, the recommended dosage of acetazolamide for AMS prophylaxis for children is 2.5 mg/kg/dose up to 125 mg total given twice daily.

Dexamethasone also prevents AMS. The lowest effective dosage is 4 mg every 12 hours.[46,47] Some patients experience the rapid onset of AMS after dexamethasone is discontinued. Dexamethasone does not facilitate acclimatization but rather reduces nausea and enhances mood; therefore, in most cases, dexamethasone use should be reserved for treatment of AMS rather than prophylaxis. Military or rescue personnel rapidly ascending to high altitude and individuals with sulfa allergies or acetazolamide intolerance are candidates for prophylaxis with dexamethasone. The combination of acetazolamide and dexamethasone may be more effective than either drug alone.[48]

Oxygen is an effective prophylactic modality for rescue personnel. Adequate supplies must be available to ensure the safety of all team members for the entire duration of the rescue. Air drops of oxygen can be life-

BOX 142-3. High-Altitude Pulmonary Edema

Incidence	0.01% to 15%, varies with rate of ascent; rare below 8000 feet but more common above 14,500 feet; usually occurs 2 to 4 days after arrival at high altitude
Signs and symptoms	Dyspnea at rest, cough, fatigue, headache, anorexia, cyanosis, rales, tachypnea, tachycardia
Treatment	Patients with mild cases may recover with bed rest; moderate cases can be treated with bed rest and supplemental oxygen if clinical monitoring is available; severe cases require descent; hyperbaric therapy if available; nifedipine 10 mg SL, then 30 mg SR bid if no descent or oxygen is available
Prevention	Gradual ascent and recognition of early AMS symptoms so that ascent is stopped before HAPE develops; with previous HAPE history, use nifedipine during ascent, then continue for 3 days; acetazolamide may be effective

AMS, acute mountain sickness; HAPE, high-altitude pulmonary edema; SL, sublingual; SR, slow release.

saving when weather or terrain prevents the immediate arrival of rescue personnel.

HIGH-ALTITUDE PULMONARY EDEMA

High-altitude pulmonary edema is the most common fatal manifestation of severe high-altitude illness (Box 142-3). Although HAPE is uncommon below 10,000 feet, it can occur, and even be fatal, at altitudes as low as 8000 feet. Episodes occurring between 8000 and 10,000 feet are usually related to heavy exercise, but at higher altitudes pulmonary edema can also occur at rest or with light activity.[49]

Some individuals are susceptible and experience HAPE with each ascent to altitude. Rarely, the congenital absence of a pulmonary artery exaggerates the pulmonary vascular response to hypoxia, resulting in recurrent HAPE at elevations lower than expected.[25] Many patients, however, have a single episode of HAPE and subsequently are able to return to high altitude without a recurrence. Conversely, those with previously uneventful high-altitude exposures may have HAPE develop in a future ascent.

Individuals who have been residents at high-altitude locations for extended periods may have pulmonary edema develop on re-ascent from a trip to low altitude. This phenomenon has been termed *re-entry HAPE.* The incidence of re-entry HAPE is not established; however, there seems to be an increased risk for children and young adults and possibly a greater incidence compared with HAPE experienced by low-altitude residents during their initial ascent.[50,51] This apparent increased susceptibility among children to develop HAPE is probably the result of developmental changes in pulmonary vascular reactivity and tone.

Clinical Presentation

The initial symptoms of HAPE usually begin insidiously 2 to 4 days after arrival at high altitude. Most cases occur during the second night, but HAPE may develop rapidly, with early symptoms apparent after just a few hours at high altitude. Marked dyspnea on exertion, fatigue with minimal to moderate effort, and dry cough are early manifestations of the disease. The symptoms of AMS usually occur concurrently with the development of HAPE.

As the HAPE patient deteriorates, usually through the night, the dyspnea intensifies with effort and is unrelieved by rest. *Dyspnea at rest must be recognized as a red flag that warns of the development of a serious pulmonary problem.* The cough becomes productive of copious amounts of clear, watery sputum, and in severe cases hemoptysis may be seen. As the condition intensifies, cerebral edema or simply severe hypoxemia causes central nervous system dysfunction, such as ataxia and altered mentation. Coma may follow and precede death in a few hours if oxygen therapy or descent is not instituted.

The physical examination reveals a few rales in patients with mild HAPE, usually found in the region of the right middle lobe, progressing to unilateral or bilateral rales, and then to diffuse bilateral rales and audible rhonchi and gurgles that can be heard without the stethoscope. Cyanosis of the nail beds alone may progress to severe central cyanosis as the patient's condition deteriorates. Tachypnea and tachycardia become more pronounced as severity increases. Elevated temperatures are common, and a concurrent respiratory tract infection is occasionally seen, especially in children.[29]

Ancillary Tests

Chest radiographs can help elucidate the nature of the illness. The infiltrates seen in HAPE victims are alveolar and patchy in distribution, with areas of clearing between the patches. Unilateral infiltrates may be present in mild cases; however, bilateral infiltrates are seen in more advanced cases, with involvement of the right midlung field most common (see Figure 142-4). Pleural effusion is rare but may be present in severe cases. The extent of the edema present on the chest radiograph roughly parallels the clinical severity. Of note, the radiographic findings of cardiomegaly, batwing distribution of infiltrates, and Kerley B lines, which are typical of cardiogenic pulmonary edema, are absent in cases of HAPE.

Radiographic evidence for HAPE clears rapidly after initiation of treatment; some mild cases may clear in 4 to 6 hours and most clear by 24 hours. Radiographs of patients with severe HAPE may reveal infiltrates that persist for as long as 2 weeks, even though the clinical symptoms have resolved.

An electrocardiogram reveals tachycardia and evidence of right heart strain, including right axis deviation, P wave abnormalities, tall R waves in the precordial leads, and S waves in the lateral leads.[49] Hemodynamic studies reveal increased pulmonary vascular resistance, elevated pulmonary artery pressures, and normal pulmonary wedge pressures. Echocardiography studies demonstrate high estimated pulmonary artery pressures, pulmonary vascular resistance, and normal left ventricular function.[22]

Differential Diagnosis

Pneumonia can be misdiagnosed in the setting of HAPE because the symptoms and signs of pneumonia are similar to those of HAPE. The incidence of pneumonia and the common organisms responsible for pneumonia at high altitude are unknown, but visitors to high altitudes may be predisposed to acquiring bacterial infections because of impaired T lymphocyte function.[52] Patients who present with symptoms compatible with pneumonia at high altitude should be treated for HAPE. If any doubt exists regarding the diagnosis of HAPE versus pneumonia, empiric antibiotic therapy should be initiated. Because of the mild immunosuppression coincident with high-altitude exposure, the treatment of any serious infectious illness at high altitude requires oxygen and descent in addition to local wound care and antibiotics.[52]

High-altitude bronchitis and pharyngitis are common problems among climbers. They may result from the increased ventilation of cold, dry air across the upper airway mucosa, causing mucosal inflammation. Copious sputum production is sometimes seen, and antibiotic therapy usually is not helpful. Coughing spasms may be severe and require codeine. Other therapeutic measures include hydration, lozenges, and steam inhalation. Any signs or symptoms of respiratory distress should alert the clinician to consider HAPE.

Death from pulmonary embolism at high altitude is described.[53] Hypercoagulability of the blood resulting from altitude effects, hyperviscosity caused by elevation in hematocrit and dehydration, and venous stasis caused by immobility when confined to a sleeping bag inside a tent are predisposing factors for deep venous thrombosis. The symptoms and signs of pulmonary embolism can mimic those of HAPE; however, embolic disease tends to have a more rapid onset, and pleuritic chest pain is a more prominent feature.

Management

If HAPE is recognized early, death usually can be avoided. Descent to a lower altitude, bed rest, and supplemental oxygen are most effective. In remote settings, where oxygen and medical expertise may be unavailable, immediate descent is a life-saving measure and should be a primary goal after diagnosing HAPE. Delaying descent while HAPE progresses or waiting for rescue personnel to initiate evacuation can prove fatal. Descents of 1500 to 3000 feet should be adequate to allow for a rapid recovery. After recovery, the victim may be able to re-ascend in 2 or 3 days.

Resting and keeping warm are important in HAPE therapy to avoid cold- or exercise-induced pulmonary hypertension. Mild cases of HAPE can be treated without descent or oxygen with 1 or 2 days of bed rest. Oxygen administration increases the rate of improvement. Moderate cases can be treated without descent if bed rest and adequate supplies of supplemental oxygen are available. At ski resorts in Colorado, with immediate cessation of further ascent, many victims of mild HAPE are administered supplemental oxygen in their hotel rooms, and with careful monitoring are able to recover, avoid descent, and continue their ski holidays. Any treatment plan that does not include descent mandates serial examinations by clinicians with experience in managing high-altitude illness. If any deterioration is noted, prompt descent to a lower altitude is indicated.

On difficult terrain or in weather conditions that prevent or slow efforts to descend, oxygen administration (or hyperbaric therapy) is a life-saving measure. Rescue personnel should air drop oxygen supplies if immediate evacuation to lower altitudes will be delayed. High-flow rates of oxygen (6-8 L/min) by mask should be delivered initially to victims with severe HAPE until improvement is seen. Lower flow rates can then be used until recovery or descent is completed. Delivering oxygen with a continuous positive airway pressure mask improves oxygenation in HAPE victims, as compared with normal oxygen delivery.[54]

Patients with AMS and HAPE are treated successfully in hyperbaric chambers, which simulate descent, without the administration of supplemental oxygen. Hyperbaric therapy is equivalent to oxygen therapy for these conditions.[55] Several portable, lightweight (14.9-lb), fabric hyperbaric chambers are available that are pressurized manually (Figure 142-5). These chambers generate 103 mm Hg (2 psi) above the ambient pressure; this can simulate a descent of 4000 to 5000 feet at moderate altitudes and at the summit of Mt. Everest would simulate a descent of approximately 9000 feet. These devices can be lifesaving in patients with HAPE and HACE. Some nonambulatory patients are able to descend under their own power after a few hours in hyperbaric chambers.

In treating HAPE, agents that lower pulmonary artery pressure, pulmonary blood volume, and pulmonary vascular resistance would intuitively seem to be useful. Furosemide, 80 mg twice daily, is beneficial in treating HAPE and, when combined with morphine for the initial dose, results in even greater diuresis and clinical improvement. Some authors caution that deleterious dehydration may result from furosemide therapy and that the potential ventilatory depression caused by morphine can further increase the severity of the underlying hypoxemia that lies at the root of AMS.[49] Others argue that during the state of antidiuresis found with severe AMS, furosemide may be useful and that no documented reports of deleterious effects from this treatment exist.[56] Furosemide may also be useful in the setting in which both oxygen therapy and descent are not available options. Nifedipine, a pulmonary vasodilator, may prove to be a useful adjunct for HAPE,

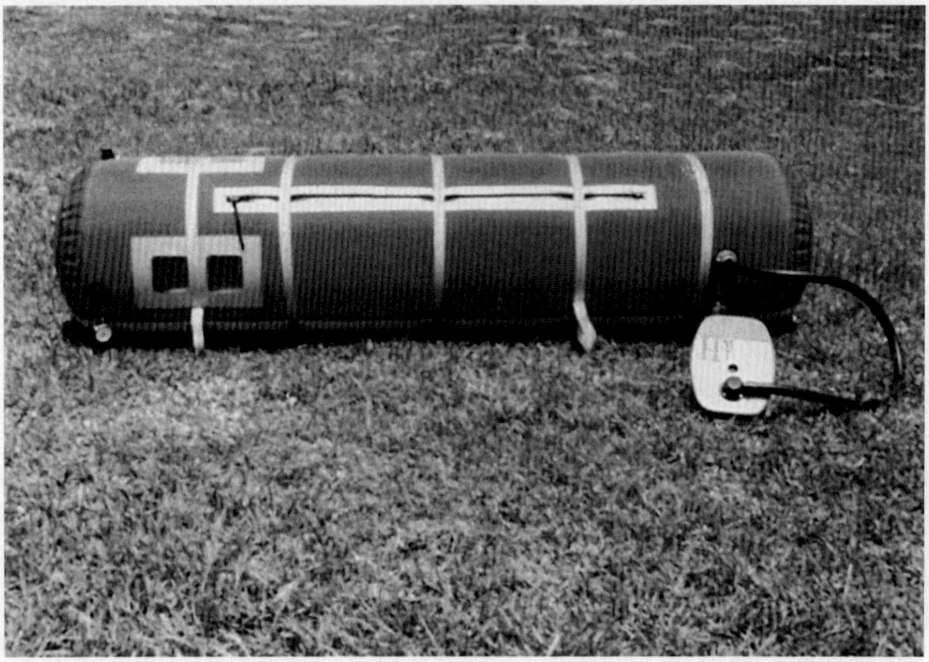

Figure 142-5. Gamow bag: lightweight, portable hyperbaric chamber. Note the attached foot-operated pressure pump. (Courtesy of Portable Hyperbarics, Ilion, NY.)

especially when oxygen is unavailable or descent is impossible.[22,57] Nifedipine does not improve pulmonary hemodynamics as much as oxygen and does not have an additive effect when administered with oxygen.[22] Treatment with 10 mg of nifedipine sublingually every 4 to 6 hours or 30 mg of a slow-release preparation administered once or twice daily is effective. A response to treatment with improvement in symptoms is usually noted within 15 to 30 minutes after the first sublingual dose.[57] Patients should be monitored for the development of hypotension during nifedipine administration.

Disposition

Rapid recovery is usually seen after descent to lower altitudes, and observation of the patient in the emergency department to ensure adequate room air oxygenation is generally adequate. Occasionally, admission to the hospital is indicated to maintain the SaO_2 greater than 90%. Hypocapnia, alkalosis, and radiographic evidence of HAPE may persist for several days. After oxygen saturation remains greater than 90% on room air and clinical improvement is apparent, the patient can be discharged. If the patient requires air travel to return home (cabin pressures equal approximately 8000 feet), additional recovery time before travel or arrangement for supplemental oxygen administration is advised. Detection of a heart murmur in a patient with HAPE should lead to an evaluation looking for cardiac structural anomalies that may increase pulmonary vascular resistance.

Prevention

Individuals with a prior history of HAPE are candidates for prophylactic therapy. Nifedipine, 20 mg three times daily, taken before ascent and continued at altitude for 3 days, is effective in preventing a recurrence of HAPE.[58] Individuals with a prior history of HAPE should also avoid extreme exertion during the first 2 days at altitude. As with all forms of serious altitude illness, a gradual ascent that allows time to acclimatize and immediate cessation of further ascent at the onset of symptoms are the most effective means of prevention.

BOX 142-4. High-Altitude Cerebral Edema

Incidence	Lower than 1% to 2%, uncommon as a pure entity; usually associated with the presence of severe AMS and HAPE
Signs and symptoms	Ataxia, severe headache, nausea and vomiting, altered mentation, seizures, coma
Treatment	Immediate evacuation to a lower altitude; oxygen, bed rest, dexamethasone, and hyperbaric therapy while awaiting descent

AMS, acute mountain sickness; HAPE, high-altitude pulmonary edema.

HIGH-ALTITUDE CEREBRAL EDEMA

High-altitude cerebral edema is the least common yet most severe form of high-altitude illness. Death from HACE at as low as 8200 feet has been reported, although most cases occur above 12,000 feet. Mild AMS can progress to severe HACE with coma in as little as 12 hours. The usual time course is 1 to 3 days for the development of severe symptoms. In some cases, the severe symptoms and coma take 5 to 9 days to develop (Box 142-4).[59]

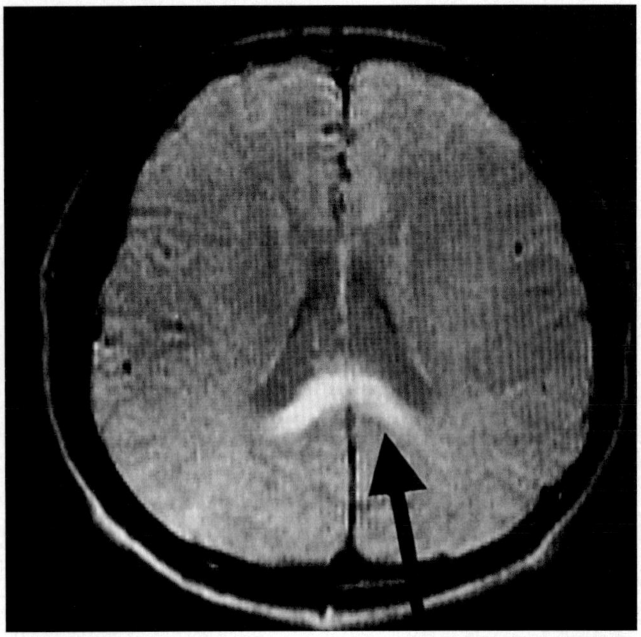

Figure 142-6. Axial proton-weighted magnetic resonance imaging scan of a mountain climber with high-altitude cerebral edema. *Arrow* demonstrates the markedly increased signal (edema) in the splenium of the corpus callosum. (Courtesy of Dr. Peter Hackett.)

Clinical Presentation

High-altitude cerebral edema is characterized by evidence of global cerebral dysfunction and represents the most severe manifestation of AMS. The symptoms of severe AMS (headache, fatigue, vomiting), as well as those of HAPE (cough and dyspnea), are usually present. HACE-specific signs include ataxia, generalized seizures, slurred speech, rare focal neurologic deficits, and altered mentation. The latter can range from mild emotional lability or confusion to hallucinations and ultimately decreased levels of consciousness that may proceed to coma and death.[59] Magnetic resonance imaging of patients with HACE reveals white matter changes consistent with vasogenic edema (Figure 142-6).[31]

Cerebellar ataxia is the most sensitive sign for early recognition of HACE. This early appearance of ataxia reflects the particular sensitivity of the cerebellum to hypoxia. Ataxia alone is an indication for immediate descent.

Retinal hemorrhages are common but often occur as an isolated finding. Papilledema and occasionally cranial nerve palsy can also be found in the setting of increased intracranial pressure. The presence of focal neurologic signs warrants an investigation into the possibility of a vascular lesion. Although rare, the occurrence of cerebral thrombosis and transient ischemic attacks, in the absence of high-altitude illness, has been documented at high altitude.[60,61] Differentiating between HACE and stroke may be difficult. The absence of any other evidence for high-altitude illness, or signs that persist despite adequate treatment of high-altitude illness, suggests the presence of a vascular lesion.

Management

Early recognition and initiation of descent are the keys to successful therapy for HACE. High-flow oxygen should be administered, if available. Steroid therapy is recommended and may result in recovery from HACE without neurologic deficits. The initial dose of dexamethasone is 8 mg parenterally, or orally in mild cases, followed by 4 mg every 6 hours.

Patients with severely altered levels of consciousness require tracheal intubation and hyperventilation to control elevated intracranial pressures. Diuretics (e.g., furosemide) and hypertonic solutions (e.g., mannitol) decrease intracranial pressure. Many patients with HACE are already volume depleted from poor fluid intake, and care must be taken to ensure adequate intravascular volumes if a diuretic agent is used.

Hyperbaric treatment of HACE is also effective and may result in temporary improvement, allowing for self-rescue. Conversely, coma may persist for several days after descent to lower altitudes, so placement of HACE patients in a hyperbaric device may only delay the more comprehensive care available in the hospital setting.

Long-term neurologic deficits, such as ataxia and cognitive impairment, are reported after recovery from acute episodes of HACE. Both transient and long-lasting neurobehavioral impairments can occur in mountaineers after climbing to extreme altitude without experiencing clinical HACE.[62] Some of these sequelae can persist for 1 year. Because of the potential for long-lasting neurologic injury, the clinician who treats high-altitude illness must be extremely sensitive to the early manifestations of HACE. Early treatment for HACE generally results in good outcomes, but after coma is present, the mortality rate exceeds 60%.[63]

HIGH-ALTITUDE RETINAL HEMORRHAGE

High-altitude retinal hemorrhage (HARH) is the most common type of retinopathy in visitors to high altitude.[64] These hemorrhages are common at altitudes over 17,500 feet, although they can occur at lower levels.[65]

The exact incidence of HARH is unknown because most patients are asymptomatic, with HARH noted only on retinoscopy. HARH is not generally related to the presence of mild AMS but does seem to be related to strenuous exercise at high altitude. At any altitude, in the setting of severe cases of HAPE or HACE, retinal hemorrhages are commonly noted.[65]

Hemorrhages generally are seen in the peripapillary area and throughout the fundus but usually spare the macula (Figure 142-7). Retinal hemorrhages usually are self-limited, do not produce any long-term effects, and resolve without treatment in 2 to 3 weeks. With macular involvement, central scotomata may be

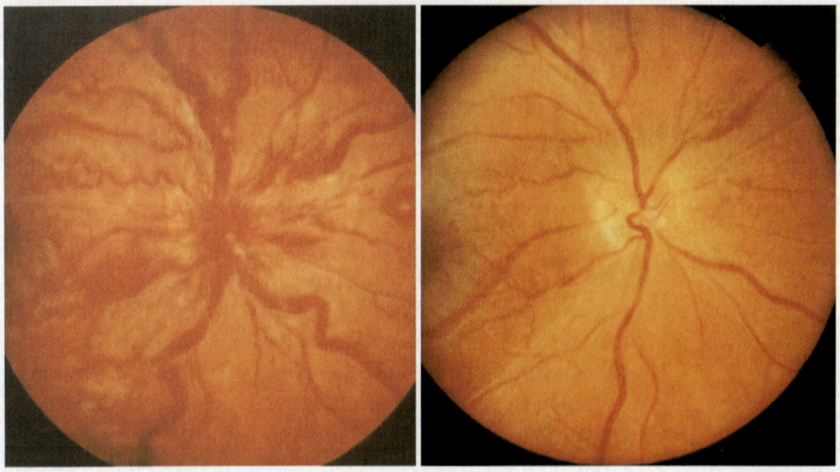

A B

Figure 142-7. High-altitude retinal hemorrhages. **A,** Acute. **B,** After 1 week of resolution. (Courtesy of Dr. Charles Houston.)

noticed for several years, gradually resolving. In some cases, however, these visual defects are permanent. HARH is more likely to occur among individuals with a previous history of HARH; however, because of the generally benign nature of the problem, this does not pose a contraindication to return to high altitude unless the macular region is involved.

ALTITUDE AND UNDERLYING MEDICAL CONDITIONS

Individuals with underlying, chronic medical conditions may be especially sensitive to the potential deleterious effects of high-altitude exposure. This interrelationship is not well studied, yet empiric evidence suggests that individuals with diseases such as moderate to severe chronic obstructive pulmonary disease (COPD) and coronary artery disease have these illnesses aggravated by the relatively hypoxic atmosphere at high altitude and may have a higher predisposition for the development of high-altitude illness.

Respiratory Illnesses

Travelers with COPD to moderate altitudes have underlying anatomic and physiologic changes that predispose them to develop hypoxemia, sleep apnea, pulmonary hypertension, and ventilation disorders. It is not surprising that COPD is a risk factor for the development of AMS.[4] Although oxygen saturation remains more than 90% in a healthy, awake individual until an altitude of 8000 feet, patients with COPD may desaturate below 90% at lower altitudes. Travel to 5000 feet, however, did not result in significant desaturation below 90% in one group of COPD patients and did not produce significant adverse effects on the systemic circulation in another group at 8000 feet.[66]

A nomogram predicts the arterial oxygen partial pressure at the expected high-altitude exposure (Figure 142-8). Patients with asthma, on the other hand, may have fewer problems at altitude, due to decreased allergies, pollutants, and decreased airflow turbulence. There have been no descriptions of worsening hypoxemia or exacerbations of asthma attacks at altitude. In addition, AMS incidence is not increased in asthmatic persons.[67]

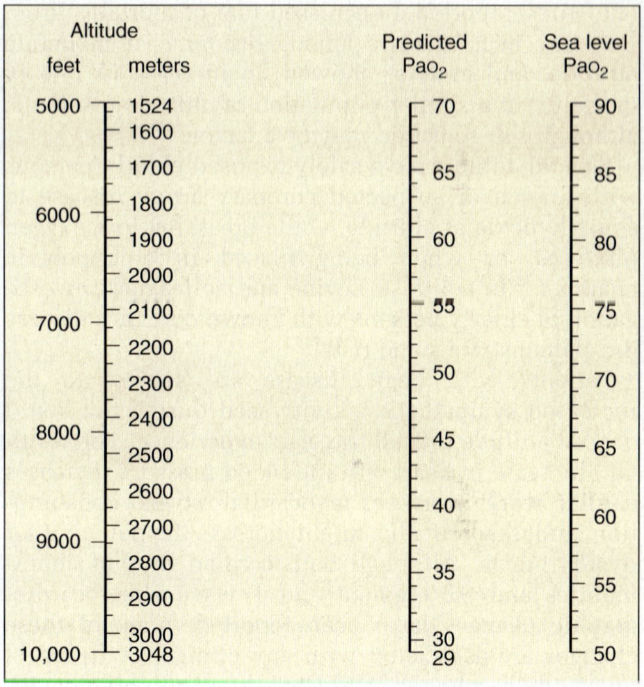

Figure 142-8. Nomogram for prediction of oxygenation at high altitude, based on sea level arterial partial pressure of oxygen (Pa_{O_2}). Find sea level Pa_{O_2} and lay a straightedge across to altitude to find the predicted Pa_{O_2}. (Redrawn from Hackett PH, Roach RC, Sutton JR: high-altitude medicine. In Auerbach P, Geehr E (eds): *Management of Wilderness and Environmental Emergencies*, 2nd ed. St. Louis, Mosby, 1989, p 27.)

High altitude increases hypoxic pulmonary vasoconstriction and may potentiate the development of cor pulmonale, which is known to adversely affect survival at sea level.[68] Colorado, for example, has a relatively low incidence of COPD but a higher mortality rate than expected from emphysema.[69]

Individuals with symptomatic pulmonary hypertension, a known complication of COPD, should avoid even moderate altitudes because the primary underlying disease can be exacerbated and susceptibility to HAPE can occur. Any person with chronic COPD should be advised of the potential need for oxygen supplementation when traveling to moderate altitude, especially if dyspnea becomes worse.

Cardiovascular

Individuals with a history of congestive heart failure, angina, dysrhythmias, or coronary bypass surgery are rarely studied in this setting. The theoretical argument of decreased environmental oxygen availability to a diseased myocardium results in advice to avoid trips to high altitude; however, no studies report increased mortality in visitors to these locations. To the contrary, one study reported a decreased rate of mortality from ischemic heart disease among residents at moderate altitude, and another showed no increase in rate of mortality in a similar population of altitude residents, although self-selection may be a factor.[70,71]

Several authors have safely exposed elderly persons with known or suspected coronary artery disease to acute hypoxia at altitude, while breathing low oxygen mixtures, or when being placed in a hypobaric chamber.[72] In contrast, Levine and colleagues' investigation of elderly persons with known coronary disease did demonstrate some risk.[73]

Patients with heart disease are subject to the increased sympathetic activity seen during the first 3 days at altitude that all travelers experience. The resultant increase in heart rate and blood pressure increases cardiac work, increases myocardial oxygen consumption, and, theoretically, might increase the potential for dysrhythmias. Although both cardiac rhythm abnormalities and ST segment and T wave electrocardiographic changes have been reported, none of these changes are associated with any clinical evidence of myocardial ischemia.[72,74] Even when individuals with stable angina were exercised, there is conflicting evidence as to the probability of inducing malignant dysrhythmias or untoward cardiac events.[73,75] Anecdotal reports indicate that many people who have had coronary artery bypass grafts travel successfully to very high altitudes (higher than 17,000 feet) without ill effects; however, these individuals were asymptomatic and had normal exercise stress test results at sea level. Travelers with heart disease who ascended to moderate altitudes did not appear to have an increased incidence of AMS.[4,9]

Recommendations for travelers with mild stable coronary artery disease should include gradual ascent, limitation of activity, and continuation of antianginal and antihypertensive medications. Individuals who have more severe, symptomatic coronary disease or those in a high-risk group (low ejection fraction, abnormal stress test results, high-grade ventricular ectopy) should be cautioned against travel to high altitudes, but ascent to moderate elevations can be undertaken on an individual basis with the above precautions. If the anticipated workload at altitude is greater than the individual is accustomed to at sea level, exercise stress testing at this increased workload before ascent should be considered.[76]

Hypertension

High-altitude travel produces a mild increase in blood pressure and heart rate in healthy individuals because of increased catecholamine activity and resultant sympathetic tone. This increase begins in the first few days after ascent, is maximal at 2 to 3 weeks, and returns to baseline values over time at high altitude or on descent to sea level.[77]

The incidence of hypertension in sea level dwellers traveling to high altitude is 10% to 25%.[78] One study showed no difference in blood pressure readings, in either normotensive or hypertensive individuals, when measured at low altitudes (3000 feet), but significant increases in both blood pressure and heart rate at altitudes greater than 9800 feet.[79] This would suggest that people with severe hypertension should travel only to moderate altitudes. Although individual variability exists, patients with hypertension should be monitored frequently in the first few days at altitude. Antihypertensive medications should be continued for those travelers who take them.

Sickle Cell Disease

Patients with sickle cell disease are affected by the hypoxemia occurring at low to moderate altitudes (5000 to 6500 feet). Up to 20% of patients with hemoglobin sickle cell and sickle cell–thalassemia disease experienced vaso-occlusive crises, even under pressurized aircraft conditions.[80] Oxygen is therefore advised for air travelers who have sickle cell disease.

Although most people with sickle cell trait remain asymptomatic, this subgroup can experience the development of left upper quadrant pain as a result of splenic ischemia or infarction. Nonblacks, usually of Mediterranean origin, who have sickle cell trait may be more prone to splenic infarctions developing than blacks. Treatment is similar to that for other vasoocclusive crises.

Pregnancy

Studies of permanent high-altitude residents in Colorado and Peru have shown an increased incidence of complications in maternal, fetal, and neonatal life.[1] Babies born at high altitude have a lower birth weight compared with babies born at sea level. Fetal growth retardation at high altitude is believed to be the result of a reduction in uterine artery blood flow.

Pregnancy-induced hypertension, proteinuria, and peripheral edema (manifestations of toxemia and preeclampsia) are more common at high altitude and may also be related to maternal hypoxemia.[81] Although hypertension in pregnancy is more common at high altitudes, no evidence exists for an increase in spontaneous abortions, abruptio placentae, or placenta previa.

Travel by pregnant women to moderate altitudes appears to be safe, but caution is advised for lowland women with normal pregnancies who wish to travel above 13,000 feet, for pregnant women who wish to remain at high altitude for a prolonged period, and for women with complicated pregnancies.

Radial Keratotomy

Individuals who have had radial keratotomy may experience visual changes with ascent to altitude. This results from corneal swelling from ambient hypoxia because the cornea obtains its oxygen almost entirely by diffusion from the atmosphere. In normal corneas, this swelling is uniform but is exacerbated and nonuniform after the incisions previously made with the radial keratotomy procedure.[82] Photorefractive keratotomy, which uses a laser technique that does not produce incisions but instead shaves the cornea, does not result in similar problems. Patients with radial keratotomy may need to bring glasses of increasing refraction if they ascend to altitudes above 9000 feet.[83]

KEY CONCEPTS

- The symptoms of AMS can resemble a viral syndrome and include headache, nausea, anorexia, fatigue, and insomnia. Unlike other antiemetics, prochlorperazine beneficially stimulates the HVR.
- The management of altitude illness must include adherence to the principle that, after the symptoms occur and until symptoms resolve, further ascent is contraindicated.
- Dyspnea at rest is an early symptom of HAPE. As the HAPE patient's condition deteriorates, the dyspnea intensifies with effort and is unrelieved by rest.
- Cerebellar ataxia must be recognized as an early symptom of HACE, and descent is mandatory.
- Effective prophylaxis options for altitude illness include acetazolamide for AMS and nifedipine for HAPE. Dexamethasone should be reserved for acetazolamide intolerance, or to facilitate descent with severe AMS.

REFERENCES

1. Moore LG: Altitude aggravated illness: Examples from pregnancy and prenatal life. *Ann Emerg Med* 16:965, 1986.
2. Larson EB, et al: Acute mountain sickness and acetazolamide. Clinical efficacy and effect on ventilation. *JAMA* 288:328, 1982.
3. Hackett PH, Rennie ID, Levine HD: The incidence, importance, and prophylaxis of acute mountain sickness. *Lancet* 2:1149, 1976.
4. Honigman B, et al: Acute mountain sickness in a general tourist population at moderate altitudes. *Ann Intern Med* 118:587, 1993.
5. Singh I, et al: High altitude pulmonary oedema. *Lancet* 1:229, 1965.
6. Yaron M, et al: Physiologic response to moderate altitude exposure among infants and young children. *High Altitude Med Biol* 2:101, 2001.
7. Yaron M, et al: The diagnosis of acute mountain sickness in preverbal children. *Arch Pediatr Adolesc Med* 152:683, 1998.
8. Theis MK, et al: Acute mountain sickness in children at 2835 meters. *Am J Dis Child* 147:143, 1993.
9. Roach RC, et al: How well do older persons tolerate moderate altitude? *West J Med* 162:32, 1995.
10. Roach RC: The role of the hypoxic ventilatory response in performance at high altitude. In Wood SC, Roach RC (eds): *Sports and Exercise Medicine*. New York, Dekker, 1994, pp 211-224.
11. Matsuzawa Y, et al: Hypoxic ventilatory response and pulmonary gas exchange during exposure to high altitude in subjects susceptible to high altitude pulmonary edema (HAPE). In Sutton JR, Houston CS, Coates G (eds): *Hypoxia and the Brain*. Burlington, Vt, Queen City Press, 1995.
12. Pugh LG: High altitudes. In Edholm OG, Bacharach AL (eds): *The Physiology of Human Survival*. New York, Academic Press, 1965, pp 121-152.
13. Winslow RM: High altitude polycythemia. In West JB, Lahiri S (eds): *High Altitude and Man*. Bethesda, Md, American Physiological Society, 1984, pp 163-172.
14. Sutton JR, et al: Effects of acclimatization on sleep hypoxemia at altitude. In West JB, Lahiri S (eds): *High Altitude and Man*. Bethesda, Md, American Physiological Society, 1984, pp 141-146.
15. Bärtsch P, et al: Enhanced exercise-induced rise of aldosterone and vasopressin preceding mountain sickness. *J Appl Physiol* 71:136, 1991.
16. Krasney JA: A neurogenic basis for acute altitude illness. *Med Sci Sports Exerc* 26:195, 1994.
17. Bärtsch P, et al: Aldosterone, antidiuretic hormone and atrial natriuretic peptide in acute mountain sickness. In Sutton JR, Coates G, Houston CS (eds): *Hypoxia and Mountain Medicine*. Burlington, Vt, Queen City Press, 1992.
18. Westendorp RG, et al: Atrial natriuretic peptide improves pulmonary gas exchange in subjects exposed to hypoxia. *Am Rev Respir Dis* 148:304, 1993.
19. Roach RC, et al: Exercise exacerbates acute mountain sickness at simulated high altitude. *J Appl Physiol* 88:581, 2000.
20. Durand J, et al: Hypoxic pulmonary vasoconstriction and ambient temperature. In Brendel W, Zink RA (eds): *High Altitude Physiology and Medicine*. New York, Springer-Verlag, 1982, pp 263-265.
21. Duplain H, et al: Augmented sympathetic activation during short-term hypoxia and high-altitude exposure in subjects susceptible to high-altitude pulmonary edema. *Circulation* 99:1713, 1999.
22. Hackett PH, et al: The effect of vasodilators on pulmonary hemodynamics in high altitude pulmonary edema: A comparison. *Int J Sports Med* 13:S68, 1992.
23. Scherrer U, et al: Inhaled nitric oxide for high-altitude pulmonary edema. *N Engl J Med* 334:624, 1996.
24. Maggiorini M, et al: High altitude pulmonary edema is initially a hydrostatic, not a permeability edema. *Circulation* 103:2078, 2001.
25. Hackett PH, et al: High altitude pulmonary edema in persons without the right pulmonary artery. *N Engl J Med* 302:1070, 1980.
26. West JB, Mathieu-Costello O: Stress failure in pulmonary capillaries: A mechanism for high altitude pulmonary edema. In Sutton JR, Coates G, Houston CS (eds): *Hypoxia and Mountain Medicine*. Burlington, Vt: Queen City Press, 1992, pp 229-240.
27. Swenson ER, et al: Pathogenesis of high-altitude pulmonary edema: Inflammation is not an etiologic factor. *JAMA* 287:2228, 2002.
28. Scherrer U, et al: High-altitude pulmonary edema: From exaggerated pulmonary hypertension to a defect in transepithelial sodium transport. *Adv Exp Med Biol* 474:93, 1999.

29. Durmowicz AG, et al: Inflammatory processes may predispose children to high-altitude pulmonary edema. *J Pediatr* 130:838, 1997.
30. Hackett PH: High altitude cerebral edema and acute mountain sickness: A pathophysiology update. In Roach RC, Wagner PD, Hackett PH (eds): *Hypoxia: Into the Next Millennium*, vol 474. New York, Plenum/Kluwer Academic Publishing, 1999, pp 23-46.
31. Hackett PH, et al: High-altitude cerebral edema evaluated with magnetic resonance imaging: Clinical correlation and pathophysiology. *JAMA* 280:1920, 1998.
32. Lassen NA: Increase of cerebral blood flow at high altitude: Its possible relation to AMS. *Int J Sports Med* 13:S47, 1992.
33. Sanchez del Rio M, Moskowitz MA: High altitude headache: Lessons from headaches at sea level. *Adv Exp Med Biol* 474:145, 1999.
34. Levine BD, Zhang R, Roach RC: Dynamic cerebral autoregulation at high altitude. *Adv Exp Med Biol* 474:319, 1999.
35. Severinghaus JW: Hypothetical roles of angiogenesis, osmotic swelling, and ischemia in high-altitude cerebral edema. *J Appl Physiol* 79:375, 1995.
36. Clark IA, et al: Can excessive iNOS induction explain much of the illness of acute mountain sickness [abstract] In Roach RC, Wagner PD, Hackett PH (eds): *Hypoxia: Into the Next Millennium*, vol 474. New York, Plenum/Kluwer Academic Publishing, 1999, p 373.
37. Schilling L, Wahl M: Mediators of cerebral edema. In Roach RC, Wagner PD, Hackett PH (eds): *Hypoxia: Into the Next Millennium*, vol 474. New York, Plenum/Kluwer Academic Publishing, 1999, pp 123-141.
38. Ross RT: The random nature of cerebral mountain sickness. *Lancet* 1:990, 1985.
39. Zavasky D, Hackett P: Cerebral etiology of acute mountain sickness: MRI findings [abstract]. *Wilderness Environ Med* 6:229, 1995.
40. Roach RC, Loeppky JA: Does hypobaria play a role in the development of the high altitude illnesses? In Sutton JR, Houston CS, Coates G (eds): *Hypoxia and the Brain*. Burlington, Vt, Queen City Press, 1995, pp 277-283.
41. Roach RC, et al: The Lake Louise acute mountain sickness scoring system. In Sutton JR, Houston CS, Coates G (eds): *Hypoxia and Molecular Medicine*. Burlington, Vt, Queen City Press, 1993, pp 272-274.
42. Grissom CK, et al: Acetazolamide in the treatment of acute mountain sickness: Clinical efficacy and effect on gas exchange. *Ann Intern Med* 116:461, 1992.
43. Hackett PH, et al: Respiratory stimulants and sleep periodic breathing at high altitude: Almitrine versus acetazolamide. *Am Rev Respir Dis* 135:896, 1987.
44. Beaumont M, et al: Effect of zolpidem on sleep and ventilatory patterns at simulated altitude of 4,000 meters. *Am J Respir Crit Care Med* 153:1864, 1996.
45. Levine BD, et al: Dexamethasone in the treatment of acute mountain sickness. *N Engl J Med* 321:1707, 1989.
46. Johnson TS, et al: Prevention of acute mountain sickness by dexamethasone. *N Engl J Med* 310:683, 1984.
47. Hackett PH, et al: Dexamethasone for prevention and treatment of acute mountain sickness. *Aviat Space Environ Med* 59:950, 1988.
48. Bernhard WN, et al: Acetazolamide plus low-dose dexamethasone is better than acetazolamide alone to ameliorate symptoms of acute mountain sickness. *Aviat Space Environ Med* 69:883, 1998.
49. Hultgren HN: High altitude pulmonary edema. In Staub NC (ed): *Lung Water and Solute Exchange*. New York, Dekker, 1978, pp 437-469.
50. Hultgren HN, Marticorena E: High altitude pulmonary edema: Epidemiologic observations in Peru. *Chest* 74:372, 1978.
51. Scoggin CH, et al: High-altitude pulmonary edema in the children and young adults of Leadville, Colorado. *N Engl J Med* 297:1269, 1977.
52. Meehan RT: Immune suppression at high altitude. *Ann Emerg Med* 16:974, 1987.
53. Shlim DR, Papenfus K: Pulmonary embolism presenting as high-altitude pulmonary edema. *Wilderness Environ Med* 6:220, 1995.
54. Schoene RB, et al: High altitude pulmonary edema and exercise at 4400 meters on Mt. McKinley: Effect of expiratory positive airway pressure. *Chest* 87:330, 1985.
55. Kasic JF, et al: Treatment of acute mountain sickness: Hyperbaric versus oxygen therapy. *Ann Emerg Med* 20:1109, 1991.
56. Hackett PH, Roach RC: Medical therapy of altitude illness. *Ann Emerg Med* 16:980, 1987.
57. Oelz O, et al. Prevention and treatment of high altitude pulmonary edema by a calcium channel blocker. *Int J Sports Med* 13:S65, 1992.
58. Bärtsch P, et al: Prevention of high-altitude pulmonary edema by nifedipine. *N Engl J Med* 325:1284, 1991.
59. Houston CS, Dickinson JG: Cerebral form of high altitude illness. *Lancet* 2:758, 1975.
60. Song S-Y, et al: Cerebral thrombosis at altitude: Its pathogenesis and the problems of prevention and treatment. *Aviat Space Environ Med* 57:71, 1986.
61. Wohns RN: Transient ischemic attacks at high altitude. *Crit Care Med* 14:517, 1986.
62. Hornbein TF, et al: The cost to the central nervous system of climbing to extremely high altitude. *N Engl J Med* 321:1714, 1989.
63. Clarke C: High altitude cerebral oedema. *Int J Sports Med* 9:170, 1988.
64. Frayser R, et al: Retinal hemorrhage at high altitude. *N Engl J Med* 282:1183, 1970.
65. Honigman B, et al: High altitude retinal hemorrhages in a Colorado skier. *High Altitude Med Biol* 2:539, 2001.
66. Berg BW, et al: Hemodynamic effects of altitude exposure and oxygen administration in chronic obstructive pulmonary disease. *Am J Med* 94:407, 1993.
67. Matsuda S, Onda T, Iikura Y: Bronchial responses of asthmatic patients in an atmosphere-changing chamber. *Int Arch Allergy Immunol* 107:402, 1995.
68. Coultas DB, Samet JM, Wiggins CL: Altitude and mortality from chronic obstructive lung disease in New Mexico. *Arch Environ Health* 39:355, 1984.
69. Moore LG, Rohr AL, Maisenbach JK: Emphysema mortality is increased in Colorado residents of high altitude. *Am Rev Respir Dis* 126:225, 1985.
70. Mortimer EA, Monson RR, MacMahon B: Reduction in mortality from coronary heart disease in men residing at high altitude. *N Engl J Med* 296:581, 1977.
71. Morton WE: Coronary heart disease at high altitudes [letter]. *N Engl J Med* 297:60, 1977.
72. Yaron M, Hultgren HN, Alexander JK: Low risk of myocardial ischemia in the elderly visiting moderate altitude. *Wilderness Environ Med* 6:20, 1995.
73. Levine BD, Zuckerman JH, deFilippi CR: Effect of high-altitude exposure in the elderly: The Tenth Mountain Division study. *Circulation* 96:1224, 1997.
74. Halhuber M, et al: Does altitude cause exhaustion of the heart and circulatory system. In Rivolier J, Cerretelli P, Foray J, Segantini P (eds): *High Altitude Deterioration*, vol 19. Basel, Karger, 1985, pp 192-202.
75. Morgan BJ, et al: The patient with coronary heart disease at altitude: Observations during acute exposure to 3100 meters. *J Wilderness Med* 1:147, 1990.
76. Alexander JK: Coronary heart disease at altitude. *Texas Heart Inst J* 21:261, 1994.
77. Mazzeo RS, Wolfel EE, Butterfield GE, et al: Sympathetic response during 21 days at high altitude (4,300 m) as deter-

mined by urinary and arterial catecholamines. *Metabolism* 43:1226, 1994.
78. Kamat SR, Banerji BC: Study of cardiopulmonary function on exposure to high altitude: Acute acclimatization to an altitude of 3500 to 4000 meters. *Am Rev Respir Dis* 106:404, 1972.
79. Palatini P, Businaro R, Berton G, et al: Effects of low altitude exposure on 24-hour blood pressure and adrenergic activity. *Am J Cardiol* 64:1379, 1989.
80. Mahoney BS, Githens JH: Sickling crisis and altitude: Occurrence in the Colorado patient population. *Clin Pediatr* 18:431, 1979.
81. Moore LG, et al: The incidence of pregnancy-induced hypertension is increased among Colorado residents at high altitude. *Am J Obstet Gynecol* 144:423, 1982.
82. Mader TH, White LJ: Refractive changes at extreme altitude after radial keratotomy. *Am J Ophthalmol* 119:733, 1995.
83. Mader T: Refractive changes during 72-hour exposure to high altitude after refractive surgery. *Ophthalmology* 103:1188, 1996.

CHAPTER 143 Submersion

Andrew L. Knaut and Kim M. Feldhaus

PERSPECTIVE: EPIDEMIOLOGY

Unintentional drowning accounted for 3281 deaths in the United States in 2001.[1] Worldwide, it is estimated that submersion kills 500,000 people per year, although the accuracy of this figure is questionable because of inconsistent reporting.[2] Drowning is the fourth most common cause of accidental death in the United States. Among children 1 through 14 years old, drowning is second only to motor vehicle crash as the leading cause of injury mortality.[1,3] Toddlers and older teenagers are at greatest risk of death by drowning, with annual incidences of 2.71 and 1.59 per 100,000.[1] Boys account for almost 80% of victims older than age 12 months, and race plays a decided, although incompletely understood, role: Black boys between ages 15 and 19 years have the highest annual incidence of drowning mortality (5.21 per 100,000), and black boys between ages of 10 and 19 years drown at 12 to 15 times the rate of white boys of the same age.[1,4]

The incidence of nonfatal submersion injuries is less well known. The Centers for Disease Control and Prevention estimates that for every child who dies by drowning in the United States, six receive emergency department care for a submersion event, and half of these children require hospitalization.[5] Among all age groups, it is estimated that one to four hospitalizations secondary to nonfatal submersions occur for every drowning death.[6-8]

Submersion injuries occur in domestic settings such as swimming pools, hot tubs, bathtubs, and large buckets and in all forms of natural bodies of water. A review of all drowning deaths among individuals younger than 20 years old in the United States over a 1-year period revealed that 55% of infants younger than 1 year old who drowned did so in bathtubs, and nearly 16% drowned in large household buckets.[4] Most (56%) children 1 to 4 years old drown in artificial pools, whereas most (63%) deaths among older children occur in natural bodies of freshwater.[4] Drowning in the United States follows clear temporal patterns; two thirds of pediatric deaths occur between the months of May and August, and most submersion injuries occur on weekends between the hours of noon and 8:00 P.M.[6]

PRINCIPLES OF DISEASE

Definitions

Traditionally the terminology used to describe submersion injuries has been confusing and impractical. In the past, *drowning* referred to death within 24 hours of suffocation from submersion in a liquid, whereas *near-drowning* described victims who survived at least 24 hours past the initial event regardless of the outcome. The American Heart Association and the European Resuscitation Council recommend a clearer definition of terms. *Drowning* connotes a terminal outcome from a submersion event whether the death occurs in the field, in the emergency department, or in the hospital. The term *near-drowning* should not be used. Instead, *submersion victim* defines anyone who has some submersion distress requiring medical support and transport to an emergency facility. The patient remains a submersion victim until either recovery or death. In the latter instance, the term *drowning* then applies.[15]

Immersion syndrome refers specifically to syncope resulting from cardiac dysrhythmias on sudden contact with water that is at least 5° C less than body temperature. Vagal stimulation leading to asystole and ventricular fibrillation secondary to Q-T prolongation and a massive release of catecholamines on contact with cold water are proposed as mechanisms for the syndrome. The resultant loss of consciousness leads to secondary drowning. The risk of immersion syndrome is proportional to the difference between body and water temperature. Wetting the face and head before entering the water may prevent the inciting sequence of events.[2]

Risk Factors

Alcohol use in proximity with water is a major risk factor for submersion injury or death. Acute ethanol intoxication may be a contributing factor in 30% to 50% of drownings among adults and adolescents.[3,6] In one study of boating fatalities, most of which were due to drowning, a blood alcohol concentration greater than 100 mg/dL conveyed a 16-fold increase in the risk of mortality compared with sober case controls.[16]

The relationship between swimming ability and the risk of drowning is unclear. No direct evidence exists to suggest that inexperienced swimmers are more likely to drown. On the contrary, skilled swimmers have greater exposure to water and may be more prone to submersion incidents.[17]

Numerous medical conditions confer an increased likelihood of drowning or submersion injury. Seizure disorders sharply increase the chance of drowning among children and adolescents, and autism and other developmental and behavioral disorders increase risk in children.[10,18-20] Prolonged Q-T syndrome also is a risk factor for drowning. Laboratory studies show that immersion in cold water extends the Q-T interval. Interrogation of the automated internal cardiac defibrillator of a 12-year-old girl with prolonged Q-T syndrome who had a cardiac arrest on diving into the ocean revealed immediate further prolongation of the Q-T interval followed by a premature ventricular complex and subsequent ventricular tachycardia within 5 seconds.[21,22] This phenomenon may account for a significant proportion of immersion syndrome events and otherwise unexplained submersion injuries.

Pathophysiology

Unexpected submersion triggers breath holding, panic, and a struggle to surface. Air hunger and hypoxia develop, and the victim begins to swallow water. As breath holding is overcome, involuntary gasps result in aspiration. The quantity of fluid aspirated rather than the composition determines subsequent pulmonary derangement. The historical emphasis on pathophysiologic differences between freshwater and saltwater aspiration with respect to resultant electrolyte imbalance, hemolysis, and fluid compartment shifting was based on animal studies conducted early in the 20th century.

Subsequent investigations revealed that significant intravascular abnormalities do not occur until the amount of aspirated water exceeds 11 mL/kg of body weight, and autopsy studies show that most drowning victims aspirate less than 4 mL/kg.[23] In one review of the hospital treatment of 91 submersion victims, no patient required emergent intervention for a significant electrolyte abnormality.[24] Aspiration of 1 to 3 mL/kg of either freshwater or saltwater destroys the integrity of pulmonary surfactant, leading to alveolar collapse, atelectasis, noncardiogenic pulmonary edema, intrapulmonary shunting, and ventilation-perfusion mismatch.[2] Profound hypoxia and metabolic and respiratory acidosis ensue, leading to cardiovascular collapse, neuronal injury, and, ultimately, death.

The classic hypothesis was that 10% to 15% of drowning victims die without aspirating a significant amount of water. Death from such "dry" drowning putatively results from severe laryngospasm causing hypoxia, convulsion, and death without fluid entering the lungs. An exhaustive review of the literature fails to corroborate this hypothesis [25] Dry drownings more appropriately reflect deaths from causes other than simple submersion.

Many factors may influence the pathophysiologic sequence of events in submersion injury and affect the chance of survival, including age, water temperature, duration and degree of hypothermia, the diving reflex, and the effectiveness of resuscitative efforts. Because of a lower ratio of body mass to surface area, children develop hypothermia more quickly and to a greater degree after immersion in cold water than adults. Hypothermia lowers cerebral metabolic rate and is neuroprotective to some extent for victims of submersion injury.[26] Despite dramatic case reports of patients surviving prolonged submersion in cold water with full neurologic recovery, however, in general hypothermia is a poor prognostic finding. Cold water immersion speeds the development of exhaustion, altered consciousness, and cardiac dysrhythmia. The *diving reflex* also may play a protective role in infant and child submersions. Activation of the diving reflex by fear or immersion of the face in cold water shunts blood centrally to the heart and brain. Apnea and bradycardia ensue, prolonging the duration of submersion tolerated without central nervous system damage.[27]

CLINICAL FEATURES

Symptoms and Signs

Many submersion injuries are witnessed. Toddler drownings are an important exception, however, often occurring because of a lapse in supervision. Occasionally the history of coughing, choking, or vomiting in a patient found near a body of water suggests the diagnosis. Signs of *pulmonary injury* may be obvious in a submersion victim who is hypoxic, cyanotic, and in obvious respiratory distress or arrest. More subtle clues, such as increased respiratory rate and audible rhonchi, rales, or wheezes, should alert the clinician to evolving respiratory compromise. Submersion victims swallow a significantly greater volume of water than is aspirated, and gastric distention from positive-pressure ventilation during rescue is common. As a result, 60% of patients vomit after a submersion event.[2] Aspiration of gastric contents greatly compounds the degree of pulmonary injury and increases the likelihood that acute respiratory distress syndrome will ensue. Additionally, aspiration of particulate contaminants, such as mud, sewage, and bacteria, may obstruct the smaller bronchi and bronchioles and greatly increase the risk of infection.[28]

Victims with *central nervous system injury* may present with symptoms ranging from mild lethargy to coma with fixed and dilated pupils. Adverse neurologic findings on initial presentation do not preclude full neurologic recovery, although in general patients whose duration of submersion or resuscitation exceeds 25 minutes have an unfavorable outcome.[29] Central nervous system injury results from the initial hypoxic or ischemic insult and from the cascade of reperfusion injury that follows re-establishment of cerebral blood flow after an arrest. The release of inflammatory mediators and the generation of oxygen free radicals in the postresuscitative period contribute to cytotoxic cerebral edema, compromise of the blood-brain barrier, and increased intracranial pressure. Cerebral arteriolar vasospasm and enhanced platelet aggregation impede cerebral perfusion at the macrocirculatory and microcirculatory levels.[27]

Cardiac dysrhythmias may incite a submersion injury or develop as its consequence. Hypoxemia, acidosis, and potentially hypothermia are the primary factors responsible for dysrhythmias ranging from ventricular tachycardia and fibrillation to bradycardia-asystole. Electrolyte disturbances are rarely significant enough to be dysrhythmogenic.[24]

Other clinical sequelae of submersion injury may include acute *renal impairment,* present in approximately 50% of patients as the result of lactic acidosis; prolonged hypoperfusion; and, in some instances, rhabdomyolysis.[30] *Coagulopathy* as a consequence of associated hypothermia or disseminated intravascular coagulation also may occur.

Prognostic Factors

Many factors may help predict patients who will survive a submersion injury neurologically intact. Submersion victims who arrive in the emergency department alert with normal hemodynamics are unlikely to experience neurologic impairment. Circumstantial variables that portend a poor outcome include victim age younger than 3 years, submersion for longer than 5 minutes, and initiation of cardiopulmonary resuscitation (CPR) more than 10 minutes after rescue.[2,31] With the exception of victim age, however, such measurements are generally either unknown or inaccurately estimated at the time of a patient's arrival in the emergency department. Objective findings on emergency department arrival that are associated with an unfavorable prognosis include hypothermia, severe acidosis, unreactive pupils, a Glasgow Coma Scale score of 3, and asystole or the need for ongoing CPR.[2,32-35] Neurologically intact survival is reported for individual patients when any of these factors are present, and none of several proposed scoring systems using combinations of these variables shows 100% predictive power.[9,31,33,36]

DIFFERENTIAL CONSIDERATIONS

The precipitants of a submersion injury, such as drug or alcohol intoxication, cardiac arrest, hypoglycemia, seizure, and attempted suicide or homicide, should be considered in a patient who is found unresponsive in the water. For pediatric victims, child abuse or neglect also must be considered as a potential etiology.

Potential head or cervical spine injury is an important consideration when a history of trauma is associated with the submersion. A review of 2244 cases of submersion injury in King, Pierce, and Snohomish counties in Washington State identified only 11 (0.5%) patients with a cervical spine injury, however. Each patient had either clinical signs of serious trauma or a history of motor vehicle crash, fall from height, or diving into the water.[37] Unless such factors are present, routine cervical spine immobilization for submersion victims is not warranted.

DIAGNOSTIC STUDIES

Cardiac monitoring and an electrocardiogram must be obtained to determine the presence of significant dysrhythmias or Q-T prolongation. Pulse oximetry, capnography, and arterial blood gases should be monitored closely in all submersion victims for signs of hypoxemia, hypercarbia, and acidosis. Blood glucose, serum creatinine, and electrolytes should be obtained, although serum creatinine and electrolytes are usually normal on initial presentation. Similarly, complete blood count is often normal with the exception of leukocytosis. Screening for alcohol or other drugs of abuse may be appropriate depending on the circumstances of the submersion. Subsequently, evidence of renal failure, hepatic dysfunction, and disseminated intravascular coagulation may be noted on laboratory testing.

The initial chest radiograph may underestimate the severity of pulmonary injury, although infiltrates or pulmonary edema may be evident within hours. Cranial computed tomography is rarely contributory initially, unless significant trauma or other pertinent pathology is suspected. Magnetic resonance imaging of the brain may predict neurologic outcome after submersion injury, but its prognostic value is not optimal until 3 or 4 days elapse.[9,38]

MANAGEMENT

Salient details of the events surrounding the accident should be ascertained rapidly. Resuscitation of pulseless and apneic patients should be attempted initially in most cases because bystander estimates of total submersion time are often inaccurate. The clinical presentation of severe hypothermia often mimics death, and case reports exist of functional recovery for individuals submerged for 66 minutes.[39,40]

For a victim without vital signs, outcome depends on the interval preceding CPR. Mouth-to-mouth assisted ventilation should begin immediately, even before the victim is extricated from the water. Chest compressions are impractical before extrication but should be initiated as soon as the individual is placed on a solid surface. Maneuvers such as those proposed by Heimlich and Patrick to remove fluid from the lungs are ineffective and dangerous in a victim at risk for aspiration and may delay ventilation. Use of such maneuvers is not recommended unless there is reason to suspect airway occlusion by a foreign body.[41]

On arrival in the emergency department, cardiac monitoring and continuous pulse oximetry should be established. A core temperature obtained with a low-reading probe is indicated for any unstable or lethargic patient. Rewarming a hypothermic patient may suffice for hemodynamic stabilization and improvement in mental status. Bedside blood glucose measurement and empirical naloxone administration likewise are warranted. In a spontaneously breathing patient, monitoring for signs of developing pulmonary injury should be established. Initial chest radiographs are often unremarkable even in the setting of serious and evolving pathology. Frequent arterial blood gas determinations are essential in submersion victims.

The decision regarding tracheal intubation should be based on clinical impression and objective determination of the adequacy of oxygenation and ventilation. Apparent or developing respiratory distress, absence of protective airway reflexes, and significant associated head or chest injuries are indications. A $PaCO_2$ greater than 50 mm Hg mandates intubation and mechanical ventilation. Patients unable to maintain an oxygen saturation greater than 90% or a PaO_2 greater than 60 mm Hg on high-flow oxygen require positive airway pressure to increase functional residual capacity, decrease intrapulmonary shunting, and reduce ventilation-perfusion mismatch. In an awake patient, this may be accomplished by face or nasal mask (continuous positive airway pressure), but the risk of potential gastric distention, vomiting, and aspiration must be considered. Otherwise, tracheal and mechanical ventilation with positive end-expiratory pressure is necessary. The hemodynamic consequences of positive end-expiratory pressure must be monitored carefully because increased intrathoracic pressure may compromise venous return and cardiac output. Decreased cranial venous return may impede cerebral perfusion.

No consensus exists with regard to the appropriate length of resuscitative effort for hypothermic submersion victims in the emergency department. The safest parameter is to continue until the core temperature reaches at least 30° C to 35° C because cerebral death cannot be diagnosed accurately in hypothermic patients with temperatures below this level. This parameter may not always be practical, however, because brain-dead patients are often poikilothermic.

The administration of corticosteroids in the setting of submersion injury and potential acute respiratory distress syndrome does not improve outcome.[2,9] Similarly, empirical antibiotics do not increase survival and should be administered only to the rare patient who was submerged in grossly contaminated water or who shows signs of infection or sepsis.[2]

Interventions such as induced or permissive hypothermia aimed at attenuating reperfusion injury after anoxic brain insult are the focus of intense investigative effort, but at present no consensus exists regarding their use in submersion injury. Corticosteroid administration, barbiturate-induced coma, aggressive diuresis, neuromuscular blockade, and hyperventilation have not been shown to improve neurologic outcome and, particularly in the case of hyperventilation, may be harmful.[27]

DISPOSITION

Symptomatic patients must be admitted for treatment. Patients with a history of apnea, unconsciousness, or hypoxia and any patients who manifest dysrhythmia or an abnormal chest radiograph also require admission. Patients who are asymptomatic on presentation to the emergency department, maintain a normal room air oxygen saturation, and have no chest radiograph or arterial blood gas abnormalities can be discharged safely after an observation period of 6 hours.[9,42] Careful instructions regarding symptoms or signs of delayed pulmonary complications are necessary, and the patient should be discharged in the care of a competent relative or friend.

Preventive Efforts

The mortality rate from drowning has decreased steadily since the 1990s in the United States.[1,3,9] A similar downward trend in submersion injuries is reported in Great Britain.[10] Although the exact causes of this decline are unknown, an increased public awareness of preventive measures and an emphasis on public education with regard to CPR and the dangers of alcohol use in conjunction with water-related activities likely have contributed significantly to the reduction in fatalities. A longitudinal study of drownings over a 21-year period in King County, Washington, notes that the incidence of death attributable to alcohol use has decreased by 81%.[3]

Parental education regarding the danger of pediatric drowning is an important focus of preventive effort. Inadequate supervision of children playing in or near water is one of the most common causes of pediatric submersion death, underscoring the importance of increasing awareness of the need for constant oversight of children in this setting.[8,11] Most pediatric submersion injuries in swimming pools occur at the victim's home.[9] In most cases, the child was last seen in the house, was left unattended for a moment, and entered the pool on an unfenced side closest to the home with no audible splash or screaming.[4] Adequate and fully circumferencial fencing of residential pools is a current recommendation of the American Academy of Pediatrics. A meta-analysis of the literature regarding the efficacy of this preventive step reports an odds ratio of 0.27 for drowning or submersion in a properly fenced compared with a nonfenced pool.[11,12]

Pool covers are inadequate and potentially dangerous as barriers. Solar blankets do not support the weight of a child and can enmesh and obscure a struggling victim from view. A rigid pool cover may convey a false sense of stability to a child tempted to walk across its surface and is considered an insufficient substitute for effective four-sided fencing.[11]

Medical care providers are a vital resource for enhancing public awareness of the importance of these measures. The literature supports the concept that education in the emergency department with regard to drowning prevention can have a positive impact on patient and family awareness of steps to lessen the likelihood of catastrophic drowning or submersion injury.[13,14]

KEY CONCEPTS

- The fluid medium in which a submersion injury occurs (freshwater versus saltwater) is usually of little clinical relevance; all significant submersions induce pulmonary injury and hypoxia based on the amount of water aspirated and the duration of submersion, not the water content.
- Aggressive pulmonary support is essential to optimizing the victim's chances for a favorable outcome.
- In submersion incidents, the Heimlich maneuver is reserved for patients with a suspected airway occlusion by a foreign body.
- No prognostic scale or clinical presentation accurately predicts long-term neurologic outcome; normal neurologic recovery is documented in patients with prolonged submersions, persistent coma, cardiovascular instability, and fixed and dilated pupils.
- Hyperventilation, steroids, dehydration, barbiturate coma, and neuromuscular blockade do not seem to improve outcome.

REFERENCES

1. National Center for Injury Prevention and Control, Centers for Disease Control and Prevention: Web-based injury statistics query and reporting system [database]. Available at: http://www.cdc.gov/ncipc/wisqars. Accessed December 2, 2003.
2. Orlowski JP, Szpilman D: Drowning: Rescue, resuscitation, and reanimation. *Pediatr Clin North Am* 48:627, 2001.
3. Cummings P: Trends in unintentional drowning: The role of alcohol and medical care. *JAMA* 281:2198, 1999.
4. Brenner RA, et al: Where children drown, United States, 1995. *Pediatrics* 108:85, 2001.
5. National Center for Injury Prevention and Control, Centers for Disease Control and Prevention: Water-related injuries [fact sheet]. Available at: http://cdc.gov/ncipc/factsheets/drown.htm. Accessed December 2, 2003.
6. Brenner RA, and the Committee on Injury, Violence, and Poison Prevention: Prevention of drowning in infants, children, and adolescents. *Pediatrics* 112:440, 2003.
7. Ellis AA, Trent RB: Hospitalizations for near drowning in California: Incidence and costs. *Am J Public Health* 85:1115, 1995.
8. Quan L, et al: Ten-year study of pediatric drownings and near-drownings in King County, Washington: Lessons in injury prevention. *Pediatrics* 83:1035, 1989.
9. Ibsen LM, Koch T: Submersion and asphyxial injury. *Crit Care Med* 11:S402, 2002.
10. Sibert JR, Lyons RA, Smith BA: Preventing deaths by drowning in the United Kingdom: Have we made progress in 10 years? Population-based incidence study. *BMJ* 324:1070, 2002.
11. American Academy of Pediatrics, Committee on Injury, Violence, and Poison Prevention: Prevention of drowning in infants, children, and adolescents. *Pediatrics* 112:437, 2003.
12. Thompson DC, Rivara FP: Pool fencing for preventing drowning in children. *Cochrane Database Syst Rev* 2:CD001047, 2000.
13. Quan L, et al: Do parents value drowning prevention information at discharge from the emergency department? *Ann Emerg Med* 37:382, 2001.
14. Barkin S, Gelberg L: Sink or swim-clinicians don't often counsel on drowning prevention. *Pediatrics* 104:1217, 1999.
15. International ECC and CPR Guidelines 2000, Part 8, Section 3. *Circulation* 102(Suppl I):I-229, 2000.
16. Smith GS, et al: Drinking and recreational boating fatalities: A population-based case-control study. *JAMA* 286:2974, 2001.
17. Brenner RA, Saluja G, Smith GS: Swimming lessons, swimming ability, and the risk of drowning. *Inj Control Saf Promot* 10:211, 2003.
18. Diekema DS, Quan L, Holt VL: Epilepsy as a risk factor for submersion injury in children. *Pediatrics* 91:612, 1993.
19. Shavelle RM, Strauss DJ, Pickett J: Causes of death in autism. *J Autism Dev Disord* 31:569, 2001.
20. Brehaut JC, et al: Childhood behavior disorders and injuries among children and youth: A population-based study. *Pediatrics* 111:232, 2003.
21. Ackerman MJ, Tester DJ, Porter CJ: Swimming: A gene-specific arrhythmogenic trigger for inherited long QT syndrome. *Mayo Clin Proc* 74:1088, 1999.
22. Baktra AS, Silka MJ: Mechanism of sudden cardiac arrest while swimming in a child with the prolonged QT syndrome. *J Pediatr* 141:283, 2002.
23. Modell JH, Davis JH: Electrolyte changes in human drowning victims. *Anesthesiology* 30:414, 1969.
24. Modell JH, Craves SA, Ketover A: Clinical course of 91 consecutive near-drowning victims. *Chest* 70:231, 1976.
25. Modell JH, Bellefleur M, Davis JH: Drowning without aspiration: Is this an appropriate diagnosis? *J Forensic Sci* 44:1119, 1999.
26. Biggart MJ, Bohn DJ: Effect of hypothermia and cardiac arrest on outcome of near-drowning accidents in children. *J Pediatr* 117:179, 1990.
27. Sachdeva RC: Near drowning. *Crit Care Clin* 15:281, 1999.
28. Ender PT, Dolan MJ: Pneumonia associated with near-drowning. *Clin Infect Dis* 25:896, 1997.
29. Jacinto SJ, Gieron-Korthals M, Ferreira JA: Predicting outcome in hypoxic-ischemic brain injury. *Pediatr Clin North Am* 48:647, 2001.
30. Spicer TS, et al: Acute renal impairment after immersion and near-drowning. *J Am Soc Nephrol* 10:382, 1999.
31. Suominen P, et al: Impact of age, submersion time, and water temperature on outcome in near-drowning. *Resuscitation* 52:247, 2002.
32. Habib DM, et al: Prediction of childhood drowning and near-drowning morbidity and mortality. *Pediatr Emerg Care* 12:255, 1996.
33. Christensen DW, Jansen P, Perken RM: Outcome and acute care hospital costs after warm water near drowning in children. *Pediatrics* 99:715, 1997.
34. Graf WD, Cummings P, Quan L: Predicting outcome in pediatric submersion victims. *Ann Emerg Med* 26:312, 1995.

35. Zuckerman GB, Gregory PM, Santos-Damiani SM: Predictors of death and neurologic impairment in pediatric submersion injuries. The Pediatric Risk of Mortality Score. *Arch Pediatr Adolesc Med* 152:134, 1998.
36. Gonzalez-Luis G, et al: Use of the Pediatric Risk of Mortality Score as predictor of death and serious neurologic damage in children after submersion. *Pediatr Emerg Care* 17:405, 2001.
37. Watson RS, et al: Cervical spine injuries among submersion victims. *J Trauma* 51:658, 2001.
38. Dubowitz DJ, et al: MR of hypoxic encephalopathy in children after near drowning: Correlation with quantitative proton MR spectroscopy and clinical outcome. *AJNR Am J Neuroradiol* 19:1617, 1998.
39. Bolte RG, et al: The use of extracorporeal rewarming in a child submerged for 66 minutes. *JAMA* 260:377, 1988.
40. Hughes SK, et al: Neurodevelopmental outcome for extended cold water drowning: A longitudinal case study. *J Int Neuropsychol Soc* 8:588, 2002.
41. Rosen P, Stoto M, Harley J: The use of the Heimlich maneuver in near drowning: Institute of Medicine report. *J Emerg Med* 13:397, 1995.
42. Causey AL, Tilelli JA, Swanson ME: Predicting discharge in uncomplicated near-drowning. *Am J Emerg Med* 18:9, 2000.

CHAPTER 144

Radiation Injuries

Vincent Markovchick

HISTORICAL PERSPECTIVE AND EPIDEMIOLOGY

The technology of the 20th and 21st centuries has ushered in the nuclear age. Nuclear energy has peaceful industrial and medical uses, but it poses great potential destructive hazards. Although the safety record involving the use of radiation and radioisotopes is excellent overall, the hazards involved are well known as a result of the serious potential for disaster that occurred at Three Mile Island in Pennsylvania in 1979, the disastrous accident at the Chernobyl Nuclear Power Station in the former Soviet Union in 1989, and the potential for disaster that occurred at a uranium processing plant in Tokaimura, Japan, in 1999.[1,2] The potential exposure and contamination of large numbers of people have and will continue to stress the capabilities of existing emergency medical systems.

The only wartime use of atomic and nuclear energy was the detonation of atomic bombs over Hiroshima and Nagasaki in 1945. With dissemination of technical information and raw materials, many nations now have nuclear weapons in their arsenals; the possibility of terrorist groups obtaining and using such weapons also exists. Because the spent fuel from a nuclear power reactor can be reprocessed into plutonium, which can be used to produce nuclear weapons, more countries are acquiring the raw material to produce nuclear weapons. The technology is available for the production and use of small, low-yield, tactical nuclear weapons and for megaton-yield, strategic nuclear weapons. Delivery systems have become sophisticated as a result of the nuclear arms race.

Proliferation of nuclear weapon technology and materials from Pakistan to other nations, including North Korea, and the proliferation of global terrorism raise new concerns about the possibility of a nuclear weapon being used by a rogue nation or terrorist group. A more likely scenario is the production and detonation of a "dirty bomb" by a terrorist group. In contrast to a nuclear weapon, which is difficult to produce, a dirty bomb can be produced and detonated with relative ease. The real threat from such a bomb lies in its potential to cause widespread terror from fear of radioactive contamination. Although the number of deaths and injuries should not exceed those of a conventional explosion, the panic over radioactivity and evacuation measures and the prolonged cleanup efforts that would ensue would wreak havoc for months or years.

A dirty bomb can be produced from existing strontium-90 or cobalt-60 radioactive materials, such as radium and cesium-137 isotopes that are used in cancer therapy and found in many hospitals, university laboratories, and industry. Such a weapon can be produced by combining radioactive materials in solid or powder form with a conventional explosive that on detonation would send radioactive material into the area of the explosion and downwind. Even though minimal to no harm would come from these sources of radiation, there would be tremendous psychological effects.[3,4]

It is technically much more difficult to produce a nuclear weapon than it is to manufacture a chemical or a biologic weapon. Use of a nuclear weapon by terrorists is highly unlikely unless they obtained such a weapon from existing stockpiles.

Injury from a nuclear explosion initially involves the mechanical effects of the blast wave that result in large-scale conventional types of blunt and penetrating trauma. Second, the thermal or burn effects occur. Third, the effects of ionizing radiation injury occur in proportion to the blast and thermal effects. In addition,

Table 144-1. Approximate Distance from the Detonation Site at which a 50% Fatality Rate Might Be Expected, According to the Size of a Nuclear Weapon

Yield (kt)	Shock Wave	Thermal Radiation (m)	Ionizing Radiation	
			Initial	*Residual**
0.01	60	60	350	1270
0.1	130	200	460	2750
1	275	610	790	5500
10†	590	1800	1200	9600

*Data are for residual radiation (mostly fallout) in the first hour.
†At yields exceeding 10 kT, the lethal range of the fireball extends several times farther than the lethal range of either the blast or the initial radiation.
Data from the National Council on Radiation Protection and Measurements: Management of Persons Accidentally Contaminated with Radionucleotides (NCRP Report No. 65). Washington DC, 1980.

Table 144-2. Prognosis According to the Lymphocyte Count within the First 48 Hours after Acute Exposure to Penetrating, Whole-Body Radiation

Minimal Lymphocyte Count per mm²	Approximate Absorbed Dose (Gy)	Extent of Injury	Prognosis
1400-3000 (normal range)	0-0.4	No clinically significant injury	Excellent
1000-1499	0.5-1.9	Clinically significant but probably nonlethal	Good
500-999	2-3.9	Severe	Fair
100-499	4-7.9	Very severe	Poor
<100	≥8	Most severe	High incidence of death even with hematopoietic stimulation

radioactive fallout results from a nuclear weapon detonation at or above ground. Detonation of a nuclear weapon produces unimaginable devastation and injury from its immediate and long-term effects (Table 144-1).[5]

Accidents involving peacetime nuclear energy include exposure to and contamination by radioactive sources. The sources of this exposure are medical, industrial, and laboratory accidents that expose people to unacceptably high doses of radiation. The increased need to transport such materials results in an increased risk of accidents during transport. Emergency physicians are concerned primarily with the acute effects of exposure and contamination. A paucity of information about the chronic or long-term effects still exists. The long-term effects continue to be studied on the large numbers of the populace exposed to radiation as a result of the Chernobyl accident.[1]

Nuclear Reactor Incidents

A nuclear weapon, as distinguished from a nuclear reactor, is designed to be autocatalytic (i.e., rather than being self-sustaining, the power grows without bounds after the chain reaction is initiated). The water-cooled nuclear reactors in U.S. power plants are designed to operate in their most reactive configuration. Any material or geometric change (except for removal of the control rods) renders them subcritical. In the graphite-moderated, steam-cooled reactors operating in the former Soviet Union, a nuclear excursion or accident can occur on loss of coolant. This is what happened at Chernobyl.[6]

Every nuclear reactor should be housed within a containment structure to prevent the release of radioactivity in the event of an accident. The Three Mile Island reactor has five layers of defense; in 1979, very little radiation was released into the environment. At Chernobyl, however, the containment structure failed, and all the radioactive material from the core of the reactor escaped into the environment. Even though the release of radioactive materials from the core at Chernobyl was only about 3 times that released from the core at Three Mile Island, failure of containment resulted in a 5000-times greater dose of radiation to people within a 10-mile radius of Chernobyl (40,000 mrem) compared with Three Mile Island (8 mrem).[1] In addition, the large amount of radioactive material released into the atmosphere at Chernobyl was carried aloft by prevailing winds, causing increased radiation exposure at long distances.

As a result of human error at a uranium processing plant in Tokaimura, Japan, 49 people were exposed to radiation, 2 of whom received a potentially lethal dose. Enriched uranium was mixed with nitric acid in an open vessel, resulting in Cherenkov radiation. This radiation is released when the speed of a charged particle in a transport medium is so high that it exceeds the velocity of light in that medium. Then part of the energy is emitted as Cherenkov radiation—which is manifest as a visible flash—from radiation emitted when the uranium reaches a critical mass and sets off an uncontrolled chain reaction for 20 hours.

A terrorist attack on a nuclear reactor may result in an atmospheric plume of radioactive iodine and noble gases released through a breach in the reactor core. These gases could have immediate health effects nearby and long-term effects from radioactive iodine at great distances from the reactor.

Radon Exposure

Radon gas is a major source of radiation exposure in the general public. Radon and its breakdown products are in the decay chain of uranium-238. Because uranium-238 has a long half-life and is distributed throughout the earth's rocks and soil, its decay products are ubiquitous. Radon is a noble gas—colorless, odorless, and chemically nonreactive. Its decay scheme results in the production of four heavy metal isotopes with short half-lives termed *radon daughters* (Figure 144-1). These isotopes include alpha-emitting solids that can be inhaled and deposited in the tracheobronchial tree.

Because radon is a gas, it moves by diffusion and pressure flow into basements and buildings, where concentrations may reach hazardous levels. Radon daughters can be collected on filters, and alpha activity can be measured. The major source of radon gas is soil containing high levels of radon, such as uranium tailings used for landfill beneath buildings. Radon gas entry can be decreased by sealing basement cracks; its removal can be enhanced by proper ventilation systems.[7]

Because radon and radon daughters result from the decay of uranium-238, uranium miners sustain some of the highest levels of occupational exposure. These individuals have an increased incidence of lung cancer and diffuse interstitial pulmonary fibrosis secondary to radon progeny exposure from inhalation of alpha particles.[8] Each year, 15,000 lung cancer deaths in the United States may result from indoor radon exposure; radon in homes may be a significant public health problem.[9]

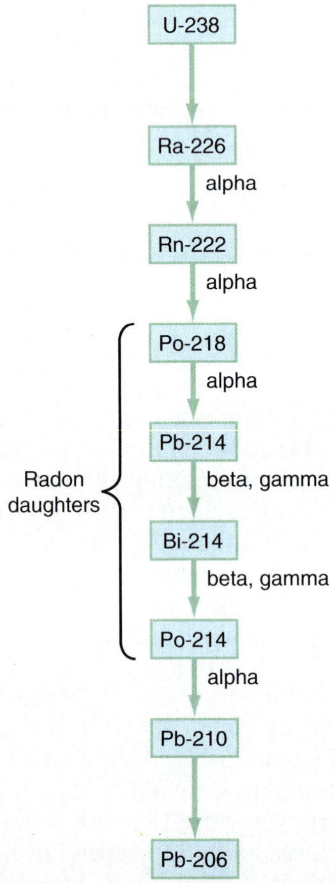

Figure 144-1. Radon and radon daughters in the major decay path of uranium-238. (Redrawn from Hart BL, Mettler FA Jr, Harley NH: Radon: Is it a problem? *Radiology* 172:593, 1989.)

PATHOPHYSIOLOGY OF RADIATION EXPOSURE

The electromagnetic spectrum (Figure 144-2) encompasses a range from gamma rays to microwaves. The frequency and length of these waves determine the energy, measured in units called *photons*. *Frequency* is the number of times per second the crest of a wave passes a given point, whereas *wavelength* is the distance between crests.

Ionizing versus Nonionizing Radiation

The term *radioactivity* refers to the loss of particles (e.g., alpha or beta) or energy (e.g., x-rays, gamma rays) from an unstable atom that is spontaneously decaying. To understand the effects of radiation exposure on humans requires a distinction between ionizing and nonionizing radiation. *Nonionizing radiation* refers to all forms of the electromagnetic spectrum, with the exception of x-rays and gamma rays. Nonionizing (in contrast to ionizing) radiation has a long wavelength, low frequency, and low energy. Examples of nonionizing radiation include visible light, radar, radio and television broadcasting, garage door openers, microwave ovens, relay stations, medical diathermy, and satellite communications.

The primary adverse effects of nonionizing radiation are related to local heat production because the energy

Figure 144-2. Electromagnetic spectrum.

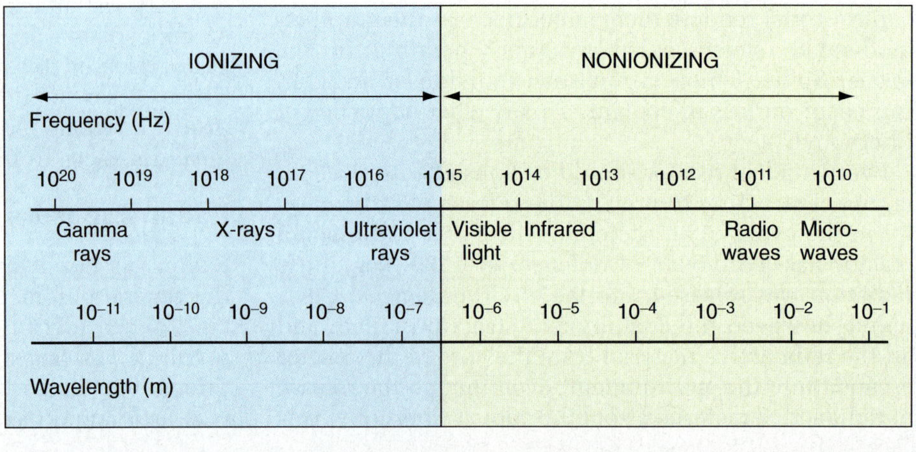

of nonionizing radiation is practically all expended in heat. This effect depends directly on the intensity of the source, the distance from the source to the person exposed, and the duration of exposure.[5] Long-term exposure to microwave irradiation at some distance from the source has received extensive study. The most thoroughly researched example involves U.S. State Department employees exposed to long-term microwave irradiation in the U.S. chancery in Moscow. This building was subjected to a direct beam, which resulted in exposed rooms having a higher power density than that usually found on the ground near transmission towers. After extensive study, it was concluded that no adverse health effects occurred from this exposure. This and other studies performed on various groups of workers exposed to radiofrequency radiation concluded that the present exposure levels (including microwaves) to the general public do not cause significant adverse health effects; specifically, there is no evidence of either decreased longevity or an increased incidence of cancer. The possibility of hazardous health effects resulting from low-level microwave exposure remains, however; this is an area of ongoing study.[10]

A microwave oven generates 2450-MHz microwaves. This megahertz wavelength can produce hyperthermia above a 25-mW level with a penetration of several centimeters. If a microwave oven has a door leak, a person can be exposed to the thermal effect of microwaves only by placing a body part in direct contact with the area. Electromagnetic waves dissipate at a rate directly related to the square of the distance from the source; exposure is one fourth at twice the distance from the source. No thermal effect exists at a distance of several feet, but a potential exists for deleterious effects on electronic devices that are sensitive to the wavelength of this electromagnetic radiation.

Ionizing radiation has a short wavelength, high frequency, and high energy. The photons of ionizing radiation carry 1 billion times more energy than the photons of nonionizing radiation.

Irradiation versus Contamination and Incorporation

Irradiation

A radioactive substance is one that emits ionizing radiation. It is referred to as a radionucleotide or radioisotope. If such radiation passes through a nearby object, the object is said to have been irradiated. With the exception of direct exposure to neutrons, the object that has been irradiated only does not become radioactive. When a person has been irradiated only, but not contaminated, no hazard exists to medical personnel, and the patient may be handled as any other emergency patient. An example of this concept is a post–radiation therapy patient.

Contamination

Radioactive contamination of a patient or an object presents some special considerations. Contamination is essentially radioactive particulate matter (alpha and beta particles) covering an exposed surface. Contamination is not an acute threat to life, and its presence should not preclude instituting lifesaving measures for associated trauma. This radioactive particulate matter may emit radiation with an effect that is directly related to the time of exposure, distance from the source, and type of contamination. Four types of radiation exist with different hazards (Figure 144-3): alpha, beta, gamma, and neutron radiation.

Alpha particles are helium nuclei, and with external contamination penetration is limited to the thickness of the epidermis. Alpha particles are produced by alpha emission from many of the heavy radioactive elements, such as plutonium and uranium decay. Alpha particles cannot be detected with the standard Geiger-Mueller counter, which is excellent for detecting beta and gamma radiation. Because of alpha particles' low penetrating ability, a proportional alpha counter with a special window must be used.

Beta particles have a tissue penetration of about 8 mm. On the skin surface, significant burns can result. Most radioisotopes decay by beta emission. Because clothing effectively shields covered areas, the primary danger is to exposed skin. Standard skin-cleansing procedures remove most of this contamination. Burns are not visible immediately after exposure; the only means of detection is a radiation-sensing instrument (Geiger-Mueller counter), which all hospitals should have. If exposure to beta particles is allowed to continue, significant exposure to gamma radiation may occur in the following manner. Alpha or beta decay may proceed directly to the ground (lowest energy) state of the daughter nucleus without gamma emission, but it also may proceed wholly or partly to higher energy (excited) states of the daughter nucleus. In the latter case, gamma emission may occur as the excited states transform to the lower energy states of the same nucleus.

Gamma rays penetrate tissue deeply, with a fraction of the rays interacting with every layer of tissue. Gamma rays are emitted from radioisotopes after beta decay and are the primary cause of the acute radiation syndrome.

Neutrons are unique. When they are stopped, or "captured," after emission, they commonly cause a previously stable atom to become radioactive. This is the source of radioactive fallout. A surface burst of a thermonuclear weapon instantly vaporizes tons of surface soil, transforming it into highly radioactive material by the intense neutron bombardment. This cloud rises with the fireball and is carried away by the prevailing winds at high altitudes. Its radioactive particles ultimately descend as fallout.

Some gamma exposure also occurs with neutron exposure. In peacetime accidents, significant neutron exposure can occur only around nuclear reactors and accelerators. Quantitation of the radioactive material induced by neutron irradiation is helpful in estimating neutron exposures and, sometimes indirectly, the dose of gamma radiation. The induced radioactivity is primarily sodium-24, which can be detected by a whole-body counter or in blood samples. If neutron exposure

TYPE OF RADIATION	SYMBOL	USUAL SOURCE	PENETRATION OF EXTERNAL RADIATION	PRINCIPLE TYPES OF INTERACTION
X-rays Gamma rays	x γ	X-ray machines and accelerators Most radioisotopes emit a gamma ray following beta decay	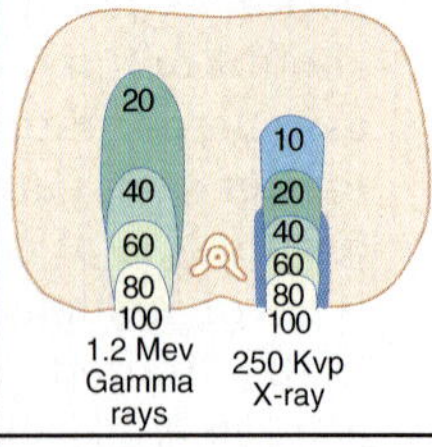 X- and γ rays penetrate deeply, for only a fraction of the rays interact with each layer of tissue	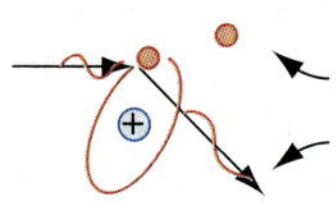 Ejected electron loses energy by causing additional ionization Deflected x- or γ ray may interact again some distance away Ionized atom formed after electron ejection
Neutrons	n	Neutrons are generally produced by critical assemblies, nuclear reactors, or accelerators	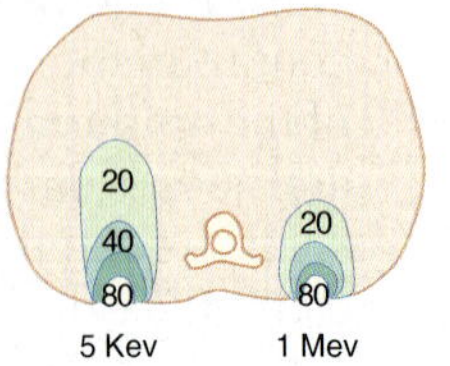 Neutrons penetrate deeply, for only a fraction of the neutrons interact with each layer of tissue	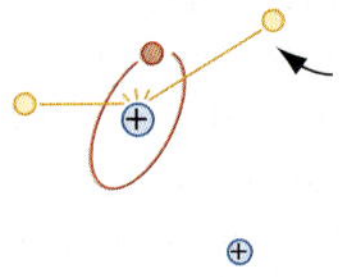 Deflected neutron may interact again some distance away Recoil proton loses energy by causing ionization
Beta particles	β	Most radioisotopes decay by beta emission, usually followed by gamma emission	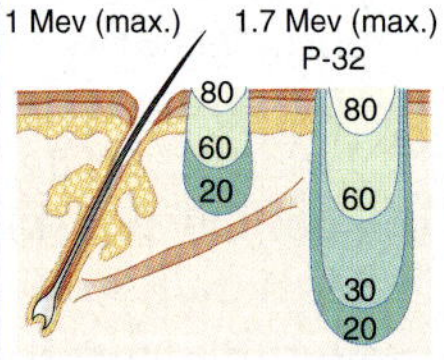 Penetration depends on energy of beta but is usually limited to less than 8 mm in tissue	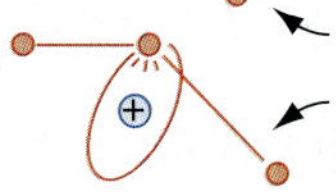 Ejected electron loses energy by causing additional ionization Deflected electron or beta particle causes additional ionization Ionized atom formed after electron ejection
Alpha particles	α	Many of the heavy radioactive elements such as plutonium decay by alpha particle emission	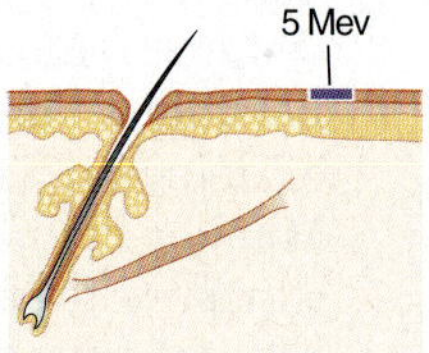 Penetration is limited to about the thickness of the epidermis	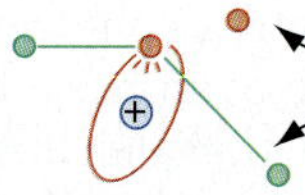 Ejected electron loses energy by causing additional ionization Deflected alpha goes on to cause additional ionization Ionized atom formed after electron ejection
Protons	p	Energetic protons are found only near particle accelerators	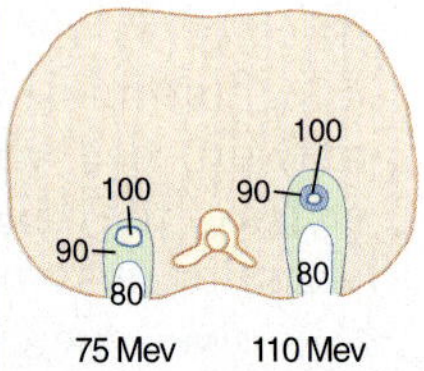 Penetration depends on energy of the proton	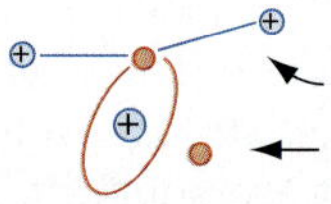 Deflected proton causes additional ionization Ejected electron loses energy by causing additional ionization Ionized atom formed after electron ejection

Figure 144-3. Types of radiation and possible external hazards. (Redrawn from Gould A, Cloutier RJ: Arch Environ Health 10:499, 1965.)

is suspected, all feces and urine should be refrigerated and saved. All clothing, especially items containing metal parts, such as belt buckles, also should be saved for analysis of neutron-induced radioisotopes.

Incorporation

Incorporation occurs when a radioactive material is ingested, inhaled, or absorbed through an open wound.

TYPES OF EXPOSURE

- *External radiation* exposure results from partial-body or whole-body irradiation from an outside source. The patient may have received a lethal dose but presents no radioactive hazard to other people or the environment. Examples include accidental irradiation of personnel working with fissionable materials in laboratories or with nuclear reactors in nuclear power plants.
- *Incorporation and internal contamination* usually result from inhalation or ingestion of radioactive substances, but also can occur from absorption of radioactive substances through open wounds. When this occurs, alpha particles, which normally present no real health hazard with external exposure, may have long-term effects, such as the development of lung cancer. The treatment of this type of exposure is often similar to that of acute poisoning with heavy metals.
- *External contamination* involves surface exposure to radioactive dirt or liquids. Care must be taken to confine this contamination. Emergency treatment consists of removal of clothing and careful cleansing of exposed parts.

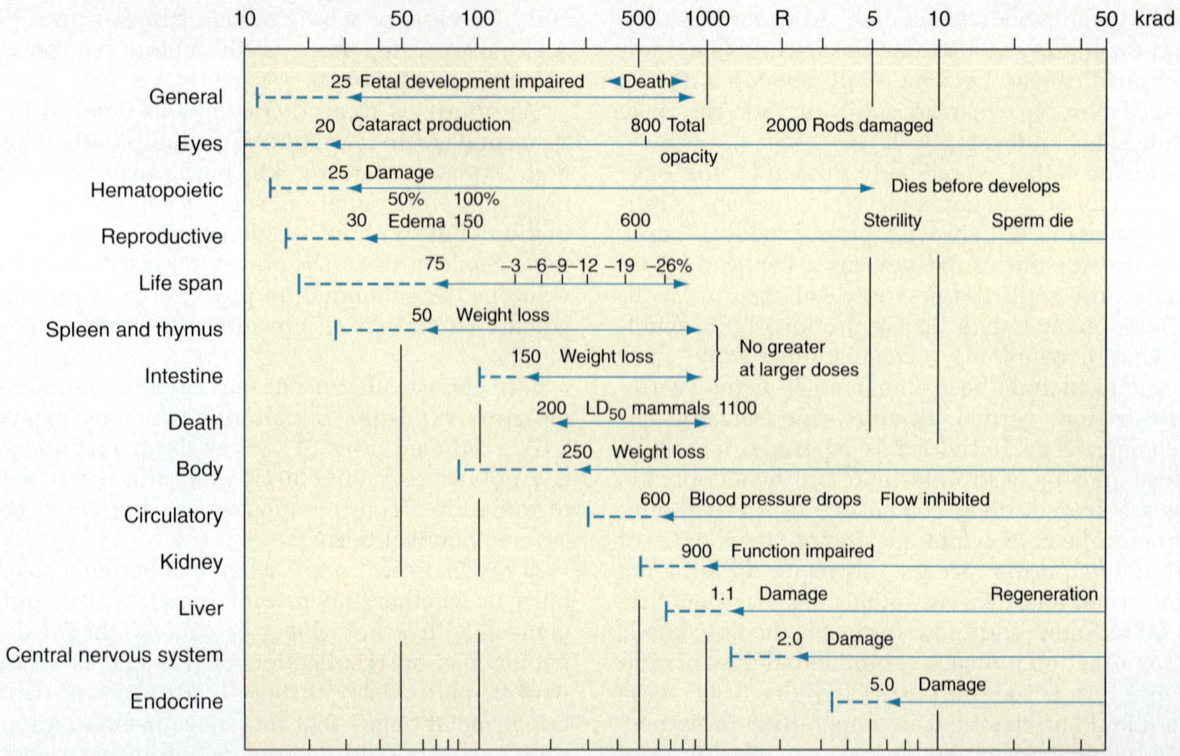

Figure 144-4. Organ and tissue sensitivity in mammals. The dose values are for whole-body, acute, x-ray, or gamma ray exposures. For low-intensity or fractionated exposure, the lines would be moved toward the right (higher doses). Radiosensitivity is directly related to the proliferative rate of the cells of the organs. (Redrawn from Auerbach PS, Gehr EC: *Management of Wilderness and Environmental Emergencies*. New York, Macmillan, 1983.)

- *Wound contamination* involves exposure of an open wound to radioactive solids or liquids and results in varying degrees of internal contamination depending on the specific circumstances.

Combinations of these types of radiation accidents can occur. The traumatic blast effects after a thermonuclear explosion may result in exposure to all types of radioactivity in addition to causing radioactively contaminated wounds.

CLINICAL FEATURES AND DIAGNOSTIC STRATEGIES

Symptoms and Signs

The *acute radiation syndrome* is a symptom complex that occurs after whole-body irradiation. It varies in nature and severity depending on dose, dose rate, dose distribution, and individual susceptibility. This syndrome results from external or internal exposure to radiation over a short period.

The principal units used for expressing the dose of radiation absorbed in living tissue are the *gray* (Gy) (1 Gy = 1 joule of radiation absorbed per kilogram of tissue) and the *radiation absorbed dose* (rad) (1 rad = 100 erg per gram of tissue = 0.01 Gy). The *roentgen-equivalent-man* (rem) is the dosage of ionizing radiation equal to 1 rad of x-radiation (100 rem = 1 sievert). A chest radiograph equals 45 mrem, and flying 3000 miles in a jet at 35,000 ft results in 4 mrem of exposure.

The relative sensitivity of organ systems exposed to the radiation determines the clinical symptoms. Because it is often difficult or impossible to quantitate rad accurately, the symptoms and signs become important in determining the diagnosis, therapy, and prognosis. In many radiation accidents, exposed individuals are not wearing a monitoring device that can measure high doses of radiation. In these instances, the radiation dose must be measured from its biologic effects. The earliest indicator is the decrease in the absolute lymphocyte count, which can occur within 48 hours after exposure (see Table 144-2).[5]

With exposures greater than 3 Gy, peripheral granulocyte analysis is a more accurate estimator. The nadir in the granulocyte count, which occurs 8 to 30 days after exposure, should be followed closely. Higher dose exposure results in increasingly severe granulocytopenia with a shorter time from exposure to the nadir level. The severity of thrombocytopenia and reticulocytopenia is also an indicator of radiation dose. Finally, cytogenetic studies (i.e., analysis of the presence and number of dicentric chromosomes in blood and bone marrow) are relatively accurate dose estimators.[6,11]

Tissues with greater rates of cellular division are more radiosensitive (Figure 144-4). Organ systems that have the greatest cellular division rates are the hematopoietic and gastrointestinal systems. In intense irradiation exposure, however, central nervous system (CNS) symptoms result, even though the CNS has a low cellular turnover rate. Invariably, all organ systems are involved in whole-body irradiation. At doses less than 1 Gy, most cells survive but may be susceptible to radiation-induced cancer. Leukemia can develop within 2 years of exposure, whereas solid tumors can take several decades to develop.[5,12,13]

The median lethal whole-body dose (i.e., the dose that is lethal for 50% of test subjects) for humans is estimated to be about 4.5 Gy with proper medical care.[6] Whole-body exposure of 10 Gy seems to be the maximal survivable dose with the best medical therapy available.[5] Doses greater than 20 Gy produce CNS symptoms. These symptoms occur immediately after exposure and include headache, mental status aberration, prostration, vertigo, tinnitus, and sensory and motor changes. If the individual is exposed to a nonuniform dose and the gastrointestinal and hematopoietic systems are spared, there is a chance of survival after resolution of the CNS symptoms. If more than 20 Gy of whole-body exposure occurs, however, fulminating gastrointestinal and CNS symptoms ensue, sometimes within 30 minutes, and in all instances the outcome is fatal. This situation indicates a supralethal dose of radiation, and for triage purposes, the death of these patients should be classified as "impending" or "expectant." If medical resources are scarce, sedation and analgesia should be the only therapies. With whole-body exposure of more than 10 Gy, mortality is nearly 100%. Death results from hematopoietic system complications if the patient survives the CNS and gastrointestinal system involvement.

The gastrointestinal syndrome is seen regularly at doses higher than 1 Gy. In general, the higher the dose received, the sooner the onset of symptoms after exposure. In its mildest form, nausea and vomiting of less than 20 hours' duration are seen. More protracted nausea and vomiting are seen with higher exposures. The onset of high fever and persistent bloody diarrhea is an ominous sign. Even if intense fluid and electrolyte therapy results in early survival, death from hematopoietic system failure may result.

Generally, a latent period, lasting 2 days to 4 weeks from exposure, occurs before the signs of hematopoietic system involvement develop, specifically pancytopenia resulting from marrow suppression. This syndrome includes leukopenia and thrombocytopenia with fever, increased susceptibility to infection, petechiae, and hemorrhagic tendencies. Protective isolation is important during this period. The absolute lymphocyte count 48 hours after exposure is a good predictor of hematopoietic involvement (see Figure 144-4). If the absolute lymphocyte count is greater than 1200/μL, it is unlikely that the patient has received a clinically significant dose of radiation. If the absolute lymphocyte count falls between 100/μL and 500/μL at 48 hours, the possibility of exposure to a lethal dose of radiation should be suspected. A level in this range is an indication for hospitalization. Levels less than 500/μL are critical, and heroic procedures such as the use of hematopoietic growth factors may be helpful.[5,14] If a patient is symptomatic, serial complete blood counts should be performed in the hospital. Hemorrhagic complications should be treated with platelet concentrates and, if necessary, whole blood or fresh frozen plasma. Anemia resulting from erythropoietic suppression is usually not a problem.

Skin burns with erythema may be delayed in onset. If secondary to penetrating radiation, they indicate high exposure. Severe skin burns may be a result of nonpenetrating radiation, such as beta particle contamination, but without accompanying systemic symptoms. Such burns can be prevented or tempered by early vigorous decontamination procedures. If present, they should be treated as any other thermal or chemical burn.

Skin changes that occur may be used to quantify the radiation exposure. Epilation occurs after exposure to 3 Gy; erythema, after 10 Gy; wet desquamation, after 20 Gy; and necrosis, after 30 Gy of localized skin exposure to radiation.[5] These responses are similar to those of severe chemical burns.

A key historical point when evaluating a suspicious burn is whether the patient remembers coming into contact with a hot object or caustic chemical. If the patient has no recollection of this and is a radiation worker, particularly if there is a history of carrying a bright metal object that may have been a radioisotope source, the possibility of a radiation burn should be considered. The patterns of symptoms and signs of acute radiation syndrome overlap and contain many variables (see Figure 144-4).

MANAGEMENT

Prehospital Care

The history obtained from field personnel is crucial. The exact type of exposure (external versus internal, whole body versus partial body) should be ascertained. If internal exposure is suspected, the portal of entry (inhalation versus ingestion) and the radioactive material involved should be ascertained.

Decontamination

If the patient's condition permits, decontamination should be initiated at the scene because many emergency departments are not designed for this procedure. In the case of an industrial or laboratory accident, each facility should have a specific protocol and equipment available to initiate the decontamination process. Prehospital personnel who are inexperienced in such procedures should follow the direction of the on-site personnel who have been trained in the decontamination process. Ambulance personnel should wear protective clothing, including rubber gloves, shoe covers, and respirators if airborne contamination is suspected.

The patient's clothing should be removed and placed in plastic bags. If possible, soap and water cleansing of exposed skin should be performed. All materials, including wash water, should be placed in containers and labeled as radioactive waste. Performing these tasks at the scene minimizes contamination of the ambulance and the emergency department.

If the patient is unstable, rapid, initial, and partial decontamination procedures, such as clothing removal, should be done at the scene before expeditious transportation to an emergency department. Radio contact with the receiving hospital should provide the available history. If the community disaster plan has a designated hospital for radiation-contaminated victims, they should be transported directly to that facility. Physicians wishing to establish a comprehensive plan to manage radiation accident victims are referred to the National Council on Radiation Protection Report No. 65, *Management of Persons Accidentally Contaminated with Radionucleotides*.[15]

Emergency Department

Every emergency department designated as a decontamination facility should have a radiation accident protocol. An excellent prototype was published by Leonard and Ricks.[16] This protocol should be in the policy and procedures manual and posted in the decontamination facility.

Preparation

The chaos that ensued in the wake of the Three Mile Island experience suggests that a community disaster plan should be developed with a predetermined individual empowered to make decisions regarding evacuation and other issues concerning the at-risk population. On notification of the numbers and types of patients involved in a radiation exposure accident, a decision should be made regarding implementation of a full disaster plan versus a limited response. The radiation control officer, usually a radiologist or pathologist, should be called immediately. The radiation control officer should monitor all patients and medical personnel with a radiation counter and should supervise the "cleanup" and the routing of patients to minimize "tracking," or spread, of contamination. Timely and accurate information and instructions should be given to a public relations person for dissemination to the news media to minimize the chaos and paranoia that inevitably would result from such incidents.

Decontamination

Contaminated patients should be decontaminated in the field, but if they are not and arrive at the emergency department, they should enter through a separate, protected entrance or be isolated until a decontamination tent can be erected (Figure 144-5). All medical personnel should wear protective, disposable clothing, including surgical gloves and shoe covers. Respirators are not required at the hospital, but should be used by first responders who are entering a highly contaminated area.[5] The emergency suite should contain all equipment necessary for a major resuscitation. If decontamination occurs inside the emergency department, it should have a closed drainage and ventilation system to prevent the spread of water-borne or airborne radioactive contamination. In many hospitals, the only area equipped with such facilities is the autopsy room or morgue. The radiation disaster plan may necessitate taking resuscitation equipment to this area and providing decontamination and initial care there if this cannot be done in a decontamination facility outside of the emergency department.

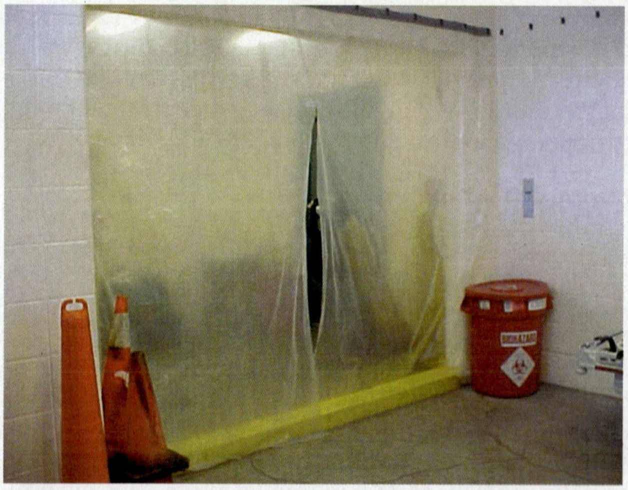

Figure 144-5. Protected entrance in the emergency department.

The patient should be undressed immediately, and all clothing should be placed in sealed containers labeled "radioactive waste." Exposed skin should be cleansed with soap and water. Hair should be shampooed. All waste water, washcloths, and towels should be saved in properly labeled containers. The cleansing process should be repeated as many times as necessary depending on the dosimeter readings received and interpretations made by the radiation control officer. The hair may have to be cut. The nails should be trimmed and meticulously scraped to remove contamination.

Wound Management

If the patient has open wounds, the surrounding skin should be decontaminated by scrubbing with soap and water. Adhesive, disposable, surgical drapes should be applied, and the wounds should be prepared and irrigated with copious amounts of saline. Frequent monitoring for radioactive contamination determines when irrigation can be discontinued. Surgical debridement should be performed according to the usual indications of dirt and nonviable tissue or continued high readings of radioactive contaminants. The normal principles of wound closure should be followed for contaminated wounds. The wounds in patients who have received whole-body radiation greater than 1 Gy should be closed, primarily so that they do not become a portal for lethal infection.[5]

Any surgery needed should be performed immediately because a delay may be complicated by the fluid and electrolyte problems resulting from acute radiation syndrome. Longer delays may be complicated by the increased risk of infection and hemorrhage caused by the hematopoietic effects of acute radiation syndrome.

Ancillary Tests

If the history is one of possible neutron exposure, all vomitus, urine, and feces should be saved for possible analysis and an estimation of dosage received. Laboratory studies should include a baseline complete blood count and platelet count. Particular attention should be paid to the absolute lymphocyte and neutrophil counts obtained on arrival and at 48 hours after exposure.

Internal Contamination

Oral ingestion of radionucleotides presents some special considerations. After ingestion, there is usually a variable time period before absorption and uptake by the cells. It is important to determine exactly what radionucleotides are involved because therapy with blocking or chelating agents is determined by the elements involved. A *blocking agent* is a chemical that saturates a tissue with a nonradioactive element, reducing the uptake of the radionucleotide. An example of this is the use of potassium iodine (Lugol's iodine solution) to reduce the uptake of radioactive iodine. *Chelating agents* bind metals into complexes, preventing tissue uptake and allowing urinary excretion. Two examples are calcium disodium edetate and penicillamine, both recommended for treating radioactive lead poisoning. Ideally, these agents should be administered soon after exposure, before significant uptake of the radionucleotide can occur. A poison information center should be contacted to determine the current recommendations and dosages of chelating and blocking agents and other recommended treatment modalities.[17]

In addition, the standard therapeutic maneuvers for poison ingestion, such as induced emesis, cathartics, activated charcoal, and lavage, may be useful. All excretions (urine, feces, vomitus, and lavage fluid) should be saved in specially labeled containers for proper disposal and for possible dosimetry.

Acute inhalation of radionucleotides presents a difficult problem. Early bronchopulmonary lavage may be effective in partial removal of the radioactive contaminants. Chelating and blocking agents also may be used. Chronic low-level inhaled contaminants are more common, and long-term sequelae are reported. Extensive cutaneous radiation fibrosis occurred in some long-term survivors of the Chernobyl accident, and interferon therapy is reported to be of benefit.[18]

Triage Classification, Further Treatment, and Disposition

Patients can be classified for triage purposes by presenting symptoms into three categories: survival probable, survival possible, and survival improbable. The *survival probable group* consists of patients having either no initial symptoms or mild symptoms, such as nausea and vomiting, which subside within a few hours. Exposure in this group is estimated to be less than 2 Gy. The initial laboratory studies and serial complete blood counts reveal no depression of the leukocyte count. It is not necessary to hospitalize these patients unless subsequent laboratory studies or symptoms indicate a need for in-hospital treatment.

The *survival possible group* includes patients in whom nausea and vomiting are relatively brief (lasting 24 to 48 hours), followed by an asymptomatic period. After the initial symptoms, these patients exhibit the typical hematologic changes of thrombocytopenia, granulocytopenia, and lymphopenia. The severity of these changes depends on individual susceptibility and the level of the initial radiation dose. These patients should be admitted for fluid and electrolyte therapy if vomiting is severe. Antiemetics may be ineffective. Also, protective isolation precautions are indicated, particularly if there is significant granulocytopenia at 48 hours.

The exposure dosage range for patients in the survival possible group is estimated to be 2 to 10 Gy, with the median lethal dose (LD_{50}) for humans estimated to be 3 to 5 Gy. The LD_{50} varies depending on the vigor of supportive therapy. In mass casualty situations, the LD_{50} is probably in the range of 3.5 Gy; it is probably 4.5 Gy in other situations. The concept of calculating the LD_{10} versus LD_{90} for human radiation exposure is a means of determining what level of therapeutic intervention is indicated. A patient who has received an LD_{90} exposure may survive only if hematopoietic growth factors are used, whereas a patient with an LD_{10} exposure may need only low-risk supportive care, such as reverse isolation and intravenous fluids.

Therapy for the survival possible group is based on the exact hematologic derangements present. Platelet concentrates are recommended if the count falls below 25,000/mm^3. Treatment with appropriate broad-spectrum antibiotics should be considered only if clinical signs of infection appear. Prophylactic antibiotics may be indicated if serious gastrointestinal symptoms, such as vomiting and diarrhea, are present. Prophylactic antifungal agents, such as amphotericin B, also may be indicated. Acyclovir may be useful in treating or preventing oral herpes simplex infection. Hematopoietic growth factors may have substantial benefit with little risk in victims predicted to have moderate or severe bone marrow failure. Intravenous hyperalimentation may be necessary for the successful treatment of the gastrointestinal syndrome.

The third group is the *survival improbable group*. The exposed dose range in this group is estimated to be greater than 10 Gy whole-body exposure. These patients experience rapid onset of fulminating nausea, vomiting, and diarrhea. Intense fluid and electrolyte and hyperalimentation therapy may result in initial survival for these patients. They later experience the sequelae of bone marrow aplasia and pancytopenia that is uniformly fatal. If CNS symptoms appear early, it can be assumed that the patient has received a very large dose of radiation. In mass casualty situations, these patients should be made comfortable with narcotics and sedatives. They should be triaged into the "impending" or "expectant" death category. In isolated situations, vigorous supportive therapy may be used, but the prognosis is dismal.

Consultative Resources

For questions about radiation exposure and injuries, the U.S. Department of Energy can be contacted 24 hours a day at the Radiation Emergency Assistance

Center/Training Site (REAC/TS) in Oak Ridge, Tennessee (telephone number, 865-576-1005; interactive website, http://www.orau.gov/reacts). For information about the training of physicians, REAC/TS can be contacted at 865-576-3131. The *Medical Management of Radiological Casualties Handbook* is available online at http://www.afrri.usuhs.mil. The Chemical/Biological Hotline of the National Response Center is 800-424-8802.

KEY CONCEPTS

- Contaminated patients are "radioactive"; irradiated patients are not.
- No danger to medical personnel from contaminated patients should exist if proper precautions and decontamination procedures are carried out.
- Careful evaluation of initial symptoms and signs is the most reliable indicator of the radiation dose received and the patient's prognosis.
- Most therapy is supportive and symptomatic except for exposures involving the ingestion or inhalation of radioactive material, when specific therapy with blocking or chelating agents may be indicated.
- Detonation of a "dirty bomb" would cause psychological terror and little or no radiation injuries.
- Formal consultation is available 24 hours a day and should be obtained when any patient with radiation injuries is evaluated.

REFERENCES

1. Gale RP, Thompson MA, Crawford MA: Recent radiation accidents: Chernobyl and Boiania: Their impact and global implications. *Ala J Med Sci* 25:439, 1988.
2. *One Decade after Chernobyl, Summing up the Consequences of the Accident. Proceedings of an International Conference, Vienna, April 8-12, 1996.* Vienna, International Atomic Energy, 1996.
3. *Terrorism: Questions and Answers: "Dirty Bombs."* Council on Foreign Relations, revised June 23, 2003.
4. *Radiation Emergencies/Dirty Bombs.* CDC Emergency Preparedness and Response, revised July 28, 2003.
5. Mettler FA, Voelz G: Major radiation exposure—what to expect and how to respond. *N Engl J Med* 346:20, 2002.
6. Champlin HE, Kastenberg WE, Gale RP: Radiation accidents and nuclear energy: Medical consequences and therapy. *Ann Intern Med* 109:730, 1988.
7. Hart BL, Mettler FA Jr, Harley NH: Radon: Is it a problem? *Radiology* 172:593, 1989.
8. Archer VE, Renzetti AD, Doggett RS: Chronic diffuse interstitial fibrosis of the lung. *J Occup Environ Med* 40:460, 1998.
9. Little JB: What are the risks of low-level exposure to a radiation from radon? *Proc Natl Acad Sci U S A* 24:5996, 1997.
10. Goldsmith JR: Epidemiologic evidence relevant to radar (microwave) effects. *Environ Health Perspect* 105:1579, 1997.
11. Baranov A, et al: Bone marrow transplantation after the Chernobyl nuclear accident. *N Engl J Med* 321:205, 1989.
12. United Nations Scientific Committee on the Effects of Atomic Radiation: *Sources and Effects of Ionizing Radiation: UNSCEAR 2000 Report to the General Assembly, with Scientific Annexes.* New York, United Nations, 2000.
13. Pierce DA, Preston D: Radiation-related cancer risks at low doses among atomic bomb survivors. *Radiat Res* 154:178, 2000.
14. MacVitte TJ, Weiss JF, Browne D (eds): *Advances in Treatment of Radiation Injuries. Advances in the Biosciences,* vol 94. New York, Pergamon Press, 1996.
15. National Council on Radiation Protection and Measurements: *Management of Persons Accidentally Contaminated with Radionucleotides* (NCRP Report No. 65). Washington, DC, 1980.
16. Leonard RB, Ricks RC: Emergency department radiation accident protocol. *Ann Emerg Med* 9:462, 1980.
17. *Management of Internally Deposited Radionuclides* (Report No. 65). Bethesda, Md, National Council on Radiation Protection and Measurements, 1985.
18. Peter RU, et al: Interferon gamma in survivors of the Chernobyl power plant accident: New therapeutic option for radiation-induced fibrosis. *Int J Radiat Oncol Biol Phys* 45:147, 1999.

Section II **TOXICOLOGY**

CHAPTER 145 General Approach to the Poisoned Patient

Ken Kulig

PERSPECTIVE

Most poisoned patients seen in the emergency department are adults with acute, oral drug overdoses. Other common clinical scenarios include accidental poisoning in children; parenteral drug abuse; chronic poisoning, usually from environmental, industrial, and agricultural chemical exposure; medication reactions or interactions; and envenomation. Management requires both a general approach and specific actions directed at the particular toxin or toxins involved, as outlined in the various chapters in this section. Clinical studies have modified the management of poisoned patients, such as the use of gastric decontamination, but much of the toxicology literature, especially with unusual poisonings, remains case based.

INITIAL APPROACH TO THE POISONED PATIENT

With rare exception, the priorities of care for a poisoned patient are identical to those for all patients coming to the emergency department. Patients who are contaminated with an agent that might injure health care personnel require decontamination before treatment to avoid disabling the hospital staff or the entire health care facility. Except for specific lifesaving antidotes against certain toxins, most poisoned patients require only supportive therapy for recovery. The initial workup should determine whether a specific patient has been exposed to an agent for which an antidote (or other specific treatment) exists.[1] A thorough poisoning history and toxicologic physical examination are followed by the selective use of laboratory tests.

After initial stabilization of a critically ill patient, specific antidote therapy is administered while a detailed history and physical examination are performed. Hypoglycemia must always be considered in a patient with altered mental status or seizures and should be evaluated by bedside glucose testing rather than empiric administration of hypertonic glucose solution.[2] *Naloxone* can be given to patients with respiratory depression while preparations are made to secure the airway because a positive response may obviate the need for intubation. *Flumazenil* is not indicated in an undifferentiated overdose patient, and its use should be limited to confirmed acute benzodiazepine overdose in a patient known to not be a regular benzodiazepine user (e.g., an adolescent who impulsively ingests a parent's benzodiazepine). Indiscriminate use may force a chronic benzodiazepine user into severe benzodiazepine withdrawal. Likewise, the patient may have ingested tricyclic antidepressants or other drugs likely to cause seizures. In either case, the use of flumazenil can carry a substantial risk of seizures. Patients with benzodiazepine overdose respond well to supportive care. *Thiamine* should be administered when dextrose is given to nutritionally compromised, alcoholic patients with altered mental status (100 mg in the maintenance intravenous line is sufficient and safe).[3]

A complete *overdose history* is required, particularly when the ingested agent is unknown or the patient is suicidal (Box 145-1). Valuable clues often come from unexpected sources, such as the patient's previous medical records, the pharmacy where prescriptions were filled, or the prescribing physician as listed on the patient's prescription bottles. Field personnel, whenever possible, should bring the patient's medications to the hospital with them. If the ingested agent is a hazardous chemical (e.g., pesticide) that might endanger hospital personnel, it should be brought to the hospital in an airtight container or secured at the scene. Precise product identification information must be ascertained so that a hazardous materials reference system can be consulted. When it is suspected that the contents of the container are not the original product, the substance should be checked against the product label. It is easy to confuse the different types of chemical agents with similar names found in many homes, and some may have specific properties that affect treatment. In rare cases, overdose patients may deliberately attempt to deceive caregivers by hiding the ingested agents.

BOX 145-1. Obtaining an Overdose History

- Obtain all prescription bottles and other containers when possible. Perform a pill count. Be sure that the bottles contain the medications listed. Identify any unknown tablets.
- Contact the prescribing physician(s) or the pharmacy as listed on the bottles to determine previous overdoses or other medications that the patient may have available. Identify underlying medical and psychiatric disorders and medication allergies. Review past medical records.
- Talk to the patient's family and friends in the emergency department. If necessary, call the patient's home to ask questions of others. The persons providing the important elements of the history should be identified in the chart.
- Search the patient's belongings for drugs or drug paraphernalia. A single pill hidden in a pocket, for example, may provide *the* most important clue to the diagnosis.
- Have family members (or the police) search the patient's home, including the medicine cabinet, clothes drawers, closets, and garage: such searches may also provide clues that make the diagnosis. This has the added benefit of involving the family in the patient's care.
- Always look for track marks on the patient. Consider body packing or body stuffing.

Vital signs, including pulse oximetry, are important in the diagnosis of poisoning and should be measured accurately and repeated as indicated. At least one measurement of temperature must always be included. Respirations should be counted, not estimated. A cardiac monitor or 12-lead electrocardiogram should be evaluated for QRS and QT intervals, morphology, and rhythm. The physical examination in a comatose patient should ensure that concomitant treatable conditions (e.g., intracranial hemorrhage, central nervous system [CNS] infection) are not missed. Focal neurologic findings could be possible indicators of intracranial catastrophe or severe head trauma.

The pupillary examination may give misleading information. Some opioid agonists, especially propoxyphene and pentazocine, may not produce the characteristic miosis of opioid intoxication. When multiple drugs are ingested, the expected pupillary findings related to any particular agent may be modified or absent.

Physical stigmata of intravenous drug use (track marks) should be sought in both usual (e.g., antecubital fossa) and unusual (e.g., under the tongue, top of the feet) locations. A critical condition of unknown cause may be a result of "body packing" or "body stuffing," complicated by rupture of packets of cocaine, heroin, or amphetamines (see Chapter 152). Rectal, vaginal, and radiographic examination of the abdomen should be performed in these circumstances.

Other important physical findings are evidence of aspiration or noncardiogenic pulmonary edema on chest auscultation. Bowel sounds may be increased or decreased if agents affecting the cholinergic nervous system have been ingested. A rectal examination to detect melena or hematochezia may also provide evidence of suicidal ingestion of anticoagulant medication.

Unusual odors of the patient's breath, skin, clothing, vomitus, or nasogastric aspirate may also provide useful diagnostic clues (Table 145-1).[4] The absence of such odors, however, should not be taken as evidence that the agents listed are not present.

TOXIC SYNDROMES AND ANTIDOTES

The term *toxidrome* refers to a constellation of physical findings that can provide important clues to narrow the differential diagnosis.[1] The general rules outlined here have many exceptions, and polydrug overdoses may result in overlapping and confusing mixed syndromes. Nevertheless, this approach may confirm the history, provide the clinician with a starting point for management, and suggest useful laboratory tests. The most common toxidromes are the anticholinergic syndrome, sympathomimetic syndrome, opioid/sedative/ethanol syndrome, and cholinergic syndrome (Table 145-2).

The *anticholinergic syndrome* occurs frequently because many common medications and plants have anticholinergic properties. Anticholinergic CNS poisoning causes mild temperature elevation and acute delirium with mumbling speech and typical "picking movements" of the fingers. Suppression of cholinergic inhibition of the heart rate leads to tachycardia. Inhibition of the secretory functions of the integument causes dry mouth and skin, and the face is typically flushed. Unopposed sympathetic drive of the ciliary apparatus causes wide papillary dilation. Most patients recover with supportive therapy, but the delirium may last a day or more. *Physostigmine* may be a useful antidote in carefully selected patients and quickly resolves the delirium. It should not be used with a possible cyclic antidepressant overdose where it is associated with asystole. The *sympathomimetic syndrome* is usually seen after acute or chronic abuse of cocaine, amphetamines, or decongestants (e.g., phenylpropanolamine). Patients may be delusional; amphetamine, in particular, may cause complicated, intricate, and paranoid delusions. Seizures may occur, and the postictal state can contribute to the altered mental status. Blood pressure is usually elevated, the pulse is rapid (except with pure α-adrenergic agonists such as phenylpropanolamine, which can cause reflex bradycardia), the pupils are dilated, and piloerection may be seen. In massive overdoses of sympathomimetic agents,

Table 145-1. Odors in Overdose History

Odor	Possible intoxicant
Bitter almonds	Cyanide
Carrots	Water hemlock (cicutoxin)
Fishy	Zinc or aluminum phosphide
Fruity	Ethanol, acetone, isopropyl alcohol, chlorinated hydrocarbons (e.g., chloroform)
Garlic	Arsenic, dimethyl sulfoxide (DMSO), organophosphates, yellow phosphorus, selenium, tellurium
Glue	Toluene, other solvents
Pears	Chloral hydrate, paraldehyde
Rotten eggs	Disulfiram, hydrogen sulfide, *N*-acetylcysteine, dimercaptosuccinic acid (DMSA)
Shoe polish	Nitrobenzene
Wintergreen	Methyl salicylate

Table 145-2. Common Toxic Syndromes (Toxidromes)

Anticholinergic	
Common signs	Delirium with mumbling speech, tachycardia, dry flushed skin, dilated pupils, myoclonus, slightly elevated temperature, urinary retention, decreased bowel sounds. Seizures and dysrhythmias may occur in severe cases
Common causes	Antihistamines, antiparkinsonians, atropine, scopolamine, amantadine, antipsychotics, antidepressants, antispasmodics, mydriatics, muscle relaxants, many plants (e.g., jimson weed, *Amanita muscaria*)
Sympathomimetic	
Common signs	Delusions, paranoia, tachycardia (or bradycardia with pure α-agonists), hypertension, hyperpyrexia, diaphoresis, piloerection, mydriasis, hyperreflexia. Seizures, hypotension, and dysrhythmias may occur in severe cases
Common causes	Cocaine, amphetamine, methamphetamine and its derivatives, over-the-counter decongestants (phenylpropanolamine, ephedrine, pseudoephedrine). In caffeine and theophylline overdoses, similar findings, except for the organic psychiatric signs, result from catecholamine release
Opioid/Sedative/Ethanol	
Common signs	Coma, respiratory depression, miosis, hypotension, bradycardia, hypothermia, pulmonary edema, decreased bowel sounds, hyporeflexia, needle marks. Seizures may occur after overdoses of some narcotics (e.g., propoxyphene)
Common causes	Narcotics, barbiturates, benzodiazepines, ethchlorvynol, glutethimide, methyprylon, methaqualone, meprobamate, ethanol, clonidine, guanabenz
Cholinergic	
Common signs	Confusion, central nervous system depression, weakness, salivation, lacrimation, urinary/fecal incontinence, gastrointestinal cramping, emesis, diaphoresis, muscle fasciculations, pulmonary edema, miosis, bradycardia/tachycardia, seizures
Common causes	Organophosphate and carbamate insecticides, physostigmine, edrophonium, some mushrooms

Modified from Kulig K: Initial management of ingestions of toxic substances, *N Engl J Med* 326:1677, 1992.

cardiovascular collapse can occur with the development of shock and wide-complex dysrhythmias. This clinical picture can mimic that of overdose of cardioactive drugs or cyclic antidepressants. In contrast to the diaphoresis seen with anticholinergic syndrome, the skin in sympathomimetic syndrome is dry.

All sedative/hypnotic agents, when taken in sufficient dosage, cause general anesthesia with a complete loss of awareness and reflex activity. The CNS depressant (opioid/sedative/ethanol) syndrome is the most common toxic syndrome seen in the emergency department, and a depressed sensorium is its hallmark. Mixing agents in this class (e.g., ethanol and benzodiazepines) is common. As the drugs are absorbed at higher doses, the patient becomes increasingly obtunded, the deep tendon reflexes diminish, and finally, the vital signs deteriorate as medullary drive of respiration and cardiovascular function is attenuated.

Respiratory depression is particularly pronounced with opioid overdose, and the respiratory rate is often diminished before decreases in blood pressure or pulse occur. The diagnosis of opioid overdose is confirmed by the use of naloxone (Narcan) or nalmefene (Revex) in adequate doses.[2,5,6] *Naloxone* has an elimination half-life of 1.1 hours, whereas that of nalmefene is 10.8 hours. *Nalmefene* is especially useful when the offending opioid has a very long elimination half-life itself (e.g., methadone, with a half-life of 15 to 40 hours).[5] Close observation, investigation of alternative causes of depressed mental status when suggested by the clinical course, and airway intervention when indicated are the keys to successful management.

The *cholinergic syndrome* is uncommon, but important to recognize because lifesaving treatment is available. Cholinergic syndrome causes the patient to be "wet," as opposed to the anticholinergic syndrome, which causes the patient to be "dry." The wetness is manifest by profuse sweating and excessive activity of virtually the entire exocrine system, often accompanied by vomiting, diarrhea, and urinary incontinence. The mnemonic "SLUDGE" is used to recall the specific elements of the syndrome: *s*alivation, *l*acrimation, *u*rination, *d*efecation, *g*astrointestinal cramping, and *e*mesis. The CNS (e.g., confusion, coma, seizures) and the skeletal muscles (e.g., weakness, fasciculations) can also be involved. The pupils are often miotic. Cholinergic syndrome is most frequently caused by organophosphate or carbamate pesticide exposure, which may be through unsuspected dermal contamination. Anticholinergic agents are also the foundation of "nerve agents" such as sarin, which was used in the Tokyo subway attack. Recognition of the syndrome led to the use of atropine and cholinesterase regenerators, with a subsequent good outcome in many patients.[7]

Serotonin syndrome ensues when there is a drug interaction involving the selective serotonin reuptake inhibitors (SSRIs) or an overdose of an SSRI.[8] Fluoxetine (Prozac), sertraline (Zoloft), paroxetine (Paxil), fluvoxamine (Luvox), and citalopram (Celexa) are commonly used SSRIs. Other drugs that are serotonin reuptake inhibitors (SRIs) also inhibit the reuptake of other neurotransmitters and are therefore not specific. These drugs include venlafaxine (Effexor), nefazodone (Serzone), and mirtazapine (Remeron). Drug interactions between many drugs can cause the serotonin syndrome described in Chapter 159. These drugs include the SSRIs, SRIs, monoamine oxidase inhibitors (MAOIs), tryptophan, sympathomimetics, tricyclic and other antidepressants, meperidine, dextromethorphan, and lithium. Because of the long-lasting effects of the SSRIs, the syndrome can occur when one of the active agents is ingested even weeks after use of an SSRI has been discontinued.

Serotonin syndrome is characterized by altered mental status, fever, agitation, tremor, myoclonus, hyperreflexia, ataxia, incoordination, diaphoresis, shivering, and sometimes diarrhea.[8] The diagnosis relies on the drug history, and it is difficult to distinguish serotonin syndrome from an overdose of cocaine, lithium, or MAOIs; the neuroleptic malignant syndrome; or thyroid storm. Patients may deteriorate slowly and become critically ill after an apparently benign manifestation.

As possible toxidromes are investigated, the use of specific antidotes should be considered (Table 145-3).

TOXICOLOGY LABORATORY

A toxicology screen (usually urine, sometimes blood and urine, and occasionally including gastric contents) only rarely results in identification of the ingested agent for three major reasons. First, the laboratory does not even attempt to screen for many substances, even commonly ingested agents that are capable of causing critical illness (Box 145-2).[9]

BOX 145-2. Drugs, Chemicals, and Groups *Not Detected* by a Comprehensive Toxicology Screen

Ammonia	Laxatives
Anesthetic gases	Lithium
Antibiotics	Metals
Anticoagulants	Monoamine oxidase inhibitors
β-Blockers	Most antihypertensives
Borates	Most cardiac medications
Bromides	Muscle relaxants
Caustics/corrosives	Mushrooms
Colchicine	Newer antidepressants (e.g., fluoxetine, sertraline, paroxetine, bupropion, buspirone)
Cyanide	Nitrates/nitrites
Digitalis glycosides	NSAIDs
Disulfiram	Paraquat
Ergot alkaloids	Pesticides
Ethylene glycol	Phenol
Fentanyl and its derivatives	Plants
Fluorides	Solvents
H_2 antagonists	Thyroid hormone
Hallucinogens (e.g., LSD)	Vitamins
Herbicides	
Household products	
Hypoglycemics	
Insect repellents	
Isoniazid	

NSAIDs, nonsteroidal anti-inflammatory drugs.

Table 145-3. Antidotes Used in the Emergency Department

Toxin Used For	Antidote	Dose and Comments
Acetaminophen	*N*-acetylcysteine	140 mg/kg po, then 70 mg/kg q4h for up to 17 doses or 150 mg/kg IV load over 1 hr with 50 mg/kg over 4 hr followed by 100 mg/kg over 16 hr
Anticholinergics	Physostigmine	1-2 mg IV in adults, 0.5 mg in children over 2 min for anticholinergic delerium, seizures, or dysrhythmias
Arsenic, lead, and mercury	BAL	3-5 mg/kg IM only
	D-Penicillamine	20-40 mg/kg/day; 500 mg tid in adults; may cross-react with penicillin in allergic patients
Benzodiazepines	Flumazenil	0.2 mg, then 0.3 mg, then 0.5 mg, up to 5 mg; not to be used if patient has signs of TCA toxicity; not approved for use in children, but probably safe
Black widow spider bite	*Latrodectus* antivenin	1 vial by slow IV infusion is usually curative; may cause anaphylaxis
β-Blockers	Glucagon	5-10 mg in adults, then infusion of same dose per hour
	Insulin and glucose	10 U insulin with dextrose 25 g initially, then 0.1-1.0 U/kg/hr, 10-30 g/hr
Calcium channel blockers	Calcium	1 g calcium chloride IV in adults, 20-30-mg/kg/dose in children, over a few minutes with continuous monitoring. Repeat as needed
	Glucagon	5-10 mg in adults, then infusion of same dose per hour
	Insulin and glucose	10 U insulin with dextrose 25 g initially, then 0.1-1.0 U/kg/hr with 10-30 g/hr
Cyanide, hydrogen sulfide	Sodium thiosulfate	50 mL of 25% (12.5 g; 1 ampule) in adults; 1.65 mL/kg IV in children
	Sodium nitrate	10 mL of 3% (300 mg; 1 ampule) in adults; 0.33 mL/kg slowly IV in children
Digitalis glycosides	Digoxin-specific Fab fragments	10-20 vials if patient in ventricular fibrillation; otherwise dose based on serum digoxin concentration or amount ingested
Ethylene glycol	Fomepizole	15 mg/kg × 1, then 10 mg/kg q12h × 4, until ethylene glycol < 20 mg/dL. Adjust dose during dialysis
	Pyridoxine	100 mg IV daily
	Thiamine	100 mg IV
Hydrofluoric acid	Calcium gluconate	3.5 g in 5 oz of KY jelly topical; apply liberally to affected skin
Iron	Deferoxamine	15 mg/kg/hr IV; higher doses reported to be safe
Isoniazid, hydrazine, and monomethylhydrazine	Pyridoxine	5 g in adults, 1 g in children, if ingested dose unknown; antidote may cause neuropathy in very large doses
Lead	DMSA (succimer)	Reported useful for arsenic and lead as well; one 100-mg capsule per 10-kg body weight tid for 1 wk then bid, with chelation breaks
	EDTA	75 mg/kg/day by continuous infusion; watch for nephrotoxicity, best done in hospital
Methanol	Folate or leucovorin	50 mg IV q4h in adults while patients has serious toxicity
	Ethanol	Loading dose, 10 mL/kg of 10%; maintenance dose, 0.15 mL/kg/hr of 10%; double rate during dialysis
	Fomepizole	15 mg/kg × 1, then 10 mg/kg q12h × 4, until methanol < 20 mg/dL. Adjust dose during dialysis
Methemoglobin-forming agents	Methylene blue	1-2 mg/kg IV, one 10-mL dose of 10% solution (100 mg) is typical for an adult without anemia
Opioids	Nalmefene	2 mg; much longer half-life than naloxone
	Naloxone	2 mg; less to avoid narcotic withdrawal, more if inadequate response; same dose in children
Organophosphates and carbamates	Atropine	Test dose, 1-2 mg IV in adults, 0.03 mg/kg in children; titrate to drying of pulmonary secretions
	Protopam	Loading dose, 1-2 g IV in adults, 25-50 mg/kg in children; adult maintenance, 500 mg/hr or 1-2 g q4–6h
Rattlesnake bite	*Cro-Fab* antivenin	5 vials minimum dose by infusion in normal saline; increases in rate dependent on patient tolerance; may cause anaphylaxis
Serotonin syndrome	Cyproheptadine	4 mg PO as needed; no parenteral form available; antidote may cause anticholinergic effects
Sulfonureas	Octreotide	50 µg SC q12h, 5-10 µg/kg/24 hr IV
Tricyclic antidepressants	Bicarbonate	44-88 mEq in adults, 1-2 mEq/kg in children; best used by IV push and not by slow infusion
Valproic acid	Carnitine	100 mg/kg IV or PO loading dose with 25 mg/kg q6h

BAL, British anti-Lewisite; DMSA, dimercaptosuccinic acid; EDTA, ethylenediaminetetraacetic acid; TCA, tricyclic antidepressant.

Second, the urine screen is often performed soon after the ingestion, when the drug concentration is too low for a positive result. Even the drug responsible for life-threatening symptoms (e.g., tricyclic antidepressant) may be negative on the urine screen soon after ingestion. Other drugs, such as γ-hydroxybutyrate, need to be collected in the first urine sample to be detected.

Third, drugs found on screening may not be those responsible for the initial symptoms, especially if the drugs are not quantified (e.g., benzodiazepines, cocaine parent compound). In such cases, a positive screen may not relate to the patient's current findings and symptoms. Drugs with a large volume of distribution or high fat solubility may be detected in urine for a long time after the last dose. Cocaine metabolites may be detected for days and marijuana for weeks after the last exposure.

In addition, the results of toxicology screens are not usually available until many hours after most of the important treatment decisions are made. Screening results rarely change the clinical management of patients.[9] Toxicology screens are often very expensive ($300 or more), and their use is not warranted in most routine drug overdoses.

Alternatives to a full toxicology screen include obtaining (1) discrete drug levels (e.g., acetaminophen, which should be considered in almost all adult intentional ingestions), (2) a qualitative urine screen for drugs of abuse, or (3) no toxicology tests.[9,10] Several commercial urine testing kits have a rapid turnaround time, primarily for drugs of abuse. The full toxicology screen is most useful in patients who are critically ill for an unknown reason when identification of an otherwise unsuspected toxin may change management. Electrolyte levels help identify metabolic acidosis by the carbon dioxide content ("bicarbonate level"), which should be repeated if low to ensure that the acidosis is resolving. A persistent, unexplained metabolic acidosis should prompt urine examination for oxalate crystals (suggestive of ethylene glycol poisoning,) a serum salicylate level, and methanol and ethylene glycol levels. Arterial blood gas measurement is rarely helpful. A normal arterial blood gas or electrolyte measurement does not rule out such ingestion because metabolic acidosis is delayed and does not appear until after metabolism of the acids from ethylene glycol/methanol or until after erratic and slow absorption of salicylate.

Rhabdomyolysis is evaluated, when indicated, with a urinary dipstick for blood (myoglobin) and determination of serum creatine kinase. Rhabdomyolysis and its treatment are discussed in Chapter 125. Noncardiogenic pulmonary edema on a chest radiograph suggests opioid or salicylate overdose. Selective abdominal radiographs can detect smuggled packets. Some drugs are radiopaque (e.g. heavy metals, phenothiazines, potassium, calcium, and chlorinated hydrocarbons such as chloral hydrate), but radiography is rarely helpful in the evaluation of a poisoned patient except to monitor the decontamination of iron, lead, or body packets.[11]

DECONTAMINATION

Gastric decontamination rarely affects the clinical outcome in poisoned patients.[12,13] In the occasional situations in which decontamination may be helpful, activated charcoal (AC) may be beneficial if given early after an ingestion or for drugs that may have delayed emptying, including drugs with an anticholinergic effect, opioids, sustained-release drugs, or drug packets in "body stuffers." For patients who are initially seen hours after ingestion, AC is usually unnecessary and should not be given. Administration of AC only in the small number of circumstances in which it is truly indicated also avoids rare complications such as pulmonary aspiration of the charcoal slurry.[12-14]

If charcoal is used, 50 g of an oral slurry of AC is usually sufficient. If the patient is obtunded or uncooperative and the benefits of AC administration are thought to outweigh the risks (principally aspiration), intubation should be considered, and the AC can be administered through a nasogastric tube. A cathartic such as sorbitol is often used to speed AC transit through the gut, but cathartics have never been shown to be of benefit and, in general, should be avoided. Agents that do not adsorb to charcoal include ions (e.g., acids and alkalies, lithium, borates, bromides), hydrocarbons, metals (e.g., iron), and ethanol.

Whole-bowel irrigation with a polyethylene glycol solution may be useful in certain cases of severe, recent ingestion of lithium or metals such as iron or lead or in patients with massive ingestion of sustained-release formulations of highly toxic drugs. Whole-bowel irrigation has also been used to aid in the evacuation of drug packets from body packers.[15]

Gastric lavage is rarely, if ever, indicated (and should be considered only when a patient is seen within a few minutes [less than an hour] after the ingestion of a highly toxic substance [e.g., calcium channel blocker, cyclic antidepressant]). Gastric lavage has not been shown to improve the clinical course or outcome of most poisoned patients.[16] In the rare circumstances in which gastric lavage is performed, a large (30-French or greater) orogastric tube is used, and specially designed lavage systems with large-bore tubes are available for this purpose. In 2004, the Federal Drug Administration withdrew approval of syrup of ipecac because of its abuse by patients with bulimia.

Exposure of the eye to caustic chemicals and irritants requires immediate irrigation with large amounts of water or readily available fluid, as outlined in Chapter 151. Exposure to a gas does not require decontamination because the patient and rescuers are not at risk once the patient is removed from the toxic environment. The exception is when the patient's skin or clothing is contaminated with a liquid that is evaporating. The most important intervention to limit dermal exposure is to remove all clothing as soon as possible

DISPOSITION AND CONSULTATION

The decision to admit a patient is not difficult when the patient manifests serious toxicity. When the patient is minimally symptomatic but has ingested a potentially dangerous substance, the decision is more difficult. Identification of a agent that causes a particular risk for the patient, especially cardiovascular instability, seizures, or respiratory depression, generally mandates admission to the hospital or to an observation unit in the emergency department. A 6-hour period of observation for a minimally symptomatic patient is usually sufficient, except for some extended-release preparations. Patients with cardiac dysrhythmia, conduction disturbance, altered mental status requiring intubation, or the need for frequently titrated agents (e.g., pressors) should be admitted to the intensive care unit or a monitored inpatient unit. If the patient is acutely suicidal, a sitter or secure environment may be required.

Poison control centers and medical toxicologists can provide specific, current advice, especially for more esoteric or unfamiliar poisons. Consultation with a medical toxicologist is particularly helpful when an uncommon agent has been ingested, the patient is not following the anticipated clinical course, or specific interventions such as administration of antibody therapy or dialysis are contemplated.

KEY CONCEPTS

- A thorough history from many sources is the key to toxicologic diagnosis.
- Common toxidromes should guide judicious use of antidotes.
- Minimally symptomatic patients do not benefit from toxicology screening or extensive laboratory investigation.
- Good supportive care is the key to management.
- Activated charcoal is rarely indicated in overdose, and other methods of gut decontamination (gastric lavage, whole-bowel irrigation) are virtually never helpful. Activated charcoal may decrease absorption of many drugs, but its use should be carefully weighed against potential complications.

REFERENCES

1. Kulig K: Initial management of ingestion of toxic substances. *N Engl J Med* 326:1677, 1992.
2. Hoffman RS, Goldfrank LR: The poisoned patient with altered consciousness: Controversies in the use of a "coma cocktail." *JAMA* 274:562, 1995.
3. Wrenn K, Murphy F, Slovis C: A toxicity study of parenteral thiamine hydrochloride. *Ann Emerg Med* 18:867, 1989.
4. Goldfrank L: Teaching the recognition of odors. *Ann Emerg Med* 11:684, 1982.
5. Glass PJ, Jhaver RM, Smith LR: Comparison of potency and duration of action of nalmefene and naloxone. *Anesth Analg* 78:536, 1994.
6. Doyon S, Roberts JR: Reappraisal of the "coma cocktail." *Emerg Med Clin North Am* 12:301, 1994.
7. Suzuki T, et al: Sarin poisoning in a Tokyo subway. *Lancet* 345:980, 1995.
8. Boyer EW, Shannon M: The serotonin syndrome. *N Engl J Med* 352:1112, 2005.
9. Kulig K: The appropriate utilization of toxicology screens. In *Cost-Effective Diagnostic Testing in Emergency Medicine.* Dallas, American College of Emergency Physicians, 2000.
10. Mahoney JD, et al: Quantitative serum toxic screening in the management of suspected drug overdose. *Am J Emerg Med* 8:16, 1990.
11. Craig SA: Radiology. In Ford MD, et al (eds): *Clinical Toxicology.* Philadelphia, WB Saunders, 2001, pp 61-72.
12. Chyka PA, Seger D: Position statement: Single-dose activated chavcoal. American Academy of Clinical Toxicology; European Association of Poisons Centres and Clinical Toxicologists. *J Toxicol Clin Toxicol* 35:721, 1997.
13. Bond GR: The role of activated charcoal and gastric emptying in gastrointestinal decontamination: A state-of-the-art review. *Ann Emerg Med* 39:273, 2002.
14. Osterhoudt KC, et al: Activated charcoal in a pediatric emergency department. *Pediatr Emerg Care* 20:493, 2004.
15. Tennenbein M: Position statement: Whole bowel irrigation. American Academy of Clinical Toxicology; European Association of Poisons Centres and Clinical Toxicologists. *J Toxicol Clin Toxicol* 35:753, 1997.
16. Vale JA: Position statement: Gastric lavage. American Academy of Clinical Toxicology; European Association of Poisons Centres and Clinical Toxicologists. *J Toxicol Clin Toxicol* 35:711, 1997.

CHAPTER 146 Acetaminophen

Kenneth E. Bizovi and Robert Hendrickson

PERSPECTIVE

Acetaminophen is one of the most common analgesic-antipyretic medications. More hospitalizations occur after acetaminophen overdose than after overdose of any other pharmaceutical agent.[1] In addition to recognized acetaminophen overdose, the widespread availability and the multitude of combination products make acetaminophen toxicity a concern in cases of unknown ingestion, drug abuse, and therapeutic misadventures.

Despite established protocols for assessment and management of acute acetaminophen exposure, variations in treatment strategies exist, and controversy remains regarding indications, route, and duration of antidotal treatment. The indications and endpoints for treatment after chronic excessive acetaminophen exposure are almost completely undefined, and the importance of ethanol use, malnutrition, drug interactions, and individual differences in metabolism remains unresolved.[2]

PRINCIPLES OF DISEASE

Most acetaminophen absorption occurs within 2 hours, even after overdose. Peak plasma concentrations generally occur within 4 hours. Once acetaminophen is absorbed, hepatic metabolism normally accounts for up to 90% of its elimination. Acetaminophen is primarily metabolized in the liver through three routes: (1) conjugation with glucuronide (40-67%), (2) conjugation

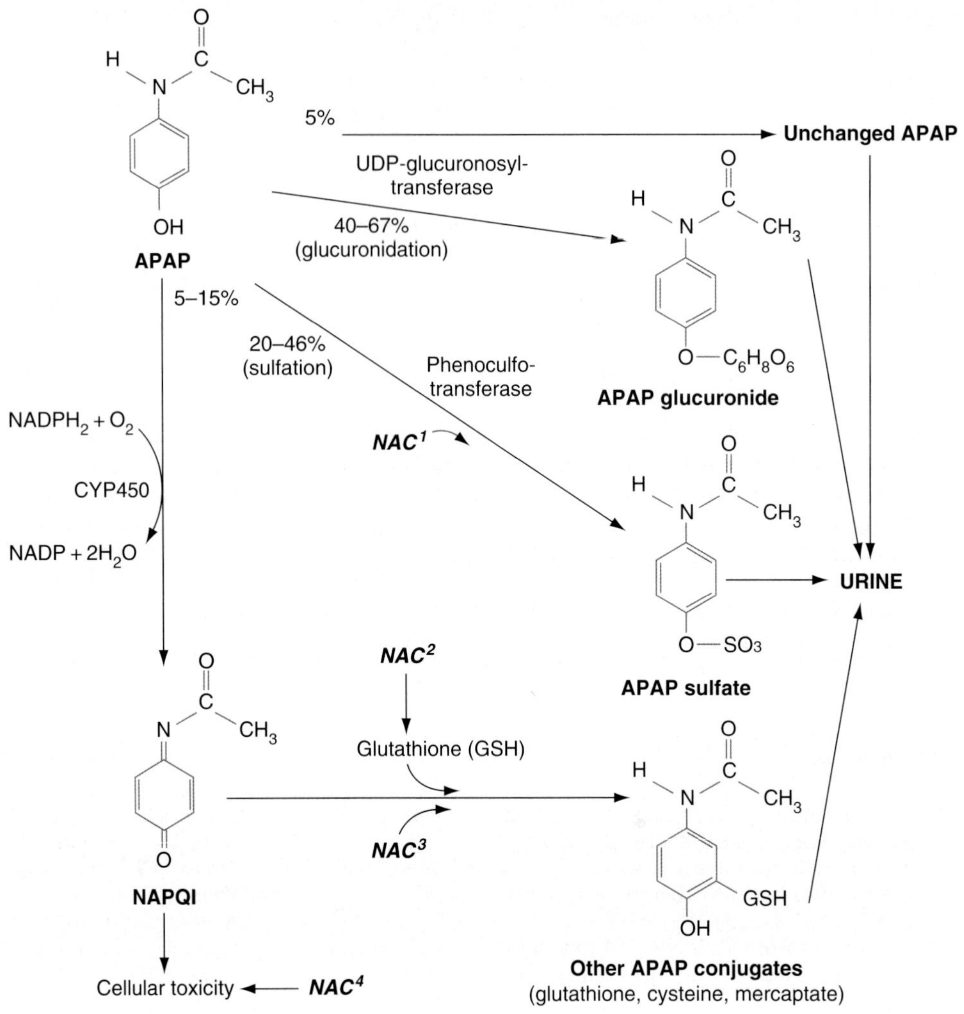

Figure 146-1. Acetaminophen (APAP) metabolism and *N*-acetylcysteine (NAC) mechanisms of action. NAC[1] enhances sulfation; NAC[2] serves as a glutathione (GSH) precursor; NAC[3] is a GSH substitute; NAC[4] may reduce systemic toxicity. NAPQI, *N*-acetyl-*p*-benzoquinoneimine. (Modified from Smilkstein MJ. Acetaminophen. In Goldfrank LR, et al (eds): *Goldfrank's Toxological Emergencies*, 6th ed, Stamford, Conn, Appleton & Lange, 1998, p 547.)

with sulfate (20-46%), or (3) oxidation via the cytochrome P450 (CYP450) mixed-function oxidase system (CYP2E1, CYP1A2, and CYP3A4)[3] with subsequent conjugation (Figure 146-1).

The oxidation of acetaminophen by CYP450 subfamilies, predominantly CYP2E1[4,5] results in the formation of the highly reactive electrophile, *N*-acetyl-*p*-benzoquinoneimine (NAPQI).[3] NAPQI combines rapidly with glutathione and other thiol-containing compounds, forming nontoxic conjugates, which are eliminated in urine. When NAPQI formation exceeds glutathione supply, free NAPQI binds to hepatocyte intracellular proteins, causing toxicity. Inducers (e.g., ethanol, isoniazid, anticonvulsants) and inhibitors (e.g., cimetidine) of CYP450 enzymes may affect the NAPQI formation, but their clinical significance is controversial. Renal injury may occur with or without hepatic injury[6] and may be mediated by the presence of CYP450 enzyme species[7,8] and the activation of prostaglandin synthase within the kidneys.[9,10]

Most oxidative metabolism is concentrated in hepatic zone III, which is affected most via acetaminophen toxicity. In cases of severe toxicity, necrosis can extend into zones I and II, destroying the entire liver parenchyma. The sequelae of severe acetaminophen toxicity are those of fulminant liver failure, rather than direct acetaminophen effects, and the pathophysiology of these complex multisystem problems is well described (see Chapter 89).[11]

As treatment for acetaminophen toxicity, *N*-acetylcysteine (NAC) serves as both a glutathione precursor and a glutathione substitute (see Figure 146-1). In addition, NAC may decrease NAPQI formation by augmenting nontoxic sulfation.[12] Unlike its early acetaminophen-specific actions, other NAC mechanisms are suggested by the surprising finding that intravenous NAC improves survival in patients with acetaminophen-induced fulminant hepatic failure, even long after completion of acetaminophen metabolism.[13] Possible mechanisms include improving oxygen delivery and uptake by tissues, changes in hepatic microcirculation, scavenging of reactive species, and diminishing cerebral edema.[14] The ability of NAC to ameliorate multiorgan failure suggests that extrahepatic mechanisms not specific to acetaminophen are of benefit.

CLINICAL FEATURES

The progression of acetaminophen-induced hepatic injury occurs in four stages. Stage 1 is the preinjury period, usually the first 24 hours after ingestion. Nonspecific symptoms, including nausea, vomiting, anorexia, diaphoresis, and malaise, are common in the first 8 hours after ingestion, usually resolving thereafter. Patients may be asymptomatic during this stage.

Stage 2 is the onset of liver injury, usually 24 hours after ingestion but possibly 12 to 36 hours after overdose. In extraordinary cases, liver injury is evident as early as 8 hours after ingestion. Signs and symptoms of hepatic injury include nausea, vomiting, and right upper quadrant and epigastric pain or tenderness.

Stage 3 is maximum liver injury, usually 3 to 4 days after ingestion, with a wide variety of clinical manifestations, depending on severity of the injury. Signs and symptoms of hepatic injury can persist or progress. Fulminant hepatic failure can develop during this stage, with encephalopathy, coma, and clinical evidence of coagulopathy. Patients with hepatic failure sometimes develop hypoglycemia and metabolic acidosis. Death with hepatic failure can occur from hemorrhage, adult respiratory distress syndrome, sepsis, multiorgan failure, or cerebral edema.[2,15] The risk of renal injury increases with severity of hepatic injury, occurring in less than 2% of patients without hepatotoxicity and in 25% of patients with severe hepatotoxicity.[16–18]

Stage 4 is the recovery period. Hepatic enzymes return to baseline by 5 to 7 days but may take longer with severe hepatic injury. Complete histologic resolution of hepatic insult can take months. Regeneration of the liver is complete, without chronic hepatic dysfunction.[19]

DIAGNOSTIC STRATEGIES

The primary goals of patient assessment after acetaminophen exposure are to identify risk for acetaminophen-induced hepatotoxicity and to initiate timely treatment with NAC. The history and physical examination establish potential risk of toxicity, but because early symptoms are unreliable indicators of toxicity, and late symptoms occur long after NAC should be started, laboratory evaluation is essential. Once a patient is determined to be at risk for acetaminophen toxicity, treatment with NAC should be initiated. Additional diagnostic testing of these patients involves evaluation for hepatic injury and hepatic failure in select patients.

Acetaminophen exposures can be categorized as acute or chronic. Acute overdose is usually considered to be a single ingestion, arbitrarily defined as occurring within a single 4-hour period.[2] All other repeated ingestions of greater than recommended doses are considered to be chronic exposure. The initial management of most single acute overdoses in adults is well established. Liver failure and death are completely preventable if NAC is administered early after ingestion.[20] Factors that complicate evaluation and management decisions after acute exposures include inability to establish the time of ingestion, presentation longer than 24 hours after ingestion, new formulations of acetaminophen, age younger than 5 years, and pregnancy. Management of chronic excessive acetaminophen dosing is much more controversial and includes widely accepted approaches to uncomplicated acute overdose, as well as our approach to complicated acute and chronic acetaminophen exposures (Boxes 146-1 and 146-2).

BOX 146-1. Risk Assessment and Treatment Recommendations for Acute Acetaminophen Ingestion

I. Laboratory evaluation
   A. Serum acetaminophen concentration 4 hours after ingestion or as soon as possible thereafter
   B. Aspartate transaminase (AST) measurement if:
      1. Patient has signs or symptoms of hepatic injury.
      2. Acetaminophen concentration is on or above nomogram treatment line.
      3. Time of ingestion is completely unknown.
   C. Prothrombin time, electrolytes, glucose, blood urea nitrogen, and creatine kinase if AST greatly elevated
II. *N*-acetylcysteine (NAC) treatment if:
   A. Acetaminophen concentration is on or above nomogram treatment line.
   B. AST is elevated.
   C. Acetaminophen concentration is greater than 10 μg/mL, and time of ingestion is unknown.*

*NAC treatment should not be delayed more than 8 hours after ingestion. If the patient presents after this time, NAC should be started as soon as possible.

Careful, reliable history with the assumption that the patient has ingested the greatest amount possible will lead to appropriate laboratory evaluation of patients with potential risk. Dosing history should not be used to rule out risk for cases involving uncertain history, self-harm, or drug abuse.[21] Ingestions estimated to be greater than 7.5 g in an adult or 150 mg/kg in a child indicate potential risk and require laboratory evaluation.[2,22,23]

Once potential risk has been established, the next step is to determine acetaminophen concentration 4 hours after the ingestion, or as soon as possible after 4 hours. In many cases acetaminophen concentration alone will be adequate to define risk. When the physical findings are consistent with hepatic injury, or the timing of the ingestion cannot be established, aspartate transaminase (AST) should also be measured to establish the presence or absence of hepatic injury. Patients at risk for acetaminophen-induced hepatotoxicity on the basis of acetaminophen concentration, or with evidence of hepatic injury, should be treated with NAC.

Risk Assessment Using Treatment Nomogram

Risk of hepatotoxicity is best established by plotting acetaminophen concentration on the acetaminophen treatment nomogram, which is an adaptation of the Rumack-Matthew nomogram (Figure 146-2).[24] Acetaminophen concentration must be measured between 4 and 24 hours after ingestion and then plotted on the nomogram. The treatment line currently used in the

BOX 146-2. Risk Assessment and Treatment Recommendations for Chronic Acetaminophen Ingestion*

I. Indications for laboratory evaluation
  A. Signs or symptoms of hepatic injury
  B. Children
    1. Ingestion of >75 mg/kg in 24-hour period associated with acute febrile illness, malnourishment, or chronic use of medications that induce CYP450 system (e.g., anticonvulsants, isoniazid)
    2. Ingestion of >150/kg in 24-hour period
  C. Adults
    1. Ingestion of >4 g in 24-hour period associated with malnourishment, chronic alcohol consumption, or chronic use of medications that induce CYP450 system (e.g., anticonvulsants, isoniazid)
    2. Ingestion of >7.5 g in 24-hour period

II. Laboratory evaluation: acetaminophen concentration, AST

III. Risk classification
  A. Higher risk
    1. Acetaminophen concentration < 10 μg/mL
      a. AST > twice normal
      b. AST > normal; patient symptomatic
    2. Acetaminophen concentration > 10 μg/mL and as expected for appropriate dose[†]
      a. AST > normal
    3. Acetaminophen concentration greater than expected for appropriate dose[†]
  B. Low risk
    1. Acetaminophen concentration < 10 μg/mL; AST normal to twice normal; patient asymptomatic
    2. Acetaminophen concentration as expected for appropriate dose[†]; AST normal
  C. Minimal risk: acetaminophen concentration < 10 μg/mL; AST normal

IV. Treatment based on risk classification
  A. Higher risk
    1. Admit to hospital.
    2. Treat with NAC.
  B. Low risk
    1. Give instructions to return immediately for signs or symptoms of hepatic injury.
    2. Phone or clinic follow-up in 24 hours.
    3. If first two cannot be accomplished, admit and treat with NAC.
  C. Minimal risk
    1. Discharge from hospital.
    2. Provide instructions to return immediately for signs or symptoms of hepatic injury.

*The approach outlined represents the authors' opinion of a logical evaluation, coupled with conservative thresholds for the initiation of treatment.

[†]After peak level of last dose, Acetaminophen concentration should not exceed 30 μg/mL (30-90 minutes after dose), with rapid decline to <10 μg/mL (4-6 hours after dose).

AST, aspartate transaminase; CYP450, cytochrome P-450; NAC, *N*-acetylcysteine.

United States is 25% lower than the original line to increase sensitivity.[2,25] Patients with acetaminophen concentration on or above the treatment line should be treated.

The acetaminophen treatment nomogram is well established as a sensitive screening tool. To maintain sensitivity, the earliest possible time of ingestion should be used to plot the acetaminophen concentration. Using this approach, patients with acetaminophen concentration that plots below the treatment line do not need NAC, regardless of variability in acetaminophen metabolism and factors that may predispose patients to hepatotoxicity.[2,25,26]

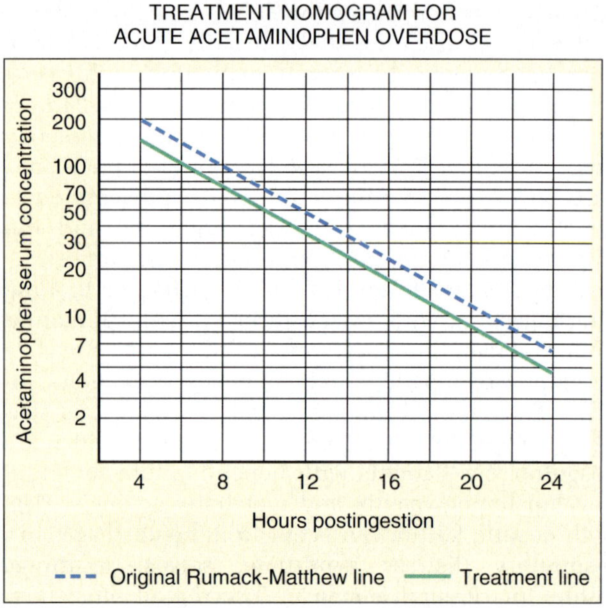

Figure 146-2. Treatment nomogram for acute overdose. The lower treatment line should be used for treatment decisions. (Modified from Rumack BH, Matthew H: Acetaminophen poisoning and toxicity. *Pediatrics* 55:871, 1975.)

Patients who present later than 8 hours after ingestion should have NAC started as soon as possible and continued if indicated by the acetaminophen concentration plotted on the nomogram.

Contraindications

The treatment nomogram cannot be used when the acetaminophen concentration cannot be obtained, the time of ingestion cannot be established, or the patient is evaluated more than 24 hours after the ingestion. When the acetaminophen concentration is not available, treatment is recommended for adults who ingest more than 7.5 g, children who ingest more than 150 mg/kg, and patients for whom the reliability of the history is in question. If time of ingestion cannot be established to a degree permitting the use of the nomogram, measurement of acetaminophen concentration and AST is recommended. In most circumstances, a time window of ingestion can be established. If not, NAC should be administered if the AST level is above normal or if the acetaminophen concentration is above detectable limits. In patients with an unknown ingestion time and acetaminophen concentration below detectable limits with normal AST, NAC is not recommended.

Hepatic Injury

The presence of right upper quadrant or epigastric pain or tenderness in a patient with a history of acetaminophen ingestion suggests hepatic injury, which mandates AST measurement as a screening test. Treatment is often indicated based on the treatment nomogram. In some cases, however, an elevated AST level will indicate hepatic injury, and acetaminophen concentration will plot below the treatment line. Possible causes of this presentation include inaccurate timing of the ingestion or another source of hepatic injury. These patients merit review of the history, further workup for hepatic failure, and consideration of other sources of hepatic injury in addition to treatment with NAC.

Extended-Release Preparations

Extended-release preparations have given rise to concerns over the use of the nomogram.[27] The packaging of the extended-release product allows for an immediate release of one half of the acetaminophen dose, followed by sustained release of the other half over several hours.[28] Initially, recommendations were made to obtain both a 4-hour concentration measurement and an 8- to 10-hour concentration measurement to rule out delayed elevations of acetaminophen concentration and resulting liver disease.[28] However, evaluation of patients with nontoxic[29,30] and toxic ingestions[28] of extended-release formulations has demonstrated that peak plasma acetaminophen concentration occurs within 4 hours, although some absorption can continue for up to 8 hours. For this reason, unless unusual circumstances are evident, a single acetaminophen concentration plotted on the nomogram is sufficient to determine the need for antidotal therapy.

Pediatric Ingestion

Acute exposures to acetaminophen in children younger than 5 years have resulted in severe hepatotoxicity and hepatic failure,[31–34] but these cases are infrequent, making analysis of pediatric data or comparison with adult exposures exceedingly difficult. Less aggressive management has been proposed,[35–38] but until studies documenting safety are done with adequate power, ingestion of 150 mg/kg should be used as the threshold for laboratory evaluation, with risk determination based on the current treatment line (see Figure 146-2).

Chronic Exposure

Evaluation after chronic acetaminophen overdose should follow a similar pattern of establishing potential risk based on history and physical examination findings and further risk assessment through laboratory studies. The primary problem with evaluation of chronic acetaminophen overdose is the lack of a rigorously studied screening test to establish the risk of hepatotoxicity. The need for laboratory testing with a history of chronic overuse is based on symptoms, physical findings, factors that may predispose patients to hepatotoxicity, and greatest amount ingested in any 24-hour period (see Box 146-2). Any patient with signs and symptoms of hepatic injury after chronic use of acetaminophen merits laboratory evaluation.[39,40]

Factors that have been reported to predispose patients to hepatic injury after chronic overuse include malnourishment,[41] chronic alcohol use,[42–45] medications that induce the CYP450 system[46] (e.g., isoniazid[47,48]), and febrile illness in children younger than 5 years.[49–56] Until the role of these factors can be validated and quantified, it is prudent to use a lower threshold for laboratory evaluation in patients with these potentially predisposing factors. Laboratory evaluation of patients with potentially predisposing factors is recommended after ingestion of more than 90 mg/kg of acetaminophen concentration in a child or 4 g in an adult during a 24-hour period. Patients without these factors should undergo laboratory evaluation after ingestion of greater than 150 mg/kg (child) or 7.5 g (adult) during any 24-hour period.

The AST level and acetaminophen concentration are used to assist in determining the risk of hepatotoxicity. Logical categories of risk can be established, based on evidence of hepatic injury, as indicated by AST level, and the potential for ongoing production of toxic APAP metabolite, as indicated by acetaminophen concentration (see Box 146-2). The potential for production of consequential toxic metabolite is present when acetaminophen concentration is greater than would be expected for an appropriate acetaminophen dose. After normal dosing, the peak acetaminophen concentration should be less than 30 μg/mL, 30 to 90 minutes after the dose, and decline to less than 10 μg/mL by 4 to 6 hours after ingestion.

Patients are at higher risk for hepatotoxicity if (1) their AST level is twice normal or they are symptomatic with an AST level that is greater than normal; (2) acetaminophen concentration is greater than 10 μg/mL and AST level is greater than normal; or (3) acetaminophen concentration is greater than expected for appropriate dose. Hospital admission and treatment with NAC are recommended.

Criteria for low risk include (1) acetaminophen concentration less than 10 μg/mL, with AST between normal and twice normal, and no symptoms of hepatic injury, and (2) acetaminophen concentration as expected for appropriate dose with normal AST level. Recommended management includes follow-up (telephone or repeat visit) in 24 hours and discharge instructions to return immediately if any increase in symptoms are noted that are consistent with hepatic injury. Treatment is not recommended for low-risk patients unless adequate follow-up cannot be arranged.

Patients with acetaminophen concentration less than 10 μg/mL and normal AST have minimal risk, and treatment with NAC is not indicated. Discharge is recommended, with instructions to return immediately if symptoms of hepatic injury arise.

MANAGEMENT

The goals in managing acetaminophen overdose are to (1) limit gastrointestinal absorption when appropriate; (2) initiate NAC in a timely manner, within 8 hours of ingestion; (3) control symptoms; and (4) provide supportive and follow-up care.

Activated Charcoal

Gastric lavage is rarely indicated in cases of isolated acetaminophen overdose because of the very rapid gastrointestinal absorption of acetaminophen and the availability of an effective antidote. Activated charcoal effectively adsorbs acetaminophen,[57] but its ability to favorably influence outcome in cases of acute overdose is not proven. Activated charcoal might also adsorb oral NAC and limit its efficacy. Unlike NAC, there is no evidence that the use of activated charcoal decreases subsequent need for NAC or improves outcome in terms of hepatic injury or enzyme elevations. When there is conflict between apparent need for activated charcoal and demonstrated need for NAC, the NAC must always take priority, and activated charcoal should not be given or should be delayed for at least 2 hours after the NAC. In most cases, there is no conflict because administration of activated charcoal within the first 2 to 3 hours need not overlap with NAC, which can be given up to 8 hours after ingestion. Rarely, because of co-ingestants and timing of presentation, there may be consideration of the need to administer NAC and activated charcoal simultaneously. In such cases, unless there is believed to be an overwhelming need for the activated charcoal, the NAC should be administered alone, and the activated charcoal delayed or not given at all, since the NAC is a proven antidote, and the activated charcoal is of theoretical benefit only. In the very rare circumstances in which it is determined that the two agents should be given together, however, reassurance can be drawn from the fact that there is no evidence to prove that activated charcoal limits the clinical effectiveness of NAC.[58]

N-Acetylcysteine

Once the need for NAC is determined, it can be given orally in a dilute solution (3-5%) from a covered container through a straw or gastric tube. The loading dose is 140 mg/kg, followed by a maintenance dose of 70 mg/kg every 4 hours. Emesis from the noxious odor is common, and any dose vomited within 1 hour of administration should be given again. Starting NAC any time within the first 8 hours appears to be equally efficacious. Antiemetics (e.g., ondansetron) may be needed for the patient to tolerate the first dose within 8 hours of ingestion.

Intravenous Administration

A parenteral NAC preparation was approved by the Food and Drug Administration in 2004, but until it becomes universally available, administration of the oral compound by the intravenous route is beneficial and safe in several situations. Intravenous NAC has been responsible for anaphylactoid reactions, including flushing, urticaria, angioedema, bronchospasm, hypotension, and death,[59–64] but these serious reactions are dose, rate, and concentration dependent.[62–64] When NAC is diluted and given slowly, approximately 4% to 14% of patients develop a transient rash during the loading dose. More serious sequelae of wheezing and hypotension are reported with an incidence of 0.05% or less.[62,64] Flushing can be managed without stopping the infusion.[65] Other serious reactions can be managed with standard therapy such as a fluid bolus, diphenhydramine, and slowing the infusion rate if necessary. These reactions merit assessment of risk and benefit but do not preclude subsequent doses and rarely recur during maintenance dosing.

Intravenous NAC should be infused as a 3% solution (30 g of NAC in D_5W to a total volume of 1 L). The initial bolus of intravenous NAC is 140 to 150 mg/kg IV over 1 hour. Subsequent doses can be given on the same schedule as oral NAC,[62,63] or continuous infusion protocols. For acute acetaminophen overdose treated within 8 hours of exposure, the continuous infusion is run at 15 mg/kg/hr for 4 hours followed by 7.5 mg/kg/hr for 16 hours. For patients treated more than 8 hours after exposure, chronic ingestion, or hepatic failure the continuous infusion is 15 mg/kg/hr for 44 hours.[64] Properly administered, intravenous NAC is very safe; however, it is more complicated to give than by the oral route, a potential source of medical error.

Indications

Fulminant Hepatic Failure. The most important indication for intravenous NAC is probably fulminant hepatic failure. Only the intravenous route has been systematically studied in liver failure. In a prospective, randomized trial, British investigators found that even when started after fulminant hepatic failure was evident, patients treated with intravenous NAC required less vasopressor support and had a lower incidence of cerebral edema and death.[13]

Oral Intolerance. A more common indication for intravenous NAC is the patient with a very high acetaminophen concentration at 8 hours or longer since ingestion who is unable to tolerate oral NAC after a brief, aggressive trial of antiemetic therapy. Once nausea and vomiting have abated, oral administration can be resumed.

Pregnancy

Fetal acetaminophen toxicity is rare, and a causal relationship remains unproven, but adverse outcomes have been reported at all stages of pregnancy.[66] Acetaminophen is capable of crossing the placenta and may be present in concentrations in the fetus that are as high, or higher than, those in the mother.[66] In the early gestational period, acetaminophen toxicity can be associated with fetal death.[66] CYP450 enzymes appear in the fetus during the second trimester and activity increases with gestational age,[67] which may put the maturing fetus or newborn at risk for hepatotoxicity.

Treating the mother with NAC is safe and effective, but data are inadequate to evaluate efficacy in the fetus. Fetal outcome has generally been excellent after maternal treatment with oral NAC,[66] but concern exists about those at greatest risk. Oral NAC may reach the fetus, and fetal serum levels may approach maternal levels.[68] It is unlikely, however, that equivalent serum NAC concentrations correspond to equivalent hepatic protection. Unlike the mother, who achieves a given NAC concentration after hepatic first-pass clearance of oral NAC, the fetal serum NAC concentration follows transplacental dosing and may not be accompanied by high intrahepatic NAC concentration.

Intravenous NAC has theoretical advantages in treating acetaminophen exposure during pregnancy, particularly in the later stages of pregnancy, to achieve the highest possible maternal-fetal NAC gradient. Since lack of maternal toxicity may or may not exclude fetal toxicity, intravenous NAC can be continued for the full 17-dose oral protocol to maximize any benefit to the fetus. Consultation with a medical toxicologist is advised if uncertainty exists.

Duration of Treatment

The treatment course of oral NAC is an oral loading dose followed by 17 doses at 4-hour intervals. A 20-hour intravenous NAC protocol in the United Kingdom,[69] a 48-hour intravenous NAC protocol studied in the United States,[62] and other short-course dosing protocols[70,71] suggest that a shorter duration of NAC therapy is safe and effective.

All durations of NAC administration are effective when started within 8 hours of ingestion, indicating that shorter courses of treatment are appropriate when NAC is used for its preventive actions. In contrast, protocol comparisons and series involving late NAC administration suggest that a longer duration of treatment may be needed when treating established liver injury.[13] Rather than a single duration of therapy for all patients, it may be appropriate to use different treatment protocols on the basis of clinical course or other markers.[2,72]

Complications and Supportive Care

Management of hepatic injury, renal dysfunction, and the other rare manifestations is based on general principles and is not acetaminophen dependent. Treatment of hypoglycemia due to liver failure is critical but straightforward. Once hepatic injury is established by elevations in AST, prothrombin time and international normalized ratio should be serially measured. Coagulopathy can be treated with vitamin K or fresh frozen plasma. The effect of vitamin K is dependent on hepatic function and may be limited. Administration of fresh frozen plasma should be based on clinical indications rather than on the prothrombin time or international normalized ratio alone. Parenteral NAC, other advances in supportive care, and successful liver transplantation programs have improved survival.[15]

DISPOSITION

Asymptomatic patients who fit criteria for treatment should be treated with NAC and can be admitted to a medical ward or emergency department observation unit. The motivation behind any ingestion needs to be evaluated, and psychiatric consultation should be obtained when appropriate. In rare instances of unintentional ingestions, outpatient treatment with close follow-up has been used. This practice should be discouraged, however, since vomiting is likely, and achieving compliance even in motivated patients is difficult.

Patients showing evidence of severe hepatotoxicity, and those at risk for fulminant hepatic failure may need to be admitted to a monitored bed in an intensive care unit. These patients require frequent neurologic checks, monitoring of vital signs, and laboratory studies, including bedside blood glucose measurement. Early contact with a regional poison center and transplant center is important to guide treatment strategies and to coordinate transplantation when needed. It is especially important to obtain psychiatric consultation early, before encephalopathy, to help determine transplantation eligibility. Absolute indications for transplantation vary and should be discussed early with local transplant centers and hepatologists. Patients with a serum pH less than 7.30 after appropriate resuscitation are unlikely to recover without transplantation.[13] Any patient with fulminant hepatic failure, as evidenced by encephalopathy, severe coagulopathy, or refractory metabolic acidosis, should prompt immediate consultation with a transplant center.

KEY CONCEPTS

- Acetaminophen concentration should be measured in cases of unknown or mixed overdoses. Acetaminophen is relatively clinically silent until serious hepatotoxicity ensues.
- Excessive repeated dosing of therapeutic acetaminophen can lead to life-threatening toxicity.
- The treatment nomogram applies only to acute ingestions; the earliest possible time of ingestion is used to plot acetaminophen concentration.
- For maximum benefit, NAC treatment should not be delayed beyond 8 hours after ingestion. If more than 8 hours has passed since ingestion, treatment should be started immediately.
- Late administration of NAC is beneficial even after hepatotoxicity is evident.

REFERENCES

1. Watson WA, et al: 2002 annual report of the American Association of Poison Control Centers Toxic Exposure Surveillance System. *Am J Emerg Med* 21:353, 2003.
2. Bizovi KE, Smilkstein MJ: Acetaminophen. In Goldfrank LR, et al (eds): *Goldfrank's Toxicologic Emergencies*, 7th ed. New York, McGraw-Hill, 2002, pp 480-501.
3. Corcoran GB, Mitchell JR, Vaishnav YN, Horning EC: Evidence that acetaminophen and N-hydroxyacetaminophen form a common arylating intermediate, N-Acetyl-p-benzoquinoneimine. *Mol Pharmacol* 18:536, 1980.

4. Manyike PT, Kharasch ED, Kalhorn TF, Slattery JT: Contribution of CYP2E1 and CYP3A to acetaminophen reactive metabolite formation. *Clin Pharmacol Ther* 67:275, 2000.
5. Hazai E, Vereczkey L, Monostory K: Reduction of toxic metabolite formation of acetaminophen. *Biochem Biophys Res Comm* 291:1089, 2002.
6. Boutis K, Shannon M: Nephrotoxicity after acute severe acetaminophen poisoning in adolescents. *J Toxicol Clin Toxicol* 39:441, 2001.
7. Emeigh Hart SG, et al: Acetaminophen nephrotoxicity in CD-1 mice. I. Evidence of a role for in situ activation in selective covalent binding and toxicity. *Toxicol Appl Pharmacol* 126:267, 1994.
8. Breen K, Wandscheer JC, Peignoux M, Pessayre D: In situ formation of the acetaminophen metabolite covalently bound in kidneys and lung: Supportive evidence provided by total hepatectomy. *Biochem Pharmacol* 31:115, 1982.
9. Prescott LF, Mattison P, Menzies DG, Manson LM: The comparative effects of paracetamol and indomethacin on renal function in health female volunteers. *Br J Clin Pharmacol* 29:403, 1990.
10. Walker RJ, Fawcett JP: Drug nephrotoxicity: The significance of cellular mechanisms. *Prog Drug Res* 41:51, 1993.
11. Lee WM: Acute liver failure. *N Engl J Med* 329:135, 1993.
12. Slattery JT, Wilson JM, Kalhorn TF, Nelson SD: Dose-dependent pharmacokinetics of acetaminophen: Evidence for glutathione depletion in humans. *Clin Pharmacol Ther* 41:413, 1987.
13. Keays R, et al: Intravenous acetylcysteine in paracetamol induced fulminant hepatic failure: A prospective controlled trial. *Br Med J* 303:1026, 1991.
14. Jones AL: Mechanism of action and value of *N*-acetylcysteine in the treatment of early and late acetaminophen poisoning: A critical review. *J Toxicol Clin Toxicol* 36:277, 1998.
15. Makin AJ, Wendon J, Williams R: A 7-year experience of severe acetaminophen-induced hepatotoxicity (1987-1993). *Gastroenterology* 109:1907, 1995.
16. Davenport A, Finn R: Paracetamol (acetaminophen) poisoning resulting in acute renal failure without hepatic coma. *Nephron* 50:55, 1988.
17. Makin AJ, Williams R: The current management of paracetamol overdosage. *Br J Clin Prac* 48:144, 1994.
18. Prescott LF, Proudfoot AT, Cregeen RJ: Paracetamol-induced acute renal failure in the absence of fulminant liver damage. *Br Med J* 284:421, 1982.
19. Mathew J, Hines JE, James OFW, Burt AD: Non-parenchymal cell responses in paracetamol (acetaminophen)-induced liver injury. *J Hepatol* 20:537, 1994.
20. Smilkstein MJ, Knapp GL, Kulig KW, Rumack BH: *N*-Acetylcysteine in the treatment of acetaminophen overdose. *N Engl J Med* 320:1418, 1989.
21. Lucanie R, Chiang WK, Reilly R: Utility of acetaminophen screening in unsuspected suicidal ingestions. *Vet Hum Toxicol* 44:171, 2002.
22. Anker AL, Smilkstein MJ: Acetaminophen: Concepts and controversies. *Med Clin North Am* 12:335, 1994.
23. Linden CH, Rumack BH: Acetaminophen overdose. *Emerg Med Clin North Am* 2:102, 1984.
24. Rumack BH, Mathew H: Acetaminophen poisoning and toxicity. *Pediatrics* 55:871, 1975.
25. Rumack BH, Peterson RG, Koch GG, Amara IA: Acetaminophen overdose: 662 cases with evaluation of oral acetylcysteine treatment. *Arch Intern Med* 141:380, 1981.
26. Smilkstein MJ, Douglas DR, Daya MR: Acetaminophen poisoning and liver function. *N Engl J Med* 330:1310, 1994.
27. Temple AR: *Guidelines for Management of Acute Acetaminophen Overdose.* Fort Washington, Pa, McNeil Consumer Products Company, 2002.
28. Cetaruk EW, et al: Tylenol Extended Relief overdose. *Ann Emerg Med* 30:104, 1997.
29. Douglas DR, Sholar JB, Smilkstein MJ: A pharmacokinetic comparison of acetaminophen products (Tylenol Extended Relief vs regular Tylenol). *Acad Emerg Med* 3:740, 1996.
30. Stork CM, et al: Pharmacokinetics of extended relief vs regular release Tylenol in simulated human overdose. *J Toxicol Clin Toxicol* 34:157, 1996.
31. Lieh-Lai MW, et al: Metabolism and pharmacokinetics of acetaminophen in a severely poisoned young child. *J Pediatr* 105:125, 1984.
32. Arena JM, Rourk MHJ, Sibrack CD: Acetaminophen: Report of an unusual poisoning. *Pediatrics* 61:68, 1978.
33. Rumack BH: Acetaminophen overdose in young children: Treatment and effects of alcohol and other additional ingestants in 417 cases. Am J Dis Child 138:428, 1984.
34. American Academy of Pediatrics: Acetaminophen toxicity in children. *Pediatrics* 108:1020, 2001.
35. Anderson BJ, Holford NHG, Armishaw JC, Aicken R: Predicting concentrations in children presenting with acetaminophen overdose. *J Pediatr* 135:290, 1999.
36. Bond GR, et al: Acetaminophen ingestion in childhood: Cost and relative risk of alternative referral strategies. *J Toxicol Clin Toxicol* 32:513, 1994.
37. Caravati EM: Unintentional acetaminophen ingestion in children and the potential for hepatotoxicity. *J Toxicol Clin Toxicol* 38:291, 2000.
38. Mohler CR, et al: Prospective evaluation of mild to moderate pediatric acetaminophen exposures. *Ann Emerg Med* 35:239, 2000.
39. Heubi JE, Barbacci MB, Zimmerman HJ: Therapeutic misadventures with acetaminophen: Hepatotoxicity after multiple doses in children. *J Pediatr* 132:22, 1998.
40. Kozer E, McGuigan M: Approaches toward repeated supratherapeutic doses of paracetamol in children: A survey of medical directors of poison centres in North America and Europe. *Drug Safety* 25:613, 2002.
41. Whitcomb DC, Block GD: Association of acetaminophen hepatotoxicity with fasting and ethanol use. *JAMA* 272: 1845, 1994.
42. Seeff LB, et al: Acetaminophen hepatotoxicity in alcoholics: A therapeutic misadventure. *Ann Intern Med* 104:309, 1986.
43. Zimmerman HJ, Maddrey WC: Acetaminophen (paracetamol) hepatotoxicity with regular intake of alcohol: Analysis of instances of therapeutic misadventure. *Hepatology* 22:767, 1995.
44. Schiodt FV, Rochling FA, Casey DL, Lee WM: Acetaminophen toxicity in an urban county hospital. *N Engl J Med* 337:1112, 1997.
45. Lauterburg BH, Velez ME: Glutathione deficiency in alcoholics: Risk factor for paracetamol hepatotoxicity. *Gut* 29:1153, 1988.
46. Rumack BH: Acetaminophen hepatotoxicity: The first 35 years. *J Toxicol Clin Toxicol* 40:3, 2002.
47. Epstein MM, et al: Inhibition of the metabolism of paracetamol by isoniazid. *Br J Clin Pharmacol* 31:139, 1991.
48. Murphy R, Swartz R, Watkins PB: Severe acetaminophen toxicity in a patient receiving isoniazid. *Ann Intern Med* 113:799, 1990.
49. Chao TC: Adverse drug reactions: Tales of a forensic pathologist. *Ann Acad Med Singapore* 22:86, 1993.
50. Clark JH, Russell GJ, Fitzgerald JF: Fatal acetaminophen toxicity in a 2-year-old. *J Indiana State Med Assoc* 76:832, 1983.
51. Day A, Abbott GD: Chronic paracetamol poisoning in children: A warning to health professionals. *N Z Med J* 107:201, 1994.
52. Douidar SM, Al-Khalil I, Habersang RW: Severe hepatotoxicity, acute renal failure, and pancytopenia in a young child after repeated acetaminophen overdosing. *Clin Pediatr* 33: 42, 1994.
53. Henretig FM, et al: Repeated acetaminophen overdosing: Causing hepatotoxicity in children. *Clin Pediatr* 28:267, 1989.

54. Nogen AG, Bremner JE: Fatal acetaminophen overdosage in a young child. *J Pediatr* 92:832, 1978.
55. Smith DW, Isakson G, Frankel LR, Kerner JA: Hepatic failure following ingestion of multiple doses of acetaminophen in a young child. *J Pediatr Gastroenterol Nutr* 5:822, 1986.
56. Swetnam SM, Florman AL: Probable acetaminophen toxicity in an 18-month-old infant due to repeated overdosing. *Clin Pediatr* 23:104, 1984.
57. Rose SR, et al: Simulated acetaminophen overdose: Pharmacokinetics and effectiveness of activated charcoal. *Ann Emerg Med* 20:1064, 1991.
58. Spiller HA, et al: A prospective evaluation of the effect of activated charcoal before oral *N*-acetylcysteine in acetaminophen overdose. *Ann Emerg Med* 23:519, 1994.
59. Bateman DN, Woodhouse KW, Rawlins KW: Adverse reactions to *N*-acetylcysteine. *Hum Toxicol* 3:393, 1984.
60. Dawson AH, Henry DA, McEwan J: Adverse reactions to *N*-acetylcysteine during treatment for paracetamol poisoning. *Med J Aust* 150:329, 1989.
61. Mant TGK, Tempowski JH, Volans GN, Talbot JCC: Adverse reactions to acetylcysteine and effects of overdose. *Br Med J* 289:217, 1984.
62. Smilkstein MJ, et al: Acetaminophen overdose: A 48-hour intravenous N-acetylcysteine treatment protocol. *Ann Emerg Med* 20:1058, 1991.
63. Yip L, Dart R, Hurlbut KM: Intravenous administration of oral *N*-acetylcysteine. *Crit Care Med* 26:40, 1998.
64. Kao LW, et al: What is the rate of adverse events after oral *N*-acetylcysteine administered by the intravenous route to patients with suspected acetaminophen poisoning? *Ann Emerg Med* 42:741, 2003.
65. Bailey B, McGuigan MA: Management of anaphylactoid reactions to intravenous *N*-acetylcysteine. *Ann Emerg Med* 31:710, 1998.
66. Riggs BS, et al: Acute acetaminophen overdose during pregnancy. *Obstet Gynecol* 74:247, 1989.
67. Rollins DE, et al: Acetaminophen: Potentially toxic metabolite formed by human fetal and adult liver microsomes and isolated fetal liver cells. *Science* 205:1414, 1979.
68. Horowitz RS, et al: Placental transfer of *N*-acetylcysteine following human maternal acetaminophen toxicity. *J Toxicol Clin Toxicol* 35:447, 1997.
69. Prescott LF, Illingworth RN, Critchley JAH: Intravenous N-acetylcysteine: The treatment of choice for paracetamol poisoning. *Br Med J* 2:1097, 1979.
70. Yip L, Dart RC: A 20-hour treatment for acute acetaminophen overdose. *N Engl J Med* 348:2471, 2003.
71. Woo OF, et al: Shorter duration of oral *N*-acetylcysteine therapy for acute acetaminophen overdose. *Ann Emerg Med* 35:363, 2000.
72. James LP, Wells E, Beard RH, Farrar HC: Predictors of outcome after acetaminophen poisoning in children and adolescents. *J Pediatr* 140:522, 2002.

CHAPTER 147

Aspirin and Nonsteroidal Agents

Donna L. Seger and Lindsay Murray

ASPIRIN

Perspective

The incidence of aspirin (acetylsalicylic acid [ASA]) overdose and related childhood deaths has decreased significantly in recent years. Reasons include pediatricians' preference for acetaminophen preparations, the Food and Drug Administration's mandate limiting 36 tablets of baby ASA to each bottle, and the use of child-resistant caps.

Unfortunately, lack of familiarity with the clinical picture of this poisoning causes the severity of the poisoning to be underestimated. Salicylate toxicity can cause metabolic acidosis, seizure, hyperthermia, pulmonary edema, cerebral edema, renal failure, and death. Morbidity and mortality are increased by delayed diagnosis in elderly patients with chronic medical problems and in young patients diagnosed with an acute illness.[1]

Principles of Disease

Pharmacokinetics

Salts of salicylic acid are rapidly absorbed intact from the gastrointestinal tract, with appreciable serum concentrations in 30 minutes. Two thirds of a therapeutic dose is absorbed in 1 hour, and peak levels occur in 2 to 4 hours. Serum concentrations may rise for more than 12 hours after large ingestions (which may delay gastric emptying) or ingestions of enteric capsules.[2]

In the intestinal wall, liver, and red blood cells, aspirin is hydrolyzed to free salicylic acid, which reversibly binds to albumin (which contains a variable number of salicylate binding sites). In the liver, salicylate is conjugated with glucuronic acid and glycine (Figure 147-1). A small fraction is hydroxylated. Free salicylate and conjugates are eliminated by renal excretion. At therapeutic salicylate concentrations, elimination follows first-order kinetics, and excretion

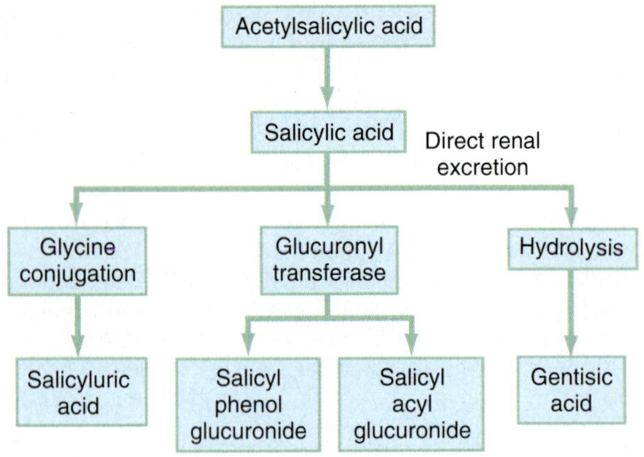

Figure 147-1. Aspirin metabolism.

is proportional to salicylate concentration. When serum salicylate concentrations are greater than 30 mg/dL, however, elimination follows zero-order kinetics, and the metabolic rate is constant. The metabolic pathways become saturated, and the pH-sensitive urinary excretion of salicylic acid determines the half-life (which may approach 15 to 30 hours with toxic doses).[3]

Pathophysiology

Acid-Base Disturbances and Metabolic Effects

Salicylate stimulates the medullary respiratory center and increases the sensitivity of the respiratory center to pH and carbon dioxide partial pressure (PCO_2). Prolonged high serum concentrations eventually depress the respiratory center. Respiratory alkalosis is compensated for by buffering of the hemoglobin-oxyhemoglobin system, the exchange of intracellular hydrogen ions for extracellular cations, and the urinary excretion of bicarbonate. Loss of bicarbonate decreases buffering capacity and intensifies the metabolic acidosis.[4,5]

Salicylates inhibit the Krebs dehydrogenase cycle, increasing production of lactic and pyruvic acids. Lipid metabolism is increased and ketone bodies are produced. Uncoupling of oxidative phosphorylation increases the body's metabolic rate and temperature and causes increased production of tissue carbon dioxide and increases oxygen consumption. Uncoupling also increases tissue glycolysis, which predisposes patients to hypoglycemia. Hepatic gluconeogenesis and release of adrenaline may cause the less common hyperglycemia.

Only nonionized particles can cross the cell membrane and accumulate in the brain and other tissues. Because ASA has a low pK_a (3.5), the majority of salicylate is ionized and little salicylate enters tissues at physiologic pH of 7.4. However, as pH decreases, more particles become un-ionized and cross the cell membrane, markedly increasing movement of salicylate into the tissues and central nervous system (CNS).[4,5]

Fluid and Electrolyte Abnormalities

Significant potassium loss in salicylate toxicity is caused by (1) vomiting, secondary to stimulation of the medullary chemoreceptor trigger zone; (2) increased renal excretion of sodium, bicarbonate, and potassium as a compensatory response to the respiratory alkalosis; (3) salicylate-induced increased permeability of the renal tubules with further loss of potassium; (4) intracellular accumulation of sodium and water; and (5) inhibition of the active transport system, secondary to uncoupling of oxidative phosphorylation. The net result is rapid depletion of potassium stores.[4]

A salicylate-induced decrease in renal blood flow or direct nephrotoxicity may cause acute nonoliguric renal failure. Salicylate-induced secretion of inappropriate antidiuretic hormone secretion may also affect renal function.[6]

Pulmonary and Cerebral Edema

The exact mechanism by which salicylate increases alveolar-capillary membrane permeability is unknown. Theories include inhibition of prostacyclin, changes in platelet-vessel interaction, and neurogenic influences. In adults, the risk factors for salicylate-induced pulmonary edema include age older than 30 years, cigarette smoking, chronic salicylate ingestion, metabolic acidosis, neurologic symptoms, and serum salicylate concentration greater than 40 mg/dL. Risk factors in children include high serum salicylate levels, large anion gap, decreased serum potassium concentration, and low PCO_2.[7]

Any alteration in sensorium is evidence of cerebral edema and is a grave prognostic sign. Factors causing cerebral edema are unknown. Patients with cerebral or pulmonary edema require immediate dialysis.

Chronic Ingestion Physiology

Physiologic changes of aging predispose elderly patients to toxicity from chronic therapeutic ingestion. Decreased liver blood flow rates decrease biotransformation of salicylate, and decreased renal function decreases salicylate clearance. Chronic ingestion of free aspirin decreases albumin binding, which increases free salicylate. The free salicylate enters the cell, causing significant clinical illness with a relatively low serum salicylate concentration. A patient with chronic salicylate toxicity and a serum concentration of 40 mg/dL may be more ill than a patient with an acute ingestion and serum concentration of 80 mg/dL.[8]

Pediatric salicylism from overaggressive dosing may be more serious than acute ingestion. Sweating, fever, and tachycardia caused by salicylism may be attributed to underlying infection. Other sources of salicylate exposure include breast milk, teething gels, and percutaneous absorption of skin ointments, which have high concentrations of methyl salicylate.

CLINICAL FEATURES

A toxic dose of aspirin is 200 to 300 mg/kg, and ingestion of 500 mg/kg is potentially lethal. The initial manifestations of acute salicylate toxicity include tinnitus, impaired hearing, hyperventilation, vomiting, dehydration, and hyperthermia. Salicylate-induced hyperpnea may manifest as increased respiratory depth without commensurate increase in rate. Hyperventilation is more common in adults, who usually have an initial respiratory alkalosis. Young children are predisposed to toxicity due to the metabolic acidosis, which increases tissue and CNS salicylate concentrations. Vomiting can occur 3 to 8 hours after ingestion. Serious dehydration can occur from hyperpnea, vomiting, and hyperthermia. CNS manifestations are usually associated with acidemia.

Shortness of breath and altered sensorium are caused by pulmonary and cerebral edema, respectively. Noncardiac pulmonary edema may be more common in children than scattered case reports suggest.[9] Failure to recognize salicylate toxicity as the cause of pulmonary edema increases the morbidity and mortality of these patients.

Salicylates can depress the hepatic synthesis of factor VI and decrease platelet aggregation. Although prothrombin times may be slightly increased as salicylates compete with vitamin K, gastrointestinal bleeding and significant hemorrhage are rare.

DIAGNOSTIC STRATEGIES

A serum salicylate concentration should be measured 6 hours or more after ingestion. A second sample should be obtained 2 hours later. If the second concentration is greater than the first, serial concentrations should be obtained. Special caution is required in interpreting the salicylate level after chronic ingestion or the ingestion of enteric-coated tablets.[2,8]

Prognosis and treatment of the acutely poisoned patient should be determined by the serum salicylate concentration, the dose of salicylate ingested, and the patient's age, clinical features, and acid-base status. Acid-base status can change quickly, and frequent monitoring of arterial pH is necessary to guide treatment.[10] The Done nomogram should not be used.

Differential Considerations

The symptoms of salicylism (hyperthermia, altered mental status or coma, pulmonary edema, and shock) mimic the symptoms of many other diseases (Box 147-1). This is especially true with chronic ingestion, when the patient does not recognize the cause, serum salicylate concentration is low, and the severity of the poisoning is not recognized.[11] Death is caused by CNS depression and cardiovascular collapse.

Management

Treatment of salicylate toxicity has three objectives: to prevent further absorption, to correct fluid deficits and acid-base abnormalities, and to increase excretion (Box 147-2).

BOX 147-1. Symptoms of Salicylate Toxicity

Asymptomatic: occasional subjective but no objective manifestations
Mild: mild to moderate hyperpnea tinnitis, sometimes with lethargy
Moderate: severe hyperpnea, prominent neurologic disturbances, such as marked lethargy or excitability, but no coma or convulsions
Severe: severe hyperpnea, coma, or semicoma, sometimes with convulsions

BOX 147-2. Treatment of Acute Salicylate Poisoning

1. Treat dehydration; maintain urine output at 2–3 mL/kg/hr with 5% dextrose (D_5) in lactated Ringer's solution or normal saline.
2. Correct potassium depletion.
3. Alkalinize urine.
   a. Obtain baseline arterial blood gas values.
   b. Administer 1-2 mEq/kg sodium bicarbonate initially, then as needed (50 mL bicarbonate increases serum pH by 0.1).
   c. Infuse intravenous fluids: D_5 with 100 mEq bicarbonate/L.
   d. Monitor serum pH; do not cause systemic alkalosis.
   e. Do not attempt forced diuresis.
4. Monitor for dialysis indications:
   a. Coma, seizure
   b. Renal hepatic, or pulmonary failure
   c. Pulmonary edema
   d. Severe acid-base imbalance
   e. Deterioration in condition
   f. Serum salicylate concentration ≥ 100 mg/dL

Initial Evaluation

In addition to general physical examination, including vital signs (especially respiratory rate), assessment of the minute volume of respiration, auscultation of the chest, and assessment of skin temperature, arterial blood gases can be used to rapidly assess severity of illness.

Activated Charcoal

Early administration of activated charcoal reduces salicylate absorption, although an improved outcome has not been demonstrated in overdose patients after a single dose of activated charcoal. Single-dose activated charcoal can be considered if a toxic dose of salicylate is ingested and the patient presents within 1 hour of ingestion, but there is no evidence that this will result in any improvement in outcome, avoidance of toxicity, or alteration of therapy or course.[12]

Intravenous Fluids

Dehydration occurs early in salicylate intoxication because of the hypermetabolic state and should be treated with intravenous fluid. Potassium depletion must be corrected. Fluid administration should be guided by the patient's apparent deficit and should not exceed the estimated replacement, because excessive fluid administration can worsen cerebral and pulmonary edema. Urine output should be maintained at 2 to 3 mL/kg/hr.

Additionally, the metabolic rate is increased in these cases. Intravenous fluid should contain dextrose, and the serum glucose level should be frequently monitored. In animal studies, hypoglycemia consistently occurs with death. Intracerebral glucose levels may be low even with serum euglycemia.

Urinary Alkalinization

Because salicylates have a low pK_a and are renally excreted, alkaline urine traps the salicylate ion and increases excretion. Urinary alkalinization should be considered in patients with salicylate levels greater than 35 mg/dL, acid-base abnormalities, or rapidly increasing salicylate levels. A urine pH of 7.5 to 8.0 is necessary to increase excretion. Sodium bicarbonate (1-2 mEq/kg) can be administered over 1 to 2 hours, with subsequent dosage adjustment determined by urinary and serum pH.

Urinary alkalinization is difficult to achieve because the excretion of salicylic acid in the urine decreases urinary pH. Additionally, potassium depletion must be corrected to attain an alkaline urine. Alkaline urine should not be produced at the cost of systemic acidosis. Forced diuresis does not increase salicylate excretion and may potentiate cerebral and pulmonary edema. Salicylate clearance varies in direct proportion to flow rate, but exponentially with pH.[13]

Hemodialysis

Hemodialysis should be considered in patients with the following: serum salicylate levels greater than 100 mg/dL in acute cases and 40 mg/dL in chronic cases of poisoning; altered mental status; coma; renal or hepatic failure; pulmonary edema; severe acid-base imbalance; rising serum salicylate level; and failure to respond to more conservative treatment. Exchange transfusion can be considered in young infants or unusual cases of congenital salicylism.[14]

Pregnancy

Greater salicylate concentration on the fetal side of the placenta and relative fetal acidemia contribute to fetal distress from maternal salicylate poisoning. Salicylate poisoning during pregnancy is associated with fetal demise, and delivery of the distressed fetus should be considered if the fetus is viable.[15]

Disposition

In patients with acute intoxication, hospital admission is required for pulmonary edema, CNS symptoms other than tinnitus, seizures, acidosis, electrolyte disorders, dehydration, renal insufficiency, or increasing serum levels. In patients with chronic intoxication, remarkably low serum salicylate concentrations may accompany severe salicylism. Any indication of infant salicylism requires hospital admission. The mortality rate of chronic salicylate intoxication is 25%, compared with a mortality rate of 1% following acute salicylate intoxication.

In patients with acute ingestion, a second serum salicylate concentration measurement is essential to determine whether the peak serum concentration has been attained. As in any case of intentional overdose, psychiatric evaluation is essential.

NONSTEROIDAL AGENTS

Perspective

The nonsteroidal anti-inflammatory drugs (NSAIDs) are a heterogeneous group of agents with variable analgesic, anti-inflammatory, and antipyretic activities. They are usually classified according to chemical structure, although classification based on cyclooxygenase (COX) selectivity may be more clinically relevant. NSAIDs are prescribed for a wide variety of conditions, and more than 13 million Americans use them daily.[16] Ibuprofen and naproxen are common over-the-counter NSAIDs.

Principles of Disease

Physiology

The therapeutic anti-inflammatory effect of the NSAIDs is achieved by inhibition of COX and consequent blockade of prostaglandin production. Of the two discrete COX isoenzymes, COX-1, the constitutive enzyme, is concentrated in platelets, vascular endothelial cells, gastric mucosal cells, and renal collecting tubules. It is a physiologic maintenance enzyme, producing the prostaglandins critical for the autocrine/paracrine responses to circulating hormones and the maintenance of normal renal function, gastric mucosal integrity, and hemostasis. COX-2, the inducible enzyme, is expressed only in response to certain inflammatory stimuli. The benefits of NSAIDs are thus believed to result from COX-2 inhibition, whereas the principal gastrointestinal and renal adverse effects are attributed to inhibition of COX-1.

Traditional NSAIDs are nonselective and inhibit both COX-1 and COX-2. Newer, specific COX-2 inhibitors (e.g., celecoxib, rofecoxib, meloxicam) have fewer side effects than traditional NSAIDs while maintaining analgesic and anti-inflammatory efficacy.

Pharmacokinetics

The NSAIDs are almost completely absorbed from the upper small intestine after oral administration. The presence of food may alter the site and timing of drug uptake. As weak organic acids (pK_a, 4-5), NSAIDs are largely un-ionized in the stomach and readily diffuse across the bipolar layer lipid membrane of gastric-lining cells. Once intracellular, the drug can become ionized again at the relatively high pH of normal cytoplasm and become trapped within the mucosal cell. This relatively high local concentration of drug contributes to the frequent gastrointestinal symptoms associated with NSAIDs.

The NSAIDs are highly bound to plasma proteins, mainly albumin, and therefore have small volumes of distribution (0.10-0.17 L/kg). They are eliminated by hepatic biotransformation, principally oxidation and glucuronidation, with the metabolites excreted in the urine. Metabolites are inactive, except for those of sulindac, nabumetone (inactive parent drugs metabolized to active agent in vivo), and phenylbutazone. Plasma half-lives are short (1-4 hours), except for naproxen (12-15 hours), oxaprozin (25-50 hours), piroxicam (45 hours), and phenylbutazone (50-100 hours). Elimination half-lives are not substantially prolonged in overdose.[17]

Clinical Features

Most NSAID overdoses, even with large amounts, are asymptomatic or cause only minor CNS or gastrointestinal disturbances. Experience with overdose of the newer COX-2 inhibitors is limited but significant toxicity is not reported.

Ibuprofen is the most common NSAID ingested in overdose and is representative of the propionic acid derivatives. Despite case reports of coma, seizure, hypotension, hypothermia, upper gastrointestinal tract bleeding, acute renal failure, and metabolic acidosis, the vast majority of ibuprofen overdoses follow a benign, rapidly self-limiting course. About 50% of adults and 7% of children develop symptoms. Symptomatic overdose requires ingestion of at least 100 mg/kg, and all those who develop symptoms will do so within 4 hours of ingestion. Life-threatening symptoms or signs are rare, and most toxicity is a mild gastrointestinal or CNS disturbance that resolves in 24 hours.[18-22] Less common clinical effects include mild metabolic acidosis, muscle fasciculations, mydriasis, chills, diaphoresis, hyperventilation, mildly elevated systolic blood pressure, asymptomatic bradycardia, hypotension, dyspnea, tinnitus, and rash.

Reversible renal dysfunction is seen only after massive acute overdose and in association with a period of relative hypovolemia with hypotension.[18-23] It usually responds to supportive measures. Serum ibuprofen concentrations do not predict toxicity.[18]

Overdose with mefenamic acid, a fenamate, is associated with a relatively high incidence of seizures, which occur 2 to 7 hours after ingestion.[24] Rapid recovery is the rule with supportive care and intravenous benzodiazepines. Serum mefenamic acid concentrations correlate with seizures but do not aid in acute management.

Phenylbutazone, a pyrazolone, is now rarely used because of its association with aplastic anemia and agranulocytosis. Although rare, phenylbutazone overdose is much more severe than overdose with other NSAIDs.[25] Mild poisoning consists of nausea, abdominal pain, and drowsiness. Severely poisoned patients have early onset of abdominal pain, nausea, vomiting, hematemesis, diarrhea, restlessness, dizziness, coma, convulsions, hyperpyrexia, electrolyte disturbances, hyperventilation, alkalosis or acidosis, respiratory arrest, hypotension, cyanosis, edema, electrocardiographic abnormalities, or cardiac arrest. Late sequelae of severe poisoning (2-7 days) include renal, hepatic, and hematologic dysfunction. The clinical course is prolonged compared with other NSAIDs, reflecting the prolonged elimination half-lives of phenylbutazone and its principal metabolite, oxyphenbutazone.

Diagnostic Strategies

The diagnosis and assessment of severity and risk are based on history and clinical features. Plasma NSAID concentrations are not useful, but screening for acetaminophen should be done. Baseline electrolyte levels, renal and hepatic function tests, serum salicylate level, urinalysis, and chest radiograph may be helpful only with significant signs or symptoms.

Management

The management of NSAID overdose is supportive, and there is no specific antidote. Pyrazolone and fenamate overdoses are associated with significantly higher morbidity and should be managed more aggressively.

Children with ingestions of less than 100 mg/kg of ibuprofen do not require medical evaluation. Those who ingest more than 300 mg/kg should be evaluated. With ingestion of 100 to 300 mg/kg, children need treatment only if symptoms develop. Adults who deliberately overdose on NSAIDs should be observed until 6 hours after ingestion before psychiatric evaluation.

All patients with pyrazolone and fenamate ingestions should be evaluated in the emergency department. For other agents, emergency department evaluation is indicated if the amount ingested is greater than five times the maximum daily therapeutic dose, the patient is symptomatic, or a suicide attempt is suspected.

There is no evidence supporting the use of gastric emptying or activated charcoal in cases of NSAID overdose, although activated charcoal is often used. In general, if activated charcoal is to be used, it should be reserved for patients presenting within 1 hour of the ingestion of a massive quantity of an NSAID. Regardless of whether activated charcoal is administered, all patients should be monitored for at least 4 hours and until asymptomatic. Aggressive management of hypotension is mandatory because maintenance of good renal perfusion during acute toxicity reduces the risk of renal failure as a complication.

Because of high protein binding and rapid metabolism, urinary alkalinization, hemodialysis, or hemoperfusion is not clinically useful. Multidose activated charcoal reduces the elimination half-life of phenylbutazone by 30% and may be of benefit in cases of severe intoxication.[26]

Disposition

Patients who remain asymptomatic more than 4 hours after an NSAID overdose do not require further medical surveillance. It is prudent to observe those who have ingested a pyrazolone or fenamate for another 4 hours. Patients who develop significant symptoms or signs of toxicity requiring supportive care should be admitted to hospital or an emergency department observation unit for ongoing medical management. Patients with only gastrointestinal or neurologic symptoms may be observed in the emergency department until asymptomatic. All patients for whom the ingestion represented a suicidal gesture need to undergo psychiatric assessment before hospital discharge.

KEY CONCEPTS

- ASA intoxication, especially chronic salicylism should be considered in the differential diagnosis of altered mental status in the elderly
- Potassium stores are rapidly depleted in patients with salicylate intoxication.
- The acute toxic dose of ASA is 300 mg/kg, and 500 mg/kg is potentially lethal.
- Acidosis signifies severe salicylism as unbound salicylate is moving into the cell.
- Signs of pulmonary or cerebral edema, coma, hepatic failure, circulatory collapse, refractory acidosis, or levels greater than 100 mg/dL require immediate hemodialysis.
- Hyperthermia, altered mental status, coma, pulmonary edema, and shock may be presenting signs of salicylism.
- Serial salicylate concentrations should be obtained after acute ingestion to ensure that the salicylate concentration is decreasing.
- Consider dialysis in patients with coma, seizures, renal failure, hepatic failure, pulmonary failure, or refractory acidosis, or in acute cases in which serum levels are greater than 100 mg/dL.
- NSAID overdose, other than ASA, is usually self-limited, with predominantly gastrointestinal toxicity.

REFERENCES

1. Chapman BJ, Proudfood AT: Adult salicylate poisoning: Deaths and outcome in patients with high plasma salicylate concentrations. *Q J Med* 72:699, 1989.
2. Wortzman DI, Grunfeld A: Delayed absorption following enteric-coated aspirin overdose. *Ann Emerg Med* 16:434, 1987.
3. Roberts LJ, Morrow JD: Analgesic-antipyretic and anti-inflammatory agents and drugs employed in the treatment of gout. In Hardman J, Limbird L (eds): *Goodmans and Gillman's The Pharmacologic Basis of Therapeutics.* New York, McGraw Hill, 2001, pp 687-729.
4. Krause DS, Wolf BA, Shaw LM: Acute aspirin overdose: Mechanisms of toxicity. *Ther Drug Monit* 14:441, 1992.
5. Dromgoole S, Furst D: Salicylates. In Evans WE, Schentag JJ, Jusko WJ (eds): *Applied Pharmacokinetics: Principles of Therapeutic Drug Monitoring.* Vancouver, Wash, Applied Therapeutics, 1992.
6. Pemeger TV, Whelton PK: Risk of kidney failure associated with the use of acetaminophen, aspirin, and nonsteroidal anti-inflammatory drugs. *N Engl J Med* 331:1675, 1994.
7. Gonzolea E, et al: Recurrent ARDS in a 39-year-old woman with migraine headaches. *Chest* 114:919, 1998.
8. Gaudreault P, Temple AR, Lovejoy FH: The relative severity of acute versus chronic salicylate poisoning in children: A clinical comparison. *Pediatrics* 70:566, 1982.
9. Fisher CJ, Albertson TE, Foulke GE: Salicylate-induced pulmonary edema: Clinical characteristics in children. *Am J Emerg Med* 3:33, 1985.
10. Dugandzic R, et al: Evaluation of the validity of the Done nomogram in the management of acute salicylate intoxication. *Ann Emerg Med* 18:1186, 1989.
11. Lamesh RA: Accidental chronic salicylate intoxication in an elderly patient: Major morbidity despite early recognition. *Vet Hum Toxicol* 35:34, 1993.
12. Chyka PA, Seger DL: Single-dose activated charcoal. *Clin Toxicol* 35:721, 1997.
13. Prescott L, et al: Diuresis or urinary alkalinization for salicylate poisoning? *BMJ* 285:1383, 1982.
14. Krenzelok E, Derr F, Proudfoot AT: Salicylate toxicity. In *Clinical Management of Poisoning and Drug Overdose,* 3rd ed. Philadelphia, WB Saunders, 1998.
15. Palatnick W, Tenenbein M: Aspirin poisoning during pregnancy: Increased fetal sensitivity. *Am J Perinatol* 15:39, 1998.
16. McCarthy D: Nonsteroidal anti-inflammatory drug-related gastrointestinal toxicity: Definitions and epidemiology. *Am J Med* 105(Suppl 3A):3S, 1998.
17. Hall AH, et al: Ibuprofen overdose: 126 cases. *Ann Emerg Med* 15:1308, 1986.
18. McElwee NE, et al: A prospective, population-based study of acute ibuprofen overdose: Complications are rare and routine serum levels not warranted. *Ann Emerg Med* 19:652, 1990.
19. Perry SJ, Streete PJ, Volans GN: Ibuprofen overdose: The first two years of over-the-counter sales. *Hum Toxicol* 6:173, 1987.
20. Halpern SM, Fitzpatrick R, Volans GN: Ibuprofen toxicity: A review of adverse reactions and overdose. *Adverse Drug React Toxicol Rev* 12:107, 1993.
21. Hall AH, et al: Ibuprofen overdose in adults. *Clin Toxicol* 30:23, 1992.
22. Le HT, Bosse GM, Tsai Y: Ibuprofen overdose complicated by renal failure, adult respiratory distress syndrome, and metabolic acidosis. *J Toxicol Clin Toxicol* 32:315, 1994.
23. Perazella MA, Buller GK: Can ibuprofen cause acute renal failure in a normal individual? A case of acute overdose. *Am J Kidney Dis* 18:600, 1991.
24. Balali-Mood M, et al: Mefenamic acid overdosage. *Lancet* 1:1354, 1981.
25. Court H, Volans GN: Poisoning after overdose with non-steroidal anti-inflammatory drugs. *Adverse Drug React Acute Poison Rev* 3:1, 1984.
26. Neuvonen PJ, Elonen E: Effect of activated charcoal on absorption and elimination of phenobarbitone, carbamazepine and phenylbutazone in man. *Eur J Clin Pharmacol* 17:51, 1980.

CHAPTER

148 Anticholinergics

Wilfredo Rivera and Larissa I. Velez

PERSPECTIVE

In 1676, a group of British soldiers in Jamestown, Virginia, became ill after ingesting a boiled salad made of a local plant now known as Jamestown, or "jimson," weed. Its stimulatory and amnesic central nervous system (CNS) effects were well documented, as follows:

"Some of them did eat plentifully of it, the effect of which was a very pleasant Comedy; for they turned natural Fools upon it for several Days. . . . In this frantic Condition they were confined, lest they in their Folly should destroy themselves . . . after Eleven Days, [they] returned themselves again, not remembering anything that had passed."[1]

Since then, numerous descriptions of the effects induced by plants and plant extracts that contain anticholinergic alkaloids have been recorded.[1,2] In 1923, fever, widely dilated pupils, and a deep-red flush were noted in some of the 30 children who caused pandemonium in an orphanage after a group experience with jimson weed.[3] Prisoners cleaning an infirmary in 1864 were the first to be treated with physostigmine after ingesting atropine.[4]

Anticholinergic agents are divided into three main groups: antimuscarinics, affecting the muscarinic acetylcholine receptors; neuromuscular blockers, blocking nicotinic acetylcholine receptors (Figure 148-1); and ganglionic blockers, affecting acetylcholine sympathetic and parasympathetic nicotinic ganglia. This chapter refers only to antimuscarinic agents, and the terms *anticholinergic* and *antimuscarinic* will be used interchangeably. The prototypical anticholinergic agents are the naturally occurring belladonna alkaloids—atropine, scopolamine (L-hyoscine), and hyoscyamine—found in many plant members of the Solanaceae family (Table 148-1). Atropine is the major alkaloid of *Atropa belladonna,* an important pharmaceutical source of that drug. *Datura stramonium,* or jimson weed, contains scopolamine, grows in almost all climates, and is often involved in plant-related belladonna poisoning.[3,5,6]

Physicians have used belladonna alkaloids for hundreds of years as mydriatics and antiparkinsonian agents and for the treatment of asthma (Box 148-1).[4,5,7] The belladonna alkaloids and their synthetic congeners are used today as pupillary dilators (atropine, homatropine, tropicamide, cyclopentolate), as antispasmodics (dicyclomine), to decrease gastric secretions (propantheline), to prevent motion sickness (scopolamine), and to treat asthma (ipratropium) and bradycardia (atropine). Atropine or scopolamine is used to dry airway secretions and block vagal responses to laryngoscopy and endotracheal intubation. The significant central nervous system (CNS) effects of scopolamine facilitate the induction of perioperative amnesia.[7]

The anticholinergic antiparkinsonian agents are synthetic tertiary amine congeners of atropine and include benztropine (Cogentin) and trihexyphenidyl (Artane).[7] They are used as second-line antiparkinsonian agents and to counteract the extrapyramidal side effects of neuroleptics. These agents readily cross the blood-brain barrier and exhibit antimuscarinic effects similar to those of belladonna alkaloids.

Methantheline (Banthine) and propantheline (Pro-Banthine) are synthetic quaternary ammonium congeners of atropine commonly used for urinary incontinence. They also exhibit significant anticholinergic effects at nicotinic, ganglionic, and neuromuscular junction acetylcholine receptors, leading to postural hypotension and impotence at high therapeutic doses, and a curare-like paralysis in overdose.[7] These agents do not penetrate the blood-brain barrier and thus do not cause significant CNS effects.

Many other drugs possess anticholinergic activity besides their main pharmacologic action. Some examples are the tricyclic antidepressants, the phenothiazines, and the antihistamines (H_1 blockers). Drugs that are structurally related to the tricyclics, such as carbamazepine (Tegretol) and cyclobenzaprine (Flexeril), also exhibit antimuscarinic effects.[8]

In patients with significant toxicity from any of these drugs, the antimuscarinic effects provide valuable diagnostic clues (Boxes 148-1 and 148-2).

Inadvertent and intentional poisoning by anticholinergic drug overdoses occurs commonly with readily available over-the-counter agents such as pyrilamine (Sominex), diphenhydramine (Nytol, Benadryl), and cyclizine (Marezine). Antihistamine and anticholinergic overdoses have a 1% incidence of serious effects or fatalities, compared with 7% for a similar number of antidepressant overdoses.[9] Poisoning from drugs with toxicity limited to anticholinergic effects rarely results in death when adequate supportive care is provided. However, thermoregulatory dysfunction caused by impairment of sweating may result in fatal hyperthermia in the agitated or seizing patient with an anticholinergic overdose.[10-13] Heat stroke fatalities have occurred in heat-exposed or exercising patients taking therapeutic doses of anticholinergics.[14,15] Deaths from trauma or drowning caused by perceptual distortion can also be attributed to anticholinergics.[5]

Table 148-1. Plants with Anticholinergic Toxins

Scientific Name	Common Name
*Atropa belladonna**	Deadly nightshade
*Brugmansia X candia**	Angel's trumpet
Cestrum nocturnum	Night-blooming jessamine (jasmine)
Cestrum diurnum	Day-blooming jessamine
Datura arborea	Trumpet lily
Datura meteloides	Sacred datura
*Datura stramonium**	Jimson weed
*Hyocyamus niger**	Henbane
Lycium halimifolium	Matrimony vine
Mandragora officinarum	Mandrake
Solandra spp.*	Chalice vine, cup-of-gold

*Solanaceae species.

BOX 148-1. Drugs Exhibiting Primarily Anticholinergic Toxicity

Belladonna Alkaloids and Representative Synthetic Congeners
Atropine
Scopolamine
Homatropine
Cyclopentolate
Tropicamide
Propantheline (Pro-Banthine)
Ipratropium (Atrovent)

Antiparkinsonlans
Benztropine (Cogentin)
Trihexyphenidyl (Artane)
Procyclidine (Kemadrin)
Biperiden (Akineton)
Ethopropazine (Parsidol)

Prototypical H_1-Receptor Blockers
Diphenhydramine (Benadryl)
Chlorpheniramine (Chlor-Trimeton)
Brompheniramine (Dimetane)
Cyclizine (Marezine)
Meclizine (Antivert)
Hydroxyzine (Atarax, Vistaril)
Dimenhydrinate (Dramamine)

Phenothiazine
Promethazine (Phenergan)

Poisonings with belladonna alkaloids are common. Deliberate ingestion of seeds or teas of the ubiquitous jimson weed for its hallucinogenic effects has occurred in many cultures. In modern times, military recruits, adolescents, and children have experimented with this plant and required medical attention.[6] An Internet search of the term *Datura stramonium* will reveal that its use as a recreational stimulant remains a problem among teenagers. Inadvertent poisonings have resulted from ingestion of commercially available herbal teas contaminated with atropine and from smoking herbal cigarettes.[2,16,17] A cluster of nonfatal scopolamine poisonings was described in New York City, when the tasteless, difficult to detect drug was added to tourists' drinks in an attempt to facilitate robbery.[10] The combination of heroin with anticholinergics leading to a complex toxidrome has also been reported in drug users in several states on the East Coast of the United States.[11,12]

BOX 148-2. Drugs Exhibiting Anticholinergic Effects as Part of Toxic Manifestations

Tricyclics or Related Drugs
Cyclobenzaprine (Flexeril)
Carbamazepine (Tegretol)
Amitriptyline
Imipramine
Doxepin
Amoxapine
Desipramine
Nortriptyline
Glutethimide (Doriden)

Phenothiazines
Chlorpromazine (Thorazine)
Prochlorperazine (Compazine)
Mesoridazine (Serentil)
Thioridazine (Mellaril)

PRINCIPLES OF DISEASE

Atropine and atropine-like drugs inhibit muscarinic acetylcholine receptors both centrally and peripherally at the end-organ sites of the parasympathetic nervous system (see Figure 148-1). Although the term *anticholinergic* is commonly used, the most appropriate term to describe the pharmacologic action of these drugs is *antimuscarinic*. These drugs do not block the effects of acetylcholine on nicotinic receptors in the ganglia or at the neuromuscular junction, with the exception of the synthetic quaternary amines. Muscarinic receptors affect smooth muscle function in the eye, intestinal tract, and urinary bladder. They also regulate sweat, salivary, and mucosal gland activity. Cardiac cholinergic receptors associated with vagal nerve fibers affect heart rate and conduction through the atrioventricular node.[7] Muscarinic receptors in the CNS appear to be involved in new information storage, general perceptive and cognitive modalities, and motor coordination.[13,18-20]

Generalized inhibition of muscarinic receptors by atropine results in tachycardia, pupillary dilation, loss of accommodation, inability to sweat, drying of mucosal surfaces, gastrointestinal paralysis, and urinary retention. In the CNS, muscarinic inhibition causes stimulation, seizures, coma, choreoathetosis, memory impairment, and perceptual and cognitive dysfunction.[13,18-24] "Hot as a hare, red as a beet, blind as a bat, dry as a bone, mad as a hatter," aptly characterizes the more florid manifestations of the antimuscarinic syndrome. The toxic effects of atropine are dose dependent (Table 148-2). With increasing doses, CNS depression follows the initial stimulation.[7] In adults, the CNS depression can predominate without stimulation.[25]

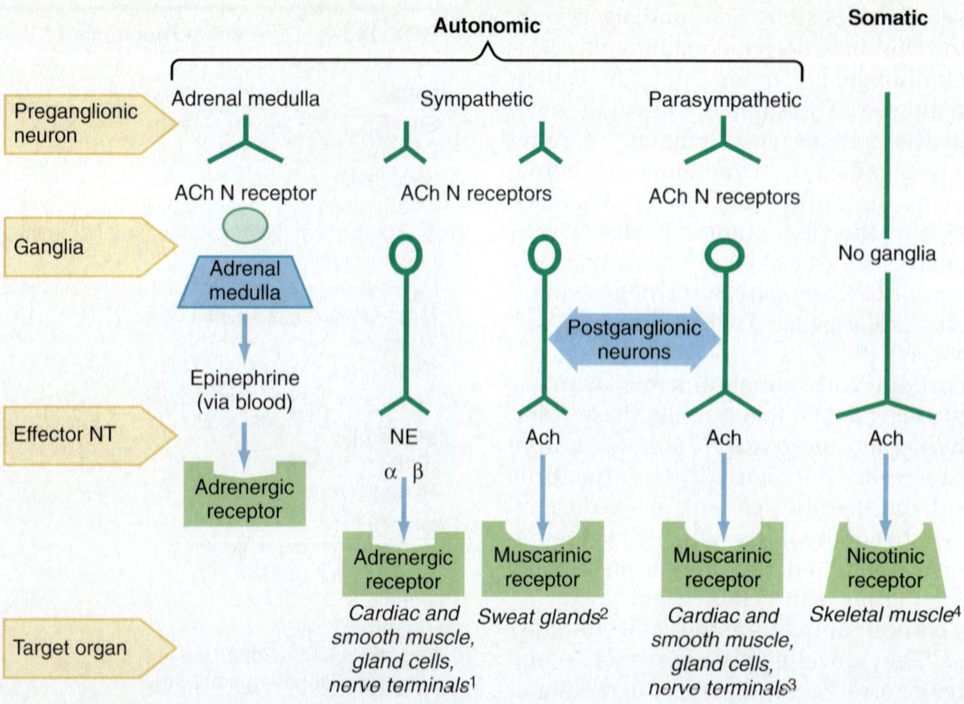

Figure 148-1. The sites of nicotinic and muscarinic acetylcholine receptors. Ach, acetylcholine; N, nicotinic; NE, norepinephrine; NT, neurotransmitter. [1]Causing tachycardia, hypertension, diaphoresis, mydriasis. [2]Causing diaphoresis. [3]Causing bradycardia, diarrhea, diaphoresis, urination, miosis, bronchospasm, bronchorrhea, lacrimation, salivation. [4]Causing fasiculations.

Table 148-2. Dose-Related Effects of Atropine

Dose (mg)	Pupils	CNS	Heart	Gastrointestinal	Skin	Mucosa	Bladder
0.5	None	None	Slower	None	+	++	None
1.0	+	None	++	None	++	++	None
2.0	++	None	+++	None	+++	+++	+
5.0	+++	++	++++	++	++++	++++	+++
>10	++++	++++	++++	++++	++++	++++	++++

Modified from Weiner N: Muscarinic receptor agonist and antagonists. In Goodman L, et al (eds): *Goodman and Gilman's The Pharmacological Basis of Therapeutics*, 7th ed. New York. Macmillan, 1985.

Different end-organs manifest different but predictable sensitivities to these drugs. Salivation, bronchial secretion, and sweating are suppressed by small doses of atropine, followed by pupillary dilation, inhibition of accommodation, and tachycardia. Larger doses are required to inhibit micturition and decrease intestinal tone and motility. Only very large doses of anticholinergic agents affect gastric acid secretion and gastric motility. Thus, therapeutic use of an anticholinergic to decrease gastric motility invariably leads to pupillary dilation, problems with accommodation, and the possibility of urinary retention.[7]

Anticholinergics are generally rapidly absorbed from the gastrointestinal tract and are widely distributed in the body. The onset of action of therapeutic doses occurs within 30 minutes, and maximum effect is seen within 1 hour. If the anticholinergic agent is smoked or ingested as a tea, the onset is also rapid. However, with plant and seed ingestions, the onset of symptoms can be delayed.[3] In the overdose setting, symptoms typically develop within a few hours of ingestion, although serious symptoms may not occur for several hours.[26] Death associated with seizures and cardiogenic shock has occurred within hours of ingestion.[27] Prolonged anticholinergic toxicity has been reported, which may indicate that anticholinergic effects on the bowel slow gastrointestinal absorption of the ingested drug and prolong its toxicity.[22,28,29] Poisoning from dermal absorption of topical antihistamines has been reported in children.[30]

CLINICAL PRESENTATION

The diagnosis of acute anticholinergic poisoning is suggested by the characteristic anticholinergic toxidrome.[10,23] Mydriasis, dry mucous membranes, the absence of axillary sweat, flushed skin, fever, tachycardia, decreased or absent bowel sounds, and bladder distention from urinary retention constitute peripheral evidence of muscarinic blockade. The presence of only one or two of these findings does not exclude the diagnosis of an anticholinergic poisoning.[24,31-33] The patient is often alert and may be silly, agitated, violent, or incoherent. Visual hallucinations are common.[34] Central motor effects may manifest as myoclonus or choreoathetoid movements in adults and children. Children are more sensitive to the CNS stimulant effects than adults and are more likely to have seizures, typically preceded by signs of CNS irritability or depression.[35] Massive ingestions are associated with coma and cardiovascular collapse.[10,26, 27,29]

The agitated patient with anticholinergic overdose may have a greatly elevated temperature. In these cases, significant morbidity and the possibility of death from hyperthermia supersede the morbidity of the drug effects.[15,31] The hyperthermic patient may develop hepatic necrosis, rhabdomyolysis with myoglobinuric renal failure, cerebral edema, and disseminated intravascular coagulation with hemorrhage.[36]

Patients with chronic anticholinergic poisoning are often overlooked. They develop organic mental symptoms that may be incorrectly attributed to dementia or underlying psychiatric illness. Significant peripheral signs of anticholinergic excess are typically absent. Two likely settings are (1) the elderly patient taking anticholinergic drugs for parkinsonism or another chronic disease and (2) the psychiatric patient receiving neuroleptic therapy and an anticholinergic or tricyclic antidepressant.[18,24] Resolution of behavioral or cognitive symptoms after withdrawal of the offending drug will confirm the diagnosis.

DIFFERENTIAL DIAGNOSIS

The differential diagnosis of the comatose, psychotic, delirious, or febrile patient is extensive, and serious alternative diagnoses should be considered and excluded (Box 148-3).[23,37] Salicylism, sedative-hypnotic withdrawal, and poisoning with commonly abused sympathetic drugs (e.g., cocaine, phencyclidine, and amphetamines) must be considered. In the elderly patient, almost any medication can be implicated in the presentation of delirium.[38]

The physical examination findings can be helpful. As in cases of anticholinergic poisoning, patients with excessive sympathetic stimulation secondary to cocaine or amphetamine poisoning also exhibit fever, tachycardia, and dilated pupils. The finding of diaphoresis helps distinguish patients with sympathetic overload from those with anticholinergic effects; however, this finding can be absent in severely dehydrated patients. Marked nystagmus, diaphoresis, small pupils, and extreme agitation suggest phencyclidine poisoning. Lithium or monoamine oxidase inhibitor toxicity should also be considered. These patients usually have tremors and significant hyperreflexia or clonus, which are not characteristic of anticholinergic poisoning. Patients with serotonin syndrome often present with agitation. These patients are often diaphoretic and have a tremor that is more prominent in the lower extremities. Neuroleptic malignant syndrome and malignant hyperthermia can also manifest similarly, but these patients will have rigidity as a main physical examination feature.

BOX 148-3. Differential Diagnosis of Delirium

Toxic
Steroids
Lithium
Salicylates
Anticholinergics
Sympathomimetics (cocaine, amphetamines)
Phencyclidine
Mushrooms containing muscimol/ibotenic acid (*Amanita* spp.)
Monoamine oxidase inhibitors
Solvents
Carbon monoxide
Sedative-hypnotic withdrawal

Metabolic
Sodium disorders
Hypoglycemia
Hypercarbia
Hypoxia, severe anemia
Calcium disorders
Uremia
Thyrotoxicosis
Hepatic encephalopathy
Hypertensive encephalopathy
Shock
Sepsis

Infectious/Inflammatory
Meningoencephalitis
Meningitis
Vasculitis

Neurologic/Neurosurgical
Cerebrovascular accident
Subarachnoid hemorrhage
Subdural/epidural hematoma
Frontal contusion
Postictal state
Temporal lobe seizures

The nontoxicologic differential diagnosis of acute agitated delirium should consider metabolic, endocrine, infectious, neurologic, and neurosurgical emergencies. Nuchal rigidity or focality on neurologic examination or physical signs of systemic infection, hepatic failure, or thyroid disease suggests alternative diagnoses. A positive response to empiric administration of 50% dextrose or the demonstration of hypoxia, uremia, glucose, or calcium abnormalities also suggests a nontoxic diagnosis.

Except for sinus tachycardia, electrocardiographic abnormalities from a pure anticholinergic overdose are unusual and should suggest a cardiotoxic agent with antimuscarinic side effects, such as a tricyclic antidepressant, carbamazepine, or a phenothiazine. In the presence of hyperkalemia due to rhabdomyolysis, peaked T waves can be observed.

DIAGNOSTIC STRATEGIES

Mildly symptomatic patients with well-established histories and consistent symptoms do not benefit from routine laboratory testing. Laboratory investigation of the seriously poisoned patient should include measurement of serum electrolytes, renal function, creatinine phosphokinase level, and glucose level. Arterial blood gas measurements document disorders of oxygenation and ventilation and allow early detection of metabolic acidosis. Clinical responses to administration of 50% dextrose, thiamine, oxygen, and naloxone (in the comatose patient) provide clues to common metabolic disturbances that could mimic the anticholinergic toxidrome.

Broad, nonspecific toxicologic screening is rarely useful in the acute setting, although it may retrospectively confirm a diagnosis in a seriously ill patient. Patients with significant infectious or neurosurgical problems will often have evidence of an incidental toxin. A positive toxicology screen should not distract the physician from ruling out a more serious diagnosis.

Quantitative measurements of specific suspected agents may be helpful. In the agitated or convulsing patient, salicylate, theophylline, or lithium levels may be critical and significantly alter management. In any case of intentional ingestion, serum acetaminophen levels should be obtained to exclude this common co-ingestant, especially because many over-the-counter products contain acetaminophen with the antihistamine that causes the anticholinergic symptoms.

Computed tomography of the brain and a lumbar puncture will exclude neurologic and neurosurgical emergencies in the patient who deteriorates, who fails to improve, or for whom the history or examination suggests a nontoxic problem.

MANAGEMENT

In the emergency department, many patients with anticholinergic poisoning have no clear history of exposure. The patient is often unable to provide a history owing to the delirium. The diagnosis is often suspected on the basis of the physical examination. The general management proceeds with consideration of the broader differential diagnosis of the acutely agitated, febrile, or comatose patient.[23] Intubation is not usually indicated, unless cyclic antidepressants have been ingested, or the anticholinergic or a co-ingested agent has resulted in significantly depressed mental status with failure of airway protection. Intubation is not indicated for agitation, which should be managed with intravenous benzodiazepines.

Agitation

The need for aggressive sedation with a benzodiazepine, cooling, and hydration takes precedence over specific toxicologic concerns in these critically ill patients. Physical restraint alone is detrimental.[39] Agitation should be controlled by titrating intravenous benzodiazepines to sedation. Benzodiazepines, such as intravenous midazolam or diazepam, are recommended over phenothiazines and butyrophenones because exacerbation or induction of hypotension is unlikely, the possibility of seizures is decreased, and anticholinergic effects are absent.[40] Pharmacologic intervention in the agitated patient prevents self-injury, severe hyperthermia, and the development of myoglobinuric renal failure from muscle injury. Control of the agitation also allows for a more thorough physical examination and for airway and imaging procedures to take place.

Hyperthermia

Many deaths of agitated patients are associated with undetected or untreated hyperthermia. The patient's temperature should be measured with a flexible rectal probe. Aggressive temperature reduction with ice water or evaporative cooling should be the first priority in the severely hyperthermic patient. Evaporative cooling with mist and fans is highly efficient, but if the equipment required to do this adequately is not available, ice is widely available and effective. The use of dantrolene, a drug that decreases rigidity caused by abnormal calcium fluxes in muscle tissue, has no role in the treatment of hyperthermic patients who do not have muscle rigidity.[41] Antipyretic agents and simple cooling blankets are also ineffective.

Seizures

Seizures should be treated with intravenous benzodiazepines such as lorazepam or diazepam. In the absence of an intravenous line, the intramuscular route can be effectively used.

Drug Removal

Decontamination of the patient with documented or strongly suspected anticholinergic poisoning must be individualized, based on time since exposure, type of anticholinergic agent involved, route of exposure, probable amount ingested, and severity of the clinical condition. Early gastric emptying (within 1 hour) should be considered for large ingestions (e.g., suicidal adult) of an initially asymptomatic patient. In intubated patients who are comatose after large ingestions, gastric lavage should also be considered, regardless of the time of ingestion. In most agitated patients, the risks of gastric lavage outweigh its potential benefit, especially in the absence of a history or hospital course suggestive of massive ingestion.

Activated charcoal has been shown to be efficacious in binding diphenhydramine, tricyclic antidepressants, and phenothiazines, and administration through a nasogastric tube is reasonable.[42,43] Decreased gastrointestinal motility may make activated charcoal more useful in these overdose cases than in cases with other poisons, but repeated oral therapy with activated charcoal occasionally causes gastric distention and aspiration in the nonintubated patient. Therefore, poor bowel motility is a contraindication to repeated activated charcoal administration. Patients who have smoked anticholinergic agents or ingested teas do not require any gastrointestinal decontamination.[44]

Physostigmine

Physostigmine is a naturally occurring acetylcholinesterase inhibitor, similar to neostigmine, pyridostigmine, and edrophonium. These agents block the metabolism of acetylcholine, which then accumulates in the synaptic space and antagonizes the effects of acetylcholine receptor blockade. Physostigmine is the only agent that can cross the blood-brain barrier and antagonize both central and peripheral muscarinic blockade.

The role of physostigmine in the management of anticholinergic overdoses has been controversial.[45] In the absence of anticholinergic blockade, physostigmine itself has significant toxicity. It can cause seizures, muscle weakness, bradycardia, lacrimation, salivation, bronchorrhea, and diarrhea, and exacerbate asthma. Even in documented cases of anticholinergic toxicity, seizures have been reported after rapid administration.[46] Asystole has occurred after the administration of physostigmine for tricyclic antidepressant overdose,[47] so a conduction delay (QRS > 0.10 sec) or suspicion of tricyclic antidepressant ingestion should be a contraindication to physostigmine administration.[48]

With anticholinergic overdose, physostigmine reverses delirium in 96% of patients.[49] Patients treated with benzodiazepines have control of agitation, but without reversal of delirium. Physostigmine has been used successfully to treat anticholinergic symptoms such as coma, severe agitation, and symptomatic supraventricular tachycardia.[22,23,32,50] To minimize toxicity, physostigmine should be infused over 5 minutes in an initial dose of 1 to 2 mg for adults and 0.02 mg/kg (max 0.5 mg) for children to control severe anticholinergic manifestations; this dose can be repeated as needed. Atropine should be available at the bedside and the infusion immediately stopped if signs of cholinergic excess develop.

Physostigmine can be used diagnostically in patients with obvious anticholinergic signs or suspected anticholinergic poisoning.[33,51] Reversal of coma or severe agitation and normalization of mental status avoid the need for further diagnostic evaluation. Physostigmine should not be used in patients with known or suspected tricyclic antidepressant ingestion or as an empiric "coma" therapy.

DISPOSITION

Most patients with anticholinergic overdoses recover rapidly with sedation, temperature control, hydration, activated charcoal, and observation. Patients with hyperthermia, agitation, coma, or seizures should be admitted to an intensive care unit. Patients who are alert, or have symptoms and vital signs that improve during observation in the emergency department, do not require hospital admission.

The onset of symptoms after antihistamine ingestion is rapid; 4 hours of observation is adequate to exclude significant toxicity in an asymptomatic patient. Patients who have ingested *Datura stramonium* seeds or cyclobenzaprine should be observed for 8 hours.[44] Predischarge measures include psychiatric assessment, documentation of a nontoxic acetaminophen level, and assessment of a child's home situation.

KEY CONCEPTS

- Anticholinergic effects from medications and plants are extremely common.
- Lack of sweating is common with an anticholinergic and rare in a sympathomimetic toxidrome.
- Hyperthermia and agitation should be aggressively treated with cooling and benzodiazepines.
- Physostigmine may be helpful in cases of severe toxicity with a known anticholinergic origin, but it has intrinsic toxicity and is not necessary in the vast majority of cases.

REFERENCES

1. Beverly R: *History and Present State of Virginia.* Richmond, Va, JW Randolph, 1855.
2. Gopel C, Laufer C, Marcus A: Three cases of angel's trumpet tea-induced psychosis in adolescent substance abusers. *Nordic J Psychiatry* 56:49, 2002.
3. Garvin J, Ruh H: Acute poisoning due to eating the seeds of the Jimson weed (*Datura stramonium*). *Arch Pediatr* 40:827, 1923.
4. Nickalls RW, Nickalls EA: The first use of physostigmine in the treatment of atropine poisoning: A translation of Kleinwachter's paper entitled 'Observations on the effect of Calabar bean extract as an antidote to atropine poisoning'. *Anaesthesia* 43:776, 1988.
5. Gowdy JM: Stramonium intoxication: Review of symptomatology in 212 cases. *JAMA* 221:585, 1972.
6. Shervette RE 3rd, Schydlower M, Lampe RM, Fearnow RG: Jimson "loco" weed abuse in adolescents. *Pediatrics* 63:520, 1979.
7. Brown J, Taylor P: Muscarinic receptor agonist and antagonists. In Goodman LS, et al (eds): *Goodman & Gilman's the Pharmacological Basis of Therapeutics.* New York, McGraw-Hill Health Professions Division, 1996.
8. Fisher RS, Cysyk B: A fatal overdose of carbamazepine: Case report and review of literature. *J Toxicol Clin Toxicol* 26:477, 1988.
9. Watson WA, et al: 2002 annual report of the American Association of Poison Control Centers Toxic Exposure Surveillance System. *Am J Emerg Med* 21:353, 2003.
10. Goldfrank L, et al: Anticholinergic poisoning. *J Toxicol Clin Toxicol* 19:17, 1982.
11. Hamilton RJ, et al: A descriptive study of an epidemic of poisoning caused by heroin adulterated with scopolamine. *J Toxicol Clin Toxicol* 38:597, 2000.
12. Wang HE: Street drug toxicity resulting from opiates combined with anticholinergics. *Prehosp Emerg Care* 6:351, 2002.
13. Drachman DA: Memory and cognitive function in man: Does the cholinergic system have a specific role? *Neurology* 27:783, 1977.

14. Torline RL: Extreme hyperpyrexia associated with central anticholinergic syndrome. *Anesthesiology* 76:470, 1992.
15. Zelman S, Guillan R: Heat stroke in phenothiazine-treated patients: A report of three fatalities. *Am J Psychiatry* 126:1787, 1970.
16. Rhoads PM, Tong TG, Banner W Jr, Anderson R: Anticholinergic poisonings associated with commercial burdock root tea. *J Toxicol Clin Toxicol* 22:581, 1984.
17. Cheng SW, Hu WH, Hung DZ, Yang DY: Anticholinergic poisoning from a large dose of Scopolia extract. *Vet Hum Toxicol* 44:222, 2002.
18. Katz IR, et al: Screening for cognitive toxicity of anticholinergic drugs. *J Clin Psychiatry* 46:323, 1985.
19. Tune LE, et al: Association of postoperative delirium with raised serum levels of anticholinergic drugs. *Lancet* 2:651, 1981.
20. Tune LE, et al: Serum levels of anticholinergic drugs and impaired recent memory in chronic schizophrenic patients. *Am J Psychiatry* 139:1460, 1982.
21. Potamianos G, Kellett JM: Anti-cholinergic drugs and memory: The effects of benzhexol on memory in a group of geriatric patients. *Br J Psychiatry* 140:470, 1982.
22. Stern TA: Continuous infusion of physostigmine in anticholinergic delirium: Case report. *J Clin Psychiatry* 44:463, 1983.
23. Jones J, Dougherty J, Cannon L: Diphenhydramine-induced toxic psychosis. *Am J Emerg Med* 4:369, 1986.
24. Moreau A, Jones BD, Banno V: Chronic central anticholinergic toxicity in manic depressive illness mimicking dementia. *Can J Psychiatry* 31:339, 1986.
25. Monane M, Avorn J, Beers MH, Everitt DE: Anticholinergic drug use and bowel function in nursing home patients. *Arch Intern Med* 153:633, 1993.
26. Hestand HE, Teske DW: Diphenhydramine hydrochloride intoxication. *J Pediatr* 90:1017, 1977.
27. Krenzelok EP, Anderson GM, Mirick M: Massive diphenhydramine overdose resulting in death. *Ann Emerg Med* 11:212, 1982.
28. Fahy P, Arnold P, Curry SC, Bond R: Serial serum drug concentrations and prolonged anticholinergic toxicity after benztropine (Cogentin) overdose. *Am J Emerg Med* 7:199, 1989.
29. Freedberg RS, Friedman GR, Palu RN, Feit F: Cardiogenic shock due to antihistamine overdose: Reversal with intra-aortic balloon counterpulsation. *JAMA* 257:660, 1987.
30. Shawn DH, McGuigan MA: Poisoning from dermal absorption of promethazine. *Can Med Assoc J* 130:1460, 1984.
31. Goldstein MR, Kasper R: Hyperpyrexia and coma due to overdose of benztropine. *South Med J* 61:984, 1968.
32. Magera BE, Betlach CJ, Sweatt AP, Derrick CW Jr: Hydroxyzine intoxication in a 13-month-old child. *Pediatrics* 67:280, 1981.
33. Sopchak CA, Stork CM, Cantor RM, Ohara PE: Central anticholinergic syndrome due to Jimson weed physostigmine: Therapy revisited? *J Toxicol Clin Toxicol* 36:43, 1998.
34. O'Grady TC, Brown J, Jacamo J: Outbreak of Jimson Weed abuse among Marine Corps personnel at Camp Pendleton. *Mil Med* 148:732, 1983.
35. Reyes-Jacang A, Wenzl JE: Antihistamine toxicity in children. *Clin Pediatr (Phila)* 8:297, 1969.
36. Delaney K, Goldfrank L: Metabolic aspects of hyperthermia. In Cohen RD (ed): The metabolic and molecular basis of acquired disease. Philadelphia, Bailliere Tindall, 1990.
37. Perrone J, Chu J, Stecker MM: Viral encephalitis masquerading as a fulminant anticholinergic toxidrome. *J Toxicol Clin Toxicol* 35:627, 1997.
38. Cooper JW: Adverse drug reaction-related hospitalizations of nursing facility patients: A 4-year study. *South Med J* 92:485, 1999.
39. Hick JL, Smith SW, Lynch MT: Metabolic acidosis in restraint-associated cardiac arrest: A case series. *Acad Emerg Med* 6:239, 1999.
40. Dubin WR, Feld JA: Rapid tranquilization of the violent patient. *Am J Emerg Med* 7:313, 1989.
41. Amsterdam JT, et al: Dantrolene sodium for treatment of heatstroke victims: Lack of efficacy in a canine model. *Am J Emerg Med* 4:399, 1986.
42. Guay DR, Meatherall RC, Macaulay PA, Yeung C: Activated charcoal adsorption of diphenhydramine. *Int J Clin Pharmacol Ther Toxicol* 22:395, 1984.
43. Neuvonen PJ, Olkkola KT: Oral activated charcoal in the treatment of intoxications: Role of single and repeated doses. *Med Toxicol Adverse Drug Exp* 3:33, 1988.
44. Salen P, Shih R, Sierzenski P, Reed J: Effect of physostigmine and gastric lavage in a Datura stramonium-induced anticholinergic poisoning epidemic. *Am J Emerg Med* 21:316, 2003.
45. Teoh R, Page AV, Hardern R: Physostigmine as treatment for severe CNS anticholinergic toxicity. *Emerg Med J* 18:412, 2001.
46. Newton RW: Physostigmine salicylate in the treatment of tricyclic antidepressant overdosage. *JAMA* 231:941, 1975.
47. Pentel P, Peterson CD: Asystole complicating physostigmine treatment of tricyclic antidepressant overdose. *Ann Emerg Med* 9:588, 1980.
48. Schmidt W, Lang K: Life-threatening dysrhythmias in severe thioridazine poisoning treated with physostigmine and transient atrial pacing. *Crit Care Med* 25:1925, 1997.
49. Burns MJ, et al: A comparison of physostigmine and benzodiazepines for the treatment of anticholinergic poisoning. *Ann Emerg Med* 35:374, 2000.
50. Rumack BH: Anticholinergic poisoning: Treatment with physostigmine. *Pediatrics* 52:449, 1973.
51. Arnold SM, Arnholz D, Garyfallou GT, Heard K: Two siblings poisoned with diphenhydramine: A case of factitious disorder by proxy. *Ann Emerg Med* 32:256, 1998.

CHAPTER

149 Antidepressants

Elisabeth F. Bilden and Frank G. Walter

PERSPECTIVE

Antidepressants include a wide variety of drugs: cyclic antidepressants (CAs), selective serotonin reuptake inhibitors (SSRIs), monoamine oxidase inhibitors (MAOIs), and miscellaneous agents (Table 149-1). Antidepressants can be classified based on structure or major mechanism of action.[1,2] Antidepressants account for only 4.2% of poisonings; however, they cause 12% of poisoning deaths and are the second most common cause of death from poisoning. The case-fatality rate is second only to stimulants and street drugs. Overdoses with SSRIs result in lower morbidity and mortality than overdoses with tricyclic antidepressants (TCAs) and MAOIs.[3-5] Toxicity with miscellaneous antidepressants occurs less frequently than with TCAs and usually involves coingestants.

CYCLIC ANTIDEPRESSANTS

Principles of Disease

TCAs and the tetracyclic antidepressant maprotiline have similar properties and are called CAs. The CAs are well absorbed from the gastrointestinal tract and reach peak plasma concentrations in 2 to 4 hours after therapeutic doses.[1] Absorption is prolonged in overdose because the anticholinergic effect delays gastrointestinal motility and absorption. These pharmacokinetic data are compatible with the recommended 6-hour observation period in management of CA overdose (Figure 149-1).[6,7] CAs are highly lipophilic, are extensively bound to plasma proteins, and have large volumes of distribution. CAs are metabolized predominantly by the liver.[1]

TCAs and their active metabolites have two basic structures, tertiary amines and secondary amines. All tertiary-amine TCAs are metabolized to secondary amines that are active. Amitriptyline forms nortriptyline, and imipramine forms desipramine. Amoxapine, a secondary amine, is metabolized to active intermediates by hepatic hydroxylation. Hydroxylation of other secondary-amine TCAs results in inactive metabolites.[1] The parent compound and the active metabolites may undergo enterohepatic circulation.

Seven major pharmacodynamic effects of CAs result in characteristic signs and symptoms of toxicity and are manifested mainly in the cardiovascular and nervous systems (Box 149-1). Phase 0 myocardial depolarization is prolonged when sodium conductance is blocked through fast sodium channels.[8] This results in decreased conduction with a prolonged QRS complex (>100 msec) and negative inotropic effects.[8,9] Impaired excitation-contraction coupling within myocardial cells and diminished release of calcium from sarcoplasmic calcium stores decrease contractility.[8] α_1-Adrenoreceptor blockade can result in vasodilation in all vascular beds, causing hypotension from decreased preload and afterload. α_1-Blockade can decrease systemic vascular resistance, widen pulse pressure, and decrease pupillary size.

Serotonin and norepinephrine reuptake inhibition within the central nervous system (CNS) predisposes to agitated delirium and seizures. Peripheral inhibition of catecholamine reuptake results in increased circulating catecholamines and initial hypertension.[10] Eventual metabolism of peripheral catecholamines by catechol *O*-methyltransferase results in late hypotension and bradycardia.

Anticholinergic and antihistaminic effects are associated with peripheral autonomic nervous system antimuscarinic effects (Box 149-2) and CNS effects of delirium, seizures, sedation, and coma (Box 149-3).[1] Potassium efflux blockade prolongs phase 3 of the myocardial action potential, repolarization, resulting in an increased duration of the Q-T interval. This increases the risk for developing torsades de pointes. CAs promote CNS excitation and seizures because of their indirect inhibition of γ-aminobutyric acid (GABA), the primary cerebral inhibitory neurotransmitter. CAs bind to the picrotoxin site of the $GABA_A$ receptor–chloride ionophore complex.

Clinical Features

CA poisoning initially presents with anticholinergic symptoms, including sinus tachycardia and early hypertension (see Chapter 148). Severe poisoning is characterized by subsequent convulsions, coma, and cardiovascular collapse. CA toxicity should be considered in all patients with a decreased level of consciousness and prolonged QRS complex. Mental status changes do not predict the occurrence of seizures, and 23% of patients are awake and alert immediately before a seizure.[11]

Hypotension caused by CA poisoning can occur with or without QRS prolongation (>100 msec).[12] Hypotension can result from myocardial depression or peripheral vasodilation. Catastrophic cardiovascular collapse closely follows seizures in 13% of patients with CA-induced seizures.[11] Cardiovascular collapse is attributed to lactic acidosis, which impairs myocardial sodium conduction.

Table 149-1. Antidepressants Approved by U.S. Food and Drug Administration

Generic Name	Trade Name	Mechanism of Action
Tricyclics		
Amitriptyline	Elavil	5-HT and NE reputake inhibition
Amoxapine	Asendin	NE reuptake inhibition DA_2 receptor inhibition
Clomipramine	Anafranil	5-HT and NE reuptake inhibition
Desipramine	Norpramin	NE reuptake inhibition
Doxepin	Sinequan	5-HT and NE reuptake inhibition
Imipramine	Tofranil	Same
Nortriptyline	Pamelor	NE reuptake inhibition
Protriptyline	Vivactil	Same
Trimipramine	Surmontil	5-HT and NE reuptake inhibition
Tetracylic		
Maprotiline	Ludiomil	NE reuptake inhibition
Selective Serotonin Reuptake Inhibitors		
Citalopram	Celexa	Selective 5-HT reuptake inhibition
Escitalopram	Lexapro	Same
Fluoxetine	Prozac	Same
Paroxetine	Paxil	Same
Sertraline	Zoloft	Same
Miscellaneous		
Bupropion	Wellbutrin	DA and NE reuptake inhibition
Mirtazapine	Remeron	α_2-Adrenoreceptor antagonism* $5\text{-}HT_2$ and $5\text{-}HT_3$ receptor antagonism
Nefazodone		5-HT reuptake inhibition $5\text{-}HT_2$ receptor antagonism
Trazodone	Desyrel	Same
Venlafaxine	Effexor	5-HT and NE reuptake inhibition
Monoamine Oxidase Inhibitors		
Phenelzine	Nardil	Monoamine oxidase inhibition
Tranylcypromine	Parnate	Same

*With disinhibition of serotonin and norepinephrine neurotransmission (i.e., increased neurotransmission).
5-HT, serotonin; NE, norepinephrine; DA, dopamine.

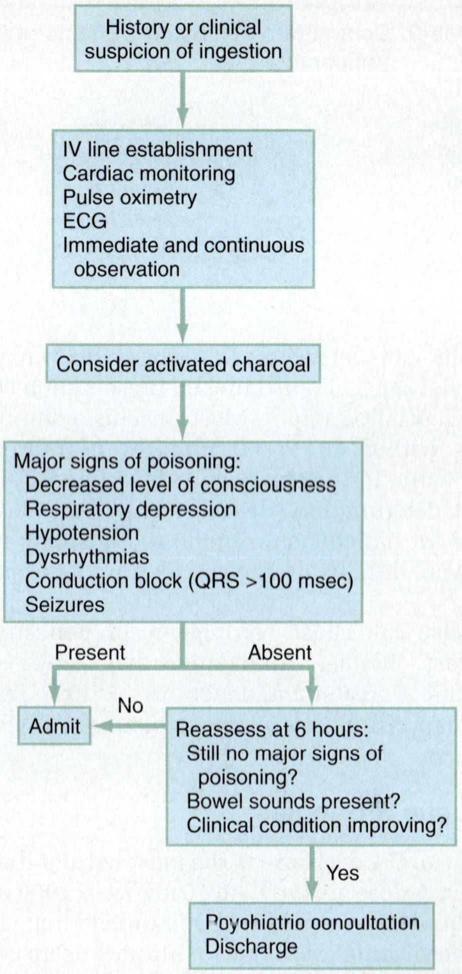

Figure 149-1. Algorithm for managemnt of cyclic antidepressant overdose. (Modified from Cyclic antidepressant (CA) overdose. In Callaham M [ed]: *Current Therapy in Emergency Medicine*. Philadelphia, BC Decker, 1991.)

BOX 149-1. Major Pharmacodynamic Effects of Cyclic Antidepressants (CAs)

1. Sodium channel blockade (quinidine-like membrane-stabilizing effects)
2. α_1-Adrenoreceptor blockade
3. Inhibition of reuptake of biogenic amines (e.g., norepinephrine, serotonin)
4. Muscarinic receptor blockade (anticholinergic effects)
5. Histamine receptor blockade (antihistaminic effects)
6. Potassium efflux blockade
7. Indirect $GABA_A$ antagonism caused by binding at picrotoxin receptor

BOX 149-2. Peripheral Nervous System Effects of Cyclic Antidepressants

Anticholinergic
Tachycardia caused by vagolysis
Hyperthermia
Mydriasis
Anhydrosis
Red skin
Decreased bowel sounds
Ileus
Urinary retention
Distended bladder

α_1-Blockade
Reflex tachycardia
Miosis or midrange pupils (inhibition of dilatory radial muscle of iris)

BOX 149-3. Central Nervous System Effects of Cyclic Antidepressants

Excitation
Agitation
Delirium
Myoclonic jerks
Hyperreflexia
Clonus
Seizures
Hyperthermia

Inhibition
Sedation
Coma

Patients can deteriorate rapidly, and even patients with trivial signs of poisoning on presentation can have a 50% mortality rate.[13] Most serious complications develop within 30 to 60 minutes of presentation, usually while in the emergency department.[12] Because of rapid deterioration, death rates of 44% have been reported for patients en route to the hospital, many of whom were initially awake and alert with normal sinus rhythm.[13]

CAs also can cause cardiogenic or noncardiogenic pulmonary edema. Amoxapine has fewer cardiac effects but a greater incidence of seizures. The tetracyclic maprotiline has more cardiac and CNS effects than TCAs.

Diagnostic Strategies

A history of CA overdose is the most helpful diagnostic indicator. A dose greater than 10 mg/kg or 1000 mg in an adult should be considered life-threatening. Patients who have an anticholinergic toxidrome, decreased level of consciousness, QRS prolongation (>100 msec), or rightward deviation of the terminal 40-msec QRS axis (R wave in aVR >3 mm or R/S_{aVR} ratio of ≥0.7) should be considered to have CA poisoning until proved otherwise (Figure 149-2).[14,15] With QRS prolongation greater than 100 msec in the limb leads, 30% of patients experience seizures; for prolongation greater than 160 msec, 50% develop dysrhythmias. CAs can induce an electrocardiogram (ECG) pattern consistent with the Brugada syndrome, a genetic disorder resulting in sodium channel dysfunction. A right bundle branch block and ST segment elevation in the right precordial leads (V_1 through V_3) are seen.[16] CA toxicity is not fully excluded with normal ECG findings.

Quantitative serum toxicology tests for CAs are not usually available in a timely fashion and do not predict adequately the degree of toxicity. Qualitative laboratory tests may document only exposure. Neither serum toxicology tests nor laboratory tests are useful for clinical decision making. Diagnosis, treatment, and disposition are determined on a clinical basis and with ECG and cardiac monitoring.[6,7] Determining which patients require admission has been simplified with a management algorithm for CA overdose (see Figure 149-1).

Differential Considerations

The differential diagnosis of CA poisoning is extensive and includes intoxications by anticholinergic, psychiatric, and cardiac medications, especially type I antidysrhythmics. Many conditions cause sinus tachycardia and hypotension with a wide pulse pressure; however, QRS widening, seizures, or coma suggests CA poisoning.

Table 149-2. Treatment of Neurologic Complications of Antidepressant Poisoning

Complication	Treatment
Coma	Endotracheal intubation
	Mechanical ventilation
	Supportive care
Seizures	Lorazepam or diazepam
	Phenobarbital, continuous intravenous midazolam infusion, or propofol
Hyperthermia	Cessation of seizures with benzodiazepines and phenobartital
	Neuromuscular blockade with vecuronium during phenobarbital loading
	General anesthesia with continuous EEG monitoring
	Evaporative cooling
	Ice water bath

EEG, electroencephalogram.

Management

Treatment begins with assessment of airway and breathing. Endotracheal intubation should be performed if the patient is exhibiting a markedly decreased level of consciousness or if the level of consciousness is rapidly deteriorating. Respiratory depression, with attendant hypoxia and hypercarbia, significantly increases morbidity and mortality of CA poisoning. Patients with overdoses severe enough to require admission to the intensive care unit (ICU) have a high incidence of airway and breathing complications, with aspiration pneumonitis reported in 13% to 18% of patients.[17] The initial benign appearance of the patient's presentation may be deceptive; rapid deterioration with cardiac dysrhythmias, generalized seizures, and death can occur despite appropriate management.

Ventilatory support to avoid respiratory acidosis is crucial because acidosis inhibits conductance through fast sodium channels. Any patient with a significant CA overdose should have continuous pulse oximetry. Arterial blood gas determination or capnography may be helpful when ventilatory function is questionable despite normal oxygen saturations on pulse oximetry. Patients assessed clinically to be ventilating adequately have been shown to have low minute volumes, hypoxia, and acidosis.

Gastric lavage and administration of activated charcoal within 60 minutes from time of significant ingestion is theoretically appealing, but there is no evidence that gastrointestinal decontamination improves clinical outcome. Physostigmine is contraindicated in CA overdose. Seizures, cardiac arrest, and death have occurred when physostigmine has been used in CA overdose.[18] No clinically effective method exists to change the metabolism or distribution of CAs.

Hypertension is usually mild and transient and requires no treatment (see Table 149-3). Treatment of

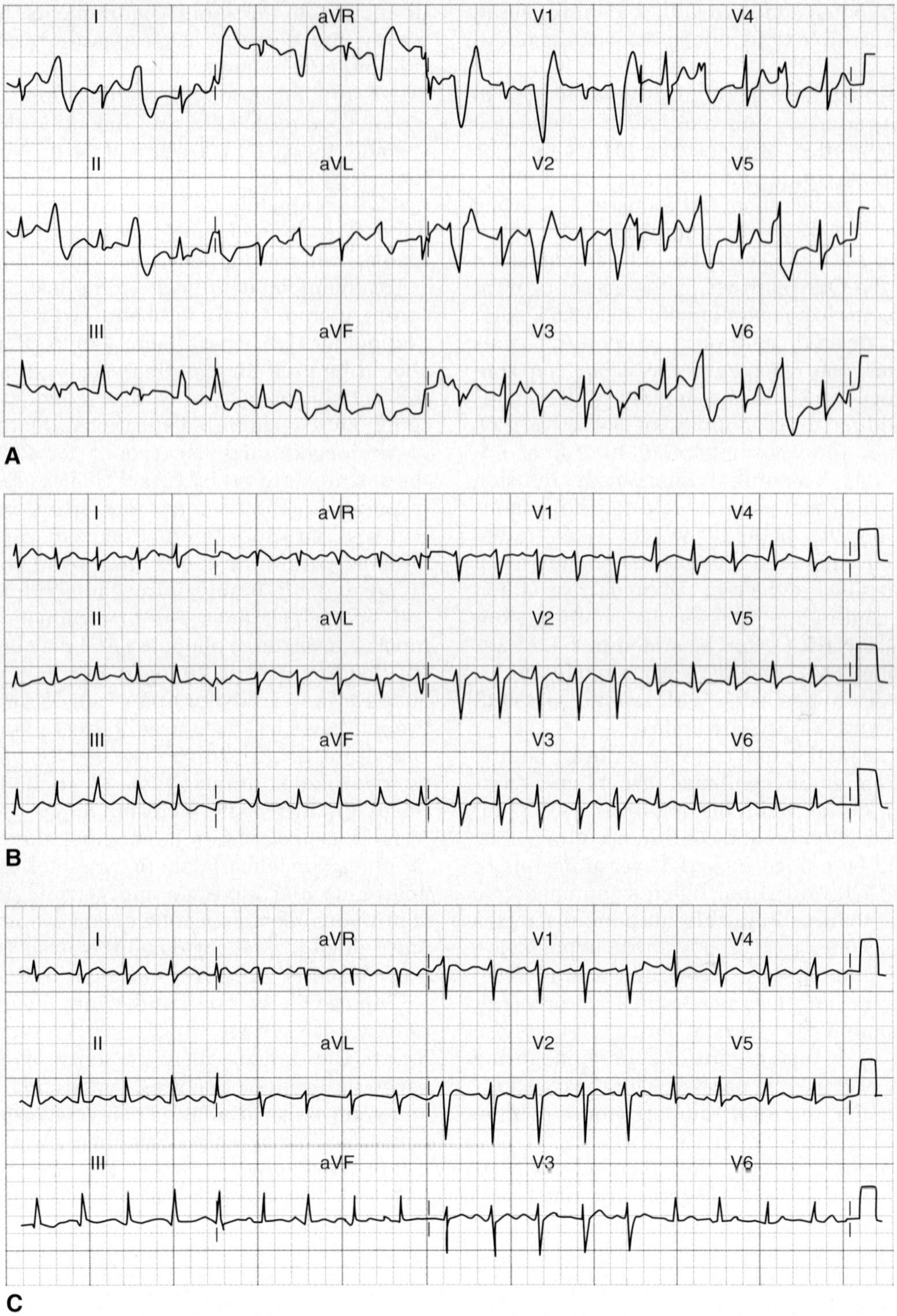

Figure 149-2. Electrocardiogram (ECG) changes in cyclic antidepressant poisoning. **A,** ECG of a 24-year-old woman who ingested 2.5 g of desipramine shows ventricular bigeminy, right axis deviation, wide QRS complex, long Q-T_c interval, and right deviation of terminal 40-msec QRS vector in limb leads, with prominent R wave in aVR. **B,** ECG of same patient after receiving bolus and continuous intravenous infusion of sodium bicarbonate shows sinus tachycardia, 90-degree axis, slight prolongation of QRS and Q-T_c intervals, and persistent right axis deviation of terminal 40 msec in limb leads. **C,** ECG of same patient 25 hours after ingestion and 4 hours after termination of sodium bicarbonate infusion shows persistent but improved sinus tachycardia, normalization of QRS axis and width, normalization of Q-T_c interval, and resolution of prominent R wave in aVR.

hypotension begins with isotonic crystalloids. If the QRS is greater than 100 msec, and the patient is symptomatic, with hypotension or a dysrhythmia, or if the patient is acidemic, intravenous sodium bicarbonate ($NaHCO_3$) also should be administered.[19] $NaHCO_3$ produces an alkaline pH and provides a sodium load and hypertonicity that increase sodium conductance through myocardial fast sodium channels.[8] Hyperventilation and hypertonic sodium chloride also enhance sodium conduction.[20] Hypertonic sodium chloride has been used for hypotension with QRS widening caused by CA-induced cardiotoxicity unresponsive to standard therapies.[21]

Serum alkalinization is clinically effective in decreasing CA-induced intraventricular conduction delays. The major effect of increasing pH seems to be increased sodium conductance through myocardial sodium channels rather than the increase in plasma protein binding.[8] $NaHCO_3$ is administered by intravenous boluses of 1 to 2 mEq/kg until hypotension improves and the QRS narrows to 100 msec, or until serum pH increases to a maximum of 7.50 to 7.55. After obtaining the desired endpoint with intravenous $NaHCO_3$ boluses, the emergency physician can consider initiating continuous isotonic intravenous infusion by adding three ampules of 8.4% $NaHCO_3$ (50 mEq/ampule, 100 mOsm/ampule) to 1 L of 5% dextrose in water. The initial intravenous infusion is started at a usual maintenance rate for intravenous fluids, based on the patient's weight. This initial $NaHCO_3$ infusion rate often must be maintained for at least 4 to 6 hours before the rate can be decreased. For a hypertonic continuous intravenous solution, four ampules of 8.4% $NaHCO_3$ can be added to 1 L of 5% dextrose in water. This infusion is occasionally necessary for refractory hypotension with a prolonged QRS or refractory ventricular dysrhythmias.

Excess $NaHCO_3$ and saline can worsen heart failure. Excessive alkalemia from combined use of hyperventilation and $NaHCO_3$ can result in complications, including death.[22] Repeat boluses and continuous intravenous infusion should be guided by serial measurements of arterial pH and QRS duration. When symptoms were refractory, hypertonic sodium chloride administered as an intravenous bolus was used to treat hypotension and wide QRS interval with ventricular ectopy in an adult.[21] If hypotension does not resolve, norepinephrine or dopamine is recommended.[8] High-dose dopamine (20 to 30 μg/kg/min) and norepinephrine (0.1 to 1 μg/kg/min) may be necessary for the direct α_1-agonist effect.[23] For inotropic support alone, dobutamine is controversial.[8]

Sinus tachycardia is usually well tolerated and does not require specific therapy. β-Receptor antagonists and physostigmine are contraindicated.[19] Wide-complex tachycardia is not always ventricular tachycardia and can represent sinus tachycardia with aberrant conduction. Determining the specific type of wide-complex rhythm is unnecessary because treatment in either case is intravenous $NaHCO_3$.[8] Lidocaine has not been consistently effective.[24] Phenytoin has been shown to increase the frequency and duration of episodes of ventricular tachycardia and is not recommended as an antidysrhythmic agent.[25] Type IA antidysrhythmics (quinidine, disopyramide, procainamide) and type IC antidysrhythmics (flecainide, moricizine, propafenone) are contraindicated because they also inhibit fast sodium channels. A transvenous pacemaker and overdrive pacing can be used for CA-associated polymorphic ventricular tachycardia (torsades de pointes) not responsive to magnesium. Bradydysrhythmias are rare and late in CA overdose. CA poisoning can result in increased threshold requirements for ventricular pacing and decrease electric cardioversion and defibrillation effectiveness.

Q-T prolongation, PR prolongation, and rightward terminal 40-msec QRS axis deviation do not mandate specific therapy.[8,19] Treatment with $NaHCO_3$, hypertonic sodium chloride, and hyperventilation does not resolve completely Q-T prolongation, which involves not only sodium channel blockade, but also protracted repolarization from potassium efflux blockade.

Treatment of neurologic complications of CA poisoning includes early intubation with mechanical ventilation for coma (see Table 149-2). Benzodiazepines should be used for agitation because they do not have the anticholinergic or cardiac conduction effects of some antipsychotic medications. Status epilepticus or prolonged seizures account for 20% to 30% of the seizures caused by CAs.[11,26] These seizures usually respond to intravenous lorazepam or diazepam.[11] Seizures refractory to other benzodiazepines have terminated with intravenous midazolam boluses of 2.5 to 10 mg and continuous intravenous infusions.[27]

If benzodiazepines fail to terminate prolonged or repetitive seizures, phenobarbital may be administered in a loading dose of 20 mg/kg, given at a rate of up to 50 mg/min in adults or up to 1 mg/kg/min in children. Propofol also has been used to treat refractory seizures successfully.[28] A loading dose of 2.5 mg/kg is followed by continuous infusion of 25 to 200 μg/kg/min.[28] Phenytoin may cause more and longer episodes of ventricular tachycardia.[25] If maximal doses of benzodiazepines, phenobarbital, or propofol are ineffective, neuromuscular blockade and general anesthesia with continuous electroencephalogram monitoring are recommended to prevent rhabdomyolysis and hyperthermia caused by excessive muscle activity.

Flumazenil is contraindicated, even if benzodiazepines are known coingestants.[29,30] Flumazenil counteracts the anticonvulsant activity of the coingested benzodiazepines. Seizures, ventricular tachycardia, and ventricular fibrillation can occur when flumazenil is used in mixed benzodiazepine/CA overdoses.[30]

Life-threatening hyperthermia (rectal temperature >40° C) is best treated with control of seizures and neuromuscular blockade. A nondepolarizing neuromuscular blocker (e.g., rocuronium) is recommended if rhabdomyolysis and hyperkalemia with ECG changes are present. Evaporative cooling should be used until core temperature reaches 38.5° C. Forced diuresis, hemodialysis, and hemoperfusion are not indicated because CAs have large volumes of distribution, are highly bound to plasma proteins, and are minimally eliminated by the kidneys.

Disposition

Patients with known or suspected CA overdoses require 6 hours of observation with continuous cardiac monitoring and pulse oximetry. After 6 hours of observation, patients may be discharged for psychiatric evaluation if they do not develop (1) ventilatory insufficiency, (2) desaturation on pulse oximetry, (3)

Table 149-3. Cardiovascular Complications of Cyclic Antidepressant Toxicity and Treatments

	Mechanism: Cause		
Complication	***Cardiac***	***Peripheral Vascular***	**Treatment**
Hypertension (early and transient)	Positive chronotropism: anticholinergic vagolytic effects Positive inotropism: increased circulating catecholamines caused by reuptake inhibition	Initial vasoconstriction: increased circulating catecholamines caused by reuptake inhibition	Not indicated
Hypotension	Negative inotropism: fast sodium channel inhibition with impairment of excitation-contraction coupling	Vasodilation: α_1-adrenoreceptor blockade	IV isotonic crystalloid IV $NaHCO_3$ if QRS >100 msec Norepinephrine or dopamine
Sinus tachycardia	Positive chronotropism: anticholinergic vagolytic effects Positive chronotropism: increased circulating catecholamines caused by reuptake inhibition	Reflex tachycardia: α_1 adrenoreceptor blockade	Not indicated
Ventricular tachycardia (monomorphic)	Negative dromotropism: fast sodium channel inhibition with QRS prolongation		IV $NaHCO_3$ Synchronized cardioversion Overdrive pacing
Ventricular tachycardia (polymorphic) (torsades de pointes)	Negative dromotropism: fast sodium channel inhibition with QRS prolongation and resultant Q-T prolongation, and potassium efflux inhibition		Magnesium sulfate for torsades de pointes
Bradydysrhythmias (late and uncommon)	Negative dromotropism: fast sodium channel inhibition Negative chronotropism: impaired automaticity from threshold voltage elevation and slowing of phase 4 depolarization		ACLS algorithm for bradycardia
QRS prolongation, Q-T prolongation	Negative dromotropism: fast sodium channel inhibition (potassium efflux inhibition), PR prolongation, rightward terminal 40-msec QRS axis deviation		IV $NaHCO_3$ for symptomatic QRS prolongation

IV $NaHCO_3$, intravenous sodium bicarbonate; ACLS, advanced cardiac life support.

QRS greater than 100 msec, (4) sinus tachycardia greater than 120 beats/min, (5) dysrhythmias, (6) hypotension, (7) decreased level of consciousness, (8) seizures, or (9) abnormal or inactive bowel sounds. Patients who exhibit any of these findings should be admitted to an ICU (see Figure 149-1).[6,7]

SELECTIVE SEROTONIN REUPTAKE INHIBITORS

SSRIs approved in the United States for treatment of depression are fluoxetine (Prozac), paroxetine (Paxil), sertraline (Zoloft), citalopram (Celexa), and escitalopram (Lexapro). Fluvoxamine (Luvox) is approved in the United States for treating obsessive-compulsive disorder.

Principles of Disease

SSRIs are well absorbed from the gastrointestinal tract and reach peak plasma concentrations 3 to 8 hours after therapeutic doses. Controlled-release paroxetine reaches peak serum concentration 6 to 10 hours after ingestion. Because SSRIs have no significant anticholinergic effects, they are less likely than CAs to have delayed absorption. SSRIs are highly lipophilic, are extensively bound to plasma proteins, and have large volumes of distribution (12 to 97 L/kg).[31]

SSRIs are metabolized predominantly by the liver. The elimination half-life is about 15 hours for fluvoxamine, about 1 day for paroxetine and sertraline, 27 hours for escitalopram, 35 hours for citalopram, and 1 to 4 days for fluoxetine. Fluoxetine, sertraline, citalopram, and escitalopram have active metabolites that increase the duration of their effect. Fluoxetine is demethylated to its clinically active metabolite, norfluoxetine, with a half-life of 4 to 9 days.[31] The long half-lives of the SSRIs and their active metabolites explain the long interval necessary between stopping SSRI treatment and beginning MAOI treatment to avoid the life-threatening serotonin syndrome. MAOI therapy should not be initiated until at least 5 weeks after stopping fluoxetine and for at least 2 weeks after stopping the other SSRIs. Likewise, none of the SSRIs should be used for at least 2 weeks after stopping MAOI treatment. Minimal amounts of SSRIs are eliminated in the urine as unchanged drugs; forced diuresis is of no benefit.

Enterochromaffin cells of the gastrointestinal tract contain 90% of the total serotonin in adults. Most remaining serotonin is in platelets and the CNS. In the CNS, serotonin is involved with mood, depression, anxiety, obsession, compulsion, perception of pain, migraine headaches, sleep, circadian rhythms, temperature regulation, and regulation of blood pressure.[32] Serotonin's roles in the periphery involve regulating gastrointestinal motility and facilitating hemostasis by

Table 149-4. Clinical Manifestations of Acute Fluoxetine Overdoses in Adults

Neuromuscular System Manifestations	%	Cardiovascular System Manifestations	%	Gastrointestinal System Manifestations	%
Drowsiness	21	Sinus tachycardia	22	Nausea	6
Tremor	8	Hypertension	6	Emesis	6
Euphoria	2	Trigeminy	2	Abdominal pain	2
Headache	2	Junctional rhythm	2		

From Borys DJ, et al: Acute fluoxetine overdose: A report of 264 cases. *Am J Emerg Med* 10:115, 1992.

promoting vasoconstriction and platelet aggregation. The antidepressant effects of SSRIs are thought to be due to the blockade of presynaptic reuptake of serotonin at the 5-hydroxytryptamine type 1 (5-HT_1) autoreceptors, resulting in increased intrasynaptic serotonin.

Clinical Features

Overdose

The signs, symptoms, morbidity, and mortality of SSRI poisoning are much less than for CA poisoning. The organ systems most affected by excessive serotonin are the gastrointestinal tract, cardiovascular system, and CNS (Table 149-4). Overdose can cause sedation, agitation, tremor, hyperreflexia, tachycardia, bradycardia, nausea, vomiting, abdominal pain, facial flushing, and dizziness. More severe overdoses can cause seizures and cardiac toxicity. The frequency of severe symptoms increases with coingestants.[33]

Fluoxetine

About 45% of adults and 90% of children who overdose on fluoxetine alone develop no symptoms.[3,34,35] Common symptoms of fluoxetine overdose include agitation, anxiety, restlessness, confusion, and hypomania.[36] Other milder symptoms are tachycardia, drowsiness, tremor, nausea, and vomiting. In children, 5% develop diarrhea, and 5% develop sleepiness.[3] Q-T_c prolongation, torsades de pointes, QRS widening, ventricular bigeminy, ventricular tachycardia, and seizures, with delayed onset 10 hours after ingestion, have been observed with fluoxetine overdose.[36-38]

Fluvoxamine

Tachycardia, bradycardia, hypotension, ECG abnormalities, seizures, liver function abnormalities, coma, and death have been reported with fluvoxamine.[36] Status epilepticus and refractory hypotension also have been described with fluvoxamine toxicity.[39]

Citalopram

Gastrointestinal upset; mild CNS changes, such as dizziness and somnolence; and mild autonomic symptoms, such as tachycardia, are observed with ingestions of citalopram less than 600 mg.[40] Q-T_c prolongation has been observed after an ingestion of 400 mg.[40] At higher doses, Q-T_c prolongation, QRS widening, ventricular fibrillation, seizures, and death have been reported.[40-42] Seizures have been reported to start 14 hours after a citalopram and fluoxetine overdose.[43]

BOX 149-4. Clinical Manifestations of Serotonin Toxicity

Neuromuscular
Agitation
Akathisia
Anxiety
Ataxia
Bilateral Babinski signs
Clonus
Coma
Confusion
Delirium
Diaphoresis
Dysarthria
Euphoria
Headache
Hyperreflexia
Hyperthermia
Hypomania
Insomnia
Mania
Mydriasis
Myoclonus
Nystagmus
Piloerection
Rhabdomyolysis
Rigidity
Seizures
Shivering
Tremor

Cardiovascular
Cutaneous flushing
Hypertension
Hypotension
Sinus tachycardia
Ventricular tachycardia (rare)

Gastrointestinal
Abdominal cramps
Diarrhea
Salivation

Escitalopram

Limited information is available about this new drug. In one review, ingestion of 600 mg was associated with only minor effects, including drowsiness, agitation, and tachycardia. No seizures were reported.[44]

Sertraline and Paroxetine

Mild symptoms after sertraline or paroxetine overdose are similar to symptoms with other SSRIs. Seizures and death have been reported with large doses of sertraline.[45,46] In general, deaths attributed to SSRI overdose usually are associated with polydrug poisonings involving significant coingestants.[41,42,45,46]

Serotonin Syndrome

Serotonin syndrome is a constellation of signs and symptoms manifesting autonomic, neuromuscular, and mental status changes (Box 149-4).[1,47] Various drugs increase serotonin concentrations and serotoninergic neurotransmission (Box 149-5). Serotonin syndrome can occur when (1) a serotoninergic agent is added to an established medication regimen, (2) the dose of a serotoninergic agent is increased, or (3) high but usually therapeutic doses of a serotoninergic agent are taken.[47] Sternbach[48] suggested diagnostic criteria for

BOX 149-5. Drugs Associated with Serotonin Toxicity

Increase Serotonin Synthesis
L-Tryptophan*

Increase Serotonin Release
Amphetamines
Cocaine
Codeine
Dextromethorphan
Fenfluramine
Levodopa
Pentazocine
Reserpine

Decrease Serotonin Degradation (Monoamine Oxidase Inhibitors)
Amphetamine metabolites*
Clorgyline*
Iproniazid*
Isocarboxazid*
Moclobemide*
Pargyline*
Phenelzine
Selegiline
Tranylcypromine

Decrease Serotonin Reuptake
Amphetamines
Carbamazepine
Citalopram
Cyclic antidepressants
Cocaine
Dextromethorphan
Fluoxetine
Fluvoxamine
Meperidine
Methadone
Paroxetine
Sertraline
Trazodone
Venlafaxine

Direct or Indirect Serotonin Receptor Agonists
Buspirone
Electroconvulsive therapy
Lithium
LSD and other indoles*
Mescaline and other phenylalkylamines*
Sumatriptan

*Not marketed in the United States.

BOX 149-6. Sternbach's Diagnostic Criteria for Serotonin Syndrome

1. Adding a serotoninergic agent to a patient's established medication regimen or increasing the dose of a patient's serotoninergic agent.
2. At least three of the following signs and symptoms:
   a. Agitation
   b. Ataxia
   c. Diaphoresis
   d. Diarrhea
   e. Hyperreflexia
   f. Hyperthermia
   g. Mental status changes (e.g., confusion, hypomania)
   h. Myoclonus
   i. Shivering
   j. Tremor
3. A neuroleptic has not been started or increased in dosage before the onset of the above signs and symptoms.
4. Other etiologies have been ruled out, such as infections, intoxications, metabolic derangements, and withdrawal.

From Sternbach H: The serotonin syndrome. *Am J Psychiatry* 148:705, 1991.

BOX 149-7. Hunter Serotonin Toxicity Criteria: Decision Rules

In the presence of a serotonergic agent:
1. IF (spontaneous clonus = yes) THEN serotonin toxicity = YES
2. ELSE IF (inducible clonus = yes), AND [(agitation) OR (diaphoresis = yes)] THEN serotonin toxicity = YES
3. ELSE IF (ocular clonus = yes) AND [(agitation = yes) OR (diaphoresis = yes)] THEN serotonin toxicity = YES
4. ELSE IF (tremor = yes) AND (hyperreflexia = yes) THEN serotonin toxicity = YES
5. ELSE IF (hypertonic = yes) AND (temperature $>$ 38° C) AND [(ocular clonus = yes) OR (inducible clonus = yes)] then serotonin toxicity = YES
6. ELSE serotonin toxicity = NO

From Dunkley EJC, et al: The Hunter serotonin toxicity criteria: Simple and accurate diagnostic decision rules serotonin toxicity. *QJM* 96:635, 2003.

the serotonin syndrome (Box 149-6); these also could include signs and symptoms of severe disease, such as muscle rigidity, clonus, hypertension, and tachycardia.[47] The Hunter criteria are diagnostic decision rules for diagnosis of serotonin toxicity (Box 149-7).[49]

Diagnostic Strategies

A history of SSRI dosage increase, SSRI overdose, or SSRI use with an incompatible drug is the most helpful diagnostic indicator. Urine and blood toxicology tests for SSRIs are neither readily available nor clinically useful.

Differential Considerations

The differential diagnosis of SSRI poisoning includes intoxications and pathologic conditions that cause sinus tachycardia, hypertension or hypotension, gastrointestinal upset, and seizures. In addition to these signs and symptoms secondary to SSRI overdose, SSRIs can produce serotonin syndrome (see Boxes 149-6 and 149-7). CNS and other infections, intoxications (e.g., methamphetamine, cocaine, other sympathomimetics), metabolic derangements (e.g., thyroid storm), sedative-hypnotic withdrawal, and strychnine poisoning should be considered in the differential diagnosis of serotonin syndrome. Clinically, serotonin syndrome can be difficult to distinguish from neuroleptic malignant syndrome. A history of precipitating medication use (SSRI versus neuroleptic), more rapid onset of symptoms, and presence of clonus helps differentiate serotonin syndrome from neuroleptic malignant syndrome (Table 149-5).

Management

Activated charcoal may be considered, but is of no proven benefit and should not be used if there is risk of aspiration. Hemodialysis and hemoperfusion are not indicated because SSRIs have large volumes of distribution and are highly bound to plasma proteins.[31]

Table 149-5. Comparison of Serotonin Toxicity and Neuroleptic Malignant Syndrome

Factor	Serotonin Toxicity	Neuroleptic Malignant Syndrome
Dopamine antagonists	No	Yes
Serotonin agonists	Yes	No
Onset of symptoms	Within minutes to hours	Usually over days to weeks, may occur immediately
Hyperthermia, altered level of consciousness, autonomic dysfunction, muscle rigidity	Present in varying degrees	Almost universal for each sign
Leukocytosis, metabolic acidosis	Unusual	Very common
Elevated creatine kinase	Present in varying degrees	Very common
Hyperreflexia, myoclonus	Present in varying degrees	Unusual
Treatment	Benzodiazepines, cyproheptadine	Bromocriptine
Resolution of symptoms	Resolution of symptoms begins but not complete in < 24 hours; usually 24-48 hours to complete	Usually over days to weeks

Table 149-6. Treatment of Cardiovascular Coplications of Selective Serotonin Reuptake Inhibitor Overdose and Serotonin Toxicity

Complication	Treatment
Hypertension	Not usually indicated Sodium nitroprusside if clinical signs of hypertensive emergency
Hypotension	Intravenous isotonic crystalloid, then norepinephrine or dopamine
Sinus tachycardia	Not usually indicated
Ventricular tachycardia	ACLS algorithm for ventricular tachycardia (lidocaine, synchronized cardioversion) IV $NaHCO_3$ if symptomatic with wide QRS complex
Bradydysrhythmias (rare)	ACLS algorithm for bradycardia

ACLS, advanced cardiac life support; IV $NaHCO_3$, intravenous sodium bicarbonate.

Forced diuresis is not indicated because minimal amounts of SSRIs and their active metabolites are eliminated in the urine.

Cardiovascular complications of serotonin toxicity include hypertension, sinus tachycardia, hypotension, and, rarely, ventricular dysrhythmias (see Box 149-4).[47] Hypertension and tachycardia are usually mild and transient and require no treatment.[3] Hypotension is treated with intravascular volume repletion with isotonic crystalloids. Vasopressors are rarely necessary. Ventricular dysrhythmias should be treated with standard antidysrhythmic agents (e.g., lidocaine) (Table 149-6).[3] QRS prolongation in the setting of fluoxetine toxicity narrowed with intravenous $NaHCO_3$ treatment.[37]

Neurologic complications of SSRI overdose and serotonin syndrome are treated similarly to neurologic complications of CAs (see Table 149-2). The mainstay of therapy is benzodiazepines. Cyproheptadine, methysergide, chlorpromazine, and propranolol have been proposed as therapies, but have inconsistent instead of multiple effects. They have been used in isolated case reports of serotonin syndrome; however, none of these should be considered a proven therapy or diagnostic modality.[47,50] Consultation with a medical toxicologist or regional poison center may be advisable before initiating therapy with these agents. Cyproheptadine is available as a convenient liquid that can be given through a nasogastric tube, beginning with an adult dose of 4 to 8 mg followed by 4-mg doses every 1 to 4 hours as needed to a maximum of 32 mg/day. For children, 0.25 mg/kg/day is given in divided doses every 6 hours to a maximum of 12 to 16 mg/day depending on the child's age and weight. For children 2 to 6 years old, 2-mg doses can be given to a maximum of 12 mg/day based on the child's weight. For children 7 to 14 years old, 4-mg doses can be given to a maximum of 16 mg/day. Complications are rare, but cyproheptadine should be avoided in anticholinergic overdoses. Methysergide is not available as a liquid preparation.

Disposition

Patients with known or suspected SSRI overdose should have a 6-hour observation period with cardiac monitoring. Asymptomatic patients who have not overdosed on citalopram may receive psychiatric evaluation and disposition. ECG abnormalities and seizures have been reported later in the course of citalopram overdoses. These overdoses warrant a longer observation period of up to 12 hours.[43]

Patients with known or suspected serotonin syndrome should be admitted to a monitored inpatient unit for 24 hours of observation. The clinical course and treatment of serotonin syndrome is less defined than that of SSRI overdose. Serotonin syndrome can be fatal and may require ICU admission for potential complications (e.g., ventricular tachycardia, hypotension, coma, hyperthermia, rhabdomyolysis).

MISCELLANEOUS ANTIDEPRESSANTS

Bupropion (Wellbutrin, Zyban), trazodone (Desyrel), venlafaxine (Effexor), and mirtazapine (Remeron) are the four antidepressants approved by the U.S. Food and Drug Administration that constitute the miscellaneous category. Serzone was withdrawn because of liver toxicity. The structures and mechanisms of action of the miscellaneous antidepressants are unique and unrelated to the CAs, SSRIs, and MAOIs.

Table 149-7. Clinical Manifestations of Bupropion Overdose

Neuromuscular System Manifestations	%	Cardiovascular System Manifestations	%	Gastrointestinal System Manifestations	%
Lethargy	41	Sinus tachycardia	43	Emesis	14
Tremors	24	Other dysrhythmias	0		
Seizures	21	Hypertension	0		
Confusion	14	Hypotension	0		
Lightheadedness	10	Conduction delays (e.g., wide QRS)	0		
Hallucinations	9				
Coma	0				

Modified from Spiller HA, et al: Bupropion overdose: A three year multi-center retrospective analysis. *Am J Emerg Med* 12:43, 1994.

Bupropion

Bupropion is available in immediate-release, sustained-release, and newer extended-release formulations. A sustained-release formulation of bupropion is approved for use in smoking cessation. Bupropion is well absorbed from the gastrointestinal tract, reaches peak concentrations in 2 hours for immediate-release formulations, and has a maximal serum concentration of metabolites at 3 to 4 hours. The sustained-release peak concentration occurs at 3 hours for the parent compound and at 5 to 6 hours for the metabolites. The extended-release parent compound peak concentration occurs at 5 hours and at 7 to 8 hours for the metabolites. Bupropion is highly lipophilic, is extensively bound to plasma proteins, has a large volume of distribution (20 to 30 L/kg), and is metabolized predominantly by the liver. It has a half-life of 10 to 21 hours. Bupropion has three metabolites; two are active and clinically significant, with half-lives longer than 20 hours. Bupropion inhibits dopamine reuptake and enhances dopaminergic neurotransmission. To a lesser extent, bupropion also enhances noradrenergic neurotransmission by inhibition of norepinephrine reuptake.[2]

Clinical Features

Bupropion's most significant toxic effect is seizure activity, which occurs not only with overdose, but also when the maximal daily dose is exceeded.[51] At the recommended daily dose of 450 mg of immediate-release bupropion, the seizure incidence is 0.4%.[52] Incidence increases to 4% with dosages of 450 to 600 mg/day.[1] The incidence of seizure with the sustained-release formulation is 0.1%. Seizures cannot be predicted from ECG or cardiac monitoring, and there is no correlation between seizures and the presence of other symptoms.[53]

Patients who overdose on bupropion alone do not usually develop hypotension or coma, but concomitant overdose with benzodiazepines can lead to coma or respiratory failure. The rare deaths associated with bupropion overdose usually involve coingestants.[54] Deaths due to bupropion alone have been reported, however.[55] Tachycardia, vomiting, agitation, lethargy, tremor, confusion, and drowsiness are the most common symptoms in adults and teenagers; vomiting is the most common symptom in children (Table 149-7).[55] Seizures are usually single and self-limited, but about 5% of patients develop status epilepticus.[55] Delayed onset of seizures has been recorded, including one case with seizure onset 32 hours after ingestion of a sustained-release product.[56] Another case of a delayed seizure occurred at 19 hours after an overdose of Zyban, a sustained-release bupropion formulation.[57] These seizures were thought to be caused by the slow-release nature of the parent product and accumulation of its active metabolites.[57] Cardiovascular complications, including hypotension, bradycardia, intraventricular conduction delays, asystole, and death, have been reported.[56] A pharmacobezoar was noted in one fatal sustained-release bupropion overdose.[56]

Management

Bupropion-induced seizures should be treated with an intravenous benzodiazepine (e.g., lorazepam, diazepam). Patients who have recurrent seizures or status epilepticus should be loaded with phenobarbital. Phenytoin is not indicated. ECG conduction delays (e.g., QRS/Q-T_c prolongation) have resolved without specific treatment.[53] Activated charcoal has no proven clinical efficacy and is not indicated in an isolated bupropion ingestion, considering the often benign course and the risk of aspiration during a seizure. Forced diuresis, hemodialysis, and hemoperfusion have no role for enhanced elimination. Patients with an immediate-release bupropion overdose require 8 hours of observation because seizures have occurred 8 hours after this overdose in the absence of other signs and symptoms.[51] With a sustained-release preparation, observation should be at least 12 hours. Because of limited data about overdose with the extended-release formula, a 24-hour observation period seems reasonable. All of these observation periods should be extended if patients are otherwise symptomatic or experience a seizure during the observation period because of the risk of subsequent seizures.

Trazodone

Trazodone is well absorbed from the gastrointestinal tract, reaches peak concentration in 1 to 2 hours, is extensively bound to plasma proteins, and is metabolized predominantly by the liver. The half-life of trazodone is about 6 hours.[1,58] The major action of trazodone is inhibition of reuptake of serotonin, but it is not an SSRI.[2] It does not have antimuscarinic or antihistaminic effects.[2,36] Other pharmacodynamic effects include α_1-adrenoreceptor blockade, inhibition of norepinephrine reuptake, and postsynaptic serotonin$_2$-receptor blockade.[2] Hypotension in trazodone overdose is caused by α_1-adrenoreceptor blockade.[58] Trazodone overdoses are less toxic than CA and MAOI overdoses.[56,58,59]

Clinical Features

Clinical presentation of trazodone overdose is similar to SSRI overdose.[58] Cardiac toxicity has been reported with trazodone, but is rare. Trazodone also has been implicated in serotonin syndrome.[47,49] The most common manifestations of trazodone overdose are orthostatic hypotension with lightheadedness, drowsiness, lethargy, ataxia, nausea, and vomiting.[58] There are isolated reports of priapism, respiratory arrest, prolonged Q-T_c, ventricular dysrhythmias including torsades de pointes, bradycardia, hypotension, seizures, coma, and death. When trazodone overdose occurs with coingestants, morbidity and mortality are increased.[58,59]

Management

Hypotension responds to boluses of intravenous crystalloids and usually does not require vasopressors.[58] Rare ventricular dysrhythmias with trazodone overdose should be treated with standard advanced cardiac life support therapy. Neurologic complications of trazodone poisoning are treated similarly to neurologic complications of CAs (see Table 149-2). There is no proven efficacy of activated charcoal, and this is usually a more benign ingestion. Based on the pharmacokinetic data, forced diuresis, hemodialysis, and hemoperfusion have no role. After 6 hours of observation, asymptomatic overdose patients can receive psychiatric evaluation and disposition.

Venlafaxine

Venlafaxine is well absorbed from the gastrointestinal tract, reaches peak concentrations in 2 hours, has a large volume of distribution (about 7.5 L/kg), and undergoes extensive hepatic metabolism to form the active metabolite *O*-desmethylvenlafaxine (ODV). The half-life of venlafaxine is about 5 hours, and the half-life of ODV is about 11 hours.[1] The extended-release preparation, Effexor XR, reaches a peak concentration 6 to 7 hours after therapeutic dosing.[56] Venlafaxine and ODV inhibit reuptake of serotonin to a greater extent than norepinephrine and dopamine.[1,56,60] There is a dose-dependent blockade of sodium channels.[56]

Clinical Features

Most venlafaxine overdose patients are asymptomatic. Somnolence and sinus tachycardia are the most common symptoms.[56] Seizures and prolonged Q-T_c are rarer.[56] Neuromuscular signs and symptoms were most common in one study, but patients recovered without permanent sequelae (Table 149-8).[61]

Table 149-8. Clinical Manifestations of Venlafaxine Overdose

Clinical Manifestations	%
Drowsiness	39
Tremor	5
Seizures	5
Responsive only to pain	4
Unresponsive	3
Lightheadedness	3
Nervousness	1
Headache	1

From Setzer SC, et al: Acute venlafaxine overdose: A multicenter study. *J Toxicol Clin Toxicol* 33:496, 1995.

Seizures, life-threatening hypotension, QRS and Q-T_c prolongation, and death from venlafaxine overdose have been reported, but occur more often in combination with coingestants.[56,62] Venlafaxine may not be as safe in overdose, however, as other serotoninergic drugs.[45,56] Massive venlafaxine overdose has resulted in arrhythmogenic death.[63] Serotonin syndrome has occurred when venlafaxine was used with MAOIs.[56,64]

Management

Standard supportive care is the foundation of venlafaxine overdose treatment. There is no antidote. Cyproheptadine has been used in serotonin syndrome associated with venlafaxine. The rare instances of hypotension are treated successfully with intravenous fluids, dopamine, and norepinephrine.[62] Benzodiazepines have been effective for venlafaxine-associated seizures. Forced diuresis, hemodialysis, and hemoperfusion have no role. After 6 hours of observation, asymptomatic overdose patients can receive psychiatric evaluation and disposition.

Mirtazapine

Mirtazapine is well absorbed from the gastrointestinal tract, reaches peak concentrations within 2 hours after therapeutic doses, and is highly protein bound. It is extensively metabolized in the liver to one active and two inactive metabolites. The elimination half-life of mirtazapine is 20 to 40 hours; the half-life for the active demethylated metabolite, normirtazapine, is about 19 hours.[56,65] Mirtazapine blocks presynaptic α_2-adrenergic receptors, increasing release of 5-HT and norepinephrine.[2,65,66] Mirtazapine blocks 5-HT_2 and 5-HT_3 receptors with high potency but has little effect on 5-HT_1 receptors; this results in fewer gastrointestinal effects compared with SSRIs.[2,66] To a lesser extent, mirtazapine antagonizes H_1 (histaminic), muscarinic, and peripheral α_1-adrenergic receptors; this can cause sedation, tachycardia, and hypotension.[2] Mirtazapine has fewer anticholinergic, antihistaminic, and antiadrenergic effects than CAs.

Clinical Features

In the few cases reported, somnolence, dizziness, anxiety, confusion, moderate hypotension, slight

BOX 149-8. FDA-Approved and Other Monoamine Oxidase Inhibitors (MAOIs)

MAOI Antidepressants
Phenelzine (Nardil)
Tranylcypromine (Parnate)

Antimicrobial
Furazolidone (Furoxone)

Antiparkinsonian
Selegiline (Eldepryl)

Antineoplastic
Procarbazine (Matulane)

Not Marketed in United States
Brofaromine
Cimoxatone
Clorgyline
Iproniazid
Isocarboxazid
Mebanazine
Moclobemide
Nialamide
Pargyline
Safrazine

FDA, Food and Drug Administration; MAOI, monoamine oxidase inhibitor.

BOX 149-9. Monoamine Oxidase Inhibitors Grouped by Inhibitory Activity

Irreversible Nonselective Inhibitors of MAO-A and MAO-B
Furazolidone
Iproniazid
Isocarboxazid
Mebanazine
Nialamide
Phenelzine
Procarbazine
Safrazine
Tranylcypromine

Relatively Selective MAO-A Inhibitors

Reversible	*Irreversible*
Brofaromine	Clorgyline
Cimoxatone	
Moclobemide	

Relatively Selective MAO-B Inhibitors

Reversible	*Irreversible*
None	Pargyline
	Selegiline

MAO-A, monoamine oxidase type A; MAO-B, monoamine oxidase type B.

increase in systolic blood pressure, and mild tachycardia have occurred and resolved without specific treatment. No seizures or significant ECG changes have been reported in isolated mirtazapine overdoses, and all reported patients have recovered fully.[67,68] Sedation, tachycardia and cognitive disorganization have been observed, but without permanent sequelae.[36]

Management

Hypotension may require intravenous fluids. A 6-hour observation period is reasonable.

MONOAMINE OXIDASE INHIBITORS

Many drugs inhibit monoamine oxidases (MAOs).[1] Five drugs with significant MAO inhibition are marketed in the United States: the antidepressants phenelzine and tranylcypromine, the antiparkinsonian agent selegiline, the antimicrobial furazolidone, and the antineoplastic procarbazine (Box 149-8).[1] MAOIs are well absorbed from the gastrointestinal tract, reach peak concentrations in 0.5 to 2.5 hours, are extensively bound to plasma proteins, and have relatively large volumes of distribution.[69] Tranylcypromine and selegiline have active metabolites that include significant amounts of amphetamine and methamphetamine.[70] Minimal amounts of MAOIs are eliminated in the urine as unchanged drugs.

The MAO isoenzymes, MAO-A and MAO-B, inactivate direct-acting, endogenous, biogenic amines, such as epinephrine, norepinephrine, and serotonin. The MAO isoenzymes also inactivate indirect-acting exogenous biogenic amines, such as tyramine.[69-71] Effects of MAOIs include (1) inhibition of MAO; (2) MAOI effect on indirect sympathomimetics, such as amphetamine and methamphetamine, with the potential for enhanced CNS and peripheral nervous system sympathomimetic toxicity; (3) eventual depletion of norepinephrine stores; and (4) inhibition of pyridoxine phosphokinase and pyridoxine (vitamin B_6)-containing enzymes (Box 149-9).[69,70]

Clinical Features

The three presentations of MAOI toxicity are (1) MAOI overdose, (2) MAOI-food or MAOI-beverage interactions, and (3) MAOI-drug interactions.[69] These three presentations are differentiated by precipitating events, time to onset of symptoms, duration of symptoms, and major sign and symptom complexes (Table 149-9). All three presentations involve excessive sympathetic activity. The most common cardiovascular complications of interactions between foods, beverages, or drugs and MAOIs are hypertension and tachycardia. Reflex bradycardia can occur with severe hypertension.

Overdose

The clinical course of severe MAOI overdose occurs in four phases: (1) asymptomatic or latent, (2) neuromuscular and cardiovascular excitation with sympathetic hyperactivity, (3) CNS depression and cardiovascular collapse with hypotension and bradycardia late in severe overdoses, and (4) secondary complications caused by previous phases.[69] Onset of signs and symptoms after acute overdose usually occurs in 6 to 12 hours, but may be delayed 24 hours. Symptoms in acute MAOI overdose last for days (Table 149-10).

Seizures, coma, and muscular rigidity impair patients' abilities to keep airways patent, decrease ventilatory drive, and can produce rigid chest walls. Seizures, agitated delirium, myoclonus, muscular rigidity, and hyperthermia can result in rhabdomyolysis.[69] An overdose of 2 mg/kg (170 mg in an adult) can be lethal. Occasionally, hypotension, bradycardia, and

Table 149-9. Three Major Types of Monoamine Oxidase Inhibitor Toxicity

Toxicity	Onset	Duration	Major Symptom Complexes
MAOI overdose	Delayed for hours	Days	CNS sympathomimetic storms
MAOI-food or MAOI-beverage interaction	Minutes to hours	Hours	CNS and PNS sympathomimetic storms
MAOI-drug interaction	Minutes to hours	Hours to days	CNS and PNS sympathomimetic storms; serotonin syndrome

MAOI, monoamine oxidase inhibitor; CNS, central nervous system; PNS, peripheral nervous system.

Table 149-10. Clinical Manifestations of Acute Monoamine Oxidase Inhibitor Overdose

Neuromuscular System Manifestations	%	Cardiovascular System Manifestations	%
Agitation	67	Sinus tachycardia	67
Mydriasis	58	Hypertension	17
Rigidity	58	Hypotension	17
Hyperthermia	50		
Coma	50		
Hyperreflexia	33		
Nystagmus	33		
Writhing	25		
Seizures	17		
Hallucinations	8		
Papilledema	8		

From Meredith TJ, Vale JA: Poisoning due to psychotropic agents. *Adverse Drug React Acute Poisoning Rev* 4:83, 1985.

asystole have been reported late in severe poisonings.[69] Initial release of norepinephrine can result in a decrease in the amount available for subsequent discharge from presynaptic vesicles. This situation may explain late CNS depression and cardiovascular collapse after earlier stimulatory phases of MAOI overdose.[69] Another potential cause of late bradycardic dysrhythmias is hyperkalemia from rhabdomyolysis. Long-term use of phenelzine has been associated with a sensorimotor peripheral neuropathy, probably from pyridoxine depletion.[72,73]

Monoamine Oxidase Inhibitor–Food or Monoamine Oxidase Inhibitor–Beverage Interactions

Onset of sympathetic signs and symptoms with MAOI-food or MAOI-beverage interactions occurs in minutes to hours because ingested tyramine acts on the adrenal medulla to release endogenous biogenic amines (Box 149-10). These interactions last only a few hours because of tyramine's short duration of action.

BOX 149-10. Foods and Beverages Associated with Monoamine Oxidase Inhibitor Toxicity

Foods

Aged, fermented, pickled, smoked, or tenderized meats and fish
Aged cheeses
Decayed or spoiled foods
Broad beans
Fava beans
Bean curd
Sauerkraut
Yeast and meat extracts
Ripe avocados
Ginseng
Chocolate
Figs
Raisins
Bananas
Soy sauce
Miso soup

Undistilled Alcoholic Beverages

Ales
Beers
Wines
Sherry
Vermouth

Monoamine Oxidase Inhibitor–Drug Interactions

Signs and symptoms of MAOI-drug interactions are sympathetic storm or the serotonin syndrome and begin minutes to hours after ingesting precipitating drugs (see Boxes 149-4 to 149-7 and Table 149-9). Most MAOI-drug interactions occur in patients who are taking MAOIs regularly on an ongoing basis and ingest incompatible drugs, such as indirect-acting and mixed-acting (direct/indirect–acting) sympathomimetics, methylxanthines, antidepressants, opioids (e.g., meperidine), and other drugs that can cause serotonin syndrome (Box 149-11). These drugs produce excessive concentrations of endogenous biogenic amines that are not degraded because of MAO inhibition. Duration of MAOI-drug interactions is hours to days, depending on the precipitant's duration of effect, half-life, and formulation (e.g., sustained release, delayed release).

Differential Considerations

A history of MAOI ingestion is the most helpful diagnostic indicator. Urine and blood toxicology tests for MAOI levels are not readily available and are of little clinical value. The differential diagnosis of MAOI poisoning includes illnesses (e.g., thyroid storm, meningitis) and sympathomimetic intoxications (e.g., cocaine, amphetamines, theophylline, nicotine). Hypertensive emergencies, malignant hyperthermia, and heatstroke also are considerations in the differential diagnosis.

BOX 149-11. Drugs That Interact with Monoamine Oxidase Inhibitors to Produce Toxicity

Sympathomimetics
Indirect Acting
Amphetamines
Bretylium
Cocaine
Fenfluramine
Guanethidine
Ketamine
Methyldopa
Methylphenidate
Pemoline
Phencyclidine
Phentermine
Phenylpropanolamine
Pseudoephedrine
Reserpine
Ritodrine
Tyramine

Indirect Acting Mixed (Direct/Indirect Acting)
Dopamine
Ephedrine
Mephentermine
Metaraminol

Methylxanthines
Aminophylline
Caffeine
Oxtriphylline
Theophylline

Serotonin Toxicity
See Box 149-5

Effects of MAO inhibition persist for weeks after cessation of MAOIs because MAO enzyme activity must be regenerated by synthesis of new MAO isoenzymes. Significant potential for MAOI toxicity can persist long after the drug has left the body.

Management

There is no antidote for MAOI toxicity, and forced diuresis, hemodialysis, and hemoperfusion are not effective.[69] Sinus tachycardia does not require treatment. β-Blockers can cause unopposed α_1-adrenoreceptor stimulation of the peripheral vasculature with vasoconstriction and worsening of the hypertension. β-Blockers also can exacerbate the hypotension and bradycardia that can occur later in severe MAOI poisonings. Calcium channel blockers also are relatively contraindicated because of the potential for hypotension and bradycardia.[69]

Hypertension associated with MAOI toxicity can range from mild to life-threatening hypertensive emergencies. Mild hypertension does not require treatment. Hypertension with signs of impending or ongoing target-organ damage or with reflex bradycardia mandates treatment with sodium nitroprusside or phentolamine; both have rapid onset, easy titratability, and rapid resolution of effect when stopped, if hypotension develops later. An initial 5-mg bolus (adults) or 0.02 mg/kg to 0.1 mg/kg (children) of phentolamine is given over 1 minute.[69] The initial intravenous bolus can be repeated at 5- to 10-minute intervals as needed to lower the blood pressure to the desired range, followed by a phentolamine infusion to maintain the pressure. The initial dose of nitroprusside is 0.3 μg/kg/min, titrated to effect with a maximum rate of 10 μg/kg/min. Sodium thiosulfate can be used with continuous infusions of nitroprusside to prevent cyanide toxicity.

Reflex bradycardia is a beneficial compensatory response to significant, acute hypertension and decreases cardiac output; bradycardia should not be treated, unless it is associated with significant hypotension. Hypotension caused by MAOI toxicity usually occurs late in severe intoxications. If hypotension is associated with bradycardia, intravenous atropine should be administered until the bradycardia and hypotension resolve or a vagolytic dose of atropine has been reached (3 mg in adults or 0.04 mg/kg in children, with a minimum dose of 0.1 mg in children). Hypotension without bradycardia should be treated with intravenous isotonic crystalloids. A pacemaker is necessary for symptomatic bradycardia with accompanying hypotension that does not respond to atropine or agents such as epinephrine, dobutamine, or norepinephrine.[69] Initially a transcutaneous pacemaker can be used. Symptomatic, treatment-resistant bradycardia is often prolonged, however, and a transvenous pacemaker is optimal. Lidocaine is the drug of choice for ventricular dysrhythmias associated with MAOI toxicity. Bretylium is contraindicated in patients taking MAOIs and during acute MAOI toxicity because it releases endogenous biogenic amines.

Neurologic complications of MAOI toxicity are treated similarly to neurologic complications of CA toxicity (see Table 149-2). Dantrolene, 2.5 mg/kg intravenously initially and repeated every 6 hours for 24 hours, seemed to be useful in a phenelzine overdose accompanied by life-threatening hyperthermia.[74] Intravenous benzodiazepines may be used to control agitation.

Disposition

The severity of acute MAOI overdoses is easily underestimated because signs and symptoms usually are not evident during the first 6 to 12 hours and may be delayed in onset for 24 hours. Patients with significant MAOI overdose or suspected serotonin syndrome should be observed for 24 hours. Symptomatic patients with known or suspected MAOI interactions with food, beverages, or drugs should be admitted to an ICU for at least 24 hours. Patients with suspected food or drug interactions can be discharged if they remain asymptomatic for 6 hours.

DISCONTINUATION SYNDROME

Discontinuation syndromes with MAOIs, CAs, SSRIs, and various atypical antidepressants including venlafaxine and mirtazapine have been described.[75] A discontinuation syndrome has not yet been described for citalopram.[36] Symptoms depend on the agent and its mechanism of active action. With some SSRIs, insomnia, nausea, headache, sensory disturbances, hyperarousal, anxiety, agitation, tachycardia, and tremor have been reported.[75]

Restarting the drug and instituting a gradual taper over days to weeks generally reverses the discontinuation syndrome. Augmenting a drug that has a short half-life with another that has a long half-life may help to overcome the discontinuation syndrome.[75] Confusion and psychotic symptoms caused by stopping MAOIs may require hospital admission, restarting the MAOI, or treating with an antipsychotic medication.[75] Atropine and benztropine can help treat CA discontinuation symptoms because these symptoms reflect cholinergic rebound.[75]

A neonatal discontinuation syndrome, after in utero exposure to an SSRI in the third trimester of pregnancy, was described.[75] Symptoms included irritability, constant crying, shivering, increased tonus, eating and sleeping difficulties, and seizures.[76] Signs and symptoms began within a few days after birth and have lasted 1 month.[76]

KEY CONCEPTS

- A patient with CA poisoning can deteriorate quickly.
- When in doubt, it is better to perform endotracheal intubation to prevent aspiration, hypoxia, or hypercarbia that can increase significantly the morbidity and mortality of CA poisoning.
- $NaHCO_3$ treats cardiac conduction abnormalities and negative inotropic effects of CA poisoning that result in ventricular dysrhythmias and hypotension with a wide QRS complex.
- The case-fatality rate for SSRI overdose is much lower than for CA overdose.
- If serotonin syndrome is suspected, the patient should be admitted to a monitored unit for 24 hours of observation.
- Medication lists should be scrutinized for serotonin-enhancing drugs, and medications such as meperidine should be avoided in patients with SSRI overdose.
- Although the case-fatality rate for overdoses with miscellaneous antidepressants is much lower than for CA overdoses, fatal poisoning can occur, even without coingestants.
- Bupropion poisoning should be considered when seizures occur.
- Trazodone toxicity should be considered in a patient with priapism.
- If MAOI overdose is suspected or diagnosed, admission for 24 hours of observation is indicated, even if the patient is initially asymptomatic.
- Differential considerations of MAOI toxicity include etiologies for hyperthermia, altered mental status, and muscular rigidity, such as meningitis, thyroid storm, neuroleptic malignant syndrome, malignant hyperthermia, and heatstroke.
- Hyperthermia must be treated aggressively to limit morbidity and mortality.
- The source of a food, beverage, or drug interaction with an MAOI should be identified to avoid recurrence and future complications.

REFERENCES

1. Baldessarini RJ: Drugs and the treatment of psychiatric disorders: Depression and anxiety disorders. In Hardman JG, et al (eds): *Goodman and Gilman's the Pharmacological Basis of Therapeutics,* 10th ed. New York, McGraw-Hill, 2001.
2. Stahl SM: Basic pharmacology of antidepressants: Part 1. Antidepressants have seven distinct mechanisms of action. *J Clin Psychiatry* 59:5, 1998.
3. Borys DJ, et al: Acute fluoxetine overdose: A report of 264 cases. *Am J Emerg Med* 10:115, 1992.
4. Stoner SC, et al: Antidepressant overdoses and resultant emergency department services: The impact of SSRIs. *Pharmacol Bull* 33:667, 1997.
5. Phillips S, et al: Fluoxetine vs. tricyclic antidepressants: A prospective multicenter study of antidepressant overdoses. *J Emerg Med* 15:439, 1997.
6. Tokarski GF, Young MJ: Criteria for admitting patients with tricyclic antidepressant overdose. *J Emerg Med* 6:121, 1988.
7. Banahan BF, Schelkun PH: Tricyclic antidepressant overdose: Conservative management in a community hospital with cost-saving implications. *J Emerg Med* 8:451, 1990.
8. Pentel PR, Benowitz NL: Tricyclic antidepressant poisoning: Management of arrhythmias. *Med Toxicol* 1:101, 1986.
9. Heard K, et al: Tricyclic antidepressants directly depress human myocardial mechanical function independent of effects on the conduction system. *Acad Emerg Med* 8:1122, 2001.
10. Schwartz R, Esler M: Catecholamine levels in tricyclic antidepressant self-poisoning. *Aust N Z J Med* 4:479, 1974.
11. Ellison DW, Pentel PR: Clinical features and consequences of seizures due to cyclic antidepressant overdose. *Am J Emerg Med* 7:5, 1989.
12. Shannon M, Merola J, Lovejoy FH: Hypotension in severe tricyclic antidepressant overdose. *Am J Emerg Med* 6:439, 1988.
13. Callaham M, Kassel D: Epidemiology of fatal tricyclic antidepressant ingestion: Implications for management. *Ann Emerg Med* 14:1, 1985.
14. Foulke G, Albertson T: QRS interval in tricyclic antidepressant overdosage: Inaccuracy as a toxicity indicator in emergency settings. *Ann Emerg Med* 16:160, 1987.
15. Emerman C, Connors A, Burma G: Level of consciousness as a predictor of complications following tricyclic overdose. *Ann Emerg Med* 16:326, 1987.
16. Goldgran-Toledano D, Sideris G, Kevorkian J: Overdose of cyclic antidepressants and the Brugada syndrome. *N Engl J Med* 346:1591, 2002.
17. Roy TM, et al: Pulmonary complications after tricyclic antidepressant overdose. *Chest* 96:852, 1989.
18. Pentel P, Peterson CD: Asystole complicating physostigmine treatment of tricyclic antidepressant overdose. *Ann Emerg Med* 9:588, 1980.
19. Shannon M, Liebelt EL: Toxicology reviews: Targeted management strategies for cardiovascular toxicity from tricyclic antidepressant overdose: The pivotal role for alkalinization and sodium loading. *Pediatr Emerg Care* 14:293, 1998.
20. Bessen HA, Niemann JT: Improvement of cardiac conduction after hyperventilation in tricyclic antidepressant overdose. *J Toxicol Clin Toxicol* 23:537, 1986.
21. McKinney PE, Rasmussen R: Reversal of severe tricyclic antidepressant induced cardiotoxicity with intravenous hypertonic saline solution. *Ann Emerg Med* 42:20, 2003.
22. Wrenn K, Smith BA, Slovis CM: Profound alkalemia during treatment of tricyclic antidepressant overdose: A potential hazard of combined hyperventilation and intravenous bicarbonate. *Am J Emerg Med* 10:553, 1992.

23. Vernon DD, et al: Efficacy of dopamine and norepinephrine for treatment of hemodynamic compromise in amitriptyline intoxication. *Crit Care Med* 19:544, 1991.
24. Bain DJG, Turner T: Imipramine poisoning. *Arch Dis Child* 46:887, 1971.
25. Callaham M, Schumaker H, Pentel P: Phenytoin prophylaxis of cardiotoxicity in experimental amitriptyline poisoning. *Pharmacol Exp Ther* 245:216, 1988.
26. Olson KR, et al: Seizures associated with poisoning and drug overdose. *Am J Emerg Med* 11:565, 1993.
27. Kumar A, Black TS: Intravenous midazolam for the treatment of refractory status epilepticus. *Crit Care Med* 20:483, 1992.
28. Merigian KS, Browning RG, Leeper LV: Successful treatment of amoxapine induced refractory status epilepticus with propofol (Diprivan). *Acad Emerg Med* 2:128, 1995.
29. Mordel A, et al: Seizures after flumazenil administration in a case of combined benzodiazepine and tricyclic antidepressant overdose. *Crit Care Med* 20:1733, 1992.
30. Geller E, et al: Risks and benefits of therapy with flumazenil (Anexate) in mixed drug intoxications. *Eur Neurol* 31:241, 1991.
31. Preskorn SH: Clinically relevant pharmacology of selective serotonin reuptake inhibitors: An overview with emphasis on pharmacokinetics and effects on oxidative drug metabolism. *Clin Pharmacokinet* 32:1, 1997.
32. Briley M, Moret C: Neurobiological mechanisms involved in antidepressant therapies. *Clin Neuropharmacol* 16:387, 1993.
33. Whyte IM, Dawson AH, Buckley NA: Relative toxicity of venlafaxine and selective serotonin reuptake inhibitors in overdose. *QJM* 96:369, 2003.
34. Myers LB, Krenzelok EP: Paroxetine (Paxil) overdose: A pediatric focus. *Vet Hum Toxicol* 39:86, 1997.
35. Spiller HA, Morse S, Muir C: Fluoxetine ingestion: A one year retrospective study. *Vet Hum Toxicol* 32:153, 1990.
36. Goldberg JF: New drugs in psychiatry. *Emerg Med Clin North Am* 18:211, 2000.
37. Graudins A, Vossler C, Wang R: Fluoxetine-induced cardiotoxicity with response to bicarbonate therapy. *Am J Emerg Med* 15:501, 1997.
38. Braitberg G, Curry S: Seizure after isolated fluoxetine overdose. *Ann Emerg Med* 26:234, 1995.
39. Hahn I, et al: Fluvoxamine overdose producing status epilepticus [abstract]. *J Toxicol Clin Toxicol* 38:573, 2000.
40. Catalano G, et al: QTc interval prolongation associated with citalopram overdose: A case report and literature review. *Clin Neuropharmacol* 24:158, 2001.
41. Personne M, Persson H, Sjöberg G: Citalopram toxicity. *Lancet* 350:518, 1997.
42. Grundemar L, et al: Symptoms and signs of severe citalopram overdose. *Lancet* 349:1602, 1997.
43. Grover J, Caravati EM: Right bundle branch block and delayed seizure associated with citalopram and fluoxetine ingestion [abstract]. *J Toxicol Clin Toxicol* 39:491, 2001.
44. Lindgren KN, et al: Escitalopram, a review of adverse effects in overdose reported to select regional poison centers. *J Toxicol Clin Toxicol* 41:658, 2003.
45. Buckley NA, McManus PR: Fatal toxicity of serotoninergic and other antidepressant drugs: Analysis of United Kingdom mortality data. *BMJ* 325:1332, 2002.
46. Lau GT, Horowitz Z: Sertraline overdose. *Acad Emerg Med* 3:132, 1996.
47. Mills KC: Serotonin syndrome: A clinical update. *Crit Care Clin* 13:763, 1997.
48. Sternbach H: The serotonin syndrome. *Am J Psychiatry* 148:705, 1991.
49. Dunkley EJC, et al: The Hunter serotonin toxicity criteria: Simple and accurate diagnostic decision rules for serotonin toxicity. *QJM* 96:635, 2003.
50. Bodner RA, et al: Serotonin syndrome. *Neurology* 45:219, 1995.
51. Spiller HA, et al: Bupropion overdose: A three-year multi-center retrospective analysis. *Am J Emerg Med* 12:43, 1994.
52. Dunner DL, et al: A prospective safety surveillance study for bupropion sustained-release in the treatment of depression. *J Clin Psychiatry* 59:366, 1998.
53. Paris PA, Saucier JR: ECG conduction delays associated with massive bupropion overdose. *J Toxicol Clin Toxicol* 36:595, 1998.
54. Harris CR, Gualtieri J, Stark G: Fatal bupropion overdose. *J Toxicol Clin Toxicol* 35:321, 1997.
55. Belson MG, Kelley TR: Bupropion exposures: Clinical manifestations and medical outcome. *J Emerg Med* 23:223, 2002.
56. Buckley NA, Faunce TA: "Atypical" antidepressants in overdose: Clinical considerations with respect to safety. *Drug Saf* 26:539, 2003.
57. Falkland M, et al: Bupropion SR in overdose: Subsidized poisoning. *J Toxicol Clin Toxicol* 40:275, 2002.
58. Gamble DE, Peterson LG: Trazodone overdose: Four years of experience from voluntary reports. *J Clin Psychiatry* 47:544, 1986.
59. Goeringer KE, Raymon L, Logan BK: Postmortem forensic toxicology of trazodone. *J Forensic Sci* 45:850, 2000.
60. Patat A, et al: Absolute bioavailability and electroencephalographic effects of conventional and extended-release formulations of venlafaxine in healthy subjects. *J Clin Pharmacol* 38:256, 1998.
61. Setzer SC, et al: Acute venlafaxine overdose: A multicenter study. *J Toxicol Clin Toxicol* 33:496, 1995.
62. Kokan L, Dart RC: Life-threatening hypotension from venlafaxine overdose. *J Toxicol Clin Toxicol* 34:559, 1996.
63. Cumpston K, Chao M, Pallasch E: Massive venlafaxine overdose resulting in arrhythmogenic death. *J Toxicol Clin Toxicol* 41:659, 2003.
64. Daniels RJ: Serotonin syndrome due to venlafaxine overdose. *Hum Exp Toxicol* 16:14, 1997.
65. Caccia S: Metabolism of the newer antidepressants: An overview of the pharmacological and pharmacokinetic implications. *Clin Pharmacokinet* 34:281, 1998.
66. De Boer T: The pharmacologic profile of mirtazapine. *J Clin Psychiatry* 57:19, 1996.
67. Holzbach R, et al: Suicide attempts with mirtazapine overdose without complications. *Biol Psychiatry* 44:925, 1998.
68. Bremner JD, Wingard P, Walshe TA: Safety of mirtazapine in overdose. *J Clin Psychiatry* 59:233, 1998.
69. Linden CH, Rumack BH, Strehlke C: Monoamine oxidase inhibitor overdose. *Ann Emerg Med* 13:1137, 1984.
70. Youdim MBH, et al: Tranylcypromine (Parnate) overdose: Measurement of tranylcypromine concentrations and MAO inhibitory activity and identification of amphetamines in plasma. *Psychol Med* 9:377, 1979.
71. McDaniel KD: Clinical pharmacology of monoamine oxidase inhibitors. *Clin Neuropharmacol* 9:207, 1986.
72. Goodheart RS, Dunne JW, Edis RH: Phenelzine associated peripheral neuropathy: Clinical and electrophysiologic findings. *Aust N Z J Med* 21:339, 1991.
73. Heller CA, Friedman PA: Pyridoxine deficiency and peripheral neuropathy associated with long-term phenelzine therapy. *Am J Med* 75:887, 1983.
74. Kaplan RF, et al: Phenelzine overdose treated with dantrolene sodium. *JAMA* 255:642, 1986.
75. Haddad PM: Antidepressant discontiunuation syndromes, clinical relevance, prevention and management. *Drug Saf* 24:183, 2001.
76. Nordeng H, et al: Neonatal withdrawal syndrome after in utero exposure to selective serotonin reuptake inhibitors. *Acta Paediatr* 90:288, 2001.

CHAPTER

150 Cardiovascular Drugs

David J. Roberts

Cardiovascular drugs rank among the most common causes of poisoning fatalities, both in children (third leading cause) and in adults (fifth leading cause). Of the scores of cardiovascular drugs, three—digitalis, propranolol, and verapamil—account for the majority of fatalities.

DIGITALIS

Perspective

Digitalis is derived from the foxglove plant (Figure 150-1). Despite centuries of experience with digitalis, chronic and acute poisonings remain common. Dr. Benjamin Rush wrote in 1797, "I suspect the cases in which [digitalis preparations] were useful to have been either so few or doubtful and that the cases they had done harm were so much more numerous and unequivocal as justly to banish them from the *Materia Medica*."[1] Medication errors and toxic effects account for the most common causes (44%) of preventable iatrogenic cardiac arrests.[2] Digoxin is the most common offending drug, and although its use is now generally limited to treatment of congestive heart failure and atrial fibrillation, digitalis remains a commonly prescribed drug in the United States.

Principles of Disease

Pathophysiology

In therapeutic doses, digitalis has two effects: (1) increasing the force of myocardial contraction to increase cardiac output in patients with heart failure; and (2) decreasing atrioventricular (AV) conduction to slow the ventricular rate in atrial fibrillation. The biochemical basis for its first effect is an inhibition of membrane sodium-potassium adenosine triphosphatase (ATPase), which increases intracellular sodium and calcium and increases extracellular potassium. At therapeutic doses, the effects on serum electrolyte levels are minimal. With toxic levels, digitalis paralyzes the Na-K pump, potassium cannot be transported into cells, and serum potassium can rise as high as 13.5 mEq/L.[3] Because intracellular levels of calcium are already high, administering calcium, a common treatment for hyperkalemia, can be dangerous in the digitalis-intoxicated patient.

Digitalis exerts direct and indirect effects on sinoatrial (SA) and AV nodal fibers. At therapeutic levels, digitalis indirectly increases vagal activity and decreases sympathetic activity. At toxic levels, digitalis can directly halt the generation of impulses in the SA node, depress conduction through the AV node, and increase sensitivity of the SA and AV nodes to catecholamines. Catecholamines, whether endogenous or administered by physicians to treat bradydysrhythmias or hypotension, probably play an important role in digitalis toxicity. It is unclear how much iatrogenic interventions may contribute to digitalis toxicity. Because bradydysrhythmias and tachydysrhythmias can appear and alternate in the same patient, administering one class of drugs to treat tachycardias may later contribute to more refractory bradycardias and AV block.

Digitalis also exerts three primary effects on Purkinje's fibers: (1) decreased resting potential, resulting in slowed phase 0 depolarization and conduction velocity; (2) decreased action potential duration, which increases sensitivity of muscle fibers to electrical stimuli; and (3) enhanced automaticity resulting from increased rate of phase 4 repolarization and delayed after depolarizations. These mechanisms account for the most common manifestation of digitalis toxicity, an increase in premature ventricular contractions. At toxic extremes, these effects result in a dangerous sensitivity to mechanical and electrical stimulation. Iatrogenic interventions with pacemaker catheters and cardioversion can result in asystole, ventricular tachycardia, and ventricular fibrillation.[4]

Unlike most cardiovascular drugs, digitalis can produce virtually any dysrhythmia or conduction block, and bradycardias are as common as tachycardias (Box 150-1). Unfortunately, none is peculiar to digitalis, and they can all occur in the setting of ischemic and other heart disease in the absence of digitalis. Digitalis intoxication remains a clinical rather than an electrocardiographic diagnosis.

The volume of distribution (V_d), or apparent body volume into which digoxin distributes, is 5 L/kg for adults but varies from 3.5 L/kg in premature infants to 16.3 L/kg in older infants.[5] This indicates that only a small fraction of digitalis remains in the intravascular space, and the drug is highly concentrated in cardiac tissue. The myocardial-to-serum ratio at equilibrium ranges from 15:1 to 30:1.[6] The V_d for digitoxin is 0.5 L/kg.

The elimination half-life of digoxin, which is primarily excreted in the urine, is 30 hours, and the half-life of digitoxin, which is metabolized in the liver, is 7 days.[6] Whereas digoxin undergoes only a small enterohepatic circulation, that for digitoxin is large, and multiple-dose charcoal treatment is clearly indicated for the latter.

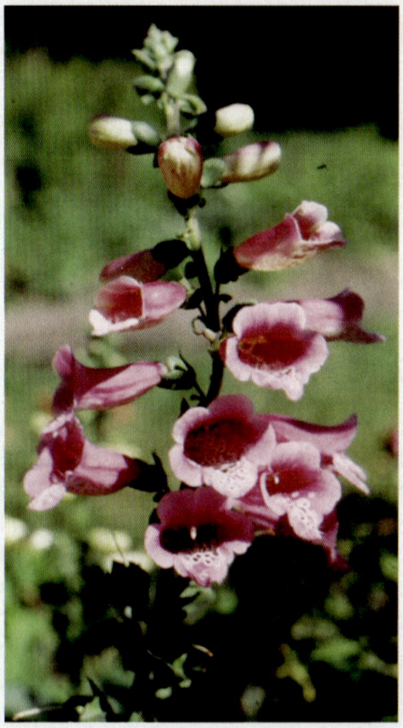

Figure 150-1. The foxglove plant, from which digitalis is derived.

BOX 150-2. Factors Associated with Increased Risk of Digitalis Toxicity

Renal insufficiency
Heart disease
- Congenital heart disease
- Ischemic heart disease
- Congestive heart failure
- Myocarditis

Electrolyte imbalance
- Hypokalemia or hyperkalemia
- Hypomagnesemia
- Hypercalcemia

Alkalosis
Hypothyroidism
Sympathomimetic drugs
Cardiotoxic coingestants
- β-Blockers
- Calcium channel blockers
- Tricyclic antidepressants

Drug interactions
- Quinidine, amiodarone
- Erythromycin
- Verapamil, diltiazem, nifedipine
- Captopril

Elderly woman

BOX 150-1. Dysrhythmias Associated with Digitalis Toxicity

Nonspecific
PVCs, especially bigeminal and multiform
First-, second- (Wenckebach), and third-degree AV block
Sinus bradycardia
Sinus tachycardia
Sinoatrial block or arrest
Atrial fibrillation with slow ventricular response
Atrial tachycardia
Junctional (escape) rhythm
AV dissociation
Ventricular bigeminy and trigeminy
Ventricular tachycardia
Torsades de pointes
Ventricular fibrillation

More Specific, but not Pathognomonic
Atrial fibrillation with slow, regular ventricular rate (AV dissociation)
Nonparoxysmal junctional tachycardia (rate 70 to 130 beats/min)
Atrial tachycardia with block (atrial rate usually 150 to 200 beats/min)
Bidirectional ventricular tachycardia

AV, atrioventricular; PVC, premature ventricular contraction.

Protein binding varies from 25% for digoxin to 95% for digitoxin.[6] Both significant protein binding and a large volume of distribution suggest that hemodialysis, hemoperfusion, and exchange transfusion are ineffective. The long half-lives suggest that temporizing measures such as pacemakers, atropine, and antidysrhythmic drugs might in the end cost more time, money, and lives than simply giving Fab fragments initially.

Multiple drugs and disease states can negatively alter absorption, volume of distribution, protein binding, and elimination and render the heart more susceptible to digitalis toxicity. The factors listed in Box 150-2 are especially important in evaluating suspected cases of chronic intoxication.

Clinical Features

The symptoms and signs of digitalis intoxication are nonspecific. The most common symptoms—reported in more than 80% of cases—are nausea, anorexia, fatigue, and visual disturbance, but a variety of gastrointestinal, neurologic, and ophthalmic disturbances have been linked to digitalis (Box 150-3). One should consider digitalis intoxication in any patient on maintenance therapy who develops consistent symptoms, especially with new conduction disturbances or dysrhythmias.

Significant differences exist between acute and chronic intoxication (Table 150-1). Chronic poisoning has an insidious onset and is accompanied by a higher mortality rate. In cases of chronic intoxication, the LL_{50} (the level with a 50% mortality) is only 6 ng/mL.[7] The LL_{50} for acute intoxication is not known, but it is certainly much higher, especially in children. Chronically intoxicated patients almost always have underlying heart disease, which contributes to both morbidity and mortality.

Diagnostic Strategies

It is the steady state, rather than peak level, that correlates with tissue toxicity and is used to calculate antidote dosages. Peak levels after an oral dose of digoxin

BOX 150-3. Noncardiac Symptoms of Digitalis Intoxication in Adults and Children

General
Weakness
Fatigue
Malaise

Gastrointestinal
Nausea and vomiting
Anorexia
Abdominal pain
Diarrhea

Ophthalmologic
Blurred or snowy vision
Photophobia
Yellow-green chromatopsia (also red, brown, blue)
Transient amblyopia, diplopia, scotomata, blindness

Neurologic
Dizziness
Headache
Confusion, disorientation, delirium
Visual and auditory hallucinations
Paranoid ideation, acute psychosis
Somnolence
Abnormal dreams
Paresthesias and neuralgia
Aphasia
Seizures

Table 150-1. Chronic Versus Acute Digitalis Intoxication

Chronic	Acute
Higher mortality (LL_{50} = 6 ng/mL)	Lower mortality
Potassium level normal or low	Potassium level normal or high
Ventricular dysrhythmias more common	Bradycardia and atrioventricular block more common
Usually elderly patients	Usually younger patients
Often need Fab fragment therapy	Often do well without Fab (*caution:* many exceptions)
Underlying heart disease increases morbidity and mortality	Absence of heart disease decreases morbidity and mortality

occur in 1.5 to 2 hours, with a range of 0.5 to 6 hours.[6,8] Steady-state serum concentrations are not achieved until after distribution, or 6 to 8 hours after a dose or overdose, and may be only one fourth to one fifth of the peak level. Serum steady-state digoxin levels of 1.6 to 3.0 ng/mL are equivocal; that is, levels as low as 1.6 ng/mL have been associated with toxicity, and patients with levels up to 3.0 ng/mL can be asymptomatic.[9] A level drawn too soon after the last maintenance dose will falsely suggest toxicity, especially in cases of chronic intoxication, in which significant morbidity and mortality can occur at levels of 2 to 6 ng/mL.[7] After an acute massive overdose in a patient who is rapidly becoming symptomatic, however, it may be impractical to wait 6 to 8 hours for the first reading.[10,11] It is unlikely that early levels exceeding 10 to 20 ng/mL will fade to clinical insignificance at 6 to 8 hours after ingestion.

Patients taking digitalis therapeutically often take diuretics as well, and they often have low serum and total body potassium levels. The acutely poisoned patient, in contrast, may have life-threatening hyperkalemia, and empiric potassium administration is contraindicated.

Differential Considerations

No sign or symptom, including dysrhythmias, is unique to digitalis poisoning, so the differential diagnosis is broad. Intrinsic cardiac disease as well as other cardiotoxic drugs must be considered. Central nervous system (CNS) depression or confusion may be secondary to various drugs and toxins as well as infection, trauma, inflammation, and metabolic derangements. Visual disturbances, which should be binocular, are often not reported by the patient, and the clinician should ask directly about them. Gastrointestinal disturbances are common and nonspecific and may be misdiagnosed as gastritis, enteritis, or colitis.

Management

With the availability of digoxin-specific Fab fragment antibodies (Digibind and DigiFab), all other therapies, except for mild cases, must be considered temporizing.

There is no evidence to support gastric emptying for the treatment of digoxin overdose. Oral overdoses can be treated with activated charcoal if it can be administered within 1 hour of ingestion, but no improvement in outcome has been proven. Similarly, although not proven to improve outcome, multidose charcoal has historically been used for digitoxin toxicity because of its prominent 26% enterohepatic circulation. The benefit, if any, of multidose charcoal may largely be irrelevant with the widespread availability of antidigoxin antibody treatment as a specific antidote.

Electrolyte Correction

Potassium replacement is one of the first steps taken to treat chronic intoxication. In cases of chronic intoxication, often exacerbated by hypokalemia, most authorities recommend raising the serum potassium level to 3.5 to 4 mEq/L. Potassium can be administered orally (which is safer) or intravenously. Infusing potassium intravenously more rapidly than 10 to 40 mEq/hr is dangerous.

In cases of acute poisoning, when serum potassium may begin to rise rapidly after 1 to 2 hours, potassium should be withheld, even if mild hypokalemia is measured initially. A serum potassium level greater than 5 mEq/L warrants consideration of digitalis antibody treatment. If digitalis antibodies are not immediately available, severe hyperkalemia must be treated with infusions of glucose, insulin, and sodium bicarbonate. Calcium, as noted earlier, should be avoided.

Many patients on diuretic therapy are also magnesium depleted, even when the serum magnesium level is normal. If significant magnesium depletion is suspected, 1 to 2 g of magnesium sulfate can be given over 10 to 20 minutes (child: 25 mg/kg), followed by a constant infusion of 1 to 2 g/hr. Patients must be closely monitored for respiratory depression, which is usually preceded by progressive loss of deep tendon reflexes. Hypermagnesemia can exacerbate digitalis toxicity, but magnesium has been reported to reverse digoxin-induced tachydysrhythmias. It is prudent to infuse magnesium slowly and stop the infusion if heart block or bradycardia develops. Avoid magnesium in patients with renal failure. The role of magnesium in bradydysrhythmias and conduction blocks is less clear but probably dangerous because hypermagnesemia can actually impair impulse formation and AV conduction.

Atropine

Atropine is generally used for severe bradycardia and advanced AV block, with mixed results. Generally, an external or transvenous pacemaker should be readied when bradycardia or AV block appears.

Pacing

Transvenous pacing has been a mainstay of treatment for several decades, but the catheter may induce ventricular tachydysrhythmias in a myocardium made irritable by digitalis. Iatrogenic accidents of cardiac pacing are frequent (14/39, 36%) and often fatal (5/39, 13%).[12] It may be safer to temporize with an external rather than a transvenous pacemaker while waiting for Fab fragments to take effect. Cardioversion and defibrillation can also be dangerous, with asystole after attempts to treat tachydysrhythmias. Lower energy settings, such as 25 to 50 J, may be less hazardous.

Carotid Sinus Massage

Carotid sinus massage is dangerous in the setting of digitalis toxicity and may result in bradyasystole and cardiac arrest.

Phenytoin and Lidocaine

Phenytoin and lidocaine are believed to be the safest of the antidysrhythmic drugs for controlling tachydysrhythmias in the setting of digitalis intoxication. Phenytoin may enhance AV conduction. Phenytoin has been infused at 25 to 50 mg/min to a loading dose of 10 to 15 mg/kg. Lidocaine can be given initially at a dosage of 1 to 3 mg/kg over several minutes, followed by an infusion of 1 to 4 mg/min (30 to 50 μg/kg/min).[13] Most other cardiac drugs (isoproterenol, procainamide, amiodarone, β-blockers, calcium antagonists) may worsen dysrhythmias or depress AV conduction. Digoxin immune Fab fragments are the preferred therapy for dysrhythmias.

Fab Fragments

The rate of mortality before Fab fragment therapy was 23% despite all of the interventions decribed.[14,15] Fab fragment treatment is well established in both chronic and acute poisonings with a 90% response rate.[12,14-16] Nonresponders usually received too little antibody or received it too late. Other nonresponders were compromised by underlying heart or multisystem disease.

Digitalis antibodies are derived from sheep immunized with digoxin. Because the more antigenic Fg fragments are discarded, allergic reactions are less than 1% and routine skin testing is uneccessary.[16,17] Reactions have included erythema, urticaria, and facial edema, all of which have responded to the usual treatment. Other adverse reactions to Fab fragment neutralization of digitalis include hypokalemia, exacerbation of congestive heart failure, or increase in ventricular rate with atrial fibrillation.

Because of its expense, Fab fragment treatment is best reserved for cases of life-threatening toxicity rather than for routine or prophylactic administration. The primary indication for antibody treatment in cases of acute poisoning is hyperkalemia with a serum potassium level greater than 5.5 mEq/L or electrocardiographic changes. Although toxicity increases with greater body load, there is no clear correlation with amount ingested, especially in children, and many patients with large ingestions or high serum levels become only mildly symptomatic.[5] Fab fragment therapy should be used before transvenous pacing, which carries significant risk.

The median time to initial response is 19 minutes *after* completion of the Fab infusion, but complete resolution of digitalis-toxic rhythms may require hours.[15,18] Late administration of Fab fragments has resuscitated 54% of patients who have suffered cardiac arrest.[15,19] This antidote should be considered whenever hemodynamic compromise attends a digitalis-toxic dysrhythmia or heart block (Box 150-4).[20]

Current formulas for calculating Digibind dosages are found in the package insert. There are at least three approaches. The first is empiric. A patient has a history of digitalis ingestion, consistent symptoms, and life-threatening dysrhythmias. There is no time to assess serum digoxin levels, either at 1 hour or in steady state. In such a situation, 10 vials should be administered over 30 minutes through a 0.22-μm filter for the average acute ingestion, and 4 to 6 vials for the average chronic ingestion. In patients in cardiac arrest, 20 vials of Digibind can be administered undiluted by intravenous bolus. The second approach uses a simple calculation when the ingested dose is known with reasonable certainty. One vial of Digibind contains 38 mg of Fab fragments, which bind 0.5 mg of digoxin or digitoxin (Box 150-5). A third approach is to base the dosage on the steady-state serum digoxin or digitoxin level after 6 to 8 hours (Boxes 150-6 and 150-7). Once Fab fragments have been administered, it is no longer fruitful to measure digitalis levels for up to 1 week because most assays will measure both bound and unbound drug, with values greater than 100 ng/mL common. Newer methods can measure free digoxin, but it is more meaningful to follow the patient clinically.

BOX 150-4. Recommendations for Administration of Digitalis Antibody Fragments

Adults

1. Severe ventricular dysrhythmias
2. Progressive and hemodynamically significant bradydysrhythmias unresponsive to atropine
3. Serum potassium greater than 5 mEq/L
4. Rapidly progressive rhythm disturbances or rising serum potassium level
5. Co-ingestion of cardiotoxic drug such as β-blockers, calcium channel blockers, or tricyclic antidepressants
6. Ingestion of plant known to contain cardiac glycosides *plus* severe dysrhythmias (rare)
7. Acute ingestion greater than 10 mg *plus* any one of factors 1 through 6 above
8. Steady-state serum digoxin greater than 6 ng/ml *plus* any one of factors 1 through 6 above

Children

1. Ingestion of greater than 0.1 to 0.3 mg/kg or steady-state digoxin greater than 5 ng/mL *plus* rapidly progressive symptoms or signs of digitalis intoxication *or* potentially life-threatening dysrhythmias or conduction blocks *or* serum potassium greater than 6 mEq/L
2. Co-ingestion of other cardiotoxic drugs with additive or synergistic toxicity
3. Ingestion of plant known to contain cardiac glycosides *plus* severe dysrhythmias (rare)

BOX 150-5. Sample Calculation of Digibind Based on Ingested Dose of Digoxin or Digitoxin*

Case: A toxic 40-year-old woman has ingested 50 0.25-mg digoxin tables

Body load = amount ingested × 0.8 (bioavailability of digoxin tablets)

= 12.5 mg × 0.8 = 10 mg

Dose of Digibind (in vials) = 10 mg ÷ 0.5 mg bound per vial

= 20 vials

*Formula from GlaxoSmithKline 2005.

Pediatric Considerations

Children at greatest risk are those on chronic digitalis therapy for heart disease. Children with healthy hearts have been known to tolerate massive acute oral ingestions without digitalis antibody treatment.[12] This excludes therapeutic errors, children taking digitalis therapeutically, and children with heart disease.

Dosage calculation and administration errors probably account for more pediatric digitalis intoxication and death than accidental oral ingestion. Therapeutic errors—especially accidental intravenous overdoses—are often catastrophic, with death within 1 to 4 hours.

Signs and symptoms in children with digitalis poisoning are somewhat different (Table 150-2). Somnolence or obtundation is more common than in adults.[11,14] A CNS depression, in the absence of a history, might lead the clinician to suspect narcotic or sedative-hypnotic overdose, or even nontoxicologic causes such as head injury, metabolic disorder, or CNS infection. Vomiting is probably more common than in adults. Conduction disturbances and bradycardias are more common than ventricular dysrhythmias in children, especially in cases of acute ingestion.[6,11]

BOX 150-6. Sample Calculation of Digibind Based on Steady-State Digoxin Concentration*

Case: A toxic 4-year-old child weighing 20 kg has a digoxin level of 16 ng/mL 8 hours after ingestion of an unknown number of digoxin tablets

Dose (in number of vials) = (serum digoxin concentration × weight in kg) ÷ 100

= (16 × 20) ÷ 100

= approximately 3 vials

*Formula from GlaxoSmithKline 2005; assumes V_d = 5 L/kg.

BOX 150-7. Calculation Based on Steady-State Digitoxin Concentration*

Case: A toxic 70-year-old man weighing 80 kg has a digitoxin level of 200 ng/mL (therapeutic = 10 to 35 ng/mL)

Dose (in number of vials) = (serum digitoxin concentration × weight in kg) ÷ 1000

= (200 × 80) ÷ 1000

= 16 vials

*Formula from GlaxoSmithKline 2005, V_d = 5 L/kg.

Table 150-2. Age Differences in Digitalis Intoxication

Adult	Pediatric
Toxic at lower levels	Asymptomatic at higher levels
Nausea, fatigue, and visual disturbances most common	Obtundation and vomiting more common than in adults
Tachydysrhythmias as common as blocks and bradydysrhythmias	Bradydysrhythmias and block most common
Allergic reactions to Fab fragments uncommon (<1%)	Allergic reactions extremely rare
V_d less variable (5-7.5 L/kg)	V_d more variable 3.5-6.0 L/kg in premature infants 8.0-16.3 L/kg in infants 2-24 mo

Disposition

All cases of symptomatic digitalis intoxication with hyperkalemia, dysrhythmia, AV block, or significant comorbidity should be admitted to the hospital or the emergency department observation unit for at least 12 hours of continuous cardiac monitoring. Patients with a history of acute ingestion of a large quantity of digoxin should be treated with Fab and admitted to an intensive care unit or coronary care unit until stabilized. All patients treated with antibodies require admission to an intensive care unit or a coronary care unit until their toxicity resolves.

KEY CONCEPTS

- Consider digitalis intoxication in any patient with gastrointestinal or visual disturbance who presents with a new dysrhythmia or conduction disturbance.
- Dose digitalis Fab antibody fragments by body load of digitalis, not by body weight of patient.
- Use digitalis antibodies before pacing or other antidysrhythmic drugs, which may unnecessarily complicate treatment.
- Avoid treatment of hyperkalemia in digitalis toxicity with calcium, but other traditional hyperkalemia treatments can be used while obtaining Fab.

β-ADRENERGIC BLOCKERS

Perspective

β-Adrenergic blocking drugs became widely used in Europe in the 1960s for treatment of dysrhythmias. Their antihypertensive effects were later appreciated, and by the 1970s they were one of the most widely prescribed classes of drugs in the United States. Their use continues to expand as more applications are discovered. Current indications include supraventricular dysrhythmias, hypertension, angina, thyrotoxicosis, migraine, and glaucoma. Overdose of propranolol causes the most deaths, followed by acebutolol, oxprenolol, and alprenolol.[21]

Principles of Disease

Pathophysiology

β-blockers structurally resemble isoproterenol, a pure β-agonist. They competitively inhibit endogenous catecholamines such as epinephrine at the β-receptor. Catecholamine stimulation of β-receptors results in the activation of adenyl cyclase, converting adenosine monophosphate (AMP) to cyclic AMP, which augments myocardial contraction (inotropy), enhances cardiac conduction (dromotropy), and accelerates heart rate (chronotropy). These are all β_1 effects. Complex β_2 effects include vascular (smooth muscle relaxation and vasodilation), liver (glycogenolysis, gluconeogenesis), lungs (bronchodilation), adipose tissue (release of free fatty acids), and uterus (smooth muscle relaxation) effects. Equally important properties, which vary from one β-blocker to another, include cardioselectivity, membrane-stabilizing effect, lipophilicity, and intrinsic sympathomimetic activity (Table 150-3). Although cardioselectivity is lost in overdose, cardioselective β-blockers such as atenolol, metoprolol, and esmolol are associated with a lower mortality rate than propranolol, the oldest β-blocker.

β-Blockers are rapidly absorbed after oral ingestion, and the peak effect of normal-release preparations occurs in 1 to 4 hours.[22] Hepatic metabolism on first pass results in significantly less bioavailability than with intravenous injection (1:40 for propranolol). Volume of distribution for various β-blockers generally exceeds 1 L/kg, meaning tissue concentrations exceed those of serum. Therefore, hemodialysis is not efficacious for most β-blockers. Protein binding varies from 0% for sotalol to 93% for propranolol. Elimination half-lives vary from 8 to 9 minutes for esmolol to as long as 24 hours for nadolol and others (see Table 150-3).

Table 150-3. Selected Characteristics of Common β-Blockers

	V_d (L/kg)	ISA	Lipophilic	Elimination Half-life (hr)	Protein Binding (%)	MSE	Comments
Nonselective β Blockers							
Propranolol	4		+	4	93	+	Most fatalities
Nadolol	1.9			10-20	20		Dialyzable
Timolol	1.4-3.5		+	3-5	10		Dialyzable
Pindolol	3-6	+	+	3-4	51	+	
Labetalol	10			4-6	50	+	α Blockade also
Oxprenolol	1.3	+	+	2	78	+	
Sotalol	1.6-2.4		+	7-18	0		Class III and class II antidysrhythmic; torsades de pointes; dialyzable
Carvedilol	1.5-2		+	6-10	95		
Selective β Blockers							
Metoprolol	5.5		+	3-4	12		
Atenolol	0.7			5-8	5		Dialyzable
Esmolol	2			0.13	55		
Acebutolol	1.2	+	+	2-4	26	+	QT prolongation, VT
Practolol	1.6	+	+	10-11			
Bisoprolol	2.9			10-12	30		
Betaxolol	5-13			12-22	55		

ISA, intrinsic sympathomimetic activity; MSE, membrane-stabilizing effect; V_d, volume of distribution; VT, ventricular tachycardia.

BOX 150-8. Manifestations and Complications of β-Blocker Overdose in Order of Decreasing Frequency*

1. Bradycardia (65/90 cases)
2. Hypotension (64/90)
3. Unconsciousness (50/90)
4. Respiratory arrest or insufficiency (34/90)
5. Hypoglycemia (uncommon in adults)
6. Seizures (common only with propranolol, 16/90)
7. Symptomatic bronchospasm (uncommon)
8. VT or VF (6/90)
9. Mild hyperkalemia (uncommon)
10. Hepatotoxicity, mesenteric ischemia, renal failure (rare or single case reports)

VF, ventricular fibrillation; VT, ventricular tachycardia.
Intoxication with beta-sympatholytics.

Clinical Features

The most common initial sign remains bradycardia, which should draw attention to the possibility of cardiac drug overdose. Hypotension and unconsciousness are the second and third most common signs (Box 150-8). Unlike with digitalis, tachydysrhythmias, especially ventricular tachycardia and ventricular fibrillation, are rare. Much of propranolol's toxicity derives from its lipophilic nature and membrane-stabilizing effect that allow it to penetrate the CNS, leading to obtundation, respiratory depression, and seizures. Other β-blockers do not have these effects. Seizures probably result from a combination of hypotension, hypoglycemia, hypoxia, and direct CNS toxicity. Surprisingly, bronchospasm has not been problematic in cases of β-blocker overdose, even with nonselective β-blockers. The few cases of symptomatic bronchospasm respond to the usual bronchodilator nebulizations.

Propranolol's membrane-stabilizing (or quinidine-like) effect impairs SA and AV node function and leads to bradycardia and AV block. Ventricular conduction is also depressed, leading to QRS widening and occasional ventricular dysrhythmias.[23] Nadolol and acebutolol also have a significant membrane-stabilizing effect. These β-blockers, like the tricyclic antidepressants, can cause ventricular dysrhythmias such as ventricular tachycardia, ventricular fibrillation, and torsades de pointes as well as the bradydysrhythmias more characteristic of β-blockers in general. The intrinsic sympathomimetic activity of some β-blockers such as pindolol and carteolol has led to some unusual presentations such as sinus tachycardia instead of bradycardia and ventricular dysrhythmias. Labetalol is unique in that it also blocks α-adrenergic receptors, yielding an additional mechanism for hypotension. However, labetalol's β blockade is three to seven times more potent than its α blockade.[24] In contrast to digitalis, β-blocker toxicity has a more rapid onset: life-threatening CNS and cardiovascular effects can occur 30 minutes after oral overdose. Patients ingesting delayed-release preparations may remain asymptomatic for several hours, affording a valuable therapeutic window.

Diagnostic Strategies

Blood levels of β-blockers correlate poorly with severity of intoxication and are not readily available or clinically useful. Most urine toxicology screens do not identify antidysrhythmic drugs and are not helpful.[25] Hypoglycemia is common in children, and bedside glucose determination should be done with obtundation. Known access of the patient to a β-blocker and consistent clinical features such as obtundation, seizures, bradydysrhythmias, and occasionally tachydysrhythmias should lead the clinician to consider β-blocker intoxication.

Differential Considerations

The combination of bradycardia and hypotension suggests β blockade or calcium channel blockade. Without a history of β-blocker ingestion, the diagnosis can be challenging, especially when noncardiac effects such as CNS depression and seizures predominate. The differential diagnosis includes sedative-hypnotic drug overdose, hypoglycemic drug ingestion, opiate overdose, CNS injury or infection, endocrine-metabolic disorder, sepsis, and acute myocardial infarction.

Management

Immediate measures include intravenous fluids, supplemental oxygen, and monitoring rhythm and respirations. Activated charcoal has been recommended in the first hour after overdose, but its benefit is not proven. Although multiple-dose charcoal (0.5 g/kg every 4 hours) has been recommended for β-blockers that undergo enterohepatic or enteroenteric circulation, there is no evidence to support its use. Similarly, whole-bowel irrigation has been advocated with a polyethylene glycol solution (OCL, GoLytely, CoLyte), administered orally or per nasogastric tube at 1 to 2 L/hr in adults or 20 mL/kg initially in children, but evidence for improved outcome is similarly lacking. Onset of toxicity is so uniformly early that absence of symptoms 4 hours after ingestion implies a low risk for subsequent morbidity unless a delayed-release preparation is involved.

Hypotension, Bradycardia, and Atrioventricular Block

Because bradycardia and heart block are usually attended by hypotension, catecholamines with chronotropic and dromotropic as well as inotropic and vasopressor effects should be chosen. Although therapeutic doses of β-blockers may exacerbate Raynaud's phenomenon through an unopposed α effect, extreme peripheral vasodilation is the rule in cases of overdose. It is uncommon for one catecholamine to be equally effective against all four toxic effects, so combinations of drugs are often used in severe cases.

The first step in the treatment of β-blocker overdose is bolus administration of atropine, glucagon, and crystalloid fluids. A dose of atropine may quickly wear off or be ineffective, so infusion of more potent drugs or cardiac pacing is usually necessary. Atropine (0.5 mg for adults, 0.02 mg/kg for children, minimum 0.10 mg) should be given before vagal stimuli such as tracheal or gastric intubation. Glucagon, which does not depend on β-receptors for its action, has both inotropic and chronotropic effects.[26] Furthermore, it helps to counteract the hypoglycemia induced by β-blocker overdose. Glucagon is given as a 5- to 10-mg intravenous bolus. Because of its short 20-minute half-life, an infusion of 2 to 5 mg/hr (or for children, 0.05 to 0.1 mg/kg bolus, then 0.05 to 0.1 mg/kg/hr) should be started immediately after the bolus. With cumulative large doses, glucagon should be diluted in 5% glucose in water for constant infusion.[26] Side effects include nausea, vomiting, mild hyperglycemia, hypokalemia, and allergic reactions. The response to glucagon alone is often inadequate.

Initially, 20 to 40 mL/kg of normal saline or Ringer's lactate solution can be infused and repeated. If hypotension or bradycardia persists, other cardioactive drugs are indicated. A single drug of choice after glucagon has not emerged, but many clinicians favor isoproterenol (isoprenaline in Europe), dopamine, or epinephrine.[27-29] Other catecholamines that have been successfully used include norepinephrine, dobutamine, prenalterol, metaraminol, and phenylephrine. Often, norepinephrine or dopamine is added to β-agonists such as isoproterenol that lack vasopressor activity. Because patients are resistant to these drugs, the initial dose should be high and the infusion rates should be rapidly titrated to effect. A common mistake with catecholamine infusions in cases of β-blocker overdose is to timidly titrate within previously familiar ranges. In the setting of massive β blockade, much higher doses are usually needed, such as isoproterenol up to 200 μg/min.

Phosphodiesterase inhibitors such as aminophylline, amrinone, and milrinone have also been used to treat β-blocker overdose in experimental animals and in humans. Like glucagon, they also help raise intracellular cyclic AMP levels and stimulate contractility.[30,31] Bradycardia usually responds to glucagon and high-dose catecholamine infusions, but refractory cases may respond to an external or transvenous pacemaker.

Calcium

Because deleterious effects on calcium transport may contribute to β-blocker toxicity, intravenous calcium salts have been suggested for treating hypotension.[32,33] In animals, hypercalcemia as well as hypocalcemia can inhibit the action of glucagon,[34] and until more is known, calcium should be given cautiously and less aggressively than for cases of calcium channel blocker overdose. Constant infusions are safer than boluses. Give 1 to 2 grams over 5 to 10 minutes, monitoring closely for effect.

Ventricular Dysrhythmias

Although uncharacteristic, ventricular tachydysrhythmias do occur sometimes. Cardioversion and defibrillation are indicated for ventricular tachycardia and ventricular fibrillation, respectively, following American Heart Association guidelines. Pulsatile ventricular tachycardia or frequent ventricular ectopy can most safely be treated with lidocaine. Other antidysrhythmic drugs, especially of class IA and IC, should be avoided because they may potentiate AV block or be prodysrhythmic because of an additive membrane stabilizing effect. Sotalol, unlike other β-blockers, has class III as well as class II effects; that is, it prolongs the QT interval and can cause torsades de pointes and other ventricular dysrhythmias. Overdrive pacing with isoproterenol or a pacemaker and magnesium sulfate are specific therapies for torsades de pointes.

Extracorporeal Elimination and Circulatory Assistance

Hemodialysis or hemoperfusion may be beneficial for β-blockers with lower V_d, lower protein binding, and greater hydrophilicity: atenolol, nadolol, sotalol, and timolol.[35]

Unlike other overdoses such as acetaminophen and iron, cardiovascular drugs do not destroy tissue, and if circulation can be supported, complete recovery can be expected. An intra-aortic balloon pump or cardiopulmonary bypass can be lifesaving in cases of refractory hypotension.[36,37] The relatively short half-lives (hours rather than days) of β-blocking and calcium-blocking drugs fall within the temporal range of such interventions. To be successful, such heroic measures must be taken before prolonged hypotension leads to multiorgan ischemic injury (Box 150-9). Because most patients recover from most overdoses, these expensive and invasive interventions should be reserved for drugs and circumstances associated with higher rates of mortality, such as propranolol, verapamil, and mixed cardiotoxic overdoses.

BOX 150-9. Treatment of β-Blocker Poisoning

Phase I (Resuscitation)
Boluses of atropine, glucagon, fluids

Phase II (Stabilization)
Infusions of
- Glucagon
- Catecholamines (epinephrine, norepinephrine, isoproterenol, dobutamine, dopamine, metaraminol)
- Phosphodiesterase inhibitors (amrinone)

Early cardiac pacing if no prompt response to chronotropic or dromotropic drugs
Peripheral arterial and pulmonary artery catheter monitoring if refractory hypotension
Consider hemodialysis of hydrophilic β-blockers with low protein binding and low V_d

V_d, volume of distribution.

Pediatric Considerations

Compared with adult cases, pediatric poisonings are rare. In the cases reported, CNS, cardiac, and metabolic toxicities are similar.[38] However, symptomatic hypoglycemia is much more common in children, especially in those who have been fasting, and occurs even after therapeutic doses. Therefore, serum glucose concentration should be measured in children. Risk factors include young age, fasting state, and diabetes mellitus. Obtunded children should receive empiric glucose, 1 to 2 mL/kg of 25% glucose IV. Generally, 5% glucose infusions have been sufficient to maintain euglycemia, especially with concomitant use of glucagon and catecholamines, which stimulate glucose release. Because glycogen mobilization is a β_2 effect, hypoglycemia may be less common with the cardioselective (β_1) blockers.

Seizures also occur in cases of pediatric β-blocker overdose, but hypoglycemia is probably an important contributing factor. They are more common with the lipid-soluble β-blockers propranolol and oxprenolol. Diazepam is effective.[21]

Children generally fare well after β-blocker ingestion. Belson and colleagues[38] reported symptoms in only 8 of 378 (2%) potential β-blocker exposures in children.

Disposition

Most patients who remain completely asymptomatic for 6 hours after an oral overdose of normal-release preparations can be safely triaged to psychiatry evaluation, with medical consultation for the first 24 hours. Patients ingesting sustained-release preparations should be admitted to a medical or toxicology service, but those who remain asymptomatic 8 hours after ingestion are very unlikely to develop toxicity. Those who have been hypotensive, who have more than first-degree heart block, or who have hemodynamically significant dysrhythmias should be admitted to the intensive care unit.

KEY CONCEPTS

- β-Blocker intoxication usually causes AV block and bradydysrhythmias.
- Noncardiac symptoms such as obtundation, seizures, and hypoglycemia may predominate, especially early in the course and particularly with propranolol.
- Volume expansion, atropine, and glucagon are early measures used to restore normal heart rate and cardiac output.

CALCIUM CHANNEL BLOCKERS

Perspective

Verapamil and nifedipine, the earliest calcium channel antagonists, were introduced in Europe in the 1970s and in the United States in the early 1980s. Calcium antagonists have found many clinical applications: angina pectoris, hypertension, supraventricular dysrhythmias, hypertrophic cardiomyopathy, and migraine prophylaxis. Over the last several years, more than 2000 cases of poisoning have been reported annually to American poison centers. Most fatalities occur with verapamil, but severe toxicity and death have been reported for most drugs of this class.

Pathophysiology

Calcium channel antagonists block the slow calcium channels in the myocardium and vascular smooth muscle, leading to coronary and peripheral vasodilation. They also reduce cardiac contractility, depress SA nodal activity, and slow AV conduction. In cases of overdose, verapamil has the deadliest profile, combining severe myocardial depression and peripheral vasodilation. Both verapamil and diltiazem act on the heart and blood vessels, whereas nifedipine causes primarily vasodilation. As with β-blockers, selectivity is lost in cases of overdose, and toxicity is fourfold, with negative effects on inotropy, chronotropy, dromotropy, and vasotropy.

All calcium channel blockers are rapidly absorbed, although first-pass hepatic metabolism significantly reduces bioavailability (Table 150-4). Onset of action and toxicity ranges from less than 30 minutes to 60 minutes, which has important implications for therapy. Peak effect of nifedipine can occur as early as 20 minutes after ingestion, but peak effect of sustained-release verapamil can be delayed for many hours. High protein binding and V_d greater than 1 to 2 L/kg make hemodialysis or hemoperfusion ineffective. Fortunately (except with sustained-release preparations), their half-lives are relatively short, limiting toxicity to 24 to 36 hours.

Clinical Features

Severe calcium antagonism eventually affects multiple organ systems, but cardiovascular toxicity is primarily responsible for morbidity and mortality. Hypotension and bradycardia occur early, and other rhythm disturbances include AV block of all degrees, sinus arrest, AV dissociation, junctional rhythm, and asystole. Nifedipine overdose more commonly causes reflex sinus tachycardia from peripheral vasodilation. Calcium channel blockade has little effect on ventricular conduction, so QRS widening is not seen early on. Ventricular dysrhythmias are also uncommon except with bepridil, which has class I antidysrhythmic properties. This drug prolongs the QT interval in a dose-related fashion, and intervals greater than 520 msec are associated with increased risk of ventricular tachycardia, especially torsades de pointes (Box 150-10).

Diagnostic Strategies

Serum levels of calcium antagonists are not readily available, nor will urine toxicology screens reliably detect this class of drugs. Blood samples should be obtained for measurement of glucose and electrolytes (including calcium and magnesium). Hyperglycemia secondary to insulin inhibition occurs occasionally, but the elevation is usually mild (150 to 300 mg/L), is

Table 150-4. Selected Characteristics of Some Calcium Channel Blockers

	V_d (L/kg)	Half-life (hr)	Protein Binding (%)	Comments
Verapamil	4	3-12	90	Most fatalities; impairs contractility and cardiac conduction more than most other calcium antagonists
Diltiazem	1.7-5.3	3-7.9	70-80	Suppression of atrioventricular node similar to verapamil; myocardial depression otherwise less
Nifedipine	1.4-2.2	1-5	92-98	Vasodilation greatest effect
Nicardipine	0.64	8-9	95	Vasodilation
Nimodipine	0.94-2.3	1-2	95	No reports of oral overdosage (2005 *PDR*)
Amlodipine	21	30-50	98	Vasodilation
Bepridil	8	33-42	99	Class I as well as class IV antidysrhythmic; prolongs QT: torsade de pointes
Felodipine	10	10	99	Vasodilation
Isradipine	3	1.9-16	95	Vasodilation
Nisoldipine	4-5	7-12	99	Vasodilation

V_d, volume of distribution.

BOX 150-10. Manifestations and Complications of Calcium Channel Blocker Poisoning

Cardiovascular: hypotension, sinus bradycardia, sinus arrest, AV block, AV dissociation, junctional rhythm, asystole; ventricular dysrhythmias uncommon except with bepridil
Pulmonary: respiratory depression, apnea; pulmonary edema; adult respiratory distress syndrome
Gastrointestinal: nausea, vomiting, bowel infarction (rare)
Neurologic: lethargy, confusion, slurred speech, coma; seizures (uncommon); cerebral infarction (rare)
Metabolic: metabolic (lactic) acidosis; hyperglycemia (mild); hyperkalemia (mild)
Dermatologic: flushing, diaphoresis, pallor, peripheral cyanosis

AV, atrioventricular.

usually short lived (less than 24 hours), and generally requires no treatment.[39] A metabolic (lactic) acidosis is often observed with hypotension and hypoperfusion.

An electrocardiogram should be promptly obtained, with special attention to atrial and ventricular rates and PR, QRS, and QT intervals. A prolonged QRS or QT interval suggests bepridil or a co-ingested cardiac toxin such as a tricyclic antidepressant.

Differential Considerations

Differential diagnosis is similar to that of β-blocker cases. Until characteristic rhythm disturbances supervene, many other toxic, metabolic, traumatic, and cardiovascular disorders are considered. Like the β-blockers, calcium antagonists cause early toxicity, and symptoms can be expected within 6 hours of ingestion of normal-release preparations.[40] Toxicity can be delayed 12 to 24 hours with sustained-release preparations.

As with β-blockade, CNS-depressive effects are common and include lethargy, confusion, and coma. Unlike β-blockers, calcium antagonists seldom induce seizures. Pulmonary effects include noncardiogenic pulmonary edema. Apnea can also occur. As with digitalis and β-blocker overdose, nausea and vomiting are common.

Management

Initial management includes rapid establishment of vascular access, supplemental oxygen, cardiac monitoring, and frequent blood pressure measurement. Because of the rapid onset of toxicity with normal-release preparations, induction of emesis is dangerous and contraindicated. Vomiting is a powerful vagal stimulus that can exacerbate bradycardia and heart block. Gastric emptying or activated charcoal are similarly of no benefit because of the rapid absorption of these drugs.

Hypotension and Bradycardia

Hypotension can be caused by myocardial depression, inadequate heart rate, or peripheral vasodilation. Atropine can be administered in the usual American Heart Association's recommended doses (0.5 to 1 mg, up to 3 mg for adults, and 0.02 mg/kg for children, minimum 0.1 mg). Atropine's effect has often been disappointing and short-lived, and multiple doses risk anticholinergic poisoning.[41] If symptomatic bradycardia or heart block persists, the next step is a pacemaker or chronotrope such as isoproterenol. A bolus of crystalloid fluid, 20 mL/kg or more, should also be infused early. Intravenous calcium salts have traditionally been given to most patients. Their effect on contractility is considerable, but their effect on bradycardia, AV block, and peripheral vasodilation is often poor. The optimal dose of calcium is unknown. A reasonable dose is 6 g of calcium chloride, but some practitioners advocate aggressive calcium infusions, administering up to 30 g and raising the total serum calcium level to as high as 23.8 mg/dL.[42] Adverse effects of hypercalcemia include lethargy, coma, anorexia, nausea, vomiting, pancreatitis, polyuria, dehydration, and nephrocalcinosis. Most of these effects have been reported after weeks or months of hypercalcemia from malignancy or hyperparathyroidism. It is doubtful that hours or days of acutely induced hypercalcemia would be detrimental in the setting of massive calcium channel blockade. However, with *rapid* intravenous injection in animals and humans, bradycardia, AV block, AV dissociation, junctional tachycardia, ventricular ectopy, and ventricular fibrillation have been reported.[43] Extravasation of calcium salts can cause severe tissue necrosis. Administration through a central venous catheter is safer than through a peripheral intravenous line. Infiltration of calcium gluconate is less destructive than calcium chloride, but larger doses are necessary because it provides fewer calcium ions.

It is prudent to raise the total serum calcium level no higher than 14 mg/dL, which the endocrine and oncology literature define as the threshold of "severe" hypercalcemia. If ionized calcium levels are followed, it is probably wise not to exceed twice-normal levels. Adults should receive 10 to 20 mL of 10% calcium chloride slowly over 5 to 10 minutes, followed by a constant infusion of 5 to 10 mL/hr. Children can receive 10 to 30 mg/kg (0.1 to 0.3 mL/kg) of 10% CaCl initially. The serum calcium level can be as high as 18.2 mg/dL within 15 minutes after a bolus of just 5 mL of 10% CaCl, so levels should be measured later during the constant infusion.

As with β-blocker poisoning, a monotherapeutic approach will probably succeed only for trivial overdoses. Most severely poisoned patients will require addition of catecholamines to accelerate the heart rate (chronotropy), enhance AV conduction (dromotropy), and restore tone to peripheral vessels (vasotropy). Most experience and success have been reported with isoproterenol and dopamine, often in combination.[41] Isoproterenol infusion can begin at 2 to 10 μg/min (0.1 μg/kg/min in children), but much higher rates may be needed. Unlike β-blocker overdose, however, the β-adrenergic receptor remains intact, and lower catecholamine infusion rates have generally been effective (e.g., dopamine 5 to 30 μg/kg/min). Epinephrine, norepinephrine, and dobutamine have also led to successful outcomes.[44] Isoproterenol or dobutamine alone may not reverse or may even exacerbate peripheral vasodilation; therefore, it is logical to add a vasopressor such as norepinephrine, metaraminol, phenylephrine, or high-dose dopamine.

Glucagon has also been used for its inotropic and chronotropic effects, in doses similar to those advocated for β-blocker poisoning. Bailey recently reviewed 30 controlled animal studies (no controlled human studies exist) of glucagon use in β-blocker and calcium channel blocker overdose.[26] The results were somewhat disappointing: although it possibly increased cardiac out-put in β-blocker overdose, its effect on survival was unclear; it increased heart rate and cardiac output in calcium antagonist overdose in animals, but it did not increase mean arterial pressure and appeared to have no effect on survival.

Insulin (0.5 to 1 μ/kg/hr) infusion has demonstrated efficacy in both animal trials and human cases.[45,46] Glucose is infused concurrently to maintain serum glucose at 100 mg/dL (usually 10 to 30 g/hr). Insulin euglycemia is thought to act by improving myocardial carbohydrate metabolism. Finally, phosphodiesterase inhibitors such as amrinone (5 μg/kg/min) have been used to treat both calcium antagonist and β-blocker poisoning.[47]

If hypotension persists despite the preceding interventions, peripheral arterial and pulmonary arterial catheters should be inserted to precisely measure and coordinate effects on blood pressure, pulmonary capillary wedge pressure, cardiac output, and peripheral resistance. Without such measurements, the clinician risks overtreatment with fluid and undertreatment with pressors, which may be needed in doses hitherto not encountered. As long as dysrhythmias are not aroused, cardiotonic infusions should be aggressively titrated to effect (Box 150-11).

BOX 150-11. Treatment of Calcium Channel Blocker Intoxication

Phase 1
Boluses of atropine, calcium, fluids

Phase 2
Catecholamine infusions
Calcium infusion
Insulin glucose infusion
Glucagon infusion
Phosphodiesterase infusion
Transcutaneous or transvenous cardiac pacing
Invasive monitoring

Phase 3
Consider intra-aortic balloon counterpulsation, cardiac bypass

Pediatric Considerations

Nifedipine, and probably other drugs in its class, joins the short list of medications that can kill a child with ingestion of a single tablet.[48,49] Seizures may be more common in children than adults and should be treated with diazepam, lorazepam, or calcium. Recommendations for CaCl administration in children range from 10 to 30 mg/kg (0.1 to 0.3 mL/kg of 10% CaCl) over 5 to 10 minutes, followed by an infusion.

Overall, death following calcium antagonist ingestion in children is uncommon. French poison centers reported 51 cases of pediatric diltiazem ingestion over 10 years without a single fatality.[50] The intravenous route of administration, as with digitalis, is much more dangerous. Even therapeutic doses of intravenous verapamil are considered contraindicated in infants with supraventricular tachycardia because of case reports of cardiovascular collapse and cardiac arrest after injection.[51]

Hyperglycemia occasionally occurs in children, but the elevation is usually short lived. Although insulin has been administered in a handful of cases, it is generally not necessary, because the hyperglycemia usually resolves spontaneously within 24 to 36 hours.

A small number of children in refractory shock secondary to drug toxicity have been treated with intra-aortic balloon counterpulsation or cardiac bypass. The common thread is a toxin with a reasonably short half-life that, although lethal, does not directly cause irreversible tissue damage. Circulatory support during the day or two required for hepatic or renal elimination of the drug is potentially beneficial. However, expense, invasiveness, and complications restrict its application.

In summary, aside from the differences previously noted, the presentation in children is similar to the presentation in adults: rapid onset of toxicity with CNS depression, bradydysrhythmias, hypotension, and metabolic acidosis.

Disposition

Because the peak effect of normal-release calcium channel blockers commonly occurs in 90 minutes to 6 hours, patients who are totally asymptomatic for 6 hours after an ingestion can be safely discharged according to psychiatric needs. Symptomatic patients or those who ingested delayed-release preparations should be admitted to a medical or toxicology service for at least 24 hours of continuous cardiac monitoring.

KEY CONCEPTS

- Signs and symptoms of calcium channel blocker intoxication occur early after overdose.
- CNS depression is common; seizures are not.
- AV block and bradydysrhythmias predominate, except with bepridil.
- Volume expansion, calcium, and vasopressors have been the mainstays of treatment, but insulin-glucose infusion probably offers the most therapeutic benefit in cases of severe intoxication.

REFERENCES

1. Rush B: *Medical Enquiries and Observations.* Philadelphia, T Dobson, 1797.
2. Bedell SE, et al: Incidence and characteristics of preventable iatrogenic cardiac arrests. *JAMA* 265:2815, 1991.
3. Reza MJ, et al: Massive intravenous digoxin overdose. *N Engl J Med* 291:771, 1974.
4. French JH, et al: Magnesium therapy in massive digoxin intoxication. *Ann Emerg Med* 13:562, 1984.
5. Wells TG, Young RA, Kearns GL: Age-related differences in digoxin toxicity and its treatment. *Drug Saf* 7:135, 1992.
6. Hardman JG, Limbird LE (eds): *Goodman and Gilman's The Pharmacological Basis Of Therapeutics,* 10th ed. New York, McGraw-Hill, 2001.
7. Ordog GJ, et al: Serum digoxin levels and mortality in 5,100 patients. *Ann Emerg Med* 16:32, 1987.
8. Lewander WJ, et al: Acute pediatric digoxin ingestion: A ten-year experience. *Am J Dis Child* 140:770, 1986.
9. Smith TW, Haber E: Digoxin intoxication: The relationship of clinical presentation to serum digoxin concentration. *J Clin Invest* 49:2377, 1970.
10. Piergies AA, Worwag EM, Atkinson AJ: Pharmacoepidemiology and drug utilization: A concurrent audit of high digoxin levels. *Clin Pharmacol Ther* 55:353, 1994.
11. Lilley B, Nolan T, Tibballs J (eds): *Paediatric Pharmacopoeia.* Melbourne, Australia, Royal Children's Hospital, 1989.
12. Taboulet P, et al: Acute digitalis intoxication: Is pacing still appropriate? *Clin Toxicol* 31:261, 1993.
13. Hazinski MF, Cummins RO, Field JM (eds): *Handbook of Emergency Cardiovascular Care for Healthcare Providers.* Dallas, American Heart Association, 2002.
14. Smolarz A, Abshagen U: Digitalis-antikörper-fragmente (Fab) bei 90 schweren Glykosidvergiftungen: Klinische Erfahrungen aus einer multizentrischen Studie. *Herz/Kreislauf* 6:261, 1986.
15. Antman EM, et al: Treatment of 150 cases of life-threatening digitalis intoxication with digoxin-specific Fab antibody fragments: Final report of a multicenter study. *Circulation* 81:1744, 1990.
16. Hickey AR, et al: Digoxin immune Fab therapy in the management of digitalis intoxication: Safety and efficacy results of an observational surveillance study. *J Am Coll Cardiol* 17:590, 1991.
17. Kirkpatrick CH: The Digibind study advisory panel: Allergic histories and reactions of patients treated with digoxin immune Fab (ovine) antibody. *Am J Emerg Med* 9:7, 1991.
18. Schaumann B, et al: Kinetics of the Fab fragments of digoxin antibodies and of bound digoxin in patients with severe digoxin intoxication. *Eur J Clin Pharmacol* 30:527, 1986.
19. Schneider AP II, Nelson DJ, Brown DD: In-hospital cardiopulmonary resuscitation: A 30-year review. *J Am Board Fam Pract* 6:91, 1993.
20. Woolf AD, et al. The use of digoxin-specific Fab fragments for severe digitalis intoxication in children. *N Engl J Med* 326:1739, 1992.
21. Langemeijer JJM, et al: Intoxication with beta-sympatholytics. *Neth J Med* 40:308, 1992.
22. Weinstein RS, et al: Beta-blocker overdose with propranolol and with atenolol. *Ann Emerg Med* 14:161, 1985.
23. Kenyon CJ, et al: Successful resuscitation using external cardiac pacing in beta-adrenergic antagonist-induced bradyasystolic arrest. *Ann Emerg Med* 17:711, 1988.
24. Louis WJ, McNeil JJ, Drummer OH: The pharmacology of combined alpha-beta blockade I. *Drugs* 28:16, 1984.
25. Maurer JJ: Identification of antiarrhythmic drugs and their metabolites in urine. *Arch Toxicol* 64:218, 1990.
26. Bailey B: Glucagon in β-blocker and calcium channel blocker overdoses: A systematic review. *J Toxicol Clin Toxicol* 41:595, 2003.
27. Taboulet P, et al: Pathophysiology and management of self-poisoning with beta-blockers. *Clin Toxicol* 31:531, 1993.
28. Strubelt O: Evaluation of antidotes against the acute cardiovascular toxicity of propranolol. *Toxicology* 31:261, 1984.
29. Hicks PR, Rankin PN: Massive adrenaline doses in labetalol overdose. *Anaesth Intensive Care* 19:447, 1991.
30. Sato Tsuji, Okubo N, Naito H: Milrinone versus glucagon: Comparative hemodynamic effects in canine propranolol poisoning. *Clin Toxicol* 32:277, 1994.
31. Love JN, et al: A comparison of amrinone and glucagon therapy for cardiovascular depression associated with propranolol toxicity in a canine model. *Clin Toxicol* 30:399, 1992.
32. Kerns W, et al: Mechanism of propranolol cardiotoxicity. *Vet Hum Toxicol* 36:347, 1994.
33. Brimacombe J, Scully M, Swainston R: Propranolol overdose: A dramatic response to calcium salts. *Med J Aust* 155:267, 1991.

34. Chernow B, et al: Glucagon's chronotropic action is calcium dependent. *J Pharm Exp Ther* 241:833, 1987.
35. Saitz R, Williams BW, Farber HW: Atenolol-induced cardiovascular collapse treated with hemodialysis. *Crit Care Med* 19:116, 1991.
36. Lane AS, Woodward AC, Goldman MR: Massive propranolol overdose poorly responsive to pharmacologic therapy: Use of the intraaortic balloon pump. *Ann Emerg Med* 16:1381, 1987.
37. McVey FK, Corke CF: Extracorporeal circulation in the management of massive propranolol overdose. *Anaesthesia* 46:744, 1991.
38. Belson MG, Sullivan K, Geller RJ: Beta-adrenergic antagonist exposures in children. *Vet Hum Toxicol* 43:361, 2003.
39. Ramoska EA, Spiller HA, Myers A: Calcium channel blocker toxicity. *Ann Emerg Med* 19:649, 1990.
40. Ramoska EA, et al: A one-year evaluation of calcium channel blocker overdoses: Toxicity and treatment. *Ann Emerg Med* 22:196, 1993.
41. Erickson FC, et al: Diltiazem overdose: Case report and review. *J Emerg Med* 9:357, 1991.
42. Buckley NA, Whyte IM, Dawson AH: Overdose with calcium channel blockers [letter]. *BMJ* 308:1639, 1994.
43. Chin RL, Garmel GM, Harter PM: Development of ventricular fibrillation after intravenous calcium chloride administration in a patient with supraventricular tachycardia. *Ann Emerg Med* 25:416, 1995.
44. Chimienti M, et al: Acute verapamil poisoning: Successful treatment with epinephrine. *Clin Cardiol* 5:219, 1982.
45. Kline JA, Leonova E, Raymond RM: Beneficial myocardial metabolic effects of insulin during verapamil toxicity in the anesthetized canine. *Crit Care Med* 23:1251, 1995.
46. Yuan TH, et al: Insulin-glucose as adjunctive therapy for severe calcium channel antagonist poisoning. *J Toxicol Clin Toxicol* 37:463, 1999.
47. Wolf LR, Spadafora MP, Otten EJ: Use of amrinone and glucagon in a case of calcium channel blocker overdose. *Ann Emerg Med* 22:1225, 1993.
48. Koren G: Medications which can kill a toddler with one tablet or teaspoonful. *Clin Toxicol* 31:407, 1993.
49. Passal DB, Crespin FH Jr: Verapamil poisoning in an infant. *Pediatrics* 73:543, 1984.
50. Lambert H, Weber M, Renaud D: Intoxications aigues par diltiazem (DTZ). Bilan des Centres Anti-Poisons Français. Travail cooperatif des Centres Anti-Poison Français et de l'A.R.I.T. *J Toxicol Clin Exp* 10:229, 1990.
51. Hazinski MF (ed): *PALS Provider Manual.* Dallas, American Heart Association, 2002.

CHAPTER 151 Caustics

Paul M. Wax and Sandra M. Schneider

PERSPECTIVE

Caustic agents are a diverse group of substances that have the potential to cause tissue burns on contact with the gastrointestinal tract, airway and lungs, eye, and dermis. This chapter discusses oral exposure; dermal exposure is discussed in Chapter 61 and inhalational exposure in Chapter 157. Agents capable of causing chemical injury include alkalis (e.g., NaOH, KOH, NH_3), acids (e.g., HCl, H_2SO_4), and other chemicals, such as phenol, formaldehyde, iodine, and concentrated hydrogen peroxide. Hydrofluoric acid is a relatively weak acid, but it causes necrotizing injury and life-threatening systemic toxicity because fluoride chelates endogenous calcium. In this chapter, *caustic* refers to any agent capable of causing tissue injury on contact. *Lye* refers to hydroxide, usually sodium hydroxide or potassium hydroxide.

In 2002, more than 60,000 caustic exposures were reported to poison centers in the United States.[1] Before 1950, strong lyes (concentration >50%) made up the majority of caustic ingestions in the United States. Ingestion led to respiratory compromise, severe esophageal burns, perforation of the esophagus and stomach, mediastinitis, late stricture, and sometimes death. The first major poison prevention legislation in the United States (Federal Caustic Poison Act, 1927) was directed at decreasing the occurrence of these terrible burn injuries, most of which occurred in children.[2]

Some household liquid drain cleaners continue to have high concentrations of alkali (30% KOH) or acid (93% H_2SO_4) (Table 151-1). Commercial industries, farms (dairy pipeline cleaners containing liquid NaOH and KOH in concentrations of 8% to 25%), and swimming pool chemicals also contain caustics in high concentrations.[3]

Ingestion of crystals and solid particles results in prolonged tissue contact and more severe burns. Fortunately, most crystal lye ingestions are limited by immediate oral pain. The ingestion of granular automatic dishwashing detergents has been associated with devastating injuries.[4] Crystal drain cleaners have lye concentration as high as 74% NaOH and may cause proximal esophageal injury. Liquid dishwashing detergents and laundry detergents have a pH greater than 12, but because the titratable base content is significantly less, there is less risk of injury after ingestion.

Liquid household bleach typically contains dilute (5.25%) sodium hypochlorite (NaHClO), and ingestion rarely causes injury. Industrial strength bleach may contain significantly higher concentrations of sodium hypochlorite, leading to esophageal necrosis. Toilet

Table 151-1. Sampling of Currently Manufactured Household Cleaning Products that Contain Caustic Chemicals

Application	Product (Manufacturer)	Chemical
Drain cleaner—liquid	Heavy Duty Liquid Drain Opener (Share)	H_2SO_4 93%
	Drain Out Extra (Iron Out)	KOH 30%
	Liquid-Plumr (Clorox)	NaOH 0.5-2%, NaOCl 10%
	Maximum Strength Drain Opener (Enforcer)	KOH 5-15%
Drain cleaner—crystals	Crystal Drain Opener (Rohyme)	NaOH 74%
	Crystal Drain Out (Iron Out)	NaOH 55%
	Drano Pipe Cleaner (Johnson)	NaOH 54%
Oven cleaner	Easy Off Heavy Duty Oven Cleaner (Reckitt Benckiser)	NaOH <5%
Rust remover	Rust Stain Remover (Whink)	HF 2.5-3%
	Rust Stripper (Certified)	NaOH 50-75%
	Naval Jelly Rust Remover (Loctite)	Phosphoric acid 25-30%
Toilet bowl cleaner	Instant Power Toilet Bowl Cleaner (Scotch)	HCl 26%
	Bowl and Porcelain Cleaner (Cleanline)	HCl <10%
Swimming pool cleaner	Muriatic Acid, Aqua Chem (Recreational Water)	HCl 31%

bowl cleaners contain hydrochloric acid as high as 26% HCl. General purpose anticorrosive cleaners, such as 31% muriatic acid (HCl), are sold in gallon containers for home use and as swimming pool cleaners.

Hair perm relaxers (sodium hydroxide) can cause facial and oral burns, as well as esophageal burns, if ingested. The alkali powder in air bags has caused ocular burns.[5] Perfumes accidentally sprayed into the eyes can be caustic. Cement is alkaline and causes topical burns, typically on the knees.[6]

More than 70 different pills can cause damage when in contact with esophageal mucus for prolonged periods.[7] Patients who take medications in the supine position, or who take pills without water, are at higher risk. Pills most likely to adhere are doxycycline, tetracycline, potassium chloride, and aspirin. Potassium chloride is particularly dangerous and has caused perforation into the aorta, left atrium, and bronchial artery.[7]

At least 85% of reported caustic ingestions are unintentional.[8] Transfer and storage of cleaners in alternative containers, such as soda bottles and jars, contribute to unintentional ingestion. Contact with the mucosa causes immediate severe pain that usually limits large ingestion; however, a swallowed mouthful may be enough to cause permanent injury. Among suicidal patients who ingest caustic agents, more than half have a history of psychiatric illness.[9]

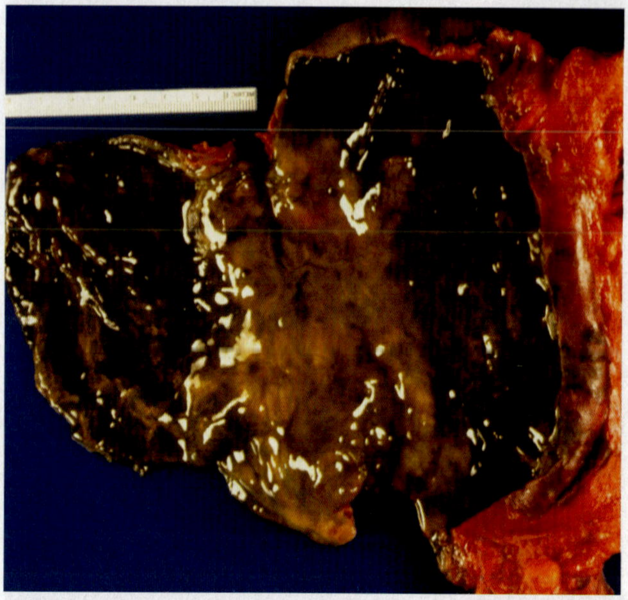

Figure 151-1. Gastric mucosa after ingestion of 35% potassium hydroxide.

PRINCIPLES

Factors that influence the extent of injury from a caustic exposure include type of agent, concentration of solution, volume, viscosity, duration of contact, pH, and presence or absence of food in the stomach. The titratable alkaline reserve of an alkali or acid may be particularly correlative with its propensity to cause burn injury.[10]

When strong acid contacts epithelium, a coagulum or eschar is created, limiting the further spread of the acid. Alkaline contact causes liquefaction necrosis, fat saponification, and protein disruption, allowing further penetrance of the alkaline into the tissue. A concentrations of 30% sodium hydroxide in contact with tissue for 1 second results in a full-thickness burn.[11] The depth of the necrosis is dependent on the concentration of the lye. Acids cause a similar incidence of esophageal and gastric injury and may also cause laryngeal burns. Alkalis may cause gastric necrosis (Figures 151-1 and 151-2) and perforation, as well as small intestine injury and esophageal injury (Figure 151-3).[12,13]

Classically, the damage occurs in four steps. Initially, necrosis occurs, with invasion by bacteria and polymorphonuclear leukocytes. Vascular thrombosis occurs, increasing the damage. Over the next 2 to 5 days, superficial layers of injured tissue begin to slough. The tensile strength of the healing tissue may be quite low for up to 3 weeks following the caustic exposure, greatly increasing the chance of delayed perforation in some cases. Between 1 week and several months, granulation tissue forms, collagen is deposited, and a re-epithelization occurs in the area.

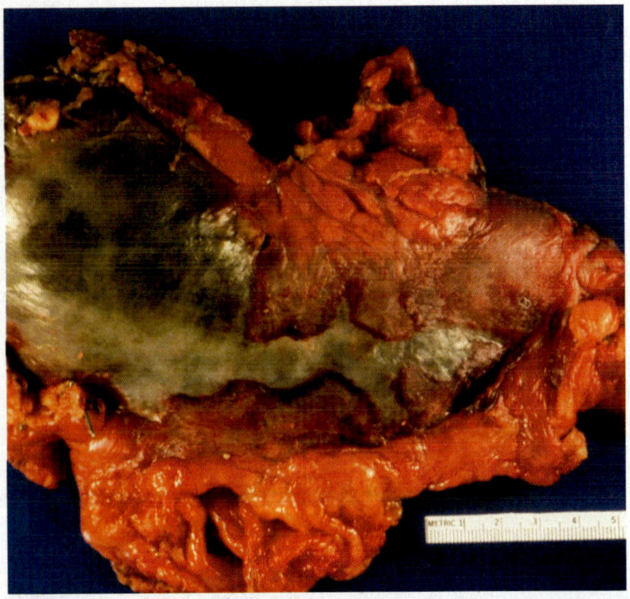

Figure 151-2. Gastric serosa after ingestion of 35% potassium hydroxide.

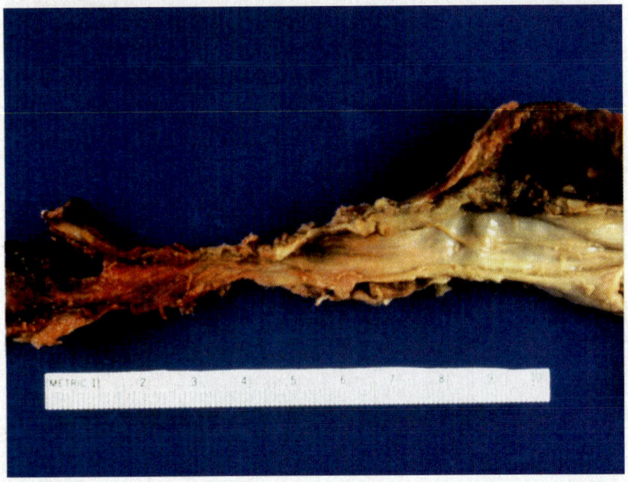

Figure 151-3. Esophagus after ingestion of 35% potassium hydroxide.

Esophageal stricture may form over a period of weeks to years from contraction of the scar.

Caustic injury is categorized as first-, second-, and third-degree, similar to a thermal burn, based on appearance at endoscopy. The initial depth of injury found on esophagoscopy correlates with the risk of stricture formation. First-degree burns (also known as grade 1) consist of edema and hyperemia. Second-degree burns (grade 2) are characterized by superficial ulcers, whitish membranes, exudates, friability, and hemorrhage. Although grade 1 injuries do not progress to stricture, 15% to 30% of all grade 2 burns, and up to 75% of circumferential grade 2 injuries of the esophagus, develop strictures.[14] With full-thickness third-degree burns (grade 3), 90% result in stricture. Whether heat from the exothermic reaction increases the injury has never been quantified, but it has led to concerns regarding initial dilution or gastric lavage.[15,16]

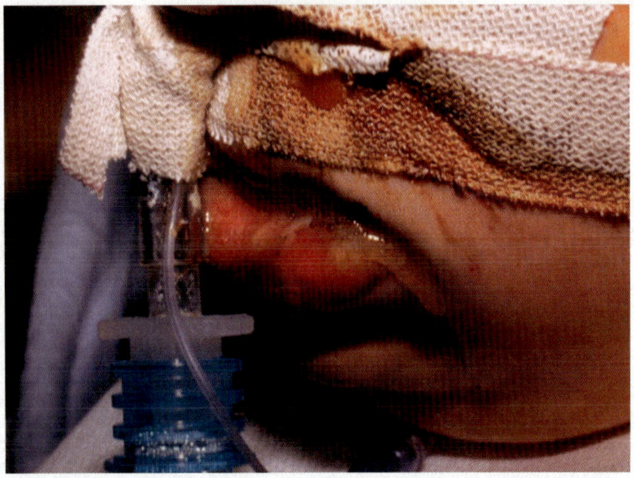

Figure 151-4. Labial burn after exposure to 35% potassium hydroxide.

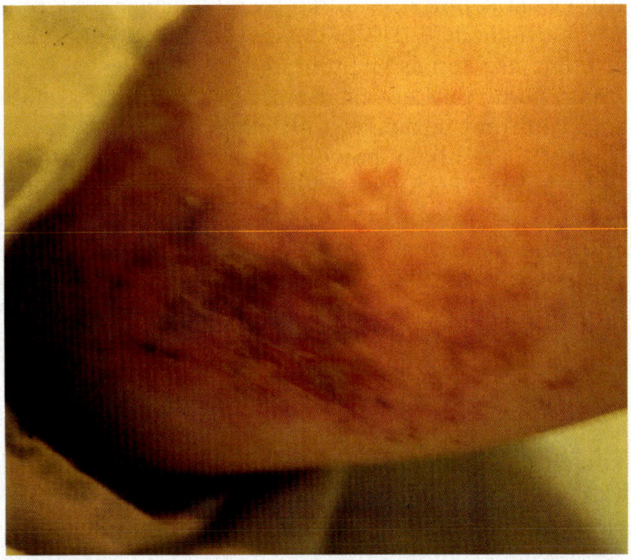

Figure 151-5. Upper arm burn after secondary contamination from vomit after 35% potassium hydroxide ingestion.

CLINICAL FEATURES

Airway edema and esophageal/gastric perforation are the most emergent issues. Laryngeal edema occurs over a matter of minutes to hours. Systemic toxicity, hypovolemic shock, and hemodynamic instability with hypotension, tachycardia, fever, and acidosis are ominous findings. Small ingestions of potent substances can be as serious as larger ingestions. More than 40% of patients reporting to have "only taken a lick" will have esophageal burns.[17] Patients present with oral pain (41%), abdominal pain (34%), vomiting (19%), and drooling (19%).[8] Many patients have wheezing and coughing. Others present with stridor and dysphonia. Chest pain is common. Visible burns to the face, lips, and oral cavity may be seen (Figure 151-4). Skin burns can occur from spillage or secondary contamination after vomiting (Figure 151-5). Peritoneal signs suggest hollow viscous perforation or contiguous extension of the burn injury to adjoining visceral areas. Tracheal necrosis is one of the most frequent causes of death after caustic ingestion.[18]

Studies have presented conflicting data correlating clinical symptoms with the severity of esophageal burns.[8,14,19] Oropharyngeal burns alone do not appear predictive of more distal injury, but prolonged drooling and dysphasia predicted significant lesions with 100% sensitivity and 90% specificity.[20] Vomiting and stridor may also be more predictive of burn injury.

Dysphasia usually subsides in 3 to 4 days. Patients with significant esophageal burns, particularly those that are circumferential, may develop esophageal stricture; 80% of strictures become apparent in 2 to 8 weeks. Symptoms include dysphagia and food impactions. Strictures that become symptomatic early are generally more severe. In one study of 86 adults admitted to the hospital after caustic ingestion, 18 developed complications and 6 died.[9]

Patients have an increase in esophageal cancer (1000-fold to 3000-fold increases) that develops 40 to 50 years after the caustic ingestion.[21] A recent long-term study showed that 1.8% of patients who ingested caustic soda developed esophageal cancer.[22] Nearly 3% of esophageal cancer patients have a history of caustic ingestion.[21]

Significant acid ingestions may also be devastating and result in a higher mortality rate than alkali ingestions. The more fulminant course of some acid ingestions may be due to systemic absorption of the acid, resulting in metabolic acidosis (which may also be the result of extensive tissue necrosis), hemolysis, and renal failure. In Russia, concentrated acetic acid ingestions account for 64% of caustic ingestions.[23]

DIAGNOSTIC STRATEGIES

The goal is to identify the extent and severity of the burn. Patients with chest and abdominal pain should have a chest radiograph and decubitus or upright abdominal studies to identify peritoneal and mediastinal air, denoting perforation or pleural effusion. Any suspicion of abdominal involvement should prompt abdominal computed tomography or ultrasonography.[24] Arterial blood gas determination may be particularly useful after significant acid ingestions to monitor systemic metabolic acidosis. In cases of intentional overdose, co-ingestants should be considered. Hydrofluoric acid exposures, either inhalational, ingestion, or dermal (hand size or larger), require immediate cardiac monitoring to assess for QTc prolongation, torsades de pointes, or other ventricular dysrhythmias. Rapid cardiac deterioration should be expected in these unusual cases.[25] Serum calcium and magnesium levels should also be determined, but empiric intervention with high-dose intravenous calcium chloride may be required for life-threatening dysrhythmias before confirmatory laboratory data are available.

The depth of burns cannot be predicted based on signs or symptoms. Noninvasive techniques (barium swallow) do not gauge the depth of burn injury. Patients with signs and symptoms (vomiting, drooling, stridor, or dyspnea) or intentional ingestion should undergo endoscopy early. Wound softening makes late endoscopy (after 24 hours) more hazardous. A soft feeding tube or silk string can be placed in the esophagus, when burns are present, for future dilation. With the current flexible endoscopes, endoscopy should be continued past the area of burn and into the stomach, if possible.

According to the results of endoscopy, patients can be divided into four groups: no esophageal/gastric injury, gastric injury, linear burns of the esophagus, and circumferential burns.

MANAGEMENT

After a caustic ingestion, little can be done to attenuate the severity of the tissue injury. The most important task is to monitor the patient and intervene as necessary to treat complications, such as perforation. Early endotracheal intubation is warranted when airway compromise is suspected with hoarseness, throat pain, drooling, or edema. Intubation should be undertaken early if significant exposure is suspected, before edema and secretions both threaten the airway and make intubation difficult or impossible. Blind nasotracheal intubation is contraindicated. When oral intubation is anticipated to be difficult or impossible because of edema and anatomic distortion, rapid-sequence intubation should be avoided and awake fiberoptic intubation or primary surgical cricothyrotomy may be necessary. Patients should have intravenous access and vigorous fluid resuscitation. In alert patients who are not vomiting and can tolerate liquids, small volumes (1 to 2 cups) of water or milk can be considered within the first few minutes after ingestion. Because injuries occur almost immediately, later dilution is not warranted. Forcing fluids is never indicated. Emesis induction and activated charcoal administration have no place in the treatment of patients with these ingestions. Gastric and esophageal lavage are not warranted. Careful nasogastric aspiration may be useful in the setting of significant acid ingestions, but given the ominous natural history of many of these ingestion cases and the somewhat lower risk of esophageal perforation, compared with alkali ingestion, consultation with a toxicologist or poison center may be helpful in this situation. The patient's history should be obtained early, including amount and substance ingested, time of ingestion, and presence of suicidal ideation.

Immediate surgical exploration is indicated for free air, peritonitis, increasing and severe chest and abdominal pain, and hypotension. Early and continuous hemodynamic monitoring is essential. The patient should be fully examined for evidence of dermal and ocular caustic exposures. Contaminated clothing should be treated as hazardous waste and disposed of using proper precautions.

Emesis, activated charcoal, and lavage have no place in the treatment of these ingestions. Careful nasogastric aspiration may be useful for significant large-volume acid ingestions, given the ominous outcome of these ingestions and the somewhat lower risk of esophageal perforation.

Corticosteroid therapy remains controversial. Its use has been advocated to potentially prevent stricture formation. Despite the lack of proven efficacy in prospective clinical trials,[26] corticosteroids are still recommended by some authorities in the treatment of circumferential second-degree burn injuries of the esophagus.[27] If steroid treatment is elected, prednisolone 2 mg/kg/day in children or 40 mg three times a day in adults for 14 to 21 days is recommended, followed by a taper. Infectious prophylaxis with antibiotics that treat oral pathogens and anaerobic bacteria (e.g., ampicillin, clindamycin, or piperacillin/tazobactam) should be initiated only if corticosteroid therapy is utilized. Prophylactic antibiotics may potentially mask evidence of impending perforation.

DISPOSITION

Surgical intervention is required in cases of hollow viscous perforation; early exploration may also be warranted in cases of suspected full-thickness burns.[13] Asymptomatic patients can undergo endoscopy in the emergency department or discharged home with close follow-up monitoring. Psychiatric evaluation is indicated in patients with intentional ingestion. Symptomatic patients require admission to the intensive care unit.

SPECIAL CASES

Ocular alkali exposures are true ophthalmologic emergencies. Immediate and aggressive lavage with at least 2 L of normal saline per eye is indicated in all cases except for frank perforation. Management is described in Chapter 70.

Dermal caustic exposures can also result in significant burn injuries (see Chapter 57). Clothing removal, copious irrigation, and local wound debridement are the most important initial treatment measures. Hydrofluoric acid burns warrant special attention. Although this is a relatively weak acid compared with HCl or H_2SO_4, the dissociated fluoride anion is problematic because of its extreme electronegativity. Fluoride avidly binds to cations, such as calcium and magnesium, disrupting cellular function and integrity and resulting in significant necrosis. The hallmark of a hydrofluoric acid dermal burn is pain disproportionate to physical findings. Deaths from hydrofluoric acid exposure have occurred after skin contact with concentrated hydrofluoric acid and after inhalation of hydrofluoric acid vapor.[28] Systemic toxicity is characterized by immediate and profound hypocalcemia and dysrhythmias. Because systemic toxicity from profound hypocalcemia has been seen in cases in which dermal exposure is limited to the face or hands in areas as small as 1% of the body surface area, cardiac monitoring and serum calcium monitoring are warranted except in all but the most limited fingertip exposures. Hemodialysis to remove fluoride may be effective in cases of severe hydrofluoric acid poisoning when the conventional treatment of fluoride-induced cardiotoxicity proves insufficient.[29] Treatment of dermal hydrofluoric acid exposures requires the provision of exogenous cations to chelate the fluoride ions with topical calcium gluconate gel[30] or benzalkonium chloride (Zephiran) until pain relief. Ten grams of powdered calcium gluconate can be mixed with K-Y jelly and placed in a glove with the affected hand. In refractory cases, intradermal injection, intraarterial infusion, or regional intravenous infusions of 10% calcium gluconate solution is recommended.[31] Calcium chloride should be avoided because it causes tissue necrosis if extravasated.

Povidone-iodine (Betadine) is used as a surgical scrub and is not a caustic agent, but ingestion of tincture of iodine can cause severe gastrointestinal injury and is potentially life threatening. Gastric irrigation with starch or milk in these cases may convert iodine to the much less toxic iodide.

Ingestion of phenol or formaldehyde can also cause severe caustic injury to the gastrointestinal tract.[32,33] Both phenol and formaldehyde are general protoplasmic poisons and can cause protein denaturation and coagulation necrosis. Systemic symptoms, including dysrhythmias, hypotension, seizures, and coma, may also result from phenol ingestion. Acidosis may be quite prominent after formaldehyde ingestion with its metabolism to formic acid. Phenol is well absorbed through the skin, and dermal exposure may result in burns and systemic toxicity. Although dermal decontamination of phenol exposures with low-molecular-weight polyethylene glycol has been suggested, irrigation with water may prove just as useful.

Ingestion of concentrated hydrogen peroxide (H_2O_2) may cause gastrointestinal burn injury and the formation of gas emboli.[34] Radiographic evaluation for the presence of gas in the chest or abdominal cavities, including the portal system, should be performed in symptomatic patients or those who ingest concentrated H_2O_2. Hyperbaric oxygen has been used successfully to treat gas emboli from hydrogen peroxide ingestion.[35]

Button (disk) batteries and conventional alkaline cylindrical batteries pose potential obstructive and chemical hazards if ingested. Ingestion of large 25-mm wafer-sized button batteries was a problem in the past. The smaller button batteries of today are less likely to cause esophageal obstruction. Button batteries are usually made of a metallic salt (lithium, mercury, nickel, zinc, cadmium, or silver) bathed in NaOH or KOH. Obstruction can cause pressure necrosis, caustic injury due to leakage of alkaline medium, or electrical injury. Ulceration, perforation, and possible fistula formation occur but are uncommon. Heavy metal absorption can also occur, but clinical heavy metal toxicity in this setting has not been reported.[30]

Evaluation of button battery ingestions requires radiography to assess the position of the foreign body. Batteries lodged in the airway or esophagus require expeditious removal. Gastric or intestinal batteries can be observed.[36] Checking the stool for passage of the batteries is recommended. Follow-up radiographs should be obtained in 1 week if the battery has not passed.

KEY CONCEPTS

- Ingestion of very small amounts of a caustic material (even a lick) can cause serious esophageal injury.
- All symptomatic patients should undergo endoscopy and be considered for admission.
- Asymptomatic patients can undergo endoscopy in the emergency department or be discharged with very close follow-up monitoring.
- Caustic ingestions can lead to esophageal stricture and a lifelong increased risk of esophageal cancer.

REFERENCES

1. Watson WA, et al: 2002 annual report of the American Association of Poison Control Centers Toxic Exposure Surveillance System. *Am J Emerg Med* 21:353, 2003.
2. Boyd A: Chevalier Jackson: The father of American bronchoesophagoscopy. *Ann Thorac Surg* 57:502, 1994.
3. Neidich G: Ingestion of caustic alkali farm products. *J Pediatr Gastroenterol Nutrition* 16:75, 1993.
4. Kynaston JA, et al: The hazards of automatic-dishwasher detergent. *Med J Aust* 151:5, 1989.
5. White JE, et al: Ocular alkali burn associated with automobile air-bag activation. *CMAJ* 153:933, 1995.
6. Spoo J, Elsner P: Cement burns: A review 1960-2000. *Contact Dermatitis* 45:68, 2001.
7. Kikendall JW: Pill-induced esophageal injury. *Gastroenterol Clin North Am* 20:835, 1991.
8. Gorman RL, et al: Initial symptoms as predictors of esophageal injury in alkaline corrosive ingestions. *Am J Emerg Med* 10:189, 1992.
9. Christesen HB: Prediction of complications following caustic ingestion in adults. *Clin Otolaryngol* 20:272, 1995.
10. Hoffman RS, et al: Comparison of titratable acid/alkaline reserve and pH in potentially caustic household products. *J Toxicol Clin Toxicol* 27:241, 1989.
11. Krey H: On the treatment of corrosive lesions in the oesophagus. *Acta Otolaryngol* S102:1, 1952.
12. Zargar SA, et al: Ingestion of corrosive acids: Spectrum of injury to upper gastrointestinal tract and natural history. *Gastroenterology* 97:702, 1989.
13. Thompson JN: Corrosive esophageal injuries. I. A study of nine cases of concurrent accidental caustic ingestion. *Laryngoscope* 97:1060, 1987.
14. Christesen HB: Prediction of complications following unintentional caustic ingestion in children: Is endoscopy always necessary? *Acta Paediatr* 84:1177, 1995.
15. Maull KI, et al: Liquid caustic ingestions: An in vitro study of the effects of buffer, neutralization, and dilution. *Ann Emerg Med* 14:1160, 1985.
16. Homan CS, et al: Thermal characteristics of neutralization therapy and water dilution for strong acid ingestion: An in-vivo canine model. *Acad Emerg Med* 5:286, 1998.
17. Andreoni B, et al: Esophageal perforation and caustic injury: Emergency management of caustic ingestion. *Dis Esophagus* 10:95, 1997.
18. Christesen HB: [Ingestion of caustic agents: Epidemiology, pathogenesis, course, complications and prognosis]. *Ugeskr Laeger* 155:2379, 1993.
19. Gaudreault P, et al: Predictability of esophageal injury from signs and symptoms: A study of caustic ingestion in 378 children. *Pediatrics* 71:767, 1983.
20. Nuutinen M, et al: Consequences of caustic ingestions in children. *Acta Paediatr* 83:1200, 1994.
21. Isolauri J, Markkula H: Lye ingestion and carcinoma of the esophagus. *Acta Chir Scand* 155:269, 1989.
22. Mamede RC, de Mello Filho FV: Ingestion of caustic substances and its complications. *Sao Paulo Med J* 119:10, 2001.
23. Kirichenko AS, Sentzov VG, Wax PM: Caustic ingestions in Russia: A perpetual problem demanding further study. *J Toxicol Clin Toxicol* 35:514, 1997.
24. Guth AA, et al: Combined duodenal and colonic necrosis: An unusual sequela of caustic ingestion [see comment]. *J Clin Gastroenterol* 19:303, 1994.
25. Kao WF, et al: Ingestion of low-concentration hydrofluoric acid: An insidious and potentially fatal poisoning. *Ann Emerg Med* 34:35, 1999.
26. Anderson KD, et al: A controlled trial of corticosteroids in children with corrosive injury of the esophagus [see comment]. *N Engl J Med* 323:637, 1990.
27. Howell JM, et al: Steroids for the treatment of corrosive esophageal injury: A statistical analysis of past studies. *Am J Emerg Med* 10:421, 1992.
28. Blodgett DW, et al: Fatal unintentional occupational poisonings by hydrofluoric acid in the U.S. *Am J Ind Med* 40:215, 2001.
29. Bjornhagen V, et al: Hydrofluoric acid-induced burns and life-threatening systemic poisoning: Favorable outcome after hemodialysis. *J Toxicol Clin Toxicol* 41:855, 2003.
30. Burkhart KK, et al: Comparison of topical magnesium and calcium treatment for dermal hydrofluoric acid burns. *Ann Emerg Med* 24:9, 1994.
31. Graudins A, et al: Regional intravenous infusion of calcium gluconate for hydrofluoric acid burns of the upper extremity [see comment]. *Ann Emerg Med* 30:604, 1997.
32. Horch R, et al: Phenol burns and intoxications. *Burns* 20:45, 1994.
33. Hawley CK, Harsch HH: Gastric outlet obstruction as a late complication of formaldehyde ingestion: A case report. *Am J Gastroenterol* 94:2289, 1999.
34. Humberston CL, et al: Ingestion of 35% hydrogen peroxide. *J Toxicol Clin Toxicol* 28:95, 1990.
35. Mullins ME, Beltran JT: Acute cerebral gas embolism from hydrogen peroxide ingestion successfully treated with hyperbaric oxygen. *J Toxicol Clin Toxicol* 36:253, 1998.
36. Litovitz T, Schmitz BF: Ingestion of cylindrical and button batteries: An analysis of 2382 cases [see comment]. *Pediatrics* 89:747, 1992.

CHAPTER

152 Cocaine and Other Sympathomimetics

Rama B. Rao and Robert S. Hoffman

PERSPECTIVE

Cocaine, a naturally occurring plant-derived alkaloid, has been used for centuries as a medicinal product. In 2000 BC, the leaves of the cocoa plant (*Erythroxylon coca*) were chewed for treatment of various ailments. In 1860, the pure alkaloid form was isolated and became a popular constituent of various beverages, pharmaceuticals, and therapeutic tonics; inclusion of cocaine in U.S. consumer products was banned in 1914. At the peak of the cocaine epidemic in the early 1990s, it was estimated that 5 million people used cocaine regularly in the United States.[1] The drug is still popular, and the consequences of recreational cocaine use are profound. Between 1993 and 1995, 2000 unintentional cocaine-related deaths were reported in New York City.[2] Cocaine also is implicated in violent deaths; the drug was detected in 25% of autopsies of fatal injuries in adults age 15 to 44.[3]

Amphetamines are stimulant agents originally designed for use as decongestants and dietary aids that became popular as recreational drugs in the mid-20th century. Modifications of the amphetamine molecule, or "designer" amphetamines, are inexpensively and illicitly produced. The enhanced clinical effects from these alterations add to the popularity of drugs such as methylenedioxymethamphetamine (MDMA) and methamphetamines. Cocaine, amphetamines, and derivatives of amphetamines are called *sympathomimetics* (Box 152-1). These agents cause central nervous system (CNS) stimulation and a cascade of physiologic effects.

PRINCIPLES OF DISEASE

Pathophysiology of Cocaine

Acute cocaine use causes release of dopamine, epinephrine, norepinephrine, and serotonin. These neurotransmitters act on different receptor subtypes to cause many effects, but the most important are adrenergic stimulation by norepinephrine and epinephrine (see Box 152-1). Norepinephrine causes vasoconstriction by stimulating α-adrenergic receptors on vascular smooth muscle, overcoming the smooth muscle relaxation and vasodilation from β_2-adrenergic receptor stimulation. Epinephrine increases myocardial contractility and heart rate through stimulation of β_1-adrenergic receptors. In addition to causing catecholamine release, the reuptake of these stimulatory neurotransmitters from synaptic clefts is inhibited, altering the normal balance between excitatory and inhibitory tone in the CNS. Subsequent stimulation propagates peripheral catecholamine release (Figure 152-1).

Cocaine also is a local anesthetic agent, slowing nerve impulses from pain fibers by blocking the inward movement of sodium across cell membranes (phase 0 of the action potential).[4,5] Sodium channel blockade across myocardial cells, similar to the class Ia antidysrhythmic agents, is responsible for the occasional conduction abnormality with acute cocaine toxicity.

Cocaine metabolism occurs in the liver and the plasma. In the liver, the drug is metabolized primarily to the active metabolite norcocaine, which potentiates the parent drug. In the plasma, cocaine is metabolized to ecgonine methyl ester via pseudocholinesterase (plasma cholinesterase). This difference may account for the differences in duration of action with different routes of administration.[6] Ecgonine methyl ester may be protective because it is a vasodilator.[7] Genetic differences in the phenotypic expression of plasma cholinesterases may account for individual differences in susceptibility to cocaine toxicity.[8]

Benzoyl ecgonine is the metabolite identified in urine toxicology screens. Methylecgonidine and its metabolite ecgonidine are products of cocaine pyrolysis (crack).[9] Although less commonly assayed, methylecgonidine also can be identified in the urine.[9] The use of ethanol with cocaine may form cocaethylene, a metabolite that may potentiate the drug's stimulatory effects.[10]

Cocaine Formulations

Unpurified cocaine paste is converted to usable forms of cocaine. The crystallized freebase of the cocaine alkaloid is known as "crack cocaine." It is inhaled using a special "crack pipe" designed to tolerate the high temperature required to volatilize pure cocaine. The high lipid solubility and rapid transport from the lungs into the brain contribute to crack's rapid onset of action (Table 152-1). The water-soluble salts of cocaine (cocaine hydrochloride and cocaine sulfate) are available as a white crystalline powder that is taken intranasally or dissolved and injected intravenously. Gastrointestinal administration is uncommon except for patients who are smuggling or concealing drugs.

CLINICAL FEATURES

The primary clinical effect of cocaine is the excitation of the sympathetic nervous system. Patients with moderate toxicity are alert and awake but may have diaphoresis, tachycardia, mydriasis, and hypertension without signs or symptoms of organ damage. A more severely intoxicated patient may present agitated, combative, and hyperthermic. Signs and symptoms of end-organ damage also may be present; this includes acute hypertensive emergencies. Patients may present with focal, acute pain syndromes, circulatory abnormalities, delirium, or seizures.

Clinical presentation may be modified by dose, route of administration, and time to presentation after drug use. Additives, contaminants, or other drugs also may alter the classic signs of acute cocaine intoxication. Patients who are "speedballing," using intravenous heroin and cocaine together, may be initially sedated, depending on the relative absorption and metabolism of each agent. Administration of naloxone may precipitously reveal the underlying cocaine intoxication.

Environmental factors, such as ambient temperature, also may affect the presentation and outcome of an intoxicated patient. Mortality from acute cocaine overdose is significantly higher on days with ambient temperatures greater than 88° F.[11] The profound diaphoresis associated with cocaine use may be absent or limited in cooler environments or when the patient is excessively dehydrated.

BOX 152-1. Clinical Effects of Sympathomimetics

- Hypertension
- Tachycardia
- Mydriasis
- Diaphoresis
- Hyperthermia
- Central nervous system excitation

Complications

The emergency physician should focus on identification and treatment of rapidly fatal complications, specifically hyperthermia, hypertensive emergencies, and cardiac dysrhythmias.

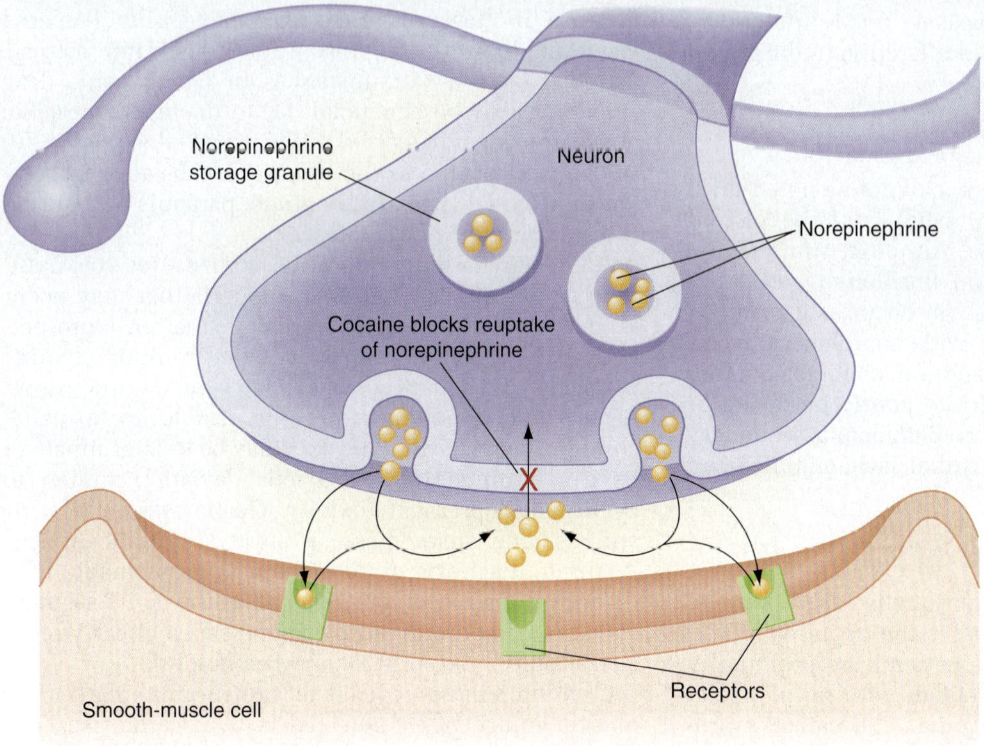

Figure 152-1. How cocaine increases sympathetic tone by increasing neurotransmitters in the synapse.

Table 152-1. Cocaine Pharmacology by Route of Administration

Route	Formula	Onset of Action	Peak Effect	Duration
Inhalation	"Crack"	8 sec	2-5 min	10-20 min
Intranasal	Cocaine HCl	2-5 min	5-10 min	30 min
Intravenous	Cocaine HCl	Seconds	10-20 min	
Oral	Cocaine HCl			
Skin popping	Cocaine HCl			

Hyperthermia

Acute psychomotor agitation with delirium increases the risk of hyperthermia.[12] Toxic patients have increased motor tone and may generate heat faster than it can dissipate. Vasoconstriction and dehydration further compromise cooling, resulting in life-threatening hyperthermia with core temperatures exceeding 106° F (41.1° C). Delay in recognition and management may increase mortality. In the setting of normal temperatures, increased motor tone can release intramuscular creatinine phosphokinase with rhabdomyolysis and its attendant renal and electrolyte complications.[13]

Hypertensive Emergencies

Acute cocaine-induced hypertension can cause serious or lethal damage to the cardiovascular system and CNS (see Chapter 83). Reported sequelae include aortic dissection,[14] pulmonary edema,[15] myocardial ischemia and infarction,[16] intracranial hemorrhage,[17] strokes,[18] and infarction of the anterior spinal artery. Locally induced hypertension and vasospasm can compromise perfusion to various organs. Intestinal infarctions and mesenteric ischemia can occur, particularly in body packers with large oral ingestions. Other local ischemic events include retinal vasospasm, renal infarctions, and placental insufficiency and infarction in the gravid uterus.[19]

Cardiac Dysrhythmias

A life-threatening dysrhythmia may not be noted until cardiac output abruptly diminishes, and the patient suddenly loses consciousness. Although sinus tachycardia is most common, atrial fibrillation and other supraventricular tachycardias can occur as a result of the surge in catecholamines. Wide-complex tachycardias from blockade of fast sodium channels on the myocardium may deteriorate into poorly perfusing or fatal ventricular rhythms.[4,20] Hyperkalemia secondary to rhabdomyolysis and myocardial ischemia also can cause dysrhythmias.

Other Complications

People who binge with continuous use over an extended time may present after the acute effects of cocaine have subsided. These patients are profoundly sleepy but arousable and oriented, with normal vital signs or a mild sinus bradycardia. The patient's prolonged state of arousal during the binge intoxication causes catecholamine depletion, dehydration, and poor nutrition, which may account for this clinical presentation.

Occasionally a patient may experience a transient choreoathetoid movement disorder after using cocaine. This is known as "crack dancing," and it is probably related to abnormalities in dopaminergic tone.[21] Deep venous thrombosis is reported in association with cocaine use, probably secondary to the drug's effects on coagulation. Paranoia, either drug induced or from underlying psychiatric illness, may occur even after the acute effects of the drug subside. The neuropsychiatric effects of cocaine can alter behavior and judgment, increasing the risk of violent injuries.

Complications may arise from the route of administration of cocaine. Inhalation of crack cocaine may cause oropharyngeal burns from the high temperature required to volatilize the drug.[22] Pneumothorax, pneumopericardium, and pneumomediastinum may occur from inhalational barotrauma. Intranasal cocaine use is associated with nasal perforation and sinusitis. Intravenous cocaine users have a high risk of local and systemic infections, including endocarditis, and an increased risk of infection with blood-borne viruses.[23] Transdermal use of injected cocaine, or "skin popping," has similar types of complications. For a chronic user, addiction, or psychological dependence, is mediated through specific neurotransmitter pathways. Although there are no well-defined syndromes constituting cocaine withdrawal, the patient may have cravings for the drug or a general feeling of dysphoria that is not physiologically life-threatening.[24]

DIAGNOSTIC STRATEGIES

Urine drug screening is unlikely to change management because it measures a cocaine metabolite (benzoyl ecgonine) that may be present for 5 days after last use. There are a few circumstances in which urine drug screening may be beneficial: (1) to document possible abuse or neglect in a child with suspected exposure, (2) to confirm cocaine as the unknown substance in body packers, and (3) to differentiate paranoia into drug-induced or psychiatric causes.

An electrocardiogram (ECG) screens for dysrhythmias, other conduction abnormalities that may occur secondary to ischemia or hyperkalemia, or, more precipitously, QRS prolongation from sodium channel blockade. This particular property of cocaine slows myocardial depolarization and results in a wide-complex tachycardia. The axis may be indeterminate or have a terminal rightward axis deviation similar to cyclic antidepressant toxicity. Cyclic antidepressants and cocaine share class Ia antidysrhythmic effects. Accurate diagnosis of chest pain is problematic. ECG diagnosis of acute myocardial infarction by ST segment elevation is confounded by the presence of early repolarization.[25,26] Serial ECGs may be helpful.

Creatine kinase (CK) is a nonspecific marker for muscle injury often elevated with cocaine use. The serum CK-MB fraction, troponin I, and troponin T are more specific in patients with atherogenic coronary disease, but it is uncertain if these same parameters can be applied to cocaine-related chest pain.[24,27] Some patients with elevations in CK-MB fail to show an elevation in either troponin I or troponin T.[27] Although the role of serum enzyme markers is still being investigated for cocaine-related chest pain, cardiac enzymes should be used as with other cardiac patients until cocaine-specific parameters are established. Severe, persistent headache despite normalization of blood pressure may occur with a subarachnoid hemorrhage and warrants cranial computed tomography scan and, if

BOX 152-2. Differential Diagnosis of Agitated Delirium

- Metabolic causes
  - Electrolyte abnormalities
  - Hypoglycemia
  - Hypoxia
  - Uremia/hyperammonemia
- Structural lesions of the CNS
  - Trauma
  - Stroke
  - Hemorrhage
  - Mass
- Endocrine disease
  - Thyrotoxicosis
- Infections
  - Bacterial/viral meningitis/encephalitis
- Toxicologic causes
  - Sympathomimetic/stimulants
    - Cocaine
    - Amphetamines and derivatives
    - Caffeine
    - Phencyclidine/ketamine
  - Anticholinergics
  - Serotonin syndrome
  - Sedative-hypnotic withdrawal
- Heatstroke
- Postictal

CNS, central nervous system.

the scan is negative, lumbar puncture. Urinalysis should be checked for myoglobin, which indicates rhabdomyolysis.

DIFFERENTIAL CONSIDERATIONS

A thorough differential diagnosis of acute cocaine intoxication considers the various causes of agitated delirium (Box 152-2). A thorough assessment of mental status, vital signs, and physical examination can help direct and narrow the differential diagnosis. Several entities may be clinically indistinguishable from cocaine intoxication. In particular, sedative-hypnotic withdrawal, intoxication from amphetamines and amphetamine derivatives, and heatstroke are similar, as is their management. Phencyclidine intoxication may be distinguished by the presence of multidirectional nystagmus, but the treatment is similar. Patients with anticholinergic poisoning typically have urinary retention, dry skin, and minimally reactive pupils as distinguishing factors. For all hyperthermic patients, infection should be considered.

MANAGEMENT

A severely poisoned patient is combative and unable to cooperate in assessment of vital signs. These first few moments are crucial (Box 152-3). Because the patient's history is not always clear, the initial goal is to identify and treat the rapidly fatal agitated delirium.

BOX 152-3. Initial Evaluation of Patients with Sympathetic Stimulation

- Rapid assessment of vital signs, especially core temperature
- Rule out hypoxia, hypoglycemia
- Pharmacologic sedation with benzodiazepines
- Electrocardiogram
- Urinalysis
- Serum creatinine phosphokinase

After initial airway assessment, patients transiently may require physical restraints to obtain complete vital signs and to secure intravenous access. If a chest restraint is used, a mesh vest is preferred to a jacket to help limit hyperthermia. The patient can receive empirical therapy with intravenous dextrose and thiamine or assessment with a bedside blood glucose monitor. Immediate pharmacologic sedation may be necessary with intravenous benzodiazepines, which, in adequate doses, restore inhibitory tone to the CNS and decrease excessive sympathetic outflow to peripheral tissues. Pharmacologic sedation also facilitates measurement of vital signs, particularly core temperature, and allows for completion of the physical examination and continuous ECG monitoring.

Pharmacologic Sedation

In adults, intravenous diazepam can be administered in increments of 10 mg every 5 minutes until sedation is achieved. Diazepam has a rapid onset of action, is easily titratable, and has active metabolites. Persistently increased motor tone reflects inadequate titration of diazepam, even if the patient appears otherwise sleepy. In wildly agitated patients in whom 20 to 30 mg of diazepam is used without notable effect, the increments may be increased carefully to 20 mg with close monitoring. Benzodiazepines also treat the choreoathetoid movements of crack dancing. Most cocaine toxic patients are salt and water depleted and require vigorous replacement with intravenous crystalloid. In patients in whom the etiology of delirium is unclear, careful attention to the patient's respiratory status avoids the respiratory depression caused by excessive benzodiazepine administration in the presence of other sedative-hypnotic agents, such as ethanol.

Phenothiazines, droperidol, and haloperidol are best avoided in patients suspected of acute sympathomimetic intoxication.[28] Although CNS sedation is achieved, the anticholinergic effects of these agents can limit cooling by impeding diaphoresis and may increase morbidity. Additionally, they may have associated dysrhythmic effects that may be additive or even synergistic with cocaine.

Hyperthermia

Cocaine-induced hyperthermia must be treated with rapid cooling (Box 152-4). Patients who sustain elevated core temperatures greater than 106° F (41° C) for more than 20 minutes are likely to stabilize transiently,

BOX 152-4. Management of Stimulant-Induced Hyperthermia

Early identification of core temperature
Large-bore intravenous access with rapid infusion of crystalloid
Sedation and muscle relaxation with benzodiazepines
Rapid cooling within 20 min*
Foley catheterization to monitor output
Fluid resuscitation
Laboratory analysis for organ function
- Serum chemistries/creatinine/CPK
- Liver function
- PT/PTT/fibrin split products
- Bacterial cultures†

Urinalysis for myoglobinuria
Paralysis and intubation if necessary

*Ideally with ice water immersion.
†Consider lumbar puncture or antibiotic therapy.
CPK, creatine phosphokinase; PT, prothrombin time; PTT, partial thromboplastin time.

then develop fatal multisystem organ failure, often heralded by disseminated intravascular coagulation. Patients should have continuous monitoring of core temperature with a rectal probe. Heat generated by agitation and increased muscle tone can be terminated by aggressive use of benzodiazepines, with neuromuscular paralysis and intubation as required. It is crucial to reduce core temperature to 102° F (38.8° C) within 20 minutes. Cooling blankets are insufficient. Ice water, wet sheets with large fans, and packing the entire body in ice with continuous monitoring of core temperature can be used. These patients require aggressive fluid resuscitation.[29]

Hypertensive Emergencies

The goal in hypertensive emergencies is to reverse promptly the vasoconstriction of norepinephrine at peripheral α-adrenergic receptors. Benzodiazepines restore the CNS inhibitory tone on the peripheral nervous system. With evidence of end-organ damage, intravenous nitroglycerin or nitroprusside can be used.[30] Phentolamine, a direct α-adrenergic antagonist, is the antihypertensive of choice. It can be titrated slowly using 1 to 5 mg intravenously; blood pressure is reassessed over 5 minutes. Repeat doses can be given until adequate control is achieved. In contrast to patients with chronic hypertension, individuals with acute cocaine hypertension have a normal blood pressure in the absence of the drug, and unless the patient's history suggests otherwise, a normal systolic and diastolic blood pressure should be the endpoint of therapy. β-Adrenergic antagonists are contraindicated with cocaine because of paradoxical hypertension, when the primary cause of cocaine-induced vasoconstriction is untreated and unopposed.[31,32] Patients undergoing cardiac catheterization show decreased coronary artery diameter in the presence of cocaine and β-adrenergic antagonists.[32,33] The treatment of cocaine-induced subarachnoid hemorrhage, myocardial infarction, or aortic

BOX 152-5. Causes of Stimulant-Induced Chest Pain

Noncardiac
- Pneumothorax
- Pneumomediastinum
- Pneumopericardium
- Aortic dissection
- Pulmonary infarction
- Infection

Cardiac chest pain
- Endocarditis
- Pericarditis
- Ischemia/infarction
  - During acute intoxication
  - After acute intoxication

dissection differs significantly from treatment for other causes of the same conditions. The combined use of phentolamine and β-adrenergic antagonists is inadequately investigated and may result in profound hypotension. Likewise, data on the use of labetalol are disappointing.

Dysrhythmias

Dysrhythmias from cocaine may be either atrial or ventricular. Atrial dysrhythmias, including atrial fibrillation, and supraventricular tachycardias are likely due to sympathetic stimulation and are less common. These dysrhythmias often respond to sedation with benzodiazepines. Other standard therapies can be considered, but β-adrenergic antagonists should be avoided.

When the etiology of a wide-complex tachycardia from cocaine is unknown, intravenous bolus administration of sodium bicarbonate, 1 to 2 mEq/kg, with closely recorded cardiac monitoring empirically treats sodium channel blockade and potential cardiotoxicity from hyperkalemia.[5,34] Lidocaine is a class Ib antidysrhythmic agent that may increase seizure risk and mortality and is best reserved for use in patients with ventricular dysrhythmias who have failed bicarbonate therapy and already have received benzodiazepines. Lidocaine may have its greatest utility for ventricular dysrhythmias that occur in the setting of cocaine-associated myocardial infarction.

Cocaine-Related Chest Pain

The etiologies of cocaine-related chest pain are diverse (Box 152-5). A chest radiograph may identify pneumothorax or pneumomediastinum from inhalational barotrauma. Fever with chest pain and shortness of breath should prompt consideration of pneumonia; pulmonary infarction[35,36]; or, in an injection drug user, endocarditis with septic pulmonary emboli.

Cocaine acutely induces coronary vasoconstriction, while increasing myocardial oxygen demand. Platelet aggregation is enhanced through prothrombogenic and antifibrinolytic pathways.[37,38] These cumulative effects can result in coronary insufficiency. Cigarette smoking acutely exacerbates these conditions. Chronic cocaine use may accelerate atherogenesis and induce left ventricular hypertrophy. All of these factors may account for myocardial ischemia or infarction in patients who use cocaine. Of nonfatal myocardial infarctions in persons age 18 to 45, 25% were attributed to cocaine, even after adjustment of other myocardial infarction risk factors.[39]

Identifying a patient with a cocaine-related coronary syndrome is difficult. Patients may present hours to days after use, possibly owing to vasoactive metabolites.[40] The patient may deny drug use and may experience atypical chest pain. Almost one third of cocaine-using patients meeting serum enzyme criteria for myocardial infarction report pleuritic chest pain.[41] There are no clear predictors for patients at risk for myocardial infarction. A prospective evaluation of patients with cocaine-related chest pain found that age, route of drug use, time to presentation, and preexisting risk factors for coronary artery disease were inadequate to identify patients sustaining myocardial infarction.[41] An investigation of patients with cocaine-related coronary syndromes found significant angiographic stenosis in individuals with positive serum enzyme markers for myocardial infarction.[42] Of patients without positive serum markers, 18% had significant disease by angiogram.[42] Other predictors of significant disease in this group included elevated cholesterol and prior diagnosis of coronary disease or myocardial infarction.[42]

As recommended for most complications of cocaine use, benzodiazepine administration decreases myocardial oxygen demand by limiting peripheral stimulation. Limited clinical investigations support early administration of benzodiazepine.[43] Aspirin and nitrates also should be administered.[40] In patients meeting ECG criteria for myocardial infarction with persistent chest pain and hypertension and a clear history of acute cocaine intoxication, coronary vasodilation with intravenous phentolamine, 1 mg, given slowly should be considered. This dose can be repeated, if needed, as long as the patient's blood pressure remains stable. Morphine sulfate also can be used to treat pain.[44]

In contrast to non–cocaine-induced myocardial ischemia or infarction, β-adrenergic antagonists, including labetalol, *are contraindicated during acute cocaine toxicity* because coronary vasoconstriction may worsen.[31,32] In patients with a suspected cocaine-related coronary syndrome without signs and symptoms of acute drug toxicity, the role of persistent cocaine metabolites and the risks and benefits of β-adrenergic blockade are not adequately studied.

Heparin can be administered, but the role of fibrinolytic therapy is not well established. Some mechanisms of cocaine-induced myocardial infarction would be expected to respond to fibrinolytic agents. Patients failing aggressive coronary vasodilation with nitrates and phentolamine who have known coronary artery disease or a previous ECG confirming new ST segment elevations may be candidates for fibrinolysis, although in this setting, cardiac catheterization is preferable. The same contraindications apply as with non–cocaine-induced myocardial infarction. Nuclear imaging studies also may provide more diagnostic information.[25,40,45]

Antiplatelet and glycoprotein IIb/IIIa inhibitors and calcium channel antagonists seem to benefit some patients with myocardial infarction or ischemia of atherosclerotic origin. Theoretically, these agents may counter some of the platelet aggregation enhanced by cocaine, but data investigating their use are lacking.

Cocaine Body Packers

Cocaine is smuggled by a variety of techniques. Before crossing international borders, body packers ingest cocaine that has been wrapped tightly into condoms or other latex products. Each packet can contain 10 g of cocaine, and packers may swallow 150 packets.[46,47] On arrival at their destination, a cathartic is taken to stimulate gastrointestinal passage of the contraband for subsequent delivery and distribution. Body packers are likely to know the exact number of packets they ingested.

A body packer may present without symptoms to the emergency department. The body packer should be placed immediately on continuous cardiac monitoring, with large-bore intravenous access. Diagnosis is made by history. An abdominal radiograph may offer qualitative confirmation of foreign bodies, but cannot be used quantitatively. Plain radiographs have limited sensitivity to detect an isolated or small number of packets. When uncertainty persists, a contrast study is warranted. Body packing also is used for transporting heroin and other illicit substances. Although heroin body packing rarely requires surgical intervention, an asymptomatic patient may refuse to identify the packet's contents. A urine toxicology may be useful because some fine quantities of drug may be directly ingested while swallowing the contraband. Body packers with a positive urine screen for cocaine metabolites should be aggressively decontaminated.

Rupture of a cocaine packet can result in death because each packet contains almost 10 times the lethal dose. As such, all cocaine body packers should be admitted to a monitored setting and be kept nothing per mouth except for treatments. These patients may die suddenly. Patients with a leaking or poorly secured packet who become symptomatic are likely to die without aggressive intervention and meet the single absolute criterion for surgical removal of packets. When evidence of cocaine toxicity is manifest, rapid transportation to the operating room may be the only way to salvage these patients from a fatal outcome. Benzodiazepines, neuromuscular blockade, or sodium bicarbonate administration may be required en route.

It is reasonable to administer activated charcoal (1 g/kg body weight) to an asymptomatic body packer whose airway is otherwise not compromised. Whole-bowel irrigation with polyethylene glycol solution facilitates gastrointestinal passage of the packets and cleanses the bowel in the event of emergent transport to the operating room.[47] Subsequent contrast studies may be required to evaluate for remaining packets. Computed tomography and contrast abdominal radiographs may fail to detect isolated packets with potentially fatal quantities of cocaine. Patients suggesting that they swallowed a larger number of packets than passed or who refuse to reveal the number ingested warrant continued bowel irrigation, observation, and repeat studies. Although endoscopic retrieval is discouraged because of concern over packet rupture during the procedure, it has been used safely in selected cases.

All packets passed by stool, endoscopic procedures, or in the operating room should be counted carefully and placed immediately with law enforcement officials if they already are involved with the case. When law enforcement is not yet involved, advocacy of hospital legal counsel or risk management and the hospital ethics committee may be helpful in determining the disposition of the packets and ultimately of the patient when he or she is medically cleared.[47]

Body Stuffers

A "body stuffer" is an individual who attempts to conceal evidence of cocaine possession by swallowing the drug while pursued by law enforcement officials. These are usually unplanned events with generally small quantities of drug intended primarily for personal use. As such, the drugs may be swallowed in poorly sealed vials or glassine packets that may not be evident on radiographs. Generally, patients ingest nonlethal doses and are asymptomatic. Activated charcoal, 50 g, can absorb any potentially released drug. Monitoring and whole-bowel irrigation should be performed if the quantity ingested is of concern or if signs of intoxication persist.[48] Rarely, stuffers can have fatal events, but these patients usually present with symptoms and have life-threatening complications in the first few hours.

DISPOSITION

Patients with acute intoxication who need only observation or respond quickly to sedation and do not develop complications can be discharged after the acute intoxication resolves. These patients may be extremely sleepy from catecholamine depletion, and it is best to discharge them with a responsible adult. Patients may be open to drug counseling and referral while in the emergency department. Patients who develop complications should be admitted to the intensive care unit for further treatment.

The disposition of patients with chest pain depends on several factors (Box 152-6). Acutely toxic patients with dynamic changes on the ECG, dysrhythmias, or congestive heart failure or patients requiring nitroglycerin, phentolamine, or reperfusion should be admitted. Cocaine exposure of this severity warrants further evaluation of the extent of preexisting reversible ischemia and intervention to encourage cessation of drug use.

The disposition of patients with chest pain who are not acutely toxic is less clear. Admission is warranted for patients with complications or ECG changes and patients requiring pharmacologic intervention. Other patients may be admitted for short-term observation to an emergency department observation unit or discharged, depending on the level of concern about underlying coronary artery disease.

BOX 152-6. Admission Criteria Cocaine-Related Chest Pain

Persistent chest pain
Electrocardiogram changes
Dysrhythmias
CHF/cardiogenic shock
Elevated enzymes
Requiring vasodilation
Preexisting CAD
Multiple risk factors for CAD

CHF, congestive heart failure; CAD, coronary artery disease.

Young patients who present after resolution of chest pain with normal, unchanging ECGs, no dysrhythmias, and few or no risks of coronary artery disease are likely to have a good outcome.[46] Complications such as congestive heart failure and ventricular dysrhythmias typically present within the first 4 hours.[16] After a 12-hour monitored observation period, patients with a benign clinical course and negative serum enzyme markers can probably be discharged.[45,49]

Body packers need to be observed until all packets have passed. Ideally, these patients have had three packet-free stools, a reliable packet count consistent with the ingestion, and a negative contrast radiographic study.[47] Body stuffers who receive activated charcoal and remain asymptomatic after 4 hours of observation may be discharged.

OTHER STIMULANTS

Amphetamines

Amphetamines enhance release of catecholamines from presynaptic nerve terminals by altering the pH of presynaptic vesicles. Amphetamines usually are administered as pills, but occasionally are crushed and injected. The subsequent CNS stimulation results in nearly identical sympathomimetic effects that occur in cocaine toxicity, but not with the same frequency or intensity (see Box 152-1). Patients are at risk for hyperthermia, hypertensive emergencies, dysrhythmias, myocardial ischemia, and hyperkalemia associated with rhabdomyolysis. In contrast to cocaine, amphetamines do not block sodium channels and only minimally affect presynaptic reuptake of catecholamines. Although urine drug screens identify amphetamines, they are of little utility in managing a toxic patient. The management follows the same guidelines as for cocaine (see Box 152-3), although the duration of toxicity tends to be longer for amphetamines.

Methylenedioxymethamphetamine

MDMA (Ecstasy, XTC, Adam) is a chemically modified amphetamine that is an orally administered drug originally used in all-night dance parties, or "raves." Patients describe the euphoria allowing "closeness to others," so it is sometimes called the "love drug." The molecular structure of MDMA confers some serotoninergic properties that may account for the "shimmering" visual effects patients report.

Along with the previously described complications of amphetamines, MDMA can precipitate a potentially life-threatening hyponatremia. MDMA or its metabolite may alter release of endogenous stores of vasopressin.[50] Although the exact mechanism is not understood, patients with MDMA-induced hyponatremia have concentrated urine samples with a relatively high urine sodium, similar to syndrome of inappropriate antidiuretic hormone. Patients usually can be treated supportively with fluid restriction, unless seizures or other neurologic events are present. Urine can be tested for specific gravity, and a sample should be sent to the laboratory for electrolyte analysis and osmolality. Normal saline or other crystalloids may worsen the hyponatremia because these patients are likely to retain more free water than sodium. They should be fluid restricted unless severe hypovolemia exists and treated with hypertonic saline for neurologic impairment. In contrast to other amphetamines, MDMA causes potentially irreversible neurologic damage to serotoninergic neurons when used chronically.[51] Other MDMA variants, such as 3,4-methylenedioxyethamphetamine (Eve), may cause similar complications (see Chapter 154).

Methamphetamine

Methamphetamine, known as "crank" and "crystal meth," is a fat-soluble, smokable, designer amphetamine. Complications are similar to the complications for other sympathomimetics. The duration of action can be significantly longer, however, with some paranoid delusions persisting for 15 hours. The production of methamphetamines requires a variety of metal salts, and lead toxicity from inappropriately produced drug is reported.[52] Injuries during illicit methamphetamine production include exposure to anhydrous ammonia, hydrochloric acid, sodium hydroxide, ether, and ephedrine and burns and explosions.

Ephedrine and Ephedra

Ephedrine is another illicitly used amphetamine-like agent associated with complications of excessive sympathomimetic stimulation. Ephedra, a plant-derived product, also known as a Chinese herbal product, *ma-huang,* has been associated with strokes and deaths in adolescents using the agent.[53] The Food and Drug Administration has banned all ephedra-containing dietary supplements.

Khat and Methcathinone

Khat is a stimulant agent naturally occurring in the leaves of the plant *Catha edulis.*[54] These leaves traditionally are chewed to extract the active compounds, cathinone and methcathinone, which are stimulants with sympathomimetic effects.[55] Smoking khat does not typically result in clinical effects because the agent degrades with pyrolysis. Illicitly manufactured methcathinone is known as "cat." Management and disposition follow the same guidelines as that of cocaine.

KEY CONCEPTS

- Rapid sedation with an intravenous benzodiazepine is the key treatment for most symptoms of toxicity resulting from cocaine and other stimulants.
- Hyperthermia is a high-risk sign, and body temperature must be reduced rapidly.
- β-Adrenergic blockade may cause paradoxical hypertension and increase coronary vasoconstriction and is generally contraindicated.
- Wide-complex rhythms secondary to cocaine ingestion may respond to intravenous bicarbonate therapy.
- Cocaine body packers who become symptomatic need immediate surgery.

REFERENCES

1. National Institute of Drug Abuse: National Household Survey on Drug Abuse: Population Estimates, 1991 (DHHS number [ADM] 92-1887). Rockville, Md, Department of Health and Human Services, 1992.
2. Marzuk PM, et al: Homicide in New York City: Cocaine use and firearms. *JAMA* 272:43, 1994.
3. Marzuk PM, et al: Fatal injuries after cocaine use as a leading cause of death among young adults in New York City. *N Engl J Med* 332:1753, 1995.
4. Bauman JL, et al: Cocaine-related sudden cardiac death: A hypothesis correlating basic science and clinical observations. *J Clin Pharmacol* 34:902, 1994.
5. Winecoff AP, et al: Reversal of the electrocardiographic effects of cocaine by lidocaine: Part 1. Comparison with sodium bicarbonate and quinidine. *Pharmacotherapy* 14:698, 1994.
6. Javaid J, Musa M, Fischman MW: Kinetics of cocaine in humans after intravenous and intranasal administration. *Biopharm Drug Dispos* 4:9, 1983.
7. Hoffman RS, Morasco R, Goldfrank LR: Administration of purified human plasma cholinesterase protects against cocaine toxicity in mice. *J Toxicol Clin Toxicol* 34:259, 1996.
8. Hoffman RS, et al: Association between life-threatening cocaine toxicity and plasma cholinesterase activity. *Ann Emerg Med* 21:247, 1991.
9. Scheidweiler KB, et al: Pharmacokinetics and pharmacodynamics of methylecgonidine, a crack cocaine metabolite. *J Pharm Exp Ther* 307:1179, 2003.
10. Perez-Reyes M: Subjective and cardiovascular effects of cocethylene in humans. *Psychopharmacology* 113:144, 1993.
11. Marzuk PM, et al: Ambient temperature and mortality from unintentional cocaine overdose. *JAMA* 279:1795, 1998.
12. Merigian KS, Roberts JR: Cocaine intoxication: Hyperpyrexia, rhabdomyolysis and acute renal failure. *J Toxicol Clin Toxicol* 25:135, 1987.
13. Herzlich BC, et al: Rhabdomyolysis related to cocaine abuse. *Ann Intern Med* 109:335, 1988.
14. Fisher A, Holroyd BR: Cocaine-associated dissection of the thoracic aorta. *J Emerg Med* 10:723, 1992.
15. Kline JN, Hirasuna JD: Pulmonary edema after freebase cocaine smoking—not due to an adulterant. *Chest* 97:1009, 1990.

16. Hollander JE, et al: Cocaine associated myocardial infarction: Mortality and complications. *Arch Intern Med* 155:1081, 1995.
17. Seaman ME: Acute cocaine abuse associated with cerebral infarction. *Ann Emerg Med* 19:34, 1990.
18. Mody CK, et al: Neurologic complications of cocaine abuse. *Neurology* 38:1189, 1988.
19. MacGregor SN, et al: Cocaine use during pregnancy: Adverse perinatal outcome. *Am J Obstet Gynecol* 157:686, 1987.
20. Crumb WJ, Clarkson CW: Characterization of sodium channel blocking properties of the major metabolites of cocaine in single cardiac myocytes. *J Pharmacol Exp Ther* 261:910, 1992.
21. Daras M, Koppel BS, Atos-Radzion E: Cocaine-induced choreoathetoid movements ("crack dancing"). *Neurology* 44:751, 1994.
22. Meleca RJ, et al: Mucosal injuries of the upper aerodigestive tract after smoking crack or freebase cocaine. *Laryngoscope* 107:620, 1997.
23. Chambers HF, Morris DL, Tauber MG, Modin G: Cocaine use and the risk for endocarditis in intravenous drug users. *Ann Intern Med* 106:833, 1987.
24. Mendelson JH, Mello NK: Management of cocaine abuse and dependence. *N Engl J Med* 334:963, 1996.
25. Hoffman RS, Hollander JE: Thrombolytic therapy in cocaine-induced myocardial infarction [editorial]. *Am J Emerg Med* 14:693, 1996.
26. Wang K, Asinger RW, Marriot HJL: Current concepts: ST-elevation in conditions other than acute myocardial infarction. *N Engl J Med* 349:2128, 2003.
27. Hennekene CH, et al: Drug therapy for acute myocardial infarction—evidence from clinical trials. *N Engl J Med* 335:1660, 1996.
28. Derlet RW, Albertson TE, Rice P: The effect of haloperidol in cocaine and amphetamine intoxication. *J Emerg Med* 7:633, 1989.
29. Crandall CG, Vonpatanasin W, Victor RG: Mechanism of cocaine induced hyperthermia in humans. *Ann Intern Med* 136:785, 2002.
30. Brogan WC, et al: Alleviation of cocaine-induced coronary vasoconstriction by nitroglycerin. *J Am Coll Cardiol* 18:581, 1991.
31. Haynes S, et al: Beta-adrenergic blockade in cocaine toxicity [letter]. *J Emerg Med* 13:537, 1995.
32. Lange RA, et al: Cocaine-induced coronary-artery vasoconstriction. *N Engl J Med* 321:1557, 1989.
33. Boehrer JD, et al: Influence of labetalol of cocaine-induced coronary vasoconstriction in humans. *Am J Med* 94:608, 1993.
34. Wilson LD, Shelat C: Electrophysiologic and hemodynamic effects of sodium bicarbonate in a canine model of severe cocaine intoxication. *J Toxicol Clin Toxicol* 41:777, 2003.
35. Delaney K, Hoffman RS: Pulmonary infarction associated with crack cocaine use in a previously healthy 23 year old woman. *Am J Med* 91:92, 1991.
36. Haim DY, Lippman ML, Goldberg SK, Walkenstein MD: The pulmonary complications of crack cocaine: A comprehensive review. *Chest* 107:233, 1995.
37. Rinder HM, et al: Platelet alpha granule release in cocaine users. *Circulation* 90:1162, 1994.
38. Togna G, et al: Platelet responsiveness and biosynthesis of thromboxane and prostacyclin in response to in vitro cocaine treatment. *Haemostasis* 15:100, 1985.
39. Qureshi AI, Suri MF, Guterman LR, Hopkins LN: Cocaine use and the likeligood of non-fatal infarction and stroke, data from the National Health and Nutrition Examination Survey. *Circulation* 103:502, 2001.
40. Hollander JE: Management of cocaine associated myocardial ischemia. *N Engl J Med* 333:1267, 1995.
41. Hollander JE, et al: Prospective multicenter evaluation of cocaine associated chest pain. *Acad Emerg Med* 1:330, 1994.
42. Kontos MC, Jesse RL, Tatum JL, Ornato JP: Coronary angiographic findings in patients with cocaine-associated chest pain. *J Emerg Med* 24:9, 2003.
43. Honderick T, et al: A prospective, randomized, controlled trial of benzodiazepines and nitroglycerine or nitroglycerine alone in the treatment of cocaine associated acute coronary syndromes. *Am J Emerg Med* 21:39, 2003.
44. Saland KE, et al: Influence of morphine sulfate on cocaine induced coronary vasoconstriction. *Am J Cardiol* 90:810, 2002.
45. Hollander JE, et al: Cocaine associated chest pain: One year follow-up. *Acad Emerg Med* 2:179, 1995.
46. McCarron MM, Wood JD: The cocaine body packer syndrome. *JAMA* 250:1417, 1983.
47. Traub SJ, Hoffman RS, Nelson LS: Current concepts: Body packing—the internal concealment of illicit drugs. *N Engl J Med* 349:2519, 2003.
48. June R, Aks SE, Keys N, Wahl M: Medical outcome of cocaine body stuffers. *J Emerg Med* 18:221, 2000.
49. Weber JE, et al: Validation of a brief observation period for patients with cocaine associated chest pain. *N Engl J Med* 348:510, 2003.
50. Henry JA, et al: Low-dose MDMA ("ecstacy") induces vasopressin secretion. *Lancet* 351:1784, 1998.
51. Ricaurte GA, et al: Aminergic metabolites in cerebrospinal fluid of humans previously exposed to MDMA: Preliminary observations. *Ann N Y Acad Sci* 600:699, 1990.
52. Alcott JV, Barnhart RA, Mooney LA: Acute lead poisoning in two users of illicit methamphetamine. *JAMA* 258:510, 1987.
53. Perotta DM, et al: Adverse events associated with ephedrine-containing products—Texas, December 1993 to September 1995. *MMWR Morb Mortal Wkly Rep* 45:689, 1996.
54. Kalix P: Pharmacological properties of the stimulant khat. *Pharm Ther* 48:397, 1990.
55. Glennon RA, et al: Metcathinone: A new and potent amphetamine-like agent. *Pharmacol Biochem Behav* 26:547, 1987.

CHAPTER

153 Toxic Alcohols

Suzanne R. White and Joseph Kosnik

METHANOL

Perspective

Methanol is a colorless, volatile, slightly sweet-tasting alcohol. It is a product of natural fermentation and originally was manufactured from the distillation of wood. Methanol currently is produced almost exclusively by synthetic pathways. Certain products found in the home may contain high concentrations of methanol, including antifreeze; windshield washer fluid; carburetor fluid; duplicator fluid; hobby engine fuel; gasohol; dry gas; Sterno; glass cleaners; and thinners for shellacs, lacquers, adhesives, and inks. Methanol is a precursor in the manufacture of plastics, films, and dyes. Methanol also is found in formalin and embalming fluid. Illicit alcohol production remains a global source of methanol poisoning from products such as chang'aa (Kenya), raki (Turkey), and tuica (Romania).

Although epidemic poisonings from methanol are reported occasionally, most exposures are sporadic. In 2002, of the 2822 cases of methanol poisoning reported to American poison centers, 86% were unintentional, 9% had moderate to major complications, and 18 resulted in fatalities. Treatment delay is associated with increased morbidity, making early recognition of clinical and laboratory clues crucial.

Principles of Disease

Pharmacology and Metabolism

Methanol is absorbed rapidly from the gastrointestinal tract, and blood levels peak 30 to 60 minutes after ingestion.[1] Transdermal and respiratory tract absorption also has resulted in toxicity, especially in infants. Certain occupations are at high risk for inhalational exposure to methanol, including painting, glazing, varnishing, lithography, and printing. At low serum concentrations, the elimination of methanol follows first-order kinetics; at concentrations after overdose, zero-order kinetics predominate. A prolonged half-life of 24 to 30 hours results, which may be extended even further by the concurrent ingestion of ethanol. First-order elimination prevails at high levels (>300 mg/dL), possibly as a result of enhanced pulmonary elimination. Small amounts of ingested methanol may be exceptionally toxic. In adults, the smallest lethal dose reported is 15 mL of 40% methanol; 4 mL of pure methanol has led to blindness. With appropriate, timely treatment, however, survival without loss of eyesight has been reported despite extremely high levels. From a pediatric perspective, the ingestion of only 1.5 mL of 100% methanol in a toddler (0.15 mL/kg) is sufficient to produce a toxic blood level of 20 mg/dL. Any suspected pediatric methanol ingestion warrants aggressive evaluation and treatment.

Methanol itself has little toxicity, producing less central nervous system (CNS) depression and inebriation than ethanol. Metabolites of the parent alcohol are extremely toxic, however. Although small amounts of methanol are eliminated via renal and pulmonary routes, 90% is metabolized hepatically. Methanol is oxidized by alcohol dehydrogenase (ADH) to formaldehyde, which is rapidly converted by aldehyde dehydrogenase to formic acid (Figure 153-1). Formic acid is the primary toxicant and accounts for much of the anion gap metabolic acidosis and ocular toxicity peculiar to methanol ingestion.[2] Through a folate-dependent pathway, formic acid is degraded to carbon dioxide and water.

Pathophysiology

Optic neuropathy and putaminal necrosis are the two main complications of severe methanol poisoning. Long-term morbidity takes the form of visual impairment, including blindness, and parkinsonian motor dysfunction, characterized by hypokinesis and rigidity. Formic acid has a high affinity for iron and, as such, inhibits mitochondrial cytochrome oxidase, halting cellular respiration.[3] Methanol metabolism, in the cytosol and mitochondria, may account for a second mechanism of adenosine triphosphate depletion.[4] Lactate accumulation resulting from hypotension or seizures further compounds the metabolic acidosis predominantly caused by formate. Other mechanisms of toxicity involve increased lipid peroxidation, free radical formation, and impaired protective antioxidant reactions.[3] Severe dysfunction of subcellular metabolism from methanol also has been linked to significant disturbance in proteolytic-antiproteolytic balance.[5]

The primary sites of ocular injury are the retrolaminar optic nerve and retina. Selective myelin damage to the retrolaminar optic nerve in patients dying as a result of methanol toxicity has been seen at autopsy. Müller cells, the principal glial cells of retinal neurons and photoreceptors, have been proposed as the initial target in methanol-induced visual toxicity. It seems that they alone harbor the enzymes necessary to metabolize methanol to formate. Histopathologic correlates suggest that retinal cells develop intra-axonal swelling, calcium influx, mitochondrial destruction, and microtubular disruption. Ultimately, interference with trans-

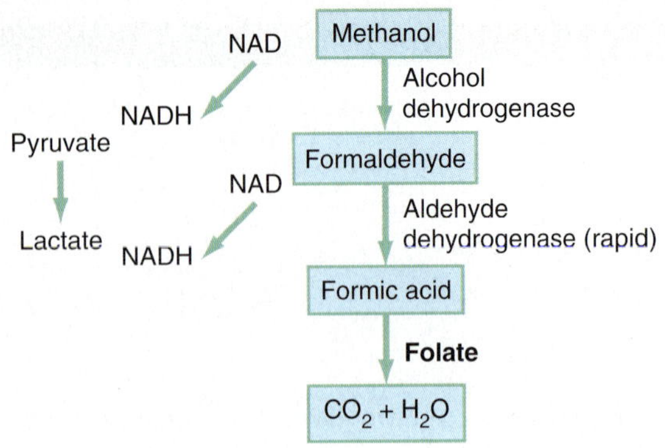

Figure 153-1. Metabolism of methanol.

port of essential proteins from the retinal neuron cell body to the nerve fiber axoplasm results. Oligodendrocyte involvement results in myelin degeneration and leads to visual decrements. Acidosis may accelerate this process, by enhancing nonionic diffusion of formic acid into neurons and further increasing lactate production.[3] This self-perpetuating cycle of acidosis, termed *circulus hypoxicus*,[6] underscores the need for aggressive correction of pH to accomplish ion trapping of formate outside the CNS.

Methanol adversely affects other areas of the CNS, specifically the basal ganglia. Bilateral, symmetric putaminal hypodensities, hemorrhages, or cystic lesions are characteristic, occurring in 13.5% of patients.[7] Necrosis is described in the subcortical white matter, spinal cord anterior horn cells, and cerebellum.[8] Acute signs and symptoms may be lacking or may take several days to develop, despite the presence of these radiographic findings. The cellular mechanisms of injury may be similar to the mechanisms of the ophthalmologic injury, but the reason for localization of neurologic damage to the basal ganglia is unknown.[7] Although some quantitative neuropathologic studies have shown high concentrations of formic acid within the putamen, others show that formate levels are not extraordinarily elevated in these areas compared with levels in the blood or other tissues. Massive edema adjacent to the putamen shown by magnetic resonance imaging (MRI) suggests a possible localized disruption of the blood-brain barrier. Other proposed mechanisms for the vulnerability of this region include the unique pattern of arterial blood supply and venous drainage and greater metabolic activity.

Clinical Features

With individual cases of methanol poisoning, the history may be unobtainable or unreliable. The diagnosis should be considered in patients with altered mental status, visual complaints, or metabolic acidosis or in patients with occupations at high risk for exposure. Because methanol is a poor substrate for ADH, a latency period exists between the time of ingestion and onset of visual or metabolic disturbance. The typical 12- to 24-hour latency may be shorter when large amounts are consumed or longer when ethanol is coingested (range 40 minutes to 72 hours).[1] In patients who present early, formate accumulation may be ongoing, with risk for significant toxicity despite being asymptomatic. When symptoms manifest, they are primarily neurologic, gastrointestinal, or ocular in nature.

Although methanol is less inebriating than ethanol, early symptoms of methanol poisoning are depressed mental status, confusion, and ataxia. Nonspecific complaints of weakness, dizziness, anorexia, headache, and nausea develop. In severe cases, coma and seizures may be seen. Although vomiting and abdominal pain commonly result from mucosal irritation, the absence of gastrointestinal complaints does not rule out a serious ingestion.[1] Abdominal tenderness may be so severe that it suggests an acute surgical abdomen.[1] This may result from pancreatitis, and elevation of serum amylase is relatively common. Other authors have noted increased salivary amylase isoenzyme without pancreatic inflammation.

Visual disturbances are seen in 50% of patients, and their development may precede or parallel that of other clinical symptoms.[6] Patients may complain of cloudy, blurred, indistinct, or misty vision or may note yellow spots or, rarely, photophobia. The most common acute field defect is a dense central scotoma.[9] Some patients compare their visual symptoms with "stepping out into a snowstorm," a complaint unique to methanol ingestion. Patients can have a complete lack of light perception and total loss of vision. On examination, optic disk hyperemia is seen at 18 to 48 hours after ingestion. Peripapillary retinal edema follows, is most striking in the nerve fiber layer along the vascular arcades, and only rarely involves the macula.[4,9] Sluggishly reactive or fixed and dilated pupils indicate a poor prognosis. Pallor and cupping, indicative of optic atrophy, are late findings suggesting a poor prognosis for visual recovery. Occasionally, the fundus may appear normal, even in patients with visual symptoms.

Compensatory tachypnea heralds the onset of metabolic acidosis, which often may be severe, with reported serum bicarbonate concentrations of less than 5 mEq/L and an arterial pH less than 7.0. Early tachycardia has been noted, but in general, cardiovascular abnormalities are rare.[1] Hypotension and bradycardia, when present, are preterminal findings.[10] Historically, death was described in association with a peculiar, abrupt cessation of respiration, rather than with cardiovascular collapse.[1,11] Rarely, multiple organ failure develops.[10]

Prognosis after methanol ingestion seems to correlate with the degree of acidosis, time to presentation, and initiation of treatment within 8 hours of exposure.[1] Poor prognosis is associated with coma, seizures, or arterial pH less than 7.0.[10,12] Patients surviving the acute phase of toxicity may be left with permanent blindness or neurologic deficits, such as parkinsonism, toxic encephalopathy, polyneuropathy, cognitive dysfunction, transverse myelitis, primitive reflexes, or seizures.

Diagnostic Strategies

A severe anion gap metabolic acidosis is the hallmark of methanol ingestion. In some cases, this anion gap metabolic acidosis may be the only diagnostic clue. Because the onset of acidosis may be delayed 12 to 24 hours, the presence of a normal anion gap does not rule out methanol exposure. Absence of high anion gap acidosis has been described in cases with concomitant ethanol, lithium, or bromide ingestion. In methanol toxicity, this anion gap is due primarily to the presence of formic acid, with a variable contribution from lactic acid. Another classic laboratory finding in methanol toxicity is an elevated osmol gap. The osmolal gap is defined as follows:

$$\text{Osmol gap} = \text{measured serum osmolality} - \text{calculated serum osmolality}$$

Serum osmolality depends on the presence of low-molecular-weight solutes, primarily sodium, chloride, glucose, and blood urea nitrogen (BUN). One formula for calculating osmolality attributable to these solutes is as follows:

$$\text{Calculated serum osmolality (mOsm/kg)} = 2(Na^+) + [BUN/2.8] + [glucose/18] + [ethanol (mg/dL)/4.6]$$

The "normal" osmol gap is often cited to be less than 10 mOsm/kg when the preceding equation is used. This is an arbitrary number, and there is considerable variability in baseline osmolal gaps in patients, particularly children.[13] If the osmol gap is significantly greater than 10 mOsm/kg, it may be a useful aid in the diagnosis of toxic alcohol ingestion. Caution should be taken, however, in ruling out toxic alcohol ingestion with a "normal" osmol gap for several reasons. First, calculated serum osmolality results may vary among laboratories and must be done by the freezing point depression method. Also, delayed presentation after toxic alcohol ingestion may be associated with prior metabolism of most of the parent alcohol. Because only the parent compound is osmotically active, and because the charged metabolites are electrically balanced by sodium, there may be little or no osmol gap elevation in this setting. Finally, a toxic level of either methanol or ethylene glycol may be present with a gap of only 10 mOsm/kg. If there is clinical suspicion of toxic alcohol ingestion, direct measurement of the serum toxic alcohol level is necessary, and if not readily available, empiric treatment is warranted.[14] In addition to methanol, ethylene glycol, and isopropanol, other low-molecular-weight solutes may cause elevated osmol gaps, such as ethanol, acetone, propylene glycol, mannitol, glycerol, and ethyl ether. In addition to severe acidosis, rhabdomyolysis, pancreatitis, and metabolic derangements, such as hypomagnesemia, hypokalemia, and hypophosphatemia, are described.

Computed tomography may be indicated in an intoxicated patient with altered mental status. The characteristic finding of bilateral putaminal lesions suggests methanol poisoning, but this finding also may be seen with Leigh's syndrome, Wilson's disease, hypoxic-ischemic insult, encephalitis, and certain metabolic disorders. Ischemic necrosis, cerebral edema, or brain hemorrhages also may be noted. Follow-up scans may have prognostic value because parkinsonian features are unlikely to develop in patients whose putaminal lesions resolve within a short time frame.[15] MRI may detect optic neuropathy or putaminal aberrations from methanol intoxication.

Differential Considerations

Methanol and ethylene glycol cause inebriation and are ingested as ethanol substitutes. The differential diagnosis of a patient with altered mental status includes hypoglycemia, head trauma, postictal state, carbon dioxide narcosis, hypoxia, infection, hepatic encephalopathy, other metabolic disorders, thiamine deficiency, endocrinopathy, drug abuse, and other poisoning. Patients who present with severe abdominal pain and altered mental status could slant the differential diagnosis toward a long list of intra-abdominal entities. When an anion gap acidosis is identified, however, the differential diagnosis must be tapered toward entities that cause this, and a primary decision must be made regarding whether the acidosis is a result of an ingested toxin or some other cause (e.g., mesenteric ischemia, diabetic ketoacidosis). Usually, the presence of an ingestion is admitted by the patient or strongly suspected by the providers, but this is not always the case, especially when the patient has depressed mental status of unknown cause. Causes of an elevated anion gap in patients without evidence of renal failure, hypotension, hypoxemia, diabetes, seizures, or alcoholism include methanol, ethylene glycol, paraldehyde, isoniazid, iron, salicylates, toluene, or lactic acidosis from myriad toxicants, including metformin, carbon monoxide, cyanide, and cocaine. Ethylene glycol and methanol may cause a "double gap" (i.e., an osmol gap in addition to the anion gap). Other substances that contribute to an elevated osmol gap include isopropyl alcohol, ethanol, propylene glycol, mannitol, glycerol, and ethyl ether. Other situations in which double-gap acidosis may be encountered include diabetic ketoacidosis; alcoholic ketoacidosis; acetonitrile, methanol, ethylene glycol, and propylene glycol toxicity; multiple organ failure; chronic renal failure; and critical illness.[16] Hyperlipidemia and hyperproteinemia, by decreasing the measured sodium concentration, can increase the osmolal gap. Characteristically, isopropanol does not cause an increased anion gap.

Certain unusual characteristics of methanol and ethylene glycol intoxication lead to the specific diagnosis. The presence of ocular complaints unique to methanol poisoning is a valuable clue. Ethylene glycol ingestion often is associated with calcium oxalate crystalluria, which is not seen in methanol ingestion. Ultimately, the definitive diagnosis depends on the identification of the parent alcohol in the blood by laboratory tests that may not be routinely available. It is often necessary to start treatment based on clinical suspicion alone. Because the initial treatment for methanol and ethylene glycol is almost identical, identification of the specific toxic alcohol is not crucial to the initiation of therapy.

Management and Disposition

See the section on ethylene glycol management.

ETHYLENE GLYCOL

Perspective

Ethylene glycol is a viscous, colorless, odorless, slightly sweet-tasting liquid. It lowers the freezing point of water, and as such, its primary utility is as a commercial antifreeze or coolant. Other sources include airplane deicing solutions, hydraulic brake fluids, and industrial solvents/precursors; it also is a component of certain paints, lacquers, and cosmetics. Most ethylene glycol poisonings occur with the ingestion of antifreeze. Unusual poisoning scenarios are described, including an epidemic after the contamination of water supplies and the intentional poisoning of an infant, presenting as a inherited metabolic disorder. In 2002, the American Association of Poison Control Centers reported 6077 exposures to ethylene glycol. Of those exposures, 85% were unintentional, and 12% resulted in moderate or severe effects; there were 40 fatalities. If treated early and aggressively, ethylene glycol poisoning is unlikely to result in death. Conversely, failure to recognize and treat ethylene glycol ingestion rapidly may result in multiorgan failure and death within 24 to 36 hours.[17]

Principles of Disease

Pharmacology and Metabolism

Absorption of ethylene glycol is rapid after ingestion. It distributes evenly to tissues with a volume similar to that of body water. Peak blood levels are reached within 1 to 4 hours after ingestion. In contrast to methanol and isopropanol, ethylene glycol is nonvolatile at room temperature; absorption via inhalation is unlikely. Reported half-lives range from 3 to 8.6 hours.[18] When metabolism is blocked by fomepizole or ethanol, the half-life increases to 11 to 15 hours or 17 hours, respectively.[19] The toxic and lethal doses of 100% ethylene glycol have been reported as 0.2 mL/kg and 1.4 mL/kg. At the other extreme, with therapeutic advances, patients who have ingested 3000 mL have survived.[20] Twenty-seven percent of ethylene glycol is excreted unchanged by the kidneys. The remainder is hepatically oxidized via ADH and other oxidative enzymes to various toxic organic aldehydes and acids (Figure 153-2).

Pathophysiology

Unmetabolized ethylene glycol has limited toxicity, yet all metabolites are toxic. In humans, 2.3% of a dose of

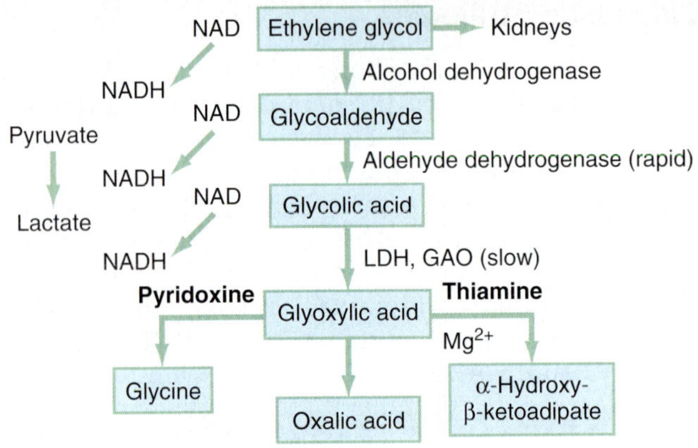

Figure 153-2. Metabolism of ethylene glycol.

ethylene glycol ultimately is converted to oxalic acid, most of which is excreted in the urine. A fraction of oxalic acid combines with calcium to form calcium oxalate crystals, which precipitate in renal tubules, brain, and other tissues. Although calcium oxalate crystals previously were thought to be the most significant cause of renal toxicity, much of ethylene glycol's nephrotoxic effect now is known to stem from the direct cytotoxic action of the organic acid metabolites themselves. When administered to rats, the ethylene glycol metabolites glycolate, glyoxylic acid, and glycolaldehyde cause significant renal toxicity in the absence of calcium oxalate crystal deposition. Persistent deposition of these crystals has been observed in serial renal biopsy specimens despite recovery. An in vitro study on human proximal tubular cells showed that toxicity occurred primarily from the direct effect of oxalic acid, despite exposure to much higher levels of glycolate.[21] Other authors suggest that glycolate levels correlate better with disruption of CNS metabolism, the development of renal failure, and mortality.[22] An intermediary of glycolic acid metabolism, glyoxylic acid, theoretically can be shunted toward pyridoxine-dependent or thiamine-dependent pathways, which generate the nontoxic products glycine and α-hydroxy-β-ketoadipate (see Figure 153-2). Based on this biochemical observation, these cofactors have found a place in therapy.

Histologically, proximal renal tubular dilation with hydropic change and vacuolar degeneration, intratubular crystal deposition, and edema of the interstitium are seen. Relative sparing of the glomeruli is typical, although glomerular interloop space crystal deposition may occur. Glomerular function is preserved, but tubular dysfunction manifest as protein leak is noted.[23] Neuropathologic changes induced by ethylene glycol include diffuse calcium oxalate deposition with petechial hemorrhages in the retina, brain, vessel walls, and perivascular spaces, with evidence of cerebral edema and chemical meningoencephalitis. Similar changes also have been noted in the liver, spleen, pancreas, pleura, lungs, pericardium, and blood vessel walls throughout the body. Myonecrosis occurs in skeletal and myocardial muscle, and rhabdomyolysis and myocardial dilation occur.[24] Fatty liver with focal necrosis has been noted.

The metabolism of ethylene glycol results in a profound anion gap metabolic acidosis caused mainly by glycolic acid.[25] Lactate elevation, triggered by the altered redox potential within cells and inhibition of the citric acid cycle by products of glyoxylate metabolism, is a minor contributing factor to the severe acidosis.[25]

Clinical Features

The clinical syndrome with ethylene glycol ingestion is divided into four stages: acute neurologic stage, cardiopulmonary stage, renal stage, and delayed neurologic sequelae stage. The severity of illness seen in each stage varies, as does progression through stages, which may be telescoped. Patients may die in any stage of ethylene glycol poisoning. Poor prognostic factors include hyperkalemia, severe acidosis, seizures, and coma. Metabolic acidosis and symptoms typically occur within 4 to 8 hours, but may be delayed for 12 hours or longer if ethanol has been co-ingested.

Stage I, the *acute neurologic stage,* occurs 30 minutes to 12 hours after ingestion. The parent alcohol causes approximately the same degree of inebriation as ethanol with CNS depression, slurred speech, nystagmus, ataxia, and vomiting. With large ingestions, more dramatic neurologic findings may be present during the early phase of intoxication, such as hallucinations, convulsions, or coma. Ocular findings, similar to findings seen with methanol intoxication, including decreased pupillary reflexes, decreased visual acuity, optic disk blurring, papilledema, and loss of color discrimination, are reported. Methanol exposure was not ruled out, however, in most of these case reports.

Stage II, the *cardiopulmonary stage,* occurs 12 to 24 hours after ingestion. Often, the patient exhibits mild hypertension and tachycardia. Tachypnea may reflect the underlying profound metabolic acidosis or may herald the onset of cardiogenic or noncardiogenic pulmonary edema.[6] The mechanism of acute respiratory distress syndrome (ARDS) is unclear, but may be related to the toxicity of glycolic and glyoxylic acids and to the deposition of calcium oxalate crystals within the lungs. Pulmonary infiltrates are described during this phase. Circulatory collapse may occur as a result of myocardial depression. Hypocalcemia, rarely associated with tetany or cardiac dysrhythmia, occurs in 30% of patients as a result of systemic chelation of calcium by oxalate.[24] Myositis with muscle tenderness and creatine phosphokinase (CPK) elevation results from skeletal muscle inflammation and necrosis.

Stage III, the *renal stage,* occurs 24 to 72 hours after ingestion. In one epidemic of 36 patients, renal damage was noted in 67%.[24] Awake patients may complain of flank pain or have costophrenic angle tenderness. Calcium oxalate monohydrate or dihydrate crystalluria is seen in only 50% of cases.[26] Hematuria and proteinuria are common, however. As with other causes of acute tubular necrosis, oliguria is not always present, but may develop 12 hours after ingestion and may progress to frank anuria. The outcome has not been well studied in patients who develop renal failure. Prolonged hemodialysis may be necessary, although recovery of renal function has been reported. Delayed onset of ARDS has been reported to occur during this stage, but more typically is seen in stage II. The degree of acidosis, delay in presentation, and glycolate levels correlate better with the development of renal failure than do ethylene glycol levels.[24,27]

Stage IV, the *delayed neurologic sequelae stage,* occurs 6 to 12 days after ingestion and typically manifests as cranial neuropathy.[28] All cases have been associated with renal failure. Facial diplegia, occasionally with deafness, is encountered most frequently. Other reported findings include dysarthria, dysphagia, tongue deviation, visual deterioration, and internal ophthalmoplegia. Delayed and persistent cognitive and motor deficits, such as ataxia, chorea, coma, and late personality changes, also are reported. Total paralysis from severe axonal peripheral polyneuropathic degeneration with oxalate deposition is reported,[29] as is polyradiculopathy from nerve root (not distal) pathology. Although some improvement in neurologic status has been noted at follow-up, most patients are left with residual neurologic deficits. Some authors have coined this delayed syndrome *facial auditory nerve oxalosis,* based on heavy calcium oxalate crystal deposition along the subarachnoid portions of the seventh and eighth cranial nerves seen at autopsy.[30] It is not clear, however, what causal role calcium oxalate deposition plays. Direct mechanical injury from crystals, inflammatory response triggered by ethylene glycol metabolites, meningitis, and pyridoxine deficiency all have been proposed as mechanisms. Because the syndrome has been reported only since 1978, it is possible that the advent of hemodialysis has allowed more patients with potentially lethal ingestions of ethylene glycol to survive to display delayed neurologic complications.

DIAGNOSTIC STRATEGIES

Useful laboratory tests for evaluating a patient with potential ethylene glycol toxicity include serum electrolytes, calcium, BUN, creatinine, serum glucose, serum osmolality, blood ethanol level, arterial blood gases, ethylene glycol level, electrocardiogram, and urinalysis. Although crystalluria is considered the hallmark of ethylene glycol ingestion, its absence does not rule out the diagnosis because less than half of patients have this finding.[26,31] Crystalluria may take the form of envelope-shaped calcium oxalate dihydrate crystals or needle-shaped calcium oxalate monohydrate crystals, occasionally mistaken for hippurate crystals.[6] Other crystal shapes and composites have been noted so that in the setting of combined anion and osmolal gap elevation, the presence of *any* type of crystalluria warrants a search for ethylene glycol. Monohydrate crystals are thought to be more specific for ethylene glycol poisoning.[26] Irrigating the urinary bladder with 50 to 100 mL of saline, centrifuging the irrigant, and examining the sediment for crystals may yield the diagnosis in patients already anuric. Other findings reflecting tubular dysfunction include decreased specific gravity, proteinuria, microscopic hematuria, pyuria, and cylindruria. Falsely elevated ethylene glycol levels may be seen in the face of elevated lactate or lactate dehydrogenase with certain enzymatic assays.

Freshly voided urine can be examined for fluorescence with a Wood's lamp. Sodium fluorescein is added to antifreeze to aid in the detection of radiator leaks. Urinary fluorescence may be seen 6 hours after ingestion of fluorescein-containing antifreeze. Gastric contents and the patient's skin or clothing also may fluoresce under Wood's lamp. The lack of fluorescence does not rule out ethylene glycol ingestion, however, because examiner sensitivity, specificity, and interrater reliability are low.[32] One study found urinary fluorescence in all specimens from children evaluated for conditions unrelated to poisoning.[33] Specimens should be collected in borosilicate glass test tubes or deposited directly onto gauze or filter paper because many plastic specimen containers and some glass tubes are fluorescent. The urine pH also should be checked and adjusted to 4.5 or greater before Wood's lamp examination.

Leukocytosis may be seen in ethylene glycol poisoning, with a typical white blood cell count of 10,000 to 40,000/μL, but is neither a sensitive nor a specific finding and is not of diagnostic value. The hematocrit and platelet count are normal. One third of patients have hypocalcemia, which is most likely caused by calcium precipitation with oxalate.[34] Q-T prolongation on the electrocardiogram leads to the early diagnosis of hypocalcemia. Rarely, profound hypocalcemia resulting in seizures and tetany may occur. The CPK can be elevated owing to toxic effects of ethylene glycol metabolites on muscle tissue.

Similar to methanol, ethylene glycol often causes a profound anion gap metabolic acidosis when the metabolites glycolic acid and glyoxylic acid (and, to some extent, lactic acid) accumulate. Artifactual elevations of lactic acid levels may occur in the presence of glycolate with certain analyzers.[35] Similar to methanol toxicity, an elevated osmolal gap as measured by freezing point depression is a clue to the diagnosis of ethylene glycol toxicity. Lethal concentrations can be associated, however, with a normal or only slightly elevated osmolal gap. The cerebrospinal fluid may be normal or may display a cloudy or bloody appearance, increased protein or, most commonly, a polymorphonuclear pleocytosis.

Imaging studies show cerebral edema with decreased attenuation in the mediobasilar portions of the brain, typically with a return to isodensity within 1 week; this does not correspond to the clinical picture.[6] MRI in one patient with delayed cranial neuropathy showed gadolinium enhancement of cranial nerve V bilaterally, possibly secondary to calcium oxalate deposition. Electroencephalographic findings have been nonspecific.

Differential Considerations

Classically, patients who ingest ethylene glycol appear intoxicated without the odor of ethanol and have an anion gap metabolic acidosis, increased osmolal gap, and calcium oxalate crystalluria. Without evidence of alcoholic ketoacidosis or diabetic ketoacidosis, the differential diagnosis of the "double gap" should include methanol and ethylene glycol. The hallmark finding with late presentation is renal toxicity. Toxicant-induced acute renal failure is extensively reviewed elsewhere; substances commonly implicated include antimicrobials, nonsteroidal anti-inflammatory drugs, acetaminophen, halogenated hydrocarbons, radiocontrast media, metals, antineoplastic agents, and myoglobin. Hypocalcemia and a prolonged Q-T interval are important diagnostic clues. Toxicant-induced hypocalcemia is unusual and may be related to aminoglycosides, calcitonin, cisplatin, loop diuretics, interferon-α, mithramycin, pentamidine, and phosphate infusions. Healthy individuals with dietary excesses of vitamin C or foods rich in oxalate, such as tomatoes, garlic, spinach, rhubarb, cocoa, and tea, may exhibit calcium oxalate crystalluria.

Management

Methanol and ethylene glycol ingestions are treated essentially the same, and the following recommendations apply to both. As in any overdose setting, resuscitation and stabilization are paramount. Specific blood levels that confirm the presence of these substances may not be readily available, and a delay in instituting therapy can lead to irreversible organ damage or death. For any significant history of exposure, treatment should be initiated pending a confirmatory toxic alcohol blood level.

Because methanol and ethylene glycol are absorbed rapidly from the gastrointestinal tract, and gastric emptying has not been shown to alter clinical course or outcome and may be associated with complications, its use is restricted to patients who have ingested a substantial volume and arrive in the emergency department within 30 to 60 minutes of ingestion. Activated charcoal is not useful unless co-ingestants are suspected. Obtunded patients should receive intravenous naloxone, dextrose, and thiamine. Forced diuresis is of no value and may cause pulmonary edema and ARDS. Early intubation may be indicated to protect the airway against aspiration and in anticipation of further deterioration in mental status.

Three treatment goals exist for patients with methanol or ethylene glycol toxicity: (1) correction of metabolic acidosis with bicarbonate; (2) ADH blockade, which inhibits the metabolism of methanol and ethylene glycol to toxic metabolites; and (3) removal of the parent alcohol and its metabolites by hemodialysis. The acidic metabolites of methanol and ethylene glycol can cause a profound bicarbonate-resistant metabolic acidosis, with several hundred milliequivalents of excess acid produced per hour.[36] In contrast to lactic acid, these acids are not metabolized to bicarbonate, and massive amounts of bicarbonate may be necessary merely for partial correction of acidosis.[6] Early correction of metabolic acidosis may be beneficial in reversing methanol-induced visual impairment,[37] most likely related to the induction of a larger fraction of dissociated formic acid, which should decrease the amount of formic acid entering the CNS. Depending on the severity of the patient's acidosis, intravenous bicarbonate can be administered by intermittent boluses, an initial bolus followed by an infusion, or infusion alone. Boluses of 1 to 2 mEq/kg to attain a target serum pH of 7.45 to 7.50 followed by an infusion of 150 mEq/L of sodium bicarbonate in 5% dextrose at 1.5 to 2 times the maintenance fluid rate are suggested. With ethylene glycol, the potential for worsened hypocalcemia during the administration of large amounts of sodium bicarbonate should be considered.

To prevent further production of the toxic and acidic metabolites of methanol and ethylene glycol, metabolism of the parent compounds by the enzyme ADH must be blocked by either ethanol or fomepizole (Antizol). After significant toxic alcohol exposure, ADH blockade should be carried out in any adult or child with symptoms or with methanol or ethylene glycol levels greater than 20 mg/dL, even if asymptomatic. If ethanol is used to block ADH, the goal is to maintain the blood ethanol level between 100 and 150 mg/dL, which completely saturates ADH.[6] The affinity of ADH for ethanol is 10 to 20 times greater than for methanol and 100 times greater than for ethylene glycol. When methanol or ethylene glycol metabolism is blocked by ethanol, their half-lives increase to more than 30 hours or 17 hours, respectively. Prevention of methanol and ethylene glycol metabolism by ethanol explains the delayed toxicity seen in patients who ingest ethanol in combination with either of these substances. When dosing ethanol, it also is important to measure the patient's initial blood ethanol level. If it is greater than 100 mg/dL, a loading dose is unnecessary, and the patient can be started on a maintenance infusion (Table 153-1). The required maintenance dose of ethanol may nearly triple during hemodialysis because ethanol also is efficiently removed. Ethanol may be given orally or intravenously. Potential side effects of intravenous administration include CNS and respiratory depression, hypotension, vomiting, hypoglycemia, and thrombophlebitis although, even in children, adverse effects are limited.[38] Oral ethanol loading may be associated with gastritis. Initial close monitoring of serum ethanol and glucose levels every 1 to 2 hours is essential until a steady-state level of 100 to 150 mg/dL is achieved. Levels should be checked every 2 to 4 hours thereafter. Monitoring of ethanol therapy ideally is accomplished in the intensive care unit.

Similar to ethanol, fomepizole blocks the metabolism of methanol and ethylene glycol by ADH and prevents the formation of toxic metabolites.[19,39] Fomepizole is a pregnancy category C drug; although not approved for use in children, its use has been reported.[40] Potential advantages of the use of fomepizole compared with ethanol include ease of administration, predictable pharmacokinetics, improved patient safety profile, a standardized and less complicated dosing regimen that does not require direct observation or frequent blood monitoring, longer duration of action, and lack of CNS depression.[41] Nonetheless, simply blocking toxic alcohol metabolism does not alter the toxicity of preformed metabolites. Neither the use of fomepizole nor the use of ethanol supplants the need for hemodialysis. The main disadvantage of the use of fomepizole is its acquisition cost. The dose is 15 mg/kg followed by 10 mg/kg every 12 hours for four doses. After five doses, the dose increases to 15 mg/kg every 12 hours until the ethylene glycol concentration is undetectable or less than 20 mg/dL *and* the patient is asymptomatic with a normal arterial pH. Dosing changes are required during hemodialysis. Side effects of fomepizole include headache, nausea, dizziness, inflammation at the site of infusion, rash, eosinophilia, and mild, reversible transaminase elevation. To date, no clinical trials have compared the relative efficacy, safety, or cost of fomepizole and ethanol in the treatment of ethylene glycol or methanol toxicity.

Rapid removal of the methanol or ethylene glycol through hemodialysis before they have been metabolized remains the cornerstone of therapy. In addition, hemodialysis, preferably using high bicarbonate–containing dialysate, corrects acidosis and uremia, aids in fluid management and cardiovascular stabilization, and removes the toxic metabolites in late presenters. Hemodialysis decreases the half-life of methanol and ethylene glycol to 2.5 to 3.5 hours. Peritoneal dialysis and hemoperfusion are much less effective.[42] Indications for hemodialysis in patients with methanol or eth-

Table 153-1. Standard Range of Therapeutic Doses of Ethanol Based on Average Pharmacokinetic Values

	Amount Absolute Ethanol*	Volume (43% Oral Solution)†	Volume (10% IV Solution)‡
Loading dose§	600 mg/kg	1.8 mL/kg	7.6 mL/kg
Standard maintenance dose (nondrinker)	66 mg/kg/h	0.2 mL/kg/h	0.83 mL/kg/h
Standard maintenance dose (chronic drinker)	154 mg/kg/h	0.46 mL/kg/h	1.96 mL/kg/h
Maintenance dose during dialysis (nondrinker)	169 mg/kg/h	0.5 mL/kg/h	2.13 mL/kg/h
Maintenance dose during dialysis (chronic drinker)	257 mg/kg/h	0.77 mL/kg/h	3.26 mL/kg/h

*Specific gravity = 0.79.
†Equivalent to 86 proof undiluted liquor (34 g ethanol/dL).
‡Equivalent to 7.9 g ethanol/dL.
§Assumes initial ethanol concentration is zero; dose is independent of chronic drinking status.
Modified from Barceloux DG, et al: American Academy of Clinical Toxicology practice guidelines on the treatment of ethylene glycol poisoning. *Clin Toxicol* 36:537, 1999.

ylene glycol toxicity are controversial. In general, however, hemodialysis is indicated in patients who have metabolic acidosis, renal compromise, visual symptoms (methanol), deterioration despite intensive supportive care, or electrolyte imbalances unresponsive to conventional therapy.[6] In addition, hemodialysis is recommended by some authorities for a blood level of either substance greater than 25 mg/dL, whereas another consensus group advocates extracorporeal elimination for an ethylene glycol or methanol level of 50 mg/dL.[41,43] Still others propose that with fomepizole use, serum creatinine concentration at presentation and creatinine clearance can be used to predict ethylene glycol elimination, and that absolute levels greater than 50 mg/dL are not independent criteria for hemodialysis.[44] Along these lines, other authors suggest that glycolic acid levels greater than 8 mmol/L, an initial anion gap greater than 20 mmol/L, or an initial pH less than 7.30 are predictive of renal failure and the need for hemodialysis during ethylene glycol intoxication.[45] Similarly, a small series of patients with methanol poisoning without pretreatment visual complaints were treated successfully with fomepizole alone.[46] Overall, "action levels" for toxic alcohols are arbitrary, generally not evidence based,[47] and must be interpreted with caution, taking into consideration the time since ingestion along with the clinical and acid-base status of the patient. A blood ethylene glycol or methanol level of 25 mg/dL drawn 1 hour after ingestion in an asymptomatic patient is much different than a level of 25 mg/dL drawn 12 hours after ingestion in a patient with metabolic acidosis who presumably has metabolized the parent alcohol and has accumulated toxic metabolites.

The endpoint for hemodialysis is an undetectable serum ethylene glycol or methanol concentration and the disappearance of acid-base abnormalities and signs of systemic toxicity. Closure of the anion gap also may serve as an endpoint for hemodialysis in situations in which levels are not available or reliable (i.e., in patients with delayed presentation).

In methanol poisoning, the rate of the final degradation reaction of formic acid to carbon dioxide and water depends on the cofactor folate in primates (see Figure 153-1). Studies in animals and limited human data suggest that formate metabolism is enhanced with the use of folate. Accordingly, 50 mg of leucovorin (folinic acid) should be given intravenously every 4 hours to adults with methanol toxicity. Likewise, the cofactors thiamine and pyridoxine have theoretical benefit based on their use in humans with primary hyperoxaluria, although no clinical trials have studied their efficacy in the treatment of ethylene glycol toxicity. Adequate cofactor levels minimize oxalic acid production by favoring the production of other, less toxic metabolites (see Figure 153-2). Because underlying deficiencies of these vitamins may not be readily apparent in patients, empiric administration is reasonable. The recommended adult doses are thiamine, 100 mg intravenously every 6 hours, and pyridoxine, 50 mg every 6 hours for 2 days. With symptomatic hypocalcemia, intravenous calcium should be supplemented, albeit cautiously, to avoid further precipitation of calcium oxalate crystals in tissues. Asymptomatic hypercalcemia need not be treated. Magnesium is a cofactor along with thiamine for the detoxification of glycolic acid and should be replaced in patients who are deficient.

Disposition

Admission is generally necessary for patients undergoing treatment for ethylene glycol or methanol exposure. In addition, all patients with clinical or laboratory findings consistent with these ingestions should be admitted, even when the history is lacking or unavailable. Early consultation with a nephrologist for possible hemodialysis is necessary in the management of patients with suspected toxic alcohol ingestion. If such services are not available, the patient should be given an ADH inhibitor and transferred to a setting where dialysis is available. A regional poison center or medical toxicologist may be contacted to guide management. An ophthalmologist can evaluate visual injury fully in patients with methanol poisoning. Neurologic consultation and follow-up monitoring of patients with either methanol or ethylene glycol toxicity are prudent given the potential for delayed or persistent neurologic sequelae.

Prevention

The addition of the bittering agent denatonium benzoate (Bitrex) to consumer automotive products containing 10% or more ethylene glycol or 4% or more methanol has been implemented in Oregon. The impact of this effort has yet to be fully determined. Another opportunity for prevention is the substitution of less toxic glycols, such as propylene glycol, into commercial antifreezes.

ISOPROPYL ALCOHOL

Perspective

Isopropyl alcohol (isopropanol) is a clear, colorless liquid with a slightly bitter taste. It is the second most commonly ingested alcohol after ethanol. In 2002, the American Association of Poison Control Centers reported 31,187 isopropanol exposures: 91% were unintentional, and 3% involved moderate or major effects; there were 4 fatalities. Rubbing alcohols, which contain 70% to 91% isopropanol or ethanol, are frequent sources of exposure and may be tinted green or blue. Other sources include skin and hair products, nail polish removers, disinfectants, window and pine household cleaners, and antifreeze. Children experience toxicity most commonly from accidental ingestion, but inhalation and transdermal absorption during sponge bathing may occur. Isopropanol and its major metabolite acetone cause twice the CNS depression as does ethanol, so intentional ingestion as an alcohol substitute is encountered frequently in adults. Iso-

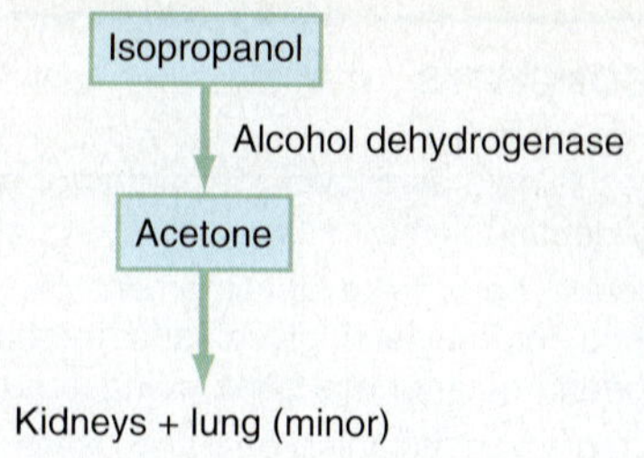

Figure 153-3. Metabolism of isopropanol.

propanol is not associated with the toxicity of ethylene glycol or methanol poisoning, and death after exposure is rare. The typical fatality involves a chronic, older alcoholic with mixed ethanol-isopropanol intoxication after a drinking binge.[48]

Principles of Disease

Pharmacology and Metabolism

Absorption of isopropanol is rapid and complete; 80% of a dose is absorbed within 30 minutes of ingestion. The kidneys excrete 20% as unchanged isopropanol. A small portion is resecreted into the stomach and saliva; the remaining 80% is metabolized in the liver to acetone by ADH (Figure 153-3). Acetone is excreted primarily by the kidneys, with small amounts expired through the lungs.

Isopropanol blood levels peak 30 minutes to 3 hours after ingestion, and elimination follows first-order kinetics with a half-life of 3 to 7 hours.[49] In children, the half-life may be slightly shorter.[50] Acetone is eliminated more slowly with a half-life of 22 hours. The rate of elimination of isopropanol may be increased by chronic ethanol abuse and decreased by hepatic damage.[48] A potentially lethal dose in adults is 150 to 240 mL (2 to 4 mL/kg), but adults have survived ingestions of 1 L (8 to 15 mL/kg).

Pathophysiology

Isopropanol is a potent CNS depressant, but the mechanism of action is unclear. Acetone is also a CNS depressant, and it has been suggested that coma may be prolonged by the extended elimination of this metabolite. The extent to which acetone contributes to coma is brought into question by the report of a patient who was awake and conversant, with acetone levels of 200 mg/dL. In large doses, isopropanol causes hypotension from peripheral vasodilation and direct myocardial depression. Topical effects include corneal de-epithelialization or dermal burns, described in premature infants as a result of skin de-esterification. Acetone does not seem to be shunted into the formation of acetoacetate or β-hydroxybutyrate; the finding of ketosis without acidosis is characteristic of isopropyl ingestion. No pathognomonic postmortem features are seen in isopropanol intoxication. Pulmonary congestion at autopsy is nonspecific and typical of deaths involving drug-induced CNS depression.[48]

Clinical Findings

Clinically, gastrointestinal and CNS complaints predominate. Intoxication may be suspected based on apparent inebriation with the odor of acetone rather than ethanol detected on the breath. The patient may have headache or dizziness and may exhibit neuromuscular incoordination, confusion, and nystagmus. Severe ingestions may result in deep coma, which is prolonged compared with ethanol. Respiratory depression or failure may occur. Patients may have a loss of deep tendon, corneal, or protective airway reflexes and have an extensor response to plantar reflex testing.[51] Pupillary size varies, but miosis is most common.[52] Isopropanol is a gastrointestinal irritant; the patient may complain of abdominal pain, nausea, and vomiting. Gastritis can occur with dermal and oral exposure.[53] Hematemesis and upper gastrointestinal bleeding stem from gastritis, but are not commonly reported.

Hypotension, although rare, signifies severe poisoning, with a mortality rate of 45%. One case series found mortality only when coma and hypotension were present.[52] Sinus tachycardia is common, but other atrial and ventricular dysrhythmias are rare and generally found only with confounding hypoxia, acidosis, or shock. Hypothermia is frequent.[52] Rarely, myoglobinuria, acute tubular necrosis, hepatic dysfunction, and hemolytic anemia have been reported. Metabolic acidosis is not present with isopropanol intoxication unless accompanied by hypotension, gastrointestinal bleeding, or co-ingestants; this is a distinguishing clinical feature. Hyperglycemia may be noted, but hypoglycemia has not previously been described, even though it should be sought in patients who have altered mental status.

Diagnostic Strategies

Useful laboratory tests for evaluating a patient with isopropanol ingestion include an isopropanol level, serum electrolytes, BUN, creatinine, osmolality, serum and urine ketones, and arterial blood gas analysis. Peak isopropanol levels occur soon after ingestion, whereas acetone levels peak later at 4 hours after ingestion.[52] The most common laboratory abnormality is ketosis with little or no acidosis and normal blood glucose levels. The ketosis is from the metabolite acetone, which can be detected in the blood 15 minutes after ingestion and in the urine 3 hours after ingestion.[52] Acetone is uncharged, and it does not elevate the anion gap. Isopropanol and acetone contribute to the increased osmol gap. In theory, a 1-mg/dL increase in blood isopropyl alcohol concentration should result in a 0.17-mOsm/kg increase in serum osmolality.

One early laboratory clue to the diagnosis of isopropanol ingestion is "pseudo–renal failure," or isolated false elevation of creatinine with a normal BUN.

This condition results from interference of acetone and acetoacetate by the colorimetric method of creatinine determination. Creatinine is expected to increase 1 mg/dL for every 100 mg/dL of acetone. A CPK level should be checked because patients with isopropanol toxicity may have coma-induced myoglobinuria and rhabdomyolysis.

Differential Considerations

Patients who ingest significant amounts of isopropanol appear intoxicated or have depressed consciousness, and the differential diagnosis includes all of the causes of altered mental status in an alcoholic patient, as discussed previously. The presence of ketosis warrants a search for diabetic ketoacidosis, alcoholic ketoacidosis, salicylism, cyanide, or starvation ketosis. A distinguishing feature of isopropanol ingestion is the presence of ketosis without acidosis. An increased osmolal gap with acidosis mandates a search for other toxic alcohols. In the setting of a high or rising creatinine and normal BUN, acute rhabdomyolysis also should be considered. Other substances that falsely elevate creatinine are cimetidine and nitroethane. Detection of isopropanol in acetonemic patients not exposed to isopropanol (i.e., the conversion of acetone to isopropanol in vivo) is well described.

Management and Disposition

Unless large amounts have been ingested recently, neither gastric emptying nor activated charcoal administration is warranted. The patient should be intubated if the patient is unable to protect the airway, if intubation is indicated on the basis of coingestants, or if the patient's mental status is poor and deteriorating. In contrast to methanol and ethylene glycol, ADH blockade with ethanol or fomepizole is not indicated. Hypotension should be managed with fluids and vasopressors as needed. If the patient remains hypotensive or has further vital sign deterioration despite these measures, dialysis is indicated. Some authors also recommend dialysis for isopropanol serum levels greater than 400 mg/dL.[47] Coma itself is not an indication for dialysis, but may necessitate mechanical ventilation. Peritoneal dialysis and hemodialysis have been successful; hemodialysis is much more effective and is preferred. Because of isopropanol's rapid absorption, patients who are hemodynamically stable without coma during the first 6 hours are at low risk for developing significant sequelae and generally do not require extracorporeal removal of isopropanol. The development of altered mental status within 2 hours is a clinical predictor of toxic blood isopropanol levels in children.[54] Care is otherwise supportive and includes rewarming, administration of thiamine, evaluation for hypoglycemia, and monitoring for gastrointestinal bleeding.

KEY CONCEPTS

- Small doses (single swallows) of methanol and ethylene glycol may cause toxicity.
- A latent period before the development of symptoms is characteristic for ethylene glycol and methanol toxicity, especially when ethanol has been coingested.
- A double-gap acidosis (anion gap and osmol gap) should suggest methanol or ethylene glycol toxicity.
- Therapy should begin immediately based on clinical suspicion of exposure to ethylene glycol or methanol. Acidosis should be corrected rapidly with bicarbonate, cofactors should be administered, and ADH should be blocked with ethanol or fomepizole.
- Because acidosis in the setting of exposure to either substance indicates toxic metabolite accumulation, immediate consultation for hemodialysis should be made, even before laboratory confirmation of toxic ethylene glycol or methanol levels.
- Toxic alcohol exposure cannot be ruled out by a "normal" osmol gap.
- The presence of an osmol gap without acidosis is characteristic of isopropanol ingestion. Prolonged coma may be seen, and hypotension portends a poor prognosis.

ACKNOWLEDGMENT

The authors thank Deborah Mouzon for her assistance with the preparation of this chapter.

REFERENCES

1. Bennett IL, Cary FH, Mitchell GL: Acute methyl alcohol poisoning: Review based on experiences of an outbreak of 323 cases. *Medicine* 32:431, 1953.
2. Martin-Amat G, et al: Methanol poisoning: Ocular toxicity produced by formate. *Toxicol Appl Pharmacol* 45:201, 1978.
3. Liesivuori J, Savolainen H: Methanol and formic acid toxicity: Biochemical mechanisms. *Pharmacol Toxicol* 69:157, 1991.
4. Martinasevic MK, et al: Folate and 10-formyltetrahydrofolate dehydrogenase in human and rat retina: Relation to methanol toxicity. *Toxicol Appl Pharmacol* 141:373, 1996.
5. Skrzydlewska E, Szmitkowski M, Farbiszewski R: Activity of cathepsin G, elastase, and their inhibitors in plasma during methanol intoxication. *J Toxicol Environ Health* 57:431, 1999.
6. Jacobsen D, McMartin KE: Methanol and ethylene glycol poisonings: Mechanism of toxicity, clinical course, diagnosis and treatment. *Med Toxicol* 1:309, 1986.
7. Chen JC, Schneiderman JF, Wortzman G: Methanol poisoning: Bilateral putaminal and cerebellar cortical lesions on CT and MR. *J Comput Assist Tomogr* 15:522, 1991.
8. Jacobsen D, McMartin KE: Antidotes for methanol and ethylene glycol poisoning. *Clin Toxicol* 35:127, 1997.
9. McKellar MJ, Hidajat RR, Elder MJ: Acute ocular methanol toxicity: Clinical and electrophysiological features. *Aust N Z J Ophthalmol* 25:225, 1997.
10. Williams GF, Hatch FJ, Bradley MC: Methanol poisoning: A review and case study of four patients from Central Australia. *Aust Crit Care* 10:113, 1997.
11. Chinard FP, Frisell WR: Methanol intoxication: Biochemical and clinical aspects. *J Med Soc N J* 73:712, 1976.

12. Liu JJ, et al: Prognostic factors in patient with methanol poisoning. *Clin Toxicol* 36:175, 1998.
13. McQuillen KK, Anderson AC: Osmol gaps in the pediatric population. *Acad Emerg Med* 6:27, 1999.
14. Glaser DS: Utility of the serum osmol gap in the diagnosis of methanol or ethylene glycol ingestion. *Ann Emerg Med* 27:343, 1996.
15. Hantson P, Duprez T, Mahieu P: Neurotoxicity to the basal ganglia shown by magnetic resonance imaging (MRI) following poisoning by methanol and other substances. *Clin Toxicol* 35:151, 1997.
16. Schelling JR, Howard RL, Winter SD: Increased osmolal gap in alcoholic ketoacidosis and lactic acidosis. *Ann Intern Med* 113:580, 1990.
17. Jacobsen D: New treatment for ethylene glycol poisoning. *N Engl J Med* 340:879, 1999.
18. Eder AF, et al: Ethylene glycol poisoning: Toxicokinetic and analytical factors affecting laboratory diagnosis. *Clin Chem* 44:168, 1998.
19. Baud FJ, et al: Treatment of ethylene glycol poisoning with intravenous 4-methylpyrazole. *N Engl J Med* 319:97, 1988.
20. Johnson B, Meggs WJ, Bentzel CJ: Emergency department hemodialysis in a case of severe ethylene glycol poisoning. *Ann Emerg Med* 33:108, 1999.
21. McMartin KE, Cenac TA: Toxicity of ethylene glycol metabolites in normal human kidney cells. *Ann N Y Acad Sci* 919:315, 2000.
22. Brent J, et al: Fomepizole for the treatment of ethylene glycol poisoning. *N Engl J Med* 340:832, 1999.
23. Niederstadt C, Lerche L, Steinhoff J: Proteinuria in ethylene glycol-induced acute renal failure. *Nephron* 73:316, 1996.
24. Karlson-Stiber C, Persson H: Ethylene glycol poisoning: Experiences from an epidemic in Sweden. *Clin Toxicol* 30:565, 1992.
25. Jacobsen D, et al: Glycolate causes the acidosis in ethylene glycol poisoning and is effectively removed by hemodialysis. *Acta Med Scand* 216:409, 1984.
26. Jacobsen D, Kesson I, Shefter E: Urinary calcium oxalate monohydrate crystals in ethylene glycol poisoning. *Scand J Clin Lab Invest* 42:231, 1982.
27. Sabeel AI, Kurkaus J, Lindholm T: Intensified dialysis treatment of ethylene glycol intoxication. *Scand J Urol Nephrol* 29:125, 1995.
28. LaKind JS, et al: A review of the comparative mammalian toxicity of ethylene glycol and propylene glycol. *Crit Rev Toxicol* 29:331, 1999.
29. Tobe TJM, Braam GB, Meulenbelt J, et al: Ethylene glycol poisoning mimicking Snow White. *Lancet* 359:444, 2002.
30. Anderson B, Adams QM: Facial-auditory nerve oxalosis. *Am J Med* 88:87, 1990.
31. Leikin JB, et al: Summertime cluster of intentional ethylene glycol ingestions. *JAMA* 278:1406, 1997.
32. Wallace KL, Suchard JR, Curry SC, et al: Diagnostic use of physicians' detection of urine fluorescence in a simulated ingestion of sodium fluorescein-containing antifreeze. *Ann Emerg Med* 38:49, 2001.
33. Casavant MJ, Shah MN, Battels R: Does fluorescent urine indicate antifreeze ingestion by children? *Pediatrics* 107:113, 2001.
34. Jacobsen D, McMartin KE: Methanol and ethylene glycol poisonings: Mechanism of toxicity, clinical course, diagnosis and treatment. *Med Toxicol* 1:309, 1986.
35. Porter WH, Crellin M, Rutter RW, et al: Interference by glycolic acid in the Beckman Syncron method for lactate: A useful clue for unsuspected ethylene glycol intoxication. *Clin Chem* 46:874, 2000.
36. Michelis MF, Mitchell B, David BB: "Bicarbonate-resistant" metabolic acidosis in association with ethylene glycol intoxication. *Clin Toxicol* 9:53, 1976.
37. Chew WB, et al: Alkali treatment of methyl alcohol poisoning. *JAMA* 130:61, 1946.
38. Roy M, et al: What are the adverse effects of ethanol used as an antidote in the treatment of suspected methanol poisoning in children? *Clin Toxicol* 41:155, 2003.
39. McMartin KE, Heath A: The treatment of ethylene glycol poisoning with intravenous 4-methylpyrazole. *N Engl J Med* 320:125, 1989.
40. Brown MJ, Shannon MW, Woolf A, et al: Childhood methanol ingestion treated with fomepizole and hemodialysis. *Pediatrics* 108:1, 2001.
41. Barceloux DG, Krenzelok EP, Olson K, Watson W: American Academy of Clinical Toxicology Practice Guidelines on the Treatment of Ethylene Glycol Poisoning. Ad Hoc Committee. *J Toxicol Clin Toxicol* 37:537, 1999.
42. Whalen JE, Richards CJ, Ambre J: Inadequate removal of methanol and formate using the sorbent based regeneration hemodialysis delivery system. *Clin Nephrol* 11:318, 1979.
43. Barceloux DG, Bond R, Krenzelok EP, et al: American Academy of Clinical Toxicology practice guidelines on the treatment of methanol poisoning. *J Toxicol Clin Toxicol* 40:415, 2002.
44. Sivilotti MLA, Burns MJ, McMartin KE, et al: Toxicokinetics of ethylene glycol during fomepizole therapy: Implications for management. *Ann Emerg Med* 36:114, 2000.
45. Porter WH, Rutter PW, Bush B, et al: Ethylene glycol toxicity: The role of serum glycolic acid in hemodialysis. *Clin Toxicol* 39:607, 2001.
46. Megarbane B, Borron SW, Trout H, et al: Treatment of acute methanol poisoning with fomepizole. *Intensive Care Med* 27:1370, 2001.
47. Kostic MA, Dart RC: Rethinking the toxic methanol level. *J Toxicol Clin Toxicol* 41:793, 2003.
48. Alexander CB, McBay AJ, Hudson RP: Isopropanol and isopropanol deaths: Ten years' experience. *J Forensic Sci* 27:541, 1982.
49. Pappas AA, et al: Isopropanol ingestion: A report of six episodes with isopropanol and acetone serum concentration time data. *J Toxicol Clin Toxicol* 29:11, 1991.
50. Parker KM, Lera TA: Acute isopropanol ingestions: Pharmacokinetic parameters in the infant. *Am J Emerg Med* 10:542, 1992.
51. Rich J, et al: Isopropyl alcohol intoxication. *Arch Neurol* 47:322, 1990.
52. LaCouture PG, et al: Acute isopropyl alcohol intoxication: Diagnosis and management. *Am J Med* 75:680, 1983.
53. Dyer S, et al: Hemorrhagic gastritis from topical isopropanol exposure. *Ann Pharmacother* 36:1735, 2002.
54. Stremski E, Hennes H: Accidental isopropanol ingestion in children. *Pediatr Emerg Care* 16:238, 2000.

CHAPTER 154

Hallucinogens

Binh T. Ly, Richard F. Clark, and Saralyn R. Williams

The term *hallucinogen* implies a single class of drugs, but these compounds have different chemical structures, mechanisms of action, and side effects. Most drugs usually do not produce actual hallucinations. Hallucinations are definitely not produced with marijuana, are possibly produced with phencyclidine (PCP), are rarely produced with sympathomimetic amines, and are produced only with high doses of serotoninergic agents. Almost any sympathomimetic compound can cause psychosis, paranoia, and other effects that some would classify as hallucinations. These effects typically are misperceptions of objects found in reality and are more accurately termed *illusions*. This chapter describes five groups of drugs: serotoninergic agents, sympathomimetic amines (entactogens), selected plants and fungi, and dissociative agents.

SEROTONIN-LIKE AGENTS

Perspective: Background and Epidemiology

Serotonin-like agents are a broad category of compounds that share chemical similarities to serotonin (5-hydroxytryptamine [5-HT]) or enhance serotoninergic tone within the body. These agents include various lysergic acid derivatives (lysergic acid diethylamide [LSD]) and tryptamines. All of these agents have a structural relationship with serotonin, specifically the indole ring. Serotonin-like agents produce changes in thought, mood, perception, and consciousness. Orientation to person, place, and time typically is preserved, but in cases of severe intoxication confusion may ensue. Patients occasionally present to the emergency department because of acute panic reactions, massive ingestions, or accidental ingestions (e.g., children or adults who have ingested the drugs unknowingly). In doses taken for consciousness alteration, only minor side effects occur except for sympathetic nervous system stimulation.[1] There is no addictive component in psychedelics and no euphoria-dysphoria cycle (as seen with cocaine) that would prompt a user to consume more. The rapid development of tolerance also limits the effect of repeated doses.

Before 1960, ingestion of psychoactive substances in the United States was limited to the Native American Church, a few botanists, and researchers. Wasson discovered the Mexican Indians' use of psilocybin mushrooms in 1955.[2] LSD was discovered by the Swiss chemist Hofmann in 1943 and was popularized by Leary in the 1960s.

LSD

LSD, or "acid," is the most potent psychoactive drug. Doses of 1 to 1.5 μg/kg produce psychedelic effects. The typical dose taken for an acid "trip" is approximately 25 to 100 μg. In terms of lethality of acute overdose, the margin of safety is tremendous with this drug, and the lethal dose of LSD has been approximated to be 14,000 μg.

LSD has been sold in tablets, liquid, powder, and gelatin squares, but the most common form of LSD sold today is "blotter" acid. Sheets of blotting paper are sprayed with LSD, dried, and perforated into small squares. Graphics are stamped onto the blotting paper in designs that include cartoon characters (e.g., Felix the Cat) or geometric designs (Figure 154-1). Each sheet contains hundreds of squares that are placed sublingually or eaten whole. Massive ingestions are rare.

In addition to synthetic LSD, several plants contain alkaloids similar in structure and action to LSD. These plants include Hawaiian baby woodrose (*Argyreia nervosa*), Hawaiian woodrose (*Merremia tuberosa*), morning glory (*Ipomoea violacea*), and ololiuque (*Rivea corymbosa*). Intoxication may result after ingestion of the seeds or an extract.[3]

Tryptamines

Substances in the tryptamines category are naturally occurring and synthesized. For centuries, Central and South American Natives have been using tryptamine-containing beverages, *Ayahoasca,* in their religious ceremonies. More recently, this plant-derived drink, which contains dimethyltryptamine (DMT) and 5-methoxy-dimethyltryptamine (5-MeO-DMT), has gained popularity in Europe and North America. Designer tryptamines also can be synthesized and possess the psychotropic effects of their natural relatives.

Psilocybin and psilocin are other naturally occurring tryptamines found in some species of *Psilocybe* mushrooms (Figure 154-2).[4] Many species of psilocybin-containing mushrooms are found worldwide except in arid regions. Psilocybin is resistant to oxidation and remains active when the mushrooms are dried or cooked into omelets or other foods. Psilocybin mushrooms are used for religious ceremonies and for alleged extrasensory perception effects by Mexican Indians. These mushrooms are the most desired psychedelic by users in Western society today. With the "back to nature" movement, most users would rather consume a mushroom than a synthetic chemical.[1] Street psilo-

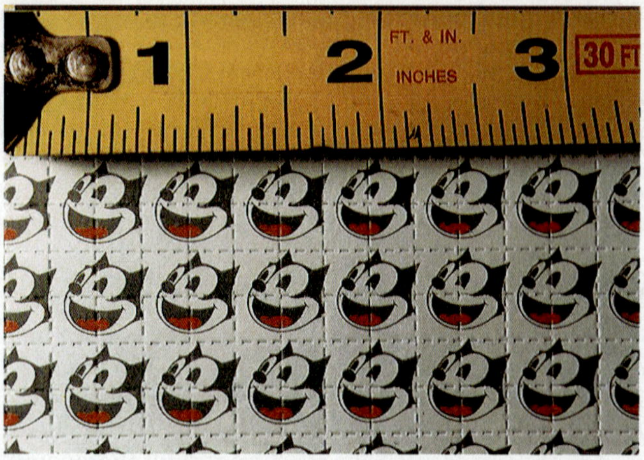

Figure 154-1. LSD blotters. (Copyright © 2001 Blotterart.com. Accessed at: http://www.erowid.org. URL = http://www.erowid.org/chemicals/show_image.php?i=lsd/lsd_blotter_felix.jpg.)

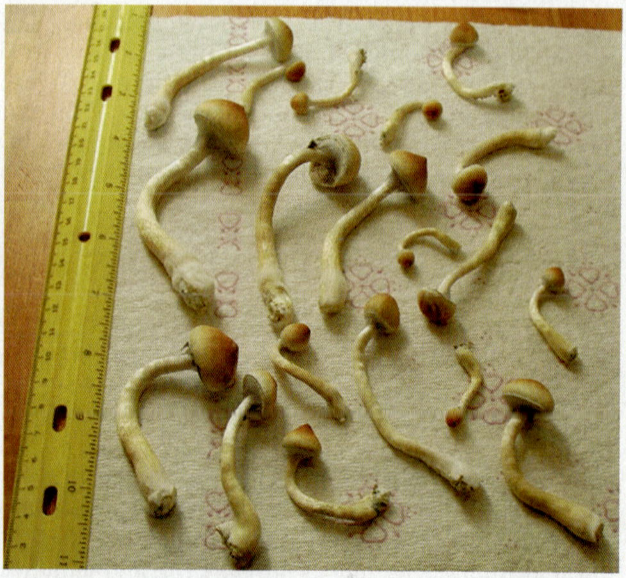

Figure 154-2. *Psilocybe cubensis* mushroom. (Anonymous photographer, Copyright © 2003 Erowid.org. Accessed at: http://www.erowid.org. URL = http://www.erowid.org/plants/show_image.php?i=mushrooms/cultivation_psilocybe_cubensis17.jpg.)

cybin sold in pills or capsules is usually substituted PCP or LSD. Misidentification and ingestion of poisonous species is a danger of consuming mushrooms.

Naturally occurring tryptamines not only are found in plants and fungi, but also in the parotid glands of the *Bufo* toad. Several tryptamines, including the aptly named compound *bufotenine,* have been isolated from these toads. Although bufotenine (found in numerous *Bufo* species) is alleged to possess hallucinogenic properties, this is highly unlikely because bufotenine does not cross the blood-brain barrier.[6] Only the venom of the Sonoran Desert toad (*Bufo alvarius*) contains a hallucinogenic substance, 5-MeO-DMT, also found in the plant-derived drink *Ayahoasca*. The venom can be extracted from *B. alvarius* without harming the toad. Smoking the dried venom results in psychoactive effects similar to those of 5-MeO-DMT.[7] Licking of these toads to achieve the hallucinogenic effects was highly sensationalized by the media in the 1980s, but is likely nothing more than mythology.

In addition to the tryptamines that occur in nature, designer tryptamines have been synthesized and are orally active.[8] Included in this group are diisopropyltryptamine and its 5-methoxy derivative, which also is known on the streets as "foxy" or "foxy methoxy."[9] The effects of these synthetic agents are similar to other tryptamines.

Principles of Disease: Pharmacology and Pathophysiology

Although the neurophysiology of the serotonergic agents may seem obvious because of their structural relationship to serotonin, understanding of these drugs is incomplete. Current evidence indicates these drugs act postsynaptically on serotonergic neurons.[10,11] One theory postulates that midbrain raphe cells send signals to higher centers via serotonin and that psychedelics change these transmissions, causing increased activity in the cerebral cortex and the limbic forebrain.[12-14]

There is cross-tolerance among LSD, mescaline, and psilocybin, but not to amphetamines.[15,16] The psychoactive effects of LSD may last for approximately 12 hours. Onset of action is approximately 30 minutes, and the most profound psychedelic effects are seen in the first 4 hours. In the last half of the 12-hour effect, irritability, increased muscle tension (especially in the face), and paranoia can be present.[1,17] Psilocybin effects begin within 30 minutes of ingestion, with the psychedelic phase lasting 30 minutes to 2 hours. The effects then wane, with resolution by 4 to 6 hours.

Clinical Features

In Western society, psychoactive agents are taken for internal mental exploration or more commonly for "recreation" (e.g., at a rock concert, at the beach, or in the woods). Changes include loss of boundaries between the user and the environment; the sensation that colors and sounds are distorted and intensified; and the perception that usual objects appear novel, fascinating, or awe inspiring. This state differs from the confusional and dissociative state produced by PCP. Users are usually aware that they are hallucinating. A sense of euphoria is typical, but may alternate with intense dysphoric experiences that are accompanied by suffering (e.g., that of dying or being born).

Acute panic reaction is the most common adverse reaction to psychedelics. Paranoid delusions and fear of impending death may be present. Behavior is either agitated or, occasionally, withdrawn. Sympathomimetic effects include dilated reactive pupils and moderate increases in blood pressure, heart rate, and, rarely, temperature. Mydriasis seems to parallel the intensity of the trip. Normal pupillary size returns as the patient regains a normal mental state.[15] In contrast to PCP, nystagmus, ataxia, muscle rigidity, and increased secretions are not present.

The patient's altered perceptions may result in lack of awareness of dangers in the environment, resulting in injury. Psychosis after LSD trips is reported, and schizophrenia (overt and borderline) may worsen. Transient depression sometimes occurs after LSD use. Flashbacks, or post-hallucinogen perceptual disorder, are transient episodes of altered consciousness that occur months or years after an LSD trip. LSD use and these episodes have not been shown convincingly to have a cause-and-effect relationship, however.

Massive ingestions may result in a person becoming comatose and unresponsive to pain. The person also may be hyperactive with marked auditory and visual hallucinations. Fixed and dilated pupils, diaphoresis, vomiting, and bleeding complications may result. Transient hypertension and convulsions may occur.[18]

Euphoria and a distortion of reality usually occur after ingesting one to five *P. cubensis* mushrooms. Transient nausea is uncommon, and in contrast to peyote, vomiting is unusual. Larger doses (5 to 20 *P. cubensis* mushrooms) produce visual hallucinations. Few adverse reactions occur, and the incidence of "bad trips" or panic reactions is lower than with LSD. There have been reports of convulsions, coma, and hyperthermia after psilocybin use, and deaths have been reported in small children.

Diagnostic Strategies

Serum and urine can be sent for toxicologic screening. Even when tests are available, however, the results are usually delayed, and diagnosis and treatment must be on clinical grounds. Mass spectrometry can identify psychedelics in serum, urine, or gastric contents.

Differential Considerations

Other drugs or mixed ingestion are a possible source of the patient's symptoms, especially with coma or marked physiologic changes. PCP, cocaine, and amphetamines must be considered because their effects may require specific treatment. Schizophrenia may appear similar to psychedelic ingestion.

Management

The basic principle of prehospital care is reassurance and supportive care. Patients may need to be restrained or preferably sedated if they are a danger to themselves or others. There is no specific antagonist to the effects of serotonergic agents. The most important therapeutic modality is sympathetic reassurance in a calm, quiet environment; the patient is "talked down." The patient may be worried about dying or being arrested. Patients should be reminded that they have ingested a drug that affects their perceptions and feelings. The effects last for hours, but when they wear off, the patient feels normal again.

Benzodiazepines, such as lorazepam (1 to 2 mg intravenously), can be given safely to decrease agitation. Phenothiazines should be avoided in case the symptoms are actually caused by an anticholinergic drug and not a psychedelic. Butyrophenones, such as haloperidol, can be useful if the patient is violent and must be sedated. Butyrophenones may be given by intramuscular or intravenous injection in doses titrated to clinical response. Monitoring during and after administration is recommended, if possible, when droperidol is used. Gastric emptying techniques are not useful because the drug already has been absorbed.

Disposition

Patients with anxiety or panic reactions can be talked down and sent home with responsible family or friends. Patients who persist with confused or paranoid behavior should be admitted. If the diagnosis is in question, the patient should be observed for several hours to see if significant changes in the condition occur. Follow-up evaluation should be provided with a psychiatrist, family physician, or drug counseling facility. Patients with massive ingestions may need admission to a monitored setting for serial reassessments.

ENTACTOGENS

Perspective: Background and Epidemiology

Entactogens, or hallucinogenic amphetamines, are structural analogues of amphetamine and mescaline and share effects in varying degrees of true stimulants and the serotonin-like hallucinogens.

Designer Amphetamines

Designer amphetamines include 3,4-methylenedioxymethamphetamine (MDMA, Ecstasy, XTC, Adam), 3,4-

methylenedioxyamphetamine (MDA), 3,4-methylenedioxyethamphetamine (Eve), paramethoxyamphetamine (PMA), and 4-methyl-2,5-dimethoxyamphetamine (serenity, tranquility, peace, STP). They have been termed *designer amphetamines* because they were developed chemically to circumvent the law before the advent of the prospective standard for the Controlled Substances Act.

MDMA is the best-known agent. It was first synthesized in 1914 as an appetite suppressant. Recreational and psychotherapeutic use began in the late 1970s and has increased in recent years, especially on college campuses, where 39% of students may have tried this drug.[5,19,20] In 1996, 9% of high school seniors in Texas had tried MDMA before graduation.[21] MDMA and MDA have been called "love drugs" because of claims from users that sexual pleasure and feelings are heightened. The sympathomimetic effects may produce erectile dysfunction, however. MDMA can produce euphoria, increase emotional awareness, and improve interpersonal communications. Overt hallucinations of the type experienced with LSD are rare; however, sensory enhancement and distortion and illusions can occur. Because of these effects, Nichols[20] suggested that these drugs represent a new class: *entactogens* (i.e., enabling the user to "touch within"). This concept is based on clinical effects in humans and on drug discrimination studies in laboratory animals.[20,22] MDMA was classified as a schedule 1 drug by the Drug Enforcement Agency in July 1985.

These agents are commonly used in three main settings: as "psychotherapeutic adjuncts," recreationally in small groups or by couples, and at dance clubs or "rave" parties. Some psychiatrists or psychotherapists use entactogens as pharmacologic adjuncts to increase emotional awareness and interpersonal closeness and introspection during psychotherapy.[23] Rave parties are all-night dances held in warehouses or dance halls. Virtual nonstop dancing occurs to loud, repetitive, electronically synthesized "techno" music, and a variety of hallucinogens and amphetamine derivatives are consumed, especially MDMA. "Herbal ecstasy," otherwise known as ma-huang or ephedra, sometimes has been substituted for MDMA at these gatherings when MDMA is scarce. Although this herb contains ephedrine, its effects are not as psychedelic as MDMA. MDMA is now widely available and is sold in clubs, on the street, and at raves for about $20 per pill (usually 50 mg). The continuous muscular activity required during these parties may combine with MDMA and other psychostimulants to produce toxicity, resulting in rhabdomyolysis and hyperthermia. Typical doses of MDMA are 1 to 2 mg/kg.[24]

A series of nine deaths in Canada associated with PMA was originally reported in 1974. More recently, clusters of multiple deaths in association with PMA exposure were reported in Europe and Australia.[25-27] Because of the popularity of MDMA, PMA is reportedly being sold under the guise of MDMA. Signs and symptoms of adrenergic excess occur before death, but whether PMA is more toxic in equipotent dosages than other amphetamines is not known.

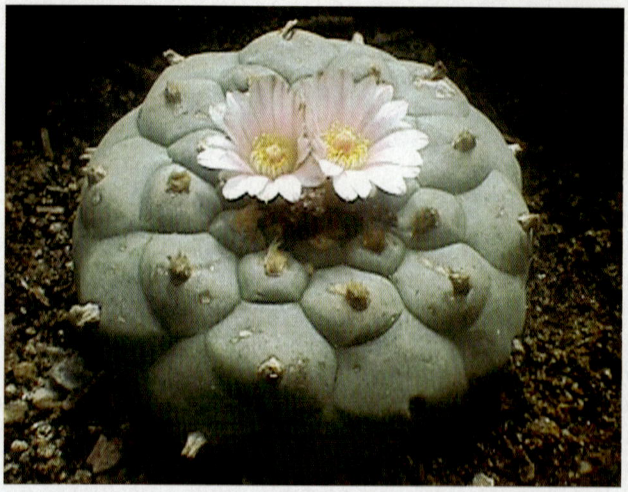

Figure 154-3. *Lophophora williamsii* (peyote cactus). (Photo by Christopher B., Copyright © 2000 Erowid.org. Accessed at: http://www.erowid.org. URL = http://www.erowid.org/plants/show_image.php?i=peyote/lophophora_williamsii24.jpg.)

Mescaline

Mescaline usually is consumed in the form of peyote "buttons," which are derived from the small blue-green cacti *Lophophora williamsii* and *Lophophora diffusa* (Figure 154-3). The cacti grow in the deserts of the southwestern United States and Mexico. The peyote buttons are the round fleshy tops, which are removed and dried. Mescaline is the active hallucinogenic alkaloid found in the buttons of the cactus.

Peyote has been used religiously and ceremonially for 8000 years. Mescaline also is contained in the San Pedro cactus (*Trichocereus pachanoi*) of South America and is used ritualistically by Andean Native Americans.[1] These cacti contain many other alkaloids, some of which also are psychoactive. The use of peyote is legal for members of the Native American Church in some states. Adverse reactions (e.g., panic) to peyote are rare in this structured religious use.[28] Mescaline has an onset of action of 45 to 60 minutes with a duration of effects of 4 to 8 hours. The central nervous system (CNS) and physiologic effects of mescaline use are similar to those of LSD, but more vid hallucinations can occur. Nausea and vomiting are pronounced and almost always precede the hallucinogenic effects.

Nutmeg

Nutmeg is a spice derived from the seed of the nutmeg tree, *Myristica fragrans*. Use of nutmeg as a natural and legal psychotropic agent was popularized in the 1960s. Despite lack of any in vivo human studies, myristicin and elemicin have been suggested as the agents responsible for intoxication because their chemical structures resemble that of mescaline. A proposed biotransformation of myristicin and elemicin would result in substances resembling known psychoactive agents, 3,4,5-trimethoxyamphetamine and 3-methoxy-4,5-methylenedioxyamphetamine.[29] Reports of intoxication are uncommon.[30,31] Ingestion of 5 to 30 g (1 to 4 tablespoons) of the spice is said to induce euphoria and hallucinations but is most likely to result in gastrointestinal distress.

Principles of Disease: Pathophysiology

The psychoactive effects of MDMA and other entactogens are thought to result from alterations in 5-HT neurotransmission at postsynaptic and presynaptic sites and a dopamine-agonist effect on the presynaptic release of dopamine. Depressed glutamate-evoked neuronal firing and increases in extracellular levels of dopamine and serotonin in the nucleus accumbens also occur in the presence of these agents. Epinephrine and norepinephrine release may produce the cardiovascular effects. MDMA and possibly other entactogens are serotonergic neurotoxins.[32-34] When MDMA is administered to nonhuman primates and laboratory animals, serotonin is released initially from serotonergic neurons followed by degradation of 5-HT projections. Magnetic resonance imaging shows significant neurodegeneration.[34] These effects may persist for weeks or longer after a single dose.[35,36] The significance of this neurotoxic effect for humans at the dosages taken is unknown.[37]

Psychostimulant-associated hyperthermia has been well described in humans. Animal models suggest that not only can exposure to entactogens cause hyperthermia by itself in the absence of physical exertion, but also animals under the influence of these drugs seem to be less capable of regulating core body temperature in response to environmental hyperthermia.[38] In addition, increasing body temperature in the presence of MDMA or other entactogens seems to enhance serotonergic neurotoxicity.[39]

Hyponatremia resulting in seizures, stupor, and death is another complication of MDMA use and has not been described with other amphetamines. Two hypotheses have been suggested as the mechanisms for hyponatremia: (1) excessive intake of free water because users of MDMA are often advised to keep well hydrated by drinking lots of water[40] and (2) MDMA-mediated release of antidiuretic hormone (ADH). Increases in ADH levels have been documented in human volunteers taking MDMA and in a case of hyponatremia associated with MDMA use.[41,42]

Clinical Features

MDMA effects last 3 to 5 hours. Blood pressure increases during the first hour and gradually returns to baseline within 6 hours. CNS effects of MDA may last 6 to 12 hours. The psychedelic and stimulant effects of MDMA are preferred over MDA by most users. Larger dosages or greater frequency dosing of MDMA may lead to more frequent unpleasant side effects, such as agitation or confusion. Recreational users rarely report dysphoria, however.

Clinical effects expected from the entactogens would be similar to clinical effects of other amphetamine derivatives (see Chapter 152). Deaths after ingestions of these compounds seem to be linked to hyperthermia. Hyperthermia is reported more often in Great Britain than in the United States. Deaths at rave parties in Great Britain typically involve seizures and hyperthermia at recreational dosages. Dehydration and high ambient temperatures during rave parties may be contributing factors. The mechanism behind psychostimulant-induced hyperthermia is still unclear, but likely combines CNS factors and factors such as seizure activity with drug effects.[39] Rhabdomyolysis can occur from a combination of direct toxic effects of the agent, extreme physical activity, and hyperthermia. Preexisting cardiac disease may contribute to sudden death, presumably from dysrhythmias.[24,43,44] MDMA can precipitate a hypertensive crisis in patients taking monoamine oxidase inhibitors.[45] MDMA analogues also have contributed to fatal overdoses.[46,47]

Diagnostic Strategies

Urine screening with immunoassay techniques can detect entactogens. Small dosages may not be detected, but larger doses test positive for amphetamine-methamphetamine.[48] Thin-layer chromatography also can detect MDMA and other designer amphetamines and their metabolites in the urine.[49]

Differential Considerations

All sympathomimetic compounds, including cocaine, amphetamine derivatives, PCP, and LSD, can present with violent and psychotic behavior, convulsion, coma, and any combination of sympathomimetic signs and symptoms. Many of these reactions may not be from overdose, but from idiopathic and unpredictable toxic reactions. Initial management is consistent for each of these compounds.

Management

Patients with panic reactions or violent psychotic episodes should be placed in a quiet environment if possible and reassured. Diazepam, 2 to 10 mg, or lorazepam, 1 to 2 mg, can be administered orally to cooperative patients. A repeat dose of intravenous diazepam, 5 to 10 mg, or intramuscular or intravenous lorazepam, 2 to 4 mg, can be used in violent subjects as necessary. Butyrophenones, such as haloperidol and droperidol, also can be used. Hypertension and tachycardia should be treated with aggressive sedation. If necessary, β-adrenergic antagonists in combination with vasodilators may be used. Dysrhythmias should be treated in the usual manner. Activated charcoal has no demonstrated value.

Because hyperthermia is a common complication, a core temperature should be obtained. If the patient's temperature is greater than 40° C to 42° C, multiple organ damage often can result in fatalities. Active cooling measures should be immediate and aggressive because the presenting temperature and length of time the patient has been hyperthermic strongly correlate with outcome. Rapid sequence intubation, paralysis with a nondepolarizing neuromuscular blocker, intravenous fluid resuscitation, and water spray and fans should be used. Rhabdomyolysis, myoglobinuric renal failure, hepatic damage, and disseminated intravascular coagulopathy all may accompany hyperthermia.[50-52] Treatment of hyponatremia should proceed in the usual fashion. Aggressive pharmacologic management of nausea and vomiting may be necessary with peyote and nutmeg ingestions.

Disposition

Most patients with a toxic reaction or overdose to an entactogen who are not hyperthermic or do not have abnormal cardiac rhythms experience resolution of symptoms in several hours. Psychiatric assessment may be necessary if psychotic or abnormal thoughts or actions persist longer than this time period. Urine screening may not be necessary for a treatment decision, but may aid the psychiatrist in counseling.

Patients with ongoing or severe toxicity to these agents require admission to the hospital. Seizures, cardiac dysrhythmias, myoglobinuric renal failure, hepatic damage, and heat-related problems should be monitored in an intensive care unit or step-down unit. Direct sympathomimetic toxicity resolves over 24 hours, but sequelae may require prolonged hospitalization.

MARIJUANA AND MISCELLANEOUS PLANTS AND FUNGI

Marijuana

Perspective: Background and Epidemiology

Marijuana is the most common illegal substance in the United States. It has been used medicinally since ancient times for conditions such as colic and asthma but has been illegal since 1937. The use of marijuana peaked in the late 1970s, with 20 million smokers, but declined during the 1980s. The National Institute of Drug Abuse suggests a new increase in its use, particularly among teenagers. Today, there are more than 12 million users in the United States and more than 300 million regular users worldwide.

Cannabis sativa and *Cannabis indica* plants are some of the earliest plants grown by humans. Bioactive substances derived from these plants are collectively called *cannabinoids.* The seedless flowering tops of the female plant are referred to as *sinsemilla* and are the commonly grown form of marijuana in the United States. The resin from the flowers is made into hashish. Marijuana is smoked or eaten blended into foods, such as brownies.

Principles of Disease: Pharmacology and Pathophysiology

Δ-9-Tetrahydrocannabinol (THC) is the main active agent of the more than 61 cannabinol compounds and approximately 300 other substances present in the cannabis plant.[53] Congeners Δ-8-tetrahydrocannabinol and Δ-9-tetrahydrocannabavarin and cannabinol are less bioactive than THC.[54] One major compound, cannabidiol, may attenuate some effects of THC.[54] Marijuana smoke also contains carbon monoxide, cyanide, acetone, and phenol, but not nicotine.[53,55]

The most efficient route of THC delivery is by inhalation. Fifty percent of smoked THC is absorbed compared with 6% by ingestion.[54] Experienced users may be able to absorb higher dosages with breath-holding techniques. Peak blood levels occur within 8 minutes of inhalation, with rapid distribution into tissues, especially tissues with high lipid content. The volume of distribution of THC is greater than 10 L/kg.[56] Experienced marijuana users report "highs" in the range of 9 ng/mL of THC in plasma after smoking, but these can increase to much higher levels with continued smoking.[57,58] Chronic or heavy users can excrete THC or metabolites in urine for 2 months.[58] The duration of perceived effects is usually 2 to 4 hours when smoked and 6 to 12 hours when ingested.

Clinical Features: Acute Signs and Symptoms

Smoking leads to rapid and more predictable signs and symptoms. Ingestion can cause delayed and sometimes unpredictable effects. The most common effects from smoking marijuana include alteration of mood and usually relaxation and euphoria. The only reliable physiologic changes produced are a mild increase in heart rate and conjunctival injection.[57] Pupillary changes usually do not occur. Other acute peripheral changes include urinary retention, decreased testosterone levels, and decreased intraocular pressure.[59,60] Short-term memory is impaired, and the ability to perform complex tasks (e.g., flying a simulated airplane) may be adversely affected.[61] Many users report excessive appetite after marijuana use.

Adverse reactions are rare. The most common adverse reaction is panic, paranoia, or acute psychosis. Individuals may believe they are dying, suffering a heart attack, or experiencing a "nervous breakdown," especially novice marijuana users or people with preexisting psychiatric disease. The patient is acutely panicked but alert and oriented, with reality testing intact, and gives a history of using marijuana. These episodes are usually transient. Even when "high-potency" marijuana is smoked continuously for hours, adverse effects are rarely seen. Patients become more sedated as they continue to smoke but never reach the point of being unarousable. No deaths have been solely attributed to marijuana.

Pediatric exposures to marijuana can lead to symptoms including hypothermia, ataxia, nystagmus, tremor, tachycardia, injected conjunctiva, and labile affect.[62,63] Oral ingestion of potent marijuana in children can produce rapid onset of drowsiness, hypotonia, and lethargy, which potentially could lead to coma and airway obstruction.[62,64]

Diagnostic Strategies

Marijuana screening is not helpful in the emergency department. Urinary metabolites of THC are detectable within 1 hour after smoking marijuana, but a positive urine test does not correlate with acute intoxication. A single marijuana cigarette can be detected for 72 hours when a 100 ng/mL cutoff level is used, and positive urine levels may persist for 3 months after chronic marijuana use.[65] Inadvertent or passive exposure to marijuana can produce positive urine testing.[66] False-positive urine screen results may be produced by nonsteroidal analgesic medications, such as ibuprofen and naproxen.[67]

Differential Considerations

The presentation that most closely resembles marijuana intoxication is an acute presentation of psychosis. Some individuals with underlying and preexisting psychiatric disorders may progress to overt psychosis after heavy or first-time marijuana consumption.

Management and Disposition

Care of patients intoxicated from marijuana consists of prevention of injury and reassurance of patients who have panic reactions. An extremely agitated patient can be sedated with oral or intravenous benzodiazepines. Patients who have an underlying psychopathologic condition when the drug effects have worn off after several hours should be referred for psychiatric evaluation. Children who are significantly symptomatic may require admission. Activated charcoal can be administered for very recent ingestions.

Salvia

Salvia divinorum has become popular more recently for its hallucinogenic potential. This plant is cultivated well outdoors in mild climates and is a member of the mint (Lamiaceae) family.[68] Common names include "the leaf or herb of Mary," "the Shepherdess," and "*Ska Maria Pastora.*" The main component of the plant is thought to be a diterpene, salvinorin A, one of the first to be associated with hallucinations in humans and the most potent plant hallucinogen discovered to date.

Salvia is usually chewed and either spit out or swallowed and seems to be absorbed better from the oral mucosa than the rest of the gastrointestinal tract. Dried leaves also can be smoked. Inhalation of smoke can produce symptoms within 1 minute that subside over 20 to 30 minutes. Sensations experienced are variable, but include distortions of color and vision. *S. divinorum* is often used in conjunction with other agents, such as marijuana and MDMA. Treatment of all of these new hallucinogen toxicities is supportive.

Absinthe

Absinthe is a bitter, emerald green liqueur derived from an extract of wormwood, *Artemisia absinthium*. The liqueur had achieved popularity in the 19th century, particularly among artists, poets, and playwrights, but it was made illegal in most countries in the early 20th century. The legal sale of absinthe has resumed in several European countries and Japan, and with the Internet, there has been resurgence in its use and popularity.

In addition to ethanol, the active ingredient of absinthe is thought to be α-thujone, an aliphatic terpenoid related to camphor and turpentine. Although the mechanism is not clear, thujone is thought to antagonize the inhibitory γ-aminobutyric acid ($GABA_A$) receptor, which explains the clinical effects observed with absinthe.[69] The acute clinical effects of absinthe are beyond the inebriation expected from ethanol alone and include confusion, delirium, euphoria, and hallucinations (auditory and visual). Thujone is a proconvulsant and may cause generalized clonic followed by tonic convulsive activity.[70] Ingestion of an essential oil of wormwood has been reported to result in convulsions complicated with renal failure secondary to rhabdomyolysis.[71] Treatment of convulsions include supportive care and benzodiazepines.

Anticholinergic Mushrooms

Anticholinergic mushrooms include *Amanita muscaria, Amanita pantherina,* and *Amanita cothurnata. A. muscaria* has a red or yellow cap with white warty structures on its surface and grows in forests of aspen, birch, fir, or pine trees (Figure 154-4). It has been used as an intoxicant by Siberians for centuries and is often described in folklore and fairy tales. Pharmacolinguistic evidence indicates that several modern religions began as *A. muscaria* cults.[2]

The active ingredients in anticholinergic mushrooms such as *A. muscaria* include ibotenic acid and its decarboxylation product, muscimol. The mechanism of

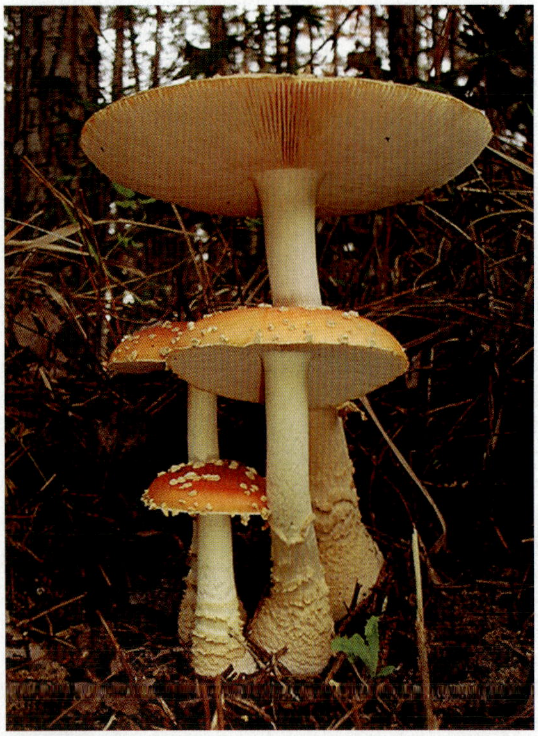

Figure 154-4. *Amanita muscaria* mushroom. (Photo by Mark Shubert, Copyright © 2004 Erowid.org. Accessed at: http://www.erowid.org. URL = http://www.erowid.org/plants/show_image.php?i=amanitas/amanita_muscaria17.jpg.)

action is thought to be as an agonist on glutamic acid and GABA receptor sites. The effects begin approximately 20 minutes after ingestion. Usually a phase of "sleep" occurs, and it may be difficult to arouse the patient. This phase is followed by elation, giddiness, hyperactivity, and muscle tremors. Visual hallucinations and manic excitement alternate with periods of deep sleep. The duration of effect is 6 to 12 hours. Anticholinergic effects may occur, and tonic-clonic seizures are reported. Deaths are rare. Prolonged sleep with *A. muscaria* ingestion requires only observation or supportive care.

There has been a high incidence of mistreatment of *A. muscaria* ingestion with atropine because the name implies that it contains muscarine with cholinergic effects. The amount of muscarine is, however, very small (<0.0002% in fresh specimens). Many textbooks recommend the use of atropine, but atropine can exacerbate the anticholinergic effects of ibotenic acid and muscimol. Central antimuscarinic effects frequently resemble delirium. Peripheral antimuscarinic effects may include mydriasis, sinus tachycardia, dry mucous membranes, dry and flushed skin, decreased intestinal motility, and urinary retention. These mushrooms should not be mistaken for other mushrooms exhibiting cholinergic activity, such as *Clitocybe dealbata*, which produce bradycardia, sweating, salivation, lacrimation, and diarrhea. These cholinergic mushrooms are not taken as psychedelics but usually are accidentally ingested and may require atropine for treatment. Also, one should not confuse the *A. muscaria* group with the cyclopeptide group, of which *A. phalloides* is a member. Mushrooms from the cyclopeptide category do not produce psychedelic effects and can cause significant hepatotoxicity, leading to death (see Chapter 162).

DISSOCIATIVE AGENTS

Perspective: Background and Epidemiology

PCP and ketamine are the two main agents included in the class of dissociative agents. They are similar in chemical structure and pharmacologic effect. PCP and ketamine are general anesthetics with analgesic and amnestic activity while lacking respiratory or cardiovascular depression by causing dissociation of the patient from the environment.

Phencyclidine

PCP was marketed for use as a general anesthetic in humans and animals. Vivid descriptions of distressing and terrifying emergence reactions and 8 days of confusion or coma in patients after PCP administration rapidly led to its recall. In 1978, PCP was classified as a schedule I drug. The use of PCP as a veterinary anesthetic also was discontinued. In the 1960s, PCP was sold as the "PeaCe Pill," which usually was consumed orally; the effects were often unpredictable and unpleasant. In the mid-1970s, PCP was the most common cause of recreational drug–related emergencies. The most common users were adolescents, but today PCP intoxication is seen most often in men age 20 to 29, often in large cities.[72] Its popularity decreased because of unpredictable effects, a long clinical course, dysphoria, and association with violence. Today, most users smoke the drug on vegetable matter (e.g., parsley or oregano) or marijuana so that the user can titrate the dose to desired effects. The smoker becomes too confused or ataxic to continue smoking, avoiding overdose and unwanted reactions.[73]

PCP often is marketed as a more expensive drug. Most drugs sold on the street as exotic psychedelics, such as mescaline or psilocybin, are PCP. PCP in the crystalline form is often sold as cocaine and in other forms is marketed as cannabinol. PCP can be manufactured easily in a basement laboratory with readily obtainable chemical precursors. The volatile chemicals used in producing PCP have led to explosive fires and burns.

Ketamine

The structural and functional similarities between PCP and ketamine virtually guaranteed the eventual abuse of ketamine. Spurred by the rave party fad and the Internet, ketamine is one of the most rapidly increasing drugs of abuse in some parts of the United States, going by the names of "vitamin K" or "special K." In some cities near the Mexican border, such as San Diego, ketamine is approaching PCP in popularity. Although more difficult to produce than PCP, users can obtain large quantities of ketamine inexpensively from veterinary pharmacies in Mexico. Preparations available on the street often are adulterated with various stimulants. The most common use of street ketamine is insufflation, but subcutaneous and intramuscular injection and even rectal infusion are also popular. The goal of using ketamine is to achieve a level of intoxication or "high" known as the "K hole." Ketamine also has been used to temper the "crash" associated with the end of cocaine and amphetamine binges. Legitimate uses of ketamine today are the same as those originally intended for PCP in human and veterinary medicine.

Dextromethorphan

Dextromethorphan is not truly a dissociative agent but does share some pharmacologic and clinical features with PCP and ketamine. It has been a popular over-the-counter cough suppressant for more than 30 years. The similarity in structure of dextromethorphan to PCP and other opioid compounds and its binding to the PCP site of the *N*-methyl-D-aspartate (NMDA) receptor caused speculation of its abuse potential, which became reality in the 1990s. Reports from poison centers suggest that individuals abusing dextromethorphan are in the high school age group (13 to 17 years).[74,75] The Internet also has played a tremendous role in popularizing the misuse of this agent. Referred to as "DXM" or "Robo," dextromethorphan predominates on many

Internet websites devoted to rave parties, drug use, and experimentation.

Principles of Disease: Pharmacology and Pathophysiology

Despite being simple molecules, the pharmacology of PCP and ketamine are complex with agonist and antagonist actions at numerous sites.[76] At clinically relevant dosages, sites of action include the NMDA receptor, dopamine/norepinephine/serotonin reuptake pump, sigma-opioid receptor, and cholinergic receptors. PCP is well absorbed from any oral, nasal, or rectal mucous membrane and can be insufflated or smoked. It can be injected intramuscularly, subcutaneously, or intravenously. Ingested PCP is well absorbed in the small bowel, with onset between 15 and 60 minutes. When smoked, PCP produces symptoms within 5 minutes, with peak activity in 15 minutes.[77] Length of intoxication with PCP usually ranges from 8 to 16 hours, but can be longer in chronic users. Although enterohepatic recirculation has been proposed, more likely causes are either gastrointestinal concretion or delayed release from lipid stores.[78]

The pharmacologic effects of ketamine are only about one tenth as potent as PCP.[76] With ketamine, the intensity of intoxication is less pronounced, although in higher dosages the effects may parallel the effects of PCP. Duration of action of ketamine is typically shorter with symptoms lasting about 1 hour after insufflation but may be prolonged to 4 to 8 hours after an oral dose. PCP and ketamine are highly lipid-soluble agents that undergo extensive metabolism in the liver and are excreted eventually in the urine.

Dextromethorphan is the dextrorotatory isomer of the synthetic opioid levorphanol. Although typically classified as an opioid, its pharmacology is complex. It is an agonist at sigma opiate receptors, inhibits the uptake of serotonin, and blocks the NMDA receptor at the PCP binding site.[79] At high dosages, dextromethorphan is an agonist at the sigma opiate receptor. Naloxone has been reported to reverse intoxication.[80] Drug interactions with selective serotonin reuptake inhibitors and monoamine oxidase inhibitors also have been reported.[81]

Clinical Features

Patients with PCP intoxication have a wide spectrum of findings, with autonomic signs and symptoms often similar to other sympathomimetic agents (Tables 154-1 and 154-2). Recognizing PCP intoxication can be challenging because the classic findings may or may not be present. Assessing a patient with potential or actual trauma is difficult because PCP is a dissociative anesthetic agent, and findings such as abdominal tenderness are not consistently present.[82-84] The major cause of death or injury from PCP is behavioral toxicity leading to suicide and provoked homicide.[85-87]

Behavior may be bizarre, lethargic, agitated, confused, or violent. A blank or catatonic stare is common. Vertical, horizontal, and rotatory nystagmus is often present. Moderate hypertension and tachycardia may be present. Pupils usually are midsized and reactive, although there may be miosis or mydriasis. Bizarre posturing, grimacing, and writhing may be seen.[82]

Table 154-1. Comparison of PCP with Other Drug Groups

Classes of Drugs	Similarities	Differences
CNS depressants	Coma Ataxia Nystagmus	Tachycardia Increased deep tendon reflexes Hypertension
Sympathomimetics	Tachycardia Hypertension	Coma Ataxia Muscle rigidity Increased secretions Nystagmus
Anticholinergics	Hypertension Tachycardia Hyperthermia Bizarre behavior Seizures Coma	Increased secretions Pupils usually normal Blank stare Muscle rigidity Nystagmus
Cholinergics	Increased secretions Miosis Seizures	Tachycardia Hypertension Increased deep tendon reflex Muscle rigidity
Psychedelics	Bizarre behavior Tachycardia	Ataxia Muscle rigidity Increased secretions Coma Nystagmus Acute brain syndrome
Opiates	Coma Miosis Hypoventilation Apnea	No response to naloxone Increased deep tendon reflex Muscle rigidity Hypertension

CNS, central nervous system.

Other variable findings include ataxia, muscle rigidity, increased deep tendon reflexes, increased secretions, bronchospasm, hyperthermia, and convulsions. The percentage of violent patients ranges from 10% to 40% for PCP, and controlling these patients may be the most challenging problem in the emergency department. "Superhuman" strength is possible because of the dissociative action of PCP. Patients have broken police handcuffs, fracturing bones in doing so, and have performed other destructive actions not normally possible. Although mild hypertension in PCP intoxication is common, hypertension requiring antihypertensive treatment is rare. Severe hypertension with PCP overdose has been reported to cause intracerebral hemorrhage, but not as commonly as with cocaine or amphetamine.[83]

Hyperthermia can range from mild to life-threatening. Core temperatures of PCP victims can exceed 40° C and often go undetected for prolonged periods in the emergency department. Severe hyperthermia with temperatures greater than 42° C resembles heatstroke and often is associated with multiple organ damage.[84] Particularly susceptible organs are the kidneys, liver, heart, and brain. High-output congestive heart failure has been

Table 154-2. Assessing PCP Toxicity: Incidence of Findings in 1000 Cases

Findings	Percentage
Hallmarks	
Nystagmus	57.4
Hypertension (>140 mm Hg systolic or >90 mm Hg diastolic)	57
Sensorium	
Alert and oriented	45.9
Acute brain syndrome	36.9
Unconscious	10.6
Lethargy/stupor	6.6
Behavior	
Violent	35.4
Agitated	34
Bizarre	28.8
Hallucinating/delusional	18.5
Mute and staring	11.7
Nudism	3.3
No behavioral effects	3.5
Motor Signs	
Generalized rigidity	5.2
Grand mal seizures	3.1
Localized dystonias	2.4
Facial grimacing	1.7
Athetosis	1.3
Cholinergic Signs	
Profuse diaphoresis	3.9
Bronchospasm	2.1
Pupils ≤1 mm	2.1
Hypersalivation	1.7
Bronchorrhea	0.6
Anticholinergic signs	
Pupils ≥4 mm	6.2
Urinary retention	2.4
Abnormal Vital Signs	
Tachycardia (>100/min)	30
Hypothermia (<36.7° C [98° F])	6.4
Apnea/respiratory arrest	2.8
Hyperthermia (>38.9° C [102° F])	2.6
Cardiac arrest	0.3
Hypotension	1.6

From McCarron MM, et al: Acute phencyclidine: Incidence of clinical findings in 1,000 cases. *Ann Emerg Med* 10:5, 1981.

reported.[84] The presumed mechanism is muscle damage from seizures, extreme muscular activity such as struggling against restraints, or prolonged immobility. Rhabdomyolysis and acute myoglobinuric renal failure are the most common serious medical complications. Renal function returns after several weeks in most cases. Among the most lethal complications of PCP are respiratory depression, apnea, and cardiac arrest.[82]

Although dextromethorphan has activity at opioid receptors, the typical triad of opioid intoxication (miosis, respiratory depression, and mental status depression) generally is not encountered.[88] Similar to meperidine, dextromethorphan intoxication may result in mydriasis through paralysis of the ciliary body.[89] More typical clinical findings as a result of misuse are lethargy, agitation, slurred speech, ataxia, diaphoresis, hypertension, and nystagmus.[90] With higher doses, nausea and vomiting is common, and intoxication resembles that of LSD with euphoria and hallucinations. Dystonic reaction has been reported in a child after therapeutic administration.[79]

Diagnostic Strategies

Most hospital laboratories can perform urine screening for PCP. These tests are frequently bedside or point-of-care evaluations with rapid results. Many radioimmunoassays now can detect urinary PCP with a detection limit of 5 ng/mL. Urine is positive for 2 to 4 days after PCP use, but this can extend for more than 1 week after chronic exposure. Serum screening for PCP is of little clinical benefit because levels correlate poorly with symptoms. Several substances may cross-react with urine screens for PCP, including dextromethorphan owing to its structural similarity. Chlorpromazine, methadone, ketamine, and diphenhydramine also may cross-react with some assays.[91] Rhabdomyolysis can be diagnosed with elevated creatinine phosphokinase (CPK) or a positive urine test for occult blood (ortho-toluidine test) with few or no red blood cells, pigmented granular casts in the urine, and urine positive for myoglobin. Because dextromethorphan typically is formulated as a hydrobromide salt, chronic use may result in spurious hyperchloremia with a low or negative anion gap. This is due to interference of chloride analysis by the bromide ion in the autoanalyzer.[92]

Differential Considerations

PCP, ketamine, and dextromethorphan intoxications can mimic such diverse entities as head trauma, meningitis, catatonia, or heatstroke. Sympathetically mediated vital sign changes can be found in numerous other agents, including cocaine, amphetamine, and LSD. Antimuscarinic compounds, such as diphenhydramine, benztropine, and tricyclic antidepressants, also can simulate the tachycardia and altered mentation found with PCP or ketamine. Salicylate poisoning, thyrotoxicosis, and sepsis should be considered. Meningitis, intracerebral hemorrhage, and viral encephalitis all can present with altered mental status of unclear etiology. Even with a urine screen positive for PCP, the diagnosis is not certain unless a definitive history of recent PCP, ketamine, or dextromethorphan use is obtained and other conditions have been eliminated.

Management

Prehospital

Life-threatening complications, such as apnea or seizures, should be stabilized before transport. The threat of violence to prehospital care providers from patients with PCP poisoning makes it dangerous, or impossible, for only two or three prehospital care providers to restrain these patients until additional help arrives. Oxygen and glucose testing should be deferred until the patient is controlled. Violent patients under the influence of PCP may have traumatic injuries.

Emergency Department

Patients with PCP toxicity can have unpredictable, violent behavior or sudden life-threatening complications, such as cardiac arrest or seizures. Violent behavior, although possible, is less common with ketamine. Most patients with minor intoxication are alert, oriented, and neurologically normal after 4 to 6 hours.[83] All patients with signs of trauma or struggle should be evaluated for injuries. Reliable assessments of these individuals are difficult, and sedation and restraint are often necessary before diagnostic tests or examinations are undertaken.

Chemical sedation or restraint usually is preferred to physical force in cases of PCP or ketamine intoxication. Although mental status may not be as reliable after chemical sedation, the benefits of protecting the staff and patient in this manner far outweigh the disadvantages. Haloperidol, 5 to 20 mg intramuscularly or intravenously, or droperidol, 2.5 to 10 mg intramuscularly or intravenously (using appropriate precautions as per the Food and Drug Administration black box warning), is usually an effective means of chemical restraint in these patients. These agents may antagonize CNS receptor sites that are responsible for much of the violent behavior in these individuals. Benzodiazepines, such as lorazepam, 2 to 4 mg intravenously or intramuscularly, or diazepam, 5 to 10 mg intravenously, may be used in aggressive dosages to calm patients with all types of sympathomimetic poisonings. A well-coordinated team may be needed to apply hard restraints simultaneously to all four extremities and the body.

Comatose patients or patients with a questionable airway should be empirically intubated to ensure adequate ventilation. Although PCP intoxication can cause mild hypotension, profound hypotension is probably the result of trauma or a mixed-drug ingestion, and the patient should be resuscitated with fluids. Seizures should be treated with intravenous benzodiazepines (diazepam or lorazepam). Phenobarbital, 20 mg/kg intravenously, should be used for refractory seizures. Tachycardia does not require additional treatment except for sedation.

Hyperthermia (temperature >40° C) is common in severe cases of PCP poisoning. All patients with significant symptoms, psychosis, or violent behavior should have rectal temperatures measured. Individuals with elevated temperatures should be treated aggressively with active cooling measures.

Renal status and CPK should be monitored to detect rhabdomyolysis and myoglobinuric renal failure. Urinary acidification has been used in the past to trap PCP in urine and aid elimination, but its use has been abandoned because of the large volume of distribution of the drug (6 L/kg), the insignificant renal clearance of the drug (10%), and the potential adverse impact of acid urine on myoglobin in renal tubules that is often present after PCP intoxication. Activated charcoal is of no value in acute intoxication, but a standard oral dose of 50 g should be administered when body stuffing is suspected.

Dextromethorphan poisoning can be managed with supportive care and measures to prevent injury to the patient. Sedation with a benzodiazepine may be needed when the patient is agitated. The patient should improve over 4 to 6 hours. Because many dextromethorphan cough and cold preparations also contain acetaminophen, levels should be measured routinely.

Disposition

For nonviolent patients with PCP intoxication, a quiet holding room is ideal for observation, with 4 to 6 hours of observation. If patients have never been hyperthermic and have no signs of trauma, laboratory or other diagnostic tests are not needed. If hyperthermia or trauma is witnessed or suspected, urinalysis, CPK, and the appropriate radiographs should be considered before discharge. Patients with violent behavior or obtundation often require admission to the hospital, where close observation and treatment of potential life-threatening complications can be accomplished. Serial chemistry evaluations, including serum creatinine and CPK, should be monitored. Most of these patients can be medically cleared the next day.

KEY CONCEPTS

- Hallucinogens include many types of drugs with different associated effects.
- Diagnosis and management are based primarily on the history and physical examination.
- Reassurance and supportive care suffice for most patients.
- Aggressive sedation is necessary in agitated and violent patients.

REFERENCES

1. Schultes RE, Hofmann A: *The Botany and Chemistry of Hallucinogens,* 2nd ed. Springfield, Ill, Charles C Thomas, 1980.
2. Wasson RC: *Soma, Divine Mushroom of Immortality.* New York, Harcourt Brace, 1968.
3. Gertsch JH, Wood C: Case report: An ingestion of Hawaiian Baby Woodrose seeds associated with acute psychosis. *Hawaii Med J* 62:127, 2003.
4. Schwartz RH, Smith DE: Hallucinogenic mushrooms. *Clin Pediatr* 27:70, 1988.
5. Cuomo MJ, Dyment PG, Gammino VM: Increasing use of "ecstasy" (MDMA) and other hallucinogens on a college campus. *J Am Coll Health* 42:271, 1994.
6. Gessner PK, Page IH: Behavioral effects of 5-methoxy-N,N-dimethyltryptamine, other tryptamines and LSD. *Am J Physiol* 203:167, 1962.
7. Weil AT: *Bufo alvarius*: A potent hallucinogen of animal origin. *J Ethnopharmacol* 41:1, 1994.
8. Shulgin AT: N,N-Diisopropyltryptamine (DIPT) and 5-methoxy-N,N-diisopropyltryptamine (5-MeO-DIPT): Two orally active tryptamine analogs with CNS activity. *Commun Psychopharmacol* 4:363, 1980.
9. Meatherall R: Foxy, a designer tryptamine hallucinogen. *J Anal Toxicol* 27:313, 2003.
10. Jacobs BL: How hallucinogenic drugs work. *Am Sci* 75:386, 1987.
11. Glennon RA, et al: Evidence for 5-HT 2 involvement in the mechanism of action of hallucinogenic drugs. *Life Sci* 35:2506, 1985.
12. Smythies JR: On the molecular mechanism of action of hallucinogens. In Stillman R, Willette R (eds): *The Psy-*

chopharmacology of Hallucinogens, Elmsford Park, NY, Pergamon Press, 1978, pp. 23-27.
13. Grinspoon L, Bakasar J: *Psychedelic Drugs Reconsidered*. New York, Basic Books, 1979.
14. Sloviter R, et al: A common mechanism for lysergic acid, indolealkylamine and phenethylamine hallucinogens: Serotonergic medication of behavioral effects in rats. *J Pharmacol Exp Ther* 214:231, 1980.
15. Freedman DX: LSD: The bridge from human to animal. In Jacobs BL (ed): *Hallucinogens: Neurochemical, Behavioral and Clinical Perspectives*. New York, Raven Press, 1984, pp 203-226.
16. Jacobs BL: Postsynaptic serotonergic action of hallucinogens. In Jacobs BL (ed): *Hallucinogens: Neurochemical, Behavioral and Clinical Perspectives*. New York, Raven Press, 1984, pp 183-202.
17. Hoolister LE: Effects of hallucinogens in humans. In Jacobs BL (ed): *Hallucinogens: Neurochemical, Behavioral and Clinical Perspectives*. New York, Raven Press, 1984, pp 19-33.
18. Klock JC, et al: Coma, hyperthermia and bleeding associated with massive LSD overdose, a report of eight cases. *J Toxicol Clin Toxicol* 8:191, 1975.
19. Peroutka SJ: Incidence of recreational use of 3,4 methylenedimethoxymethamphetamine (MDMA, ecstasy) on an undergraduate campus. *N Engl J Med* 317:1542, 1987.
20. Nichols DE: Differences between the mechanism of action of MDMA, MBDB, and the classic hallucinogens: Identification of a new therapeutic class: Entactogens. *J Psychoactive Drugs* 18:305, 1986.
21. Texas Commission on Alcohol and Drug Use: *Texas Commission of Alcohol and Drug Use 1996 Texas School Survey: Grades 7-12*. Austin, Tex, Texas Commission of Alcohol and Drug Use, 1997.
22. Leverant R: MDMA reconsidered. *J Psychoactive Drugs* 18:373, 1986.
23. Riedlinger TJ, Riedlinger JE: Psychedelic and entactogenic drugs in the treatment of depression. *J Psychoactive Drugs* 26:41, 1994.
24. Peroutka SJ, Newman H, Harris H: Subjective effects of 3,4-methylenedioxymethamphetamine in recreational users. *Neuropsychopharmacology* 1:273, 1988.
25. Voorspoels S, et al: Resurgence of a lethal drug: Paramethoxyamphetamine deaths in Belgium. *J Toxicol Clin Toxicol* 40:203, 2002.
26. Byard RW, et al: Death and paramethoxyamphetamine—an evolving problem. *Med J Aust* 176:496, 2002.
27. Ling LH, et al: Poisoning with the recreational drug paramethoxyamphetamine ("death"). *Med J Aust* 174:453, 2001.
28. Bergman R: Navajo peyote use: Its apparent safety. *Am J Psychiatry* 128:51, 1971.
29. Shulgin AT, Sargent T, Naranjo C: The chemistry and psychopharmacology of nutmeg and of several related phenylisopropylamines. *Psychopharmacol Bull* 4:13, 1967.
30. Sangalli BC, Chiang W: Toxicology of nutmeg abuse. *J Toxicol Clin Toxicol* 38:671, 2000.
31. Sjoholm A, Lindberg A, Personne M: Acute nutmeg intoxication. *J Intern Med* 243:329, 1998.
32. Cowen PJ: Serotonin receptor subtypes: Implications for psychopharmacology. *Br J Psychiatry* 12(Suppl):7, 1991.
33. Rudnick G, Wall SC: The molecular mechanism of [3,4-methylenedioxy-methamphetamine (MDMA)]: Serotonin transporters are targets for MDMA-induced serotonin release. *Proc Natl Acad Sci U S A* 89:1817, 1992.
34. Ricaurte GA, et al: (+) 3,4-Methylenedioxymethamphetamine selectively damages serotonergic neurons in nonhuman primates. *JAMA* 260:51, 1988.
35. Kleven MS, Woolverton WL, Seiden LS: Evidence that both intragastric and subcutaneous administration of methylenedioxymethylamphetamine (MDMA) produce serotonin neurotoxicity in rhesus monkeys. *Brain Res* 488:121, 1989.
36. Ricaurte GA, et al: Toxic effects of MDMA on central serotonergic neurons in the primate: Importance of route and frequency of drug administration. *Brain Res* 446:165, 1988.
37. McCann UD, Ricaurte GA: Lasting neuropsychiatric sequelae of (+) methylenedioxymethamphetamine ("ecstasy") in recreational users. *J Clin Psychopharmacol* 11:302, 1991.
38. Malberg JE, Seiden LS: Small changes in ambient temperature cause large changes in 3,4-methylenedioxymethamphetamine (MDMA)-induced serotonin neurotoxicity and core body temperature in the rat. *J Neurosci* 18:5086, 1998.
39. Farfel GM, Seiden LS: Role of hyperthermia in the mechanism of protection against serotonergic toxicity: II. Experiments with methamphetamine, p-chloroamphetamine, fenfluramine, dizocilpine and dextromethorphan. *J Pharmacol Exp Ther* 272:868, 1995.
40. O'Connor A, et al: Death from hyponatraemia-induced cerebral oedema associated with MDMA ("Ecstasy") use. *N Z Med J* 112:255, 1999.
41. Henry JA, et al: Low-dose MDMA ("ecstasy") induces vasopressin secretion. *Lancet* 351:1784, 1998.
42. Holden R, Jackson MA: Near-fatal hyponatraemic coma due to vasopressin over-secretion after "ecstasy" (3,4-MDMA). *Lancet* 347:1052, 1996.
43. Brown C, Osterloh J: Multiple severe complications from recreational ingestion of MDMA ("ecstasy"). *JAMA* 258: 780, 1987.
44. Verebey K, Alrazi J, Jaffe JH: The complications of "ecstasy" (MDMA). *JAMA* 259:1649, 1988.
45. Smilkstein MJ, Smolinske SC, Rumack BH: A case of MAO inhibitor/MDMA interaction: Agony after ecstasy. *J Toxicol Clin Toxicol* 25:149, 1987.
46. Dowling GP, McDonough ET III, Bos RO: "Eve" and "ecstasy": A report of five deaths associated with the use of MDEA and MDMA. *JAMA* 257:1615, 1987.
47. Randall T: Ecstasy-fueled "rave" parties become dances of death for English youths. *JAMA* 268:1505, 1992.
48. Kunsman GW, et al: Application of Syva EMIT and Abbott TDX amphetamine immunoassays to the detection of 3,4-methylenedioxyamphetamine (MDMA) and 3,4-methyleneethoxyamphetamine (MDEA) in the urine. *J Anal Toxicol* 14:149, 1990.
49. Schwartz RH, Miller NS: MDMA (ecstasy) and the rave: A review. *Pediatrics* 100:705, 1997.
50. Logan AS, et al: Survival following "ecstasy" ingestion with a peak temperature of 42 degrees C. *Anaesthesia* 48:1017, 1993.
51. Padkin A: Treating MDMA ("ecstasy") toxicity. *Anaesthesia* 49:259, 1994.
52. Chadwick IS, et al: Ecstasy, 3-4 methylenedioxymethamphetamine (MDMA), a fatality associated with coagulopathy and hyperthermia. *J R Soc Med* 84:371, 1991.
53. Nahas GG: Cannabis: Toxicological properties and epidemiological aspects. *Med J Aust* 145:82, 1986.
54. Mason AP, McBay AJ: Cannabis: Pharmacology and interpretation of effects. *J Forensic Sci* 30:615, 1985.
55. Taylor FM: Marijuana as a potential respiratory carcinogen. *South Med J* 81:1213, 1988.
56. Wall ME, et al: Metabolism, disposition, and kinetics of delta-9-tetrahydrocannabinol in men and women. *Clin Pharmacol Ther* 34:352, 1983.
57. Ohlsson A, et al: Plasma delta-9-tetrahydrocannabinol concentration and clinical effects after oral and intravenous administration and smoking. *Clin Pharmacol Ther* 28:409, 1980.
58. Hawks RL: The constituents of cannabis and the disposition and metabolism of cannabinoids. In Hawks RL (ed): *Analysis of Cannabinoids: NIDA Research Monograph 42*. Rockville, Md, NIDA, 1982, pp 125-137.

59. Heishman SJ, et al: Acute and residual effects of marijuana: Profiles of plasma TCH levels, physiological, subjective and performance measures. *Pharmacol Biochem Behav* 37:561, 1990.
60. Huestis MA: Pharmacology and toxicology of marijuana. *Ther Drug Monit* 14:131, 1993.
61. Janowsky DS, et al: Simulated flying performance after marijuana intoxication. *Aviat Space Environ Med* 47:124, 1976.
62. Renier S, Messi G, Orel P: Acute cannabis poisoning in a female child. *Minerva Pediatr* 46:335, 1994.
63. Weinberg D, Lande A, Hilton N: Intoxication from accidental marijuana ingestion. *Pediatrics* 71:848, 1983.
64. Macnab A, Anderson E, Susak L: Ingestion of cannabis: A cause of coma in children. *Pediatr Emerg Care* 5:238, 1989.
65. Ellis GM, et al: Excretion patterns of cannabinoid metabolites after last use in a group of chronic uses. *Clin Pharmacol Ther* 38:572, 1985.
66. Cone EJ, et al: Passive inhalation of marijuana smoke: Urinalysis and room air levels of delta-9-tetrahydrocannabinol. *J Anal Toxicol* 11:89, 1987.
67. Otten EJ: Marijuana. In Goldfrank LR, et al (eds): *Toxicologic Emergencies,* 7th ed. New York, McGraw Hill, 2002, pp 1054-1058.
68. Valdes LJ: *Salvia divinorum* and the unique diterpene hallucinogen, Salvinorin (Divinorin) A. *J Psychoactive Drugs* 26:277, 1994.
69. Hold KM, et al: Alpha-thujone (the active component of absinthe): Gamma-aminobutyric acid type A receptor modulation and metabolic detoxification. *Proc Natl Acad Sci U S A* 97:3826, 2000.
70. Arnold WN: Absinthe. *Sci Am* 260:112, 1989.
71. Weisbord SD, Soule JB, Kimmel PL: Poison online—acute renal failure caused by oil of wormwood purchased through the Internet. *N Engl J Med* 337:825, 1997.
72. Crider R: Phencyclidine: Changing abuse patterns. *NIDA Res Monogr* 64:163, 1986.
73. Siegel RK: Phencyclidine and ketamine intoxication: A study of four populations of recreational users. In Peterson RC, Stillman RC (eds): *Phencyclidine (PCP) Abuse: An Appraisal* (Department of Health, Education and Welfare Pub. No. [ADM] 78-728). Washington, DC, US Government Printing Office, 1978, pp 119–147.
74. Baker SD, Borys DJ: A possible trend suggesting increased abuse from Coricidin exposures reported to the Texas Poison Network: Comparing 1998 to 1999. *Vet Hum Toxicol* 44:169, 2002.
75. Banerji S, Anderson IB: Abuse of Coricidin HBP cough and cold tablets: Episodes recorded by a poison center. *Am J Health Syst Pharm* 58:1811, 2001.
76. Javitt DC, Zukin SR: Recent advances in the phencyclidine model of schizophrenia. *Am J Psychiatry* 148:1301, 1991.
77. Cook CE, et al: Phencyclidine and phenylcyclohexane disposition after smoking phencyclidine. *Clin Pharmacol Ther* 31:635, 1982.
78. Young JD, Crapo LM: Protracted phencyclidine coma from an intestinal deposit. *Arch Intern Med* 152:859, 1992.
79. Graudins A, Fern RP: Acute dystonia in a child associated with therapeutic ingestion of a dextromethorphan containing cough and cold syrup. *J Toxicol Clin Toxicol* 34:351, 1996.
80. Schneider SM, et al: Dextromethorphan poisoning reversed by naloxone. *Am J Emerg Med* 9:237, 1991.
81. Skop BP, et al: The serotonin syndrome associated with paroxetine, an over-the-counter cold remedy, and vascular disease. *Am J Emerg Med* 12:642, 1994.
82. McCarron MM, et al: Acute phencyclidine intoxication: Incidence of clinical findings in 1,000 cases. *Ann Emerg Med* 10:238, 1981.
83. McCarron MM: Phencyclidine intoxication. *Dig Emerg Med Care* 5:4, 1985.
84. Barton CH, et al: Rhabdomyolysis and acute renal failure associated with phencyclidine intoxication. *Arch Intern Med* 140:568, 1980.
85. Burns RS, Lerner SE: Phencyclidine deaths. *J Am Coll Emerg Physicians* 7:135, 1978.
86. Burns RS, Lerner SE, Corrado R: Phencyclidine: States of acute intoxication and fatalities. *West J Med* 123:345, 1975.
87. Schwartz RH, Einhorn A: PCP intoxication in seven young children. *Pediatr Emerg Care* 2:238, 1986.
88. Wolfe TR, Caravati EM: Massive dextromethorphan ingestion and abuse. *Am J Emerg Med* 13:174, 1995.
89. Pender ES, Parks BR: Toxicity with dextromethorphan-containing preparations: A literature review and report of two additional cases. *Pediatr Emerg Care* 7:163, 1991.
90. Nordt SP: "DXM": A new drug of abuse? *Ann Emerg Med* 31:794, 1998.
91. Osterloh JD, Snyder JW: Laboratory principles and techniques to evaluate the poisoned or overdosed patient. In Goldfrank LR, et al (eds): *Toxicologic Emergencies,* 6th ed. Stamford, Conn, Appleton & Lange, 1998, pp 63-75.
92. Ng YY, et al: Spurious hyperchloremia and decreased anion gap in a patient with dextromethorphan bromide. *Am J Nephrol* 12:268, 1992.

CHAPTER 155 Heavy Metals

Larissa I. Velez and Kathleen A. Delaney

IRON

Iron is an essential metal that can be extremely toxic, either after an overdose or from accumulation in disease states. The acute ingestion of iron is especially hazardous to children.[1] More than 100 iron-containing preparations are listed in the *Physicians' Desk Reference*, and many more are available as nonprescription drugs. Most iron exposures result from the ingestion of a pediatric multivitamin formulation (usually minimally toxic) by a child younger than 6 years of age. Life-threatening poisonings in children are associated with ingestion of more potent adult preparations, often pre-

Table 155-1. Common Iron Preparations

Compound	Percentage of Elemental Iron
Ferrous sulfate	20
Ferrous fumarate	33
Ferrous gluconate	12
Ferric pyrophosphate	30
Ferrocholinate	14
Ferroglycine sulfate	16
Ferrous sulfate, dried	33
Ferrous carbonate, anhydrous	38
Carbonyl iron	100

scribed to the mother during pregnancy. Serious iron ingestions in adults are usually the result of suicide attempts.[2-4]

Principles of Disease

Pharmacology

Iron is an essential cofactor in the function of hemoglobin, myoglobin, many cytochromes, and catalytic enzymes.[2,5] Iron absorbed from the intestine is bound to transferrin. Under normal conditions, only 15% to 35% of the iron-binding capacity of transferrin is utilized. Following a significant iron overdose, transferrin becomes completely saturated and the excess iron circulates as free iron in the serum. This unbound iron is directly toxic to target organs.[2,6] Transferrin levels vary considerable among individuals and are affected by disease states. The total iron-binding capacity (normal, 300-400 μg/dL) provides a crude measure of the extent of saturation of transferrin and the possibility of free unbound iron. Serum iron levels are normally in the range of 50 to 150 μg/dL.

The toxicity of an iron compound depends primarily on the amount of elemental iron it contains, which in turn depends on the formulation (Table 155-1). The total amount of elemental iron ingested can be approximated by multiplying the estimated number of tablets ingested by the fraction of elemental iron contained in the tablet. Ingestion of less than 20 mg/kg of elemental iron usually causes no symptoms. Ingestion of 20 to 60 mg/kg results in mild to moderate symptoms, and more than 60 mg/kg may lead to severe morbidity. Although the dose of elemental iron associated with 50% mortality (LD_{50}) is reported to be 200 to 250 mg/kg, doses as small as 130 mg of elemental iron have been lethal in children.[7]

Pathophysiology

Iron has two distinct toxic effects: (1) direct caustic injury to the gastrointestinal mucosa and (2) impairment of intracellular metabolism that primarily affects the heart, liver, and central nervous system (CNS). The caustic effects of iron on the gut cause vomiting, diarrhea, and abdominal pain. Hemorrhagic necrosis of gastric or intestinal mucosa can lead to bleeding, perforation, and peritonitis.[6-9]

Unbound (free) iron moves into cells and localizes near the mitochondrial cristae, resulting in uncoupling of mitochondrial oxidative phosphorylation and impairment of adenosine triphosphate synthesis. Cellular injury from iron is also associated with the production of free radicals that injure cell membranes by lipid peroxidation.[2,7,10]

Iron increases capillary permeability and induces both arteriolar and venodilation. It is also directly toxic to the myocardium. These effects, combined with severe gastrointestinal fluid losses, lead to the development of shock.[2,7] In addition, hydration of the iron molecule creates an excess of unbuffered protons, which contributes to the production of metabolic acidosis.[2,7] Cardiovascular collapse and death may ensue from this multitude of effects.

Clinical Features

The clinical effects of acute iron poisoning are described in five stages.[8] Phase I reflects the corrosive effects of iron on the gut. Vomiting occurs within 80 minutes of ingestion in more than 90% of symptomatic cases of ingestion. Diarrhea follows and gastrointestinal bleeding is common. Phase II represents an apparent (but not complete) recovery that lasts less than 24 hours but can extend up to 2 days. Most patients recover after this point. Phase III is characterized by the recurrence of gastrointestinal symptoms, severe lethargy or coma, anion gap metabolic acidosis, leukocytosis, coagulopathy, renal failure, and cardiovascular collapse. Serum iron levels may be normal during this phase, reflecting distribution into the tissues. Phase IV, characterized by fulminant hepatic failure, occurs 2 to 5 days after ingestion. This is relatively rare but usually fatal.[11] Phase V, the consequence of healing of the corrosive gastrointestinal mucosal effects, is characterized by pyloric or proximal bowel scarring, sometimes associated with obstruction.[2,6,8]

Metabolic derangements due to iron poisoning include hypoglycemia, leukocytosis, and severe lactic acidosis from hypoperfusion and interference with cellular respiration. Early coagulation defects are probably related to the direct effects of iron on vitamin K–dependent clotting factors.[12] Later, these coagulation defects are due to hepatic failure. Elevated aspartate and alanine transaminases, and bilirubin levels and hypoglycemia are other markers of hepatotoxicity.[11]

Diagnostic Strategies

The presence of gastrointestinal symptoms suggests a potentially serious ingestion, whereas their absence is reassuring. A serum iron level measured at its peak, 3 to 5 hours after ingestion, is the most useful laboratory test to evaluate the potential severity of an iron overdose. Sustained-release or enteric-coated preparations may have erratic absorption, so a second level 6 to 8 hours after ingestion should also be checked. Peak serum iron levels of less than 350 μg/dL are generally associated with minimal toxicity, 350 to 500 μg/dL with moderate toxicity, and greater than 500 μg/dL with severe toxicity (Table 155-2).[3] Because iron is rapidly

Table 155-2. Toxicity of Iron by Amount Ingested and Peak Serum Levels

Elemental iron (mg/kg)	Peak serum iron (μg/dL)	Toxicity
<20	50-150	None
20-40	150-300	Mild
40-60	300-500	Moderate
>60	>500	Severe

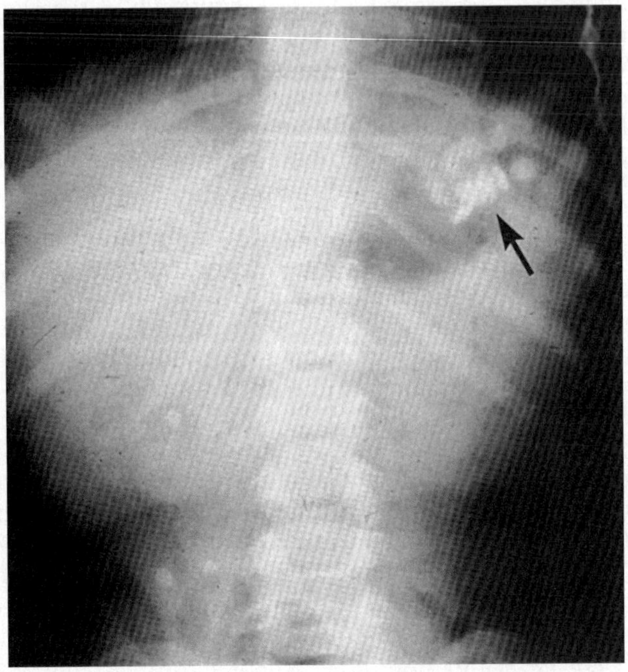

Figure 155-1. Radiopaque iron tablets seen on abdominal radiograph. (From Craig SA: Radiology. In: Ford MD, Delaney KA, Ling LJ, Erickson T (eds): *Clinical Toxicology*. Philadelphia, WB Saunders, 2001, p 62.)

cleared from the serum and deposited in the liver, iron levels may be deceptively low if measured too late after a substantial ingestion.

Although a negative radiograph does not rule out the presence of iron from chewable, liquid, and completely dissolved iron compounds, most nonchewable iron tablets are radiopaque, and the presence of tablets on a radiograph correlates with the severity of the ingestion (Figure 155-1).[13,14]

Management

Gastric Emptying

Iron is not bound to activated charcoal, and neither gastric lavage nor ipecac effectively removes large amounts of pills. Iron tablets clump together as their outer coatings dissolve. Gastrotomy has been required to remove iron from the stomach, but the success of whole-bowel irrigation generally obviates the need to consider surgery for purposes of decontamination.[15]

For significant ingestions, especially when tablets are identified on the abdominal radiograph, whole-bowel irrigation with a polyethylene glycol electrolyte lavage solution (PEG-ELS) (CoLyte, NuLytely, GoLYTELY) is indicated. The solution is either taken orally or administered through a nasogastric tube.[3,16] The usual rate of administration of PEG-ELS is 20 to 40 mL/kg/hr in young children and 1.5 to 2 L/hr for teenagers or adults, continued until the rectal effluent is clear and there is no radiographic evidence of pill fragments. This technique has been used in children, adolescents, and pregnant women without serious complications or electrolyte disturbances.[15,17] Common side effects include nausea, vomiting, abdominal cramping, and bloating. Whole-bowel irrigation is contraindicated in the presence of bowel obstruction or ileus.

Hemodialysis and hemoperfusion are not effective in removing iron, due to its large volume of distribution. Exchange transfusions should be considered in severely symptomatic patients with serum iron levels exceeding 1000 μg/dL.[18]

Deferoxamine

Deferoxamine binds with iron to form a water-soluble compound, ferrioxamine, which can be renally excreted or dialyzed. One hundred milligrams will chelate 9.35 mg of elemental iron.[7] Deferoxamine may also limit the entrance of iron into the cell and chelate intracellular iron. Because of its short half-life, it is administered as a continuous infusion at a dose of 15 mg/kg/hr for up to 24 hours. Rapid administration of deferoxamine can lead to hypotension, which is treated by reducing the rate of the infusion and slowly increasing it to the desired rate. Pregnancy is not a contraindication for deferoxamine. The presence of ferrioxamine turns the urine a "vin rosé" color, which reflects the excretion of chelated iron. Historically, the deferoxamine challenge test, which relied on detection of this color change, was used to diagnose the presence of free iron in the serum. The color change is difficult to detect, especially when the urine is dilute, resulting in false-negative results even in cases of serious poisoning. Falsely low serum iron values also occur in the presence of deferoxamine, so serum iron should be measured before its administration.[19]

Disposition

The asymptomatic patient with an ingestion of less than 20 mg/kg of elemental iron can be observed without further therapy. If the patient remains asymptomatic after 6 hours of observation, discharge is recommended.[2]

The patient who has ingested more than 20 mg/kg of elemental iron, or has pills visible on an abdominal radiograph, and is asymptomatic or exhibits evidence of mild toxicity should receive whole bowel irrigation. Abdominal radiographs can verify adequate gastrointestinal emptying. The serum iron should be checked 3 to 5 hours after ingestion, and a second iron level 6 to 8 hours after ingestion should be decreasing. Moderate gastrointestinal toxicity can be expected with peak levels of 300 to 500 μg/dL. Patients with an iron level greater than 500 μg/dL or patients with any systemic signs of toxicity require chelation with deferoxamine. If peak levels are below 300 μg/dL, are not rising, and no symptoms develop over 6 hours of observation, the patient can be discharged home.

When serum iron levels are not available on an immediate basis, elevations of the serum glucose level and leukocyte count are helpful markers of early toxicity. If results of both these tests are normal, no signs or symptoms of toxicity occur over the 6-hour period, and the abdominal radiographs do not show pills in the gastrointestinal tract, the patient can be sent home.

LEAD

The use of lead in human endeavors dates back more than 5000 years, and its toxic effects have been recognized for at least 2000 years. In 370 BC, Hippocrates attributed severe abdominal pain in a metal extractor to "lead colic." In the 1970s, the addition of lead to household paints and gasoline was banned in the United States.

Lead poisoning, a disease of industrialization, is the most common toxicologic problem of environmental origin in the United States.[20,21] Exposure usually results from ingestion or inhalation or, less often, from direct skin contact with organic lead compounds or from retained bullets.[22] Approximately 3 to 4 million children (1 in 20) in the United States have toxic blood lead levels (BLLs).[21,23] Lead-based paint is still found in 30 million homes in the United States.[23] Other sources of toxic lead ingestions include curtain weights, buckshot, fishing weights, lead-contaminated soil or water, bootleg whiskey ("moonshine"), food or beverages stored or prepared in lead-soldered cans, lead-glazed pottery, and lead crystal decanters. Herbal and folk remedies, including numerous products imported from Asia and Mexico, contain dangerous amounts of lead.[24]

Children typically present to the emergency department (1) following an ingestion of lead, (2) symptomatic with a possible exposure history, or (3) referred for management of a toxic BLL. Lead toxicity in adults most often results from inhalational exposure in the workplace, as well as from hobbies and related activities. More than 3 million workers in the United States are estimated to be at risk for toxic lead exposure in industries such as lead smelting, battery manufacture, radiator repair, bridge and ship construction or demolition, soldering or welding, cable or tin can production, stained glass manufacture, lead-glazed or crystal pottery making, glass production, firing range operation, and lead-based paint abatement.[20,21] Hobbies at risk include making glazed pottery, target shooting at indoor firing ranges, soldering lead, smelting lead in the preparation of buckshot and fishing sinkers, repairing cars or boats, and remodeling homes. Lead toxicity should be considered in adults with compatible symptoms associated with these exposures.

Principles of Disease

Pharmacology

There is no known biologic need for lead. Its absorption is highest in malnourished children (about 40%) and in pregnant women.[25] Although 90% to 95% of lead is stored in cortical bone and teeth, it is also found in the brain, liver, and kidneys. About 75% of the absorbed lead is eliminated renally, with the remainder through the skin, hair, sweat, nails, and gastrointestinal tract.[20]

Pathophysiology

Lead binds to sulfhydryl groups and other ligands, interfering with critical enzymatic reactions.[20] Its toxic effects are most prominent in the hematopoietic, neurologic, and renal systems.[25]

Anemia, the classic manifestation of toxicity in the hematopoietic system, may be either normochromic or hypochromic. The severity of the anemia correlates directly with BLLs. Inhibition of heme biosynthesis results in the accumulation of heme precursors, such as δ-aminolevulinic acid and protoporphyrin.[25] In the peripheral nervous system, the motor axons are the principal target, with segmental demyelination and axonal degeneration resulting in peripheral neuropathies.[21] Wrist drop and footdrop are characteristic of adult lead poisoning. Lead toxicity causes neuropsychiatric disorders. In children, elevated BLLs are associated with decreased intelligence (IQ) scores, hyperactivity, decreased attention span, overaggressive behavior, learning disabilities, criminal behavior, and subclinical sensorineural hearing loss.[26-31] Adults and children with acute toxicity may present with lead encephalopathy associated with increased capillary permeability and cerebral edema.[27] Lead poisoning has also been correlated with hypertension.[32]

Lead nephropathy is characterized by fibrosis in the proximal tubules, with relative sparing of the glomeruli. Hyperuricemic gout ("saturnine gout") can result from increased reuptake of uric acid by the tubular cells. Acute lead poisoning results in "lead colic," cramping abdominal pain with nausea, vomiting, constipation, and occasionally, diarrhea.[27]

Clinical Features

Chronic mild lead poisoning is slow in onset and nonspecific in symptoms. The diagnosis is suspected by obtaining an accurate and comprehensive history of exposure to lead.

Acute exposure to lead often results in symptomatic poisoning. The characteristic symptoms and signs of acute toxicity include abdominal colic, malaise, nausea, vomiting, constipation, fatigue, anemia, peripheral neuropathy, renal impairment, hepatic dysfunction, and CNS dysfunction. The CNS toxicity can range from mild headache or personality changes to full-blown encephalopathy with coma, convulsions, and papilledema. Permanent neurologic and behavioral sequelae can occur in patients who have acute lead encephalopathy.[20]

Table 155-3. Serum Lead Levels and Symptomatology

Level (μg/dL)	Symptoms: Adults	Symptoms: Children
10	None	Decreased intelligence Decreased hearing Decreased growth
20	Increased protoporphyrin No symptoms	Decreased nerve conduction velocity Increased protoporphyrin
30	Increased blood pressure Decreased hearing	Decreased vitamin D metabolism
40	Peripheral neuropathies Nephropathy Infertility (men)	Decreased hemoglobin synthesis
50	Decreased hemoglobin synthesis	Lead colic
70	Anemia	Anemia Encephalopathy Nephropathy
100	Encephalopathy	Death

Diagnostic Strategies

The most informative biomarker is a BLL.[33,34] The Centers for Disease Control and Prevention has defined a chronic BLL of greater than 10 μg/dL as toxic for a child. Acute exposure can result in levels up to 100 μg/dL (Table 155-3).[35] Other ancillary data include findings on complete blood cell count; serum glucose, blood urea nitrogen, creatinine, and electrolyte level measurements; urinalysis; and, with acute lead ingestion, liver function tests. Lead-containing paints and objects are radiopaque when present in sufficient quantities, and radiographs can confirm acute ingestion and monitor the effectiveness of whole-bowel irrigation. In cases of altered mental status, seizures, or coma, a computed tomography scan of the head will show cerebral edema associated with acute lead encephalopathy and rule out other causes for these symptoms. In children, plain radiographs of the wrist and knees may show a characteristic "lead band" or "lead line" of increased metaphyseal activity seen with chronic exposures.

Management

Acute Lead Encephalopathy

Acute lead encephalopathy can be rapidly fatal. The initial goals in management are to identify and treat all life-threatening conditions, followed by efforts to prevent further exposure to lead, minimize absorption of acutely ingested lead, enhance its elimination, and prevent or reverse cellular pathology. Standard measures to control cerebral edema, including intubation and neurosurgical consultation for invasive monitoring of intracranial pressure, are indicated. When poisoning is associated with ingestion or if radiopacities are seen on the radiograph, decontamination with gastric lavage and whole-bowel irrigation is indicated.[36,37] Activated charcoal does not bind lead.

Chelation Therapy

The use of chelation in cases of acute lead poisoning is guided by the patient's clinical status and the BLL. Any patient with a BLL greater than 70 μg/dL, or with protracted gastrointestinal symptoms or CNS toxicity from an acute lead exposure, will require parenteral chelation therapy. For these seriously poisoned patients, dimercaprol (or British antilewisite) should be the first chelator given. The dosage is 3 to 5 mg/kg (25 mg/kg/day), given by deep intramuscular injection every 4 hours for 2 days, followed by another dose every 4 to 6 hours for 2 more days, and then every 4 to 12 hours for up to 7 days. Dimercaprol forms complexes that undergo both renal and biliary excretion. Adverse reactions to dimercaprol include nausea, vomiting, urticaria, pyrexia, hypertension, and hemolysis in patients with glucose-6-phosphate dehydrogenase deficiency.[38] Since dimercaprol is diluted in peanut oil, it is contraindicated in patients allergic to peanuts. Dimercaprol is followed by calcium disodium ethylenediaminetetraacetic acid ($CaNa_2EDTA$), a highly effective lead chelator. Because of concerns that the chelated lead can cross the blood-brain barrier and worsen the encephalopathy, the first dose of $CaNa_2EDTA$ is administered with the second dose of dimercaprol. The dosage of $CaNa_2EDTA$ for patients with acute lead encephalopathy is 75 mg/kg/day or 1500 $mg/m^2/day$ given intravenously or intramuscularly in two to four divided doses, with a maximum daily dose of 1 g in children and 2 g in adults. Adverse reactions include renal tubular injury and chelation of other metals, especially iron and zinc. $CaNa_2EDTA$ should be given only with adequate urine flow or with hemodialysis in the patient with renal failure.[39]

The need for parenteral chelation therapy in asymptomatic or minimally symptomatic children is guided by the BLL. A BLL of more than 69 μg/dL mandates hospitalization and parenteral chelation therapy.[35,38] For less seriously poisoned patients, the dosage of $CaNa_2EDTA$ is 50 mg/kg/day or 1000 $mg/m^2/day$, given in two to four divided doses for up to 5 days.

Serum lead levels of 45 to 69 μg/dL in patients without vomiting or CNS symptoms can be managed in the outpatient setting using oral succimer (2,3-dimercaptosuccinic acid, DMSA, Chemet).[35,38] The initial dose of DMSA is 10 mg/kg every 8 hours for 5 days, then 10 mg/kg every 12 hours for 14 days. The most common adverse reactions include nausea, vomiting, diarrhea, and transient elevations in liver transaminase levels. Although DMSA has been approved only for children, it is also used in adults.[34,40,41] Oral D-penicillamine should be used only in patients who do not tolerate succimer. The usual oral dose of D-penicillamine is 25 mg/kg every 6 hours for 5 days. D-Penicillamine is less efficacious than succimer and has more adverse reactions. Penicillin allergy is a contraindication to the use of D-penicillamine.

The key to managing chronic lead toxicity is the identification and reduction of sources of primary exposure. Any patient treated on an outpatient basis must be discharged to a lead-free environment. A BLL between 20 and 44 μg/dL in a patient who is asymptomatic or minimally symptomatic requires a more aggressive medical and environmental evaluation. The current evidence indicates no need for chelation for children with a BLL lower than 45 μg/dL.[42] Children with lead levels of 10 to 19 μg/dL require family counseling about the symptoms and sources of lead exposure and careful follow-up, with frequent screening of BLLs.

The treatment of adults with chronic poisoning is less aggressive than for children. If gastrointestinal symptoms or CNS problems are present, hospitalization with parenteral chelation therapy is indicated. In the asymptomatic adult or the adult with only mild clinical problems, the only intervention needed is cessation of exposure. Workers with serum lead levels greater than 60 μg/dL must be removed from work and should not be allowed to return until levels are below 40 μg/dL.

Disposition

Patients who have ingested a single lead foreign body (e.g., fishing sinker) will usually pass it harmlessly.[43] If the foreign body remains in the gastrointestinal tract after 2 weeks, removal should be considered to prevent lead toxicity.

Patients who are significantly symptomatic after an acute lead exposure and children with a BLL of 69 μg/dL or greater require hospitalization and chelation therapy, as outlined previously. Patients discharged home on oral chelation therapy should not return to a contaminated environment. The health department should conduct an environmental assessment so that the primary source of lead exposure can be identified and further exposure prevented. Follow-up should be arranged with an experienced pediatrician, toxicologist, or occupational medicine physician. Basic education about hand washing, good nutritional habits, and multivitamin supplementation is also indicated.

ARSENIC

Arsenic (As), a tasteless, odorless substance that looks like sugar, has an infamous history as an agent of homicide. Arsenic has also been implicated in many incidences of epidemic poisoning. At present, arsenic exposure is primarily environmental and occupational. It is found in smelters and electric power plants that burn arsenic-rich coal. It is used in industry as a wood preservative and in the production of glass and microcircuits. Inorganic arsenicals are also used in rodenticides, fungicides, insecticides, paint, and tanning agents, and as defoliants in the cotton industry. Arsenic is still used for medicinal purposes in the treatment of trypanosomiasis, amebiasis, and leukemia.[44] It has also been found as a contaminant in herbal remedies and drugs such as opium. There are widespread reports of chronic arsenic poisoning associated with contaminated drinking water in underdeveloped countries. Arsenic poisoning should be suspected if compatible symptoms occur with the use of these products or these possible exposures.

Principles of Disease

Pharmacology

Arsenic has no metabolic or biologic function. The elemental metal is poorly water soluble and is considered nontoxic. Of the two inorganic forms, trivalent arsenite (As^{3+}) is highly lipid soluble and is 5 to 10 times more toxic than the pentavalent arsenate (As^{5+}) form. Trivalent arsenic has a lower gastrointestinal absorption but is well absorbed by the skin. Pentavalent arsenic is water soluble and readily absorbed from the gastrointestinal tract. Absorbed arsenic is bound by hemoglobin, leukocytes, and plasma proteins. It is cleared from the intravascular compartment within 24 hours and concentrates in the liver, kidneys, spleen, lungs, and gastrointestinal tract. Arsenic crosses the placenta and can accumulate in the fetus. Its affinity for sulfhydryl groups in keratin makes arsenic detectable in the hair, skin, and nails. Arsine (AsH_3), a colorless and almost odorless gas, is extremely toxic. It is immediately lethal at 250 ppm.[45] The excretion of arsenic and its metabolites occurs mainly through the kidneys.

Pathophysiology

Arsenic disrupts cellular energy production by binding avidly to sulfhydryl groups, inhibiting critical enzymes such as lactate dehydrogenase and glyceraldehyde-3-phosphate dehydrogenase, a critical step in glycolysis. It also disrupts oxidative phosphorylation by replacing phosphorus in the formation of high-energy phosphate bonds (arsenolysis).[44]

Clinical Features

Acute exposure to arsine gas is characterized by severe hemolysis that is associated with renal tubular injury. Gastrointestinal symptoms are common, and CNS and liver dysfunction can occur. The mortality rate is 25% to 30%. Exchange transfusions have been used to remove arsine, which is tightly bound to the erythrocytes. Urinary alkalinization can decrease renal deposition of hemoglobin. Chelation is not useful for arsine exposures.

Acute gastrointestinal effects—nausea, vomiting, abdominal pain, and diarrhea—predominate as the initial manifestations of acute exposure to arsenic salts.[44,46,47] These symptoms can be so severe as to result in hematemesis and hematochezia. Within 30 to 60 minutes of exposure, patients complain of a metallic or garlicky taste in the mouth. The patient can also develop encephalopathy with seizures and coma, acute respiratory distress syndrome and respiratory failure, and dysrhythmias associated with cardiac conduction disturbances.[48-50] In cases of severe poisoning, cardiovascular collapse and death ensue. Less common complications include hepatitis, rhabdomyolysis, hemolytic anemia, renal failure, unilateral facial nerve palsy, pancreatitis, pericarditis, pleuritis, and fetal

BOX 155-1. Acute Effects of Arsenic Poisoning

Gastrointestinal
Violent gastroenteritis
Hematemesis/hematochezia
Jaundice
Pancreatitis
Dysphagia
Hepatomegaly

Cardiovascular
Third spacing with shock
Sinus/ventricular tachycardia
Prolonged QT interval, ST depression, T wave inversion
Torsades de pointes
Pericarditis

Respiratory
Respiratory failure
Adult respiratory distress syndrome (ARDS)
Pulmonary edema
Pneumonia

Renal
Proteinuria
Hematuria
Oliguria
Renal failure

Neurologic
Headache
Drowsiness
Delirium
Coma
Encephalopathy
Seizures

demise (Box 155-1).[51] The syndrome may be misdiagnosed as gastroenteritis or sepsis.

Weeks to months after the initial symptoms, chronic effects of arsenic poisoning appear. These include characteristic lines in the nails (Mees' lines), painful sensorimotor neuropathy, and hyperkeratosis of the palms and soles.[44] Arsenic poisoning should also be considered in any patient with a history of severe or recurrent gastroenteritis and unexplained dermatologic lesions associated with peripheral neuropathy. Finally, arsenic is a known human carcinogen.[44]

Diagnostic Strategies

Normal arsenic levels are 5 μg/L or less in blood or less than 50 μg/day in a 24-hour urine collection. Any urine level above 100 μg/day or 50 μg/L necessitates treatment. A spot urine sample may be falsely low because urinary excretion of arsenic is intermittent. Seafood contains arsenobetaine, which can increase urinary arsenic excretion to as high as 1700 μg/L.[52] Arsenobetaine, however, does not result in arsenic toxicity.

Other laboratory results may raise the suspicion of arsenic poisoning. Anemia, leukocytosis or leukopenia, and erythrocyte basophilic stippling are seen in the complete blood cell count. The results of renal function tests may be abnormal. Proteinuria, hematuria, and pyuria are also seen. The alanine transaminase, aspartate transaminase, and bilirubin levels may be elevated. In cases of chronic arsenic poisoning, the serum and urine arsenic levels may be undetectable, and hair and nail specimens can confirm the diagnosis.

Arsenic in the gastrointestinal tract is radiopaque and can show up on a radiograph, although sensitivity is limited by arsenic's rapid absorption.[53]

Management

The initial management should address life-threatening conditions with aggressive supportive management of shock, dysrhythmias, and seizures. Activated charcoal does not bind arsenic and should be considered only if a serious co-ingestion is suspected. Orogastric lavage or whole-bowel irrigation should be considered for very recent ingestions or if radiopaque material is visualized on an abdominal radiograph. Hemodialysis removes arsenic in the setting of acute renal failure.[50]

With a known history in a symptomatic patient, chelation should start as early as possible without waiting for laboratory confirmation of the arsenic levels. Intramuscular dimercaprol is the preferred chelator in patients who are critically ill. DMSA is a water-soluble analogue of dimercaprol that can be given orally.[54] D-Penicillamine has a high side effect profile, and its ability to chelate arsenic is inferior to that of dimercaprol and DMSA.

MERCURY

Mercury is a silvery white metal, familiar to most as the only liquid metal at room temperature. It has been mined in Spain for more than 2500 years in the form of cinnabar (HgS) and has been used for many medical purposes as an antiparasitic, a diuretic, a cathartic, and an antiseptic.[55] Significant poisoning in the home has occurred when small amounts of spilled mercury, such as that contained in a sphygmomanometer, were aerosolized by vacuuming, or when mercury was heated on the kitchen stove to extract gold from ore.[56,57] Various other sources of mercury have resulted in intoxication (Box 155-2). Because of its many uses in the manufacture of batteries, polyvinyl chloride, and latex paint, mercury is a common pollutant of air and water, which has led to restrictions in the consumption of fish caught in many local waters.[58]

Principles of Disease

Pharmacology

The most familiar form of mercury is elemental mercury or metallic mercury, also known as "quicksilver." A common route of exposure to elemental mercury is the inhalation of volatilized vapor. Aspiration of elemental mercury and intentional subcutaneous and intravenous injections also cause poisoning.[59] After inhalation, 74% of the metallic mercury is retained in the lungs. This can result in severe pneumonitis and acute respiratory distress syndrome. Aspiration of elemental mercury results in

BOX 155-2. Sources of Mercury

Elemental
Spill from mercury-containing devices
Gastrointestinal exposure from ruptured Cantor or Miller-Abbott tube
Inhalational exposure in the workplace/home
Deliberate injection or ingestion
Accidental ingestion

Salts
Accidental disk battery ingestion
Deliberate ingestion
Laxative abuse

Organic
Oral/dermal exposure to mercurochrome or thimerosal
Repeated injections of drugs containing thimerosal as a preservative
Exposure from occupational or agricultural accidents
Water/soil pollution
Consumption of contaminated seafood
Exposure to paint containing mercury

Table 155-4. Mercury Intoxication Syndromes

Type of Mercury/ Route of Exposure	Signs/Symptoms
Inhalation of metallic mercury	Hypoxemia Respiratory distress, ARDS Dyspnea, chest tightness Fever, chills Burning in mouth and throat Nausea, vomiting Bloody diarrhea Renal tubular necrosis
Aspiration of metallic mercury	Aspiration pneumonitis ARDS
Subacute/chronic inhalation of metallic mercury	Metal fume fever Neuropsychiatric symptoms Renal dysfunction Skin changes
Ingestion of inorganic mercury salts	Severe hemorrhagic gastroenteritis, shock, hypovolemia, third spacing Acute tubular necrosis in 24 hours, with albuminuria and hematuria
Subacute/chronic inhalation of inorganic mercury	Neurasthenia, erethism, acrodynia
Methylmercury	Delayed neurologic problems (ataxia, tremor, dysarthria), visual field constriction, hearing loss, spasticity, hyperreflexia

ARDS, acute respiratory distress syndrome.

primary pulmonary toxicity, in addition to CNS and renal toxicities. Elemental mercury is not absorbed by the gastrointestinal tract, and ingestion does not normally lead to toxicity. Injected elemental mercury is slowly absorbed from the site of tissue deposition.

Inorganic mercury salts have two different valences, Hg^{+} (*mercurous*) and Hg^{++} (*mercuric*). Ingestion of either salt leads to significant gastrointestinal and renal toxicity.

The organic mercury compounds are categorized as either short chain (*alkyl*) or long chain (*aryl*). The major route of exposure to this type of mercury is through ingestion. These compounds are also readily absorbed through the skin. These organic forms classically result in delayed neurotoxicity with prominent ataxia, tremor, dysarthria, and tunnel vision.

Pathophysiology

Mercury binds covalently to sulfhydryl groups, disturbing cellular enzyme functions. Nephrotoxicity results from both direct damage and an immune reaction in the kidney.[57] The skin changes associated with mercury poisoning are also caused by an immune reaction. Mercury increases catecholamine levels by inhibition of catechol *O*-methyltransferase, resulting in hypertension and tachycardia.[60] Atrophy of the cerebellum, postcentral gyri, and calcarine areas of the brain correlate with the symptoms of visual field constriction, ataxia, and sensory disturbances, respectively.

Clinical Features

The clinical manifestations of mercury poisoning depend on the acuity of the exposure, route of exposure, and chemical form of mercury. The inhalation of metallic mercury vapor results in a rapid onset of shortness of breath, fever, and chills that progresses to respiratory distress and pneumonitis.[56,61] Aspiration of liquid metallic mercury during medical procedures results in tracheobronchial hemorrhage.[62]

The acute ingestion of inorganic salts typically causes a corrosive gastroenteritis with third spacing and hemorrhage. Patients complain of a metallic taste in the mouth and may have a grayish discoloration of the mucous membranes. Massive fluid loss results in shock and acute tubular necrosis. The manifestations of subacute or chronic inorganic mercury poisoning are neurologic (neurasthenia and erethism), renal (ranging from proteinuria to the nephrotic syndrome), and gastrointestinal (metallic taste, gingivostomatitis, loose teeth, burning sensation in mouth, hypersalivation, nausea).[57,63]

Exposure to organic mercury compounds does not generally cause acute toxicity. Neurologic symptoms progress slowly over weeks to months. The neurologic and teratogenic effects of chronic exposure to methyl mercury were well illustrated by the tragedy inflicted on the population of Minamata, Japan, by the contamination of fish through the release of mercury into the water. Slowly progressive and fatal CNS injury was described following a single apparently minor topical exposure to dimethylmercury in a laboratory researcher (Table 155-4).[58,64,65]

Diagnostic Strategies

Measurement of urine mercury levels is the most helpful test in confirming exposure and monitoring the effectiveness of chelation. For organic mercury compounds, which undergo little urinary excretion, serum levels must be used to confirm the diagnosis. "Normal" mercury levels are considered to be less than 10 μg/L in the blood or less than 20 μg/L in the urine. Blood levels greater than 35 μg/L and urine levels greater than 150 μg/L require intervention.[61] No information is available on chelation at levels between 20 and 150 μg/L. Injected metallic mercury is radiopaque on plain radiographs.

Management

Initial management in the acutely poisoned patient should be aggressive support and decontamination. Gastric lavage with protein-containing solutions (e.g., milk, egg whites) may be beneficial in the decontamination of the gastrointestinal tract following ingestion of mercury salts. Charcoal binds very little mercury and is not recommended. Ingested metallic mercury is generally harmless unless its passage is impaired by entrapment in a diverticulum or the appendix.

For acute inhalational exposures, the patient should be removed from the source and supportive management provided. There is no role for antibiotics or steroids. Suction and postural drainage are indicated in cases of acute aspiration of metallic mercury. Self-injection of metallic mercury often requires surgical debridement.[59]

For mercury spills, sand or mercury decontamination kits that contain calcium polysulfide, which converts mercury to mercuric sulfide, should be used. Absorbable surfaces such as carpets should be removed. Help can be obtained from the local hazardous materials (HazMat) team. Attempts to remove mercury by vacuuming can volatilize the mercury and precipitate acute inhalational toxicity. Small spills, such as the contents of a thermometer, can be scooped up with a stiff card, placed in a baggie, and ideally disposed of as hazardous waste. Mecury placed in household trash is incinerated and contributes to water pollution and fish contamination.

Chelation Therapy

Chelating agents have thiol groups that compete with the enzyme's sulfhydryl groups that bind mercury after its absorption. BAL is used for clinically significant acute inorganic mercury intoxication. Because it increases brain mercury levels in patients with methyl mercury poisoning, BAL is contraindicated for patients with organomercurial poisoning. Although DMSA is not currently approved by the U.S. Food and Drug Administration for this indication, it is used for both acute and chronic mercury poisoning and may be the best chelator for methyl mercury. D-Penicillamine is also used. It should be administered only after thorough gastrointestinal decontamination because mercury absorption from the intestinal lumen is enhanced by the penicillamines.

Disposition

In general, in cases of acute intoxication, the most toxic forms are the inorganic mercurials. Suicidal patients with such ingestions require decontamination and admission for supportive treatment. Patients who self-inject metallic mercury often need surgical debridement. Most asymptomatic individuals can be followed closely with urinary testing as outpatients.

KEY CONCEPTS

- Most ingested metals cause severe gastrointestinal pain and emesis.
- Chelation with acute iron ingestion is guided by symptoms and two serum iron levels measured between 3 and 8 hours after ingestion.
- Patients with symptomatic acute lead exposures require immediate chelation. Asymptomatic or minimally symptomatic children with elevated BLLs require close follow-up and possible outpatient chelation. Parenteral chelation is indicated in children with lead levels greater than 69 μg/dL.
- Patients with a possible chronic heavy metal exposure and compatible symptoms should have further investigation and close follow-up.

REFERENCES

1. Charney E: A fatal case of ferrous sulfate poisoning. *JAMA* 178:326, 1961.
2. Mills KC, Curry SC: Acute iron poisoning. *Emerg Med Clin North Am* 12:397, 1994.
3. Fine JS: Iron poisoning. *Curr Probl Pediatr* 30:71, 2000.
4. Olenmark M, et al: Fatal iron intoxication in late pregnancy. *J Toxicol Clin Toxicol* 25:347, 1987.
5. van Eijk HG, de Jong G: The physiology of iron, transferrin, and ferritin. *Biol Trace Elem Res* 35:13, 1992.
6. Whitten CF, Brough AJ: The pathophysiology of acute iron poisoning. Clin Toxicol 4:585, 1971.
7. Robotham JL, Lietman PS: Acute iron poisoning: A review. *Am J Dis Child* 134:875, 1980.
8. Banner W Jr, Tong TG: Iron poisoning. *Pediatr Clin North Am* 33:393, 1986.
9. Gezernik W, Schmaman A, Chappell JS: Corrosive gastritis as a result of ferrous sulphate ingestion. *S Afr Med J* 57:151, 1980.
10. Aisen P, Cohen G, Kang JO: Iron toxicosis. *Int Rev Exp Pathol* 31:1, 1990.
11. deCastro FJ, Jaeger R, Gleason WA Jr: Liver damage and hypoglycemia in acute iron poisoning. *Clin Toxicol* 10:287, 1977.
12. Evensen SA, et al: Acute iron intoxication with abruptly reduced levels of vitamin K-dependent coagulation factors. *Scand J Haematol* 29:25, 1982.
13. Chyka PA, Butler AY: Assessment of acute iron poisoning by laboratory and clinical observations. *Am J Emerg Med* 11:99, 1993.
14. Ng RC, Perry K, Martin DJ: Iron poisoning: Assessment of radiography in diagnosis and management. *Clin Pediatr (Phila)* 18:614, 1979.
15. Tennebein M, Wiseman N, Yatscoff RW: Gastrotomy and whole bowel irrigation in iron poisoning. *Pediatr Emerg Care* 7:286, 1991.
16. Tenenbein M: Whole bowel irrigation in iron poisoning. *J Pediatr* 111:142, 1987.
17. Kaczorowski JM, Wax PM: Five days of whole-bowel irrigation in a case of pediatric iron ingestion. *Ann Emerg Med* 27:258, 1996.
18. Movassaghi N, Purugganan GG, Leikin S: Comparison of exchange transfusion and deferoxamine in the treatment of acute iron poisoning. *J Pediatr* 75:604, 1969.

19. Wythe E, Osterloh J, Becker C: The reliability of serum iron levels after deferoxamine treatment: An in vitro study. *Vet Hum Toxicol* 28:478, 1986.
20. Paloucek FP: Lead poisoning. *Am Pharm* NS33:81, 1993.
21. Landrigan PJ, Todd AC: Lead poisoning. *West J Med* 161:153, 1994.
22. Akhtar AJ, Funnye AS, Akanno J: Gunshot-induced plumbism in an adult male. *J Natl Med Assoc* 95:986, 2003.
23. Markowitz G, Rosner D: "Cater to the children": The role of the lead industry in a public health tragedy, 1900-1955. *Am J Public Health* 90:36, 2000.
24. Tait PA, et al: Severe congenital lead poisoning in a preterm infant due to a herbal remedy. *Med J Aust* 177:193, 2002.
25. Markowitz M: The diagnosis and treatment of childhood lead poisoning. *Resident Staff Physician* 3:27, 1997.
26. Lidsky TI, Schneider JS: Lead neurotoxicity in children: Basic mechanisms and clinical correlates. *Brain* 126:5, 2003.
27. Nevin R: How lead exposure relates to temporal changes in IQ, violent crime, and unwed pregnancy. *Environ Res* 83:1, 2000.
28. Needleman HL, Gatsonis CA: Low-level lead exposure and the IQ of children: A meta-analysis of modern studies. *JAMA* 263:673, 1990.
29. Needleman HL, et al: The long-term effects of exposure to low doses of lead in childhood: An 11-year follow-up report. *N Engl J Med* 322:83, 1990.
30. Wang CL, et al: Relationship between blood lead concentrations and learning achievement among primary school children in Taiwan. *Environ Res* 89:12, 2002.
31. Canfield RL, et al: Intellectual impairment in children with blood lead concentrations below 10 microg per deciliter. *N Engl J Med* 348:1517, 2003.
32. Cheng Y, et al: Bone lead and blood lead levels in relation to baseline blood pressure and the prospective development of hypertension: The Normative Aging Study. *Am J Epidemiol* 153:164, 2001.
33. Gordon JN, Taylor A, Bennett PN: Lead poisoning: Case studies. *Br J Clin Pharmacol* 53:451, 2002.
34. Graziano JH: Validity of lead exposure markers in diagnosis and surveillance. *Clin Chem* 40:1387, 1994.
35. Harvey B, Campbell CC, Dolbeare CN, et al: Center for Disease Control and Prevention. Managing blood lead levels among young children: Recommendations from the Advisory Committee on Childhood Lead Poisoning Prevention, Atlanta, CDC, 2002. Available at http://www.cdc.gov/nceh/lead/ACCLPP/recommend.htm (Accessed 3/6/2005).
36. McNutt TK, et al: Bite the bullet: Lead poisoning after ingestion of 206 lead bullets. *Vet Hum Toxicol* 43:288, 2001.
37. Roberge RJ, Martin TG: Whole bowel irrigation in an acute oral lead intoxication. *Am J Emerg Med* 10:577, 1992.
38. American Academy of Pediatrics Committee on Drugs: Treatment guidelines for lead exposure in children. *Pediatrics* 96:155, 1995.
39. Chisolm JJ Jr: Safety and efficacy of meso-2,3-dimercaptosuccinic acid (DMSA) in children with elevated blood lead concentrations. *J Toxicol Clin Toxicol* 38:365, 2000.
40. Safety and efficacy of succimer in toddlers with blood lead levels of 20-44 microg/dL, Treatment of Lead-Exposed Children (TLC) Trial Group. *Pediatr Res* 48:593, 2000.
41. Torres-Alanis O, Garza-Ocanas L, Pineyro-Lopez A: Effect of meso-2,3-dimercaptosuccinic acid on urinary lead excretion in exposed men. *Hum Exp Toxicol* 21:573, 2002.
42. Rogan WJ, et al: The effect of chelation therapy with succimer on neuropsychological development in children exposed to lead. *N Engl J Med* 344:1421, 2001.
43. Durback LF, Wedin GP, Seidler DE: Management of lead foreign body ingestion. *J Toxicol Clin Toxicol* 27:173, 1989.
44. Ratnaike RN: Acute and chronic arsenic toxicity. *Postgrad Med J* 79:391, 2003.
45. Teitelbaum DT, Kier LC: Arsine poisoning: Report of five cases in the petroleum industry and a discussion of the indications for exchange transfusion and hemodialysis. *Arch Environ Health* 19:133, 1969.
46. Heyman A, et al: Peripheral neuropathy caused by arsenical intoxication: A study of 41 cases with observations on the effects of BAL (2,3,dimercapto-propanol). *N Engl J Med* 254:401, 1956.
47. Cullen NM, Wolf LR, St Clair D: Pediatric arsenic ingestion. *Am J Emerg Med.* 13(4): p. 432, 1995.
48. Bolliger CT, van Zijl P, Louw JA: Multiple organ failure with the adult respiratory distress syndrome in homicidal arsenic poisoning. *Respiration* 59:57, 1992.
49. Beckman KJ, et al: Arsenic-induced torsade de pointes. *Crit Care Med* 19:290, 1991.
50. Mathieu D, et al: Massive arsenic poisoning: Effect of hemodialysis and dimercaprol on arsenic kinetics. *Intensive Care Med* 18:47, 1992.
51. Roses OE, et al: Mass poisoning by sodium arsenite. *J Toxicol Clin Toxicol* 29:209, 1991.
52. Arbouine MW, Wilson HK: The effect of seafood consumption on the assessment of occupational exposure to arsenic by urinary arsenic speciation measurements. *J Trace Elem Electrolytes Health Dis* 6:153, 1992.
53. Hilfer RJ, Mandel A: Acute arsenic intoxication diagnosed by roentgenograms: Report of a case with survival. *N Engl J Med* 266:663, 1962.
54. Shum S, et al: Chelation of organoarsenate with dimercaptosuccinic acid. Vet Hum Toxicol 37:239, 1995.
55. Sunderman FW: Perils of mercury. *Ann Clin Lab Sci* 18:89, 1988.
56. Rennie AC, et al: Mercury poisoning after spillage at home from a sphygmomanometer on loan from hospital. *BMJ* 319:366, 1999.
57. Kazantzis G: Mercury exposure and early effects: An overview. *Med Lav* 93:139, 2002.
58. Kulig K: A tragic reminder about organic mercury. *N Engl J Med* 338:1692, 1998.
59. Soo YO, et al: Subcutaneous injection of metallic mercury. *Hum Exp Toxicol* 22:345, 2003.
60. Wossmann W, et al: Mercury intoxication presenting with hypertension and tachycardia. *Arch Dis Child* 80:556, 1999.
61. Taueg C, et al: Acute and chronic poisoning from residential exposures to elemental mercury: Michigan, 1989-1990. *J Toxicol Clin Toxicol* 30:63, 1992.
62. Zimmerman JE: Fatality following metallic mercury aspiration during removal of a long intestinal tube. *JAMA* 208:2158, 1969.
63. Rosenman KD, et al: Sensitive indicators of inorganic mercury toxicity. *Arch Environ Health* 41:208, 1986.
64. Nierenberg DW, et al: Delayed cerebellar disease and death after accidental exposure to dimethylmercury. *N Engl J Med* 338:1672, 1998.
65. Clarkson TW, Magos L, Myers GJ: The toxicology of mercury: Current exposures and clinical manifestations. *N Engl J Med* 349:1731, 2003.

CHAPTER

156 Hydrocarbons

David C. Lee

PERSPECTIVE

Human exposure to hydrocarbons is one of the most frequently reported poisonings, accounting for more than 60,000 cases annually, with most treated in an outpatient setting.[1,2] The cases of patients with hydrocarbon exposures who present to the emergency department generally can be classified into four types, as follows:

1. Accidental ingestion involving children younger than 5 years. This is the most common scenario causing fatality and usually involves significant pulmonary injury.
2. Intentional inhalational abuse of a volatile hydrocarbon. Recreational abuse has been a medical problem ever since solvent inhalation became popular during the late 1800s. Fatalities typically occur within distinct demographic groups (e.g., American Indians, homosexual males, teenagers).[2,3]
3. Accidental inhalational or dermal exposure to hydrocarbons in the household or workplace.
4. Massive oral ingestion of hydrocarbons in a suicide attempt.

PRINCIPLES OF DISEASE

Pharmacology

Hydrocarbons are a diverse group of organic compounds that contain hydrogen and carbon (Table 156-1). Most hydrocarbons are byproducts of crude oil and are therefore called *petroleum distillates* (e.g., gasoline). Some products, such as turpentine, are derived from pine oil, not petroleum. Hydrocarbons are also classified by their structure. The two main categories are straight-chain hydrocarbons (*aliphatic*; e.g., propane) and those containing a benzene ring structure (*aromatic*; e.g., toluene). Hydrocarbons can also have multiple nonorganic side chains—for example, halogenated hydrocarbons such as carbon tetrachloride. Hydrocarbons are commonly used as the solvent base for many toxic chemicals, such as insecticides and metals, which in turn can cause a separate type of poisoning. Although the range of toxicity of hydrocarbon varies widely, most human exposures are confined to petroleum distillates.

Pathophysiology

Acute hydrocarbon toxicity usually affects three main target organs: the lungs, the central nervous system (CNS), and the heart. Although certain hydrocarbons can enter the body through the skin or gastrointestinal tract, hydrocarbons cause the most acute damage in the lungs. Despite the thousands of different types of hydrocarbons, their potential for acute toxicity depends mainly on the following four characteristics[4]:

1. *Viscosity,* or the capacity to resist flow. Low viscosity allows a substance to spread rapidly; thus, the lower the viscosity, the higher the toxicity. Viscosity is measured in Saybolt seconds universal (SSU), and substances with an SSU of less than 60 have the highest potential risk of aspiration. For example, lubricants and mineral oil have high viscosity and low toxicity, whereas furniture polish has low viscosity and high risk of aspiration.
2. *Volatility,* or the capacity for a liquid to turn into a gas. High volatility enables a substance to displace alveolar oxygen. Butane and gasoline are hydrocarbon types with high volatility.
3. *Surface tension,* or the capacity for a substance to collect on a liquid surface. Low surface tension enables a substance (e.g., turpentine) to disperse easily.
4. *Chemical side chains,* which often increase toxicity. These toxic side chains include heavy metals (e.g., arsenic), halogens (e.g., carbon tetrachloride), and aromatic structures (e.g., toluene).

Pulmonary Disease

Fatalities usually occur after an ingestion that is accompanied by an aspiration. Animal studies have shown that pulmonary toxicity is caused by aspiration rather than by gastrointestinal absorption with hematogenous spread. A small amount of hydrocarbon in the trachea can be devastating, whereas a much larger amount in the stomach can be benign.[5,6]

Lung injury is mediated through several mechanisms. First, most hydrocarbons are poorly water soluble and can penetrate into the lower airways, producing bronchospasm and an inflammatory response. Second, volatilized hydrocarbon can displace oxygen in the alveolar space. Third, hydrocarbon can inhibit surfactant function, leading to alveolar instability and collapse. Fourth, hydrocarbon can damage pulmonary alveoli and capillaries causing hyperemia, diffuse hemorrhagic exudative alveolitis with granulocytic infiltration, microabscesses, and lipoid pneumonias. These effects cause alveolar dysfunction, ventilation/perfusion mismatch, hypoxemia, and respiratory failure.[7-9]

Table 156-1. Spectrum of Hydrocarbon Toxicity

Type	Example	Use	Pathophysiology	Comments
Aliphatic petroleum distillates	Methane Propane Butane	Fuels Exist as gases	Asphyxiants causing hypoxia and CNS depression Abused inhalants	Sudden death from intentional inhalation
	Gasoline Kerosene Mineral spirits Mineral oil Naphtha Mineral seal oil Diesel oil n-Hexane	Liquid fuels Solvents Furniture polish Degreasers Multiple uses in chemical industry	Pneumonitis when aspirated Abused inhalants CNS depression from fumes n-Hexane causes peripheral neuropathy	Viscosity and volatility determine spectrum of toxicity Mineral seal oil has high aspiration potential Poor gastrointestinal absorption
Aromatic petroleum distillates	Toluene Xylene Benzene	Used in plastics, pharmaceutical, rubber, chemical, and solvent industries In patients, degreasers	Highly volatile, lung aspiration Absorbed from gastrointestinal tract Abused inhalants	Inhaled toluene causes renal tubular acidosis Benzene causes aplastic anemia, leukemia
Wood distillates	Turpentine Pine oil	Solvent Household disinfectants	Well absorbed from gastrointestinal tract CNS toxicity	Gastrointestinal/CNS toxicity
Halogenated hydrocarbons	Methylene chloride Chloroform Carbon tetrachloride Trichloroethylene Freon Methylbromide Lindane DDT	Solvents Cleaning fluids Degreasers Fire extinguishers Paint strippers Fumigants	Multisystem toxicity (CNS, renal, hepatic, cardiac) Inhalant abuse Highly lipid soluble	Methylene chloride metabolized to carbon monoxide Carbon tetrachloride is radiopaque Insecticides absorbed through skin
Related chemicals	Phenol Creosols	Disinfectants Used in chemical industry	Very corrosive	Phenol causes severe skin burns

CNS, central nervous system; DDT, Dichlorodiphenyltrichloroethane.

Central Nervous System

Certain hydrocarbons can cause CNS depression (e.g., toluene, benzene, gasoline, butane, and chlorinated hydrocarbons). These hydrocarbons can have a narcotic-like effect and cause euphoria, disinhibition, confusion, and obtundation. With an isolated single exposure, patients usually have a rapid onset of intoxication and rapid recovery. For these reasons, substance abusers seek these hydrocarbons for recreational use. Inhalation of these substances avoids hepatic first-pass metabolism and generates high concentrations in the CNS. Chronic use of inhaled hydrocarbons can cause peripheral neuropathy, cerebellar degeneration, neuropsychiatric disorders, chronic encephalopathy, and dementia.[3,10] More than 50% of patients who abuse toluene for more than 10 years have cerebrocortical atrophy with histologic changes, including loss of neurons, diffuse gliosis, and axonal degeneration.[11]

Cardiac

Hydrocarbons can cause sudden death, typically with sudden physical activity during or after intentional inhalation. These compounds are thought to produce myocardial sensitization to endogenous and exogenous catecholamine, which precipitates ventricular dysrhythmias and myocardial dysfunction. This is particularly true for halogenated and aromatic hydrocarbons (e.g., trichloroethylene found in paper correction fluid).[12]

Other Systems

Various hydrocarbons have been reported to be toxic to other organ systems. Recognized syndromes include toluene-induced renal tubular acidosis, benzene-induced bone marrow toxicity and leukemia, methylene chloride–induced carbon monoxide poisoning, and chlorinated hydrocarbon–induced centrilobular hepatic necrosis and renal failure.[3,4] Direct skin exposure of certain hydrocarbons can cause extensive chemical burns. Hydrocarbons are often used as solvents for other chemicals that may have significant inherent toxicity.

CLINICAL FEATURES

There are four typical presentations of acute hydrocarbon exposures. The first scenario is a toddler who has ingested an unknown quantity of a hydrocarbon. One third of these patients will have drunk from a reused beverage container storing hydrocarbon.[9] Patients with significant life-threatening poisonings usually have early respiratory symptoms, including cyanosis, coughing, grunting, noisy respirations, or repeated bouts of vomiting. These findings suggest aspiration. A patient may initially have mild symptoms and then develop tachypnea, dyspnea, bronchospasm, wheezing, rales, and fever within 6 hours.[4,9,13] A change in mental status may be a manifestation of hypoxia or hypercapnia but may also be a direct CNS effect of hydrocarbons. In extreme cases, patients present with frank respiratory failure. Additives or solutes in the hydrocarbon base can produce other symptoms (e.g., seizures from camphorated hydrocarbons, cyanosis from nitrite-induced methemoglobinemia). Pesticides are a classic example of such a toxic substance that is often placed in a hydrocarbon base. With pesticide exposures, it can be difficult to distinguish acute respiratory distress induced by hydrocarbon aspiration from bronchorrhea induced by organophosphate exposure.

The second scenario is the solvent-abusing adolescent or adult. In extreme cases, these patients can be in cardiac arrest. Prehospital care providers often describe an individual who has inhaled solvents, performed some type of physical activity, then suddenly collapsed. This is thought to result from cardiac sensitization by endogenous catecholamines and the ensuing development of dysrhythmias. Paraphernalia is often found, including plastic bags used for "bagging" (pouring hydrocarbon in a bag or container, then inhaling deeply) or a hydrocarbon-soaked cloth used for "huffing" (inhaling through a saturated cloth). Other paraphernalia include gasoline containers, multiple butane lighters, and spray paint cans. These patients often have a distinctive odor because almost all these hydrocarbons are volatile. They may have paint or a rash over the mouth and nose (*glue-sniffer's rash*) (Figure 156-1). These patients can also present to the emergency department with CNS intoxication, euphoria, agitation, hallucinations, confusion, and bizarre behavior, which may progress to CNS depression and convulsions. Drug abusers who chronically inhale hydrocarbons may not be brought to medical attention specifically for treatment of their drug abuse but rather for behavioral problems or nonspecific medical symptoms caused by their abuse. The long-term chronic abuser may clinically appear similar to the long-term "skid-row" alcoholic, with peripheral neuropathy, cerebellar degeneration, and encephalopathy.[3]

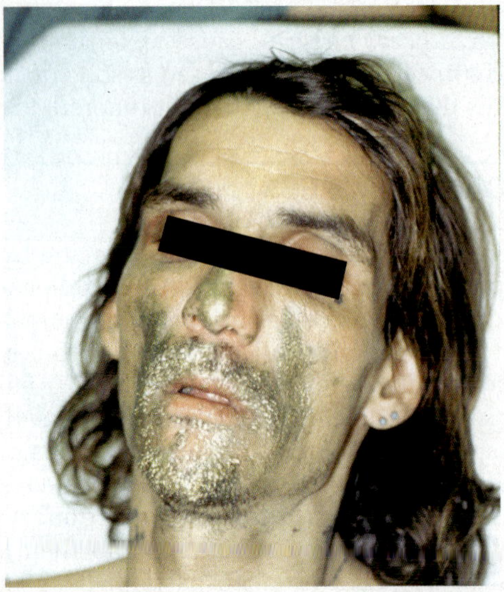

Figure 156-1. Typical presentation of paint sniffer ("huffer") with paint around the face and sedation. (Courtesy of Chris Tomaszewski, MD, Carolinas HealthCare System.)

A third common scenario is the accidental dermal or inhaled (nonaspiration) respiratory exposure to hydrocarbons in the workplace or home. This is rarely life threatening, and most patients do not seek medical care. Most are asymptomatic or have transient nonspecific symptoms, such as headache, dizziness, or nausea. Symptoms resolve with fresh air and removal from the offending environment.[1,2] Patients with significant respiratory exposure may have persistent pulmonary complaints and physical findings, such as coughing, wheezing, and cyanosis. Patients with significant acute dermal exposures may report pain and have evidence of chemical burns consisting of erythema, swelling, blistering, and dermal destruction.

A fourth scenario is the rare patient who intentionally ingests or intravenously injects a hydrocarbon in a suicide attempt. These patients can be difficult to treat because hydrocarbons are often used in combination with other substances. In the absence of aspiration or co-ingestion of another toxic substance, the massive oral ingestion of most commonly available hydrocarbons is not associated with significant morbidity or mortality.

DIAGNOSTIC STRATEGIES

The diagnosis of hydrocarbon poisoning is made on clinical grounds. Prehospital providers, family, and bystanders should be encouraged to bring the offending agent to the emergency department. The local poison control center can help identify and verify the agent. Laboratory identification of hydrocarbons is time-consuming and unhelpful in the emergency department management. Signs of a significant exposure include tachypnea, tachycardia, wheezing, and hypoxemia. Patients with a significant hydrocarbon exposure should have a chest radiograph taken. Radiographic changes can occur within 30 minutes of ingestion and may identify pathologic lesions not recognized by auscultation in more than 50% of patients (Figure 156-2).[14] Continuous pulse oximetry and arterial blood gas measurement may also be helpful. Patients who chronically abuse hydrocarbons can be similar to the intoxicated chronic alcoholic and require close scrutiny to exclude underlying or secondary diseases. For example, chronic toluene sniffing can cause acid-base disorders, so measurement of acid-base, electrolytes, blood urea nitrogen, and creatinine levels and urinalysis should be performed.

DIFFERENTIAL CONSIDERATIONS

In the most common fatal pediatric scenario, the child who ingests and then aspirates hydrocarbons, the physician should ensure that no other toxic substances are involved. Organophosphate, salicylate, and paraquat poisonings can mimic the symptoms of hydrocarbon aspiration. These poisonings mandate gastrointestinal decontamination and antidotal therapy, whereas hydrocarbon poisoning requires only good

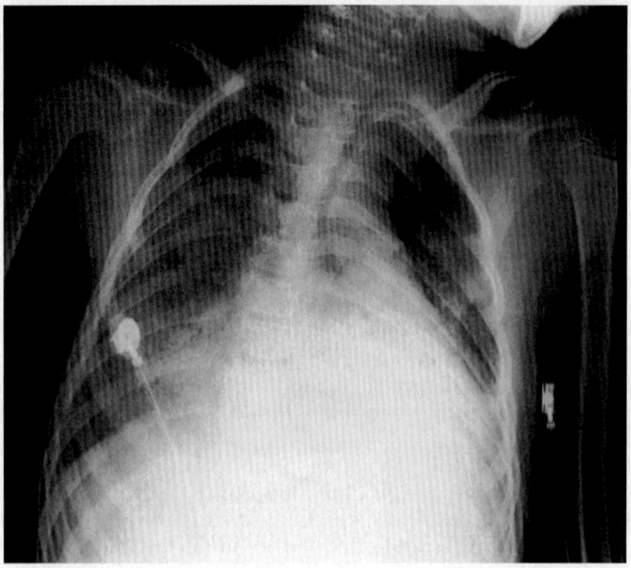

Figure 156-2. Chest radiograph of a patient with hydrocarbon ingestion 6 hours after exposure.

supportive care. In the recreational abuser, multiple drugs of abuse may be present. Behavioral disorders and confusion can result from hypoxia and respiratory compromise as well as from the drugs. In the chronic abuser, it can be difficult to differentiate between functional and organic confusional states.

MANAGEMENT

Because hydrocarbons can cause sudden decompensation in pulmonary, cardiac, and CNS functions, patients should be monitored with cardiac monitors and pulse oximeters in a well-observed area. In patients with severe aspiration, early intubation for airway control and positive airway pressure has been advocated to minimize aspiration risks and counteract hydrocarbon-induced alveoli collapse.[4] However, no studies have proven this to be more beneficial than standard respiratory care. High-frequency jet ventilation and extracorporeal membrane oxygenation have been used to treat children with respiratory failure secondary to aspiration.[4,15,16] Surfactant therapy has also been considered in these cases, but its benefit has not been proven. Corticosteroids and antibiotics have not been shown to be beneficial in cases of hydrocarbon aspiration, but the differentiation between bacterial and chemical pneumonia is difficult.[4]

The aphorism, "the safest place in the body for hydrocarbons is the duodenum," holds true for most hydrocarbons regardless of the volume ingested. Routine gastrointestinal decontamination such as gastric lavage should be avoided. This reflects the high toxicity of hydrocarbon to the lungs and the low toxicity of most hydrocarbons to the gastrointestinal tract, with low potential for systemic gastrointestinal absorption. A common complication of aggressive decontamination after the ingestion of a benign hydrocarbon is aspiration, which converts a relatively nontoxic ingestion to a toxic aspiration. In special cases, aggressive gastrointestinal decontamination is indicated because of the inherent toxicity of the hydrocarbon or the toxicity of additives to the hydrocarbon. A mnemonic to describe most of these cases is *CHAMP: c*amphor, which can cause seizures and status epilepticus; *h*alogenated hydrocarbon, which can cause dysrhythmias and hepatotoxicity; *a*romatic hydrocarbon, which can cause bone marrow suppression and cancer; *m*etals (arsenic, mercury, lead); and *p*esticides, which can cause cholinergic crises, seizures, and respiratory depression. The mode of decontamination is also controversial.[17,18] In most cases of hydrocarbon ingestion or inhalation, close observation, supportive care, and monitoring are the cornerstones of management. There are no specific antidotes for hydrocarbon poisoning.

Epinephrine and isoproterenol should be avoided unless required for cardiac resuscitation. Theoretically, exogenous catecholamine can cause dysrhythmias in hydrocarbon-sensitized myocardium.[3,4] Other β-adrenergic agonists (e.g., metaproterenol, albuterol) have not been well explored. Patients should be kept calm and sedated, if necessary, to prevent excess catecholamine release.

Dermal exposures of certain hydrocarbons can cause extensive burns. Exposed patients should be decontaminated immediately. Contaminated clothing should be removed, and the skin should be washed with soap and copious lukewarm water.

DISPOSITION

Patients with exposures to known, relatively benign hydrocarbons should receive appropriate decontamination and undergo a 4- to 6-hour period of observation. Patients who have ingested unknown hydrocarbons and do not have symptoms initially should be monitored for a minimum of 6 hours. A reassessment at the last hour of observation can include pulse oximetry, arterial blood gas measurements, and chest radiography. The presence of any signs or symptoms at this time suggests hospital admission and further observation. Asymptomatic patients with accidental exposures to hydrocarbons can be discharged after a period of observation with appropriate follow-up.

Patients who have ingested hydrocarbons and have cough, difficulty breathing, or shortness of breath suggestive of aspiration should be admitted for a minimum of 24 hours for observation. Patients who present after an episode of recreational hydrocarbon inhalation should be observed for 4 to 6 hours. Patients who chronically abuse hydrocarbons often go to the emergency department for behavioral problems or nonspecific symptoms caused by their drug addiction. All patients in this category should be offered drug addiction counseling.

KEY CONCEPTS

- Aspiration is the major effect from ingested hydrocarbons.
- Routine gastrointestinal decontamination of hydrocarbons should be avoided.
- Asymptomatic patients should be observed for delayed symptoms for a minimum of 4 hours.
- Solvent-abusing patients are at risk for sudden cardiovascular collapse and should be kept calm and quiet.
- Patients exposed to hydrocarbon vapors recover rapidly with fresh air and removal from the exposure.

REFERENCES

1. Machado B, Cross K, Snodgrass WR: Accidental hydrocarbon ingestion cases telephoned to a regional poison center. *Ann Emerg Med* 17:804, 1988.
2. Watson WA, et al: 2002 annual report of the American Association of Poison Control Centers Toxic Exposure Surveillance System. *Am J Emerg Med* 21:353, 2003.
3. Linden C: Volatile substances of abuse. *Emerg Med Clin North Am* 8:559, 1990.
4. Ellenhorn M: The hydrocarbon products. In Ellenhorn MJ, et al (eds): *Medical Toxicology, Diagnosis and Treatment of Human Poisoning*, 2nd ed. Baltimore, Williams & Wilkins, 1997, pp 1420-1426.
5. Gerarde HW: Toxicological studies on hydrocarbons. IX. The aspiration hazard and toxicity of hydrocarbons and hydrocarbon mixtures. *Arch Environ Health* 6:329, 1963.
6. Richardson J, Pratt-Thomas H: Toxic effects of varying doses of kerosene administered by different routes. *Am J Med Sci* 221:531, 1951.
7. Gross P, McNerney JM, Babyak MA: Kerosene pneumonitis: An experimental study with small doses. *Am Rev Respir Dis* 88:656, 1963.
8. Ohwada A, et al: Exogenous lipoid pneumonia following ingestion of liquid paraffin. *Intern Med* 41:483, 2002.
9. Truemper E, Reyes de la Rocha S, Atkinson SD: Clinical characteristics, pathophysiology, and management of hydrocarbon ingestion: Case report and review of the literature. *Pediatr Emerg Care* 3:187, 1987.
10. Hormes JT, Filley CM, Rosenberg NL: Neurologic sequelae of chronic solvent vapor abuse. *Neurology* 36:698, 1986.
11. Schikler KN, Seitz K, Rice JF, Strader T: Solvent abuse associated cortical atrophy. *J Adolesc Health Care* 3:37, 1982.
12. Anene O, Castello FV: Myocardial dysfunction after hydrocarbon ingestion. *Crit Care Med* 22:528, 1994.
13. Press E: Cooperative Kerosene Poisoning Study: Evaluation of gastric lavage and other factors in the treatment of accidental ingestion of petroleum distillate products. *Pediatrics* 29:648, 1962.
14. Zucker AR, Berger S, Wood LD: Management of kerosene-induced pulmonary injury. *Crit Care Med* 14:303, 1986.
15. Scalzo AJ, et al: Extracorporeal membrane oxygenation for hydrocarbon aspiration. *Am J Dis Child* 144:867, 1990.
16. Bysani GK, Rucoba RJ, Noah ZL: Treatment of hydrocarbon pneumonitis: High frequency jet ventilation as an alternative to extracorporeal membrane oxygenation. *Chest* 106:300, 1994.
17. Ng RC, Darwish H, Stewart DA: Emergency treatment of petroleum distillate and turpentine ingestion. *Can Med Assoc J* 111:537, 1974.
18. Beamon RF, Siegel CJ, Landers G, Green V: Hydrocarbon ingestion in children: A six-year retrospective study. *JACEP* 5:771, 1976.

CHAPTER 157

Inhaled Toxins

Lewis S. Nelson and Robert S. Hoffman

Airborne toxins produce local noxious effects on the airways and lungs, and the respiratory tract can also serve as a portal of entry for systemic poisons. Inhalational exposure can be covert and indolent (as in occupational exposure to asbestos or urban exposure to photochemical smog) or fulminant and obvious. The circumstances and location of the exposure, presence of combustion or odors, and number and condition of victims assist in the diagnosis. Despite the array of possible toxic inhalants, identification of a specific inhalant is generally unnecessary because therapy is based primarily on the clinical manifestations (Table 157-1).

SIMPLE ASPHYXIANTS

Perspective

The vast majority of simple asphyxiations are workplace related and typically occur during the use of liquefied gas or airline respirators or while working in confined spaces.[1] With catalytic converters, most deaths related to the intentional inhalation of automotive exhaust result from simple asphyxiation and not carbon monoxide poisoning.[2]

Table 157-1. Common Inhaled Toxins

Inhalant	Source/Use	Predominant class
Acrolein	Combustion	Irritant, highly soluble
Ammonia	Fertilizer, combustion	Irritant, highly soluble
Carbon dioxide	Fermentation, complete combustion, fire extinguisher	Simple asphyxiant; systemic effects
Carbon monoxide	Incomplete combustion, methylene chloride	Chemical asphyxiant
Chloramine	Mixed cleaning products (hypochlorite bleach and ammonia)	Irritant, highly soluble
Chlorine	Swimming pool disinfectant, cleaning products	Irritant, intermediate solubility
Chlorobenzylidenemalononitrile/ chloroacetophenone	Tear gas (Mace)	Pharmacologic "irritant"
Hydrogen chloride	Tanning and electroplating industry	Irritant, highly soluble
Hydrogen cyanide	Combustion of plastics, acidification of cyanide salts	Chemical asphyxiant
Hydrogen fluoride	Hydrofluoric acid	Irritant, highly soluble; systemic effects
Hydrogen sulfide	Decaying organic matter, oil industry, mines, asphalt	Chemical asphyxiant; irritant, highly soluble
Methane	Natural gas, swamp gas	Simple asphyxiant
Methylbromide	Fumigant	Chemical asphyxiant
Nitrogen	Mines, scuba divers (nitrogen narcosis, decompression sickness)	Simple asphyxiant; systemic effects
Nitrous oxide	Inhalant of abuse, whipping cream, racing fuel booster	Simple asphyxiant
Noble gases (e.g., helium)	Industry, laboratories	Simple asphyxiant
Oxides of nitrogen	Silos, anesthetics, combustion	Irritant, intermediate solubility
Oxygen	Medical use, hyperbaric conditions	Irritant, free radical; systemic effects
Ozone	Electrostatic energy	Irritant, free radical
Phosgene	Combustion of chlorinated hydrocarbons	Irritant, poorly soluble
Phosphine	Hydration of aluminum or zinc phosphide (fumigants)	Chemical asphyxiant
Smoke (varying composition)	Combustion	Variable, but may include all classes
Sulfur dioxide	Photochemical smog (fossil fuels)	Irritant, highly soluble

Principles of Disease

Simple asphyxiants are typically inert and produce toxicity by displacing oxygen and lowering the fraction of inspired oxygen (FIO_2). Exposed patients remain asymptomatic if the FIO_2 is normal. Carbon dioxide and nitrogen, both constituents of air, produce narcosis at elevated levels, but their predominant toxic effect is simple asphyxiation.

Clinical Features

Acute effects occur within minutes of onset of asphyxia and are the manifestations of hypoxia. A fall in the FIO_2 from normal, 0.21 (i.e., 21%), to 0.15 results in autonomic stimulation (e.g., tachycardia, tachypnea, dyspnea) and cerebral hypoxia (e.g., ataxia, dizziness, incoordination, confusion). Dyspnea is not an early finding because hypoxemia is not as potent a stimulus for this sensation as hypercarbia. Lethargy from cerebral edema is expected as the FIO_2 falls below 0.1 (10%), and life probably cannot be sustained at an FIO_2 below 0.06 (6%).[3] Since removal from exposure terminates the hypoxia and results in clinical improvement, most patients present with resolving symptoms. However, failure to improve suggests complications of ischemia (e.g., seizures, coma, cardiac arrest) and is associated with a poor prognosis.

Diagnostic Strategies and Differential Considerations

A consistent history, an appropriate spectrum of complaints, and rapid resolution on removal from exposure are generally sufficient to make the diagnosis. Minimally symptomatic or asymptomatic patients do not require chest radiography or arterial blood gas (ABG) analysis. Definitive diagnosis ultimately requires scene investigation by a trained and suitably outfitted team. Determination of the exact nature of the gas is of limited clinical value but may have important public health implications. Since the presenting complaints offered by most exposed patients are nonspecific and protean (e.g., dizziness, syncope, dyspnea), the differential diagnosis is extensive.

Management and Disposition

Management rarely requires specific therapy other than removal from exposure, supportive care, and possibly administration of supplemental oxygen. Neurologic injury or cardiorespiratory arrest should be managed with standard resuscitation protocols. Patients with manifestations of mild poisoning who recover after removal from the exposure can be observed briefly and discharged. Patients at risk for complications of hypoxia, such as those presenting with significant symptoms (e.g., coma) or with exacerbating medical conditions (e.g., cardiac disease) should be observed for the development or progression of posthypoxic complications.

KEY CONCEPTS

- Any gas can be a simple asphyxiant if it displaces sufficient oxygen from the breathable air.
- Appropriate therapy for asphyxiation includes removal from exposure, administration of oxygen, and supportive care.

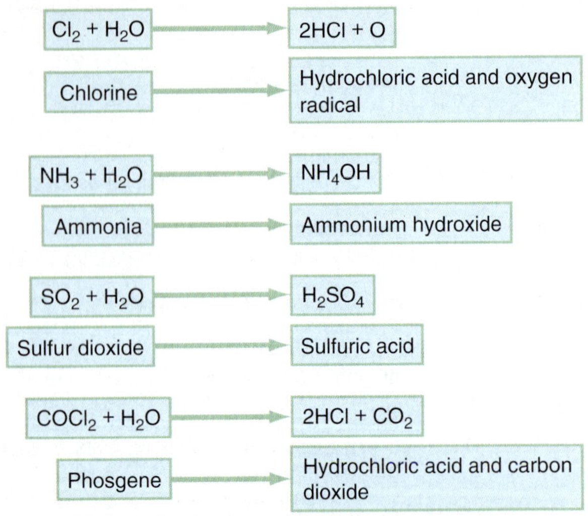

Figure 157-1. Sample reactions of pulmonary irritants reacting with water in the lung.

PULMONARY IRRITANTS

Perspective

The pulmonary irritant gases are a large group of agents that produce a common toxicologic syndrome when inhaled in moderate concentrations. Although many of these agents can be found in the home, significant poisoning from consumer products is uncommon because of restrictions designed to reduce their toxicity. Still, catastrophes such as the 1984 release of methyl isocyanate in Bhopal, India, which resulted in more than 2000 fatalities and 250,000 injuries, remain as a rare environmental risk. On a different scale, industrialization has increased ambient levels of sulfur dioxide, ozone, and oxides of nitrogen. These irritant gases frequently exacerbate chronic pulmonary disease.

Principles of Disease

Irritant gases dissolve in the respiratory tract mucus and alter the air-lung interface by invoking an irritant or inflammatory response. When dissolved, most of the gases produce an acid or alkaline product, but several generate oxygen-derived free radicals that produce direct cellular toxicity (Figure 157-1). Pulmonary irritants are grouped by their water solubilities (see Table 157-1).

Clinical Features

Highly water-soluble gases have their greatest impact on the mucous membranes of the eyes and upper airway. Exposure results in immediate irritation, with lacrimation, nasal burning, and cough. Although their pungent odors and rapid symptom onset tend to limit significant exposure, massive or prolonged exposure can result in life-threatening laryngeal edema, laryngospasm, bronchospasm, or acute lung injury (ALI), formerly known as "noncardiogenic pulmonary edema."[4] Poorly water-soluble gases do not readily irritate the mucous membranes, and some have pleasant odors (e.g., phosgene's odor is similar to that of hay). Since there are no immediate symptoms, prolonged breathing in the toxic environment allows the substance to reach the alveoli. Even moderate exposure causes irritation of the lower airway, alveoli, and parenchyma and causes pulmonary endothelial injury after a 2- to 24-hour delay. Initial symptoms consistent with ALI may be mild, only to progress to overt respiratory failure and acute respiratory distress syndrome over the ensuing 24 to 36 hours.[5]

Gases with intermediate water solubility tend to produce clinical syndromes that are a composite of the other gases, depending on the extent of exposure. Massive exposure is most often associated with rapid onset of upper airway irritation and more moderate exposure with delayed onset of lower airway symptoms.[6]

Diagnostic Strategies and Differential Considerations

The evaluation of upper airway symptoms is usually done through physical examination but may require laryngoscopy. After exposure, swelling may occur rapidly or may be delayed, so a normal oropharyngeal or laryngeal evaluation may not exclude subsequent deterioration. Radiographic and laboratory studies have little role in the evaluation of upper airway symptoms.

Oxygenation and ventilation are assessed by serial chest auscultation and pulse oximetry, supplemented by chest radiography and ABGs in patients with cough, dyspnea, hypoxia, or abnormal findings on physical examination. No clinical tests can identify the specific irritant, and identification is not generally necessary for patient care, although knowing the causative agent may allow reduction of the observation period.

Bronchospasm, cough, chest tightness, and acute conjunctival irritation frequently follow allergen exposure, but the history generally suggests the diagnosis. ALI occurs after many physiologic insults, including trauma and sepsis, again highlighting the need for accurate history taking.

Management

Signs of upper airway dysfunction (e.g., hoarseness, stridor) mandate direct visualization of the larynx and immediate airway stabilization, if necessary. Given the potential rapidity of airway deterioration, early and frequent reassessment should be performed.

Bronchospasm generally responds to inhaled β-adrenergic agonists; the role of ipratropium is not yet defined. Other than as a standard treatment for a comorbid condition, such as asthma, there is no clear indication for corticosteroids.[7]

Nebulized 2% sodium bicarbonate solution can provide symptomatic relief in patients exposed to chlorine or hydrogen chloride gas.[8] Because the inflammatory cascade is not altered, however, the component of lung injury mediated by free radicals probably continues. Thus, delayed deterioration predictably occurs based on the nature of the exposure. Patients receiving inhalational bicarbonate therapy therefore require extensive discharge instructions or admission to the hospital.

Diagnosis of ALI or acute respiratory distress syndrome indicates the need for aggressive supportive care, including manipulations of the patient's airway pressures (e.g., continuous positive airway pressure, positive end-expiratory pressure). Exogenous surfactant and nitric oxide may have a beneficial role in toxin-induced acute respiratory distress syndrome, despite little support for its use in other forms of the syndrome.

Disposition

Patients exposed to highly water-soluble agents can be discharged if they are asymptomatic or improve with symptomatic therapy. After exposure to intermediate or poorly water-soluble agents, asymptomatic patients should be observed for increasing dyspnea for several hours before final disposition. Patients with substantial exposure to these agents or those in high-risk situations (e.g., underlying pulmonary disease, extremes of age, poor follow-up) should be observed for 24 hours and may require hospitalization. All patients should be instructed to return if symptoms recur.

KEY CONCEPTS

- Highly water-soluble agents produce rapid irritation and predominantly upper respiratory tract symptoms.
- Poorly water-soluble agents often produce delayed lower respiratory tract findings.

SMOKE INHALATION

Perspective

Annually, 4000 persons are injured or die in residential fires in the United States. Many of these casualties do not suffer serious cutaneous burns, but rather die from smoke inhalation. This is a variant of irritant injury in which heated particulate matter and adsorbed toxins injure normal mucosa, similar to other irritant gases. Although carbon monoxide and cyanide are often discussed with the smoke inhalation syndrome because of their common origin, these are systemic, not pulmonary, toxins.

Principles of Disease

Even at temperatures between 350° C and 500° C, air has such a low heat capacity that it rarely produces lower airway damage. However, the greater heat capacities of steam (approximately 4000 times that of air) or heated soot suspended in air (i.e., smoke) can transfer heat and cause injury deep within the respiratory tract.

The nature of the fuel determines the composition of its smoke, and since fires involve variable fuels and burning conditions, the character of fire smoke is almost always undefined to the clinician. Irritant toxins produced by the fire are adsorbed onto carbonaceous particles that deposit in the airways. The irritant substances damage the mucosa through mechanisms similar to the irritant gases, including acid generation and free radical formation.

Clinical Features

Most smoke-associated morbidity and mortality relate to respiratory tract damage. Thermal and irritant-induced laryngeal injury may produce cough or stridor, but these findings are often delayed. Soot and irritant toxins in the airways can produce initial cough, dyspnea, and bronchospasm. Subsequently, a cascade of airway inflammation results in acute lung injury and failure of pulmonary gas exchange. The time between smoke exposure and the onset of clinical symptomatology is highly variable and dependent on the degree and nature of the exposure. Singed nasal hairs and soot in the sputum suggest substantial exposure but are not sufficiently sensitive or specific to be practical.

Carbon monoxide (CO) inhalation should be considered in these patients. Patients who are exposed to filtered or distant smoke (e.g., in a different room) or to relatively smokeless combustion (e.g., engine exhaust) inhale predominantly CO, cyanide, and metabolic poisons and do not suffer irritant exposure.

Diagnostic Strategies and Differential Considerations

Early death is caused by asphyxia, airway compromise, or metabolic poisoning (e.g., CO). Airway patency should be evaluated early, optimally with fiberoptic laryngoscopy. Signs of alveolar filling or hyperinflation on chest radiography, abnormal flow-volume loop or diffusing capacity for carbon monoxide on pulmonary function testing, or abnormal distribution and clearance of radiolabeled gas on ventilation scans can help predict lower airway injury.[8]

Metabolic acidosis, particularly when associated with a serum lactate level greater than 10 mmol/L, suggests concomitant cyanide poisoning.[9] Oxygenation should be assessed by co-oximetry because ABG analysis and pulse oximetry may be inaccurate in CO-poisoned patients.

With the obvious exposure history, the differential diagnosis is limited. Although it is often unclear whether inhalational injuries are thermal or irritant, the differentiation is clinically irrelevant. CO and cyanide should be considered in every case.

Management

The acute management of victims of smoke inhalation is identical to that of other irritant inhalational injuries. Rapid assessment of the airway and early intubation are critical because deterioration may be precipitous. Inhaled β agonists are widely used, but without evidence supporting their benefit. Optimal supportive care and maintenance of adequate oxygenation (e.g., suctioning, pulmonary toilet) are the most important aspects of care. Bronchoscopy with bronchoalveolar lavage is frequently recommended to clear debris and toxins from the distal airways. Corticosteroids, whether inhaled or systemic, are not indicated and potentially harmful in patients with cutaneous burns.[10] Ibuprofen, antioxidants, exogenous surfactant, and high-frequency ventilation yield variably improved survival in experimental and clinical trials; none is generally considered as standard care. Antibiotics should be used only in patients with suspected infection.

Disposition

After the airway is examined and stabilized, patients with worrisome clinical findings (e.g., hoarseness, respiratory distress) and those with identifiers of substantial exposure (e.g., closed-space exposure, carbonaceous sputum) should be admitted to a critical care unit or transferred to a burn center. This decision will vary based on local resources, such as hospital capabilities or availability of a burn referral center.

KEY CONCEPTS

- Smoke inhalation injury is typically irritant in nature.
- Early visualization of the airway is critical. Early intubation prior to deterioration is critical if damage is present.

CYANIDE AND HYDROGEN SULFIDE

Perspective

Hydrogen cyanide (prussic acid) is a gas with many commercial uses, particularly in synthetic fiber manufacture and fumigation, in addition to its intentionally poisonous role in capital punishment. Hydrogen cyanide is occasionally noted to have the odor of bitter almonds. Cyanide in its salt form (e.g., sodium or potassium) is important in the metallurgic (e.g., jewelry) and photographic industries and is dramatically safer to work with because of its low volatility. Cyanide salts do not have an odor under dry conditions. When cyanide salts are dissolved in water, hydrogen cyanide can leave the surface, particularly under acidic conditions. Cyanide is generated in vivo from precursors (cyanogens) such as amygdalin, found in apricot and other *Prunus* species pits, and from nitriles, a group of chemicals with many commercial uses .

Hydrogen sulfide (H_2S) poisoning most often occurs in petroleum refinery and sewage storage tank workers. Occasionally, well-intentioned would-be rescuers become victims, emphasizing the need for proper training and equipment. Hydrogen sulfide has a noxious odor similar to rotten eggs, which becomes unnoticeable with extremely high concentrations or prolonged exposure (*olfactory fatigue*).[11]

Principles of Disease

Gaseous cyanide is rapidly absorbed after inhalation and is immediately distributed to the oxygen-utilizing body tissues. Inhibition of oxidative metabolism by binding to complex IV of the electron transport chain within mitochondria occurs within seconds. The poisoned tissue rapidly depletes its adenosine triphosphate reserves and ceases to function (Figure 157-2). Cyanide has no evident effect on other oxygen-binding enzyme systems, most notably hemoglobin. This is probably explained by the oxidation state of its iron moiety; cyanide binds only to oxidized iron (Fe^{+++}), whereas deoxyhemoglobin contains reduced iron (Fe^{++}).

Hydrogen sulfide exerts its toxic effects both as a pulmonary irritant and as a cellular poison.[11] Its deadly metabolic effects are produced by a mechanism identical to that for cyanide poisoning. However, hydrogen sulfide's spontaneous dissociation from the mitochondria is rapid, allowing patients to survive after brief exposure.

Clinical Features

Tissue hypoxia occurs within seconds to minutes, depending on the route and nature of the exposure. Dysfunction of the heart and the central nervous system, the organ systems most sensitive to hypoxia, is characteristic of cyanide poisoning, manifesting as coma, seizures, cardiovascular collapse, and severe metabolic acidosis. Cyanosis is not characteristic but can be present in profoundly poisoned patients. Given the extreme toxicity of cyanide, mild acute poisoning is uncommon. Patients with acute hydrogen sulfide poisoning have similar clinical manifestations, although many are recovering by the time of arrival in the emergency department.

Since cyanide and hydrogen sulfide prevent tissue extraction of oxygen from the blood, the oxygen content of venous blood remains high, approaching that of arterial blood. Clinically, this may appear as the "arterialization," or brightening, of venous blood to resemble arterial blood. A comparison of the measured venous (ideally but impractically mixed venous) and arterial oxygen contents may assist in the diagnosis of cyanide poisoning.[12]

Patients surviving cyanide or hydrogen sulfide poisoning may have persistent[13] or delayed-onset neurologic syndromes identical to those noted in patients with CO poisoning or cardiac arrest.

Diagnostic Strategies and Differential Considerations

Obtaining a serum cyanide level is generally too slow for emergency department use but can be useful for confirmation and documentation purposes. Technology exists for immediate cyanide determination but is not widely available. Rapid tests for hydrogen sulfide are not available, but the presence of blackened copper coins in the pockets of victims may be a clue to the diagnosis.

In practice, the diagnosis must be based on the circumstances of exposure and a corroborative physical examination. Pulse oximetry and ABG analysis are accurate in cases of isolated cyanide or hydrogen

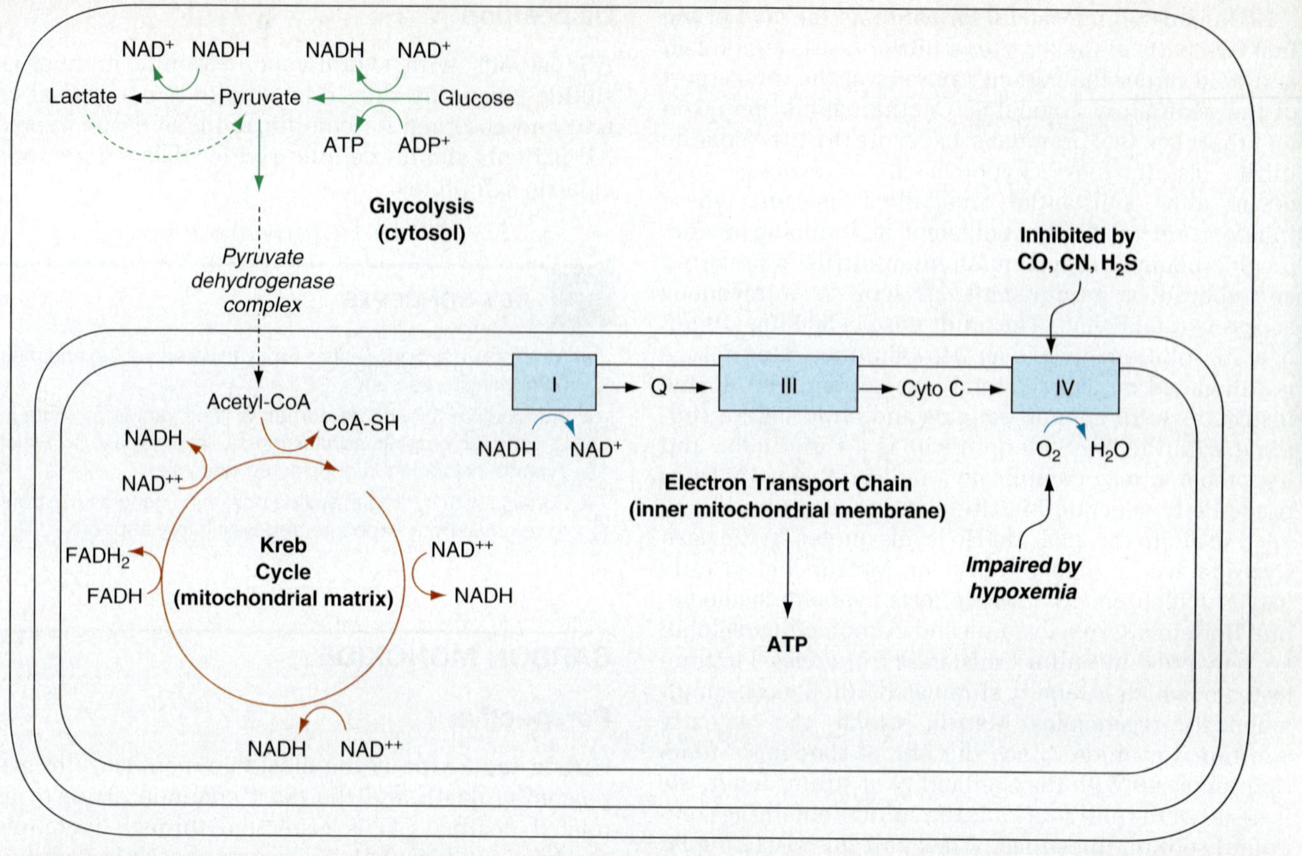

Figure 157-2. The complete metabolism of a molecule of glucose to energy is complex but occurs in two broad steps. The first step, anaerobic glycolysis, which occurs in the absence of oxygen, generates pyruvate, NADH, and adenosine triphosphate (ATP). Pyruvate then enters the Krebs cycle to create potential energy in the second step, through the reduction of NAD^+ to NADH and FADH to $FADH_2$. Similarly, fatty acid metabolism and protein metabolism produce $FADH_2$ and NADH, which also must be converted to ATP. These conversions occur in the mitochondrial membrane, where oxidative phosphorylation is linked to the electron transport chain, the last phase of which involves the transfer of electrons to molecular oxygen to form water. Cyanide (CN), hydrogen sulfide (H_2S), and carbon monoxide (CO) bind to and inhibit the last step, the Fe^{3+}-containing cytochrome aa_3 in complex IV, preventing further oxidation of NADH. This in turn hinders the Krebs cycle, since the required regeneration of NAD^+ does not occur, and glucose metabolism is forced to end at pyruvate. For energy production to continue, NADH donates its electrons to pyruvate, creating lactate, and sufficient NAD^+ is regenerated for glycolysis to progress. Ultimately, energy failure and end-organ damage occur. CoA, coenzyme A; FAD, flavin adenine dinucleotide; NAD, nicotinamide adenine dinucleotide.

sulfide poisoning. An increased anion gap metabolic acidosis and elevated serum lactate level are usually present. A lactate level greater than 10 mmol/L in a fire victim is highly predictive of cyanide poisoning.[9] Carboxyhemoglobin levels frequently correlate with the presence of cyanide poisoning but may take too long to obtain and may falsely exclude patients exposed to combustion products of substances that generate only cyanide (e.g., certain plastics).

Rapid cardiovascular collapse, ventricular dysrhythmias, and seizures are typical. Coma, acidosis, or hemodynamic instability in a fire victim should suggest cyanide poisoning, but each of these findings is also consistent with severe CO poisoning.[9] This differentiation is important given the implication of cyanide treatment.

Management

Patients exposed to cellular poisons, including hydrogen cyanide and hydrogen sulfide, require individualized and specific therapy. The diagnosis can usually not be confirmed, and therapy is almost always empiric but should not be delayed in patients with suspected acute cyanide poisoning. In uncertain situations, the cyanide antidote kit, or at least the thiosulfate component for victims exposed to fires, should be administered immediately.

Hydrogen Cyanide

Although the exact mechanism of the cyanide antidote kit is controversial, the accepted goal of therapy is to reactivate the cytochrome oxidase system by providing an alternative, high-affinity source of ferric ions (Fe^{+++}) for cyanide to bind. The kit has three components, each of which is helpful in treating cyanide poisoning. Although the best results are likely attained when the entire kit is used, this may be impractical or dangerous, particularly for prehospital providers. Since animal models and clinical evidence in humans demonstrate that sodium thiosulfate in combination with oxygen and sodium bicarbonate offers substantial protection, this should be the initial therapy administered by paramedics and during mass poisoning events. At all times, aggressive resuscitation measures including 100% oxygen and intravenous fluids should be provided simultaneously.

Methemoglobin (MetHb) formation is the goal of the first two parts of the kit. Amyl nitrite pearls are broken and held under the patient's nose or at the intake port of the ventilatory apparatus. Caution should be taken to minimize the provider's exposure to this volatile nitrite, as dizziness, hypotension, or syncope may occur after substantial inhalation. Because these inhalers are relatively inefficient at inducing methemoglobinemia, intravenous sodium nitrite is preferred and should be administered as soon as intravenous access is established. The adult dose is 300 mg (10 mL of a 3% solution) given over 2 to 4 minutes. This dosage is calculated on average total hemoglobin, and dosing instructions for anemic patients and children are supplied with the kit. Sodium nitrite is a vasodilator, and hypotension may complicate a rapid infusion. Nitrites predictably generate MetHb levels of 8%; there is no need to attain the 25% MetHb levels quoted in the past. Cyanide has a high affinity for MetHb and readily leaves cytochrome oxidase to form cyanomethemoglobin. Both free serum cyanide and cyanomethemoglobin are converted by sulfur transferase (*rhodanese*) to thiocyanate, which is renally eliminated. Rhodanese simultaneously regenerates MetHb, which can detoxify additional cyanide. Since the rate of rhodanese function increases with the availability of sulfur donor, the last part of the antidote kit is the sulfur-containing compound sodium thiosulfate. The adult dose is 12.5 g IV, which is provided as 50 mL of a 25% solution. Generally, few, if any, adverse effects are associated with proper doses. Extreme caution must be used in the administration of the nitrite component cyanide antidote kit to fire victims with possible simultaneous CO and cyanide poisoning.

Each cyanide antidote kit contains enough to treat two adults or one adult twice. The need to administer a second dose depends on the response to the first treatment and may be common in patients with ingestions of cyanide salts or cyanogenic compounds. Patients with oral cyanide exposure require prolonged therapy and aggressive gastrointestinal decontamination because of ongoing absorption. Hyperbaric oxygen therapy has been advocated but is of no proven benefit and is not routinely indicated. In selected cases, when immediately available, its apparent value may lie in its ability to superoxygenate plasma and tissues, thus permitting higher levels of methemoglobinemia, particularly when CO poisoning is also present.

Hydrogen Sulfide

Since the bond between hydrogen sulfide and cytochrome oxidase is rapidly reversible, removal from exposure and standard resuscitative techniques are usually sufficient to reverse hydrogen sulfide toxicity. The nitrite portion of the cyanide antidote kit to create MetHb is suggested for use in patients with severe or prolonged toxicity.[11] Sodium thiosulfate is unnecessary because hydrogen sulfide is not detoxified by rhodanese. There is no role for hyperbaric oxygen therapy in cases of hydrogen sulfide toxicity.

Disposition

All patients with symptomatic cyanide or hydrogen sulfide poisoning should be admitted to a critical care unit and observed for complications of tissue hypoxia. All patients should be followed for delayed neuropsychiatric symptoms.

KEY CONCEPTS

- An effective antidote exists for cyanide poisoning and must be administered early.
- The sodium thiosulfate portion of the cyanide antidote kit is safe for empiric administration in any case in which cyanide poisoning is considered possible.
- Patients with hydrogen sulfide poisoning generally respond to removal from exposure and ventilatory support.

CARBON MONOXIDE

Perspective

Carbon monoxide is the most common cause of acute poisoning death and the most common cause of fire-related death.[14] CO is generated through incomplete combustion of virtually all carbon-containing products. Structure fires (e.g., wood), clogged vents for home heating units (e.g., methane), and use of gasoline-powered generators indoors are examples of the myriad means through which patients are poisoned by CO. Appropriate public health authorities (e.g., fire department, Department of Health officials) should be informed immediately about any potential public health risks that are identified during the care of a CO-exposed patient.

Principles of Disease

Carbon monoxide interacts with deoxyhemoglobin to form carboxyhemoglobin (COHb), which cannot carry oxygen. Hemoglobin binds carbon monoxide tightly and forms a complex that is only slowly reversible. This allows the exposed individual to accumulate CO, even with exposure to low ambient concentrations. Although this is the classically described mechanism of CO poisoning, it is relevant only to patients who are profoundly CO poisoned. This is because a simple reduction in oxygen carrying capacity due, for example, to anemia would not be expected to result in similar symptoms. However, and relevant to the management of pregnant patients, the affinity of fetal hemoglobin for CO is even greater than that of adult hemoglobin, suggesting that the fetal exposure exceeds that predicted by maternal COHb levels.[15]

In addition to preventing the binding of oxygen to hemoglobin, CO also shifts the oxyhemoglobin dissociation curve to the left, interfering with the ability of normal hemoglobin to release its bound oxygen to tissues. CO also affects cellular oxygen utilization at the tissue level. In muscle, CO binds myoglobin, preventing its normal function and causing atraumatic rhabdomyolysis. CO also inhibits the final cytochrome complex involved in mitochondrial oxidative phosphorylation, similarly to cyanide. This results in a switch to anaerobic metabolism and ultimately cellular death.

Delayed-onset neurologic complications may be a manifestation of the hypoxic insult, although reperfusion injury and lipid peroxidation related to platelet-induced nitric oxide release may play a significant role.[16] By altering the platelet-associated nitric oxide cycle, the microvascular endothelium of the central nervous system undergoes free radical-mediated injury, resulting in localized inflammation and dysfunction. Animal models and human reports suggest that loss of consciousness during CO exposure may be necessary, and is certainly a risk factor, for the development of delayed neurologic sequelae.[17]

Clinical Features

Severe CO toxicity and cyanide poisoning have identical clinical presentations: altered mental status, including coma and seizures; extremely abnormal vital signs, including hypotension and cardiac arrest; and metabolic acidosis. Unlike cyanide poisoning, however, mild CO poisoning occurs frequently, with headache, nausea, vomiting, dizziness, myalgia or confusion, and other signs of hypoxia. The neurologic assessment in these patients may yield normal findings or may demonstrate focal findings or subtle perceptual abnormalities. The often-touted cherry-red skin color is a postmortem finding and is not noted in living patients.

Delayed neurologic sequelae are a well-documented phenomenon after CO exposure, although their frequency varies from 12% to 50%, depending on their definition and with the sensitivity of the test used for their detection.[18] Patients develop a variety of neurologic abnormalities after an asymptomatic period ranging from 2 to 40 days.[17] The delayed neurologic effects can be divided into those with readily identifiable neurologic syndromes (e.g., focal deficits, seizures) and those with primarily psychiatric or cognitive findings (e.g., apathy, memory deficits). Although the latter form of delayed neurologic sequelae requires formal neuropsychiatric testing for detection, the impact of these abnormalities on the patient's daily function may be significant. Since the majority of CO poisoned patients survive, prevention of delayed neurologic and neuropsychiatric sequelae is the predominant goal of therapy.

Diagnostic Strategies and Differential Considerations

Suspicion of CO poisoning relies on the history and physical examination findings. Co-oximetry, an inexpensive and readily available spectrophotometric laboratory method that can distinguish between the normal hemoglobins and COHb (and MetHb), confirms exposure to carbon monoxide. Other laboratory tests only exclude other diagnoses. Severity of poisoning may not correlate with COHb levels; prolonged exposure to low levels can result in fatality with low COHb, but a brief, high-concentration exposure can produce a high COHb level with minimal symptoms.

The ABG measurement cannot be used as a diagnostic test for CO poisoning other than to identify the presence of a metabolic acidosis and a normal partial pressure of oxygen (PO_2). CO does not affect the amount of oxygen dissolved in the serum. Since the PO_2, a measure of dissolved oxygen, is normal in patients with CO poisoning, the calculated oxygen saturation will be normal even in the presence of substantial CO poisoning. The pulse oximeter is also inadequate for the detection of CO poisoning, since COHb is essentially misinterpreted as oxyhemoglobin.

Mild to moderate CO poisoning is a difficult diagnosis to establish clinically, and patients are easily misdiagnosed as having a benign headache syndrome or viral illness. CO poisoning should be suspected in every patient with persistent or recurrent headache, especially if a group of people have similar symptoms or if the headache improves shortly after the person leaves an exposure site.

Patients with severe CO poisoning present with coma or cardiovascular collapse, both of which have a broad toxicologic, metabolic, infectious, medical, and traumatic differential diagnosis. Many diagnoses are excluded by the medical history, physical examination, or standard laboratory testing. Given the relatively protean manifestations of CO poisoning, when seriously considered, it should be excluded by co-oximetry of a venous blood sample. Misdiagnosis can be catastrophic, particularly if the patient returns to the poisoned environment.

Management

Treatment begins with oxygen therapy, which serves two purposes. First, the half-life of COHb is inversely related to the PO_2; it can be reduced from approximately 5 hours on room air to 1 hour by providing supplemental 100% oxygen. Hyperbaric oxygen therapy further reduces the half-life to approximately 40 minutes. Altering the kinetics of COHb is only applicable to patients with extremely elevated COHb levels (i.e., >50%). Even then, few patients can be treated rapidly enough that enhanced CO clearance by hyperbaric oxygen would be lifesaving. Second, under hyperbaric oxygen conditions, a sufficient PO_2 can be achieved to sustain life in the absence of adequately functioning hemoglobin, but this is also relevant only to situations in which the COHb is extremely elevated. Thus, the primary indication for hyperbaric oxygen is to prevent delayed neurologic sequelae. Risk factors that predict the development of delayed neurologic sequelae include age and loss of consciousness.

The controversy over the benefit of hyperbaric oxygen is related to the fact that for the vast majority of patients, hyperbaric oxygen is not administered as a lifesaving therapy, but rather to prevent or minimize the development of delayed neurologic sequelae. Thus, a benefit is not identified immediately (as with life and death) but rather requires close follow-up and sophisticated testing. Hyperbaric oxygen is associated with a reduction in the rate of neurologic delayed neurologic sequelae from approximately 12% without hyperbaric oxygen to less than 1%.[17] When hyperbaric oxygen administration is delayed more than 6 hours after exposure, its efficacy appears to decrease,[19] suggesting the need for rapid decision making. Similarly, evidence suggests that hyperbaric oxygen therapy positively affects the development of the neuropsychiatric delayed neurologic sequelae after CO poisoning.[19,20] A recent randomized, double-blind study found that hyperbaric oxygen was superior to normobaric oxygen at reducing the incidence of neuropsychiatric delayed neurologic sequelae at both 6 weeks and 1 year postpoisoning.[20] However, it is not universally accepted that hyperbaric oxygen is useful in preventing the development of neuropsychiatric delayed neurologic sequelae. A 1999 Australian study that compared hyperbaric oxygen to normobaric oxygen suggested that there was no benefit of hyperbaric oxygen on the development of neuropsychiatric delayed neurologic sequelae.[21] In this study, however, the majority of patients were suicidal and presumably depressed, a condition that interferes with performance on the neuropsychiatric testing needed to differentiate the two groups of patients. In addition to other methodologic flaws in the study (e.g., mean delay to hyperbaric oxygen of more than 6 hours, atypical hyperbaric regimen, unusual randomization protocol, limited neuropsychiatric testing), the alternative to hyperbaric oxygen suggested by this study is continuous 100% oxygen for 3 or 6 days. This therapeutic alternative is likely to be poorly accepted by both patients and the medical community.

Given the implications of poor tissue oxygenation due to the presence of COHb, many practitioners suggest that any patient with a neurologic abnormality or cardiovascular instability (e.g. syncope, altered mental status, myocardial ischemia, dysrhythmias) is a candidate for hyperbaric oxygen therapy.[22,23] This consideration should be relatively independent of the patient's COHb level, which correlates only weakly with toxicity. Patients with prolonged low-level exposure develop a "soaking" phenomenon, in which extremely high tissue concentrations of CO occur without the patient ever having high COHb levels.

In addition to using hyperbaric oxygen therapy in those patients with obvious signs of tissue hypoxia, some institutions have set an arbitrary conservative COHb level of 25% at which asymptomatic or minimally symptomatic patients will be referred for hyperbaric oxygen therapy. Some institutions use COHb levels of 40%, and others refrain from specifying a number. Special consideration is given for pregnancy because of the higher oxygen affinity of fetal hemoglobin and lower fetal P_{O_2}. Because fetal CO poisoning is associated with dysfunction and death, and hyperbaric oxygen therapy appears safe in pregnancy, many institutions have lowered the standard for initiating hyperbaric oxygen therapy in a pregnant patient to a COHb level of 15%.[24]

Further study is still needed to define the optimal duration, pressure, and frequency of hyperbaric oxygen therapy. In particular, although previous studies suggested that there is no benefit to multiple hyperbaric oxygen sessions, the study by Weaver and associates utilized three sessions and may ultimately become the de facto standard therapy. Patients with elevated COHb levels who do not require hyperbaric oxygen therapy should be treated with normobaric oxygen therapy delivered by a tight-fitting nonrebreather face mask, at least until the symptoms resolve and the COHb levels fall. The total duration of such therapy is undefined, and while 3 days was suggested in one study,[21] most mildly CO-poisoned patients probably require no more than 6 hours of therapy.[25]

Simultaneous Carbon Monoxide and Cyanide Poisoning (Fire Victim)

Concurrent toxicity from CO and cyanide is widely reported and a major factor in the mortality associated with exposure to fire smoke.[9,26] Smoke inhalation victims who present with coma and metabolic acidosis can have severe CO poisoning, cyanide poisoning, or both. Nitrite-induced methemoglobinemia, which further reduces the tissue oxygen delivery, may be detrimental to patients with elevated COHb levels.

Sodium thiosulfate, administered alone, is shown experimentally to be beneficial, safe, and without the risk of hypotension or decrease of oxygen-carrying capacity engendered by MetHb.[27] A standard dose of 12.5 g should be given to all adult smoke inhalation victims with coma, hypotension, acidosis, or cardiovascular collapse in whom cyanide poisoning cannot be rapidly excluded (1.65 mL/kg of 25% sodium thiosulfate in children). If the COHb level is known to be low and the patient has persistent acidosis or hemodynamic instability, the complete cyanide antidote kit, including the nitrites, can be administered. Patients with high COHb levels undergoing therapy in a hyperbaric oxygen chamber can receive nitrite therapy while pressurized, with little concern of decreasing the oxygen-carrying capacity.

Disposition

The decision to transfer a patient to a hyperbaric oxygen facility must consider the time delay to therapy, patient issues (e.g., burns, age), and potential transport-related complications.[28] At a minimum, prolonged oxygen therapy should be administered, although the benefit of this remains undefined. Hyperbaric oxygen should be administered to all patients with consequential CO poisoning, which includes patients with syncope or altered mental status independent of COHb level and patients with elevated COHb concentrations independent of clinical findings. The specific level depends on the availability of a hyperbaric chamber and local standards, as does the decision to provide hyperbaric oxygen therapy for patients with mild symptoms (e.g., headache, dizziness). All patients exposed to CO require close follow-up to evaluate for delayed sequelae.

KEY CONCEPTS

- Carbon monoxide poisoning is common and has important public health implications.
- Carbon monoxide poisoning can be obscure and should be corroborated with co-oximetry when common occupants or families present with headache and vague flulike symptoms.
- Because the role of hyperbaric oxygen therapy in CO poisoning is controversial, consultation with a hyperbaric oxygen facility or poison control system may be helpful in significant toxicity.

REFERENCES

1. Gill JR, Ely SF, Hua S: Environmental gas displacement: Three accidental deaths in the workplace. *Am J Forens Med Pathol* 23:26, 2002.
2. Shelef M: Unanticipated benefits of automotive emission control: Reduction in fatalities by motor vehicle exhaust gas. *Sci Total Environ* 146/147:93, 1994.
3. DeBehnke DJ, et al: The hemodynamic and arterial blood gas response to asphyxiation: A canine model of pulseless electrical activity. *Resuscitation* 30:169, 1995.
4. Kollef MH, Schuster DP: The acute respiratory distress syndrome. *N Engl J Med* 332:27, 1995.
5. Bernard GR, et al: The American-European Consensus Conference on ARDS: Definitions, mechanisms, relevant outcomes, and clinical trial coordination. *Am J Respir Crit Care Med* 149:818, 1994.
6. Traub SJ, Hoffman RS, Nelson LS: Case report and literature review of chlorine gas toxicity. *Vet Hum Toxicol* 44:235, 2002.
7. Wang J, Zhang L, Walther SM: Inhaled budesonide in experimental chlorine gas lung injury: Influence of time interval between injury and treatment. *Intensive Care Med* 28:352, 2002.
8. Lin WY, Kao CH, Wang SJ: Detection of acute inhalation injury in fire victims by means of technetium-99m DTPA radioaerosol inhalation lung scintigraphy. *Eur J Nucl Med* 24:125, 1997.
9. Baud FJ, et al: Elevated blood cyanide concentrations in victims of smoke inhalation. *N Engl J Med* 325:1761, 1991.
10. Nieman GF, Clark WR, Hakim T: Methylprednisolone does not protect the lung from inhalation injury. *Burns* 17:384, 1991.
11. Reiffenstein RJ, Hulbert WC, Roth SH: Toxicology of hydrogen sulfide. *Annu Rev Pharmacol Toxicol* 32:109, 1992.
12. Johnson RP, Mellors JW: Arteriolization of venous blood gases: A clue to the diagnosis of cyanide poisoning. *J Emerg Med* 6:401, 1988.
13. Snyder JW, et al: Occupational fatality and persistent neurological sequelae after mass exposure to hydrogen sulfide. *Am J Emerg Med* 13:199, 1995.
14. Girman JR, et al: Causes of unintentional deaths from carbon monoxide poisoning in California. *West J Med* 168:158, 1998.
15. Longo LD: The biological effects of carbon monoxide on the pregnant woman, fetus and newborn infant. *Am J Obstet Gynecol* 129:69, 1977.
16. Thom SR, Fisher D, Manevich Y: Roles for platelet-activating factor and *NO-derived oxidants causing neutrophil adherence after CO poisoning. *Am J Physiol Heart Circ Physiol* 281:H923, 2001.
17. Choi IS: Delayed neurologic sequelae in carbon monoxide intoxication. *Arch Neurol* 40:433, 1983.
18. Thom SR, et al: Delayed neuropsychiatric sequelae following CO poisoning. *Ann Emerg Med* 23:612, 1994.
19. Goulon M, et al: Intoxication oxy carbonee et anoxic aique par inalation de gay de charbon et d'hydvocarbure. *Ann Med Interne (Paris)* 120:335, 1969. [English translation, *J Hyperbaric Med* 1:23, 1986.]
20. Weaver LK, et al: Hyperbaric oxygen for acute carbon monoxide poisoning. *N Engl J Med* 347:1057, 2002.
21. Scheinkestel CD, et al: Hyperbaric or normobaric oxygen for acute carbon monoxide poisoning: A randomized controlled clinical trial. *Med J Aust* 170:203, 1999.
22. Hardy KR, Thom SR: Pathophysiology and treatment of carbon monoxide poisoning. *J Toxicol Clin Toxicol* 32:613, 1994.
23. Gorman D, Drewry A, Huang YL, Sames C: The clinical toxicology of carbon monoxide. *Toxicology* 187:25, 2003.
24. Elkharrat D, et al: Acute carbon monoxide intoxication and hyperbaric oxygen in pregnancy. *Intensive Care Med* 17:289, 1991.
25. Raphael JC, et al: Trial of normobaric and hyperbaric oxygen for acute carbon monoxide intoxication. *Lancet* 2:414, 1989.
26. Alarie Y: Toxicity of fire smoke. *Crit Rev Toxicol* 32:259, 2002.
27. Ivankovich AD, et al: Cyanide antidotes and methods of their administration in dogs: A comparative study. *Anesthesiology* 52:210, 1980.
28. Sloan EP, et al: Complications and protocol considerations in carbon monoxide-poisoned patients who require hyperbaric oxygen therapy: Report from a ten-year experience. *Ann Emerg Med* 18:629, 1989.

CHAPTER

158 Lithium

Keith K. Burkhart

PERSPECTIVE

Lithium has been recommended as an antidepressant since the 1870s but fell into disfavor because of its side effects. In 1949, Cade advocated lithium for acute mania, and its effectiveness for bipolar mood disorders became well recognized. In the 1940s, lithium chloride was used as a salt substitute, but the U.S. Food and Drug Administration banned its use until 1970 because of fatalities from this practice. Because of its effectiveness, however, lithium remains a mainstay for the treatment of bipolar disorders. Studies are underway to determine whether the suicide rate is lower in patients prescribed lithium, so there is the possibility that increased use of this drug will be seen in the future. Unfortunately, fatalities continue to occur because lithium has such a narrow therapeutic window.

PRINCIPLES OF DISEASE

The mechanism for lithium's antipsychotic effect is not fully understood. Competition at the sodium-potassium pump has been proposed. Changes in catecholamine and serotonergic neurotransmission may result from its cellular alterations. With more serotonergic drugs on the market, lithium therapy also places patients at risk for many drug interactions, especially the serotonin syndrome (Table 158-1).

Lithium is a group IA alkali metal smaller than, but similar to, sodium and potassium. Lithium carbonate is the most commonly prescribed formulation; the typical dose for adults is 600 to 1200 mg/day. Immediate-release and sustained-release preparations are available. In cases of acute overdose, peak serum levels usually occur within 2 to 6 hours for immediate-release preparations, but not until 6 to 24 hours and even days for some sustained-release products. Lithium has a slow alpha phase of distribution. Although the volume of distribution approximates total body water, 0.7 L/kg, lithium moves slowly across cellular membranes. Lithium's elimination from cells is also slow, with a half-life of 24 ± 12 hours. Therefore, patients can present severely toxic with levels in the therapeutic range (0.6-1.2 mEq/L). During recovery from chronic lithium toxicity, serum levels can become undetectable, but symptoms may persist.

Lithium elimination is almost entirely renal. Lithium is actively reabsorbed in the proximal tubule and to a lesser extent in the thick ascending limb and collecting duct. During volume loss or sodium depletion, the kidney increases reabsorption of sodium and lithium. Therefore, febrile illnesses, vomiting from any cause and especially gastroenteritis, and heat-related fluid losses can precipitate lithium toxicity. Excessive daily doses or renal insufficiency with stable doses can also lead to elevated lithium levels. In addition, chronic poisoning is commonly seen in patients with nephrogenic diabetes insipidus, patients older than 50 years of age, and those with thyroid dysfunction.[1]

A number of drug interactions have been reported (see Table 158-1). Many enhance the renal absorption of lithium. Lithium also has been implicated in precipitating the serotonin syndrome when used concomitantly with many psychiatric drugs, including cyclic antidepressants, the monoamine oxidase inhibitors, and possibly the atypical antipsychotic olanzapine (see Chapter 159).[2] Another report describes lithium intoxication after levofloxacin therapy.[3]

CLINICAL FEATURES

Patients present with either acute overdose or chronic toxicity from slowly increasing lithium levels (Table 158-2). Most acutely poisoned patients first have nausea, vomiting, abdominal cramping, and sometimes diarrhea. Typical progression of acute toxicity includes neuromuscular signs. Headache has been described as a manifestation of lithium intoxication.[4] Tremulousness, dystonia (e.g., cogwheel rigidity), hyperreflexia, and ataxia usually precede agitation, confusion, dysarthria, lethargy, coma, and seizures. Cardiovascular complications from acute toxicity are rare but can include ventricular dysrhythmias, sinus arrest, and asystole.[5] Lithium substitution for potassium is a presumed mechanism.

Chronic poisonings manifest primarily with neurologic signs and symptoms. Lethargy and confusion develop first, and if unrecognized, patients often continue their lithium regimen. Coma and status epilepticus can result if early symptoms are not recognized. Many severely poisoned patients develop permanent neurologic sequelae, including cognitive impairment, sensorimotor peripheral neuropathy, and cerebellar dysfunction.[6,7]

Electrocardiographic changes are common in cases of chronic poisoning. T wave changes predominate and include flattening, nonspecific ST-T wave changes, and inversion. These changes can persist for weeks after toxicity. Conduction defects include prolonged PR, QRS, and QTc intervals.

Renal toxicity is a common manifestation of chronic lithium intoxication. Lithium inhibits arginine vasopressin (antidiuretic hormone), impairing sodium and water conservation. Increased parathyroid levels may explain this inhibition.[8] Diabetes insipidus develops from both therapeutic use and toxicity. The replacement of free water at rates of 1 L per hour is sometimes required. Many chronically poisoned patients are severely dehydrated. Because of underlying diabetes insipidus from therapy, some patients drink gallons of water a day. Any illness that interferes with this water consumption can aggravate or precipitate lithium toxicity.

Lithium has an antithyroid effect. Myxedema coma has been reported as a complication of toxicity. The central nervous system effects of hypothyroidism and lithium toxicity are similar. Hypothyroidism may diminish the neuromuscular manifestations of lithium toxicity.

DIAGNOSTIC STRATEGIES

Any patient with a history of bipolar disorder or taking lithium who presents to the emergency department should be evaluated for lethargy, increased tremor, and dehydration from lithium toxicity. Symptomatic patients should have their lithium levels checked. After an acute ingestion, toxicity develops from sustained elevated lithium levels. The ingestion of immediate-release formulations can produce dramatically elevated initial levels that subsequently fall quickly without the development of significant toxicity. The patient who has ingested sustained-release preparations, however, may present with an initially therapeutic level, only to develop sustained elevations that lead to severe life-threatening toxicity days later. Because of the delay to signs and symptoms, patients must be cared for in facilities where lithium levels can be measured immediately.

Diagnostic testing should include assessment of electrolytes and renal function. A low anion gap may suggest, but is not typical for, lithium toxicity. Sodium depletion may be identified as well as renal dysfunction. Thyroid functions should also be checked, especially in the chronically poisoned patient.

DIFFERENTIAL CONSIDERATIONS

Acute gastroenteritis symptoms are common to many drug overdoses, including acute lithium intoxication. A thorough history of possible exposures may be the only initial clue to the diagnosis of lithium intoxication before neurologic symptoms develop. The broad differential diagnoses of ataxia, neuromuscular rigidity, altered mental status including central nervous system depression, and seizures must include lithium toxicity.

MANAGEMENT

Severely lithium-poisoned patients in coma or with seizures may require urgent airway interventions and anticonvulsant therapy with benzodiazepines, phenobarbital, and propofol as necessary. A recent report, however, describes a patient who had electroencephalographic evidence for status epilepticus that did not respond to lorazepam therapy.[9] Patients with chronic lithium toxicity are often volume depleted. Although frank hypotension is unusual, fluid resuscitation is needed and should include normal saline. The goal of saline administration is to restore glomerular filtration, normalize urine output, and enhance lithium clearance. Forced diuresis does not assist in lithium clearance.

Once the patient is stabilized, methods to prevent absorption should be considered. In acute overdose, induced emesis should be avoided. Most patients will already be vomiting, which may interfere with other decontamination procedures. As with most elemental

Table 158-1. Drug Interactions that Result in Lithium Toxicity

Agent	Action
ACE inhibitors	Increase Li level
Angiotensin II receptor blockers	Increase Li level
Antibiotics	Increase Li level
Spectinomycin, tetracycline, metronidazole, levofloxacin	
Benzodiazepines	Enhance Li toxicity
Clonazepam, diazepam	
Carbamazepine	Enhance Li toxicity
Diuretics: thiazide and loop	Increase Li level
α-Methyldopa	Enhance Li toxicity
Monoamine oxidase inhibitors	Serotonin syndrome
NSAIDs	Increase Li level
Olanzapine	Enhance Li toxicity
Phenothiazines	Enhance Li toxicity
SSRIs	Serotonin syndrome
Serotonin agonists*	Serotonin syndrome

ACE, angiotensin-converting enzyme; Li, lithium; NSAIDs, nonsteroidal anti-inflammatory drugs; SSRIs, selective serotonin reuptake inhibitors.
*For example, buspirone, meperidine, mirtazapine, nefazodone, tramadol, trazodone, and venlafaxine.

Table 158-2. Comparison of Acute and Chronic Lithium Toxicity

	Acute	Chronic
Cause	Overdose	Sodium loss or volume depletion
Presenting symptoms	Asymptomatic or gastrointestinal symptoms	Gastrointestinal and neurologic symptoms
Whole-bowel irrigation	Helpful acutely	Ineffective
Consider dialysis	Neurologic symptoms or levels > 4 mEq/L	Neurologic symptoms or levels > 2.5 mEq/L

cations, activated charcoal is of little benefit for patients with lithium toxicity, except in the case of coingestants. Gastric lavage is of little, if any, benefit, most likely failing a risk-benefit analysis. Whole-bowel irrigation with polyethylene glycol electrolyte lavage solution (PEG-ELS) is effective in preventing absorption from extended-release lithium and is theoretically useful in cases involving immediate-release formulations.[10] Adult patients should drink or receive PEG-ELS by nasogastric tube, approximately 1.5 L of solution per hour until effluents are clear. Adjunctive antiemetic therapy may be required. Serial levels are still necessary, because not all pills are cleared by PEG-ELS. During the whole-bowel irrigation procedure, absorption of tablets that are not eliminated may be slowed or prevented. Falling levels have occurred during whole-bowel irrigation, only to rise again when the procedure is stopped. Cationic exchange resins such as sodium polystyrene sulfonate are effective in reducing the absorption of lithium. Although multiple doses of sodium polystyrene sulfonate have been suggested in animal models, further human study is needed. Care must be taken to avoid severe life-threatening hypokalemia from sodium polystyrene sulfonate.

Lithium is readily dialyzed because of its small molecular weight, water solubility, and lack of protein binding. Although dialysis dramatically shortens the plasma half-life, outcome studies have not demonstrated its benefit in chronic toxicity. Dialysis should be used in the case of an acute overdose with decreased levels of consciousness, seizures, and renal failure and in symptomatic patients with levels greater than 4.0 mEq/L. Asymptomatic patients with higher levels have been managed without dialysis. For cases of chronic toxicity, dialysis is helpful in symptomatic patients with levels greater than 2.0 mEq/L. In critically ill patients, continuous arteriovenous and venovenous hemofiltration have been used.

DISPOSITION

Patients with any symptom more than a tremor require hospital admission. Asymptomatic patients with increasing lithium levels require admission for monitoring of serial levels after ingestions. Most patients should be admitted to an institution where dialysis, if indicated, can be performed. An observation unit is not helpful because symptoms are delayed up to 24 hours after the peak serum levels of an acute poisoning.

Chronically poisoned patients with neurologic signs, including seizures, myoclonus, hyperexcitability, or decreased level of consciousness, should be admitted to the critical care unit.

KEY CONCEPTS

- Consider lithium toxicity in the patient with altered mental status, neuromuscular hyperexcitability, myoclonus, hyperreflexia, rigidity, or seizures.
- Levels should be checked in all patients receiving lithium who present with medical symptoms. Conditions or medications that lead to dehydration or renal insufficiency can precipitate chronic toxicity.
- Dialysis should be considered for lithium levels greater than 2.0 mEq/L in symptomatic patients with chronic toxicity or for patients with decreased level of consciousness or seizure.
- Early whole-bowel irrigation after acute ingestion may prevent lithium toxicity and the need for dialysis. Lithium levels may rebound after the procedure is stopped.
- Lithium is a common comedication in the serotonin syndrome.

REFERENCES

1. Oakley PW, Whyte IM, Carter GL: Lithium toxicity: An iatrogenic problem in susceptible individuals. *Aust N Z J Psychiatry* 35:833, 2001.
2. Haslett CD, Kumar S: Can olanzapine be implicated in causing serotonin syndrome? *Psych Clin Neurosci* 56:533, 2002.
3. Takahashi H, Higuchi H, Shimizu T: Severe lithium toxicity induced by combined levofloxacin administration. *J Clin Psychiatry* 61:949, 2000.
4. Bigal ME, Bordini CA, Speciali JG: Daily headache as a manifestation of lithium intoxication. *Neurology* 57:1733, 2001.
5. Apte S, Langston W: Permanent neurologic deficits due to lithium intoxication. *Ann Neurol* 13:453, 1983.
6. Lang EJ, Davis SM: Lithium neurotoxicity: The development of irreversible neurological impairment despite standard monitoring of serum lithium levels. *J Clin Neurosci* 9:308, 2002.
7. Bartha L, Marksteiner J, Bauer G, et al: Persistent cognitive deficits associated with lithium intoxication: A neuropsychological case description. *Cortex* 38:743, 2002.
8. Carney SL, Ray C, Gillies-Alastair HB: Mechanism of lithium-induced polyuria in the rat. *Kidney Int* 50:377, 1996.
9. Gansaeuer M, Alsaadi T: Lithium intoxication mimicking clinical and electrographic features of status epilepticus: A case report and review of the literature. *Clin Electroencephalogr* 34:28, 2003.
10. Smith S, Ling L: Whole-bowel irrigation as a treatment for acute lithium overdose. *Ann Emerg Med* 20:536, 1991.

CHAPTER

159 Antipsychotics

Mary A. Wittler and Eric J. Lavonas

PERSPECTIVE

The antipsychotic medication chlorpromazine was first used effectively for the treatment of psychosis in France in 1952 and in the United States and Canada in 1954. The term *neuroleptic,* historically used because of the high degree of sedation produced by earlier antipsychotic drugs, is no longer appropriate because newer agents cause little sedation. The term *antipsychotic* is now preferred. U.S. poison control centers report more than 5000 exposures to phenothiazines and 25,000 exposures to atypical antipsychotics annually, resulting in 11 (phenothiazines) and 78 (atypical antipsychotics) deaths.[1]

PRINCIPLES OF DISEASE

Antipsychotic medications are used to treat agitation and psychosis caused by schizophrenia, mania, acute idiopathic psychosis, alcohol withdrawal hallucinosis, and Alzheimer's disease. Antipsychotic medications are often divided into three broad categories based on their receptor profiles, clinical effects, and adverse effects (Table 159-1). All antipsychotic medications effectively treat the *positive symptoms* of psychotic disorders; they reduce hallucinations, control agitation, and aid in restructuring disordered thinking. In general, the low-potency neuroleptics are the most sedating at usual clinical doses. Movement disorders, including extrapyramidal syndromes and tardive dyskinesia (TD), are significant problems with low-potency and high-potency neuroleptics. In addition to producing less sedation and fewer movement disorders, the atypical antipsychotic agents assist with the *negative symptoms* of psychotic disorders, such as flat affect, avolition, social withdrawal, and impoverished thought and speech. Although neuroleptic malignant syndrome (NMS) has occurred with all agents, it occurs least with the atypical antipsychotics.

Anatomy and Physiology

Antipsychotic drugs block dopamine receptors in several areas of the brain, including the cerebral cortex, basal ganglia, limbic system, hypothalamus, and chemoreceptor trigger zone. Traditional antipsychotic agents reduce the positive symptoms of schizophrenia by blocking the dopamine D_2 receptor subtype in the mesolimbic region of the brain. Blockade of D_2 receptors in the nigrostriatal brain region produces the undesired extrapyramidal movement disorders, and blockade of D_2 receptors in the mesocortical brain region impairs cognition and worsens the negative symptoms of schizophrenia.[2] Atypical antipsychotic agents block D_2 and serotonin (5-hydroxytryptamine type 2A [$5\text{-}HT_{2A}$]) receptors. These agents selectively bind D_2 receptors in the mesolimbic areas of the brain, with less effect on nigrostriatal D_2 receptors resulting in fewer extrapyramidal effects. The $5\text{-}HT_{2A}$ receptor antagonism is thought to reduce extrapyramidal effects and improve the negative symptoms of schizophrenia. Antipsychotic medications also block other receptor types (see Table 159-1).

The antiemetic effects of prochlorperazine, promethazine, and droperidol result from blockade of dopamine receptors in the chemoreceptor trigger zone of the medulla. Hydroxyzine reduces itching by blocking histamine (H_1) receptors. Prochlorperazine and droperidol are theorized to abort migraine headaches by preventing dopamine-mediated meningeal artery vasodilation. Chlorpromazine can treat severe hiccups. Haloperidol is used for certain movement disorders, including Tourette's syndrome and Huntington's chorea.

Pathophysiology

Extrapyramidal symptoms (EPS) can be divided into two groups based on the time of development after initiating drug therapy. Acute EPS include dystonia, akathisia, and parkinsonism. These adverse effects are caused by blockade of nigrostriatal D_2 receptors and are reduced by muscarinic receptor antagonism. The delayed-onset syndromes, including TD and tardive dystonia, develop after prolonged use of antipsychotic medications, most likely because chronic dopamine receptor blockade in the nigrostriatal area leads to D_2 receptor upregulation and hypersensitivity to dopamine.[3] NMS, an idiosyncratic reaction to antipsychotic medication, is thought to result from neuroregulatory dysfunction secondary to D_2 receptor blockade in the substantia nigra and hypothalamus.

The phenothiazines possess quinidine-like effects, resulting in Q-T prolongation and potential dysrhythmias in overdose.[4,5] Thioridazine and mesoridazine have the greatest risk of cardiac toxicity.[6] The butyrophenones can prolong cardiac repolarization, potentially causing *torsades de pointes.* Partial blockade of the delayed inward rectifier potassium current prolongs phase 3 of the cardiac action potential.[7] The atypical antipsychotics produce less cardiotoxicity than the traditional agents, although most potentially cause repolarization abnormalities in therapeutic dosing or overdose.[2,4,8]

Table 159-1. Selected Antipsychotic Agents Approved or Nearing Approval for Use in the United States

Medication	Receptors Blocked	Clinical Effects	Adverse Effects
Low potency Chlorpromazine Chlorprothixene Fluphenazine Hydroxyzine Mesoridazine Molindone Perphenazine Prochlorperazine Promethazine Thioridazine	Dopamine D_2 (moderate affinity in mesolimbic and nigrostriatal areas) Acetylcholine muscarinic (generally strong affinity) Histamine H_1 (strong affinity) α-Adrenergic (moderate affinity) Dopamine D_1, D_3, D_4, D_5 (variable affinity)	Control positive symptoms of psychotic disorders: Hallucinations Delusions Agitation Disordered thoughts	Extrapyramidal syndromes (common) Tardive dyskinesia (common) Sedation (common) Orthostatic hypotension (common) Anticholinergic symptoms (common): Dry mouth Blurred vision Impaired sweating Constipation Weight gain Urinary retention Angle-closure glaucoma
High potency Droperidol Haloperidol Loxapine Pimozide Thiothixene Trifluoperazine	Dopamine D_2 (strong affinity in mesolimbic and nigrostriatal areas) Acetylcholine muscarinic, histamine H_1. α-adrenergic (weak affinity) Dopamine D_1, D_3, D_4, D_5 (variable affinity)	Control positive symptoms of psychotic disorders	Extrapyramidal syndromes (common) Tardive dyskinesia (common) Sedation, orthostatic hypotension, and anticholingeric symptoms (uncommon in usual clinical doses)
Atypical Clozapine Olanzapine Quetiapine Risperidone Ziprasidone Aripiprazole*	Serotonin 5-HT_{2A} (strong) Dopamine D_2 (mild to moderate affinity, selective for mesolimbic areas) Dopamine D_1, D_3, D_4, D_5 (variable affinity)	Control positive symptoms of psychotic disorders Control negative symptoms of psychotic disorders: Social withdrawal Flattened affect Decreased activity Paucity of speech Pseudodementia	Extrapyramidal syndromes and tardive dyskinesia (uncommon)

*Aripiprazole has partial agonist activity at dopamine D_2 and serotonin 5-HT_{1A} receptors and antagonist activity at serotonin 5-HT_{2A} receptors.

Clozapine produces agranulocytosis in approximately 0.4% of patients even after strict adherence to labeling requirements.[9] Seizure occurs uncommonly with antipsychotic drugs, but is a risk with clozapine, perhaps related to anticholinergic effects.[10] The atypical antipsychotics have been associated with altered glucose metabolism and diabetes, especially clozapine and olanzapine, but the cause of this has not been established.

CLINICAL FEATURES

Acute Overdose

In overdose, antipsychotic medications produce signs and symptoms that are exaggerations of the clinical effects. Most patients develop symptoms within a few hours. Central nervous system (CNS) depression is universally present, ranging from mild sedation and confusion to coma, loss of brainstem reflexes, and respiratory depression. Pupils can be of any size. Mild orthostatic hypotension is a common finding secondary to α-adrenergic blockade. The most common cardiac rhythm is sinus tachycardia with a normal QRS duration. If QRS prolongation is present, coingestion of another drug should be suspected. Significant Q-T prolongation can occur, predisposing to torsades de pointes.[11-13] Overdose with low-potency antipsychotics can cause an anticholinergic delirium. EPS has been reported with the traditional and atypical antipsychotics.

Atypical antipsychotic overdose is similar to overdose with the traditional antipsychotics. Clozapine, olanzapine, quetiapine, and risperidone overdoses are characterized by CNS depression and tachycardia.[14-18,20] Miosis may be present, potentially mimicking opioid toxicity.[19] Extremity twitching is common. With the exception of clozapine, seizures rarely occur in overdose. Q-T_c prolongation has been reported in overdose, particularly with ziprasidone.[11,12,21] The clinical significance of Q-T_c prolongation and the risk of torsades are not known, however. Acute EPS has been reported for risperidone overdose. There are no reports of aripiprazole overdose published to date. Adverse effects during therapeutic use include headache, agitation, akathisia, somnolence, and dyspepsia. Aripiprazole does not seem to prolong the Q-T_c in therapeutic dosing.[22]

Acute Extrapyramidal Syndromes

Acute dystonia manifests as involuntary motor tics or spasms that most often involve the facial, neck, back, or limb muscles. Dystonic reactions usually develop within the first several doses of treatment. *Oculogyric crisis,* characterized by continuous rotatory eye movements, also has been reported. *Laryngeal dystonia* is a rare but life-threatening form of dystonia that manifests as throat tightening, difficulty breathing or swallowing, or a choking sensation.[23]

Akathisia, a subjective feeling of restlessness associated with objective motor restlessness, is often mistaken for worsening agitation, leading incorrectly to an increase in antipsychotic dose. Akathisia usually develops within the first few days of treatment. In one clinical study, 40% of patients administered 10 mg of intravenous haloperidol developed akathisia within 1 hour of the dose, and the syndrome is often seen in migraine headache patients treated with prochlorperazine.

A *parkinsonian syndrome* of bradykinesia, masked facies, shuffling gait, muscular rigidity, and resting tremor frequently develops during the first weeks of therapy with low-potency and high-potency neuroleptic-antipsychotic agents. *Perioral tremor* (rabbit syndrome), in which lip and nose movements resemble those of a rabbit, also can develop after prolonged therapy.[25]

Tardive Dyskinesia

TD is a chronic movement disorder induced by prolonged use of antipsychotic medication. Typical signs of TD include quick, involuntary movements of the face (blinking, grimaces, tongue movements, chewing), extremities, or trunk. Twenty percent of patients treated with long term traditional antipsychotics are affected. The risk of development is much lower with the atypical antipsychotics. Although anticholinergic agents may reduce the symptoms of TD, the disorder is frequently permanent and difficult to treat. Reducing the antipsychotic dose or changing to an atypical agent should be considered. TD improves in many patients switched to clozapine, but further clinical trials are needed to study all atypical antipsychotic agents.[26,27] Respiratory dyskinesia, a variant of TD, is characterized by orofacial dyskinesia, dyspnea, dysphonia, and respiratory alkalosis. This chronic disorder often goes undiagnosed and can cause repeated bouts of aspiration pneumonia.

Neuroleptic Malignant Syndrome

NMS, the most serious extrapyramidal effect, typically develops during the first 2 weeks of drug therapy but has occurred in patients on stable drug regimens. Risk factors include rapid drug loading, high dosage, increase in dosage, high-potency antipsychotics, parenteral formulations, dehydration, and previous episodes of NMS.[28] Other medications may contribute to NMS, including lithium, which inhibits dopamine secretion, and withdrawal from dopaminergic agents used to treat Parkinson's disease.[28,29] NMS develops in 0.02% to 12.2% of patients treated with the traditional antipsychotics.[28] The atypical antipsychotic agents, including clozapine, risperidone, olanzapine, and quetiapine, have been associated with NMS.[30]

Table 159-2 lists the diagnostic criteria for NMS. Other features of NMS include sialorrhea, dysarthria, opisthotonus, dyskinesia, metabolic acidosis, liver function elevations, sodium imbalance, dehydration, elevations in serum catecholamines, coagulopathy, generalized slowing on the electroencephalogram, pulmonary embolism, and renal failure.[28] Multiple case reports discuss atypical presentations that lack full diagnostic criteria for NMS.[30]

Table 159-2. Diagnostic Criteria and Clinical Features of Neuroleptic Malignant Syndrome

Criteria/Features	Prevalence
A. Development of severe muscle rigidity and elevated temperature associated with the use of a neuroleptic/antipsychotic medication	Rigidity: 97% Fever: 98%
B. Two (or more) of the following are present:	
1. Diaphoresis	98%
2. Dysphagia	
3. Tremor	
4. Incontinence	
5. Change in level of consciousness ranging from confusion to coma	97%
6. Mutism	
7. Tachycardia	88%
8. Elevated or labile blood pressure	61%
9. Leukocytosis	98%
10. Laboratory evidence of muscle injury (e.g., elevated CK)	95%
C. Symptoms in criteria A and B are not caused by another substance (e.g., phencyclidine), a neurologic or other general medical condition (e.g., viral encephalitis), or another mental disorder (e.g., mood disorder with catatonic features).	

Modified from American Psychiatric Association: *Diagnostic and Statistical Manual of Mental Disorders*, 4th ed (TR). Washington, DC, 2000; *American Psychiatric Association*, prevalence data from Caroff SN, Mann SC: Neuroleptic malignant syndrome. *Med Clin North Am* 77:185, 1993.

Most patients develop the cardinal features of altered mental status, muscle rigidity, autonomic nervous system instability, and hyperthermia within 3 days. The signs of NMS may develop gradually, however, and in any order.[31] Agitation, often mistaken for worsening psychosis, may occur first. Physicians should consider discontinuing antipsychotic drugs in a patient who has developed one or more of the major manifestations of NMS. Most episodes resolve within 2 weeks after cessation of the offending medication, but some cases have lasted 6 months.[32]

Cardiac Repolarization Abnormalities and Dysrhythmias

Q-T prolongation and torsades de pointes are well-described adverse effects of thioridazine, mesoridazine, droperidol, sertindole, and high-dose intravenous haloperidol.[4,5,33,34] Therapeutic doses of oral haloperidol, chlorpromazine, pimozide, and ziprasidone also have been associated with Q-T prolongation.[35] In a clinical study, ziprasidone prolonged the Q-T interval more than risperidone, olanzapine, or quetiapine. Q-T prolongation should be considered a "class effect" of all antipsychotic medications. Whenever possible, antipsychotic medications should not be prescribed concomitantly with other drugs known to prolong the Q-T interval. Atrioventricular nodal block is a rare reported complication of overdose with chlorpromazine, thioridazine, and other older neuroleptics.[36]

Agranulocytosis

Clozapine produces agranulocytosis, with 75% of occurrences developing within the first 18 weeks after initiation of therapy, peaking at 3 months. The concomitant use of other bone marrow–suppressing agents (e.g., carbamazepine) should be avoided. Clozapine administration must be halted if the total white blood cell count decreases to less than 3000 cells/mm^3 or if the absolute neutrophil count is less than 1500 cells/mm^3. Agranulocytosis has not been reported after an acute overdose. Olanzapine, whose chemical structure is similar to clozapine, has been associated with neutropenia and agranulocytosis. All patients recovered after discontinuation of olanzapine.[37]

Seizures

Antipsychotic medications can lower the seizure threshold and induce epileptiform electroencephalogram abnormalities in many asymptomatic patients. Antipsychotic-induced seizures are rare, however. An exception is clozapine, which causes a dose-related increased risk of seizures (approximately 5% at high doses). Antipsychotics can be prescribed for patients with known seizure disorders.[38]

DIFFERENTIAL CONSIDERATIONS

Differential diagnostic considerations include a broad list of agents and clinical conditions that produce altered mental status, orthostatic hypotension, anticholinergic syndrome, seizure, Q-T prolongation, or torsades de pointes. Although the signs of NMS are similar to serotonin syndrome and heatstroke, the etiologies of these conditions are quite different (Table 159-3). Malignant hyperthermia should be considered in patients receiving inhalational anesthetics or succinylcholine.

DIAGNOSTIC STRATEGIES

Blood levels are neither readily available nor helpful in the management of an overdose with antipsychotic medication. As with any patient who presents with altered mental status, blood glucose and pulse oximetry readings should be obtained immediately. Other testing, such as brain computed tomography, lumbar puncture, serum acetaminophen measurement, and electrolyte measurements, may be required depending on the clinical situation.

Table 159-3. Differential Diagnosis of Neuroleptic Malignant Syndrome

Disease*	Pathologic Mechanism	Differentiating Factor	Time Course	Treatment
Neuroleptic malignant syndrome	Impaired thermoregulation in hypothalamus and basal ganglia due to relative lack of dopamine activity	Antipsychotic medication use, muscular rigidity (diagnostic criteria in Table 159-2)	Gradual, progresses over several days	Stop offending medication(s) Hydration Active cooling Intravenous benzodiazepines to relax muscles and control agitation Neuromuscular blockade (nondepolarizing agents) Controversial: Bromocriptine or amantadine Dantrolene
Serotonin syndrome	Excess serotonin and dopamine levels in central nervous system	Medications (usually a combination) that increase serotonin levels (e.g., SSRIs, MAOIs, dextromethorphan, lithium, meperidine, tramadol, tryptophan); muscular rigidity	Usually rapid after introduction of new medication or increase in dose; can be gradual	Stop offending medication(s) Hydration Active cooling Cyproheptadine
Heatstroke	Environmental heat stress	Environmental exposure history; muscular rigidity rare	Rapid or gradual	Hydration Active cooling
Malignant hyperthermia	Genetic instability of sarcoplasmic reticulum, causing massive calcium release after administration of triggering medication	Occurs after administration of inhalational anesthetic or succinylcholine; muscular rigidity	Sudden, provoked by administration of anesthetic	Stop anesthetic Hydration Active cooling Dantrolene

*Other clinical entities to consider in the diagnosis of these conditions include Addison's syndrome, central nervous system infection, delirium tremens, hypoglycemia, hypoglycemia, hyponatremia, intracranial hemorrhage, lethal catatonia, poisoning (amphetamines, anticholinergics, cocaine, nicotine, salicylates, sympathomimetics, strychnine, theophylline), sedative-hypnotic drug withdrawal, sepsis, status epilepticus (including nonconvulsive status), tetanus, thalamic infarct, thyroid storm, and psychotic agitation.

SSRIs, selective serotonin reuptake inhibitors; MAOIs, monoamine oxidase inhibitors.

An electrocardiogram should be obtained in all patients with significant antipsychotic medication overdose and in symptomatic patients taking thioridazine, mesoridazine, or droperidol. Patients receiving high-dose intravenous haloperidol or droperidol for sedation require cardiac rhythm monitoring. If Q-T prolongation is present, serum potassium, calcium, and magnesium levels should be measured.

Patients who develop NMS, parkinsonism with marked muscle rigidity, or prolonged seizures are at risk for rhabdomyolysis. Measurement of serum creatinine kinase, renal function, and urine myoglobin may be indicated. A chest radiograph should be obtained if aspiration is suspected. Patients taking clozapine or olanzapine who present with infection or fever should be checked for leukopenia.

MANAGEMENT

Acute Overdose

Treatment is supportive; no specific antidote exists for antipsychotic medication overdose. Endotracheal intubation may be required to prevent aspiration or, less often, to support respiration. Hypotension is generally mild and responds to intravenous crystalloids. A vasopressor with α-adrenergic receptor agonism, such as norepinephrine, may be used if needed. If sedation and miosis suggest opioid intoxication, a trial of naloxone is warranted. Physostigmine and flumazenil are not beneficial and may precipitate seizures.

Acute Extrapyramidal Syndromes

Diphenhydramine, 25 to 50 mg intravenously, intramuscularly, or orally, or benztropine, 1 to 2 mg intramuscularly or orally, usually controls dystonic reactions. Benzodiazepines also may be effective. Akathisia can be treated with a lipophilic β-adrenergic blocker (e.g., propranolol), anticholinergic agents, or benzodiazepines.[39] Patients with EPS who respond to diphenhydramine or benztropine should continue on therapy for at least 48 hours to prevent recurrence. Benztropine, diphenhydramine, and the neuroleptic antipsychotic medications all cause anticholinergic effects, so combination therapy may worsen dry mouth, blurred vision, and urinary retention. Reducing the antipsychotic dose or changing to an atypical agent may be necessary.

Q-T Prolongation and Torsades de Pointes

Correction of hypokalemia, hypomagnesemia, and hypocalcemia shortens the Q-T interval. Treatment of torsades de pointes includes intravenous magnesium sulfate, overdrive pacing, and possibly isoproterenol (see Chapter 78). Administration of other antiarrhythmic drugs that prolong the Q-T interval should be avoided.

Neuroleptic Malignant Syndrome

Treatment of NMS revolves around supportive care and discontinuation of the offending medication. Agitation, psychomotor hyperactivity, and muscular rigidity should be treated aggressively with intravenous benzodiazepines. Lorazepam can be administered intravenously, 1 to 2 mg every 3 minutes until muscle rigidity improves, to a maximum dose of 10 mg. In refractory cases or cases at risk of aspiration, rapid sequence intubation, endotracheal intubation, and neuromuscular blockade with a nondepolarizing agent (e.g., vecuronium, pancuronium) are required. Hyperthermia should be managed aggressively with intravenous fluids and active external cooling with mist and fans (see Chapter 139). If rhabdomyolysis is present, intravenous hydration and urinary alkalization with sodium bicarbonate may be used to prevent renal damage, although the use of sodium bicarbonate is controversial (see Chapter 125).

The dopamine agonists bromocriptine and amantadine have been advocated as adjunctive treatments for NMS but do not consistently show a benefit.[40,41] Bromocriptine is administered orally or via nasogastric tube, beginning with 5 mg every 8 hours and titrated to a maximum of 20 mg per dose. The dose of amantadine is 200 mg orally every 12 hours. Response to therapy requires at least 24 hours. Bromocriptine has been linked to stroke, seizure, myocardial infarction, and severe hypertension in lactating or postpartum women, but not during treatment of NMS.[42]

Dantrolene, which inhibits the release of calcium from the sarcoplasmic reticulum, also has been advocated as an adjunctive therapy for NMS. As with the dopaminergic agents, it has no proven benefit.[31,40,41] Because the muscular rigidity of NMS is proposed to be secondary to dopamine blockade in the CNS rather than a muscle abnormality, dantrolene offers no advantage over benzodiazepines and neuromuscular blockade. Adverse effects after intravenous dantrolene include visual disturbances, dizziness, weakness, and gastrointestinal upset.[43] Pleural effusions, pneumonitis, pericarditis, and hepatitis have been reported with long-term administration.[44-46] Dantrolene can cause hyperkalemia and is contraindicated with verapamil.[47]

DISPOSITION

Patients with NMS and overdose patients who develop hypotension, coma, torsades de pointes, or airway compromise should be admitted to a critical care unit. Patients with a prolonged Q-T interval ($Q\text{-}T_c$ >460 msec) and all patients with significant ingestions of thioridazine or mesoridazine should receive at least 12 hours of cardiac monitoring. Patients with less severe signs of toxicity should be observed in the emergency department for a minimum of 4 hours from the time of ingestion. Persistent or worsening signs and symptoms mandate hospitalization. Criteria for hospital discharge include return to normal mental status and resolution of any vital sign, metabolic, and electrocardiogram abnormalities.

KEY CONCEPTS

- Extrapyramidal movement disorders are a common complication of antipsychotic medications.
- The most common finding in antipsychotic overdose is CNS depression. Treatment centers on supportive care, airway control, and cardiac monitoring.
- Q-T abnormalities and torsades de pointes are potential complications from overdose of many antipsychotic medications and can occur with therapeutic doses of some agents.
- NMS is characterized by altered mental status, hyperthermia, muscular rigidity, and autonomic instability. Aggressive supportive care includes airway management, benzodiazepines, neuromuscular blockade, and active cooling.

REFERENCES

1. Watson WA, et al: 2002 Annual report of the American Association of Poison Control Centers Toxic Exposure Surveillance System. *Am J Emerg Med* 21:353, 2003.
2. Burns MJ: The pharmacology and toxicology of atypical antipsychotic agents. *J Toxicol Clin Toxicol* 39:1, 2001.
3. Seeman P: Tardive dyskinesia, dopamine receptors, and neuroleptic damage to cell membranes. *J Clin Psychopharmacol* 18:477, 1998.
4. Haddad PM, Anderson IM: Antipsychotic-related QTc prolongation, torsades de pointes and sudden death. *Drugs* 62:1649, 2002.
5. Reilly JG, et al: QTc-interval abnormalities and psychotropic drug therapy in psychiatric patients. *Lancet* 355:1824, 2000.
6. LeBlaye I, et al: Acute overdosage with thioridazine: A review of the available clinical exposure. *Vet Hum Toxicol* 35:147, 1993.
7. Drolet B, et al: Droperidol lengthens cardiac repolarization due to block of the rapid component of the delayed rectifier potassium current. *J Cardiovasc Electrophysiol* 10:1597, 1999.
8. Drici MD, et al: Prolongation of QT interval in isolated feline hearts by antipsychotic drugs. *J Clin Psychopharmacol* 18:477, 1998.
9. Honigfeld G, et al: Reducing clozapine-related morbidity and mortality: 5 years of experience with the clozaril national registry. *J Clin Psychiatry* 59(Suppl 3):3, 1998.
10. Welch J, Manschreck T, Redmond D: Clozapine-induced seizures and EEG changes. *J Neuropsychiatry* 6:250, 1994.
11. Gajwani P, Pozuelo L, Tesar G: QT interval prolongation associated with quetiapine (seroquel) overdose. *Psychosomatics* 41:63, 2000.
12. Hustey F: Acute quetiapine poisoning. *J Emerg Med* 17:995, 1999.
13. Brown K, et al: Overdose of risperidone. *Ann Emerg Med* 22:1908, 1993.
14. Staffan H, Spigset O, Edwardson H, Bjork H: Prolonged sedation and slowly decreasing clozapine serum concentrations after an overdose. *J Clin Psychopharmacol* 10:282, 1999.
15. Sartorius A, et al: High-dose clozapine intoxication. *J Clin Psychopharmacol* 22:91, 2002.
16. Harmon T, et al: Loss of consciousness from acute quetiapine overdosage. *J Toxicol Clin Toxicol* 36:599, 1998.
17. Pollak P, Zbuk K: Quetiapine fumarate overdose: Clinical and pharmacokinetic lesions from extreme conditions. *Clin Pharmacol Ther* 68:92, 2000.
18. Cohen L, et al: Olanzapine overdose with serum concentrations. *Ann Emerg Med* 34:275, 1999.
19. O'Malley G: Olanzapine overdose mimicking opioid intoxication. *Ann Emerg Med* 34:279, 1999.
20. Acri A, Henretig F: Effects of risperidone in overdose. *Am J Emerg Med* 16:498, 1998.
21. Bryant S: A case series of ziprasidone overdoses. *Vet Hum Toxicol* 45:81, 2003.
22. Bowles T, Levin G: Aripiprazole: A new atypical antipsychotic drug. *Ann Pharmacother* 37:687, 2003.
23. Modestin J, Krapf R, Boker W: A fatality during haloperidol treatment: Mechanism of death. *Am J Psychiatry* 138:1616, 1981.
24. Drotts D, Vinson D: Prochlorperazine induces akathisia in emergency patients. *Ann Emerg Med* 34:469, 1999.
25. Levin T, Heresco-Levy U: Risperidone-induced rabbit syndrome: An unusual movement disorder caused by an atypical antipsychotic. *Eur Neuropsychopharmacol* 9:137, 1999.
26. Hubert F, Friedman J: Classification and treatment of tardive syndromes. *Neurologist* 9:16, 2003.
27. Tarsy D, Baldessarini RJ, Tarazi FI: Effects of newer antipsychotics on extrapyramidal function. *CNS Drugs* 16:23, 2002.
28. Caroff S, Mann S: Neuroleptic malignant syndrome. *Med Clin North Am* 77:185, 1993.
29. Pope HG, et al: Apparent neuroleptic malignant syndrome with clozapine and lithium. *J Nerv Ment Dis* 174:493, 1986.
30. Farver D: Neuroleptic malignant syndrome induced by atypical antipsychotics. *Expert Opin Drug Saf* 2:21, 2003.
31. Velamoor VR, et al: Progression of symptoms in neuroleptic malignant syndrome. *J Nerv Ment Dis* 182:168, 1994.
32. Legras A, et al: Protracted neuroleptic malignant syndrome complicating long-acting neuroleptic administration. *Am J Med* 85:875, 1988.
33. Buckely NA: Cardiotoxicity more common in thioridazine overdose than with other neuroleptics. *J Toxicol Clin Toxicol* 33:199, 1995.
34. Krahenbuhl S, et al: Case report: Reversible QT prolongation with torsades de pointes in a patient with pimozide intoxication. *Am J Med Sci* 309:315, 1995.
35. Taylor D: Ziprasidone in the management of schizophrenia: The QT interval issue in context. *CNS Drugs* 17:423, 2003.
36. Hulisz DT, et al: Complete heart block and torsades de pointes associated with thioridazine poisoning. *Pharmacotherapy* 14:239, 1994.
37. Tolosa-Vilella C, et al: Olanzapine-induced agranulocytosis, a case report and review of the literature. *Prog Neuropsychopharmacol Biol Psychiatry* 26:411, 2002.
38. Welch J, Manschreck T, Redmond D: Clozapine-induced seizures and EEG changes. *J Neuropsychiatry Clin Neurosci* 6:250, 1994.
39. Miller C, Fleischhacker W: Managing antipsychotic-induced acute and chronic akathisia. *Pract Drug Saf* 22:73, 2000.
40. Shalev A, Hermesh H, Munitz H: Mortality from the neuroleptic malignant syndrome. *J Clin Psychiatry* 50:18, 1989.
41. Rosebush PI, Stewart T, Mazurek MF: The treatment of neuroleptic malignant syndrome: Are dantrolene and bromocriptine useful adjuncts to supportive care? *Br J Psychiatry* 159:709, 1991.
42. Webster J: A comparative review of the tolerability profiles of dopamine agonists in the treatment of hyperprolactinaemia and inhibition of lactation. *Drug Saf* 14:228, 1996.

43. Wedel DJ, Quinlan JG, Iazzo PA: Clinical effects of intravenously administered dantrolene. *Mayo Clin Proc* 70:241, 1991.
44. Mahoney JM, Bachtel MD: Pleural effusion associated with chronic dantrolene administration. *Ann Pharmacother* 28:587, 1994.
45. Chan CH: Dantrolene sodium and hepatic injury. *Neurology* 40:1427, 1990.
46. Miller DH, Haas LF: Pneumonitis, pleural effusion and pericarditis following treatment with dantrolene. *J Neurol Neurosurg Psychiatry* 47:553, 1984.
47. San Juan AC, Wong KC, Port JD: Hyperkalemia after dantrolene and verapamil-dantrolene administration in dogs. *Anesth Analg* 67:759, 1988.

CHAPTER 160 Opioids

Christina E. Hantsch

PERSPECTIVE

Opioid is a term that applies to all natural, synthetic, and semisynthetic agents with morphine-like actions. It is more inclusive than the term *opiate,* which refers only to natural agents. Both terms are derived from *opium,* the Greek word for juice in reference to poppy juice. Poppy juice contains more than 20 distinct natural alkaloids with morphine-like activity. The term *narcotic* refers to any agent that induces sleep and is nonspecific. Although the term *narcotic* persists, primarily in legal contexts, *opioid* is more precise and is the correct medical term for the family of agents that act on opiate receptors in the body. Finally, the term *endorphin* applies to any of the peptides of the three endogenous opioid families: enkephalins, β-endorphins, and dynorphins.[1]

Pharmacologic actions of opioids involve the gastrointestinal system, genitourinary system, cardiovascular system, pulmonary system, and central nervous system (CNS) and cause characteristic clinical effects. Sedation and analgesia are the most common therapeutic goals of opioid medications, which are available alone or in combination with other agents (e.g., acetaminophen, salicylates) for these purposes. Additional therapeutic goals of opioids and combination preparations include antitussive and antidiarrheal effects.

Misuse of pharmaceutical opioid preparations and use of illicit opioids are significant problems in the United States. In 2001, 404,000 Americans age 12 and older had used heroin; 3.7 million have used heroin at least once.[2] Since the early 1990s, there has been a trend among heroin users toward inhalation rather than injection of heroin, although injection is still the more common route overall.[3] Heroin and morphine are among the most frequent drugs reported in drug-related death.[2,4]

PRINCIPLES OF DISEASE

Anatomy and Physiology

Although opioids have been used for more than 5000 years, receptors and endogenous opioids have been recognized and characterized only since the 1970s.[1,5] Opioids have an incompletely understood physiologic role.

Three established receptors, originally named *mu, kappa,* and *delta,* but now called OP_1 (delta), OP_2 (kappa), and OP_3 (mu),[5] have been cloned and genetically sequenced. Opioid receptors are distributed throughout the CNS. They are concentrated in pain pathways and in areas associated with the perception of pain (e.g., periaqueductal gray matter, locus ceruleus, limbic system, nucleus raphe magnus).[6] Systemically, opioid receptors are localized in sensory nerve endings, on mast cells, and in the gastrointestinal tract.[5,7] The role of the opioid receptors in pain perception and the analgesic effects of exogenous opioids are discussed in detail in Chapter 187.

Pathophysiology and Pharmacology

Toxicity

Opioids are a large group of drugs that include therapeutic agents and illicit substances. Opioid toxicity occurs as an adverse effect of therapeutic use, intentional overdose, or intentional abuse. Although different opioids have receptor preferences in therapeutic or low doses, this specificity is lost at higher doses.

In general, opioids are well absorbed after gastrointestinal (oral, rectal) or parenteral administration. Nasal, buccal, pulmonary, and transdermal absorption are effective, depending on the lipid solubility of the specific opioid.[1] Heroin is usually abused through intravenous and subcutaneous routes, but it also is absorbed after nasal administration because it is lipid soluble.[8,9] In general, opioid toxicity is less pronounced but more prolonged with oral ingestion than with parenteral administration.[1] Absorption of opioids after oral administration occurs in the small intestine. With therapeutic doses, absorption is complete within 1 to 2 hours. Absorption and clinical effects of toxicity may be prolonged after overdose, however, because gastric emptying is delayed.

Most opioids have a large volume of distribution. Clinical effects are influenced by the ease with which and extent to which opioids and their metabolites cross the blood-brain barrier; this also depends on lipid solubility. All opioids undergo hepatic metabolism and renal elimination. Variations in hepatic and renal function are important in opioid toxicity because metabolite activity may contribute to clinical effects and toxicity.[1] Excitatory effects (including seizures) with meperidine are caused primarily by its metabolite, normeperidine. The half-lives of meperidine and normeperidine are prolonged with cirrhosis, and the elimination of normeperidine is decreased with renal insufficiency. The likelihood of excitatory side effects is increased in these clinical settings and after multiple or large doses.

The pharmacokinetics of the specific agent involved affect the clinical course of opioid toxicity. Heroin peaks in the serum within 1 minute of intravenous injection, 3 to 5 minutes of intranasal administration, and 10 minutes of subcutaneous injection.[1,9] Heroin's lipophilic nature allows for its rapid transport across the blood-brain barrier into the CNS. In the CNS and in blood, heroin is rapidly hydrolyzed to 6-monoacetylmorphine and then morphine (less lipid soluble). In the liver, morphine undergoes conjugation with glucuronic acid to form more water-soluble compounds that are excreted by the kidneys.[9]

Withdrawal

Pharmacokinetics affect the clinical course of opioid withdrawal. Because the half-life of heroin is 0.5 hour, and the half-life of methadone is 15 to 40 hours, withdrawal symptoms occur 4 to 6 hours after discontinuation of heroin compared with 24 to 48 hours after discontinuation of methadone.[10,11] Duration of symptoms is 7 to 10 days and 2 weeks. In addition, the degree of physical dependence that has developed is important. With chronic opioid exposure, cellular adaptation results in upregulation of cyclic adenosine monophosphate (cAMP). When either the exposure is discontinued or an antagonist is administered, the result is a temporary elevation of cAMP levels and increased sympathetic activity above a normal baseline.

CLINICAL FEATURES

Toxicity

Opioid toxicity is associated with the toxidrome of CNS depression, respiratory depression, and miosis. Other potential findings in opioid toxicity are associated with toxicity from any opioid, but some features are unique to a specific agent or route of exposure.

Neurologic

CNS depression is a well-recognized manifestation of opioid toxicity, and hypoxia from CNS depression and respiratory depression causes many neurologic complications. Dysphoria and acute psychosis may occur with an agonist-antagonist opioid. Excitatory effects may occur with opioid toxicity. Hypertonicity, myoclonus, and seizures have been reported with overdose of the synthetic opioids meperidine and propoxyphene. Meperidine-related seizures probably are caused by accumulation of normeperidine, especially after multiple or large doses or in patients with hepatic or renal insufficiency. Seizures also may result from hypoxia with overdose of any opioid.

Parkinsonian symptoms in intravenous drug abusers have been attributed to 1-methyl-4-phenyl-1,2,3,6-tetrahydropyridine (MPTP), an unintended side product during synthesis of a meperidine analogue in street laboratories. MPTP injection is associated with focal lesions in the substantia nigra and a syndrome clinically indistinguishable from idiopathic parkinsonism. The syndrome is irreversible in some patients.[12] Similar syndromes have not been seen with other opioids.

Spongiform leukoencephalopathy has been associated with inhalation of heated heroin, a practice known as "chasing the dragon." Patients present with psychomotor retardation, dysarthria, ataxia, tremor, and other neurologic abnormalities.[13] This syndrome is incompletely understood but is thought to be related to a combination of mitochondrial injury and hypoxia.[14]

Serotonin syndrome is a clinical triad of mental status changes, autonomic instability, and neuromuscular changes (see Chapter 149). It results from excessive stimulation of CNS serotonin receptors and may be fatal. Most reported cases involve an interaction between a serotoninergic agent and a second agent, usually a selective serotonin reuptake inhibitor or a monoamine oxidase inhibitor.[15] Meperidine and dextromethorphan have serotoninergic properties and have been associated with serotonin syndrome.[15]

Respiratory

Opioids decrease respiratory rate and tidal volume in a dose-dependent manner by suppression of the sensitivity of the medullary respiratory center to hypercapnia.[1,16] Although it initially remains intact, the hypoxic drive is overridden in severe poisoning or when antagonistic stimuli (e.g., pain) are blocked.[16] Overdose of an agonist-antagonist agent produces less significant respiratory depression, presumably because of OP_3 receptor antagonism (Table 160-1).[1]

Bronchospasm has been reported rarely with heroin use in asthmatic and nonasthmatic patients. Bronchospasm occurs most often after inhalational exposure, but other routes also have been implicated. The bronchospasm is often severe, prolonged, and refractory to β-agonist therapy. Patients may require mechan-

Table 160-1. Select Opioid Doses and Associated Respiratory Depression

Drug	Oral Dose (mg)*	Intramuscular Dose (mg)*	Time to Onset of Respiratory Depression†
Codeine	200	120	Fast
Dextromethorphan	700	—	Fast
Dihydrocodeine	150	60	Fast
Diphenoxylate	300	—	Slow (or even more delayed)
Fentanyl	—	0.125	Very fast
Heroin	15	3	Fast
Hydrocodone	100	—	Fast
Hydromorphone	6	1.5	Fast
Levorphanol	1	2	Fast
Meperidine	250	100	Fast
Methadone	20	10	Slow (or even more delayed)
Morphine	70	10	Fast
Oxycodone	30	10	Fast
Oxymorphone	6	1	Fast
Paregoric	175	—	Fast
Propoxyphene	600	—	Fast

*Equivalent to 10 mg of intramuscular morphine.
†Varies with the drug and route of administration. In addition, the effects of a dose in any particular patient depend on multiple factors, including age, weight, and comorbid conditions. After IM administration, *very fast* means 5 to 30 minutes, *fast* means 15 to 60 minutes, and *slow* means 1 to 4 hours. After oral administration, these time definitions are approximately doubled.

ical ventilation for several days. It is unclear whether the heroin, an adulterant, or a combination triggers the bronchospasm and whether the response is histamine mediated or the result of direct irritation.[8]

Noncardiogenic pulmonary edema may occur with therapeutic opioid use but is much more common after overdose.[17] The capillary leak is likely from a hypoxic event and is not a receptor-mediated phenomenon. If present, symptoms include cough and dyspnea, and physical signs include hypoxemia, rales, rhonchi, and frothy sputum. Manifestations and radiographic findings after heroin-induced noncardiogenic pulmonary edema typically resolve within 36 hours, unless other pathology intervenes.[9] This is not the case with longer acting agents.

Ophthalmologic

Miosis is seen in more than 90% of heroin overdoses[18] and results from stimulation of OP_3 receptors in the Edinger-Westphal nuclei of the third nerve.[16] Miosis is not typically seen with meperidine, propoxyphene, or diphenoxylate-atropine (Lomotil) overdose. Toxicity from agonist-antagonists (e.g., pentazocine) or multiple agents may not produce miosis.

Cardiovascular

Opioids cause mild hypotension and relative bradycardia. Hypotension seems to result from histamine release and can be blocked by the administration of antihistamines (H_1 antagonists).[19] In addition, hypotension is typically orthostatic and resolves with supine positioning. Propoxyphene and its metabolite, norpropoxyphene, cause sodium channel blockade similar to that of type IA antidysrhythmic agents to produce widening of the QRS complex.[20]

Gastrointestinal

Nausea and vomiting are common side effects of therapeutic opioid use and are seen with overdose. Several mechanisms contribute to these symptoms, including opioid-induced delayed gastric emptying, direct stimulation of the chemoreceptor trigger zone, and vestibular stimulation. Because several mechanisms are involved, antihistamines and dopamine antagonists (e.g., chlorpromazine) may be effective in treatment.[16]

Decreased gastrointestinal motility is a common finding with therapeutic use and overdose of opioids. Severe cases may develop ileus.[1] Increased biliary tract pressures and choledochoduodenal sphincter spasm occur with therapeutic dosing of many opioids, including morphine, meperidine, and codeine.[10] Spasm is not always reproducible within the same patient, but seems related more to individual susceptibility than to a specific agent. Presenting clinical symptoms mimic biliary colic and may respond to naloxone or glucagon.[21]

Genitourinary

Opioids can cause urinary retention from urethral sphincter spasm and decreased detrusor tone. α-Adrenergic antagonists may reverse this effect.[16] Glomerulosclerosis and renal amyloidosis are seen in end-stage “heroin nephropathy” of chronic opioid addicts.[22]

Dermatologic

Pruritus, flushing, and urticaria occur after administration of certain opioids that release histamine (e.g., morphine) and do not represent a true allergy. Pruritus and erythema often are localized to the area of injection (e.g., along the vein through which the morphine was administered). Although all opioids have the potential to stimulate mast cell degranulation and histamine release, some (e.g., fentanyl) release only clinically negligible amounts of histamine and so have outstanding hemodynamic stability. Symptoms typically are controlled easily with antihistamines.

Metabolic

Hypoglycemia can occur after opioid overdose, but the mechanism is unclear. Coingestants, especially ethanol, may contribute to this finding. Hypothermia has been reported, but the mechanism is unclear. Hyperthermia should prompt a search for infectious complications, particularly in intravenous drug users, and for coingestants (e.g., cocaine) or adulterants (e.g., tripelennamine, scopolamine).[23] "Cotton fever" is reported in intravenous drug users who strain suspended drug through cotton balls or cigarette filters to remove particulates. Filters are boiled to extract residual drug when supply is low. Cotton is a known pyrogen and can cause a benign fever in patients who subsequently "shoot the cottons" or inject the extracted residue from the filters.[24]

Withdrawal

Opioid withdrawal occurs in tolerant individuals when opioid use is discontinued or an antagonist is administered. Increased sympathetic discharge and adrenergic hyperactivity are responsible for the clinical symptoms and signs. Although these can be significant, they are typically not life-threatening.[10,11] In contrast to the typical toxidrome of opioid toxicity (CNS and respiratory depression, miosis), withdrawal is associated with CNS excitation, tachypnea, and mydriasis. Pulse and blood pressure also are increased.

Neurologic manifestations are prominent in opioid withdrawal. Restlessness, agitation, and anxiety are virtually universal, and seizures rarely may occur. Cognition and mental status are unaffected. Dysphoria and drug craving may be severe and prolonged.

Nausea, vomiting, diarrhea, and abdominal cramps are common in withdrawal. They can be significant and lead to dehydration and electrolyte abnormalities. Opioid withdrawal symptoms also may include diffuse myalgias and insomnia. Additional signs are piloerection, yawning, lacrimation, rhinorrhea, and diaphoresis.

DIAGNOSTIC STRATEGIES

Toxicity

The diagnosis of opioid intoxication is usually based on history and physical examination. Diagnostic studies rarely assist in evaluation of patients suspected of opioid overdose. Other than hypoglycemia, specific abnormalities on standard hematology and chemistry studies are not seen with opioid toxicity. When the patient exhibits hypoxemia and pulmonary rales on examination, a chest radiograph should be obtained to evaluate for noncardiogenic pulmonary edema. In the appropriate circumstances, an abdominal radiograph may identify packets of opioids or other illicit substances in a body packer or body stuffer. There is a case of QRS widening thought to be associated with propoxyphene overdose, but this has not been validated.[20] If cardiac monitoring shows a prolonged QRS, a 12-lead electrocardiogram is advisable. When the patient presents with an oral ingestion of an unknown opioid preparation, acetaminophen and salicylate levels should be checked because many prescription opioids are available in combination products. Likewise, many illicit opioid users are exposed to additional drugs and contaminants.[23,24]

Although opiates are detected on most qualitative urine toxicology screens, these are rarely helpful in acute situations. On some assays, several synthetic opioids also are detected because they cross-react or because they are metabolized to opiates, which are then excreted. Other agents, such as fentanyl and its derivatives, are missed on urine screens.[25] Poppy seeds can lead to a positive opiate screen secondary to the presence of morphine and codeine; however, detection of 6-monoacetylmorphine, a specific metabolite of heroin, can confirm heroin use.[25]

Withdrawal

As with opioid toxicity, no diagnostic test exists for opioid withdrawal.

DIFFERENTIAL CONSIDERATIONS

Toxicity

The diagnosis of opioid intoxication is usually obvious, based on history and physical examination, although patients with other intoxications or nontoxicologic conditions may have a similar physical examination. Other drugs that should be considered are clonidine (or a related drug), tramadol, valproic acid, gamma hydroxybutyrate, and sedative-hypnotic agents. The differential diagnosis encompasses all causes of depressed mental status, but the coexistence of miosis and respiratory depression greatly narrows the possibilities.

Withdrawal

Opioid withdrawal is usually a straightforward diagnosis, and the patient often reveals it as the chief complaint. Simultaneous intoxication with, or withdrawal from, other classes of agents, especially CNS depressants and stimulants, may be seen.

MANAGEMENT

Toxicity

Attention to the airway, oxygenation, and ventilation are of particular importance in patients with opioid intoxication because significant CNS and respiratory depression are the most common life-threatening developments. Appropriate interventions include airway protection and ventilatory support if reversal is not achieved with antidote therapy. Patients with noncardiogenic pulmonary edema may require oxygen and positive-pressure modalities, such as bilevel positive airway pressure, continuous positive airway pressure, or mechanical ventilation with positive end-expiratory pressure. Circulatory support usually does not require more than a crystalloid infusion. Most opioids have a large volume of distribution and cannot be cleared by dialysis. There are no clinically effective techniques for enhanced elimination of opioids.

Gastrointestinal Decontamination

Gastrointestinal decontamination is unnecessary because the antidote can reverse the effects. Whole-bowel irrigation has been advocated to hasten passage of drug packets from body packers or patients with ingestions involving opioid combination products or multidrug ingestions. A single early dose of activated charcoal (1 g/kg in children, 50 to 100 g in adults) may be beneficial in some patients because gastrointestinal motility may be reduced.[26]

Antidote

Naloxone, a pure opioid antagonist, is the antidote most frequently used to reverse opioid toxicity. Naloxone has a rapid onset of action. It is ineffective after oral administration secondary to the first-pass effect, but intravenous, subcutaneous, intramuscular, and endotracheal routes can be used. Naloxone acts through competitive binding at opioid receptors and can reverse all the receptor-mediated actions of opioids. Naloxone is indicated for patients with opioid intoxication who have significant CNS or respiratory depression. The initial intravenous dose is 0.4 to 2 mg for adults and children, but 10 mg may be required to obtain a clinical response for synthetic opioids, including return of protective airway reflexes and resolution of hypoventilation and hypoxia. The endotracheal dose is 2 to 2.5 times the intravenous dose.

Naloxone can precipitate acute withdrawal in chronic opioid users. In this population, the dose should be started at 0.2 mg and slowly titrated. The duration of action of naloxone is 1 to 2 hours. Consequently, either repeat doses or a continuous infusion of two thirds of the effective initial dose per hour may be required.[1]

Naloxone has an excellent safety profile. Noncardiogenic pulmonary edema, hypertension, and dysrhythmia have been reported with use of naloxone after general anesthesia[27,28] and in patients with underlying cardiac or pulmonary disease.[27] Whether the naloxone is the cause of these complications is unproven. Idiosyncratic reactions and sympathetic discharge with precipitation of acute withdrawal have been proposed as explanations. Complete clinical recovery in response to naloxone is strongly suggestive of opioid overdose. Other intoxications may improve to lesser degrees with naloxone therapy, including valproic acid, clonidine, tramadol, captopril, and ethanol. Naloxone has been given to patients who have ingested these agents because of a presentation similar to opioid intoxication or suspicion of a mixed exposure that included opioids. The mechanism of these responses to naloxone is not established. Some of these drugs may have activity at opioid receptors.[27]

Nalmefene, another opioid antagonist, has a long half-life (8 to 11 hours) and duration of clinical effect. Intravenous nalmefene has a rapid onset of action in reversing opioid-induced CNS and respiratory depression. Alternate administration routes are oral, subcutaneous, and intramuscular. The initial intravenous dose is 0.5 to 1.5 mg (pediatric dose not established). Higher doses have been used but are associated with increased risk of adverse effects.[29,30] When a clinical response has been achieved with nalmefene, repeat doses or continuous infusions are generally not required; however, the duration of withdrawal symptoms or other rare adverse effects may be longer with nalmefene. Naloxone remains the preferred antidote in patients at risk for withdrawal or other adverse effects and in patients with anticipated short duration of opioid toxicity. Seizures associated with opioid toxicity may resolve with correction of hypoxia or may require administration of benzodiazepines.

Withdrawal

Opioid withdrawal is not life-threatening, but the potentially serious manifestations mandate attention to supportive and symptomatic care. When withdrawal is produced by administration of naloxone, the symptoms are of short duration, and replacement opioids should be avoided.[10,11] Other patients with withdrawal can receive opioid replacement or other medications to alleviate symptoms. In addition, fluid and electrolyte replacement is important for patients with dehydration from gastrointestinal symptoms.

Methadone, a long-acting opioid, and 1-α-acetyl methadol (LAAM), a newer and even longer acting opioid, are options for opioid replacement to treat or prevent withdrawal in chronic heroin users admitted for other medical conditions, but they are not indicated in the emergency department. One method uses an initial dose of methadone of either 20 mg orally or 10 mg intramuscularly, with an onset of action in 30 to 60 minutes. This initial dose typically controls significant manifestations.[10] Some symptoms, particularly drug craving, may be ongoing and require a subsequent dose after several hours. Maintenance methadone therapy requires doses every 12 to 24 hours and is tapered daily. The starting dose of LAAM is 30 mg orally, and the drug is given three times a week.[10]

Clonidine, a central α_2-agonist, is an option for treatment of opioid withdrawal without opioid replacement.[10] Clonidine controls symptoms by suppressing sympathetic hyperactivity. It also may shorten the duration of withdrawal. The initial dose is 0.1 mg orally. Repeat doses may be given every 30 to 60 minutes; relatively large total doses may be required. As with opioid replacement, clonidine therapy must be titrated to individual clinical response. Hypotension may limit the treatment but is not common in the setting of opioid withdrawal treatment. Patches for transdermal administration of clonidine are available, but onset of action is delayed 24 hours. Oral doses still must be given initially.

Buspirone is an azaspirone compound that is used to treat ethanol and nicotine addiction. Studies suggest that it also may be an option to treat withdrawal in opioid addicts, but further investigation is needed.[31]

DISPOSITION

Toxicity

Patients with manifestations of opioid toxicity usually are treated successfully in the emergency department, sometimes in conjunction with the emergency department observation unit. Patients who receive naloxone should be observed for 2 hours to assess the extent of re-sedation. Stable patients who present after an ingestion but who are asymptomatic can be observed in the emergency department until 4 hours after the ingestion, at which time they can be discharged with appropriate psychiatric evaluation or drug abuse counseling. Patients who have ingested an opioid with a longer half-life or active metabolite and patients with multiple drug ingestions involving an opioid may require longer observation periods.

Patients who have a known or potential overdose of diphenoxylate-atropine (Lomotil) should be observed in a monitored unit even if asymptomatic[32]; this includes small children who may have ingested only a single tablet (2.5 mg of diphenoxylate, 0.025 mg of atropine). The metabolite of diphenoxylate, difenoxin, has a longer half-life, is five times more active than diphenoxylate, and may cause delayed and prolonged toxicity. Delayed absorption, caused by each component of Lomotil and enterohepatic recirculation, may contribute as well.[32]

Patients who have a known or potential ingestion of packets of illicit opioid drugs should be admitted until the packets are passed. Body packers and body stuffers may remain asymptomatic until one or more of the packets leak. A poison center or medical toxicologist should be consulted if there is uncertainty about the appropriate disposition for a particular patient.

Withdrawal

Patients with opioid withdrawal may be managed in the outpatient setting. Clonidine may alleviate some of the symptoms of withdrawal but has a high incidence of postural hypotension. Patients with refractory complications (e.g., vomiting, dehydration, electrolyte abnormalities) and patients with an uncertain diagnosis may require hospitalization. Some patients may need to be detoxified before entering chemical treatment programs. Substance abuse counseling and establishment of outpatient program referral should be completed before discharge.

KEY CONCEPTS

- Diagnosis of opioid intoxication is based on history, physical examination, and response to naloxone.
- The opioid toxidrome includes three prominent findings—CNS depression, respiratory depression, and miosis—but may not be present in every patient.
- Early administration of reversal agents and airway management and attention to oxygenation and ventilation are crucial to management of patients with opioid toxicity.
- The duration of action of many opioids, especially after overdose, is significantly longer than that of naloxone. Patients responsive to naloxone should be observed for recurrence of opioid toxicity after the effect of naloxone has resolved.
- Opioid withdrawal syndrome does not include altered cognition. Patients with known or suspected opioid withdrawal who also have altered cognition should be evaluated for another etiology of the altered cognition.

REFERENCES

1. Reisene T, Pasternak G: Opioid analgesics and antagonists. In Hardman JG, Limbird LE (eds): *Goodman and Gilman's the Pharmacologic Basis of Therapeutics,* 9th ed. New York, McGraw-Hill, 1996, pp 521-555.
2. National Institute on Drug Abuse: Heroin InfoFacts. Available at: www.drugabuse.gov/pdf/Infofacts/heroin.
3. Office of Applied Studies, Substance Abuse and Mental Health Services Administration: The Dasis Report: Heroin—changes in how it is used. Available at: http://oas.samsha.gov/2k1/HeroinRT/HeroinRT.cfm.
4. Watson WA, et al: 2002 annual report of the American Association of Poison Control Centers Toxic Exposure Surveillance System. *Am J Emerg Med* 21:353, 2003.
5. Dhawan BN, et al: International Union of Pharmacology XII classification of opioid receptors. *Pharmacol Rev* 48:567, 1996.
6. Pasternak GW: Pharmacological mechanisms of opioid analgesics. *Clin Neuropharmacol* 16:1, 1993.
7. Pleuvry BJ: Opioid receptors and their relevance to anaesthesia. *Br J Anaesth* 71:119, 1993.
8. Cygan J, Trunsky M, Corbridge T: Inhaled heroin-induced status asthmaticus: Five cases and a review of the literature. *Chest* 117:272, 2000.
9. Sporer KA: Acute heroin overdose. *Ann Intern Med* 130:584, 1999.
10. Olmedo R, Hoffman RS: Withdrawal syndromes. *Emerg Med Clin North Am* 18:273, 2000.
11. Jenkins DH: Substance abuse and withdrawal in the intensive care unit. *Surg Clin North Am* 80:1033, 2000.
12. Ballard PA, Tetrud JW, Langston JW: Permanent human parkinsonism due to 1-methyl-4-phenyl-1,2,3,6-tetrahydropyridine (MPTP): Seven cases. *Neurology* 35:949, 1985.
13. Hill MD, Cooper PW, Perry JR: Chasing the dragon—neurological toxicity associated with inhalation of heroin vapour: Case report. *Can Med Assoc J* 162:236, 2000.
14. Vella S: Acute leukoencephalopathy after inhalation of a single dose of heroin. *Neuropediatrics* 34:100, 2003.
15. Mills KC: Serotonin syndrome: A clinical update. *Crit Care Clin* 13:163, 1997.
16. Schug SA, Zech D, Grond S: Adverse effects of systemic opioid analgesics. *Drug Saf* 7:200, 1992.
17. Soto J, Sacristan JA, Alsar MJ: Pulmonary oedema due to fentanyl. *Anaesthesia* 47:913, 1992.

18. Sporer KA, Firestone J, Isaacs SM: Out-of-hospital treatment of opioid overdoses in an urban setting. *Acad Emerg Med* 3:660, 1996.
19. Flacke JW, et al: Histamine release by four narcotics: A double-blind study in humans. *Anesth Analg* 66:723, 1987.
20. Stork CM, et al: Propoxyphene-induced wide QRS complex dysrhythmia responsive to sodium bicarbonate—a case report. *J Toxicol Clin Toxicol* 33:179, 1995.
21. Bird KJ: Narcotic-induced choledochoduodenal sphincter spasm reversed by naloxone. *Anaesthesia* 41:1120, 1986.
22. Dubrow A, et al: The changing spectrum of heroin-associated nephropathy. *Am J Kidney Dis* 5:36, 1985.
23. Perrone J, Shaw L, DeRoos F: Laboratory confirmation of scopolamine co-intoxication in patients using tainted heroin. *J Toxicol Clin Toxicol* 37:491, 1999.
24. Harrison DW, Walls RM: "Cotton fever": A benign febrile syndrome in intravenous drug abusers. *J Emerg Med* 8:135, 1990.
25. Kwong TC: Toxicology. In McClatchey KD (ed): *Clinical Laboratory Medicine*. Baltimore, Williams & Wilkins, 1994, pp 445-467.
26. American Academy of Clinical Toxicology, European Association of Poison Centres and Clinical Toxicologists: Position statements on gastrointestinal decontamination. *J Toxicol Clin Toxicol* 35:695, 1997.
27. Chamberlain JM, Klein BL: A comprehensive review of naloxone for the emergency physician. *Ann Emerg Med* 12:650, 1994.
28. Johnson C, Mayer P, Grosz D: Pulmonary edema following naloxone administration in a healthy orthopedic patient. *J Clin Anesth* 7:356, 1995.
29. Kaplan JL, et al: Double-blind randomized study of nalmefene and naloxone in emergency department patients with suspected narcotic overdose. *Ann Emerg Med* 34:42, 1999.
30. Chumpa A: Nalmefene hydrochloride. *Pediatr Emerg Care* 15:141, 1999.
31. Rose JS, et al: Effects of buspirone in withdrawal from opiates. *Am J Addict* 12:253, 2003.
32. McCarron MM, Challoner KR, Thompson GA: Diphenoxylate-atropine (Lomotil) overdose in children: An update. *Pediatrics* 87:694, 1991.

CHAPTER 161

Pesticides

Cynthia K. Aaron

PERSPECTIVE

Pesticides, a generic term to refer to all pest-killing agents, include numerous chemicals intended for use as insecticides, herbicides, rodenticides, fungicides, and fumigants. Many of these chemicals are general protoplasmic poisons affecting a wide range of organisms, including humans. Although space does not allow a comprehensive discussion of each individual chemical that may produce human toxicity, numerous chemical classes are commonly used as pesticides. These classes have associated characteristic clinical pictures that are important to recognize because patients with acute (and occasionally chronic) exposures to these agents come to the emergency department. In addition, many other pesticides with particularly unique and interesting mechanisms of toxic effects are described.

ORGANOPHOSPHATE INSECTICIDES

The organophosphate insecticide triethyl pyrophosphate was first synthesized in 1859, but was not used to replace nicotine as a pesticide until World War II. After World War II, these compounds were used as nerve agents in wars, as organophosphorus and carbamate insecticides, and as medicinal agents (Box 161-1). After the negative publicity associated with the organochlorine DDT, organophosphate insecticides soon became some of the most common pesticides for home and industrial use. In the late 1990s and in 2000, with the advent of increased awareness of terrorism, nerve agents have gained prominence as weapons of mass destruction (see Chapter 195).[1]

Principles of Disease

Pharmacology

Organophosphorus insecticides are highly lipid soluble and are readily absorbed via dermal, gastrointestinal (GI), and respiratory routes.[2] This lipid solubility results in the storage of organophosphorus compounds in body fat, making possible the gradual or rapid accumulation of toxic systemic levels from repeated low-level exposures. The parent compound and its metabolites are acetylcholinesterase inhibitors, and many parent organophosphorus compounds are less potent than their metabolites (e.g., parathion to paraoxon), resulting in delayed onset of clinical toxicity.

Pathophysiology

Organophosphorus pesticides work by persistently inhibiting the enzyme acetylcholinesterase, the enzymatic deactivator of the ubiquitous neurotransmitter acetylcholine. Because of the global penetration of organophosphorus compounds, inhibition occurs at tissue sites (true acetylcholinesterase or butyryl-

BOX 161-1. Acetylcholinesterase Inhibitors

Nerve Gases	
"G" or German agents	
GA	Tabun
GB	Sarin
GD	Tabun
"V" agents	
VX	
Organophosphate Insecticides	
Acephate	Orthene
Azinphos-methyl	Guthion
Bomyl	Swat
Bromophos	Nexion
Bromophos-ethyl	Nexagan
Carbophenothion	Trithion
Chlorfenvinphos	Birlane
Chlorpyrifos	Dursban, Lorsban
Chlormephos	Dotan
Chlorthiophos	Celathion
Coumaphos	Co-Ral
Crotoxyphos	Ciodrin
Cyanofenphos	Surecide
Cyanophos	Cyanox
Cythioate	Proban
DEF	De-Green
Demeton	Systox
Demeton-methyl	Metasystox
Dialifor	Torak
Diazinon	Spectracide
Dichlofenthion	Mobilawn
Dichlorvos	Bidrin
Dimethoate	Cygon, De-Fend
Dioxathion	Delnav
Disulfoton	Di-System
EPN	Santox
Ethion	Acithion
Ethoprop	Mocap
Ethyl parathion	Parathion
Etrimfos	Ekamet
Famphur	Warbex, Fanfos
Fenamiphos	Nemacur
Fenitrothion	Agrothion
Fenephosphon	Agritox
Fensulfothion	Dasanit
Fenthion	Baytex, Entex
Fonofos	Dyfonate
Formothion	Anthio
Heptenophos	Hostaquick
Iodofenphos	Nuvanol-N
Isofenphos	Amaze, Oftanol
Isoxathion	Karphos
Leptophos	Phosvel
Malathion	Cythion
Merphos	Folex
Methamidophos	Monitor
Organophosphate Insecticides—cont'd	
Methidathion	Supracide
Methyl parathion	Dalf
Mevinphos	Phosdrin
Monocrotophos	Azodrin
Naled	Dibrom
Phencapton	G 28029
Phenthoate	Tanone
Phorate	Thimet
Phosalone	Zolone
Phosfolan	Cyolane
Phosmet	Imidan, Prolate
Phosphamidon	Dimecron
Phoxim	Baythion
Pirimiphosmethyl	Actellic
Profenofos	Curacron
Propetamphos	Safrotin
Propylthiopyrophosphate	Aspon
Prothoate	Fac
Pyrazophos	Afugan, Curamil
Pyridaphenthion	Ofunack
Quinalphos	Bayrusil
Schradan	OMPA
Sulfotepp	Bladafum Dithione
Sulprofos	Bolstar
Temephos	Abate, Abathion
Terbufos	Gounter
Tetrachlorvinphos	Gardona, Rabon
Tetraethyl pyrophosphate	TEPP
Thiometon	Ekatin
Triazophos	Hostathion
Trichlorfon	Dylox, Neguvon
Carbamate Insecticides	
Aminocarb	Matacil
Aldicarb	Temik
Bufencarb	Bux
Carbaryl	Sevin
Carbofuran	Furadan
Dimeton	Snip Fly Bands
Formetanate	Carzol, Dicarzol
Methiocarb	Draza, Mesurol
Methomyl	Nudrin, Lannate Vydate
Oxamyl	Aphox, Pirimor
Pirimicarb	Carbamult
Promecarb	Minacide
Propoxur	Baygon
Therapeutic Agents	
Ambenonium	Mytelase
Demecarium	Humorsol
Edrophonium	Tensilon
Neostigmine	Prostigmin
Physostigmine	Antilirium
Pyridostigmine	Mestinon

EPN, ethyl-*p*-nitrophenylthionobenzeneiophosphate; OMPA, octamethyl pyrophosphoramide; TEPP, tetraethyl diphosphate.

cholinesterase and represented by erythrocyte or red blood cell [RBC] cholinesterase) and in plasma (circulating pseudocholinesterase).[3,4] Inhibition of cholinesterase results in the accumulation and subsequent prolonged effect of acetylcholine at a variety of neurotransmitter receptors, including the sympathetic and parasympathetic ganglionic nicotinic sites, postganglionic cholinergic sympathetic and parasympathetic muscarinic sites, skeletal muscle nicotinic sites, and central nervous system sites (Fig. 161-1).[2]

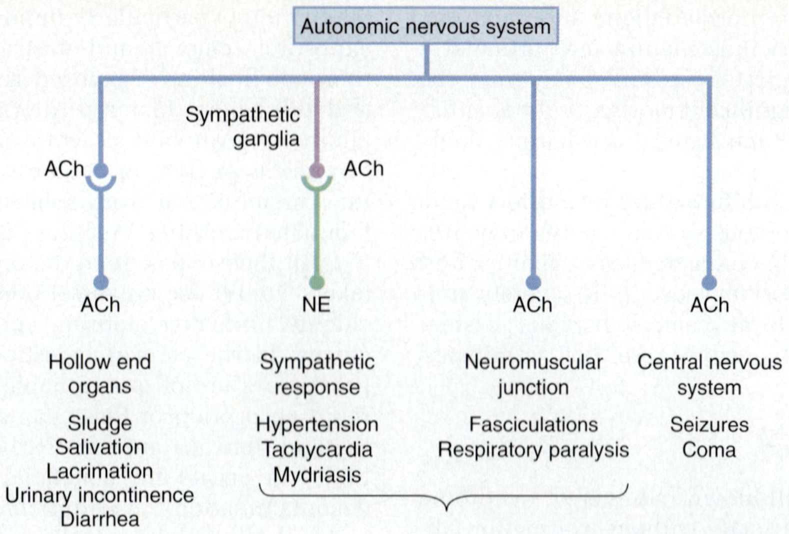

Figure 161-1. Schematic representation of the autonomic nervous system (ANS). The ANS comprises the sympathetic and parasympathetic nervous systems. The sympathetic nervous system also is known as the thoracolumbar outflow, where the cell body lies in the spinal cord and the first synapse occurs in the sympathetic ganglia. The neurotransmitter in this first synapse is acetylcholine (ACh) (preganglionic), and the neurotransmitter in the postganglionic neuron with the target organ is norepinephrine (NE). In the parasympathetic nervous system (craniosacral outflow), nerves from the medulla and sacrum use ACh as the neurotransmitter in preganglionic and postganglionic target organs. The ANS is divided further into the muscarinic and nicotinic receptors, where atropine can block the muscarinic receptors but not the nicotinic receptors. The neuromuscular junction uses ACh as the effector neurotransmitter. In the brain, ACh is just one of several active neurotransmitters.

BOX 161-2. SLUDGE Symptoms

Salivation
Lacrimation
Urinary incontinence
Defecation
Gastrointestinal cramps
Emesis

Clinical Features

Signs and Symptoms

The accumulation of acetylcholine results in a classic cholinergic syndrome, manifested by hyperactivity of cholinergic responses at the receptor sites indicated earlier. The clinical syndrome of muscarinic acetylcholinesterase inhibition is commonly called the *SLUDGE syndrome* (Box 161-2). This syndrome represents postganglionic acetylcholine-induced hollow end-organ general hypersecretion,[2] resulting in clinical findings including miotic pupils, lacrimation, rhinorrhea, sialorrhea, bronchorrhea, vomiting, diarrhea, and urinary incontinence. Bradycardia is commonly mentioned as a classic sign of acetylcholinesterase poisoning, but the increased release of norepinephrine from postganglionic sympathetic neurons precipitated by excess cholinergic activity at sympathetic ganglia may result in normal or even tachycardic heart rates (nicotinic effect). Sympathetic hyperactivity can cause diffuse diaphoresis, although this response is mediated by cholinergic receptors at preganglionic (nicotinic) and postganglionic (muscarinic) sites. The most lethal components of acetylcholinesterase inhibition occur in the brain and neuromuscular junction. A combination of sympathetic stimulation, involvement of the *N*-methyl-D-aspartate receptor, and enhanced acetylcholine concentrations can lead to seizures.[5] At the neuromuscular junction, excess acetylcholine causes hyperstimulation of the muscles with secondary paralysis. Because the diaphragm is affected, cholinesterase poisoning leads to respiratory arrest.[6]

Although the usual clinical picture of acute organophosphorus poisoning is impressive, toxicity from gradual, cumulative exposure may be much more subtle. These patients commonly exhibit vague confusion or other central nervous system complaints; mild visual disturbances; or chronic abdominal cramping, nausea, and diarrhea.[7]

Complications

Seizures and pulmonary hypersecretion, or bronchorrhea and bronchoconstriction, are prominent mechanisms of early morbidity and mortality in cases of poisoning from acetylcholinesterase inhibitors. Bronchorrhea is typically, although incorrectly, called *noncardiogenic pulmonary edema* because the origin of the excessive pulmonary fluids is from airway secretions and does not represent transudation of fluid across the alveolar-capillary membrane. The obstruction of upper and lower airways, the potential intrusion of these bronchial secretions into alveolar sacs, and bronchoconstriction produce hypoxia, which is the primary concern in the initial stages of poisoning.[2]

Nicotinic hyperstimulation of skeletal muscle determines the ultimate morbidity and mortality of acetylcholinesterase inhibitors. Signs of skeletal muscle hyperactivity include involuntary twitches, fasciculations, and hyperactive reflexes. Muscle hyperactivity eventually gives way to muscle fatigue and paralysis, including the respiratory musculature and particularly the diaphragm.[6,8] Respiratory insufficiency may be delayed and result in significant morbidity if not anticipated and corrected by mechanical or pharmacologic means.

Acetylcholinesterase inhibitors produce direct toxic effects on the central nervous system leading to neurologic signs of confusion, combativeness, seizures, and coma. Status epilepticus may occur in severely poisoned patients. Structural central nervous system damage may occur if seizures are not terminated rapidly.[9]

Diagnostic Strategies

Any patient with a full-blown cholinergic syndrome should be treated empirically without waiting for laboratory confirmation of decreased cholinesterase activity. Known or suspected exposure to cholinesterase inhibitors should be confirmed by ordering plasma and erythrocyte (RBC) cholinesterase levels. In acute exposures, the plasma cholinesterase levels fall first, with decreases in RBC cholinesterase levels lagging behind. The RBC cholinesterase level is more indicative of what is occurring at the nerve terminal.[3] Patients with chronic exposures may show only reduced RBC cholinesterase activity, and a normal plasma cholinesterase level may impart a false sense of security. The true reflection of depressed cholinesterase activity is found in the RBC activity, and even a mild acute exposure may result in severe clinical poisoning. RBC cholinesterase levels recover at a rate of 1% per day in untreated patients and take about 6 to 12 weeks to normalize, whereas plasma cholinesterase levels may recover in 4 to 6 weeks. Other studies should be geared toward the evaluation of pulmonary, cardiovascular, and renal function and fluid and electrolyte balance.

Differential Diagnosis

Few toxins or other clinical conditions produce the same symptoms as acetylcholinesterase inhibitors. One species of mushroom, *Amanita muscaria,* historically has been mentioned in the differential diagnosis, but actually contains alkaloids that usually produce an anticholinergic (antimuscarinic) syndrome. A variety of conditions that induce excessive vagal responses (e.g., inferior wall myocardial infarction) also may produce some signs suggesting acetylcholinesterase inhibition, but other symptoms should make the primary cause apparent.

Management

Treatment of poisoning with acetylcholinesterase inhibitors is directed toward four goals: (1) decontamination, (2) supportive care, (3) reversal of acetylcholine excess at muscarinic sites, and (4) reversal of toxin binding at active sites on the cholinesterase molecule. Decontamination should be started in the prehospital phase of care to prevent greater absorption and subsequent toxicity and to protect care providers. Decontamination is particularly important in cases of dermal exposure; removal and destruction of clothing and thorough flushing of exposed skin may limit absorption and subsequent toxicity. Alternatively, dermal decontamination can be done with dry agents, such as military resins or flour or bentonite. Caregivers are at risk for contamination from splashes or handling of contaminated clothing. Treating personnel may be rotated to limit their exposure to the organophosphates.[6] Caretakers should use universal precautions, including eye shields, protective clothing, and nitrile or butyl rubber gloves. In the case of ingestion, GI decontamination procedures are of questionable benefit because of the rapid absorption of these compounds. Profuse vomiting and diarrhea are seen early in ingestion and may limit[10] or negate any beneficial effect of additional GI decontamination.[11,12] Equipment may be washed with a 5% hypochlorite solution to inactivate the cholinesterase inhibitor.

Because morbidity results from airway and respiratory failure, supportive care should be directed primarily toward airway management, including suctioning of secretions and vomitus, oxygenation, and, when necessary, ventilatory support. Succinylcholine can be used for intubation but may have an extremely prolonged duration.[3] It is preferable to use a competitive neuromuscular blocking agent, such as rocuronium, for rapid sequence intubation in these patients, but increased dosing may be necessary. Although some authors have advocated the use of β-blockers to control tachycardia, this may lead to worsening cardiovascular instability.[11,13] Most cardiovascular complications that occur in this setting rarely require specific therapy.

The definitive treatment of acetylcholinesterase inhibition starts with the administration of *atropine.*[2] A competitive inhibitor of acetylcholine at muscarinic receptor sites, atropine reverses the clinical effects of cholinergic excess at parasympathetic end organs and sweat glands. Large doses of atropine may be required.[14] Data suggest that the more rapid the atropinization, the faster control is obtained.[6,11,12] Suggested dosing is 1 to 2 mg of atropine (0.02 to 0.05 mg/kg) intravenously, with doubling of each subsequent dose every 5 minutes until there is control of mucous membrane hypersecretion and the airway clears.[6,11,12] If intravenous access is not immediately available, atropine may be administered intramuscularly. Patients may require 200 to 500 mg of atropine intravenously during the first hour, followed by prolonged continuous infusions of 5 to 100 mg/hr to maintain adequate secretion control.[14] Tachycardia and mydriasis may occur at these doses, but they are not indications to stop atropine administration. The endpoint of atropinization is drying of respiratory secretions and easing of respiration. Increasing animal evidence suggests that early rapid atropinization may limit seizure propagation and, in conjunction with diazepam, prevent status epilepticus.[9,15] Atropine is not active at nicotinic sites and does not reverse the skeletal muscle effects (e.g., muscle fatigue and respiratory failure).[3,12]

The second part of acetylcholinesterase inhibition treatment is the use of an oxime, such as *pralidoxime* (2-PAM, Protopam) or *obidoxime* (Toxigonin), to break up the organophosphate-acetylcholinesterase complex and restore cholinesterase activity at muscarinic and nicotinic sites.[3,6,12,16] The usual starting dose of pralidoxime is 1 to 2 g intravenously (pediatric dose 25 to 50 mg/kg); additional doses may be given based on clinical response and serial cholinesterase levels. The medication may be given in a bolus of 1 to 2 g intravenously over 30 to 60 minutes every 4 to 8 hours or 500 mg/hr (pediatric dose 10 to 25 mg/kg/hr).[16,17] The World Health Organization recommends an initial dose of 30 mg/kg followed by 8 mg/kg/hr continued for at least 24 hours or, if an infusion cannot be used, 30 mg/kg every 4 hours.[18] The infusion may be continued for several days with no apparent adverse effects attributable to the pralidoxime; however, rapid administration has led to hypertension, vomiting, and a transient reversible neuromuscular blockade.[19] The ideal dose of pralidoxime should be determined by monitoring the clinical condition of the patient and serial cholinesterase levels; the patient may require higher doses of oxime than recommended here. The World Health Organization–recommended infusion dose of obidoxime is 4 mg/kg followed by 0.5 mg/kg/hr; alternatively, intermittent IV doses of 4 mg/kg, then 2 mg/kg, every 4 hours is given.[18] Pralidoxime and obidoxime can be administered by intramuscular injection.

It is commonly stated that pralidoxime is useful only within the first 24 hours because of aging of the organophosphate-acetylcholinesterase complex.[2] This truism has been challenged with the acknowledgment that not all organophosphates behave in a similar fashion. Dimethyl and diethyl phosphoryl insecticides react differently at variable rates with acetylcholinesterase and oxime therapy. Many organophosphates are highly lipid soluble and slowly leach out of fat stores for days to weeks, resulting in newly formed complexes that are amenable to treatment with pralidoxime. Pralidoxime also can combine with unbound organophosphates and prevent their subsequent binding to nerve terminals. The aforementioned poison leaching may occur for 6 weeks after an acute exposure, with excellent reversal of the cholinesterase inhibition exhibited clinically and by laboratory measurements of cholinesterase activity. Even with optimal treatment, seriously intoxicated patients may require long-term supportive care, including ventilator support.[6,17]

In conjunction with atropine and oxime therapy, patients with agitation, seizures, and coma should be treated with adequate doses of a benzodiazpine after the airway has been secured.[6,9,20,21] Although diazepam is most studied, midazolam and lorazepam can be used, with midazolam being the best agent for intramuscular use. Sarin, soman, tabun, and VX are nerve agents that might be used in a terrorist attack. These agents have important differences from the common organophosphorous insecticides. VX is an oily but highly toxic agent with low volatility. It does not readily vaporize, and because its risk of inhalation is low, exposure is predominately percutaneous. The other agents can be mostly dispersed into the air resulting in inhalation. These agents do not require the same extremely large doses of atropine but do require pralidoxime. The U.S. military has preloaded Mark I antidote kits containing two syringes, one with 2 mg of atropine and the other containing 600 mg of pralidoxime for intramuscular use. In mild symptomatic exposures, one kit is given, moderate exposures receive two kits, and severe exposures receive three kits. Any patient who requires three kits or has seizures also receives 10 mg of diazepam intramuscularly or equivalent dosing of another benzodiazepine.[22] Pediatric AtroPens are now available in doses of 0.5 and 1 mg per pen.

Disposition

Because of the potential prolonged effects of acetylcholinesterase inhibition, most patients with significant exposures require hospital admission. An occasional person with chronic exposure, depressed cholinesterase levels, and mild visual or GI symptoms may be followed on an outpatient basis. Although the laboratory role is limited, if cholinesterase levels are available, they may be useful for treatment and disposition decisions. Normal or minimally depressed levels in asymptomatic or minimally symptomatic patients may allow discharge with outpatient follow-up after 4 to 6 hours, to ensure that progressive toxicity is not occurring. Patients with severely depressed levels (usually associated with significant symptoms) require admission and close monitoring, usually in an intensive care unit. Patients may develop rebound toxicity several days after apparently satisfactory response to initial treatment. Rebound toxicity may occur for many reasons, including persistent release of organophosphates from lipid stores. There have been reports in the literature of an intermediate syndrome that is purportedly caused by an abnormality at the neuromuscular junction. Review of these case reports suggests, however, that it is likely these patients received inadequate initial treatment or premature discontinuation of treatment.[6,23] The syndrome of delayed neuropathy also has been reported as a different entity from the strict or pure cholinergic effects and affects an axonal enzyme.[6] Cholinesterase levels should be followed daily after pralidoxime is discontinued, with 3 consecutive days of improving cholinesterase levels, before the physician can feel comfortable that most of the toxin has been eliminated.

CARBAMATE INSECTICIDES

Carbamate insecticides (see Box 161-1) are another class of acetylcholinesterase inhibitors and are differentiated from the organophosphorus compounds by their relatively short duration of toxic effects. Carbamates inhibit acetylcholinesterase for minutes to hours, and the carbamate-cholinesterase binding is reversible.[2] Although the clinical picture of acute carbamate poisoning may closely resemble organophosphate poisoning, the toxic effects are limited in duration; patients may require only decontamination, supportive care, and treatment

BOX 161-3. Chlorinated Hydrocarbon Pesticides

Aldrin	Aldrite Drinox
Benzene	BHC
Chlordane	Chlordan
Chlordecone	Kepone
Chlorobenzilate	Acaraben
Chlorophenothane	DDT
Diclofol	Kelthane
Dieldrin	Dieldrite
Dienochlor	Pentac
Endosulfan	Thiodan
Endrin	Hexadrin
Ethylan	Perthane
Gamma hexachlorobenzene	Lindane
Heptachlor	Rhodiachlor
Methoxychlor	Marlate
Mirex	Dechlorane
Terpene polychlorinated	Strobane
Toxaphene	Toxakil

BHC, benzene hexachloride; DDT, dichlorodiphenyltrichloroethane; HCB, hexachlorobenzene.

with adequate doses of atropine. Pralidoxime usually is not needed to treat known carbamate poisoning, and animal studies suggest that pralidoxime administration may produce greater toxicity in cases of carbaryl (Sevin) poisoning.[24] Nevertheless, if doubt exists as to whether a severe poisoning is due to a carbamate or organophosphate, pralidoxime should be administered.

CHLORINATED HYDROCARBON PESTICIDES

Dichlorodiphenyltrichloroethane (DDT), the prototype of chlorinated hydrocarbon insecticides, was first used extensively during World War II for the control of typhus and malaria and was used widely in the United States as a general insecticide after the war. Environmental contamination and the development of safer chlorinated hydrocarbon pesticides led to the banning of DDT in the United States in 1972. The compounds replacing DDT (Box 161-3) are used extensively in agricultural, commercial, and residential pest control. Some, such as chlordane, have come under close scrutiny in recent years.[25] Lindane or γ-hexachlorobenzene (Kwell), a well-known and widely used scabicide, was banned in 2000 for normal human use because of concerns over toxicity.

Principles of Disease

Pharmacology

Chlorinated hydrocarbon pesticides are highly lipid soluble. They are readily absorbed through dermal, respiratory, and GI routes.[26] Dermal and GI exposures account for most clinical poisonings, including inappropriate external use of lindane or other compounds and the occasional accidental oral administration of lindane. Because they are so lipid soluble, these compounds are stored in fatty tissues, and repeated small exposures may result in accumulation and eventual clinical toxicity.[27]

Pathophysiology

Chlorinated hydrocarbon insecticides primarily affect axonal membranes, resulting in neuronal irritability and excitation. Toxicity occurs in central and peripheral neurons.[28] Chlorinated hydrocarbons induce hepatic microsomal enzymes and produce hepatic tumors in some animal models. This potential carcinogenicity is the basis for the current human health concerns, but is only theoretical at present. Chlorinated hydrocarbon insecticides, including chlorinated hydrocarbon solvents, may sensitize the myocardium to circulating catecholamines and increase susceptibility to ventricular dysrhythmias, such as tachycardia and fibrillation.[28]

Clinical Features

Signs and Symptoms

The primary clinical picture of acute or cumulative toxicity from chlorinated hydrocarbon pesticides is related to their neurotoxicity. Premonitory peripheral signs and symptoms, such as tremor or paresthesias, are unusual, and the first sign of toxicity may be the acute onset of seizure activity.[29] Additional signs include confusion, combativeness, and muscle twitching. Untreated, continued muscle activity can lead to hyperthermia, metabolic acidosis, and rhabdomyolysis with secondary acute tubular necrosis.[30] Because many of these agents are halogenated, ventricular dysrhythmias may occur from catecholamine sensitization and direct myocardial toxic effects. Immediate hepatotoxicity is unlikely without secondary hyperthermia or other metabolic complications.[28,31] Long-term exposure may result in neuropsychiatric complaints.[32] Diagnosis may be difficult in chlorinated hydrocarbon pesticide exposure because the patient may be unable to provide a history. Prehospital personnel are often in the best position to obtain information concerning pesticide availability and use and the situation surrounding the exposure. Another clue is the solvent odor and oily feel of the hydrocarbon solvent containing the highly lipid-soluble chlorinated hydrocarbon pesticides.

Diagnostic Strategies

Diagnosis must be confirmed by history or by investigation at the site of the exposure to establish the offending agent with certainty. No specific tests are readily available to confirm the diagnosis of chlorinated hydrocarbon pesticide poisoning. Some reference laboratories can measure fat and plasma levels, but results are difficult to interpret and seldom are available during the acute phase of toxicity.[27,31] Ancillary laboratory and other studies should be based on the clinical condition, complications, and consideration of alternative diagnoses on an individual basis.

Differential Considerations

The differential diagnosis includes virtually every condition that produces seizures. The specific diagnosis depends on obtaining the history of significant acute or chronic chlorinated hydrocarbon pesticide exposure.

Management

Skin decontamination with soap and water may reduce toxicity in acute dermal exposure. High lipid solubility results in rapid absorption, and delayed GI decontamination is not of benefit. The exception is the use of repeat doses of cholestyramine (4 g orally every 8 hours) for chlordane ingestions.[32-34]

The primary therapeutic objective is seizure control, best accomplished with short-acting benzodiazepines or barbiturates. Recurrent seizures or status epilepticus may require high-dose barbiturates and paralyzing agents (e.g., pancuronium or vecuronium) to prevent secondary morbidity from continuous motor activity in prolonged seizures. The seizure activity is usually self-limiting, lasting only 1 or 2 days even in severe cases.[29,33,35]

Continuous cardiac monitoring during the acute phase is indicated because of the potential for myocardial sensitization. Ventricular dysrhythmias are most likely to occur during seizure activity because of the high circulating catecholamine levels and other metabolic abnormalities present during seizures. Dysrhythmias should be treated with β-adrenergic antagonists, such as propranolol, metoprolol, or esmolol, to reduce the effect of catecholamines on the myocardium.

Additional treatment should focus on the complications of prolonged seizure activity, such as aggressive external cooling measures for hyperthermia. Metabolic acidosis is almost always transient and resolves spontaneously without treatment. Rhabdomyolysis and myoglobinuria should be anticipated. Other complications of seizures should be treated as indicated. Because of their high lipid solubility, chlorinated hydrocarbon pesticides are distributed largely in tissues and are not amenable to hemoperfusion, dialysis, or other attempts to enhance elimination.

Disposition

Patients who have acute or cumulative chlorinated hydrocarbon pesticide toxicity require hospitalization until their seizures have been controlled, complications have resolved, and they have returned to their neurologic baselines; this usually occurs within 1 or 2 days. Severe complications, such as renal failure from rhabdomyolysis, may prolong the clinical course.

SUBSTITUTED PHENOLS

The substituted phenols include dinitrophenol, pentachlorophenol (PCP), and dinitrocresol (Box 161-4). These compounds have been used since the 1930s as insecticides, termiticides, herbicides, and wood preservatives. They currently are used in agricultural, commercial, and residential applications, including over-the-counter preparations for home gardeners. Substituted phenols such as dinitrophenol (DNP) are abused as weight-reduction agents and occasionally appear in illegitimate weight-reduction operations. Ads for DNP are found on the Internet.[36]

BOX 161-4. Substituted Phenol Pesticides

Chlorinated Phenols
- Pentachlorophenol
  - Dowicide EC7
  - PCP
  - Penchlorol
  - Pentacon
  - Penwar
  - Priltox
  - Sinituho
  - Triox
- 2,4-Dichlorophenol
  - Veg-I-Kill
- 2,4,6-Trichlorophenol

Nitrophenolic Compounds
- Dinitrophenol
  - Chemox PE
- Dinobuton
  - Acrex
  - Dessin
  - Dinofen
  - Drawinol
  - Talan
- Dinocap
  - Karathane
  - Crotothane
- Dinopenton
- Dinoprop
- Dinosam
  - DNAP
- Dinoseb
  - Basanite
  - Caldron
  - Chemox General
  - Chemsect DNBP
  - Dinitro-3
  - Dynamyte
  - Elgetol d8
  - Gebutox
  - Kiloseb
  - Nitropone C
  - Premerge 3
  - Sinox General
  - Subitex
  - Unicrop DNBP
- Dinosulfon
- Dinoterb
- Dinoterbon

Nitrocresolic Compounds
- Dinitrocresol
  - DNC
  - DNOC
  - Chemsect DNOC
  - Elgetol 30
  - Nitrador
  - Selinon
  - Sinox
  - Trifocide

PCP, pentachlorophenol; DNC, dinitrocresol: DNOC, 2-methyl-4,6-dinitrophenol (dinitro-*o*-cresol).

Principles of Disease

Pharmacology

Substituted phenols are readily absorbed through the skin and GI tract, and aerosols may be absorbed through the respiratory tract. There is some potential for cumulative toxicity with repeated exposures, but much less so than with the organophosphorus and chlorinated hydrocarbon pesticides already discussed.

Pathophysiology

Substituted phenols produce their toxicity by uncoupling cellular oxidative phosphorylation; this leads to inefficient production of high-energy phosphate substrates and increased cellular use of oxygen, glucose, and water, with subsequent excessive heat production.[37] These compounds are commonly used during the summer when the external heat predisposes users to increased toxicity.[38,39] In addition, nitro-substituted phenols may produce methemoglobinemia.

Clinical Features

Patients with substituted phenol toxicity present hypermetabolic and hyperthermic, tachycardic, tachypneic, and profusely diaphoretic. They also may have a relative hypovolemia from insensible excessive fluid losses through sweating and metabolic consumption. Loss of energy production in neurologic tissues results in neurologic changes ranging from confusion to seizures and coma. Renal and hepatic injury are common, and rhabdomyolysis with myoglobinuria is commonly present.[30] Because phenols are generally corrosive, patients with dermal exposures often show evidence of irritation or chemical burn, and some substituted phenols, such as dinitrophenol, produce a characteristic yellow staining of the skin or mucous membranes at the site of absorption. This same staining can be found throughout the internal organs at autopsy.[38]

A complication of long-term exposure to these compounds is the formation of cataracts. This condition was common in patients who used substituted phenols as part of a weight-reduction regimen and was partially responsible for banning this substance. The cataracts regress spontaneously after exposure is discontinued.[40]

Diagnostic Strategies

Laboratory evaluation of patients with substituted phenol toxicity is aimed at identifying deficiency of aerobic metabolic substrates, including oxygen, glucose, and water. A complete blood count may reveal hemoconcentration and a nonspecific leukocytosis. Electrolyte abnormalities depend on the duration and severity of symptoms, environmental factors, and complications or underlying disease states. Arterial blood gas measurements show varying degrees of acidosis, depending on the extent of anaerobic metabolic activity because of oxidative phosphorylation uncoupling and associated tissue hypoperfusion from dehydration. Serum enzyme determinations document the extent of hepatic, renal, and skeletal muscle injury. The presence of phenolic compounds in the urine of a patient with this clinical picture strongly suggests substituted phenol pesticides as the causative agent.

Differential Considerations

Acute toxicity from substituted phenol poisoning is difficult to distinguish initially from typical environmental heat-related emergencies or toxicity from sympathomimetics or salicylates. Continued evidence of hypermetabolic activity and metabolic acidosis after routine cooling measures, rehydration, and other supportive care should lead to a consideration of toxin-induced states. Persistent hyperthermia and acidosis in a weightlifter should trigger concern for DNP abuse. The presence of yellow staining virtually clinches the diagnosis.[38]

Management

Initial treatment is directed toward aggressive supportive care with body temperature control; treatment of acidosis; protecting the kidneys, brain, and liver from hyperthermic damage; and providing the basic substrates for excessive metabolic activity: oxygen, glucose, and water.[38] If the chemical exposure is known or recognized, early decontamination of affected sites is important. Therapy should be directed toward prevention or minimization of the associated complications discussed previously.

Disposition

Patients with mild toxicity usually can be stabilized after a few hours and discharged from the emergency department. Patients with significant organ system injury or a high likelihood of complications, such as prolonged or recurrent seizures, significant alteration of consciousness, and rhabdomyolysis, require admission, usually to the intensive care unit.

CHLOROPHENOXY COMPOUNDS

The chlorophenoxy pesticides were developed in the early 1940s and hailed as a selective herbicide particularly effective against broad-leaf weeds. This class of herbicide developed a special notoriety during the Vietnam War as Agent Orange, a defoliant used in aerial spraying. Agent Orange consisted of a mixture of 2,4-dichlorophenoxyacetic acid (2,4-D) and 2,4,5-trichlorophenoxyacetic acid (2,4,5-T). 2,4,5-T is virtually always contaminated with isomers of tetrachlorodibenzo dioxin. This concern over dioxin exposure has led to the extensive medical investigations of Vietnam veterans and severe restrictions on the production and use of 2,4,5-T.[41] Because of the relative safety and broad-leaf selectivity of 2,4-D, however, most home gardeners find at least one of the substances listed in Box 161-5 on a shelf in their garages, and some old cans may contain 2,4,5-T or a mixture of both compounds.

Principles of Disease

Pharmacology

Chlorophenoxy compounds may be absorbed through the skin, GI tract, and respiratory tract, but almost all significant poisonings occur as a result of accidental or intentional ingestion. The lipid solubility of these compounds is low, and excretion is fairly rapid, so cumulative toxicity from repeated exposures does not occur.[42]

Pathophysiology

Although skeletal muscle is the target organ for chlorophenoxy herbicides, the exact mechanism is obscure.[28,43] Depending on severity, muscular abnormalities may range from generalized muscle weakness to acute rhabdomyolysis. Higher doses also may uncouple oxidative phosphorylation similar to that seen with the substituted phenols.[28]

Clinical Features

Similar to most organic pesticides in an organic solvent, the chlorophenoxy herbicides may produce

BOX 161-5. Chlorophenoxy Pesticides

2,4-Dichlorophenoxyacetic Acid (2,4-D)
Agrotec
Amoxone
Aqua-Kleen
Chloroxone
Crop Rider
Dacamine 4D
Ded-Weed
Desormone
Dicotox
Dinoxol
Dormone
Emulsamine BK
Emulsamine E-3
Envert DT
Esteron 99
Esteron Four
Estone
Fernesta
Fernimine
Fernoxone
Ferxone
Hedonal
Herbidal
Lawn-Keep
Lithate
Macondray
Miracle
Netagrone 600
Pennamine D
Planotox
Plantgard
Rhodia
Salvo
Superormone Concentre
Super D Weedone
Transamine
Vertron ZD
Visko-Rhap
Weed-B-Gon
Weedar
Weed-Rhap
Weed Tox
Weedtrol

2,4,5-Trichlorophenoxyacetic Acid (2,4,5-T)
Brush-Rhap
Decamine 4T
Ded-Weed Brush Killer
Esteron 245
Fence Rider
Forron
Inverton 245
Line Rider
Spontox
Super D Weedone
Tormona
Transamine
Trinoxol
Trioxone
Veon 245
Vertron 2T
Weedar
Weedone Envert T

2,4-D-2,4,5-T Mixtures
Decamine 2D-2T
Esteron Brush Killer
Transamine
Tributon
Visko-Phap LV2D-2T

BOX 161-6. Bipyridyl Compounds

Paraquat
Crisquat
Dextrone X
Esgram
Gramoxone

Diquat
Aquacide
Dextrone
Reglone
Reglox
Weedtrine-D

Paraquat-Diquat Mixtures
Preeglone
Priglone
Weedol

mild, nonspecific dermal and GI irritation with nausea, vomiting, and GI distress. Large exposures are likely to cause systemic symptoms ranging from diffuse myotonia and muscle fasciculations progressing to rhabdomyolysis, hyperthermia, and a hypermetabolic state with metabolic acidosis consistent with uncoupling of oxidative phosphorylation.[44]

Diagnostic Strategies

There are no specific tests for the detection of the chlorophenoxy compounds. Laboratory evaluation should be aimed at evaluating skeletal muscle injury and its complications. Severely poisoned patients require generalized organ system evaluation, including hepatic and renal function, because of the effects of rhabdomyolysis and hyperthermia.

Differential Considerations

Differential diagnostic possibilities include other causes of acute myopathy. This manifestation of chlorophenoxy compound toxicity is extremely rare, however, and without a definite history or strong suspicion of exposure, other explanations for acute myopathy should be pursued.

Management

Treatment consists of initial skin decontamination, activated charcoal or gastric lavage with early presentation, and basic supportive care. Serious toxic effects develop within 4 to 6 hours after ingestion, and treatment can be directed toward the specific problems of muscle weakness, airway and ventilatory support, and treatment for rhabdomyolysis. Treatment of hyperthermia and acidosis has been discussed previously.

Disposition

Asymptomatic or minimally symptomatic patients may be discharged with reassurance after 4 to 6 hours of observation. Patients with significant toxicity should be admitted for close observation and monitoring.

BIPYRIDYL COMPOUNDS

The bipyridyl (also called *dipyridyl*) compounds, paraquat and diquat (Box 161-6), were first investigated in the late 1950s and early 1960s. They are extremely effective contact herbicides that are rapidly inactivated by the surrounding soil in the event of overspray. Paraquat is activated when exposed to sunlight, which led to its use as the herbicide of choice during aerial spraying of marijuana by the U.S. and Mexican governments. After spraying, however, growers simply would harvest the crops before the plants were exposed to enough sunlight to damage the plants, resulting in an apparently healthy harvest but one contaminated with paraquat. The burning of marijuana pyrolyzes paraquat into a nontoxic form, a fact that was lost in the warning messages dispensed by the government at that time.[45]

Principles of Disease

Pharmacology

Of the two bipyridyl compounds in use, paraquat is the most clinically significant in terms of number of cases and toxic effects, and it is the primary consideration of this discussion. Paraquat use is tightly regulated in the United States but is widespread throughout the world.

Diquat is found more easily in the United States and is included in some formulations of Roundup. Paraquat is absorbed through the skin, GI tract, and respiratory tract. Almost all fatal exposures have resulted from the ingestion of paraquat, although a few case reports have involved extensive skin contamination.[46] No fatal cases have been reported from inhalation of paraquat vapor or aerosols, but toxicity has occurred from this route of exposure. Diquat is poorly absorbed through intact skin, and most cases of toxicity result from ingestion.[47]

Pathophysiology

Paraquat's toxic effect results from the production of superoxides created during cyclic oxidation-reduction reactions of the compound in tissues. Lipid peroxidation of cellular membranes seems to be one significant pathway of cellular injury.[48,49]

Paraquat selectively concentrates in the lungs because of an amine uptake mechanism in alveolar cells. In addition, high concentrations of oxygen significantly increase the extent of paraquat-induced injury, causing the lungs to be the major target organ. The pathophysiologic lesions include direct injury to the alveolar-capillary membrane followed by surfactant loss, adult respiratory distress syndrome, progressive pulmonary fibrosis, and respiratory failure.[50] Paraquat damages other major organ systems by the same cellular membrane effects, including the liver, kidney, heart, and central nervous system. Diquat has similar effects but is not preferentially accumulated in lung tissue.[47]

Clinical Features

Both agents are extremely corrosive and cause severe chemical burns of the oropharynx soon after ingestion. Patients who ingest concentrated paraquat frequently die as a result of esophageal perforation and mediastinitis before development of the characteristic progressive pulmonary injury. Patients with dermal paraquat exposures show significant skin irritation, and ocular exposures may produce severe corneal injury.[51] Other signs of GI irritation, such as nausea and vomiting, may occur.

The classic finding of paraquat-induced progressive pulmonary injury usually occurs over 1 to 3 weeks, although the clinical course varies considerably with severity of poisoning, involvement of other organ systems, and underlying medical problems.[50] This is not a factor in the emergency department, and the pulmonary injury is not discussed here. In contrast to paraquat, diquat usually spares the lungs but produces similar toxicity in all other organ systems.[47]

Diagnostic Strategies

Paraquat is measurable in the blood, and the nomogram provides a fairly accurate prognosis. In the United States, the assay is not readily available, and by the time the results are obtained, nothing more can be done about the eventual outcome in most cases. There is a qualitative bedside test using the reduction of paraquat or diquat in alkalinized urine by sodium dithionite, but the reagent frequently is not available.[44] Studies other than evaluation of caustic GI injury and pulmonary and renal damage should be directed toward secondary effects of the poisoning.

Differential Considerations

A person with acute paraquat or diquat ingestion is likely to present with the initial complaint of an acute corrosive injury; the differential diagnosis should encompass all corrosive agents. Successful therapeutic intervention for paraquat toxicity is extremely time dependent, and patient outcome depends on the history. Any patient who has evidence of pulmonary or other organ injury caused by paraquat exposure is already beyond recovery.

Management

The key to successful treatment of an acute paraquat exposure depends almost entirely on aggressive early decontamination measures to limit absorption. Thorough skin cleansing is obvious and straightforward in dermal exposures. Aggressive gastric lavage and administration of activated charcoal may be lifesaving, but these measures must be considered in the context of a corrosive ingestion. Early endoscopy and surgical intervention may be necessary if there is evidence of esophageal perforation and mediastinitis. Although Fuller's Earth and bentonite are recommended as adsorbents in paraquat ingestions, activated charcoal is readily available and has equal, if not greater, efficacy.[52]

Although controversial, many toxicologists recommend rapid initiation of charcoal hemoperfusion to lower plasma paraquat levels and to limit pulmonary and other organ system uptake of paraquat. Many also have recommended serial and combined hemoperfusion and hemodialysis, particularly during the first 24 hours after exposure.[53,54] There are multiple suggested treatment protocols for paraquat, such as *N*-acetyl cysteine and low fraction of inspired oxygen, but no single therapy has proved universally successful.[55]

Disposition

Patients who have any significant dermal paraquat exposure and all patients who have ingested paraquat should be hospitalized and started on aggressive enhanced elimination therapy as outlined earlier. These patients should be observed and treated expectantly until paraquat levels are reported to be nonexistent or nontoxic.

PYRETHRINS AND PYRETHROIDS

Pyrethrins are naturally occurring insecticides of the yellow *Chrysanthemum cinerariifolium* and *Tanacetum cinerariifolium* and are among the oldest known insecticides, first used in the 1800s. Extracts of the dried flowers contain the active compound pyrethrum, which contains six naturally occurring pyrethrins. In addition, numerous synthetic derivatives, pyrethroids, have been produced and have greater chemical stability than the natural pyrethrins (Box 161-7). Type II

BOX 161-7. Pyrethrins and Pyrethroids

Pyrethrins	Bioallethrin
Pyrethrum extract	Bioresmethrin
Pyrethrin I	Cismethrin
Pyrethrin II	Cymethrin
Cinerin I	Cypermethrin
Cinerin II	Decamethrin
Jasmolin I	Deltamethrin
Jasmolin II	Fenothrin
Pyrethroids	Fenvalerate
Allethrin	Furamethrin
Barthrin	Tetramethrin

pyrethroids contain a cyano substituent and are among the more toxic formulations of this class. These present a potential danger to humans, but type II pyrethroids are generally less toxic than many of the other classes already discussed and are being used more commonly.

Principles of Disease

Pharmacology

Because pyrethrins and pyrethroids are most commonly aerosolized, inhalation is the most likely source of exposure. The patient may not be aware of an exposure because pyrethrin and pyrethroid aerosols are used frequently as automated insect sprays in public areas. In these situations, concentrations rarely reach levels likely to produce symptoms in any but the most sensitized patient. Occasional ingestions have been reported, and significant toxicity is possible via this route. Systemic absorption via the dermal route is unlikely, but topical effects are possible. Most pyrethrins and pyrethroids are rapidly metabolized and deactivated in human exposure to the extent that cumulative toxicity is not a problem. Piperonyl butoxide, which is added as an insect "knock-down" agent, may add to the toxicity of the pyrethrum derivatives.

Pathophysiology

Pyrethrins and pyrethroids have a variety of pharmacologic effects in humans and other mammals.[56,57] Clinically the naturally occurring pyrethrins have the ability to cause sensitization and allergic phenomena. This property does not occur with the synthetic pyrethroids. Both classes are associated with sodium channel blockade, slowing the rate of activation of the sodium channel and extending the time the channel is open. In addition, both classes affect γ-aminobutyric acid receptors, inhibiting chloride channel function. Less significant effects include potentiation of nicotinic cholinergic neurotransmission, enhancement of norepinephrine release, and inhibition of calcium adenosine triphosphatase interference with sodium-calcium exchange across membranes.[56,57]

Clinical Features

Allergic manifestations, including potentially life-threatening events, may occur after acute inhalation or dermal exposure. Inhalation exposure often occurs with the use of a pyrethrin-based aerosol in an enclosed, poorly ventilated space. Local effects include lacrimation, rhinitis, rhinorrhea, sneezing, throat irritation, and pharyngeal and laryngeal edema. Lower respiratory effects include cough, shortness of breath, chest pain, and wheezing. Skin rashes consistent with a contact or allergic dermatitis have been reported, and photosensitivity may contribute to the dermatologic picture. There is potential for allergic cross-reactivity in patients who are allergic to ragweed.

Sodium channel–mediated and γ-aminobutyric acid–mediated chloride channel effects mediate neurologic signs and symptoms. Facial paresthesias have been reported, and seizures have occurred with massive ingestions.[56,57] Nonspecific symptoms, such as headache, fatigue, dizziness, and weakness, have been reported.

Diagnostic Strategies

No laboratory tests are available to measure pyrethrins or pyrethroids in a clinical setting.

Differential Considerations

The differential diagnosis of the signs and symptoms of pyrethrin or pyrethroid toxicity includes the usual causes of bronchospasm or acute neurologic complications.

Management

Decontamination, including removal from a contaminated environment or washing, should be the first step. Definitive treatment is supportive and directed at the respiratory and neurologic complications.

Disposition

Disposition of a patient with exposure to pyrethrins depends on the severity of the underlying complications. If discharge from the emergency department is anticipated, the patient should be counseled with regard to the possibility of recurrent allergic phenomena on reexposure.

GLYPHOSATE

Glyphosate (Roundup) was introduced as a broad-spectrum nonselective herbicide in 1971 by the Monsanto Agricultural Company (St. Louis, Mo). It is the isopropyl ammonium salt of a noncholinesterase-inhibiting organophosphate herbicide. It is sold mixed with the surfactant polyoxyethylene amine (POEA). Because it is effective on broad-leaf weeds and does not undergo photodecomposition, it is popular in the home market. Newer formulations of Roundup may contain diquat.

Principles of Disease

Pharmacology

Glyphosate is poorly absorbed through the skin so that most exposures result from ingestion. The concentrated solution is extremely irritating, and patients may vomit with subsequent aspiration. The concentrated solution is provided as 41% glyphosate in 15% POEA. The directions state that it should be diluted to a 1% glyphosate solution.

Pathophysiology

Glyphosate is toxic to plants by inhibition of the enzyme 5-enolpyruvylskikimate-3 phosphatase-synthetase in the shikimic acid metabolic pathway. After application of glyphosate on the leaves, it is transported to the roots where the enzyme is active. Humans lack this enzyme and so are much less likely to develop toxicity. Reported toxicity is believed to result largely from the surfactant POEA and may reflect the direct corrosive effect from the amine salt, or it may uncouple oxidative phosphorylation.[58]

Clinical Features

Most ingestions of the dilute solution cause only minimal symptoms, including GI distress. Patients ingesting large volumes of dilute solutions or moderate volumes of concentrated solutions complain of sore throat, nausea, abdominal pain, and fever. They may develop vomiting, diarrhea, respiratory distress, noncardiogenic pulmonary edema, dysrhythmias, shock, coma, and renal failure. Acidosis most likely reflects poor tissue perfusion and cardiovascular compromise.[58] Negative prognostic indicators include shock, acidosis, and persistent hyperkalemia.[58]

Diagnostic Strategies

The key element in diagnosis is history of ingestion. Laboratory analysis shows an anion gap metabolic acidosis, hypoxemia, and hyperkalemia. Elevated transaminases may occur in 30% of ill patients, and signs of renal failure may develop in persistent shock states. The electrocardiogram may show ventricular dysrhythmias and secondary signs of hypoxemia.[58]

Differential Diagnosis

The differential diagnosis includes most corrosive ingestions. The findings of hyperkalemia and metabolic acidosis may suggest hydrofluoric acid ingestions. A normal ionized calcium level may help rule out hydrofluoric acid exposure. Any cause of aspiration also should be considered. The history is the most useful in the differential diagnosis.

Management

Treatment is supportive. The patient may require positive-pressure ventilation to overcome the noncardiogenic pulmonary edema. POEA also may be a direct cardiac depressant; inotropic agents can be useful. Hyperkalemia should be treated in the usual fashion with fluids, medications to shift potassium into the cell (bicarbonate, calcium, β-adrenergic agonists), and enhanced elimination (ion-sequestering resins). If there is a suggestion of significant corrosive ingestion, early endoscopy with placement of stent, high-dose steroids, and laparotomy all may be considered.

Disposition

Patients with small ingestions of dilute substances may be observed for 6 hours and discharged if asymptomatic. Patients with complaints consistent with corrosive ingestions require admission and GI evaluation. Any patient with pulmonary complaints requires admission and intensive supportive care.

DEET

N,N-diethyl-m-toluamide or N,N-diethyl-3-methylbenzamide (DEET) is not a pesticide but an insect repellent. It is the most widely used chemical insect repellent in the United States. DEET was developed by scientists at the U.S. Department of Agriculture in 1946, patented by the U.S. Army shortly thereafter, and released to the general public in 1957.[59] Now with the prevalence of Lyme disease and other concerning arthropod-borne diseases, the use of DEET has increased greatly. Formulations containing DEET range from 5% to 100%. The U.S. Army routinely used 75% solutions until 1987 but now uses a 35% time-release, polymer-based formulation. The American Academy of Pediatrics suggests that no more than a 10% solution be used on children.[59]

Principles of Disease

Pharmacology

DEET is lipophilic and can be absorbed through the skin. Skin absorption and toxicity increase with repeated applications, increased ambient temperatures, sweating, and abraded, thin skin. Ingestion may lead to toxicity.[60]

Pathophysiology

DEET primarily affects the central nervous system. Its mechanism of action is currently unknown. It may sensitize the skin and cause allergic reactions.

Clinical Features

Prolonged skin contact may lead to contact dermatitis, and prolonged contact with high concentrations has led to skin blisters. Patients who have ingested DEET or have repeated skin applications under conditions that enhance absorption have developed liver function test abnormalities and neurologic findings, including encephalopathy, seizures, movement disorders, and coma.[60] Most exposures to DEET result in minimal toxicity and should not preclude its use in susceptible populations where significant arthropod-borne diseases are prevalent.[61]

Diagnostic Strategies

Exposure history is central to the diagnosis. Although DEET can be detected in urine, most laboratories are not able to do this testing during the acute toxicity phase. An electroencephalogram may be useful in a patient with coma or encephalopathy and seizures.

Differential Diagnosis

The differential diagnosis includes conditions that may cause encephalopathy, seizures, and movement disorders. Such conditions may include drug intoxication, infectious causes, drug interactions, and structural defects.

Management

Treatment is supportive. If DEET exposure is suspected, the skin should be thoroughly decontaminated. Oils or lipophilic agents should be avoided because they enhance skin absorption. After DEET ingestion, milk products and oil-containing foods should be avoided until the GI tract has been emptied of the offending agent. Seizures should be treated with benzodiazepines.

Disposition

Asymptomatic patients who have ingested DEET-containing repellents should be observed for 4 to 6 hours. Patients who develop neurologic symptoms should be admitted and observed.

KEY CONCEPTS

- All patients exposed to cholinesterase inhibitors should be assumed to be dermally contaminated and should be decontaminated. Emergency department personnel need to be protected during this process.
- Morbidity in cholinesterase inhibitor exposure results from early airway compromise secondary to copious secretions, status epilepticus, and late respiratory failure.
- Vital signs in cholinesterase inhibitor exposure may reflect bradycardia or tachycardia, hypertension or hypotension, and miosis or mydriasis.
- The clinical endpoint for atropine administration is drying of airway secretions.
- Pralidoxime should be given to all organophosphorus-poisoned patients who require atropine regardless of time since exposure.
- With chlorinated hydrocarbon exposures, skin decontamination with protection of personnel is indicated.
- Catecholamine administration is avoided in chlorinated hydrocarbon exposures if possible.
- Supportive care, temperature control, and seizure control must be aggressive.
- Substituted phenol toxicity is suspected in hypermetabolic patients in whom environmental conditions are not conducive to heat-related illness or in whom salicylate toxicity is not a consideration.
- Rapid cooling and substrate provision (glucose) are the two most important therapies in substituted phenol toxicity.
- Diagnosis of chlorophenoxy compound toxicity depends on a history of accidental or deliberate ingestion.
- Treatment of chlorophenoxy compound toxicity is supportive.
- Paraquat and diquat ingestions cause a severe corrosive burn to the GI tract.
- Rapid GI decontamination may be the only hope in paraquat and diquat ingestions.
- When pulmonary and renal dysfunction develop, the prognosis is poor.
- Pyrethrin and pyrethroid exposures are usually benign except for massive ingestions.
- The predominant form of pyrethrin and pyrethroid toxicity is allergic.
- Small ingestions of dilute glyphosate solutions are GI irritants. Large or concentrated ingestions may cause acidosis, hyperkalemia, and noncardiogenic pulmonary edema.
- Treatment of glyphosate toxicity is supportive.
- DEET should not be applied over abraded or raw skin.
- DEET applications to children should be restricted to 10% solutions, should not be used under occlusive clothing, and should be washed off completely between applications.
- Treatment of DEET exposure is supportive.

REFERENCES

1. The Persian Gulf experience and health. NIH Technology Assessment Workshop Panel. *JAMA* 272:391, 1994.
2. Tafuri J, Roberts J: Organophosphate poisoning. *Ann Emerg Med* 16:193, 1987.
3. Selden BS, Curry SC: Prolonged succinylcholine-induced paralysis in organophosphate insecticide poisoning. *Ann Emerg Med* 16:215, 1987.
4. Namba T, et al: Poisoning due to organophosphate insecticides: Acute and chronic manifestations. *Am J Med* 50:475, 1971.
5. Johnson PS, Michaelis EK: Characterization of organophosphate interactions at N-methyl-D-aspartate receptors in brain synaptic membranes. *Mol Pharmacol* 41:750, 1992.
6. Johnson MK, et al: Evaluation of antidotes for poisoning by organophosphorus pesticides. *Emerg Med* 12:22, 2000.
7. Clark G: Organophosphate insecticides and behavior: A review. *Aerospace Med* 42:735, 1971.
8. Gutmann L, Besser R: Organophosphate intoxication: Pharmacologic, neurophysiologic, clinical, and therapeutic considerations. *Semin Neurol* 10:46, 1990.
9. Shih TM, Duniho SM, McDonough JH: Control of nerve agent-induced seizures is critical for neuroprotection and survival. *Toxicol Appl Pharmacol* 188:69, 2003.
10. Petroianu G, Ruefer R: Poisoning with organophosphorus compounds. *Emerg Med (Fremantle)* 13:258, 2001.
11. Eddleston M, Roberts D, Buckley N: Management of severe organophosphorus pesticide poisoning. *Crit Care* 6:259, 2002.
12. Eddleston M, Singh S, Buckley N: Acute organophosphorus poisoning. *Clin Evidence* 9:1542, 2003.
13. Sungur M, Guven M: Intensive care management of organophosphate insecticide poisoning. *Crit Care* 5:211, 2001.
14. Golsousidis H, Kokkas V: Use of 19,590 mg of atropine during 24 days of treatment, after a case of unusually severe parathion poisoning. *Hum Toxicol* 4:339, 1985.
15. McDonough JH Jr, et al: Anticonvulsant treatment of nerve agent seizures: Anticholinergics versus diazepam in soman-intoxicated guinea pigs. *Epilepsy Res* 38:1, 2000.

16. Eddleston M, et al: Oximes in acute organophosphorous pesticide poisoning: A systematic review of clinical trials. *QJM* 95:275, 2002.
17. Worek F, et al: Reappraisal of indications and limitations of oxime therapy in organophosphate poisoning. *Hum Exp Toxicol* 16:466, 1997.
18. Feldmann RJ, Szajewski J: Cholinergic syndrome. In: IPIC INTOX Databank, 1998, http://www.intox.org/databank/documents/treat/treate/tr15_e.htm.
19. Medicis JJ, et al: Pharmacokinetics following a loading plus a continuous infusion of pralidoxime compared with the traditional short infusion regimen in human volunteers. *J Toxicol Clin Toxicol* 34:289, 1996.
20. Dickson EW, et al: Diazepam inhibits organophosphate-induced central respiratory depression. *Acad Emerg Med* 10:1303, 2003.
21. Shih T, McDonough JH Jr, Koplovitz I: Anticonvulsants for soman-induced seizure activity. *J Biomed Sci* 6:86, 1999.
22. Sidell FR, Borak J: Chemical warfare agents: II. Nerve agents. *Ann Emerg Med* 21:865, 1992.
23. Senanayake N, Sanmuganathan PS: Extrapyramidal manifestations complicating organophosphorus insecticide poisoning. *Hum Exp Toxicol* 14:600, 1995.
24. Kurtz PH: Pralidoxime in the treatment of carbamate intoxication. *Am J Emerg Med* 8:68, 1990.
25. National Academy of Sciences Committee on Toxicology, Commission on Life Sciences: *An Assessment of the Health Risks of Seven Pesticides Used for Termite Control.* Washington, D.C., National Academy Press, 1982.
26. Feldmann RJ, Maibach HI: Percutaneous penetration of some pesticides and herbicides in man. *Toxicol Appl Pharmacol* 28:126, 1974.
27. Hayes WJ Jr, Curley A: Storage and excretion of dieldrin and related compounds: Effect of occupational exposure. *Arch Environ Health* 16:155, 1968.
28. Hayes WJ Jr: *Pesticides Studied in Man.* Baltimore, Williams & Wilkins, 1982.
29. Jaeger U, et al: Acute oral poisoning with lindane-solvent mixtures. *Vet Hum Toxicol* 26:11, 1984.
30. Curry SC, Chang D, Connor D: Drug- and toxin-induced rhabdomyolysis. *Ann Emerg Med* 18:1068, 1989.
31. Stehr-Green PA, et al: An evaluation of serum pesticide residue levels and liver function in persons exposed to dairy products contaminated with heptachlor. *JAMA* 259:374, 1988.
32. Kilburn KH: Chlordane as a neurotoxin in humans. *South Med J* 90:299, 1997.
33. Aks SE, et al: Acute accidental lindane ingestion in toddlers. *Ann Emerg Med* 26:647, 1995.
34. Cohn WJ, et al: Treatment of chlordecone (Kepone) toxicity with cholestyramine: Results of a controlled clinical trial. *N Engl J Med* 298:243, 1978.
35. Cable GG, Doherty S: Acute carbamate and organochlorine toxicity causing convulsions in an agricultural pilot: A case report. *Aviat Space Environ Med* 70:68, 1999.
36. New York State Department of Health: State health commissioner warns of danger of weight loss product. 2001. Available at: http://www.health.state.ny.us/nysdoh/commish/2001/dinitrophenols.htm.
37. Ilivicky J, Casida JE: Uncoupling action of 2,4-dinitrophenols, 2-trifluoromethylbenzimidazoles and certain other pesticide chemicals upon mitochondria from different sources and its relation to toxicity. *Biochem Pharmacol* 18:1389, 1969.
38. Leftwich RB, et al: Dinitrophenol poisoning: A diagnosis to consider in undiagnosed fever. *South Med J* 75:182, 1982.
39. Jorens PG, Schepens PJ: Human pentachlorophenol poisoning. *Hum Exp Toxicol* 12:479, 1993.
40. Kurt TL, et al: Dinitrophenol in weight loss: The poison center and public health safety. *Vet Hum Toxicol* 28:574, 1986.
41. Kahn PC, et al: Dioxins and dibenzofurans in blood and adipose tissue of Agent Orange-exposed Vietnam veterans and matched controls. *JAMA* 259:1661, 1988.
42. Reifenrath WG, Hawkins GS, Kurtz MS: Percutaneous penetration and skin retention of topically applied compounds: An in vitro-in vivo study. *J Pharm Sci* 80:526, 1991.
43. Berwick P: 2,4-dichlorophenoxyacetic acid poisoning in man: Some interesting clinical and laboratory findings. *JAMA* 214:1114, 1970.
44. Bradberry SM, et al: Mechanisms of toxicity, clinical features, and management of acute chlorophenoxy herbicide poisoning: A review. *J Toxicol Clin Toxicol* 38:111, 2000.
45. Landrigan PJ, et al: Paraquat and marijuana: Epidemiologic risk assessment. *Am J Public Health* 73:784, 1983.
46. Smith JG: Paraquat poisoning by skin absorption: A review. *Hum Toxicol* 7:15, 1988.
47. Jones GM, Vale JA: Mechanisms of toxicity, clinical features, and management of diquat poisoning: A review. *J Toxicol Clin Toxicol* 38:123, 2000.
48. Fukushima T, et al: Mechanism of cytotoxicity of paraquat: I. NADH oxidation and paraquat radical formation via complex I. *Exp Toxicol Pathol* 45:345, 1993.
49. Yasaka T, et al: Further studies of lipid peroxidation in human paraquat poisoning. *Arch Intern Med* 146:681, 1986.
50. Smith LL: Mechanism of paraquat toxicity in lung and its relevance to treatment. *Hum Toxicol* 6:31, 1987.
51. Manoguerra AS: Full thickness skin burns secondary to an unusual exposure to diquat dibromide. *J Toxicol Clin Toxicol* 28:107, 1990.
52. Okonek S, et al: Successful treatment of paraquat poisoning: Activated charcoal per os and "continuous hemoperfusion." *J Toxicol Clin Toxicol* 19:807, 1982.
53. Proudfoot AT, Prescott LF, Jarvie DR: Haemodialysis for paraquat poisoning. *Hum Toxicol* 6:69, 1987.
54. Suzuki K, et al: Effect of aggressive haemoperfusion on the clinical course of patients with paraquat poisoning. *Hum Exp Toxicol* 12:323, 1993.
55. Honore P, et al: Paraquat poisoning: "State of the art." *Acta Clin Belg* 49:220, 1994.
56. Ray DE, Forshaw PJ: Pyrethroid insecticides: Poisoning syndromes, synergies, and therapy. *J Toxicol Clin Toxicol* 38:95, 2000.
57. Soderlund DM, et al: Mechanisms of pyrethroid neurotoxicity: Implications for cumulative risk assessment. *Toxicology* 171:3, 2002.
58. Ling HL, et al: Clinical presentations and prognostic factors of a glyphosate-surfactant herbicide intoxication: A review of 131 cases. *Acad Emerg Med* 7:906, 2000..
59. Fradin MS: Mosquitoes and mosquito repellents: A clinician's guide. Ann Intern Med 128:931, 1998.
60. Tennenbein M: Severe toxic reactions and death following the ingestion of diethyltoluamide-containing insect repellents. *JAMA* 258:1509, 1987.
61. Koren G, Matsui D, Bailey B: DEET-based insect repellents: Safety implications for children and pregnant and lactating women. *Can Med Assoc J* 169:209, 2003.

CHAPTER 162 Plants, Mushrooms, and Herbal Medications

Richard D. Shih

PERSPECTIVE

Botanicals such as plants, herbal products, and mushrooms have a long-standing and important place in medical history. Their use as therapeutic agents has been documented in the earliest of medical writings. The extraction of alkaloids from the opium poppy in the 1800s was a forerunner of modern pharmacology. The general public increasingly is using herbal products for medicinal purposes. Despite the tremendous growth in popularity of herbal products, data on herbal efficacy and toxicity are limited. This chapter does not focus on the medicinal benefits of natural products, but rather the toxicology related to their exposure or utility.

Epidemiology

Although plants, mushrooms, and herbal products all are derived naturally, they have different exposure patterns and epidemiology.

Unintentional Childhood Exposure

Unintentional childhood exposure occurs most commonly with plants. Approximately 5% of all poison center calls involve plants. Of these, about 75% involve children younger than age 6. Most of these cases involve household plants with a limited amount of plant or toxin ingested resulting in little or no toxicity.

Misidentification of Botanical

Natural plant and mushroom gathering for personal ingestion is a popular activity. Mistakes while foraging occur commonly, with the potential for serious toxicity and numerous fatalities. In contrast to unintentional childhood exposures, foraging accidents usually involve adults and plants or mushrooms and are associated with a much larger toxin burden because a larger quantity of the botanical is ingested. Another type of botanical misidentification occurs with herbal products when plants used for herbal manufacture are misidentified by the manufacturer and incorrectly packaged and marketed.

Drugs of Abuse

Many plants and mushrooms are abused for their mind-altering potential, including hallucinogenic mushrooms and anticholinergic plants, such as jimsonweed.

BOTANICAL IDENTIFICATION

Identification of the botanical in question is most useful, but most patients do not have any knowledge of botany or plant identification. The name of the plant or mushroom is often confusing because the scientific name is not typically known, and common names often overlap. Most emergency department personnel cannot identify common plants, such as mistletoe, holly berries, philodendron, and others. Several resources may be helpful, including plant atlases, CD-ROM plant databases, a local botanical expert, botanical garden personnel, or a poison center. With herbal products, the product name or herbal plant may be known. Because of the limited Food and Drug Administration (FDA) regulation, however, the purported herb might have been harvested from the wrong plant or contaminated with other toxic material.

Plants

Among more than 100,000 plant exposures reported to U.S. poison centers annually, most plant exposures occur in children (<6 years old) and involve household plants, and 80% of exposed individuals never develop any toxicologic symptoms. Hospitalizations owing to plant poisoning are rare, with fatalities occurring in less than 1 in 1 million exposures. Of thousands of different plant species, only a few are dangerously toxic.

Abrus precatorius

Abrus precatorius (Figure 162-1), known as the jequirity pea, rosary pea, prayer bean, Seminole bean, Indian bean, and crab's eye, contains the toxin abrin, which affects protein synthesis, leading to cell death. The toxin is found in highest concentration in the seeds, which are used in jewelry or decoration. Because of their attractiveness, the seeds often are ingested by children. The hard, shiny coat causes most seeds to pass through the gastrointestinal tract without being digested. If the seeds are chewed or do not pass through the bowel rapidly and become digested, abrin is released; nausea, vomiting, and abdominal pain can be severe, and fluid and electrolyte balance is disturbed.[1] Systemic absorption of the toxin is limited because the protein is enzymatically digested. Rare parenteral exposure of small amounts is associated with severe toxicity and possible death. Treatment is supportive, with attention to fluid rehydration and electrolytes. Asymptomatic patients should be treated with acti-

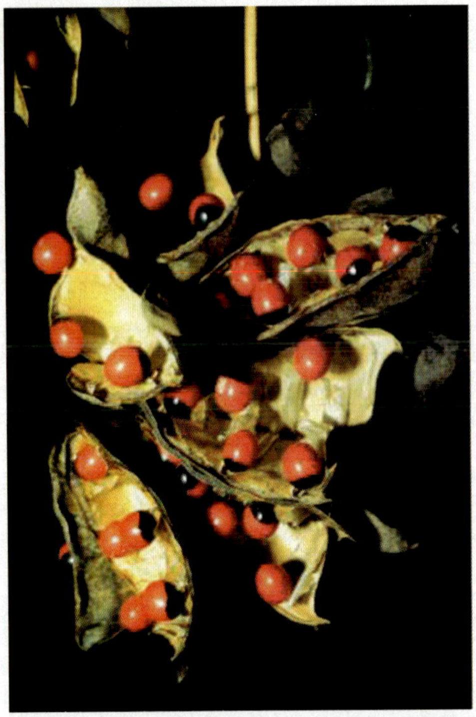

Figure 162-1. *Abrus precatorius* (jequirity pea or rosary pea). (Courtesy of Steven Setzer.)

vated charcoal, and whole-bowel irrigation may be helpful in moving numerous seeds more rapidly through the gastrointestinal tract.

Brassaia

The *Brassaia* is a popular indoor plant known as schefflera, umbrella tree, Australian umbrella tree, dwarf schefflera, rubber tree, and starleaf. This plant contains calcium oxalate crystals, which can cause mouth pain, but most ingestions cause mild or no symptoms.

Capsicum annum

Capsicum annum includes many types of peppers (e.g., chili pepper, red pepper, bell pepper) and contains the active toxin capsaicin. This alkaloid releases and depletes selected nerve terminals of substance P, causing a severe local inflammatory response, manifested by swelling, fluid exudation, and pain, which resolves rapidly as capsaicin depletes substance P.[7] Capsaicin is not absorbed well through intact skin, but symptoms rarely can occur with prolonged and intense exposure.[2] Ingestions often cause gastrointestinal symptoms depending on the amount of toxin exposure.[3] Most capsaicin exposures involve a pepper spray product causing chemical conjunctivitis.[4] Keratitis can occur and is assessed with fluorescein. Treatment consists of local irrigation and analgesics. Despite their often dramatic appearance, cases resolve rapidly over several hours without sequelae.[5] Inhalation of capsaicin-containing powders is less common but can cause severe pulmonary exudation and potential acute respiratory distress syndrome. Deaths have been reported. Treatment is supportive, but extracorporeal

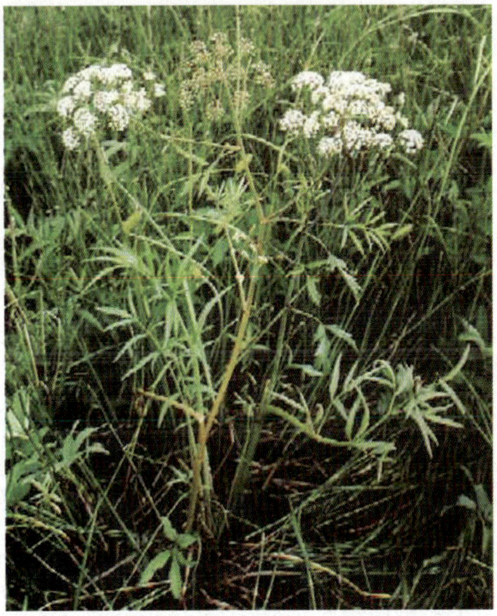

Figure 162-2. *Cicuta maculata* (water hemlock). (Courtesy of Steven Setzer.)

membrane oxygenation may be useful for acute respiratory distress syndrome.

Cicuta maculata

Cicuta maculata (Figure 162-2), commonly known as water hemlock, contains the potent neurotoxin cicutoxin. Deaths from water hemlock are among the most commonly reported plant exposure fatalities reported in the United States. Water hemlock has small white flowers at the ends of umbrella-like stems. They resemble *Daucus carota* (Queen Anne's lace) and *Heracleum lanatum* (cow parsnip). Mistaking water hemlock for one of these edible plants has been a common cause for exposure.[7] Ingestion of any part of the plant can lead to nausea, vomiting, and abdominal cramping. Severe toxicity is manifested by seizures, occurring within the first hour, which often are intractable and are a common cause of death. The toxic mechanism may be due to γ-aminobutyric acid (GABA) receptor antagonism. Fatality rates are 70%.[8] Aggressive supportive care is necessary, and asymptomatic suspected exposures should be treated aggressively with gastric lavage and activated charcoal. Patients often arrive in the emergency department with active seizures and should receive benzodiazepines and barbiturates.

Conium maculatum

Conium maculatum (Figure 162-3), or poison hemlock, was purported to be used in the execution of Socrates. It is mistaken for several edible plants, such as *Daucus carota* (Queen Anne's lace) and *Heracleum lanatum* (cow parsnip). Poison hemlock contains the toxin coniine, which is similar to nicotine in structure and toxicity. The clinical picture and management resemble tobacco poisoning (see section on *Nicotiana tabacum*).[9]

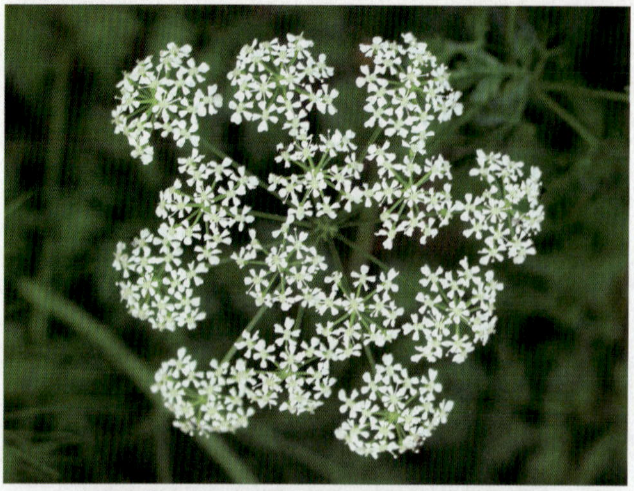

Figure 162-3. *Conium maculatum* (poison hemlock). (Courtesy of Steven Setzer.)

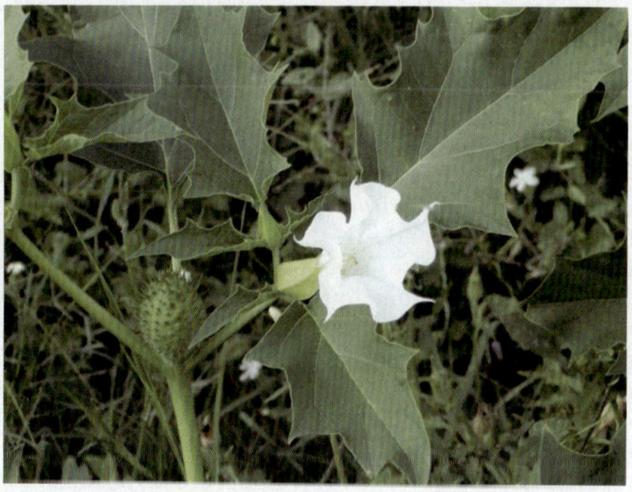

Figure 162-4. *Datura stramonium* (jimsonweed). (Courtesy of Steven Setzer.)

Datura stramonium

Datura stramonium (jimsonweed) (Figure 162-4) is one of numerous plants with alkaloids that have anticholinergic effects (see Chapter 148). The fruit is spiny and when opened contains 50 to 100 black seeds. All parts (including the seeds) contain the toxins atropine, hyoscyamine, and scopolamine, which are all potent anticholinergic agents. One hundred seeds are equivalent to 6 mg of atropine. Exposures are most commonly a result of abuse for hallucinogenic effects, usually by smoking dried leaves or ingesting the seeds.[10] The clinical picture is that of anticholinergic toxidrome.[11] The symptoms can be prolonged several days if the overdose is due to ingestion of seeds. It is unclear if activated charcoal and gastric emptying measures are effective at decreasing the course of toxicity.[10] Physostigmine reverses the clinical symptoms.[10] Anticholinergic symptoms typically return as the effects of physostigmine wear off (see Chapter 148).

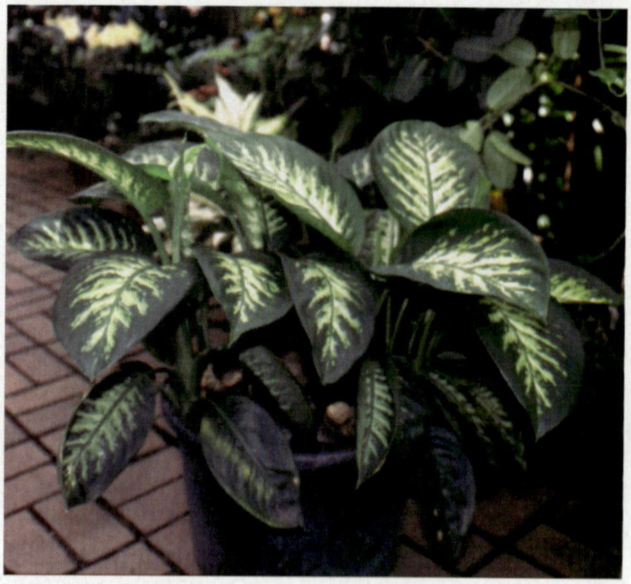

Figure 162-5. *Dieffenbachia*. (Courtesy of Steven Setzer.)

Dieffenbachia

Dieffenbachia (Figure 162-5) has more than 30 different species, including dumbcane, mother-in-law's tongue, dumb plant, and tuft root. Some of these names refer to the inability to talk that can occur after biting into parts of this plant. Typically the mucous membranes of the mouth are affected immediately with severe pain, swelling, and the sensation of biting into glass. Most cases are limited to the mucous membranes of the oropharynx. Rare cases of airway compromise have been reported.[12] The local effects are due to calcium oxalate crystals, packaged into bundles called *raphides,* which are found in cellular structures called *idioblasts.*[13] These idioblasts also contain proteolytic enzymes that are ejected out of the idioblasts with the oxalate crystals when plant parts are chewed. Because of the immediate pain, further exposure typically is limited. Treatment is aimed at pain relief and local supportive measures, typified by feeding a symptomatic infant ice cream.

Epipremnum aureum

Epipremnum aureum is a common household plant also known as pothos ivy, devil's ivy, hunter's robe, and golden pothos. Toxicity is due to calcium oxalate crystals,[14] the same toxin found in the *Dieffenbachia,* and the toxicity and treatment are similar.

Eucalyptus

Eucalyptus plants are the silver dollar, lemon-scented gum, cider gum, and blue gum. These plants are not toxic. The plants are used, however, to produce concentrated (approximately 70%) eucalyptus oil. Ingestion of small amounts (1 to 3 mL) has been reported to cause severe toxicity.[15] The predominant symptoms are neurologic, including mental status alteration, headache, ataxia, and seizures. Treatment for severe toxicity is supportive.

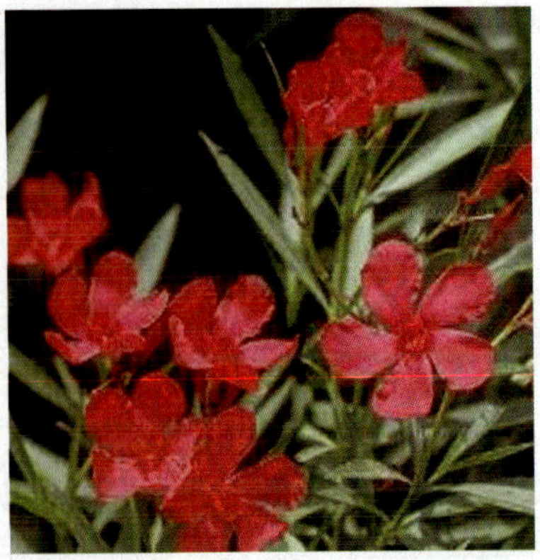

Figure 162-6. *Nerium oleander*. (Courtesy of Steven Setzer.)

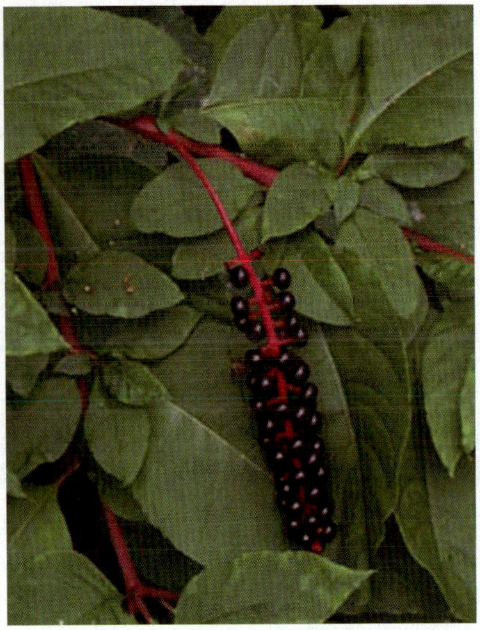

Figure 162-7. *Phytolacca americana* (pokeweed). (Courtesy of Steven Setzer.)

Euphorbia pulcherrima

E. pulcherrima (poinsettia) is a popular ornamental plant with a false reputation for being poisonous. Contact dermatitis is relatively common, however, with skin exposure.[16]

Ilex

Ilex (holly) contains more than 400 different species. The plant's red and black berries are attractive to children and contain numerous toxins that are potent gastrointestinal irritants. Symptoms include nausea, vomiting, abdominal cramping, and diarrhea.

Nerium oleander

N. oleander (Figure 162-6), or oleander, is one of many plants that contain toxic cardiac glycosides[17] structurally similar to digoxin. Ingestions of several leaves are unlikely to cause serious symptoms.[18] Large exposures from suicide attempts or misidentification of plants used for teas or herbal products can lead to severe toxicity or death.[19] The cardiac glycosides are potent sodium-potassium adenosine triphosphatase inhibitors, and the symptoms they cause are similar to those of digoxin poisoning (see Chapter 150). Measurement of an abnormal digoxin level is only qualitative proof of exposure because the serum digoxin test can falsely measure nondigoxin cardiac glycosides. Conversely a negative digoxin measurement does not rule out exposure because the level of cardiac glycoside cross-reactivity varies.[18] Treatment for suspected oleander ingestion includes activated charcoal and digoxin-specific Fab antibodies (see Chapter 150)[20-22]; however, larger doses of Fab fragments generally are needed than for comparable digoxin poisonings. Initial empirical doses of 10 to 20 vials of digoxin-specific Fab fragments have been suggested.[18]

Nicotiana tabacum

Nicotiana tabacum is widely grown in the southeastern United States as a source for cigarette and cigar tobacco. Several *Nicotiana* species contain nicotine as their major toxin, which activates and subsequently blocks acetylcholine receptors in the central nervous system (CNS) and peripheral autonomic nervous system. Most exposures are ingestion of cigarettes or cigars by young children. Dermal exposure to workers harvesting plants and ingestion of wild plants mistaken for edible plants also have led to poisoning.[23]

The ingestion of one to two cigarettes has the potential to cause moderate poisoning in children. Most children ingesting cigarettes do not manifest toxicity. Patients not experiencing nausea and vomiting do not seem to be at risk for more severe toxicity.[24] Dermal exposure in tobacco workers has been called *green tobacco sickness*.[25] Nicotine is absorbed through the skin and occurs most severely when the skin or plant is wet. Exposure can be avoided by using proper protective equipment.

Symptoms begin shortly after absorption. Nausea, vomiting, salivation, lacrimation, diarrhea, hypertension, tachycardia, diaphoresis, agitation, and fasciculation are seen initially. More severe toxicity is manifested by seizures, respiratory depression (muscle weakness), and hyperthermia. Treatment for ingestion is aimed initially at limiting absorption with activated charcoal. Gastric lavage is of questionable value. Other treatments are supportive in nature because no specific antidote for nicotine is available. Benzodiazepines can be used for seizures and agitation. If severe salivation and lacrimation occur, atropine in 1-mg doses may be repeated until symptoms improve.

Phytolacca americana

Found in the eastern United States, *Phytolacca americana* (Figure 162-7) is commonly known as pokeweed, poke, pokeberry, inkberry, scoke, American cancer, garget, phytolacca, and pigeonberry. Although the plant is poisonous, it can be detoxified by boiling it in water twice before use in salads or other recipes. Toxicity is seen when the plant is inadequately detoxified, or raw parts of the plant are eaten.[26] Symptoms begin shortly after ingestion and include severe nausea, vomiting, abdominal cramping, and diarrhea. Treatment is supportive.

Pyracantha

Pyracantha, commonly known as the firethorn, has small red, orange, or yellow fruit attractive to and commonly ingested by children. The plant is not toxic, but the thorny parts can penetrate skin deeply and are difficult to remove. Injury in a joint can lead to a chronic debilitating synovitis.[27]

Rhododendron

Rhododendron includes more than 1000 species of azaleas and rhododendrons, including mountain laurel, dwarf laurel, rose bay, western Labrador tea, and Japanese pieris. Numerous structurally related toxins (diterpene polyalcohols) have been identified from these plants, including grayanotoxin, rhodojaponin, asebotoxin, and others. These toxins bind to sodium channels and increase permeability (sodium channel openers), causing cardiovascular (bradycardia and hypotension) and gastrointestinal (nausea, vomiting, and abdominal pain) effects. Although ingestion of a few leaves of these plant species is unlikely to cause symptoms, larger exposures can cause severe toxicity. No deaths have been reported, however. Treatment is supportive; atropine has been used for bradycardia in rare cases. Sodium channel–blocking agents, such as quinidine and procainamide, may have theoretical value in severe cases, although their efficacy is unclear.[28]

Spathiphyllum

Spathiphyllum includes the peace lily, Mauna Loa, white anthurium, and snowflower. These plants contain calcium oxalates and have similar toxicity and treatment as *Dieffenbachia.*

Taxus

Taxus (yew trees) (Figure 162-8) have a hard seed surrounded by a fleshy red cup (the aril). The aril portion is not poisonous, and the seed has a hard coat that limits toxin release in the gastrointestinal tract so that most ingestions are nontoxic. If the seed is masticated or leaves are ingested, cardiac (bradycardia and hypotension) and gastrointestinal symptoms (nausea, vomiting, and abdominal pain) may occur. Deaths from this plant have been reported, usually in the setting of a suicide and secondary to cardiac manifestations.[29]

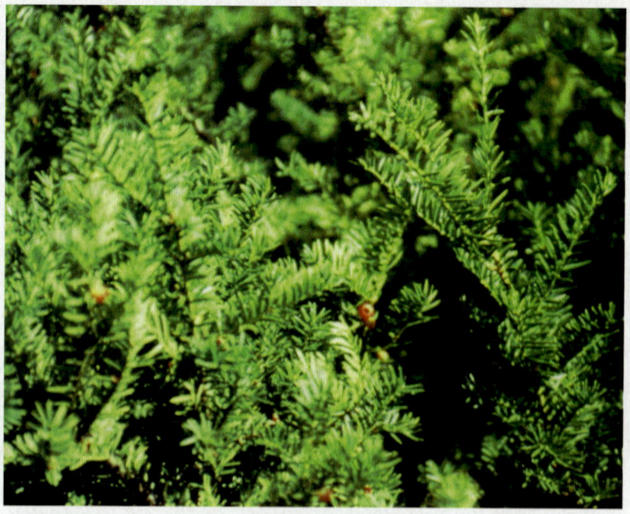

Figure 162-8. *Taxus* (yew). (Courtesy of Steven Setzer.)

HERBAL MEDICINES

Herbal products have gained an extraordinary amount of popularity over the past several decades. Although the highest usage is among immigrants and patients with difficult-to-treat diseases, such as advanced cancer and acquired immunodeficiency syndrome, these products are used by 30% of the general population.[30] One study of pregnant patients documented 45% herbal medicine usage during some point of their pregnancy.[31] Studies in emergency department patients also document the frequent use of herbal products.[32]

Herbal products are classified as dietary supplements and are not regulated as medicines. Regulation of dietary supplements is limited. Safety, quality, and efficacy for medicines are the responsibility of manufacturers. For herbal products used as dietary supplements, of which there are thousands to hundreds of thousands of potential products, the burden of proving efficacy and safety lies with the FDA.[33,34] Additionally, herbals generally are used for their medicinal value and not as dietary supplements.

Studies looking at the efficacy of herbal products are limited. Few randomized control studies address efficacy. Herbal manufacturers are not required to conduct these studies. Studies evaluating side effects, drug interactions, and toxicity are even less available.

Most herbal products have some direct pharmacologic action. The potency of these agents is usually limited, however. As a result, toxicity and side effects from the direct actions of herbal products are relatively uncommon.[35,36]

The lack of manufacturing quality control accounts for most toxicologic problems associated with their use. Four major types of toxicologic problems have been associated with herbal product use, including (1) the misidentification of an herbal plant and toxicity resulting from a substituted plant, (2) contamination with nonherbal toxic material, (3) overdose of the herbal product, and (4) drug-herbal interaction (Table 162-1).

Misidentification of Herbal Plant

Incorrect plant identification and subsequent use in the production of herbal products have occurred on numerous occasions, leading to epidemic exposures with tragic outcomes. The following examples illustrate this problem.

Table 162-1. Common Herbal Medications and Adverse Effects

Herbal Name	Botanical Name	Uses	Adverse Effect
Bee pollen	*Apis mellifera*	General tonic	Allergic reactions
Betel nut	*Areca catechu*	Stimulant	Bronchospasm
Blue cohosh	*Caulophyllum thalictroides*	Menstrual cramps	Nicotinic effects
Chaparral	*Larrea tridentata*	Cancer, aging, general tonic	Hepatotoxicity
Chamomile	*Matricaria chamomilla*	Fever, cough, colds, wounds	Allergic reactions
Comfrey	*Symphytum officinale*	Contusions and sprains	Hepatotoxicity
Echinacea	*Echinacea pupurea*	Common cold	Fever, nausea and vomiting
Fennel	*Foeniculum vulgare*	GI illnesses, cough	Allergic reactions
Feverfew	*Tanacetum parthenium*	Migraines, antipyretic	Post–feverfew syndrome, rebound migraine
Juniper	*Juniperus communis*	UTI, kidney stones, appetite	Renal toxicity
Germander	*Teucrium chamaedrys*	Gout, fever, dietary aid	Hepatotoxicity
Ginkgo	*Ginkgo biloba*	General tonic, depression, anxiety, memory	GI effects, bleeding effects, drug interactions
Ginger	*Zingiber officinale*	Motion sickness, GI illness	None reported
Ginseng	*Panax ginseng*	General tonic, depression, stress, anxiety, fatigue	Ginseng abuse syndrome
Goldenseal	*Hydrastis canadensis*	Cutaneous wounds	GI, CNS, and pulmonary effects in overdose
Larkspur	*Delphinium consolida*	Diuretic, sedative	Lethargy, muscle paralysis
Licorice	*Glycyrrhiza glabra*	Cough, GI illnesses	Hypokalemia, drug interactions
Ma-huang	*Ephedra sinica*	General tonic, common cold	Sympathomimetic
Milk thistle	*Silybum marinum*	General tonic, GI disorders	None
Parsley	*Petroselinum crispum*	UTI, kidney stones	Contact dermatitis
Pennyroyal	*Mentha pulegium*	Abortifacient, GI illnesses	Hepatotoxicity
Rue	*Ruta graveolens*	Menstrual disorders	Contact dermatitis, GI and CNS effects in overdose
St. John's Wort	*Hypericum perforatum*	Depression, anxiety	Drug interactions
Saw palmetto	*Serenoa repens*	Benign prostatic hypertrophy	GI effects
Shepherd's purse	*Capsella bursa pastoris*	Hypertension, CHF, headaches, menstrual disorders	None
Siberian ginseng	*Eleutherococcus senticosus*	General tonic	None
Scullcap	*Scutellaria lateriflora*	Nervous disorders, bitter tonic	Hepatotoxicity
Tonka bean	*Dipteryx odorata*	Whooping cough	Anticoagulant effect
Valerian	*Valeriana officinalis*	Sleep, anxiety, general tonic	Hepatoxicity
Woodruff	*Galium odorata*	Diuretic, anxiety, menstrual disorders	Anticoagulant effect, CNS effects, hepatoxicity
Wormwood	*Artemisia cima*	Worm infection, anxiety	Seizures, CNS effects
Yarrow	*Achillea millefolium*	Poor appetite, GI illnesses	Allergic reactions
Yohimbine	*Pausinystalia yohimbe*	Sexual disorders, aphrodisiac	Hypertension, agitation, CNS effects

GI, gastrointestinal; UTI, urinary tract infection; CNS, central nervous system; CHF, congestive heart failure.

Paraguay Tea, 1994

The South American herbal tea Paraguay tea is made from *Ilex paraguariensis,* used for urinary tract infections, cardiac insufficiency, and "lack of stamina." In 1994, several individuals had anticholinergic poisoning from Paraguay tea, after the manufacturer had purchased and mistakenly used other plant materials containing the belladonna alkaloids atropine, scopolamine, and hyoscyamine directly from farmers before packaging.[37]

Digitalis lanata, 1997

An herbal dietary supplement used for "internal cleansing" contained 14 herbal ingredients. Two patients developed complete heart block because one of the herbal ingredients, plantain, contained *Digitalis lanata* (a cardiac glycoside–containing plant).[38]

Herbal Slimming Regimen, 1992

During the early 1990s, the Chinese herbs *Stephania tetrandra* and *Magnolia officinalis* were used for weight loss in Belgium. Many cases of interstitial fibrosis of the kidney occurred with the use of these herbal compounds. Analysis found that *S. tetrandra,* which was substituted for *Aristolochia fangchi,* contains the nephrotoxin aristolochic acid.[36,39]

Contamination with Nonherbal Toxic Material

Contamination with nonherbal toxic material as a mechanism of herbal toxicity may be due to contamination of the products at the time of manufacture or consumer fraud. Because of the limited FDA regulation of herbal manufacturers, one of the main risks of herbal usage is the use of a product contaminated with a toxic substance. A study of Asian herbal patent medications sold in California found that 32% of these products were contaminated with heavy metals or undeclared pharmaceuticals.[40]

Lead, mercury, arsenic, cadmium, aluminum, tin, zinc, and copper all have been found in herbal products. The most common undeclared pharmaceuticals include ephedrine, chlorpheniramine, methyltestosterone, and phenacetin.[40,41] It is not clear why heavy metals are found in herbal products. Metal shavings have been added to herbal preparations to increase selling price when the herbals are sold by weight. Some herbal products use the metal as an active ingredient with a purported medicinal benefit (i.e., lead in azarcon or mercury in cinnabar). Other cases involve contamination with the metals during the manufacturing process.[42,43] Consumer fraud in the herbal industry has been well documented on numerous occasions. Typically an FDA-controlled pharmaceutical product is mixed in with an herbal product, or the label did not list the pharmaceutical agent.

Chuifong Toukuwan was an herbal preparation that was associated with several cases of agranulocytosis. Analysis revealed that it contained phenylbutazone, indomethacin, and aminopyrine.[44] Gan Mao Tong was an herbal product found to contain phenylbutazone, causing aplastic anemia.[45] An undefined herbal preparation that was used "to avoid taking other medicine" was found to contain triamcinolone. A patient using the product for more than 1 year had several manifestations of steroid excess: thoracic compression fractures, proximal muscle weakness, and osteoporosis.[46] Tung shueh was an herbal product that was found to contain mefenamic acid and diazepam, causing gastrointestinal bleeding and acute interstitial nephritis.[47] Another herbal product was found to contain mefenamic acid, which caused acute renal failure necessitating hemodialysis. Dr Tong Shap Yee's asthma pills were found to contain theophylline.[48] Leng Pui Kee herbal cough remedy was found to contain bromhexine.[48]

Some herbal preparations can cause allergic reactions ranging from contact dermatitis to anaphylactic shock (Box 162-1).[49,50] Other herbal products are associated with uncommon idiosyncratic reactions, particularly hepatic toxicity (see Table 162-1). Herbal products often are taken in overdose. Not controlled by a prescription system, herbal medicines often are seen as natural and safe so that "if one is good, then two or three is better." Direct toxicity is often due to this overuse. Herbs associated with specific toxicities and side effects are listed in Table 162-1.

Concurrent herbal and pharmaceutical use is common and can cause drug interactions. Of U.S. adults, 18% who take prescription medications also use an herbal or mineral supplement, and 60% who use alternative therapies are unlikely to report this to their physicians.[30] Individuals often do not consider the herb a potential interactant with conventional medicines, and serious drug reactions associated with an herbal product are less likely to be reported than reactions that occur with a conventional medicine. Common herbal-drug interactions are listed in Table 162-2.[51,52]

BOX 162-1. Herbals Associated with Allergic Reactions

- Agnus castus
- Angelica
- Aniseed
- Apricot
- Aristochol
- Arnica
- Artichoke
- Asafoetida
- Balxum of Peru
- Bee pollen
- Bee venom
- Black cumin oil
- Boneset
- Camphor
- Capsaican
- Cassia
- Cedar wood oil
- Celery
- Chamomile
- Chrysanthemum
- Cinnamon
- Cowslip
- Curcumin
- Dandelion
- Echinacea
- Elecampane
- Euphorbia
- Fennel
- Feverfew
- French marigold
- Fucus
- Garlic
- Gingko
- Gravel root
- Guaiacum
- Holy thistle
- Hops
- Hydrangea
- Hydrocotyle
- *Inula helenium*
- Jasmine
- Juniper
- Kava
- Lady's slipper
- Lavender
- Mai-Meu-Dong-Tang
- Meadowsweet
- Motherwort
- Paprika
- Parsley
- Peppermint oil
- Pilewort
- Plantain
- Pulsatilla
- Rosemary
- Rosewood
- Royal jelly
- Rue
- Slippery elm
- Tansy
- Tea tree oil
- Tung seed
- Wild carrot
- Yarrow
- Ylang-ylang

MUSHROOMS

U.S. poison center data estimate that five exposures take place for every 100,000 population per year. These exposures occur in three types of situations: (1) accidental ingestion of wild mushrooms by young children playing outdoors (which usually results in a small exposure), (2) mistaken selection of poisonous mushrooms while foraging for edible wild mushrooms intended for a meal (which leads to a larger toxin exposure and most of the severe cases of mushroom poisoning, including deaths), and (3) abuse of certain mushrooms for their mind-altering potential.[53] Mushrooms of abuse typically involve a young population that often abuses other drugs. Most of these cases do not come to medical attention and often involve other substances added to the mushrooms. Despite the potential for severe toxicity and death, most exposures are relatively benign. Approximately 5% result in moderate poisoning, with only a few deaths reported per year.

Management of Mushroom Exposure

The prognosis depends on the specific species. Identification of the mushroom is probably the most helpful factor in deciding on a treatment plan. Techniques for mushroom identification are described in most mycology and toxicology textbooks. Local mycologists or a poison center may helpful. If a specimen is available, it can be stored in a paper bag at room temperature. Vomitus can be collected because mushroom parts may be recovered. Despite these measures, the species is unknown in more than 90% of ingestions. *Amanita* species are responsible for most deaths. A clinical strategy for differential diagnosis and management is most often used to identify the highest risk ingestions.

Table 162-2. Common Herbal-Drug Interactions

Herbal	Drug	Type of Interaction
Betel nut	Fluphenazine	Extrapyramidal effects
	Prednisone and salbutamol	Bronchospasm
Chili pepper	ACE inhibitors	Cough
	Theophylline	Increased drug absorption
D-400	Oral hypoglycemics	Increased drug concentration and decreased serum glucose
Devil's claw	Warfarin	Increased INR
Dong quai	Warfarin	Increased INR
Garlic	Warfarin	Increased INR
Ginkgo	Blood thinners	Bleeding side effects
	Thiazide diuretics	Hypertension
Ginseng	Warfarin	Decreased INR
	Ethanol	Increased ethanol clearance
Guar gum	Many drugs	Decreased absorption of numerous drugs
Karela	Chlorpropamide	Decreased serum glucose
Licorice	Oral contraceptives	Hypertension, edema, hypokalemia
	Prednisolone	Alteration of pharmacokinetics
Ma-huang	Guanethidine	Sympathomimetic effects
	MAO inhibitors	Sympathomimetic effects
Papaya	Warfarin	Increased INR
Psyllium	Lithium	Decreased drug concentrations
Siberian ginseng	Digoxin	Increased digoixn levels
St. John's Wort	Selective serotonin reuptake inhibitors	Serotonin syndrome
	Theophylline	Decreased drug concentration
	Digoxin	Decreased drug concentration
	Cyclosporine	Decreased drug concentration
	Indinavir	Decreased drug concentration
Tamarind	Aspirin	Increased drug absorption
Yohimbine	Tricyclic antidepressants	Hypertension

ACE, angiotensin-converting enzyme; INR, international normalized ratio; MAO, monoamine oxidase.

Table 162-3. Mushroom Groups

Group/Toxin	Representative Example	Clinical Effects
Early onset of symptoms		
Coprine	*Coprinus atramentarius*	Disulfiram reaction with alcohol
GI toxin	Many species	Nausea, vomiting, diarrhea, abdominal pain
Ibotenic acid and muscimol	*Amanita muscaria*	Diverse CNS effects, including hallucinations, seizures, delirium, coma, agitation
Muscarine	*Clitocybe dealbata*	Peripheral cholinergic toxidrome
Psilocybin	*Psilocybe cubensis*	CNS effects, including hallucinations and euphoria
Late onset of symptoms		
Cyclopeptides	*Amanita phalloides*	GI effects followed by hepatotoxicity
Gyromitrin	*Gyromitra esculenta*	GI effects followed by seizures
Orellanine	*Cortinarius orellanus*	GI effects followed by renal toxicity

GI, gastrointestinal; CNS, central nervous system.

Mushroom Groups

Nine general groupings have been found to be useful for clinical management (Table 162-3). These groups can be classified into mushrooms with early onset of symptoms (0 to 4 hours postingestion), late onset of symptoms (>6 hours postingestion), or no symptoms (edible). Mushrooms with serious toxicity and potential for death are in the group that have late onset of symptoms. Particular attention should be paid to the timing of initial symptoms.[54] Mushroom species often grow together, and foragers frequently pick and eat more than one species of mushroom. The onset of early symptoms does not preclude the diagnosis of a more serious poisoning.

Early Onset of Symptoms

Gastrointestinal symptoms of nausea, vomiting, diarrhea, and abdominal cramps are common among many of the mushroom groupings (see Table 162-3). These symptoms are most predominant, however, in the gastrointestinal toxin group. This group contains numerous diverse mushrooms, many with unknown toxins. They cause symptoms rapidly (0.5 to 3 hours) after ingestion, and symptoms typically last 24 hours. Treatment is supportive, with good outcome expected.

CNS effects are associated with two groups of mushrooms, ibotenic acid/muscimol, and psilocybin.[55] Psilocybin is structurally related to serotonin and lysergic acid diethylamide (LSD). Similar to LSD, hallucinations and CNS effects are prominent. This mushroom is most often used as a drug of abuse.[56] Ibotenic acid and muscimol are toxins that are structurally related to glutamic acid and GABA. Glutamic acid is an excitatory neurotransmitter, whereas GABA is an inhibitory one. Lethargy, hallucinations, seizures, or severe agitation begins within 1 to 2 hours after ingestion. Treatment for seizures and supportive care are given.

The cholinergic toxidrome is associated with muscarine-containing mushrooms. Muscarine is structurally related to acetylcholine. Because of muscarine's quaternary structure, it does not cross the blood-brain barrier. Symptoms include salivation, lacrimation, urination, defecation, gastroenteritis, and emesis (*SLUDGE*). Atropine can be used for severe symptoms. Pralidoxime is not indicated because acetylcholinesterase inhibition is not involved.

The final mushroom group that causes early onset of symptoms occurs only with simultaneous ingestion of ethanol.[57] These coprine-containing mushrooms cause a disulfiram-like reaction by blocking acetaldehyde dehydrogenase.[57] The symptoms include flushing, nausea, vomiting, and headache. The onset of this reaction associated with ethanol can occur 30 minutes to several days after mushroom ingestion.[57] Treatment is supportive and similar to disulfiram reactions owing to other causes.

Late Onset of Symptoms

Three groups of mushrooms cause late onset of symptoms (>6 hours postingestion): cyclopeptide, gyromitrin, and orelline/orellanine. The cyclopeptide group is responsible for most mushroom-related deaths in the United States. The orelline/orellanine-containing mushrooms have not been reported to cause toxicity in the United States.

The cyclopeptide mushrooms contain many species, of which *Amanita phylloides* is the most well known. Several cyclopeptide toxins have been identified (e.g., amatoxins, virotoxins, phallotoxins) that are thought to be responsible for toxicity.[58] Initial manifestations, such as severe nausea, vomiting, diarrhea, and abdominal cramping, begin 6 to 24 hours postingestion. Hydration and supportive care often lead to relief of symptoms and a relatively quiescent period. Hepatic toxicity followed by other end-organ involvement may ensue over the next several days to weeks. Progressive elevation of hepatic transaminases, jaundice, and hepatic encephalopathy can lead to death.

Many cases are misdiagnosed as gastroenteritis. Numerous noninvasive therapies have been suggested, including silibinin, thioctic acid, activated charcoal, high-dose penicillin, dexamethasone, vitamin C, cytochrome *c*, cimetidine, *N*-acetyl cysteine, kutkin, and aucubin.[59,60] None of these therapies has been rigorously tested in human-controlled studies. Repetitive administration of activated charcoal seems to be reasonable because of its ability to bind the toxins, availability, and relative safety.

Numerous invasive therapies also have been proposed for use in cyclopeptide poisoning, including forced diuresis, hemodialysis, hemoperfusion, hemofiltration, plasmapheresis, and hepatic transplantation.[61] Similar to the noninvasive modalities, it is not clear what efficacy these therapies have. There have been several reports of successful transplantation in severe cases of poisoning[62]; however, it is uncertain what criteria should be used for selecting candidates. Patients developing hepatic signs and symptoms should be considered for transfer to a transplant center.

Gyromitrin-containing mushrooms commonly are mistaken for edible mushrooms. The metabolites of this toxin cause GABA neurotransmitter depletion similar to isoniazid toxicity, leading to excitatory CNS effects, such as headaches, agitation, and seizures. Effects also include nausea, vomiting, and possible hepatotoxicity. The onset of symptoms is at least 6 hours after ingestion. Because of its similarity to isoniazid toxicity, pyridoxine has been proposed as an antidote. It is unclear how effective this antidote is, but it is useful for gyromitrin-induced CNS effects because of its availability and safety profile.

Orelline/orellanine-containing mushrooms have been found in North America.[63] There have been no reports of toxicity associated with cases in the United States, however, with most reported cases in Europe. Symptoms begin 1 to 2 days after ingestion, with nausea, vomiting, abdominal pain, and headache. Renal toxicity manifests days to weeks after these initial symptoms and can progress to chronic renal failure.

Disposition

Initial management is aimed at ruling out mushroom groups associated with early onset of symptoms. If the patient remains asymptomatic after a period of observation, the patient should be discharged with instructions to return if any symptoms manifest over the next 72 hours.

KEY CONCEPTS

- Plant exposures occur commonly in children and most commonly involve household plants. Most exposures cause little or no toxicity.
- Plants and mushrooms often are ingested for their mind-altering properties.
- Misidentification of plants and herbal products is a common cause for plant-induced and herbal product–induced toxicity.
- Natural plant and mushroom gathering for personal ingestion is a popular activity. Mistakes while foraging occur commonly, with the potential for serious toxicity and numerous fatalities.
- Herbal medicines increasingly are being used by the general public. Limited information is available regarding the efficacy and toxicity of these products.
- In the assessment of a patient exposed to a mushroom, the timing of initial symptoms and the assessment for associated symptoms constitute the most important data needed to make a differential diagnosis.
- A patient who has eaten or been exposed to a wild mushroom may have another medical condition actually responsible for the symptoms.

REFERENCES

1. Kinamore PA: Abrus and ricinus ingestion: Management of three cases. *Clin Toxicol* 17:401, 1980.
2. Jones LA, et al: Household treatment for "chile burns" of the hands. *J Toxicol Clin Toxicol* 25:483, 1987.
3. Vogl TP: Treatment of Hunan hand. *N Engl J Med* 306:178, 1982.
4. Forrester MB, et al: The epidemiology of pepper spray exposures reported in Texas in 1998-2002. *Vet Hum Toxicol* 45:327, 2003.
5. Watson WA, et al: Oleoresin capsicum (Cap-Stun) toxicity from aerosol exposure. *Ann Pharmacother* 30:733, 1996.
6. Tanaka T, et al: Occupational dermatitis with simultaneous immediate and delayed allergy to chrysanthemum. *Contact Dermatitis* 15:152, 1987.
7. Heath KB: A fatal case of apparent water hemlock poisoning. *Vet Hum Toxicol* 43:35, 2001.
8. Mitchell MI, Routledge PA: Hemlock water dropwort poisoning: A review. *Clin Toxicol* 12:417, 1978.
9. Rizzi D, et al: Clinical spectrum of accidental hemlock poisoning: Neurotoxic manifestations, rhabdomyolysis and acute tubular necrosis. *Nephrol Dial Transplant* 6:939, 1991.
10. Salen P, et al: Effect of physostigmine and gastric lavage in a *Datura stramonium*-induced anticholinergic poisoning epidemic. *Am J Emerg Med* 21:316, 2003.
11. Parissis D, et al: Neurological findings in a case of coma secondary to *Datura stramonium* poisoning. *Eur J Neurol* 10:745, 2003.
12. Cumpston KL, et al: Acute airway compromise after brief exposure to a *Dieffenbachia* plant. *J Emerg Med* 25:391, 2003.
13. Mrvos R, et al: Philodendron/dieffenbachia ingestions: Are they a problem? *Clin Toxicol* 29:485, 1991.
14. Mitchell JC, Rook A: *Scindapsus* dermatitis. *Contact Dermatitis* 2:125, 1976.
15. Tibballs J: Clinical effects and management of eucalyptus oil ingestion in infants and young children. *Med J Aust* 163:177, 1995.
16. Krenzelok EP, et al: Poinsettia exposures have good outcomes…just as we thought. *Am J Emerg Med* 14:671, 1996.
17. Eddleston M, et al: Epidemic of self-poisoning with seeds of the yellow oleander tree (*Thevetia peruviana*) in northern Sri Lanka. *Trop Med Int Health* 4:266, 1999.
18. Clark RF, et al: Digoxin-specific Fab fragments in the treatment of oleander toxicity in a canine model. *Ann Emerg Med* 20:1073, 1991.
19. Monzani V, et al: Acute oleander poisoning after a self-prepared tisane. *Clin Toxicol* 35:667, 1997.
20. de Silva HA, et al: Multiple-dose activated charcoal for treatment of yellow oleander poisoning: A single-blind, randomised, placebo-controlled trial. *Lancet* 361:1935, 2003.
21. Dasgupta A, et al: Activated charcoal is effective but equilibrium dialysis is ineffective in removing oleander leaf extract and oleandrin from human serum: Monitoring the effect by measuring apparent digoxin concentration. *Ther Drug Monit* 25:323, 2003.
22. Eddleston M, Persson H: Acute plant poisoning and antitoxin antibodies. *J Toxicol Clin Toxicol* 41:309, 2003.
23. Rao P, et al: Hispanic farmworker interpretations of green tobacco sickness. *J Rural Health* 18:503, 2002.
24. McGee D, et al: Four year review of cigarette ingestions in children. *Pediatr Emerg Care* 11:13, 1995.
25. Ghosh SK, et al: Intervention studies against "green symptoms" among Indian tobacco harvesters. *Arch Environ Health* 46:316, 1991.
26. Hamilton RJ, et al: Mobitz type I heart block after pokeweed ingestion. *Vet Hum Toxicol* 37:66, 1995.
27. Hawkins SJ, et al: Rheumatoid arthritis developing after plant thorn synovitis. *BMJ* 285:1620, 1982.
28. Lampe KF: Rhododendrons, mountain laurel and mad honey. *JAMA* 259:2009, 1988.
29. van Ingen G, et al: Sudden unexpected death due to taxus poisoning: A report of five cases with review of the literature. *Forensic Sci Int* 56:81, 1992.
30. Eisenberg DM, et al: Trends in alternative medicine use in the United States, 1990-97. *JAMA* 280:1569, 1998.
31. Glover DD, et al: Prescription, over-the-counter, and herbal medicine use in a rural, obstetric population. *Am J Obstet Gynecol* 188:1039, 2003.
32. Hung OL, et al: Herbal preparation among urban emergency department patients. *Acad Emerg Med* 4:209, 1997.
33. De Smet PAGM: Drug therapy: Herbal remedies. *N Engl J Med* 347:2046, 2002.
34. Marcus DM, Grollman AP: Botanical medicines—the need for new regulations. *N Engl J Med* 347:2073, 2002.
35. Fugh-Berman A: Herb-drug interactions. *Lancet* 355:134, 2000.
36. Pui-Hay But P: Need for correct identification of herbs in herbal poisoning. *Lancet* 341:637, 1993.
37. Meggs WJ, et al: Anticholinergic poisoning associated with an herbal tea—New York City, 1994. *MMWR Morb Mortal Wkly Rep* 44:193, 1995.
38. Slifman NR, et al: Brief report: Contamination of botanical dietary supplements by *Digitalis lanata*. *N Engl J Med* 339:806, 1998.
39. Vanherweghem JL, et al: Rapidly progressive interstitial renal fibrosis in young women: Association with slimming regimen including Chinese herbs. *Lancet* 341:387, 1993.
40. Ko RJ: Adulterants in Asian patent medicine. *N Engl J Med* 339:847, 1998.
41. Ernst E: Adulteration of Chinese herbal medicine with synthetic drugs: A systematic review. *J Intern Med* 252:107, 2002.
42. Hill GJ: Lead poisoning due to Hai Be Fen. *JAMA* 273:24, 1995.
43. Espinoza EO, et al: Arsenic and mercury in traditional Chinese herbal balls. *N Engl J Med* 333:803, 1995.
44. Ries CA, Sahud MA: Agranulocytosis caused by Chinese herbal medicines. *JAMA* 231:352, 1975.
45. Nelson L, et al: Aplastic anemia induced by an adulterated herbal preparation. *J Toxicol Clin Toxicol* 33:467, 1995.
46. Capobianco DJ, et al: Proximal-muscle weakness induced by herbs. *N Engl J Med* 329:1430, 1993.
47. Diamond J, Pallone PL: Acute interstitial nephritis following use of Tung Shueh pills. *Am J Kidney Dis* 24:219, 1994.
48. Chan TYK, Critchley JAJH: Usage and adverse effects of Chinese herbal medicines. *Hum Exp Toxicol* 15:5, 1996.
49. Wong HCG: Allergic reactions associated with Chinese herbal medicine. *Allergy Asthma* 13:13, 2000.
50. Ernst E: Adverse effects of herbal drugs in dermatology. *Br J Dermatol* 143:923, 2000.
51. Fugh-Berman A: Herb-drug interactions. *Lancet* 355:134, 2000.
52. Smolinske SC: Dietary supplement-drug interactions. *J Am Med Womens Assoc* 54:191, 1999.
53. Jacobs J, et al: Serious mushroom poisonings in California requiring hospital admission, 1990 through 1994. *West J Med* 165:283, 1996.
54. Lampe KF, McCann MA: Differential diagnosis of poisoning by North American mushrooms, with particular emphasis on *Amanita phalloides*-like intoxication. *Ann Emerg Med* 16:956, 1987.
55. Michelot D, Melendez-Howell LM: *Amanita muscaria*: Chemistry, biology, toxicology, and ethnomycology. *Mycol Res* 107:131, 2003.
56. Schwartz RH, Smith DE: Hallucinogenic mushrooms. *Clin Pediatr (Phila)* 27:70, 1998.

57. Michelot D: Poisoning by *Coprinus atramentarius*. *Nat Toxins* 1:73, 1992.
58. Vetter J: Toxins of *Amanita phalloides*. *Toxicon* 36:13, 1998.
59. Montanini S, et al: Use of acetylcysteine as the life-saving antidote in *Amanita phalloides* (death cap) poisoning: Case report on 11 patients. *Arzneimittel-Forschung* 49:1044, 1999.
60. Schneider SM, et al: Cimetidine protection against alpha-amanitin hepatotoxicity in mice: A potential model for the treatment of *Amanita phalloides* poisoning. *Ann Emerg Med* 16:1136, 1987.
61. Aji DY, et al: Haemoperfusion in *Amanita phalloides* poisoning. *J Trop Pediatr* 41:371, 1995.
62. Skaare VK: Mushroom poisoning: An indication for liver transplantation. *J Transplant Coor* 7:141, 1997.
63. Horn S, et al: End-stage renal failure from mushroom poisoning with *Cortinarius orellanus*: Report of four cases and review of the literature. *Am J Kidney Dis* 30:282, 1997.

CHAPTER 163 Sedative Hypnotics

Leon Gussow and Andrea Carlson

BARBITURATES

Perspective

Barbiturates are discussed in do-it-yourself suicide manuals and have been implicated in the high-profile deaths of Marilyn Monroe, Jimi Hendrix, Abbie Hoffman, Margaux Hemingway, and the mass suicide of 39 members of the Heaven's Gate cult in 1997. Although barbiturates are still prescribed for the treatment of seizure disorders, their use as sedatives has declined significantly with the availability of safer alternatives, such as the benzodiazepines. There has been a concomitant decline from approximately 1500 reported barbiturate deaths per year in the 1950s to only nine fatalities in 1998.

Barbiturates are addicting, producing physical dependence and a withdrawal syndrome that can be life-threatening. Tolerance to the mood-altering effects of barbiturates develops rapidly with repeated use. Unfortunately, tolerance to the lethal effects does not develop as quickly, and the risk of severe toxicity increases with continued use.

Principles of Disease

Barbiturates depress the activity of all excitable cells, especially those in the central nervous system (CNS). They enhance the activity of γ-aminobutyric acid (GABA), the major central inhibitor of nerve excitability. In cases of acute overdose, barbiturates decrease transmission in autonomic ganglia and the activity of the myocardium and gastrointestinal tract. Barbiturates also inhibit the excitatory response to acetylcholine at autonomic neuroeffector and skeletal neuromuscular junctions.

The $GABA_A$ receptor is a protein complex found on postsynaptic membranes in the CNS. Structurally, it consists of distinct receptor sites for a number of endogenous and exogenous depressive chemicals with sedative and hypnotic properties, surrounding a chloride ion (Cl^-) channel (Figure 163-1). GABA opens the chloride channel. The resulting flow of Cl^- into the cell increases the negative resting potential, hyperpolarizing and stabilizing the membrane. There are separate receptor sites for barbiturates and for benzodiazepines, and a site that binds GABA, ethanol, and meprobamate. Barbiturates hold Cl^- channels longer in an open position, whereas benzodiazepines cause them to open more often. Although barbiturates and ethanol can directly increase Cl^- conductance, benzodiazepines require the presence of GABA to affect Cl^- flow. This may account for the relative safety of benzodiazepines in comparison with barbiturates.

Barbiturates produce the gamut of depressive effects, from mild sedation to coma, respiratory arrest, and death. In the early stages of intoxication, some patients experience euphoria. Barbiturates have no analgesic effect and can paradoxically increase the reaction to pain at low doses.

Barbiturates act directly on the medulla to produce respiratory depression. In therapeutic doses, this respiratory depression mimics that seen in normal sleep. Starting with doses approximately three times therapeutic, the neurogenic, chemical, and hypoxic respiratory drives are progressively suppressed. Laryngospasm can occur at low doses, because airway reflexes are not inhibited until general anesthesia is achieved.

Therapeutic oral doses of barbiturates produce only mild decreases in pulse and blood pressure, similar to those seen in sleep. With toxic doses, more significant hypotension occurs from direct depression of the myocardium and pooling of blood in a dilated venous system. Peripheral vascular resistance is usually normal or increased, but since barbiturates interfere with autonomic reflexes, these compensatory changes are inadequate for the decrease in blood pressure. In patients whose reflexes are already maximally stimulated, such as those with heart failure or hypovolemic

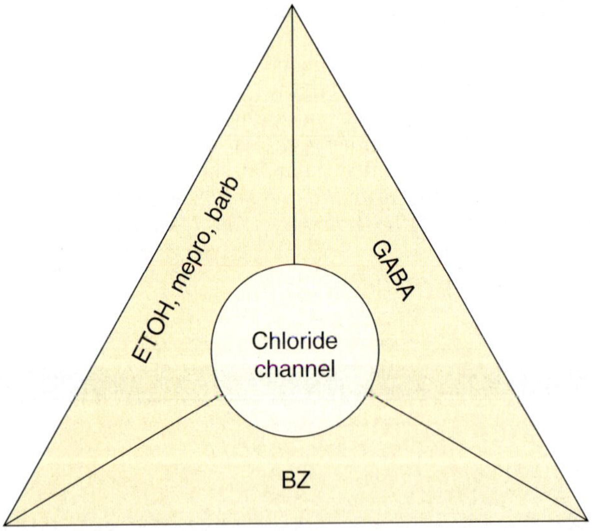

Figure 163-1. The γ-aminobutyric acid (GABA) receptor complex. BZ, benzodiazepine binding site; GABA, GABA binding site; ETOH, mepro, barb, binding site for ethanol, meprobamate, and barbiturates.

BOX 163-1. Barbiturates

Ultrashort-Acting
Methohexital (Brevital)
Thiopental (Pentothal)

Short- and Intermediate-Acting
Pentobarbital (Nembutal)
Secobarbital (Seconal)
Amobarbital (Amytal)
Aprobarbital (Alurate)
Butabarbital (Butisol)
Butalbital (Fiorinal)

Long-Acting
Phenobarbital (Solfoton, Luminal)
Mephobarbital (Mebaral)

shock, barbiturates can precipitate severe hypotension. Barbiturates also decrease cerebral blood flow and decrease intracerebral pressure. Although hypnotic doses of barbiturates do not affect gastric emptying, higher doses can decrease gastrointestinal smooth muscle tone and peristaltic contractions.

Barbiturates are classified according to their onset and duration of action: (1) ultrashort-acting (onset immediate after intravenous dose, duration minutes), (2) short-acting (onset 10 to 15 minutes after oral dose, duration 6 to 8 hours), (3) intermediate-acting (onset 45 to 60 minutes, duration 10 to 12 hours), and (4) long-acting (onset 1 hour, duration 10 to 12 hours) (Box 163-1). Only long-acting preparations have anticonvulsant effects in doses that do not cause sedation. The highly lipid-soluble, short-acting barbiturates are rapidly absorbed and quickly distributed to tissues with high perfusion, especially the brain, while phenobarbital, the least lipid-soluble barbiturate, has a slow onset.

Short- and intermediate-acting preparations are almost completely metabolized to inactive metabolites in the liver, but 25% of a phenobarbital (long-acting) dose is excreted unchanged through the kidney. Because phenobarbital is a weak acid (pK_a 7.2), alkalinizing the urine will increase the amount of drug present in ionized form, minimizing tubular reabsorption. Phenobarbital is 95% ionized at pH 7. Short- and intermediate-acting barbiturates are not significantly affected by pH changes in this range; for example, secobarbital (pK_a 7.9) is 98% nonionized at pH 7.4.

Barbiturates cross the placenta, and fetal levels approach those of the mother. They are also excreted in breast milk, but at much lower concentrations than those found in maternal plasma. Use during pregnancy is associated with birth defects (category D).

Clinical Features

Mild barbiturate toxicity mimics ethanol intoxication, with drowsiness, slurred speech, ataxia, unsteady gait, nystagmus, emotional lability, and impaired cognition (e.g., memory, judgment, and attention).

In cases of severe acute intoxication, CNS depression progresses from stupor to deep coma and respiratory arrest. Although pupils are usually normal or small but reactive, hypoxia can cause pupil dilation and loss of reactivity. Corneal and gag reflexes can be diminished or absent. Muscle tone can be flaccid, with absent reflexes and a positive Babinski sign. Flexor (decorticate) and extensor (decerebrate) posturing can occur in patients comatose from barbiturate intoxication. These neurologic signs are variable and do not always correlate with severity of intoxication or depth of coma. Fluctuating level of consciousness is common. High barbiturate levels depress gastrointestinal motility, delaying drug absorption. However, as the drug is metabolized and blood levels drop, peristalsis and drug absorption increase again and levels rise.

The threat to life in cases of severe barbiturate toxicity is respiratory depression. The degree of hypoventilation may not be readily apparent on clinical examination, because respirations can be rapid but shallow. Pulse oximetry is used to assess for hypoxemia. Cheyne-Stokes breathing may precede respiratory arrest. Delayed complications include pneumonia.

Hypotension is common in patients with severe intoxication, with a normal or increased heart rate. Barbiturate overdose can be associated with noncardiogenic pulmonary edema. Altered pulmonary capillary permeability can result from hypoperfusion or hypoxia or be a direct effect of the drug.

Hypothermia (31° to 36.6° C) occurs in patients with short-acting barbiturate intoxication or can result from exposure in any comatose patient.

A withdrawal syndrome includes tremors, hallucinations, seizures, and delirium (similar to the delirium tremens of ethanol withdrawal). However, severe withdrawal occurs only following dependence on short- or intermediate-acting barbiturates (e.g., pentobarbital, secobarbital, amobarbital, and butalbital). Because these drugs have few medical uses, this syndrome is now rare.

Diagnostic Strategies

Qualitative and quantitative tests detect barbiturates in urine and blood; however, a positive urine screen establishes the presence of the drug but does not prove that it is present in toxic amounts. The therapeutic level of phenobarbital is 15 to 40 μg/mL (65 to 172 μmol/L). A serum level greater than 50 μg/mL can be associated with coma, especially in a patient who is not a chronic barbiturate user. Levels greater than 80 μg/mL are potentially fatal. Serial phenobarbital levels may be helpful in monitoring effectiveness of treatment. Because barbiturates other than phenobarbital have high volumes of distribution, serum levels do not accurately reflect CNS concentrations or correlate with clinical severity.

In more severe overdose cases, chest radiographs can show noncardiogenic pulmonary edema or pneumonia. Computed tomography of the head can be performed in comatose patients with evidence of trauma, focal neurologic signs, papilledema, or uncertain diagnosis.

Other causes of stupor and coma must be considered and ruled out. Since the electroencephalogram may be silent as a result of barbiturate overdose, no patient should be declared "brain dead" if barbiturates are present at therapeutic levels or greater.

Management

Barbiturates have no specific antidote, and management is based on supportive care, particularly with respect to the cardiovascular and respiratory systems. Severely intoxicated patients are unable to protect their airway adequately, and ventilatory drive is decreased, with ensuing hypoxemia. Supplemental oxygen may suffice for patients with mild to moderate overdose, but intubation is often required as the patient's level of consciousness becomes progressively depressed with accompanying respiratory depression. When intubation is required, and in the absence of an identified difficult airway, a rapid-sequence technique is preferred, using a barbiturate (sodium pentothal) or benzodiazepine (midazolam) induction agent with succinylcholine for neuromuscular blockade. Long-term paralysis is rarely necessary, and the patient's own ingestion will generally provide sufficient sedation for mechanical ventilation. Cardiovascular support involves careful but adequate fluid replacement to maintain a systolic blood pressure above 90 mm Hg and adequate urine output. Patients must be monitored for signs of fluid overload and pulmonary edema. If vasopressors are necessary, dopamine is preferable to norepinephrine because of its renal vasodilating effects. Active warming should be initiated if the rectal temperature is less than 30° C.

Gastrointestinal Decontamination

Although there is no evidence proving that activated charcoal reduces the morbidity or mortality of barbiturate overdose, several studies have demonstrated enhanced clearance of specific barbiturates, so charcoal administration is generally recommended. A single dose of activated charcoal (50-100 g for an adult) can be given if ingestion has occurred recently. In addition, multiple doses of activated charcoal will increase the clearance and decrease the half-life of phenobarbital, since it has the longest half-life.[1,2] Multidose activated charcoal may adsorb the drug as it continues to be released from a bezoar and interrupt "enterohepatic" circulation, where phenobarbital is excreted in the bile and then reabsorbed from the gastrointestinal tract. Finally, multidose activated charcoal will bind the drug as it diffuses into the gastrointestinal tract, increasing both the concentration gradient across the gastrointestinal mucosal surface and drug clearance. An adult dose of multidose activated charcoal is 25 g every 2 hours; the pediatric dose is 0.5 g/kg every 2 hours. If vomiting interferes with administering multidose activated charcoal, a smaller dose or antiemetics should be used. Multidose activated charcoal can also be administered slowly through a nasogastric tube.

Although alkalinizing the urine with $NaHCO_3$ has been recommended in the past in place of or in addition to multidose activated charcoal for treating phenobarbital overdose, a recent nonrandomized study suggested that multidose activated charcoal alone is most effective at increasing the drug's clearance.[3] The authors hypothesize that alkalinization may interfere with the ability of multidose activated charcoal to clear the drug across the intestinal mucosa.

Hemodialysis or charcoal hemoperfusion is rarely needed but may increase clearance of phenobarbital in the presence of renal or cardiac failure, acid-base or electrolyte abnormalities, unstable cardiorespiratory status, or inadequate response to less invasive measures. Because phenobarbital is 40% to 60% protein-bound, hemoperfusion is sometimes advocated over hemodialysis; however, newer, high-efficiency dialyzers using high blood flow rates may provide drug clearance greater than that achieved by hemoperfusion.[4]

Disposition

An asymptomatic patient who arrives in the emergency department after ingesting barbiturates should be observed for at least 6 hours and monitored for mental status changes, slurred speech, ataxia, hypotension, and respiratory depression. Onset of symptoms generally occurs within 1 hour. Patients who remain asymptomatic and have no significant complicating co-ingestants or medical problems can be discharged or referred for psychiatric care. Patients who are still symptomatic 6 hours after arrival should be admitted for observation.

BENZODIAZEPINES

Perspective

Prior to 1950, treatment of anxiety was limited. Meprobamate, synthesized in 1950, ultimately proved no safer than the barbiturates, but its commercial success inspired the development of other nonbarbiturate anxiolytics. With the introduction of chlordiazepoxide

Table 163-1. Benzodiazepines

Generic Name	Brand Name	Usual Dose	Oral Peak (hr)	Half-Life (hr) Parent	Metabolite Activity
Alprazolam	Xanax	0.25-0.5 mg	1-2	6-27	Inactive
Clonazepam	Klonopin	0.25-0.5 mg	1-2	18-50	Inactive
Clorazepate	Tranxene	7.5-15 mg	1-2	1-3	Active
Chlordiazepoxide	Librium	5-25 mg	0.5-4	5-30	Active
Diazepam	Valium	2-10 mg	0.5-1	20-50	Active
Estazolam	ProSom	1-2 mg	2	8-28	Inactive
Flurazepam	Dalmane	15-30 mg	0.5-1	2-3	Active
Halazepam		20-40 mg	1-3	14	Active
Lorazepam	Ativan	0.5-2 mg	2-4	10-20	Inactive
Midazolam	Versed	0.025-0.1 mg/kg	1-2	1.5-3	Active
Oxazepam	Serax	10-30 mg	2-4	5-20	Inactive
Quazepam	Doral	7.5-15 mg	2	39-41	Active
Temazepam	Restoril	7.5-30 mg	1-2	3-19	Inactive
Triazolam	Halcion	0.125-0.25 mg	1-2	1.5-5.5	Inactive

in 1960 and diazepam in 1963, benzodiazepines emerged as the principal agents in the treatment of anxiety. Cardiac effects and fatalities from pure benzodiazepine overdose are rare, and respiratory depression is less pronounced than with barbiturates. Additionally, drug-drug interactions involving benzodiazepines are uncommon.

Benzodiazepines remain among the most widely prescribed class of drugs (Table 163-1). With nearly 50 individual agents available worldwide, they account for two thirds of all prescriptions for psychotropic drugs.[5] Benzodiazepines are the most common prescription drugs used by individuals attempting drug-assisted suicide. Despite such frequent misuse, the vast majority of benzodiazepine overdoses follow a relatively benign clinical course. Children make up 10% of benzodiazepine overdose cases.

Principles of Disease

Benzodiazepines produce sedative, hypnotic, anxiolytic, and anticonvulsant effects by enhancing the inhibitory actions of GABA. Binding of a benzodiazepine to a specific benzodiazepine receptor potentiates GABA effects on the chloride channel at the $GABA_A$ receptor, increasing intracellular flux of chloride ions and hyperpolarizing the cell. The net effect is a diminished ability of the nerve cell to initiate an action potential, resulting in inhibition of neural transmission.

Three unique benzodiazepine receptors have been identified. The distribution of these receptors varies throughout the central and peripheral nervous systems. Classic benzodiazepines are nonselective, producing a broad range of clinical effects. Newer benzodiazepines interact selectively with a single receptor subtype to achieve a desired result, such as sedation, while minimizing unnecessary effects.

Pharmacokinetics

Oral benzodiazepines are rapidly absorbed. Intramuscular use of chlordiazepoxide and diazepam is limited by erratic absorption, but both lorazepam and midazolam are predictably absorbed intramuscularly. Following absorption, benzodiazepines distribute readily. Penetration of the blood-brain barrier is facilitated by their highly lipophilic structure. In plasma, benzodiazepines are highly protein-bound.[5]

Metabolism of all benzodiazepines occurs in the liver. Oxazepam, temazepam, and lorazepam are directly conjugated to an inactive, water-soluble glucuronide metabolite that is excreted by the kidney. Other benzodiazepines must first be metabolically converted by the hepatic cytochrome P-450 system. Chlordiazepoxide, diazepam, flurazepam, and clorazepate are metabolized to active derivatives that are then slowly conjugated and excreted. The long elimination half-lives of these intermediates can result in their accumulation in the body with repeated dosing. Triazolam, alprazolam, and midazolam are converted to hydroxylated intermediates that, although active, are very rapidly conjugated and excreted and do not contribute significantly to the drug's overall pharmacologic effect.[5]

Cytochrome P-450 processes may be significantly impaired in elderly patients or those with liver disease, leading to prolonged elimination of some benzodiazepines. Co-ingestion of drugs that also undergo cytochrome P-450 metabolism (e.g., cimetidine, ethanol) prolongs the half-lives of these benzodiazepines. The clinical significance of these interactions is unclear.[6]

Clinical Features

Central nervous system depression is common in patients with benzodiazepine poisoning and ranges from mild drowsiness to coma. Respiratory depression can be seen with large oral overdoses or with intravenous conscious sedation. The latter is particularly pronounced when the benzodiazepine is combined with an opioid such as fentanyl.[7] Hypotension is uncommon. Other complications include aspiration pneumonia and pressure necrosis of skin and muscles.

The vast majority of children develop symptoms within 4 hours of benzodiazepine ingestion. Ataxia is the most common sign of toxicity, occurring in 90% of patients. In children, respiratory depression occurs in less than 10% of cases and hypotension has not been reported. The duration of physical findings averages 18 hours, with a range of 4 to 48 hours.

Diagnostic Strategies

Rapidly determine the blood glucose level. Qualitative immunoassays for benzodiazepines in urine are readily available but do not aid management decisions. Many of these tests detect only benzodiazepines that are metabolized to oxazepam glucuronide. Therefore, benzodiazepines that do not produce this metabolite (clonazepam, lorazepam, midazolam, alprazolam) are not detected on a urine drug screen.[8] Serum drug concentrations are not routinely available on an emergency basis and do not correlate with clinical severity.

The benzodiazepine antagonist flumazenil should not be administered to patients with coma of unknown origin or suspected benzodiazepine overdose. Any possibility of concomitant tricyclic overdose contraindicates flumazenil use.[7]

Differential Considerations

Benzodiazepine overdose is usually suspected or diagnosed because of the clinical setting in which the patient presents. Many patients are rousable and can provide supporting information. Because signs and symptoms of benzodiazepine intoxication are nonspecific, atypical findings can be clues to the presence of other conditions. For example, profound coma or cardiopulmonary instability with pure benzodiazepine overdose is rare, and the presence of either should prompt the search for a co-ingestant. Nontoxicologic causes of CNS depression should also be considered.

Management

General

Respiratory compromise is the primary life threat in benzodiazepine overdose. Initial stabilization, including endotracheal intubation if warranted, must not be delayed by attempts at antidote administration. The vast majority of benzodiazepine overdoses can be managed expectantly. Activated charcoal is generally of no benefit in benzodiazepine overdose cases. Whole-bowel irrigation is unwarranted because sustained-release preparations are rarely used clinically. Neither multidose activated charcoal nor hemodialysis is effective.

Antidote

Flumazenil, a nonspecific competitive antagonist of the benzodiazepine receptor, can be used for reversal of benzodiazepine-induced sedation after general anesthesia, conscious sedation, and overdose. Seizures and cardiac dysrhythmias can occur with flumazenil administration.[9-11] Although the majority of these effects are well tolerated, fatalities have been reported.[10] Co-ingestion of drugs with proconvulsant properties is associated with an increased risk of seizures, presumably due to loss of the benzodiazepine's protective anticonvulsant effect when the antagonist is administered. Combined overdose of benzodiazepines with tricyclic antidepressants accounts for 50% of these seizures.[9] Co-ingestants possessing prodysrhythmic properties, such as carbamazepine or chloral hydrate, may increase the likelihood of cardiac effects by a similar mechanism.[7] Other risk factors are summarized in Box 163-2. A recent observational study found that 12% of patients receiving flumazenil after known pure or mixed benzodiazepine overdose actually had a contraindication to its use.[12]

BOX 163-2. Use of Flumazenil

Indications
Isolated benzodiazepine overdose in nonhabituated user (e.g., accidental pediatric exposure)
Reversal of conscious sedation

Absolute Contraindications
Known or suspected co-ingestant that lowers seizure threshold
Tricyclic antidepressants, cocaine, lithium, methylxanthines, isoniazid, propoxyphene, monoamine oxidase inhibitors, bupropion, diphenhydramine, carbamazepine, cyclosporine, chloral hydrate
Patient taking benzodiazepine for control of a potentially life-threatening condition (e.g., seizures)
Concurrent sedative hypnotic withdrawal
Seizure activity or myoclonus
Hypersensitivity to flumazenil or benzodiazepines
Patient with neuromuscular blockade

Relative Contraindications
Chronic benzodiazepine user, not taking for control of life-threatening condition
Known seizure disorder not treated with benzodiazepines
Head injury
Panic attacks
Alcoholic patients

The initial adult dose of flumazenil is 0.2 mg given intravenously over 30 seconds. A second dose of 0.3 mg may be given, followed by 0.5-mg doses at 1-minute intervals, to a total of 3 mg. Most patients respond to less than 3 mg. In children, the initial dose is 0.01 mg/kg (up to 0.2 mg). Because the duration of action of flumazenil is short (0.7-1.3 hours), resedation occurs in up to 65% of patients and requires either redosing or continuous infusion (0.25-1.0 mg/hr). Although flumazenil reverses benzodiazepine-induced sedation, it does not consistently reverse respiratory depression.

In summary, benzodiazepine overdose requires only supportive care (including, in some cases, intubation), and flumazenil should generally not be used because of the risk of precipitating seizures or acute withdrawal. It is most useful in highly selected cases, such as small children with accidental poisoning or others who are known to not be chronic benzodiazepine users. When flumazenil is used, careful monitoring is necessary for persistent respiratory depression and for resedation. Use of flumazenil has not consistently altered outcome,

BOX 163-3. Benzodiazepine Withdrawal Symptoms

Nonspecific
Anxiety, depression, insomnia, tremor, tachycardia, sweating

Severe (rare)
Visual hallucinations, delirium, seizures

complication rate, number of costly procedures performed, or duration of hospital stay.[12]

Disposition

Patients remaining asymptomatic after 4 to 6 hours of emergency department observation may be medically cleared after appropriate psychiatric consultation.

Withdrawal Syndrome

Abrupt discontinuation of a benzodiazepine in a chronic user results in a unique constellation of symptoms (Box 163-3). Risk for withdrawal is a function of both the dose of benzodiazepine and the duration of its use. Continuous treatment for more than 4 months is generally required before a patient is at risk for withdrawal. With abrupt discontinuation of a short acting benzodiazepine, the most severe withdrawal symptoms are expected within 2 to 3 days. For longer acting agents, the peak of withdrawal may be delayed up to 7 days.[13] Use of flumazenil can precipitate immediate withdrawal symptoms. Treatment of withdrawal consists of reinstitution of long-acting benzodiazepines. If discontinuation of the drug is the ultimate goal, a gradual taper should be performed over several weeks.[13]

FLUNITRAZEPAM

Flunitrazepam (Rohypnol) has been used in Europe, Asia, and Latin America for insomnia and preoperative sedation since 1975. Although never manufactured or sold in the United States, recurrent reports of its use in "date rape" prompted the U.S. Drug Enforcement Agency to classify flunitrazepam as a Schedule I drug. Flunitrazepam has been an active agent in the illicit drug market, where it is used to alter the effects of other drugs, including heroin and cocaine.[14]

Flunitrazepam has 10 times more affinity than diazepam for $benzodiazepine_2$ receptors. Onset of marked CNS depression occurs within 30 minutes. The drug is most frequently ingested with alcohol, producing disinhibition and amnesia. Despite marked CNS depression, patients can usually be aroused with noxious stimuli. The half-life of the drug is 16 to 35 hours, but the resulting coma can be prolonged for up to 48 hours.[14] Despite many years of concern over flunitrazepam as a "date rape" agent, its use in such cases has rarely been documented.[15] Nevertheless, this drug remains easily obtainable outside the United States. Flunitrazepam is not detected on routine urine drug screens but, if needed as evidence, urine should be collected, refrigerated, or frozen and the local or state police crime laboratory contacted to arrange testing. Metabolites of flunitrazepam are detectable in the urine up to 72 hours after exposure.[15]

BUSPIRONE

Buspirone (BuSpar) has been approved for treatment of generalized anxiety since 1986. Unlike benzodiazepines, buspirone does not have any significant effect on the actions of GABA. Rather, it acts as a partial serotonin ($5\text{-}HT_{1A}$) agonist. To a lesser extent, it also antagonizes dopamine (D_2) receptors. Buspirone has no hypnotic, anticonvulsant, or muscle relaxant effects.

The use of buspirone has several advantages over benzodiazepines. The drug causes minimal CNS depression, even in combination with ethanol. Dosage adjustment is not needed for elderly patients. Chronic administration does not cause tolerance. Additionally, dependence does not occur. A withdrawal state after discontinuation has not been reported.

Only one case of isolated buspirone overdose has been published. That patient was lethargic and had a tonic-clonic seizure but recovered fully.[16]

ZOLPIDEM AND ZALEPLON

Zolpidem (Ambien) and zaleplon (Sonata) differ in structure from both the benzodiazepines and buspirone. They act selectively at the benzodiazepine receptor, producing sedation without many of the other effects seen with benzodiazepines. They have modest anxiolytic, muscle relaxant, and anticonvulsant properties. Significant drug interactions are uncommon. Compared with zolpidem, zaleplon causes less memory loss and sedation at therapeutic doses and is more rapidly eliminated.[17] Transient visual disturbances and hallucinations can occur in patients with normal levels of consciousness with use of both zolpidem and zaleplon.[17,18] Abuse of zolpidem is limited by vomiting, which may occur after a supratherapeutic dose. Both zolpidem and zaleplon have rapid elimination and lack active metabolites.[19]

Patients with zolpidem overdose generally do well with supportive care alone. Zolpidem is antagonized by flumazenil. Fatalities from isolated zolpidem overdose are rare; all published cases involve individuals found dead at home. Fatalities are often associated with co-ingestants, particularly other sedative hypnotics or antipsychotics.[20] Drowsiness is by far the most common manifestation of toxicity. Development of coma and respiratory failure are rare, despite overdoses of up to 40 times the normal dose.[21] Zolpidem overdose in children follows a similarly benign course. Drowsiness, ataxia, and hallucinations resolve within 10 hours.[22]

Overdose information for zaleplon is limited. In a case series, patients manifested CNS depression and mild hypotension. In one patient, arousal was temporally associated with flumazenil administration.[23] To date, the only published fatality involved a mixed drug intoxication (unknown quantities of zaleplon and butalbital). In this case, the postmortem serum zaleplon concentration was found to be approximately 40 times greater than what is reported following therapeutic use.[24] Adverse effects with therapeutic use include headache, anterograde amnesia, and transient visual hallucinations.[19]

CHLORAL HYDRATE

Perspective

Deaths related to chloral hydrate overdose were first reported in the medical literature in 1890. Incorrectly thought of as safe, chloral hydrate actually has a low therapeutic ratio and can produce significant, potentially fatal, toxicity. Chloral hydrate use is rare today, but it is still occasionally prescribed as a sedative in the elderly and for sedation in children undergoing medical procedures. The hyprotic oral adult dose is 0.5 to 1.0 g. The toxic oral dose in adults is approximately 10 g and may be as little as 1.5 g in a child.[25]

The toxic effects of chloral hydrate include CNS depression, gastrointestinal irritation, cardiovascular instability, hepatitis, and proteinuria. The primary active metabolite of chloral hydrate, trichloroethanol, has a barbiturate-like effect on $GABA_A$ receptors and is responsible for most of the CNS depression seen with significant overdose.

Chloral hydrate is rapidly absorbed from the gastrointestinal tract and almost immediately metabolized to trichloroethanol by the enzyme alcohol dehydrogenase. Onset of action is 20 to 30 minutes.[26] Trichloroethanol is long-acting, with a half-life (8-12 hours after a single therapeutic dose) that is significantly prolonged after overdose (up to 35 hours) as metabolic pathways become saturated.

The combination of chloral hydrate and ethanol (the so-called Mickey Finn) can produce rapid loss of consciousness. Both agents are CNS depressants and potentiate each other's action. Chloral hydrate increases the half-life of ethanol by competitively inhibiting the enzyme alcohol dehydrogenase, and the metabolism of ethanol will generate NADH, a cofactor for the conversion of chloral hydrate to the long-acting trichloroethanol.

Clinical Features

Chloral hydrate toxicity causes CNS and respiratory depression, gastrointestinal irritation, and cardiovascular instability and dysrhythmias. The combination of deep coma and cardiac dysrhythmia without hypoxia is characteristic of severe cases.

Mild chloral hydrate toxicity can look like intoxication from ethanol or barbiturates, with drowsiness, ataxia, and lethargy. A pearlike odor on the patient's breath or gastric contents may suggest the diagnosis. With more severe toxicity, findings can include miosis, muscle flaccidity, diminished deep tendon reflexes, hypoventilation, hypotension, and hypothermia.[25] Chloral hydrate is corrosive and causes nausea, vomiting, esophagitis, hemorrhagic gastritis and, more rarely, gastrointestinal perforation, gastric necrosis, or esophagitis with stricture formation.[25] Transient hepatic or renal dysfunction can occur.

Dysrhythmias from chloral hydrate toxicity correlate with fatal outcome. Chloral hydrate decreases myocardial contractility, shortens the cardiac refractory period, and increases the sensitivity of myocardium to catecholamines. Specific cardiac dysrhythmias include atrial fibrillation, supraventricular tachycardia, ventricular tachycardia, multifocal premature ventricular contractions, torsades de pointes, ventricular fibrillation, and asystole.[26] Hypotension results from inhibition of central neurovascular regulatory centers and impaired myocardial contractility.

Management

The management of the patient severely intoxicated with chloral hydrate includes support of cardiorespiratory function. Intubation may be required for airway protection or to support ventilation and oxygenation. Naloxone and flumazenil may precipitate ventricular dysrhythmias.[25] Because chloral hydrate sensitizes myocardium to the effects of catecholamines, epinephrine and norepinephrine should be avoided. Standard antidysrhythmic agents such as lidocaine do not appear effective against chloral hydrate-induced cardiac ectopy. The treatment of choice is a β-blocker.[27] Intravenous propranolol can be given in adult doses of 0.5 mg until ectopy is suppressed, followed by an infusion of 1 to 2 mg/hr, titrated to a heart rate of 80 to 100 beats per minute. A short-acting agent such as esmolol can also be used. Torsades de pointes should be treated with intravenous magnesium or overdrive pacing. Type I antidysrhythmic agents should be avoided. Unstable patients not responding to conservative therapy can be treated with hemoperfusion or hemodialysis.[25]

OVER-THE-COUNTER SLEEP AIDS

Perspective

In the past, most over-the-counter (OTC) sleep aids contained a combination of an antihistamine (either methapyrilene or pyrilamine) and scopolamine. Some preparations also contained a bromide. For safety concerns, these products were reformulated in the late 1980s to contain diphenhydramine or doxylamine, now the only two drugs found in nonprescription hypnotics. Many preparations contain acetaminophen or aspirin, added to create a "nighttime" pain reliever (Table 163-2). The availability and frequent use of these agents may explain in part why overdose is so common.

Principles of Disease

Diphenhydramine and doxylamine are antihistamines that also have hypnotic, anticholinergic, and weak

Table 163-2. Nonprescription Sedative Hypnotics, United States

Brand Name	Active Ingredient(s)
Alka-Seltzer PM effervescent tablets	38 mg diphenhydramine citrate 325 mg aspirin
Bayer PM Aspirin Plus Sleep Aid caplets	25 mg diphenhydramine hydrochloride 500 mg aspirin
Excedrin PM tablets, caplets or geltabs	38 mg diphenhydramine citrate 500 mg acetaminophen
Goody's PM powder	38 mg diphenhydramine citrate 500 mg acetaminophen
Nytol QuickCaps caplets	25 mg diphenhydramine hydrochloride
Maximum Strength Nytol QuickGels softgels	50 mg diphenhydramine hydrochloride
Simply Sleep caplets	25 mg diphenhydramine hydrochloride
Sleepinal Night-Time Sleep Aid capsules and softgels	50 mg diphenhydramine hydrochloride
Sominex Night-Time Sleep Aid tablets	25 mg diphenhydramine hydrochloride
Unisom SleepTabs tablets	25 mg doxylamine succinate
Unisom Maximum Strength SleepGels	50 mg diphenhydramine hydrochloride

local anesthetic properties. They act as competitive antagonists of H_1 histamine receptors and cause sedation by inhibiting the actions of acetylcholine on muscarinic receptors in the CNS.

Pharmacologic profiles of diphenhydramine and doxylamine are similar. Both are rapidly absorbed, with peak plasma levels occurring at 1 to 2 hours after administration. In the systemic circulation, they are highly protein-bound, with large volumes of distribution. Extensive metabolism occurs in the liver by the cytochrome P-450 system. The elimination half-life for diphenhydramine is 4 hours and for doxylamine 9 hours.

Clinical Features

Impaired consciousness is the most frequent finding with diphenhydramine overdose. Somnolence, psychotic behavior, and agitation are common.[28] Anticholinergic effects may be apparent, as noted in Chapter 148. Apart from a lower incidence of psychosis, doxylamine has toxicity similar to that of diphenhydramine.[29] Seizures and rhabdomyolysis may occur with severe toxicity. Despite recognized membrane-stabilizing effects, serious cardiotoxicity from poisoning with these agents is rare.

Diagnostic Strategies

Some comprehensive urine drug immunoassays will detect diphenhydramine. Quantitative serum levels of diphenhydramine or doxylamine are neither routinely available nor clinically useful. Serum acetaminophen and salicylate concentrations should be measured in patients with OTC sleep aid overdoses, because some preparations contain both a hypnotic and an analgesic. Serum creatine phosphokinase and urinary myoglobin assessments may detect myoglobinuria.

BOX 163-4. γ-Hydroxybutyrate Street Names

GHB	Liquid ecstasy
Grievous bodily harm	Liquid G
GBH	Somatomax
Georgia home boy	Soap
Gib	Salty water
Natural sleep-500	Scoop
Gamma-OH	Sodium oxybate
Gamma hydrate	Easy lay
Liquid X	Cherry menth
Organic Quaalude	Fantasy
Liquid E	G-Riffick

Management

Management of mild to moderate toxicity from OTC sleep aid overdose is generally supportive.

Prolongation of the QRS interval has been reported after massive diphenhydramine overdoses. This is most likely due to a quinidine-like effect of the drug on the myocardial conduction system. $NaHCO_3$ has been used successfully to overcome this effect, and administration of 1 to 2 mEq/kg intravenously should be considered.[30] In cases of extremely large overdoses, $NaHCO_3$ alone may not be effective. Physostigmine can be used in patients manifesting severe anticholinergic toxicity (e.g., delirium, refractory seizures, cardiac instability) (see Chapter 148).

Disposition

Patients who remain asymptomatic throughout a 4- to 6-hour emergency department observation can be medically cleared for psychiatric evaluation. Patients with minor sedation or anticholinergic effects can also be cleared when symptoms are clearly resolving. All other patients require inpatient observation in a monitored setting.

γ-HYDROXYBUTYRATE

Perspective

Originally synthesized in the 1960s, γ-hydroxybutyrate (GHB) was first used as an anesthetic in Europe and Japan. Researchers later discovered that GHB was a naturally occurring metabolite of GABA. Since 1970, GHB has been used to treat narcolepsy and alcohol addiction, as well as alcohol and opiate withdrawal.

A 1977 report that GHB may enhance the effects of steroids and the release of growth hormone resulted in marketing of the agent as a natural aid for increasing muscle mass. Numerous reports of adverse effects followed. In 1989, the U.S. Food and Drug Administration called for a voluntary withdrawal of the drug from store shelves. Its sale and manufacture were banned in 1990; however, illicit use of GHB increased along with the emergence of GHB precursors, γ-butyrolactone (GBL) and 1,4-butanediol (1,4-B) (Box 163-4). On February 18, 2000, President Clinton signed "The Hillory J. Farias and Samantha Reid Date-Rape Drug Prohibition Act of 2000," making GHB a Schedule I controlled substance. Recently, GHB has been approved for the treatment of narcolepsy, under the trade name Xyrem (sodium oxybate, 0.5 mg/mL). When used with a legitimate prescription, it is a Schedule III drug in many states.

γ-Hydroxybutyrate remains a popular drug of abuse. Recipes for home synthesis are widely available. Some individuals take GHB for its purported muscle-building and fat-burning properties, others for its psychoactive effects. The drug's euphoria-producing properties make it popular at "raves" (large, crowded youth parties with energetic dancing to rhythmic music for many hours).[31-33] Self-treatment of insomnia with GHB has been reported and can cause dependence.[34] The CNS depression, amnesia, and disinhibition that occur with GHB, especially mixed with ethanol, make this combination a potential agent of sexual assault, especially in date rape situations.

Chemical precursors to GHB are also commonly abused. GBL is rapidly converted to GHB by plasma lactonases. 1,4 Butanediol is metabolized to γ-hydroxybutyraldehyde by the enzyme alcohol dehydrogenase, and then to GHB by aldehyde dehydrogenase.[35,36]

Principles of Disease

γ-Hydroxybutyrate binds to specific GHB receptors found primarily in the hippocampus, cortex, and striatum; it also binds weakly to $GABA_B$ receptors.[37] The drug stimulates dopamine synthesis but inhibits its release, causing dopamine to concentrate in the nerve terminal. With higher doses of GHB, dopamine release is triggered. GHB also has effects through the endogenous opioid system, increasing dynorphin levels, which may explain its euphoria-producing properties.

γ-Hydroxybutyrate is available in a powder or granular form that, when dissolved in water, produces a colorless, odorless liquid with a mildly salty taste. Underground home-based laboratories often synthesize liquid GHB by mixing and heating butyrolactone and sodium hydroxide. Careless preparation can result in residual unreacted base, causing significant caustic injury when the liquid is ingested.

γ-Hydroxybutyrate is rapidly absorbed. It is lipophilic and readily enters the CNS. Peak plasma levels occur within 20 to 60 minutes after ingestion.[34] Onset of symptoms is within 15 to 30 minutes of ingestion. Unlike GABA, it readily crosses the blood-brain barrier. The half-life of GHB is 27 minutes but may increase at higher doses. A characteristic feature of GHB intoxication is that the patient may awaken from deep coma suddenly, sometimes with self-extubation. Supportive therapy usually results in complete recovery within 7 hours of ingestion.

γ-Butyrolactone is an industrial solvent that is rapidly absorbed after ingestion and metabolized within minutes to GHB by peripheral and hepatic lactonases.[36] It produces a clinical syndrome similar to that of GHB ingestion, but its effects are greater and more prolonged.[36,37] In fact, GBL is more efficient at delivering GHB to the central nervous system than GHB itself.[36] GBL is available under a number of street names (Box 163-5).

BOX 163-5. γ-Butyrolactone Street Names

Blue Nitro
Enliven
Gamma G
GH Revitalizer
GHRE (growth hormone release extract)
Nitro
NRG3
Renewtrient
Revitalize Plus
Revivarant
SomatoPro
Verve 5.0

BOX 163-6. Butanediol Street Names

Inner G
Pine needle extract
Pine needle oil
Revitalize Plus
Serenity
Thunder nectar
Weight belt cleaner
Zen

1,4-Butanediol (1,4-B), an aliphatic alcohol normally present in the body in trace amounts, is converted after ingestion to GHB by the enzyme alcohol dehydrogenase.[35] Like GBL, it is used as an industrial solvent. A recent series of cases of 1,4-B toxicity reported nine episodes in eight patients, with two deaths.[36] Clinical findings included dizziness, confusion, unconsciousness, vomiting, incontinence, bradycardia, respiratory depression, myoclonus, and ataxia. When 1,4-B and ethanol are ingested together, ethanol acts as a competitive inhibitor of alcohol dehydrogenase so the toxic effects of 1,4,-B are delayed and prolonged, and the risk of fatality is increased.[36] 1,4,-B is available under a number of street names (Box 163-6).

Clinical Features

Diagnosis of GHB intoxication is based on the history, or retrospectively on the patient's rapid recovery. Signs and symptoms are generally consistent with poisoning by other sedative hypnotic agents. Hypothermia may be noted,[32] as well as Cheyne-Stokes breathing. In the presence of coma, bradycardia with or without hypotension may also be seen, which occasionally responds to stimulation alone.[32] Eye examination may reveal miosis with or without nystagmus. Behavioral changes are most common and range from aggression and delirium to coma.[32] A distinctive feature of GHB intoxication is respiratory depression with apnea, interrupted by periods of agitation and combativeness, especially following attempts at intubation. Emesis occurs in nearly 50% of cases.[32] Generalized seizures have been reported and may appear as random myoclonic movements of the face and extremities. The severity of the signs and symptoms caused by GHB is dependent on the dose and the concurrent use of alcohol or other psychoactive drugs.[34] The dose-response curve of GHB is steep. An oral dose of 10 mg/kg results in hypotonia and amnesia, whereas 25 mg/kg induces sleep. A dose of 50 to 60 mg/kg produces anesthesia, and higher doses may cause coma associated with bradycardia, respiratory depression, vomiting, and myoclonic activity.

Diagnostic Strategies

γ-Hydroxybutyrate is not detected on most urine toxicology screens. If laboratory confirmation is required, gas chromatography–mass spectroscopy must be performed. Because GHB is metabolized to endogenous substances, specimens must be collected early, ideally the first urine sample, to capture the parent compound. The drug is detectable in urine up to 12 hours after ingestion.

Poisoning with another sedative hypnotic can produce a clinical picture identical to that seen with GHB. Unique to GHB, however, is the relatively rapid resolution of symptoms. In the absence of a co-ingestant such as ethanol, most patients will awaken within 3 to 4 hours. Nearly all patients recover fully within 8 hours. Thus, the presence of prolonged coma should prompt a search for another cause. Cardiac effects and refractory seizures are uncommon, and either of these findings suggests the presence of an-other agent.

Management

Because of the high incidence of emesis in cases of GHB overdose, intubation for airway protection is essential in patients with significant CNS depression. Bradycardia unresponsive to stimulation should be treated with atropine. Treatment of isolated GHB ingestion is supportive. Patients should be protected from self-injury and observed for resolution of symptoms. Although physostigmine had been used to reverse the effects of GHB when used as an anesthetic agent, it does not follow that its use would be safe in the less controlled emergency setting when unknown co-ingestants might be present. Since good supportive therapy is very effective and spontaneous recovery rapid, the use of physostigmine as an antidote to GHB toxicity is not recommended.[35]

Withdrawal

Patients who suddenly stop ingestion of GHB or its precursors after chronic, frequent use can experience a severe and potentially life-threatening withdrawal syndrome, similar to withdrawal from other sedatives and hypnotics.[38,39] Because of the short half-life of GHB, symptoms of withdrawal usually begin within several hours of the last dose. The typical patient will have been using these products for weeks or years, and taking them every 1 to 3 hours around the clock in an effort to avoid withdrawal symptoms.

Mild withdrawal consistently manifests with anxiety, tremor, and insomnia. This can progress to confusion, delirium, overt psychosis, paranoid ideation, hallucinations (visual, aural, and/or tactile), and autonomic instability. Diagnosis relies on a history of symptoms beginning after abruptly ceasing use of these products, following a period of chronic frequent ingestion. The differential diagnosis includes withdrawal from other sedatives or hypnotics, delirium tremens, sympathomimetic toxicity, serotonin syndrome, neuroleptic malignant syndrome, CNS infection, and thyroid storm.

Initial treatment usually begins with high-dose benzodiazepines. However, GHB withdrawal may involve depleted levels of GABA.[38] Since benzodiazepines require the presence of GABA, they may not be effective in controlling GHB withdrawal. Barbiturates, which open chloride channels directly and do not need GABA to be effective, are often required in cases of severe intoxication. Pentobarbital has been used successfully in the treatment of severe GBL withdrawal.[40]

These patients often require intensive care unit admission for high-dose sedatives to manage agitation and to monitor fluctuating vital signs. Rhabdomyolysis and severe hyperthermia should be ruled out. Deaths are reported, sometimes many days after presentation and after apparent improvement.[38]

Disposition

Because of GHB's short half-life, symptoms sometimes resolve while the patient is still in the emergency department. The patient generally regains consciousness spontaneously. No delayed toxicity is expected. Patients should be counseled about the seriousness of their intoxication because they will be amnesic for the event.

KEY CONCEPTS

- Most patients with barbiturate intoxication will recover with observation and meticulous supportive care. The vast majority will not require gastric lavage, hemodialysis, or hemoperfusion.
- A urine toxicology screen positive for barbiturates does *not* prove that the patient's clinical condition is caused by the drug. Quantitative levels confirm the diagnosis. Serum barbiturate levels do not necessarily correlate with depth of coma or clinical outcome.
- Flumazenil is rarely indicated and can be dangerous. Administering flumazenil to reverse conscious sedation in the emergency department does not permit early discharge, because the patient must be monitored for the occurrence of resedation.
- Chloral hydrate–induced dysrhythmia should be treated with β-blockade.
- Endotracheal intubation to protect against emesis and respiratory depression should be strongly considered for patients with GHB overdose and significant CNS depression.
- Withdrawal from GHB or its precursors can manifest mildly with anxiety, tremor, and insomnia, but can progress to a severe syndrome characterized by delirium and autonomic instability. Management of this syndrome often requires admission to the intensive care unit for high-dose benzodiazepines or barbiturates.

REFERENCES

1. Frenia ML, et al: Multiple-dose activated charcoal compared to urinary alkalinization for the enhancement of phenobarbital elimination. *J Toxicol Clin Toxicol* 34:169, 1996.
2. Pond SM, et al: Randomized study of the treatment of phenobarbital overdose with repeated doses of activated charcoal. *JAMA* 251:3104, 1984.
3. Ebid AI, et al: Pharmacokinetics of phenobarbital during certain enhanced elimination modalities to evaluate their clinical efficacy in management of drug overdose. *Ther Drug Monitor* 23:209, 2001.
4. Palmer BF: Effectiveness of hemodialysis in the extracorporeal therapy of phenobarbital overdose. *Am J Kidney Dis* 36:640, 2000.
5. Chouinard G, et al: Metabolism of anxiolytics and hypnotics: Benzodiazepines, buspirone, zoplicone, and zolpidem. *Cell Mol Neurobiol* 19:533, 1999.
6. Tanaka E: Clinically significant pharmacokinetic drug interactions with benzodiazepines. *J Clin Pharm Ther* 24:347, 1999.
7. Weinbroum AA, et al: A risk-benefit assessment of flumazenil in the management of benzodiazepine overdose. *Drug Saf* 17:181, 1997.
8. Perry HE, Shannon MW: Diagnosis and management of opioid and benzodiazepine-induced comatose overdose in children. *Curr Opin Pediatr* 8:243, 1996.
9. Spivey WH: Flumazenil and seizures: Analysis of 43 cases. *Clin Ther* 14:292, 1992.
10. Haverkos GP, et al: Fatal seizures after flumazenil administration in a patient with mixed overdose. *Ann Pharmacother* 28:1347, 1994.
11. Davis CO, Wax PM: Flumazenil associated seizure in an 11-month-old child. *J Emerg Med* 14:331, 1996.
12. Mathieu-Nolf M, et al: Flumazenil use in an emergency department: A survey. *Clin Toxoicol* 39:15, 2001.
13. Molle HJ: Effectiveness and safety of benzodiazepines. *J Clin Psychopharmacol* 19:2, 1999.
14. Waltzman ML: Flunitrazepam: A review of "Roofies." *Pediatr Emerg Care* 15:59, 1999.
15. ElSohly MA, Salamone SJ: Prevalence of drugs used in cases of alleged sexual assault. *J Anal Toxicol* 23:141, 1999.
16. Catalano G, et al: Seizures associated with buspirone overdose: Case report and literature review. *Clin Neuropharmacol* 21:347, 1998.
17. Drover DR: Comparative pharmacokinetics and pharmacodynamics of short acting hypnosedatives: Zaleplon, zolpidem and zopiclone. *Clin Pharmacokinet* 43:227, 2004.
18. Tsai MJ, et al: A novel clinical pattern of visual hallucinations after zolpidem use. *J Toxicol Clin Toxicol* 41:869, 2003.
19. Weitzel KW, et al: Zaleplon: A pyrazolopyrimidine sedative-hypnotic agent for the treatment of insomnia. *Clin Therapeut* 22:1254, 2000.
20. Gock SB, et al: Acute zolpidem overdose: Report of two cases. *J Anal Toxicol* 23:559, 1999.
21. Garnier R, et al: Acute zolpidem poisoning: Analysis of 344 cases. *J Toxicol Clin Toxicol* 32:391, 1994.
22. Kurta D, et al: Zolpidem (Ambien): A pediatric case series. *J Toxicol Clin Toxicol* 35:453, 1997.
23. Hojer J, et al: Zaleplon-induced coma and bluish-green urine: Possible antidotal effect by flumazenil. *Clin Toxicol* 40:571, 2002.
24. Moore KA, et al: Mixed drug intoxication involving zaleplon ("Sonata"). *Forensic Sci Intern* 134:120, 2003.
25. Stracciolini A: Chloral hydrate. *Clin Tox Rev* 21:1, 1998.
26. Sing K, et al: Chloral hydrate toxicity from oral and intravenous administration. *J Toxicol Clin Toxicol* 34:101, 1996.
27. Zahedi A, et al: Successful treatment of chloral hydrate cardiac toxicity with propranolol. *Am J Emerg Med* 17:490, 1999.
28. Koppel C, et al: Clinical symptomatology of diphenhydramine overdose: An evaluation of 136 cases in 1982 to 1985. *J Toxicol Clin Toxicol* 25:53, 1987.
29. Koppel C, et al: Poisoning with over-the-counter doxylamine preparations: An evaluation of 109 cases. *Hum Toxicol* 6:355, 1987.
30. Clark RF, Vance MV: Massive diphenhydramine poisoning resulting in a wide-complex tachycardia: Successful treatment with sodium bicarbonate. *Ann Emerg Med* 21:318, 1992.
31. Williams SR: γ-Hydroxybutyric acid poisoning. West J Med 168:187, 1998.
32. Chin RL, et al: Clinical course of γ-hydroxybutyrate overdose. *Ann Emerg Med* 31:716, 1998.
33. Li J, et al: A tale of novel intoxication: Seven cases of γ-hydroxybutyric acid overdose. *Ann Emerg Med* 31:723, 1998.
34. Galloway GP, et al: γ-Hydroxybutyrate: An emerging drug of abuse that causes physical dependence. *Addiction* 92:89, 1997.
35. Mason PE, Kerns WP: Gamma hydroxybutyric acid (GHB) intoxication. *Acad Emerg Med* 9:730, 2002.
36. Zvosek DL, et al: Adverse events, including death, associated with the use of 1,4-butanediol. *N Engl J Med* 344:87, 2001.
37. Wong C, et al: From the street to the brain: Neurobiology of the recreational drug γ-hydroxybutyric acid. *Trends Pharmacol Sci* 25:29, 2004.
38. Dyer J, et al: Gamma-hydroxybutyrate withdrawal syndrome. *Ann Emerg Med* 37:147, 2001.
39. Schneir AB, et al: A case of withdrawal from the GHB precursors gamma-butyrolactone and 1,4-butanediol. *J Emerg Med* 21:31, 2001.
40. Sivilotti MLA, et al: Pentobarbital for severe gamma-butyrolactone withdrawal. *Ann Emerg Med* 38:660, 2001.

PART FIVE

Special Populations

CHAPTER 164

General Approach to the Pediatric Patient

Robert A. Wiebe

PERSPECTIVE

Background

Assessment of pediatric patients from the newly born through adolescence offers unique and varied challenges to the emergency care provider. Approximately 30% of all visits to a general emergency department are for issues related to pediatric patients. The vast majority of children in crisis are not seen in pediatric specialty hospitals, but in community hospital emergency departments. Although most pediatric visits to an emergency room are not serious, it is not uncommon to see true emergencies in infants and young children. Serious and life-threatening pediatric emergencies result from a wide variety of causes and require the health care provider to understand the unique anatomic, physiologic, immunologic, and developmental differences that make serious problems often difficult to recognize and the differential diagnosis dependent on the age of the patient.

Emergency care does not stop or start in the emergency department. An integrated emergency medical system that is capable of responding to the needs of children is a critical part of pediatric emergency care. Likewise, many critically ill or injured children cannot receive definitive care in small community hospitals. Therefore, a support network that includes interfacility transport resources and definitive care for pediatric patients must be part of an integrated system of emergency care for children. This chapter focuses on the role of the emergency physician in recognizing and assessing children needing emergency care.

Epidemiology

According to the National Center for Health Statistics, an estimated 107,490,000 emergency department visits took place during the year 2001; 20.7% were for the care of children younger than 15 years.[1] Less than 50% of these visits were for children triaged as emergent or urgent.[2] The National Hospital Ambulatory Medical Care Survey documented that only 6.4% of 24-hour emergency departments had more than one separate emergency service area. Of emergency departments with more than one emergency service area, a specialty area for the care of children was the most common separate service area. Data suggest that health insurance status is not a significant cause of emergency department overcrowding.[3] The convenience of the emergency department, access without appointment, and lack of understanding by parents of the meaning of an emergency are the major factors related to pediatric nonurgent visits.[1]

Respiratory emergencies and trauma are the most common reasons for visits to an emergency department. Table 164-1 lists the 20 most common triage complaints at a pediatric specialty emergency department. Injury is the most common cause of serious morbidity and mortality in children younger than 15 years and is responsible for 13.5 emergency department visits per 100 persons per year. In the pediatric age group, approximately 95% of these visits are for unintentional injuries that are largely predictable and preventable. Although the reasons for pediatric emergency department visits are many and varied, the care of critically ill or injured children should always focus on two physiologic events: shock and respiratory failure.

PRINCIPLES OF DISEASE

Pathophysiology

Anatomic and Physiologic Differences

Physical assessment of a pediatric patient requires attention to a variety of anatomic, physiologic, and developmental differences that vary with the age of the patient. It is sometimes difficult to separate anatomic and physiologic issues; for example, the large surface area–to–weight ratio in young infants can result in heat loss and temperature instability. Thus, it is important to maintain a neutral thermal environment during the physical assessment and stabilization process.

The relatively large head-to-body ratio and the small, weak neck of infants and young children make them particularly prone to head injuries. Blunt trauma to the chest and abdomen often results in injury to internal organs with minimal or no external signs of trauma. The elasticity of growing bones creates unique problems in pediatrics. Soft and pliable growing ribs will bend rather than break and transmit the forces of blunt trauma to the thoracic and upper abdominal organs. The weakest part of growing bones is the physeal plate or growth plate, and this area is injured more frequently than the surrounding ligaments are. In a growing child, sprains are uncommon and physeal fractures result in nearly 20% of pediatric fractures. Recognition of growth plate injuries in children is critical to avoid imbalance in bone growth.

Anatomic differences between the pediatric and adult airway are important to understand for appropri-

Table 164-1. Chief Pediatric Complaints from Emergency Department Triage

Complaint	No. of Patients	Percentage of Total Visits
Fever	19,754	19.3
Trauma/injury	11,650	11.4
Breathing difficulty	9,979	9.7
Upper respiratory symptom	9,004	8.8
Vomiting/diarrhea	7,657	7.5
Abdominal pain	4,460	4.4
Rash	4,287	3.3
Ear complaint	3,428	3.3
Genitourinary problem	3,235	3.2
Soft tissue infection	1,754	1.7
Seizure	1,745	1.7
Eye complaint	1,712	1.7
Sore throat	1,562	1.5
Oral/dental complaint	1,236	1.2
Headache	1,229	1.2
Irritability	780	0.8
Chest pain	707	0.7
Foreign body	547	0.5
Behavior issue	392	0.4
Sexual abuse suspected	354	0.3
Total visits to triage	102,453	
Top 20 visits		82.6%

From Children's Medical Center of Dallas: 2003 ED Triage Statistics.

Table 164-2. Normal Pediatric Vital Signs for Age*

Age (yr)	Respiratory Rate (breaths/min)	Heart Rate (beats/min)
<1	30-60	100-160
1-2	24-40	90-150
2-5	22-34	80-140
6-12	18-30	70-120
>12	12-16	60-100

Lower limits of systolic blood pressure†
0-28 days: 60 mm Hg
1-12 months: 70 mm Hg
1-10 years: 70 mm Hg + (2 × age in years)

*From Dieckmann R, Brownstein D, Gausche-Hill M (eds): *Pediatric Education for Prehospital Professionals.* Sudbury, Mass, Jones & Bartlett, American Academy of Pediatrics, 2000, pp 43-45.
†From American Heart Association ECC Guidelines, 2000.

ate assessment and emergency support of the airway when required. The small airways of infants and young children are more prone to obstruction from secretions, which can result in relatively rapid deterioration ranging from respiratory distress to failure. Simple maneuvers such as deep suction of the upper airway can frequently have dramatic results in improving air movement in small infants. Because infants are often preferential nose breathers, nasal obstruction from secretions can result in significant airway compromise. An irritable and crying infant may just be learning to mouth breath when the nose is obstructed.

Vital Signs

Table 164-2 provides normal ranges of vital signs by age. The normal heart rate varies significantly with age, and the first sign of compensated shock is an increase in heart rate. However, tachycardia is a very nonspecific finding in pediatric patients and may be related to fever, anxiety, pain, or fear. When measuring the heart rate, the quality of the pulse can be extremely helpful, as well as a comparison of the strength of the central and peripheral pulses in the same extremity. The quality of the brachial and radial pulses or the femoral and dorsalis pedis pulses palpated concurrently provides important information to differentiate shock from benign causes of tachycardia.

The lack of cooperation by infants and small children can often make determination of blood pressure difficult. Whenever possible, blood pressure should be obtained in an infant or child younger than 3 years; however, time should not be wasted when cooperation is a problem. An alert, crying infant with good peripheral pulses and normal mental status can be assumed to have adequate blood pressure.

Infants and young children have excellent compensatory measures for maintaining blood pressure in the presence of significant loss of circulatory volume. Compensatory mechanisms include an increase in heart rate and systemic vascular resistance. When these compensatory mechanisms fail and blood pressure drops below normal, the patient moves from a state of compensated to decompensated shock. The lower limit for acceptable blood pressure in children older than 1 year can be quickly estimated by using the following formula: systolic blood pressure = 70 + (2 × age [in years]). The pulse oximetry waveform can also be used to determine systolic blood pressure. Observing for the return of a plethysmographic waveform of the pulse oximeter as the blood pressure cuff is deflated has been shown to correlate closely with conventional methods of blood pressure measurement.[5]

The respiratory rate must be interpreted carefully in infants younger than 12 months. It is not at all unusual for infants to have periodic breathing with episodes of apnea lasting up to 20 seconds. To be considered normal, periodic breathing must not be associated with a drop in heart rate or oxygen saturation. The respiratory rate is dependent on the age of the patient, as well as other physiologic factors. In a febrile infant, the respiratory rate will increase by up to 5 respirations per minute for every degree centigrade in temperature elevation. Either a slow or rapid respiratory rate can be a sign of impending respiratory failure. A normal respiratory rate alone cannot be used to determine adequacy of ventilation. The respiratory rate must be compared with the adequacy of air exchange and work of breathing when assessing ventilation in a pediatric patient.

Vital signs at one given point in time may be quite difficult to interpret. Repeated measurement of the respiratory rate, heart rate, and blood pressure over time will provide a more accurate assessment of a patient's physiologic condition.

Developmental Issues

Knowledge of basic behavioral and developmental differences by age is important when assessing a pediatric patient. Table 164-3 summarizes age-related pediatric

Table 164-3. Developmental Milestones

Age	Gross Motor	Visual-Motor and Problem Solving	Language	Social and Adaptive
1 mo	Raises head slightly from prone position, makes crawling movements	Birth: visually fixes 1 mo: has tight grasp, follows to midline	Alerts to sound	Regards face
2 mo	Holds head in midline, lifts chest off table	No longer clenches fist tightly, follows object past midline	Smiles socially (after being stroked or talked to)	Recognizes parent
3 mo	Supports on forearms in prone position, holds head up steadily	Holds hands open at rest, follows in circular fashion, responds to visual threat	Coos (produces long vowel sounds in musical fashion)	Reaches for familiar people or objects, anticipates feeding
4 mo	Rolls front to back, supports on wrists and shifts weight	Reaches with arms in unison, brings hands to midline	Laughs, orients to voice	Enjoys looking around environment
5 mo	Rolls back to front, sits supported	Transfers objects	Says "ah-goo," orients to bell (localizes laterally)	
6 mo	Sits unsupported, puts feet in mouth in supine position	Unilateral reach, uses raking grasp	Babbles	Recognizes strangers
7 mo	Creeps	7-8 mo: inspects objects	Orients to bell (localized indirectly)	7-9 mo: finger-feeds
8 mo	Comes to sit, crawls		"Dada" indiscriminately	
9 mo	Pivots when sitting, pulls to stand, cruises	Uses pincer grasp, probes with forefinger, holds bottle, throws objects	"Mama" indiscriminately, gestures, waves bye-bye, understands "no" 10 mo: "Dada" and "Mama" discriminately, orients to bell (directly) 11 mo: 1 word other than "Dada" and "Mama," follows 1-step command with gesture	Starts to explore environment, plays gesture games (e.g., patty cake)
12 mo	Walks alone	Uses mature pincer grasp, releases voluntarily, marks paper with pencil	Uses 2 words other than "Dada" and "Mama," immature jargoning (runs several unintelligible words together) 13 mo: uses 3 words 14 mo: follows 1-step command without gesture	Imitates actions, comes when called, cooperates with dressing
15 mo	Creeps up stairs, walks backward	Scribbles in imitation, builds tower of 2 blocks in imitation	Uses 4-6 words 17 mo: uses 7-20 words, points to 5 body parts, uses mature jargoning (includes intelligible words in jargoning)	15-18 mo: uses spoon, uses cup independently
18 mo	Runs, throws objects from standing without falling	Scribbles spontaneously, builds tower of 3 blocks, turns 2-3 pages at a time	Uses 2-word combinations 19 mo: knows 8 body parts	Copies parent in tasks (sweeping, dusting), plays in company of other children
21 mo	Squats in play, goes up stairs	Builds tower of 5 blocks	Uses 50 words, 2-word sentences	Asks to have food and to go to toilet
24 mo	Walks up and down steps without help	Imitates stroke with pencil, builds tower of 7 blocks, turns pages 1 at a time, removes shoes, pants, etc.	Uses pronouns (I, you, me inappropriately), follows 2-step commands	Parallel play

Modified from Gunn KL, Nechyba C (eds): *The Harriet Lane Handbook*, 16th ed. St. Louis, CV Mosby, 2003.

differences in motor function, problem-solving, language, and social/adaptive milestones during the first 2 years.

Neonates

During the neonatal period and early infancy, normal behavior consists of sleeping, feeding, and crying when hungry or experiencing discomfort. There is little or no eye contact and no social smile. Discomfort is usually nonspecific, and the cause of the irritability or crying may be difficult to interpret.

Infants (12 Months or Younger)

As infants grow, they become more interactive and increase their behavioral repertoire such that failure to achieve or loss of specific behavioral milestones can be a sign of serious illness or injury. By 2 to 3 months an infant has a social smile and responds to a friendly voice. Lack of appropriate social interaction can be worrisome. An infant with a glassy-eyed, "nobody home" stare can be easily distinguished from a normal infant who tracks lights or has a smiling face. Beyond 6 months of age, separation (stranger) anxiety is a predictable behavior. A 6-month-old infant will cry when taken from the safety of the caretaker's arms. Infants at this age have little or no understanding of language, but they will certainly respond to a calm and soothing voice. Of concern is a 6-month-old who does not acknowledge your presence. Normal behavior for this age includes any expression of curiosity or anxiety, such as crying. Children older than 6 months should be approached with caution. The emergency physician should anticipate stranger anxiety and examine the patient, whenever possible, in the lap of the caregiver. Distractions such as toys and penlights are useful to provide emotional control of the infant during the examination.

Toddlers (13 Months to 3 Years of Age)

During the toddler age, as language develops, it is important to talk directly to the child. Praise and reassurance during the examination can go a long way in maintaining control. It is important to realize that toddlers and preschoolers usually have more extensive receptive language even when their expressive language is limited. Misconceptions about illness and injury may be picked up from communications with parents and result in illogical fears.

Preschool Children (4 to 5 Years of Age)

Preschool children often fantasize, and such fantasies may result in irrational assumptions and even nightmares. The cause of injuries or illnesses in preschoolers or loved ones may be misinterpreted as being a result of their own misbehavior.

School-Age Children (6 to 12 Years of Age)

As children reach school age, it becomes particularly important to explain procedures, answer questions, and address fears and concerns honestly. Privacy and modesty should be respected. Whenever possible, the child should be included in conversations, and historical information should be taken from both the child and parent. The powers of reasoning begin to mature, and a school-age child will often attempt to negotiate control over having painful or distasteful procedures performed. Choices and behavior limits should be given only when they do not compromise care. A child may be given the choice to have blood drawn from the left arm or the right arm or be told that it is OK to cry but that it is important to keep the arm still.

Adolescents (13 to 19 Years of Age)

With adolescence comes independence and autonomy. Peer pressure becomes far more important than the behavior boundaries provided by the caretaker. Adolescents are risk takers and often have no fear of danger or injury. They rarely anticipate consequences and may lack common sense. Privacy and confidentiality should always be respected, and it is wise to separate adolescents from the caregiver when obtaining information and performing the physical examination.

CLINICAL FEATURES

Recognition of early and compensated shock may be a challenge to a health care provider forced to multitask in a busy emergency department. An infant in respiratory distress who begins to tire and slip slowly into failure may even be interpreted as improving until it is too late. Surgically correctable problems such appendicitis, intussusception, and volvulus can be difficult to recognize early, and delay in diagnosis will predictably increase morbidity and mortality. Infections that could be life threatening must be diagnosed by the history and physical examination. The clinician cannot rely on a blood count to rule out a serious bacterial illness. The possibility of child abuse should always be considered whenever injuries are inconsistent with the reported cause. Signs of increased intracranial pressure may suggest intracranial bleeding, infection, or tumors.

Pediatric Assessment Triangle

A "hands-off" assessment of infants and young children can allow the examiner to gather critical information from a distance before upsetting the child with an invasive physical examination. The pediatric assessment triangle (PAT) offers a sensible, orderly approach that can be used to assess children of all ages, identify abnormal physiology, and define the urgency and need for lifesaving interventions. Before touching the patient, observe the child from a distance for visual and auditory clues. Figure 164-1 defines the three arms of the PAT: appearance, work of breathing, and circulation to the skin. This brief assessment rarely takes more than 30 seconds and adds to the initial discernment of "sick from well" (Table 164-4).[6,7]

Appearance

From a distance, quickly determine the general appearance of the child. Is the child interacting normally with

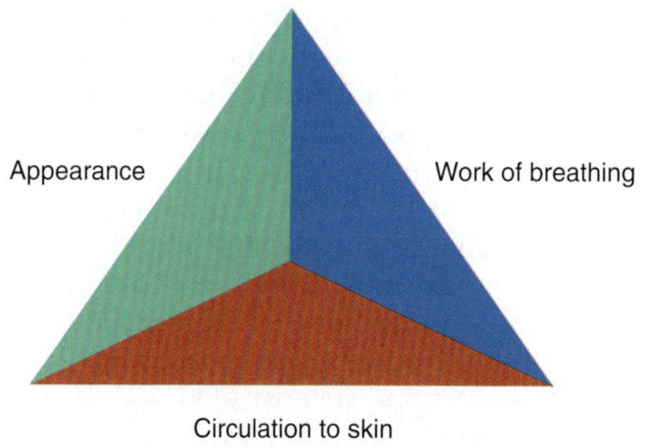

Figure 164-1. Pediatric assessment triangle.

Table 164-4. PAT—Initial Assessment

Appearance	Work of Breathing	Circulation to the Skin
Tone Irritable, interactive Consolable Look/gaze Speech/cry	Abnormal sounds: stridor, grunting, snoring, wheezing Abnormal positioning: sniffing, tripoding, refusal to lie down Retractions Head bobbing Nasal flaring	Pallor Mottling Cyanosis Petechiae

PAT, pediatric assessment triangle.
Modified from Dieckmann R, Brownstein D, Gausche-Hill M (eds): *Pediatric Education for Prehospital Professionals.* Sudbury, Mass, Jones & Bartlett, American Academy of Pediatrics, 2000, pp 36-40.

the environment? When the brain is not being adequately perfused for any reason, irritability is usually the first sign, followed by alternating irritability and lethargy. This situation is typified by an infant who sleeps quietly but, when touched or stimulated, immediately begins to shake and become irritable; when the stimulation is removed, the infant immediately returns to sleep. Alternating lethargy and irritability will progress to lethargy and ultimately coma if the causative condition is not reversed. The glassy-eyed, "nobody home" stare of a septic or brain-injured infant is not difficult to recognize. A high-pitched or cephalic cry is characteristic of any insult to the central nervous system. When in doubt, the parent can usually confirm that the cry is atypical. Simple observation of older children for proper tone, motor movements, and reaction to environmental stimulation is a good assessment of the appearance arms of the PAT. Appearance, when normal, can ensure that ventilation, oxygenation, and brain perfusion are at least adequate.

Work of Breathing

Assessment of the work of breathing in infants and young children is best done from a distance. Once an infant begins to cry, it is difficult to make any reasonable interpretation of oxygenation and ventilation or to interpret breath sounds. Listening carefully for audible abnormal airway sounds such as grunting, wheezing, stridor, and snoring can be quickly assessed without the use of a stethoscope. Grunting is an infant's or child's way of providing self-administered positive end-expiratory pressure to recruit collapsed or fluid-filled alveoli. The presence of inspiratory stridor alerts the examiner to upper airway obstruction. Muffled, hoarse, or abnormal speech can occur with trauma to the larynx or from a peritonsillar or peripharyngeal abscess. Assessment of wheezing should determine whether the sounds occur during both inhalation and exhalation and whether there is a prolonged expiratory phase. Observing for abnormal positioning can help determine the cause and severity of airway obstruction. A child assuming the "sniffing position" is attempting to best position the airway to overcome obstruction.

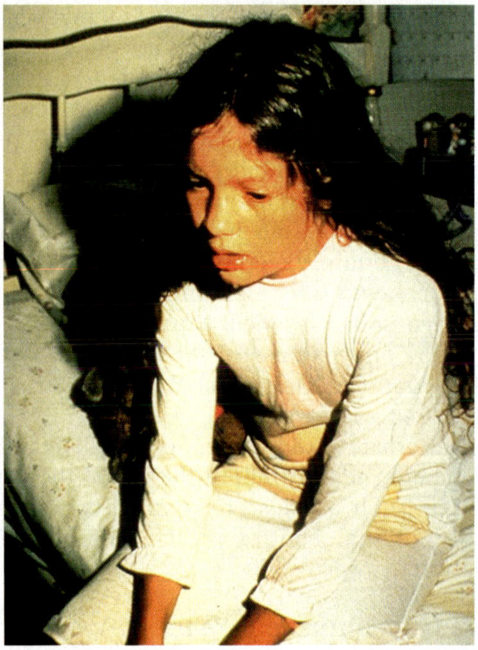

Figure 164-2. Tripod position in a child with airway obstruction.

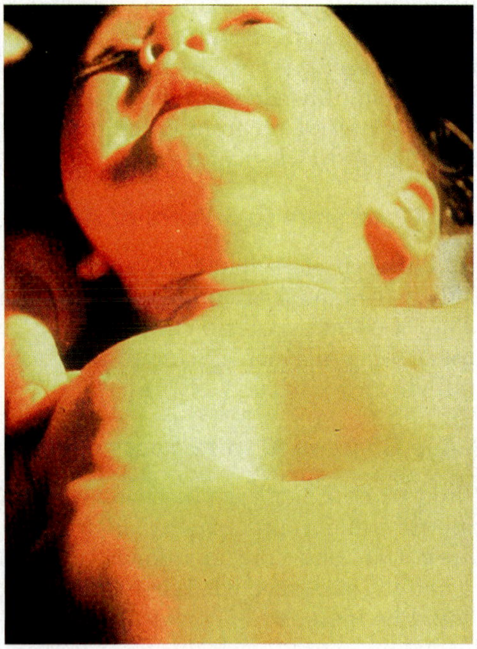

Figure 164-3. Intercostal retractions in a child with respiratory distress.

Tripoding is often seen with severe respiratory distress in an attempt to maximize use of the accessory muscles of breathing (Figure 164-2). The presence of intercostal, supraclavicular, and substernal retractions indicates an increased work of breathing (Figure 164-3). Infants, for the first several months of life, may normally demonstrate abdominal breathing. Seesaw movements of the chest and abdomen are always abnormal. A child with a retropharyngeal abscess may have torticollis or may just refuse to extend the neck with loss of upward gaze. Nasal flaring and head bobbing can be seen in infants

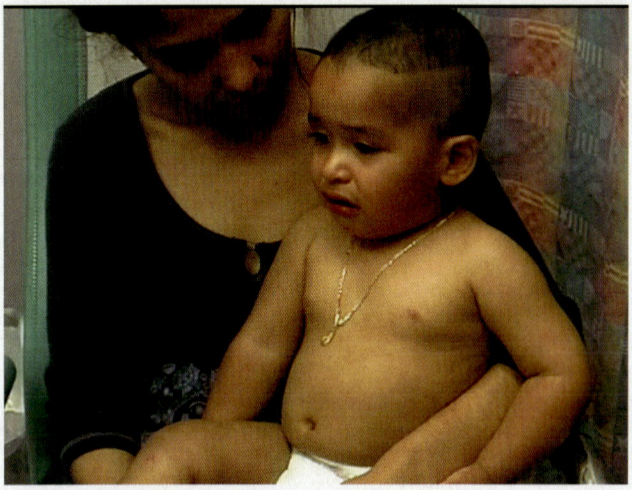

Figure 164-4. Nasal flaring in a child with respiratory distress from lower airway obstruction.

and young children with significantly increased work of breathing (Figure 164-4).

Effortless tachypnea, or rapid respirations with no increased work of breathing, is characteristic of a child in compensated or decompensated shock. It reflects a physiologic response to metabolic acidosis by increasing the respiratory drive and driving the pH toward normal. Irregular respirations in a child with an abnormal appearance may suggest increased intracranial pressure. It is important to remember that as a patient slips from respiratory distress to respiratory failure, work of breathing and the respiratory rate may both decrease. When this occurs, the appearance will change and a decrease in the level of consciousness will be evident.

Circulation to the Skin

Visual inspection of the skin can be used to quickly assess peripheral perfusion. Young children have excellent compensatory reserves, and with early and compensated shock, blood is shunted from the skin to vital organs. Compensated shock can be recognized by the presence of pallor. A pale child with a rapid heart rate should always be considered to be in shock until proved otherwise. As cardiac output is further compromised and perfusion to vital organs is decreased, the skin may become mottled. Mottling is manifested by areas of vasoconstriction and vasodilation in a random pattern on the skin. It reflects loss of small vessel integrity and may be similar to what is seen in vital organs during multiple organ system failure. Mottling is usually an ominous sign. It is important to not confuse cutis marmorata with mottling in young infants (Figure 164-5). Cutis marmorata is a lacy marbling of the skin caused by vascular instability. It is a normal finding and is commonly seen in infants in a cool ambient environment. Cyanosis may occur in the late stages of shock or with respiratory failure. Unless the child is cyanotic as a result of chronic primary cardiopulmonary problems or congenital heart disease, the development of cyanosis is an indication of respiratory failure or decompensated shock.

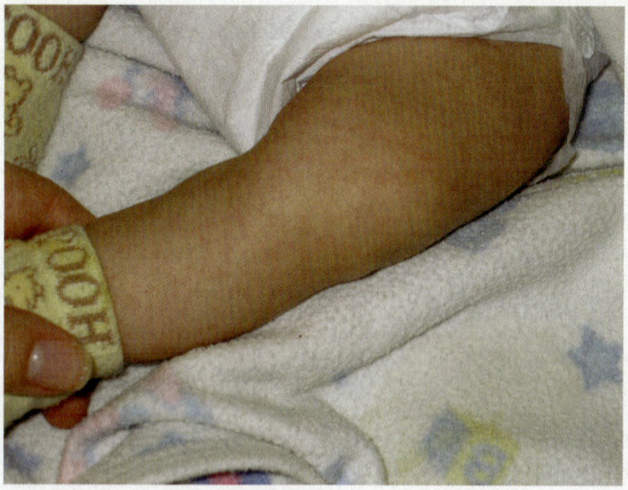

A

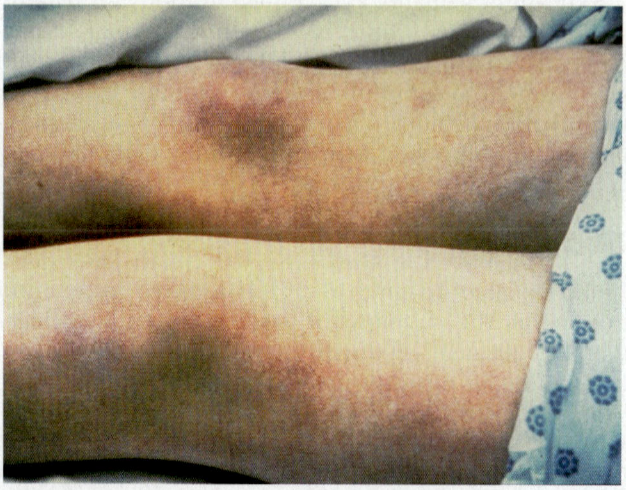

B

Figure 164-5. Cutis marmorata **(A)** and mottling of the skin **(B)**.

Table 164-5 summarizes how the PAT can be used to interpret specific physiologic abnormalities and the clinical condition of the patient.

Hands-on Initial Assessment

Two critical issues should be remembered when interpreting vital signs in children: first, remember to use age-appropriate standards (see Table 164-2); second, changes in vital signs over time are far more important than any single recording. A monitored and sleeping infant with an increasing heart rate cannot be ignored.

The initial hands-on assessment should be done in an orderly fashion by performing a stepwise assessment of airway, breathing, and circulation and resolving issues related to each before progressing to the next step.

Assessment of neurologic status or disability provides an opportunity for a more detailed objective measure of the child's appearance from the PAT. The Glasgow Coma Scale or its pediatric modification provides methods for assessing disability that can be used to monitor changes in mental status over time. The AVPU (alert, verbal, painful, unresponsive) scale is a

Table 164-5. Interpretation of the Pediatric Assessment Triangle

Physiologic State	Appearance	Work of Breathing	Circulation to the Skin
Respiratory distress	Normal	Abnormal	Normal
Respiratory failure	Abnormal	Abnormal	Normal
Compensated shock	Normal	Normal	Abnormal
Decompensated shock	Abnormal	Normal	Abnormal
Brain injury/dysfunction	Abnormal	Normal	Normal
Cardiopulmonary failure	Abnormal	Abnormal	Abnormal

Modified from Dieckmann R, Brownstein D, Gausche-Hill M (eds): *Pediatric Education for Prehospital Professionals.* Sudbury, Mass, Jones & Bartlett, American Academy of Pediatrics, 2000, pp 30-57.

simple alternative to assess whether the child is alert, responsive to verbal commands, responsive only to painful stimuli, or unresponsive.

Exposure of infants and young children can usually be performed more effectively with the parent's assistance. Make every effort to maintain a neutral thermal environment to avoid unnecessary heat loss during the examination. Modesty can be preserved and cooperation can be improved by exposing body parts one area at a time.

Triage

The purpose of triage is to rapidly assess a patient and determine the urgency of evaluation and management. A number of triage scores have been devised, including the recently developed Canadian Pediatric Triage and Acuity Scale.* This triage tool uses a five-level system. Table 164-6 uses a similar triage tool to list the 10 most common signs, symptoms, or problems categorized as triage level I in a busy inner-city emergency department in the United States. A triage level I patient is defined as one in shock or respiratory failure, nonresponsive, or with absent or unstable vital signs. Traumatic injuries rank first for triage level I visits and rank third for triage level II visits. The second most common cause for a triage level I emergency department visit is seizures, which represent 16% of all triage level I visits. Respiratory failure is responsible for nearly 10% of all triage level I emergency department visits, and respiratory distress is the most common cause of triage level II visits.

Table 164-7 lists the 10 most common causes for triage level II visits. A triage level II patient is one who is considered to be an emergency with a potential threat to life, limb, or function; one who is lethargic, with significant respiratory distress; or one with severe pain. A level II patient requires physician assessment within 15 minutes of arrival to triage.

Table 164-6. Triage Level I Emergency Department* Visits

Category	No. of Patients	Percentage of Level I Visits
Trauma	369	56.3
Seizures	107	16.3
Respiratory failure	64	9.8
Altered consciousness	19	2.9
Sepsis	15	2.3
Cardiac problem	15	2.3
Diabetic ketoacidosis	11	1.7
Toxic ingestion	9	1.4
SIDS/CPR	8	1.2
Hypovolemic shock	4	0.6
Percentage of total		94.8
Total level I visits	655	64.0

*Children's Medical Center of Dallas, 2003; *N* = 102,453 visits.
CPR, cardiopulmonary resuscitation; SIDS, sudden infant death syndrome.

Table 164-7. Triage Level II Emergency Department* Visits

Category	No. of Patients	Percentage of Level II Visits
Respiratory distress	4,132	33.0
Suspected sepsis/meningitis	881	7.0
Trauma/injury	786	6.3
Sickle cell disease complications	727	5.8
Diabetes complications	447	3.6
Genitourinary complaints	413	3.3
Ventriculoperitoneal shunt complications	388	3.1
Seizures	332	2.6
Hypovolemic dehydration	309	2.5
Oncology patient with fever	255	2.0
Percentage of total		69.2
Total level II visits	12,540	(12.2)

*Children's Medical Center of Dallas, 2003; *N* = 102,453 visits.

Clinical Interview

The initial contact with the child and parent will often determine the ultimate level of cooperation received and parent satisfaction with the visit. Parents who bring children to an emergency department for care usually perceive that their child has an emergency. Treating a family with respect, gentleness, and kindness goes a long way. Never resent the patient for a visit. If the family has been waiting a long time to see

*See *Canadian Journal of Emergency Medicine,* October 2001, vol 3, no 4 (suppl). www.caep.ca

BOX 164-1. Focused "Sample" History

Signs/symptoms
Allergies
Medications
Past medical problems
Last food or liquid
Events leading to injury/illness

Modified from Dieckmann R, Brownstein D, Gausche-Hill M (eds): *Pediatric Education for Prehospital Professionals.* Sudbury, Mass, Jones & Bartlett, American Academy of Pediatrics, 2000, p 51.

the doctor, start the conversation with a simple apology that expresses regret for the long wait. Introducing oneself to both the parents and child will facilitate a relaxed atmosphere for the interview.

Toddlers and early school-age children may be expected to say little during the interview process, but they should be allowed to provide answers to questions when appropriate. In an emergency setting, the chief complaint and present illness are the main focus for information gathering, but the past, family, and social history pertinent to the child's condition must also be explored. It is wise to not begin the interview with "What's the problem?" Parents do not like to consider their children or their conditions as "problems." A better approach would be "What brings you and your child to the emergency department today?" The "SAMPLE" mnemonic may be used to systematically obtain a focused history (Box 164-1). *Signs and symptoms* that describe the onset and nature of the chief complaint should be detailed. *Allergies* or drug reactions are recorded with information describing the characteristics of the reaction. *Medications* that the patient is currently taking are recorded, including the time and amount of the last dose. *Past medical problems* and special health care needs are detailed, including information about the pregnancy, labor and delivery, and current immunization status. Knowledge of the *last food and liquid given* is important if sedation, analgesia, airway management, or surgery is necessary. *Events* leading up to the injury or illness should be recorded. Gentle and soothing conversation throughout the physical examination often improves information gathering and reduces anxiety. The history is generally obtained while performing the secondary assessment.

Physical Examination

In infants and young children, the physical examination is not a stepwise process. It is neither a head-to-toe nor a toe-to-head evaluation. The examination should be performed in the least traumatic fashion by leaving painful or frightening components until the end and concentrating on high-value components initially. Children in late infancy through the toddler age should be left in the caretaker's lap during the majority of the examination.

BOX 164-2. Historical Indicators of Child Abuse

Unexplained delay in seeking medical care
History does not explain the injury
History changes with time
History is not consistent with the child's developmental abilities
Child has "magical" injuries

Specific Disorders

Trauma

A careful and detailed secondary trauma survey is necessary to identify subtle, but life-threatening injuries. A systematic approach to pediatric trauma that includes a continuum of care from first responders through emergency department stabilization, interfacility transport, and definitive care will save lives.[8] Attention to assessment of the cervical spine is a critical part of pediatric assessment. Because of the elasticity of the cervical spine in young children, spinal cord injuries without radiographic abnormalities (SCIWORA) can occur. These injuries result in ligamentous instability, which if ignored, may result in significant morbidity or mortality. A history of neck pain, paresthesias, numbness, tingling, or focal neurologic findings must not be ignored even if cervical spine films are normal.[9] Because most prehospital emergency medical systems require out-of-hospital providers to transport patients in complete spinal immobilization, it is important to obtain information from the transport professionals before they leave. Was the immobilization simply a precautionary measure? Was the child up, walking, and moving the neck before immobilization? Was there any history of pain, paresthesias, or evidence of neurologic injury? Such information can be helpful in determining whether the child needs radiographic imaging or can be clinically cleared from cervical spine immobilization.

As the secondary trauma survey is systematically performed, continued attention to the PAT and primary survey is critical to identify ongoing bleeding or progressing respiratory problems. A pale trauma victim should have vascular access and blood available before or during the secondary survey.

Intentional injuries to children still result in more than 1200 deaths per year. Because these injuries are most commonly associated with blunt trauma, it is possible that no external evidence of injury will be apparent.[10] When historical indicators suggest possible child abuse, consultation with child protective services is mandatory. Box 164-2 lists historical indicators that should alert the heath care provider to the possibility of child abuse.[11] Examination of the skin for burns or bruises consistent with child abuse should be a part of any trauma survey. Box 164-3 summarizes bruises typically found in abused infants and children. See Chapter 64 for a more extensive discussion of these issues.

BOX 164-3. Bruises Suggestive of Child Abuse

- Multiple bruises of different ages
- Pattern injuries
  - Hand prints
  - Belt marks
  - Cord loop marks
  - Linear marks from rigid objects
  - Bite marks
- Unusual distribution of bruises
  - Neck
  - Groin
  - Inner aspect of thigh
- Restraint marks on wrists or ankles

BOX 164-4. Clinical Croup Score

Stridor	
None	0
Audible with stethoscope (at rest)	1
Audible without stethoscope (at rest)	2
Retractions	
None	0
Mild	1
Moderate	2
Severe	3
Air Entry	
Normal	0
Decreased	1
Severely decreased	2
Cyanosis	
None	0
With agitation	4
At rest	5
Level of Consciousness	
Normal	0
Altered	5

From Westley CR, Cotton EK, Brooks JG: Nebulized racemic epinephrine by IPPB for the treatment of croup. *Am J Dis Child* 132:484, © 1978. Reprinted by permission of Wiley-Liss, a division of John Wiley & Sons, Inc.

Medical Disorders

Seizures

Seizures are a common initial sign in the emergency department. Although most seizures in children are benign and self-limited, assessment must include attention to the airway and ventilation. An actively convulsing child must be quickly assessed for adequacy of oxygenation and ventilation. A nasal airway properly inserted can dramatically relieve airway obstruction and allow for assisted bag/mask ventilation when appropriate. As a part of the secondary survey, the emergency physician should observe carefully for the character of the seizure and the presence or absence of any focal findings. Fever, central nervous system infections, and brain injury must always be considered in children with seizures and no history of childhood epilepsy. Other less common problems to rule out include intoxication, metabolic derangements, intracranial vascular anomalies, and tumor. Neonatal seizures can be very subtle and difficult to recognize. A seizure in this age group may be manifested as lack of an appropriate response to environmental stimuli, nystagmus, blinking eyes, or any fine repetitive movements.[12]

The Difficult Airway and Airway Obstruction

Recognition of a "difficult airway" can be a critically important issue in the assessment of seriously ill and injured children. Although scientific evidence for defining a difficult airway in children is limited, certain critical observations may be helpful. Dysmorphic features or physical conditions in special health care needs children that limit the ability to completely open the mouth or that reduce neck mobility should suggest the possibility of a difficult airway. Although Mallampati grades have not been well studied in children, if the uvula cannot be visualized when opening the mouth, the patient should be considered high risk. Any evidence of upper airway obstruction in a child who is in impending respiratory failure should indicate the need for potential surgical airway support.[13]

Scores that quantify the severity of upper and lower airway obstruction and disease are helpful tools to monitor response to therapeutic interventions. An example of a clinical croup score is detailed in Box 164-4.[15] The pediatric asthma severity score seen in Table 164-8 has been shown to be reliable, reproducible, and valid for assessing the severity of acute asthma in children aged 1 to 18 years.[15]

Altered Level of Consciousness

Altered level of consciousness accounts for approximately 3% of all critical emergency department visits. An orderly approach to the assessment of an altered level of consciousness is important to minimize organ damage and provide timely initial management. Quick assessment of the respiratory pattern can identify the irregular appearance of a Cheyne-Stokes breathing pattern, which consists of alternating periods of hyperpnea, followed by slowing ventilatory effort and periods of apnea. This respiratory pattern is typically found in children with increased intracranial pressure. Midbrain dysfunction will generally cause hyperventilation that is regular and rapid with normal oxygen saturation and low $PaCO_2$.

Examination of the eyes is helpful in sorting out causes of an altered level of consciousness. Pupils that are fixed and dilated in an unresponsive patient are always suggestive of serious intracranial pathology and are never seen in patients unresponsive because of metabolic derangements. A unilaterally dilated pupil is usually secondary to increased intracranial pressure from mass lesions causing uncal compression on the third cranial nerve. With significantly increased intracranial pressure, transtentorial herniation will

Table 164-8. Pediatric Asthma Severity Score

Clinical Finding	Definition	0	1	2
Wheezing	High-pitched expiratory sound heard by auscultation	None or mild	Moderate	Severe wheezing or absent wheezing because of poor air exchange
Air entry	Intensity of inspiratory sounds by auscultation	Normal or mildly diminished	Moderately diminished	Severely diminished
Work of breathing	Observed use of accessory muscles, retractions, or in-breathing	None or mild	Moderate	Severe
Prolongation of expiration	Ratio of duration of expiration to inspiration	Normal or mildly prolonged	Moderately prolonged	Severely prolonged
Tachypnea	Respiratory rate above normal for age	Absent	Present	
Mental status	Observation of the child's state of alertness	Normal	Depressed	

From Gorelick MH, Stevens MW, Shultz TR, Scribano PV: Performance of a novel clinical score, the Pediatric Asthma Severity Score (PASS), in the evaluation of acute asthma. *Acad Emerg Med* 11:10, 2004.

increase pressure on the brainstem and result in asymmetric pupils that become fixed and dilated. The doll's eye reflex can be performed by rapidly rotating the head from side to side while observing for a normal doll's eye response; the eyes of a child with a positive response remain fixed forward as the head is turned. Observe closely for equality of extraocular movements, nystagmus, and deviation of the eyes at rest. Funduscopic examination is helpful in identifying papilledema and retinal hemorrhages.

Assessment of motor movements and tone is an important part of the secondary assessment for altered consciousness. Observe closely for symmetry of movements and the presence or absence of abnormal posturing, and assess muscle strength and tone.

Shock

Patients with trauma, sepsis, cardiac problems, diabetic ketoacidosis, hypovolemic shock, and ingestion of toxic substances may arrive at the emergency department in shock. The secondary survey will help differentiate causes of the shock state. Assessment of four organ systems in systematic fashion will help determine the etiology and severity of the shock and monitor response to treatment. The heart is the first organ to respond to a shock state and does so with an increased rate. Cardiac output is a function of stroke volume and heart rate, and when stroke volume decreases for any reason, the heart rate will increase. Careful examination of the heart by listening closely for a gallop rhythm, murmurs, indistinct or muffled heart sounds, or any dysrhythmia will help identify cardiogenic shock as the cause. Tachycardia may be absent in patients with distributive shock. In the late stages of decompensated shock, bradycardia will occur as the shock progresses.

The second organ to respond to shock is the skin. In addition to the manifestations covered in the PAT, observe for skin temperature and signs of dehydration. The reverse thermometer sign can be of assistance in roughly judging the degree of hypovolemic shock. The examiner assesses skin temperature by running the fingers up the extremity to determine the point of cool/warm demarcation. During resuscitation, as reperfusion of the skin occurs, this point of warm/cold demarcation progresses peripherally. With early septic shock, the skin may appear warm and flushed. Look closely for signs of dehydration, including tenting of the skin, a hollow-eyed appearance, or dry mucous membranes, which suggest hypovolemic shock. Capillary refill must be measured at or above the level of the heart to avoid erroneous results from venous flushing. In a neutral thermal environment, capillary refill longer than 2 seconds will be present in all forms of shock.

The third organ that objectively responds to the shock state is the brain. Irritability or a decrease in mental status is consistent with progressing shock.

The lungs respond to shock with tachypnea and hyperpnea. Hypovolemic shock will often be manifested as effortless tachypnea when the patient has become acidotic. Cardiogenic shock, distributive shock, and septic shock may also give rise to increased work of breathing, crackles, or wheezing (or any combination of the three).

Close and repeated monitoring of these four organ systems must be continued throughout the secondary survey and stabilization processes.

Children With Special Health Care Needs

Children with special health care needs account for a large number of emergency and urgent emergency department visits. In a child with developmental delay, encephalopathy, or significant neurologic problems, it may be difficult to establish a normal baseline functional level. The caretaker is usually quite experienced and can provide valuable information to assist in assessment. Children with life-sustaining hardware such as ventriculoperitoneal shunts commonly come to the emergency department with nonspecific findings such as vomiting and headache. A behavior change that is recognized by the caretaker is a valuable clue suggestive of shunt obstruction.

It is important to engage the parent to assist with baseline information and to seek specialty consultation from providers who are familiar with children who have special health care needs.

DIAGNOSTIC STRATEGIES

Noninvasive Monitoring

Noninvasive monitoring techniques such as oxygen saturation and end-tidal carbon dioxide measurements have become a routine part of pediatric assessment for a variety of illnesses and injuries. Pulse oximetry provides a valuable noninvasive and continuous measurement of arterial hemoglobin oxygen saturation, which has rapidly become a new "vital sign" for many illnesses. The role of pulse oximetry in monitoring children with respiratory distress and failure has been well defined. The use of pulse oximetry in children with cardiorespiratory problems is a valuable assessment tool and helps the clinician titrate the need for oxygen supplementation and respiratory support.

End-tidal carbon dioxide measurement is a noninvasive method of monitoring a variety of critically ill children that helps avoid repeated blood gas analysis. Studies have demonstrated that analysis of exhaled end-tidal CO_2 can be used to monitor respiratory failure and perfusion to peripheral tissues during the resuscitation of patients in shock. Measurement of end-tidal CO_2 and pulse oximetry can provide valuable assistance in monitoring children in both shock and respiratory failure and is a critical component of assessing correct placement of a tracheal tube after endotracheal intubation has been performed.

The Pediatric-Ready Emergency Department

Emergency department preparedness for the care of children is a special need that requires limited additional resources, but significant professional support and advocacy from both physicians and nursing staff. It is quite clear that the majority of hospitals with emergency departments will serve as pediatric receiving facilities for emergency care independent of size, volume, or availability of comprehensive resources. Hospitals without all the necessary resources must clearly be prepared to stabilize critical pediatric illnesses and injuries within their limitations and ensure timely transfer to facilities with available necessary resources. Guidelines for preparedness for the care of children in the emergency department are available.[16] The availability of protocols and policies that ensure timely transfer of critically ill and injured patients after stabilization is a part of the pediatric assessment process.

KEY CONCEPTS

- The physical and developmental stages of growth in pediatric patients provide challenges to the assessment of children in crisis.
- An understanding of age-related developmental issues and differences is important for performing an adequate pediatric assessment.
- Establishing good rapport with pediatric patients is necessary to get cooperation in performing the examination process.
- The pediatric assessment triangle provides a rapid assessment of severity and physiologic status and will thus provide a road map for the initial assessment of all pediatric patients.
- A neutral thermal environment should be maintained during the physical examination to avoid heat loss in infants who are critically ill.
- The presence of a difficult airway can be assessed in seriously ill or injured children by determining whether they are able to open their mouths wide enough for visualization of the uvula and normally extend and flex their neck.
- Special needs children: The caregiver can assist in determining baseline status when attempting to assess children with special needs who have significant developmental delays.
- Beware the pale child: Pallor is a consistent and objective early sign of shock that cannot be ignored, especially in those with blunt trauma.
- Cervical spine: A large head with an elastic cervical spine may result in SCIWORA. Patients with this condition may not have any neurologic deficits, and cervical spine images may be normal. A history of transient paresthesia, numbness, tingling, or any focal neurologic findings, even if radiographs are normal, should be interpreted in this light.
- Emergency department preparedness for pediatric emergencies: Guidelines for having a pediatric-ready emergency department are available through the American College of Emergency Physicians and the American Academy of Pediatrics.

REFERENCES

1. U.S. Department of Health and Human Services, Centers for Disease Control and Prevention. National Center for Health Statistics, Division of Data Services. Available at www.cdc.gov/nchs/fastats/ervisits.htm.
2. McCaig LF, Burt CW: National Hospital Ambulatory Medical Care Survey: 2001 emergency department summary. *Adv Data* 335:1, 2003.
3. Luo X, et al: Children's health insurance status and emergency department utilization in the United States. *Pediatrics* 112:314, 2003.
4. Doobinin KA, et al: Nonurgent pediatric emergency department visits: Care-seeking behavior and parental knowledge of insurance. *Pediatr Emerg Care* 19:10, 2003.
5. Gilmore B, et al: Determination of systolic blood pressure via pulse oximeter in transported pediatric patients. *Pediatr Emerg Care* 15:183-186, 1999.
6. Dieckman R, Brownstein D, Gausche-Hill M (eds): *Pediatric Education for Prehospital Professionals.* Sudbury, Mass, Jones & Bartlett, American Academy of Pediatrics, 2000.

7. Gausche-Hill M, Fuchs S, Yamamoto L (eds): *APLS: The Pediatric Emergency Medicine Resource.* Sudbury, Mass, Jones & Bartlett, American Academy of Pediatrics and American College of Emergency Physicians, 2004.
8. Morrison W, Wright JL, Paidas CN: Pediatric trauma systems. *Crit Care Med* 30(11 Suppl):S448, 2002.
9. Patel JC, et al: Pediatric cervical spine injuries: Defining the disease. *J Pediatr Surg* 36:373, 2001.
10. Cabinum-Foeller E, Perkin RM: Non-accidental injury: Recognizing child abuse in the pediatric trauma patient. *Trauma Rep* 4:1, 2003.
11. Block RW: Child abuse: Controversies and imposters. *Curr Probl Pediatr* 29:253, 1999.
12. Haafiz A, Kissoon N: Status epilepticus: Current concepts. *Pediatr Emerg Care* 15:119, 1999.
13. Caplan RA, et al: Practice guidelines for management of the difficult airway. An updated report by the American Society of Anesthesiologists Task Force on Management of the Difficult Airway. *Anesthesiology* 98:1269, 2003.
14. Westley CR, Cotton EK, Brooks JG: Nebulized racemic epinephrine by IPPB for the treatment of croup. *Am J Dis Child* 132:484, 1978.
15. Gorelick MH, et al: Performance of a novel clinical score, the Pediatric Asthma Severity Score (PASS), in the evaluation of acute asthma. *Acad Emerg Med* 11:10, 2004.
16. American College of Emergency Physicians and American Academy of Pediatrics: Care of children in the emergency department: Guidelines for preparedness (policy statement). *Ann Emerg Med* 37:423, 2001.

CHAPTER 165 Fever

Roger M. Barkin and D. Demetrios Zukin*

The evaluation and treatment of fever may vary dramatically with the patient's age and preexisting conditions. Management generally varies by age group: neonates and infants less than 1 month of age, infants 2 to 3 months of age, infants 3 months to 3 years of age, children 3 to 7 years of age, and children 7 to 18 years of age.[1,2]

Recommendations reflect the child's chief complaint, underlying conditions, community epidemiology, and anticipated compliance and follow-up. Enhanced flexibility may be used in children over 1 month of age for whom care givers' compliance and communication are anticipated.

PRINCIPLES OF DISEASE

Pathophysiology

Fever in normal infants and toddlers is a rectal temperature of 38° C (100.4° F) or higher. During the first 3 months of life any fever may have a particularly great clinical importance. An oral temperature above 37° C (98.6° F) reflects a fever in teenagers.

The thermoregulatory center in the body lies in the hypothalamus. The use of a rectal thermometer or temperature probe remains the most reliable method of measuring temperature in infants and toddlers; epidemiologic data on fever and most protocols for care are based upon a rectal temperature assessment.

Temperature is maintained near normal (euthermia) via physiologic mechanisms (sweating and hyperventilation to lower temperature, vasoconstriction and shivering to raise temperature) and environmental measures (seeking shelter from a storm, increasing or decreasing the amount of protective clothing). Complex cascades of circulating interleukins, prostaglandins, and prostacyclin mediate the febrile response to infection.

In most cases fever is a sign of infection. Other processes that can lead to an elevated temperature are environmental (e.g., the mild temperature elevation that occurs when an infant is swaddled with too many clothes or the severe fever that occurs in heat stroke), physiologic (e.g., the temperature elevation that normally occurs in school-age children after vigorous running and play), toxicologic (e.g., from aspirin ingestion), and hypothalamic (the abnormal temperature control that may occur secondary to damage to the central nervous system [CNS]).

SPECIAL CONSIDERATIONS

Occult Bacteremia[1-15]

In the early 1970s, McGowan found a high incidence of bacteremia in infants and toddlers with fever.[3] Children under 36 months of age with a rectal temperature of 39° C (102.2° F) and no obvious source for the fever have an incidence of bacteremia of 3% to 5%. Most do not appear toxic. The most common pathogen is *Streptococcus pneumoniae,* accounting for more than 85% of the positive cultures. The remaining 15% of infections are *Haemophilus influenzae* type b, *Neisseria meningitidis, Salmonella* spp., and other pathogens. *H. influenzae* type b vaccine has decreased the incidence of this pathogen. A new vaccine for *S. pneumoniae* may also change the epidemiology. *(Reviewer suggests The vaccine for* S. pneumoniae *[pneumococcal conjugate vaccine] has also decreased the incidence of this pathogen [Black S, Shinefield H, Fireman B, et al. Efficacy, safety, and immunogenicity of heptavalent conjugate pneumococcal vaccine in children. Pediatr Infect Dis J 2001; 19:187-195].)*

*Material new to this chapter in this edition was prepared by Marianne Gausche-Hill, MD, Department of Emergency Medicine, Harbor-UCLA Medical Center, Torrance, CA, and is indicated in bracketed italic type.

Children 24 to 36 months of age are less likely than younger infants to have bacteremia. Each degree of temperature elevation above 39° C (102.2° F) increases the risk of bacteremia. Harper and Fleisher report that those with a temperature of 39.5° to 39.9° C (103° F to 103.8° F) have approximately a 3% incidence of bacteremia, 40° to 40.9° C (104° F to 105.6° F) a 4% risk, and above 41° C (105.8° F) a 10% risk.[5] A drop in temperature after administration of acetaminophen does not reflect any change in risk of developing bacteremia.[12]

The greater the white blood cell (WBC) count, the larger the risk of bacteremia. Obtaining a blood culture only in patients with a WBC count above 20,000/mm^3 will fail to identify some infants with bacteremia. This is particularly true with *H. influenzae* and *N. meningitidis* bacteremias. In the case of *H. influenzae,* one third of bacteremic patients have a WBC count under 15,000/mm^3. Of patients with meningococcemia who initially appear well enough to go home, more than 50% have a WBC count under 15,000/mm^3. Of those with pneumococcal bacteremia only one fourth have a WBC count below 15,000/mm^3.[6]

With pneumococcal bacteremia, most children become afebrile within 3 or 4 days with or without antibiotic coverage. However, *H. influenzae* and *N. meningitidis* may cause persistent bacteremia, pneumonia, meningitis, and sepsis. Approximately 33% of those with meningococcal bacteremia die or de-velop meningitis, compared with 7% experiencing *H. influenzae* bacteremia and 4% having pneumococcal bacteremia.

Children who receive prophylactic antibiotics at the time of their febrile illness appear to do better than those who receive placebo. In retrospective reviews of both *H. influenzae* and *N. meningitidis* bacteremias, patients sent home on oral antibiotics did better than those discharged without therapy. Oral amoxicillin hastened defervescence and clinical improvement but failed to prevent major morbid events such as meningitis in a prospective evaluation. Harper compared children who received antibiotics for suspected bacteremia with those who were not treated prior to discharge. Treated children were more likely to be improved and less febrile on follow-up, and had persistent bacteremia or required hospitalization less frequently.[13] Fleisher's examination of 6733 children with temperatures below 39° C (102.2° F) *(Reviewer suggests Fleisher's study included children between 3 and 36 months of age with temperatures greater than or equal to 39° C [102.2° F].)* compares patients given ceftriaxone 50 mg/kg intramuscularly with subjects given six doses of oral amoxicillin 20 mg/kg. Blood cultures were positive in 195. All five children with definite bacterial infections at follow-up (three meningitis, one pneumonia, and one sepsis) were in the amoxicillin group.[14] Of children with occult pneumococcal bacteremia, 10% to 25% will develop some complication, including 3% to 6% who have meningitis.[15]

Hyperpyrexia[16-19]

True hyperpyrexia, defined as a temperature greater than 41° C (105.8° F), is an uncommon but serious problem. Extreme elevations of temperature account for fewer than 1% of pediatric visits. The main concern about hyperpyrexia is that it may indicate a serious underlying disease (e.g., meningitis or Kawasaki syndrome). In addition, the high fever itself can threaten the child. Approximately 20% of children with fevers above 41° C (105.8° F) will have convulsions.[18] With fevers above 42° C (107.6° F), direct end-organ damage may occur.[16]

Overall, infectious diseases far outweigh all other causes of hyperpyrexia. High fever can follow almost any infectious disease but is particularly common in certain viral infections, such as roseola, rubeola, and enteroviral infections.[18] At temperatures of 39° C (102.2° F) and above, children are at increasing risk for occult bacteremia, as well as localized bacterial infections. This tendency becomes exaggerated at very high temperatures. Children with temperatures greater than 41.1° C (106° F) have a 10% risk of bacterial meningitis, and an additional 7% have bacteremia without meningitis. Marcinak found that of children with fever above 40° C (104° F), 40% had a viral cause and 45% had a bacterial cause.[17] The bacterial illnesses, such as otitis media and sinusitis, tend to be benign. Other reviews, however, show a higher incidence of serious illness in children with extreme elevations of temperature. Press and Fawcett found that 8 of 15 (53%) children with fevers above 41.1° C (106° F) had serious diseases: two with bacterial meningitis, two with bacteremia, two with pneumonia, one with pericarditis, and one with Kawasaki syndrome.[18]

Many entities other than infection can cause hyperpyrexia. Temperatures greater than 42° C (107.6° F) are most often noninfectious in origin. Causes of such dramatically elevated temperatures include head injury, ingestion of psychotropic agents, heatstroke, and malignant hyperthermia secondary to anesthetic agents.[16]

An unusual and often fatal illness consisting of profound hyperpyrexia, hemorrhagic shock, and encephalopathy has been reported.[16,20] Children with this illness have sudden temperature spikes to as high as 43.9° C (111° F) and a rapidly progressive deterioration characterized by cerebral edema, shock, azotemia, anemia, and usually death. No etiology, infectious or environmental, has yet been determined.

Management should consist of an aggressive search for the etiology of the fever. The fever can generally be controlled with acetaminophen 15 mg/kg every 4 hours or ibuprofen 10 mg/kg every 6 to 8 hours. These agents may sequentially or concurrently be used for slowly responsive fevers. Sponging with lukewarm water may be useful.

Hyperpyretic children should all be evaluated with at least a complete blood count (CBC), blood culture, urinalysis, and urine culture. When no source is found, a chest radiograph and a lumbar puncture (LP) should be obtained, unless the patient is smiling and playful once the temperature comes down.

Because of the high incidence of bacterial infection, these patients are generally treated parenterally with antibiotics (ceftriaxone 50 mg/kg every 12 hours or cefotaxime 50 mg/kg every 6 hours; plus ampicillin 50 mg/kg every 6 hours if the child is under 3 months of age) pending culture results. Age-specific management considerations discussed in this chapter must also be implemented.

Febrile Seizure

Febrile seizures are common but generally benign events occurring in infants, toddlers, and young children. Approximately 2% to 5% of all children are affected. The convulsions are usually generalized and tonic-clonic, last less than 10 to 15 minutes, and occur during the up-slope of the fever curve. The peak incidence occurs between 8 and 20 months of age; febrile seizures are uncommon after 5 to 6 years of age.

The main entity in the differential diagnosis is meningitis, which can cause fever and convulsions. In the past, many believed that all patients with febrile seizures required an LP to exclude meningitis. Patients at greatest risk for meningitis are those under 18 months of age, having a seizure in the ED, having a focal or prolonged seizure, and who have seen a physician within the past 48 hours. The American Academy of Pediatrics recommends that an LP should be "strongly considered" in infants under 12 months of age with a first febrile seizure. Most children over 12 to 18 months of age who have brief, generalized convulsions and who appear playful and nontoxic after the postictal period can be treated without an LP. Children experiencing a first-time febrile seizure should have an LP if there are any concerns about follow-up. Prior treatment with antibiotics should inspire enhanced concern.

Fever of Unknown Origin[21]

The term *fever of unknown origin (FUO)* is traditionally used to refer to a febrile illness of unknown etiology lasting 14 days or more.

Most children with a chief complaint of a febrile illness lasting longer than 2 weeks simply have had two or three febrile illnesses, one after the other. Careful questioning usually reveals a period of relative wellness during the time period in question. Miller's review of 40 children with fevers persisting over 1 month in whom an evaluation was inconclusive revealed that these children usually have a benign course.[22]

True prolonged fever is a more serious matter. The causes include inflammatory bowel disease, Hodgkin's disease, other neoplasms, juvenile rheumatoid arthritis, systemic lupus erythematosus, infectious mononucleosis, Kawasaki syndrome, and tropical infections such as malaria. In one study of 100 children with FUO, 62 had infections, 20 had collagen-inflammatory disease, 6 had malignancies, and 12 were undiagnosed.[21] Box 165-1 presents a list of the various causes of FUO. A systematic approach to evaluation is essential, usually in collaboration with appropriate consultants.

BOX 165-1. Causes of Prolonged Fever of Unknown Origin

Infection

Bacterial
- Adenitis
- Endocarditis
- Mastoiditis
- Occult abscess
- Pyelonephritis
- Sinusitis
- Tuberculosis

Viral
- Cytomegalovirus
- Hepatitis A, B, or C
- Infectious mononucleosis

Chlamydial
- Lymphogranuloma venereum
- Psittacosis

Mycoplasmal

Fungal
- Blastomycosis
- Cysticercosis
- Histoplasmosis

Rickettsial
- Q fever
- Rocky Mountain spotted fever

Parasitic
- Malaria
- Toxoplasmosis

Collagen Vascular
- Juvenile rheumatoid arthritis
- Lupus erythematosus
- Regional enteritis
- Rheumatic fever
- Ulcerative colitis
- Vasculitis

Malignancy
- Leukemia
- Lymphoma
- Neuroblastoma
- Wilms' tumor

Drug-Induced Fever
- Antibiotics
- Anticonvulsants
- Antituberculous agents
- Procainamide
- Propylthiouracil
- Quinidine
- Serum sickness

Miscellaneous
- Acquired immunodeficiency syndrome (AIDS)
- Central nervous system and hypothalamic
- Environmental
- Factitious
- Familial dysautonomia
- Kawasaki syndrome
- Pulmonary embolus
- Serial infections
- Thyrotoxicosis

Fever and Petechiae

One of the most devastating illnesses in pediatric or adult medicine is overwhelming meningococcal sepsis. Afflicted patients commonly develop a downward spiral of disseminated intravascular coagulation (DIC) and irreversible shock despite aggressive antibiotic administration and treatment in the intensive care unit.

Selecting which patients with petechiae are at risk for meningococcal or other bacterial sepsis is not an easy task. Several relatively benign viral infections and other conditions can also cause fever and petechiae. Furthermore, early in the course of meningococcal disease the child commonly appears minimally ill.

In a study of 190 pediatric patients with fever and petechiae, Baker et al found that 15 had invasive bacterial diseases, half of which were meningitis.[23] The most common invasive pathogen is *N. meningitidis*, accounting for 13 of the 15 cases. Of those without invasive bacterial disease, the most common documented causes were group A streptococcal pharyngitis (10%), respiratory syncytial virus (RSV), or other viruses (12%). The remaining causes are nonspecific viral syndrome (50%), otitis media (15%), pneumonia (5%), and rare cases of Henoch-Schönlein purpura, acute leukemia, and Rocky Mountain spotted fever. Children with a normal LP, CBC, associated neutrophil and band counts, and a temperature greater than 40° C *(Reviewer suggests A temperature less than 40° C.)* (104° F) are less likely to have a bacterial infection.

Patients with invasive bacterial disease often appear toxic and have elevations of both the WBC count and total band count. Of note, all patients in this study with invasive bacterial diseases had petechiae above and below the nipple line.

CLINICAL FEATURES

History

Parents should be questioned about the length and duration of the illness, the height of the fever, dosage and frequency of antipyretics, pertinent past medical problems (including immunocompetence, drug allergies, immunization status, recurrent infections), and possible exposure to a communicable disease. Is the patient acting normally at home in terms of feeding, playing, speech (when appropriate), and elimination of feces and urine? Explore whether the child has been exposed to other children with communicable diseases such as chicken pox, measles, viral croup, bacterial pneumonia, or meningitis. In young infants the birth history is relevant. The immunization status should be determined, and when appropriate, a travel history obtained.

Has the child displayed symptoms consistent with common causes of pediatric fever? For example, children with otitis media typically rub or pull at the affected ear and appear irritable. Infants and toddlers with stomatitis commonly refuse feedings because of oral inflammation. Those with an upper respiratory infection will have sneezing, nasal discharge, and usually night cough. Pneumonia causes fever, cough, and sometimes grunting, flaring, and retracting. Gastroenteritis usually causes vomiting and diarrhea. Inability to walk in older patients points to cellulitis, osteomyelitis, or arthritis of the lower extremity.

Temperature Determination[24]

Despite many recent technical advances in temperature measurement, the glass-mercury thermometer remains the gold standard for accuracy. However, the relatively long dwell time (2 to 3 minutes) and the risk of cross-contamination and potential breakage have led many practitioners to use newer technologies.

Electronic thermometers are as accurate as glass-mercury. They have the advantages of a shorter dwell time and disposable sheaths.

Tympanic membrane (TM) thermometers measure the infrared radiation emitted by the TM, yielding an almost instantaneous temperature reading. Unfortunately, TM thermometers commonly yield a falsely low value.[25-27] In a recent study the TM thermometer was 76% sensitive in detecting fever above 100.4° F but only 57% sensitive for fever of 103° F or above.[25] The correlation between tympanic and rectal temperatures in patients over 3 months of age is good, but the correlation in those under 3 months of age is poor.[28] Many recommend against the use of electronic thermometers in children under 3 to 6 months of age. Technique is important when using the tympanic thermometer; tugging down on the earlobe during measurement improves the accuracy.[29]

In older children, eating, drinking, hyperventilating, and smoking can falsely raise or lower the oral temperature.[30]

Liquid crystal forehead strips are inconsistent.[31]

Axillary temperatures are also unreliable, often being falsely low. One third of patients with fever will have a normal axillary temperature, even with correction.

In infants and toddlers the preferred route for taking the temperature is rectal, because most algorithms defining risk of serious illness in this age group are based on the rectal temperature. In older children and adolescents the temperature may be taken by the oral route, if the patient has not recently been eating, drinking, or smoking.

After the initial rectal or oral temperature is documented, axillary or TM temperatures may be adequate to follow the subsequent course of the fever.

Physical Examination

The physical examination is the key to determining the workup of a febrile child. Vital signs should be noted. Tachycardia out of proportion to the degree of fever occurs with dehydration, septicemia, and primary cardiac conditions such as myocarditis and pericarditis. Tachypnea out of proportion to the degree of fever occurs with respiratory infections such as laryngotracheitis, bronchiolitis, and pneumonia.

Box 165-2 presents various illnesses to keep in mind during the physical examination. Box 165-3 lists the causes of fever and altered sensorium.

Ancillary[11,32-34]

Numerous laboratory tests are available to help differentiate serious from nonserious illness and to help locate the source of infection.

Despite the guidelines that are presented later, there is tremendous variability among clinicians in the types of diagnostic tests they order. Hospital-based subspecialists are more likely to order diagnostic tests than community-based physicians. Children seen by a physician with more than 10 years of experience are less likely to have tests than those seen by more junior colleagues. The presence of trainees tends to increase the likelihood of doing tests.[35,36]

White Blood Cell Count

Both high (>15,000/mm^3) and low (<5000/mm^3) WBC counts can indicate serious disease. In meningococcemia, for example, an abnormally low WBC count can be a harbinger of a poor outcome.

An increased proportion of polymorphonuclear (PMN) leukocytes and immature forms (bands) occurs with bacterial illness and sometimes early in the course of viral disease. The presence of toxic granulations or vacuolization of PMN leukocytes correlates with bacterial disease.

With viruses, as time passes there is a shift to a predominance of lymphocytes and monocytes (right shift); in bacterial disease, the left shift usually persists. A high WBC count with a left shift, common in serious

BOX 165-2. Common Illnesses to Screen for During the Physical Examination

Meningitis
Look for meningismus (unreliable under 12 months of age), irritability, and altered sensorium.

Otitis Media
Note that just as the forehead flushes red in a febrile, screaming infant, so does the tympanic membrane (TM). Therefore TM redness alone is not a sufficient criterion to make the diagnosis of otitis media. In one study, none of the infants with red TMs but normal landmarks had otitis media based on direct aspiration of the middle ear.

Upper Respiratory Infection (URI)
Nasal congestion and nasal discharge are so common in children that the diagnosis of URI should not be used to explain a high fever until more serious causes have been ruled out.

Pharyngitis
Keep in mind that tonsillar hypertrophy (*without* exudate or erythema) is a common normal finding in children 1½ to 3 years of age.

Croup and Epiglottitis
Both cause inspiratory stridor. Children with croup typically have a gradual onset of symptoms over 2 to 3 days, do not appear systemically toxic, and respond to mist or cool air. Children with epiglottitis generally have a more rapid onset of symptoms (12 to 24 hours), appear toxic and apprehensive, and sit upright, drooling, with the head tilted forward.

Bronchiolitis
Wheezing and tachypnea are seen in infants and toddlers.

Pneumonia
The child will usually cough during the examination and display rales on auscultation. Auscultatory findings of pneumonia may be absent in younger children.

Appendicitis
Abdominal tenderness and guarding may be seen. Note that these signs are absent as often as present in children under 3 to 4 years of age.

Intussusception
Intermittently irritable infant or toddler, heme-positive stool, and (commonly but not always) a palpable abdominal mass are seen. Lethargy with altered mental status also may be seen.

Septic Arthritis
Check for range of motion of the joints and feel for overlying warmth. Logroll the leg with the child supine. This maneuver will elicit tenderness in the case of a septic hip.

Meningococcemia
Petechial skin rash (early) and purpuric rash (late) are seen.

Chicken Pox
This may be difficult to diagnose before true pox occurs. Early lesions consist of a 2- to 3-mm clear vesicle on a ½- to ¾-cm erythematous base ("teardrop on a rose petal"). Children who have defervescence early with rise of temperature on day 4 or remain febrile at 5 days or beyond should have an in-depth evaluation for bacteremia, especially group A streptococcus.

Measles
Salmon-colored maculopapular exanthem with cough, coryza, palpebral conjunctivitis, and (early) Koplik spots may be seen. Stridor may also be present.

BOX 165-3. Causes of Fever and Altered Sensorium

- Bacterial sepsis, other than meningitis
- Febrile seizure
- Hypoglycemia, secondary to poor oral intake plus vomiting and diarrhea
- Hyponatremic dehydration
- Intussusception
- Meningitis or encephalitis
- Shigella gastroenteritis
- Toxic ingestion
- Unsuspected head trauma, including shaken-baby syndrome with central nervous system bleeding

conditions such as bacteremia, pneumococcal pneumonia, and meningitis, also occurs in benign conditions such as group A streptococcal pharyngitis.

Sedimentation Rate

The erythrocyte sedimentation rate (ESR) is sensitive for well-localized bacterial infections such as osteomyelitis, septic arthritis, and pelvic inflammatory disease and is a good screen for collagen vascular diseases, inflammatory bowel disease, and children with FUO. It also is a sensitive marker for bacteremia, comparing favorably with more traditional measures such as the WBC count, differential, and height of fever. Unfortunately, the test is not specific and is elevated in a legion of minor viral illnesses.

As a general screen, the standard ESR has the disadvantage of requiring 1 hour to be completed.

Blood Culture

Blood cultures for aerobic and anaerobic organisms should be obtained in any patient suspected of having bacteremia. After appropriate antisepsis of the skin (alcohol prep followed by povidone iodine that is allowed to dry), venipuncture should be performed and blood transferred immediately to blood culture bottles or vials, generally changing the needle after venipuncture and before transfer.[37] Culture techniques provide reliable results with even small amounts of blood, often as little as 0.5 to 1.0 ml. As in adults, yield is proportional to volume, so it is best to obtain the maximum amount for a particular culture system whenever possible. Drawing cultures from an intravenous catheter during placement is an acceptable procedure provided the skin has been aseptically prepared.

Urine Collection and Analysis

Examination of the urine is essential in infants, toddlers, and young children who are to receive antibiotics while bacteremia is being excluded without a clear source of infection. The antibiotic will usually eradicate the urinary pathogens, and therefore the diagnosis of a urinary tract infection (UTI) will not be made, even if the urine is examined at the follow-up visit. In some studies, up to 7.5% of infants under 8 weeks of age being treated at an ED without an identified source for their fevers are later found to have a UTI.[38] Often this is due to an obstructive urologic anomaly, which if uncorrected can result in hydronephrosis. Many recommend that urine cultures be obtained from all febrile boys under 6 months of age and all acutely febrile girls under 2 years of age who are to be treated with antibiotics.

Because of the great potential for morbidity, accurate documentation of a UTI is paramount. The presence of a documented UTI in these patients mandates a subsequent radiographic evaluation of the genitourinary tract to exclude anomalies and reflux. During infancy the only reliable methods to obtain a urine sample are straight catheterization or suprapubic aspiration of the bladder.[33,38] The urine obtained by these methods should always be cultured. A urinalysis should also be performed, keeping in mind the significant limitations of its sensitivity in identifying a true UTI. Even in the presence of infection, an infant may not mount a pyuric response, the urine may be too dilute to allow identification of bacteria on the slide, or the organisms may not reduce nitrate to nitrite.[39] On the other hand, urine dipsticks positive for both nitrites and leukocyte esterase have a higher correlation with a UTI. In the neonatal period, the urinalysis may be unremarkable in up to 50% of children with a documented positive culture. Twenty percent of older children with UTIs have a normal urinalysis, including a negative leukocyte esterase, nitrite, or both. A Gram's stain of a smear of the urine sediment is the most sensitive screening test (99%).[40] Urine samples obtained by securing a bag over the genitalia are appropriate when used to document degree of hydration or the presence of hematuria or glucosuria. In general, urine collection should precede the other invasive steps of the fever workup in an infant; noxious stimuli will often prompt the baby to void.

In children who are toilet trained, meticulous cleaning of the external genitalia with a mild soap and subsequently rinsing with copious water usually allows the collection of urine samples that can be cultured and analyzed, if they are obtained as a midstream specimen. Special care must be taken in the preparation of uncircumcised boys, a group that even in early infancy appears to have a special predilection for UTIs. The foreskin should be gently retracted as much as possible (most can be completely retracted by 5 years of age) and the glans cleaned before obtaining the sample, regardless of the collection method used.

Once obtained, urine samples should be sent to the laboratory for culture without delay. Common bladder pathogens have multiplication times of approximately 20 minutes. Keeping a sample unrefrigerated for longer than that may confound the interpretation of the culture results.

Stool Examination[41]

A stool examination for PMN leukocytes helps differentiate viral from bacterial gastroenteritis. The presence of PMN leukocytes in the stool indicates a possible bacterial infection. A stool culture should be considered in cases of diarrhea with fever or altered mental status, because *Shigella* infection can cause both.[42] Stool can be obtained by rectal swab, by collection cup in older children, or from the diaper in infants.

The stool should be checked for occult blood using a Hemoccult card. A methylene blue slide can be examined for WBCs. The presence of either blood or white cells in the stool sample of a febrile child is an indication to send the sample for culture and sensitivity to rule out *Shigella, Salmonella, Campylobacter,* toxigenic *Escherichia coli,* and *Yersinia* spp.[43]

Chest Radiographic Study

A chest radiograph is indicated in children with cyanosis, intercostal retractions, persistent cough, or tachypnea out of proportion to the degree of fever. A respiratory rate in children less than 6 months of age greater than 59 per minute, in those 6 to 11 months of age over 52 per minute, and in children 1 to 2 years of age over 42 per minute suggests an increased risk of pneumonia.

In cases in which the physical examination is highly consistent with pneumonia (dullness to percussion and rales), many pediatricians make the diagnosis of "clinical pneumonia" in the nontoxic child and begin therapy *without* first obtaining a chest radiograph.

Especially in young children, pneumonia may be present without auscultatory abnormalities on chest examination and even with a normal respiratory rate.[31] Therefore the radiographic chest film is a reasonable addition to the workup of an ill-appearing young child with fever and no evident source of infection.

UNCOMMON SYNDROMES

Heat Exhaustion and Heatstroke

Heat exhaustion and heat cramps cause malaise, muscle cramps, and temperatures generally below 39° C (102.2° F).

With heatstroke, the ability to sweat is lost. The temperature often exceeds 40° C (104° F), the skin is hot and dry, tachycardia and frank hypotension commonly occur, and the patient commonly has altered mental status. Laboratory studies show hemoconcentration with an elevated hematocrit and often hypernatremia. Rhabdomyolysis with an elevated creatine phosphokinase and myoglobinuria is also common.

Toxic Ingestion

The most common agents causing hyperpyrexia are aspirin, anticholinergics, and β-adrenergics. These agents are common ingredients in over-the-counter cold remedies. Other agents causing fever include glutethimide, general anesthetics, lithium carbonate, lysergic acid diethylamide (LSD), amphetamines, cocaine, phencyclidine (PCP), phenothiazines, and tricyclic antidepressants.

Septic Shock

Septic shock can be caused by numerous bacterial infections, the most common being *N. meningitidis, H. influenzae,* and *S. pneumoniae.* Early in septic shock the blood pressure is maintained, but the pulse rate is rapid. Arteriovenous shunting at the microcirculatory level can cause the skin to feel warm; however, the tissue perfusion is decreased, as evidenced by hyperpnea and a low serum bicarbonate (HCO_3^-). Patients typically appear confused. Laboratory data may reveal a normal or even a depressed WBC count secondary to bone marrow suppression. Later in the course, DIC may occur associated with abnormal serum clotting findings.

Toxic Shock Syndrome[44]

Toxic shock occurs secondary to a toxin produced by *Staphylococcus aureus.* The syndrome occurs most commonly in menstruating women, classically in association with tampon use. However, the syndrome also may occur in male children and premenstrual girls.

The syndrome causes high fever, rapid pulse, diarrhea, and an erythematous rash. Patients commonly become lethargic and disoriented. Systemic hypotension occurs. Laboratory abnormalities include leukocytosis, thrombocytopenia, elevated serum alanine aminotransferase (SGPT) and serum aspartate aminotransferase (SGOT), and abnormal clotting studies (prothrombin time [PT], partial thromboplastin time [PTT], fibrin split products [FSP]). The diagnostic criteria for the diagnosis of toxic shock are listed in Box 165-4.

BOX 165-4. Toxic Shock Syndrome: Specific Diagnostic Findings

Fever of 40° C (104° F) or greater
Diffuse, blanching, erythematous rash; may progress to erythroderma
Skin desquamation, 1 to 2 weeks after the onset of the illness, particularly of palms and soles
Hypotension (systolic blood pressure less than fifth percentile for age, or an orthostatic increase in the pulse rate of at least 20 beats per minute or an orthostatic drop in systolic blood pressure of ≥20 mm Hg)
Involvement of three or more of the following organ systems:
- Gastrointestinal (vomiting or diarrhea)
- Muscular (severe myalgia)
- Mucous membrane (vaginal, oropharyngeal, or conjunctival hyperemia)
- Renal (BUN or creatinine two times normal or ≥5 WBC/hpf without UTI)
- Hepatobiliary (bilirubin, SGOT, or SGPT at least two times normal)
- Hematologic (platelet count <100,000/mm^3)
- Central nervous system (disorientation or altered level of consciousness without lateralizing signs)

Negative serologies (if obtained) for the following:
- Rocky Mountain spotted fever
- Leptospirosis
- Rubeola (measles)

BUN, Blood urea nitrogen; *WBC/hpf,* white blood cells per high-power field; *UTI,* urinary tract infection; *SGOT,* serum glutamic oxaloacetic transaminase; *SGPT,* serum glutamic pyruvic transaminase.

Kawasaki Syndrome (Mucocutaneous Lymph Node Syndrome)[45-47]

Kawasaki syndrome is a vasculitis that causes a prolonged fever (more than 5 days). The fever usually will exceed 39.5° to 40° C (103° to 104° F). The clinical findings include conjunctival injection without exudate; red, peeling lips; strawberry tongue; and pharyngitis. Early on there may be painful swelling of the hands and feet; peeling of the skin of the fingers occurs late in the course. A salmon-colored maculopapular rash may be present. Cervical adenopathy in excess of 5 cm *(Reviewer suggests 1.5 cm.)* is common. Cardiac involvement can lead to a pericar-dial friction rub, summation gallop, and cardiomegaly during the acute phase of the syndrome, and coronary artery aneurysm during the convalescent period. Initial laboratory findings classically include leukocytosis, thrombocytosis, and an elevated ESR.

The treatment of Kawasaki syndrome is directed toward the amelioration of symptoms and the prevention of coronary aneurysms. γ-Globulin 2 gm/kg intravenously should be administered over 12 hours, followed by high-dose aspirin therapy (100 mg/kg/24 hr PO given in divided doses every 6 hours for 14 days). *(Reviewer suggests The dose should be 80 to 100 mg/kg/24 hr PO given in divided doses every 6 hours for 4 to 5 days after fever is controlled.)* Low-dose aspirin therapy (3 to 5 mg/kg/24 hr PO) should continue until acute phase reactants return to normal over 3 to 5 months. *(Reviewer suggests And there is no evidence of coronary artery damage by 6 to 8 weeks after the illness began.)* Children should be followed by a pediatric cardiologist to monitor cardiac status.

Box 165-5 lists the specific diagnostic criteria for making the diagnosis.

MANAGEMENT OF THE FEBRILE CHILD

Prehospital Care

Because the main concern with a febrile, toxic-appearing child is a serious infection (e.g., meningitis, pneumonia, or meningococcemia) or accompanying dehydration, the focus of the paramedic should be on rapid transport to the ED for evaluation and the early institution of antibiotics. Field interventions such as establishing intravenous access or sponging with tepid water are usually not necessary.

The administration of a single dose of acetaminophen (15 mg/kg) to children under 6 years of age, especially those with a history of febrile seizures, is appropriate.

BOX 165-5. Diagnostic Criteria of Kawasaki Syndrome

Principal Clinical Findings*

Fever above 38.5° C (101.3° F) for at least 5 days' duration† *and* presence of four of the following principal features:
- Changes in extremities, including edema, erythema, desquamation
- Polymorphous exanthem
- Bilateral conjunctival injection
- Changes in the lips and oral cavity, including an injected pharynx, cracked lips, strawberry tongue
- Cervical lymphadenopathy, >1.5 cm in diameter, usually unilateral

Exclusion of other diseases with similar findings

Other Clinical and Laboratory Findings

Cardiac findings

Pancarditis, in the early stages of disease

Coronary artery abnormalities, usually beyond 10 days of onset of illness

Noncardiac findings

Musculoskeletal system
- Arthritic, arthralgia

Gastrointestinal tract
- Diarrhea, vomiting
- Abdominal pain
- Hepatic dysfunction
- Hydrops of the gallbladder

Cervical nervous system
- Extreme irritability
- Aseptic meningitis

Respiratory tract
- Pulmonary infiltrates

Other findings
- Testicular swelling
- Peripheral gangrene
- Aneurysms of medium-sized noncoronary arteries

Laboratory findings

Neutrophilia with immature forms

Elevated erythrocyte sedimentation rate

Positive C-reactive protein

Anemia

Hypoalbuminemia

Thrombocytosis

Proteinuria

Sterile pyuria

Elevated serum transaminase

*Patients with fever and fewer than four principal clinical features can be diagnosed as having Kawasaki syndrome when coronary artery disease is detected by two-dimensional echocardiography or coronary angiography.

†Many experts believe that in the presence of classic features, the diagnosis of Kawasaki syndrome can be made by experienced practitioners before the fifth day of fever.

ED CARE

Infants from Birth to 12 Weeks of Age[48-52]

Neonates and young babies with fever are of special concern. Despite having some protective immunity from maternal antibodies, young infants do not have the immunocompetence of older children, being relatively deficient in immune functions such as chemotaxis, phagocytosis, intracellular killing, and serum levels of various immune globulins.[48,49]

The evaluation of young infants is complicated by many factors. The first several weeks of life are a period of tremendous developmental change, making a 3-week-old infant very different from an 8-week-old infant, who is in turn very different from a 12-week-old infant. During the first 4 weeks of life, many activities (e.g., sucking, eye opening, and grasping) are reflex in origin and can persist even in the face of serious diseases. In one study, one in nine young babies with serious bacterial infections appeared clinically well even to experienced physicians.[50] Infants with meningitis do not have stiff necks.

There are no specific and reliable laboratory studies that can identify or exclude all children with serious disease.[51,53]

The causes of infection also change greatly with increasing age. As the infant is discharged from the nursery and exposed to a variety of community-acquired pathogens at home, the spectrum of agents changes from maternal vaginal flora (*E. coli,* group B streptococci, *Listeria monocytogenes,* herpes virus, and *Chlamydia trachomatis*) to community-acquired viruses and bacteria (enterovirus, *S. pneumoniae,* and *H. influenzae*). During the first month of life, 73% of cases of bacteremia or bacterial meningitis are due to group B streptococci and 8% to *E. coli* infections.[52]

Fever, especially high fever in young infants, is rare but suggests the possibility of a serious infection.[53,54] The reported incidence of bacterial infection varies, with early reports suggesting that bacteremia may be as common as 12% to 14% during the first 8 weeks of life. Others estimate a lower risk, on the order of 3% to 4%.[53] Combining the data from multiple studies of infants less than 12 weeks of age with a temperature of 38° C (100.4° F) or greater, Baskin estimates the prevalence of serious bacterial infections (including pneumonia, pyelonephritis, and aseptic meningitis) to be approximately 7%, and the incidence of bacteremia or bacterial meningitis to be 2% to 3%.[52]

Clinical and Ancillary Data

The relative immaturity of infants under 8 weeks of age makes clinical evaluation difficult at best.[50,55] For example, studies find that the presence of a normal smile is a good predictor of the absence of serious illness in most age groups, but a social smile is not in the developmental repertoire of a 4-week-old infant and may not appear in some infants until 8 weeks of age.

Although the absence of certain signs does not rule out disease, their presence indicates infants who are at risk for serious infection. These signs include overall impression of toxicity, abnormal or decreased feeding pattern, irritability, lack of consolability, and pale or mottled skin. High fever has a high correlation with serious illness. However, the lack of fever does not rule out the presence of bacterial or other serious disease.

Unfortunately, laboratory evaluation is less helpful in this age group than in older children. Several studies have attempted to demonstrate the efficacy of one test or another, but as yet no single test or combination of tests can prospectively predict the presence or absence of serious illness with assurance.[48,53] During the first week of life, the WBC count is commonly lower in the bacteremic than in the nonbacteremic patient.

Overall, the CBC is useful as a guide to the degree of illness. In general, a WBC count either above 15,000/mm^3 or below 5000/mm^3 and increased numbers of immature (band) forms correlate with the presence of serious infection.[48,53]

Evaluation

Febrile infants under 8 to 12 weeks of age require a complete septic workup including a CBC with differential, platelet count, blood culture, chest radiograph, urinalysis and urine culture (obtained by catheterization), and LP. In infants 8 to 12 weeks of age with normal feeding, normal activity, a good social smile, excellent follow-up, and a normal CBC, the LP may be omitted.

Management and Admission Criteria

Infants from Birth to 4 Weeks of Age

Infants under 4 weeks of age with fever require admission for parenteral antibiotics and apnea monitoring until cultures prove negative. Admission is the rule for all infants under 4 weeks of age, even when an identifiable source of fever, such as otitis media, is discovered. Ferrera attempted to apply a modification of the low-risk criteria delineated in Box 165-6 and demonstrated that 3 of 48 meeting these guidelines had serious bacterial infections.[56]

Infants from 4 to 12 Weeks of Age

Ill-appearing infants between 4 and 12 weeks of age require hospital admission for parenteral antibiotics and apnea monitoring.

For well-appearing febrile infants between 4 and 12 weeks of age, studies support the safety of outpatient management.[48,49,57,58] Baraff et al have established a list of low-risk criteria that must be met for these infants to be treated as outpatients.[59-62] The parents or caretakers must be deemed reliable, and the infant must have no underlying medical diseases or acute bacterial infections excluding otitis media. The WBC count should be between 5000/mm^3 and 15,000/mm^3 with a total band count under 1500/mm^3. The urinalysis is normal (<5 WBC per high-power field [WBC/hpf]). When diarrhea is present, there are fewer than 5 WBC/hpf in the stool (see Box 165-6).

Patients may be given a single injection of ceftriaxone (Rocephin), and the infant's parents or caretakers told to bring the infant for a recheck within 24 hours

BOX 165-6. Low-Risk Criteria for Infants 4 to 12 Weeks of Age[59-62]

Clinical Criteria
Previously healthy
Nontoxic clinical appearance
No focal bacterial infection (except otitis media)
Good social situation

Laboratory Criteria
WBC count 5000/mm^3 to 15,000/mm^3 with <1500 bands/mm^3
Normal urinalysis <5 WBC/hpf
When diarrhea present, <5 WBC/hpf in stool

WBC, White blood cell; *WBC/hpf,* white blood cells per high-power field.

or to call earlier if signs and symptoms change. A full sepsis evaluation including LP is appropriate if antibiotics are given empirically. Do not use ceftriaxone during the first 30 to 60 days of life if there is clinical jaundice; the antibiotic displaces bilirubin from its serum binding sites.

Baker identified 64 of 65 children 29 to 56 days of age who had serious bacterial infections by having the following criteria: WBC >15,000/mm^3, urinalysis >10 WBC/hpf, cerebrospinal fluid (CSF) >8 WBC/mm^3, and a chest radiograph with an infiltrate.[63] Infants 8 to 12 weeks of age who have obvious signs of an upper respiratory infection (nasal congestion, discharge, and sneezing) but who smile and appear well and have only a low-grade fever of 38° to 38.2° C (100.4° to 100.8° F) and normal vital signs can be discharged to home without a septic workup, without medications but with follow-up within 24 hours after extensive instructions have been given to the parents.

Inpatient Antibiotics for Infants from Birth to 12 Weeks of Age

The choice of inpatient antibiotics varies with age because of the changing spectrum of etiologies as the child grows older. Empiric treatment for the infant under 4 weeks of age traditionally consists of ampicillin 100 mg/kg/24 hr intravenously given in divided doses every 4 to 6 hours, plus an aminoglycoside (gentamicin 5 mg/kg/24 hr given in divided doses every 8 hours IV). *(Reviewer suggests The dose should be administered every 8 to 12 hours IV.)* This combination provides excellent coverage for the typical pathogens in neonates (group B streptococci, *E. coli, L. monocytogenes,* and enterococci). The combination of ampicillin and cefotaxime ([Claforan] 50 to 150 mg/kg/24 hr given in divided doses every 6 to 8 hours IV), *(Reviewer suggests The dose should be 150 mg/kg/24 hr given in divided doses every 8 hours IV.)* a third-generation cephalosporin, is also acceptable. Advantages to using a cephalosporin rather than an aminoglycoside include no need for time-consuming, expensive serum aminoglycoside levels, little or no associated otic or nephric toxicity, excellent penetration into the meninges, and superior coverage against *H. influenzae.*

After 4 weeks of age, ampicillin (50 mg/kg every 6 hours IV) *(Reviewer suggests The dose should be 50 to 100 mg/kg every 6 hours IV.)* and cefotaxime (Claforan 50 mg/kg every 8 hours IV) are the first-line agents, because they provide excellent coverage for both the neonatal pathogens and community-acquired pathogens such as *H. influenzae, N. meningitidis,* and *S. pneumoniae.* Ampicillin is needed in addition to a cephalosporin until at least 6 to 12 weeks of age in order to treat *L. monocytogenes* and enterococci. Vancomycin should be considered in children with suspected *S. pneumoniae* until sensitivities are defined. Vancomycin may be given in children over 1 month of age in a dose of 10 to 15 mg/kg IV every 6 to 8 hours. *(Reviewer suggests The dose should be 40 to 60 mg/kg/24 hr given in divided doses IV every 6 to 8 hours.)* (Neonates require a lower dose.) Therapeutic levels of vancomycin and gentamicin should be monitored. Modifications of both agent and dosage may be required in toxic children and those with underlying disease or suspected meningitis.

Note: Here and throughout this chapter the dose of antibiotics listed is the same for both the intravenous and the intramuscular routes. In most cases, the intravenous route is preferred. However, delays in instituting antibiotic therapy may occur because of inability to establish intravenous access. In such cases one should not hesitate to give the first doses of antibiotics intramuscularly.

Children from 3 to 36 Months of Age

Children from 3 to 36 months of age are those most likely to be brought to the ED for evaluation of fever. Common causes of fever in this age group include viral nasopharyngitis and bronchitis, otitis media, herpes stomatitis, hand-foot-and-mouth disease (coxsackievirus), pharyngitis (including herpangina, group A β-hemolytic streptococcus pharyngitis, and adenovirus pharyngoconjunctival fever), croup (paramyxovirus), bronchiolitis (RSV), pneumonia, acute gastroenteritis, and occult bacteremia. With increasing age, sinusitis becomes more common, at times associated with ipsilateral periorbital cellulitis. Another common disease is roseola. With roseola, despite a high fever, the infant generally remains playful and nontoxic. A pink morbilliform rash appears coincident with defervescence.

More serious illnesses include epiglottitis, retropharyngeal abscess, pyelonephritis, intussusception, meningococcemia, and meningitis.

The triage evaluation should include temperature, respiratory rate, and pulse rate. The preferred initial temperature should be a rectal reading, because most algorithms for the risk of serious illness in this age group are based on the rectal temperature. Those who have a temperature above 38.5° C (101.3° F) should be given acetaminophen 15 mg/kg orally or rectally if they have not had a dose within the past 4 hours to facilitate evaluation.

During the physical examination, the emergency physician should first observe the child from a distance, noting whether the child smiles, plays, babbles, interacts normally with parents, is listless, or cries irritably. The Yale Observation Scale and other similar systems of determining a child's responsiveness are reflective of serious illness. A sleeping patient must be awakened. In most cases the infant who smiles, plays, and coos will not be a candidate for LP.

After the initial observation, the next step is to cautiously approach, waving an enticing toy or flashlight. With the infant on the lap of one of the parents, the emergency physician should gently flex the neck to check for meningismus and then auscultate the chest, listening for abnormal breath sounds and heart murmur, gallop, or rub. The abdomen should be examined for tenderness, masses, hepatosplenomegaly, and quality of bowel sounds. The last part of the examination with the infant still on the parent's lap is to palpate the extremities for bone and joint tenderness or warmth, and to logroll the legs at the thigh to exclude a septic hip.

The parts of the examination requiring patient cooperation completed, the child can then be transferred to the stretcher for evaluation of the TMs (with pneumatic otoscopy), eyes, nose, and throat. The skin is then examined for the presence of petechiae or viral exanthems such as measles and chicken pox.

Infants who remain irritable during the entire physical examination must be considered for LP. In infants and toddlers the absence of a stiff neck does *not* rule out meningitis. If the temperature is still high despite an appropriate dose of acetaminophen (15 mg/kg), lowering the temperature by means of ibuprofen (10 mg/kg PO) may convert an irritable infant into a playful one. Adding a 15-minute tepid sponge bath to antipyretics does not make a significant difference in temperature over the subsequent 2 hours and leads to greater discomfort of the child.[65] A bolus of 20 ml/kg of normal saline may make a dehydrated, lethargic infant become more alert and playful. If the infant remains irritable despite these measures, an LP is necessary.

The infant who initially appears septic with marked lethargy, stiff neck, weak cry, poor perfusion, or a purpuric rash requires a prompt septic workup followed by broad-spectrum antibiotics. Treatment should not be delayed in such infants to see whether they improve when the temperature is lowered. The workup should include blood, urine, and CSF cultures, and a chest radiograph. Appropriate antibiotic regimens when there is no apparent source include cefotaxime (Claforan) 50 mg/kg every 6 hours *(Reviewer suggests The dose should be 50 mg/kg every 6 to 8 hours.)* or ceftriaxone (Rocephin) 50 mg/kg every 12 hours by the intravenous or intramuscular routes. If *S. pneumoniae* is a potential pathogen, vancomycin 10 to 15 mg/kg *(Reviewer suggests The dose should be vancomycin 40 to 60 mg/kg/24 hr given in divided doses IV every 6 to 8 hours.)* every 6 to 8 hours should also be initiated pending sensitivities.

In nontoxic patients in whom a source of fever is found, the child should be treated appropriately. For example, otitis media can be safely treated with outpatient antibiotics, without the need for CBC, blood culture, or any other tests. Periorbital cellulitis, however, often requires CBC, blood culture, and hospital admission.

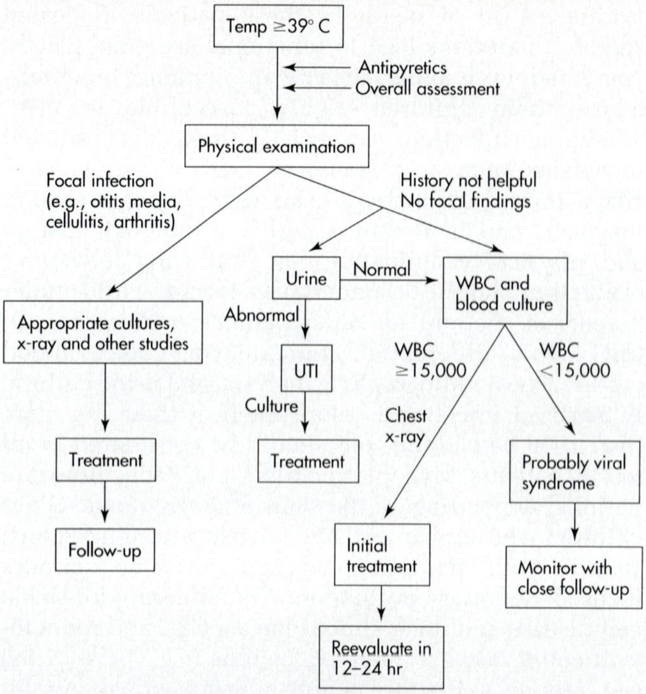

Figure 165-1. Evaluation of the febrile child 3 months to 3 years of age. See text for discussion. *Modified from Barkin RM, Rosen P: Emergency pediatrics, ed 5, St Louis, 1999, Mosby.*

When there is no obvious source of infection on the initial examination and the child is not so irritable as to require prompt LP and septic workup, the height of the temperature can serve as a guide to the subsequent workup. One protocol uses a rectal temperature of 39° C (102.2° F) as the cutoff for working up children 3 to 36 months of age with fever without a source (Figure 165-1); many clinicians have established different guidelines, while others follow a more case-by-case approach.[36,59,66,67]

If the rectal temperature is below 39° C (102.2° F) and the patient is nontoxic, the patient should be discharged with instructions to take acetaminophen (not aspirin) 15 mg/kg every 4 hours for continued fever and to contact the primary health care provider the next day.

If the temperature is 39° C (102.2° F) or greater, a CBC should be considered. If the WBC count is less than 15,000/mm^3, the patient should be discharged with instructions to control the fever with acetaminophen and to contact the primary health care provider the next day. If the WBC count is 15,000/mm^3 or greater, a blood culture should be obtained, and the patient should be treated with a single dose of ceftriaxone 50 mg/kg intravenously or intramuscularly. For patients receiving antibiotics, a blood culture and a urine specimen obtained by bladder catheterization for urinalysis and culture should be obtained before the first dose. The urinalysis and culture may be omitted if the patient is a boy older than 6 months of age or a girl older than 2 years of age. Urinalysis and culture should also be obtained if the fever has persisted for 3 days or more or if the temperature is 40° C (104° F) or greater. A chest radiograph should be obtained if there are respiratory signs or symptoms. A stool culture is recommended if there is blood or mucus in the stool or 5 or more WBC/hpf on microscopic examination. The parents are instructed to have the child seen by the primary care physician the next day.

Bearing in mind that the WBC count is relatively insensitive for *H. influenzae* and *N. meningitidis* infections, it is also advisable to obtain blood cultures and administer ceftriaxone to patients who appear clinically ill but who are not sick enough to warrant an immediate septic workup, even when the WBC count is normal.

Because bacteremia becomes less common after 24 months of age, a CBC and blood culture should not be routinely obtained unless the child has a fever of 40° C (104° F) or greater or is ill-appearing.

(Reviewer suggests The incidence of bacteremia is significantly lower in children who have received the primary series of the pneumococcal conjugate vaccine, usually by the age of 6 months. Because of this change in epidemiology, laboratory screening and empiric antibiotic therapy may not be necessary in the highly febrile, well-appearing 6- to 36-month-old child who has received the primary series of this vaccine [Kuppermann N. The evaluation of young febrile children for occult bacteremia: time to reevaluate our approach. Arch Pediatr Adoles Med 2002; 156:855-857].)

Children from 3 to 7 Years of Age

The incidence of occult bacteremia decreases dramatically after 3 years of age. Pharyngitis caused by group A β-hemolytic streptococci becomes more common during the preschool years and increases dramatically after school entry. After children reach approximately 5 years of age, *Mycoplasma hominis* is a common nonviral cause of lower respiratory tract infections.

Although a child who is febrile and toxic in appearance should have a thorough evaluation, most patients in this age group will have either a viral or a localized bacterial infection and can receive a more focused evaluation. A thorough history and physical examination, supplemented by selected laboratory testing, are often sufficient.

Children from 7 to 18 Years of Age

Visits for fever are less common in this age group, and the evaluation becomes easier because these children are better able to cooperate with the physical examination and laboratory testing.

Infections continue to be the most common cause of temperature elevations after 7 years of age, although the spectrum of organisms changes with age. Although routine viral illnesses predominate, other organisms, such as Epstein-Barr virus, mycoplasma, and group A streptococci, become more common causative agents in older children and adolescents.

These patients can be evaluated with a history, physical examination, and selected laboratory testing. Except for those found to have serious systemic illnesses (pyelonephritis, pelvic inflammatory disease, appendicitis) or other reasons for admission (hypoxia, dehydration), most of these patients can be managed as outpatients with appropriate therapy.

FEVER IN CHILDREN WITH UNDERLYING ILLNESSES

Oncology Patients

Children with cancer, especially those undergoing cytotoxic chemotherapy, are at special risk of overwhelming sepsis.[68,69] When febrile, these children should be promptly evaluated with a CBC and differential and a blood culture. Chest radiographs, evaluation of the urine, and an LP should be performed as clinically indicated. The emergency physician should *not* perform a rectal examination on a patient with neutropenia. Patients with an indwelling vascular device such as a Broviac catheter should have central and peripheral blood cultures taken.

Neutropenia requires intravenous antibiotics without delay once the blood cultures are obtained. Appropriate antibiotics should include coverage for *Pseudomonas* and other gram-negative organisms. A combination of tobramycin 7.5 mg/kg/24 hr in divided doses every 8 hours (every 24 hours for neonates) *(Reviewer suggests Neonates require a lower dose.)* intravenously and ceftazidime 150 mg/kg/24 hr in divided doses every 8 hours intravenously provides good initial coverage for most cases.

For patients with suspected sepsis in an indwelling vascular catheter, the emergency physician should avoid flushing the device until well after initial antibiotic doses have been given via a peripheral intravenous line, and then only in consultation with the child's physician. An antistaphylococcal antibiotic such as vancomycin 30 to 45 mg/kg/24 hr in divided doses every 6 to 8 hours (every 12 hours in neonates) *(Reviewer suggests The dose should be vancomycin 40 to 60 mg/kg/24 hr in divided doses every 6 to 8 hours [every 8 to 12 hours in neonates].)* should be added to the regimen of tobramycin and ceftazidime to cover gram-positive cocci.[68]

Acquired Immunodeficiency Syndrome[70]

Children with acquired immunodeficiency syndrome (AIDS) often have repeated episodes of infections with common bacterial pathogens. Children with either acquired or inherited immune deficiency are also at risk from otherwise relatively innocuous organisms such as *Pneumocystis carinii.* Other causes of fever in these children include mycobacterial infections (*Mycobacterium avium intracellulare*), cryptococcosis, cytomegalovirus, Epstein-Barr virus, lymphomas or other malignancies, focal bacterial infections such as sinusitis, and pneumonia.

The child with AIDS, fever, and a low CD4 lymphocyte count warrants an approach similar to that of the neutropenic cancer patient, with aggressive diagnosis followed by treatment with broad-spectrum parenteral antibiotics.

Sickle Cell Anemia

Children with sickle cell disease require special attention during episodes of fever.[71,72] Infection is the leading cause of death in these patients. Repeated splenic infarctions lead to functional asplenia, which, combined with other defects in immune functions, leaves these children highly susceptible to overwhelming infections, especially from encapsulated organisms such as pneumococci and *H. influenzae.* Hence these patients require an aggressive approach to diagnosis and treatment.[71,72] After a thorough history and physical examination, the following laboratory evaluation should be undertaken for any child under 2 years of age and for older patients who appear ill: CBC with differential, reticulocyte count, blood culture, chest radiograph, urinalysis, and urine culture. A bacterial infection is more likely if there are more than 1000 bands/mm^3 but should be considered in all febrile patients. Mycoplasma titers and stool culture are optional depending on the signs and symptoms. Older children who appear well and have localized infections such as otitis media or pharyngitis may have a more focused laboratory evaluation. All children with sickle cell disease and fever should have a CBC and reticulocyte count because many infections (e.g., parvovirus) can induce a life-threatening aplastic crisis. An LP should be performed whenever meningitis is clinically suspected; criteria are the same as for children without sickle cell disease.

Osteomyelitis should be suspected in the child with fever and localized bone pain. The evaluation of such a child includes a CBC, sedimentation rate, and plain radiographs. A bone scan may be necessary to localize the infection and differentiate osteomyelitis from a vasoocclusive crisis. If the scan is positive, aspiration of material from suspicious areas for culture and sensitivities should be performed. Because *Salmonella* is often the causative organism, a stool sample should be obtained and may be the only source of a positive culture.

Most patients under 2 years of age, and those over 2 years of age who appear ill or have an identified bacterial infection (e.g., pneumonia, UTI), should promptly receive parenteral antibiotics and be admitted to the hospital for further care. Appropriate antibiotic choices include a second-generation (cefuroxime 50 to 240 mg/kg/24 hr in divided doses every 6 to 8 hours IV) *(Reviewer suggests The dose should be cefuroxime 50 to 150 mg/kg/24 hr in divided doses every 6 to 8 hours IV.)* or third-generation cephalosporin (ceftriaxone). If an infection with *Salmonella (Reviewer suggests If meningitis is suspected, a third generation cephalosporin should be used)* is suspected, a third-generation cephalosporin or other antibiotic active against *Salmonella* spp. should be used.

Patients over 2 years of age who appear well and have either no focus of infection or have a minor, localized process such as pharyngitis may be discharged after receiving an initial parenteral dose of ceftriaxone (50 mg/kg IV or IM). Outpatient treatment of low-risk patients is prudent.[73-75] The initial dose of ceftriaxone can be followed by appropriate oral antibiotics or a subsequent dose of ceftriaxone after 24 hours. The most crucial aspects of outpatient management are the availability and reliability of follow-up. All patients should be reevaluated within 24 to 36 hours.

Vancomycin should be initiated if *S. pneumoniae* is a potential pathogen.

Congenital Heart Disease

Children with congenital heart disease often have ongoing congestive heart failure that is only tenuously controlled by medications. This balance is easily upset by even relatively benign viral respiratory infections.

Children with valvular heart disease are at risk for infective endocarditis. In such patients, fever without an obvious source, especially when associated with a new or changing cardiac murmur, generally warrants hospital admission for serial blood cultures, echocardiography, and parenteral antibiotics effective against *Streptococcus viridans, S. aureus, S. faecalis, S. pneumoniae,* enterococci, *H. influenzae,* and other gram-negative rods. A good initial regimen when the causative organism is unknown is nafcillin 200 mg/kg/24 hr intravenously in divided doses every 6 hours (every 12 hours for neonates), plus gentamicin 7.5 mg/kg/24 hr in divided doses every 8 hours intravenously (every 12 hours for neonates). *(Reviewer suggests The dose should be nafcillin 200 mg/kg/24 hr IV in divided doses every 6 hours [100 mg/kg/24 hr every 6 hours for neonates], plus gentamicin 7.5 mg/kg/24 hr in divided doses every 8 hours IV [5 mg/kg/24 hr every 8 to 12 hours for neonates].)*

Ventriculoperitoneal Shunts

Patients with ventriculoperitoneal shunts and fever must be evaluated for shunt infection. Especially in cases in which the patient displays headache, stiff neck, vomiting, or irritability, the shunt reservoir should be aspirated under sterile conditions and after appropriate consultations. Fluid is examined for pleocytosis and bacteria. The most common bacterial pathogen is *Staphylococcus epidermidis.* A computed tomography (CT) scan of the head is also warranted.

DISPOSITION

The evaluation and treatment of the febrile infant or child are not simple. A large percentage of life-threatening pediatric emergencies initially cause fever. In patients under 3 years of age, a high fever may indicate occult bacteremia, most commonly from *S. pneumoniae,* but also from *N. meningitidis* and *H. influenzae.* Unusually high fever at any age may indicate a serious infectious disease, such as meningitis or pyelonephritis, as well as such conditions as heatstroke, anticholinergic poisoning, Kawasaki syndrome, and toxic shock syndrome.

Most febrile children can be treated as outpatients. Exceptions include infants under 1 month of age and any child with a serious infection regardless of age. Admission is also indicated in patients with infections of only moderate severity when the home environment may not ensure good follow-up.

KEY CONCEPTS

- Management of the febrile child must consider the age and toxicity of the patient, fever, and ancillary data.
- Special considerations modify the clinical approach.
- Underlying illnesses enhance the potential of serious illness and progression.

REFERENCES

1. Slater M, Krug SE: Evaluation of the infant with fever without source: an evidence based approach, *Emerg Med Clin North Am* 17:97-126, 1999.
2. McCarthy PL et al: Fever without apparent source on clinical examination, infectious diseases, and lower respiratory infections in children, *Curr Opin Pediatr* 10:101-116, 1998.
3. McGowan JE Jr et al: Bacteremia in febrile children seen in a "walk-in" pediatric clinic, *N Engl J Med* 288:1309, 1973.
4. Anderson AB et al: *Haemophilus influenzae* type b unsuspected bacteremia, *Pediatr Emerg Care* 3:82, 1987.
5. Harper MB, Fleisher GR: Occult bacteremia in the 3-month-old to 3-year-old age group, *Pediatr Ann* 22:484, 1993.
6. Jaffe DM, Fleisher GR: Temperature and total white blood cell count as indicators of bacteremia, *Pediatrics* 87:670, 1991.
7. Jaffe DM et al: Antibiotic administration to treat possible occult bacteremia in febrile children, *N Engl J Med* 317:1175, 1987.
8. Kline MW, Lorin MI: Bacteremia in children afebrile at presentation to an emergency room, *Pediatr Infect Dis J* 6:197, 1987.
9. Kramer MS et al: Should blood cultures be obtained in the evaluation of young febrile children without evident focus of bacterial infection? A decision analysis of diagnostic management strategies, *Pediatrics* 84:18, 1989.
10. Liu CH et al: Early detection of bacteremia in an outpatient clinic, *Pediatrics* 75:827, 1985.
11. Mellors JW et al: A simple index to identify occult bacterial infection in adults with acute unexplained fever, *Arch Intern Med* 147:666, 1987.
12. Baker RC et al: Severity of disease correlated with fever reduction in febrile infants, *Pediatrics* 83:1016, 1989.
13. Harper MD: Effect of antibiotic therapy on the outcome of out patients with unsuspected bacteremia, *Pediatric Infect Dis J* 14:760-767, 1995.
14. Fleisher GR et al: Intramuscular versus oral antibiotic therapy for the prevention of meningitis and other bacterial sequelae in young, febrile children at risk for occult bacteremia, *J Pediatr* 124:504, 1994.
15. Kupperman N et al: Predictors of occult pneumococcal bacteremia in young febrile children, *Ann Emerg Med* 31:679-687, 1998.
16. Caspe WB et al: Extreme hyperpyrexia in childhood: presentation similar to hemorrhagic shock and encephalopathy, *Clin Pediatr* 28:76, 1989.
17. Marcinak JF: Evaluation of children with fever 104° F in an emergency department, *Pediatr Emerg Care* 4:92, 1988.
18. Press S, Fawcett NP: Association of temperature greater than 41.1 degrees C (106 degrees F) with serious illness, *Clin Pediatr* 24:21, 1985.
19. Surpure JS: Hyperpyrexia in children: clinical implications, *Pediatr Emerg Care* 3:10, 1987.
20. Zuckerman GB et al: Hemorrhagic shock and encephalopathy syndrome and heatstroke: a physiologic comparison of two entities, *Pediatr Emerg Care* 10:172, 1994.
21. Pizzo PA et al: Prolonged fever in children: review of 100 cases, *Pediatrics* 55:468, 1975.

22. Miller LC et al: Prolonged fevers of unknown origin in children: patterns of presentation and outcome, *J Pediatr* 129:419-423, 1996.
23. Baker RC et al: Fever and petechiae in children, *Pediatrics* 84:1051, 1989.
24. Ward L et al: A comparison of tympanic and rectal temperatures in the emergency department, *Ann Emerg Med* 17:435, 1988.
25. Brennan DF et al: Reliability of infrared tympanic thermometry in detection of rectal fever in children, *Ann Emerg Med* 25:21, 1995.
26. Freed GL, Fraley JK: Lack of agreement of tympanic membrane temperature assessment with conventional methods in a private practice setting, *Pediatrics* 89:384, 1992.
27. Ros SP: Evaluation of a tympanic membrane thermometer in an outpatient clinical setting, *Ann Emerg Med* 18:1004, 1989.
28. Stewart JV, Webster D: Re-evaluation of the tympanic thermometer in the emergency department, *Ann Emerg Med* 21:158, 1992.
29. Terndrup TE, Rajk J: Impact of operator technique and device on infrared emission detection tympanic thermometry, *J Emerg Med* 10:683, 1992.
30. Terndrup TE et al: A comparison of oral, rectal, and tympanic membrane-derived temperature changes after ingestion of liquids and smoking, *Am J Emerg Med* 7:150, 1989.
31. Ellis GL et al: Liquid crystal thermometer strips (letter), *J Emerg Med* 7:675, 1989.
32. Anbar RD et al: Difficulties in universal application of criteria identifying infants at low risk for serious bacterial infection, *J Pediatr* 109:483, 1986.
33. Bonadio WA: Urine culturing technique in febrile infants, *Pediatr Emerg Care* 3:75, 1987.
34. Zukin DD et al: Correlation of pulmonary signs and symptoms with chest, *Ann Emerg Med* 15:792, 1986.
35. McGillivray DL et al: Diagnostic test ordering in the evaluation of febrile children. Physician and environmental factors, *Am J Dis Child* 147:870-874, 1993.
36. Egland AG, McGuirk TD: Survey of clinical management of febrile infants and children. Birth to 24 months of age, *Ann Emerg Med* 34:397, 1999.
37. Sommit D et al: Effect of needle changing and intravenous cannula collection in blood culture contamination rates, *Ann Emerg Med* 22:1164, 1993.
38. Crain E, Gershel J: Urinary tract infections in febrile infants younger than 8 weeks of age, *Pediatrics* 86:363, 1990.
39. Goldsmith B, Campo J: Comparison of urine dipstick, microscopy, and culture for the detection of bacteriuria in children, *Clin Pediatr* 29:214, 1990.
40. Lockhart GR: Use of urinary Gram stain for detection of urinary tract infection in infants, *Ann Emerg Med* 25:31, 1995.
41. Barkin RM: Acute infectious diarrheal disease in children, *J Emerg Med* 3:1, 1985.
42. Huskins W et al: Shigellosis in neonates and young infants, *J Pediatr* 122:14, 1994.
43. Sondheimer JM: Office stool examination—a practical guide, *Contemp Pediatr* 63, 1990.
44. Resnick SD: Toxic shock syndrome: recent developments in pathogenesis, *J Pediatr* 116:321, 1990.
45. Rowley AH, Shulman ST: Current therapy for acute Kawasaki syndrome, *J Pediatr* 118:987, 1991.
46. Shackelford PG, Srauss AW: Kawasaki syndrome (editorial), *N Engl J Med* 324:1664, 1991.
47. Newburger JW et al: A single intravenous infusion of γ-globulin as compared with four infusions in the treatment of acute Kawasaki syndrome, *N Engl J Med* 324:1633, 1991.
48. Berkowitz CD et al: Fever in infants less than two months of age: spectrum of disease and predictors of outcome, *Pediatr Emerg Care* 1:128, 1985.
49. Berkowitz CD et al: Variability in the management of the febrile infant under 2 months of age, *J Emerg Med* 3:345, 1985.
50. Roberts KB, Borzy MS: Fever in the first 8 weeks of life, *Johns Hopkins Med J* 141:9, 1977.
51. Roberts KB: "Hot babies": managing the very young, febrile infant, *Contemp Pediatr* 4:14, 1987.
52. Baskin MN: The prevalence of serious bacterial infections by age in febrile infants during the first 3 months of life, *Pediatr Ann* 22:462, 1993.
53. Crain EF, Gershel JC: Which febrile infants younger than two weeks of age are likely to have sepsis? A pilot study, *Pediatr Infect Dis J* 7:561, 1988.
54. Klein JO et al: Management of the febrile infant 3 months of age or younger, *Pediatr Infect Dis J* 3:75, 1984.
55. Baker MD et al: Failure of infant observation scales in detecting serious illness in febrile, 4 to 8 week old infants, *Pediatrics* 85:1040, 1990.
56. Ferrera PC et al: Neonatal fever: utility of the Rochester criteria in determining low risk for serious bacterial infections, *Am J Emerg Med* 15:299-302, 1997.
57. Dagan R et al: Ambulatory care of febrile infants younger than 2 months of age classified as being at low risk for having serious bacterial infections, *J Pediatr* 112:355, 1985.
58. Dagan R et al: Identification of infants unlikely to have serious bacterial infection although hospitalized for suspected sepsis, *J Pediatr* 107:855, 1985.
59. Baraff LJ et al: Practice guideline for the management of infants and children 0 to 36 months of age with fever without source, *Pediatrics* 92:1, 1993.
60. Baraff LJ et al: Practice guideline for the management of infants and children 0 to 36 months of age with fever without source. Agency for Health Care Policy and Research, *Ann Emerg Med* 22:1198, 1993. (Erratum, *Ann Emerg Med* 22:1490, 1993.)
61. Baraff LJ et al: Probability of bacterial infections in febrile infants less than 3 months of age: a meta-analysis, *Pediatr Infect Dis J* 11:257, 1992.
62. Baraff LJ: Management of febrile neonates: what to do with low risk infants, *Pediatr Infect Dis J* 13:943, 1994.
63. Baker MD et al: Outpatient management without antibiotics of fever in selected infants, *N Engl J Med* 329:1437-1441, 1993.
64. Bonadio WA: The history and physical assessments of the febrile infant, *Pediatr Clin North Am* 45:65-77, 1998.
65. Sharber J: The efficacy of tepid sponge bathing to reduce fever in young children, *Am J Emerg Med* 15:188-192, 1997.
66. Baraff LJ: Management of infants and children 3 to 36 months of age with fever without source, *Pediatr Ann* 22:497, 1993.
67. Baraff LJ, Lee SI: Fever without source: management of children 3 to 36 months of age, *Pediatr Infect Dis J* 11:146, 1992.
68. Langley J, Gold R: Sepsis in febrile neutropenic children with cancer, *Pediatr Infect Dis J* 7:34, 1988.
69. Pizzo PA et al: The child with cancer and infection. 1. Empiric therapy for fever and neutropenia, and preventive strategies, *J Pediatr* 119:679, 1991.
70. Kline M: Fever in human immunodeficiency virus—infected infants and children, *Semin Pediatr Infectious Dis* 4:65, 1993.
71. Vichinsky E, Lubin BH: Suggested guidelines for the treatment of children with sickle cell anemia, *Hematol Oncol Clin North Am* 1:483, 1987.
72. Pearson HA: Sickle cell diseases: diagnosis and management in infancy and childhood, *Pediatr Rev* 9:121, 1987.
73. Platt OS, Dover GJ: Sickle cell disease. In Nathan DG, Oski FA, editors: *Hematology of infancy and childhood,* ed 4, Philadelphia, 1993, WB Saunders.
74. Williams JA et al: A randomized study of outpatient treatment with ceftriaxone for selected febrile children with sickle cell disease, *N Engl J Med* 329:472, 1993.
75. West TB et al: The presentation, frequency and outcome of bacteremia among children with sickle cell disease and fever, *Pediatr Emerg Care* 10:141, 1994.

CHAPTER 166

Pediatric Respiratory Emergencies: Upper Airway Obstruction and Infections

Mariann Manno

PERSPECTIVE

Respiratory distress from upper airway obstruction is a common emergency in young children. It may be caused by a number of different processes, including an acute infectious process, a complex congenital anomaly, or a foreign body in the airway or esophagus. A working knowledge of the anomalies and diseases of the upper airway is of primary importance in pediatric emergency medicine. Classification of airway pathology can be based on the anatomic location, the patient's age, the urgency of the symptoms, and whether it is a congenital or acquired lesion or an infectious or noninfectious process. The starting point for any classification is an appreciation of the unique aspects of pediatric airway anatomy.

PRINCIPLES OF DISEASE

A number of differences between the adult and pediatric airway are important in airway management (Figure 166-1). An infant's tongue is disproportionately large in relation to the mouth and protrudes back into the posterior of the pharynx. The tongue is a formidable obstacle when performing bag/mask ventilation and visualizing the airway. In the setting of hypotonia, posterior displacement of the tongue is the most common cause of functional upper airway obstruction. The infant larynx is more anterior and caudad, or higher in the neck relative to the cervical spine (at C3-4), than in an adult (at C4-5). The anterior aspect of the vocal cords is tipped inferiorly. The narrowest site of the infant airway is at the cricoid ring rather than the cords as in an adult. A child's epiglottis is relatively larger, longer, and omega shaped. It extends vertically beyond the opening of the cords, thus making a complete view of the airway difficult. The caliber of all airway structures is small; newborn tracheal length is 57 mm and laryngeal diameter is 4 mm. All cartilaginous supporting structures are soft, pliable, and prone to collapse. Finally, a prominent occiput allows passive flexion of the head and neck on the cervical spine. In aggregate, these anatomic features of the pediatric airway predispose infants and young children to functional upper airway obstruction and make airway intervention technically challenging.

The type and size of equipment required for management of the pediatric airway are derived from the anatomy just discussed. A face mask should be sized so that the top and bottom rims fit on the bridge of the nose (below the eye) and in the cleft of the chin. A straight (Miller) blade is generally used for endotracheal intubation in infants and young children because the tip of the straight blade lifts the epiglottis up and out of the line of vision of the airway. Endotracheal tube size is a function of the patient's size. For children older than 1 year, endotracheal tube size (internal diameter in millimeters) can be estimated by the formula (age in years/4) + 4. Alternatively, endotracheal tube size can be estimated by comparing the endotracheal tube with the width of the child's fifth fingernail or, more reliably, by using a length-based measuring system such as the Broselow tape. Uncuffed endotracheal tubes may be used in children younger than 8 years because the cricoid is the narrowest part of the airway and acts as a physiologic cuff.

The spectrum of clinical findings in children who arrive at the emergency department with symptoms related to upper airway pathology is broad and includes the following general categories.

- The signs and symptoms of acute infections of the upper airway range from mild distress in a child with benign, self-limited disease to the abrupt onset of rapidly progressing distress and obstruction in a toxic-appearing child.
- Undiagnosed congenital anomalies of the airway and surrounding structures may be manifested as chronic or progressive stridor or difficulty feeding.
- An infant with a congenital airway anomaly in whom an acute airway infection develops is at higher risk for decompensation and respiratory failure.
- Upper airway obstruction from a foreign body in the airway or esophagus can cause partial or complete airway obstruction and may require advanced airway management skills.

STRIDOR

Stridor is the classic sound associated with upper airway obstruction. It is derived from the Latin *stridulus*, meaning harsh or grating. Stridor is caused by partial airway obstruction and the resultant turbulent airflow through a portion of the airway from the nose to the trachea. It is not a diagnosis in itself, but an important symptom that must be thoroughly investigated.[1-3] Stridor should be timed in the respiratory cycle (inspiratory, expiratory, biphasic) and assessed in terms of quality (coarse, high pitched).

The airway can be artificially divided into four regions: the nose and pharynx, the supraglottic struc-

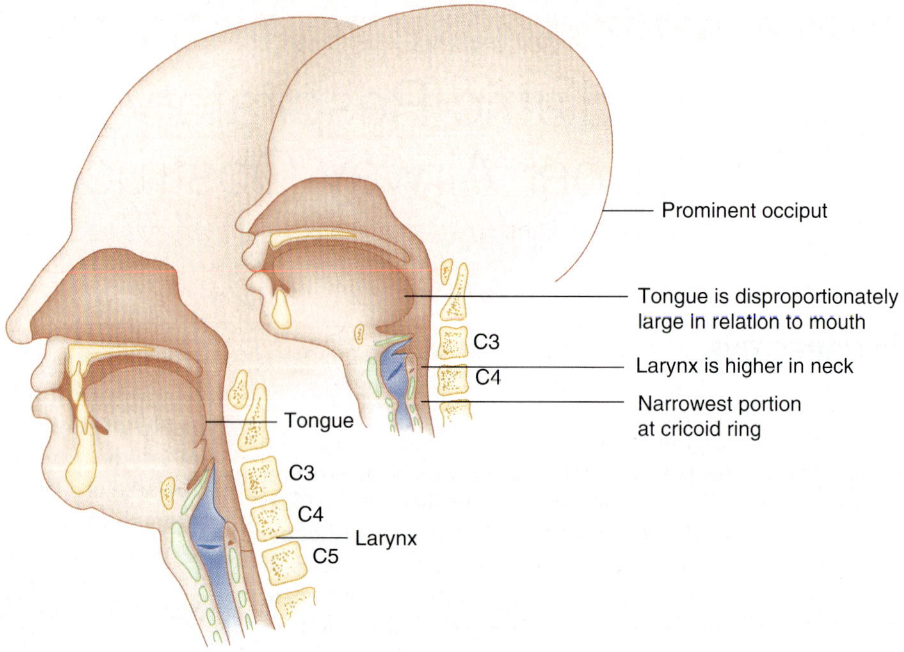

Figure 166-1. Comparison of adult and pediatric airways. (From Finucane BT: *Principles of Airway Management.* Philadelphia, FA Davis, 1988.)

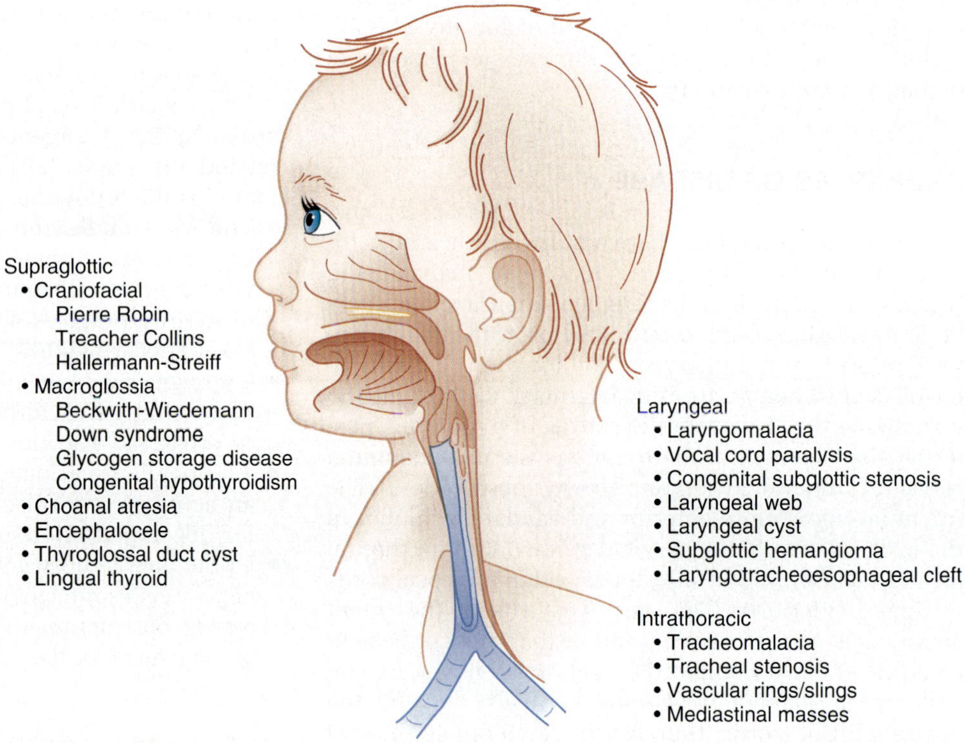

Figure 166-2. Regions and associated pathology of the pediatric upper airway. (From Simon NP, Simon N: Evaluation and management of stridor in the newborn. *Clin Pediatr [Phila]* 30:211, 1991.)

tures, the glottis and immediate subglottic area, and the intrathoracic trachea (Figure 166-2). Stridor has different characteristics, depending on its exact origin in the airway (Table 166-1).

Stridor from the nose and pharynx has a sonorous, gurgling, and coarse quality. The voice may have a muffled or "hot potato" quality. An example is a retropharyngeal abscess. High-pitched, inspiratory stridor comes from the supraglottic and immediate subglottic trachea. Inspiratory stridor is heard with pathology in this region because the extrathoracic airway narrows with inspiration as a result of atmospheric pressure outside the airway being slightly higher than that inside the airway. The voice may sound hoarse or weak. Examples include viral croup and laryngomalacia.

Biphasic stridor is heard with inspiration and expiration and usually suggests a fixed lesion that does not change in size at the glottis or cricoid ring with respiration. Examples of conditions resulting in biphasic stridor are a laryngeal web and vocal cord paralysis. Stridor from the lower part of the trachea is usually expiratory. Bacterial tracheitis and a foreign body are examples.

Table 166-1. Causes of Stridor: Anatomic Location, Sound, and Etiology

Features	Supraglottic	Glottic	Subglottic Trachea
Sound	Sonorous Gurgling Coarse Expiratory stridor	Biphasic stridor	High-pitched stridor Inspiratory stridor
Structures	Nose Pharynx Epiglottis	Larynx Vocal cords	Subglottic trachea
Congenital	Micrognathia Pierre Robin syndrome Treacher Collins syndrome Macroglossia Down syndrome Storage diseases Choanal atresia Lingual thyroid Thyroglossal cyst	Laryngomalacia Vocal cord paralysis Laryngeal web Laryngocele	Subglottic stenosis Tracheomalacia Tracheal stenosis Vascular ring Hemangioma cyst
Acquired	Adenopathy Tonsillar hypertrophy Foreign body Pharyngeal abscess Epiglottitis	Papillomas Foreign body	Croup Bacterial tracheitis Subglottic stenosis Foreign body

OVERVIEW OF THE EVALUATION AND MANAGEMENT OF A CHILD WITH AN UPPER AIRWAY OBSTRUCTION

Evaluation of a child with signs of airway obstruction begins with careful observation of the child at rest (work of breathing, respiratory rate, alertness, color) and during activity (crying, feeding). In most cases, observation and a carefully obtained history will provide most clues to the correct diagnosis. Important items to be elucidated in the history include the following:

- Onset and duration (acute, chronic)
- Associated symptoms (respiratory distress, fever, toxicity, drooling, cyanosis)
- Progression with age (number of bouts/severity of "croup" with increasing age)
- Exacerbations (supine versus prone position, upper respiratory infection [URI], crying)
- Feeding pattern (dysphagia, feeding abnormalities)
- Airway procedures (intubation in the neonatal period)
- Choking episode
- Baseline noises, quality of cry and voice

The initial physical examination includes assessment of the severity of respiratory distress (respiratory rate, retractions, flaring, heart rate) and the presence of respiratory failure (extreme distress, hypoventilation, altered mental status, dusky skin color, cyanosis, hypotonia). The character and timing of stridor, as well as the symmetry and quality of breath sounds, are important observations.

Definitive airway management always takes precedence over laboratory and diagnostic tests in a patient with an acute airway emergency. In a stable patient with an uncertain diagnosis, an individualized diagnostic evaluation is important.

Radiographs of the soft tissues of the neck should include both lateral and anteroposterior views. These views are helpful to assess adenoid and tonsillar size, the contour of the epiglottis, the thickness of the retropharyngeal soft tissue space, the vallecula, the aryepiglottic folds, and the tracheal air column (Figure 166-3).[4,5] Optimally, the child's head should be positioned in extension and the film taken during inspiration. Views of the chest may be helpful to assess heart size, location of the aortic arch, pulmonary pathology, and the trachea and bronchi.

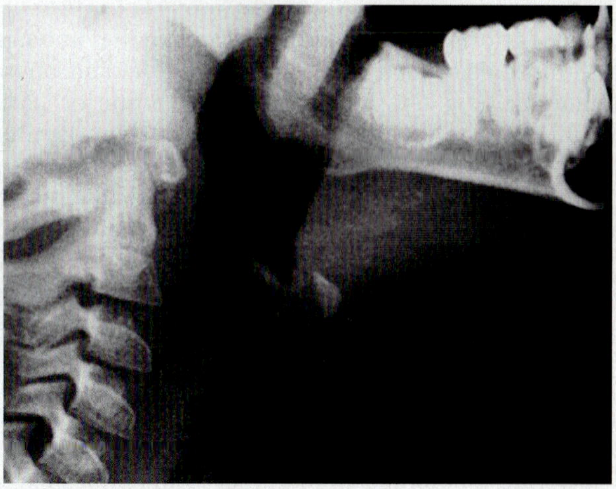

Figure 166-3. Normal appearance of upper airway structures on a lateral neck radiographic study. Note the hyoid bone, epiglottis, retropharyngeal space, and tracheal air column.

Additional studies may be indicated in specific settings. Bedside fiberoptic nasopharyngoscopy can be performed without anesthesia and allows visualization and movement of the supraglottic structures and vocal cords. An esophagogram may help define lesions compressing the airway and trachea. Computed tomography (CT), magnetic resonance imaging (MRI), and fiberoptic and rigid bronchoscopy should be considered on an individual basis.

SPECIFIC DISORDERS

Supraglottic Airway Diseases

Perspective

The supraglottic portion of the airway includes the nose, pharynx, epiglottis, and surrounding structures. Pathology of the nose and pharynx is commonly associated with noisy, congested breathing and respiratory distress. Congenital lesions involving these structures may cause mild symptoms at baseline but dramatic distress when the patient is stressed with a superimposed infectious process. Among the congenital lesions with which the emergency physician should be familiar are choanal atresia, macroglossia, micrognathia, thyroglossal duct cyst, and lingular thyroid. Important acquired causes include a nasal foreign body, nasal polyps, hypertrophic tonsils and adenoids, epiglottitis, retropharyngeal or peritonsillar abscess, pharyngitis, mononucleosis, and an upper airway foreign body. The most common ones are discussed in the following sections.

Congenital Lesions

Choanal atresia, the most common congenital anomaly of the nose, is caused by persistence of the bucconasal membrane or a bony septum in the posterior naris. Infants are "preferential nose breathers" because they breath through their nose when their mouth is closed at rest and in order to suck and swallow. This breathing preference is a result of the posterior aspect of the soft palate extending downward and contacting the tip of the epiglottis. Bilateral choanal atresia is a life-threatening emergency that is identified shortly after birth. Infants with bilateral choanal atresia become acutely distressed and cyanotic at birth and are managed with an oral airway that opens the mouth to allow a passage for breathing. Surgical correction of the obstructing membrane is required. Unilateral choanal atresia may go undetected in the nursery and become apparent only when the normal, patent nares are obstructed by swelling or secretions, most frequently from an upper respiratory infection.

Macroglossia is associated with a number of conditions, including Down syndrome, glycogen storage disease, and congenital hypothyroidism. The tongue is abnormally large and protrudes posteriorly into the hypopharynx. The increased secretions and swelling associated with a URI exacerbate the underlying obstruction, and stridor or labored breath sounds are produced.

Micrognathia is associated with syndromes such as Pierre Robin and Treacher Collins. A small mandible posteriorly displaces the normally sized tongue. Signs of obstruction often worsen when the patient is supine.

Retropharyngeal Abscess

Perspective

A retropharyngeal abscess is a potentially life-threatening airway emergency resulting from infection of the retropharyngeal soft tissue space. The retropharyngeal space is a potential space between the posterior pharyngeal wall and the prevertebral fascia that extends from the base of the skull to the level of T2. It is rich in lymph tissue that drains the nose, pharynx, sinuses, and ears. An abscess may result from direct trauma, suppuration of lymph nodes, or hematogenous spread. Most cases are seen in children younger than 3 years. In one study, 7 of 17 patients, including 2 neonates who required intubation, had traumatic perforations of the hypopharynx or esophagus caused by objects such as an airplane propeller, turkey bone, open safety pin, pencil, and metal tube as a result of the common tendency of toddlers to put objects in their mouths.[6] *Staphylococcus aureus*, group A *Streptococcus*, and anaerobes are the organisms most commonly responsible for this infection.[7]

Clinical Features

The variable manifestations of a retropharyngeal abscess may make it a challenging diagnosis. Common signs and symptoms include fever, sore throat, neck stiffness/nuchal rigidity, torticollis, trismus, neck swelling, drooling, stridor, and a muffled voice. In a prospective study of 17 patients, stridor and airway obstruction were observed in more than half (56%) of the patients.[6] The common finding of acute airway obstruction in children is a function of the high position of the larynx in the neck. Such anatomy places the airway proximate to and easily compressed by the bulging retropharyngeal mass. In patients with airway compression, the clinical appearance may resemble epiglottitis. With less obvious signs of airway obstruction, patients can exhibit a mixture of symptoms (fever, neck stiffness, generalized toxicity) suggesting meningitis or sepsis. Complications of a retropharyngeal abscess can be serious: generalized sepsis, aspiration pneumonia, mediastinitis, and empyema.

Diagnostic Strategies

Careful evaluation of airway patency should take precedence in managing a child with a presumed retropharyngeal abscess.[8-17] Examination of the pharynx may reveal bulging of the posterior pharyngeal wall. A soft tissue lateral view of the neck may be helpful to evaluate the fullness of the retropharyngeal soft tissues. The width of the retropharyngeal space should not exceed the diameter of the adjacent vertebral body (Figure 166-4). An air-fluid level is more commonly seen with perforations and anaerobic infections. Redundant soft tissue of the retropharyngeal space complicates interpretation of lateral neck films in young infants with a retropharyngeal abscess. Artifactual widening of a normal retropharyngeal space is commonly seen when the radiograph is taken with the head and neck in flexion or during exhalation (or both). CT may be beneficial in selected cases.

Management

The size of the abscess, the degree of airway obstruction, and the overall toxicity of the patient dictate management. The need for intubation or surgical drainage is determined on an individual basis, and these

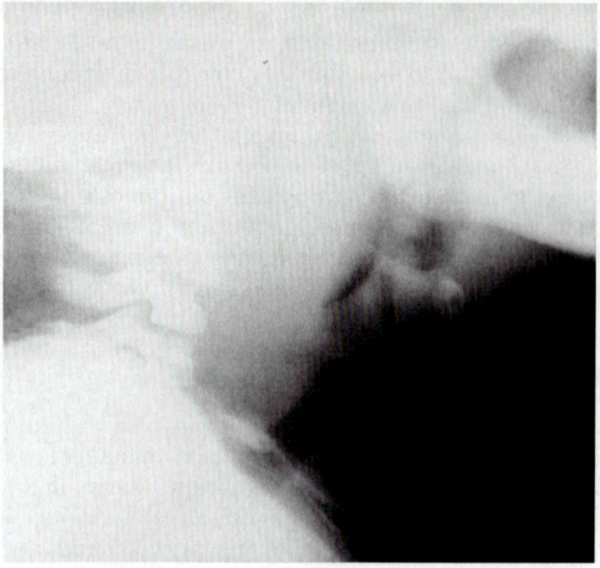

Figure 166-4. Retropharyngeal abscess. Note the widened retropharyngeal soft tissue space.

patients generally benefit from involvement of an ear, nose, and throat specialist.

Epiglottitis

Perspective

Although it remains among the most feared pediatric emergencies, the incidence of acute epiglottitis has declined markedly over the last 15 years[18-20] after the widespread use of *Haemophilus influenzae* type b vaccine. First licensed in 1985 for children 24 months old, the vaccine became available for immunization of infants 2 months of age in 1990. A study that compared epiglottitis before and after 1990 revealed a drop in the annual incidence of epiglottitis from 10.9 to 1.8 per 10,000 admissions.[21]

Principles of Disease

Typical epiglottitis caused by *H. influenzae* type b affects children between 3 and 7 years of age and occurs year-round. It is an invasive bacterial disease that causes inflammation and edema of the epiglottis, aryepiglottic folds, and surrounding supraglottic tissues. As these structures become inflamed and distended, they protrude downward and over the glottic opening. Several studies and case reports describe a change in this traditional profile.[21-24] In a survey of patients with epiglottitis since 1990, the average patient is older (80 versus 35 months) with varying microbiology. *H. influenzae* type b is seen in a small minority of patients, and organisms such as group A beta-hemolytic *Streptococcus*, *S. aureus*, and *Streptococcus pneumoniae*[21] are more common. Noninfectious causes are rare and include thermal injury from swallowing hot liquids.[25,26]

Clinical Features

Epiglottitis is classically an acute condition, without an extended prodrome. It is marked by high fever, intense sore throat, toxicity, and rapid progression. In one study, 85% of children with epiglottitis were symptomatic for less than 24 hours.[27] Children with epiglottitis appear anxious and maintain themselves in a "sniffing" or "tripod" position with the jaw jutting forward and the neck extended to maximize airway patency. As symptoms worsen, cough and phonation are usually absent. Drooling is prominent because of an inability to swallow. A study of children 2 to 18 years of age revealed that fever, difficulty breathing, irritability, change in voice or cry, stridor, and retractions were common initial symptoms that occurred in more than 80% of patients.[27] Singer and colleagues showed that in children younger than 24 months, toxicity, altered mental status, dyspnea, stridor, retractions, and fever were common initial symptoms.[28] Losek and coworkers in a study of 236 patients reported that 7 patients (3%) died.[27] The correct diagnosis of epiglottitis was not made in 11 of 58 (19%) children younger than 2 years and in 49 of 178 (28%) children between 2 and 18 years old. Incorrect diagnoses in patients who died included croup, summer virus, and pharyngitis. Croup is the most commonly assigned misdiagnosis and is more often made in the setting of very young children or those in whom drooling or difficulty swallowing were not prominent.[28]

A majority of patients with *H. influenzae* epiglottitis have bacteremia (50% to 75%).[27] Pneumonia is occasionally a coexisting finding. Uvulitis has been reported to coexist with epiglottitis,[29] but alone it is rarely a cause of serious airway obstruction.

Diagnostic Strategies

Direct examination of the pharynx with a tongue depressor or fiberoptic scope should be reserved for stable patients in whom the diagnosis is in doubt. It should be performed only in a setting in which both the equipment and personnel required for emergency intubation are at hand. Stimulation of the posterior of the pharynx with subsequent contraction of the pharyngeal muscles may increase airway obstruction. In adult patients this is rarely a concern because of the relatively larger upper airway. A lateral neck radiograph can be helpful to confirm the diagnosis and should be evaluated for an enlarged epiglottis ("thumbprint sign"; Figure 166-5), thickened aryepiglottic folds, lack of air in the vallecula, and a dilated hypopharynx. Careful observation of a child with suspected epiglottitis is essential. Laboratory tests, intravenous fluids and antibiotics, blood and epiglottis cultures, and sedation are all important considerations once the airway has been secured.

Management

The clinical features of classic epiglottitis are usually sufficiently characteristic that diagnostic tests are not necessary and should be avoided. The importance of securing the airway takes precedence over diagnostic evaluation. A "stable" patient who is maintaining a patent airway and adequate oxygenation should not be moved or repositioned for examination, laboratory tests, or radiography. Such patients should be carefully transported to a setting where definitive airway management can be achieved in a controlled fashion. If diagnostic studies are needed, constant and close observation is vital.

Careful decision making is essential when a child with epiglottitis requires transport. A survey of pediatric intensive care and emergency physicians found that 49% recommended intubation before interhospital transport in all cases. The remainder individualized the recommendation for pretransport intubation based in part on the referring physician's perceived ability to intubate the child.[30] Close observation without intubation has been reported.[31,32] However, this observation occurred in the selective setting of a pediatric intensive care unit (ICU) where several physicians with advanced training in anesthesia and pediatric critical care were on site at all times. Clearly, this is not the environment of most emergency departments and critical care units, and expeditious controlled intubation remains optimal management.

Unstable patients with respiratory failure require assisted ventilation. Bag/mask ventilation should be attempted first and, if successful, continued until intubation can be performed. If neither bag/valve/mask ventilation nor intubation are successful, more aggressive techniques such as needle cricothyroidotomy or tracheostomy may be indicated.

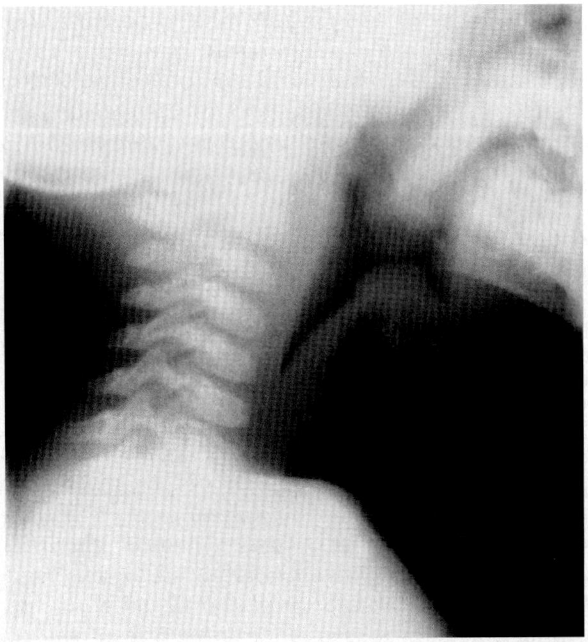

Figure 166-5. Epiglottitis. Note the "thumb sign" of the epiglottis and thickened aryepiglottic folds.

Diseases of the Larynx

The larynx and vocal cords occupy an important region in the airway that is often associated with airway pathology causing obstruction. Many of these obstructing conditions are congenital lesions, including laryngomalacia, a laryngeal web, and vocal cord paralysis. Acquired lesions include laryngeal papillomas.

Congenital Lesions

Laryngomalacia, the most common cause of chronic stridor in infants,[33,34] is a result of incomplete development of the supporting cartilage of the larynx. With inspiration, the long, floppy epiglottis, arytenoids, and aryepiglottic folds are drawn into the larynx and create a partial obstruction (Figure 166-6). Baseline inspiratory stridor begins shortly after birth and worsens with supine positioning and increased respiratory effort (crying, URI). Laryngomalacia is rarely associated with significant respiratory distress, feeding difficulties, or failure to thrive. Most patients experience complete resolution of symptoms by 2 years of age. Fiberoptic bronchoscopy has been used to confirm the diagnosis and exclude coexisting anomalies such as vocal cord paralysis and subglottic stenosis, which are found in approximately 20% of patients.

Vocal cord paralysis is the second most common cause of chronic stridor in infants. Bilateral vocal cord

Figure 166-6. Laryngomalacia. Note the progressive obstruction with inspiration as the epiglottis and surrounding structures collapse into the glottic opening.

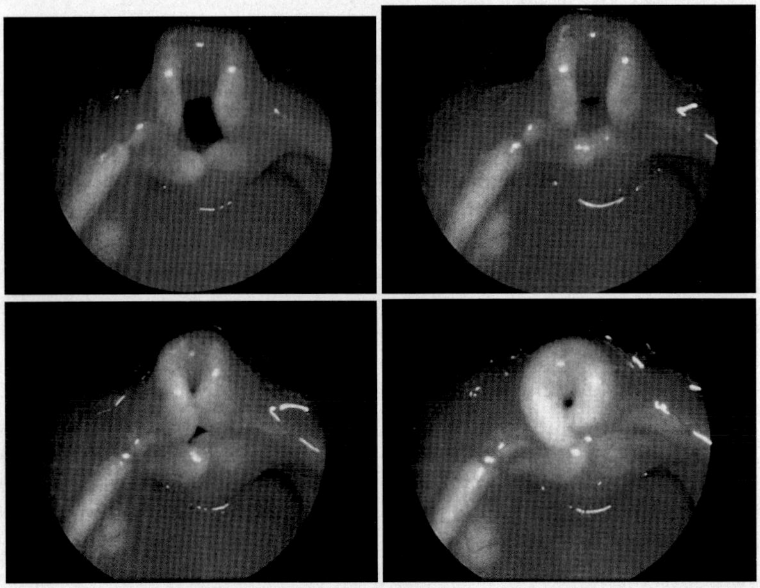

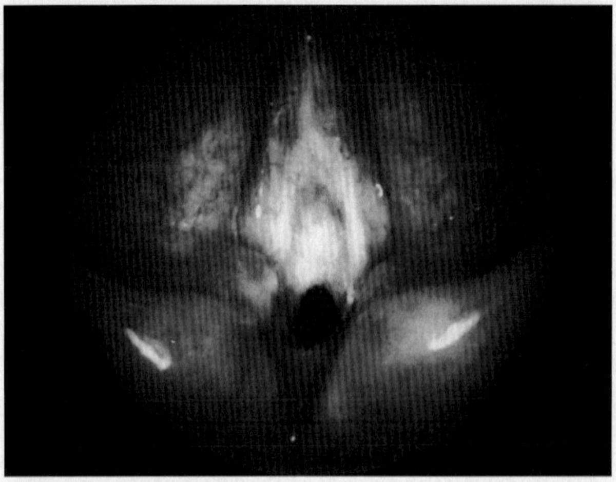

Figure 166-7. Large laryngeal web.

paralysis results in severe respiratory distress and stridor and is usually associated with serious central nervous system abnormalities such as Arnold-Chiari malformation. Unilateral vocal cord paralysis is most commonly left-sided and related to traction on the left recurrent laryngeal nerve at birth or compression from mediastinal structures. Infants with unilateral vocal cord paralysis have a hoarse, weak cry. Stridor often worsens with distress and improves with positioning of the affected side down.

A *laryngeal web* results from failure of complete canalization of the airway.[35] Most webs lie between the cords and appear as a partial anterior fusion (Figure 166-7). The spectrum of symptoms reflects the size of the web. Small webs may cause a hoarse, weak cry and mild stridor. Larger, more complete webs are associated with aphonia and severe distress.

Laryngeal Papillomas

Laryngeal papillomas arise from the laryngeal epithelium and may result from perinatal or postnatal exposure to human papillomavirus. When acquired in the prenatal period, hoarseness, abnormal cry, and inspiratory stridor commonly occur by 3 to 4 years of age. Symptoms can progress to severe respiratory distress as the lesions enlarge and obstruct the larynx.

Subglottic Tracheal Diseases

The subglottic trachea is the origin of the high-pitched inspiratory sound commonly associated with upper airway obstruction. The subglottic space is the narrowest part of the airway in children younger than 8 years and is completely surrounded by the cricoid ring. Such anatomy predisposes this part of the airway to obstruction. Subglottic narrowing or stenosis can result from a congenital anomaly, inflammation from infection, and trauma associated with prolonged intubation.

Congenital Lesions

Congenital laryngotracheal ("subglottic") stenosis is a result of a congenital defect in canalization of the subglottic trachea. Deformity of the cricoid ring is usually seen. Infants with severe stenosis have stridor at birth. Milder lesions may be asymptomatic until additional obstruction from infection or inflammation occurs. Subglottic stenosis is also an acquired condition that occurs after prolonged intubation or blunt trauma to the neck.

A *subglottic hemangioma* is a less common cause of stridor and subglottic airway obstruction in infants. The infant is usually asymptomatic at birth, but stridor (which may be biphasic) and cough develop within the first few weeks to months of life. Symptoms generally peak at 6 months as a result of rapid growth of the infant and the hemangioma during the first months of life. Respiratory symptoms worsen with crying and agitation. Cutaneous hemangiomas are seen in approximately half of cases. Hemangiomas of the airway may be seen on plain film as an asymmetric lesion along the tracheal air column.

Viral Croup

Principles of Disease

Croup (laryngotracheobronchitis) is the most common cause of upper respiratory obstruction in childhood, with a peak incidence at 2 years (range, 6 months to 6 years) and most commonly occurring in late fall, early winter, and spring. Rarely, viral croup is seen in older (9 and 10 years), healthy children. Parainfluenza virus type 1 accounts for about half of cases, with parainfluenza virus types 2 and 3, respiratory syncytial virus, influenza A and B virus, and rhinovirus responsible for the remainder.[36] Croup is caused by inflammation, exudate, and edema of the loosely adherent mucosal and submucosal tissues of the subglottic space. The inflamed mucosa expands into the airway lumen because the cricoid forms a complete cartilaginous (nonexpanding) ring in this part of the trachea.

The true incidence of croup is uncertain. Most children with croup have an uncomplicated course, and many cases are managed without medical intervention. Only a small percentage of those who receive urgent care require hospitalization. Croup is recurrent in a small number of patients. A subset of children with croup have involvement of the lower airway and exhibit bronchoconstriction, lower airway edema, and atelectasis.

Clinical Features

Croup can generally be diagnosed clinically. Children with typical croup have a constellation of symptoms, including a barky cough, hoarse voice, and high-pitched, inspiratory stridor. These findings usually follow a prodrome of mild fever and URI symptoms lasting several days.

Scoring systems have been developed for assessment of croup and include an evaluation of worsening stridor, retractions, cyanosis, heart rate, and respiratory rate. Although a formal croup score is often not assigned in many clinical settings, determination of mild, moderate, or severe croup should be based on careful evaluation of these five signs, as well as mental

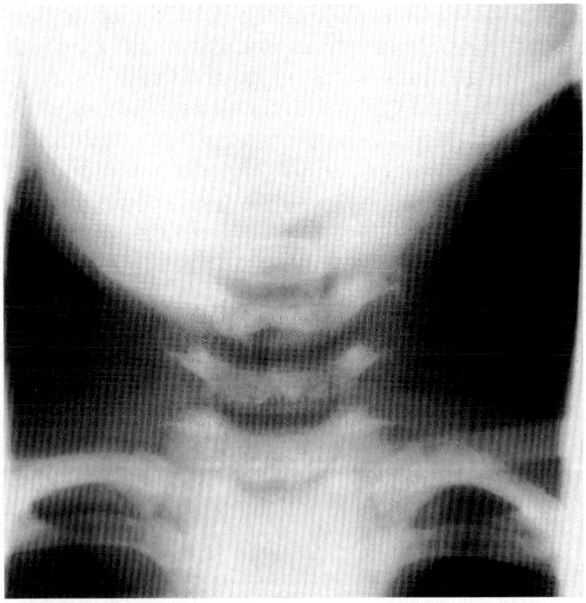

Figure 166-8. Croup. Note the "steepling" of the subglottic trachea.

status and air movement. Mild croup is characterized by an intermittent barky cough, stridor with agitation but not at rest, mild tachypnea, and tachycardia. A child with mild croup is minimally distressed and well hydrated and has normal mental status. Moderate croup is characterized by audible stridor at rest, worsening stridor with agitation, a barky cough, and increased work of breathing (retractions, tachypnea, tachycardia). A patient with moderate croup may be fussy but is alert, interactive, and comforted by parents. Hypoxia is atypical in mild or moderate croup. When seen, it may signify concomitant lower respiratory disease, another disease process, or severe croup.

Laboratory tests are nondiagnostic. Radiographic studies of the neck are useful when the diagnosis is in doubt, but they do not change management. The classic finding in croup is a tapered narrowing of the normal shouldered appearance of the subglottic trachea such that it has the appearance of a pencil or steeple (Figure 166-8).

Management

The mainstays of treatment of mild and moderate to severe croup are cool mist, aerosolized epinephrine, and glucocorticoids. Cool mist may act by moistening thickened secretions, thereby making them easier to mobilize out of the airway; however, mist does not reduce subglottic edema. A randomized trial of mist therapy in moderate croup showed no clear benefit in improving oxygen saturation, respiratory rate, or assessment times.[37] Its use in mild croup has not been studied, but other therapy is prudent in moderate to severe croup.

Aerosolized epinephrine, either racemic epinephrine (containing *d* and *l* isomers) or *l*-epinephrine, acts on α-adrenergic receptors in the subglottic mucosa.[38] Through vasoconstriction, epinephrine reverses edema and relieves acute symptoms in a subset of patients. It is a temporizing measure with a quick onset of action (within 10 minutes). Racemic epinephrine has traditionally been preferred over *l*-epinephrine because the racemic mixture has been thought to be associated with fewer cardiovascular side effects, and it is still widely used. It is now clear, however, that the *l* form of epinephrine is the active isomer and has the same degree of safety and efficacy as racemic epinephrine[41]; either form may be used. The "rebound" phenomenon of epinephrine is defined as recurrence or worsening of the patient's pretreatment symptoms when aerosolized epinephrine wears off. This rebound is rarely clinically significant if steroids are given early in management.[42] Many patients with moderate croup benefit from aerosolized epinephrine. It has been demonstrated that a subset of these patients can be safely discharged from the emergency department after a posttreatment observation period of 2 to 4 hours.[38,43,44] A retrospective study evaluating the policy of discharging selected patients after treatment with racemic epinephrine yielded favorable results. Of 50 patients discharged after the administration of epinephrine, none were subsequently hospitalized and only 1 required retreatment within 48 hours as an outpatient. Importantly, 92% were discharged on a regimen of steroids. The authors recommend that children with moderate croup who have received aerosolized epinephrine can be safely discharged (1) after 2 hours of observation subsequent to the administration of epinephrine, (2) if they are free of stridor and retractions, and (3) if they have access to follow-up care. They also recommend administration of steroids in these patients.[43] The decision to discharge after administration of aerosolized epinephrine should also be based on the patient's symptoms. Did symptoms worsen during the several hours of observation? Are there other factors (dehydration, preexisting airway pathology, other congenital anomalies) that would increase the risk for complications?

The role of oral, parenteral, and inhaled steroids in the treatment of croup has been debated for decades.[39] In 1989, a meta-analysis of nine studies investigating steroid use in hospitalized patients with moderate croup suggested that (1) steroid therapy resulted in faster improvement in hospitalized patients, (2) steroids decreased the incidence of intubation, and (3) higher doses (>0.3 mg/kg dexamethasone) were more effective than lower doses.[40] Subsequent to this study, Geelhoed and Macdonald[45] compared the effect of different doses of dexamethasone in hospitalized children in sequential clinical trials. In trial A, children were given either 0.6 or 0.3 mg/kg. In trial B, patients received either 0.3 or 0.15 mg/kg. These studies demonstrated that oral dexamethasone in doses as small as 0.15 mg/kg was as effective as higher doses in decreasing the duration of symptoms and hospitalization time.

Budesonide is an inhaled steroid with potent topical anti-inflammatory properties and compares favorably with dexamethasone. It was chosen for study because the nebulized route avoids the pain of needle injection (in patients unable/unwilling to take oral medication) and the theoretical risk of gastrointestinal complications. A single dose (2 mg) of nebulized budesonide was shown to shorten emergency department stay, decrease the rate of hospitalization, and cause a more rapid improvement in symptoms in children with mild to moderate croup evaluated in the emergency department.[46] Inhaled budesonide (2 mg per dose) was shown to be as effective as oral dexamethasone (0.6 mg/kg) in decreasing the duration of hospital stay, improving clinical symptoms, and decreasing the ongoing requirement for aerosolized epinephrine.[47] Subsequently, the combination of dexamethasone and nebulized budesonide was reported to be superior to dexamethasone alone in emergency department patients with moderate croup, although the added improvement was small.[48]

A study by Klassen and colleagues[49] attempted to define the actual benefit of budesonide over dexamethasone. Oral dexamethasone (0.6 mg/kg) was compared with nebulized budesonide (2 mg per dose) and with both dexamethasone and budesonide. Similar outcomes were reported in all three groups.

A more compelling piece of evidence for the use of routine steroids in croup was Geelhoed and MacDonald's comparison[47] of the experience at Princess Margaret Hospital for Children before and after steroids became mandatory in the treatment of croup in patients in the ICU. Before 1989, less than 5% of ICU patients received steroids. At that time, 11% (yearly average) were intubated, and the total ICU days amounted to 129 (yearly average). Beginning in 1989, every child admitted to the ICU received 0.6 mg/kg dexamethasone intramuscularly. The intubation rate declined to 1% (yearly average), and total ICU days dropped to 21 (yearly average). The dose of dexamethasone was later decreased to 0.15 mg/kg.

Overall, steroids are recommended for the management of croup. Children with suspected croup should receive oral or intramuscular dexamethasone. The effective dose is as low as 0.15 mg/kg.

A small percentage of patients with croup are admitted to the hospital. The decision to admit a child with moderate croup is based on a number of factors: the severity of symptoms at initial evaluation, persistence of respiratory distress, stridor at rest, oxygenation, response to treatment (humidification and aerosolized epinephrine), hydration, history suggesting airway pathology or recurrent croup, young age (<6 months), high fever, overall toxicity, and parental reliability (Box 166-1).

BOX 166-1. Croup: Indications for Admission

- Severe respiratory distress or failure
- Unusual symptoms (hypoxia, hyperpyrexia)
- Dehydration
- Persistence of stridor at rest after aerosolized epinephrine and steroids
- Persistence of tachycardia, tachypnea
- Complex past medical history (prematurity, pulmonary, cardiac disease)

Severe croup is rare and associated with signs of impending airway obstruction and respiratory failure: fatigue, hypoxia, hypercapnia, abnormal mental status, extreme respiratory distress, and stridor. Since the advent of steroid administration, only an estimated 1% to 2% of patients with croup require intubation. Ideally, intubation should be performed under controlled circumstances. Orotracheal intubation with an endotracheal tube at least a half-size smaller than expected for the child's size is often necessary. If the tube that can be passed is too small to allow adequate ventilation, tracheostomy may be required. The decision to extubate a child with severe croup is complex; age, coexisting congenital lesions, and length of intubation are all variables that should be considered.

Spasmodic Croup

Spasmodic croup is a somewhat indistinct clinical entity in which many of its features overlap those of viral coup. It is characterized by the sudden onset of severe stridor and a barky cough without a viral prodrome. It may be recurrent and has been associated with allergy and gastroesophageal reflux. Previous parainfluenza infection has been postulated as a predisposing condition for a hypersensitivity reaction on later exposure to the virus. There is little in the literature to delineate the difference between spasmodic and viral croup.

Diseases of the Trachea

Obstruction of the trachea distal to the subglottic space can be a result of both congenital and acquired lesions.

Congenital Lesions

Tracheomalacia results from abnormally soft, undeveloped supporting cartilage of the tracheal rings. This diagnosis should be suspected in patients with a history of stridor that increases over the first few weeks of life and worsens with agitation, supine positioning, and infection. Plain radiographs are usually nondiagnostic, but dynamic studies such as fluoroscopy or ultrafast CT may be helpful.

Tracheal stenosis is a congenital anomaly that results from complete tracheal rings. Infants have persistent stridor and respiratory distress. Because the trachea is "fixed," symptoms worsen with agitation and age.

A *vascular ring* is an anomaly of the aortic arch and related vessels in which a ring is formed that encircles the trachea, esophagus or both. Examples of "vascular rings" include a double aortic arch, right-sided aortic arch with a persistent left ligament, aberrant right subclavian artery, and a pulmonary sling. These conditions are rare and are often manifested in infancy with a variety of symptoms related to breathing and feeding. However, the nonspecific nature of the infant's symptoms and the low prevalence of these lesions often result in an initial incorrect diagnosis of croup or URI. In a retrospective review of 38 patients, the diagnosis was made in the first year of life in 87%. Stridor (50%), wheezing (53%), and dyspnea (45%) were the most

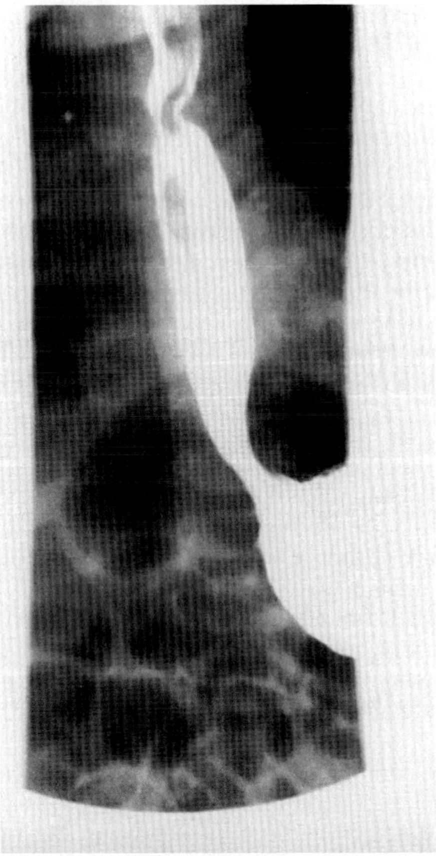

Figure 166-9. Barium esophagogram. Note the indentation of the esophagus caused by an encircling vascular ring.

common initial symptoms, followed by cough (34%), recurrent URI (32%), and dysphagia (32%). Sixty-three percent of these patients had associated cardiovascular anomalies.[50]

This diagnosis should be considered in any infant with persistent, unexplained respiratory and feeding problems. A chest radiograph revealing an abnormal (right-sided) location of the aortic arch may suggest the diagnosis in the emergency department. Definitive diagnosis requires further investigation. Traditionally, a barium esophagogram has been considered to be the single most important diagnostic procedure in patients with complete vascular rings (Figure 166-9).[51] The need for additional studies such as CT, MRI, angiography, or bronchoscopy should be individualized. Importantly, the common association of congenital cardiac anomalies is a consideration in the workup of these patients.

Bacterial Tracheitis

Principles of Disease

Bacterial tracheitis (membranous croup, bacterial croup, pseudomembranous croup) is a relatively rare but serious cause of stridor and airway obstruction in children. Bacterial tracheitis was "reintroduced" by Jones and associates in 1979 after a period of almost 4 decades when it seemed to disappear as a clinical entity.[52] It generally affects younger children, with a peak incidence at approximately 3 to 4 years of age. However, bacterial tracheitis has been reported in patients well beyond this age group, thus making it a diagnosis seen in adolescence and young adulthood as well.

The pathogenesis of bacterial tracheitis is severe inflammation of the tracheal epithelium and the production of thick mucopurulent secretions. The lining of the trachea forms a loosely adherent membrane that sloughs into the lumen. Traditionally, *S. aureus* has been the organism primarily responsible for bacterial tracheitis. More recently, the microbiology of bacterial tracheitis has been better defined. In a review of bacterial tracheitis in 14 children, Brook reported that aerobic bacteria (43%), anaerobic bacteria (20%), and mixed anaerobic and aerobic flora (36%) were cultured. The predominant organisms recovered in tracheal secretions were *S. aureus* (5), *H. influenzae* type b (4), *Moraxella catarrhalis* (2) *Peptostreptococcus* species (4), *Prevotella* and *Porphyromonas* (4), and *Fusobacterium* species (2).[53] Others have reported *S. pneumoniae*, alpha-hemolytic and group A streptococci, and *Candida albicans*.

Bacterial tracheitis is a secondary bacterial infection complicating a preexisting viral infection In 1983, Edwards and coauthors published two cases of *S. aureus* bacterial tracheitis in which influenza B was also cultured in one case and parainfluenza 2 was demonstrated in the other.[54] In a later series of 46 patients with bacterial tracheitis, concomitant viral respiratory cultures were positive in 72%.

Clinical Features

The clinical features of bacterial tracheitis overlap the symptoms of both croup and epiglottitis (Table 166-2). Patients experience a viral prodrome of fever, barky cough, and stridor. These symptoms typically intensify. The child appears toxic, and signs of airway obstruction and respiratory failure may develop acutely. Differentiating bacterial tracheitis from severe croup or epiglottitis on clinical grounds alone can be difficult. In a combined analysis of three studies, the correct initial diagnosis of bacterial tracheitis was made in only 4 of 26 patients. The admitting diagnoses in the remaining 22 patients were viral croup, epiglottitis, and aspiration.[55] In another report of 16 patients with bacterial tracheitis, an initial diagnosis of croup was made in 7 and acute epiglottitis in 2.[56] Features that suggest bacterial tracheitis include a viral prodrome followed by acute decompensation, symptoms atypical for croup (high fever, cyanosis, and severe distress), a poor response to usual treatment of croup (steroids and aerosolized epinephrine), and the presence of both inspiratory and expiratory stridor.

Diagnostic Strategies

Evaluation of a toxic-appearing child with bacterial tracheitis should be conducted expeditiously. Laboratory tests are nondiagnostic. The white blood cell count is normal or slightly elevated. Blood cultures are usually negative. Lateral and anteroposterior views of the neck and chest may be helpful. Findings on plain radiographs include subglottic narrowing, a ragged edge of the usually smooth tracheal air column, and a hazy density within the tracheal lumen. The epiglottis and supraglottic structures appear normal. In addition, the

Table 166-2. Comparison of Croup, Epiglottitis, and Bacterial Tracheitis

	Croup	Epiglottitis	Bacterial Tracheitis
Peak age	6 months-3 years	3-7 years	3-5 years, but seen throughout childhood
Pathology	Subglottic inflammation, edema	Inflammation and edema of the epiglottis, aryepiglottic folds	Bacterial superinfection with inflammation of the tracheal mucosa, copious mucopurulent secretions obstructing the trachea
Organisms	Parainfluenzavirus, RSV, adenovirus	*Haemophilus influenzae*	*Staphylococcus aureus* or mixed flora
Clinical features	Onset follows URI prodrome consisting of croupy cough, hoarse voice, low-grade fever, inspiratory stridor	Rapid progression of high fever, toxicity, drooling, stridor	Several-day prodrome of crouplike illness progressing to toxicity, inspiratory/expiratory stridor, marked distress
Laboratory and radiographic findings	Steeple sign on PA view of the neck	Thumb sign on lateral aspect of the neck, thickened aryepiglottic folds, loss of air in the vallecula	Normal upper airway structures, shaggy tracheal air column
Management	Steroids; uncommon, aerosolized epinephrine; rare, intubation	Intubation, antibiotics	Intubation common, antibiotics

PA, posteroanterior; RSV, respiratory syncytial virus; URI, upper respiratory infection.

chest radiograph may reveal coexisting pneumonia. Bronchoscopy is both diagnostic and therapeutic and should be performed on an emergency basis. This procedure should allow for visualization of the supraglottic structures and larynx, exclusion of other pathology, suctioning of tracheal secretions and debris, and establishment of an artificial airway.

Management

In relatively few cases, severe distress requires immediate intubation and suctioning in the emergency department. Airway management in the setting of the operating room is preferred. These patients require hospital admission, intensive care, supplemental oxygen, fluid resuscitation, and broad-spectrum antibiotics.

Intubation has been required in the majority of patients. In six of eight series, intubation rates exceeded 70%. The remaining two reported intubation rates of only 30%.[55] The authors postulated that the absence of aspiration pneumonia[57] and older age[58] are factors that may account in part for the decreased need for active airway management in some patients. Overall, recovery is slow. The duration of intubation in patients with bacterial tracheitis is reported to be 4 to 5 days, as opposed to 48 hours for croup and 54 hours for epiglottitis.[56] Reintubation after elective extubation was reported to be necessary in 4 of 10 patients because of recurrence of severe respiratory distress.[55]

Rare complications that have been reported in association with bacterial tracheitis include toxic shock syndrome, septic shock, postintubation pulmonary edema, and acute respiratory distress syndrome.[59]

Aeroesophageal Foreign Bodies

Airway Foreign Body

Perspective

Asphyxia after foreign body aspiration is a common cause of death in children. The majority of cases and deaths occur in toddlers younger than 3 years. A foreign body can lodge in any part of the airway and can move. Round-shaped foods are the most frequently aspirated objects: grapes, raisins, peanuts, and hot dogs.[60] Nonfood objects include a whole host of items. Conformable objects are the most difficult to manage and remove, and balloons, including those made from examination gloves found in physicians' offices, are the objects most likely to result in death.[61]

In general, objects that pass through the subglottic space will lodge in a bronchus, usually the right main stem bronchus, or in a more terminal part of the airway. Large objects that lodge in the upper airway and trachea tend to cause obvious and dramatic signs of upper airway obstruction: dyspnea, drooling, stridor, and cyanosis. They also carry the worst prognosis.

Clinical Features

An upper airway foreign body can cause partial or complete obstruction. A patient who is adequately oxygenated and is moving air should be initially allowed to maintain a preferred position, continue coughing to clear the obstruction, and breathe spontaneously.

Clinical signs of complete obstruction include poor air exchange, ineffective cough, severe distress, and cyanosis. The response to complete obstruction will be determined by the setting and available equipment. Outside a setting in which laryngoscopy and airway equipment are available, relief of a complete obstruction should follow the American Heart Association age-specific guidelines for obstruction by a foreign body.[62]

Diagnostic Strategies

In a child with an aspirated foreign body in the upper airway, there is often no time nor is it prudent to obtain diagnostic imaging. In a stable patient, a portable lateral neck radiograph and a chest radiograph may be obtained as long as the patient is allowed to maintain a position of comfort.

Management

Basic life support maneuvers to remove a foreign body in children include back blows and chest thrusts in infants and abdominal thrusts in children and adolescents. Choking infants younger than 1 year should receive a series of five back blows delivered between the shoulder blades, followed by five chest thrusts. Chest thrusts should be performed with two to three fingers on the midsternum in a manner similar to chest compressions. The infant's head should be held below the trunk. Abdominal thrusts should not be performed in infants because of the possibility of injury to abdominal organs. Blind finger sweeps are not performed in infants or children because this maneuver may push the object further into the airway.[62]

In children older than 1 year, the Heimlich maneuver or subdiaphragmatic thrusts are used. The rescuer places the fist of one hand in the other hand and against the abdomen of the victim. Five thrusts are delivered between the waist and rib cage. The rescuer's hands should not be placed on the xiphoid. This maneuver is performed in the standing position in a conscious victim. An unconscious child should be placed supine with the rescuer kneeling astride the victim. In the hospital setting, the airway should be open with a jaw thrust and the patient assessed for respirations. If there is no chest rise, assisted ventilation with a bag/mask device (manual resuscitator) is indicated. If there is still no chest rise, laryngoscopy should be performed to visualize and remove the foreign body with pediatric Magill forceps.[63] If the foreign body cannot be seen in the pharynx or larynx, it may be located in the esophagus where it could be pushing on the soft cartilage of the trachea and causing the obstruction. In this case, basic life support maneuvers may dislodge the foreign body into the mouth where it can be removed. If it appears within the subglottic space or trachea and cannot be removed, basic life support maneuvers may dislodge it into the oropharynx, or an attempt to push it into a main stem bronchus with an endotracheal tube may allow ventilation of the other lung but may result in irreversible airway obstruction. Recruiting additional expertise in the form of an ear, nose, and throat specialist, anesthesiologist, or general surgeon may be valuable.

Emergency needle cricothyroidotomy is a procedure of last resort to access the airway in an obstructed patient who cannot be intubated or ventilated. A large intravenous catheter (14 to 18 gauge) is passed through the midline of the inferior edge of the cricothyroid membrane. When air is aspirated, the plastic catheter is advanced and connected to the adapter of a 3-0 endotracheal tube and then connected to a manual resuscitator. Needle cricothyrotomy kits are also commercially available. Jet ventilation devices or the use of wall oxygen flow may allow for greater ventilation than possible with a self-inflating manual resuscitator.[64] This is generally considered a temporizing measure that allows for oxygenation until another airway can be established.

KEY CONCEPTS

- *Retropharyngeal abscess.* A potentially life-threatening emergency in young children with signs of upper airway obstruction or meningismus, a retropharyngeal abscess is often related to oral trauma. It is most frequently caused by *Staphylococcus aureus*, group A streptococci, and anaerobes.
- *Epiglottitis.* In the post–*Haemophilus influenzae* type b (Hib) vaccine era, the typical profile of epiglottitis has changed to include older patients. Group A *Streptococcus* causes the majority of infections; Hib is the infectious agent in a minority of cases. The clinical features of epiglottitis are usually sufficiently characteristic that diagnostic tests are not necessary to make the diagnosis.
- *Croup.* Viral croup is the most common infection of the upper airway in young children and is often mild. The mainstays of managing moderate to severe croup include vaporized epinephrine and glucocorticoids. These patients can be discharged from the emergency department after a posttreatment observation period of several hours if they remain free of stridor and distress and have access to follow-up care.
- *Bacterial tracheitis.* The clinical features of bacterial tracheitis represent a progression from a viral upper respiratory illness to acute toxicity and marked respiratory distress. *Staphylococcus aureus* is the most common cause of this infection. Bronchoscopy is both diagnostic and therapeutic and should be performed on an emergency basis.
- *Airway foreign body.* Children with an airway foreign body are managed with basic, followed by advanced, life support procedures for removal of the foreign body. Emergency cricothyroidotomy is reserved for obstructed patients who cannot be intubated or ventilated.

REFERENCES

1. Leung AKC, Cho H: Diagnosis of stridor in children. *Am Fam Physician* 60:2289, 1999.
2. Simon N: Evaluation and management of stridor in the newborn. *Clin Pediatr (Phila)* 30:211, 1991.
3. Tunkel DE, Zalzal GH: Stridor in infants and children: Ambulatory evaluation and operative diagnosis. *Clin Pediatr (Phila)* 31:48, 1992.
4. Walner DL, et al: Utility of radiographs in the evaluation of pediatric upper airway obstruction. *Ann Otol Rhinol Laryngol* 108:378, 1999.
5. Goodman TR, McHugh K: The role of radiology in the evaluation of stridor. *Arch Dis Child* 81:456, 1999.
6. Morrison JE, Pashley NRT: Retropharyngeal abscesses in children: A 10-year review. *Pediatr Emerg Care* 4:9, 1988.
7. Asmar BI: Bacteriology of retropharyngeal abscess in children. *Pediatr Infect Dis J* 9:595, 1990.
8. Brechtelsbauer PB, et al: Retropharyngeal abscess: Pitfalls of plain films and computed tomography. *Am J Otolaryngol* 18:258, 1997.
9. Coulthard M: Neonatal retropharyngeal abscess. *Pediatr Infect Dis J* 10:547, 1991.
10. DeLorenzo RA, Singer JI, Matre WM: Retropharyngeal abscess in an afebrile child. *Am J Emerg Med* 11:151, 1993.
11. Gaglani JM, Edwards MS: Clinical indicators of childhood retropharyngeal abscess. *Am J Emerg Med* 13:333, 1995.

12. Goldenberg D, Golz A, Joachims HZ: Retropharyngeal abscess: A clinical review. *J Laryngol Otol* 111:545, 1997.
13. Greene JS, Asher IM: Retropharyngeal abscess: A previously unreported symptom. *Ann Emerg Med* 13:615, 1984.
14. Harries PG: Retropharyngeal abscess and acute torticollis. *J Laryngol Otol* 111:1183, 1997.
15. Hartmann RW: Recognition of retropharyngeal abscess in children. *Am Fam Physician* 46:193, 1992.
16. Machida BK, Hawkins DB: Idiopathic retropharyngeal abscess in a neonate. *Otolaryngol Head Neck Surg* 97:396, 1987.
17. Thompson JW, Cohen SR, Reddix P: Retropharyngeal abscess in children: A retrospective and historical analysis. *Laryngoscope* 98:589, 1988.
18. Adams WG, et al: Decline of childhood *Haemophilus influenzae* type b (Hib) disease in the Hib vaccine era. *JAMA* 269:221, 1993.
19. Broadhurst LE, Erickson RL, Kelley PW: Decreases in invasive *Haemophilus influenzae* disease in US army children, 1984 through 1991. *JAMA* 269:227, 1993.
20. Murphy TV, et al: Declining incidence of *Haemophilus influenzae* type b disease since introduction of vaccination. *JAMA* 269:246, 1993.
21. Gorelick MH, Baker MD: Epiglottitis in children, 1979 through 1992. *Arch Pediatr Adolesc Med* 148:47, 1994.
22. Balsam D, Sorrano D, Barax C: *Candida* epiglottitis presenting as stridor in a child with HIV infection. *Pediatr Radiol* 22:235, 1992.
23. Bogger-Goren S: Acute epiglottitis caused by herpes simplex virus. *Pediatr Infect Dis J* 6:1133, 1987.
24. Narasimhan N, et al: Acute supraglottitis caused by varicella. *Pediatr Infect Dis J* 12:619, 1993.
25. Harjacek M, et al: Thermal epiglottitis after swallowing hot tea. *Pediatr Emerg Care* 8:342, 1992.
26. Kulick RM, et al: Thermal epiglottitis after swallowing hot beverages. *Pediatrics* 81:441, 1988.
27. Losek JD, et al: Epiglottitis: Comparison of signs and symptoms in children less than 2 years old and older. *Ann Emerg Med* 19:55, 1990.
28. Singer JI, McCabe JB: Epiglottitis at the extremes of age. *Am J Emerg Med* 6:228, 1988.
29. Wynder SG, Lampe RM, Shoemaker ME: Uvulitis and *Haemophilus influenzae* b bacteremia. *Pediatr Emerg Care* 2:23, 1986.
30. Waisman Y, et al: Management of children with epiglottitis during transport: Analysis of a survey. *Pediatr Emerg Care* 9:191, 1993.
31. Arndal H, Andreassen UK: Acute epiglottitis in children and adults. Nasotracheal intubation, tracheostomy or careful observation? Current status in Scandinavia. *J Laryngol Otol* 102:1012, 1988.
32. Butt W, et al: Acute epiglottitis: A different approach to management. *Crit Care Med* 16:43, 1988.
33. Lis G, Szczerbinski T, Cichocka-Jarosz E: Congenital stridor. *Pediatr Pulmonol* 20:220, 1995.
34. Nussbaum E, Maggi JC: Laryngomalacia in children. *Chest* 98:942, 1990.
35. Cohen SR: Congenital glottic webs in children: A retrospective review of 51 patients. *Ann Otol Rhinol Laryngol Suppl* 121:2, 1985.
36. Marx A, et al: Pediatric hospitalizations for croup (laryngotracheobronchitis): Biennial increases associated with human parainfluenza virus I epidemics. *J Infect Dis* 176:1423, 1997.
37. Neto GM, Kentab O, Klassen TP, Osmond MH: A randomized controlled trial of mist in the acute treatment of moderate croup. *Acad Emerg Med* 9:873, 2002.
38. Cornell HM, Bolte RG: Outpatient use of racemic epinephrine in croup. *Am Fam Physician* 46:683, 1992.
39. Geelhoed GC: Sixteen years of croup in a western Australian teaching hospital: Effects of routine steroid treatment. *Ann Emerg Med* 28:621, 1996.
40. Kairys SW, Olmstead EM, O'Connor GT: Steroid treatment of laryngotracheitis: A meta-analysis of the evidence from randomized trials. *Pediatrics* 83:683, 1989.
41. Waisman Y, et al: Prospective randomized double-blind study comparing L-epinephrine and racemic epinephrine aerosols in the treatment of laryngotracheitis (croup). *Pediatrics* 89:302, 1992.
42. Prendergast M, Jones JS, Hartman D: Racemic epinephrine in the treatment of laryngotracheitis: Can we identify children for outpatient therapy? *Am J Emerg Med* 12:613, 1994.
43. Kelley PB, Simon JE: Racemic epinephrine use in croup and disposition. *Am J Emerg Med* 10:181, 1992.
44. Ledwith CA, Shea LM, Mauro RD: Safety and efficacy of nebulized racemic epinephrine in conjunction with oral dexamethasone and mist in the outpatient treatment of croup. *Ann Emerg Med* 25:331, 1995.
45. Geelhoed GC, Macdonald WBG: Oral dexamethasone in the treatment of croup: 0.15 mg/kg versus 0.3 mg/kg versus 0.6 mg/kg. *Pediatr Pulmonol* 20:362, 1995.
46. Klassen TP, et al: Nebulized budesonide for children with mild-to-moderate croup. *N Engl J Med* 331:2859, 1994.
47. Geelhoed GC, Macdonald WBG: Oral and inhaled steroids in croup. *Pediatr Pulmonol* 20:355, 1995.
48. Klassen TP, et al: The efficacy of nebulized budesonide in dexamethasone-treated outpatients with croup. *Pediatrics* 97:463, 1996.
49. Klassen TP, et al: Nebulized budesonide and oral dexamethasone for treatment of croup. *JAMA* 279:1629, 1998.
50. Bakker DAH, Berger RM, Witsenburg M, Bogers AJ: Vascular rings: A rare cause of common respiratory symptoms. *Acta Paediatr* 88:947, 1999.
51. Backer CL, et al: Vascular anomalies causing tracheoesophageal compression. *J Thorac Cardiovasc Surg* 97:725, 1989.
52. Donnelly BW, McMillan JA, Weiner LB: Bacterial tracheitis: Report of eight new cases and review. *Rev Infect Dis* 12:729, 1990.
53. Brook I: Aerobic and anaerobic microbiology of bacterial tracheitis in children. *Pediatr Emerg Care* 13:16, 1997.
54. Edwards KM, Dundon MC, Altemeier WA: Bacterial tracheitis as a complication of viral croup. *Pediatr Infect Dis* 2:390, 1983.
55. Eckel HE, et al: Airway endoscopy in the diagnosis and treatment of bacterial tracheitis in children. *Int J Pediatr Otorhinolaryngol* 27:147, 1993.
56. Damm M, et al: Management of acute inflammatory childhood stridor. *Otolaryngol Head Neck Surg* 121:633, 1999.
57. Friedman EM, et al: Bacterial tracheitis—two year experience. *Laryngoscope* 95:9, 1985.
58. Bernstein T, Brilli R, Jacobs B: Is bacterial tracheitis changing? A 14-month experience in a pediatric intensive care unit. *Clin Infect Dis* 27:458, 1998.
59. Britto J, et al: Systemic complications associated with bacterial tracheitis. *Arch Dis Child* 74:2490, 1996.
60. Rimell FL, et al: Characteristics of objects that cause choking in children. *JAMA* 274:1763, 1995.
61. Lifschultz BD, Donoghue ER: Deaths due to foreign body aspiration in children: The continuing hazard of toy balloons. *J Forensic Sci* 41:247, 1996.
62. Guidelines 2000 for cardiopulmonary resuscitation and emergency cardiovascular care. Part 9: Pediatric basic life support. *Circulation* 102:I253, 2000.
63. Guidelines 2000 for cardiopulmonary resuscitation and emergency cardiovascular care. Part 10: Pediatric advanced life support. *Circulation* 102:I291, 2000.
64. Marr JK, Yamamoto LG: Gas flow rates through transtracheal ventilation catheters. *Am J Emerg Med* 22:264, 2004.

CHAPTER 167

Pediatric Respiratory Emergencies: Lower Airway Obstruction

Christine D. Darr

ASTHMA

PERSPECTIVE

Background

Asthma is a chronic inflammatory disorder of the airways. Airway inflammation increases the existing airway hyperresponsiveness to a variety of stimuli. In addition, the inflammation results in widespread but variable airflow obstruction, which is often reversible spontaneously or with treatment. This inflammation causes recurrent episodes of wheezing, breathlessness, chest tightness, and coughing in susceptible individuals.[1] This working definition of asthma, which was presented by the National Asthma Education Program Expert Panel in their 1997 report, has led to therapeutic strategies that focus on managing chronic inflammation by avoidance of precipitants and long-term anti-inflammatory medications. Aggressive use of bronchodilation medications and corticosteroids is recommended for acute bronchospasm.[1,2]

Epidemiology

Asthma is estimated to affect the lives of 4.8 million children younger than 18 years of age in the United States and 1.3 million children younger than 5 years[3]; 570,000 asthmatic children under the age of 15 visit the emergency department every year.[4] Asthma exacerbation is the most frequent pediatric diagnosis requiring hospital admission in the United States. Children younger than 5 years are admitted most frequently for asthma. Between 1980 and 1995, the incidence of asthma increased by more than 160% and asthma hospitalizations increased by 45% in children less than 4 years old. During the same time period, reported asthma increased approximately 74% in children 5 to 14 years old and asthma hospitalizations increased 13%.[5,6] In 2000, the prevalence rates for childhood asthma were 7.7% for African Americans, 5.3% for whites, and 4.2% for Hispanics. In 2000, African American children with asthma had exacerbations 44% more frequently than white asthmatic children.[7]

It has been shown that children living in impoverished urban areas are at greater risk for morbidity and mortality from asthma. Trending over the past two decades has revealed that African American children are two to three times more likely to experience significant impairment in daily activities than white children with asthma,[8,9] 2.9 times more likely to visit the emergency department, 3.8 times more likely to be hospitalized, and 4.6 times more likely to die.[7,9] In a study of 1528 inner-city children aged 4 to 9 years with asthma, the participants had limited asthma problem-solving skills, multiple adults managing their asthma, high levels of life stress, increased numbers of child behavior problems, and caretaker psychological symptoms.[10] Children whose caretakers had clinically significant mental health problems had twice the hospitalization rate of children whose caretakers did not have mental health problems.[11]

Data from 1987 until 1994 demonstrate that in the United States, hospitalization rates for asthma increased to 2.95 in 1000 in patients younger than 14 years old.[12] Approximately 10% of children with asthma have severe disease, and they account for 35% of the asthma hospitalizations and 77% of the hospital days in that group. Peak hospitalizations seem to occur in the fall. The annual health care cost of pediatric asthma approaches $2 billion in the United States.[4]

Between 1980 and 1998, the asthma death rate in children increased by an average of 3.4% per year. In 1998, the asthma mortality rate was 3.5 per 1,000,000 children. Children 11 to 17 years old had asthma death rates approximately twice the rate of younger children.[7]

PRINCIPLES OF DISEASE

Pathophysiology

Most of the symptoms of asthma result from airway obstruction and inflammation caused by airways that are hyperresponsive to stimuli. Two recent large studies following children with wheezing through adulthood suggest that there are three categories of pediatric patients who wheeze. It is thought that these three phenotypes have different pathophysiology.[13,14]

The first category, which is the most common phenotype, is the child who has intermittent symptoms in the presence of a viral respiratory infection. Despite the fact that these patients account for substantial morbidity and hospitalizations before the age of 5, their ultimate prognosis is very favorable. They are commonly asymptomatic between episodes and have low risk of long-term sequelae.[15] These have been categorized as "transient early or infant wheezers." The causes of wheezing in infancy are thought to be different than those later in childhood and in adulthood.[16] These children typically do not wheeze after the third year of life. Eighty percent of children who wheeze in the first year of life, 60% who wheeze during the second year, and

30% to 40% who wheeze during the third year of life fall into this category. The main risk factors are low levels of lung function before illness, maternal smoking during pregnancy, and a younger mother.[14] Initial lung function is affected by prematurity, development of bronchopulmonary dysplasia, and sequelae of mechanical ventilation. The second category of children are defined as those who continue to wheeze after 3 years of age. They initially present with a lower respiratory illness during the first 2 years of life. The most common etiologic infectious agent for these lower respiratory infections are respiratory syncytial virus (RSV).[14] Parainfluenza 3 and influenza A have been implicated as well.[17] These children are three to five times more likely to wheeze at 6 and 11 years of age; however, by age 13 most have an insignificant risk of wheezing. This group has lower levels of lung function at 6 and 11 years of age. At age 11, their lower levels of lung function completely reverse with a bronchodilator. These children are hypothesized to have airway tone that is more likely to develop airway obstruction with viral infection. The cause of this alteration in airway tone is not known.[14]

The third category consists of children with atopic disease who wheeze. The children in this group who had onset of wheezing prior to age 3 show the lowest level of lung function and the highest levels of immunoglobulin E (IgE) at ages 6 and 11. These are the children who are persistent wheezers and who most likely will continue to have symptoms into adulthood.[14] Viral infections, atopy or family history of atopy, and perinatal exposure to smoke are factors associated with persistence of asthma throughout childhood. Atopy, the genetic susceptibility to produce IgE in response to exposure to environmental allergens, is one of the strongest predisposing factors in the development of asthma.[10] Several studies suggest that higher levels of serum IgE predispose to an increase in bronchial hyperresponsiveness; however, the clinical expression of this bronchial hyperresponsiveness in the form of asthma in part depends on environmental exposure to allergens. An early exposure to house dust mite antigen may increase sensitization and increase clinical reactivity to these allergens, resulting in later asthma.[20]

The pathophysiology of atopy as it relates to asthma is critical to the understanding of the disease and its management. In atopic patients with asthma, the allergen binds to IgE to stimulate the mast cell. This triggers a release of numerous mediators, such as histamine, eosinophil and neutrophil chemotactic factors, leukotrienes, cytokines, prostaglandins, and platelet-activating factor from lung mast cells. These mediators produce a variety of "early phase reactions," the most prominent being smooth muscle constriction. Histamine has been shown to create mucosal edema and mucus secretion as well. Leukotrienes have significant effects on bronchoconstriction, mucociliary function, microvascular permeability, and airway edema. Platelet-activating factor helps induce immediate bronchoconstriction and airway hyperreactivity, airway edema, and cellular inflammatory response. Within hours, macrophages, eosinophils, and neutrophils enter the airways, resulting in the secretion of additional chemotactic and vasoconstrictive products. This leads to a further increase in bronchial hyperresponsiveness and a breakdown of respiratory epithelium, partially mediated by thromboxane A_2. This late asthmatic phase occurs 4 to 12 hours after the initial insult and is now thought to be better treated with anti-inflammatory medications, rather than β-agonists alone.

Subpopulations of T lymphocytes (Th2) have been identified as cells that may regulate allergic inflammation in the airway through the release of selective cytokines and also establish disease chronicity.[4,21] In children who develop atopic asthma, Th2 cell immunity is not converted to Th1 immunity. The fetal Th2 persists and is thought to contribute to the susceptibility of allergic airway inflammation. Postnatal upregulation of Th1 is triggered by microbial stimulation. In fact, studies have shown that infants of large families,[22] those with early daycare exposure,[23] and those with early exposure to farm animals and cats and dogs[24] are less likely to develop atopic asthma. Environmental exposure to microbial antigens is thought to stimulate Th1 cells or suppress Th2, or both. This leads to immune tolerance and helps to prevent allergic disease in children.[25]

Fibroblasts, endothelial cells, and epithelial cells also contribute to the allergic airway inflammation process by releasing cytokines and chemokines. These factors are thought to be important in initiating and maintaining the level of airway inflammation.[4] The airway inflammation is composed of microvascular leakage of proteins into the subepithelial space, leading to edema and airway narrowing and exacerbating airway hyperresponsiveness. It occurs in allergic and nonallergic forms of asthma. Airway inflammation is hypothesized to be acute, subacute, and chronic. Chronic airway inflammation is characterized by a persistent level of cell damage and cell repair. The process leading to airway inflammation, airway hyperresponsiveness, and airflow limitation is multicellular, redundant, and amplifying.[4] This has major implications for treatment of asthma.

Factors Associated with Asthma

The development of asthma in an individual is complex and multifactorial, dependent on genetics, viral infection, and exposure to environmental precipitants. Asthma frequently begins during childhood. A total of 50% to 80% of children with asthma present with their first episode of symptoms before 5 years of age. Approximately 25% of children wheeze before 3 years of age, but only a minority develop asthma. Factors associated with the onset of asthma symptoms are atopy, family history of asthma or allergy, in utero and perinatal exposure to smoking, viral respiratory infections, smaller airways in early life, male gender, and low birth weight.[4] Infectious, allergic, and other physical stimuli (Box 167-1) can trigger the cascade of events leading to an asthma exacerbation in suscepti-

BOX 167-1. Precipitants of Asthma Exacerbations in Children

- Infection (usually viral)
- Environmental allergens
  - Passive smoking (cigarette, marijuana)
  - House dust mites
  - Pollens
  - Grasses
  - Molds/fungi
  - Pets
  - Cockroaches
- Exercise
- Cold air
- Stress/strong emotion
- Untreated aggravating conditions (rhinitis, sinusitis, gastroesophageal reflux)

BOX 167-2. History to be Collected in a Patient with Asthma

1. Duration and severity of exacerbation
2. Associated symptoms and fluid intake
3. Previous attacks, their frequency, severity, and response to specific therapies
4. Previous hospitalizations or intensive care unit admissions, history of intubations
5. Usual precipitants of exacerbations
6. Use of steroids in past year or any recent change in steroid dosage
7. Current medications (type, amount, and time of last dose)
8. Other underlying cardiopulmonary illnesses (e.g., congenital heart disease, bronchopulmonary dysplasia, gastroesophageal reflux, aspiration, recurrent pneumonias)
9. Other atopic illnesses
10. Previous adverse drug reactions

ble individuals. Viral upper respiratory infections cause 85% of childhood asthma exacerbations. RSV is the most common viral etiologic agent in children less than 2 years old, whereas rhinovirus is more common in older children and adults.[17]

CLINICAL FEATURES

Patient History

Parents or patients may report cough, wheezing, and dyspnea, which are the hallmark symptoms of reactive airway disease. Some children have only prolonged cough and no wheezing, although they may wheeze if challenged with exercise. Others have a history of frequent pneumonias or "bronchitis." Most children have a history of wheezing. History should include frequency of symptoms, triggers of symptoms (exercise, smoke, viral infection, cold air), severity of symptoms (hospitalization and intensive care unit care), and use of medications including steroids. History of conditions that complicate asthma such as sinusitis, gastroesophageal reflux, allergic bronchopulmonary aspergillosis, pregnancy, and sleep disorders should also be obtained (Box 167-2).

Physical Examination

The National Institute of Health guidelines for the treatment of asthma has divided acute exacerbations into mild, moderate, and severe, based on presenting signs and symptoms and limited diagnostic studies. This division is important in that recognition of the asthmatic child's degree of respiratory distress is key to determining treatment and preventing progression of respiratory failure (Table 167-1).

The physical signs important in determining the degree of respiratory distress are respiratory rate, heart rate, use of accessory muscles, presence of nasal flaring, quality of air entry, presence of wheezing, length of inspiratory and expiratory phase, pulsus paradoxus, diminished level of consciousness, and presence of cyanosis. Infants and young children become dehydrated more quickly than adults; hydration status should also be assessed. As infants become more ill with respiratory distress, they may become less responsive toward their parents, stop feeding, have chest retractions when moderate airway obstruction develops, and cry weakly. Cyanosis is a sign of severe asthma and portends respiratory arrest.

Of the physical signs used to evaluate the degree of respiratory distress, use of accessory muscles correlates best with the degree of obstruction (forced expiratory volume in 1 second [FEV_1] or peak expiratory flow rate [PEFR]) and oxygen saturation (SaO_2).[26] The accessory use of the sternocleidomastoid muscles correlates with a PEFR or FEV_1 less than 50%. Vital signs vary with age and the activity level of the child (see Table 167-1). Tachycardia occurs with respiratory distress. The alertness or level of consciousness can be assessed by observing the patient's interaction with parents and familiar objects. Agitation and irritability may signal hypoxia. Lethargy, somnolence, and fatigue are seen with hypercarbia and may signal the beginning of respiratory failure, defined as a PaO_2 less than 50 mm Hg and a $PaCO_2$ greater than 50 mm Hg. Dyspnea can be assessed by asking the patient to count to 10 or to speak a sentence. Assessment of degree of shortness of breath by parents or the patient can be helpful. Pulsus paradoxus is the measure of difference in systolic blood pressure during inspiration and expiration. A pulsus paradoxus greater than 20 mm Hg is associated with moderate to severe obstruction. In children with rapid respiratory rates, the phase of respiration is difficult to correlate with the systolic pressure. Wheezing is one of the most unreliable signs in evaluating the degree of distress. Its absence may represent severe obstruction and with improvement, wheezing may become more prominent. Cyanosis is usually a late sign. Bradypnea is ominous.

Infants may be at higher risk of respiratory failure because of increased peripheral airway resistance, deficient collateral channels of ventilation, the unique character of their airway smooth muscle, decreased

Table 167-1. Classifying Severity of Asthma Exacerbations

	Mild	Moderate	Severe	Respiratory arrest imminent
Symptoms				
Breathlessness	While walking	While talking (infant: softer shorter cry; difficulty feeding)	While at rest (infant: stops feeding)	
	Can lie down	Prefers sitting	Sits upright	
Talks in . . .	Sentences	Phrases	Words	
Alertness	May be agitated	Usually agitated	Usually agitated	Drowsy or confused
Signs				
Respiratory rate	Increased	Increased	Often >30/minute	
	Guide to rates of breathing in awake children			
	Age		Normal rate	
	<2 months		<60/minute	
	2-12 months		<50/minute	
	1-5 years		<40/minute	
	6-8 years		<30/minute	
Use of accessory muscles; suprasternal retractions	Usually not	Commonly	Usually	Paradoxical thoracoabdominal movement
Wheeze	Moderate, often only end-expiratory	Loud: throughout exhalation	Usually loud: throughout inhalation and exhalation	Absence of wheeze
Pulse/minute	<100	100-120	>120	Bradycardia
	Guide to normal pulse rates in children			
	Age		Normal rate	
	2-12 months		<160/minute	
	1-2 years		<120/minute	
	2-8 years		<110/minute	
Pulsus paradoxus	Absent <10 mm Hg	May be present 10-25 mm Hg	Often present >25 mm Hg (adult) 20-40 mm Hg (child)	Absence suggests respiratory muscle fatigue
Functional assessment				
PEF % predicted or % personal best	>80%	Approximately 50-80% or response lasts <2 hrs	<50% predicted or personal best	
PaO_2 (on air) and/or	Normal (test not usually necessary)	>60 mm Hg (test not usually necessary)	<60 mm Hg: possible cyanosis	
PCO_2	<42 mm Hg (test not usually necessary)	<42 mm Hg (test not usually necessary)	≥42 mm Hg: possible respiratory failure (see text)	
SaO_2 (on air) at sea level	>95% (test not usually necessary)	91-95%	<91%	
	Hypercapnia (hypoventilation) develops more readily in young children than in adults and adolescents.			

Note:
- The presence of several parameters, but not necessarily all, indicates the general classification of the exacerbation.
- Many of these parameters have not been systematically studied, so they serve only as general guides.

Modified from the National Asthma Education Program Expert Panel Report 2: *Guidelines for the Diagnosis and Management of Asthma*. National Institutes of Health Publication 97-4051. Bethesda. Md. NIH, 1997.

airway elastic recoil, and a reliance on diaphragmatic movement for respiration. Close monitoring is vital.

In all infants and children, serial examinations are imperative in monitoring the effect of treatment.

Complications

In 1998, the asthma mortality incidence was 3.8 per 1,000,000 children in the United States younger than 15 years of age.[7] Death occurs as a result of one of two situations. The first situation, which is extremely rare, is sudden unexpected deterioration. The second situation, which is much more common, is delayed presentation associated with inadequate use of steroids. Risk factors for asthma fatality (Box 167-3) are a history of previous life-threatening exacerbation, age (trend of increasing death in the 5- to 34-year age group), African American race (4:1), hospital admission in the previous year, poor access to medical care, inadequate medical care, psychological problems, and family dysfunction. Patients with more than two hospitalizations for asthma despite long-term oral steroid therapy are at highest risk of death. Patients who over-rely on frequent repetitive inhaled β_2-agonists at home may temporarily relieve symptoms but mask continued airway inflammation and hyperresponsiveness. This may result in sudden, severe deterioration. Depression has a high correlation with fatality in asthma, especially in children. Children with asthma whose severity is underestimated and thus inadequately treated are at risk of respiratory failure and death.

Status asthmaticus is present in the patient with moderate to severe respiratory distress who does not respond to repeated initial β-agonist nebulizations. In this situation, complications such as mucus plugging, atelectasis, and segmental collapse must be considered.

BOX 167-3. Risk Factors for Death from Asthma

- Past history of sudden severe exacerbations
- Prior intubation for asthma
- Prior admission for asthma to an intensive care unit
- Two or more hospitalizations for asthma in the past year
- Three or more emergency care visits for asthma in the past year
- Hospitalization or an emergency care visit for asthma within the past month
- Use of more than two canisters per month of inhaled short-acting β_2-agonist
- Current use of systemic corticosteroids or recent withdrawal from systemic corticosteroids
- Difficulty perceiving airflow obstruction or its severity
- Comorbidity, as from cardiovascular diseases or chronic obstructive pulmonary disease
- Serious psychiatric disease or psychosocial problems
- Low socioeconomic status and urban residence
- Illicit drug use
- Sensitivity to *Alternaria*

Modified from the National Asthma Education Program Expert Panel Report 2: *Guidelines for the Diagnosis and Management of Asthma*. National Institutes of Health Publication 97-4051. Bethesda, Md. NIH; 1997.

These children may be tachypneic but have little or no wheezing. These complications may also be a reason for sudden worsening of symptoms in an asthmatic child, but the condition improves with increased use of bronchodilators and chest physiotherapy. Pneumothorax is a rare complication. Pneumomediastinum is rare as well and usually does not require treatment but does require admission and observation. Inappropriate secretion of antidiuretic hormone can be seen on rare occasions with severe hypoxemia. Seizures may accompany severe hypoxemia, underlying central nervous system disease, and theophylline toxicity. Protracted vomiting can occur from the asthma itself or theophylline toxicity. Cardiac dysrhythmias are very uncommon in children but can be seen with severe theophylline toxicity, usually resulting from β_2-agonists.

DIAGNOSTIC STRATEGIES

The most important function of laboratory data is the detection of actual or impending respiratory failure. Laboratory data can also be used to detect complicating conditions.[1]

In children more than 5 years old, pulmonary function tests should be used to evaluate and monitor the response to asthma therapy. The children must be cooperative and consistent in their respiratory maneuvers to obtain an accurate FEV_1 or PEFR. The FEV_1 is measured with a spirometer and is the volume of air expired in 1 second from maximum inspiration. The PEFR is measured using a peak flow meter. The PEFR is the maximum flow rate that can be generated during a forced expiratory maneuver and requires maximum effort for accuracy. The FEV_1 and PEFR values are then compared with tables of standard values based on height, sex, and race or with the patient's personal best obtained when well. A moderate exacerbation has been correlated with a PEFR of 50% to 80% predicted or personal best and a severe exacerbation correlates with a PEFR of less than 50% predicted or personal best. Peak flow by age can be estimated by the following formula: $(30 \times \text{age in years}) + 30$. However, charts based on height are the most accurate (Figure 167-1).

Figure 167-1. TruZone and peak expiratory flow figures commercially recommended by the distributor. (From *Int Pediatr* 16:89, 2001.)

PEAK EXPIRATORY FLOW AT SEA LEVEL

Children and teenagers 6 to 25 years old: male

Height in.		44	48	52	56	60	64	68	72	76
Height cm.		112	122	132	142	152	163	173	183	193
Age	6	99	146	194	241	289	336	384	431	479
	8	119	166	214	261	309	356	404	451	499
	10	139	186	234	281	329	376	424	471	519
	12	159	206	254	301	349	396	444	491	539
	14	178	226	274	321	369	416	464	511	559
	16	198	246	293	341	389	436	484	531	579
	18	218	266	313	361	408	456	503	551	599
	20	238	286	333	381	428	476	523	571	618
	22	258	306	353	401	448	496	543	591	638
	24	278	326	373	421	468	516	563	611	658
	25	288	336	383	431	478	526	573	621	668

Children and teenagers 6 to 20 years old: female

Height in.		42	46	50	54	57	60	64	68	72
Height cm.		107	117	127	137	145	152	163	173	183
Age	6	134	164	193	223	245	268	297	327	357
	8	153	182	212	242	264	287	316	346	376
	10	171	201	231	261	283	305	335	365	395
	12	190	220	280	280	302	324	354	384	414
	14	209	239	269	298	321	343	373	403	432
	16	228	258	288	317	340	362	392	421	451
	18	247	277	306	336	358	381	411	440	470
	20	266	295	325	355	377	400	429	459	

Transcutaneous pulse oximetry is a reliable method for measuring oxygen saturation that should be performed on all asthmatic patients presenting to the emergency department with respiratory complaints. Hypoxia occurs as a result of ventilation/perfusion mismatches in the lungs. The ventilation/perfusion characteristic of the infant lung can lead to hypoxemia much more quickly than in the older child or adult.[1] An oxygen saturation less than 91% (sea level) correlates with a need for hospitalization.[25] Pulse oximetry has replaced assessment of arterial blood gases in patients in whom ventilation is considered adequate. Measurement of arterial blood gas values are indicated in patients with moderate to severe respiratory distress who are not responding to therapy, that is, patients with a PEFR or FEV_1 less than 50% predicted. Patients with a rising $PaCO_2$ or one with a PCO_2 that is greater than 40 mm Hg require aggressive monitoring and therapy and may rarely require invasive airway management. Chest x-ray studies are not routinely indicated in the known asthmatic patient. They are indicated in the child with fever not responding to treatment, worsening respiratory symptoms, or poor response to therapy. They are often obtained in children presenting with their first episode of wheezing, particularly if there is suspicion of foreign body aspiration, pneumonia, or pneumothorax. The chest x-ray study often demonstrates hyperinflation, peribronchial thickening, and sometimes atelectasis or infiltrate. It can be difficult to differentiate between atelectasis and infiltrate; however, atelectasis is associated with loss of lung volume (Figure 167-2). A complete blood cell count, optimally obtained before β-adrenergic therapy, is not routinely recommended but can be obtained as part of the evaluation of the febrile patient. Theophylline levels should be checked if the patient is taking chronic theophylline. Therapeutic levels are 5 to 15 μg/mL, with toxic levels being greater than 20 μg/mL. Children who are on prolonged, frequent β-agonist therapy should have their serum potassium levels checked. Patients with severe asthma should have electrolytes measured to exclude syndrome of inappropriate secretion of antidiuretic hormone.

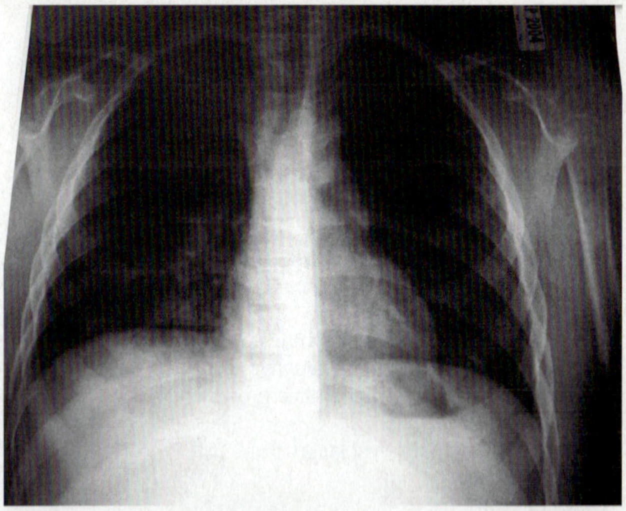

A

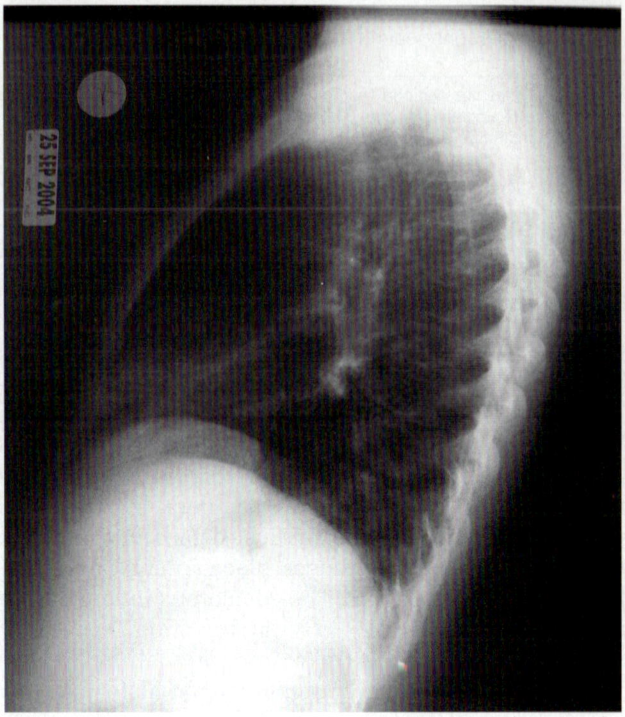

B

Figure 167-2. Posteroanterior (A) and lateral (B) chest radiographs revealing right middle lobe atelectasis. (Courtesy of Marianne Gausche-Hill, MD.)

DIFFERENTIAL CONSIDERATIONS

Recurrent episodes of cough with wheezing are usually a result of asthma; other entities must be considered in the differential diagnosis (Box 167-4). Some of these entities will be suggested by concomitant findings on history and physical examination, such as heart murmur, failure to thrive, recurrent emesis, or diarrhea. These should be pursued in wheezing children who have unusual or persistent symptoms or other associated atypical findings. Vocal cord dysfunction, hydrocarbon ingestion, toxic gas inhalation, hyperventilation syndrome, habit cough, ciliary dyskinesia, and antitrypsin deficiency can also mimic asthma. A more common problem is the underdiagnosis of asthma, especially in infants who wheeze only when they have respiratory infections.

MANAGEMENT

Prehospital

The asthmatic patient in mild distress usually requires oxygen during transport. The child in moderate or severe distress should receive a β-agonist nebulization at the scene or en route. This may be given continuously in children with respiratory distress. Intravenous access should be established in the asthmatic patient in severe distress. Epinephrine is reserved for patients in impending respiratory failure or those with possible anaphylaxis.

BOX 167-4. Differential Diagnostic Possibilities for Asthma

Upper airway diseases
- Allergic rhinitis and sinusitis

Obstructions involving large airways
- Foreign body in trachea or bronchus
- Vocal cord dysfunction
- Vascular rings or laryngeal webs
- Laryngotracheomalacia, tracheal stenosis, or bronchostenosis
- Enlarged lymph nodes or tumor

Obstructions involving small airways
- Viral bronchiolitis or obliterative bronchiolitis
- Cystic fibrosis
- Bronchopulmonary dysplasia
- Heart disease

Other causes
- Recurrent cough not due to asthma
- Aspiration from swallowing mechanism dysfunction or gastroesophageal reflux

Modified from the National Asthma Education Program Expert Panel Report 2: *Guidelines for the Diagnosis and Management of Asthma*. National Institutes of Health Publication 97-4051. Bethesda, Md. NIH, 1997.

Emergency Department

The patient or parents are usually the best indicators of the severity of an asthma exacerbation and the treatment modalities that have succeeded in the past. The lungs of infants have greater peripheral airway resistance, fewer collateral channels of ventilation, more airway smooth muscle in the peripheral airways, less elastic recoil, and the mechanical disadvantage of the diaphragm. These differences place infants at greater risk of respiratory failure. The edematous inflammatory response of the airway to viral infection, especially RSV, can lead quickly to respiratory failure.[1] Close monitoring is essential. Patients with a history of risk factors for mortality (see Box 167-3) require particularly aggressive treatment. Initial assessment of all patients with respiratory distress should include the pediatric assessment triangle (appearance, work of breathing [retractions and use of accessory muscles of ventilation], and circulation to the skin) (see Figure 167-1) and the ABCDEs (Airway, Breathing, Circulation, Disability, and Exposure). Vital signs, pulse oximetry, and auscultation of the chest should follow. In children more than 5 years old, an FEV_1 or PEFR should be obtained on presentation. Oxygen should be administered to all patients with significant wheezing or respiratory distress. In infants and children, it is given by nasal cannula or face mask. It can be titrated to achieve a pulse oximetry greater than 94% (at sea level). Patients with moderate to severe respiratory distress receiving frequent nebulizers or theophylline should be placed on a cardiac monitor.

Infants and young children become dehydrated more quickly as a result of increased respiratory rate and decreased oral intake. Their fluid status should be assessed and treated appropriately.

β-Adrenergic Agonists

β_2-Agonists given by inhalation are the initial treatment of choice for acute exacerbations of asthma and are recommended for all patients. β_2-Agonists act on β_2-adrenergic receptors to relax smooth muscle and decrease mediator release from mast cells and eosinophils. Albuterol (Proventil, Ventolin 0.5% solution, 5 mg/mL) is the most commonly used β_2-agonist. Others are terbutaline, pirbuterol, and bitolterol (Table 167-2). Three doses of nebulized β_2-agonist should usually be administered during the first 45 to 90 minutes in the emergency department (Figure 167-3).[28] The patient in severe distress can be given albuterol nebulizations every 15 to 20 minutes or continuously. Nebulized inhalation is generally more effective than parenteral or oral therapy. The nebulizer treatments usually are delivered using 6 to 8 L/min flow in a total volume of 3 to 4 mL over 15 minutes. The β-agonist onset of action is within a few minutes, and its duration of action is 3 to 6 hours. Repeated dosing produces incremental bronchodilation.[28] High-dose administration of nebulized albuterol, 0.15 mg/kg with a maximum of 5 mg (1.0 mL), has been shown to be more effective than low dose, 0.05 mg/kg with a maximum of 2.5 mg (0.5 mL), in the treatment of acute moderate and severe asthma.[29] The high-dose administration, however, is not recommended for home use. Continuous β_2-agonist nebulization may be more effective in children.[30] The dose of continuous albuterol is 0.15 mg/kg/hr by nebulization with a maximum dose of 20 mg/hr.

Levalbuterol, R-albuterol (Xopenex), is a bronchodilator that contains R and S isomers of albuterol. The R-albuterol is responsible for the bronchodilator effect. The S-albuterol provides no benefit and may be responsible for the albuterol side effects. Several pediatric studies have supported the use of levalbuterol over racemic albuterol.[31-33] The study by Gawchik and associates[32] found an increase in FEV_1 comparable to or greater than that achieved with racemic albuterol. The study by Milgrom and associates[33] demonstrated a more favorable safety profile with fewer side effects. Two additional pediatric studies do not support these findings.[34,35] Overall, a review of levalbuterol for the treatment of asthma in children found no clinically significant advantage over racemic albuterol.[36]

A Cochrane library review suggests metered dose inhalers (MDIs) with spacers and nebulizers achieve equally effective delivery of β-agonists in mild and moderate asthma exacerbations[37] and have comparable rates of improvement.[38,39] The nebulizer, however, does not require consistently good inhalation, as the MDI with spacer does. This may be difficult to ensure in a busy emergency department, even though children as young as 2 to 3 years old with stable asthma have been shown to have effective bronchodilation with MDIs and spacers. During an acute exacerbation, a nebulizer with face mask should be used to deliver inhalation therapy

Table 167-2. Dosages of Drugs for Asthma Exacerbations in Emergency Medical Care or Hospital

Medications	Dosages: Adult Dose	Dosages: Child Dose	Comments
Inhaled Short-Acting β_2-Agonists			
Albuterol			
Nebulizer solution (5 mg/mL)	2.5-5 mg every 20 minutes for three doses, then 2.5-10 mg every 1-4 hours as needed, or 10-15 mg/hour continuously	0.15 mg/kg (minimum dose 2.5 mg) every 20 minutes for three doses, 0.15-0.3 mg/kg up to 10 mg every 1-4 hours as needed, or 0.5 mg/kg/hour by continuous nebulization (maximum 15 mg/hr)	Only selective β_2-agonists are recommended. For optimal delivery, dilute aerosols to minimum of 4 mL at gas flow of 6-8 L/min
MDI (90 mcg/puff)	Four to eight puffs every 20 minutes up to 4 hours, then every 1-4 hours as needed	Four to eight puffs every 20 minutes for three doses, then every 1-4 hours inhalation maneuver; use spacer/holding chamber	As effective as nebulized therapy if patient is able to coordinate
Bitolterol			
Nebulizer solution (2 mg/mL)	See albuterol dose	See albuterol dose; thought to be half as potent as albuterol on mg basis	Has not been studied in severe asthma exacerbations. Do not mix with other drugs
MDI (370 mcg/puff)	See albuterol dose	See albuterol dose	Has not been studied in severe asthma exacerbations
Pirbuterol			
MDI (200 mcg/puff)	See albuterol dose	See albuterol dose; thought to be half as potent as albuterol on mg basis	Has not been studied in severe asthma exacerbations
Systemic (Injected) β_2-Agonists			
Epinephrine 1:1000 (1 mg/mL)	0.3-0.5 mg every 20 minutes for 3 doses SQ	0.01 mg/kg up to 0.3-0.5 mg every 20 minutes for 3 doses SQ	No proven advantage of systemic therapy over aerosol
Terbutaline (1 mg/mL)	0.25 mg every 20 minutes for three doses SQ	0.01 mg/kg every 20 minutes for three doses, then every 2 to 6 hours as needed SQ	No proven advantage of systemic therapy over aerosol
Anticholinergics			
Ipratropium bromide			
Nebulizer solution (0.25 mg/mL)	0.5 mg every 30 minutes for three doses then every 2-4 hours as needed.	0.25 mg every 20 minutes for three doses, then every 2 to 4 hours	May mix in same nebulizer with albuterol. Should not be used as first-line therapy; should be added to β_2-agonist therapy
MDI (18 mcg/puff)	Four to eight puffs as needed	Four to eight puffs as needed	Dose delivered from MDI is low and has not been studied in asthma exacerbations
Corticosteroids			
Prednisone Methylprednisolone Prednisolone	120-180 mg/day in three or four divided doses for 48 hours, then 60-80 mg/day until PEF reaches 70% of predicted or personal best	1 mg/kg every 6 hours for 48 hours then 1-2 mg/kg/day (maximum = 60 mg/day) in two divided doses until PEF 70% of predicted or personal best	For outpatient "burst" use 40-60 mg in single or two divided doses for adults (children: 1-2 mg/kg/day, maximum 60 mg/day) for 3-10 days

Note: No advantage has been found for higher dose corticosteroids in severe asthma exacerbations, nor is there any advantage for intravenous administration over oral therapy provided gastrointestinal transit time or absorption is not impaired. The usual regimen is to continue the frequent multiple daily dosing until the patient achieves an FEV_1 or PEF of 50% of predicted or personal best and then lower the dose to twice daily. This usually occurs within 48 hours. Therapy following a hospitalization or emergency department visit may last from 3 to 10 days. If patients are then started on inhaled corticosteroids, studies indicate there is no need to taper the systemic corticosteroid dose. If the follow-up systemic corticosteroid therapy is to be given once daily, one study* indicates that it may be more clinically effective to give the dose in the afternoon at 3 PM, with no increase in adrenal suppression.

*Data from Beam WR, Weiner DE, Martin RJ: Timing of prednisone and alterations of airways inflammation in nocturnal asthma. *Am Rev Respir Dis* 146:1524, 1992.

MDI, metered dose inhaler; PEF, peak expiratory flow.

Modified from the National Asthma Education Program Expert Panel Report 2: *Guidelines for the Diagnosis and Management of Asthma*. National Institutes of Health Publication 97-4051, Bethesda, Md, NIH, 1997.

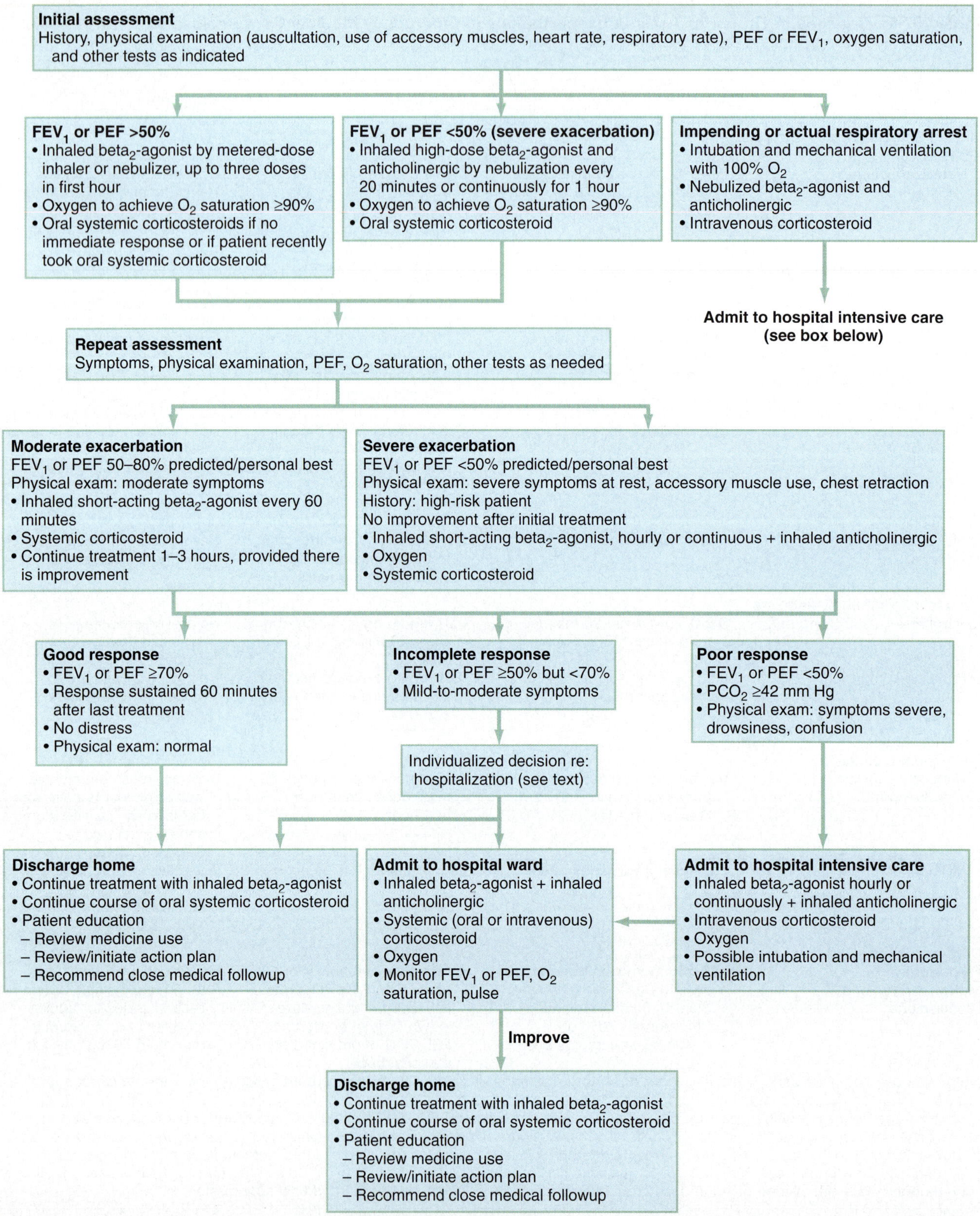

Figure 167-3. Management of asthma exacerbations: emergency department and hospital-based care. FEV_1, forced expiratory volume in 1 second; PEF, peak expiratory flow. (Modified from the National Asthma Education Program Expert Panel Report 2: *Guidelines for the Diagnosis and Management of Asthma*. National Institutes of Health Publication 97-4051. Bethesda, MD, NIH, 1997.)

in children less than 3 years old. For children 3 years old and older, a nebulizer with face mask or mouthpiece or an MDI with spacer can be used. Blow-by nebulization delivers medication poorly and is not recommended at any time.

Treatment of asthma-related respiratory arrest with endotracheal administration of albuterol can be effective. Endotracheal delivery of albuterol is given as 0.5 mL diluted in 2.5 mL of saline and is followed by five insufflations with a mechanical ventilation device.

Clinically significant tolerance to β_2-agonist nebulizers does not typically occur, and its use at home should not preclude use in the emergency department.

Terbutaline (Brethine 0.1% solution, 1 mg/mL) has been used as an inhalation agent but is more commonly given subcutaneously as an adjunct to albuterol nebulizers in the severe asthmatic patient who has little or no air movement, or if nebulizers are not readily available. Its peak onset occurs in 30 minutes, and duration of action is 3 to 4 hours. In severe exacerbations unresponsive to treatment, terbutaline can also be given as a parenteral drip, although its usefulness is debated. The dose of a terbutaline drip is a 10 μg/kg bolus over 10 minutes, followed by a 0.5 μg/kg/min infusion. Every 30 minutes, the infusion can be increased 0.3 to 0.5 μg/kg/min as needed to a maximum of 5 μg/kg/min. Risks of intravenous terbutaline include muscle tremors, dysrhythmias, hypertension, and myocardial ischemia.[40]

Epinephrine (1:1000) can also be used subcutaneously if a parenteral form is needed. Its efficacy is less than that of inhaled agents, and it has significant β_1-agonist side effects. Intramuscular epinephrine is reserved for patients with possible anaphylaxis or those presenting with signs of cardiopulmonary failure. Sus-Phrine, a derivative of epinephrine, has a longer duration of action but is inconsistently administered unless the patient is large enough to tolerate an entire ampule.

Oral agents are sometimes used in chronic asthma management but have no role in the management of acute exacerbations.

Anticholinergics

Anticholinergics block the muscarinic receptors of airway smooth muscle, inhibiting vagal tone and thereby causing bronchodilation. They are less effective than the β-agonists and thus should always be used in conjunction with β-agonists but have a place in the management of acute asthma. Ipratropium bromide (Atrovent), a derivative of atropine, is not absorbed well systemically; dry mouth, blurred vision, tachycardia, and urinary retention, which are side effects of atropine, are not seen with its administration. Ipratropium has been shown to be effective during acute exacerbations when used together with adrenergic nebulizer agents. Some studies have shown that adding high doses of ipratropium bromide (0.5 mg in children) to an albuterol nebulization causes additional bronchodilation and improvements in FEV_1, especially in patients with moderate or severe exacerbations.[41-43] In several studies, combined β_2-agonist and anticholinergic therapy reduced the risk of hospitalization by 25% in moderate and severe exacerbations.[44] In another study, pediatric patients with moderate or severe exacerbations, treated with albuterol and ipratropium nebulizer therapy every 20 minutes during the first hour in the emergency department, had shorter emergency department stays and required fewer total nebulizer treatments prior to discharge.[45] The ipratropium can be added to the β-agonist nebulizer and given every 20 minutes for three doses and then every 2 to 4 hours.

Corticosteroids

Corticosteroids are the most effective anti-inflammatory agents in the treatment of asthma. Steroids are thought to interfere with the production of arachidonic acid metabolites, thereby preventing the formation of prostaglandins and leukotrienes, which are bronchoconstrictors and chemotactic agents. Steroids also prevent the migration and activation of inflammatory cells, especially eosinophils and neutrophils, which are involved in the late asthmatic response. They also stabilize vessel walls and decrease mucosal edema. In addition, steroids increase the number of β-adrenergic receptors on bronchial smooth muscles, increasing patient responsiveness to β-agonists.

The use of oral or parenteral steroids is indicated in patients who have moderate to severe exacerbations such as in patients who do not respond well after initial bronchodilator therapy (PEFR remains <80% or patient continues to wheeze), those who are currently on or who have recently discontinued steroids, those who have a high risk of asthma death (see Box 167-2), those with a long history of symptoms before presentation, children with asthma exacerbation resulting from viral illness, and those who require hospitalization.[4]

Several studies have demonstrated equal efficacy of oral and parenteral administration of steroids.[46] Patients who are unable to drink, are vomiting, are in severe respiratory distress, are obtunded, or are intubated should be given parenteral therapy. The dosage of prednisone, methylprednisolone, and prednisolone in children is 1 mg/kg every 6 hours for the first 48 hours (maximum 60 mg/day) and then 1 to 2 mg/kg/24 hr twice a day until the peak expiratory flow is 70% of predicted or personal best (see Table 167-2).[4] The onset of action begins at 3 hours and peaks in 6 to 12 hours. Two recent studies have demonstrated no difference in efficacy between oral or intramuscular dexamethasone and prednisone in the treatment of outpatient asthma exacerbations in children. The dose of oral dexamethasone used was 0.6 mg/kg (maximum 16 mg) given once in the emergency department and repeated once in 24 hours.[47,48]

The use of steroids in the treatment of an acute moderate or severe exacerbation has been shown to decrease the number and duration of hospitalizations, the need for additional intervention, the period of hypoxia, the morbidity rate, and the number of returns to the emergency department.[49] The major adverse effects of short-term systemic steroid therapy include reversible increased appetite, fluid retention, changes in glucose metabolism, mood changes, hypertension, peptic ulcer, and aseptic necrosis of the femur. Children treated with more than four short bursts of steroids per year show prolonged adrenal suppression and thus should receive a burst of steroids for stresses such as surgery.[50]

Recently, several studies have suggested that the early use of inhaled corticosteroids in the emergency department may reduce hospitalizations and improve pulmonary function.[51] Another study, however, suggests that inhaled corticosteroids are not a replacement for systemic corticosteroid treatment in patients with acute asthma but are an adjunctive treatment.[52,53]

Magnesium Sulfate

Magnesium sulfate has been used in the treatment of severe asthma exacerbations with some success. Several reviews, which included pediatric and adult studies, concluded that the early use of magnesium sulfate in the treatment of severe asthma exacerbations is safe and can result in a higher percentage of improvement in PEFR, FEV_1, and forced vital capacity, as well as a decreased hospitalization rate.[54-56] Loading doses range from 25 to 100 mg/kg with a maximum of 2 g given over 20 minutes.[54] Nausea, vomiting, tachycardia, and facial flushing can occur. More serious side effects such as cardiac arrest and respiratory insufficiency can occur with serum magnesium levels greater than 10 mg/dL.[57] Magnesium sulfate can be included in the treatment of the severe asthma exacerbation, but should not delay intubation if it is needed.

Other Agents

The routine addition of theophylline to β-agonist and steroid therapy in the emergency department management of asthma has not been shown to be of any benefit.[58] These studies do not include children in impending respiratory failure. Its use is recommended only for patients unresponsive to other controller medications or who are on chronic theophylline therapy. In these patients, a theophylline level should be drawn to exclude toxicity. Antibiotics are generally not recommended for asthma unless the patient has evidence of pneumonia or bacterial sinusitis on physical examination or by diagnostic studies. Although viral respiratory infections are often associated with asthma exacerbations, bacterial, chlamydial, and mycoplasma respiratory infections infrequently contribute to exacerbations.[1,59]

Chest physical therapy and mucolytics are not indicated for the treatment of asthma. Sedation is contraindicated in ill asthma patients because of the respiratory depressant effect.[1]

Heliox, a mixture of helium and oxygen, can be used in a 70:30 ratio at 10 L/min to aerosolize albuterol via a nebulizer. Two studies suggest it to be beneficial.[61,62] More studies are required to evaluate its place in the treatment of asthma exacerbations. It cannot be used in patients requiring more than 30% oxygen.

Medications Used to Manage Chronic Asthma (Table 167-3)

Cromolyn (Intal) is an anti-inflammatory agent that inhibits the early asthmatic response by stabilizing mast cells and decreases the migration of eosinophils during the late phase of allergic asthma. It is used in the chronic management of asthma, often in conjunction with β-agonists.[1] It has been shown to be less effective than inhaled corticosteroids in the chronic management of asthma.[59]

Salmeterol (Serevent) is a long-acting β_2-agonist used in the chronic management of asthma. It should not be used for an acute exacerbation because of a delayed onset of action and long duration of action. The leukotriene modifiers, zafirlukast and zileuton, improve lung function and decrease asthma symptoms and the need for short-acting β_2-agonists.[60] They are used in the chronic management of mild to moderate asthmatics and are not indicated for acute exacerbations. Zileuton is not used in pediatric patients.

Intubation

Any asthmatic patient who has apnea requires immediate intubation. β-Agonists are given immediately by nebulization or direct instillation through the endotracheal tube, or they can be given parenterally (terbutaline preferred parenterally). Other indications for intubation are less clear. The general recommendations are to intubate patients with worsening or no response to therapy or with signs of respiratory fatigue (lethargy, declining mental clarity, bradypnea, or paradoxical inward movement of the abdomen with inspiration). Patients with significantly elevated $Pa{CO_2}$ or rising $Pa{CO_2}$ as reflected by respiratory acidemia, particularly in the presence of these other clinical indications, likely warrant intubation. Once intubation is thought to be necessary, it should not be delayed. Intubation is best done semi-electively. Once the patient is intubated, nebulizer treatments should be given continuously and then decreased in frequency.

DISPOSITION

Those patients with a good response to the first hour of therapy (nebulizations every 20 minutes, O_2 as needed) are most likely to be discharged home safely without relapse. A good response is the absence of shortness of breath and wheezing, normal oxygen saturation, and, in children older than 5 years, a PEFR or FEV_1 greater than 70% predicted. All patients should be observed for 30 to 60 minutes after the last β-agonist nebulizers before being discharged.

Patients in the high-risk category (see Box 167-3) should receive a 3- to 10-day course of steroids (typically, a 5-day course is prescribed). All asthmatic patients should be discharged with an intensification of their previous asthma therapy before emergency department arrival (increased nebulizer frequency, or addition of steroids). If patients are sent home with MDIs, spacers should be provided. If children are to be treated with a course of steroids, the first dose should be given in the emergency department. It is essential to determine whether the prescriptions can be filled immediately on discharge from the emergency department. If not, a prescription prepack should be provided. A recent study suggests that if a patient has symptoms consistent with mild, moderate, or severe persistent asthma (see Table 167-3), inhaled corticosteroids should be added upon discharge from the emergency department.[63] The inhaled corticosteroids do not replace systemic steroids but rather are adjuvant

Table 167-3. Asthma Pharmacology for Infants and Children: Long-Term Control

Medication	Dosage Form	Child Dose	Comments
Systemic Corticosteroids	(Applies to all three systemic corticosteroids)		
Methylprednisolone	2, 4, 8, 16, 32 mg tablets	■ 0.25-2 mg/kg daily in single dose or qod as needed for control ■ Short course "burst"; 1-2 mg/kg/day, maximum 60 mg/day, for 3-10 days	■ For long-term treatment of severe persistent asthma, administer single dose in AM either daily or on alternate days (alternate-day therapy may produce less adrenal suppression). If daily doses are required, one study suggests improved efficacy and no increase in adrenal suppression when administered at 3:00 PM (Beam et al, 1992). ■ Short courses or "bursts" are effective for establishing control when initiating therapy or during a period of gradual deterioration. ■ The burst should be continued until patient achieves 80% PEF personal best or symptoms resolve. This usually requires 3-10 days but may require longer. There is no evidence that tapering the dose following improvement prevents relapse.
Prednisolone	5 mg tablets, 5 mg/5 cc, 15 mg/5 cc		
Prednisone	1, 2.5, 5, 10, 20, 25 mg tablets; 5 mg/cc, 5 mg/5 cc		
Cromolyn and Nedocromil			
Cromolyn	MDI 1 mg/puff Nebulizer solution 20 mg/ampule	1-2 puffs tid-qid 1 ampule tid-qid	■ One dose prior to exercise or allergen exposure provides effective prophylaxis for 1-2 hours.
Nedocromil	MDI 1.75 mg/puff	1-2 puffs bid-qid	■ See cromolyn.
Long-Acting Beta$_2$-Agonists			
Salmeterol	*Inhaled* MDI 21 mcg/puff, 60 or 120 puffs DPI 50 mcg/blister	 1-2 puffs q12 hours 1 blister q12 hours	 ■ May use one dose nightly for symptoms. ■ Should not be used for symptom relief or for exacerbations.
Sustained-Release Albuterol	*Tablet* 4 mg tablet	0.3-0.6 mg/kg/day, not to exceed 8 mg/day	
Methylxanthines			
Theophylline	Liquids, sustained-release tablets, and capsules	Starting dose 10 mg/kg/day; usual max: ■ <1 year of age: 0.2 (age in weeks) + 5 = mg/kg/day ■ ≥1 year of age: 10 mg/kg/day	■ Adjust dosage to achieve serum concentration of 5-15 mcg/mL at steady-state (at least 48 hours on same dosage). ■ Due to wide interpatient variability in theophylline metabolic clearance, routine serum theophylline level monitoring is important.
Leukotriene Modifiers			
Zafirlukast	20 mg tablet		■ For zafirlukast, administration with meals decreases bioavailability; take at least 1 hour before or 2 hours after meals.
Zileuton	300 mg tablet 600 mg tablet		■ For zileuton, monitor hepatic enzymes (ALT).

Modified from National Institutes of Health: *Guidelines for the Diagnosis and Management of Asthma*, NIH Publication No. 97-4051, July 1997, p 92.

therapy. Inhaled corticosteroids should be considered in infants and children who (1) require symptomatic treatment more than two times per week, (2) have experienced severe exacerbations less than 6 weeks apart, or (3) have had more than three episodes of wheezing in the past year that lasted more than 1 day, affected sleep, and have risk factors for the development of asthma (atopic dermatitis or family history of asthma, or two of the following: allergic rhinitis, wheezing apart from colds, peripheral blood eosinophilia).[59]

Patients with an incomplete response and continued symptoms of shortness of breath and wheezing and a PEFR or FEV$_1$ of 50% to 70% can be given a second hour of nebulizers every 20 minutes; steroids should be started (intravenously or orally) and oxygen continued if emergency staffing allows. In these patients, the decision to admit or discharge should be individualized, with factors listed in Box 167-3 taken into consideration. At 2 hours, the nebulizer administrations should be decreased to once every hour. If little or no improvement is seen at the end of 4 hours, PEFR/FEV$_1$ is less than 70%, or retracting, wheezing, tachypnea, or tachycardia is noted, hospitalization is usually needed for continuation of therapy, especially if the patient is in the high-risk category.

Patients with poor response to the initial hour of nebulizers applied every 20 minutes usually require hospitalization for continued frequent nebulizer treatments, steroids, oxygen, and monitoring.

An initial PEFR or FEV$_1$ less than 30% predicted or an oxygen saturation less than 91% (at sea level) on presentation has been correlated with the need for admission. Studies show that the initial FEV_1 or SaO_2 alone cannot predict the need for admission. The clinical assessment is of major importance (dyspnea, accessory muscle use, wheezing, respiratory rate, pulsus paradoxus, heart rate, and persistent hypoxia less than 94% on room air) in making the admission decision, and this decision is individualized.

The treatment of an asthma exacerbation does not end with discharge from the emergency department. All patients with asthma exacerbations who are discharged home from the emergency department should be sent home with a 5- to 10-day therapy plan, preferably in collaboration with their primary care physician. All patients should be evaluated by their primary care physician within 48 to 72 hours. If no primary care physician is involved, follow-up monitoring needs to be arranged by the emergency department physician. If poor compliance is anticipated, earlier hospitalization may be necessary.

BRONCHIOLITIS

PERSPECTIVE

Background

Bronchiolitis is the most common acute lower respiratory infection seen in pediatrics. It causes inflammation of the small airways, which results in airway edema and accumulation of mucus and cellular debris in the bronchioles, leading to airway obstruction.

Epidemiology

Bronchiolitis is seen primarily in children less than 2 years old, with 80% of cases occurring in children less than 1 year old and a peak incidence between 2 and 6 months of age. Bronchiolitis is a seasonal illness, with peak activity between mid-December and mid-March in the United States. Between 1980 and 1996, approximately 1.65 million children younger than 5 were hospitalized for bronchiolitis. Infants younger than 6 months of age accounted for 57% and children younger than 1 year of age accounted for 81% of these hospitalizations. During this same time period, rates of hospitalization for infants with bronchiolitis increased 239%, from 12.9 to 31.2 per 1000. The hospitalization rate increased less substantially in children 1 to 4 years of age, increasing from a rate of 1.3 per 1000 in 1980 to 2.3 per 1000 in 1996.[64] Bronchiolitis is rarely fatal in healthy infants. Hospitalization occurs in only 2% to 3% of cases, but bronchiolitis accounts for approximately 17% of all infant hospitalizations.[65] Those infants at increased risk of RSV bronchiolitis are those born between April and September; those attending daycare; those exposed to school-age siblings, crowded living conditions, or passive cigarette smoke; those who are multiple birth cohorts or were born prematurely; and those whose caregivers are uneducated.[66]

PRINCIPLES OF DISEASE

Pathophysiology

Respiratory syncytial virus is the major cause of bronchiolitis in infancy, especially in epidemics. Approximately 70% of bronchiolitis infections and 50% of infant pneumonias are caused by RSV. At least 50% of children are infected by RSV during their first year of life. By 2 years of age, almost 100% of children have been infected with RSV for the first time.[66] Parainfluenza (types 1, 2, and 3) is the second most common bronchiolitis etiologic agent and is usually seen in fall and spring. Other etiologic pathogens are adenovirus, rhinovirus, influenza, *Mycoplasma pneumoniae*, and, rarely, enterovirus, herpes simplex, and mumps. Human metapneumovirus was identified in 2001 by van den Hoogen as another paramyxovirus, along with RSV and parainfluenza, that causes bronchiolitis in young children.[67,68] Bronchiolitis is virtually never caused by a bacterial agent, and bacterial superinfection is rare.

Respiratory syncytial virus is spread primarily by direct contact with infected nasal secretions or infected contaminated objects. The primary means of transmission are large particle aerosols (from sneezes) and hand-to-hand or hand-to-nose transmission after contact with infectious secretions. Infected individuals can shed the virus 1 to 2 days before symptoms and for 1 to 2 weeks after. Secretion of virus can last 3 to 4 weeks, especially in infants less than 6 months old. Reinfection is common, even within a few weeks of an initial infection. The incubation period ranges from 2 to 8 days.[66]

Viral replication in the small bronchioles is thought to cause necrosis of the ciliated respiratory epithelium. The regenerated epithelium is nonciliated and thus cannot effectively move secretions out of the smaller airways into the larger airways, resulting in small airway obstruction. As epithelial cells are destroyed, they release cytokines and chemokines. The cytokines cause increased capillary permeability and secretion production. The chemokines attract macrophages, neutrophils, eosinophils, and natural killer cells to the site of the infection. As a result, an interstitial pneumonitis consisting of lymphocytic infiltration of the peribronchial tissues and edema often occurs. This process also inhibits pulmonary surfactant function. Patchy areas of hyperinflation and focal atelectasis also occur. Immunologic hypersensitivity to viral antigens may also play a role in bronchiolitis. Production of virus-specific IgE stimulates the release of bronchoconstrictive mediators, such as histamine and leukotriene C_4. Leukotriene C_4 can also stimulate airway mucus secretion.[66]

Infection with RSV induces a weak serum immune response and humoral antibody response, which consists primarily of mucosal IgA in infants younger than 6 months of age. Resistance to RSV reinfection has been correlated to serum antibody titers. The body also mounts a cell-mediated response to RSV infection that consists of the release of interleukin-1, tumor necrosis factor-alpha, interleukin-6, interleukin-8, macrophage-inflammatory protein 1-alpha, and RANTES (regulated upon activation, normal T cell expressed and secreted).[67]

Children may have either single or recurrent episodes of bronchiolitis. Children younger than 3 years of age who develop a lower respiratory tract illness with RSV have an increased risk of recurrent wheezing and asthma, which may persist until age 13 years.[67,69] Studies do suggest that infants with high levels of IgE at the time of the initial bronchiolitis are more likely to develop asthma. These are also the children who often have a history of atopy, which is associated with increased risk of developing asthma.[70]

Infants are at higher risk for respiratory failure resulting from airway obstruction because of small airway diameter, very high airway resistance, poor elastic recoil, and high rib cage compliance. Air trapping, high resistance, and atelectasis produce ventilation-perfusion mismatch leading to hypoxemia. As minute ventilation decreases, the infant becomes fatigued and severe airway involvement results in hypercarbia and respiratory failure.

CLINICAL FEATURES

A 3- to 5-day history of nasal congestion and cough often accompanies bronchiolitis. The cough becomes more pronounced and symptoms of increasing respiratory distress begin. The parents may note that the patient is fussy and not eating well. Fever is usually low-grade or absent, although at times the infant has a fever greater than 38.6° C (101.5° F). As respiratory distress becomes more prominent, tachypnea, tachycardia, intercostal retractions, and a prolonged expiratory phase develop. On auscultation, wheezing and coarse rales may be heard. Many infants remain alert and playful despite increased respiratory effort. Nasal flaring, suprasternal retractions, and grunting can occur with severe distress. Irritability or lethargy can be a signal of hypoxia or hypercarbia. Cyanosis is a late and unreliable sign of respiratory distress. The duration of the illness extends from days to several weeks.[66]

Complications

Many patients have an accompanying otitis media or viral pneumonia, especially with RSV infections. In a study done by Andrade and colleagues,[71] bacterial pathogens were found in all cases of acute otitis media in children (<2 years old) with bronchiolitis; thus, acute otitis media in children with bronchiolitis requires antibiotic therapy. This bacterial infection may be a secondary pathogen because more than 50% of middle ear aspirates also had RSV detected by polymerase chain reaction.

The mortality rate for bronchiolitis usually is less than 1%. Those at highest risk of severe disease and mortality are infants with cyanotic or complex heart disease, underlying pulmonary disease (bronchopulmonary dysplasia, cystic fibrosis, tracheoesophageal fistula, recurrent aspiration pneumonitis), a history of prematurity, immunodeficiency, or neurologic and genetic disorders that hinder secretion clearance.[66] The best method of preventing death in patients with bronchiolitis is early recognition of respiratory distress and failure.

Apnea may occur, especially in infants less than 6 months old. Atelectasis can occur, causing rapid deterioration. Bronchiolitis fibrosa obliterans rarely results from progressive fibrotic reaction that obliterates the bronchioles and is initially distinguished from acute bronchiolitis by lack of response to therapy and severity of symptoms.

DIAGNOSTIC STRATEGIES

Bronchiolitis is primarily a clinical diagnosis. Pulse oximetry is very useful. An initial SaO_2 less than 95% (at sea level) is found to be the single best predictor of severe bronchiolitis. A low SaO_2 is not always clinically apparent. Infants with severe disease who do not respond to aggressive management or whose condition continues to deteriorate should have an arterial blood gas assessment. The $PaCO_2$ is usually between 30 and 35 mm Hg. A $PaCO_2$ of 45 to 55 mm Hg is ominous, and respiratory failure may be imminent.

A chest x-ray study is unnecessary in cases of mild to moderate disease[72,73]; however, it may be helpful in one or more of the following situations: (1) moderate to severe respiratory distress, (2) recurrence of wheezing, (3) toxic appearance, (4) sudden deterioration, and (5) a prolonged course. The chest x-ray study can show hyperinflation, increased bronchial markings, interstitial infiltrates, or atelectasis that may be difficult to distinguish from infiltrate. The radiograph may be normal. A complete blood cell count is not helpful. Nasopharyngeal RSV antigen testing is not routinely necessary but may be useful in febrile children to identify the cause of the fever.

DIFFERENTIAL CONSIDERATIONS

The most common considerations in the differential diagnosis are pneumonia, asthma, and foreign body aspiration. Asthma should be considered in those children with a history of recurrent wheezing, especially if there is a history of familial atopy. A chest x-ray study is helpful in diagnosing pneumonia, and a normal expiratory chest film makes a foreign body less likely. Other diagnoses to consider are congestive heart failure, cystic fibrosis, vascular ring, neoplasm, and aspiration syndrome. If paroxysmal coughing is present, pertussis should be excluded by obtaining a rapid fluorescent antibody test and culture for pertussis.

MANAGEMENT

Infants should be assessed quickly for the degree of respiratory distress. Oxygen and hydration are the mainstays of bronchiolitis therapy. The oxygen can be delivered by nasal cannula, mask (infant or pediatric size), or hood. The general alertness, ability to feed, respiratory rate, use of accessory muscles, and presence of wheezing or rales should be determined. Hydration status should be clinically assessed. An intravenous line should be placed in those infants with severe disease or evidence of dehydration (poor feeding, decreased wet diapers, dry mucous membranes, lethargy). Sequential examinations are essential.

The use of β-agonists in bronchiolitis has been controversial. Since 1996, four meta-analyses have evaluated β-agonist therapy use in bronchiolitis.[66,74-77] A meta-analysis by Kellner and associates[74] evaluated the use of all bronchodilators in the treatment of bronchiolitis. When restricted to only β-agonists and using clinical scores to measure improvement, patients were found to experience some benefit, but the study did not demonstrate a significant increase in oxygen saturation from presenting values, or reduction in the hospitalization rate with the use of β-agonists. Two of these studies suggested that a subset of bronchiolitis patients do improve with β-agonists.[74,75] There is no known method for identifying these patients prospectively; thus, a trial of one or two β-agonists may be used. If no improvement occurs, using objective measures such as pulse oximetry, respiratory rate, accessory muscle use, inspiratory/expiratory ratio, wheezing, the β-agonists should be discontinued. If a β-agonist is given, a response should be seen within 60 minutes. If no improvement occurs, nebulization can be discontinued. The conclusion of the other two meta-analyses was that β-agonist therapy offered short-term benefits but no long-term advantage in the treatment of bronchiolitis.[76,77] Ipratropium was not recommended by any of the four meta-analyses.[66]

Epinephrine nebulization therapy has been shown to be helpful, both racemic and L-epinephrine. The L-epinephrine is less expensive. Menon and associates[78] compared nebulizer therapy with salbutamol to L-epinephrine. The epinephrine group had a significantly higher oxygen saturation 60 minutes after therapy, lower heart rate 90 minutes after therapy, a faster rate of discharge from the emergency department, and a markedly reduced admission rate (33% versus 81%). Other studies have supported a significant response to racemic epinephrine and some have suggested that it be used as a first line of therapy.[79,80] If an epinephrine nebulization is given, a response should be seen within 60 minutes. If no improvement occurs, nebulization may be discontinued.

The use of steroids in the treatment of bronchiolitis has been controversial. The majority of studies performed demonstrated no benefit from the use of steroids; however, a meta-analysis done by Garrison and colleagues[81] found that pooled data from six studies demonstrated a small but significant reduction in the length of hospitalization (0.43 days) in the steroid-treated group. In this study, the mean length of stay ranged from 2.8 to 8.3 days in the placebo groups and from 3.2 to 7.1 in the treatment groups. In addition, van Woensel and associates[82] demonstrated a reduction in hospital stay by 6 days in mechanically ventilated bronchiolitis patients treated with prednisolone rather than placebo, suggesting that steroids may be of benefit in patients with severe bronchiolitis.

Antibiotics are not recommended for the treatment of uncomplicated viral bronchiolitis. Chest physical therapy has not been shown to be of benefit. Cool mist therapy is not recommended.[65] Nasopharyngeal suctioning has been shown to be helpful as a palliative measure.[66] A study by Martinon-Torres and associates[83] found heliox (70% He, 30% O_2) delivered by a nonrebreather reservoir face mask to produce a beneficial response in infants with moderate to severe bronchiolitis. The heliox produced a response within 1 hour of initiation that was defined as an improvement in the patients' clinical scores and a decrease in their tachycardia and tachypnea.

DISPOSITION

Generally, infants with underlying cardiopulmonary disease or immunodeficiency and those who are on immunosuppressive therapy should be hospitalized. Patients with moderate to severe distress who are unresponsive to bronchodilators or those who are unwilling to feed should also be hospitalized. Factors associated with more severe disease and a need for hospitalization are a toxic appearance, initial oxygen saturation less than 95% (at sea level), gestational age less than 34 weeks, respiratory rate of 70 or greater, atelectasis on chest x-ray examination, and age less than 3 months. Increased risk of hospitalization of premature infants for RSV occurred with (1) gestational age of 32 weeks or less, (2) a perinatal oxygen requirement of 28 days or more, and (3) discharge from the neonatal intensive care unit in the 3 months before RSV season. These infants are candidates for RSV immunoglobulin (RespiGam) prophylaxis or palivizumab (Synagis).[84]

Infants with mild disease and those who are feeding well can be discharged home with close follow-up monitoring (usually 24 hours). If they responded to β-agonist nebulizations, they should be discharged home with albuterol nebulizations. Epinephrine nebulization is currently not recommended for home therapy. The parents should be alerted to signs of increasing distress, such as irritability, lethargy, poor feeding, retractions, and tachypnea. If respiratory distress increases, the parents should be instructed to call their physician or return to the emergency department.

ANAPHYLAXIS

PERSPECTIVE

Background

Anaphylaxis is a systemic reaction to an allergen, which is mediated by IgE. Portier and Richet initially introduced the term *anaphylaxis* in 1902.[85] At the time, they were attempting to immunize dogs to sea anemone toxin. Upon re-exposure to the toxin several weeks later, some of the dogs died within minutes. The term *anaphylaxis* is derived from the Greek word *ana* meaning "backward" and *phylaxis* meaning "protection." Anaphylactoid reactions are clinically indistinguishable from anaphylaxis but are not IgE mediated.[86]

Epidemiology

The exact incidence of anaphylaxis is unknown; however, recent articles suggest that the incidence is increasing. It may occur as often as 1 in 3000 people.[87] Antibiotics and radiographic contrast agents, respectively, are the two most common known causes of anaphylaxis and anaphylactoid reactions. The incidence approaches 1 in 5000 exposures. Penicillins are the most frequent cause of drug anaphylaxis. The carbapenems are cross-reactive with penicillin, whereas the cephalosporins have less than 10% cross-reactivity with penicillin. Vancomycin, ciprofloxacin, aspirin, and nonsteroidal anti-inflammatory drugs are associated with anaphylactoid reactions.[88] Overall, less than 10% of these reactions are fatal; however, anaphylaxis to antibiotics and radiographic contrast agents account for the majority of deaths associated with anaphylaxis. In the United States, hymenoptera stings are the next most common cause of anaphylaxis and they account for fewer than 100 deaths per year.[86] Fire ant and snake bites can also result in anaphylaxis. Food allergies are becoming increasingly common and often result in anaphylaxis. The most common foods are peanuts, other legumes, walnuts, pecans, fish, shellfish, milk, and eggs. In addition, exercise induced food allergy can lead to anaphylaxis as well. Latex allergy is also becoming a more common cause of anaphylaxis. People at highest risk for latex allergy are health care workers, children with spina bifida and genitourinary abnormalities, and those who are exposed to latex in the workplace. Latex-allergic patients also have a higher likelihood of anaphylaxis to kiwi, bananas, chestnuts, and avocado. These foods share cross-reactive antigens with latex proteins.[88] Anaphylactic reactions to vaccines are rare.[89]

The overall incidence of anaphylaxis and anaphylactoid reactions is reported to be higher in adults than in children, although children and even infants have anaphylactic reactions. Typically, the rate of anaphylaxis and anaphylactoid reactions is not affected by gender except in certain cases. Females have a higher incidence of reactions to muscle relaxants, aspirin, and latex. Anaphylaxis secondary to insect stings has been reported to be more common in males. These variations in gender are thought to be secondary to higher incidence of exposure to the allergens mentioned. Anaphylaxis can occur by any route of administration or exposure; however, parenteral administration of an allergen is associated with more acute and severe anaphylactic reactions. Constancy of administration plays a role as well. Re-exposure after an interval without an agent, such as insulin, can result in anaphylaxis. These reactions tend to decrease in severity as the length of time to re-exposure increases.[90]

Atopy can also affect the incidence of anaphylaxis and anaphylactoid reactions. Atopic individuals have a higher incidence of anaphylaxis and anaphylactoid reactions to latex, radiographic contrast agents, and food. They also have a higher incidence of idiopathic anaphylaxis and anaphylactoid reactions. Atopy does not appear to increase the risk of reactions to penicillin, hymenoptera stings, and insulin.[90]

PRINCIPLES OF DISEASE

Pathophysiology

Anaphylaxis is an immediate (type 1) hypersensitivity reaction. It requires previous sensitization to an allergen, which upon re-exposure produces an antigen–cell surface IgE interaction. This leads to mast cell and basophil degradation resulting in the release of histamine, tryptase, cytokines, prostaglandins, and platelet activating factor.

The more common *anaphylactoid* reaction also results from the release of inflammatory mediators from mast cells and basophils; however, it is not activated by an IgE immune response. In an anaphylactoid reaction, the immune response can be mediated by direct action on the mast cells and basophils (exercise, radiographic contrast agents), by a disruption of the arachidonic acid metabolism pathway (aspirin, nonsteroidal anti-inflammatory drugs), or by an immune complex–mediated activation of complement. Anaphylactoid reactions do not require prior sensitization.[88]

Histamine, a component released from the mast cell, is thought to be responsible for the early signs of anaphylaxis and anaphylactoid reaction. Stimulation of histamine receptors can result in smooth muscle contraction, increased endothelial permeability, increased viscosity of mucus, vasodilation, and decreased rate of atrioventricular conduction. Prostaglandins, leukotrienes, thromboxane, platelet activating factor, and kinins are more active in the later reaction than in the immediate phase. The leukotrienes contribute to the bronchoconstriction and edema in the lungs and can also be cardiotoxic. Prostaglandins can also cause bronchoconstriction and vasodilation. Platelet activating factor also stimulates bronchoconstriction and increases vascular permeability, airway inflammation, and chemotaxis.

The complement pathway may be stimulated during anaphylaxis and anaphylactoid reactions, releasing C3A, C4A, and C5A. These complements result in increased vascular permeability, mast cell degradation, smooth muscle contraction, and macrophage stimulation. In addition, nitric oxide synthesis is stimulated during anaphylaxis. Nitric oxide also increases vascular permeability and bronchoconstriction.[87]

The release of these chemical mediators is responsible for the clinical symptoms that are present during anaphylaxis or an anaphylactoid reaction.

CLINICAL FEATURES

Symptoms of anaphylaxis typically occur within 5 to 30 minutes of exposure to the allergen, but occasionally will occur hours after exposure to the allergen. Urticaria and angioedema are the most frequent manifestations of anaphylaxis and anaphylactoid reactions, occurring in 90% of the cases.[90] If a child is taking histamine antagonists, the initial skin manifestations may be absent and can result in a delay in diagnosis.[87] Pruritus occurs often as a result of sensory nerve stimulation and can occur without a rash in 5% of cases. Other systemic symptoms occur as well. Upper airway edema manifested by stridor, hoarseness, dysphagia, or barky or staccato cough occurs in 56% of episodes; dyspnea or wheeze occurs in 47%; flushing in 46%; dizziness, hypotension, orthostasis, or syncope occur in 33%; gastrointestinal symptoms, such as nausea, vomiting, diarrhea, or crampy abdominal pain, occur in 30%; rhinitis in 16%; headache in 15%; and seizure in 1.5%.[90] The first symptoms in patients with food anaphylaxis are often a metallic taste, pruritus, edema of the lips and oropharynx, and a tingling sensation. Young children may scratch their tongue, palate, anterior neck, and ear canals. Skin symptoms may not occur with food anaphylaxis.[91]

Cardiovascular collapse and hypotensive shock can also occur. The first cardiac symptom is often tachycardia. The release of chemical mediators leads to increased vascular permeability and vasodilation, which can progress to hypovolemic shock. The increased vascular permeability can result in a loss of up to 50% of the intravascular volume within 10 minutes. The fall in blood pressure will often stimulate the compensatory release of catecholamines with variable results.[90] Patients with underlying cardiac disease are at increased risk for fatal cardiac arrhythmias. The most common cardiac arrhythmia in patients with no cardiac disease is supraventricular tachycardia.[88]

Biphasic reactions, in which a second anaphylactic reaction occurs, can develop 1 to 28 hours after the first reaction. In a study by Lee and Greenes,[92] 6% of children had biphasic anaphylactic reactions and 3% of the reactions were significant, requiring epinephrine. The biphasic reactions were more likely to occur in patients who had not received epinephrine within 48 minutes of development of initial symptoms.

Complications

Laryngeal edema, manifested as hoarseness and stridor, can quickly lead to a life-threatening upper airway obstruction. Cardiovascular collapse and pulmonary compromise are most often responsible for fatal anaphylactic reactions. Patients with a history of cardiac or pulmonary manifestations of anaphylaxis are at higher risk for death. Upper airway edema can be found in up to 60% of the deaths secondary to anaphylaxis.[90] Sampson and associates[93] described some of the characteristics of children who experienced a fatal or near-fatal anaphylactic reaction to food. None of the children were aware that the allergen was in the food that they ate, all of the children had asthma, all had had previous reactions to the food allergen, and if parents were present, they often did not appreciate the potential severity of allergic reactions to food. No patient who died received epinephrine before severe respiratory symptoms developed, whereas all of those with nonfatal reactions received epinephrine before or within 5 minutes of the development of severe symptoms. Although atopy does not increase an individual's risk of anaphylaxis, atopic patients with a history of asthma or prior allergic reaction to a food are at higher risk for severe or fatal anaphylaxis when exposed to the food allergen.[93,94] In asthmatic persons, even inhalation of the food allergen can be fatal.[94]

DIAGNOSTIC STRATEGIES

Anaphylaxis is primarily a clinical diagnosis. A history should be obtained to determine exposure to new or previous allergens. It should be determined whether exercise preceded the anaphylaxis. If the source of the anaphylactic allergen is unknown, a careful dietary history should review all recently ingested foods.[91] Laboratory tests to confirm anaphylaxis are not timely enough to be helpful during the acute treatment. Tryptase and histamine levels, which can be elevated in anaphylaxis, are not routinely measured in many laboratories. Histamine is elevated only briefly. Tryptase is elevated in cases of hymenoptera and drug-induced anaphylaxis but not typically in food-induced anaphylaxis.[91] Beta-tryptase,[88] histamine, and specific IgE antibody levels[90] can be used to confirm anaphylaxis during a prolonged episode that is not responding to treatment. The best time to measure serum tryptase is 1 to 2 hours after the onset of symptoms, but no longer than 6 hours after onset. The best time to measure plasma histamine levels is between 10 and 60 minutes after the onset of symptoms. Tryptase or specific IgE antibody levels can help to confirm the cause of death in a fatal episode of anaphylaxis.

DIFFERENTIAL CONSIDERATIONS

Diagnoses that can mimic the presentation of anaphylaxis are numerous. Diagnoses that can cause sudden loss of consciousness and are in the differential diagnosis include vasovagal syncopal episodes, seizures, myocardial infarction, and cardiac arrhythmias. Diseases that can cause acute respiratory compromise and can mimic anaphylaxis include status asthmaticus, epiglottitis, foreign body aspiration with airway obstruction, and pulmonary embolus. Diseases that can have cutaneous manifestations and can mimic anaphylaxis include mastocytosis (α-tryptase levels are elevated), carcinoid syndrome, hereditary angioedema, and adverse drug reactions.[86] Flushing can occur with sulfonylurea or chlorpropamide intake and concurrent intake of alcohol, niacin intake, medullary carcinoma of the thyroid, or autonomic epilepsy and can also be idiopathic. A group of postprandial syndromes, also known as *the restaurant syndromes*, can mimic anaphylaxis. These syndromes have been linked to the ingestion of sulfites, monosodium glutamate, and spoiled fish. In sensitive individuals, sulfites cause bronchospasm, flushing, and hypotension. Ingestion of monosodium glutamate causes flushing, diaphoresis, chest pain, facial burning, paresthesias, dizziness, headaches, palpitations, nausea, and vomiting. Sensitive children experience shivering, irritability, chills, screaming, and delirium. *Klebsiella pneumoniae* and

Proteus morganii are thought to precipitate the spoiled fish reaction, also known as *scrombroidosis.* They release a chemical saurine, which has histamine-like properties. Its symptoms are headache, flushing, urticaria, nausea, and vomiting.[90]

Vasodepressor reactions are in the differential diagnosis; however, skin manifestations are rare. These patients also tend to have bradycardia, which is unusual in patients with anaphylaxis. In addition, these patients are often cool and clammy, as opposed to anaphylactic patients who are flushed and warm. Psychiatric disorders such as panic attacks, vocal cord dysfunction, and Munchausen's stridor can mimic anaphylactic symptoms as well.[90]

MANAGEMENT

Anaphylaxis can be fatal, and thus, immediate recognition and treatment are paramount. It should be remembered that even mild symptoms could progress to a severe reaction. Rapid evaluation of airway, breathing, circulation, and level of consciousness should be the first steps in assessment. Oxygen should be given via nonrebreather mask if the patient demonstrates hypoxia or any symptoms of respiratory distress. If the offending allergen is still present, it should be removed immediately. Close monitoring of vital signs, cardiac rhythm, and pulmonary function is required. Evidence of impending airway obstruction such as stridor portends great difficulty in obtaining an airway. As such, active airway intervention should be undertaken as early as possible and alternative airway techniques may be required.

Epinephrine should be administered with the initial assessment. Indications for epinephrine include symptoms of bronchospasm, laryngeal edema, dysrhythmias, any hypotension, cardiac or respiratory arrest, or loss of consciousness.[86] Epinephrine can also be used to treat urticaria and angioedema, especially in children with a history of a previous severe reaction or a history of asthma.[91] Delay in the recognition of severe anaphylaxis and subsequent delay in the administration of epinephrine has been linked to poor outcome and subsequent mortality.[93,95] Intramuscular administration of epinephrine has been shown to be superior to subcutaneous administration. Intramuscular administration of epinephrine in the lateral thigh provides the most efficient absorption profile in children and adults.[96,97] The dose of intramuscular epinephrine is 0.01 mg/kg (maximum 0.3 mg) of the 1:1000 in children and 0.3 to 0.5 mg (0.3-0.5 mL) in adults. The initial dose can be repeated at 10- to 15-minute intervals if needed. In a study by Korenblat and associates,[98] more than 35% of patients with anaphylactic reactions required multiple doses of epinephrine to reverse the symptoms. The more severe the reaction is, the more likely it is that the second and third doses of epinephrine will be required.

In addition to epinephrine, hypotension should be treated with the rapid infusion of intravenous crystalloids. In children, if intravenous access is difficult, an intraosseous route of administration should be established. The initial bolus of crystalloids in children is 20 mL/kg and can be repeated. Hypotensive patients should also be placed in modified Trendelenburg position. Hypotensive patients who are unresponsive to intravenous fluid administration can be given intravenous epinephrine as a 1:10,000 concentration. Intravenous epinephrine is not routinely used, because it can be associated with cardiac ischemia and arrhythmias. The intravenous dose of epinephrine is 0.01 mL/kg of the 1:10,000 with a maximum of 0.3 mL for children and 0.5 mL for adults.[87] Constant infusion of dopamine, dobutamine, and epinephrine may be required for persistent hypotension.

Antihistamines are used in the treatment of anaphylaxis after the use of epinephrine and once cardiorespiratory symptoms have been stabilized. Antihistamines are especially helpful in the treatment of cutaneous symptoms. Studies suggest that administration of H_1 and H_2 antihistamines may be more effective than the administration of either alone.[91] Oral routes can be used for mild symptoms, intramuscular for moderate reactions, and intravenous for any patient with either severe reactions or hypotension. The most commonly used H_1 blocker is diphenhydramine. The dose of diphenhydramine is 1 to 2 mg/kg up to 75 mg. The intravenous route is necessary for rapid and effective absorption. The addition of an H_2 blocker may provide additional relief of symptoms. Cimetidine, ranitidine, and famotidine have all been shown to be helpful.[90] The intravenous dose for cimetidine is 4 mg/kg up to 300 mg, for ranitidine 1 mg/kg/dose, and for famotidine 0.5 mg/kg/dose.

Steroids are also second-line therapy for anaphylaxis. They may be helpful in reducing a late-phase anaphylaxis, though this is controversial.[92] Prednisone 1 mg/kg can be given orally for mild to moderate reactions. Methylprednisolone is given most frequently for severe reactions. The dosage is 1 to 2 mg/kg intravenously. If wheezing is present, nebulized β agonists (albuterol) and intravenous aminophylline can be given.

Patients who are on β-blockers can develop bradycardia, refractory hypotension, and relapsing symptoms. Atropine can be used to treat the bradycardia in these patients. Glucagon is probably the drug of choice for treating anaphylaxis in a patient on β-blockers. Glucagon can be given to increase cardiac output by increasing inotropic and chronotropic effects.[87,90]

DISPOSITION

Patients who have had an anaphylactic reaction should be monitored in the emergency department or in an observation unit for a minimum of 4 to 8 hours. Patients who required multiple doses of epinephrine or had a severe reaction should be monitored for 12 to 24 hours.[87] In Lee and Greenes' study of biphasic pediatric anaphylactic reactions, the late phase occurred 1.3 to 28.4 hours after the initial phase, with the majority occurring in less than 12 hours.[92] Patients with severe reactions requiring intubation and cardiopulmonary resuscitation should be admitted to an intensive care unit for further management.

Prevention of future anaphylaxis depends on avoidance of the instigating allergen. Patients and their parents must be instructed in ways to avoid the allergen causing the anaphylaxis. They must recognize the potential severity of re-exposure and the importance of prompt treatment with epinephrine. Upon discharge home, all patients who had an anaphylactic reaction should be discharged with an EpiPen (0.3 mL) or EpiPen Jr (0.15 mL). The EpiPen Jr is typically prescribed for patients weighing 10 to 20 kg. The EpiPen is prescribed for patients weighing more than 27 kg. Patients weighing between 21 and 28 kg should be given an EpiPen if they have had a severe reaction or are at risk for a severe reaction (history of asthma, allergy to peanut, tree nut, or seafood). An EpiPen Jr can be prescribed if patients have only had a mild reaction.[91] Parents and patients must be instructed to recognize the symptoms of anaphylaxis and to use the EpiPen if symptoms of respiratory distress or cardiac compromise occur. Studies have shown that even when a patient has a known history of anaphylaxis, epinephrine is often not given when indicated, either by parents or in physicians' offices or hospitals, often with dire consequences.[99,100]

FOREIGN BODY ASPIRATION

PERSPECTIVE

Background

Aspiration of foreign bodies into the airways in pediatric patients can lead to serious morbidity and even death if not recognized and treated quickly.

Epidemiology

In 1995, the National Safety Council statistics stated that foreign body suffocation accounted for 5% of all accidental deaths in children less than 4 years old, and 10% of deaths in children younger than 1 year of age.[101] The deaths were primarily associated with foreign bodies obstructing the glottis, resulting in asphyxia and a mortality rate of more than 40%.[102]

Children between the ages of 1 and 2 years have the highest incidence of foreign body aspiration, and children under the age of 3 account for 80% of cases of foreign body aspiration.[102-105] Younger children are thought to be at higher risk for aspiration for several reasons. They lack posterior dentition (molars) and thus chew less well; they frequently explore their world using their mouths; they have episodes of inspiration when startled, laughing, or crying; and their swallowing reflex is still incomplete. Several studies have demonstrated a 2:1 male-to-female ratio in the incidence of foreign body aspiration.[103,104] This is thought to be secondary to boys' more impulsive and adventurous play.[104] In one study, 75% of the accidents occurred in the home, but only 40% were witnessed by a parent.[102]

Throughout the world, the most commonly aspirated foreign bodies are organic or food matter. In North America, the most commonly aspirated food is the peanut.[101,102] Commonly aspirated foods are popcorn, seeds, hot dogs, grapes, and vegetable matter. Other commonly aspirated objects include small bones, toy parts, crayons, pen tops, pins, tacks, nails, screws, and bullets.[101]

PRINCIPLES OF DISEASE

Clinical Features

Clinical symptoms of complete upper airway obstruction are coughing followed by inability to cough, cry, or speak. The clinical findings of more distal foreign body aspiration can be fairly nonspecific. A history of a choking episode, perhaps with perioral cyanosis, followed by cough, wheezing, or stridor is classic of the initial symptoms. Unfortunately, even in the home, only 40% of choking episodes are witnessed. In addition, an asymptomatic child and normal examination findings can often accompany a good history for aspiration. Five to 40% of children have normal examination findings.[104] If a child has a reliable history for aspiration, it is important to evaluate him or her thoroughly, even in the presence of a normal examination findings.[101]

Signs and symptoms of foreign body aspiration in the lower airway can be divided into three stages. The initial stage consists of choking, followed by coughing, gagging, and sometimes airway distress. The second stage is usually asymptomatic. The third stage is manifested by symptoms of complications.[103] Ninety percent of children who have aspirated foreign bodies will have a history of initial choking, coughing, and wheezing or stridor.[101]

Physical examination findings, if present, include fever, cough, tachypnea, unequal breath sounds, wheezing, stridor, dyspnea, cyanosis, absence of breath sounds, and suprasternal retractions. Thirty to 60% of children have absence of breath sounds on auscultation. This finding is suggestive of total airway obstruction.[101] The presence of a fever may be suggestive of a contaminated or chemically irritating foreign body. In the presence of fever, one also has to consider the possibility that a foreign body has been present in the airways for a longer period of time and has caused obstructive pneumonia.[101,104]

Complications

The most serious complication of foreign body aspiration is complete airway obstruction, which results in cardiac arrest and death if not treated immediately. Prior to the availability of bronchoscopy in the early 1900s, the mortality rate for foreign body aspiration was nearly 50%. Current mortality rates are less than 1%. If a foreign body remains lodged in an airway undetected, secretions are retained, which leads to bacterial overgrowth and subsequent pulmonary infection. Recurrent pneumonia or a lung abscess should cause one to suspect an airway foreign body. A retained airway foreign body may also act as a ball-valve, causing air trapping, asymmetric wheezing, and eventual pneumothorax. More unusual complications are

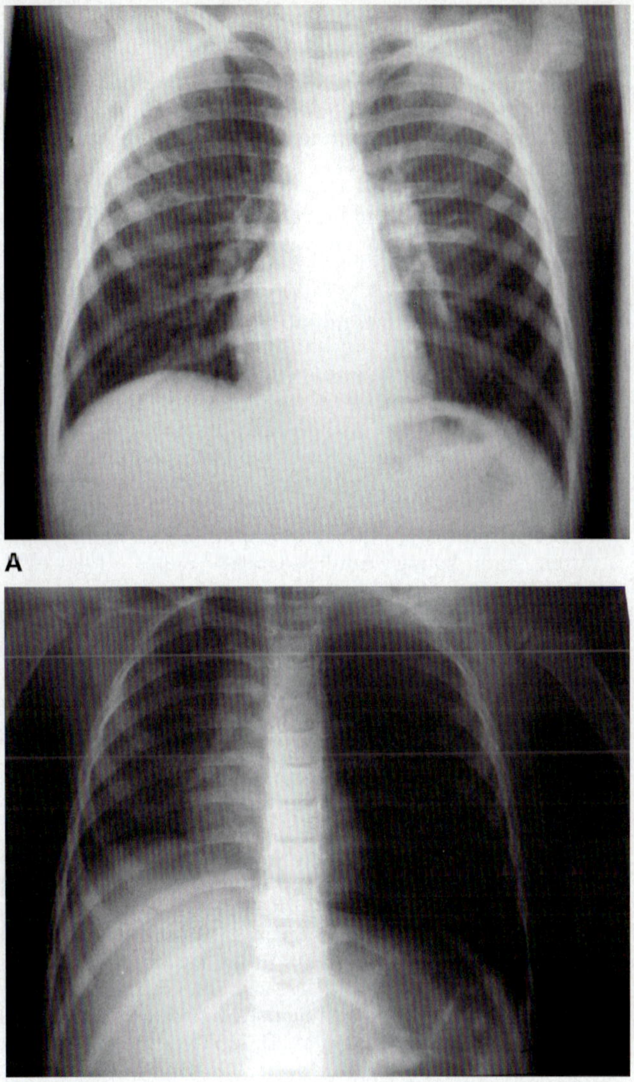

A

B

Figure 167-4. **A,** Chest radiograph demonstrating hyperinflation of the left lung typically of a foreign body with a ball-valve effect; the mediastinum is mobile and shows slight shift to the right with inspiration. **B,** Chest radiograph demonstrating marked hyperinflation on the left lung due to a trapped lower airway foreign body. (Courtesy of Marianne Gausche-Hill, MD.)

pneumomediastinum, and perforation of the bronchial tree with fistula formation.[101] A study by Reilly and coworkers[106] found that the most common complications of delayed diagnosis are croup, pneumonia, pneumothorax, atelectasis, stricture, and perforation.

DIAGNOSTIC STRATEGIES

Diagnostic radiographs may be helpful in some cases; however, 66% to 94% of aspirated foreign bodies are radiolucent organic material.[104] Posteroanterior and lateral chest x-rays can initially be normal in those cases. If the foreign body is obstructing significant airflow, x-ray findings such as air trapping, mediastinal shift, or atelectasis may be present. Inspiratory and expiratory anteroposterior chest x-rays can help to lateralize a foreign body by demonstrating unilateral air trapping (Figure 167-4A and B). Left and right lateral decubitus chest films can be used to demonstrate unilateral air trapping in infants and children who are unable to cooperate with obtaining inspiratory and expiratory x-rays.[101-104] Foreign bodies can be found anywhere from the nose to the lung parenchyma; thus, chest radiographs should include the anteroposterior and lateral views of the upper airway. In children, it is only slightly more common for the aspirated foreign body to be found in the right lung. This is because in children less than 15 years old, there is no difference in the angle at which the right and left main stem bronchi branch off from the trachea.[102,104] A study by Tan and associates[103] suggests that fluoroscopy is helpful in increasing the rate of correct diagnosis in the event of a normal chest x-ray. Fluoroscopic findings, however, may be falsely negative with small, unobstructive foreign bodies. Computed tomography and magnetic resonance imaging studies have not been shown to improve diagnosis of foreign body aspiration.

DIFFERENTIAL CONSIDERATIONS

Foreign body aspiration should be considered in the differential diagnosis of any child who has unusual pulmonary symptoms, new-onset asthma, bronchiolitis, recurrent pneumonia, lung abscess, pneumothorax, pneumomediastinum, or recurrent croup.[101]

MANAGEMENT

Any child who has signs of lower airway obstruction should be taken to the operating room for removal of the foreign body using general anesthesia and rigid bronchoscopy. The anesthesiologist should be skilled in pediatric airway management. Pediatric surgeons, pediatric otolaryngologists, or pediatric pulmonologists trained in the rigid bronchoscopy may perform the procedure. When physicians skilled in pediatric bronchoscopy perform the procedure, the removal is successful in more than 95% of cases and the complication rate is less than 1%.[101] A recent study by Swanson and associates[107] suggests that flexible bronchoscopy can be safely used to remove foreign bodies if provisions are available to use rigid bronchoscopy if the initial procedure fails at removal. If lower airway foreign body removal is unsuccessful via rigid bronchoscopy, then thoracotomy is indicated for removal and prevention of long-term complications.

DISPOSITION

Infants and children with suspected foreign body should undergo bronchoscopy in the operating room. If the foreign body was in the airway for only a brief period of time, it is likely that patients will be discharged home once they have recovered from general anesthesia. Children who presented with persistent or recurrent symptoms because of a lower airway foreign body that was retained for days, weeks, or even months may require a longer hospitalization for management and treatment of complications.

KEY CONCEPTS

Asthma

- Asthma is now defined as a chronic inflammatory disorder of the airways in susceptible individuals. This definition has major implications for therapy.
- Cough, wheezing, and tachypnea are the hallmark symptoms of asthma. Recognizing the degree of an asthmatic child's respiratory distress and initiating treatment are key to preventing progression to respiratory failure.
- Pulse oximetry and PEFR measurements are valuable diagnostic tools to aid in the evaluation of asthmatic patients.
- Oxygen, β-agonist (albuterol) inhalation therapy, and steroids are the key components of asthma treatment in the emergency department. Ipratropium can be used as well.
- Asthma patients who are discharged home from the emergency department should be sent home with a 5- to 10-day therapy plan, preferably in collaboration with their primary care physician.

Bronchiolitis

- Bronchiolitis occurs primarily in children younger than 2 years, with 80% of cases occurring in children younger than 1 year.
- The majority of children with first-time bronchiolitis do not go on to develop asthma.
- Bronchiolitis is primarily a clinical diagnosis. Pulse oximetry is very helpful. Chest radiograph, complete blood cell count, and RSV nasal wash are not routinely necessary.
- Oxygen and hydration are the key components of bronchiolitis therapy. β-Agonist and epinephrine inhalation can be tried. If no response is noted in 30 to 60 minutes, the nebulizations should be discontinued.

Anaphylaxis

- Anaphylaxis and anaphylactoid reactions have identical clinical presentations. Anaphylaxis requires previous exposure to the allergen, anaphylactoid reactions do not.
- Symptoms of anaphylaxis typically occur within 5 to 30 minutes of exposure and can include urticaria, angioedema, symptoms of upper airway edema, gastrointestinal symptoms, cardiac symptoms, hypotension, and shock.
- Patients with cardiac symptoms, hypotension, bronchospasm, laryngeal edema, or loss of consciousness require immediate treatment with intramuscular epinephrine.
- Hypotension should be treated with rapid infusion of crystalloids.
- Second-line therapy for anaphylaxis includes H_1 and H_2 antihistamines and steroids.

Foreign Body Aspiration

- The majority of foreign body aspirations occur in children younger than 3 years of age.
- Organic food matter is the most commonly aspirated foreign body and is radiolucent.
- The history is the most important component in establishing the diagnosis.
- Physical examination and diagnostic studies may yield normal results.
- Inspiratory and expiratory chest radiographs may be helpful.
- Bronchoscopy is indicated for children with a strong history for aspiration, despite normal examination findings and normal radiographs, to prevent serious sequelae.

REFERENCES

1. National Asthma Education Program Expert Panel Report 2: *Guidelines for the Diagnosis and Management of Asthma*. National Institutes of Health Publication 97-4051. Bethesda, NIH, 1997.
2. Emond SD, Camargo CA, Nowak RM: 1997 National Asthma Education and Prevention Program Guidelines: A practical summary for emergency physicians. *Ann Emerg Med* 31:579, 1998.
3. Adams PF, Marano MA: Current estimates from the National Health Interview survey, 1994. *Vital Health Stat* 10:94, 1995.
4. Pediatric Asthma: *Promoting Best Practice Guide for Managing Asthma in Children*. Milwaukee, The American Academy of Allergy, Asthma, and Immunology, 1999.
5. Rachelefsky G: Treating Exacerbations of Asthma in Children: The Role of Systemic Corticosteroids. *Pediatrics* 112:382, 2003.
6. CDC: Asthma Mortality and Hospitalization among Children and Young Adults—United States, 1980-1993. *MMWR Morb Mortal Wkly Rep* 45:350, 1996.
7. Akinbami LJ, Schoendorf KC: Trends in childhood asthma: Prevalence, health care utilization, and mortality. *Pediatrics* 110:315, 2002.
8. Akinbami LJ, et al: Racial and income disparities in childhood asthma in the United States. *Ambul Pediatr* 2:382, 2002.
9. Federico MJ, Liu AH: Overcoming childhood asthma disparities of the inner-city poor. *Pediatr Clin North Am* 50:655, 2003.
10. Wade S, et al: Psychosocial characteristics of children with asthma: A description of the NCICASS psychosocial protocol. *J Pediatric Pulmonol* 24:263, 1997.
11. Weil CM, et al: The relationship between psychosocial factors and asthma morbidity in inner city children with asthma. *Pediatrics* 104:1274, 1999.
12. National Center for Health Statistics, Healthy People 2000 Review, 1995-96. Washington, D.C., Public Health Service, 1996.
13. Phelan PD, et al: The Melbourne Asthma Study: 1964-1999. *J Allergy Clin Immunol* 109:189, 2002.
14. Taussig LM, et al: Tuscon Children's Respiratory Study: 1980 to present. *J Allergy Clin Immunol* 111:661, 2003.
15. Weinberger M: Clinical patterns and natural history of asthma. *J Pediatr* 142:S115, 2003.
16. Duffal, et al: Risk factors for acute wheezing in infants and children: Viruses, passive smoke, and IgE antibodies to inhalant allergens. *Pediatrics* 92:535, 1994.
17. Lemanske RF Jr: Is asthma an infectious disease? Thomas A. Neff Lecture. *Chest* 1223:385S, 2003.
18. Martinez FD, et al: Asthma and wheezing in the first six years of life. *N Engl J Med* 332:133, 1995.
19. Larsen GL: Asthma in children. *N Engl J Med* 326:1540, 1992.
20. Sears M, et al: Relation between airway responsiveness and serum IgE in children with asthma and in apparently normal children. *N Engl J Med* 325:1067, 1991.
21. Robinson DS,, et al: Predominant TH2-like bronchoalveolar T-lymphocyte population in atopic asthma. *N Engl J Med* 326:298, 1992.
22. Strachan DP: Family size, infection and atopy: The first decade of the "hygiene hypothesis." *Thorax* 55(Suppl 1):S2, 2000.
23. Ball, et al: Siblings, day-care attendance, and the risk of asthma and wheezing during childhood. *N Engl J Med* 343:538, 2000.
24. Gereda JE, et al: Levels of environmental endotoxin and prevalence of atopic disease. *JAMA* 284:11652, 2000.

25. Babu KS, Arshad SH: The role of allergy in the development of airway inflammation in children. *Paediatric Respir Rev* 4:40, 2003.
26. Kerem E, et al: Clinical physiologic correlations in acute asthma of childhood. *Pediatrics* 87:481, 1991.
27. Mayefsky JH, El-Shinawasay Y: The usefulness of pulse oximetry in evaluating acutely ill asthmatics. *Pediatr Emerg Care* 8:262, 1992.
28. Rudnitsky G, et al: Comparison of intermittent and continuously nebulized albuterol for treatment of asthma in an urban emergency department. *Ann Emerg Med* 20:456, 1991.
29. Schuh S, et al: High vs. low dose frequently administered, nebulized albuterol in children with severe, acute asthma. *Pediatrics* 83:513, 1989.
30. Paps MC, et al: A prospective, randomized study of continuous vs. intermittent nebulized albuterol for severe status asthmaticus in children. *Crit Care Med* 21:1479, 1993.
31. Nelson HS, et al: Improved bronchodilation with levalbuterol compared with racemic albuterol in patients with asthma. *J Allergy Clin Immunol* 102:943, 1998.
32. Gawchik SM, et al: The safety and efficacy of nebulized levalbuterol compared with racemic albuterol and placebo in the treatment of asthma in pediatric patients. *J Allergy Clin Immunol* 103:615, 1999.
33. Milgrom H, et al: Low-dose levalbuterol in children with asthma: Safety and efficacy in comparison with placebo and racemic albuterol. *J Allergy Clin Immunol* 108:938, 2001.
34. Slattery D, et al: Levalbuterol hydrochloride. *Pediatr Pulmonol* 33:151, 2002.
35. Ahrens R, Weinberger M: Levalbuterol and racemic albuterol: Are there therapeutic differences? *J Allergy Clin Immunol* 1008:681, 2001.
36. Levalbuterol for asthma. *Med Lett* 41:511, 1999.
37. Cates CJ, Rowe BH: Holding chambers versus nebulisers for β-agonist treatment of acute asthma. In: The Cochrane Library. Oxford, Update Software 3, 2001.
38. Kerem E, et al: Efficacy of albuterol administered by nebulizer vs. spacer device in children with acute asthma. *J Pediatr* 123:313, 1993.
39. Idris AH, et al: Emergency department treatment of severe asthma: MDI plus holding chamber is equivalent in effectiveness to nebulizer. *Chest* 103:665, 1993.
40. Scarfone RJ, Friedlander EY: β_2-Agonists in acute asthma: The evolving state of the art. *Ped Emerg Care* 18:442, 2002.
41. Schuh S, et al: Efficacy of frequent nebulized ipratropium bromide added to frequent high-dose albuterol therapy in severe childhood asthma. *J Pediatr* 126:639, 1995.
42. Plotnik LH, Ducharme FM: Should inhaled anticholinergics be added to beta$_2$ agonists for treating acute childhood and adolescent asthma: A systematic review. *BMJ* 317:971, 1998.
43. Stoodley RG, et al: The role of ipratropium bromide in the emergency management of acute asthma exacerbation: Meta-analysis of randomized clinical trials. *Ann Emerg Med* 34:8, 1999.
44. Qureshi F, et al: Effect of nebulized ipratropium on the hospitalization rates of children with asthma. *N Engl J Med* 339:1030, 1998.
45. Zorc JJ, et al: Ipratropium bromide added to asthma treatment in the pediatric emergency department. *Pediatrics* 103:748, 1999.
46. Becker JM, et al: Oral versus intravenous corticosteroids in children hospitalized with asthma. *J Allergy Clin Immunol* 103:586, 1999.
47. Qureshi F, et al: Comparative efficacy of oral dexamethasone versus oral prednisone in acute pediatric asthma. *J Pediatr* 139:20, 2001.
48. Gries DM, et al: A single dose of intramuscularly administered dexamethasone acetate is as effective as oral prednisone to treat asthma exacerbations in young children. *J Pediatr* 136:298, 2000.
49. Rachelefsky G: Treating exacerbations of asthma in children: The role of systemic corticosteroids. *Pediatrics* 112:382, 2003.
50. Dolan LM, et al: Short-term high-dose systemic steroids in children with asthma: The effect on the hypothalamic-pituitary-adrenal axis. *J Allergy Clin Immunol* 80:81, 1987.
51. Edmonds ML, et al: Early use of inhaled corticosteroids in the emergency department treatment of acute asthma (Cochrane Review). In The Cochrane Library. Oxford, Update Software 3, 2001.
52. Schuh S, et al: A comparison of inhaled fluticasone and oral prednisone for children with severe acute asthma. *N Engl J Med* 343:689, 2000.
53. Rowe BH, et al: Evidence-based treatments for acute asthma. *Respir Care* 46:1380, 2001.
54. Rowe BH, et al: Intravenous magnesium sulfate treatment for acute asthma in the emergency department: A systematic review of the literature. *Ann Emerg Med* 36:181, 2000.
55. Alter HJ, et al: Intravenous magnesium as an adjuvant in acute bronchospasm: A meta-analysis. *Ann Emerg Med* 36:191, 2000.
56. Ciarallo L, et al: Intravenous magnesium therapy for moderate to severe pediatric asthma: Results of a randomized, placebo-controlled trial. *J Pediatr* 129:809, 1996.
57. Pabon H, Monem G, Kissoon N: Safety and efficacy of $MgSO_4$: Infusions in children with status asthmaticus. *Pediatr Emerg Care* 10:200, 1994.
58. Rodrigo C, Rodrigo G: Treatment of acute asthma: Lack of therapeutic benefit and increase of the toxicity from aminophylline given in addition to high doses of salbutamol delivered by metered dose inhaler with a spacer. *Chest* 106:1071, 1994.
59. NAEPP Expert Panel Report: Guideline for the Diagnosis and Management of Asthma—Update on Selected Topics 2002. National Institutes of Health Publication 02-5075. Bethesda, MD, NIH, 2002.
60. Gaddy JN, et al: Bronchodilation with a potent and selective leukotriene d4 (ltd4) receptor antagonist (mk-571) in patients with asthma. *Am Rev Respir Dis* 146:358, 1992.
61. Henderson SO: Use of heliox-driven nebulizer therapy in the treatment of acute asthma. *Ann Emerg Med* 33:141, 1999.
62. Piva JP, et al: Heliox versus oxygen for nebulized aerosol therapy in children with lower airway obstruction. *Pediatr Crit Care Med* 3:6, 2002.
63. Rowe BH, et al: Inhaled budesonide in addition to oral corticosteroids to prevent asthma relapse following discharge from the emergency department. *JAMA* 281:2119, 1999.
64. Shay DK, et al: Bronchiolitis-associated hospitalizations among US children, 1980-1996. *JAMA* 282:1440, 1999.
65. Penlstein PH, et al: Evaluation of an evidence-based guideline for bronchiolitis. *Pediatrics* 104:1334, 1999.
66. Black PC: Systematic review of the biology and medical management of respiratory syncytial virus infection. *Respir Care* 48:209, 2003.
67. Welliver RC: Respiratory syncytial virus and other respiratory viruses. *Pediatr Infect Dis J* 22:S6, 2003.
68. Van den Hoogen BG, et al: A newly discovered human pneumovirus isolated from young children with respiratory tract disease. *Nat Med* 7:719, 2001.
69. Stein RT, et al: Respiratory syncytial virus in early life and risk of wheeze and allergy by age 13 years. *Lancet* 354:541, 1999.
70. Ehlenfield DR, et al: Eosinophilia at the time of respiratory syncytial virus bronchiolitis predicts childhood reactive airway disease. *Pediatrics* 105:79, 2000.
71. Andrade MA, et al: Acute otitis media in children with bronchiolitis. *Pediatrics* 101:617, 1998.
72. Roback MG, Dreitlin DA: Chest radiograph in the evaluation of first time wheezing episodes: Review of current

clinical practice and efficacy. *Pediatr Emerg Care* 14:181, 1998.
73. Swingler GH, et al: Randomized controlled trial of clinical outcome after chest radiograph in ambulatory acute lower respiratory infection in children. *Lancet* 351:404, 1998.
74. Kellner JD, et al: Efficacy of bronchodilator therapy in bronchiolitis: A meta-analysis. *Arch Pediatr Adolesc Med* 150:1166, 1996.
75. Kellner JD, et al: Bronchodilators for bronchiolitis (Cochrane Review). In The Cochrane Library. Oxford, Update Software 4, 2002.
76. Flores G, Horwitz RI: Efficacy of β_2-agonists in bronchiolitis: A reappraisal and meta-analysis. *Pediatrics* 100(2 Pt 1):233, 1997.
77. Schindler M: Do bronchodilators have an effect on bronchiolitis? *Crit Care* 6:111, 2002.
78. Menon K, et al: A randomized trial comparing the efficacy of epinephrine with salbutamol in the treatment of acute bronchiolitis. *J Pediatr* 126:1004, 1995.
79. Sanchez I, et al: Effect of racemic epinephrine and salbutamol on clinical score and pulmonary mechanics in infants with bronchiolitis. *J Pediatr* 122:145, 1993.
80. Reijonen T, et al: The clinical efficacy of nebulized racemic epinephrine and albuterol in acute bronchiolitis. *Arch Pediatr Adolesc Med* 149:686, 1995.
81. Garrison MM, et al: Systemic corticosteroids in infant bronchiolitis: A meta-analysis, *Pediatrics* 105:E44, 2000.
82. van Woensel JM, et al: Randomised double blind placebo controlled trial of prednisolone in children admitted to hospital with respiratory syncytial virus bronchiolitis. *Thorax* 52:634, 1997.
83. Martinon-Torres F, et al: Heliox therapy in infants with acute bronchiolitis. *Pediatrics* 109:68, 2002.
84. Joffe S, et al: Rehospitalization for respiratory syncytial virus among premature infants. *Pediatrics* 104:894, 1999.
85. Portier P, Richet C: De l'action anaphylactique de certains venins. *C R Soc Biol (Paris)* 54:170, 1902.
86. Bochner BS, Lichtenstein LM: Anaphylaxis. *N Engl J Med* 324:1785, 1991.
87. Uram R: What every pediatrician should know about anaphylaxis and anaphylactoid reactions. *Pediatr Ann* 29:737, 2000.
88. Murrant T, Bihari D: Anaphylaxis and anaphylactoid reactions. *ICJP* 54:322, 2000.
89. Bohlke K, et al: Risk of anaphylaxis after vaccination of children and adolescents. *Pediatrics* 112:815, 2003.
90. Winberry SL, Lieberman PL: Anaphylaxis. *Immunol Allergy Clin North Am* 15:447, 1995.
91. Sampson HA: Anaphylaxis and emergency treatment. *Pediatrics* 111:1601, 2003.
92. Lee JM, Greenes DS: Biphasic anaphylactic reactions in pediatrics. *Pediatrics* 106:762, 2000.
93. Sampson HA, et al: Fatal and near-fatal anaphylactic reactions to food in children and adolescents. *N Engl J Med* 327:380, 1992.
94. Wütrich B: Lethal or life-threatening allergic reactions to food. *Invest Allergol Clin Immunol* 10:59, 2000.
95. Simons FE, et al: Epinephrine absorption in children with a history of anaphylaxis. *J Allergy Clin Immunol* 101(1 Pt 1): 33, 1998.
96. Simons FE, et al: Epinephrine absorption in adults: Intramuscular versus subcutaneous injection. *J Allergy Clin Immunol* 108:871, 2001.
97. Yunginger JW, et al: Fatal food-induced anaphylaxis. *JAMA* 260:1450, 1988.
98. Korenblat P, et al: A retrospective study of epinephrine administration for anaphylaxis: How many doses are needed? *Allergy Asthma Proc* 20:383, 1999.
99. Novembre E, et al: Anaphylaxis in children: Clinical and allergologic features. *Pediatrics* 101:e8, 1998.
100. Dibs SD, Baker MD: Anaphylaxis in children: A 5-year experience. *Pediatrics* 99:e7, 1997.
101. Rovin JD, Rodgers BM: Pediatric foreign body aspiration. *Pediatr Rev* 21:86, 2000.
102. Lima JA, Fischer GB: Foreign body aspiration in children. *Pediatr Resp Reviews* 3:303, 2002.
103. Tan HK, et al: Airway foreign bodies (FB): A 10-year review. *Int J Pediatr Otorhinolaryngol* 56:91, 2000.
104. Schmidt H, Manegold BC: Foreign body aspiration in children. *Surg Endosc* 14:644, 2000.
105. Baharloo F, et al: Tracheobronchial foreign bodies: Presentation and management in children and adults. *Chest* 115:1357, 1999.
106. Reilly J, et al: Pediatric aerodigestive foreign body injuries are complications related to timeliness of diagnosis. *Laryngoscope* 107:17, 1997.
107. Swanson KL, et al: Flexible bronchoscopic management of airway foreign bodies in children. *Chest* 121:1695, 2002.

CHAPTER 168

Pediatric Respiratory Emergencies: Disease of the Lungs

Susan Kirelik and Brian Alverson

PNEUMONIA

PERSPECTIVE

Background

Acute infections of the respiratory tract are among the most common infections of the human host. Although most of these infections involve the upper respiratory tract, physicians caring for children in the emergency department commonly encounter lower respiratory infections, notably bronchiolitis and pneumonia. Pneumonia is an inflammation of the lung tissue; it most often is due to an infection, but occasionally may follow a noninfectious insult. Although the diagnosis of pneumonia may be suggested by clinical signs and symptoms, pneumonia is defined practically by an abnormal chest radiograph showing pulmonary infiltrates. The clinical picture of pneumonia is variable and may range from a mild illness to life-threatening disease. Given the multiplicity of agents that can cause pneumonia and the limitations of diagnostic testing, determining a precise etiologic diagnosis may be difficult. Clinical, laboratory, and radiographic findings sometimes suggest a specific organism, but often the etiology is unclear.

Epidemiology

Attack rates for pneumonia in children vary inversely with age, averaging 40 per 1000 in preschool-age children and decreasing gradually to 9 per 1000 in 9- to 15-year olds, with a male predominance ranging from 1.2:1 to 2:1.1 to 3. Three fourths of all deaths from pneumonia result from bacterial infections.[1]

The causative organisms also vary with the age of the child. Because the organism is not definitively identified in most pneumonia cases, it is difficult to determine the incidence of the specific etiologic agents.[2] Overall, it has been estimated that viral agents cause 60% to 90% of pneumonias.[3] Viral agents are more common in younger children. Bacteria predominate in neonates, but are a less common causative agent in toddlers and older children. Outside of the neonatal period, the incidence of bacterial agents is stable throughout different age groups.[3] Mixed viral and bacterial infections or concomitant bacterial infections may occur in one third of pneumonias.[3-5] *Chlamydia trachomatis* is a unique cause of pneumonia in infants 3 to 19 weeks old. *Bordetella pertussis* classically occurs in children younger than 1 year old, but also occurs in older children and adolescents.[6,7] *Mycoplasma pneumoniae* is one of the most common causes of pneumonia among children older than 5 years old and may play a role in younger children.[5,8] *Chlamydia pneumoniae* is more common in children older than 5 years, but also may cause infection in younger children.[8,9]

Among bacteria, group B streptococci and gram-negative bacilli predominate in neonates. *Ureaplasma urealyticum* and *Listeria monocytogenes* may cause illness in infants younger than 3 months old.[2] *Streptococcus pneumoniae* is the leading bacterial cause of pneumonia in all age groups beyond the newborn period; *Haemophilus influenzae* and *Staphylococcus aureus* are less common etiologic agents most often seen in the first years of life. The incidence of *H. influenzae* type B disease has decreased by 90% since the onset of immunization of infants and young children.[10] The heptavalent pneumococcal conjugate vaccine, Prevnar (Lederle Laboratories/Wyeth-Ayerst Pharmaceuticals, Wayne, NJ) was licensed by the U.S. Food and Drug Administration in 2000 and is recommended as a primary series at 2, 4, and 6 months, with a fourth booster dose given at 12 to 15 months. Clinical trials suggested 85% protection against serotype-specific cases of bacteremic pneumonia.[11] Studies have shown a decrease in carriage rates of the serotypes included in the daycare setting.[12] Pneumococcal polysaccharide vaccines have been recommended for children older than 2 years at high risk for pneumococcal disease since 1985, but they are not immunogenic in younger patients. Other, less common bacterial agents include group A streptococci, *Neisseria meningitidis,* and anaerobic bacteria, the last-mentioned being particularly common in the setting of aspiration pneumonia. Unusual causes of pneumonia include *Pseudomonas aeruginosa, Legionella pneumophila, Pneumocystis carinii,* and rickettsial infections. The incidence of *Mycobacterium tuberculosis* is increasing in the United States, particularly in urban and low-income areas and among nonwhite racial/ethnic groups.[13] Infants and adolescents are at highest risk in the United States.

Respiratory syncytial virus (RSV) and parainfluenza are the most common viral agents in infants younger than 1 year old. Viruses that may be responsible for neonatal pneumonia include rubella, cytomegalovirus (CMV), and herpes simplex virus. Other viral agents include influenza, adenovirus, rhinovirus, enterovirus, measles, varicella, and Epstein-Barr virus. The immunocompromised host is susceptible to all the aforementioned causes of pneumonia and mixed and opportunistic infections, including bacterial, viral (CMV, varicella), protozoan (*P. carinii*), and fungal disease.

PRINCIPLES OF DISEASE

Pathophysiology

The lung is protected from infection by a variety of local and systemic immune mechanisms. Passively acquired maternal antibodies are important in protection against *S. pneumoniae* and *H. influenzae* infections during the first few months of life. Children with altered protective mechanisms are at an increased risk of developing pneumonia; this includes children with congenital anatomic abnormalities (cleft palate, tracheoesophageal fistulae, pulmonary sequestration), immune deficiencies, neurologic alterations that predispose to aspiration (coma, seizures, cerebral palsy, general anesthesia), and alterations in quality of secreted mucus (cystic fibrosis [CF]).

Bacterial pneumonia and mycoplasmal infections are transmitted most often person to person by droplet aspiration. Asymptomatic upper airway colonization commonly occurs in children and may spread infection to other children.[14] Less commonly; bacterial pneumonia also may result from hematogenous spread from a distant focus or during primary bacteremia. Viral agents that cause pneumonia proliferate in the upper respiratory tract and spread contiguously to involve the lower respiratory tract. Viruses such as varicella, CMV, herpes simplex, Epstein-Barr, measles, and rubella also may infect the lung through hematogenous spread.

CLINICAL FEATURES

Symptoms and Signs

History

Clinical symptoms and signs of pneumonia in pediatric patients vary with the age of the patient, specific pathogen, and severity of the disease. Infants younger than 3 months old generally have respiratory symptoms, such as tachypnea, cough, retractions, and grunting, and nonlocalizing symptoms, including isolated fever or hypothermia, vomiting, poor feeding, irritability, and lethargy. Toddlers with *S. pneumoniae* may have nonspecific symptoms, such as high fever and lethargy, without respiratory symptoms. In general with increasing age, signs and symptoms in children become more specific and are manifestations of generalized infection, lower respiratory tract disease, and associated extrapulmonary disease, although pneumonia in any child may have only a few or subtle manifestations. General symptoms related to the infection include fever and chills, headache, rigors, and malaise. Symptoms of lower respiratory tract disease may include cough and wheezing. Pleural irritation may cause chest pain, abdominal distress, or neck pain and stiffness. Vomiting or poor oral intake can be seen with pneumonia of any cause and may imply more severe disease or dehydration.

Other important points that should be elicited in the history include birth and immunization history (particularly *H. influenzae* type B vaccine), sickle cell status, history of previous pneumonia or frequent infections, and presence of underlying chronic disease. Children with known respiratory (e.g., bronchopulmonary dysplasia or CF) or cardiac disease tend to tolerate pneumonia less well; children with primary or acquired immune deficiencies are prone to more severe and fulminant disease from common, uncommon, and opportunistic pathogens.

Physical Examination

Physical examination of a child with suspected pneumonia should begin by noting the general appearance and breathing pattern. Vital signs and oxygen saturation also should be evaluated immediately. Important findings include toxicity, level of alertness and interactiveness, color, and state of hydration and perfusion. Fever most often is present with bacterial pneumonia but may be low grade or absent in neonates and patients with nonbacterial disease. Cardiovascular parameters may indicate dehydration or, rarely, shock. Tachypnea, although not universal, seems to be the best indicator of pneumonia and may be the only manifestation in a young child.[15] The World Health Organization has published guidelines for the clinical diagnosis of pneumonia in developing countries and cites tachypnea and retractions as indicators of lower respiratory disease. Tachypnea is defined by the World Health Organization as a respiratory rate of greater than 50 breaths/min in infants younger than 1 year old and greater than 40 breaths/min in children older than 1 year.[16] Other manifestations of lower airway disease may include cough, wheezing, nasal flaring, retractions, and use of accessory muscles. The characteristics of the cough may aid the diagnosis; a staccato and paroxysmal cough in an infant may indicate pneumonia caused by *C. trachomatis* or *B. pertussis*. A hacking quality is often present with mycoplasmal disease. Auscultatory examination of an older child may reveal rales, wheezing, and diminished breath sounds, often with dullness to percussion and associated decreased fremitus. Although these findings may be present, in a younger child the clinical findings are much less consistent; rales may be masked by poor inspiratory effort or noisy upper airway sounds.

Pleural irritation may cause abdominal tenderness or meningismus, and pulmonary hyperinflation may cause downward displacement of the liver and spleen. Extrapulmonary findings may include rhinorrhea, pharyngitis, stridor, or exanthems with viral infections; conjunctivitis with chlamydial disease; pharyngitis and exanthems with mycoplasmal pneumonia; or extrapulmonary infections, such as soft tissue abscesses, otitis media, sinusitis, meningitis, and pericarditis, with bacterial pathogens.

SPECIFIC DISORDERS

Bacterial Pneumonia

Perspective

S. pneumoniae is one of the most common bacterial agents causing pneumonia in children.[13] Children at increased risk of developing infection from *S. pneumoniae* are children with immune deficiency, chronic renal disease, or functional or anatomic asplenia and Native Americans.[11] *S. aureus* pneumonia, although less common, tends to cause a more severe pneumonia, with more than 70% of all cases occurring in the first year of life.[18] Children with foreign body aspiration, immunosuppression, or skin infections may be at increased risk of *S. aureus* pneumonia. Progression of the disease is rapid, and empyema (90%), pneumatocele (50%), pneumothorax (25%), and bacteremia are common complications (Figure 168-1).[23] Since the mid-

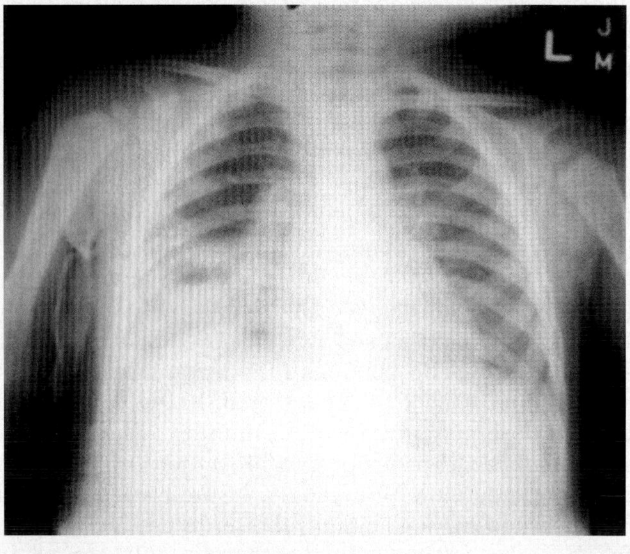

Figure 168-1. Radiograph shows staphylococcal pneumonia with empyema and abscess on right. (Courtesy of Brianna Enriquez, MD, and Marianne Gausche-Hill, MD.)

1990s, community-acquired methicillin-resistant *S. aureus* has been identified as an agent that may cause pneumonia in children. In contrast to classically described methicillin-resistant *S. aureus,* which is typically broadly resistant and nosocomially acquired, this agent is resistant to fewer antibiotics.[24]

Before immunization, *H. influenzae* was the second most common bacterial cause of pneumonia. Its incidence has decreased by 90% since the onset of effective immunization.[10] Although *H. influenzae* previously was considered a disease of younger children, most cases now occur in older children.[25] Although often clinically indistinguishable from *S. pneumoniae, H. influenzae* pneumonia has a higher incidence of associated pleural effusions (25% to 75%) and bacteremia (75% to 95%).[26] Other foci of infection are more common and include meningitis, epiglottitis, septic arthritis, pericarditis, soft tissue infection, and otitis media.[26]

Although still uncommon, the incidence of group A streptococcal pneumonia may have increased since the 1980s. One study reported an increase in the incidence from 0.16 per 100,000 in 1992 to 0.35 per 100,000 in 1999 in Canada, whereas another study suggested stable rates since the 1980s.[27,28] Group A streptococcal pneumonia may occur sporadically and may occur as a complication of varicella.[27] It is typically a severe illness with abrupt onset and rapid progression to toxicity and a high fatality rate (30% to 60% fatality rate reported in a study of all ages).[27]

Clinical Features

Bacterial pneumonia beyond the neonatal period generally has a sudden onset; fever is almost universal (most >39° C). Patients may or may not have a cough and often appear relatively toxic with tachypnea disproportionate to the fever. Confined rales or wheezes and localized decreased or tubular breath sounds commonly occur in older children, although the physical examination in a younger child may be completely unrevealing.

Diagnostic Considerations

Patients with pneumococcal infections often have a preceding dramatic presentation with high white blood cell (WBC) counts with associated pleural effusion and bacteremia in 10% to 30% of children.[18] Radiographic findings may show an alveolar infiltrate in a patchy or consolidated lobar (Figure 168-2) or subsegmental distribution, although patients with bacterial pneumonia may have an interstitial infiltrate.[17] Bilateral involvement, pleural effusion, pneumatocele, and pneumothorax may occur with more severe disease. Although the WBC count may be normal with bacterial pneumonia, leukocytosis often occurs, sometimes exceeding 20,000/mm^3. Uncomplicated bacterial pneumonia often has a rapid response to institution of chemotherapy; a stagnant or worsening clinical picture should prompt further investigation.

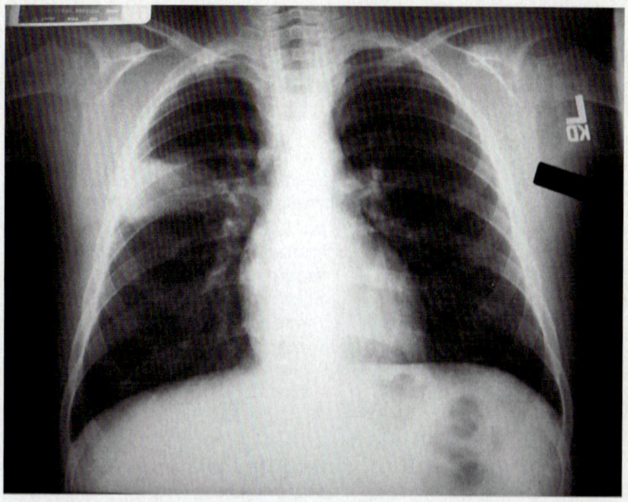

Figure 168-2. Radiograph shows pneumococcal pneumonia with infiltrate in right upper lobe. (Courtesy of Marianne Gausche-Hill, MD.)

Management

Of concern is the emergence of resistance to penicillin and cephalosporins.[19] The clinical significance of resistant pneumococcal pneumonia in children is unclear. At this time, it seems that presentation and outcome of otherwise healthy children with pneumonia secondary to resistant pneumococcus may not differ significantly from the outcome of children with pneumonia secondary to penicillin-sensitive pneumococcus.[19-21] Pneumonia caused by *S. pneumoniae* may be complicated by empyema, pleural effusion, lung abscess, or necrotizing pneumonia. Since the 1990s, there seems to have been an increase in the incidence of such complications, with one study noting an increase from 22.6% in 1994 to 53% in 1999 in children hospitalized with pneumococcal pneumonia.[22] It does not seem that this increased incidence is related to intermediate resistant organisms. It is unclear if highly resistant organisms play a role.[22] High-dose amoxicillin is recommended for initial outpatient treatment of suspected pneumococcal pneumonia in children younger than 4 years old; a standard dose may be used in older children who are immunocompetent (Tables 168-1 and 168-2).

VIRAL PNEUMONIA

Viral pneumonia occurs more commonly in the winter and generally has a gradual onset over several days, often with associated cough, coryza, and low-grade fever. Tachypnea may be the only physical finding; however, retractions, rales, and wheezing are common, with grunting, cyanosis, lethargy, dehydration, and apnea apparent in more severely affected children. The diagnosis of viral pneumonia is often made clinically. Rapid antigen testing may be useful in the diagnosis of RSV or influenza A and B. Other viral agents may be diagnosed with culture of nasopharyngeal secretions. Although in the past the use of viral cultures was limited by the time required to grow viruses, improved

Table 168-1. Antibiotics for Treatment of Pediatric Pneumonia

Age Group	Agents	Outpatient Treatment	Inpatient Treatment
0-12 wk	Group B streptococcus Gram-negative bacilli (*Listeria monocytogenes*)		Ampicillin + cefotaxime *or* Ceftriaxone*
	Bordetella pertussis or *Chlamydia trachomatis*	Erythromycin estolate	Erythromycin estolate
12 wk–preschool age	*Streptococcus pneumoniae,* (*Haemophilus influenzae, Staphylococcus aureus,* Group A streptococcus, *Neisseria meningitidis*)	Amoxicillin *or* Amoxicillin-clavulanic acid *or* Cefuroxime axetil *or* Azithromycin *or* Clarithromycin	Cefuroxime *or* Cefotaxime *or* Ceftriaxone *or* Clindamycin
	Mycoplasma pneumoniae or *Chlamydia pneumoniae*	Add erythromycin *or* Azithromycin *or* Clarithromycin	Add erythromycin (IV or PO) *or* Azithromycin (IV or PO) *or* Clarithromycin (PO)
	MRSA or critically ill		Add vancomycin
School age–adolescent	*M. pneumoniae* or *C. pneumoniae*	Erythromycin *or* Azithromycin *or* Clarithromycin *or* Tetracycline (>8 yr old) or fluoroquinolone (>16 yr old)	Cefuroxime *or* Cefotaxime *or* Ceftriaxone *or* Clindamycin *and* Macrolide
	MRSA or critically ill		Add vancomycin

*Ceftriaxone contraindicated in infants <1 month old.
MRSA; methicillin-resistant *Staphylococcus aureus*.

Table 168-2. Antibiotics for the Treatment of Bacterial Pneumonia: Daily Dosage

Agent	Daily Dosage*
Oral	
Amoxicillin (standard dose)	20-50 mg/kg div tid
Amoxicillin (high dose)	80-100 mg/kg div bid
Amoxicillin–clavulanate	25-45 mg/kg div bid†
Azithromycin	10 mg/kg day 1, then 5 mg/kg q day on days 2-5
Cefuroxime axetil	30 mg/kg div q12h
Clarithromycin	15 mg/kg div q12h
Erythromycin	40-50 mg/kg div q6h
Penicillin V	25-50 mg/kg div q6–8h
Trimethoprim-sulfamethoxazole	8-12 mg/kg div q12h
Parenteral	
Ampicillin	150 mg/kg div q6h
Ampicillin-sulbactam	150 mg/kg div q6h
Cefotaxime	150-200 mg/kg div q8h
Ceftriaxone	100 mg/kg div q12h
Cefuroxime	150 mg/kg div q8h
Chloramphenicol	50 mg/kg div q6h‡
Clindamycin	40 mg/kg div q6h
Gentamicin	5-7.5 mg/kg div q8h‡
Methicillin-nafcillin	150-200 mg/kg div q4–6h
Oxacillin	200 mg/kg div q4–6h
Penicillin G (aqueous)	100,000-400,000 U/d div q4–6h

*Dosages and intervals may differ in neonates.
†Use 875-mg tablet, 200-mg or 400-mg chewable tablets or 200 mg/5 mL, 400 mg/5 mL, 600 mg/5 mL suspensions for twice-daily dosing.
‡Must monitor serum levels.

culture techniques may yield results within 2 days and prove useful in a patient in whom cause needs to be established.

The WBC count is variable, but tends to be less than 15,000/mm^3 with lymphocyte predominance. Radiographic findings typically include hyperinflation and peribronchial thickening with diffuse increase in interstitial findings. Patchy areas of consolidation may be present, representing lobular atelectasis or alveolar pneumonia. Although lobar consolidation and small pleural effusions may occur in viral pneumonia, these findings are more consistent with a bacterial cause.

Most viral pneumonias resolve without specific therapy. Because of the likelihood of bacterial superinfection and the difficulty in differentiating between bacterial and viral pneumonia, antibiotics may be prudent in a more severely ill child. Potential complications include dehydration, local progression of the disease, bronchiolitis obliterans, and apnea (most commonly in the first 3 months of life).[29]

Mycoplasmal Pneumonia

Mycoplasmal pneumonia accounts for 10% to 20% of all pneumonias and was thought to occur most commonly in 5- to 18-year-olds. It is now clear that it also may play a significant role in younger children.[5] Mycoplasmal pneumonia is rare in infants less than 1 year old.[30] Classically the onset is gradual and insidious, but some patients also may present with abrupt onset of symptoms similar to its bacterial counterpart.[5] Prodromal symptoms include fever, headache, and malaise followed several days later by a nonproductive, hacking cough. Patients also may present with pertussis-like illness. Other symptoms of infection may include hoarseness, sore throat, and chest pain; coryza is unusual. Children with mycoplasmal pneumonia generally appear nontoxic. Patients may have rales, with wheezing occurring less often. Pharyngitis, cervical lymphadenopathy, conjunctivitis, and otitis media occur occasionally. Bullous myringitis, although rare, is believed to be indicative of *Mycoplasma*.[30] Rash is present in 10% of patients and may be urticarial, erythema multiforme, maculopapular, or vesicular.[31] The course may be complicated by pneumatocele, pleural effusion, pneumothorax, or bronchiectasis. *Mycoplasma,* typically thought to be a benign and self-limited infection, has been shown to play a significant role in exacerbating asthma.[5] *Mycoplasma* may cause chronic pulmonary structural abnormalities.[5]

Physical findings generally are less impressive than the radiographic picture; involvement is usually unilateral and in the lower lobes. The radiographic findings are protean, however, and may show lobar consolidation, scattered segmental infiltrates, or interstitial disease. Pleural effusions may occur, but are uncommon. The WBC count is usually normal; the erythrocyte sedimentation rate tends to be elevated.

Laboratory diagnosis is problematic. Although used in the past, bedside cold agglutination testing is a poor indication of infection, especially in patients younger than 12 years old.[30] Infection often is diagnosed clinically and treated empirically. Diagnosis may be confirmed with acute and convalescent antibody titers; however, patients may take 4 to 6 weeks to seroconvert, and some patients may fail to mount an immune response.[5] Culture is not routinely available; polymerase chain reaction diagnosis at this time is available only from research laboratories.[3] Complications are varied but unusual and include hemolytic anemia, myopericarditis, neurologic disease (meningoencephalitis, Guillain-Barré syndrome, transverse myelitis, cranial neuropathy), arthritis, and rash.

Chlamydial Pneumonia

C. trachomatis is a common sexually transmitted infection, causing cervical infection in 2% to 30% of pregnant women.[9] It can be transmitted from the genital tract of infected mothers to their newborn infants, resulting in conjunctivitis in 22% to 44% and pneumonia in 5% to 20%.[9] An infant with pneumonia caused by *C. trachomatis* presents at 3 to 19 weeks old after colonization with the organism at birth. The illness usually begins with nasal congestion followed by cough. In half of cases, conjunctivitis precedes the onset of respiratory symptoms. The infant is often afebrile, alert, and tachypneic, with a repetitive staccato cough. The cough may interfere with feeding or sleeping. It can resemble the paroxysms of pertussis and occasionally precipitates episodes of alarming respiratory distress. Mild retractions and diffuse inspiratory crepitant rales are noted on chest examination, with expiratory wheezing usually absent or minimal. Middle ear abnormalities are present in half of cases.

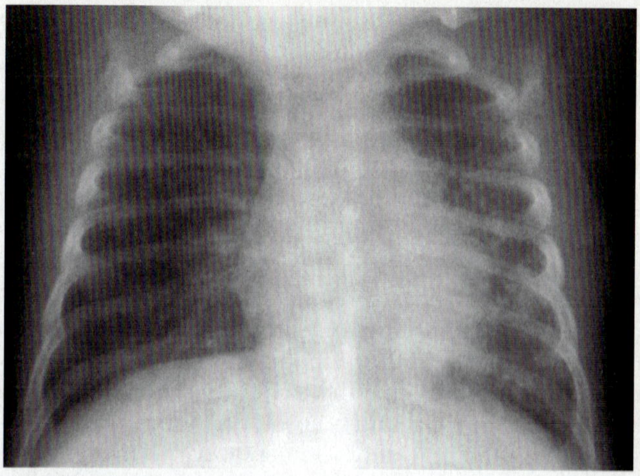

Figure 168-3. Radiograph shows chlamydial pneumonia in an infant. Note the symmetrical interstitial infiltrates. (Courtesy of Michael Diament, MD.)

The radiograph usually shows hyperinflation with bilateral and symmetrical diffuse interstitial infiltrates (Figure 168-3). The total WBC count is usually normal but often with an eosinophilia of more than 400/mm^3.[9] Definitive diagnosis is made by isolating the organism in the tissue culture; diagnostic tests based on polymerase chain reaction are more sensitive than fluorescent antibody stain or tissue culture, but may not be as specific.[13] Although often a mild illness, chlamydial pneumonia may be complicated by apnea and hypoxemia. Treatment with erythromycin may shorten the course; however, the disease tends to be protracted with cough and tachypnea often requiring weeks to clear.

C. pneumoniae is a species of *Chlamydia* that is antigenically, genetically, and morphologically distinct from other *Chlamydia* species. *C. pneumoniae* infection is readily transmitted from person to person. *C. pneumoniae* may play a role in respiratory tract infections in infants and young children and may cause mild illness or asymptomatic infection in children and adults. As with *Mycoplasma, C. pneumoniae* may play a much greater role in pediatric pneumonia than previously thought. It also commonly may be present as a mixed bacterial infection.[5] *C. pneumoniae* has been reported to cause sore throat, fever, headache, pertussis-like cough, pneumonia, and influenza-like illness.[32] Outbreaks have been reported in schools, daycare centers, military camps, adolescents, and families.[33] Infection with *C. pneumoniae* can trigger acute episodes of wheezing in children with asthma.

Pertussis

Pertussis, or whooping cough, is a respiratory tract infection seen most commonly in infants younger than 6 months old (38% of cases are in children <6 months old, and 71% of cases are in children <5 years old). The incidence of pertussis increased in the 1980s and

1990s, especially in adolescents and adults.[34] Despite high immunization rates, 77 infants died of pertussis in the 1980s.[34]

The disease is characterized by three clinical stages: catarrhal stage, paroxysmal stage, and convalescent stage.[13] In infants, the disease begins with mild upper respiratory tract symptoms and cough; this catarrhal stage usually lasts 1 to 2 weeks. The disease progresses to severe paroxysms of a staccato cough followed by post-tussive emesis and may be accompanied by periods of cyanosis and apnea in infants younger than 6 months of age.[7] Classic whoop is rare, occurring only in 6% of patients, generally in children older than 2 to 3 years old. Fever is often absent, and between paroxysms the examination is remarkably normal. Paroxysms sometimes may be induced on physical examination by gagging the patient. The paroxysmal stage lasts 2 to 4 weeks and is followed by a convalescent stage during which symptoms gradually wane. The duration of the illness in complicated cases may be 6 to 10 weeks.[7]

Immunization is only 80% effective in providing immunity after three doses: Pertussis still must be considered in an immunized infant, although the illness may be mild.[13] The WBC count is usually elevated, exceeding 15,000/mm^3 and occasionally 40,000/mm^3, with a marked lymphocytosis, although this finding may not be present in infants younger than 3 to 6 months old. The chest radiograph may show a "shaggy" right heart border or have clear lung fields. The organism is most easily recovered in the catarrhal or early paroxysmal stages and is rarely found after the fourth week of illness.[13] *B. pertussis* can be cultured from nasopharyngeal secretions. Cultures may be negative during the first week or after the fourth week of illness in immunized patients or patients treated with antibiotics.[13] Direct fluorescent antibody staining may be used, but this test has low specificity and variable sensitivity.[13] Diagnosis made by direct fluorescent antibody should be confirmed by culture.

Polymerase chain reaction may be more sensitive and specific, but availability is variable. Pertussis is a particularly severe disease in the first year of life; complications are common and include apneic episodes, seizures, secondary bacterial pneumonia, encephalopathy, and death. Pertussis has been increasing in incidence among immunized children and young adults who have waning immunity.[6] Adults are believed to be a significant source for the disease within the community. The illness in these patients does not follow the classic stages as described here. These patients have a mild but prolonged course. A dry cough is the predominant symptom, often lasting 3 weeks or more. All children younger than 6 months old with presumed pertussis should be observed in the hospital for monitoring and supportive care and should be treated with erythromycin. Other macrolides and trimethoprim-sulfamethoxazole are other possible alternatives.[13] Antimicrobials have no effect on the disease progress after the paroxysmal stage is established but may be beneficial because they limit the spread of organism.

Aspiration Pneumonia

Aspiration pneumonia may be due to mechanical, chemical, or bacterial causes. Bacterial aspiration occurs in children with anatomic abnormalities and central nervous system disturbances that impair normal swallowing or protective airway reflexes. Pulmonary damage results from chemical (e.g., stomach acid) and bacterial (gastrointestinal and upper respiratory organisms) insults. Within several hours of the aspiration, the child may have onset of cough, tachypnea, and fever. Physical examination commonly reveals rales and wheezing with cyanosis as the disease progresses. Radiographic findings include localized and diffuse infiltrates, which are often bilateral.

Pneumonia in an Immunocompromised Host

Children with chronic disease and congenital, acquired, and iatrogenic immune deficiencies are susceptible to the aforementioned respiratory pathogens and to a multitude of opportunistic organisms, including *P. carinii,* CMV, and fungi. Presenting symptoms may be similar to normal hosts; however, the course tends to be more severe and fulminant. Rigorous attempts to identify a pathogen are warranted, and patients should be hospitalized while awaiting the results of cultures for monitoring, supportive therapy, and treatment with antibiotics active against a broad spectrum of organisms. If the patient fails to improve after initial therapy, obtaining tissue for diagnosis of potentially treatable organisms is necessary.

DIAGNOSTIC STRATEGIES

Not every child suspected to have pneumonia requires laboratory or radiographic evaluation. A well-appearing child with cough and rales may be diagnosed clinically and treated as an outpatient. A child who appears ill or in whom the diagnosis is unclear requires further evaluation. Young children with high fever and a leukocytosis may have an occult pneumonia. A chest radiograph should be considered in these patients.[35]

Laboratory Studies

Any child with pneumonia is at risk for hypoxemia and should have pulse oximetry to determine oxygen saturation. An arterial blood gas study may be considered in a child with severe respiratory distress. Serum electrolytes, blood urea nitrogen, and creatinine are useful in assessing the degree of dehydration and guiding fluid management when clinically relevant.

Further laboratory studies are obtained only as warranted to help identify the disease process and potential complications. The leukocyte count may be useful in differentiating causes of pneumonia; peripheral WBC counts greater than 15,000/mm^3, with predominance of mature and immature granulocytes, suggest bacterial infection, with pneumococcal pneumonia typically producing the highest WBC counts.[36] Marked leukocytosis and toxic granulation of WBCs also may help identify a child at risk for bacteremia and its potential complications. Normal to elevated WBC counts with lymphocytosis may be seen in viral infections, and eosinophilia suggests chlamydial disease. Increased WBC counts with extreme lymphocytosis typically are associated with pertussis, but this hematologic finding may be absent in infants younger than 6 months old. Blood cultures may grow pathogens in only 1% to 10% of cases of bacterial pneumonia. In a well-appearing child with an uncomplicated pneumonia, blood culture is unlikely to be helpful.[2,37] When blood culture is positive, however, it identifies the specific pathogen and should be considered in an ill patient in whom hospitalization with bacterial pneumonia is likely. Sputum cultures may be useful in adolescents, but are technically impossible and not useful in younger children.[38,39]

Patients with pleural effusions should have lateral decubitus radiographs to assess effusion size and loculation. Computed tomography scan is useful to provide greater detail of effusions and lung abnormalities.[40] Patients with significant effusions should have thoracentesis for diagnostic and therapeutic purposes. Although most suggestive of bacterial infection, parapneumonic effusions also occur with mycoplasmal and occasionally with viral infections.[41] The fluid should be sent for Gram stain and culture (anaerobic and aerobic bacterial) and cell count and differential, total protein, pH, and glucose determinations. Interpretation of pleural fluid in children follows adult guidelines (see Chapter 76). Cultures for rare pathogens may be considered if initial assessment is not diagnostic. Bronchoscopy with bronchoalveolar lavage may be useful in a severely ill child.

Nasopharyngeal viral cultures, antigen detection for specific viral or bacterial agents, and serum antibodies for specific agents may be helpful in determining certain etiologic agents. Although most pediatric patients with tuberculosis do not have pulmonary symptoms, skin testing for tuberculosis should be considered for patients with lobar pneumonia, pulmonary effusions, or hilar adenopathy. Acid-fast bacilli often may be shown on an early morning gastric aspirate.[42] Sputum specimens generally are not helpful in a child younger than 8 years old because of contamination by organisms of the upper respiratory tract.

Bacterial cultures of upper respiratory secretions are of no value and usually grow either normal flora or organisms that reflect only colonization. Although transtracheal sampling and direct aspiration from the lung may permit a more precise diagnosis, the invasiveness of these tests limits their usefulness. Evaluation of potential additional infectious foci should be guided clinically with particular attention to the meninges, pericardium, epiglottis, soft tissue, and joints to identify the offending pathogen and to delineate the disease process fully.

Radiology

A chest radiograph may be obtained to confirm or rule out an infiltrate. Rarely a dehydrated child with pneumonia may have a normal study. The radiograph also may provide clues as to the underlying disease process. Although great variability exists, bacterial pathogens classically produce alveolar infiltrates in a lobar distribution, but may produce diffuse interstitial infiltrates.[43] Viral and chlamydial infections tend to appear as diffuse interstitial infiltrates, commonly with hyperinflation and atelectasis. Chest radiographs also identify multilobar disease, pleural effusions, pneumatoceles, and pneumothorax (Figure 168-4). Hilar adenopathy may indicate tuberculosis or malignancy.

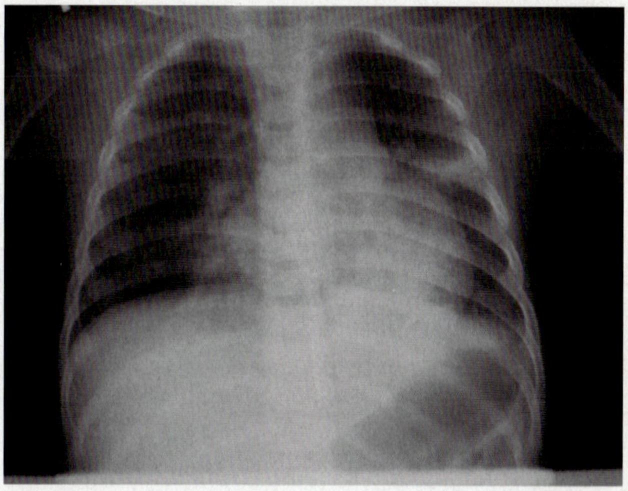

Figure 168-4. Radiograph shows multilobar pneumonia in a child with respiratory distress. (Courtesy of Marianne Gausche-Hill, MD.)

DIFFERENTIAL CONSIDERATIONS

The major conditions to be differentiated in children with pneumonia include bacterial pneumonias amenable to conventional antibiotics, viral disease, other unusual infectious causes (mycobacterial, protozoal, fungal), and noninfectious pathologic conditions (Box 168-1). Certain features help differentiate the common infectious causes (Table 168-3). As detailed previously, each disease entity has certain classic historical, clinical, and laboratory findings. At the extremes of presentation, these diseases can be distinguished easily; however, the broad spectrum of illness for each process may make accurate diagnosis in an individual patient difficult. No specific feature reliably differentiates patients with bacterial infection from children with nonbacterial pneumonia. Because of limitations of reliably detecting bacterial pneumonia by culture technique, one should presume a bacterial cause in a child with a temperature greater than 39° C, clinical toxicity, lobar infiltrate, or pleural effusions. Although it is often difficult to make a precise etiologic diagnosis, consideration of host factors, epidemiology, and the clinical picture with judicious use of laboratory tests generally points the clinician toward the likely diagnosis and allows for effective patient management.

BOX 168-1. Noninfectious Causes That May Present as Pneumonia

Radiologic Technique
Inadequate inspiration
Breast shadow
Thymus
Uneven grid on film
Underpenetrated film

Primary Pulmonary
Asthma
Bronchiectasis
Atelectasis
Bronchopulmonary dysplasia
Cystic fibrosis
Pulmonary sequestration
α_1-Antitrypsin deficiency

Aspiration
Foreign body
Chemical
Recurrent caused by anatomic or physiologic disorders

Primary Cardiac
Congenital heart disease
Congestive heart failure

Pulmonary Infarction
Sickle cell vaso-occlusive crisis
Pulmonary embolism

Collagen Vascular Disorders
Acute Respiratory Distress Syndrome
Pleural Effusion
Neoplasm

From Boyer KM, Cherry JD: Nonbacterial pneumonia. In Feigin RD, Cherry JD (eds): *Textbook of Pediatric Infectious Diseases*, 2nd ed. Philadelphia, WB Saunders, 1987.

Complications

Several complications of pneumonia result from local and systemic effects of the infection. Pleural effusions or empyemas accumulate most often with bacterial pathogens (notably *S. pneumoniae, H. influenzae,* and *S. aureus*) but are occasionally associated with mycoplasmal, viral, and tuberculous pneumonia. An increase in the occurrence of such complications seemed to have occurred in the 1990s for reasons unknown.[44] Similarly, lung abscess, pneumatocele, and pneumothorax are local complications primarily seen with bacterial disease, particularly with *S. aureus.* Extensive pulmonary involvement of any cause may lead occasionally to hypoxia and progressive respiratory failure with multiple organ failure. Apnea without other symptoms is seen most often in viral, chlamydial, and pertussis infections in infants younger than 3 months. The most common systemic complication of pneumonia is dehydration, which occurs as a result of decreased intake from malaise and excessive respiratory effort and increased losses of fluid caused by vomiting, fever, and tachypnea. Another systemic complication of bacterial disease is the development of additional infectious foci resulting from bacteremia (e.g., meningitis, epiglottitis, pericarditis, septic arthritis, and soft tissue infections). Mycoplasmal pneumonia rarely is associated with meningitis, encephalitis, arthritis, and hemolytic anemia.

MANAGEMENT AND DISPOSITION

Treatment of pneumonia in a pediatric patient consists of appropriate antimicrobial use and supportive therapy (see Table 168-1). Because of the difficulty in identifying an etiologic agent, antibiotic choice is generally empirical. The three most important factors in directing management are the patient's age, likely pathogen, and degree of illness. An infant younger than 2 months old with pneumonia should be admitted to the hospital. This age group is immunologically immature, and signs of sepsis may be subtle. Blood, urine, and cerebrospinal fluid cultures generally are indicated before initiation of antibiotics.

In an infant 2 to 3 months old, blood and urine cultures are appropriate. The decision to perform a lumbar puncture depends on clinical suspicion of central nervous system infection. Ampicillin plus an aminoglycoside or ampicillin and a third-generation cephalosporin would be appropriate initial antibiotic choices for an infant younger than 1 month old (although ceftriaxone is contraindicated in infants <1 month old). Ampicillin and a third-generation cephalosporin are reasonable for an infant 1 to 3 months old. If *C. trachomatis* or *B. pertussis* is suspected, the infant also should be treated with erythromycin after appropriate diagnostic samples have been obtained; other macrolides or sulfonamides (trimethoprim-sulfamethoxazole) may be an alternative in older infants and children.[13] Supportive therapy in this age group consists of fever control and intravenous hydration. A trial of inhaled β-agonists may be indicated if the patient is wheezing or in significant respiratory distress; supplemental oxygen and respiratory support should be provided as needed. All infants should be monitored with continuous pulse oximetry because apnea and respiratory failure may be precipitous.

An older child with pneumonia should be categorized into likely bacterial, viral, or mycoplasmal disease if possible. Because no single pathognomonic test exists to differentiate bacterial from viral infection, the physician must base the presumptive etiologic diagnosis on clinical, radiographic, and laboratory findings. Although the categorization is not always clear, a toxic child with high fever, lobar consolidation, and leukocytosis is likely to have a bacterial process, whereas a child with a disease of gradual onset, low-grade fever, and interstitial infiltrate with air trapping is more likely to have a viral process.

If a viral agent is suspected and the child is not ill, antibiotics may be withheld. Uncomplicated bacterial pneumonia in immunocompetent children is safe to treat as an outpatient disease. A well-appearing infant

Table 168-3. Pneumonia Syndromes

	Bacterial	Viral	*Chlamydia*	*Mycoplasma*
Historical				
Age	Any	Any	4-16 wk	5-18 yr
Fever	High (>39° C)	Low grade	Usually none	Low
Onset	Abrupt Often after upper respiratory infection	Gradual	Gradual	Gradual
Cough	Productive	Nonproductive	Staccato	Hacking
Associated symptoms	Chest pain Focal infarct	Myalgias Rash Sore throat Coryza	Conjunctivitis	Headache Sore throat Rash
Physical	Toxic appearance			
Lungs	Confined rales	Diffuse rales Wheeze Stridor	Diffuse rales Rare wheeze	Unilateral rales
Chest radiograph				
Infiltrate	Lobar or segmental	Interstitial	Diffuse Interstitial	Lobar or diffuse
Pleural effusion	Occasional	Rare	None	Rare
Other	Pneumatocele Abscess	Hyperinflation Atelectasis	Hyperinflation	
Laboratory	Increased WBC granulocytosis	Normal or increased WBC Lymphocytosis	Normal WBC Eosinophilia	Normal WBC
Pathogens (common)	*Streptococcus pneumoniae* *Haemophilus influenzae* *Staphylococcus aureus* <2 mo: Group B streptococcus Gram-negative enterics *L. monocytogenes*	RSV Parainfluenza Influenza Adenovirus Enterovirus	*C. trachomatis*	*M. pneumoniae*

WBC, white blood cell; RSV, respiratory syncytial virus.

or preschool-age child with isolated pneumonia may be treated with oral antibiotics on an outpatient basis. In an infant beyond the neonatal period or a preschool-age child, amoxicillin and amoxicillin–clavulanic acid are considered appropriate first-line agents. Cefuroxime axetil or high-dose amoxicillin (80 to 100 mg/kg/day) may be used when resistant *S. pneumoniae* is suspected. Azithromycin or clarithromycin also are considered appropriate first-line oral agents in this age group by some authors.[2,39] One study of the treatment of pediatric community-acquired pneumonia showed no difference in clinical cure rate when azithromycin, erythromycin estolate, and amoxicillin–clavulanic acid were compared.[45] A macrolide is the first-line antibiotic choice in a school-age child or adolescent in whom *M. pneumoniae* and *C. pneumoniae* are more common. Every child with bacterial pneumonia treated as an outpatient should be re-evaluated within 24 hours. Patients who are not afebrile, clinically improved, and well hydrated should be evaluated at this time for possible admission to the hospital for parenteral antibiotic therapy. For patients in whom signs of bacteremia are present, a single dose of intramuscular ceftriaxone followed by outpatient oral therapy is recommended. In these cases, close follow-up monitoring is crucial.

For a patient who is admitted to the hospital, intravenous therapy with cefuroxime, cefotaxime, or ceftriaxone is appropriate. Addition of a macrolide should be considered if *M. pneumoniae* is a possible etiologic agent. Vancomycin should be added if methicillin-resistant *S. aureus* is suspected.[27] If an organism has been identified, an antibiotic with a more specific spectrum might be indicated.

Since the 1980s, *S. pneumoniae* has been developing increasing resistance to penicillin and other antibiotics; in general, this has not been clinically relevant because higher doses overcome the relative resistance. Clinical outcomes with intermediate resistance levels seem to be unchanged.[46] These patients still respond to penicillin and the cephalosporins at higher doses. If the patient does not respond clinically after a trial of these agents or if the patient is critically ill, use of vancomycin with or without rifampin is recommended.[47]

Supportive therapy includes hydration and fever control with antipyretics. Appropriate laboratory testing should be performed to attempt identification of more virulent pathogens. The child should be examined for development of an additional infectious focus, and a repeat radiograph may be considered to determine spread or development of a pleural effusion.

Indications for hospitalization at the time of diagnosis include toxic appearance, vomiting or dehydration, respiratory compromise (distress, hypoxia, or inadequate ventilation), multilobar disease, pleural effusions, impaired immune function, and unstable social environments. Strong consideration should be given to hospitalizing children younger than 6 months old because they are less tolerant of bacterial pneumonia than are older children. Supportive therapy for the inpatient should include maintenance of fluid and electrolyte balance and fever control, supplemental oxygen, inhaled bronchodilators, ventilatory assistance, and pleural fluid drainage as indicated. Parenteral antibiotic therapy should be administered until clinical improvement occurs. Other factors that influence duration of parenteral antibiotic treatment include the age of the patient, specific pathogen, presence of bacteremia, and any additional infectious foci.

A trial of bronchodilators may be worthwhile (aerosolized β_2-adrenergic agent) even in the absence of wheezing and always should be considered in a patient with respiratory distress. Although this treatment is not always successful, if the child responds with diminished wheezing, improved aeration, or reduced work of breathing, one may continue with nebulized bronchodilators.

Children with neurologic or anatomic abnormalities who aspirate oral or gastric contents are susceptible to pneumonia predominantly from anaerobes. Penicillin and clindamycin are appropriate first-line antibiotic choices. In seriously ill patients, agents such as chloramphenicol, metronidazole, and cefoxitin may be more useful. Nosocomial infections should be treated with antibiotics also active against aerobes and gram-negative bacilli. Children with significant aspiration should be admitted to the hospital, and supportive therapy should include hydration, supplemental oxygen, oropharyngeal suctioning, and intubation of the trachea if airway reflexes are impaired or respiratory failure is manifest.

Long-term management of a child with pneumonia should include a clinical re-evaluation 2 to 3 weeks after diagnosis. If the child had a prompt response to therapy and is entirely well at follow-up evaluation with a normal physical examination, a repeat radiograph is unnecessary.[48] If the child has undergone a complicated disease course (e.g., pleural effusion), has residual symptoms, or manifests any abnormality on examination, or if the illness is not the child's first episode of pneumonia, a chest radiograph should be obtained to ensure complete resolution of the disease. The follow-up radiograph should be performed 6 to 8 weeks after diagnosis.

In managing a child with pneumonia, it is essential to consider the age and clinical presentation of the child in delineating specific etiologic agents. Common pathogens may be treated as an outpatient disease in nontoxic patients; infants and children who exhibit some respiratory compromise may require parenteral antibiotics, support, and hospitalization. Over the past several years, the patterns of etiologic organisms have been changing. The spectrum of antimicrobial sensitivities also has changed, particularly with the emergence of penicillin-resistant *S. pneumoniae*.

OTHER RESPIRATORY EMERGENCIES

CYSTIC FIBROSIS

Perspective

CF is an autosomal recessive disease caused by a mutation in the CF transmembrane conductance regulator (*CTFR*) gene. In whites, approximately 1 in 25 are carriers, and the disease has an incidence of 1 in 2500 births.[49] The disease also is present (in decreasing incidence) in Hispanics, Native Americans, African Americans, and Asians. Progressive lung disease and infection accounts for most of the morbidity and nearly all of the mortality in CF. Defects in chloride transport across the airway epithelium result in reduced ciliary clearance of thickened mucus, decreased antimicrobial effect of the airway surface, increased bacterial adherence, and innate secretion of inflammatory cytokines. All of these factors result in a unique sensitivity to bacterial infection of the airway.[50,51]

Diagnostic Strategies

Chest radiograph findings of CF include emphysema, peribronchial thickening, bronchiectasis, and focal infiltration, which may be linear or nodular in nature (Figure 168-5). Crucial to the effective treatment of pulmonary infections in CF patients is the identification of pathogens involved, usually through sputum culture. Early childhood pneumonias in patients with CF are predominantly caused by *S. aureus* and *H. influenzae*.

Management

With the emergence of methicillin-resistant *S. aureus*, careful attention should be paid to antibiotic coverage. Patients on antistaphylococcal prophylaxis may be at increased risk for pseudomonal infections.[49] There is emerging evidence that CF patients also are at increased risk of hospitalization by nonbacterial pathogens.[52]

By 18 years of age, 80% of patients are colonized with *P. aeruginosa*. When colonization is established, it is generally considered permanent.[53] Acute infective exacerbations generally are managed by oral and intravenous antimicrobial drugs, typically a penicillin (e.g., ticarcillin or piperacillin) or ceftazidime combined with an aminoglycoside for purposes of synergy.[6] If a patient's previous sputum culture is available, care should be taken to ensure coverage of the last known bacterial pathogens. Resistant strains may benefit from imipenem or meropenem. Patients routinely are hospitalized for 10 to 14 days for the course of therapy.[49]

Burkholderia cepacia, a significant pathogen in CF patients, has been associated with an accelerated decline in clinical status and increased mortality. Generally, antimicrobial coverage is similar to that for *Pseudomonas*. Resistance is common, however, and the existence of differing colonization and resistance pat-

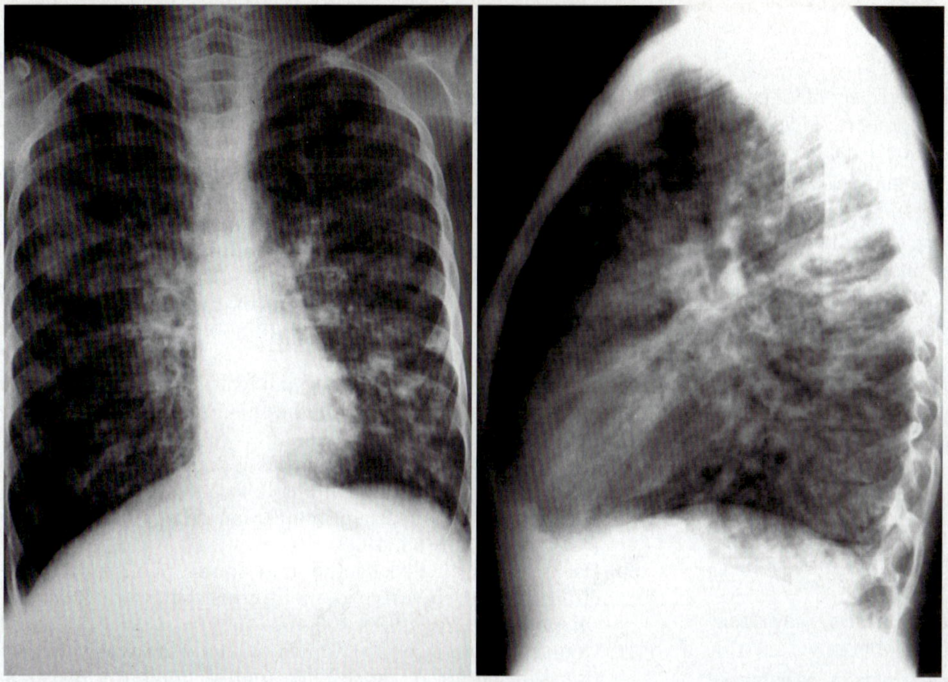

A B

Figure 168-5. Posteroanterior (A) and lateral (B) radiographs of a teenager with cystic fibrosis. Note emphysema and nodular infiltrates. (Courtesy of Michael Diament, MD.)

terns of patients with CF necessitates respiratory isolation from other susceptible individuals.[54]

Clearance of thick mucoid secretions is vital for treatment. Patients may respond favorably to bronchodilator therapy and to mucolytics, such as inhaled *N*-acetyl cysteine, in the acute setting.[55] Chest physiotherapy often is provided by a high-frequency oscillator device. A flutter valve or a positive expiratory pressure mask also may be of assistance for improved mucoid clearance. Short-term control of inflammation may be obtained by inhaled corticosteroids.[56]

CHRONIC LUNG DISEASE

Chronic lung disease of infancy (CLD), also called *bronchopulmonary dysplasia,* is extremely common in premature infants and affects 40% of children with a birth weight of less than 1000 g.[57] The severity of disease is related to several factors, including degree of prematurity, use of peripartum steroids, damage incurred by ventilation in the neonatal period, and nutritional status.[58] Infants with CLD have greatly increased rates of hospitalization because of respiratory illness in the first year of life, approaching 65% in infants born weighing less than 1000 g.[59]

Immunizations are vital to the prevention of pneumonia in patients with CLD. All infants 6 to 23 months old should receive the influenza vaccine during the appropriate season. The heptavalent pneumococcal vaccine (Prevnar) and *H. influenzae* type B vaccine are especially vital for prevention of bacterial pneumonia.[60] In addition, monthly prophylaxis against RSV is administered to carefully selected patients with the monoclonal immunoglobulin palivizumab, which reduces the incidence of RSV disease and risk of subsequent hospitalization.[13,61]

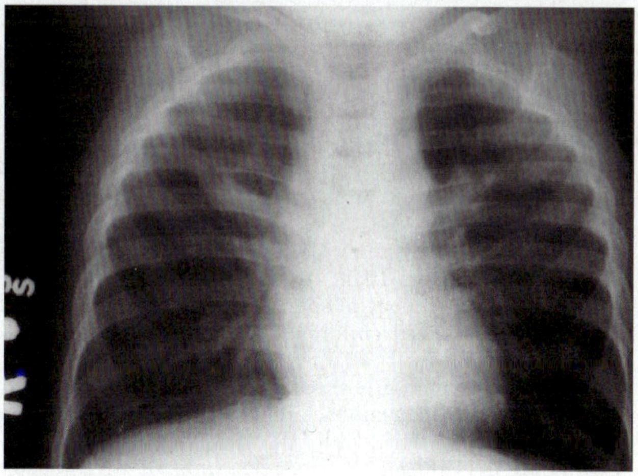

Figure 168-6. Radiograph of a child with bronchopulmonary dysplasia shows findings of chronic lung disease and hyperinflation. (Courtesy of Michael Diament, MD.)

Patients with CLD have increased airway resistance, decreased lung compliance, and obstructive lung disease. Pneumonia in patients with CLD may be complicated by a reactive airways component. Radiographs show marked hyperinflation and infiltrates if complicated by pneumonia (Figure 168-6). Inhaled bronchodilators may be efficacious, although these medications may worsen air exchange in patients with concomitant airway malacia. Hypoxia and hypercarbia are common, despite an increased respiratory effort. Patients with severe CLD may be receiving long-term diuretic therapy to improve lung mechanics; care should be taken not to confuse pneumonia with cor pulmonale, which is especially prevalent in younger infants with chronic supplemental oxygen requirements.[57]

KEY CONCEPTS

- It may be difficult to determine the etiologic agent for pneumonia by clinical presentation, radiographic findings, or laboratory studies. Mixed infections occur commonly.
- Infants and younger children with pneumonia may have subtle or nonspecific signs and symptoms on presentation.
- Pertussis should be considered in a young infant with a lower respiratory tract infection, staccato cough, or episodes of cyanosis.
- *M. pneumoniae* and *C. pneumoniae* may play a role in pneumonia in a younger child.
- In patients with CF, defects in chloride transport across the airway epithelium result in reduced ciliary clearance of thickened mucus, which results in increased likelihood for pneumonia.
- CF may respond favorably to bronchodilator therapy and to mucolytics, such as inhaled *N*-acetyl cysteine.
- Patients with CF are at risk for pneumonia caused by *P. aeruginosa.*
- CLD, also called *bronchopulmonary dysplasia,* may occur in 40% of low-birth-weight premature infants.
- Patients with CLD have increased airway resistance, decreased lung compliance, and obstructive lung disease; reactive airway disease and pneumonia are common in these patients.

REFERENCES

1. Lob-Levyt J: Prevention of pneumonia in children. *Lancet* 341:821, 1993.
2. Ruuskanen O, Mertsola J: Childhood community-acquired pneumonia. *Semin Respir Infect* 14:163, 1999.
3. Juven T, et al: Etiology of community acquired pneumonia in 254 hospitalized children. *Pedatr Infect Dis J* 10:293, 2000.
4. Korppi M: Community-acquired pneumonia in children: issues in optimizing antibacterial treatment. *Paediatr Drugs* 12:821, 2003.
5. Principi N, Esposito S: Emerging role of *Mycoplasma pneumoniae* and *Chlamydia pneumoniae* in paediatric respiratory-tract infections. *Lancet Infect Dis* 1:334, 2001.
6. Yaari E, et al: Clinical manifestations of *Bordetella pertussis* infection in immunized children and young adults. *Chest* 115:1254, 1999.
7. Mink CA, et al: Outbreak of pertussis in a fully immunized adolescent and adult population. *Arch Pediatr Adolesc Med* 148:153, 1994.
8. Principi N, et al: Role of *Mycoplasma pneumoniae* and *Chlamydia pneumoniae* in children with community-acquired lower respiratory tract infections. *Clin Infect Dis* 32:1281, 2001.
9. Darvielle T: Chlamydia. *Pediatr Rev* 19:85, 1998.
10. CDC: Progress toward elimination of *Haemophilus influenzae* type b disease infants and children—United States, 1987-1993. *MMWR Morb Mortal Wkly Rep* 43:144, 1994.
11. American Academy of Pediatrics Committee on Infectious Disease: Technical report: Prevention of pneumococcal infections, including the use of pneumococcal conjugate and polysaccharide vaccines and antibiotic prophylaxis. *Pediatrics* 106:367, 2000.
12. Dagan R, et al: Effect of a noncovalent conjugate vaccine on carriage of antibiotic-resistant *Streptococcus pneumoniae* in day-care centers. *Pediatr Infect Dis* 22:532, 2003.
13. American Academy of Pediatrics: *Red Book: Report of the Committee on Infectious Diseases,* 24th ed. Elk Grove Village, Ill, American Academy of Pediatrics, 2003.
14. Loda FA, et al: Occurrence of *Diplococcus pneumoniae* in the upper respiratory tract of children. *J Pediatr* 87:1087, 1975.
15. Leventhal JM: Clinical predictors of pneumonia as a guide to ordering chest roentgenograms. *Clin Pediatr* 21:730, 1982.
16. The WHO Young Infants Study Group: Serious infections in young infants in developing countries: Rationale for a multicenter study. *Pediatr Infect Dis J* 18(Suppl):S4, 1999.
17. Korppi M, et al: Comparison of radiological findings and microbial aetiology of childhood pneumonia. *Acta Paediatr* 82:360, 1993.
18. Todd JK: Pneumonia. In Behrman RE (ed): *Nelson Textbook of Pediatrics,* 16th ed. Philadelphia, WB Saunders, 2000, pp 1432-1435.
19. Tan QT, et al: Clinical characteristics and outcome of children with pneumonia attributable to penicillin-susceptible and penicillin-nonsusceptible *Streptococcus pneumoniae. Pediatrics* 102:1369, 1998.
20. Deeks SL, et al: Risk factors and course of illness among children with invasive penicillin-resistant *Streptococcus pneumoniae. Pediatrics* 103:409, 1999.
21. Gomez-Barreto D, et al: Clinical outcome of invasive infections in children caused by highly penicillin-resistant *Streptococcus pneumoniae* compared with infections caused by penicillin-susceptible strains. *Arch Med Res* 31:592, 2000.
22. Tan T, et al: Clinical characteristics of children with complicated pneumonia caused by *Streptococcus pneumoniae. Pediatrics* 110(1 Pt 1):1, 2002.
23. Jain A, Ben-Ami T, Daum RS: Staphylococcal infections in children: Part 2. *Pediatr Rev* 20:219, 1999.
24. Marcinak J, Frank A: Treatment of community-acquired methicillin-resistant *Staphylococcus aureus* in children. *Curr Opin Infect Dis* 16:265, 2003.
25. Melville CAS, Flaurenson JF, Augrow JA: Invasive disease due to *Haemophilus influenzae* infection [letter]. *BMJ* 309:58, 1994.
26. Ginsburg CM, Howard JB, Nelson JD: Report of 65 cases of *Haemophilus influenzae* b pneumonia. *Pediatrics* 64:283, 1979.
27. Muller M, et al: Clinical and epidemiologic features of group A streptococcal pneumonia in Ontario, Canada. *Arch Intern Med* 163:467, 2003.
28. O'Brien K, Beall B, Barrett N: Epidemiology of invasive group A streptococcus disease in the United States, 1995-1999. *Clin Infect Dis* 35:268, 2002.
29. Bruhn FW, Mokrohisky ST, McIntosh K: Apnea associated with respiratory syncytial virus infection in young infants. *J Pediatr* 90:382, 1977.
30. Cimolai N: *Mycoplasma pneumoniae* respiratory infection. *Pediatr Rev* 19:327, 1998.
31. Cherry JD, Hurwitz ES, Welliver RC: *Mycoplasma pneumoniae* infections and exanthems. *J Pediatr* 87:369, 1975.
32. Hagiwara K, et al: An epidemic of pertussis-like illness caused by *Chlamydia pneumoniae. Pediatr Infect Dis J* 18:271, 1999.
33. Ekman MR, et al: An epidemic of infections due to *Chlamydia pneumoniae* in military conscripts. *Clin Infect Dis* 17:420, 1993.
34. Vitek, C, et al: Increase in deaths from pertussis among young infants in the United States in the 1990's. *Pediat Infect Dis J* 22:628, 2003.
35. Bachur R, Perry H, Harper MB: Occult pneumonias: Empiric chest radiographs in febrile children with leukocytosis. *Ann Emerg Med* 33:166, 1999.
36. Harrison DD: Viral and bacterial pneumonias. In Tintinalli JE, Krome RL, Ruiz E (eds): *Emergency Medicine,* 2nd ed. New York, McGraw-Hill, 1988.

37. Hickey RW, Bowman MJ, Smith GA: Utility of blood cultures in pediatric patients found to have pneumonia in the emergency department. *Ann Emerg Med* 27:721, 1996.
38. Bradley J: Management of community-acquired pediatric pneumonia in an era of increasing antibiotic resistance and conjugate vaccines. *Paediatr Infect Dis J* 21:592, 2002.
39. McCracken G: Diagnosis and management of pneumonia in children. *Pediatr Infect Dis J* 19:924, 2000.
40. Hodina M, et al: Imaging of cavitary necrosis in complicated childhood pneumonia. *Eur Radiol* 12:391, 2002.
41. Givan DC, Eigen H: Disease of the pleura: Common pleural effusions in children. *Clin Chest Med* 19:363, 1998.
42. Driver CR, et al: Tuberculosis in children younger than 5 years old: New York City. *Pediatr Infect Dis* 14:112, 1995.
43. Virkii R, et al: Differentiation of bacterial and viral pneumonia in children. *Thorax* 57:438, 2002.
44. Byington C, et al: An epidemiological investigation of a sustained high rate of pediatric parapneumonic empyema: Risk factors and microbiological associations. *Clin Infect Dis* 34, 2002.
45. Wubbel L, et al: Etiology and treatment of community-acquired pneumonia in ambulatory children. *Pediatr Infect Dis J* 18:98, 1998.
46. Kaplan S, et al: Outcome of invasive infections outside the central nervous system caused by *Streptococcus pneumoniae* isolates nonsusceptible to ceftriaxone in children treated with beta-lactam antibiotics. *Pediatr Infect Dis J* 20:392, 2001.
47. American Academy of Pediatrics Committee on Infectious Diseases: Therapy for children with invasive pneumococcal infections. *Pediatrics* 99:289, 1997.
48. Gibson NA, Holloman AS, Paton JY: Value of radiological follow-up of childhood pneumonia. *BMJ* 307;117, 1993.
49. Brennan AL, Geddes DM: Cystic fibrosis. *Curr Opin Infect Dis* 15:175, 2002.
50. Conese M, Assael BM: Bacterial infections and inflammation in the lungs of cystic fibrosis patients. *Pediatr Infect Dis J* 20:207, 2001.
51. Hanutcu R, Woo MS: Advanced cystic fibrosis lung disease in children. *Curr Opin Pulm Med* 7:448, 2001.
52. Meissner HC: Selected populations at increased risk from respiratory syncytial virus infection. *Pediatr Infect Dis J* 22(2 Suppl):S40, 2003.
53. Rajan S: Pulmonary infections in patients with cystic fibrosis. *Semin Respir Infect* 17:47, 2002.
54. Garau J, Gomez L: Pseudomonas aeruginosa pneumonia. *Curr Opin Infect Dis* 16:135, 2003.
55. Ramsey BW: Management of pulmonary disease in patients with cystic fibrosis. *N Engl J Med* 335:179, 1996.
56. van der Schans C, et al: Chest physiotherapy compared to no chest physiotherapy for cystic fibrosis (Cochrane Review). In: *The Cochrane Library,* Issue 1, Chichester, UK, John Wiley & Sons, Ltd, 2004.
57. Marshall DD: Primary care follow-up of the neonatal intensive care unit graduate. *Clin Fam Pract* 5:243, 2003.
58. Jobe AJ: The new BPD: An arrest of lung development. *Pediatr Res* 46:641, 1999.
59. Davis PG, et al: Evaluating "old" definitions for the "new" bronchopulmonary dysplasia. *J Pediatr* 140:555, 2002.
60. American Academy of Pediatrics Committee on Infectious Diseases: Immunization of preterm and low birth weight infants. *Pediatrics* 112:193, 2003.
61. Welliver RC: Review of epidemiology and clinical risk factors for severe respiratory syncytial virus (RSV) infection. *J Pediatr* 143(5 Suppl):S112, 2003.

CHAPTER

169 Cardiac Disorders

Alson S. Inaba

PERSPECTIVE

Cardiac disorders in infants and children are not as common as in adults; therefore, understanding of the underlying pathophysiology of some of the more common and potentially life-threatening cardiac disorders is imperative in the emergency department evaluation and management of these patients.

Pediatric cardiac disease has typically been divided into congenital versus acquired disorders, with a further subdivision of the congenital heart disorders into cyanotic versus acyanotic lesions. From a purely clinical standpoint, however, children with cardiac disorders present to the emergency department in one of two scenarios. In the first scenario, the child has signs and symptoms that may represent an exacerbation or complication of an already known underlying cardiac disorder. In cases with a known underlying cardiac disorder, early consultation with the child's cardiologist, along with comparisons of the child's previous and most recent diagnostic cardiac studies such as chest radiographs, electrocardiograms, and echocardiograms would also be extremely useful in the evaluation and management phases.

The second scenario represents more of a challenge to the emergency physician in that a child with either an undiagnosed congenital cardiac disorder or an undiagnosed acquired cardiac disorder presents to the emergency department with signs and symptoms that may not be intuitively thought of as being due to a cardiac disorder. A wide array of signs and symptoms can be the presenting chief complaint of an underlying cardiac disorder (Box 169-1). This chapter focuses on some of the more common and life-threatening cardiac disorders in infants and children who present to the emergency department, with an emphasis on rapid evaluation, stabilization, and management of these disorders.

BOX 169-1. Common Presenting Signs and Symptoms of Cardiac Disorders in Infants and Children

General
Fussiness
Lethargy
Poor feeding (with or without associated diaphoresis)
Poor growth

Respiratory
Respiratory distress
Wheezing
Apnea

Cardiovascular
Tachycardia
Shock
Paleness
Mottling
Cyanosis
Palpitations
Chest pain
Syncope
Various dysrhythmias

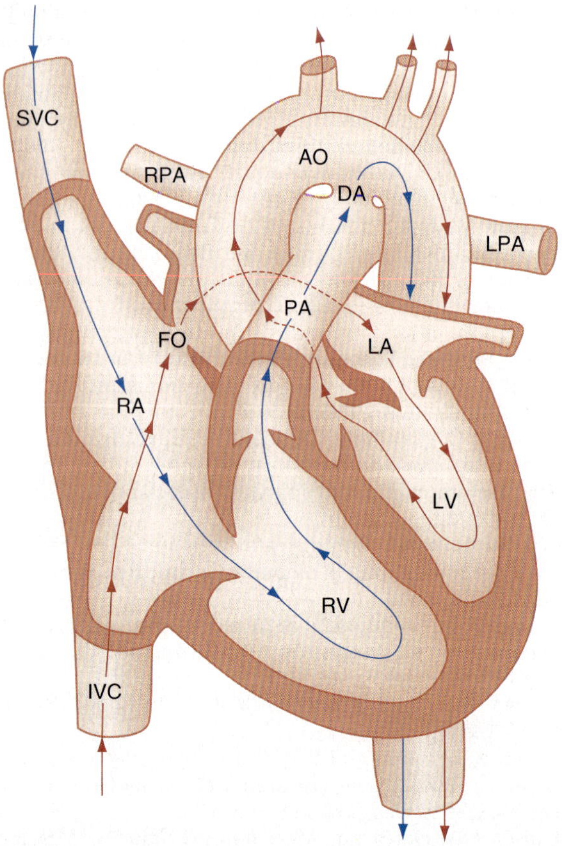

Figure 169-1. Normal intracardiac fetal circulation: Physiologic shunting through the patent foramen ovale **(**FO**)** and the patent ductus arteriosus **(**DA**)**. Oxygenated blood from the placenta (*red arrows*) reaches the right atrium (RA) via the inferior vena cava (IVC). This well-oxygenated blood is preferentially shunted from the RA across to the left atrium (LA) through the FO and is then ejected out the left ventricle (LV) to the ascending aorta (AO). Deoxygenated blood (*blue arrows*) returning from the superior vena cava (SVC) preferentially travels from RA into the RV, then out through the main pulmonary artery (PA). Because of the high pulmonary vascular resistance in the fetal lungs, this deoxygenated blood bypasses lungs and enters the descending aorta via the DA. Thus, the areas of the fetal body that are perfused by arteries proximal to the DA receive well-oxygenated blood, whereas those areas of the body that are perfused by arteries distal to the DA receive blood with a mixed oxygenation.

PRINCIPLES OF DISEASE

Fetal and Neonatal Circulation

Some of the key features of the fetal circulation that differ from that of a child are the presence of the ductus venosus, ductus arteriosus, and a patent foramen ovale. During fetal development, oxygenation of the fetal circulation bypasses the fetal lungs and is accomplished via the placenta. Blood that is oxygenated by the placenta is carried to the fetus via the umbilical vein, bypasses the fetal liver via the ductus venosus, and returns to the fetal heart via the inferior vena cava. Blood returning from the inferior vena cava then enters the right atrium and is preferentially shunted across to the left atrium via the patent foramen ovale (Figure 169-1). The blood in the left atrium is then pumped out of the aorta via the left ventricle. This oxygenated blood that is ejected through the ascending aorta is preferentially directed to the fetal coronary and cerebral circulations.

In contrast to this, deoxygenated blood that returns to the right atrium via the superior vena cava crosses the tricuspid valve and is pumped into the fetal pulmonary artery via the right ventricle. Because the fetal pulmonary vascular resistance (PVR) is higher than the fetal systemic vascular resistance (SVR), this deoxygenated blood bypasses the nonoxygenated fetal lungs via the patent ductus arteriosus (see Figure 169-1). This less oxygenated blood enters the aorta via the patent ductus arteriosus and then mixes with the well-oxygenated blood in the descending aorta. This mixed-oxygenated blood in the descending aorta then returns to the placenta for oxygenation via the two umbilical arteries.

Once the infant is delivered and the umbilical cord is cut, expansion and aeration of the lungs causes a decrease in the infant's PVR with a concomitant increase in pulmonary blood flow. This increased oxygenation causes a physiologic closure of the umbilical arteries, umbilical vein, ductus venosus, and ductus arteriosus. An increase in the pulmonary blood flow to the infant's left atrium also promotes closure of the foramen ovale. Complete anatomic closure of the foramen ovale does not occur until about 3 months of life. Although the ductus arteriosus functionally closes at about 10 to 15 hours of life, complete anatomic closure does not occur until about 2 to 3 weeks of life.

In the absence of any congenital cardiac defects, these transitional circulatory changes pose no physiologic problems to the infant. However, closure of the ductus arteriosus can pose life-threatening complications in neonates with specific congenital cardiac

BOX 169-2. Etiologies of Decreased Stroke Volume in Infants and Children

- Hypovolemia (most commonly secondary to dehydration)
- Congestive heart failure (acquired or secondary to underlying congenital cardiac defects)
- Myocarditis
- Hypertrophic cardiomyopathy with decreased diastolic filling
- Dilated cardiomyopathy with decreased systolic ejection
- Pericarditis or pericardial effusion with cardiac tamponade
- Tachydysrhythmias with decreased diastolic filling times

defects that are dependent on the patency of the ductus arteriosus for survival.

Pathophysiology of Cardiovascular Compensatory Responses

There are two fundamental and clinically useful physiologic formulas to keep in mind during the clinical assessment and management of cardiac disorders:

$$\text{Cardiac Output} = (\text{Stroke Volume}) \times (\text{Heart Rate})$$

$$\text{Blood Pressure} = (\text{Cardiac Output}) \times (\text{SVR})$$

Infants and children primarily rely on an increase in their heart rate to increase their cardiac output because of a very limited capacity to increase their stroke volume. Therefore, bradycardia in infants and young children can severely compromise cardiac output. Children develop the adult capacity to increase their stroke volume to improve overall cardiac output by 8 to 10 years of age.[1]

Based on the first physiologic formula, as stroke volume decreases, a compensatory increase in the heart rate will be necessary to preserve a normal cardiac output. A decrease in stroke volume can be produced by a "weak pump" or "decreased fluid in the circulation," or both. The most common cause of decreased stroke volume in children is hypovolemia due to dehydration. Other causes of decreased stroke volume in children may be responsible (Box 169-2). Thus, tachycardia is the first compensatory cardiovascular response when the stroke volume is decreased. If tachycardia alone is not enough to maintain a normal cardiac output, the next compensatory physiologic mechanism to preserve perfusion is an increase in the SVR. This increase in SVR is exhibited as an increase in the diastolic blood pressure, which in turn accounts for a narrowed pulse pressure. The clinical examination of the extremities of a child with an increased SVR includes paleness, mottling, coolness, a delayed capillary refill time (>2 seconds), and weak or thready distal pulses.

Pathophysiology of Cyanosis

Perspective

Cyanosis is a clinical sign caused by the presence of deoxygenated blood in the capillary beds. This accumulation of desaturated blood creates the blue discoloration of the mucous membranes, conjunctiva, nail beds, and skin. The presence of cyanosis usually means that there is at least 4 to 5 g/dL of deoxyhemoglobin in the blood, which correlates to an oxygen saturation of about 80% to 85%.[2] Pathophysiologically, cyanosis results from a decrease in pulmonary ventilation/oxygenation, a decrease in pulmonary perfusion, shunting of deoxygenated blood directly into the systemic circulation, or the presence of abnormal hemoglobin. Cyanosis in the neonate can be due to a variety of cardiac, pulmonary, or hematologic causes. Cardiac causes of cyanosis include congenital lesions with right-to-left shunts as well as cardiac lesions with decreased or increased pulmonary blood flow. Common pulmonary causes of cyanosis include bronchiolitis, pneumonia, and pulmonary edema. Methemoglobinemia can be one of the hematologic causes of cyanosis.

Table 169-1. Clinical Clues to Help Distinguish Between Cardiac and Pulmonary Etiologies of Central Cyanosis

	Cardiac Etiology	Pulmonary Etiology
Respiratory status	May be "comfortably blue"	Respiratory distress
Response to crying	Worsening cyanosis	Improved cyanosis
Response to oxygen	Minimal to no improvement	Improvement with oxygen

Note: Cyanosis due to severe pulmonary disease (i.e., severe pneumonia, tension pneumothorax, acute chest syndrome of sickle cell disease, etc.) may not show significant improvement with supplemental oxygen, but these children will also typically exhibit severe respiratory distress along with clinical cyanosis.

Clinical Features of Cyanosis

The region of the body that is cyanotic can provide important clinical clues as to the cause of the cyanosis. Central cyanosis involves the lips, tongue, and mucous membranes, whereas peripheral cyanosis (acrocyanosis) involves the hands and feet. Acrocyanosis is a common phenomenon in neonates secondary to cold stress and peripheral vasoconstriction. Central cyanosis reflects a pathologic origin and is therefore a more ominous sign. Infants with cyanosis secondary to a congenital heart defect may not exhibit as much respiratory distress as compared to the infant with cyanosis due to a pulmonary cause. Thus, a cardiac cause for central cyanosis may be more likely than a purely pulmonary cause when confronted with the child who appears "comfortably blue." Another important clinical clue to the cause of central cyanosis is that cyanosis of cardiac origin usually worsens with crying, whereas cyanosis due to a pulmonary cause may improve when the infant cries.[3] Cyanotic congenital heart defects with right-to-left shunting will demonstrate a minimal improvement with supplemental oxygen, whereas cyanosis of a purely pulmonary origin typically exhibits a significant improvement with supplemental oxygen (Table 169-1).

BOX 169-3. Key Elements to Elicit in the History of a Child with a Known Cardiac Disorder

Cardiac Diagnosis
- Congenital or acquired disorder?
- Any episodes of previous decompensation (if so, are the current signs and symptoms similar or different from those previous episodes)?

Oxygen Issues
- Currently on home oxygen supplementation (continuous or only during feedings and sleep)?
- Baseline oxygen saturation (room air or while on home oxygen)?
- Any recent need for increasing the amount of supplemental oxygen?

Medications
- Names and dosages of all current medications (cardiac and noncardiac medications)?
- Were any of these cardiac medications stopped recently (by the cardiologist or parental noncompliance)?
- Any recent increases in the cardiac medications (reasons for the increase, previous dosage versus the current dosage, and the date this dosage was increased)?
- Any new cardiac medications added recently and the reason for these additions?
- Recent digoxin level if the patient is on daily digoxin therapy?

Results of Most Recent Studies (CXR, ECG, Echocardiogram and Cardiac Catheterization)
- When were the last studies performed and what were the results?
- Why were those studies performed (routine follow-up studies or obtained because of decompensation from baseline, or a planned evaluation for an upcoming surgical procedure)?

Surgical Procedures
- Previous procedures and complications?
- Any planned future procedures?

CLINICAL FEATURES AND DIAGNOSTIC STRATEGIES: THE CARDIAC EVALUATION

The key elements that should be elicited in the history of a child with a known underlying cardiac disorder are listed in Box 169-3. Early consultation with the child's cardiologist or cardiac surgeon is extremely useful. The other important points to elicit in the history of a child with a potential or suspected cardiac disorder are covered in the subsequent sections of this chapter.

In addition to a well-focused history and physical examination, a chest radiograph and an electrocardiogram (ECG) should be obtained on any child with a known or suspected cardiac disorder. Other ancillary studies that can also be useful include an arterial blood gas analysis, hemoglobin/hematocrit levels, digoxin levels in those patients on daily digoxin, serum electrolytes in those patients on daily diuretic therapy, and the 100% oxygen (hyperoxia) challenge.

History

Certain maternal infections as well as medication and drug use during the first trimester are associated with a higher incidence of congenital cardiac disorders. The presence of certain maternal medical conditions have also been associated with a higher incidence of cardiac disorders. For example, congenital heart blocks have been associated with maternal systemic lupus erythematosus and other collagen vascular disorders, and infants of diabetic mothers have a higher incidence of cardiomyopathy.

Infants with an underlying congenital heart disorder may exhibit diaphoresis during feeds and poor weight gain secondary to congestive heart failure (CHF). The presence of cyanosis, the age of onset of the cyanosis, and the conditions under which the cyanosis is noticed by the parents may provide valuable clues to the cause of an infant's cyanosis (i.e., cardiac or pulmonary).

Respiratory tract infections are common during childhood and could serve as a critical factor in causing an acute deterioration in a child with an underlying cardiac disorder. Children with congenital heart diseases with large left-to-right shunts and increased pulmonary blood flow tend to have a higher incidence of lower respiratory tract infections. Acute respiratory distress in these patients may be from a combination of pulmonary and cardiac factors (i.e., CHF).

Chest Pain

The majority of pediatric chest pain cases are noncardiac in origin and benign in nature. Common causes include musculoskeletal/chest wall pain, costochondritis, asthma exacerbations, pneumonia, pleurisy, gastritis, and gastroesophageal reflux. An unusual cause of acute, nonradiating, left-sided chest pain in the adolescent is referred to as the *precordial catch syndrome* (also known as *Texidor's twinge*). The pain, which is located in the left periapical area of the chest wall, occurs suddenly, can be exacerbated during inspiration, and usually resolves within a few minutes. The cause is unknown and findings on physical examination, chest radiograph, ECG, and echocardiogram are all normal in these patients.

Chest pain or syncope that occurs during exertion may be due to an underlying cardiac condition and deserves a more thorough investigation, especially if there is also a positive family history of sudden unexplained death in young adulthood. Myocardial involvement secondary to drug abuse (e.g., cocaine, amphetamines, crystal methamphetamine) or drug overdoses (e.g., cyclic antidepressants) should always be considered as a potential cause in any adolescent patient who presents with chest discomfort or pain. Pulmonary embolism should be considered as a possible cause of chest pain in pregnant adolescent females or those who are taking oral contraceptive agents. The rare though life-threatening condition of aortic dissection must always be considered as a cause of chest pain in a patient with physical examination stigmata that are suggestive of Marfan's syndrome. Patients with a

Table 169-2. Pediatric Vital Signs and Pertinent Formulas for Estimating Blood Pressure

Simplified pediatric vital signs:[4]		
Age group	*Heart rate*	*Respiratory rate*
Newborn to 1 year old	140	40
1 year old to 4 years old	120	30
4 years old to 12 years old	100	20
>12 years old	80	15
Formulas to calculate the estimated normal blood pressures in children ≥1 year of age:		
Estimated systolic blood pressure (SBP): [age in years × 2] + 90 mm Hg		
Estimated diastolic blood pressure (DBP): 2/3 × [estimated SBP]		
Minimum acceptable SPBs for age:		
Newborn to 1 month old:	60 mm Hg	
1 month to 1 year old:	70 mm Hg	
>1 year old to 10 years old:	[age in years × 2] + 70 mm Hg	
>10 years old:	90 mm Hg	

known congenital heart defect or an acquired cardiac disorder (e.g., Kawasaki disease, acute rheumatic heart disease, myocarditis, cardiomyopathies) who present with chest pain also deserve a more thorough diagnostic evaluation.

Physical Examination

General Appearance and Pulses

All four extremities should be palpated for the presence and quality of pulses. The brachial and femoral pulses are the easiest to feel in infants. Bounding pulses are typically present in infants with a patent ductus arteriosus. Coarctation of the aorta should be suspected in any child with strong pulses in the upper extremities but weak pulses in the lower extremities. The pulse may be weak and thready in all extremities in a child who presents with CHF and shock.

Vital Signs and Blood Pressures

A mild resting tachypnea or tachycardia may be the only clinical clue to an underlying cardiovascular disorder. Because of the age-related variables in heart rates, respiratory rates, and blood pressures, pediatric vital signs often serve as a source of frustration and confusion to those clinicians who do not manage pediatric patients on a routine basis. Although there are numerous tables of pediatric vital signs with variations based on sleep or awake states, one can easily recall a rough estimate of the normal pediatric heart rates and respiratory rates based on a simplified table of pediatric vital signs (Table 169-2).[4] The methods to calculate the normal expected blood pressures and hypotensive blood pressures are also listed in Table 169-2.[5]

An accurate blood pressure reading is dependent on using a cuff that covers two thirds of the upper arm or thigh. A cuff that is too narrow will overestimate the patient's true blood pressure and a cuff that is too large will underestimate the true blood pressure. Any child with a suspected cardiac disorder should have blood pressures measured in both arms. If the blood pressure in the left arm is significantly lower than the blood pressure in the right arm, a coarctation of the aorta proximal to the origin of the left subclavian artery should be suspected. Blood pressures must also be measured in the thighs in any child with a suspected aortic coarctation or documented hypertensive blood pressures in the upper extremities. The mere presence of femoral pulses does not clinically rule out the possibility of a coarctation of the aorta. Even with an appropriately sized cuff, the blood pressures in the thighs can be 10 to 20 mm Hg higher than the blood pressures in the upper extremities due to the lack of well-designed blood pressure cuffs for the legs. Therefore, if the measured blood pressure in the lower extremities is lower than the blood pressures in the upper extremities, coarctation of the aorta should be suspected. Pulse oximetry readings that are lower in the legs than in the upper extremities are also suggestive of either a coarctation of the aorta or a right-to-left shunt across a patent ductus arteriosus.[6]

Cardiac Auscultation

The intensity and degree of splitting of the S2 heart sound (which reflects closure of the pulmonic and aortic valves) is extremely important in a pediatric cardiologic evaluation. In normal children, both components (aortic closure and pulmonic closure) of S2 should be heard along the left upper sternal border (the pulmonic area). A widely split and fixed S2 suggests a physiologic problem resulting from either a constant volume overload to the right side of the heart (e.g., atrial septal defect) or a pressure overload to the right side of the heart (e.g., pulmonic stenosis). The classic congenital heart defect that is associated with a widely split and fixed S2 is the atrial septal defect. The intensity of the S2 component may be louder than normal in the child with pulmonary hypertension.

The third heart sound (S3), which is best heard along the lower left sternal border or the apex, can be a normal finding in children and young adults. S3 is produced by a rapid filling of the ventricles and is heard during early diastole, just after the S2 sound. A loud S3 is always pathologic and is due to dilated ventricles with decreased compliance (e.g., CHF and large ventricular septal defects). The fourth heart sound (S4) occurs late in diastole, just before the S1 sound. The finding of an S4 is due to a decrease in ventricular compliance or CHF.

Cardiac murmurs are produced by turbulent blood flow through the heart. The presence of a cardiac murmur may not be associated with an underlying cardiac defect, however. The location, intensity, quality, timing, and radiation of the murmur determine whether the murmur is suggestive of underlying cardiac pathologic condition. Although systolic murmurs can be present without any underlying anatomic abnormalities, diastolic murmurs are always considered pathologic in nature. Some of the other criteria that would suggest an underlying anatomic cardiac abnormality are listed in Box 169-4. Murmurs may be very difficult to appreciate in the noisy emer-

BOX 169-4. A Pathologic Etiology of a Heart Murmur Should Be Suspected with Any of the Following Criteria

- Diastolic murmurs
- Systolic murmurs that are louder than a grade 3/6, continuous or associated with a thrill
- Murmurs that are associated with abnormal heart sounds (clicks, rubs, or gallop rhythms)
- Presence of cyanosis or respiratory distress
- Bounding pulses or weak pulses
- Abnormalities on the ECG
- An abnormal cardiac silhouette, abnormal pulmonary vascularity or cardiomegaly on the CXR

BOX 169-5. Auscultation Locations of Common Systolic Murmurs in Children

Left Upper Sternal Border (Pulmonic Area)
Pulmonic valvular stenosis
Atrial septal defects (due to an increased pulmonic flow)
Innocent pulmonic ejection murmur
Neonate pulmonic flow murmur
Patent ductus arteriosus (a continuous, "machinery" sounding murmur)

Left Lower Sternal Border
Innocent vibratory Still's murmur
Ventricular septal defects
Endocardial cushion defects
Tetralogy of Fallot
Hypertrophic cardiomyopathy

Apex
Innocent vibratory Still's murmur
Mitral regurgitation
Aortic stenosis
Hypertrophic cardiomyopathy

Right Upper Sternal Border (Aortic Area)
Aortic valvular stenosis
Coarctation of the aorta

gency department setting, given the degree of tachycardia that is often present even in normal infants. However, the location of the murmur may be a valuable clinical tool in determining the underlying anatomic origin of the murmur (Box 169-5).

Murmurs without any underlying anatomic abnormalities or hemodynamic significance are termed *innocent* or *functional* murmurs. All innocent murmurs are associated with normal ECGs and normal chest radiographs. Two of the most common innocent murmurs encountered in the pediatric population are the neonatal pulmonic flow murmur (also known as the peripheral pulmonic stenosis murmur) and Still's murmur. The pulmonic flow murmur of the neonate is due to the relative hypoplasia and angulation of the right and left pulmonary arteries at birth. This systolic murmur is best heard at the left upper sternal border with radiation throughout the entire chest, axilla, and back. This murmur usually disappears by 3 to 6 months of age. Persistence of a systolic murmur in the pulmonic area beyond this period should raise the possibility of a pathologic pulmonary arterial stenosis. Another common innocent murmur in children is Still's murmur, which is a systolic murmur that typically occurs in children between 2 and 6 years of age. This systolic murmur is best heard along the left midsternal border. The distinctive quality of this murmur has been described as being "vibratory," "musical," "zippy," and "twanging," and results from turbulent flow. The distinct quality of this murmur helps to distinguish Still's murmur from a ventricular septal defect murmur, which has a more "harsh" quality. The intensity of Still's murmur can be increased due to fever, excitement, exercise, or anemia.

The Hyperoxia Test

In general, infants with a cardiac origin for their cyanosis exhibit a worsening of their cyanosis with crying.[7] Administration of 100% oxygen (also known as the *hyperoxia test*) can be used as a bedside diagnostic tool to help differentiate between cardiac and pulmonary causes of central cyanosis. This test consists of assessing the rise in arterial oxygenation with the administration of 100% oxygen. The response to 100% oxygen can either be determined by the pulse oximeter or by actually measuring an arterial blood gas. According to one reference, if the patient's oxygen saturation increases by more than 10% or the PaO_2 rises by more than 20% to 30%, then the most likely origin for the cyanosis is pulmonary rather than cardiac. If the oxygen saturation does not increase and the cyanosis does not improve with supplemental oxygen, then a cardiac origin for the patient's cyanosis should be suspected.[3] The measured PaO_2 in patients with a pulmonary origin for cyanosis should rise well above 200 mm Hg unless the degree of pulmonary disease that is present is severe. PaO_2 values that do not rise above 100 mm Hg in cyanotic patients are highly suggestive of a cardiac defect. A PaO_2 that remains lower than 100 mm Hg despite 100% oxygen is suggestive of a congenital heart defect with decreased pulmonary blood flow and/or right-to-left shunting. Those congenital heart defects with an increased pulmonary blood flow may exhibit a rise in their PaO_2 (up to 150 mm Hg) in response to 100% oxygen.[2] Prolonged administration of 100% oxygen may cause some theoretical problems, such as closing the ductus arteriosus in those infants with critical left heart obstructions or by causing pulmonary vasodilation (which would potentially worsen pulmonary vascular congestion).[2]

Arterial Blood Gases

Patients with CHF exacerbations can exhibit respiratory acidosis (low pH and high $PaCO_2$) in addition to a low PaO_2. In contrast to this, children with compensated cyanotic congenital heart defects may have a normal pH despite a low PaO_2. Patients with congenital heart defects who are not experiencing respiratory failure are unlikely to exhibit elevations in their $PaCO_2$ values. Any cardiac condition that results in inade-

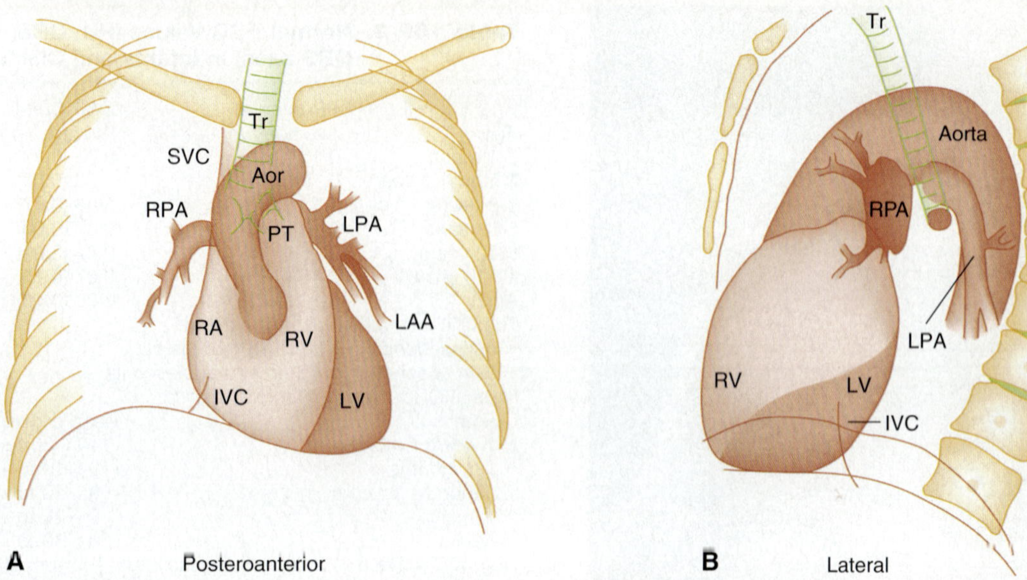

Figure 169-2. Diagrammatic representations of the anatomy of the chest radiograph. **A,** Normal heart in a young man. Posteroanterior projection. Aor, aorta; IVC, inferior vena cava; LAA, left atrial appendage; LPA, left pulmonary artery; LV, left ventricle; PT, pulmonary trunk; RA, right atrium; RPA, right pulmonary artery; RV, right ventricle; SVC, superior vena cava; Tr, trachea. **B,** Right lateral projection of a normal heart in a young man. IVC, inferior vena cava; LPA, left pulmonary artery; LV, left ventricle; RPA, right pulmonary artery; RV, right ventricle; Tr, trachea.

quate tissue perfusion (i.e., any of the acyanotic congenital heart defects that manifest in CHF) will exhibit a metabolic acidosis with or without a respiratory compensation.

Hemoglobin/Hematocrit Levels and Serum Electrolytes

The hemoglobin and hematocrit levels may reveal a compensatory physiologic elevation (i.e., polycythemia) in children with cyanotic congenital heart defects. Any concurrent medical illness or blood loss that produces an acute anemia could potentially precipitate an acute deterioration by compromising the oxygen-carrying capacity in these children with an underlying congenital heart defect. A hematocrit level would also be helpful in evaluating whether a child's pallor is due to CHF or anemia. Serum electrolytes may be helpful when evaluating children with acute dysrhythmias or suspected metabolic acidosis and those children who are on chronic diuretic therapy.

Chest Radiograph (Figure 169-2)

The three items to pay special attention to when evaluating the chest radiograph of a child with a known or suspected cardiac disorder are (1) the cardiac size (cardiothoracic ratio), (2) the cardiac shape (silhouette), and (3) the degree of pulmonary vascular markings. The easiest method to determine the heart size in children is to determine the cardiothoracic ratio, which is obtained by relating the largest transverse diameter of the cardiac shadow on the posteroanterior view of the chest radiograph to the widest internal diameter (measured from the inside rib margin to the widest point above the costophrenic angle) of the chest. The normal cardiothoracic ratio in children is approximately 50%. The cardiothoracic ratio is not very accurate in newborns and small infants, in whom a good inspiratory view is rarely obtained.[8] A cardiac silhouette that is larger than normal may be due to a shunt lesion, CHF, or a pericardial effusion.[9] An enlarged heart shadow on a chest radiograph more reliably reflects a problem with volume overload rather than pressure overload. Problems with pressure overload are better represented on the ECG.

The cardiac size can be falsely increased in infants because of the presence of the thymus, which can be seen in the mediastinum on the chest radiograph from birth until about 5 years of age. The thymic borders are typically wavy in appearance and sometimes can be seen as the classic "sail sign" along the superior right heart border (Figure 169-3). The thymic shadow may not be radiographically visible in infants during times of physiologic stress but should reappear when the infant recovers.

The three classic cardiac silhouettes seen in patients with congenital heart defects are (1) the "boot-shaped" heart of tetralogy of Fallot (Figure 169-4), (2) the "egg-on-a-string silhouette" of transposition of the great vessels, and (3) the "snowman-shaped" or "figure of 8 heart" of total anomalous pulmonary venous return.

The degree of pulmonary vascular markings is one of the key factors to consider when working through the differential diagnosis of congenital heart defects. An increase in pulmonary vascularity is present when the pulmonary arteries appear enlarged and extend into the lateral third of the lung fields or if there is an increased vascularity to the lung apices. Another criterion that suggests an increased pulmonary vascularity is if the diameter of the right pulmonary artery in the right hilum on the posteroanterior view of the chest is wider than the internal diameter of the trachea. The differential diagnosis of a cyanotic infant with decreased vascular markings includes tetralogy of Fallot, pulmonary

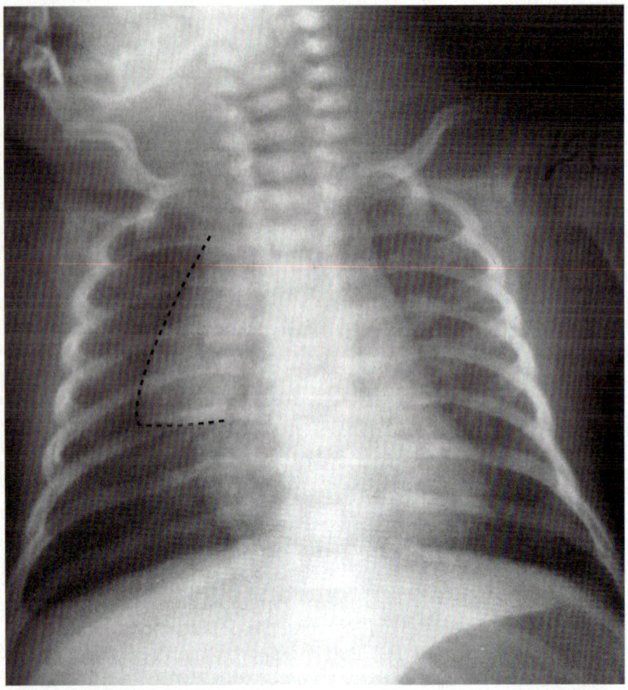

Figure 169-3. Thymic shadow demonstrating the "sail sign" along the right cardiac border (*dotted line*).

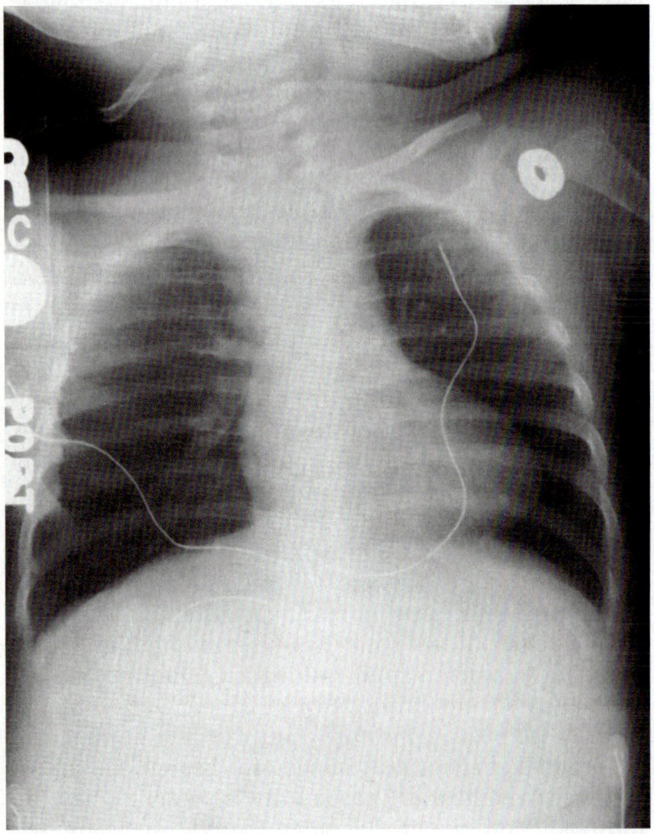

Figure 169-4. The classic boot-shaped heart of tetralogy of Fallot.

Table 169-3. Normal ECG Values (PR, QRS, QTc and QRS axes) in Infants and Children[5]

Age	*PR Interval Average (upper limit)*	*QRS Duration Average (upper limit)*	
0-1 month	0.10 (0.12)	0.05 (0.07)	
1 month-1 year	0.10 (0.14)	0.05 (0.07)	
1-3 years	0.11 (0.15)	0.06 (0.07)	
3-8 years	0.13 (0.17)	0.07 (0.08)	
8-12 years	0.15 (0.18)	0.07 (0.09)	
12-16 years	0.15 (0.19)	0.07 (0.10)	
Adult	0.16 (0.21)	0.08 (0.10)	
The QTc interval should not exceed:			
0.45 seconds in infants <6 months old			
0.44 seconds in children and adolescents			
Normal QRS axes in infants and children:			
Age		Mean degrees (range)	
1 week-1 month		+110 (+30 to +180)	
1-3 months		+70 (+10 to +125)	
3 months-3 years		+60 (+10 to +110)	
>3 years		+60 (+20 to +120)	
Adults		+50 (−30 to +105)	
Normal T wave axis in infants and children: (+) = upright T wave and (−) = inverted T wave			
	Leads V1 and V2	*Lead aVF*	*Leads I, V5, and V6*
Birth to 1 day old	+/−	+	+/−
1-4 days old	+/−	+	+
4 days to adolescent	−	−	+
Adolescent to adult	+	+	+

atresia, or tricuspid atresia. The cyanotic infant with increased vascular markings may have transposition of the great vessels, total anomalous pulmonary venous return, or truncus arteriosus. Increased vascular markings in an acyanotic infant are suggestive of an endocardial cushion defect, ventricular septal defect, atrial septal defect, or a patent ductus arteriosus.

In a normal left-sided aortic arch, the aorta descends to the left of the midline and displaces the tracheal air shadow slightly toward the right of midline above the level of the carina. In contrast to this, the tracheal air shadow may be midline or deviated toward the left in the presence of a right-sided aortic arch.[2] This finding is important to note, since a right-sided aortic arch is found in up to 25% of the children with tetralogy of Fallot.[8] Rib notching secondary to increased collateral blood flow along the intercostal vessels can sometimes be appreciated between the fourth and eighth ribs in older children with undiagnosed coarctation of the aorta but is rarely visualized in children with coarctation of the aorta who are younger than 5 years of age.[8]

Electrocardiogram

The ECG findings in infants and children can sometimes be problematic because various components of the ECGs change according to the child's age (Table 169-3).[5] At birth, the muscle mass of the right ventricle is greater than that of the left ventricle. By the end of the first month of life, the left ventricle assumes dominance. By 6 months of age, the left ventricular to right ventricular mass ratio is 2:1, which then reaches the adult ratio of 2.5:1 by adolescence. The durations of the PR interval, QRS complex, and QT intervals all increase with age.

Left axis deviation is present when the QRS axis is less than the lower limit of normal for the child's age and occurs with left ventricular hypertrophy and left bundle branch block. Right axis deviation is present when the QRS axis is greater than the upper limit of normal for the child's age and occurs with right ventricular hypertrophy and right bundle branch block. A "superior" QRS axis (0 degrees to −180 degrees with an S wave in aVF greater than the R wave) may be suggestive of an endocardial cushion defect or tricuspid atresia.

Some of the more common indications for obtaining an ECG in a pediatric patient include chest pain, dyspnea, syncope, palpitations, and suspected dysrhythmias. Other indications for obtaining an ECG are in those children with known cardiac disorders who present with signs and symptoms that could reflect an acute decompensation of their underlying disorder. A rare but potentially fatal congenital cardiac abnormality that will demonstrate ECG abnormalities (i.e., ischemic changes) is the condition of the anomalous origin of the left coronary artery. These infants have a history of poor feeding, irritability, and failure to thrive, then suddenly present with cardiogenic shock secondary to myocardial ischemia.

Biochemical Markers

The utility and clinical accuracy of cardiac biochemical markers such as creatinine phosphokinase MB and cardiac troponin-T in the emergency department setting is currently limited in the pediatric population. Plasma homocysteine levels have been studied recently as a possible link to CHF in adults; however, there are currently no studies regarding plasma homocysteine levels in pediatric cardiac disorders.[9] Several recent studies have evaluated the use of plasma B-type natriuretic peptide levels in the assessment and management of CHF in adults.[10] Studies of B-type natriuretic peptide levels in children have demonstrated a similar correlation of elevated levels in children with CHF, and these also correlated to the clinical symptoms of heart failure and the ejection fraction as measured by echocardiography.[11]

Table 169-4. Incidence of Specific Congenital Heart Defects (CHDs)

Defect	Percent of CHD
Acyanotic CHDs	
Ventricular septal defect (VSD)	20-25%
Atrial septal defect (ASD)	5-10%
Patent ductus arteriosus (PDA)	5-10%
Coarctation of the aorta (CoA)	8%
Pulmonic stenosis (PS)	5-8%
Aortic stenosis (AS)	5%
Cyanotic CHDs	
Tetralogy of Fallot (TOF)	10%
Transposition of the great arteries (TGA)	5%
Tricuspid atresia (TriA)	1-2%
Total anomalous pulmonary venous return (TAPVR)	1%
Truncus arteriosus (TA)	<1%
Pulmonary atresia (PA)	<1%
Ebstein's anomaly (EA)	<1%
Hypoplastic left heart syndrome (HLHS)	<1%
Hypoplastic right heart syndrome (HRHS)	<1%

Table 169-5. Symptomatic Presentation of Congenital Heart Defects (CHDs) and Time of Presentation

Defect	Time of Presentation
CHDs that Present with Cyanosis	
Transposition of the great arteries	Birth to 2 weeks of life
Total anomalous pulmonary venous return	Birth to 2 weeks of life
Tricuspid atresia	Birth to 2 weeks of life
Ebstein's anomaly of the tricuspid valve	Birth to 2 weeks of life
Truncus arteriosus	Birth to 2 weeks of life
Pulmonary atresia	Birth to 2 weeks of life
Hypoplastic right heart syndrome	Birth to 2 weeks of life
Hypoplastic left heart syndrome	Birth to 2 weeks of life
Tetralogy of Fallot	Birth to 12 weeks of life
CHDs that Present with Shock	
Coarctation of the aorta	From 1st week of life on
Aortic stenosis	From 1st week of life on
CHDs that Present with CHF	
Ventricular septal defects	From 4 weeks of life on
Patent ductus arteriosus	From 4 weeks of life on

SPECIFIC DISORDERS

CONGENITAL HEART DISEASE

Perspective

The incidence of congenital heart disease (CHD) in the United States has remained fairly constant at approximately 1%, or 8 to 10 cases per 1000 live births. This equates to approximately 32,000 infants born each year with some form of CHD[12] (Table 169-4). Although a large percentage of CHDs are now detected with prenatal ultrasonograms, one recent study also recommended using the pulse oximeter to routinely screen all newborns prior to discharge from the nursery as an additional inexpensive screening tool for CHDs.[13]

Clinical Features

The age, severity of symptoms, and time of presentation of a child with CHD varies depending on the specific defect, complexity and severity of the defect, and the timing of the normal physiologic changes that occur as the fetal circulation transitions to that of a neonate (Table 169-5). The more severe or complex CHDs may not be clinically apparent immediately after birth. However, as the ductus arteriosus begins to close in the first several weeks of life, those cardiac defects with obstructive lesions of the pulmonary or systemic circulations will be unmasked, and these infants will clinically present with acute cyanosis or shock, or both. The harsh systolic murmur of even a large, isolated ventricular septal defect may not be heard until about the 4th to 6th week of life when the left-to-right shunt across the ventricular septal defect increases due to the decrease in the pulmonary vascular resistance. In general, the more severe the anatomic defect is (i.e.,

BOX 169-6. Clinical Clues to Aid in the Diagnosis of Congenital Heart Disease (CHD)

- Presence or absence of central or peripheral cyanosis?
  - Central cyanosis with minimal respiratory distress ("comfortably blue") is more suggestive of a CHD rather than a purely pulmonary etiology
- Abnormalities in cardiac auscultation?
  - Murmurs: systolic-vs-diastolic, location, and radiation
  - Quality of S1, S2, and the presence of any clicks or gallops
- Change in the degree of central cyanosis with crying?
  - Worsening of cyanosis with crying suggests a cardiac rather than a purely pulmonary etiology
- Response of the PaO_2 to the hyperoxia challenge (administering 100% oxygen)?
  - Purely pulmonary causes of cyanosis:
    - PaO_2 should rise to levels above 200 mm Hg
  - Cyanotic CHDs associated with an increased pulmonary blood flow:
    - PaO_2 may occasionally reach as high as 150 mm Hg
  - Cyanotic CHDs associated with a decreased pulmonary blood flow:
    - PaO_2 will not rise over 100 mm Hg
- CXR abnormalities?
  - Cardiac size and shape (one of the three classic cardiac silhouettes)?
    - Boot-shaped heart: TOF
    - Egg on a string heart: TGA
    - Snowman-shaped or figure-eight heart: TAPVR
  - Degree of pulmonary blood flow?
    - Increased (acyanotic): ASD, ESM, VSD, PDA, ECD
    - Increased (cyanotic): TGA, TAPVR, HLHS, TruncA
    - Decreased or normal (acyanotic): PS, AS, CoA
    - Decreased (cyanotic): TOF, severe PS, EA, TriA, PA, HRHS
- ECG abnormalities?
  - Evidence of chamber enlargement: RVH, LVH, BVH, RAH, or LAH
  - An abnormal superior QRS axis is suggestive of ECD or TriA

lack of pulmonary blood flow or lack of systemic blood flow), the earlier in life these conditions will manifest with cyanosis and shock.

Although CHD has been classically subdivided into cyanotic and acyanotic conditions, not all CHDs will fit neatly into a single category, and some of the more complex defects have mixed pathophysiologic effects. Although the exact anatomic diagnosis of a CHD is dependent on echocardiography or cardiac catheterization, being able to establish the exact anatomic diagnosis is not entirely necessary in the emergency department setting.

Diagnostic Strategies

The emergency physician must rely on several key elements of the clinical examination in addition to chest radiograph and ECG findings (Box 169-6) to narrow down the diagnostic possibilities. For example, using the data in Box 169-6, the presence of cyanosis, a grade 3/6 systolic-ejection murmur best heard at the mid-left sternal border, a boot-shaped heart, and decreased pulmonary blood flow on the chest radiograph with evidence of right ventricular hypertrophy on the ECG suggests tetralogy of Fallot. Only a brief discussion of some of the more common CHDs is presented in this chapter.

BOX 169-7. Ductal-Dependent Cardiac Lesions in the Neonate

CHDs that require a patent ductus arteriosus to preserve blood flow from the aorta to the pulmonary circulation:

- Tetralogy of Fallot
- Tricuspid atresia
- Pulmonary atresia
- Hypoplastic right heart syndrome
- Transposition of the great vessels

CHDs that require a patent ductus arteriosus to preserve blood flow from the main pulmonary artery to the systemic circulation:

- Severe coarctation of the aorta
- Severe aortic stenosis
- Hypoplastic left heart syndrome

Management

The majority of the children who present to the emergency department with shock due to dehydration and hypovolemia are typically given intravenous fluids in 20 mL/kg boluses. However, if a child with a suspected CHD presents to the emergency department in possible cardiogenic shock, one could consider using smaller 10 mL/kg boluses to prevent an iatrogenic complication of fluid overload. Frequent reassessments should be performed and the child's response after each 10 mL/kg bolus monitored to determine whether additional fluid boluses or inotropic agents are necessary.

One unique pharmacologic intervention that can be lifesaving in infants involves the use of prostaglandin E1 (PGE1) to maintain the patency of the ductus arteriosus. CHDs that manifest within the first 2 to 3 weeks of life with a sudden onset of cyanosis or cardiovascular collapse are typically due to ductal-dependent cardiac lesions (Box 169-7).[3]

Closure of the ductus arteriosus in patients with these specific cardiac lesions causes life-threatening situations due to either an interruption of blood flow to the lungs producing cyanosis (i.e., tricuspid atresia) or a disruption of blood flow to the systemic circulation producing shock (i.e., hypoplastic left heart syndrome).[3] Box 169-8 details one suggested method to prepare this potentially lifesaving PGE1 infusion. The PGE1 infusion is typically started at 0.05 μg/kg/minute (which is equal to 5 mL/hour based on the method of preparation described in Box 169-8). Because one of the adverse reactions of a PGE1 infusion is apnea, one should consider intubating these infants prior to the initiation of the PGE1 infusion. Not only will intubation provide a secure airway, but controlled ventilation

BOX 169-8. Prostaglandin E1 (PGE1) Infusion Preparation for Ductal-Dependent CHDs

- Infusion rate: 0.01 to 0.1 µg/kg/minute
- Available PGE1 solution: 500 µg/mL (Alprostadil)
- [0.06] × [infant's weight in kg] = number of mg of PGE1 to add to enough diluent fluid to bring the total volume of the infusion to 100 mL. When the PGE1 drip is prepared in this manner, 1 mL/hour will provide exactly 0.01 µg/kg/minute
- Example: 0.18 mg (which equals 180 µg) of PGE1 would be required to prepare a drip for a 3 kg infant who presents with a suspected ductal-dependent cardiac defect. This solution will deliver 0.01 µg/kg/minute of PGE1 when run at 1 mL/hour. Therefore, 5 mL/hour will deliver 0.05 µg/kg/min
- The amount (µg) of PGE1 that would be required to prepare a PGE1 infusion as described in the method above is as follows:

2 kg infant	120 µg of PGE1
2.5 kg infant	150 µg of PGE1
3 kg infant	180 µg of PGE1
3.5 kg infant	210 µg of PGE1
4 kg infant	240 µg of PGE1
4.5 kg infant	270 µg of PGE1
5 kg infant	300 µg of PGE1

will also help decrease the infant's work of breathing. Other adverse reactions of a PGE1 infusion include fever, seizures, bradycardia, hypotension, flushing, and decreased platelet aggregation.

Acyanotic Congenital Heart Defect

Acyanotic CHD can be further subdivided (Figure 169-5) into obstructive lesions (i.e., pulmonic stenosis, aortic stenosis, and coarctation of the aorta) and lesions characterized by left-to-right shunts with an associated increase in pulmonary blood flow (i.e., ventricular septal defects, atrial septal defects, patent ductus arteriosus, and endocardial cushion defects). These acyanotic lesions usually manifest within the first 6 months of life with symptoms of CHF; however, atrial septal defects can remain asymptomatic until adulthood.

Ventricular Septal Defect

Perspective

Ventricular septal defects are the most common congenital cardiac defects and account for 20% to 25% of all cases of CHDs. Spontaneous closure occurs in 30% to 40% of all ventricular septal defects overall and in 50% to 70% of smaller ventricular septal defects.[14]

Clinical Features

The degree of symptoms is dependent on the size of the ventricular septal defects and the degree of PVR. Most ventricular septal defects are clinically asymptomatic (minimal to no left-to-right shunting) immediately after birth because of the high PVR. When the PVR decreases to the normal levels at 6 to 8 weeks after birth, left-to-right shunting can then occur and the typical systolic murmur of a ventricular septal defect will then be

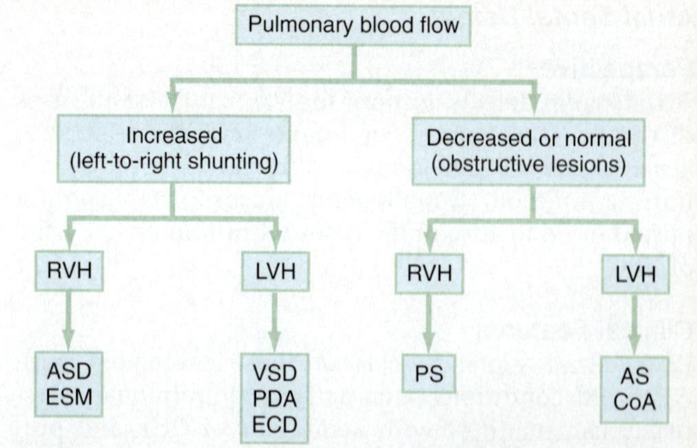

Figure 169-5. Clinical clues to diagnosing acyanotic congenital heart defects. AS, aortic stenosis; ASD, atrial septal defect; CoA, coarctation of the aorta; ECD, endocardial cushion defect; ESM, Eisenmenger's syndrome; LVH, left ventricular hypertrophy; PDA, patent ductus arteriosus; PS, pulmonic stenosis; RVH, right ventricular hypertrophy; VSD, ventricular septal defect.

appreciated. Small ventricular septal defects may remain completely asymptomatic throughout childhood. Approximately 10% of the infants with large ventricular septal defects will eventually develop signs and symptoms of CHF (e.g., poor feeding and poor growth) by 2 to 3 months of age because of the increased pulmonary blood flow. Older children with ventricular septal defects may exhibit signs of decreased exercise tolerance and recurrent pulmonary infections. If moderate-to-large ventricular septal defects are not surgically corrected, irreversible changes in the pulmonary vasculature may begin to occur as early as 6 to 12 months of age, which will result in an elevation of the PVR and pulmonary hypertension. This in turn can lead to a reversal of the shunt direction across the ventricular septal defect to now become a right-to-left shunt, the Eisenmenger syndrome, with resultant cyanosis.

Diagnostic Strategies

The chest radiograph in children with small ventricular septal defects may be entirely normal, but cardiomegaly with increased pulmonary vascular markings is usually present with untreated moderate-to-large ventricular septal defects. The ECG of moderate-sized ventricular septal defects typically reveals left ventricular hypertrophy, but biventricular hypertrophy may be present in ventricular septal defects with large left-to-right shunting.

Management

All ventricular septal defects, regardless of the size of the defect, are at risk for bacterial endocarditis due to the high velocity of turbulent blood flow through them.

Traditional closure of ventricular septal defects required open heart surgery. Today, however, a transcatheter closure technique that avoids the inherent risks and complications of open heart surgery and cardiopulmonary bypass has supplanted traditional methods.[15-17]

Atrial Septal Defect

Perspective

Atrial septal defects account for 5% to 10% of all cases of CHDs. The majority of infants and children with atrial septal defects remain clinically asymptomatic until adulthood. Spontaneous closure has been reported in up to 40% of the cases within the first 5 years of life.[14]

Clinical Features

Large atrial septal defects or those associated with comorbid conditions such as bronchopulmonary dysplasia can manifest with symptoms of CHF and pulmonary overcirculation (e.g., dyspnea with feedings, poor weight gain, and frequent lower respiratory tract infections).[2] The majority of atrial septal defects are discovered when a suspicious murmur is detected on a routine physical examination. A widely split and fixed S2 is a characteristic finding of atrial septal defects.

Diagnostic Strategies

The chest radiograph of children with atrial septal defects will reveal varying degrees of cardiomegaly, right atrial and right ventricular enlargement, and a prominent main pulmonary artery segment and increased pulmonary vascular markings. The ECG will reveal varying degrees of right axis deviation and right ventricular hypertrophy. All patients with unrepaired atrial septal defects will develop symptoms if pulmonary hypertension ensues. Patients with large atrial septal defects that are not detected and repaired are at risk for development of the Eisenmenger's syndrome. Unlike ventricular septal defects, uncomplicated atrial septal defects are not associated with high risk for bacterial endocarditis because of the lower turbulence and velocity of blood flow through the atrial septal defects.

Management

Like ventricular septal defects, the traditional closure of atrial septal defects required open heart surgery to place a patch over the septal defect. Newer therapies involving closures with septal occluder devices placed via the transcatheter approach have been described.[18,19] Antiplatelet therapy during the 6-month period after placement of the device is also utilized and is safe and effective in preventing thrombus formation on the surface of the septal occluder device.

Eisenmenger's Syndrome

Eisenmenger's syndrome can occur in any large left-to-right shunt defect that is not surgically corrected. When large left-to-right shunts are left untreated (i.e., large ventricular septal defects and atrial septal defects that are not surgically corrected), irreversible changes can occur in the pulmonary arterioles leading to pulmonary vascular obstruction and pulmonary hypertension. As the degree of pulmonary hypertension increases, the PVR may then begin to exceed the SVR, which will then promote right-to-left shunting. This reversal in the direction of shunt flow can then produce cyanosis. Clinical features of patients who have developed Eisenmenger's syndrome include chest pain, dyspnea on exertion, and hemoptysis.[20]

Coarctation of the Aorta

Perspective

Coarctation of the aorta accounts for approximately 8% of all CHDs, and up to 50% of patients with coarctation of the aorta also have an associated bicuspid aortic valve.[21] The area of coarctation can occur proximal to the insertion of the ductus arteriosus (preductal type) or distal to the insertion of the ductus arteriosus (postductal type). The majority of cases (89%) are of the postductal type.[21]

Clinical Features

The severity of the symptoms and the age at time of presentation are dependent on the location of the coarctation, the degree of narrowing, and the presence of any other associated cardiac defects. Infants with the preductal type of coarctation of the aorta may also exhibit differential cyanosis if the ductus arteriosus remains open.[22] The upper half of their body is perfused with well-oxygenated blood supplied by the left ventricle and the ascending aorta. However, the lower half of their body will appear cyanotic, as it is largely perfused via right-to-left shunting of deoxygenated blood from the patent ductus arteriosus into the descending aorta.

Infants with the rarer preductal type of coarctation of the aorta will present with signs of circulatory failure and shock when the ductus arteriosus begins to close. Weaker pulses and lower blood pressures in the lower extremities as compared with the upper extremities are the classic physical examination findings in infants and children with coarctation of the aorta.

Most of the asymptomatic postductal cases of coarctation of the aorta are diagnosed as a result of a cardiology referral for a systolic murmur or a hypertension workup, but infants with severe postductal coarctation of the aorta can also present during the first few weeks of life with signs of circulatory failure and shock. If a child is discovered to have hypertension on a routine physical examination, it is mandatory to obtain blood pressure measurements in the lower extremities to rule out the possibility of coarctation of the aorta. A systolic blood pressure in the right arm that is 15 to 20 mm Hg greater than that in the legs is sufficient evidence to suspect coarctation of the aorta because the systolic blood pressures in the legs are normally higher than that in the arms.[22] If the systolic pressure in the right arm is higher than that in the left arm, the area of coarctation is probably preductal and located proximal to the origin of the left subclavian artery.

Diagnostic Strategies

The chest radiograph will most often reveal a normal-sized cardiac silhouette and normal pulmonary vascular markings, but in children older than 5 years of age, it may exhibit notching along the lower borders of the posterior fourth to eighth ribs due to the pressure of the

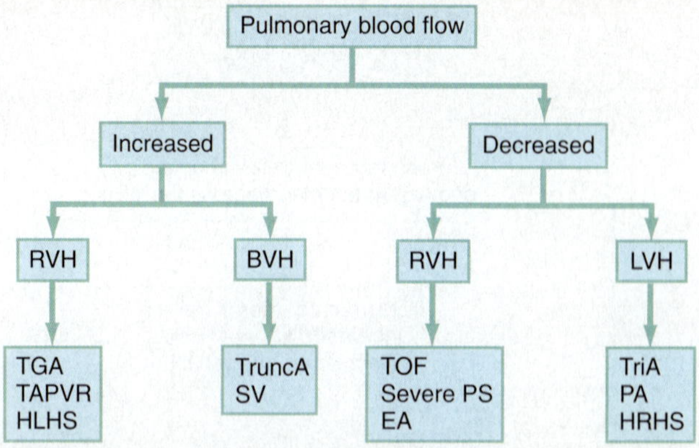

Figure 169-6. Clinical clues to diagnosing cyanotic congenital heart defects. BVH, biventricular hypertrophy; EA, Ebstein's anomaly; HLHS, hypoplastic left heart syndrome; HRHS, hypoplastic right heart syndrome; LVH, left ventricular hypertrophy; PA, pulmonary atresia; PS, pulmonary stenosis; RVH, right ventricular hypertrophy; SV, single ventricle; TAPVR, total anomalous pulmonary venous return; TGA, transposition of the great arteries; TOF, tetralogy of Fallot; TriA, tricuspid atresia; TruncA, truncus arteriosus.

dilated collateral vessels. The absence of rib notching, however, does not rule out the possibility of coarctation of the aorta. The ECG typically reveals a left axis and left ventricular hypertrophy.

Management

Definitive surgical repair of coarctation of the aorta involves resection of the narrowed section of the aorta with an end-to-end anastomosis. Complications of undiagnosed cases are related to the resultant hypertension and can include heart failure, hypertensive encephalopathy, and intracranial hemorrhages.

Cyanotic Congenital Heart Diseases

Cyanotic CHDs are a result of either decreased pulmonary blood flow to the lungs or right-to-left shunting of desaturated blood directly into the systemic circulation. These cyanotic CHDs can be further subdivided into those conditions with an increased pulmonary blood flow and those lesions with decreased pulmonary blood flow (Figure 169-6). The classic cyanotic CHDs can be remembered by the "five T's": truncus arteriosus, transposition of the great vessels, tricuspid atresia, tetralogy of Fallot, and total anomalous pulmonary venous return. Other forms of cyanotic CHDs include Ebstein's anomaly, pulmonary atresia, severe pulmonary stenosis, hypoplastic left heart syndrome, and hypoplastic right heart syndrome. Because many of these cyanotic heart lesions are usually detected either on prenatal ultrasonographic examinations or in the nursery, only tetralogy of Fallot is covered in this section.

Tetralogy of Fallot

Perspective

Tetralogy of Fallot accounts for approximately 10% of all cases of CHD and is the most common cause of cyanotic CHD beyond infancy. Tetralogy of Fallot is often associated with other cardiac defects, such as a right-sided aortic arch (25% of patients), atrial septal defect (10% of patients), and anomalous origin of the left coronary artery.[23] Tetralogy of Fallot arises from a single embryologic defect in which the subpulmonic conus fails to expand, resulting in the four abnormalities (Figure 169-7): (1) right ventricular outflow tract obstruction; (2) a large, unrestrictive, malaligned ventricular septal defect; (3) an overriding aorta that receives blood flow from both ventricles; and (4) right ventricular hypertrophy secondary to the high pressure load placed on the right ventricle by the right ventricular outflow tract obstruction. These anatomic defects collectively result in decreased pulmonary blood flow and varying degrees of right-to-left shunting of deoxygenated blood across the ventricular septal defect.

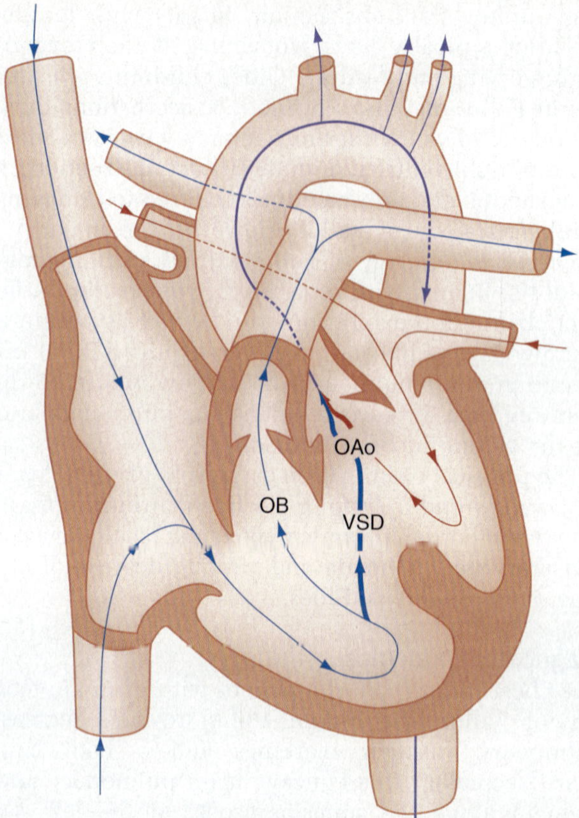

Figure 169-7. Diagrammatic representation of the right-to-left shunting that occurs in tetralogy of Fallot. Some of the deoxygenated blood (*thick blue arrow*) in the right ventricle is shunted across the ventricular septal defect (VSD) into the left ventricle. This deoxygenated blood mixes with the well-oxygenated blood from the lungs (*red arrow*). The blood that is ejected out through the overriding aorta (OAo) therefore contains blood of mixed oxygenation (*purple arrows*). The amount of deoxygenated blood that is shunted through the VSD (*thick blue arrow*) is dependent on a combination of factors, including the severity of right ventricular outflow tract obstruction (OB), the size of the VSD, and the degree of systematic vascular resistance (SVR). When the SVR falls (as occurs during a tet spell), more deoxygenated blood from the right ventricle will be shunted across the VSD into the systemic circulation, which results in hypoxia, metabolic acidosis, and worsening cyanosis.

Clinical Features

The degree of cyanosis and the age of presentation are directly dependent on the degree of right ventricular outflow tract obstruction. Infants with tetralogy of Fallot typically have worsening of their cyanosis during crying and feeding. Older children with tetralogy of Fallot may have cyanotic exacerbations during periods of physical exertion. Infants who have milder forms of right ventricular outflow tract obstruction may be acyanotic and are sometimes referred to as having a "pink" tetralogy of Fallot. However, the majority of the cases of tetralogy of Fallot exhibit some degree of cyanosis. Infants with severe right ventricular outflow tract obstruction exhibit profound cyanosis within the first few days of life and may even require a PGE1 infusion to preserve pulmonary blood flow via left-to-right shunting from the aorta into the main pulmonary artery via the patent ductus arteriosus.

The physical examination can reveal varying degrees of cyanosis and a systolic ejection murmur along the left sternal border. Chronic hypoxemia results in a compensatory polycythemia and varying degrees of clubbing of the fingers and toes.

Diagnostic Strategies

The chest radiograph of a patient with cyanotic tetralogy of Fallot (see Figure 169-4) reveals decreased pulmonary vascular markings and a boot-shaped heart (secondary to a concave main pulmonary artery segment along the superior aspect of the left heart border). The heart size in tetralogy of Fallot is normal, and a right-sided aortic arch may be seen in 25% of the cases. The ECG of cyanotic tetralogy of Fallot reveals right ventricular hypertrophy and a right axis deviation. Children with "pink" tetralogy of Fallot may not initially exhibit any degree of right ventricular hypertrophy, but these acyanotic forms of tetralogy of Fallot gradually develop the cyanotic form by 1 to 3 years of age.

A potentially life-threatening complication of tetralogy of Fallot that can be seen in a patient who presents to the emergency department is the so-called "tet spell," which has also been referred to as the "hypercyanotic spell" or the "hypoxic spell." Although these hypoxic spells can occur in children with other forms of CHDs, they are most commonly seen in infants and children with tetralogy of Fallot, and hence the term *tet spells.* These episodes occur most commonly in infants, with a peak incidence between 2 and 4 months of age.[23]

Any event that suddenly lowers the SVR, such as crying or defecation, will produce a large right-to-left shunt across the ventricular septal defect, beginning the vicious cycle of a hypoxic spell. Acute hypovolemia and tachycardia can also precipitate tet spells. The large right-to-left shunt through the ventricular septal defect bypasses the lungs, which then causes a decrease in the Pa_{O_2}, an increase in the P_{CO_2}, and a fall in the arterial pH. These metabolic changes then stimulate the respiratory centers in the brain to produce hyperpnea (deep and rapid respirations), which increases the negative intrathoracic pressure during inspiration, causing an increase in the systemic venous blood return to the right side of the heart. This

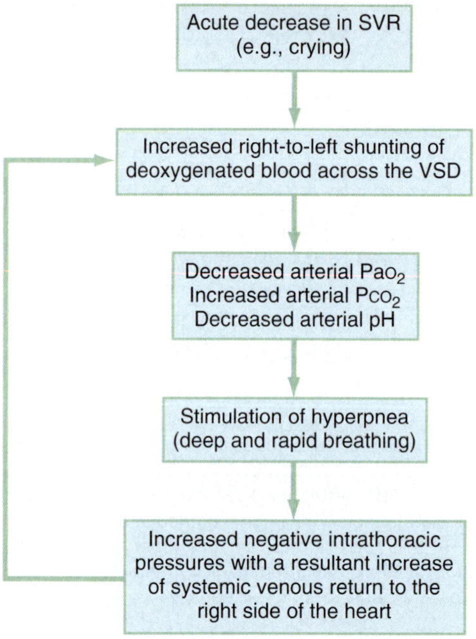

Figure 169-8. Pathophysiologic mechanisms of a hypoxic (tet) spell. SVR, systematic vascular resistance; VSD, ventricular septal defect.

increased volume of blood in the right ventricle is then shunted through the ventricular septal defect through the combination of the existing right ventricular tract outflow obstruction and the acute decrease in the SVR. This in turn further decreases the arterial oxygen saturation, perpetuating the hypoxic spell (Figure 169-8).

Clinically, these hypoxic spells are characterized by periods of hyperpnea (rapid and deep respirations), uncontrollable crying, and worsening cyanosis. Limpness, seizures, cerebrovascular accidents, and even death have been reported with more severe tet spells. During a tet spell, the intensity of the murmur decreases because of less blood flow through the right ventricular tract obstruction and more blood being shunted from the right ventricle to the left ventricle through the ventricular septal defect.

Management

The overall treatment goals for tet spells (Box 169-9) are (1) increasing the SVR, (2) abolishing the hyperpnea, and (3) correcting the metabolic acidosis. Although supplemental oxygen should be provided, this alone will not reverse a tet spell, since there is a decrease in the amount of pulmonary blood flow and an increase in the amount of right-to-left shunting across the ventricular septal defect. The infant should be picked up and placed in a knee-to-chest position. Older children can be placed in the squatting position. Both of these maneuvers are believed to increase the SVR and decrease the amount of systemic venous blood return to the right side of the heart. Morphine (0.1-0.2 mg/kg) has been traditionally given intramuscularly to suppress the respiratory center and thereby abolish the hyperpnea. A theoretical adverse affect of morphine, however, is that it can cause systemic vasodila-

BOX 169-9. Management of TOF Hypoxic Spells

- Place the infant in the knee-to-chest position to increase the SVR, which decreases the right-to-left shunt across the VSD.
- Provide supplemental oxygen (limited value by itself).
- Morphine: 0.1-0.2 mg/kg IV or IM
- Sodium bicarbonate: 1 mEq/kg IV
- Consider ketamine: 1-2 mg/kg IV or IM
- Consider propanolol: 0.01-0.2 mg/kg IV[5]
- Consider phenylephrine: 0.01-0.02 mg/kg IV[5]

tion (further decreasing the SVR) via endogenous histamine release.[24] Although there are no current studies evaluating the use of other medications that may also suppress the respiratory centers, fentanyl and midazolam could be utilized for the same effect without the potential risk of endogenous histamine release. Ketamine (1-2 mg/kg IV or IM) has also been suggested for its sedative effect as well as for its effect on increasing the SVR.[23] Sodium bicarbonate can be given to correct any metabolic acidosis and reduce the respiratory center stimulating effects of acidosis. Most infants respond to these measures and exhibit an improvement in their oxygenation and a decrease in their degree of cyanosis. Those infants whose condition does not improve with the above measures may require a vasopressor such as phenylephrine to increase the SVR and thereby decrease the degree of right-to-left shunting across the ventricular septal defect. An intravenous fluid bolus may also be considered to increase the volume of blood flow through the pulmonary artery. Propanolol has also been used as an adjunct to break the cycle of a tet spell. Although the exact pharmacophysiologic mechanisms by which propanolol accomplishes this is uncertain, it is thought to increase the SVR and perhaps promote an increase in the pulmonary blood flow by reducing spasms of the right ventricular outflow tract obstruction.

Palliative surgical procedures to temporarily increase the amount of blood flow to the pulmonary arteries are performed in infants with severe cyanotic tetralogy of Fallot. The most commonly performed shunting procedure is with the Blalock-Taussig shunt, in which an anastomosis is created between the subclavian artery and the ipsilateral pulmonary artery. Definitive surgical repair of tetralogy of Fallot consists of closing the ventricular septal defect and opening the right ventricular outflow tract obstruction by resection of the infundibular tissue. The mortality rate is 5% to 10% within the first 2 years after definitive surgical repair in uncomplicated tetralogy of Fallot cases. Complications that can occur after definitive surgical repair include complete heart block, ventricular dysrhythmias, and right bundle branch block (secondary to the right ventriculotomy). Bacterial endocarditis prophylaxis is still recommended after the definitive surgical repair of tetralogy of Fallot.

Postoperative Complications of Congenital Heart Defects

A variety of postoperative complications can be seen in patients who present to the emergency department weeks to months after cardiac surgery. The types of complications that could occur in each case depend on the original underlying cardiac defect as well as on the surgical procedure that was used to correct that defect. Some of the complications that may be seen in the emergency department include thrombosis of a shunt-conduit with decreased flow, increased shunt-conduit flow with resultant CHF, atrial and ventricular dysrhythmias, heart blocks, myocardial ischemia, and endocarditis. The size of the cardiac silhouette and the degree of pulmonary blood flow visualized on the chest radiograph may provide valuable clues as to whether there is an increased or decreased blood flow through a surgical conduit that was created to provide an improvement in blood flow to the pulmonary system.[25] Comparison of the child's other postoperative chest radiographs can help to determine whether there has been a change in the heart size and pulmonary vascularity.

The post-pericardiotomy syndrome is an inflammatory pericarditis that can occur 1 to 6 weeks after any surgical procedure that involved a pericardiotomy. This immunologic phenomenon is believed to occur as a sequela of blood in the pericardial sac. This syndrome is characterized by fever, chest pain, and a pericardial effusion. A pericardial friction rub may be heard, depending on the amount of fluid that accumulates in the pericardial sac. The chest radiograph may reveal an enlarged cardiac silhouette, and the echocardiogram will confirm the diagnosis. Pericardiocentesis is rarely required but may be necessary if the amount of pericardial effusion is significant enough to cause a pericardial tamponade. The majority of cases will resolve within 2 to 3 weeks with bed rest and nonsteroidal anti-inflammatory medication.

Many of the above-mentioned postoperative complications, including the post-pericardiotomy syndrome, can be avoided in children who undergo closure of patent ductus arteriosus, atrial septal defects, and ventricular septal defects via the transcatheter placement of various occluder devices.

Respiratory Syncytial Virus Infections in Infants and Children with Congenital Heart Defects

Respiratory syncytial virus (RSV) is the most common cause of lower respiratory tract infections in infants and children worldwide, with the majority of children being infected at least once by 2 years of age. Reinfection occurs commonly throughout life.[26] RSV lower respiratory tract infections account for more than 125,000 pediatric admissions annually in the United States, with a fatality rate of 6.3 deaths per 100,000 patients up to 4 years of age (Box 169-10).[27,28] Children with CHDs who develop RSV infections tend to have a

BOX 169-10. Conditions Associated with an Increased Risk of Severe or Fatal RSV Infections

- Cyanotic or complex congenital heart defects
- Pulmonary hypertension
- Prematurity (especially those infants with bronchopulmonary dysplasia or chronic lung disease)
- Immunodeficiency states

BOX 169-11. Recommendations for Palivizumab Administration in Children with Congenital Heart Defects (CHDs)

CHD conditions that would benefit from palivizumab administration (15 mg/kg IM q 30 days during the RSV season only):
- Cyanotic or complex CHDs
- Congenital heart failure requiring medications
- Moderate to severe pulmonary hypertension

Children with hemodynamically insignificant CHDs who do not require palivizumab administration:
- Secundum ASDs
- Small VSDs
- Pulmonic stenosis
- Uncomplicated aortic stenosis
- Mild coarctation of the aorta
- Patent ductus arteriosus

higher rate of intensive care unit admissions and require mechanical ventilation more frequently than those children who do not have CHDs. Children with CHDs who require hospitalization for RSV have a fatality rate that is two to six times greater than that of children without CHDs.[27,28] RSV is responsible for a mortality rate of 40% in infants with CHDs and up to 70% in infants with CHDs and associated pulmonary hypertension.

Currently, there are two products that can be used to prevent RSV infections. Both of these preparations must be administered monthly prior to the onset of the peak RSV season, which typically runs from November through March in most states. The two currently available preparations are (1) palivizumab (Synagis), which is a humanized monoclonal antibody administered intramuscularly at a dose of 15 mg/kg and (2) RSV immunoglobulin (RespiGam), which requires intravenous administration at a dose of 750 mg/kg (which is equal to 15 mL/kg) and must be administered over a 4-hour period.[26] The use of palivizumab in the prevention of RSV infections in high-risk infants and children has largely replaced RSV immunoglobulin because palivizumab can be given intramuscularly, requires a 100-fold lesser volume, and has a 50-fold smaller protein load than RSV immunoglobulin.[29]

In 1998, the Food and Drug Administration gave approval for the use of palivizumab in preventing RSV lower tract respiratory tract infections in selected infants and children who were deemed to have a higher risk of severe infections. During the 4-year period from 1998 to 2002, several multicenter studies involving more than 24,000 subjects (including data from the Palivizumab Outcomes Registry) have demonstrated the efficacy of palivizumab in preventing hospitalizations of high-risk infants and children.[30] During this same 4-year period, another multicenter study involving six countries demonstrated a 45% relative reduction in hospitalization of 1287 high-risk children younger than 2 years of age with CHDs who were given 15 mg/kg monthly intramuscular injections of palivizumab over a 5-month period.[29] This study also demonstrated a significant reduction in the total number of hospital days, supplemental oxygen requirements, total number of days in the intensive care unit, and total number of days requiring intubation in the group that received the monthly palivizumab intramuscular injections. Based on these results, the Food and Drug Administration in September of 2003 gave approval for the use of palivizumab in infants and children with hemodynamically significant CHDs (Box 169-11). The American Academy of Pediatrics emphasizes that prophylaxis with palivizumab should be initiated prior to the onset of RSV season. Since RSV can persist on environmental surfaces for several hours, the best method to prevent the spread of RSV-contaminated secretions within the emergency department setting is meticulous hand washing and wearing a mask when caring for children with a documented or suspected RSV infection.

CONGESTIVE HEART FAILURE

Perspective

Congestive heart failure is physiologically defined as a clinical syndrome in which the cardiac output is unable to meet the hemodynamic and metabolic demands of the body. Although there are a wide array of causes of CHF, the primary cause in infants and children is CHD, which results in a problem of volume overload or of pressure overload. Other causes of CHF include the anomalous left coronary artery in infants, myocarditis, endocarditis, rheumatic heart disease, pericardial effusions, anemia, cardiomyopathies, systemic hypertension, hypothyroidism, electrolyte imbalances, cardiac toxins, and dysrhythmias that compromise cardiac output.

Congestive heart failure can result from a derangement in one of the four primary determinants of normal cardiac function: (1) excessive preload (i.e., large left-to-right shunts and severe chronic anemia); (2) decreased cardiac contractility (i.e., myocarditis); (3) excessive afterload (i.e., left-sided obstructive lesions); and (4) rhythm abnormalities that compromise cardiac output or stroke volume (i.e., paroxysmal supraventricular tachycardia and severe forms of heart block). The treatment of CHF depends on which of these four primary determinants of normal cardiac function are compromised. For example, inotropic agents and diuretics may be required in a child with volume overload and decreased cardiac contractility, whereas vasodilating agents may be required in a child with CHF due to an increased afterload.

Clinical Features

Although the clinical manifestations of CHF depend on the exact pathophysiologic cause of the CHF, common presenting signs and symptoms include tachycardia, a gallop rhythm, tachypnea with rales, hepatomegaly, peripheral edema, and decreased peripheral perfusion of the extremities. Wheezing and a chronic cough may also be the presenting symptoms of CHF.

Diagnostic Strategies

The chest radiograph typically reveals an enlargement of the cardiac silhouette and varying degrees of pulmonary congestion. An echocardiogram will be able to visualize the effectiveness of cardiac contractility in addition to visualizing any underlying anatomic defects that could be contributing to the condition. Other diagnostic studies to consider are case specific and depend on the suspected cause of the child's CHF.

Management

Acute stabilization of any child who presents with CHF includes administration of supplemental oxygen and agents to augment cardiac contractility and improve cardiac output. Children who present in severe respiratory distress secondary to pulmonary edema may require intubation to support oxygenation and ventilation. Children with respiratory distress and air hunger secondary to pulmonary congestion may also benefit from elevation of the head and upper torso in addition to morphine sulfate (0.05-0.1 mg/kg/dose) administration. Continuous positive airway pressure or biphasic positive airway pressure ventilation may be useful and avert the need for endotracheal intubation. Plasma B-type natriuretic peptide levels have been shown to be elevated in children with CHF and have also been used to monitor the response to treatment regimens in patients with CHF.[11]

Diuretics and inotropics agents are the mainstay of treatment for the majority of children with CHF. Furosemide (Lasix) in a dose of 1 mg/kg is the most common loop diuretic used to increase renal perfusion and improve urine output. Digoxin has remained as the most widely used inotropic agent to treat CHF in children (Table 169-6). With the proper use of furosemide and digoxin, most children with CHF will demonstrate a favorable response. The narrow therapeutic index of digoxin requires that levels be monitored very closely to prevent iatrogenic digoxin toxicity, which could cause a worsening of the preexisting CHF.

Other inotropics agents that have been used for the treatment of CHF in infants and children are dopamine, dobutamine, and epinephrine (Table 169-7). Box 169-12 describes "the Rule of Six," a simple method to prepare any pediatric drip. Dopamine is an endogenous catecholamine with complex cardiovascular effects. Dopamine can increase renal blood flow in low doses (2-5 μg/kg/min) and will increase the cardiac contractility and heart rate in moderate doses (5-10 μg/kg/min). Dopamine stimulates cardiac β_1-adrenergic receptors both directly and indirectly through the release of endogenous norepinephrine stored in the cardiac sympathetic nerves. Because of this, some of the inotropic effects of dopamine may be reduced in those patients with decreased endogenous myocardial norepinephrine stores (i.e., patients with chronic CHF and neonates). At higher doses (10-20 μg/kg/min), dopamine will also increase the SVR, but excessive vasoconstriction may compromise end-organ perfusion at infusion rates greater than 20 μg/kg/min. If additional inotropic effects are required, the addition of either dobutamine

Table 169-6. Digoxin Dosing for Infants and Children with Congestive Heart Failure[5]

Age	Total Digitalizing Dose (Oral)*	Daily Maintenance Dose (Oral)
Premature	20 mcg/kg/24 hours	5 mcg/kg/day
Full term	30 mcg/kg/24 hours	8-10 mcg/kg/day
<2 years	40-50 mcg/kg/24 hours	10-12 mcg/kg/day
2-10 years	30-40 mcg/kg/24 hours	8-10 mcg/kg/day
>10 years	0.75-1.25 mg/24 hours	0.125-0.25 mg/day

*The IV dose of digoxin is equal to 75% of the oral dose (except in children >10 years old in which the IV dose is the same as the oral dose).

The total daily digitalizing dose (TDD) is given as follows: ½ of the TDD given initially, followed by ¼ of the TDD given at q 8-12 hours x 2 doses after the initial dose.

The daily maintenance dose is divided into a BID dosing regimen (except in children >10 years of age in which the maintenance dose can be given as a single daily dosing regimen).

IV digoxin is supplied as 100 mcg/mL and 250 mcg/mL solutions.

Oral digoxin suspension is supplied as a 50 mcg/mL elixir.

Therapeutic range: 0.8-2.0 mcg/L.

A lower dosing regimen may be required in those patients with renal failure since digoxin is excreted by the kidneys.

Table 169-7. Inotropic and Load Altering Agents Used in the Treatment of Congestive Heart Failure

	Inotrope	Chronotrope	Vascular Effects	Infusion Ranges
Dopamine	+	+	Pressor	2-20 mcg/kg/min
Dobutamine	+	+/−	Vasodilator	2-20 mcg/kg/min
Epinephrine	+	+	Pressor	0.1-1.0 mcg/kg/min
Amrinone	+	No	Vasodilator	0.5-2 mg/kg bolus over 5 minutes followed by 5-10 mcg/kg/min
Nitroprusside	No	No	Potent vasodilator	0.5-10 mcg/kg/min

BOX 169-12. The Rule of Six: Preparation of Pediatric Drips

The basic formula or "recipe" used to prepare pediatric drips is to multiply the child's weight (in kg) times 6: (kg) × 6 = # mg of the medication used to prepare the drip.

This resulting number is equal to the amount of medication (in mg) that you would draw up and add to enough diluent fluid to bring the TOTAL volume (medication + diluent fluid) to 100 mL.

Any solution prepared in this fashion will deliver 1 μg/kg/min when run at 1 mL/hour.

Example: Prepare a dopamine drip to run at 14 μg/kg/min in a 10 kg child.

(10 kg) × 6 = 60 mg of dopamine added to enough NS to bring the total volume up to 100 mL. Since 1 mL/hour of this solution delivers 1 μg/kg/min, simply run the IV at 14 mL/hour to deliver the desired infusion of 14 μg/kg/min.

BOX 169-13. Conditions Associated with a High Risk for Developing Dysrhythmias

- Congenital heart defects (uncorrected defects and postoperative complications)
- Congenital complete heart blocks (i.e., maternal systemic lupus erythematosus)
- Myocarditis
- Rheumatic heart disease
- Kawasaki disease with involvement of the coronary arteries
- Cardiomyopathy
- Prolonged QT syndrome
- Aberrant atrioventricular conduction pathways (i.e., WPW syndrome)
- Electrolyte abnormalities (i.e., potassium, calcium, and magnesium disturbances)
- Commotio cordis
- Profound hypothermia
- Hypoxia

or epinephrine infusions may be preferable to increasing the dopamine infusion greater than 20 μg/kg/min. The major toxicities of dopamine are tachycardia, vasoconstriction, and ventricular ectopy.

Dobutamine is a synthetic catecholamine with more selective cardiac inotropic effects and some β_2-adrenergic vasodilatory effects. It is most useful in the treatment of low cardiac output states that are secondary to poor myocardial function. Dobutamine may have an advantage over dopamine in that it has fewer arrhythmogenic effects than dopamine and may also have a more direct effect on the enhancement of coronary blood flow. The main toxicities of dobutamine are tachycardia, ventricular ectopy, and hypotension.

Epinephrine is a potent inotrope and chronotrope and also increases the SVR. Therefore, epinephrine is useful in scenarios in which poor cardiac output is also associated with diminished systemic vascular tone. Toxicities associated with epinephrine include tachydysrhythmias, severe hypertension, hyperglycemia, lactic acidosis, and hypokalemia.

Amrinone and milrinone are newer inotropic agents that also have peripheral vasodilatory effects. These agents have been used in improving cardiac index in septic shock and in prevention of low cardiac output states for children with CHD. Side effects of these medications include profound hypotension, dysrhythmias, hypersensitivity reactions, fever, hepatotoxicity, and thrombocytopenia.

Another vasodilating medication that has been used for arterial and venous dilatory effects is nitroprusside. Nitroprusside has potent vasodilatory effects on both the systemic and pulmonary circulatory systems. This medication has a prompt onset of action and a short duration of action. Nitroprusside must be used cautiously in patients with either hepatic and/or renal impairment to avoid cyanide toxicity (severe metabolic acidosis and coma) or thiocyanate toxicity (irritability, seizures, abdominal pain, and vomiting).

PEDIATRIC DYSRHYTHMIAS

Perspective

Dysrhythmias are not as common in children as they are in adults. The most common cause of cardiopulmonary arrest in infants and children is the untreated progression of respiratory failure or shock rather than a primary cardiac dysrhythmia.[31] As a result of this, the most common arrest rhythm that will confront the emergency physician will be asystole and bradyasystole rather than ventricular fibrillation or ventricular tachycardia. Therefore, when confronted with a child with a primary cardiac dysrhythmia, the physician must very quickly and systematically identify and treat the underlying cause. Children who are at risk for developing dysrhythmias are listed in Box 169-13. Various medications, drugs and toxins can also precipitate dysrhythmias in children. Even those medications that are used to treat underlying cardiac problems such as digoxin, amiodarone, and procainamide can in themselves precipitate dysrhythmias. Drugs of abuse (i.e., cocaine and crystal methamphetamine) and overdose of prescription medications (i.e., cyclic antidepressants) should always be considered when evaluating any previously healthy adolescent patient who presents with an acute dysrhythmia.

Pediatric dysrhythmias can be divided into three broad categories of rhythms based on their effect on the child's pulse: SLOW/bradycardia (sinus bradycardia and heart blocks), FAST/tachycardia (supraventricular tachycardia or ventricular tachycardia with a pulse) and those rhythms with ABSENT pulses (ventricular fibrillation, ventricular tachycardia, pulseless electrical activity, asystole).[32] The most common dysrhythmia in children is supraventricular tachycardia, which occurs most commonly in infants and young children. Although supraventricular tachycardia can spontaneously occur in infants without any underlying structural cardiac defects, ventricular tachycardias typically are due to an underlying myocardial abnormality.

Clinical Features

Rhythm disturbances in infants can manifest with symptoms such as fussiness, lethargy, poor feeding, pallor, respiratory distress, or cardiogenic shock. Older children present with chest pain, palpitations, difficulty breathing, or syncope. The type and degree of severity of the presenting signs and symptoms must be taken into account when considering the evaluation and management of the specific dysrhythmia in each case.

Management

Not every child who exhibits a rhythm disturbance requires emergency interventions. Emergency treatment and stabilization of any dysrhythmia depend on two key clinical factors: (1) Does the child have a pulse? and (2) If a pulse is present, is it slow or fast and is the child hemodynamically stable or unstable? Children who have a pulse with good perfusion parameters (i.e., an alert child with strong distal pulses, warm extremities, and brisk capillary refill times) do not require emergency interventions unless they exhibit a rhythm that has the potential to rapidly degenerate into a more serious condition. Children who exhibit ECG evidence of conduction abnormalities (i.e., Mobitz type II second-degree heart blocks, complete heart blocks, prolonged QT intervals, or aberrant conduction such as the Wolff-Parkinson-White syndrome) may also warrant more emergency treatment.

A summary of the treatment algorithms for pediatric dysrhythmias and the most commonly utilized medications in treating these dysrhythmias are listed in Box 169-14. Although some medications can only be used to treat atrial tachycardias (i.e., the use of adenosine for supraventricular tachycardia) or ventricular tachycardias (i.e., the use of lidocaine for ventricular tachycardia), amiodarone and procainamide can be used for a wide array of both atrial and ventricular dysrhythmias, including supraventricular tachycardia and ventricular tachycardia.[33,34]

Bradydysrhythmias

Sinus Bradycardia

Bradycardia is defined as a heart rate that is slower than the lower limit of normal for a child's age. Based on the current definition by the American Heart Association guidelines in Pediatric Advanced Life Support, clinically significant bradycardia in children is defined as a heart rate slower than 60 beats per minute that is associated with poor systemic perfusion.[32] Bradycardia is poorly tolerated in infants and children because they are not physiologically capable of increasing their stroke volume to maintain an adequate cardiac output in the face of significant bradycardia.

The most common cause for symptomatic bradycardia in infants and children is hypoxia. Therefore, the first step in the management of symptomatic bradycardia in children is to ensure adequate oxygenation and ventilation before automatically reaching for medications or pacing. Epinephrine is the first-line medication when treating symptomatic bradycardia in children that is not responsive to appropriate oxygenation and ventilation. This is in contrast to the treatment of bradycardia in adults, in which atropine is considered to be the first-line medication. If additional doses of IV or IO epinephrine are required when treating symptomatic bradycardia, the dose should remain at standard dosing (0.01 mg/kg) and not increased to the high dose (0.1 mg/kg) according to AHA PALS guidelines. Atropine will have no effect on the denervated heart. If vascular access is not available, both epinephrine and atropine can be administered via the tracheal tube.

Other causes of bradycardia include hypothermia, increased intracranial pressure, heart blocks (congenital and acquired), a denervated heart status-post cardiac surgery, hypothyroidism, sick sinus syndrome, and various medications and toxins (i.e., digoxin, β-blockers, calcium channel blockers, and cholinergic agents). Consider emergency pacing for Mobitz type II second-degree atrioventricular block, complete third-degree heart block, or sick sinus syndrome.

Athletic adolescent patients may have resting baseline heart rates slower than 60 beats per minute and do not require emergency treatment if they are completely asymptomatic.

Tachydysrhythmias

Supraventricular Tachycardia

Perspective

Supraventricular tachycardia is the most common symptomatic dysrhythmia in infants and children.[32] In children younger than 12 years of age, the most common cause of supraventricular tachycardia is a reentry mechanism due to an accessory atrioventricular pathway.[36] No cardiac abnormalities are found in approximately half of the cases and the Wolff-Parkinson-White syndrome is present in only 10% to 20% of the cases.[37] The QRS complex is narrow (<0.08 seconds) in up to 90% of the cases of pediatric supraventricular tachycardia.[38] The type of supraventricular tachycardia that occurs most commonly in infants and children involves a reentrant mechanism that utilizes an accessory pathway and the atrioventricular node. The orthodromic reentry phenomenon involves the normal antegrade conduction from the atria to the ventricles down the atrioventricular node with retrograde conduction back from the ventricles to the atria via the accessory pathway. Orthodromic conduction will produce a narrow QRS complex supraventricular tachycardia. The less common form of reentry mechanism is the antidromic form in which conduction from the atria to the ventricles first goes antegrade down the accessory pathway then retrograde back to the atria via the atrioventricular node. Antidromic conduction will produce a wide QRS complex supraventricular tachycardia. Supraventricular tachycardia in a

BOX 169-14. Summary of Pediatric Dysrhythmia Treatment Options and Defibrillation, Cardioversion, and Medication in Resuscitation

Simplified Summary of Dysrhythmia Treatment Options

Asystole and PEA

CPR and intubation

Epinephrine

Consider and manage treatable causes ("P-A-T2-H4" mnemonic)

Ventricular Fibrillation and Pulseless Ventricular Tachycardia

Defibrillation × 3 attempts (2 joules/kg for the 1st defibrillation followed by 4 joules/kg for all subsequent defibrillations)

Epinephrine followed by 4th defibrillation at 4 joules/kg (repeat epinephrine followed by defibrillation q 3-5 minutes)

Antidysrhythmic agents: amiodarone or lidocaine or magnesium followed by defibrillation at 4 joules/kg

Ventricular Tachycardia (with a Pulse)

Unstable:

- Immediate cardioversion (start at 0.5-1 joule/kg then 2 joules/kg)

Stable:

- Amiodarone or lidocaine or procainamide (Note: Avoid concurrent use of amiodarone and procainamide)

Supraventricular Tachycardia (SVT)

Unstable:

- If IV access is immediately available administer adenosine while preparing for cardioversion, otherwise perform immediate cardioversion if IV access is not available and/or if the patient is hemodynamically very unstable

Stable:

- Vagal maneuvers (ice water slurry to the face, Valsalva maneuver, blowing on an occluded straw or blowing on the tip of a syringe in an attempt to blow the plunger out)
- Adenosine if vagal maneuvers fail

Bradycardia (Hypoxia Is the Most Common Etiology)

Unstable:

- Assure adequate oxygenation and ventilation.
- Epinephrine
- Atropine (if suspicion of increased vagal tone or cholinergic toxicity)
- Cardiac pacing

Stable:

- No emergent treatment required.

Defibrillation, Cardioversion, and Medications in Resuscitation

Cardioversion

- Start at 0.5-1 joules/kg then may double the dose up to 2 joules/kg

Defibrillation

- Start at 2 joules/kg then double the dose to 4 joules/kg for all subsequent attempts

Adenosine

- Start at 0.1 mg/kg (maximum = 6 mg) then may repeat at 0.2 mg/kg × 2 doses (maximum = 12 mg/dose)

Epinephrine

- Standard dose = 0.01 mg/kg (equals 0.1 mL/kg of the 1:10,000 solution) IV or IO
- High dose = 0.1 mg/kg (equals 0.1 mL/kg of the 1:1,000 solution) IV, IO, or TT
- TT (tracheal dose) = 0.1 mg/kg (equals 0.1 mL/kg of the 1:1,000 solution)
- Neonatal doses: Always use the 1:10,000 solution as 0.01 mg/kg IV, IO, or UVC or 0.02-0.03 mg/kg via the TT

Atropine

- 0.02 mg/kg with minimum of 0.1 mg/dose to avoid paradoxical bradycardia. Maximum single dose is 0.5 mg in a child or 1 mg in an adolescent with an overall dosage total maximum of 1 mg in a child or 2 mg in an adolescent

Amiodarone

- 5 mg/kg IV bolus for ventricular fibrillation or slowly over 20-60 minutes for stable ventricular tachycardia to avoid the hypotensive effects of amiodarone
- Can be used to treat a wide array of both atrial and ventricular dysrhythmias in children due to its ability to slow conduction both through the AV node and within the ventricles
- Avoid concurrent use of other medications (i.e., procainamide) that can also prolong the QT interval

Procainamide

- 15 mg/kg IV slowly over 30-60 minutes
- Can be used to treat a wide array of both atrial and ventricular dysrhythmias in children due to its ability to slow conduction both through the AV node and within the ventricles
- Avoid concurrent use of other medications (i.e., amiodarone) that can also prolong the QT interval

Lidocaine

- 1 mg/kg IV
- Does not cause QT prolongation like amiodarone and procainamide

Magnesium

- 25-50 mg/kg (maximum of 2 gm) IV bolus for ventricular fibrillation or pulseless ventricular tachycardia (if suspect hypomagnesemia or torsades de pointes)

P-A-T2-H4, pneumothorax, acidosis, tamponade, toxins, hypovolemia, hypoxemia, hyper/hypokalemia.

child with a preexisting bundle branch block can also result in a wide-complex supraventricular tachycardia. The ECG in Figure 169-9 reveals a case of a wide-complex supraventricular tachycardia in a child with Ebstein's anomaly of the tricuspid valve who also presented in CHF (Figure 169-10).

Clinical Features and Diagnostic Strategies

The width of the QRS interval in patients with pediatric supraventricular tachycardia is most commonly narrow-complex, with heart rates in infants usually greater than 220 beats per minute (Figure 169-11). It

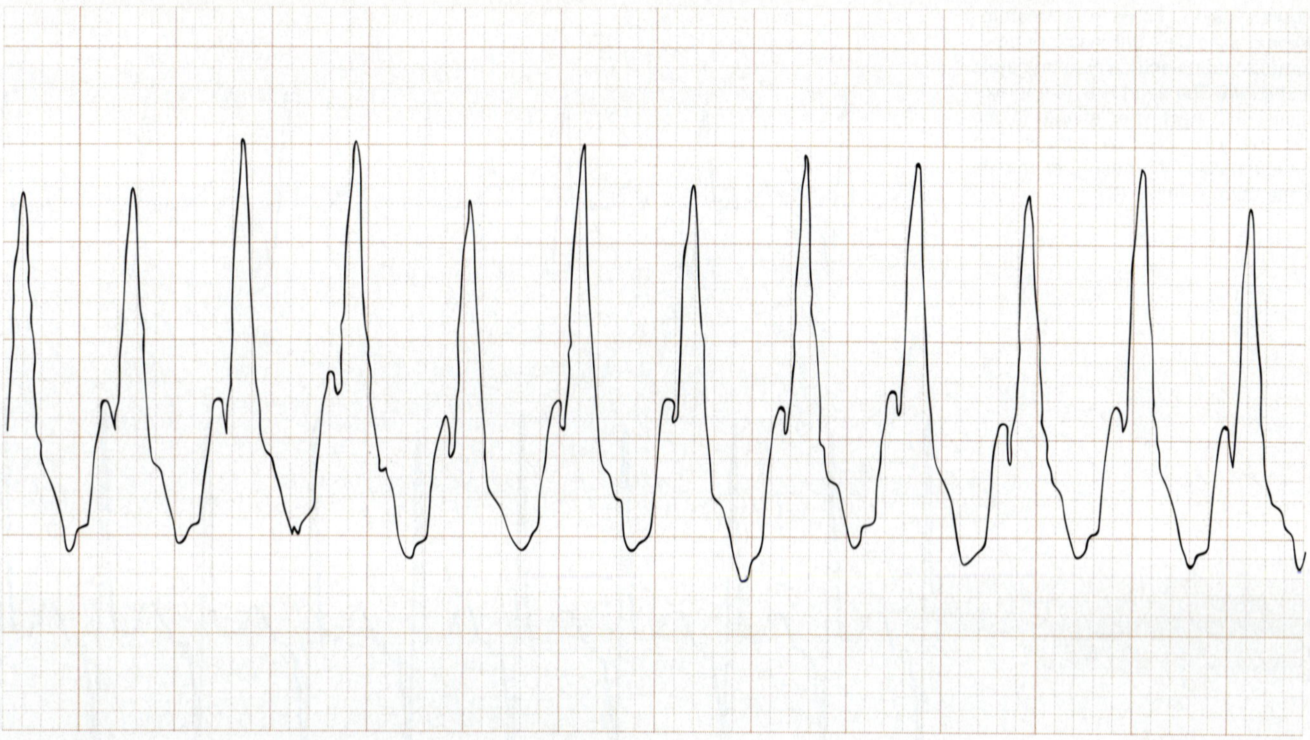

Figure 169-9. An example of an electrocardiogram showing a wide complex supraventricular tachycardia at a rate of approximately 270 beats per minute in an infant with Ebstein's anomaly of the tricuspid valve. This infant was in supraventricular tachycardia for approximately 2 days and presented with an acute exacerbation of her congestive heart failure, as evidenced by the cardiomegaly on the chest radiograph (see Figure 169-10). Note that the cardiothoracic ratio in this infant is approximately 70%.

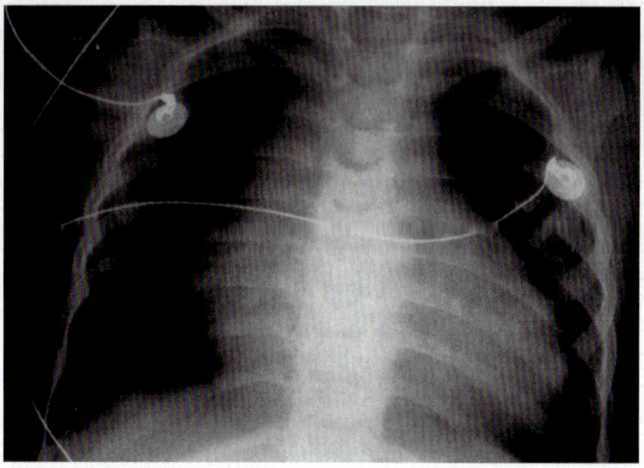

Figure 169-10. Chest radiograph of same infant as in Figure 169-9.

Table 169-8. Clinical and ECG Features to Differentiate Sinus Tachycardia from Supraventricular Tachycardia in Children[32]

	Sinus Tachycardia	Supraventricular Tachycardia
Precipitating event(s)	Dehydration, fever, pain	No precipitating event
P waves on ECG	Present	Absent
Heart rate varies with activity	Yes	No
Beat-to-beat variability	Yes	Constant R-R intervals
Heart rate in infants	Usually <220	Usually >220
Heart rate in children	Usually <180	Usually >180

is sometimes difficult to distinguish between sinus tachycardia and supraventricular tachycardia (Table 169-8).

Infants with supraventricular tachycardia typically present with very nonspecific symptoms, such as fussiness and difficulty feeding. Although healthy infants can generally tolerate supraventricular tachycardia with heart rates approaching 300 beats per minute, if left untreated supraventricular tachycardia may begin to produce signs of CHF and shock. Older children with supraventricular tachycardia commonly present with palpitations, difficulty breathing, and chest discomfort.

Management

Management of supraventricular tachycardia depends on the hemodynamic stability of the child. If the child with supraventricular tachycardia is hemodynamically unstable and intravenous access in not available, immediate cardioversion starting at 0.5 to 1 joules/kg is the treatment of choice. If the child does not convert with this initial cardioversion attempt, the energy dose can be doubled up to 2 joules/kg on subsequent attempts. If the child is hemodynamically stable, vagal maneuvers or adenosine, or both, can be attempted initially before cardioversion, depending on the individual case scenario. Regardless of the method selected to

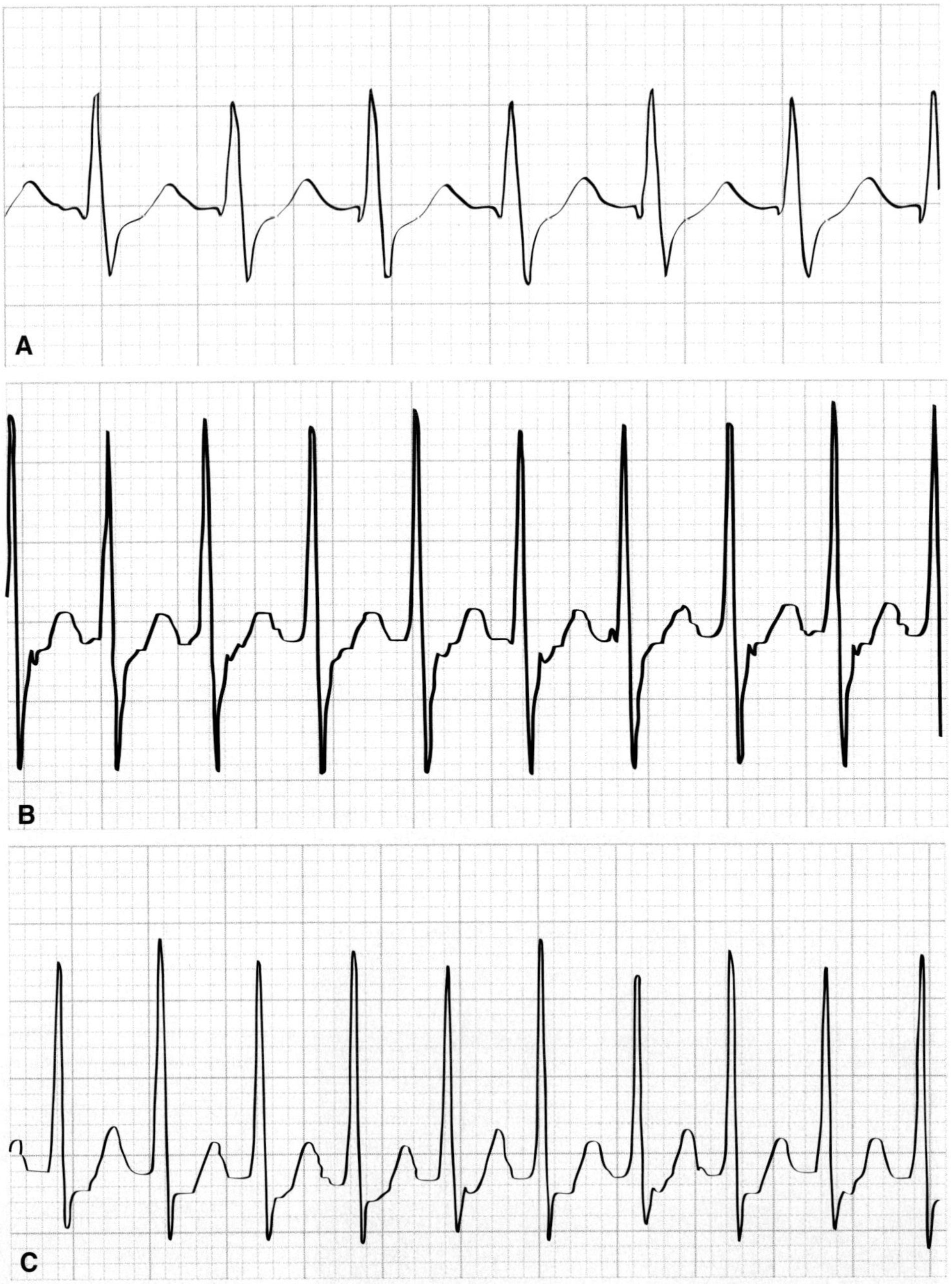

Figure 169-11. Three electrocardiographic examples of classic narrow-complex supraventricular tachycardia in children. The heart rate is approximately 240 beats per minute in the first two examples (**A** and **B**) and approximately 270 beats per minute in the third example (**C**).

convert the supraventricular tachycardia, a continuous rhythm strip should always be run to document the response to each conversion attempt. Vagal maneuvers (i.e., a bag containing a slurry of crushed ice and water to the face, blowing on an occluded straw, or blowing on the tip of a syringe) can be attempted before adenosine administration only in the child with hemodynamically stable supraventricular tachycardia. Application of ice to the face has been demonstrated to be a fairly effective method of converting supraventricular tachycardia in infants and children.[39] One method to perform this maneuver is to fill a plastic bag or surgical glove with a slurry of crushed ice and water, which is then placed over the infant's forehead, eyes, and bridge of the nose for 10 to 15 seconds. Care must be taken not to occlude the nose or mouth with the bag of ice water. External ocular pressure should be avoided, as it can be dangerous in children because excessive pressure can lead to a ruptured globe. Carotid massage is less effective and is not recommended as a vagal maneuver in infants or children.[32]

The initial dose of adenosine in children is 0.1 mg/kg with a maximum initial dose of 6 mg. If this initial dose of adenosine fails to convert the supraventricular tachycardia, the dose is then doubled to 0.2 mg/kg with a maximum of 12 mg/dose. This 0.2 mg/kg dose of adenosine can be attempted once more during the third adenosine dose. Elective cardioversion or esophageal overdrive pacing under conscious sedation may be required in children who fail to convert with adenosine. Complications of adenosine administration include asystole and various dysrhythmias, including adenosine-induced wide-complex tachycardia (secondary to an occult accessory conduction pathway) (Figure 169-12). The use of verapamil to convert supraventricular tachycardia in infants and younger

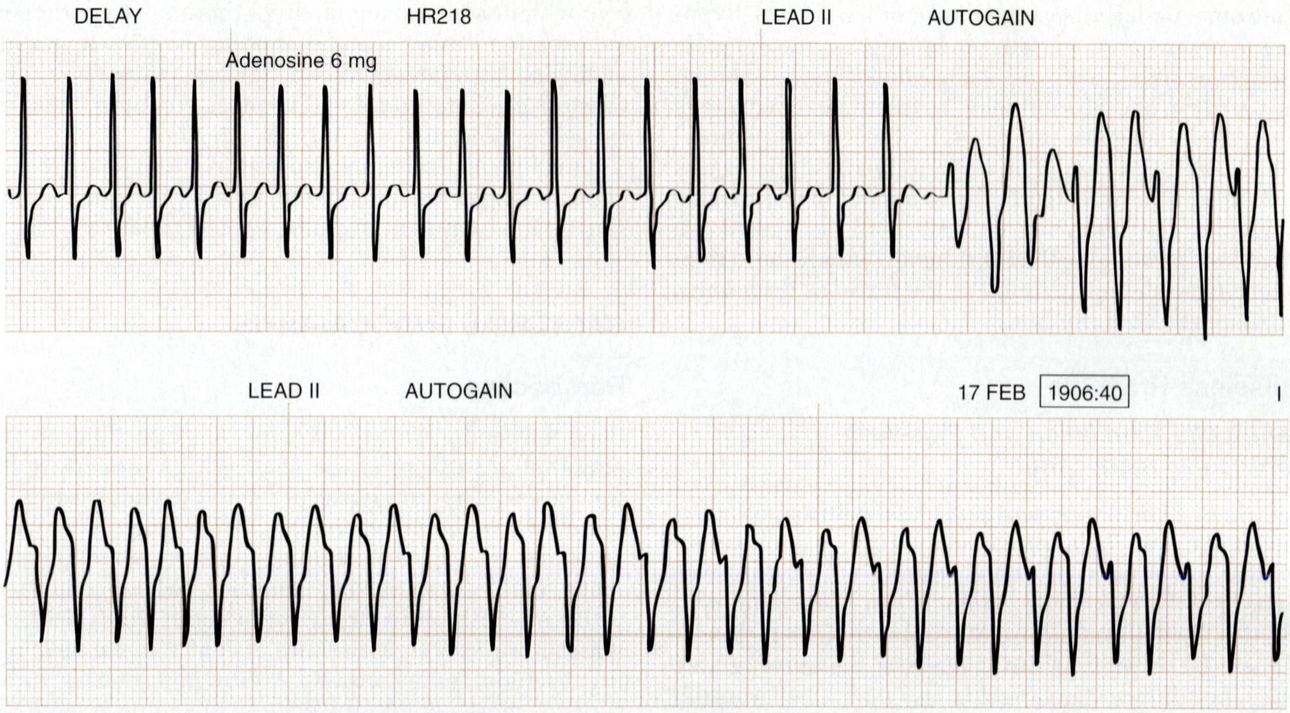

Figure 169-12. An example of adenosine-induced wide-complex tachycardia. A dose of 6 mg of adenosine was administered to this previously healthy 15-year-old girl who presented with a 6-hour history of palpitations. She had no previous cardiac problems except for intermittent palpitations in the past that always resolved spontaneously without any medical interventions. Once adenosine blocked the conduction through the atrioventricular node, a wide-complex tachycardia appeared on the electrocardiogram (ECG), which was probably due to antegrade conduction through an accessory pathway. During the 30 seconds of this wide-complex tachycardia, the patient remained alert with excellent perfusion parameters. This wide-complex tachycardia then spontaneously converted to normal sinus rhythm. Although the patient's post-conversion ECG did not reveal an accessory pathway, Holter monitoring 1 month later detected the classic ECG findings of the Wolff-Parkinson-White syndrome.

children should be avoided because of the high incidence of profound hypotension and cardiovascular collapse when this medication is administered in this age group.[32]

Once the patient has been converted to sinus rhythm, a 12-lead ECG should be obtained to assess for the possibility of Wolff-Parkinson-White syndrome or any other underlying conduction abnormalities that may have predisposed the child to developing the supraventricular tachycardia.

Atrial Flutter and Atrial Fibrillation

Both atrial flutter and atrial fibrillation are rare in children and are usually associated with underlying heart conditions (i.e., CHD, status–post open heart surgical procedures that involved the atria, myocarditis, and digoxin toxicity). Hemodynamic stability of these two dysrhythmias depends on the rate of the ventricular response. Cardioversion is the treatment of choice for children who present with hemodynamically unstable atrial flutter or atrial fibrillation. The initial treatment priority in patients with hemodynamically stable atrial flutter and atrial fibrillation is to first slow down the rate of the ventricular response with medications such as digoxin, β-blockers, or diltiazem. Once the ventricular rate is controlled, the rhythm can then be converted and suppressed with amiodarone, procainamide, or elective cardioversion. If the patient who presents with atrial flutter and atrial fibrillation is known to have an underlying Wolff-Parkinson-White syndrome, the four medications that should be avoided are the "A-B-C-D" medications (adenosine, β-blockers, calcium-channel blockers, and digoxin), since all of these medications only block conduction down the atrioventricular node while leaving the accessory pathway wide open to conduct the atrial tachycardia to the ventricles at a potentially lethal rate.[40] Under these circumstances, amiodarone, procainamide, or cardioversion would be the safer alternative. Consultation with the cardiologist and initiation of anticoagulation should also be considered before conversion of either of these two atrial dysrhythmias in the hemodynamically stable patient to prevent a thromboembolic complication.

Ventricular Tachycardia

Ventricular tachycardia is not a common dysrhythmia in children. The majority of children with ventricular tachycardia have an underlying condition such as status postoperative cardiac surgery, myocarditis, prolonged QT syndrome, drug or toxin exposures (i.e., cyclic antidepressants), or electrolyte abnormalities. The treatment of ventricular tachycardia will depend on whether a pulse is present and on the hemodynamic status of the patient (see Box 169-14). Torsades de pointes is a unique type of polymorphic ventricular tachycardia that is characterized by QRS complexes that change in polarity and amplitude. Prolonged QT syndrome, underlying congenital cardiac defects, hypomagnesemia, and various medications (i.e., cyclic antidepressants) have all been identified as known causes of torsades de pointes. The treatment of choice is intravenous magnesium. Class IA (i.e., procainamide) and class III (i.e., amiodarone) antidysrhythmic agents are both contraindicated in the treatment of torsades de pointes, since these two antidysrhythmic agents are capable of prolonging the QT interval, which could then precipitate the degeneration of the torsades de pointes into a more lethal rhythm.

Pulseless Rhythms

Ventricular Fibrillation and Pulseless Ventricular Tachycardia

Ventricular fibrillation and pulseless ventricular tachycardia account for approximately 10% of prehospital cardiac arrest cases in which a terminal rhythm was recorded.[41,42] The survival rate for out-of-hospital ventricular fibrillation and pulseless ventricular tachycardia can be as high as 30%, whereas the survival rate from asystolic cardiac arrest is less than 1%.[31] Ventricular fibrillation should also be suspected as the arrest rhythm in cases of commotio cordis. Because the current arrhythmia detection algorithms for automated external defibrillators (AEDs) appear to have a high sensitivity and specificity for detecting shockable rhythms in children, the American Heart Association gave their approval for the use of AEDs in children 1 to 8 years of age (class IIB recommendation), provided that the AED unit that is used has the appropriate-sized pediatric pads and attenuator device, which will deliver a pediatric dose of defibrillation.[43,44]

The treatment algorithm and medication dosages for ventricular fibrillation and pulseless ventricular tachycardia are listed in Box 169-14. Although biphasic defibrillators can convert ventricular fibrillation at lower dosages than the previous monophasic defibrillators in adults, until more data are gathered on biphasic defibrillation dosages in children, the current American Heart Association recommendation for pediatric defibrillation with biphasic defibrillators remains the same as for monophasic defibrillators (i.e., starting at 2 joules/kg followed by 4 joules/kg).

Asystole and Pulseless Electrical Activity

Asystole is the most common rhythm found in cases of out-of-hospital cardiac arrest in children and is associated with a less than 1% chance of survival.[45-47] The use of high-dose epinephrine has been de-emphasized in the current Pediatric Advanced Life Support guidelines. The treatment algorithm and medication dosages for asystole and pulseless electrical activity are listed in Box 169-14. Pulseless electrical activity can either be a slow or fast rhythm and have a narrow or wide QRS complex.

The key to survival from any pulseless electrical activity rhythm is to rapidly identify and correct the underlying cause. The etiologies for pulseless electrical activity can be remembered by the "4 Hs and 4 Ts": hypovolemia, hypoxemia, hypothermia, hypo/hyperkalemia (and other metabolic abnormalities including acidosis), thromboembolism, toxins, tamponade, and tension pneumothorax.[32] The most common cause of pulseless electrical activity in children is profound hypovolemia. Therefore, an intravenous fluid bolus should always be considered as a therapeutic option during the treatment of pulseless electrical activity.

BACTERIAL ENDOCARDITIS

Perspective

Bacterial endocarditis involves an infection of the endothelial surfaces of the heart with a propensity for the valves. The incidence of bacterial endocarditis in children may be increasing slightly owing to the many advances in surgical technology that are now allowing many children with very complex CHDs to survive. Children with indwelling intravenous lines with or without underlying CHDs are also at risk for developing bacterial endocarditis. Although bacterial endocarditis most commonly occurs in children with an underlying CHD or an acquired cardiac lesion (i.e., acute rheumatic valvular heart disease), it can also occur in patients with no underlying anatomic defects of the valves or endocardium. In a series of 62 children with bacterial endocarditis, 19 (30%) of the children had normal cardiac anatomy.[48]

Factors that predispose children with underlying anatomic cardiac defects to bacterial endocarditis include dental procedures and other surgical procedures involving the respiratory, gastrointestinal, or genitourinary tracts. Those cardiac lesions with a more turbulent blood flow or a higher flow velocity are more prone to developing bacterial endocarditis secondary to a greater risk of endothelial surface damage, which then increases the risk for platelet deposition and vegetation formation. Cardiac lesions that carry this higher risk include ventricular septal defects, aortic valvular stenosis, tetralogy of Fallot, single ventricle states, prosthetic valves, and postoperative systemic-to-pulmonary shunts. Isolated secundum atrial septal defects carry a much lower risk for bacterial endocarditis because the shunt flow through the atrial septal defect is typically of a much lower velocity.

Clinical Features and Diagnostic Strategies

The early clinical manifestations of bacterial endocarditis may be very nonspecific. The child may simply present with only fever and tachycardia. However, bacterial endocarditis should be suspected in any child with an anatomic cardiac defect who presents with an unexplained fever. This diagnosis must always be considered in any child with a known CHD or an acquired cardiac lesion who presents with any of the conditions listed in Box 169-15. A new heart murmur is present in fewer than 50% of the bacterial endocarditis cases.[49] Box 169-16 contains a summary of

BOX 169-15. Clinical Conditions in Which Bacterial Endocarditis Should Be Suspected in a Child with an Underlying Anatomic Cardiac Defect

- Fever of unknown etiology
- A change in the quality of the pre-existing heart murmur or the presence of a new heart murmur
- Development of a neurologic deficit (secondary to central nervous system emboli)
- New onset microscopic hematuria
- Splenomegaly
- Petechiae
- Splinter hemorrhages involving the conjunctiva, nail beds, palms, or soles
- Myalgias

BOX 169-16. Cardiac Conditions Requiring Bacterial Endocarditis Prophylaxis

High Risk for Endocarditis
Prosthetic cardiac valves
Complex cyanotic CHDs
Surgically constructed systemic-to-pulmonary shunts
Previous episode of endocarditis

Moderate Risk for Endocarditis
Most other complex CHDs
CHDs with high velocity and turbulent flow (VSD, CoA, AS, and PS)
Rheumatic heart disease with valvular dysfunction
Other acquired cardiac conditions with valvular dysfunction
Mitral valve prolapse with valvular regurgitation or thickened leaflets
Hypertrophic cardiomyopathy

Negligible Risk for Endocarditis
Innocent, functional, or physiologic murmurs
Isolated secundum ASDs
Surgically repaired ASD, VSD, or PDA without residua in infants older than 6 months of age
Mitral valve prolapse without valvular regurgitation or thickened leaflets
Kawasaki disease or rheumatic heart disease without valvular dysfunction
Cardiac pacemakers and implanted defibrillators

those cardiac conditions with the highest risk for bacterial endocarditis.[50]

Diagnostic studies to perform in a child with suspected bacterial endocarditis include a complete blood cell count, C-reactive protein assessment, measurement of erythrocyte sedimentation rate, three blood cultures, chest radiography, and ECG. Cultures from scrapings of cutaneous emboli can also aid in the diagnosis. Although the definitive diagnostic study is the echocardiogram, it is only 80% sensitive in detecting the nidus of infection on the endocardium or valves.[51] *Streptococcus viridans* and *Staphylococcus aureus* are the two most common offending organisms recovered from the blood cultures of children with bacterial endocarditis.

Management

Antibiotics should be started immediately after blood culture samples have been obtained. Although the choice of intravenous antibiotics depends on the suspected source of seeding and the child's immune status, a common recommended regimen includes an aminoglycoside plus a penicillinase-resistant penicillin such as oxacillin. If methicillin-resistant staphylococci are suspected, vancomycin should also be included in the initial empirical antibiotic regimen.[52]

Bacterial endocarditis in the preantibiotic era was nearly always a fatal disease. Although the survival rate in patients with bacterial endocarditis has improved with the initiation of antibiotics, the current mortality rate is still 6% to 14%.[53] Complications of bacterial endocarditis include systemic septic emboli, pulmonary emboli, central nervous system emboli with resultant neurologic deficits, dysrhythmias, CHF, myocarditis, myocardial abscesses, and valvular obstruction. Despite appropriate antibiotic treatment, surgical interventions to remove septic vegetations or valve replacements is sometimes necessary.

MYOCARDITIS

Perspective

Myocarditis is an inflammatory condition of the myocardium with various infectious and noninfectious origins. In the United States, the most common cause is viral, with coxsackie B and enteroviruses accounting for the majority of cases. Other viral causes include echoviruses, influenza A, influenza B, adenovirus, varicella-zoster virus, Epstein-Barr virus, cytomegalovirus, and hepatitis B virus. Bacterial causes include *Corynebacterium diphtheriae*, *Streptococcus pyogenes*, *Staphylococcus aureus*, *Mycoplasma pneumoniae*, *Borrelia burgdorferi*, and *Meningococcus*. Noninfectious causes include Kawasaki disease, acute rheumatic fever, collagen vascular disorders (e.g., systemic lupus erythematosus), toxins (e.g., cocaine and adriamycin), endocrine disorders (e.g., hyperthyroidism), and drug-induced hypersensitivity (e.g., penicillins, sulfonamides, phenytoin, carbamazepine).

Clinical Features

Myocarditis usually has a gradual onset with preceding upper respiratory tract infection symptoms. The presenting signs and symptoms of a child with myocarditis depend on the cause of the myocarditis, the age of the patient, and the degree of myocardial inflammation. The key to diagnosing myocarditis in infants and children is to suspect the diagnostic entity in the appropriate clinical setting. In mild cases, the only sign of myocarditis may be tachycardia. Tachycardia that is disproportionate to the degree of fever should alert the clinician to the possibility of myocarditis.[54] Other presenting signs and symptoms include fever, myalgias, fatigue, tachypnea, wheezing, and chest pain. More severe cases of myocarditis can even present with signs and symptoms of acute CHF and various dysrhythmias. The physical examination may reveal a new murmur, a gallop rhythm, or a pericardial friction rub with muffled heart tones (if the myocarditis is also accompanied by pericarditis).

Diagnostic Strategies and Management

The evaluation and management of the child with myocarditis depend on the suspected cause and the presenting signs and symptoms. Blood cultures and viral titers should be considered in infectious and postinfectious cases. Appropriate antibiotics should be immediately initiated in cases with suspected bacterial origins. The chest radiograph in very mild cases may be normal, but in more advanced cases cardiomegaly will be evident. The ECG findings are usually nonspecific and can include low-voltage, nonspecific ST segment abnormalities, T wave inversions, atrioventricular blocks, and various other dysrhythmias. Creatine phosphokinase-MB, cTnT, and C-reactive protein levels and erythrocyte sedimentation rate may be elevated. The echocardiogram is an essential component of the workup of any child with suspected myocarditis. The echocardiogram will not only be useful to assess the degree of left ventricular function, but it will also be able to detect any associated pericardial effusion that may accompany the myocarditis. Although an endomyocardial biopsy is rarely required, it is the definitive method to confirm the diagnosis and origin of myocarditis. If the endomyocardial biopsy is performed, it will typically demonstrate a myocardial inflammation with lymphocytic and monocytic infiltrates. The mainstay of treatment is to maintain adequate cardiac output and to control any associated dysrhythmias. Children who present in CHF may require inotropic support and diuretics. Digoxin and the various pressors must be used very cautiously in children with myocarditis because the inflamed myocardium is very sensitive to the dysrhythmogenesis of these medications. The use of β-blockers is contraindicated,[54] and the routine use of immunosuppressive agents remains controversial.[55] Although the majority of children with acute viral myocarditis make a full recovery, a few patients will progress to develop dilated cardiomyopathy, which is characterized by dilated ventricles and impaired systolic contractility.

PERICARDITIS

Perspective

Pericarditis is an inflammatory process within the pericardial sac, which may not be associated with a pericardial effusion. The majority of cases of pericarditis in children are self-limited and follow a benign clinical course. In children, there is normally about 10 to 15 mL of fluid within the pericardial sac. A sudden increase in or a large amount of fluid within this pericardial sac can cause a tamponade-induced decrease in stroke volume, which will cause a diminished cardiac output and hypotension.

Although the most common causes of pericarditis include bacterial and viral infections, other causes include acute rheumatic fever, systemic lupus erythematosus, uremia, post-pericardiotomy syndrome, leukemia, lymphoma, and tuberculosis. Approximately 30% of pericarditis cases are due to bacteria such as *Pneumococcus*, *Staphylococcus aureus*, *Meningococcus*, and *Haemophilus influenzae*.[1] Approximately 30% of the purulent bacterial pericarditis cases occur in children younger than 6 years of age.[24] Although viral causes are common, a viral pathogen is recovered in only 20% to 30% of the cases.[24] Common viral causes include coxsackie viruses, ECHO viruses, adenovirus, Epstein-Barr virus, and influenza viruses.

Clinical Features

The presenting signs and symptoms of pericarditis depend on the cause of the pericarditis as well as on the amount of fluid that has accumulated within the pericardial sac. Chest pain that varies with position is a common complaint with pericarditis. The chest pain that is classically associated with pericarditis is exacerbated with inspiration and the supine position but relieved when the patient sits up or leans forward. Tachycardia is also a common finding in patients with pericarditis. Other physical examination findings that have been associated with pericarditis include fatigue, tachypnea, and neck vein distention, pulsus paradoxus, hepatomegaly, lower extremity edema, and thready distal pulses if heart failure is present. The cardiac auscultatory findings in a patient with pericarditis can include a harsh-sounding friction rub or diminished or muffled heart tones if there is a significant amount of fluid within the pericardial sac. The pericardial friction rub, if present, is best heard when the patient sits up and leans forward. This friction rub of pericarditis can be distinguished from a pleural friction rub by having the patient hold his or her breath during auscultation. The friction rub of pericarditis will remain present during breath-holding while the pleural friction rub will no longer be heard while the patient holds the breath.

The chest radiograph in a child with pericarditis may not reveal an enlarged cardiac silhouette, depending on the amount of fluid that has accumulated within the pericardial sac. If there is a large collection of fluid within the pericardial sac, the heart shadow on the chest radiograph will resemble a "water-bottle" silhouette. Approximately 50% of pericarditis cases also have an associated pleural effusion.[1]

The classic ECG findings of pericarditis include diffuse ST segment elevation and diffuse T wave inversions in all leads. The classic ECG changes associated with pericarditis evolve through four phases (Figure 169-13). During the initial phase, there is diffuse ST segment elevation in all leads secondary to subepicardial inflammation; PR segment depression may also be seen. During the second phase, the previously elevated ST segments begin to return to isoelectric baseline and

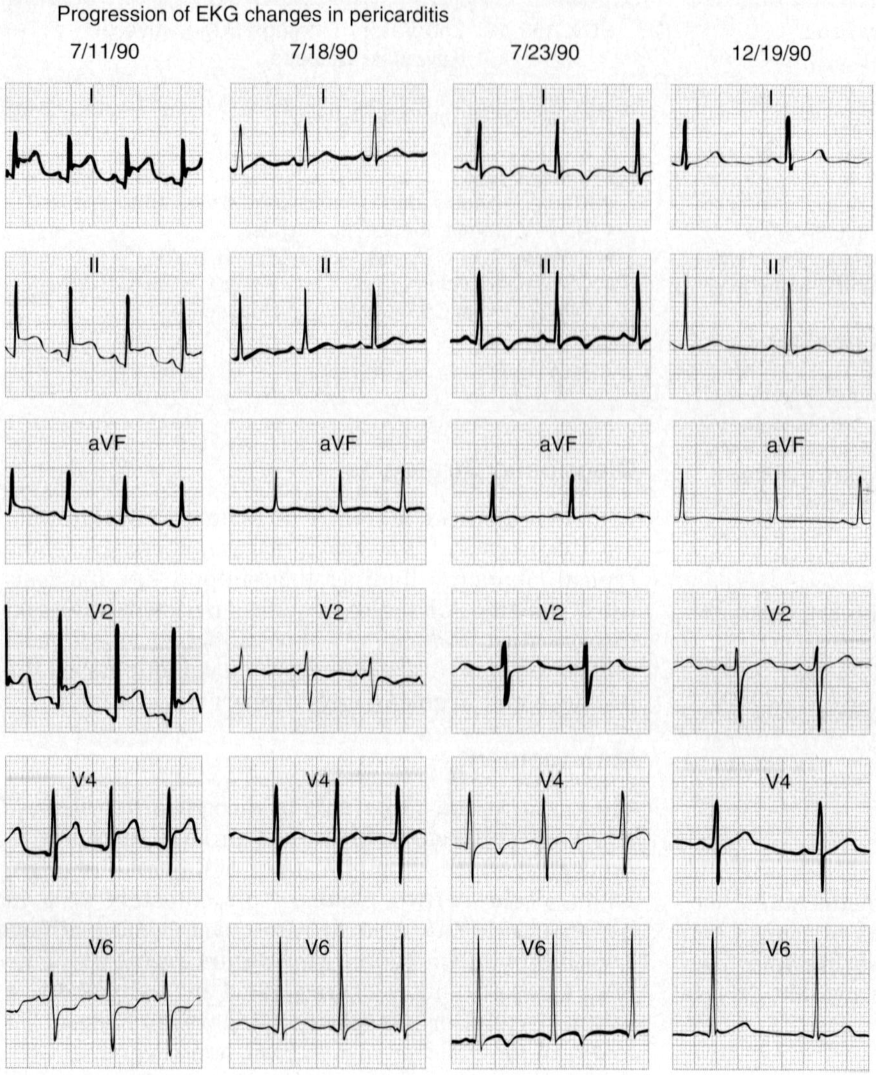

Figure 169-13. The classic electrocardiographic (ECG) progression of a patient with pericarditis. First phase: Diffuse ST segment elevation. Second phase: ST segments back to isoelectric, but decreased T wave amplitude. Third phase: T wave inversion. Fourth phase: Complete resolution. Notice that the first three phases of the ECG abnormalities of pericarditis in this patient are evident during the first 2 weeks of his illness. A follow-up electrocardiogram obtained 5 months later reveals a complete resolution of all the previous ECG abnormalities.

the T wave amplitudes begin to decrease with flattening of the T waves. During the third phase, although the ST segments are now back to isoelectric baseline, the T waves are now inverted. The fourth and final phase demonstrates complete resolution of the ST segment and T wave abnormalities. Diminished ECG voltages in all leads can also occur if there is a significant amount of fluid accumulated within the pericardial sac.

The diagnostic procedure of choice in any patient with suspected pericarditis is the echocardiogram, because this study will confirm both the presence and the amount of accumulated fluid within the pericardial sac. Although echocardiography cannot accurately quantify the exact amount of fluid that has accumulated within the pericardial space, the presence of an anterior and posterior fluid collection is suggestive of a large collection.

Management

The management of a child with pericarditis depends on both the suspected cause and the amount of fluid that has accumulated within the pericardial space. An emergency pericardiocentesis will be required in those patients who develop signs of acute cardiac tamponade. Any fluid that is aspirated from the pericardial space should be sent for routine cell counts, Gram stain, and cultures. Anti-inflammatory agents and appropriate antibiotics should also be initiated based on the suspected cause.

KAWASAKI DISEASE

Perspective

Kawasaki disease, which was originally described as the mucocutaneous lymph node syndrome by Dr. Kawasaki in 1967, has become a significant cause of acquired cardiac disease in children in the United States. An estimated 3000 to 5000 cases of Kawasaki disease are diagnosed annually in the United States. Up to 20% of untreated children develop some degree of coronary artery abnormalities.[56] This febrile, exanthematous, multisystem vasculitis is seen most commonly in children younger than 5 years of age with a male-to-female ratio of 1.5:1. The incidence is higher in Asian children and in certain geographic locations such as Hawaii. Although the exact cause of this vasculitis of

BOX 169-17. Diagnostic Criteria for Kawasaki Disease (KD)

I. Fever >5 days
II. At least four of the five following physical examination findings:
   1. Bilateral, nonexudative bulbar conjunctival injection (bilateral scleral injection with perilimbic-sparing)
   2. Oropharyngeal mucous membrane changes (pharyngeal erythema, red/cracked lips, and a strawberry tongue)
   3. Cervical lymphadenopathy (with at least one node >1.5 cm in diameter).
   4. Peripheral extremity changes (diffuse erythema and swelling of the hands and feet during the acute phase or periungual desquamation during the convalescent phase of the illness). This diffuse palmar erythema seen in KD is in contrast to the discrete macular lesions of various viral illnesses (i.e., measles) that can sometimes be seen on the palms and soles
   5. A polymorphous generalized rash (nonvesicular and nonbullous). There is no specific rash that is pathognomonic for KD

Note: If the above mentioned physical examination findings suggestive of KD are present in an irritable child who presents with fever that is <5 days in duration, KD must be still considered and appropriate treatment initiated in order to prevent the potential cardiovascular complications of KD.

small and medium-sized vessels remains unknown, early clinical recognition and initiation of aspirin and intravenous immunoglobulin therapies has improved the morbidity and mortality rates of Kawasaki disease in children.

Clinical Features

The key to preventing the coronary artery complications of Kawasaki disease is to be able to first recognize the clinical signs and symptoms of this disease. In addition to fever, the physical examination of a child with Kawasaki disease will reveal the typical findings listed in Box 169-17. Photographic examples of these physical examination findings are illustrated in Figure 169-14.

Differential Considerations

Measles can mimic Kawasaki disease but is rare (i.e., a febrile illness with red eyes, a rash, and erythema of the oropharynx). The classic location, distribution, and progression of a measles rash starts on the head and face and progresses caudally. The rash of Kawasaki disease typically begins on the trunk and then spreads to the face and extremities. The palmar lesions of measles are discrete macular lesions (see Figure 169-14F), whereas the palmar findings in children with Kawasaki disease is diffuse erythema without discrete lesions (see Figure 169-14C).

Streptococcal disease, including pharyngitis and scarlet fever, can be confused with Kawasaki disease, but conjunctivitis and swelling of the hands and feet are unusual for streptococcal disease.

BOX 169-18. Laboratory Findings Suggestive of Kawasaki Disease

- Leukocytosis with a left shift
- Elevated CRP and ESR
- Sterile pyuria
- Thrombocytosis (during the second week of the illness)
- Normochromic normocytic anemia
- Elevated liver enzymes (ALT, AST, and GGT)
- CSF mononuclear pleocytosis (usually <100 WBCs/hpf) with a normal CSF protein and glucose

Diagnostic Strategies

Although there are currently no laboratory studies that are diagnostic of Kawasaki disease, there are some typical laboratory findings that support the diagnosis (Box 169-18). All children with suspected Kawasaki disease must undergo an echocardiogram to delineate the degree of myocardial involvement and to detect the presence and degree of any coronary aneurysms.

Management

The main reason to be able to recognize this disease entity in children is to initiate prompt therapies to prevent the cardiac complications of Kawasaki disease, which occur in two phases. Approximately 25% of patients with Kawasaki disease develop mild diffuse myocardial inflammation. This occurs during the acute febrile period and is characterized by tachycardia, a gallop rhythm, or nonspecific ST-T wave changes. Up to 5% of the children also exhibit some degree of CHF during this acute phase of their illness. This carditis usually resolves when the fever resolves. Pericardial effusions also occur in up to 20% to 40% of cases. Mild mitral and aortic regurgitation is also seen in 1% to 2% of untreated cases on echocardiographic examinations. This phase of the disease is mild and self-resolving. Therapy during this phase of the illness is primarily supportive.

The second phase of the disease involves coronary artery dilation, which usually peaks 2 to 4 weeks from the onset of the illness and is seen in 15% to 25% of the untreated patients with Kawasaki disease.[57] Without the appropriate treatment, 15% to 20% of children with Kawasaki disease go on to develop coronary aneurysms within 1 to 3 weeks from the onset of their illness.[1] These coronary aneurysms can then lead to myocardial infarction and a variety of ischemia-induced dysrhythmias. Significant risk factors for coronary aneurysmal formation include male gender, age younger than 1 year or greater than 8 years, a prolonged febrile period greater than 10 to 14 days, early myocarditis, anemia (Hgb <10 g/dL), white blood cell count greater than 30,000, an increased band count, elevated erythrocyte sedimentation rate, elevated C-reactive protein level, low serum albumin levels, and aneurysms involving the renal, axillary, or iliac arteries and giant coronary aneurysms (>8 mm in diame-

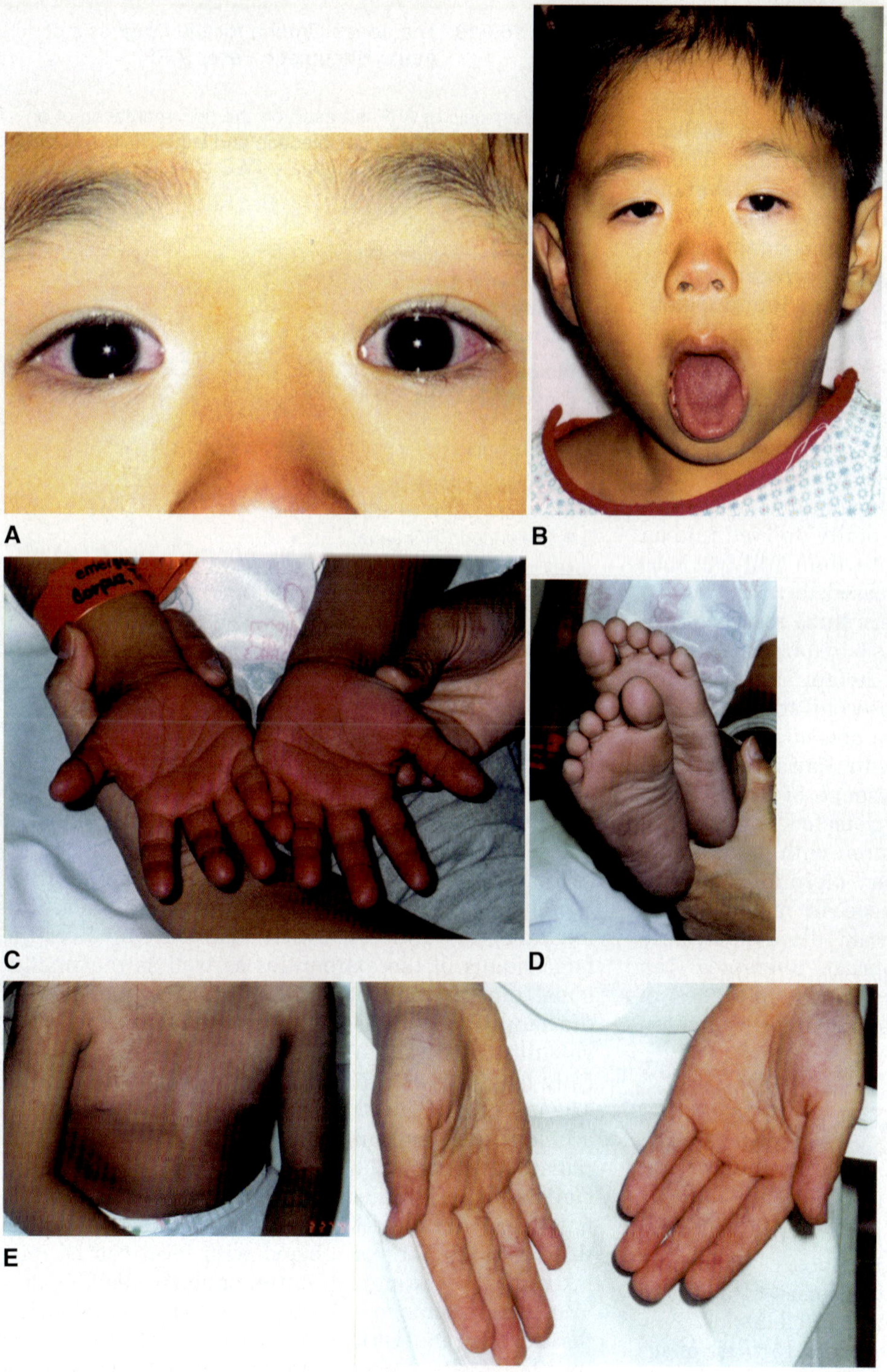

Figure 169-14. Classic physical examination findings of Kawasaki disease. Note the bilateral nonexudative scleral injections **(A)** with perilimbic sparing (the thin margin of white sclera around the cornea), red-cracked lips with a strawberry tongue **(B)**, diffuse palmar erythema **(C)**, red soles **(D),** and the polymorphous exanthem **(E)**. The diffuse palmar erythema of Kawasaki disease **(C)** is distinct from the palmar findings seen in other viral illnesses such as the discrete macular lesions on the palms in this child with measles **(F)**.

ter). Death from Kawasaki disease is primarily due to myocardial infarction secondary to coronary artery occlusion. Giant coronary artery aneurysmal rupture is rare. Although most of the fatalities that occur with Kawasaki disease occur within 6 weeks from the onset of the illness, sudden death can also occur many years after the illness. Prompt recognition and treatment has decreased this mortality rate from 2% to less than 0.01%.[56]

The main goals of treatment during the acute febrile phase of Kawasaki disease are to provide supportive care and to decrease the inflammation of the myocardium and coronary arteries. The two major components of treatment include immunoglobulin infusion and aspirin therapy. This combination of intravenous immunoglobulin and aspirin, when initiated within 10 days from the onset of the illness, can substantially decrease the progression to coronary artery dilation and aneurysm formation as compared with aspirin therapy alone and results in a more rapid resolution of fever and the other indicators of acute inflammation.[56] However, despite prompt treatment with intravenous immunoglobulin and aspirin, 2% to 4% of the children still develop coronary artery abnormalities.[56]

The current intravenous immunoglobulin regimen involves an infusion of 2 g/kg over 10 to 12 hours. Side effects of intravenous immunoglobulin include hypotension, nausea, vomiting, and seizures. Therefore, close cardiac monitoring during the intravenous immunoglobulin infusion is mandatory. The 5% to 10% of children who receive intravenous immunoglobulin who experience a persistence or recurrence of fever after the initial dose of intravenous immunoglobulin may be given a second infusion at the same dose. Approximately two thirds of those children who fail to respond to the initial dose of intravenous immunoglobulin will improve with the second infusion.

The anti-inflammatory and antithrombotic effects of aspirin are used in treating Kawasaki disease in addition to intravenous immunoglobulin. Aspirin is initiated at 80 to 100 mg/kg/day orally divided into an every-6-hour dosing regimen until the child becomes afebrile. This dose is then decreased to 3 to 5 mg/kg orally each day until the laboratory study results return to normal, which typically occurs 6 to 8 weeks after the onset of the disease. Aspirin therapy is continued beyond this period only in those children in whom coronary artery abnormalities are present.

The follow-up of children with Kawasaki disease depends on the degree and presence of carditis and coronary artery abnormalities detected on the initial echocardiogram. Those children with more severe cardiac abnormalities require very close follow-up by a cardiologist who is experienced in managing the cardiac complications of Kawasaki disease. Overall, prompt diagnosis and appropriate therapies can prevent coronary aneurysm formation in up to 95% of the cases as well as rapid symptomatic improvement in up to 90% of the cases.[58]

ACUTE RHEUMATIC FEVER

Perspective

Acute rheumatic fever (ARF) is the result of a delayed immune sequela of a group A streptococcal infection. ARF is one of the most common causes of acquired heart disease in children. In the United States, ARF most commonly occurs in children 5 to 15 years of age and has an attack rate of 0.3% to 3% in children with an untreated streptococcal infection. Although this disease affects multiple organ systems, carditis is the most serious complication.

Clinical Features and Diagnostic Considerations

The diagnosis of ARF is based on the Jones criteria (Box 169-19). In addition to the Jones criteria, there must also be evidence of an antecedent streptococcal infection, which can be documented with either a positive throat culture, a positive rapid streptococcal antigen test finding, or an elevated antistreptolysin O titer. The streptozyme test is not as reliable and therefore should not be used as a definitive test for evidence of an antecedent group A streptococcal infection.[59] The diagnosis of ARF is made in a patient with a documented antecedent streptococcal infection who exhibits either two major criteria or one major plus two minor criteria. The most common presenting major criterion is the migratory polyarthritis, which commonly involves the larger joints of the extremities as well as the smaller tarsal joints in the foot and the smaller carpal joints in the hand. The carditis of ARF most commonly involves valvulitis of the mitral and aortic valves, which clinically manifests as occult mitral or aortic insufficiency. The murmur of mitral insufficiency is characterized as a holosystolic murmur best heard over the apex with radiation to the axilla. The murmur of aortic insufficiency is characterized as a diastolic murmur that is best heard over the base of the heart. Innocent murmurs that are normally exacerbated with fever can be mistaken for the murmurs of mitral or aortic insufficiency. The other cardiac manifestations of ARF include CHF, pericarditis, and various degrees of heart blocks. The two dermatologic major criteria (erythema marginatum and subcutaneous nodules) and chorea occur less commonly than the migratory polyarthritis and carditis. Chorea may occur as the only manifestation of ARF. If arthritis is used as a major component, arthralgia cannot be used as a minor component to make the diagnosis. Likewise, if carditis is used as a major component, then a prolonged PR interval cannot be used as a minor component.[59]

In addition to the ECG, C-reactive protein level, erythrocyte sedimentation rate, and documentation of an antecedent streptococcal infection, the diagnostic workup of ARF should also include a chest radiograph as well as an echocardiogram to evaluate the degree of cardiac involvement.

BOX 169-19. The Jones Criteria for the Diagnosis of Acute Rheumatic Fever (ARF)

The diagnosis of ARF is based on the documentation of an antecedent streptococcal infection and either TWO MAJOR criteria or ONE MAJOR criteria + TWO MINOR criteria.

Major Criteria
- Carditis
- Migratory polyarthritis
- Erythema marginatum
- Subcutaneous nodules
- Chorea

Minor Criteria

Clinical Findings
- Fever
- Arthralgia

Laboratory Findings
- Elevated CRP or ESR
- Prolonged PR interval

Supporting evidence of an antecedent group A streptococcal infection with either:
- A positive throat culture or a rapid streptococcal antigen test
- An elevated antistreptolysin (ASO) titer

BOX 169-20. Cardiovascular Etiologies of Sudden Death in Young Athletes

- Hypertrophic cardiomyopathy
- Various congenital coronary artery anomalies
- Prolonged QT interval syndrome
- Various pre-excitation syndromes (i.e., Wolff-Parkinson-White syndrome)
- Commotio cordis
- Aortic rupture secondary to Marfan's syndrome
- Idiopathic dilated cardiomyopathy
- Myocarditis
- Coronary artery disease secondary to Kawasaki disease
- Aortic stenosis
- Mitral valve prolapse

Differential Considerations

The differential diagnosis of ARF includes myocarditis, bacterial endocarditis, Lyme disease, systemic lupus erythematosus, juvenile rheumatoid arthritis, serum sickness, and septic arthritis.

Management

The acute management of ARF should first focus on stabilizing and treating any of the symptomatic cardiac manifestations of the illness, such as CHF or tamponade due to a pericardial effusion. Additional goals in ARF management include appropriate antibiotic therapy to eradicate the streptococcal infection, bed rest, and anti-inflammatory agents for the arthritis. The use of steroids in the treatment of carditis should only be employed under direction of a cardiologist. Another important aspect in the management of ARF is the prevention of recurrent attacks through the prophylactic use of penicillin, which can be given as monthly injections of 1.2 million units of benzathine penicillin G. Alternative prophylactic regimens include oral penicillin administered twice daily or twice daily oral erythromycin dosing in patients who are allergic to penicillin. This prophylaxis with penicillin or erythromycin is required until 18 years of age at the minimum but can be continued for life, depending on the degree of cardiac involvement and the risk for recurrence.

CARDIAC CAUSES OF SUDDEN DEATH IN YOUNG ATHLETES

Perspective

The most common cause of sudden, unexplained death in athletes is various cardiac conditions, with only 15% of the cases stemming from noncardiovascular causes (Box 169-20).[60] The most common cardiovascular cause of sudden death in the athlete is hypertrophic cardiomyopathy, which accounts for up to 36% of the cardiovascular-related cases.[61]

Specific Disorders

Congenital Coronary Artery Anomalies

An additional 24% of the cases of sudden death are due to various anomalies of the coronary arteries.[61] Congenital coronary artery anomalies are difficult to detect from a clinical standpoint, but 37% of those individuals who died from congenital coronary artery anomalies did exhibit previous symptoms of exercise-induced syncope or chest pain.[62] The exact pathophysiologic mechanism of sudden death in individuals with congenital coronary anomalies is unknown. Although there are a variety of congenital coronary artery anomalies, the most common potentially lethal anomaly is the anomalous left coronary artery in which the left main and right coronary arteries both arise from the right sinus of Valsalva. Individuals with this particular anomaly have a 46% incidence of sudden death, with more than 85% of the known cases of sudden death occurring during exercise.[63] Congenital coronary artery hypoplasia is another uncommon cause of exercise-induced sudden death. Any athlete with exertional syncope or chest pain should be evaluated by a cardiologist for the possibility of congenital coronary artery anomalies. If an anomaly is detected and surgically corrected, the athlete may resume full activity and participation in competitive sports.

Marfan's Syndrome

Individuals with Marfan's syndrome should be evaluated for potential cardiac abnormalities before being allowed to participate in competitive sports. Clinical manifestations of the disease include tall, slender habitus, striae atrophicus of the skin (multiple stretch marks on skin), disproportionately long extremities as compared to the trunk, scoliosis, pectus excavatum or carinatum, and dislocated lenses of the eye. Approximately 50% of patients with Marfan's syndrome have cardiac manifestations such as mitral valve prolapse or aortic dilation. The most serious cardiac complication of Marfan's syndrome is the progressive dilation of the aorta with the potential risk of aortic rupture, which most commonly involves the descending portion of the aorta. Therefore, patients with Marfan's syndrome should be prohibited from participation in contact sports. Those individuals who are known to have aortic dilation should also be prohibited from participation in any competitive sports regardless of the degree of contact involved.[61] All patients with Marfan's syndrome with or without cardiac involvement on their initial evaluation should be followed by a cardiologist with serial imaging studies of their aorta using echocardiography, magnetic resonance imaging, or computed tomography.

Hypertrophic Cardiomyopathy

Perspective

Although the nonobstructive form of hypertrophic cardiomyopathy is an uncommon cardiac malformation that occurs in only 0.2% of the general population, it is the single most common cardiac cause of sudden death in the young athlete.[63-65] Hypertrophic cardiomyopathy is a familial disease that is inherited in an autosomal dominant fashion with variable penetrance. The hypertrophy of the left ventricle in this condition is idiopathic in nature and not due to chronic pressure overload conditions such as systemic hypertension or aortic stenosis. The systolic left ventricular contractile function is vigorous but the thickened muscle of the left ventricle is stiff, resulting in impaired ventricular relaxation and high diastolic filling pressures.[66]

Sudden death in previously asymptomatic individuals with hypertrophic cardiomyopathy occurs during moderate or severe physical exertion. The proposed pathophysiologic mechanisms of sudden death during exertion in these individuals is thought to be due to a transient decrease of blood flow out through the aorta or to dysrhythmias secondary to the hypertrophied ventricular myocardium.

Clinical Features

Some individuals with hypertrophic cardiomyopathy have experienced previous "warning" episodes of chest pain, dyspnea, syncope, or palpitations during vigorous activities. A family history of sudden unexplained death in young adults should also alert the clinician to the possibility of hypertrophic cardiomyopathy. Because the majority of young athletes who die from this condition have the nonobstructive form of hypertrophic cardiomyopathy, the classic loud systolic ejection murmur that is present with the obstructive form is not heard during the routine pre-sports physical examinations.[67] Therefore, the standard pre-sports screening physical examination may fail to detect the presence of nonobstructive hypertrophic cardiomyopathy in young athletes. If a systolic murmur along the lower left sternal border is heard on the routine screening physical examination of a young athlete, a Valsalva maneuver may help to differentiate the murmur of aortic stenosis from the systolic murmur associated with the obstructive form of hypertrophic cardiomyopathy. During the Valsalva maneuver, the venous blood return to the heart is decreased, which in turn transiently reduces the left ventricular size. This transient reduction in the size of the left ventricle will increase the degree of obstruction and thus cause an increase in the intensity of the systolic murmur heard with the obstructive form of hypertrophic cardiomyopathy. In contrast to this, the systolic murmur of aortic stenosis will decrease in intensity during a Valsalva maneuver due to the transient reduction of blood flow through the stenotic aortic valve.

Individuals who are suspected of having hypertrophic cardiomyopathy based on the above-mentioned exertional symptoms or a positive family history, or both, should be referred to a cardiologist for a more extensive workup.

Diagnostic Studies

The ECG findings in individuals with hypertrophic cardiomyopathy typically reveal various degrees of left ventricular hypertrophy and left atrial enlargement. Other ECG findings include prominent Q waves in the inferolateral leads or diffuse T wave inversions. The most accurate study to make the diagnosis of HSM is the echocardiogram, which will demonstrate various degrees of left ventricular hypertrophy most commonly involving the ventricular septum in up to 90% of the cases.[66] Those patients who have echocardiographic evidence of hypertrophic cardiomyopathy should be followed with serial echocardiographic examinations to monitor the progression of their condition.

Management

Although β-blockers have been used in patients with hypertrophic cardiomyopathy, they have not been shown to prevent sudden death in these patients. The use of digoxin is contraindicated in patients with hypertrophic cardiomyopathy because its positive inotropic effect may worsen the left ventricular outflow obstruction. Sudden death in these patients with hypertrophic cardiomyopathy is thought to be due to exertion-induced ventricular fibrillation or pulseless ventricular tachycardia. Therefore, the current recommendation is that all individuals who are diagnosed with hypertrophic cardiomyopathy, as well as those individuals with an equivocal diagnosis of hypertrophic cardiomyopathy, should not participate in vigorous activities and competitive sports.

Prolonged QT Syndrome

Perspective

In 1957, Jervell and Lange-Nielsen first described the association of recurrent syncope, sudden death, and long QT interval in a series of deaf patients. Later, in 1963, Romano reported a similar association of symptoms with long QT intervals in patients with normal hearing. Both the Jervell-Lange-Nielsen and the Romano-Ward syndrome are inherited disorders with variable penetrance, characterized by a prolonged QT interval that has been associated with sudden death. The corrected QT interval (QTc) in normal individuals should never exceed 0.44 seconds in children or 0.42 seconds in adolescents. Individuals with QTc intervals greater than 0.55 seconds have a higher risk of sudden death. Prolongation of the QT interval predisposes the individual to ventricular tachycardia, torsades de pointes, and ventricular fibrillation, which is often initiated by a premature ventricular contraction occurring during the prolonged repolarization phase. In addition to the inherited syndromes of prolonged QT intervals, other causes of prolonged QT intervals include hypocalcemia, hypokalemia, hypomagnesemia, myocarditis, medications (i.e., procainamide, erythromycin, cyclic antidepressants, phenothiazines, quinidine, organophosphates).

Clinical Features

Symptoms in the young athlete that are suggestive of QT prolongation include exercise-induced palpitations, chest pains, syncope, dizziness, or atypical seizures. Therefore, any young athlete who develops any of these symptoms should immediately be evaluated by a cardiologist, especially if the family history is positive for sudden unexplained death, cardiac problems, syncope, or deafness. Any young athlete who has been diagnosed with a prolonged QT syndrome should be prohibited from participation in competitive sports and vigorous activities. The growing popularity and presence of AEDs in public places and at sporting events can potentially save the lives of those athletes who suddenly collapse due to an underlying prolonged QT syndrome-induced nonperfusing ventricular dysrhythmia.

Management

Treatment of a prolonged QT interval depends on the cause. Correction of any underlying metabolic disorder or discontinuing a medication that induced the prolongation of the QT interval are the easiest conditions to correct. Magnesium sulfate is the drug of choice in the treatment of torsades de pointes. Antidysrhythmic agents that also can prolong the QT interval, such as procainamide and amiodarone, should be avoided. Therefore, the safest medication to use in a patient with prolonged QT interval–induced ventricular tachycardia or fibrillation would be lidocaine. β-Blockers have been used to prevent sudden ventricular dysrhythmias in those patients with the familial forms of QT prolongation. Adjunctive treatment in these selected patients also includes the insertion of pacemakers or internal defibrillators.

Commotio Cordis

The phenomenon of commotio cordis occurs when an object such as a baseball strikes the chest and produces sudden death. This phenomenon most commonly occurs in children between 5 and 15 years of age with no known predisposing cardiac conditions.[61,68] Although commotio cordis most commonly occurs in baseball, it has also been reported to occur in ice hockey, lacrosse, softball, and fist fights.[69] In a few cases in which the cardiac rhythm was documented after the blunt trauma to the chest, the most common rhythm documented was ventricular fibrillation.[69] The majority of patients who sustain commotio cordis do not survive, especially if they are not rapidly treated with defibrillation. If an AED is not immediately available and the patient is completely unresponsive with no pulse after sustaining a direct blow to the chest, some practitioners have proposed that performing chest thumps during cardiopulmonary resuscitation may be of some benefit under this particular circumstance.

KEY CONCEPTS

- The possibility of a congenital heart defect should be considered in an infant who presents with central cyanosis that does not respond to 100% supplemental oxygen (hyperoxia challenge).
- Neonates with ductal-dependent cardiac lesions typically present within the first 2 to 3 weeks of life with either acute cyanosis or shock. Initiation of a PGE1 infusion (0.01-0.1 μg/kg/minute) will be lifesaving in these neonates.
- Treatment of a hypoxic tet spell first includes placing the infant in the knee-to-chest position and providing supplemental oxygen. Sedative agents can be used to decrease the infant's hyperpnea. Various medications can be used as adjunctive treatment to increase the SVR and thereby decrease the degree of right-to-left shunting across the ventricular septal defect.
- Prompt recognition of the clinical findings and symptoms of Kawasaki disease along with the rapid initiation of aspirin and intravenous immunoglobulin infusion can prevent the formation of coronary aneurysms.
- Acute bacterial endocarditis should always be considered in a child with a known congenital heart defect or an acquired cardiac defect who presents with either a fever of unknown origin, the development of acute neurologic deficits, new-onset microscopic hematuria, myalgias, splenomegaly, petechiae, or other signs of systemic embolization.
- Oxygen, diuretics (furosemide), and inotropic agents (digoxin) are the mainstay of treatment for infants and children who present in congestive heart failure.
- If vagal maneuvers fail to convert stable paroxysmal supraventricular tachycardia in children, rapid adenosine administration (0.1 mg/kg for the first dose followed by 0.2 mg/kg on repeat doses) is the treatment of choice. Verapamil should be avoided in children younger than 1 year of age due to its profound hypotensive effects.
- One should consider the use of lidocaine instead of amiodarone in cases of ventricular fibrillation or ventricular tachycardia due to medications (e.g., cyclic antidepressants) or toxins that prolong the QT interval.
- Young athletes with a positive family history of sudden unexplained death or exertion-induced symptoms such as chest pain, dyspnea, palpitations, or syncope should be evaluated by a cardiologist prior to their resumption of vigorous activity.
- The increased presence of automated external defibrillators in public places and at sporting events can potentially save the lives of more young athletes who suddenly collapse secondary to hypertrophic cardiomyopathy, prolonged QT syndromes, and commotio cordis.

REFERENCES

1. Fitzmaurice L, Gerardi MJ: Cardiovascular system. In Gausche-Hill M, Fuch S, Yamamoto L (eds): *APLS: The Pediatric Emergency Medicine Resource*, 4th ed. Sudbury, Mass, Jones and Bartlett, 2004, pp 106-145.
2. Woolridge DP, Love JC: Congenital heart disease in the pediatric emergency department. Part I: Pathophysiology and clinical characteristics. *Pediatr Emerg Med Rep* 7:69, 2002.
3. Sharieff GQ, McCollough M: The nightmare neonate: Life-threatening events in the first month of life. *Emerg Med Pract* 5:1, 2003.

4. Inaba AS: A simple way to remember pediatric vital signs. *Contemp Pediatr* 19:16, 2002.
5. Siegfried BH, Henderson TO: Cardiology. In Gunn VL, Nechyba C (eds): *The Harriet Lane Handbook: A Manual for Pediatric House Officers*, 16th ed. Philadelphia, Mosby, 2002, pp 123-168.
6. Park MK: Physical Examination. In Park MK (ed): *Pediatric Cardiology for Practitioners*, 4th ed. St. Louis, Mosby, 2002, pp 10-33.
7. Flynn PA, Engle MA, Ehlers KH: Cardiac lesions in the pediatric emergency room. *Pediatr Clin North Am* 39:955, 1992.
8. Park MK: Chest roentgenography. In Park MK (ed): *Pediatric Cardiology for Practitioners*, 4th ed. St. Louis, Mosby, 2002, pp 52-59.
9. Vasan RS, Beiser A, D'Agostino RB: Plasma homocysteine and risk for congestive heart failure in adults without prior myocardial infarction. *JAMA* 289:1251, 2003.
10. Maisel A: B-type natriuretic peptide in the diagnosis and management of congestive heart failure. *Cardiol Clin* 19:557, 2001.
11. Mir TS, et al: Plasma concentrations of N-terminal pro-brain natriuretic peptide in control children from the neonatal to adolescent period and in children with congestive heart failure. *Pediatr* 110:e76, 2002.
12. Hoffman JI: The incidence of congenital heart disease. *J Am Coll Cardiol* 39:12, 2002.
13. Koppel RI, et al: Effectiveness of pulse oxymetry screening for congenital heart disease in asymptomatic newborns. *Pediatr* 111:451, 2003.
14. Park MK: Left-to-right shunt lesions. In Park MK (ed): *Pediatric Cardiology for Practitioners*, 4th ed. St. Louis, Mosby, 2002, pp 129-154.
15. Thanopoulos BD, et al: Transcatheter closure of perimembranous ventricular septal defects with the Amplatzer asymmetric ventricular septal defect occluder: Preliminary experience in children. *Heart* 89:918, 2003.
16. Chessa M, et al: Transcatheter closure of congenital and acquired muscular ventricular septal defects using the Amplatzer device. *J Invasive Cardiol* 14:322, 2002.
17. Arora R, et al: Transcatheter closure of congenital ventricular septal defects: Experience with various devices. *J Interv Cardiol* 16:83, 2003.
18. Brandt RR: Transcatheter closure of atrial septal defect and patent foramen ovale in adult patients using the Amplatzer occlusion device: No evidence for thrombus deposition with antiplatelet agents. *J Am Soc Echocardiogr* 15:1094, 2002.
19. Wilkinson JL: Interventional pediatric cardiology: Device closures. *Indian J Pediatr* 67:S30, 2000.
20. Niwa K, et al: Eisenmenger syndrome in adults: Ventricular septal defects, truncus arteriosus, univentricular heart. *J Am Coll Cardiol* 34:223, 1999.
21. Park MK: Obstructive lesions. In Park MK (ed): *Pediatric Cardiology for Practitioners*, 4th ed. St. Louis, Mosby, 2002, pp 155-173.
22. Chen YB, Liberthson RR, Freed MD: Congenital heart disease. In Lilly L (ed): *Pathophysiology of Heart Disease: A Collaborative Project of Medical Students and Faculty*, 3rd ed. Baltimore, Lippincott Williams & Wilkins, 2003, pp 347-370.
23. Park MK: Cyanotic congenital heart defects. In Park MK: *Pediatric Cardiology for Practitioners*, 4th ed. St. Louis, Mosby, 2002, pp 174-240.
24. Gewitz MH, Vetter V: Cardiac emergencies. In Fleisher GR, Ludwig S (eds): *Textbook of Pediatric Emergency Medicine*, 4th ed. Baltimore, Lippincott Williams & Wilkins, 2000, pp 659-700.
25. Woods WA, Schutte DA, McCulloch MA: Care of children who have had surgery for congenital heart disease. *Am J Emerg Med* 21:318, 2003.
26. American Academy of Pediatrics: Respiratory syncytial virus. In Pickering LK, et al (eds): *Red Book: 2003 Report of the Committee on Infectious Diseases*, 26th ed. Elk Grove Village, Ill, American Academy of Pediatrics, 2003, pp 523-528.
27. Shay DK, et al: Bronchiolitis-associated hospitalizations among US children. *JAMA* 282:1140, 1999.
28. Shay DK, et al: Bronchiolitis-associated mortality and estimates of respiratory syncytial virus-associated deaths among US children. *J Infect Dis* 183:16, 2001.
29. Feltes TF, et al: Palivizumab prophylaxis reduces hospitalization due to respiratory syncytial virus in young children with hemodynamically significant congenital heart disease. *J Pediatr* 143:523, 2003.
30. Romero JR: Palivizumab prophylaxis of respiratory syncytial virus disease from 1998 to 2002: Results from four years of palivizumab usage. *Pediatr Infect Dis J* 22:S46, 2003.
31. Young KD, Seidel JS: Pediatric cardiopulmonary resuscitation: A collective review. *Ann Emerg Med* 33:195, 1999.
32. Hazinski MF, et al: Rhythm disturbances. In *PALS Provider Manual*. Dallas, American Heart Association, 2002, pp 185-228.
33. Naccarelli GV, et al: Amiodarone: Clinical trials. *Curr Opin Cardiol* 15:64, 2000.
34. Perry JC, et al: Pediatric use of intravenous amiodarone: Efficacy and safety in critically ill patients from a multicenter protocol. *J Am Coll Cardiol* 27:1246, 1996.
35. Inaba AS: Don't wait for weight. *Emerg Med* 32:59, 2000.
36. Case CL: Diagnosis and treatment of pediatric arrhythmias. *Pediatr Clin North Am* 46:347, 1999.
37. Park MK: Cardiac arrhythmias. In Park MK: *Pediatric Cardiology for Practitioners*, 4th ed. St. Louis, Mosby, 2002, pp 333-348.
38. Kugler JD, Danford DA: Management of infants, children, and adolescents with paroxysmal supraventricular tachycardia. *J Pediatr* 129:324, 1996.
39. Aydin M, et al: Application of ice water to the face in initial treatment of supraventricular tachycardia. *Turk J Pediatr* 37:15, 1995.
40. Cummins RO: Stable tachycardias. In *ACLS Provider Manual*. Dallas, American Heart Association, 2001, pp 167-185.
41. Hickey RW, et al: Pediatric patients requiring CPR in the prehospital setting. *Ann Emerg Med* 25:495, 1995.
42. Mogayzel C, et al: Out-of-hospital ventricular fibrillation in children and adolescents: Causes and outcomes. *Ann Emerg Med* 25:484, 1995.
43. Samson RA, Berg RA, Bingham R: Use of automated external defibrillators for children: An update (an advisory statement from the Pediatric Advanced Life Support Task Force, International Liaison Committee on Resuscitation). *Circulation* 107:3250, 2003.
44. Jun K (ed): AEDs and children: Evidence for safe use now sufficient. *Currents* 14:11, 2003.
45. Hickey RW, Zuckerbraun NS: Pediatric cardiopulmonary arrest: Current concept and future directions. *Pediatr Emerg Med Rep* 8:1, 2003.
46. Kochanek PM, et al: Cerebral resuscitation after traumatic brain injury and cardiopulmonary arrest in infants and children in the new millennium. *Pediatr Clin North Am* 48:661, 2001.
47. Sirbaugh PE, et al: A prospective, population-based study of the demographics, epidemiology, management, and outcome of out-of-hospital pediatric cardiopulmonary arrest. *Ann Emerg Med* 33:174, 1999.
48. Saiman L, Prince A, Gersony WM: Pediatric endocarditis in the modern era. *J Pediatr* 122:847, 1993.
49. Brook MM: Pediatric bacterial endocarditis treatment and prophylaxis. *Pediatr Clin North Am* 46:275, 1999.
50. Dejani AS, et al: Prevention of bacterial endocarditis: Recommendations by the American Heart Association. *JAMA* 277:1794, 1997.

51. Ferrieri P, et al: Unique features of infective carditis in childhood. *Pediatr* 109:931, 2002.
52. American Academy of Pediatrics: Antimicrobial prophylaxis. In Pickering LK, et al (eds): *Red Book: 2003 Report of the Committee on Infectious Diseases*, 26th ed. Elk Grove Village, Ill, American Academy of Pediatrics, 2003, pp 782-786.
53. Bezold LI, Brisker JT: Advances in acquired pediatric heart disease. *Curr Opin Cardiol* 10:78, 1995.
54. Li MM, Klassen TP, Watters LK: Cardiovascular disorders. In Barkin RM, et al (eds): *Pediatric Emergency Medicine: Concepts and Clinical Practice*, 2nd ed. St. Louis, Mosby, 1997, pp 631-637.
55. Matson JW, et al: A clinical trial of immunosuppressive therapy for myocarditis. *N Engl J Med* 333:269, 1995.
56. American Academy of Pediatrics: Kawasaki syndrome. In Pickering LK, et al (eds): *Red Book: 2003 Report of the Committee on Infectious Diseases*, 26th ed. Elk Grove Village, Ill, American Academy of Pediatrics, 2003, pp 392-394.
57. Durongpistikul K, et al: The prevention of coronary aneurysm in Kawasaki disease: A meta-analysis on the efficacy of aspirin and immunoglobulin treatment. *Pediatr* 96:1057, 1995.
58. Sundel RP: Rheumatologic emergencies. In Fleisher GR, Ludwig S (eds): *Textbook of Pediatric Emergency Medicine*, 4th ed. Baltimore, Lippincott Williams & Wilkins, 2000, pp 1191-1220.
59. Park MK: Rheumatic Fever. In Park MK (ed): *Pediatric Cardiology for Practitioners*, 4th ed. St. Louis, Mosby, 2002, pp 304-310.
60. Maron BJ, Shirani J, Poliac LC: Sudden death in young competitive athletes: Clinical demographics and pathological profiles. *JAMA* 276:199, 1996.
61. Washington RL: Most sudden deaths in adolescent athletes caused by cardiac conditions. *Pediatr Ann* 32:751, 2003.
62. Basso C, et al: Clinical profile of congenital coronary artery anomalies with origin from the wrong aortic sinus leading to sudden death in young competitive athletes. *J Am Coll Cardiol* 35:1493, 2000.
63. Taylor A, Rogan KN, Varmani R: Sudden cardiac death associated with isolated congenital coronary artery anomalies. *J Am Coll Cardiol* 20:640, 1992.
64. Maron BJ, et al: Assessment of the prevalence of hypertrophic cardiomyopathy in a general population of young athletes: Echocardiographic analysis of 4,111 subjects in the CARDIA study. *Circulation* 92:785, 1995.
65. Liberthson RR: Sudden death from cardiac causes in children and young athletes. *N Engl J Med* 334:1039, 1996.
66. Chen YB, Dec GW, Lilly LS: The cardiomyopathies. In Lilly L (ed): *Pathophysiology of Heart Disease: A Collaborative Project of Medical Students and Faculty*, 3rd ed. Baltimore, Lippincott Williams & Wilkins, 2003, pp 237-258.
67. Spirito P, et al: The management of hypertrophic cardiomyopathy. *N Engl J Med* 26:775, 1997.
68. Maron BJ, et al: Blunt impact to the chest leading to sudden death from cardiac arrest during sports activities. *N Engl J Med* 33:337, 1995.
69. Link MS, et al: An experimental model of sudden death due to low-energy chest wall impact (commotio cordis). *N Engl J Med* 338:1805, 1998.

CHAPTER 170 Gastrointestinal Disorders

Mark A. Hostetler

NEONATAL JAUNDICE

Perspective

Many infants become jaundiced during the newborn period, most often as a result of a benign self-limited process. *Physiologic jaundice of the newborn* is the most common cause of neonatal jaundice and occurs in approximately 60% of normal newborns during the first week of life. *Breast milk jaundice* is the second most common cause of jaundice in the newborn period.

Principles of Disease

Bilirubin is formed by the breakdown of heme-containing proteins, primarily hemoglobin. Heme protoporphyrin is sequentially degraded into biliverdin and unconjugated bilirubin. Unconjugated bilirubin binds to albumin in the blood and is carried to the liver, where it is conjugated by glucuronyl transferase and excreted into bile. Jaundice may be caused by increased amounts of either unconjugated or conjugated bilirubin and becomes clinically apparent when the total bilirubin level reaches approximately 5 mg/dL. Conjugated hyperbilirubinemia occurs when the direct reacting portion exceeds 2 mg/dL or is greater than 20% of the total.

The exact mechanism of breast milk jaundice is uncertain. Breast milk jaundice may be hormonally mediated or related to intestinal excretion and resorption of bile. Other causes of jaundice vary significantly depending on the percent conjugation and age of the infant (Tables 170-1 and 170-2). Although jaundice in adults is usually the direct result of primary liver disease, infantile causes include a variety of extrahepatic causes—genetic, metabolic, infectious, and obstructive. The list of differential considerations in neonatal jaundice is extensive and requires careful consideration because the morbidity and mortality associated with many of these entities are high.

Table 170-1. Differential Considerations for Hyperbilirubinemia in Infants

	Unconjugated (Indirect)	Conjugated (Direct)
Benign/physiologic	Physiologic jaundice of the newborn Breast milk jaundice	
Hemolysis	ABO incompatibility Physiologic breakdown of birth trauma hematomas (cephalhematoma) Intraventricular/intracranial hemorrhage Spherocytosis, elliptocytosis Sickle cell Thalassemia Glucose-6-phosphate dehydrogenase deficiency Pyruvate kinase deficiency	
Infectious	TORCHS infections (toxoplasmosis, rubella, CMV, herpes, syphilis) Urinary tract infection Sepsis	TORCHS infections (toxoplasmosis, rubella, CMV, herpes, syphilis) Urinary tract infection Gram-negative sepsis Listeriosis Tuberculosis Hepatitis B Varicella Coxsackievirus Echovirus HIV
Obstructive	Meconium ileus Hirschsprung's disease Duodenal atresia Pyloric stenosis	Biliary atresia Choledochal cyst Bile duct strictures Inspissated bile syndrome Neonatal hepatitis Alagille syndrome Byler's disease Congenital hepatic fibrosis
Metabolic/genetic	Galactosemia Congenital hypothyroidism Crigler-Najjar syndrome Gilbert's syndrome	Galactosemia Tyrosinemia Glycogen storage disease type IV Niemann-Pick disease Wolman's disease Gaucher's disease Cholesterol ester storage disease α_1-antitrypsin deficiency Cystic fibrosis Dubin-Johnson syndrome Neonatal hypopituitarism Zellweger's syndrome Donohue syndrome (leprechaunism) Rotor syndrome
Miscellaneous		Drugs/toxins Parenteral nutrition

CMV, cytomegalovirus; HIV, human immunodeficiency virus.

Clinical Features

Physiologic jaundice of the newborn is the most common cause of neonatal jaundice and occurs in approximately 60% of normal newborns during the first week of life. Affected infants are born with normal bilirubin levels that gradually increase to a peak level of 6 mg/dL on the third day of life, then decline to normal within 2 weeks. Breast milk jaundice is the next most common cause of hyperbilirubinemia in newborns. Affected infants exhibit the same gradual increase seen with physiologic jaundice. Levels continue to increase, however, and reach a higher peak level at 10 days to 3 weeks of life. Elevated levels may persist for 3 to 10 weeks, then gradually subside.

Toxic levels (>20 mg/dL and dependent on age) of bilirubin may be associated with neurotoxicity, encephalopathy, and the development of kernicterus. Kernicterus is characterized by yellow staining in areas of the brain, including the basal ganglia. Symptoms begin with poor feeding and lethargy and may progress to muscular rigidity, opisthotonos, seizures, and death. Survivors may have residual problems with coordination, hearing, and learning disabilities.[1] The cornerstone of therapy is phototherapy and exchange transfusion.

Diagnostic Strategies

Although physiologic jaundice of the newborn and breast milk jaundice are most common, it is important to identify truly pathologic causes of jaundice. Initial testing requires determination of fractionated levels of total and direct bilirubin. Box 170-1 lists indications for workup in infants presenting with hyperbilirubinemia. Conjugated (direct) hyperbilirubinemia is always

Table 170-2. Differential Considerations for Hyperbilirubinemia in Older Children

	Unconjugated (Indirect)	Conjugated (Direct)
Obstructive		Gallstones Tumor Choledochal cyst Bile duct stricture
Infectious		Hepatitis Sepsis Urinary tract infection
Genetic	Sickle cell Thalassemia Spherocytosis, elliptocytosis Glucose-6-phosphate dehydrogenase deficiency Pyruvate kinase deficiency Criglor-Naijar syndrome Gilbert's syndrome	Dubin-Johnson syndrome Rotor syndrome Wilson's disease Cystic fibrosis α_1-antitrypsin deficiency Glycogen storage disease
Other	Drug-induced hemolytic anemia Autoimmune hemolytic anemia Microangiopathic hemolytic anemia Hypersplenism	Cirrhosis Sclerosing cholangitis Cholestatic jaundice of pregnancy Drugs/toxins (acetaminophen, estrogens)

BOX 170-1. Indications for Workup in Jaundiced Infants

1. Jaundice appearing within 24 hours of birth
2. Elevated direct (conjugated) bilirubin level
3. Rapidly rising total serum bilirubin unexplained by history or physical examination
4. Total serum bilirubin approaching exchange level or not responding to phototherapy
5. Jaundice persisting beyond age 3 weeks
6. Sick-appearing infant

pathologic. In such cases, a minimal workup should include a complete blood count (CBC) with peripheral smear and a Coombs' test for immune-mediated major blood group incompatibility. Ill-appearing infants also require tests for finger-stick blood glucose, electrolytes, urine for reducing substances, and serum ammonia to rule out inborn errors of metabolism.[2]

Differential Considerations

Birth history should be obtained to elicit any history of trauma because large, resolving hematomas can be associated with jaundice. Family history should focus on other children or relatives with a history of jaundice or genetic or metabolic disorders and any unexplained infant deaths. Tables 170-1 and 170-2 contain full lists of differential considerations for jaundiced children.

Infants with direct hyperbilirubinemia represent a special subset of patients. All infants with direct hyperbilirubinemia require admission and an evaluation for the cause of the jaundice based on history and presenting signs and symptoms. This evaluation may include any or all of the following: sepsis evaluation, TORCHS titers (toxoplasmosis, rubella, cytomegalovirus, herpes, syphilis), basic metabolic studies, α_1-antitrypsin, sweat test for cystic fibrosis, ultrasound, nuclear medicine (HIDA/DISIDA) scan, and liver biopsy. In children, hemolytic anemias, infection, and drugs are the most common causes of jaundice. History should focus on travel; exposures; medications; and associated symptoms, such as fever, malaise, weight loss, and fever. Gentle palpation of the liver is useful to estimate size, firmness, and tenderness and to distinguish hepatomegaly from liver inflammation.

Management

Treatment of infants with hyperbilirubinemia is based on the prevention of kernicterus. Guidelines for using phototherapy and exchange transfusion have been recommended by the American Academy of Pediatrics (Figure 170-1).[3] Feeding should be continued as much as possible because it stimulates enterohepatic circulation and decreases bilirubin levels. Unless the infant is severely jaundiced, breast-feeding should be continued and supplemented with formula as needed. Infants who are premature or who have significant comorbidity require treatment at lower levels. Phototherapy is often now readily available on an outpatient basis.

Disposition

In general, infants with bilirubin levels greater than 18 to 20 mg/dL require admission and phototherapy. All infants with direct hyperbilirubinemia require admission and workup.

HYPERTROPHIC PYLORIC STENOSIS

Perspective

Hypertrophic pyloric stenosis (HPS) is the most common cause of infantile gastrointestinal (GI) obstruction beyond the first month of life. HPS occurs in 1 of every 250 live births.[4] Boys are affected at four times the rate of girls. HPS tends to run in families; however, the exact pattern of inheritance is unclear. There is an incidence rate of 1 in 14 if the father was affected; the rate is even higher if the mother was affected.[4] Whites are affected more often than African Americans, and the disease is rare in Asian Americans.

Principles of Disease

Infants are born with a normal pylorus and develop hypertrophy only as time progresses. The exact etiology is unknown. As the pylorus continues to hypertrophy, there is progressive gastric outlet obstruction. As vomiting continues, the infant loses hydrogen and chloride ions through emesis of gastric juices. As this metabolic derangement worsens, the kidney attempts

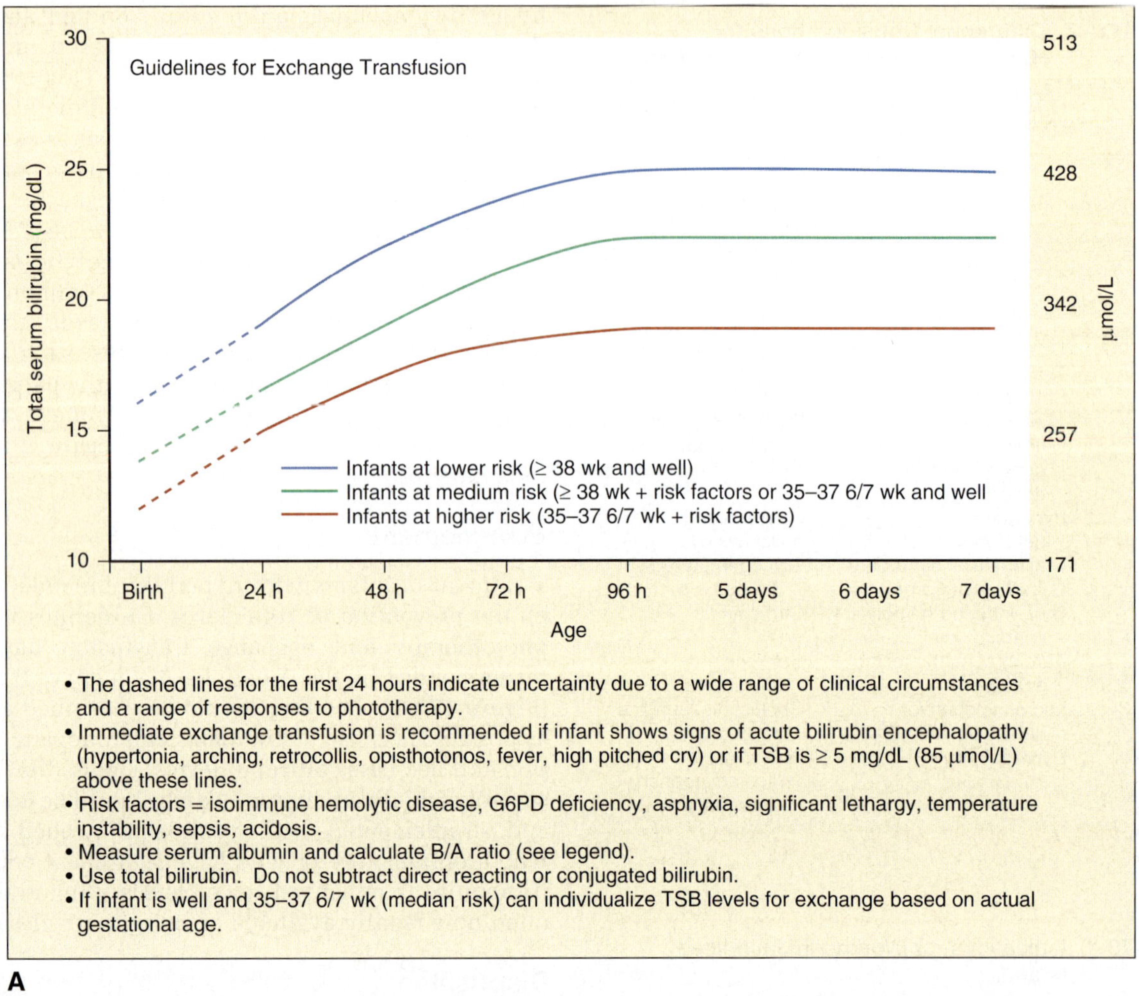

Figure 170-1. A, Guidelines for exchange transfusion in infants 35 or more weeks' gestation. Note that these suggested levels represent a consensus of most of the committee but are based on limited evidence, and the levels shown are approximations. During birth hospitalization, exchange transfusion is recommended if the TSB rises to these levels despite intensive phototherapy. For readmitted infants, if the TSB level is above the exchange level, repeat TSB measurement every 2 to 3 hours and consider exchange if the TSB remains above the levels indicated after intensive phototherapy for 6 hours.

to retain hydrogen ions by substituting potassium, resulting in a hypochloremic, hypokalemic, metabolic alkalosis.

Clinical Features

Infants classically present at 2 to 6 weeks old with gradually progressive emesis that becomes projectile and remains nonbilious. Infants remain vigorous with a ravenous appetite. They rapidly finish an entire feeding only to regurgitate the entire volume in a projectile fashion. In the later stages of the disease, children may exhibit visible waves of abdominal peristalsis in response to intense contractions against an obstruction. Children in the later stages of disease may exhibit marasmus, protein-calorie malnutrition as a result of impaired nutrient absorption.

Diagnostic Strategies

Children may have a palpable pylorus, commonly referred to as an "olive" in the right epigastrium, on abdominal examination. Placing a nasogastric tube and emptying the stomach or placing the infant in the prone position often facilitates palpation. Identification of the classic olive on physical examination is pathognomonic, and no further workup is required. HPS may be confirmed by ultrasound or upper GI series. Ultrasound is probably the diagnostic modality of choice, but both modalities have reported accuracies of greater than 95%. Ultrasound examinations reveal a thickened pylorus, which is diagnostic.[5] The upper GI tract has a characteristic "string sign" that results from the contrast material narrowly passing through the pyloric sphincter. In advanced stages with complete obstruction at the pylorus, plain films may reveal a modified "double-bubble sign," indicating an enlarged body of the stomach and pylorus (Figure 170-2).

Differential Considerations

Etiologic possibilities vary depending on whether the course of vomiting has been sudden in onset, gradually progressive, or chronic. Details such as the frequency and volume of emesis also are important because they may have important implications on the severity of

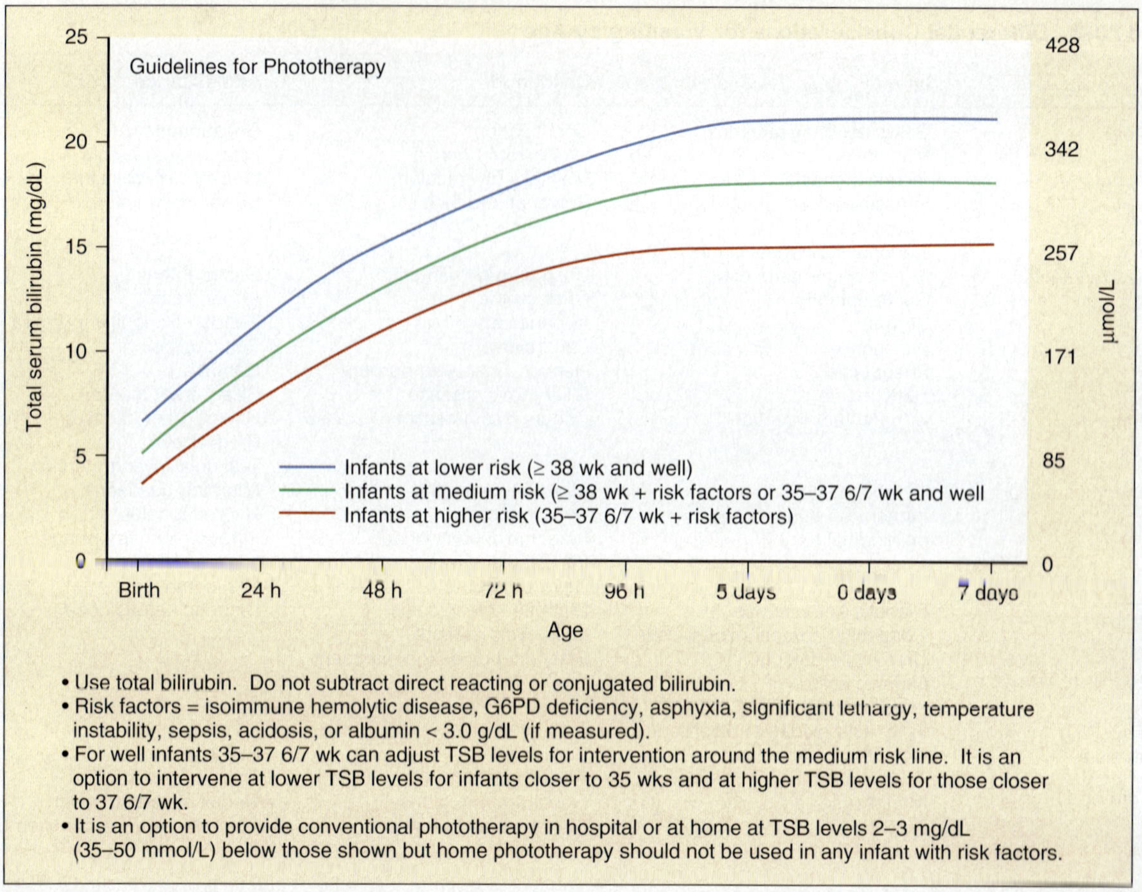

B

Figure 170-1—cont'd. B, Guidelines for phototherapy in hospitalized infants of 35 or more weeks' gestation. Note that these guidelines are based on limited evidence and the levels shown are approximations. The guidelines refer to the use of intensive phototherapy which should be used when the TSB exceeds the line indicated for each category. Infants are designated as "higher risk" because of the potential negative effects of the conditions listed on albumin binding of bilirubin, the blood-brain barrier, and the susceptibility of the brain cells to damage by bilirubin. (From American Academy of Pediatrics Clinical Practice Guidelines: Management of hyperbilirubinemia in the newborn infant 35 or more weeks of gestation. *Pediatrics* 114:305, 2004.)

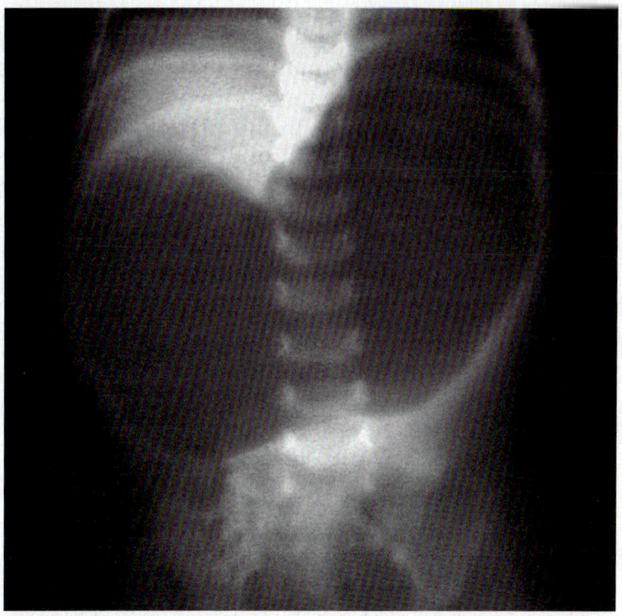

Figure 170-2. Plain radiograph of the abdomen revealing a modified double-bubble sign as seen in advanced stages of hypertrophic pyloric stenosis, in which there is complete obstruction at the pylorus. The "double bubbles" in this case represent the enlarged body and pyloric portions of the stomach. (Courtesy of Mark A. Hostetler, MD)

disease and the potential risk for dehydration or electrolyte disturbance. In infants, other major diagnoses in the differential include gastroesophageal reflux (GER) and malrotation. The age of the child and the timing of vomiting provide important clues as to the etiology. GER classically begins early in life, usually shortly after birth, and remains relatively constant. Pyloric stenosis does not begin until 2 to 3 weeks of age, then becomes increasingly severe and projectile. Acute obstruction of pyloric stenosis causes sudden-onset vomiting, which is rarely, if ever, bilious. In neonates, bilious vomiting requires careful consideration to rule out the possibility of malrotation with volvulus.[6]

Many causes of vomiting do not have a true GI origin, including sepsis, increased intracranial pressure, middle ear disturbances, inborn errors of metabolism, pain, medications, and drug intoxications. Differential considerations for vomiting in children vary by age (Table 170-3).

Management

Treatment consists of fluid and electrolyte replacement and surgical consultation. Fluid resuscitation should begin with a 20 mL/kg bolus of normal saline, followed

Table 170-3. Differential Considerations for Vomiting by Age

	Infancy	Childhood	Adolescence
Mechanical	Gastroesophageal reflux Malrotation with midgut volvulus Pyloric stenosis Intussusception Incarcerated hernia Tracheoesophageal fistula	Constipation Incarcerated hernia Meckel's diverticulum Bowel obstruction	Constipation Incarcerated hernia Meckel's diverticulum Bowel obstruction
Inflammatory/infectious	Necrotizing enterocolitis Gastroenteritis Sepsis Meningitis Pneumonia Otitis media	Gastritis/gastroenteritis Otitis media Appendicitis Pancreatitis Henoch-Schönlein purpura Biliary tract disease	Gastroenteritis Appendicitis Henoch-Schönlein purpura Pancreatitis Gastritis Biliary tract disease
Genitourinary	Urinary tract infection	Urinary tract infection	Urinary tract infection Pregnancy Testicular/ovarian torsion
Central nervous system	Hydrocephalus Intracranial hemorrhage Intracranial tumor	Migraine headache Hydrocephalus Intracranial hemorrhage Intracranial tumor Reye syndrome	Migraine headache Hydrocephalus Intracranial hemorrhage Intracranial tumor Glaucoma
Metabolic	Diabetic ketoacidosis Congenital adrenal hyperplasia Urea cycle defects Organic acidurias Amino acidopathies Fatty acid oxidation disorders	Diabetic ketoacidosis Urea cycle defects Fatty acid oxidation disorders	Diabetic ketoacidosis
Other/atypical	Occult trauma (abuse) Toxic ingestions Munchausen by proxy	Sickle cell Toxic ingestions Occult trauma (abuse) Munchausen by proxy	Sickle cell Toxic ingestions Occult trauma (abuse) Munchausen/Munchausen by proxy

by additional boluses as necessary to treat signs of shock. When the patient is stable and shows no signs of shock, 5% dextrose and half-normal saline at 1.5 to 2 times maintenance may be administered. Potassium supplementation is often necessary. IHPS is a chronic, progressive disease, not an acute ischemic process. Confirmatory radiographic diagnosis with ultrasound may be done on a semiurgent basis as symptoms warrant. Pediatric surgical consultation is mandatory, although usually not emergent. The definitive corrective surgical procedure is the Ramstedt pyloromyotomy and has an excellent track record of safety.[7] More recently, laparoscopic pyloromyotomy has gained increasing acceptance as being safe and effective.[8] Mortality is rare.

Disposition

Most children may be admitted to the hospital for rehydration and correction of electrolyte abnormalities, with imaging and surgical consultation done on a semielective basis.

MALROTATION WITH MIDGUT VOLVULUS

Perspective

Malrotation occurs in 1 in 500 live births and has a male predominance of at least 2:1.[9] Of infants with malrotation, approximately 75% eventually develop volvulus, and 75% of these infants present within the first month of life. Ninety percent of patients present within the first year of life, although cases of adult midgut volvulus have been reported.[9] Bilious emesis is the hallmark presentation and occurs in greater than 75% of cases.[6,9,10] Malrotation with volvulus has a mortality rate of 3% to 15%.[9]

Principles of Disease

During embryologic development, the GI tract rotates around the superior mesenteric artery. As it completes the rotation, the duodenum forms a C-loop and is fixed to the retroperitoneum in the left upper quadrant at the ligament of Treitz. The cecum becomes similarly fixed in the right lower quadrant. The duodenum and cecum normally come to reside widely separated and loosely connected by a broad-based mesentery. They are fixed firmly in position by peritoneal attachments called *Ladd's bands.* In cases of malrotation, the duodenum and the cecum do not rotate completely but end up in close proximity to each other suspended in the midgut region by their vascular attachment containing the superior mesenteric artery. This unusually close proximity of the intervening mesentery results in a short stalk of mesentery that easily twists on itself, resulting in obstruction of the distal duodenum and compression of the superior mesenteric artery. Vascular compression results in ischemia of the bowel and, if not rapidly reversed, necrosis of the bowel wall in 1 to 2 hours.[9,12] Twisting of the pedicle also results in varying degrees of obstruction secondary to Ladd's bands that are malpositioned and straddling the duodenum. Bilious emesis is the hallmark presentation and occurs as a result of severe obstruction. Any pigmented staining of the vomitus suggests the presence of bile. When initially produced, bile is bright yellow and turns green only with time and oxidative exposures. Differential coloring of bile-stained emesis, yellow versus green, is not predictive of surgical pathology.

Clinical Features

Infants classically present with sudden-onset bilious emesis and abdominal distention.[13] The obstruction may be relatively high, however; consequently, a distended abdomen may not always be present. Infants usually appear quite ill and may present in shock.[14,15] Infants also may present with a history of intermittent, relatively mild episodes of emesis that suddenly become more intense. Although bilious emesis in a neonate always suggests the possibility of acute obstruction and volvulus, children may present with nonspecific signs, such as abdominal distention or ill appearance.[13,14]

Diagnostic Strategies

Diagnostic strategies may include obtaining a plain film of the abdomen, an upper GI series, or a computed tomography (CT) scan of the abdomen. Findings on plain abdominal films may include air-fluid levels suggesting obstruction, dilated loops overlying the liver, and a paucity of small bowel gas distally (Figure 170-3).[12] In addition, a double-bubble sign may be present, representing a dilated stomach and obstructed proximal duodenum. Three different conditions are associated with seeing a double-bubble sign on plain abdominal films. The classic double bubble represents a dilated stomach and obstructed proximal duodenum and is seen in duodenal atresia and malrotation with midgut volvulus. Duodenal atresia is limited to the newborn nursery and presents within 24 hours of life. Malrotation with midgut volvulus typically presents with bilious vomiting within the first month of life. The modified double-bubble sign seen with HPS represents a dilated body of the stomach and pylorus and is associated with nonbilious emesis.

The diagnostic procedure of choice to determine midgut volvulus is the upper GI series, which reveals abnormal position of the duodenal C-loop (Figure 170-4) and small bowel with a characteristic corkscrew appearance (Figure 170-5).[12] An ultrasound scan may be obtained because of abdominal pain and may reveal abnormal positioning of the duodenal C-loop and superior mesenteric artery. The place of ultrasound in the evaluation of children with midgut volvulus has yet to be determined, however.[10,11]

Differential Considerations

Vomiting in childhood is common and occurs across a wide spectrum of illnesses (see Table 170-3). Causes vary depending on the age of the child and whether the course of vomiting has been sudden in onset, gradually progressive, or chronic. GER classically begins early in

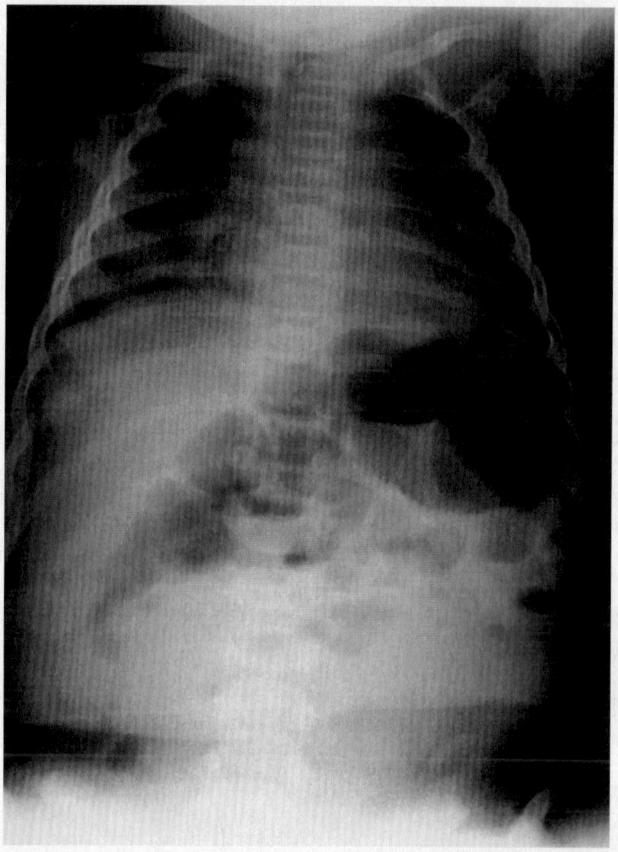

Figure 170-3. Upright abdominal radiograph of an infant with bilious vomiting illustrates dilated loops of small bowel and a paucity of bowel gas distally consistent with proximal obstruction secondary to malrotation with midgut volvulus. (Courtesy of Mark A. Hostetler, MD)

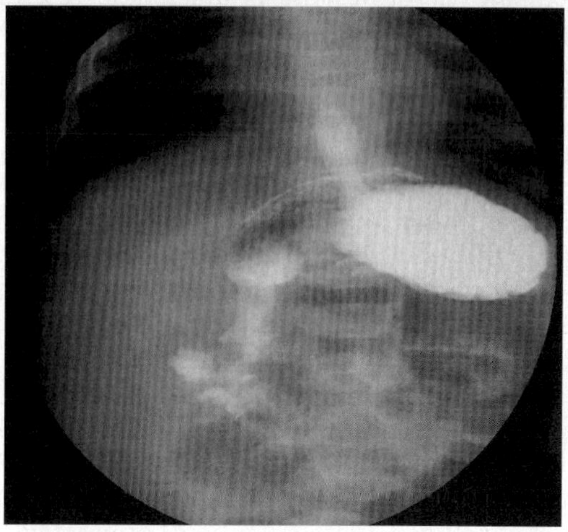

Figure 170-4. This is the infant from Figure 170-2. The upper gastrointestinal film reveals abnormal positioning of the duodenal C-loop to the right of the spinal column consistent with malrotation. (Courtesy of Mark A. Hostetler, MD)

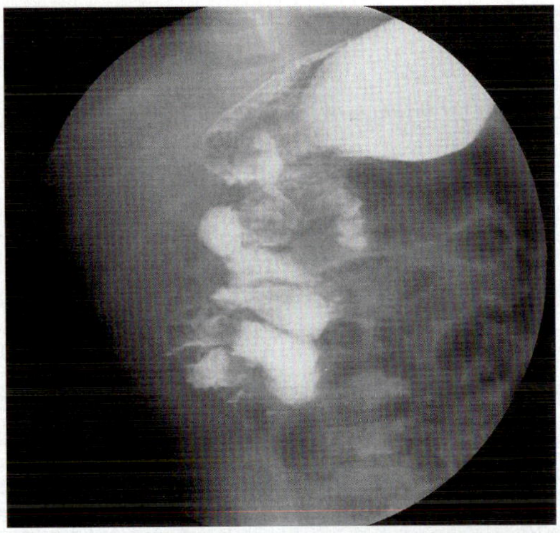

Figure 170-5. Another spot film from the upper gastrointestinal series of the infant in Figure 170-2. This radiograph shows the characteristic corkscrew appearance seen on small bowel follow-through in patients with malrotation. (Courtesy of Mark A. Hostetler, MD)

life, usually shortly after birth, and remains relatively constant. Pyloric stenosis does not begin until 2 to 3 weeks of age, then becomes increasingly severe and projectile. Acute obstruction causes sudden-onset vomiting, which may be bilious. In a neonate, bilious vomiting requires careful consideration to rule out the possibility of malrotation with volvulus.[13,14] Necrotizing enterocolitis (NEC) is another consideration because this life-threatening disease also presents with obstructive symptoms, including bilious emesis and abdominal distention. Although malrotation usually exhibits a paucity of small bowel air, NEC has diffusely dilated loops of small bowel. In addition, the presence of pneumatosis intestinalis is diagnostic of NEC and not present in cases of malrotation.

Management

Infants with sudden onset of bilious emesis who appear ill or have a distended abdomen require emergency consultation with a pediatric surgeon.[16] Intravenous access should be obtained and laboratory studies sent for CBC, electrolytes, and liver function tests. Repeated fluid boluses of normal saline, 20 mL/kg, are necessary until adequate circulation has been obtained. A fingerstick blood glucose and cultures of blood and urine should be obtained. A nasogastric or orogastric tube should be placed to decompress the abdomen. After consultation with a pediatric surgeon, an upper GI series may be needed emergently. Ill-appearing infants require broad-spectrum, triple-antibiotic coverage with ampicillin, gentamicin, and either clindamycin or metronidazole. Time is of the essence in the evaluation and operative management of these patients. Rapid pediatric surgical consultation should be obtained in any neonate or infant with bilious vomiting, especially infants who are ill appearing. In contrast with HPS, in which surgery does not need to be immediate, operative management must occur quickly to save the bowel from necrosis.

Disposition

Patients suspected to have malrotation require definitive imaging and an immediate surgical evaluation. If the diagnosis is confirmed or equivocal, surgical management and admission are required.

NECROTIZING ENTEROCOLITIS

Perspective

NEC is the most common GI emergency occurring in neonates, affecting 2000 to 4000 infants in the United States every year.[17] NEC is also the most common cause of intestinal perforation occurring during the newborn period.[17] Considering that most of the infants are premature and develop NEC in the neonatal intensive care unit, NEC is usually not considered an emergency department disease. Many of these infants may be discharged relatively early, however, because they are "feeding and growing" and present in the first month of life. Ten percent of infants with NEC are full-term births.[18] Development of NEC is related closely to gestational age. Infants of 24 to 28 weeks' gestation develop NEC within 2 to 4 weeks of life.[19] Infants of 29 to 32 weeks' gestation develop NEC within 1 to 3 weeks of life. More mature, or full-term, infants tend to develop NEC in the first week of life.[17] Children who survive NEC may develop complications, including strictures (10% to 20%), fistulae, and short gut syndrome.

Principles of Disease

The exact mechanism is unclear, but seems to be multifactorial. Proposed risk factors include prematurity, aggressive enteral feedings, birth-related hypoxic-ischemic insults, and infectious causes. Prematurity is the most common and universally accepted risk factor and occurs in 90% of all affected infants.[18,19] Rapid advancement of feedings also has been associated with increased rates of NEC.[20] Infection has been implicated as an important causative mechanism.[21] Evidence suggests that hypoxic-ischemic insults are not an independent risk factor for the development of NEC.[18] The primary pathologic event may be inflammation or injury to the intestinal wall, which begins in the mucosa, then extends transmurally. The distal ileum and proximal colon are more commonly affected, and the involvement may be continuous or patchy.[22]

Clinical Features

Infants with NEC present with feeding intolerance and emesis. Emesis may be either nonbilious or bilious. Occasionally, individual loops of bowel become distended with air and are palpable on abdominal examination. In the more severe stages of the disease, infants may be extremely ill-appearing and have hematemesis,

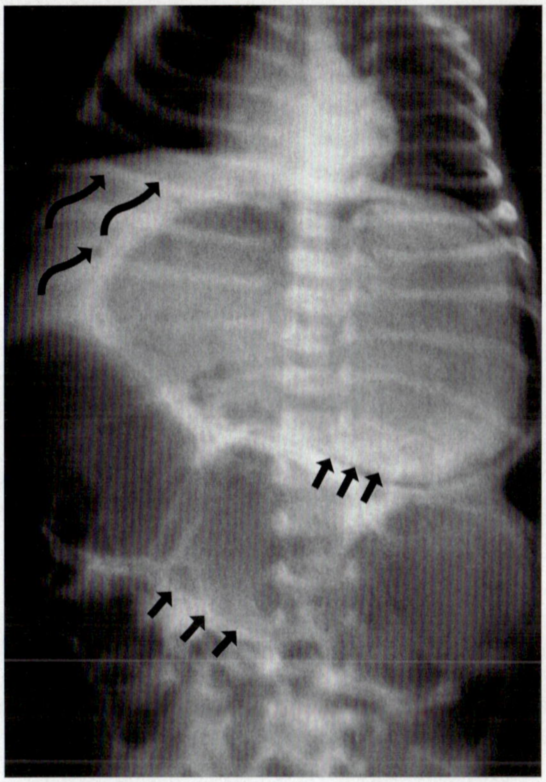

Figure 170-6. Plain radiograph of an infant with necrotizing enterocolitis. Shorter arrows indicate air within the wall of the small bowel and gastric mucosa (pneumatosis intestinalis and gastralis). Curved arrows indicate air in the biliary tree (portal venous gas). (Courtesy of Mark A. Hostetler, MD)

hematochezia, and shock. NEC commonly is placed into one of three clinical stages based on criteria developed by Bell.[23] Stage I represents early or suspected NEC based on feeding intolerance, vomiting, or ileus. Stage II represents definite NEC as proved by abdominal radiographs showing intestinal dilation and pneumatosis intestinalis. Stage III represents advanced disease and is associated with perforation. Infants in this stage are acutely ill with marked abdominal distention, metabolic acidosis, disseminated intravascular coagulation, and shock.

Diagnostic Strategies

Dilated loops of bowel are a common but nonspecific finding in stage I. Another early and more specific radiographic sign is the loss of a normal symmetric gas pattern and replacement with an asymmetric pattern of bowel gas that has varying degrees of dilation. Intramural air (pneumatosis intestinalis) is specific for NEC and is present in stage II (Figure 170-6).[23] Pneumatosis is present in 75% of patients with NEC.[18] Air also may be seen within the biliary tract (portal venous gas) or occasionally in the gastric wall (pneumatosis gastralis) (see Figure 170-5). Portal venous gas is present in 10% to 30% of cases.[18] Ultrasonography and barium enema, which have been described as an adjunct to diagnostic imaging of patients suspected to have NEC, are rarely helpful in the emergency department. No individual laboratory features are diagnostic or specific for NEC.

Differential Considerations

Etiologic possibilities vary depending on whether the emesis is bilious and whether the course of vomiting has been sudden in onset, gradually progressive, or chronic (see Table 170-3). GER classically begins early in life, usually shortly after birth, and remains relatively constant. Pyloric stenosis does not begin until 2 to 3 weeks of age, then becomes increasingly severe and projectile. In neonates, bilious vomiting requires careful consideration to rule out the possibility of malrotation with volvulus. Malrotation usually has a paucity of small bowel air, whereas NEC usually has diffusely dilated loops of small bowel. In addition, the presence of pneumatosis is diagnostic of NEC and not present in cases of malrotation.

Management

Patients suspected to have NEC should be kept nothing by mouth (NPO) and have their stomach and small bowel decompressed with either an orogastric or a nasogastric tube. These patients frequently appear quite ill and may have periods of apnea or significant respiratory distress. The airway should be secured as indicated. Intravenous access should be obtained and routine laboratory studies sent for CBC, electrolytes, type and screen, and coagulation studies (prothrombin time/partial thromboplastin time [PT/PTT]). A bedside blood glucose value should be obtained. Cultures of the blood and urine should be obtained. Careful attention should be given to managing fluids and electrolytes because considerable third spacing of fluids may occur. Repeated fluid boluses at 20 mL/kg of normal saline should be administered until adequate circulation is obtained. These boluses may be augmented with dopamine or epinephrine drips as necessary for patients in refractory shock when euvolemia has been achieved. Fluids should be continued with 5% dextrose in water and half-normal saline at a minimum of 1.5 to 2 times maintenance. Ill-appearing infants require broad-spectrum, triple-antibiotic coverage with ampicillin, gentamicin, and either clindamycin or metronidazole. Emergent consultation should be obtained from a pediatric surgeon. Patients with evidence of perforation, peritonitis, or gangrenous bowel require surgical intervention. Only one half to three quarters of patients with perforation have free air detectable on x-ray.[23]

Disposition

Ill-appearing children suspected to have NEC require admission to the hospital and pediatric surgical consultation.

GASTROESOPHAGEAL REFLUX

Perspective

GER is one of the most common causes of vomiting during infancy and refers to the regurgitation of stomach contents into the esophagus.

Principles of Disease

GER occurs as a result of an incompetent lower esophageal sphincter. Chronic reflux of gastric contents into the esophagus may result in esophagitis, aspiration, and, if severe, failure to thrive.

Clinical Features

Symptoms occur along a wide spectrum of disease, from occasional episodes of spitting up to severe, persistent vomiting and failure to thrive. GER generally responds to conservative measures and resolves with age. GER may be associated with stereotyped opisthotonic movements (Sandifer's syndrome). In Sandifer's syndrome, children exhibit extension and stiffening of the arms and legs, extension of the head, and often a shrill or guttural cry. It may be associated with a brief period of apnea and pallor as formula is refluxed into the esophagus. Sandifer's syndrome occurs most commonly shortly after feeding and usually is not associated with cyanosis.

Diagnostic Strategies

In the emergency department, the diagnosis of GER is made based on a careful history and physical examination. There are a variety of ways in which to diagnose GER, including esophageal pH probes checking for reflux of acid, barium swallow, and direct visualization via endoscopy.

Differential Considerations

Children with GER exhibit nonbilious emesis that begins shortly after birth and is relatively constant over time. There is usually not a sudden starting or ending point as would be suggested by an acute obstruction. Vomiting is usually neither gradually progressive nor projectile as seen with pyloric stenosis. Most children with milder severities of GER continue to gain weight.

Management

Most infants respond to conservative measures, such as smaller feedings, frequent burpings, thickening of formula with cereal, and maintaining a semiupright position for 45 minutes to 1 hour after feeding. Pharmacologic regimens are reserved for more severe cases. Weight loss is an important historical feature and necessitates referral for evaluation. Children exhibiting failure to thrive or esophagitis are often placed on medical management with ranitidine and metoclopramide. Ranitidine, a histamine blocker, reduces gastric acid secretion. Metoclopramide increases lower esophageal tone, reduces pyloric sphincter tone, and increases gastric motility. Patients not responding to medical management occasionally require surgical intervention with a Nissen fundoplication, which involves wrapping a portion of the stomach around the esophagus.

Disposition

Most children can be discharged home safely with conservative measures. Children with failure to thrive should be referred to a pediatrician or pediatric gastroenterologist for consideration of pharmacologic management. Children with dehydration and children with questionable diagnoses yet to be excluded may benefit from admission and further evaluation.

INTUSSUSCEPTION

Perspective

Intussusception is the most common cause of intestinal obstruction in children younger than 2 years old and occurs most commonly in infants 5 to 12 months old.[12,23] There is an estimated incidence of 1 per 2000 children younger than age 15 years with a male predominance.[23] Siblings of affected children have a relative risk 15 to 20 times higher than the general population. Mortality for untreated intussusception is high.

Principles of Disease

The exact etiology of intussusception is unclear, but the most prevalent theory relates to a lead point that causes telescoping of one segment of intestine into another.[23] As the process continues and intensifies, edema develops and obstructs venous return, resulting in ischemia of the bowel wall. As ischemia of the bowel wall continues, peritoneal irritation ensues, and perforation may occur.

In younger children, lead points are most often the result of enlarged Peyer's patches secondary to a recent viral infection. In children older than 5 years, an underlying lesion is found in more than 75% of cases; lesions include Henoch-Schönlein purpura (HSP) vasculitis, Meckel's diverticulum, lymphoma, polyps, postsurgical scars, celiac disease, and cystic fibrosis.[24-28] Intussusceptions may occur at any point along the GI tract. Ileocolic intussusceptions are most common. Ileoileal intussusceptions may occur in children with HSP.

Clinical Features

The classic triad of symptoms in intussusception is abdominal pain, vomiting, and bloody stools. All three symptoms occur in less than one third of patients, however. Three quarters of patients with intussusception have two findings, and 13% have either none or only one.[28] In a typical presentation, the child presents with cyclical episodes of severe abdominal pain. The pain typically lasts 10 to 15 minutes and has a periodicity of 15 to 30 minutes. During the painful episodes, the child is inconsolable, often described as drawing the legs up to the abdomen and screaming in pain. Children occasionally present without a history of pain and instead present with profound lethargy. Children may have vomiting or diarrhea associated with their presentation. Blood may be present in either the stool or the emesis. Diarrhea containing mucus and blood constitutes the classic "currant jelly" stool most often associated with intussusception, although in actuality it occurs relatively infrequently. Children often have had a viral illness recently. Palpation of the abdomen may reveal a sausage-like mass in the right upper quad-

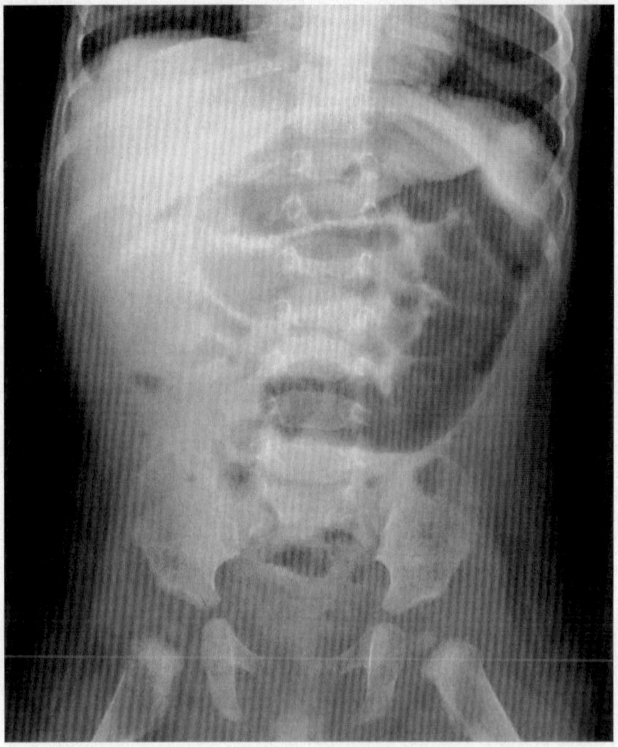

Figure 170-7. Plain radiograph of a child with crampy abdominal pain and vomiting later confirmed to have intussusception. Findings include a poorly defined soft tissue density in the right upper quadrant, obscuration of the liver edge, and focally dilated loops of small bowel consistent with an acute obstructive process (intussusception).

rant representing the actual intussusception and an empty space in the right lower quadrant representing the movement of the cecum out of its normal position. This is called *Dance's sign* and is considered pathognomonic for intussusception. Its occurrence is relatively uncommon, however. Intussusception usually is not associated with a high fever; however, low-grade fevers may occur.

Diagnostic Strategies

Initial screening films should be obtained with a minimum of two views of the abdomen. Attention should be focused on visualizing the entire colon and in particular the cecum. Films also should be examined for evidence of a soft tissue mass or mass effect, obstruction, and free air (Figure 170-7). Normal radiographs of the abdomen revealing complete visualization of the entire colon, including the cecum, essentially exclude the possibility of intussusception. Indeterminate or nonspecific films in which the entire colon cannot be visualized do not rule out intussusception and require additional imaging. Ultrasound is the least invasive and most commonly used modality for visualizing intussusceptions.[29] Ileocolic intussusceptions are most common and easily detected by ultrasound, even in inexperienced hands.[30] The exception may be in patients with HSP and severe abdominal pain. In HSP, ileoileal intussusceptions may occur, and the imaging modality of choice should be a CT scan. Barium enemas historically have been the gold standard and can be diagnostic and therapeutic. Contrast enemas reveal a sharp cutoff at the point where the intussusceptum meets the contrast material (Figure 170-8). Air contrast enemas are equally efficacious, have success rates averaging greater than 60%, and are preferred by some physicians over barium contrast studies.[29-33] Both enemas require readily available backup by a pediatric surgeon in the event of failure to reduce or perforation. Before sending the patient to radiology, the patient should have intravenous access obtained, at least one 20 mL/kg bolus of normal saline, and parenteral pain relief.

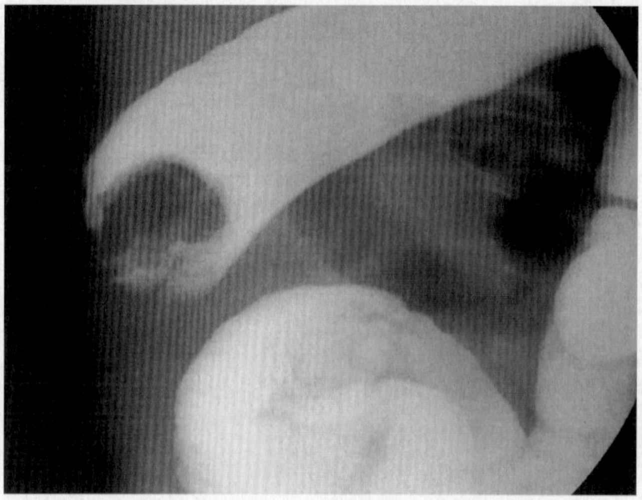

Figure 170-8. Contrast enema of a child with intussusception shows a sharp cutoff where the contrast material meets the intussusceptum and the acute obstruction.

Differential Considerations

Differential considerations for abdominal pain in children by age are listed in Table 170-4. Slow, progressive onset of pain is more likely associated with appendicitis, constipation, or pancreatitis. Children with peritoneal irritation invariably lie still, often on their sides with their knees bent, and refrain from all extraneous movement. Sudden onset of severe pain is associated most often with acute obstruction or vascular occlusion as seen with intussusception, volvulus, or torsion. Children with intussusception have severe colicky pain and often rock back and forth, frequently moaning or crying with pain. Children with ischemic pain exhibit symptoms out of proportion to their examination. They may appear diaphoretic, clammy, or pale and complain of excruciating abdominal pain, although having only mild tenderness to palpation and no localizing findings.

Management

Patients require intravenous access and screening CBC and electrolytes. Intravenous fluids are given in boluses of 20 mL/kg of normal saline until adequate vascular volume is achieved. Children should be maintained NPO. Nasogastric tube decompression may be necessary if there is evidence of significant gaseous distention. Prompt surgical consultation is required.

Table 170-4. Differential Considerations for Abdominal Pain by Age

	Infancy	Childhood	Adolescence
Mechanical	Malrotation with midgut volvulus Intussusception Incarcerated hernia Meckel's diverticulum Hirschsprung's disease	Constipation Incarcerated hernia Meckel's diverticulum Bowel obstruction	Constipation Incarcerated hernia Meckel's diverticulum Bowel obstruction
Inflammatory/infectious	Necrotizing enterocolitis	Gastroenteritis Appendicitis Henoch-Schönlein purpura Pancreatitis Gastritis Biliary tract disease	Gastroenteritis Appendicitis Henoch-Schönlein purpura Pancreatitis Gastritis Biliary tract disease
Genitourinary	Urinary tract infection	Urinary tract infection	Urinary tract infection Nephroureterolithiasis Pregnancy, ectopic Pelvic inflammatory disease Testicular/ovarian torsion
Other/atypical	Colic Occult trauma (abuse) Toxic ingestions Munchausen by proxy	Pneumonia Diabetic ketoacidosis Sickle cell Toxic ingestions Occult trauma (abuse) Munchausen by proxy	Pneumonia Diabetic ketoacidosis Sickle cell Toxic ingestions Occult trauma (abuse) Munchausen/Munchausen by proxy

Ill-appearing or febrile children require broad-spectrum, triple-antibiotic coverage with ampicillin, gentamicin, and either clindamycin or metronidazole. Diagnostic and therapeutic interventions depend on location and resources available. Patients may undergo an initial ultrasound or go straight to either air or hydrostatic barium enema. Surgical intervention is required if the reduction is unsuccessful or if perforation occurs. Intussusception may recur in 7% to 10% of radiologic reductions and 2% to 5% of surgical reductions, usually within 24 hours. Admission for observation usually is recommended for all patients after reduction.[31]

Disposition

Children with suspected intussusception require definitive imaging with ultrasound. Children with documented intussusception require reduction with either enema or surgery. Admission is recommended for all patients after reduction.

HIRSCHSPRUNG'S DISEASE

Perspective

Hirschsprung's disease accounts for approximately 20% of cases of partial intestinal obstruction in early infancy. Hirschsprung's disease occurs at a rate of 1 in 5000 live births and is four to five times more common in boys. It is usually sporadic, but may be associated with Down syndrome or a variety of other anomalies of the GI, genitourinary, or nervous systems.[34]

Principles of Disease

Hirschsprung's disease represents congenital aganglionosis of the colon and is characterized by an absence of ganglion cells in the myenteric plexus of the distal colon.[34] The anus is invariably involved with the disease, usually extending proximally 4 to 25 cm. Absence of colonic ganglion cells interferes with that segment's ability to relax, creating a functional obstruction. Stool accumulates proximal to the level of obstruction and produces dilation of the colon, the so-called megacolon.

Clinical Features

Neonates with Hirschsprung's disease often present in the nursery with failure to pass meconium. Infants may present with a history of constipation and obstipation. Vomiting, irritability, and abdominal distention may occur. Symptoms may be subtle and involve a history of chronic constipation and poor weight gain or failure to thrive. Hirschsprung's disease usually is diagnosed in infancy; however, there is a spectrum of disease, and presentations may occur later in life. Children who are ill appearing with fever should be evaluated for enterocolitis and toxic megacolon. Enterocolitis is characterized by abdominal distention, bloody stools, fever, and an elevated white blood cell count.

Diagnostic Strategies

Plain films of the abdomen may reveal evidence of fecal impaction with proximal obstruction, air and fluid levels, and dilated colon. A barium enema revealing a narrowed aganglionic segment with proximal dilation is highly suggestive of Hirschsprung's disease.[34,35] The diagnosis is confirmed by biopsy or manometry.

Differential Considerations

Constipation is one of the most common causes of abdominal pain and vomiting in children.[35,36] Children in the process of potty training occasionally become pathologic in their ability to delay defecation. Pathologic causes of constipation are uncommon. In addition to Hirschsprung's disease, considerations include cystic fibrosis, infantile botulism, and hypothyroidism. An acquired variant of the disease also may occur in which other factors produce similar dilated colonic findings, resulting in acquired megacolon. Risk factors include anal fissures; fecal impaction; toilet training issues; and neuromuscular dysfunction secondary to neurologic disease, drugs, or metabolic causes.

The exact definition of constipation is elusive because it varies with age and diet. Infants during the first few months of life may have stool frequencies that vary from one per feeding to one every other day, with breast-fed infants having more frequent stools than formula-fed infants. Frequency continues to decrease with age such that during the first year of life infants may average two to three stools per day, and from 1 to 5 years of age, one or two per day. Defecation occurs as a combination of physiologic, behavioral, and psychological factors. Relaxation of the external sphincter required for defecation is under voluntary control, whereas relaxation of the internal sphincter is involuntary. Children with a history of unpleasant or painful experiences associated with defecation may contract the external sphincter voluntarily in an effort to delay defecation for as long as possible. Accumulation of stool over time causes the rectum to dilate and decrease its propulsive activity, resulting in an increasing capacity for stool and chronic constipation. Acute episodes may occur as a result of dietary changes, travel, lack of normal exercise, or stress.

Management

Initial management is focused on ensuring adequate fluid and electrolyte status. Abdominal films should be obtained. If there is acute obstruction as evidenced by marked dilation, decompression may be necessary. Decompression usually can be accomplished easily with a rectal tube. Children who are ill appearing with fever should be evaluated for enterocolitis and toxic megacolon. Enterocolitis is characterized by abdominal distention, bloody stools, fever, and an elevated white blood cell count. Patients with enterocolitis require broad-spectrum, triple-antibiotic coverage with ampicillin, gentamicin, and either clindamycin or metronidazole. Urgent consultation should be made with a pediatric surgeon. Definitive therapy is surgical with resection of the aganglionic segments. Acquired megacolon is managed by decompressing the colon and addressing the underlying problems.

Management of *constipation* requires three considerations: cleanout, maintenance, and behavior modification. Acute constipation is easier to manage because there are fewer functional problems. The acute management of constipation is usually relatively easy and requires primarily the cleaning out of stool. Most recommend an approach that includes stool softeners or laxatives from above and suppositories or enemas from below. In milder cases, only the administration of enemas is necessary to soften feces and stimulate defecation. Tap water, Castile soap, and oil enemas all are generally equally efficacious. Maintenance includes keeping the stool soft for as long as necessary using stool softeners or laxatives. Dietary modifications include increasing fiber and water in the diet and avoiding foods that may be constipating. Management of chronic constipation is more difficult and usually requires a multidisciplinary approach with attention to behavior modification. Children with underlying pathology, such as cystic fibrosis, may benefit from more intense measures, such as large volumes of polyethylene glycol (GoLYTELY).

Disposition

Unless children are ill appearing, most can be managed safely as outpatients.

MECKEL'S DIVERTICULUM

Perspective

Meckel's diverticulum is the most common congenital malformation of the small intestine and follows the *rule of 2s*. It occurs in 2% of the population, and only 2% of affected patients ever become symptomatic.[37] Approximately half of all patients with the condition become symptomatic by age 2 years, and most present by age 20.[37] The diverticulum is 2 cm wide, 2 cm long, and usually located within 2 feet of the ileocecal valve.

Principles of Disease

Diverticula are remnants of the omphalomesenteric duct and contain bowel wall with 60% containing heterotopic tissue.[38] This tissue most commonly involves gastric mucosa, but other types include pancreatic, duodenal, and endometrial tissue.[36-38] Bleeding occurs when acid secretion from ectopic gastric mucosa causes ulceration and erosion.

Clinical Features

Patients are classically boys younger than age 5 who present with an acute onset of massive, painless rectal bleeding. Some children may have some complaints of abdominal cramping. The bleeding often is described as brick red in color. Complications may include intussusception, obstruction, perforation, and peritonitis.

Diagnostic Strategies

A technetium scan, also known as a Meckel's scan, is the diagnostic modality of choice and has an accuracy of 90% when ectopic gastric mucosa is present.[39] Administering pentagastrin, cimetidine, or glucagon may increase the sensitivity of the test.[39] Definitive diagnosis is confirmed by laparoscopy or laparotomy.

Differential Considerations

GI bleeding is uncommon in childhood. The first step in evaluating a child with suspected GI bleeding is to determine whether the substance is actually blood. Children commonly eat or drink substances containing dyes that lead to factitious changes in the stool's color. A simple Hemoccult test of the stool or Gastroccult test of the emesis can document the presence of hemoglobin. False-positive results may occur with red meat and iodine. Patients consuming products with bismuth (Pepto-Bismol), iron, and spinach may have black stools falsely appearing as melanotic; they test Hemoccult negative.

After it has been determined that the substance is blood, the second step is to determine its origin. The location of bleeding is often difficult to determine, but may be theorized based on the appearance of the blood. Hematemesis implies bleeding proximal to the ligament of Treitz. Blood exposed to gastric acids for any period of time develops the classic coffee-ground appearance. Bright red upper GI bleeding implies either more proximal bleeding, such as varices or esophagitis, or brisk gastric or duodenal bleeding. Bleeding that originates beyond the ligament of Treitz but proximal to the ileocecal valve results in melena. Hematochezia, visibly red to maroon in appearance, implies bleeding from the descending colon. Distal lesions, such as fissures or hemorrhoids, result in bright red blood. Endoscopic examination has the highest rate of determining the location of bleeding. Barium contrast studies of the upper and lower GI tract sometimes are helpful; however, nuclear scans (Meckel's scan) are the procedure of choice in detecting Meckel's diverticulum.

In neonates, the most common cause of bleeding is idiopathic. Careful examination of the rectum should be performed because the most identifiable cause for bleeding is a fissure or excoriation of the perirectal area. In young neonates, an Apt test may be performed to determine if the blood is maternal or fetal. One percent sodium hydroxide is added to the bloody stool. Fetal hemoglobin resists oxidation and remains pinkish red, whereas maternal hemoglobin changes to a dark brown color.

Another common cause for GI bleeding in infancy is milk protein allergy. Affected children typically are younger than 6 months old with a history of sudden-onset mucoid, blood-streaked stools. Children otherwise appear well. Although the most well-described occurrence is with milk protein, GI bleeding may occur with any protein and has been described in relation to soybean-based products. Children with persistent perianal excoriations and fissures refractory to standard emollients may be infected with group A streptococci and may benefit by treatment with an oral penicillin. Table 170-5 lists the differential considerations for GI bleeding in children by age.

Management

Management of GI bleeding begins with assessing and ensuring adequate circulatory status. Screening laboratory studies should include a CBC, coagulation studies (PT/PTT), and a type and screen. Two views of the abdomen should be obtained to rule out obstruction or perforation. A technetium scan is the imaging modality of choice to evaluate for Meckel's diverticulum. Consultation with a pediatric surgeon should be obtained.

Disposition

Children with suspected Meckel's diverticulum should undergo a Meckel's scan. Children with minor bleeding and normal screening laboratory studies may be fol-

Table 170-5. Differential Considerations for Gastrointestinal Bleeding by Age

	Infancy	Childhood	Adolescence
Factitious	Swallowed maternal blood Dyes in foods/beverages Vaginal origin Urinary origin	Dyes in foods/beverages Swallowed nasopharyngeal blood Vaginal origin Urinary origin	Dyes in foods/beverages Swallowed nasopharyngeal blood Vaginal origin Urinary origin
Upper GI	Necrotizing enterocolitis Intussusception Gastroenteritis Gastritis Esophagitis/varices (rare)	Esophagitis Gastroenteritis Gastritis Peptic ulcer disease Esophageal varices	Esophagitis Gastroenteritis Gastritis Peptic ulcer disease Esophageal varices
Lower GI	Necrotizing enterocolitis Intussusception Gastroenteritis Milk allergy Vascular malformation	Gastroenteritis Intussusception Meckel's diverticulum Inflammatory bowel disease Vascular malformation Henoch-Schönlein purpura Hemolytic uremic syndrome Colitis	Gastroenteritis Intussusception Meckel's diverticulum Inflammatory bowel disease Vascular malformation Henoch-Schönlein purpura Hemolytic uremic syndrome Polyps Colitis
Rectal	Rectal fissure	Rectal fissure	Rectal fissure Hemorrhoids Trauma
Other/atypical	Bleeding dyscrasia Occult trauma (abuse) Toxic ingestions Munchausen by proxy	Bleeding dyscrasia Toxic ingestions Occult trauma (abuse) Munchausen by proxy	Bleeding dyscrasia Toxic ingestions Occult trauma (abuse) Munchausen/Munchausen by proxy

GI, gastrointestinal.

lowed closely as outpatients. Children with more active bleeding should be admitted and followed by either a pediatric surgeon or a pediatric gastroenterologist.

HENOCH-SCHÖNLEIN PURPURA

Perspective

HSP, also known as anaphylactoid purpura, is a systemic vasculitis commonly associated with abdominal pain and rash. It is most common in children age 4 to 11 years, but also may occur in adults. HSP occurs most commonly in the spring after a viral upper respiratory infection. It also has been associated with insect stings and drugs.[41]

Principles of Disease

HSP is a hypersensitivity vasculitis with immune complex deposition with immunoglobulin A mainly affecting the arterioles and capillaries. Although it is most well known for its characteristic petechial-to-purpuric rash, HSP is a systemic vasculitis and may affect any blood vessel. Less common manifestations occur when the disease is more severe or widespread.

Clinical Features

Symptoms include abdominal pain, nausea, vomiting, and diarrhea. Patients most often are diagnosed clinically based on the appearance of a classic rash, abdominal pain, microscopic hematuria, and mild arthralgias. The classic rash is palpable purpura located on the buttocks and lower extremities (Figure 170-9). Seventy percent of patients with HSP have GI complaints. Microscopic hematuria occurs in 50%.[42] Intussusception may occur and may be atypical in that ileoileal intussusception is more common than the ileocolic intussusception that normally occurs. The syndrome is often relapsing and remitting over several weeks and may be associated with arthralgias. HSP may have associated nervous system involvement, although it is uncommon in children.[43]

Diagnostic Strategies

Patients most often are diagnosed clinically based on the appearance of a classic rash, abdominal pain, microscopic hematuria, and mild arthralgias. Screening studies should include a CBC with differential and platelets, urinalysis, blood culture, and sedimentation rate. Children with severe abdominal pain require CT to rule out ileoileal intussusception.

Differential Considerations

The most important entity in the differential diagnosis for this type of a rash is meningococcemia, in which the patient has a fever and is toxic appearing often with an abnormally elevated white blood cell count and leftward shift. The clinician must ensure that meningococcemia is excluded from the differential diagnosis because the condition is life-threatening and requires an entirely different management with intravenous antibiotics. The classic triad of palpable purpura, abdominal pain, and hematuria in an otherwise well-appearing child virtually ensures the diagnosis. Erythema nodosum occasionally is confused with the rash of HSP; however, in erythema nodosum the rash is described most often as subcutaneous purplish red nodules with the appearance of a bruise located on the extensor surfaces of the distal extremities. Erythema nodosum usually involves only the shins, but in more severe cases also may involve the forearms, hands, and feet.

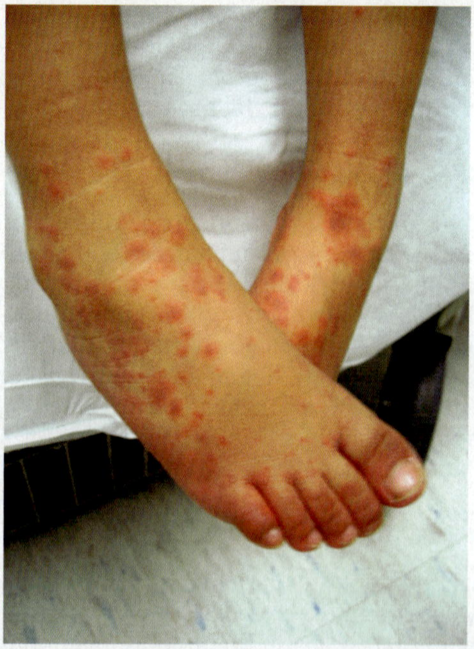

Figure 170-9. Henoch-Schönlein purpura in a 7-year-old child. Note typical red-purple rash in the lower extremities. (Courtesy of Marianne Gausche-Hill, MD.)

Management

Most children with HSP can be managed with close follow-up and require no treatment other than symptomatic. Patients with severe abdominal pain should be suspected of having intussusception and have imaging done with a CT scan because ileoileal intussusception may occur and is not detected easily by ultrasound. Management with steroids is controversial. Steroids, 1 mg/kg/day (maximum 60 mg), are reserved for patients on the more severe end of the spectrum with abdominal pain, hematuria, or arthralgias.

Disposition

Indications for admission include uncertain diagnosis to exclude the possibility of meningococcemia, severe abdominal pain, or vomiting. Most patients can be managed safely with close outpatient follow-up.

INFLAMMATORY BOWEL DISEASE

Perspective

The two major entities included within inflammatory bowel disease (IBD) are Crohn's disease and ulcerative colitis. Approximately 20% of patients present before age 20.[44] Most patients do not present until adolescence, although childhood presentations occur. IBD is rare in children younger than age 1 year.[45]

Principles of Disease

Ulcerative colitis is an inflammatory disease primarily involving the mucosa and submucosa of the rectum and distal colon. Crohn's disease is a transmural inflammatory disease that may involve any portion of the intestinal tract. The singularly most common area of involvement is distal ileum; however, multiple segments in different areas may be involved. Chronic inflammation may result in the formation of abscess, fistula, and stricture.

Clinical Features

Although patients experiencing complications frequently present to the emergency department, the diagnosis is rarely made there. More commonly, children with known disease present in the midst of a flare, usually with bloody diarrhea and abdominal pain. Extraintestinal manifestations also occur and include fever, anemia, oral ulcerations, erythema nodosum, pyoderma gangrenosum, uveitis, liver dysfunction, and failure to thrive.[45] Some of these manifestations may even occur before the child has had any GI symptoms. The most feared complication is toxic megacolon, which classically presents with abdominal pain, fever, and bloody diarrhea.

Diagnostic Strategies

Flares are diagnosed by the presence of increased frequency of diarrheal or bloody stools and abdominal pain. Patients who are ill appearing require plain films of the abdomen to rule out toxic megacolon. Patients with toxic megacolon usually have a fever, appear volume depleted, and have significant abdominal tenderness. X-rays reveal dilation of the transverse colon greater than 6 to 7 cm in diameter. Free air also should be looked for because perforation may occur. Screening laboratory studies should be obtained to evaluate for hematologic, fluid, and electrolyte abnormalities and include a CBC with differential and platelets, type and screen, coagulation studies (PT/PTT), and electrolytes.

Differential Considerations

There are a wide number of differential considerations for abdominal pain and GI bleeding (see Tables 170-4 and 170-5). Gastroenteritis is the most common consideration. Children with their first episode are much more likely to be misdiagnosed as having an acute gastroenteritis. Children outside of the usual age of presentation also are more likely to be misdiagnosed as having gastroenteritis. Children with recurrent symptoms or a family history of IBD should be referred to a pediatric gastroenterologist for further evaluation.

Management

Steroids are the mainstay of treatment for acute exacerbations. Prednisone at a dose of 1 mg/kg/day (maximum 60 mg/day) usually is recommended and should be provided in consultation with a pediatric GI specialist. Other agents commonly used include sulfasalazine, azathioprine, and a host of other immunosuppressive agents. Management begins with attention to volume status and resuscitation with boluses of 20 mL/kg of normal saline until the volume status is adequate. Patients with suspected toxic megacolon require intravenous broad-spectrum triple antibiotics (ampicillin, gentamicin, metronidazole) and surgical consultation.

Disposition

Indications for admission include children who are dehydrated, febrile, or ill appearing. Children with ongoing bloody diarrheal stools usually benefit from intravenous fluids until the flare has been controlled. Children with evidence of toxic megacolon require surgical consultation and admission.

GASTROINTESTINAL FOREIGN BODIES

Perspective

Most GI foreign bodies occur in toddlers, as they experience life by first putting it in their mouths. Children younger than 3 years are particularly at risk because of inappropriate mouthing of objects and a general lack of coordination in swallowing. Although food is the most common esophageal foreign body in adults, coins are most common in children.[46,47] Children with mental retardation swallow a variety of objects. Adolescents occasionally swallow objects in an attempt at suicide. Rectal foreign bodies are uncommon in the pediatric age group.

Principles of Disease

Most swallowed foreign bodies pass without difficulty. Foreign bodies may become lodged in any of three areas of normal physiologic narrowing: upper esophageal sphincter (cricopharyngeus muscle)/thoracic inlet (C6-T1), the aortic arch/tracheal bifurcation (T4-6), and the lower esophageal sphincter/diaphragmatic hiatus (T10-11). In general, 80% to 90% of objects that have made it into the stomach are passed without difficulty.[48]

Clinical Features

The classic example is a child who is seen from across the room putting coins in his or her mouth. Children frequently gag and sputter as they attempt to swallow the object. Aspirated objects generally produce persistent coughing, wheezing, or increased work of breathing. Objects that have been swallowed may result in the child remaining asymptomatic or produce symptoms ranging from persistent gagging to drooling and continuous dry heaves. Larger foreign bodies may compress the airway and cause significant respiratory distress.

Rapidly progressive symptoms of dysphagia, pain, respiratory distress, or fever raise the possibility of a perforation. Perforation is uncommon, even with sharp objects such as straight pins. The ileocecal valve is the most common site for perforation, and this occurs in less than 1% of patients.[48] Button batteries warrant special mention. Button batteries in the esophagus should be removed in as rapid a manner as possible because erosions and mediastinitis ultimately may occur. Button batteries in the stomach usually pass without difficulty and do not require removal unless they fail to pass the pylorus within 24 to 48 hours of ingestion.[49] Occasionally, objects pass into the stomach that are too large to pass through the pylorus; this is uncommon and heralded by persistent vomiting. Long-standing unrecognized foreign bodies may result in erosion, perforation, infection, stricture, or fistula formation.[50]

Diagnostic Strategies

Plain films are the most common method of visualizing location and are used to verify positioning past the lower esophageal sphincter into the stomach. Patients who are symptomatic after foreign body ingestion require imaging to determine location. Occasionally patients who are asymptomatic also have objects remaining in the esophagus.[51] Radiographs should include anteroposterior and lateral films of the chest and neck (Figure 170-10). The lateral film helps to delineate soft tissues in the hypopharynx and evaluate for swelling, particularly if the foreign body is either unknown or of a nonradiopaque material. Often a single view of the neck, chest, and upper abdomen can be performed easily on the pediatric patient in one film. Unless the patient becomes symptomatic, repeat films are otherwise never necessary. Patients presenting with button batteries are the exception in that they require repeat films to document passage beyond the pylorus. Rather than using standard radiography, some institutions have noted success with in-department fluoroscopy or hand-held metal detectors.[51-53] Contrast studies may be helpful to delineate nonradiopaque foreign bodies or to evaluate for perforations.

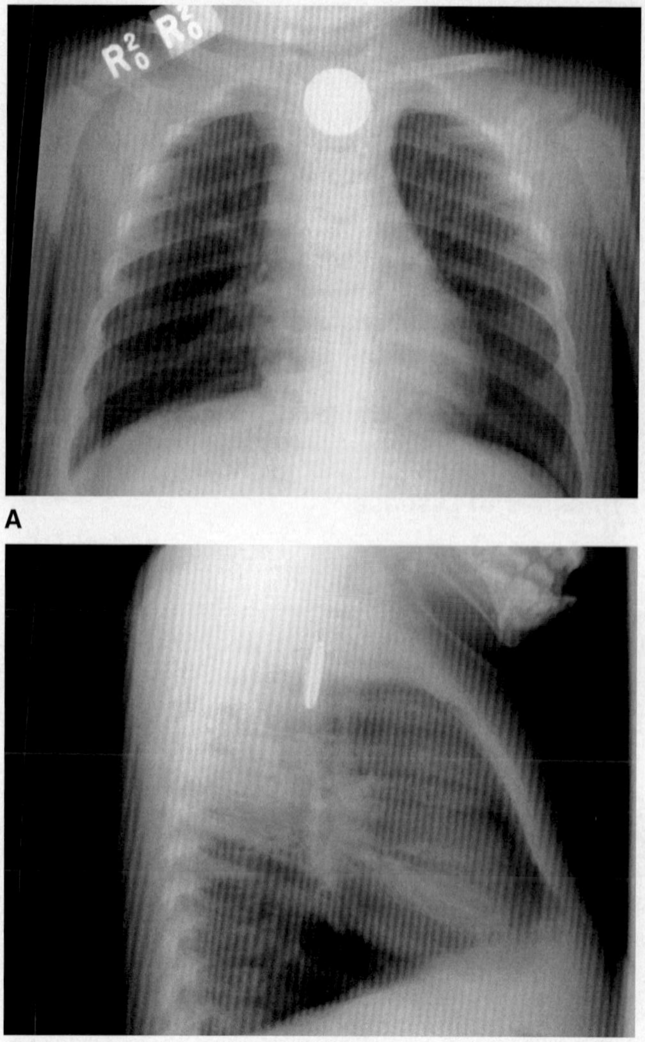

Figure 170-10. Plain radiographs of a child with an esophageal coin foreign body. Posteroanterior **(A)** and lateral **(B)** radiographs show the expected orientation for coins lodged in the esophagus. (Courtesy of Mark A. Hostetler, MD)

Differential Considerations

Not all foreign bodies are radiopaque and visible with standard radiography. Patients who remain symptomatic require further contrast-enhanced imaging or direct visualization.

Management

If the object has made it into the stomach, usually no further symptoms occur, and no further treatment is necessary. If the foreign body is in the esophagus, most authors recommend removal within 24 hours to decrease the risk of aspiration and esophageal erosion. The preferred method by which to remove esophageal foreign bodies is controversial and varies by institution. Options include fluoroscopic Foley catheter removal, bougienage advancement into the stomach, endoscopic removal in the emergency department, and removal by rigid bronchoscopy under general anesthesia in the operating room. Foley catheter removal and bougienage do not require sedation in cooperative patients, but young children invariably require sedation in the operating room. The latter two methods actually hold onto the foreign body and—at least theoretically—decrease the chance of inadvertent aspiration. They also have the additional benefit of directly visualizing the integrity of the mucosa and evaluating for perforation. Gastric foreign bodies generally do not require removal. Indications for surgical removal of gastric foreign bodies include objects that are greater than 2 cm in width, objects that are greater than 5 cm in length, and objects that are sharp.

Disposition

Esophageal foreign bodies require removal as described previously. After foreign bodies have made it into the stomach, most pass without difficulty and require no further follow-up. Button batteries are the exception and require follow-up films to document passage beyond the pylorus.

PANCREATITIS

Perspective

Pancreatitis is uncommon in childhood, especially in children younger than age 10. Pancreatitis has an incidence of approximately 1 in 50,000 in children and a mortality of 14%.[54,55] In adults, pancreatitis is associated most commonly with alcohol and biliary tract disease. In children, there is a fairly equal association of approximately 10% to 20% each for trauma, infection, structural disease, systemic disease, and drugs or toxins.[55] Mumps is the most common viral cause of pancreatitis and accounts for 10% to 15% of all cases.[55] Idiopathic causes account for 30% of cases.

Principles of Disease

Whether the result of trauma, obstruction, or inflammation, a series of events occurs resulting in inflammation, edema, and autodigestion of pancreatic tissue by pancreatic enzymes. In severe cases, this situation may progress to necrosis and hemorrhage, resulting in necrotizing or hemorrhagic pancreatitis. Further complications include the formation of abscesses, pseudocysts, and fistulae.

Clinical Features

Patients classically present with complaints of severe epigastric pain that radiates to the back. Pain is gradually progressive and constant and often is associated with nausea and vomiting. Pain classically is described as being worse with eating. There is usually significant abdominal tenderness in the epigastric area with voluntary guarding and hypoactive bowel sounds. The abdomen may be slightly distended.

Diagnostic Strategies

Screening laboratory studies reveal elevations in serum amylase or lipase. Plain films of the abdomen may be indicated to consider the possibility of free air or obstruction. An ileus pattern is common, often with a sentinel loop of dilated small bowel noted in the left upper quadrant. An ultrasound or CT scan may be helpful to evaluate anatomy for congenital malformations or biliary tract disease and to evaluate for pseudocyst formation. Patients with pseudocysts may develop hemorrhagic pancreatitis that may become life-threatening. For patients with respiratory distress, a chest x-ray can be helpful to evaluate for a coexistent pleural effusion caused by the pancreatitis.

Differential Considerations

Slow, progressive onset of pain is more likely associated with appendicitis, constipation, or pancreatitis. Children with peritoneal irritation invariably lie still, often on their sides with their knees bent, and refrain from all extraneous movement. Sudden onset of severe pain is associated most often with acute obstruction or vascular occlusion as seen with intussusception, volvulus, or torsion. Differential considerations for abdominal pain in children by age are listed in Table 170-4; differential considerations for the causes of pancreatitis are listed in Table 170-6.

Table 170-6. Differential Considerations for Pancreatitis in Children

Trauma	Handle-bar injury
Infectious	Viral: mumps, influenza A, EBV, CMV, hepatitis A and B, rubella, rubeola
	Bacterial: salmonellosis, leptospirosis
Structural	Choledochal cyst, duplication cyst, anomalous bile duct, duodenal stenosis
	Pancreas divisum
	Tumor
	Cholelithiasis
Systemic/genetic	Cystic fibrosis
	Glycogen storage disease
	Familial hyperlipidemias
	α_1-antitrypsin deficiency
	Sickle cell disease
Systemic/acquired	Systemic lupus erythematosus
	Kawasaki disease
	Hemolytic uremic syndrome
	Henoch-Schönlein purpura
	Crohn's disease
	Reye syndrome
	Diabetes mellitus
Drugs/toxins	Steroids, oral contraceptives
	Valproic acid
	Sulfasalazine, azathioprine
	Rifampin, pentamidine, metronidazole, tetracycline
	Thiazides, ethacrynic acid, furosemide
	Alcohol, L-asparaginase
Idiopathic	No definitive cause found

CMV, cytomegalovirus; EBV, Epstein-Barr virus.

Management

Management begins with attention to volume status and correction of electrolyte abnormalities if present. A bedside finger-stick blood glucose value should be obtained. Patients should be given adequate pain relief with parenteral narcotics. Patients should be maintained NPO and given adequate fluids. Intravenous fluids are given in boluses of 20 mL/kg of normal saline until adequate vascular volume is achieved, then followed by 5% dextrose in water and half-normal saline at 1.5 times maintenance. Antiemetics are indicated to help control nausea and vomiting. A nasogastric tube is usually not necessary or helpful, unless an ileus or persistent vomiting is present. Steroids and antibiotics are not indicated.

Disposition

Most children with pancreatitis require admission, unless they have known or recurrent disease with an adequate outpatient regimen for providing adequate analgesia and hydration.

APPENDICITIS

Perspective

Appendicitis is the most common surgical condition involving the abdomen, and the most common nontraumatic surgical emergency in children.[12] Approximately 200,000 appendectomies are performed every year, and approximately 1 of every 15 individuals develops appendicitis sometime during their lifetime.[12,23,56] The peak age of incidence of appendicitis is between 9 and 12 years old, and it is uncommon in children younger than age 5 years.[12,23,56]

Acute appendicitis has an overall mortality rate of less than 1%. For unruptured appendicitis, the mortality rate is 0.1%; the mortality rate increases to about 3% for ruptured appendicitis. In children, the rate of appendiceal perforation before surgery varies from 17% to 40% and is inversely related to age, with higher rates of perforation occurring in younger age groups. In children younger than age 2 years, 90% will have perforated by the time of surgery.

Principles of Disease

The appendix is a blind pouch that may become obstructed. After it is obstructed, a vicious cycle occurs with increasing edema, vasocongestion, inflammation, ischemia, infarction, necrosis, and perforation. In adults, a thicker appendiceal wall protects against perforation, and a well-developed omentum aids in walling off the infection to prevent its diffuse spread. Children have neither and tend to rupture earlier and develop diffuse peritonitis more readily.

Clinical Features

Patients classically present with a constellation of symptoms that includes abdominal pain, nausea, vomiting, fever, and anorexia. All of these symptoms are gradually progressive over 4 to 24 hours. Abdominal pain usually is described as vague, crampy, and periumbilical on origination, which then becomes more severe, constant, and localized to the right lower quadrant. Fever usually occurs later, sometimes not until after the patient already has presented to the emergency department. Nausea and vomiting are progressive and most often associated with anorexia. Patients occasionally may have a multiphasic course to their illness in which they begin with the classic abdominal pain; experience sudden resolution; and several days later develop fever, chills, and abdominal pain. This course represents acute appendicitis with spontaneous rupture and formation of abscess.

Physical examination may reveal several classic findings. Patients with inflammation surrounding the appendix usually develop peritoneal findings that localize to the right lower quadrant. Pain occurs with movement, so patients prefer to lie still. Patients are unable to jump up and down and complain that even rocking the bed or tapping their heels causes pain. The abdomen is usually quiet with an absence of bowel sounds. Rebound tenderness is present in the right lower quadrant. Rovsing's sign also may be present and occurs when the examiner presses in the left lower quadrant and rapidly releases the examining hand, causing severe pain in the right lower quadrant. Other findings associated with appendicitis include the psoas and obturator signs. The psoas sign is elicited by having the patient lie on his or her side and hyperextending the right thigh at the hip stretching the psoas muscle, which overlies the inflamed appendix and causes pain. The obturator sign is similarly elicited by internally rotating the flexed right thigh against resistance to elicit pain.

Diagnostic Strategies

Appendicitis may be diagnosed on the basis of history and physical findings alone. Patients with the appropriate constellation of findings consistent with appendicitis may not require any testing and proceed directly to the operating room for either laparoscopic or open exploration. Patients in whom the diagnosis is suspected usually require some diagnostic workup. Screening studies should include a CBC with differential, urinalysis, and pregnancy test. An estimated 96% of patients with appendicitis have either an elevated white blood cell count greater than 10,000/mm^3 or a left-shifted differential with more than 75% neutrophils.[57] Although an elevated white blood cell count supports the diagnosis, it is not specific for appendicitis. The appendix is in close proximity to the ureters and may induce some degree of sterile pyuria. Inflammatory changes related to appendicitis generally result in fewer than 5 to 10 white and red blood cells per high-power field and an absence of bacteria. Findings in excess of these amounts suggest a urinary tract etiology (infection, stone, mass, trauma). Consideration also may be given to adding a rapid streptococcal test in patients with red or sore throats.

Diagnostic imaging options include plain films of the abdomen, limited CT scan of the appendix, and ultrasound. Plain films help to rule out free air or obstruction and occasionally show an appendiceal fecalith, also called an *appendicolith* (Figure 170-11). Although the presence of an appendicolith is essentially pathognomonic for acute appendicitis, it is present in only 10% of cases.[56] Ultrasound findings consistent with appendicitis include an enlarged, noncompressible appendix that is painful during scanning. Ultrasound may show a fecalith inside an enlarged and inflamed appendix, the so-called target sign.[58] Appendiceal ultrasound studies have a sensitivity, specificity, and overall accuracy of 90% to 95%.[58-61] Ultrasound is particularly useful for evaluating for abscesses and fluid collections; however, there is a great deal of operator and reader variability.

CT of the appendix is the latest technology and seems to be the imaging modality of choice based on current evidence.[62-66] Limited CT scans of the appendix have sensitivities and specificities of 95% to 100%.[63-66] For patients with relatively low probability of appendicitis, CT offers a cost-effective screening tool, particularly compared with inpatient admission and observation.[62] In addition, the availability of appendiceal CT has been shown to reduce the negative laparotomy rate from 20% to 7%.[66] The highest accuracy has been reported using new focused appendiceal CT with rectal contrast. Imaging the pelvis and specifically the right lower quadrant with this technique effectively not only establishes the diagnosis of appendicitis, but also aids in

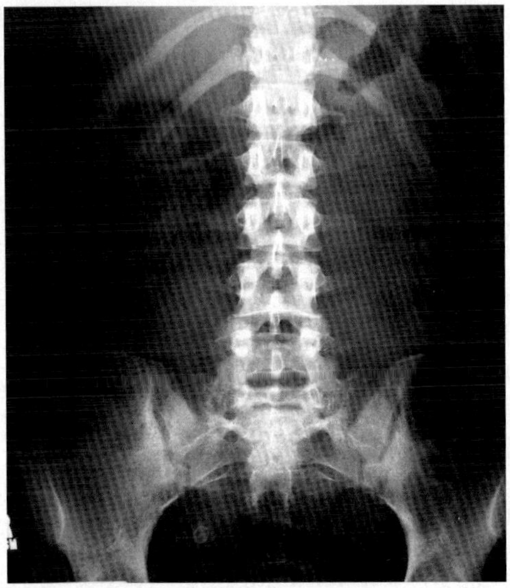

Figure 170-11. Fecalith in a child with appendicitis. (Courtesy of Marianne Gausche-Hill, MD.)

identifying the two most common differential diagnoses: IBD and mesenteric adenitis.[64-66]

Differential Considerations

Mesenteric adenitis is the most common condition associated with the signs and symptoms of appendicitis. It often has significant diffuse tenderness and may localize in the right middle to lower quadrant. Children often lack fever, however, and do not have true peritoneal signs. Mesenteric adenitis usually follows a viral illness and results from nonspecific inflammation of mesenteric lymph nodes. It is even perhaps more common than appendicitis. Differential considerations for abdominal pain by age are listed in Table 170-4. Other considerations include nonaccidental trauma (abuse), malingering, and Münchausen syndrome.[67] Girls of reproductive age require a consideration of gynecologic origin and require a pregnancy test, pelvic examination, and consideration of ovarian torsion, particularly if the pain seems to be severe and out of proportion to physical examination. Boys require an external genital examination to rule out the possibility of testicular torsion. Cryptorchidism in the face of acute abdominal pain should raise the suspicion of testicular torsion.

Management

Patients with suspected appendicitis should be maintained NPO and have an intravenous line established. Most patients have vomiting and anorexia and benefit from at least one fluid bolus of 20 mL/kg of normal saline, then 1.5 to 2 times maintenance fluids with dextrose 5% in water and half-normal saline. Screening studies should be initiated, and appropriate consultation should be made with a surgeon. Ongoing pain should be addressed adequately. Intravenous narcotics are safe and effective and should not alter the diagnostic accuracy of the physical examination. It is best to consult with a surgeon first, however, in the event that the surgeon would like to examine the abdomen before any narcotics are given. Pain relief should not be withheld indefinitely, however, pending a surgeon's examination. Patients with high fever, suspected perforation, or unusual delay to surgery require coverage with intravenous broad-spectrum antibiotics, which should be initiated in the emergency department after consulting with the surgeon.[68] Reasonable choices for antibiotics include ampicillin, gentamicin, and either metronidazole or clindamycin. Nasogastric tubes are reserved for patients with persistent nausea or vomiting related to abdominal distention or ileus.

Disposition

In the past, patients with suspected but not obvious appendicitis would be admitted and observed. The accuracy of CT is rapidly replacing this practice and may prove to be a more cost-effective alternative.

BILIARY TRACT DISEASE

Perspective

Biliary tract disease is uncommon in childhood and has causes distinct from disease in adults. In children, gallstones are associated with hemolytic disease, cystic fibrosis, total parenteral nutrition, sepsis, and dehydration.[69,70] Ceftriaxone also has been associated with sludging and biliary disease, particularly in neonates. Acute acalculous cholecystitis has been associated with Rocky Mountain spotted fever and a variety of bacterial infections ranging from *Salmonella* and *Shigella* organisms. Hydrops of the gallbladder is associated with viral upper respiratory or GI infections, Kawasaki disease, streptococcal pharyngitis, mesenteric adenitis, nephrotic syndrome, and leptospirosis.

Principles of Disease

Gallstones are classified as either cholesterol or pigment stones. Pigment stones occur in childhood, whereas cholesterol stones do not usually begin appearing until adolescence. Pigment stones result from the excess breakdown of red blood cells and are seen most commonly in hemolytic anemias, such as sickle cell disease and spherocytosis. Gallstones occurring in infants usually are associated with abdominal surgery, sepsis, necrotizing enterocolitis, or administration of total parenteral nutrition.[71] Young children most commonly develop gallstones as a result of their hemolytic disease. Adolescents form gallstones in association with oral contraceptives, pregnancy, obesity, or underlying hemolytic disease. In acute acalculous cholecystitis, the sonogram reveals evidence of gallbladder inflammation in the absence of calculi. Hydrops of the gallbladder is an acute noninflammatory, noninfectious process that results in a markedly enlarged gallbladder without evidence of calculi.

Clinical Features

Similar to adults, patients usually present with right upper quadrant pain that radiates through to the back and may be associated with fever, nausea, and vomiting. Jaundice occurs in one third of patients.[70-72]

Diagnostic Strategies

Biliary tract disease usually is associated with elevations in liver enzymes and bilirubin. Elevations in alkaline phosphatase suggest cholestasis. Elevated white blood cell counts are nonspecific, but if associated with fever may represent an acute infectious process (i.e., ascending cholangitis). Ultrasound is the imaging modality of choice. It can determine the presence of gallstones, reproduction of pain on scanning (sonographic Murphy's sign), the amount of dilation of the gallbladder and bile ducts, gallbladder wall thickness, and the anatomic configuration of the biliary and pancreatic collecting system. When ultrasound is equivocal or negative in the face of strong clinical suspicion, the gold standard for biliary tract imaging is still considered to be cholescintigraphy scanning.[71] Although only 15% of gallstones in adults are calcified and visible on plain radiographs of the abdomen, 50% of stones are visible in children.[71,72]

Differential Considerations

Biliary tract disease is uncommon in children and requires consideration of underlying or coexistent disease. Differential considerations for abdominal pain by age are listed in Table 170-4.

Management

Management of biliary tract disease begins with attention to fluid and electrolyte status. Adequate pain control should be provided, usually with a parenteral opioid. Asymptomatic patients with incidental findings of gallstones require no further emergent therapy and may be referred to a surgeon as an outpatient. Patients who are afebrile usually can be managed safely as an outpatient with adequate pain control. Febrile patients require admission and intravenous antibiotics. Reasonable choices for empiric antibiotic coverage include ampicillin and gentamicin, plus either clindamycin or metronidazole.

Disposition

Indications for admission include pain control, hydration, fever, and need for operation.

KEY CONCEPTS

- Physiologic and breast milk jaundice are the most common causes of jaundice in the neonatal period.
- Evaluation of jaundice requires fractionated levels of total and direct bilirubin.
- Direct hyperbilirubinemia in infants is always pathologic and requires a detailed workup.
- HPS presents with gradually progressive nonbilious emesis that becomes projectile.
- Infants with HPS appear vigorous and hungry.
- Hypochloremic, hypokalemic metabolic alkalosis is the classic electrolyte abnormality.
- Bilious vomiting in the neonate should immediately raise the suspicion of malrotation and volvulus.
- Infants with bilious emesis who are ill-appearing, have a distended abdomen, or show an acute obstructed pattern on abdominal radiographs represent a true surgical emergency.
- NEC occurs more commonly in premature infants, but 10% of affected infants are full-term.
- Pneumatosis intestinalis is pathognomonic for NEC.
- GER begins early after birth and remains relatively constant over time.
- GER usually responds to conservative measures (positioning, thickening of formula, smaller and more frequent feedings).
- The classic triad for intussusception is abdominal pain, vomiting, and heme-positive stools; however, the triad occurs in fewer than one third of patients.
- Children with intussusception may present without pain and with lethargy alone.
- Hirschsprung's disease is a common cause of constipation in the neonate and is usually manifested by delayed passage of meconium.
- Hirschsprung's disease may be complicated by toxic megacolon, which is a true emergency.
- Although Hirschsprung's disease is a consideration in cases of constipation, functional or acquired causes are much more common.
- Meckel's diverticulum follows the *rule of 2s*.
- Meckel's diverticulum classically presents in children younger than 5 years old with painless, brick red rectal bleeding.
- The classic presentation for HSP is a petechial or purpuric rash on the buttocks and legs associated with GI complaints and arthralgias in an otherwise well-appearing child.
- GI complaints in HSP most often include abdominal pain, nausea, vomiting, and microscopic hematuria.
- IBD is rare in infants younger than 1 year old and uncommon in children and more commonly begins in adolescence.
- Steroids are the mainstay of therapy for IBD.
- Toxic megacolon may occur as a complication and is a true emergency.
- More than 90% of foreign bodies pass without difficulty.
- Button batteries require repeat films to document passage past the pylorus.
- Pancreatitis is uncommon in childhood.
- Causes of pancreatitis include viruses, trauma, drugs, and toxins.
- The classic constellation of symptoms of pancreatitis includes abdominal pain, nausea, vomiting, anorexia, and fever.
- The imaging modality of choice for older children and adolescents who do not require surgery on clinical grounds alone is limited CT of the appendix.
- In children, pigment stones are most common secondary to hemolytic disease.
- Fifty percent of gallstones in children may be calcified and seen on plain radiographs.

REFERENCES

1. Perlman M, Frank JW: Bilirubin beyond the blood-brain barrier. *Pediatrics* 81:304, 1988.
2. Hostetler MA, et al: Hypoketotic hypoglycemic coma in a 21-month-old child. *Ann Emerg Med* 34:394, 1999.
3. American Academy of Pediatrics Clinical Practice Guidelines: Management of hyperbilirubinemia in the newborn of 35 or more weeks gestation. *Pediatrics* 114:297, 2004.
4. Zenn MR, Redo SF: Hypertrophic pyloric stenosis in the newborn. *J Pediatr Surg* 28:1577, 1993.
5. Vasavada P: Ultrasound evaluation of acute abdominal emergencies in infant and children. *Radiol Clin North Am* 42:445, 2004.
6. Kao H: Bilious vomiting during the first week of life. *Acta Paediatr Sin* 35:202, 1994.
7. Stringer MD, Brereton RJ: Current management of infantile hypertrophic pyloric stenosis. *Br J Hosp Med* 43:266, 1990.
8. Najmaldin A, Tan HL: Early experience with laparoscopic pyloromyotomy for infantile hypertrophic pyloric stenosis. *J Pediatr Surg* 30:37, 1995.
9. Torres AM, Ziegler MM: Malrotation of the intestine. *World J Surg* 17:326, 1993.
10. Leonidas JC, et al: Midgut volvulus in infants: Diagnosis with ultrasound. *Radiology* 179:491, 1991.
11. Shatzkes D, et al: Malrotation of the bowel: Malalignment of the superior mesenteric artery-vein complex shown by CT and MR. *J Comput Assist Tomogr* 14:93, 1990.
12. Felter RA: Nontraumatic surgical emergencies in children. *Emerg Med Clin North Am* 9:589, 1991.
13. Bonadio WA, Clarkson T, Naus J: The clinical features of children with malrotation of the intestine. *Pediatr Emerg Care* 7:348, 1991.
14. Seashore JH, Touloukian RJ: Midgut volvulus: An ever-present threat. *Arch Pediatr Adolesc Med* 148:43, 1994.
15. Messineo A, et al: Clinical factors affecting mortality in children with malrotation of the intestine. *J Pediatr Surg* 27:1343, 1992.
16. Spigland N, Brandt ML, Yarbeck S: Malrotation presenting beyond the neonatal period. *J Pediatr Surg* 25:1139, 1990.
17. Neu J: Pediatric gastroenterology: II. Necrotizing enterocolitis: The search for a unifying pathogenic theory leading to prevention. *Pediatr Clin North Am* 43:409, 1996.
18. Kliegman RM, Fanaroff AA: Necrotizing enterocolitis. *N Engl J Med* 310:1093, 1984.
19. Neu J, Weiss MD: Necrotizing enterocolitis: Pathophysiology and prevention. *J Parenter Enteral Nutr* 23:S13, 1999.
20. Anderson DM, Kliegman RM: The relationship of neonatal alimentation practices to the occurrence of endemic necrotizing enterocolitis. *Am J Perinatol* 8:62, 1991.
21. Larson HE: Neonatal necrotizing enterocolitis: A neonatal infection. *J Hosp Infect* 1:334, 1988.
22. Balance WA, et al: Pathology of neonatal necrotizing enterocolitis: A 10 year experience. *Pediatrics* 117:806, 1990.
23. Buchert GS: Abdominal pain in children: An emergency practitioner's guide. *Emerg Med Clin North Am* 7:497, 1989.
24. Friman S, Svanvik J, Radberg G: Intussusception at four separate locations in the small intestine: Case report. *Acta Chir Scand* 154:485, 1988.
25. Ravikumar K, Khope S, Rao P: Idiopathic colo-colic intussusception. *J Postgrad Med* 34:246, 1988.
26. McCombe AW, Orr JD: Gastric lipoma and intussusception in a child. *Scott Med J* 33:310, 1988.
27. Mir E: Surgical complications in Henoch-Schönlein purpura in childhood. *Z Kinderchir* 43:391, 1988.
28. Kim YS, Ruh JH: Intussusception in infancy and childhood: Analysis of 385 cases. *Int Surg* 74:114, 1989.
29. Bhisitkul DM, et al: Clinical application of ultrasonography in the diagnosis of intussusception. *J Pediatr* 121:182, 1992.
30. Del-Pozo G, Albillos J, Tejedor D: Intussusception: US findings with pathologic correlation—the crescent in doughnut sign. *Radiology* 121:182, 1996.
31. Hadidi AT, El Shal N: Childhood intussusception: A comparative study of nonsurgical management. *J Pediatr Surg* 34:304, 1999.
32. Meyer JS, Dangman BC, Buonomo C, Berlin JA: Air and liquid contrast agents in the management of intussusception: A controlled, randomized trial. *Radiology* 188:507, 1993.
33. Lui KW, et al: Air enema for diagnosis and reduction of intussusception in children: Clinical experience and fluoroscopy time correlation. *J Pediatr Surg* 36:479, 2001.
34. Qualman SJ, Murray R: Aganglionosis and related disorders. *Hum Pathol* 25:1141, 1994.
35. Franken EA, et al: Intestinal motility disorders of infants and children: Classification, clinical manifestations and roentgenology. *Crit Rev Diagn Imaging* 27:203, 1987.
36. Loening-Baucke V: Constipation in early childhood: Patient characteristics, treatment, and long-term follow up. *Gut* 34:400, 1993.
37. Ludtk F, et al: Incidence and frequency of complications and management of Meckel's diverticulum. *Surg Gynecol Obstet* 169:537, 1989.
38. Brown CK, Olshaker JS: Meckel's diverticulum. *Am J Emerg Med* 6:157, 1988.
39. Cooney DR, et al: The abdominal technetium scan (a decade of experience). *J Pediatr Surg* 17:611, 1982.
40. Rerksuppaphol S, Hutson JM, Oliver MR: Ranitidine-enhanced 99mtechnetium pertechnetate imaging in children improves the sensitivity of identifying heterotopic gastric mucosa in Meckel's diverticulum. *Pediatr Surg Int* 20:323, 2004.
41. Conn DL, Hunder GG, O'Duffy JD: Vasculitis and related disorders. In Kelly UN, et al (eds): *Textbook of Rheumatology*, 4th ed. Philadelphia, WB Saunders, 1993.
42. Koskimies O, et al: Renal involvement in Schonlein-Henoch purpura. *Acta Paediatr* 63:357, 1974.
43. Tervaert JWC, Kallenberg C: Neurologic manifestations of systemic vasculitides. *Rheum Dis Clin North Am* 19:913, 1993.
44. Grand RJ, Homer DR: Approaches to inflammatory bowel disease in childhood and adolescence. *Pediatr Clin North Am* 22:835, 1975.
45. Mamula P, et al: Inflammatory bowel disease in children 5 years of age or younger. *Am J Gastroenterol* 97:2005, 2002.
46. Friedman E: Caustic ingestions and foreign bodies in the aerodigestive tract of children. *Pediatr Clin North Am* 36:1403, 1989.
47. Stanley P, Law BS, Young LW: Down's syndrome, duodenal stenosis/annular pancreas, and a stack of coins. *Am J Dis Child* 142:459, 1988.
48. Binder L, Anderson WA: Pediatric gastrointestinal foreign body ingestions. *Ann Emerg Med* 13:112, 1984.
49. Sheikh A: Button battery ingestions in children. *Pediatr Emerg Care* 9:224, 1993.
50. Hernanz-Schulman M, Naimark A: Avoiding disaster with esophageal foreign bodies. *Emerg Med Rep* 4:133, 1983.
51. Sacchetti A, Carraccio C, Lichenstein R: Hand-held metal detector identification of ingested foreign bodies. *Pediatr Emerg Care* 10:204, 1994.
52. Biehler JL, Tuggle D, Stacy T: Use of the transmitter-receiver metal detector in the evaluation of pediatric coin ingestions. *Pediatr Emerg Care* 9:208, 1993.
53. Ros SP, Cetta F: Detection of ingested foreign bodies with a metal detector. *J Pediatr* 121:837, 1992.
54. Mader TJ, McHugh TP: Acute pancreatitis in children. *Pediatr Emerg Care* 8:157, 1992.
55. Haddock G, et al: Acute pancreatitis in children: A 15-year review. *J Pediatr Surg* 29:719, 1994.

56. Doherty GM, Lewis FR: Appendicitis: Continuing diagnostic challenge. *Emerg Med Clin North Am* 7:3537, 1989.
57. Dueholm S, Bagl P, Bud M: Laboratory aid in the diagnosis of acute appendicitis. *Dis Colon Rectum* 32:855, 1989.
58. Kao SCS, et al: Acute appendicitis in children: Sonographic findings. *AJR Am J Roentgenol* 153:375, 1989.
59. Sim KT, et al: Ultrasound with graded compression in the evaluation of acute appendicitis. *J Natl Med Assoc* 81:984, 1988.
60. Takada T, Yasuda H, Uchiyama K: Ultrasonic diagnosis of acute appendicitis complicated by paralytic ileus and generalized peritonitis. *J Clin Ultrasound* 16:123, 1988.
61. Amland PF, et al: Ultrasonography and parameters of inflammation in acute appendicitis. *Acta Chir Scand* 155: 185, 1989.
62. Garcia-Pena BM, et al: Effect of computed tomography on patient management and costs in children with suspected appendicitis. *Pediatrics* 104:440, 1999.
63. Rao PM, Rhea JT, Novelline RA: CT diagnosis of mesenteric adenitis. *Radiology* 202:145, 1997.
64. Rao PM, et al: Effect of computed tomography of the appendix on the treatment of patients and use of hospital resources. *N Engl J Med* 338:141, 1998.
65. Rao PM, et al: The computed tomography appearance of recurrent and chronic appendicitis. *Am J Emerg Med* 16:26, 1998.
66. Rao PM, et al: Introduction of appendiceal CT: Impact on negative appendectomy and appendiceal perforation rates. *Ann Surg* 229:344, 1999.
67. Purcell TB: Nonsurgical and extraperitoneal causes of abdominal pain. *Emerg Med Clin North Am* 7:721, 1989.
68. Elmore JR, Dibbins AW, Curci MR: The treatment of complicated appendicitis in children. *Arch Surg* 122:424, 1987.
69. Debray D, et al: Cholelithiasis in infancy: A study of 40 cases. *J Pediatr* 122:385, 1993.
70. Friesen CA, Robert CC: Cholelithiasis: Clinical characteristics in children. *Clin Pediatr (Phila)* 28:294, 1989.
71. Holcomb GW, O'Neill J, Holcomb GW: Cholecystitis, cholelithiasis and common duct stenosis in children and adolescents. *Ann Surg* 191:626, 1980.
72. Takiff H, Fonkalsrud EW: Gallbladder disease in childhood. *Am J Dis Child* 138:565, 1984.

CHAPTER 171 Infectious Diarrheal Disease and Dehydration

Roger M. Barkin and David G. Ward*

ACUTE INFECTIOUS DIARRHEA

Perspective

Worldwide, diarrhea is one of the most significant causes of morbidity and mortality and is responsible for 4 to 5 million deaths per year in children younger than 5 years of age. Variability among regions reflects resource availability, epidemiology, underlying general health status of the population, availability of safe food and water, among other factors. In the United States, acute gastroenteritis (AGE) historically accounts for 10.6% of U.S. hospital admissions of children younger than 5 years of age, estimated at 220,000 admissions per year; 300 to 400 deaths per year are caused by diarrhea, most occurring in the first year of life.[1,2] Children remain at a higher risk than adults for complications of diarrhea, fluid loss, and electrolyte abnormalities because of their physical size, physiology, an immune system that is still developing, and a dependency on adults for fluid and nutrients. Contaminated municipal water supplies and nationally distributed food sources, as well as the possibility of increasing antibiotic resistance in routine microbial agents, may affect the prevalence of diarrheal disease in the future.[3] The recognition of the role of fluids and electrolytes in the management of AGE has resulted in the widespread use of intravenous (IV) therapy for treating volume disorders in this country. In some situations, diarrhea-related volume depletion can be managed by oral replacement.

*Material new to this chapter in this edition was prepared by David Burbulys, MD, Department of Emergency Medicine, Harbor-UCLA Medical Center, Torrance, CA, and is indicated in bracketed italic type.

Epidemiology

In general, viruses are responsible for 60% of cases; bacteria, 20%; parasites, 5%; parenteral illnesses, 10%; and only 5% are in an unknown category.[4] A study of 147 children ages 2 to 11 years who were treated as outpatients documented an etiology in 60.5% of the children, 10% of whom had multiple agents identified. Rotavirus was found in 29.3% of the cases with a spring and winter peak whereas Giardia was noted in 15% of children, primarily in the spring. Hep-2 cell adherent *Escherichia coli* was isolated in 10.2% and less common etiologies identified were enteric adenoviruses, salmonella, *E. coli, Entamoeba histolytica,* and *Campylobacter jejuni.* [5] Infectious diarrhea in children is most often contracted by poor hygiene, contamination through the fecal-oral route, and poor food-handling practices. Handling diapers, fecal-oral transmission, and cleaning toys remain sources of concern in daycare centers. Causative agents may be endemic, epidemic with food- and waterborne outbreaks, or sporadic. For most agents, a large inoculum is required to transmit the disease. Individuals who have recently been hospitalized, treated with antibiotics, traveled to developing countries, are immunosuppressed, malnourished, or chronically ill are at risk of diarrheal illness and potential complications.[6]

Principles of Disease

Pathophysiology

Up to 9 L of fluid from diet and endogenous secretions enter the proximal bowel each day in the adult. In children, less total fluid enters the gut but a proportionately larger volume/weight ratio of fluid is required (e.g., 125 ml/kg/24 hr in adults versus 220 ml/kg/24 hr in a newborn). Ninety percent of the fluid is absorbed in the small bowel and the remainder in the large bowel. Water passively follows osmotic gradients created by transport of electrolytes, sugars, and amino acids. Transport includes active and passive transport-facilitated mechanisms. Glucose and certain amino acids are absorbed by active, carrier-mediated transport and coupled to the sodium exchange.

Diarrhea occurs through a variety of mechanisms: *osmotic diarrhea* is a response to the presence of poorly absorbed solutes in the colon as a result of altered bacterial gut flora, damage of the mucosal absorptive surface, or ingestion of substances.[7] These osmotically active substances alter the normal mechanisms of fluid transport by creating an osmotic gradient across the bowel lumen. This results in movement of water and electrolytes into the lumen and a hypertonic luminal fluid. Acute gastroenteritis in children produces injury to the gut epithelium, decreasing absorptive area and preventing normal fluid, electrolyte, and nutrient absorption. Diagnostic clues to an osmotic etiology are diarrhea that decreases or stops if the patient fasts, the stool pH is less than 5, and reducing substances are present in the stool.

Secretory diarrhea is the result of the presence of an enterotoxin that causes an increase in cyclic adenosine monophosphatase (cAMP) in the endothelial cell, resulting in increased chloride secretion. Enterotoxin-producing bacteria include *Salmonella* and *Shigella* organisms, *Vibrio cholera, E. coli,* and *Clostridium difficile.* Noninfectious causes are rare and include malabsorbed bile acids, fatty acids, prostaglandins, and gastrointestinal hormones. Secretory diarrhea is notable for no reduction in stool volume with fasting, a stool pH greater than 6, and no reducing substances present in the stool. Infectious agents attach directly to the gut mucosa, causing cell damage, bleeding, and mucus production. The agent may enter the systemic circulation or body tissues.[8]

Diarrhea caused by altered motility, increased or decreased transit time (diabetes, scleroderma, neuromuscular disease), reduced surface area (short gut, celiac disease), or inhibited active ion transport is uncommon in children.

Dysentery is important to recognize because of the implication that the infection has compromised the bowel wall and therefore, the risk of systemic infection is increased. Although blood loss may be clinically appreciable, it is less significant than the fluid and electrolyte losses. Systemic infection may be suspected if the total white blood count is increased or if clinical signs of prostration, chills and fever, or dysentery are present.

During childhood, children's body makeup changes with respect to the surface area to volume ratio and the fluid compartment distribution of body water. The extracellular fluid compartment begins in life as 80% of the total body water content but by adulthood makes up 50% to 55%.[9] Children have limited stores of substrate and may not tolerate fluctuations or losses of fluid, electrolytes, or nutrients that are often encountered in acute diarrheal illness.

Abnormalities of acid-base homeostasis associated with acute diarrheal illness and volume disorders may lead to metabolic acidosis with varying degrees of respiratory compensation. The metabolic acidosis usually results from the loss of HCO_3^- and Cl^- in diarrheal fluid but may also involve renal tubular acidosis, excessive acid production from poor tissue perfusion, starvation, infection, and therapeutic interventions (salicylates). The effects of metabolic acidosis may result in an increase in tidal volume and respiratory rate to correct the decreased pH by lowering the $Paco_2$. In this manner, excess acids can be eliminated by transporting the acids to the lungs by hemoglobin and other buffer systems. The maximum respiratory compensation of metabolic acidosis is a decrease in $Paco_2$ to 12 to 15 mm Hg and may occur within minutes to hours of the onset of the abnormality. Nonvolatile acids (especially sulfur and phosphoric acids) must be excreted by the kidneys and can be expected to take several hours to days to occur.

Children with intravascular volume depletion resulting in metabolic acidosis require restoration of their volume status to deliver nutrient substrate and to eliminate byproducts of cellular metabolism rather than correction of the acid-base disorder with buffer alone. Because the patient depends on the respiratory system to help eliminate acid excess in a state of poor tissue perfusion (respiratory compensation), correction of volume depletion often corrects what appears as respiratory distress in the severely volume-depleted child.

Etiology

Virus

The virus responsible for most acute viral gastroenteritis and a disproportionate amount of morbidity caused by diarrheal illness in the United States is rotavirus. It peaks in the winter and spring and can usually be managed on an outpatient basis. This virus is endemic and accounts for nearly one third of children with diarrhea.[5,9,10] Less commonly found are Norwalk agent, adenovirus, and hepatitis A virus.

Rotavirus invades the epithelium of the small intestinal mucosa and involves the villus more than the crypt. A proliferative response occurs, producing an abundance of incompletely differentiated cells on the gut mucosa. In the healthy host, repair of the epithelium and differentiation of the immature brush border take approximately 3 to 5 days and should occur without specific intervention.[10] In the chronically ill or nutritionally compromised child, this leads to high risk for malabsorption and severe complications beyond the usual brush border injury. Failure to repair the epithelium leads to progressive epithelial injury, complications, and a vicious circle of events.

Rotavirus causes acute febrile illness with vomiting and diarrhea. Severity may vary, but the diarrhea is usually watery in consistency, and the volume is large enough to cause significant and rapid intravascular volume compromise. Rotavirus may also involve symptoms of an upper respiratory tract infection. Most infections are transmitted person to person, probably through the fecal-oral route and possibly through respiratory secretions. The incubation period is 1 to 3 days. Postinfection excretion may be prolonged, ranging from 4 to 57 days.

Diagnosis is made by demonstration of the presence of antigens in stool specimens by enzyme immunoassay, many having 97% sensitivity and 97% specificity for rotavirus antigens in human stool. The test can be performed on undiluted stool without special preparation.[12] An effective vaccine was available for a short time until it was noted to be associated with increased risk of intussusception.[13]

Hepatitis A virus (HAV) infections are seen as an acute febrile illness with anorexia, nausea, vomiting, and malaise. HAV invades the hepatocytes causing immunologically mediated hepatocellular damage. In children, it may be asymptomatic, present as an anicteric illness and be misdiagnosed as a nonspecific viral gastroenteritis. HAV is not seasonal and is spread by a common food or water source with fecal-oral contamination. The incubation period is 2 to 6 weeks, and individuals shed virus for 1 to 3 weeks beginning 1 to 2 weeks before symptoms develop. Lifelong immunity is expected. Household contacts should be offered immunoglobulin prophylaxis. A vaccine for HAV has recently become available.[14]

Bacteria

The most common bacterial organisms causing acute diarrhea in the United States are, in order of frequency, *Shigella* species, *Salmonella* species, *C. jejuni,* and *Yersinia enterocolitica. Clostridium perfringens, Staphylococcus aureus, Vibrio cholerae,* and *Vibrio parahaemolyticus* each make up less than 1% of cases. Enterotoxigenic, enteroinvasive, and enterohemorrhagic *E. coli* are also found in the United States.

Shigella species consists of four antigenic groups of 40 serotypes. *S. sonnei* is the most common cause of dysentery (diarrhea with significant blood, pus, and mucus) in the United States. Shigellosis usually begins as an enterotoxin-like diarrhea with watery stools and fever that may progress to bacillary dysentery with or without systemic manifestations. Illnesses vary from mild to severe. *Shigella* species can invade the intestinal mucosa. It rarely infects infants younger than 3 months of age and is most common between 6 months and 10 years of age.[15] Because of antibiotic resistance to ampicillin, trimethoprim-sulfamethoxazole (4 to 5 mg/kg/dose TMP, 20 to 25 mg/kg/dose SMX bid orally for 7 to 10 days) is recommended for more severe illnesses.[16] *(Reviewer suggests Because of approximately 50% resistance to ampicillin and trimethoprim/sulfamethoxazole, a fluoroquinolone [such as ciprofloxacin or ofloxacin] in adults or azithromycin in children given orally for 5 days is recommended for more severe illness.)*

The 1700 serotypes of *Salmonella* species are grouped as *Salmonella enteritidis.* Clinical syndromes include a carrier state, acute gastroenteritis (AGE), bacteremia, and a disseminated abscess syndrome. It is presumed that *Salmonella* species invade the mucosa and produce a cholera-like enterotoxin and a cytotoxin. *Salmonella* species gastroenteritis is a febrile illness marked by nausea and fever, although it may vary from dysentery to a cholera-like illness. AGE occurs at any age but is most common in the first year of life. Antibiotic treatment is indicated in complicated illness, whereas AGE is treated symptomatically. Complications requiring therapy may include failure to improve within 5 to 7 days when not treated with antibiotics or focal infection in the central nervous system (CNS), bone, joint, kidney, or pericardium. Increased bacteriology and symptomatic relapse is associated with ampicillin and amoxicillin therapy.

Campylobacter species account for much of the diarrheal disease in the world. The organism is found in the gastrointestinal tract and feces of wild and domestic fowl, farm animals, and pets. Of the five types, *C. jejuni* and *E. coli (Reviewer suggests C. coli)* are the most prominent. Illness consists of abdominal cramps, diarrhea, chills, fever, a *Shigella*-like dysentery, or a presentation similar to acute appendicitis. Invasion of the mucosa with toxin production has been described. A 1- to 7-day incubation period is normal, and the illness usually lasts less than a week. *Campylobacter* species is transmitted by ingestion of contaminated food or water. Diagnosis is made by dark-field microscopy, and although erythromycin (40 mg/kg/24 hr qid orally for 7 to 10 days) *(Reviewer suggests Azithromycin [12 mg/kg daily PO for 5 days].)* may shorten the course of the illness, most children do not need antibiotic therapy.[17]

Y. enterocolitica is a relatively uncommon cause of simple self-limited AGE with diarrhea and vomiting. Diarrhea may be watery, mucoid, or bloody. Older children and adults have more nonenteric symptoms, presenting an appendicitis-like illness as a result of mesenteric adenitis. Enterotoxin production may play a role. Duration of the gastroenteritis is often 14 days or more, but antibiotics are seldom indicated.

Pseudomembranous colitis presents with diarrhea, abdominal cramps, and fever. Caused by *C. difficile,* systemic toxicity, abdominal tenderness, and dysenteric stools are often present, although asymptomatic infections and mild AGE have also been reported. It most often occurs in hospitalized patients with onset during or after antibiotic therapy. The organism is ubiquitous and transmitted by fecal-oral contamination. Incubation time is unknown. The presence of pseudomembranes, friable rectal mucosa, and *C. difficile* toxin in the stool is diagnostic. Stopping the offending agent and therapy with vancomycin, 40 mg/kg/24 hr orally, *(Reviewer suggests Metronidazole, 30 mg/kg/day, divided qid, PO for 7 days.)* is indicated.

Ingested *C. perfringens* produces an enterotoxin during sporulation in the gut that causes fluid collection in ileal loops and diarrhea. This short-lived illness is characterized by watery diarrhea, moderate to severe abdominal cramps, midepigastric pain, and an absence of fever. Vomiting is uncommon. Food source contamination, often from catered food services, is the usual source of outbreaks. The incubation time is 6 to 24 hours. Diagnosis is made by high spore counts in the stool; no specific treatment is required.

S. aureus produces the archetypal food poisoning from ingesting preformed enterotoxin, usually from contaminated food. It is short-lived and self-limited. Nausea, vomiting, abdominal cramps, and diarrhea with a notable absence of fever is the typical pattern often occurring within hours of exposure.

V. cholerae 01 (responsible for epidemic cholera) and non-01 (all other strains) is an Asian-African organism of which a uniquely subtypable strain is endemic to the Gulf Coast of the United States. Diarrhea is caused by a heat-labile enterotoxin that increases cAMP through adenyl cyclase, resulting in inhibition of sodium reabsorption with chloride and fluid secretion into the gut. This cholera toxin is mostly absent in U.S. strains.

Vibrio parahaemolyticus is commonly found in water, shellfish, and fish. It is most commonly associated with ingestion of contaminated raw foods. Diarrhea, abdominal cramps, and nausea are common, whereas vomiting, headache, fever, and chills are less common. Invasion of the mucosa is a possible mechanism of infection.

E. coli consists of several recognized categories. The enterotoxigenic form produces heat-stable and heat-labile toxins and colonization factor, which are important in the mechanism of disease. It affects travelers of all ages. The enteroinvasive form is closely related antigenically and biochemically to *Shigella* species and causes a similar dysenteric illness. *E. coli* is identified by distinct groups of either somatic or flagellar antigens that determine virulence properties. Plasmid infection usually is associated with invasive qualities. This form affects mostly adults and is often food borne. The enteropathogenic form is responsible for sporadic and endemic diarrhea in infants. It is defined by serotypes and the absence of virulent qualities, such as toxins. The enterohemorrhagic form produces bloody diarrhea without fever and is associated with a cytotoxin. Last, the enteroadherent form is related to acute and chronic diarrhea of travelers to Mexico and India. Prophylaxis with several agents is effective but difficult to achieve and not recommended. Treatment with antibiotics is helpful to shorten the course in only selected cases.[18]

The specific cause of acute diarrheal illnesses in chronically ill and immunosuppressed patients requires attention to the previously discussed agents, normal flora, and several unusual organisms. In patients with acquired immunodeficiency syndrome, clinical presentations may be acute, chronic, or recurrent and difficult to treat.[19] Unusual organisms may include *Mycobacterium avium, Cryptosporidium,* cytomegalovirus, and adenovirus. Treatment-related complications caused by *C. difficile, Candida albicans,* and *Pseudomonas aeruginosa* are more common in immune-suppressed patients because of frequent antibiotic exposure.

Clinical Features

Diagnostic Findings

Fluid and electrolyte disorders in children require meticulous diagnostic skills because serious illness may be overlooked with cursory examination or treatment. The principal concern in diarrheal illness relates to the fluid, electrolyte, acid-base, or nutrient defects that may result from vomiting, diarrhea, or decreased oral intake.

Diarrhea can be defined as an increase in liquidity, frequency, or volume of stools. It is often difficult to quantitate these characteristics from the history provided by the parents. Helping the parent describe the stool relative to usual bowel habits will provide valuable information for comparison.

History should include specific information regarding the order of presentation, duration, severity, and quantity of each symptom. It should reveal the presence or absence of fever, nausea, vomiting, hematemesis, abdominal pain, diarrhea, hematochezia, and emesis. The consistency and content of stools is important. Inquire about the relationship of symptoms to eating and drinking. It is helpful to know whether others in the household have a similar illness and whether previous episodes have occurred. A history of travel to endemic or epidemic areas may provide important information. Quantity and time of recent oral intake and information about recent preillness weight can be helpful. If the patient is old enough, information about orthostasis and the patient's activity level is desirable.

The physical examination should address the vital signs. Older children and adults may manifest symptoms at a lesser degree of volume disorder because of relatively smaller total body water and extracellular fluid volume. Important areas to emphasize are addressed in Table 171-1.

Complications

The complications of acute diarrheal illness are primarily reflected in abnormalities of fluid, electrolytes, acid-base status, and in the systemic involvement of the infection. With severe illness or illness superimposed on underlying chronic conditions, children may advance to a stage of extremis before arrival at the ED. Lethargy, weakness, respiratory distress, renal failure, shock, cardiac dysrhythmia, seizure, coma, permanent neurologic sequelae, and death can result from advanced stages of intravascular volume depletion and acidosis. Children seem to compensate for severe illness almost to the brink of disaster before they then decompensate rapidly. Often children who decompensate in the ED do so in an advanced stage of compensatory homeostatic physiology that had been unrecognized by the care givers before arrival in the ED.

Diagnostic Strategies

Stool studies usually are not indicated in most uncomplicated AGE. There may be reason to identify

Table 171-1. Clinical Assessment of Degree of Dehydration

	Mild (<5%)	Moderate (10%)	Severe (15%)
Signs and symptoms			
Dry mucous membrane	±	+	+
Reduced skin turgor (pinch retraction)	–	±	+
Depressed anterior fontanel	–	+	–
Mental status	Alert	Irritable	Lethargic
Sunken eyeballs	–	+	+
Hyperpnea	–	±	+
Hypotension (orthostatic)	–	±	+
Increased pulse	–	+	+
Capillary refill	≤2 sec	>2 sec	>2 sec
Laboratory			
Urine			
Volume	Small	Oliguria	Oliguria/anuria
Specific gravity*	≥1.020†	>1.030	>1.035
Blood			
BUN	WNL†	Elevated	Very high
pH (arterial)	7.40-7.30	7.30-7.00	<7.10

+, Present; –, absent; ±, variable.
*Specific gravity can provide evidence that confirms the physical assessment.
†Not usually indicated in mild or moderate dehydration.
From Barkin RM, Rosen P: *Emergency pediatrics*, ed 5, St Louis, 1999, Mosby.

(Reviewer suggests Depressed Anterior Fontanel should have a "+" in the Severe [15%] column and the range for pH (arterial) in the Moderate [10] column should be 7.30-7.10.)

particular infectious agents in the community because they require treatment, specific prophylaxis, or health precautions. Stool studies should be obtained if specific therapy or hospitalization is indicated, the patient has systemic involvement, underlying medical complications exist, or the illness involves dysenteric features. In immunosuppressed patients, infants less than 2 to 3 months of age or in the case of possible bacteremia, a complete blood count, stool studies, and blood and other cultures should be obtained. The stool study of primary use to the ED physician is the microscopic analysis for leukocytes and occult blood to differentiate dysentery from AGE. The presence of fecal leukocytes or blood indicates that the offending organism has crossed the mucosal barrier and that the risk of invasiveness has increased. Nearly 90% of acute diarrhea caused by *Salmonella* or *Shigella* organisms have fecal leukocytes in the stools. Fecal leukocytes are also found in patients with *Campylobacter* organisms, *Y. enterocolitica,* invasive *E. coli,* and *V. parahaemolyticus.* Stool electrolytes, fecal fat, culture, ova, and parasites are more of interest and help the follow-up physician but are of little value if the patient has already recovered. Stool culture, enzyme-linked immunoassay for rotavirus, and other testing are indicated in those who have not responded in the expected manner, have prolonged duration (more than 2 weeks), or have dysenteric features. Studies are also indicated if there is a need to identify a cause within a community outbreak. Liver enzymes, bilirubin, and hepatitis serologic studies will be useful to identify hepatitis. Urinalysis can provide an indication of hydration, the presence of urinary tract infection, hepatitis, and potential renal injury.

Table 171-2. Common Causes of Vomiting in Children

CNS	Infections, space-occupying lesion
Gastrointestinal	Obstruction, peritonitis, hepatitis, liver failure, appendicitis, pyloric stenosis, volvulus, intussusception, inborn errors of metabolism
Drug	Ingestion, overdose, drug effect
Endocrine	Addisonian crisis, diabetic ketoacidosis, congenital adrenal hypoplasia
Renal	Urinary tract infection, pyelonephritis, renal failure, renal tubular acidosis
Cardiac	Congestive heart failure of any cause
Infection	Pneumonia, acute otitis media, sinusitis, sepsis
Other	Psychogenic, respiratory insufficiency

Differential Considerations

Vomiting in children is a very common sign with an exhaustive list of causes. Young children have no social embarrassment or the personal distaste of vomiting (or diarrhea, or crying, etc.) that often forces adults to bear the relative discomfort of the symptom. Children may vomit in response to pain, anxiety, or fear, as well as the usual causes of nausea. Some causes of vomiting are given in the brief list in Table 171-2. Diarrhea is also a common reason for parents to bring their children to the ED. Most often, diarrhea is associated with other features of AGE but it may be the sole presenting complaint. Table 171-3 presents a brief list of causes of diarrhea in children.

Management

Table 171-4 lists the common infectious agents of diarrhea and the indicated treatment. Management of the fluid and electrolyte status is of primary importance.

Zinc supplement therapy may be theoretically beneficial. It has been proposed that zinc may lead to regeneration of intestinal mucosa, increased levels of brush border enzyme, and enhanced cellular immunity.[20,21]

Disposition

Most childhood diarrhea can be managed on an outpatient basis by continuing routine formula or diet specific for age. Supplemental maintenance electrolyte solutions may be given. If home oral rehydration therapy is ordered, resumption of feeding should begin as soon as vomiting subsides. Routine fasting for diarrhea illnesses is not recommended. Before discharge from the ED, careful instruction must be given to the parents or caretaker that are specific as to the signs and symptoms of expected improvement or complications (Box 171-1).[22] Instructions should address proper hygiene and hand washing techniques to prevent others from contracting the illness. Monitoring hand washing in daycare facilities had been shown to reduce bacterial contamination in children. Follow-up by the patient's primary care physician should be timely and

Table 171-3. Common Causes of Diarrhea in Children

Gastrointestinal	Malabsorption (e.g., milk intolerance, excessive juice), intussusception, inflammatory bowel disease, irritable bowel, short gut syndrome
Drug	Ingestion, overdose, drug effect
Endocrine	Thyrotoxicosis, addisonian crisis, diabetic enteropathy, congenital adrenal hypoplasia
Renal	Urinary tract infection, pyelonephritis
Infection	Pneumonia, acute otitis media, sinusitis, sepsis
Other	Parental anxiety, chronic nonspecific diarrhea

BOX 171-1. Parental Instruction Sheet for Children with Vomiting and Diarrhea

1. Give clear liquids, as much as the child wants.
   a. Children less than 2 years of age should be given a maintenance electrolyte solution, such as Pedialyte or Infalyte.
   b. Children older than 2 years of age may be given other clear fluids, such as decarbonated sodas, Gatorade, or clear soups.
2. If your child is vomiting, give clear liquids (as above) in small frequent volumes initially and advancing to normal volumes for the child's age as tolerated. It may be necessary to use teaspoons, cups, syringes, or ladles to administer the small volume. Fluid can be administered beginning 5 to 10 minutes after an episode of vomiting and should be continued despite the persistence of vomiting.
3. The child's diet may be advanced as soon as the vomiting has stopped and the child can tolerate fluids without vomiting. It is reasonable to wait 2 to 4 hours after the last episode of vomiting to resume feeding.
   a. Formula or breast feeding infants should be given their regular formula or returned to the breast.
   b. Older children should be given bland starch-containing foods (bananas, rice, applesauce, and toast are the historically popular routine) in small quantities first and advancing to larger quantities and more complex items as the child's appetite returns.
4. The child may return to a regular diet as soon as the appetite returns and foods are desired.
5. Many foods may worsen diarrhea; pectin-containing foods, such as applesauce and other fruits and fruit juices, are not recommended until the diarrhea resolves.
6. Reduce cow's milk products until the diarrhea has lessened significantly.
7. Call your child's physician or return to the ED if the following occur:
   a. The diarrhea or vomiting worsens in frequency or amount.
   b. The vomiting lasts for more than 24 hours.
   c. The stool or vomitus contains blood or the vomit becomes persistently green.
   d. The child has decreased urine output (or fewer wet diapers), fails to tear when crying, becomes less active or difficult to arouse.

Table 171-4. Etiology of Diarrhea in Children and Specific Therapy

Agent	Specific therapy beyond supportive care
Campylobacter jejuni	Erythromycin, 30-40 mg/kg/24 hr tid PO for 7-10 days
Clostridium difficile (pseudomembranous colitis)	Vancomycin, 40 mg/kg/24 hr q6hr PO, or metronidazole, 15–30 mg/kg/24 hr tid PO
Escherichia coli	Trimethoprim-sulfamethoxazole 10 mg (TMP)/kg/24 hr bid PO for 7-10 days
Giardia lamblia	Furazolidone, 6 mg/kg/24 hr qid PO for 10 days; or metronidazole, 15 mg/kg/24 hr tid PO for 5 days
Salmonella species	In toxic infants <3 mo: ampicillin, 200 mg/kg/24 hr q6hr for 7-10 days, and gentamicin 5-7.5 mg/kg/24 hr q8hr IV
Shigella species	In dysenteric illness; ampicillin, 200 mg/kg/24 hr q6hr IV 7-10 days, amoxicillin, 30 mg/kg/24 hr tid PO; or trimethoprim-sulfamethoxazole, 10 mg (TMP)/kg/24 hr bid PO for 7-10 days
Yersinia enterocolitica	If immunosuppressed, treat as presumed sepsis
Vibrio	None. Severe diarrhea or cholera may benefit from antibiotics

(Reviewer suggests a revised table 171-4, which appears at the end of this chapter.)

Table 171-5. Types of Dehydration Reflected by Serum Sodium

	Isotonic	Hypotonic	Hypertonic
Serum sodium level (mEq/L)	130-150	<130	>150
Physical signs			
Skin			
Color	Gray	Gray	Gray
Temperature	Cold	Cold	Cold
Turgor	Poor	Very poor	Fair
Feel	Dry	Clammy	Thick, doughy
Mucous membrane	Dry	Dry	Parched
Sunken eyeballs	+	+	+
Depressed anterior fontanel	+	+	+
Mental status	Lethargic	Coma/seizure	Irritable/seizure
Increased pulse	++	++	+
Decreased blood pressure	++	+++	+

+, ++, +++, Relative prominence of finding.
From Barkin RM, Rosen P: *Emergency pediatrics*, ed 5, St Louis, 1999, Mosby.

should address concerns of worsening of the condition and complications that may have developed. Hospitalization may be warranted in cases of protracted vomiting, diarrhea in excess of fluid administration, worsening condition despite therapy, underlying condition that would complicate therapy, or if systemic involvement is suspected. Very low birthweight infants are at highest risk of being admitted for AGE in the first year of life.

DEHYDRATION

Clinical Features

Children with more than 5% volume depletion can be identified by history and physical examination. Initial observation usually reveals a child who is less active than expected for age. The child may be weak or lethargic. If the fontanelle is still open, it may be sunken. The eyes appear sunken and the mucous membranes are dry (if the child has recently had something to drink, the mucous membranes may falsely appear moist). Tachycardia and tachypnea may be present, but the physician must recognize that fever, anxiety, and other factors can cause an increased heart rate. The skin over the trunk should be examined for tenting (suggesting hyponatremia) or a doughy (suggesting hypernatremia) character (Table 171-5). Stool present in the diapers should be examined visually, tested for blood, and the presence or absence of urine should be noted.

Use of laboratory tests should be reserved for patients requiring IV fluid therapy, admission, those with underlying medical conditions or toxicity, or those taking medication that might influence or be influenced by diarrheal illness and fluid therapy. Serum electrolytes, blood urea nitrogen (BUN), creatinine, osmolality, and glucose are the tests most commonly ordered. Sodium concentration is important in identifying iso/hypo/hypernatremic states for appropriate choice of therapy. A low HCO_3^- should prompt one to determine the anion gap. In some cases it may be necessary to examine urine electrolytes and osmolality.[23,24]

Table 171-6. Differential Diagnosis of Volume Depletion

Renal	Diuretics, renal tubular acidosis, renal failure, urinary tract obstruction, syndrome of inappropriate secretion of ADH, hypothyroidism, adrenal insufficiency, renal trauma, salt wasting nephritis
Extrarenal	Third spacing (pancreatitis, peritonitis, sepsis), skin loss (burns, cystic fibrosis), lung loss, congestive heart failure, liver failure, hemorrhage

Differential Considerations

Most volume depletion states result from diarrhea and vomiting in children due to infections. Table 171-6 lists some other causes of hypovolemia that should be considered when the gastrointestinal tract is not primarily involved.

FLUID AND ELECTROLYTE MANAGEMENT

Oral Rehydration Therapy

Oral rehydration therapy (ORT) has been reported as a safe and effective treatment for fluid repletion in infants and children with AGE and mild to moderate volume depletion without acute or chronic complicating conditions.[25-32]

ORT may be instituted even if the patient continues to vomit or has diarrhea. The rehydration period in the ED may cover 4 to 8 hours, and provides an opportunity to educate the family in skills of evaluating and treating childhood diarrhea. A number of oral rehydration solutions (ORS) have been shown to be effective. Rice ORS is similar to standard ORS. Hypotonic solutions (osmolality 224 mmol/l,) may be more effective.

Children with severe volume loss, shock, lethargy, acute abdomen, intestinal obstruction, sodium derangement, or significant underlying illness should be identified by a thorough physical examination and excluded from ORT. The volume of ORS is calculated in the following manner.

1. Estimate the degree of volume depletion as mild or moderate using information from the history, clinical signs, and physical examination.
2. Calculate the desired volume of ORS as 60 ml/kg for mild and 80 ml/kg for moderate volume depletion.
3. Administer 25% of the volume of ORS to be replaced each hour for the first 4 hours.
4. Monitor progress hourly and reevaluate after 4 hours.

This technique requires that the ED have the facilities and personnel to observe and monitor the patient for the 4 to 8 hours required to determine whether the patient is going to succeed or fail ORT. The child is attended by the parent or caretaker, who is also responsible for administering the fluid. Nursing personnel instruct the parent in observation skills, methods of administering the fluid, and types of fluid that are considered appropriate for children with vomiting and diarrhea. During the monitoring period, a child who is unable to tolerate the prescribed volume of fluid at the expected rate should be treated with IV fluids. It is important to determine and address whether the failure is the result of the child's inability to ingest the fluid, excessive fluid is being lost through vomiting or diarrhea, or poor technique or motivation on the parent's part. It is usually possible to maintain the fluid administration rate in children who continue to vomit by administering small volumes frequently. This may require using a spoon or syringe to slowly drip the fluid by hand; a teaspoon, syringe, graduated bottle, cup or enteral pump can be used to deliver the fluid. Common solutions used in diarrheal illness are presented in Table 171-7 for comparison. Rehydralyte is an excellent initial solution for rehydration. Emesis (volume-for-volume) and stool volume (5 ml/kg) are estimated and added to the replacement volume on an hourly basis. The patient is reassessed at the end of the first 4 hours and, if clinically volume repleted, may be discharged home with further specific instructions regarding maintenance fluid requirements. If, on the other hand, the patient is still mildly or moderately volume depleted by clinical examination, and no deterioration in status has occurred, the patient is reevaluated as if from the beginning and another 4-hour trial is attempted. During the monitoring period, a child who is unable to ingest the appropriate volume of or if at the end of 8 hours volume repletion is not achieved, IV therapy should be initiated. It is important to determine whether a failure is the result of the child's inability to ingest fluids, excessive fluid loss, poor technique, or motivation on the part of the family. Patients who do not qualify for ORT based on exclusion criteria include those with a possible acute surgical condition of the abdomen, intestinal obstruction, or underlying illness that may require special consideration. These patients should be resuscitated with IV fluid and managed as the condition dictates.

Intravenous Therapy

Patients who do not qualify for or who fail ORT and require IV fluid therapy need particular attention to their circulatory status, type and degree of fluid deficit, and nutritional status. This includes patients with circulatory collapse, shock, severe volume depletion, increasing deficit or clinical deterioration during ORT, intractable vomiting, and failure to achieve clinical rehydration within 8 hours of beginning ORT.

Patients are evaluated based on their immediate (emergency phase, phase I), short-term (repletion phase, phase II), and long-term (early refeeding phase, phase III) needs. The emergency phase is the fluid resuscitation required to reverse vascular collapse,

Table 171-7. Common Oral Hydrating Solutions

Solution	Na^+ (mEq/L)	K^+ (mEq/L)	Cl^- (mEq/L)	HCO_3^-/citrate (mEq/L)	Glucose* (gm/dl)	mOsm/L
Rehydration						
Rehydralyte	75	20	65	30	2.5	270
WHO Solution	90	20	80	10	2.0	310
Maintenance						
Lytren	50	25	45	30	2.0	
Pedialyte	45	20	35	30	2.5	270
Infalyte	50	25	45	34	1.9	200
Clear liquids						
Gatorade	20	3			2.1	
Cola	3	0.1-0.9		7-13	10.0	
Ginger ale	4	0.2			9.0	

*May be long-chain oligosaccharide subject to hydrolysis.
WHO, World Health Organization.
From Barkin RM, Rosen P: *Emergency pediatrics,* ed 5, St Louis, 1999, Mosby.

shock, cerebral, and cardiac compromise. This fluid needs to be administered rapidly to prevent imminent serious morbidity or mortality. Repletion phase refers to the fluid and electrolyte resuscitation required to reverse deficits and to maintain ongoing losses during a period of 0 to 24 hours. Early refeeding phase and long-term needs are addressed over the few days after an episode of fluid and electrolyte disorder during which the body recovers fluid, electrolyte, and nutritional homeostasis.[32] Immediate and short-term therapy are initiated in the ED, but completion is carried out by the admitting physician or therapy at home is managed by the primary care physician. This conceptualization is, in practice, a continuum of care and not three distinct, separate phases. Monitoring of serum electrolytes, BUN, and glucose is indicated for patients receiving IV fluid therapy.

Emergency Resuscitation Phase

Rapid reexpansion of the intravascular space is the goal of immediate resuscitation and can be achieved with an isotonic crystalloid solution. Administering 20 ml/kg of 0.9% saline (or other appropriate isotonic crystalloid solution) IV at a rapid rate should result in reversal of signs of shock within 5 to 15 minutes. Reevaluation at 5- to 10-minute intervals will reveal the patient with excessive deficits requiring repeat administrations of 20 ml/kg until clinical improvement occurs. Volume requirements greater than 60 ml/kg without signs of improvement suggest other conditions, such as septic shock, hemorrhage, capillary leak with third space fluid sequestration, heart failure, and others; reevaluation is required. Rate of administration should be tailored to the urgency of the patient's condition. In critical situations, interosseous routes should be used if venous access is not immediately available.

A rapid determination of serum glucose is important. Children require glucose as an energy substrate and often have marginal stores available in stress situations. If the serum glucose is low (<50 mg/dl), administration of dextrose D25 at 2 ml/kg IV (in neonates younger than 3 months of age, use D10 at 2 to 4 ml/kg) should correct the deficit. Glucose should be monitored (every 30 to 60 minutes until stable) to ensure improvement and to identify future needs.

Repletion Phase

After immediate resuscitation, the patient's fluid therapy must be reassessed to incorporate the fluids already administered and to accommodate changes in clinical condition. An accurate clinical history, physical examination, and laboratory results should confirm the type of volume deficit. Volume replacement should consider the sodium level in planning the type and amount of fluid to be administered: hypernatremic ($Na^+ > 150$ mEq/L), hyponatremic ($Na^+ < 130$ mEq/L), or isonatremic ($Na^+ = 130$ to 150 mEq/L) to allow planning of the type and amount of fluid to be administered.[33]

Isonatremic Volume Depletion

Isonatremic volume depletion is the most common form of volume depletion and results from relatively equal loss of sodium and water. No change in body fluid tonicity or redistribution of fluid between extracellular and intracellular fluid space occurs. This results in loss of fluid from the extracellular space and, therefore, intravascular volume depletion. Gastrointestinal fluid loss with or without decreased intake or increased urine loss is the most common cause. Repletion fluids are outlined in Box 171-2. Generally one half of the deficit fluids are given during the first 8 hours of repletion.

Note that the sample patient is mildly acidotic ($HCO_3^- = 12$ mEq/L) and restoring intravascular volume results in improved tissue perfusion and correction of the metabolic acidosis. These calculations account for water and electrolyte requirements (maintenance and deficit) and demonstrate that using a standard fluid preparation (0.9%, 0.45% or 0.2% saline) closely approximates calculated requirements and facilitates treatment by using readily stocked supplies. Each patient must be evaluated to determine whether a resuscitation bolus of fluid is indicated or not. Symptoms suggesting the need for a bolus of fluid include abnormal mental status, lethargy, poor muscle tone, a history of decreased urine output, decreased capillary refill, tachycardia at rest (not caused by fever, pain, or anxiety), bradycardia, or any other indication of shock. Certainly, all patients with severe and some with moderate volume depletion will require fluid bolus.

Hyponatremic Volume Depletion

Hyponatremic volume depletion results in relatively more loss of Na^+ than water, resulting in extracellular fluid shift into the intracellular fluid space trying to maintain osmolar equality. This results in a significant decrease in intravascular volume and hemodynamic problems. This type is usually caused by gastrointestinal fluid loss that has been replaced with hypotonic fluid.

A sample patient (Box 171-3) is presented as an illustration of management. If the serum sodium is 120 to 130, administer D5W 0.9% saline, one half of the daily fluid requirement in the first 8 hours, and one half of the daily fluid requirement over the following 16 hours. Monitor serum electrolytes, BUN, weight, intake, and output. Add KCl, 20 mEq/L, to the IV fluids after renal function is assessed. If the serum sodium is less than 120 mEq/dl, the patient exhibits seizures, hyperexcitability, or other symptoms; 3% saline (0.5 mEq NaCl/ml) should be administered according to the following formula.

$$3\% \text{ saline (ml)} = (10 \text{ mEq/L})(0.6)(\text{weight})/(0.5)$$

In some conditions causing hyponatremia, furosemide (1.0 mg/kg IV) or other diuretics have been recommended. The mechanism of action of the loop diuretics

BOX 171-2. Sample Calculation of Fluid and Electrolyte Requirements in a Patient with Isonatremic Volume Depletion

Isotonic Volume Depletion: Management of Moderate to Severe Deficits

1. Initial findings
   a. Pre-illness weight: 10 kg (a 1-yr-old)
   b. Degree of volume depletion, moderate (10%)
   c. Body weight on admission: 9 kg
   d. Electrolytes:

Na^+ 135 mEq/L	K^+ 5 mEq/L	Cl^- 115 mEq/L	HCO_3^- 12 mEq/L

2. Summary of fluid requirements

	H_2O (ml)	Na^+ (mEq)	K^+ (mEq)
Maintenance	1,000 (100 ml/kg)	30 (3 mEq/kg)	20 (2 mEq/kg)
Deficit (100 ml/kg)			
ECF (60%)	600	84 (140 mEq × 0.6)	
ICF (40%)	400		30 (150 mEq × 0.4 × 50% correction)
TOTAL	1000 ml	84 mEq	30 mEq
Resuscitation Fluids	200 ml	28 mEq	
Net Deficit	800 ml	56 mEq	30 mEq

3. Fluid Schedule

	Fluids	
Phase	**Calculation**	**Administered**
I (0-½ hr)	20 ml/kg	200 ml 0.9% NS or LR over 20-30 min.
II (½-9 hr)	½ net deficit: 400 ml D5W with 28 mEq NaCl and 15 mEq KCl ⅓ maintenance: 333 ml D5W with 10 mEq NaCl and 7 mEq KCl TOTAL: 733 ml with 38 mEq NaCl and 22 mEq KCl	733 ml (~90 ml/hr) of D5W 0.45% NS with 22 mEq KCl (~30 mEq/L) (this approximation facilitates care)
III (9-25 hr)	½ deficit ⅔ maintenance	1,067 ml (~67 ml/hr) of D5W 0.45% NS with 28 mEq KCl (~26 mEq/L) (this approximation facilitates care)

NOTES:

1. Fluid resuscitation is crucial during Phase I. If initial response is poor, additional infusion(s) are warranted. Generally, include the initial emergency fluid bolus as part of the deficit replacement.
2. Blood glucose should be assessed early, especially in children with prolonged vomiting, diarrhea or inadequate intake. Early glucose infusion may be warranted.
3. If a patient is acidotic with HCO_3^- of ≥10 mEq/L or a pH < 7.1 on the basis of metabolic acidosis, one third of the sodium may be administered as $NaHCO_3$.
4. In the face of acidosis, serum potassium does not reflect total body deficit.
5. Adjust for fever (add 10% for each 1°C over 37°C), stool loss (5 ml/kg) or vomiting (volume for volume).

Modified from Barkin RM, Rosen P, editors: *Emergency pediatrics*, ed 5, St Louis, 1999, Mosby.

must be considered because free water is excreted with an obligatory solute (sodium) loss. Diuretics may be used in combination with saline administration in an attempt to avoid sodium depletion.

Hypernatremic Volume Depletion

Hypernatremic volume depletion occurs when relatively more loss of water than sodium occurs. It can occur if inappropriate types of fluids are given, if the fluid or formula is mixed incorrectly, and if fever or hyperventilation complicates the illness. This is the least common type because of a generally lower content of sodium in most modern infant fluid and formulas. Because intracellular fluid shifts to the extracellular fluid space attempting to maintain osmolar balance, the resulting signs found are doughy skin and altered CNS function (irritability, seizures, high-pitched cry). Intravascular volume is relatively preserved and shock-like states are a less common finding because the primary problem is cellular dehydration. Care must be taken not to administer hypotonic fluid at too fast a rate because water will equilibrate across the cerebral blood-brain barrier almost immediately (long before the sodium is corrected), creating increased intracranial pressure. This type of volume disorder should be corrected over 48 to 72 hours. Box 171-4 provides guidelines for the calculation of fluids and electrolytes. Monitor appropriate parameters over the period of rehydration.

BOX 171-3. Sample Calculation of Fluid and Electrolyte Requirements in a Patient with Hyponatremic Volume Depletion

Isotonic Volume Depletion: Management of Moderate to Severe Deficits

1. Initial findings
   a. Pre-illness weight: 10 kg (a 1-yr-old)
   b. Degree of volume depletion, moderate (10%)
   c. Body weight on admission: 9 kg
   d. Electrolytes:
      Na^+ 110 mEq/L K^+ 5 mEq/L Cl^- 90 mEq/L HCO_3^- 12 mEq/L
2. Summary of fluid requirements

	H_2O (ml)	Na^+ (mEq)	K^+ (mEq)
Maintenance	1,000 (100 ml/kg)	30 (3 mEq/kg)	20 (2 mEq/kg)
Deficit (100 ml/kg)			
ECF (60%)	600	84 (140 mEq × 0.6)	
ICF (40%)	400		30 (150 mEq × 0.4 × 50% correction)
Sodium deficit*		125	
TOTAL	1000 ml	209 mEq	30 mEq
Resuscitation Fluids	200 ml	28 mEq	
Net Deficit	800 ml	181 mEq	30 mEq

3. Fluid Schedule

Phase	*Calculation* (Fluids)	*Administered* (Fluids)
I (0-½ hr)	20 ml/kg	200 ml 0.9% NS or LR over 20-30 min.
II (½-9 hr)	½ net deficit: 400 ml D5W with 90 mEq NaCl and 15 mEq KCl ⅓ maintenance: 333 ml D5W with 10 mEq NaCl and 7 mEq KCl TOTAL: 733 ml with 100 mEq NaCl and 22 mEq KCl	733 ml (~90 ml/hr) of D5W 0.9% NS with 22 mEq KCl (~30 mEq/L) (this approximation facilitates care)
III (9-25 hr)	½ deficit ⅔ maintenance	1,067 ml (~67 ml/hr) of D5W 0.9% NS with 28 mEq KCl (~26 mEq/L) (this approximation facilitates care)

***Sodium deficit calculation**

A. Na^+ required to correct to 135 mEq/L = 135 mEq/L – 110 mEq/L (observed Na^+) = 25 mEq/L
B. Total body water (TBW)(L/kg) = 0.6 L/kg (pre-illness TBW) – 0.1 L/kg (water loss) = 0.5 L/kg
C. Pre-illness weight = 10 kg

Sodium deficit = A × B × C = 25 mEq/L × 0.5 L/kg × 10 kg = 125 mEq

NOTES:

1. Fluid resuscitation is crucial during Phase I. If initial response is poor, additional infusion(s) are warranted. Generally, include the initial emergency fluid bolus as part of the deficit replacement.
2. If a patient is acidotic with HCO_3^- of ≤10 mEq/L or a pH ≤7.1 on the basis of metabolic acidosis, one third of the sodium may be administered as $NaHCO_3$
3. In the face of severe hyponatremia with decreased TBW in symptomatic patients, hypertonic 3% saline must be given to raise the serum sodium level to 125 mEq/L. A 3% saline solution contains approximately 0.5 mEq Na^+/ml. Patients may be given 3% saline 4 ml/kg IV over 10 minutes and the response monitored. Once seizures have stopped, half of the deficit may be corrected over the next 8 hours as outlined in the fluid schedule.
4. If excess water load is the cause, furosemide (Lasix) 1 mg/kg/dose IV may be used. During the subsequent diuresis, urinary sodium, potassium, and chloride should be measured and replaced milliequivalent for milliequivalent with 3% saline and supplemental potassium chloride.
5. Blood glucose should be assessed early, especially in children with prolonged vomiting, diarrhea or inadequate intake. Early glucose infusion may be warranted.
6. In the face of acidosis, serum potassium does not reflect total body deficit.
7. Adjust for fever (add 10% for each 1°C over 37°C), stool loss (5 ml/kg) or vomiting (volume for volume).

Modified from Barkin RM, Rosen P, editors: *Emergency pediatrics*, ed 5, St Louis, 1999, Mosby

BOX 171-4. Hypertonic Dehydration

A 2-week-old infant presents to the ED with a history of 1 day of poor breast milk intake. Weight yesterday at a well-baby visit was 4 kg; today the child weighs 3.4 kg. Laboratory studies include serum Na^+–155 mEq/L; K^+ –4.5 mEq/L; HCO_3^-–13 mEq/L.

Maintenance therapy
100 ml/day for first 10 kg = 400 ml
Na^+ requirements = 3 mEq/kg × 4 kg = 12 mEq
K^+ requirements = 2 mEq/kg × 4 kg = 8 mEq

Total fluid deficit = 4.0 – 3.4 = 0.6 L
Free water deficits = [observed Na^+ – ideal Na^+ (145 mEq/L)] × 4 ml/kg × wt (kg) = (155 − 145) × 4 ml/kg × 4 kg = 160 ml

Na^+ deficit (The illness is less than 3 days duration Therefore the fluid lost is 75% from the ECF and 25% the ICF. Primary sodium reservoir is ECF.)
Na^+ loss = (ECF Na^+ concentration) × (75% of solute fluid deficit*)
= (140 mEq/L) × (0.75 × 0.440 L)
= 46 mEq

NOTE: Solute containing deficit = Total fluid deficit – free water deficit
= 600 ml − 160 ml
= 440 ml

K^+ deficit (primary potassium reservoir is ICF):
K^+ loss = (ICF K^+ concentration) × (25% of solute fluid deficit)
= (150 mEq/L) × (0.25) × 0.440 L
= 16 mEq

48-hour requirements = maintenance + deficits
Total deficits: Fluid (ml) = (400 × 2) ml + 160 ml (free) + 440 (solute) = 1400 ml
Sodium (mEq) = 24 + 46 = 70 mEq
Potassium (mEq) = 16 + 16 = 32 mEq

Fluid schedule
The fluid is administered in a step-wise fashion over 48 hours. One half the deficit is given in the first 24 hours then the remainder in the next 24.

First day fluids = Maintenance + ½ deficits
First day fluids = (400 ml + 12 mEq Na^+ + 8 mEq K^+) + ½ (600 ml + 46 mEq Na^+ + 16 mEq K^+)
First day fluids = 700 ml D5W + 35 mEq Na^+ + 16 mEq K^+
In practice (and after the calculations are done), the usual fluid that is required to rehydrate the child with hypertonic dehydration is either D5W 0.2% NS or D5W 0.45% NS because it would appear that the *rate* not the type of fluid is most important. The volume of free water needed to lower a serum sodium concentration above 145 mEq/L is about 4 ml/kg of free water for each 1 mEq/L over 48 hours. Studies demonstrate that D5W, D5W 0.2% NS, or D5W 0.45% NS are all acceptable if infused at a conservative rate, correcting deficits over 48 hours.

Modified from Barkin R et al: *Pediatric emergency medicine,* ed 2, St Louis, 1997, Mosby.
*(600 ml fluid deficit – 160 free water deficit)

KEY CONCEPTS

- *Identification of pathogen:* Stool studies are not indicated in most uncomplicated AGE. Exceptions are those that require specific treatment, specific prophylaxis, or health precautions, and when the patient has systemic involvement or underlying medical complications, or the illness involves dysenteric features.
- *Fecal leukocytes:* The presence of fecal leukocytes or blood indicates that the offending organism has crossed the mucosal barrier and that the risk of invasiveness has increased. Nearly 90% of acute diarrhea caused by *Salmonella* or *Shigella* organisms have fecal leukocytes in the stools.
- *Oral rehydration:* With oral rehydration therapy, resumption of feeding should begin as soon as vomiting subsides. Routine fasting for diarrhea illnesses is not recommended. Instruction should address proper hygiene and hand washing techniques to prevent others from contracting the illness.
- *Dehydration assessment:* Estimate the degree of volume depletion using information from the history, clinical signs, and physical examination. Calculate the desired volume of oral rehydration solution (ORS) as 60 ml/kg for mild and 80 ml/kg for moderate volume depletion, then administer 25% of the volume of ORS to be replaced each hour for the first 4 hours.
- *Severe dehydration:* In severe dehydration, 20 ml/kg of 0.9% saline (or other appropriate isotonic crystalloid solution) IV at a rapid rate should be administered and should result in reversal of signs of shock within 5 to 15 minutes. Repeat administrations of 20 ml/kg are indicated until clinical improvement occurs, but volume requirements greater than 60 ml/kg without signs of improvement suggest other conditions, such as septic shock, hemorrhage, capillary leak with third space fluid sequestration, and heart failure.

REFERENCES

1. Ho M-S et al: Diarrheal deaths in American children: are they preventable? *JAMA* 260:3281, 1988.
2. Glass RI et al: Estimates of morbidity and mortality rates for diseases in American children, *J Pediatr* 118:S27, 1991.
3. Koopman JS et al: Patterns and etiology of diarrhea in three clinical settings, *Am* J Epidemiol 19:114, 1984.
4. Ghishan FK: Gastrointestinal diseases. In Ichikawa I, editor: *Pediatric textbook of fluids and electrolytes,* Baltimore, 1990, Williams & Wilkins.
5. Caeiro JP et al: Etiology of outpatient pediatric nondysenteric diarrhea: a multicenter study in the United States, *Pediatr Dis J* 18:94-97, 1999.
6. Barnes GL: Intestinal viral infections. In *Pediatric gastrointestinal disease,* Philadelphia, 1991, BC Becker.
7. Pickering LK, Cleary TG: Approach to patients with gastrointestinal tract infections and food poisoning. In *Textbook of pediatric infectious disease,* Philadelphia, 1992, WB Saunders.
8. Mehta DI, Lebenthal E: New developments in acute diarrhea, *Curr Probl Pediatr* 24:95, 1994.
9. Hamilton JR: Viral enteritis in pediatric gastroenterology I, *Pediatr Clin North Am* 35:89, 1988.
10. Flores J et al: The role of rotavirus in pediatric diarrhea, *Pediatr Infect Dis* 5:553, 1986.
11. Richardson S et al: Extended excretion of rotavirus after severe diarrhea in young children, *Lancet* 351:1844-1848, 1998.

12. Abbott Laboratories Diagnostic Division: *Rotazyme II: Enzyme immunoassay for the detection of Rotavirus antigens in human fecal specimens,* Abbott Park, Ill, 1989, Abbott Laboratories Diagnostic Division.
13. Offit PA: The rotavirus vaccine, *J Clin Virology* 11:155-159, 1998.
14. 1997 Redbook: *Report of the Committee on Infectious Diseases,* Elk Grove Village, Ill, American Academy of Pediatrics, 1997.
15. Rennels MB, Levine MM: Classical bacterial diarrhea: perspectives and update: *Salmonella, Shigella, Escherichia coli, Aeromonas,* and *Plesiomonas, Pediatr Infect Dis* 5:S91, 1986.
16. Schulman SK et al: Multistate outbreak of *Shigella sonnei* gastroenteritis: United States, *Morb Mortal World Rep* 36:440, 1987.
17. Pai CH et al: *Campylobacter* gastroenteritis in children, *J Pediatr* 94:589, 1979.
18. NIH Consensus Conference: Traveler's diarrhea, *JAMA* 253:2700, 1985.
19. McLoighlin LC: Gastrointestinal manifestations of pediatric HIV infection. In *Management of HIV infection in infants and children,* St Louis, 1992, Mosby.
20. Folwaczy C: Zinc and diarrhea in infants, *J Trace Elements Med Biol* 11:116-122, 1997.
21. Sazawal S et al: Efficacy of zinc supplementation in reducing the incidence and prevalence of acute diarrhea—a community based, double blind controlled trial, *Am J Clin Nutr* 66:413-418, 1997.
22. Austin PE et al: Discharge instructions: do illustrations help our patients understand them? *Ann Emerg Med* 25:317, 1995.
23. De Bruin WJ et al: Fluid resuscitation in pediatrics, *Crit Care Clin* 8:423, 1992.
24. Brewer E: Disorders of acid-base balance, *Pediatr Clin North Am* 37:429, 1990.
25. Casteel HB, Feidorek SC: Oral rehydration therapy, *Pediatr Clin North Am* 37:295, 1990.
26. Molina S et al: Clinical trial of glucose oral rehydration solution, rice dextrin ORS and rice flour ORS for the management of children with acute diarrhea and mild or moderate dehydration, *Pediatrics* 95:191-197, 1995.
27. Fayad IM et al: Comparative efficacy of rice-based and glucose-based oral rehydration salts plus early reintroduction of food, *Lancet* 342:772-775, 1993.
28. Rautanen T, EL-Radhi S, Zesikari T: Randomized double blind study of hypotonic oral rehydration solution in diarrhea, *Arch Dis Child* 76:272-274, 1997.
29. Rautanen T, Kurki S, Zesikari T: Clinical experience with a hypotonic oral rehydration solution in acute diarrhea, *Acta Paediatr* 82:52-54, 1994.
30. Faruque AS et al: Hypo-osmolar sucrose oral rehydration solution in acute diarrhea: a pilot study, *Acta Paediatr* 85:1247-1248, 1996.
31. Faruque AS et al: Randomized controlled clinical trial of rice versus glucose oral rehydration solutions, *Acta Paediatr* 86:1308-1311, 1997.
32. Snyder JD: Use and misuse of oral therapy for diarrhea: comparison of US practices with American Academy of Pediatrics recommendation, *Pediatrics* 87:28, 1991.
33. Trachtman H: Volume depletion states: dehydration or denaturation? *Pediatr Nephrol* 5:271, 1991.

***Table 171-4.* Etiology of Diarrhea in Children and Specific Therapy**

Agent	Specific therapy beyond supportive care
Campylobacter jejuni	Azithromycin 12 mg/kg/day PO for 5 days or Erythromycin 30-50 mg/kg/day divided tid PO for 5-7 days
Clostridium difficile	Metronidazole 30 mg/kg/day divided qid PO for 7-10 days or Vancomycin 40 mg/kg/day divided qid PO for 7-10 days
Escherichia coli	Azithromycin 12 mg/kg/day PO for 5 days or Trimethoprim-sulfamethoxazole 10 mg (TMP)/kg/day divided bid for 5-7 days
Giardia lamblia	No change
Salmonella species	No change
Shigella species	Azithromycin 12 mg/kg/day PO for 5 days or Trimethoprim-sulfamethoxazole 10 mg (TMP)/kg/day divided bid for 5-7 days if susceptible
Yersinia enterocolitica	No change
Vibrio	No change

Reference Red Book 26th edition, American Academy of Pediatrics, Larry K Pickering, MD, FAAP Editor, 2003 and The Harriet Lane Handbook 16th edition, Mosby, Gunn and Nechyba, 2002.

CHAPTER 172 Renal and Genitourinary Tract Disorders

Maureen McCollough and Ghazala Sharieff

PERSPECTIVE

The child with an acute scrotum or an acute renal process can be challenging for the emergency practitioner. This chapter discusses some of the more common causes of scrotal, testicular, and penile pain as well as acute renal failure, urinary tract infections, and hypertension in pediatric patients.

SPECIFIC DISORDERS

Penile Disorders

Priapism

Principles of Disease

Priapism is the engorgement of the dorsal corpora cavernosa, resulting in dorsal penile erection and ventral penile flaccidity. Sickle cell disease and leukemia are responsible for the majority of cases in children. Spinal trauma, immunosuppressive disorders, anticoagulation, and intracavernosal injections such as papaverine, phentolamine, and prostaglandin-1 can also result in priapism. Other drugs such as phenothiazines, sedative-hypnotics, selective serotonin uptake inhibitors, antihypertensives, anticoagulants, and drugs of abuse (e.g., cocaine, alcohol, and marijuana) may be contributory.

The more common *low-flow priapism* is secondary to decreased venous outflow and is characterized by prolonged, painful erection. *High-flow priapism* is usually painless and is typically associated with penile arterial laceration and excessive inflow of arterial blood, resulting in corporal engorgement. If prolonged engorgement of the corpora cavernosa occurs, stagnant, hypoxic blood results in thrombosis and ischemia. Urinary retention can also occur.

Clinical Features

Priapism is a clinical diagnosis and can be distinguished from other causes of erection by careful history and complete physical examination. The history should include past medical history with attention to previous treatment for anemia, leukemia, sickle cell disease, or drug abuse and current history of trauma or symptoms of immunosuppressive disease. Physical examination should be extensive and look for rash, lymphadenopathy, pale or jaundiced skin, or signs of a toxidrome. Priapism is a clinical diagnosis; however, laboratory studies may assist in isolating the cause of the condition. A complete blood count (CBC), hemoglobin electrophoresis, and coagulation studies may be useful in some cases. Diagnostic studies of penile blood flow include magnetic resonance imaging, color Doppler cavernosonography, and technetium-99m penile scanning. Angiography is helpful in localizing the arterial bleeding site in high-flow priapism.[1]

Differential Considerations

The differential diagnosis of priapism in children differs from that in adults. In adults, penile erection from sexual arousal, urethral foreign bodies, Peyronie's disease, spinal cord injury, and penile implants may occur, but these would be rare in children. Anticoagulation, drugs of abuse, medications, trauma (including spinal trauma), Kawasaki's disease, leukemia, and sickle cell disease are all associated with priapism in children.

Management and Disposition

Management centers on hydration, pain control, relief of urinary obstruction, and treatment of any other underlying conditions. Local anesthesia through a dorsal nerve block using 1% lidocaine without epinephrine may be beneficial. In patients with sickle cell disease, treatment is begun with oxygen, hydration, and analgesics.

In addition, cavernosal aspiration and irrigation have been effective in patients with low-flow priapism and acidosis. This procedure should be performed within the first few hours of symptom onset and is rarely beneficial after 48 hours. Phentolamine, phenylephrine (100 to 500 µg per dose, up to 10 doses; 10 to 20 mL of 20 µg/mL solution by intracavernous injection every 5 to 10 minutes), ephedrine, or 1:1,000,000 epinephrine is often added to the irrigation solution when performing corporal aspiration. Parenteral vasodilators such as papaverine, hydralazine, or terbutaline have also been used with varying success.[2]

If the priapism is not relieved, an exchange transfusion is indicated with a goal to achieve a hemoglobin level of 10 g/dL. Patients with leukemia may respond with detumescence after chemotherapy is begun.

High-flow priapism can be effectively treated by arterial embolization. If these nonsurgical approaches are unsuccessful, a cavernous-glans shunt procedure may be necessary. Interventions should be initiated within 12 hours of symptom onset to avoid long-term dysfunction and irreversible infarction.[3]

Phimosis

Principles of Disease

Phimosis is a constriction of the foreskin resulting in the inability to retract the prepuce over the glans. It can result in pain, hematuria, and urinary outlet obstruction. Most cases are physiologic, representing normal development, and do not require intervention. Most uncircumcised infants have an unretractable foreskin. Only 4% of newborn males have a fully retractable foreskin. This percentage increases with age: 25% of 6-month-olds, 50% of 1-year-olds, 80% of 2-year-olds, and 90% of 4-year-old males have fully retractable foreskins.[4] Phimosis may also result from trauma, infections, chemical irritation, or poor hygiene or be a complication of circumcision.

Clinical Features

Phimosis is a clinical diagnosis. History may reveal that the foreskin is unretractable and that there is narrowing or diversion of the urinary stream and bulging out of the foreskin with urination.

Management and Disposition

Because the ability to retract the foreskin fully is age related, parents should be advised not to retract the prepuce forcefully. Gentle retraction with good hygiene should be stressed. If there are signs of urinary outlet obstruction, dilation of the prepuce or the urethral meatus or both can be performed by gentle use of forceps. If there is vascular compromise of the glans, a dorsal split procedure, circumcision, preputial plasty, or balloon dilation may be necessary.[5,6] Topical steroid treatment (betamethasone valerate 0.6% cream) for 6 weeks was 87% effective in reducing inflammation and treating phimosis.[7,8] In patients with severe stenosis, obstructive uropathy can result. In these cases, blood urea nitrogen (BUN) and creatinine should be obtained and a renal ultrasound examination should be performed if signs of obstructive renal failure are present. Patients who are able to urinate and have no evidence of severe infection or ischemia can be discharged with outpatient urologic follow-up.

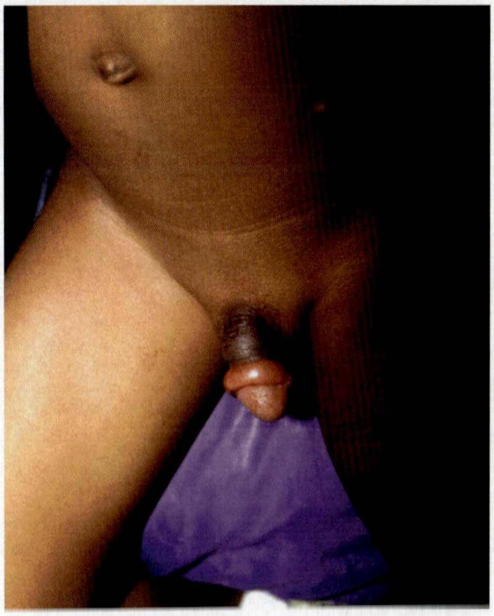

Figure 172-1. Four-year-old uncircumcised boy with paraphimosis. (Courtesy of Marianne Gausche-Hill, MD.)

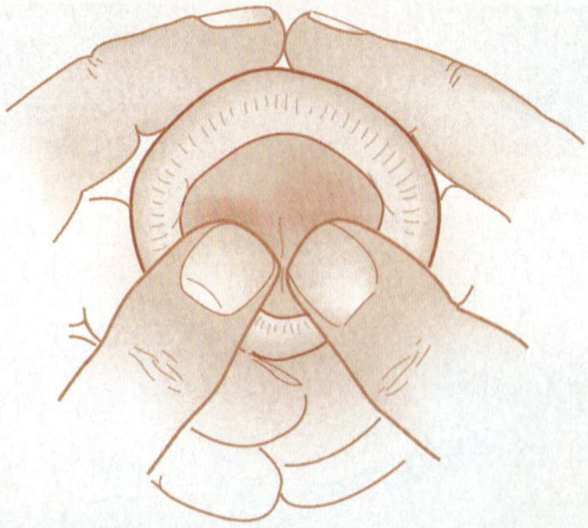

Figure 172-2. Paraphimosis reduction. (Courtesy of P.P. Kelalis.)

Paraphimosis

Principles of Disease

Paraphimosis is the inability to reduce the proximal foreskin over the glans penis, resulting in distal venous congestion and resultant inability to return the foreskin to its anatomic position. Paraphimosis can be caused by infection, masturbation, trauma, or hair or clothing tourniquets. Iatrogenic causes include failure to reduce the foreskin after a medical examination. Paraphimosis is a true urologic emergency and can result in arterial compression, penile necrosis, and gangrene.

Clinical Features

The patient is typically anxious, and the history often reveals that the parents or patient tried to retract the foreskin and then could not replace the foreskin back over the glans (Figure 172-1). One should verify by history that the patient is uncircumcised because hair tourniquet syndrome may mimic paraphimosis. Physical examination reveals a flaccid proximal penis with erythema and engorgement distal to the obstruction. The foreskin is retracted and cellulitis may be present. The diagnosis of paraphimosis is based on clinical findings, but if there is concern about possible penile foreign bodies, radiographs can be obtained after relief of the vascular occlusion.

Management and Disposition

Pain can be controlled either parenterally or by performing a local dorsal penile nerve block. Placing the tip of a rubber glove filled with ice water over the glans and foreskin can reduce the edema. Circumferential compression of the penis starting at the glans can also reduce the edema. Manual reduction may be necessary with gentle, steady pressure on the glans with both thumbs (Figure 172-2). Another method is to puncture the edematous foreskin with an 18- or 21-gauge needle.[9,10] The puncture may be followed by squeezing of the glans penis to further facilitate fluid drainage. Dorsal band traction has been performed in some cases by application of Adson forceps directly to the band formed by the retracted foreskin and applying traction and countertraction to loosen the constriction. If all attempts fail, urologic consultation and circumcision or a dorsal slit procedure may be necessary. Patients can be discharged after reduction if they are able to void spontaneously and urologic follow-up can be arranged.

Balanoposthitis

Principles of Disease

Balanoposthitis is an inflammation that involves the glans and the foreskin, occurring in up to 3% of uncircumcised males. Balanitis involves the glans penis only. The primary cause of balanoposthitis is infection; however, chemical irritation, trauma, fixed drug rash, and contact dermatitis can also be contributory. Infectious organisms include gram-negative and gram-positive organisms, including group A beta-hemolytic streptococci and rarely *Neisseria gonorrhoeae* and *Chlamydia*.[11] Recurrent cases of *Candida albicans* balanoposthitis should raise the suspicion of diabetes mellitus.

Clinical Features

Physical examination reveals penile erythema, edema, and possibly a discharge (Figure 172-3). Systemic symptoms such as fever, vomiting, and diarrhea are unusual. Diagnosis is clinical, but the offending organism can be identified by culturing any discharge.

Management and Disposition

Management includes emphasis on adequate hygiene with sitz baths to reduce inflammation. Painful urination can be relieved by having the child urinate while in a bath of warm water. In patients with cellulitis, 5 to 7 days of a first-generation cephalosporin may be required. If group A beta-hemolytic streptococcus is identified, a streptococcus-specific antibiotic is required. Inflammation can also be treated with 0.5% hydrocortisone cream applied sparingly to the area. Circumcision may be required for recurrent disease. Patients who are toxic or have evidence of cellulitis

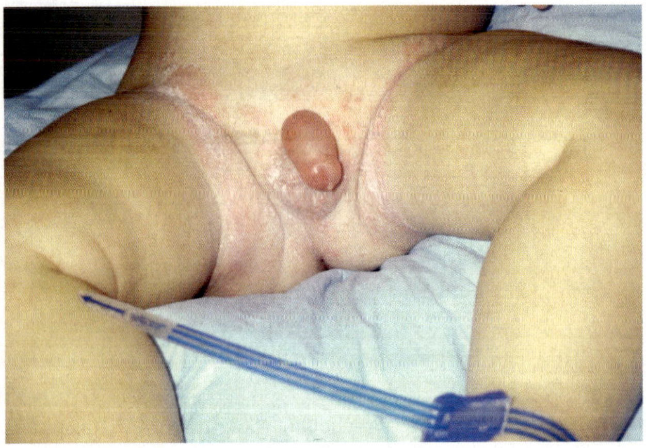

Figure 172-3. Balanoposthitis in an 8-month-old caused by candidal infection. (Courtesy of Marianne Gausche-Hill, MD.)

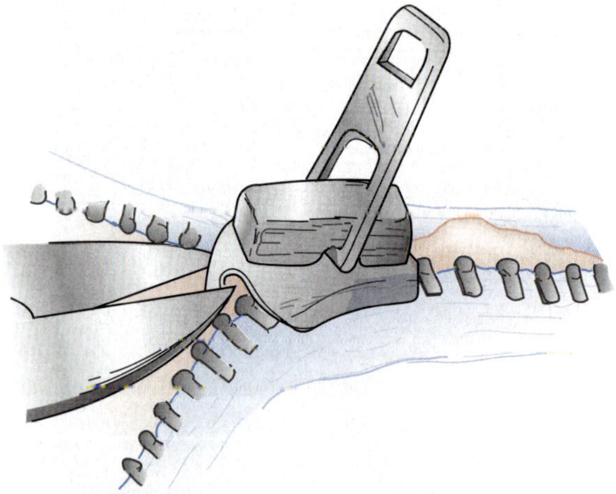

Figure 172-4. Release of zipper entrapment by cutting the median bar. (From Snyder HM III. In Fleisher GR, Ludwig S [eds]: *Textbook of Pediatric Emergency Medicine*, 4th ed. Philadelphia, Lippincott Williams & Wilkins, 2000.)

or constricting phimosis with uropathy should be admitted.

Complications of Circumcision

Principles of Disease

Circumcision is usually advocated for prevention of phimosis, paraphimosis, recurrent balanoposthitis, urinary tract infections, and penile cancer. Three techniques can be used: Plastibell or Gomco clamp, excision, or a dorsal slit procedure. The decision about which procedure is used is dependent on the person performing the circumcision. The most common complication of these procedures is hemorrhage, which is usually minor and can be controlled by direct pressure, silver nitrate application, or suture placement. Significant bleeding may be a sign of a blood dyscrasia. Localized, systemic, or urinary tract infection can also occur.

Management and Disposition

Postoperative pain usually resolves within 12 to 24 hours. Occlusive dressings can contribute to urinary retention and edema and should be removed. Stenosis of the now exposed urethral meatus may result from prolonged exposure to the ammonia in urine. Application of a Plastibell that is too small can also lead to meatal stenosis in 8% to 31% of cases.[12] Symptoms include pain with urination, bloody discharge resulting from inflamed meatus, high-velocity stream, and the need to sit while voiding. Postcircumcision phimosis may result if excess foreskin remains. If the constriction is severe and urinary outlet obstruction occurs, dilation of the stenosis can be performed using a hemostat. Surgical revision is usually necessary.[13]

Skin bridges are small fibrotic bands that attach the glans to the penile shaft and may form after circumcision. Inclusion cysts result from smegma retained in the wound or from epidermis involution along the circumcision site. Like skin bridges, these are treated by surgical resection. These complications may be prevented by proper hygiene and application of an antimicrobial ointment to the circumcision site for 7 to 10 days after the procedure.

Penile Entrapment and Tourniquet Injuries

Penile rings, string, wire, and human hair tourniquets can result in penile venous and arterial occlusion. The patient presents with swelling of the glans, wherein the offending agent may be difficult to visualize because of edema of the coronal sulcus. In addition to the vascular supply, the dorsal penile nerve supply can be occluded. Urethral obstruction can be evaluated by performing a retrograde urethrogram and Doppler ultrasonography can be performed to assess penile arterial blood flow. Once identified, the constriction is relieved and the patient should not be discharged until spontaneous voiding is assured. Urologic consultation may be necessary emergently if penile arterial flow is disrupted and the constricting object cannot be removed rapidly or signs of necrosis are present.

Zipper entrapment of the foreskin can also occur in children, typically those between 2 and 6 years of age. The zipper can be removed with bone or metal cutters to cut the median bar of the zipper (Figure 172-4). The zipper falls apart and the foreskin is freed. Although local anesthesia is not necessary, the patient may be quite anxious and require sedation before its removal. There is reported success with soaking the penis in mineral oil before zipper removal.[14] Parents should be instructed that their children be encouraged to wear underwear to decrease the risk of entrapment.

Scrotal Masses and Swelling

Epididymitis

Principles of Disease

Epididymitis results from inflammation of the epididymis, which is located along the posterior aspect of the testicle. The most common cause is infectious, and the etiology varies by age. Adolescents should be evaluated for possible sexually transmitted diseases, such as *N. gonorrhoeae* and *Chlamydia trachomatis*.

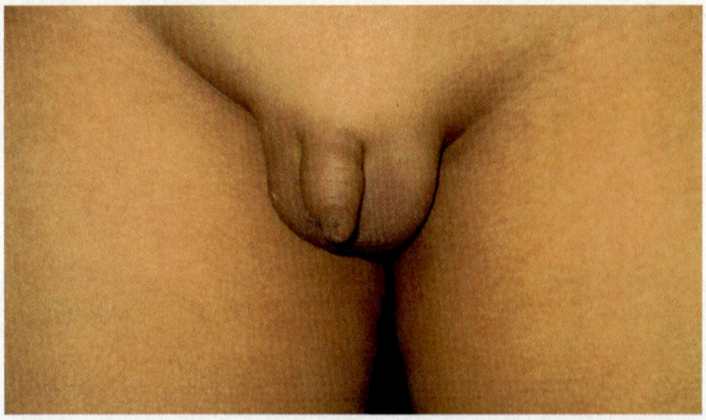

Figure 172-5. Epididymitis in a 5-year-old; note mild swelling and erythema on the left. (Courtesy of Marianne Gausche-Hill, MD.)

Patients may have a history of previous urinary tract infections, anatomic abnormalities, or prior genitourinary instrumentation. Urinary tract infections leading to epididymitis are typically caused by viruses or bacterial agents, such as *Escherichia coli, Klebsiella pneumoniae, Proteus,* or *Pseudomonas aeruginosa.*

Clinical Features

Patients present with a painful, edematous scrotum and tenderness at the epididymis (Figure 172-5). A urethral discharge may be present, particularly when the condition is secondary to a sexually transmitted disease. Systemic symptoms such as nausea, vomiting, fever, and lower abdominal, scrotal, or testicular pain may also be present. Infants and young children may present with fever without other symptoms. The emergency physician should therefore do a complete examination including a genitourinary examination on all children with fever or other systemic signs. As the edema increases, obliteration of the sulcus between the testis and epididymis occurs, making differentiation from testicular torsion extremely difficult. Relief of pain with scrotal elevation (Prehn's sign) is unreliable.

Diagnostic Strategies

A urinalysis should be obtained and a urine culture sent in all infants and children younger than 2 years. In children 2 years of age or older, a culture may be sent only if the urinalysis results indicate urinary tract infection. Lack of pyuria does not rule out epididymitis because up to 50% of patients may have normal studies. CBC may show leukocytosis, although these results are nonspecific. Any urethral discharge should be cultured and sent for Gram stain, *N. gonorrhoeae,* and *C. trachomatis* evaluation. Color-flow Doppler ultrasonography or radionuclide scintigraphy reveals a normal testis and preserved or increased vascular flow toward the side of the inflamed epididymis.[15,16]

Management and Disposition

In addition to antibiotic administration, pain control is imperative. Scrotal elevation, placement of ice packs on the swollen area as tolerated, and nonsteroidal anti-inflammatory or narcotic medications are useful. If there is urethral discharge, the adolescent patient should be treated for both *N. gonorrhoeae* and *C. trachomatis.* The treatment for sexually acquired epididymitis in children 9 years or older includes ceftriaxone 250 mg intramuscularly, followed by doxycycline 100 mg orally twice a day or tetracycline 500 mg orally four times a day. Patients younger than 9 years should be treated with erythromycin 50 mg/kg/day divided four times a day. Treatment typically ranges from 7 to 14 days depending on the antibiotic regimen. Nonsexually acquired epididymitis can be treated with trimethoprim 8 mg/kg/day divided twice a day. Other treatment options include oral erythromycin, clarithromycin, cephalexin, and azithromycin. Patients with systemic symptoms and toxicity should be admitted for intravenous antibiotics with either ceftriaxone or cefotaxime. Children need close urologic follow-up to ensure that there are no contributing anatomic abnormalities and that the antibiotic choice treats an infecting organism.

Orchitis

Orchitis is a result of a bacterial or viral testicular infection leading to diffuse edema, pain, and discoloration of the scrotum. The most common offending agent is paramyxovirus and can occur in up to 38% of postpubertal males with mumps. Other etiologic agents include *E. coli, K. pneumoniae, P. aeruginosa, Staphylococcus* or *Streptococcus* species, Epstein-Barr virus, coxsackievirus, arbovirus, enterovirus, brucellosis, granulomatous disease, and filariasis. Empirical treatment includes oral antibiotics with predominantly gram-negative organism coverage. Urologic follow-up should be arranged.

Testicular Torsion

Principles of Disease

Torsion of the spermatic cord is a common cause of an acutely painful scrotum. Delay in diagnosis and treatment can result in a loss of spermatogenesis and in severe cases necrotic, gangrenous testes. Testicular salvage rates are time dependent with a 96% success rate if detorsion is performed less than 4 hours from symptom onset, decreasing to less than 10% if there is a greater than 24-hour delay to treatment.[17] The incidence of testicular torsion is 1 in 4000 males, with a peak incidence at age 13 years. Testicular torsion has been reported in all age groups from the developing fetus to the elderly but is most common in adolescence.

The testis enters the scrotum through the inguinal canal after descent from the abdomen. The peritoneum invaginates through the canal and partially covers the testis and epididymis, forming the tunica vaginalis. Typically, the tunica vaginalis attaches to the posterior wall of the hemiscrotum and superior pole of the testes to achieve testicular fixation. If the tunica completely covers the testis and attaches higher up on the spermatic cord (bell clapper deformity), proper testicular fixation does not occur and there is a predisposition to torsion (Figure 172-6). In intravaginal torsion, the testicle may rotate within the tunica vaginalis and thereby

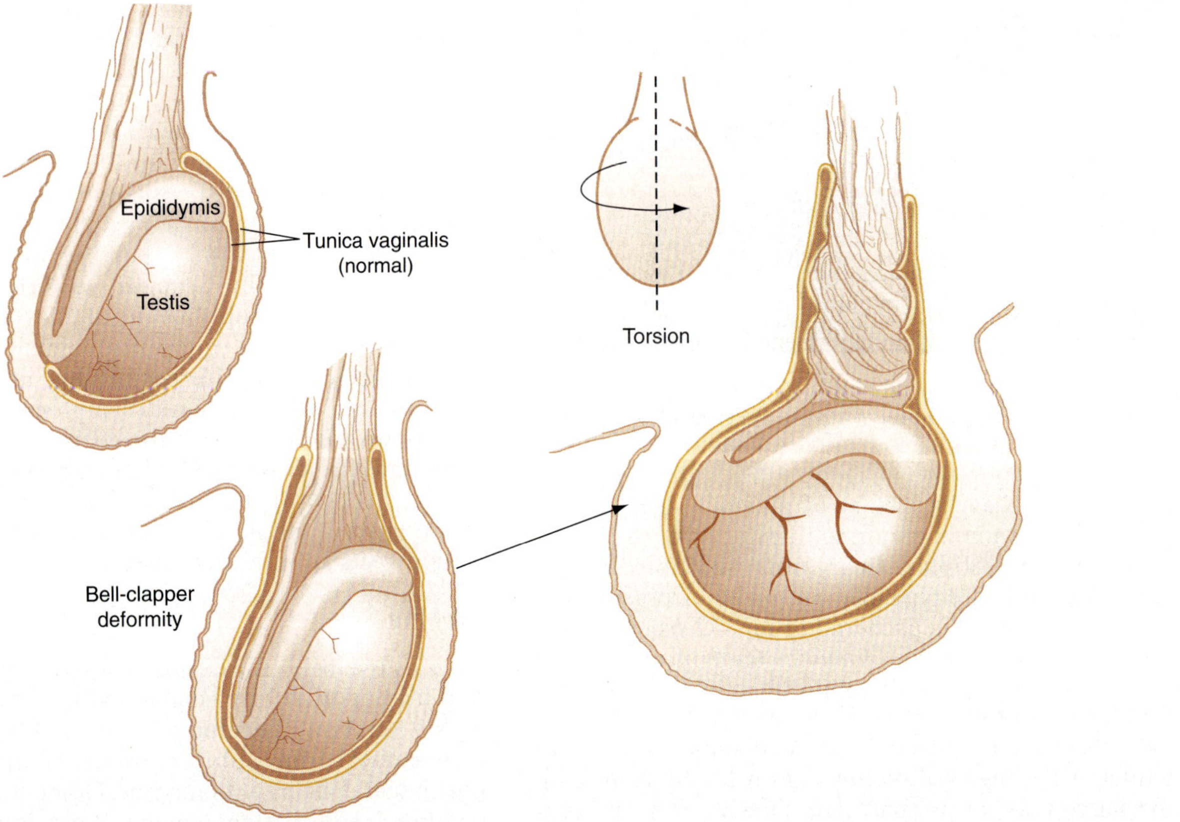

Figure 172-6. Anatomy of testicular torsion. (From Snyder HM III, et al: In Fleisher GR, Ludwig S [eds]: *Textbook of Pediatric Emergency Medicine*, 4th ed. Philadelphia, Lippincott Williams & Wilkins, 2000.)

constrict the arterial blood flow. Extravaginal torsion is seen most commonly in neonates who are premature and can also occur antenatally. If the torsion is prolonged, testicular infarction and atrophy have been reported after as little as 4 hours of ischemia.

Clinical Features

Patients present with acute scrotal pain and swelling, an elevated testicle, and, typically, an absent cremasteric reflex.[18] Although in one series, the cremasteric reflex was absent in 100% of patients with torsion and in only 14% of patients with epididymitis, the presence of the cremasteric reflex does not preclude testicular torsion. Abnormal epididymal and testicular position may also be present with left-sided torsions slightly more common than right. Nausea, vomiting, and a low-grade fever may also be seen. In the patient with an undescended testicle who presents with abdominal pain, torsion should be a consideration.[19]

Diagnostic Strategies

Unless alternative diagnoses are absolutely secure (e.g., epididymitis), it is necessary to evaluate the patient for testicular torsion. Alternatively, when there is relative to absolute confidence in the clinical diagnosis of torsion, diagnostic testing should not delay appropriate management. Results of a urinalysis are rarely helpful as pyuria can be seen in as many as 25% of cases of testicular torsion. The widely preferred diagnostic study for the prospect of torsion is color flow Doppler ultrasonography. This technique has a sensitivity of 79% to 86%, with a specificity of almost 100% for testicular torsion. As opposed to scintigraphy, it can be performed rapidly, is often available 24 hours a day, and does not require that an intravenous line be placed. Scintigraphy has a sensitivity ranging from 79% to 100% and a specificity of 89% to 100%.[20-22] In cases of indeterminate ultrasound results, the urology consultant should be notified for disposition decisions; in addition, scintigraphy may be performed as resources allow. Surgical exploration when clinical suspicion is high should not be delayed for diagnostic studies, especially in patients who present with less than 12 hours of symptoms.

Management

If the patient presents within 12 hours of symptom onset, immediate surgical exploration is indicated, predicated upon clinical findings or confirmatory clinical studies.[23] Detorsion of the affected testicle is performed followed by an elective orchiopexy of the contralateral side to avoid recurrence. Approximately 40% of patients have a bell clapper deformity of the contralateral testicle. Manual detorsion may also be performed by rotating the testicle in an open book fashion as viewed from below, from medial to lateral, until detorsion is complete.[24] Sedation and pain relief should be considered before this intervention.

Torsion of the Testicular Appendage

The appendix testis is a remnant of the müllerian duct. The appendix testis is involved in 92% of the cases of testicular appendage torsion and the appendix epididymis is involved in the remaining cases. The average age of occurrence is 10 years. Patients typically present with the sudden onset of moderate pain that is localized to the involved hemiscrotum. The pathognomonic finding of the "blue dot" sign, a small bluish hue less than 3 mm located in the upper lateral portion of the hemiscrotum, is present in less than 25% of cases and represents the cyanotic appendage below the scrotal wall. If there is any doubt about the diagnosis, a nuclear scan or color Doppler ultrasound study should be performed. Color Doppler ultrasonography reveals normal or increased flow to the affected testicle. Conservative therapy with analgesics is usually all that is indicated, with the involved appendage undergoing autoamputation within 1 week accompanied by resolution of symptoms.

Varicocele

A *varicocele* is a collection of venous varicosities of the spermatic veins in the scrotum caused by incomplete drainage of the pampiniform plexus. There is a reported incidence of 14% to 16% in adolescent males,[25] but varicoceles are rare in children younger than 10 years.[26] Left-sided varicoceles account for 85% to 95% of cases; however, bilateral varicoceles may be present in up to 22% of patients.[27] Intra-abdominal pathology should be suspected in cases of right-sided varicoceles because these are usually caused by inferior vena cava (IVC) thrombosis or compression of the IVC by tumors.[28] The sudden onset of left-sided varicocele should raise the suspicion of renal cell carcinoma with obstruction of the left renal vein. The venous dilation can be tender on physical examination, can be palpated superior and posterior to the testis, and is usually more pronounced in the upright position; therefore, the emergency physician should examine the patient in both the standing and supine positions. Patients in whom scrotal swelling persists in the supine position should be evaluated with a computed tomography (CT) scan of abdomen with oral and intravenous contrast administration for conditions obstructing the renal vein. Varicoceles have been described in appearance and on palpation as a "bag of worms." Surgical correction may be required if the patient becomes symptomatic or has bilateral varicoceles.[29]

Idiopathic Scrotal Edema

Idiopathic scrotal edema is painless erythema and induration of the scrotum, with 77% of cases occurring before 10 years of age. Two thirds of cases are unilateral and no specific allergens have been identified. Patients develop painless erythema and induration of the scrotum, which may be pruritic. There is minimal tenderness on physical examination, but the edema and erythema may extend to the phallus, groin, and abdomen. Examination of the testes and epididymis reveals no palpable masses. Systemic symptoms are rare. Patients can be discharged home with outpatient follow-up after acute pathology has been ruled out. Most cases resolve spontaneously within a few days and do not require any specific treatment. Recurrence may occur in up to 21% of patients.

Hydrocele

A *hydrocele* is a collection of fluid that accumulates in the tunica vaginalis. Communicating hydroceles occur when the upper processus vaginalis fails to obliterate and there is an open tract between the peritoneum and the scrotum. The tract is closed in noncommunicating hydroceles. Most hydroceles are right sided. They may be present at birth, but they are usually painless and often resolve spontaneously by 18 months of age. Visual examination reveals enlargement of the scrotum with transillumination. Color flow Doppler ultrasonography or radionuclide scintigraphy may be necessary to determine the cause of the hydrocele and to exclude acute pathology in patients demonstrating acute symptoms of pain; otherwise, asymptomatic patients can be discharged with urologic follow-up. Patients with a hydrocele that has persisted for more than 1 year or who are older than 18 months should undergo ultrasonography to ensure that the hydrocele is not a reactive hydrocele caused by testicular tumor or inflammation.

Inguinal Hernia

Principles of Disease

Inguinal (direct and indirect) hernias are more common in males, with bimodal peaks before 1 year of age and then again after age 40. An indirect inguinal hernia occurs when the processus vaginalis does not obliterate in infancy and abdominal contents invaginate through this patent sac. Entrapment of mesentery, bowel, intraperitoneal organs, and the hernial sac can occur and is more common with small hernias. If the contents of the hernia can be returned to their anatomic position, the hernia is reducible; if the contents remain entrapped, it is incarcerated or irreducible. Hernias that remain incarcerated can result in strangulation, with resultant necrosis of bowel or mesentery.

Clinical Features

Patients with incarcerated hernias may present with pain, edema extending to the scrotum, nausea, vomiting, and low-grade fever. Physical examination may reveal bowel sounds in the scrotal sac. If the inguinal mass can be palpated separately from the testes, it is possible to diagnose an inguinal hernia clinically. Rarely, the incarcerated and strangulated hernia can arise as a tense, blue mass in the scrotum.

Management and Disposition

The patient should be placed in the Trendelenburg position with an ice pack placed on the groin to reduce swelling; sedation may be necessary before reduction. Slow, gentle pressure should be applied to reduce the hernia.

If the hernia cannot be reduced or strangulation is suspected (fever, overlying cellulitis, peritonitis), the patient should receive fluid resuscitation, broad-spectrum parenteral antibiotics, and an emergent surgical consultation.[30]

Patients who are found to have a hernia on routine examination or who have had the hernia reduced and are without symptoms suggestive of incarceration or strangulation should be referred for surgical repair.

Carcinoma

Principles of Disease

Testicular and scrotal cancer represents approximately 1% of solid tumors in children. There is an increased incidence of testicular cancer in patients with cryptorchidism in both the undescended testicle and the contralateral descended testicle. Tumor types include teratomas, embryonal carcinomas, yolk sac, choriocarcinomas, Leydig's cell, and Sertoli cell tumors. Lymphoma and leukemia can metastasize to the testicle as well.

Patients typically present with a painless, unilateral mass palpated separately from the testis or may present with a feeling of fullness, tugging, or increased weight of the scrotum and testicular enlargement. A reactive hydrocele may be seen in 7% to 25% of patients and can lead to a delay in diagnosis. Physical examination reveals a firm mass, smooth or nodular, that is not transilluminated. A complete physical examination looking for lymphadenopathy, petechiae, abdominal mass, hepatosplenomegaly, or gynecomastia should be performed.

Diagnostic Strategies

Diagnostic evaluation includes a CBC, urinalysis, testing the urine for human chorionic gonadotropin (produced by germ cell tumors), and ultrasonography of the testis.

Management and Disposition

Management includes prompt urologic and oncologic consultation and biopsy. Admission to the hospital to facilitate the evaluation may be necessary.

Urinary Tract Infections

Perspective

Sequelae of untreated urinary tract infections (UTIs) may include sepsis and renal scarring, and accurate and early diagnosis is important. At the same time, avoiding unnecessary evaluation and treatment of children less at risk is cost effective and minimizes iatrogenic harm. Diagnosing UTIs in infants and young children can be challenging because the clinical signs are often nonspecific and obtaining urine specimens can be difficult.

Principles of Disease

The risk of developing UTIs before age 12 is approximately 3% for girls and 1% for boys. Although neonatal boys are more susceptible to UTIs than girls, beyond that period, UTIs in females prevail. Girls younger than 2 years and uncircumcised boys younger than 6 to 12 months are also especially at risk.

Seven percent of children younger than 2 years with a temperature greater than 39° C and presenting without a source of the fever have an occult UTI.[31] Moreover, up to 4% with a significant fever and an associated upper respiratory tract infection or acute otitis media may also have a UTI.[31,32] By comparison, the background prevalence of asymptomatic bacteriuria is estimated to be 1% to 2% of all children.[33]

On the basis of renal nuclear scans, it is estimated that 75% of children younger than 5 years with a febrile UTI have pyelonephritis.[31] Vesicoureteral reflux from the bladder into the ureter is a common cause of the pyelonephritis and renal scarring. A UTI in infants younger than 3 months is associated with bacteremia in up to 50% of cases; in children older than 3 months, the risk drops to 5%. Renal scarring can occur in 27% to 64% of children after pyelonephritis and may lead to renal failure and a risk of hypertension later in life.[31]

E. coli is the predominant cause of UTIs in children, with *Klebsiella* species more likely in newborn children. *Enterobacter*, *Proteus*, *Morganella*, *Serratia*, and *Salmonella* species are also important pathogens.[34] In neonates and young infants, bacteremia is considered the route of infection to the urinary tract. In older children, infection from the lower tract is often the cause of upper tract infection. A common cause of UTIs in toilet-trained females is believed to be improper wiping after urination. Young females should be taught to wipe from anterior to posterior, or front to back, after urination.

Clinical Features

Infants and Children Younger than 2 Years

Signs and symptoms are usually nonspecific and include decreased oral intake, lethargy, jaundice, fever, vomiting, abdominal pain, and irritability. Young children may not be able to verbalize when urination is painful. It is assumed that a UTI in this age group represents upper tract disease and would therefore arise with more systemic symptoms.

Children Older than 2 Years

UTIs in children older than 2 years can be either an isolated cystitis or more upper tract disease with more systemic symptoms. Cystitis is usually associated with local symptoms (i.e., suprapubic tenderness and dysuria). Pyelonephritis findings include fever, costovertebral angle tenderness, abdominal pain, vomiting, or ill appearance. New bedwetting may also be a sign of a UTI.

Diagnostic Strategies

There are various techniques for collecting urine samples from children. Because of the difficulty in cleaning the perineal area, the bag collection method poses an increased risk of contamination by periurethral flora, with false-positive results ranging from 12% to 83%.[31] Thus, the bag collection method is not recommended in infants and children who are not toilet trained. Because urethral catheterization is almost always successful, suprapubic aspiration to obtain a urine sample is rarely needed.[33,34] A suprapubic bladder aspiration is also used for young infants because the expanded bladder is located more intra-abdominally. Chances of a full bladder and successful aspiration improve if 45 to 60 minutes have elapsed since the last diaper change. The use of ultrasonography has been advocated to enhance the probability of obtaining urine by the suprapubic method.[35]

Urethral catheterization is relatively simple and poses little risk, although it may be more difficult in uncircumcised boys or in young infants. There is a slight risk of both trauma to the urethra and the introduction of bacteria into the urinary tract with this technique. A 5 French feeding tube can be used in young infants. Young male infants sometimes spontaneously urinate when the urethral meatus is cleansed; a midstream clean-catch urine specimen may then be obtained.

For a clean-catch urine sample from a toilet-trained child, the parent can clean the child with soap and water before urination. Children can be instructed to sit backward on the toilet to urinate, allowing the parent better access for obtaining the urine specimen. A urine sample with more than 10 white blood cells (WBCs) per high-power field and a large number of epithelial cells must be considered contaminated, and either an improved clean-catch method or catheterization must be tried. Females, regardless of age, with a vaginal discharge should be catheterized.

In children younger than 2 years, a urinalysis alone is not considered adequate for ruling out UTIs. As many as 10% to 50% of patients with UTIs can have a false-negative urinalysis.[36,37] Nitrite and leukocyte esterase urinalysis markers have the highest combined sensitivity and specificity for infection. If both markers are positive, the false-positive rate is less than 4%.[31] Gram staining the urine has a sensitivity of 93%.[31] Depending on the technique used to obtain the urine culture, criteria for a definite UTI vary (Table 172-1).

Renal function tests are rarely abnormal but should be performed in children with hypertension, hematuria, proteinuria, or signs of dehydration. Blood cultures, in general, are not indicated in the majority of children with UTIs. The true-positive rate of blood cultures in the presence of a UTI is low, and the organism identified is invariably the same as the organism in the urine culture.[38]

Differential Considerations

Underlying renal disease or urinary tract abnormality should be considered in a child presenting with hypertension, hematuria, or difficulty with urination or suspected in children with elevated BUN, creatinine or abnormal electrolytes, or acidosis on laboratory examination. CT of the abdomen may be necessary to delineate the extent of urinary tract abnormalities.

There are several other causes of dysuria in children (Box 172-1). Irritants such as bubble bath or soaps may cause a local irritation and dysuria. A retained foreign body in the vagina (such as toilet paper) can cause irritation or bacterial growth with associated dysuria and vaginal discharge. Pinworms in the genitourinary area can cause itching and scratching. Balanitis in uncircumcised males can also cause dysuria and pyuria.

Accidental injuries to the genital area can cause abrasions, lacerations, and subsequent dysuria. Sexual or physical abuse must be considered in any young child with a history of multiple UTIs.

Management

Infants Younger than 3 Months

Because of the risk of associated sepsis, infants younger than 3 months with a UTI should generally be admitted to the hospital for intravenous antibiotics (e.g., gentamicin and ampicillin).[39]

Children 3 Months to 2 Years

Although inpatient treatment of children with suspected pyelonephritis has traditionally been recommended, studies now show that well-appearing children without signs of toxicity may be managed as outpatients.[40] Community antimicrobial resistance patterns are important to consider when deciding

Table 172-1. Definitions of Urinary Tract Infections Based on Collection Technique

Urine Collection Technique	Infection
Suprapubic bladder aspiration	10 × 2 CFU/mL, one pathogen
Urethral catheterization	10 × 4 CFU/mL, one pathogen
Midstream clean catch	10 × 5 CFU/mL, one pathogen, two cultures*

CFU, colony-forming units.
*Suspicious for urinary tract infection if only one culture positive.
From Shaw KN, Gorelick MH: Urinary tract infection in the pediatric patient. *Pediatr Clin North Am* 46:1111, 1999.

BOX 172-1. Etiology of Dysuria in Children

Infection
Urinary tract infection including cystitis or pyelonephritis
Vaginitis resulting from *Gardnerella*, *Trichomonas, Candida,* or sexually transmitted organisms
Pinworms
Balanitis

Irritation
Bubble bath, new soaps, or douches
Vaginal foreign body, such as retained toilet paper

Trauma
Sexual or physical abuse
Straddle injury (unintentional)
Self-stimulation or masturbation

Other
Labial adhesions
Renal stones or hypercalciuria

on an appropriate antimicrobial. *E. coli* resistance to trimethoprim-sulfamethoxazole can be as high as 20% to 30% in some communities.[41] Administering the first dose of a parenteral or a double dose of an oral antibiotic appears to be equivalent. Because UTIs in this age group are considered to be upper tract disease processes, a longer course of antimicrobials is indicated (e.g., 10 to 14 days). Although a review of studies found no difference in the frequency of positive urine cultures between short-course therapy (2 to 4 days) and longer course therapy (7 to 14 days), most of these studies mixed children younger than 2 years with older children including adolescents. Thus, the recommendation for short-course therapy in children younger than 2 years is not supported at this time.[42] Follow-up in 2 to 3 days is essential to evaluate the culture and sensitivity results and to assess clinical status. The primary care physician can schedule additional follow-up and appropriate imaging studies to determine the presence of renal scarring, posterior urethral valves, or vesicoureteral reflux.[43]

Children Older than 2 Years

In older children with simple cystitis, a short 3-day course of antibiotics, such as trimethoprim-sulfamethoxazole or amoxicillin clavulanate, is adequate. Shorter courses result in higher failure rates and are not indicated. In older children with pyelonephritis, a longer course of antibiotics (generally 14 days) is recommended. In the adult population, a new study shows that a 7-day course of a fluoroquinolone is as effective as a 14-day course of trimethoprim-sulfamethoxazole.[44] In children, fluoroquinolones are still contraindicated because of the presumed effect on cartilage growth.

Disposition

Children with signs of toxicity, urinary obstruction, or inability to take oral medications should be admitted to the hospital for intravenous antibiotics.[45] Upon discharge, parents should be instructed to return if the child is unable to take the oral medication or if the symptoms worsen. The child may remain febrile for 48 hours despite adequate antimicrobial therapy. The child should be checked in 48 to 72 hours either in person or by telephone. At follow-up, the urine culture should be checked to ensure appropriate antimicrobial therapy.[46]

Hematuria

Perspective

Hematuria is common in the pediatric population. *Hematuria*, defined as two positive urine samples, has a prevalence rate of 1% to 2% in children ages 6 to 15 years old.[47] Microscopic hematuria is defined as more than 5 red blood cells (RBCs)/mm^3 and is detected using chemical reagent strips and microscopic urinalysis. Persistent hematuria is defined as three positive urinalyses over a 2- to 3-week period.[47] Macroscopic or gross hematuria is seen by the naked eye and may be associated with clots.

Principles of Disease

Hematuria results from RBCs entering the urinary tract. Inflammation, infection, trauma, or anatomic abnormalities can occur anywhere from the glomerulus to the urethra. The endothelium and basement membrane of the glomerulus are usually impervious to large proteins such as RBCs and hemoglobin, but myoglobin may pass freely. Damage to the glomerulus, however, may allow RBCs and hemoglobin to pass into the collecting system.

Urine with lysed RBCs is positive for hemoglobin, negative for RBCs, and may be pink in color. Urine containing myoglobin from muscle breakdown is positive for hemoglobin and negative for RBCs. Evaluation of creatine phosphokinase, fractionated bilirubin, and hematocrit can often help differentiate hemoglobinuria from myoglobinuria. Not all red urine contains blood. Certain drugs or foods such as phenothiazines, ibuprofen, beets, and blueberries can cause reddish-colored urine. In neonates, urate crystals can cause red-tinged urine in the diaper. *Serratia marcescens*, a fecal pathogen, can cause a red pigmentation when left in the diaper. Bleeding from the vagina or rectum can sometimes be mistaken for blood in the urine.

Clinical Features

The history and physical examination should focus on signs of infection, trauma, or bleeding disorders. Signs of renal disease (e.g., hypertension), edema, rales, or cardiac murmurs are important findings. An examination of the genitalia may reveal signs of inflammation or bleeding.

Differential Considerations

The etiologies of RBCs in the urine are diverse (Box 172-2). RBCs in the urine as a result of trauma are discussed elsewhere.

Extrarenal causes of hematuria include urethral valves and meatal stenosis. Extensive exercise can also cause hematuria as a result of both direct renal trauma and ischemic injury.

Intrarenal disorders include pyelonephritis, renal or bladder tumors, poststreptococcal acute glomerulonephritis, and basement membrane disease of the glomerulus.

Systemic illnesses that cause hematuria such as Henoch-Schönlein purpura (HSP) and hemolytic-uremic syndrome (HUS) are discussed later in this chapter. Other systemic causes of hematuria include bleeding disorders, aspirin, and anticoagulants.

Diagnostic Strategies

A urinalysis that shows more than five RBCs per high-power field indicate hematuria. The presence of WBCs or leukocyte esterase should be noted. Casts in the urine or proteinuria demonstrates a glomerular origin of the hematuria. If glomerular disease is suspected, a throat culture, antibody test for streptococcus, complement studies, an erythrocyte sedimentation rate, anti-

BOX 172-2. Etiology of Hematuria in Children

Extrarenal
Trauma
Meatal stenosis or posterior urethral valves
Exercise
Menstruation or rectal bleeding
Foreign bodies
Cystitis, urethritis, or epididymitis

Intrarenal
Pyelonephritis
Renal or bladder stones or tumors
Poststreptococcal or idiopathic glomerulonephritis
Acute interstitial nephritis
Acute tubular necrosis
Basement membrane glomerular disease
Renal vein or arterial thrombosis
Recurrent familial hematuria
Polycystic kidney disease

Systemic
Henoch-Schönlein purpura
Systemic lupus erythematosus
Hemolytic-uremic syndrome
Infectious mononucleosis
Sickle cell disease or other hemoglobinopathies
Bacterial endocarditis or artificial cardiac valves
Bleeding disorders, warfarin, or aspirin
Medications such as amitriptyline, chlorpromazine, contrast dyes
Munchausen's syndrome or factitious

nuclear antibody, or hepatitis B serology tests should be considered. If the patient has signs of hypertension, edema, or proteinuria, laboratory tests for electrolytes, total protein, and albumin should be ordered.[48]

A 24-hour urine collection for creatinine and protein should be evaluated for asymptomatic hematuria. Urine and plasma calcium levels should also be measured.

Noncontrast helical CT is the current study of choice for the identification of renal stones. It has exceptional sensitivity and specificity for calculi as small as 1 mm and can identify associated processes such as obstruction, hydroureter, hydrocalyx, and renal abscess. In addition, it has ability superior to that of intravenous pyelography to determine alternative diagnoses such as abdominal tumor.

Management

The management of the child with hematuria depends on the underlying cause. The management of a child with renal stones and renal tumors is discussed further.

Disposition

The disposition of a child with hematuria depends on the ultimate cause. Simple cystitis or pyelonephritis can be treated in the emergency department and followed by the child's primary care physician. A child diagnosed with a renal tumor or stone should be referred to a nephrologist or urologist. Children with acute renal failure, especially with those with signs of fluid overload or hyperkalemia, need admission to the hospital.

Renal Stones

Perspective

Renal stones result from a complex process of crystallization involving growth inhibitors and promoters and urine pH and flow. Congenital abnormalities, trauma, or infection can also be an inciting cause. An increased risk for hypercalciuria and the production of renal stones is often inherited.

Principles of Disease

Renal stones are uncommon in children, with approximately 1 case for every 1000 pediatric admissions.[49] Calcium-containing stones are responsible for approximately 60% of all cases, followed by struvite (infection), uric acid, and cystine stones.[49] Renal stones are three to four times more common in white children than in nonwhite children. Family history also seems to play a role in the production of kidney stones.[50]

Clinical Features

The signs and symptoms of renal stones in older children typically include colicky flank pain, vomiting, and hematuria. Younger children with renal stones can also present with less specific complaints, such as nontender abdominal pain, vomiting, or malaise. In a study from the United Kingdom, 17% of patients with pediatric renal stones were found to present only with hematuria and without flank or abdominal pain.[50] When taking histories of children with possible renal stones, previous UTIs, especially those caused by organisms such as *Proteus* species, family history of renal stones, diet (including excessive vitamin use), and fluid intake must be noted.

Obstruction of the collecting system can sometimes lead to infection, papillary necrosis, or decreasing renal function. Fever in the presence of a renal stone should be taken as an indicator of upper tract infection.

Diagnostic Strategies

Children suspected of having renal stones should have their urine checked for hematuria, leukocytes, and bacteria. The urine should be strained and any crystals should be sent for analysis. Other laboratory tests to consider are CBC, electrolytes, BUN, creatinine, uric acid, total protein, and albumin. Ninety percent of renal calculi are visible on a plain abdominal radiograph, although stool can sometimes obscure the view. Other types of calcifications appearing on plain abdominal radiographs include gallstones, phleboliths, vessel or lymph node calcifications, and calcified malignancies.

Children with suspected kidney stones should have a non–contrast-enhanced CT scan of the urinary tract, called a CT urogram. A CT urogram may be obtained to define the anatomy and other potential causes of hematuria, such as a tumor or pyelonephritis; a CT urogram also avoids the use of nephrotoxic contrast material. The intravenous pyelogram should be reserved for institutions without access to CT.

Differential Considerations

The differential diagnosis for a child with colicky flank or abdominal pain is long. Gastroenteritis and constipation are more common causes of colicky abdominal pain in young children than kidney stones. Intussusception most commonly occurs in children younger than 2 years and can arise with intermittent abdominal pain. In adolescents, biliary colic and intermittent gonadal torsion must also be considered.

Management

Initial pain management should include a narcotic analgesic in conjunction with a longer acting, nonsteroidal anti-inflammatory drug (NSAID). The analgesic effect of NSAIDs is directly related to the inhibition of prostaglandin-mediated contraction of the ureter and is characteristic of all NSAIDS (e.g., ibuprofen, naproxen, and ketorolac). Patients with signs of volume depletion or with a history of fever, vomiting, or poor fluid intake should be hydrated to improve urine flow and prevent urinary stasis, which may contribute to stone formation. Excessive fluid administration to increase urine flow to enhance movement of the stone down the urinary tract, however, has not been proved effective.

After cultures have been obtained, infected urinary tracts with stones should be treated with antibiotics; patients generally require hospitalization. Children with larger renal stones may undergo shockwave lithotripsy as a therapeutic modality.

Children with normal renal function and adequate pain control, without signs of toxicity or renal infection, can be safely discharged home with good follow-up. Follow-up with a nephrologist or urologist may include testing of parathyroid hormone, fasting urine samples for calcium/creatinine ratio, or 24-hour urine collection for calcium, magnesium, phosphorus, uric acid, oxalate, cystine, protein, and creatinine.[49,51]

Renal Tumors

Perspective

Abdominal masses in children are not uncommon, and in infants the vast majority are benign renal tumors or cysts.[52]

Principles of Disease

Renal tumors in children can range from the benign cystic nephroma to the more aggressive malignant rhabdoid tumor. The prognosis for the child depends on the type and staging of the renal tumor.

Clinical Features

The most frequent presentation for a child with a renal tumor is an abdominal mass found by the parent while the child is being bathed or dressed. Hematuria or pain is a less common presentation compared with that in the adult population.

Diagnostic Strategies

As a significant number of abdominal masses are the result of renal cysts, renal ultrasonography is the imaging study of choice. Ultrasonography can define the mass in question and is not associated with exposure to radiation. Laboratory tests should include CBC, platelet count, BUN, creatinine, urinalysis, and urine catecholamines. Urinary catecholamines are increased in 95% of neuroblastoma patients but are normal in cases of a Wilms tumor. Any solid masses found on ultrasonography should be better defined by CT of the abdomen. If the mass appears malignant, a CT scan of the chest is indicated to look for pulmonary metastases.[53]

Differential Considerations

The differential diagnosis for a renal mass includes cystic lesions such as those of polycystic kidney diseases or severe hydronephrosis resulting from obstruction or severe reflux. Solid masses include Wilms' tumor, renal cell carcinoma, mesoblastic nephromas, and cystic nephromas.

Management and Disposition

Management depends on the function of the urinary tract. Because the renal mass usually involves only one kidney, renal function is usually maintained.

A preliminary diagnosis of the etiology of the mass should be obtained before discharging the child. Well-appearing children with normal renal function who can be assured close follow-up may be managed as outpatients. Because of the potential seriousness of a renal tumor, admission should be considered for all children. Consultation with a nephrologist, urologist, and hematologist-oncologist can be coordinated during admission.

Proteinuria

Perspective

The normal glomerulus is relatively impervious to albumin, a high-molecular-weight protein. Low-molecular-weight proteins, however, pass through the glomeruli and are reabsorbed in the proximal tubule. Proteinuria can result from either increased passage through the glomeruli or decreased reabsorption by the tubules. In most cases, proteinuria is benign and asymptomatic. If the amount of protein lost is significant, such as in nephrotic syndrome, the resultant hypoalbuminemia (albumin less than 2 g/dL and protein less than 4 g/dL) may cause ascites and generalized edema.

Principles of Disease

Proteinuria is a common finding in children. Trace to mild proteinuria (1+ to 2+) can be seen in up to 85%

of children and adolescents screened, especially during the summer months.[54,55]

Clinical Features

Clinical features found in a proteinuric child depend on the etiology of the proteinuria. Recent pharyngitis, presence of hematuria, changes in weight or urine output, or family history of proteinuria should be investigated. Abnormal findings may include hypertension, edema, ascites, or palpable kidneys in infants. A butterfly rash of systemic lupus or the purpuric rash of HSP may be present.

Differential Diagnosis

Causes of proteinuria can be divided into glomerular and tubular. Glomerular causes include nephrotic syndrome, glomerulonephritis, and posttransplantation rejection. Transient causes of altered glomerular function include exercise, fever, and seizures. Tubular etiologies include heavy-metal poisoning, UTIs, diabetes, and asymptomatic proteinuria.[54,55] False-positive results for proteinuria on a urinary dipstick can occur when the urine is alkaline or when it contains mucus, blood, vaginal secretions, semen, or a significant number of inflammatory cells.

Orthostatic proteinuria is a benign condition characterized by the presence of protein in the urine collected in an upright position but not in samples collected from a supine child. Proteinuria that is persistent or associated with hematuria or other signs of renal disease is usually a sign of a more serious condition.

Diagnostic Strategies

Proteinuria 2+ or less (equivalent to 100 mg/dL or less) requires no further management unless there are signs of infection. Proteinuria 3+ or greater (equivalent to 300 mg/dL or greater) should be evaluated with laboratory tests for serum total protein and albumin, serum electrolytes, BUN, and creatinine and urine culture. A 24-hour urine collection for protein is also indicated. The urine protein/creatinine ratio (urine Pr/Cr mg/dL) in a random urine sample, however, correlates strongly with the protein levels found in a 24-hour urine collection.[54] Urine Pr/Cr of less than 0.2 mg/dL is considered normal for children older than 2 years and for adults. Children 6 months to 2 years old have a ratio of less than 0.5 mg/dL. A urine Pr/Cr greater than 3.0 mg/dL is consistent with nephrotic syndrome.

Antistreptolysin O (ASO) titer can be measured to prove a previous streptococcal infection that is causing the proteinuria. In young children, renal ultrasonography detects polycystic disease or anatomic abnormalities. Referral to primary care or pediatric nephrology for follow-up and renal biopsy is indicated. Renal biopsy may be indicated in patients with increased creatinine levels, low complement levels, or hematuria.[56]

Management

The management of a child found to have proteinuria depends on the ultimate cause. Management of children with poststreptococcal glomerulonephritis and nephrotic syndrome is discussed further.

Disposition

A child with significant edema and ascites from the loss of albumin needs to be hospitalized. Children with significant hypertension as a result of glomerulonephritis or with marked impairment of renal function also need to be hospitalized. Well-appearing children who can be assured good follow-up can be discharged from the emergency department.

Poststreptococcal Glomerulonephritis

Perspective

Poststreptococcal glomerulonephritis (PSGN) is one of the sequelae of streptococcal pharyngitis. Treatment of streptococcus pharyngitis with antibiotics has not been shown definitively to decrease the incidence of PSGN, as opposed to acute rheumatic fever, another sequela of streptococcal pharyngitis.

Principles of Disease

This disease is not well understood but probably results from circulating immune complexes deposited in the kidney.[57] These result in decreased glomerular filtration, allowing proteins to flow freely into the urine.

Clinical Features

PSGN occurs most commonly in children 3 to 7 years of age, usually with a history of pharyngitis with fever 2 weeks before the onset of glomerulonephritis. Symptoms can be either localized to the urinary tract, arising as hematuria or flank pain, or appear less specific, including lethargy or generalized edema. Some children may present with more significant symptoms such as pulmonary edema, cardiac arrhythmias, or significant hypertension. Renal failure is found in 2% of these patients.[58,59]

Diagnostic Strategies

Urinalysis shows significant blood and protein, with RBC casts in 60% of cases. Pyuria with granular or hyaline casts may also be found.

The ASO and immunoglobulin G levels should be elevated. Total complement levels, especially C3, are decreased in most patients during the first 2 weeks of the illness. The complement levels should return to normal within 3 to 4 weeks. The BUN is elevated; hyponatremia and hyperkalemia may also be present.[59]

Differential Considerations

The differential diagnosis includes the entities previously mentioned regarding proteinuria, including nephrotic syndrome and UTI.

Management and Disposition

Management includes restricting fluid and salt intake and sometimes using diuretics. A child with significant hypertension, congestive heart failure, or uremia requires inpatient management. Significant hypertension should be managed as outlined in the section on hypertension.

Children with mild symptoms who can be assured good follow-up can be managed on an outpatient basis.

Nephrotic Syndrome

Perspective

Nephrotic syndrome is characterized by hypoproteinemia, proteinuria, and edema. Primary nephrotic syndrome applies to diseases limited to the kidney; renal biopsy is used to categorize patients and determine therapeutic and prognostic decisions. Secondary nephrotic syndrome results from systemic illnesses such as PSGN.

Principles of Disease

From 2 to 7 cases of nephrotic syndrome per 100,000 children are discovered each year.[56] Boys are affected twice as often as girls, but the distribution equalizes by adulthood. Primary nephrotic syndrome occurs more commonly in children younger than 5 years and secondary nephrotic syndrome more often in older children. Ninety percent of nephrotic children have the primary disease, with 85% having minimal change nephrotic syndrome, 10% focal sclerosis, and 5% mesangial proliferation (referring to the thin membrane supporting capillaries surrounding the tubule of nephrons).

The etiology of primary nephrotic syndrome is thought to be idiopathic, but various theories involving bacterial or viral infections, allergic reactions (pollens, poison ivy), or drug ingestions (heroin, mercury) have been investigated.[56]

Clinical Features

Characteristics of nephrotic syndrome include edema, hypoalbuminemia, proteinuria, and hyperlipidemia. The onset of edema may be insidious, beginning with periorbital edema. As weight increases, pants and shoes may not fit. The edema progresses but the child usually does not appear ill unless pulmonary edema or ascites is present. Anorexia, nausea, and vomiting may be present because of edema of the intestine. Hypertension, hematuria, or oliguria may be present. Acute renal failure is rare in primary nephrotic syndrome.

Nephrotic children are also at risk for thrombosis, with 2% of nephrotic children having thromboembolic complications.[60] Renal veins are particularly vulnerable to thrombosis, as characterized by flank pain, hematuria, and worsening renal function. Nephrotic children should not undergo punctures to deep vessels because of this risk of thrombosis.

Children with nephrotic syndrome taking corticosteroids are also at risk for side effects of corticosteroid use. Acute mood changes, from depression to mania, are associated with steroids. Irritability, excessive crying, and sleeping difficulties can result.

Because of steroid therapy and decreased levels of immunoglobulins, nephrotic children are at risk for bacterial infections, such as *E. coli* and *Streptococcus pneumoniae*.

Diagnostic Strategies

Proteinuria in nephrotic syndrome is defined as greater than 3.5 g of protein per 1.73 m^2 per 24 hours or greater than 50 mg/kg per 24 hours. This corresponds to 3+ or 4+ on the dipstick reading. Specific gravity may be high because of the proteinuria. Microscopic hematuria may also be present. Total serum protein is usually low at 4.5 to 5.5 g/dL and serum albumin is less than 2 g/dL.

Hyperlipidemia may occur because of the increased serum cholesterol. Hyponatremia may be present, but other electrolytes are usually normal. If an elevated cholesterol level is present, the lowered sodium level may be a combination of true and pseudo-hyponatremia. BUN and creatinine are also usually normal, and hemoglobin and hematocrit levels may be elevated because of hemoconcentration.

Chest radiographs sometimes show pleural effusions or pulmonary edema. The heart appears normal or small because of hypovolemia. An abdominal radiograph may reveal ascites, and ultrasonography may show a renal abnormality.

Renal biopsy is important for diagnostic and therapeutic decisions and should be obtained in older children or if there is evidence of hematuria, elevated BUN, persistent hypertension, or failure to respond to steroids.

Differential Considerations

Other renal diseases that cause edema include glomerulonephritis and renal failure. A vasculitis or acute thrombosis of the renal vessels must also be considered. Gastrointestinal causes that produce hypoproteinemia include cirrhosis, cystic fibrosis, and protein-losing enteritides.

Management

Despite the edema, children with signs of hypovolemia or shock need to be resuscitated with crystalloid. Hypertension may result from the intrinsic disease. Prompt recognition and treatment for the hypertension are important.

After consultation with a pediatric nephrologist, patients between 12 months and 5 years of age with no gross hematuria and no large loss of protein or complement can be treated with corticosteroids. After the initial evaluation is completed, including a tuberculin test, prednisone at 2 mg/kg per 24 hours orally divided twice or three times a day can be initiated. Relapses or steroid resistance may necessitate a second course of steroids.[56]

Diuretics such as furosemide 1 to 2 mg/kg per 24 hours orally or IV in divided doses may be necessary if respiratory distress or significant ascites is present. Salt restriction may be required. Fluid intake should be restricted only if edema is present despite salt restriction or if the child exhibits hyponatremia because of an impaired ability to excrete excess water.

The relatively immunocompromised state of nephrotic children increases the risk of infection. A fever or signs of peritonitis must be evaluated thoroughly. A paracentesis should be performed and fluid sent for cell count and differential, Gram stain, and culture. Admission and antibiotics with activity against *S. pneumoniae* and *E. coli* are appropriate.[56]

Disposition

Newly diagnosed patients should be admitted for initial evaluation, treatment, and education of both patient and parents. Patients with signs of shock or respiratory distress should be admitted to the hospital after initial stabilization. Other patients with suspected bacterial infections, peritonitis, edema refractory to therapy, or evidence of renal insufficiency should also be admitted.

Acute Renal Failure

Perspective

Acute renal failure results from a decrease in the glomerular filtration rate. Blood pressure, acid-base balance, removal of nitrogen waste, and fluid management may all be affected. The incidence of acute renal failure is unknown, but large children's hospitals may see 30 to 50 new cases each year.

Principles of Disease

Acute renal failure can be divided into three categories: prerenal, which involves decreased renal perfusion; renal, which is caused by parenchymal damage; and postrenal, which involves obstruction of the urinary tract (Box 172-3).

Causes of prerenal failure include hypovolemia resulting from a variety of factors (e.g., dehydration, burns, or hemorrhage), shock (e.g., sepsis or anaphylaxis), and congestive heart failure (e.g., decreased cardiac output). Obstruction of the renal artery or thrombosis of the renal vein can also cause acute renal failure.

Intrarenal causes result from damage to the nephron. Glomerular damage most commonly results from PSGN. Systemic lupus erythematosus, HUS, and sepsis with hypoperfusion are systemic causes of renal failure. Tubular damage can result from heavy-metal poisonings or hemoglobin-myoglobin in the tubules from a crush injury, burn, or hemolytic crisis. Cases of acute renal failure in dehydrated children after NSAID use have been reported.[61] Postrenal failure resulting from an obstruction in the urinary tract may be caused by infection, tumor, renal stones, or posterior urethral valves. Bilateral obstruction of the kidneys is usually necessary for renal failure.

Clinical Features

A child with acute renal failure has an increase in nitrogen wastes shown by an increase in BUN and creatinine levels. A decrease in urine output is sometimes seen. Urinary output of 1 mL/kg/hr is usually considered adequate, but the output may be lower if the patient is dehydrated. Nephrotoxic agents such as certain aminoglycosides can actually increase the urinary output because of renal tubular damage, but an elevated BUN and creatinine are still present.

Acute renal failure can result in life-threatening complications that must be recognized and treated promptly. These include severe hyperkalemia, pulmonary edema or fluid overload, hypertensive encephalopathy, septic shock from renal obstruction and infection, and seizures from metabolic abnormalities or encephalopathy.[62]

Diagnostic Strategies

Preliminary laboratory tests should include CBC, electrolytes, calcium, phosphorus, BUN, creatinine, and a urinalysis with microscopy and culture. Diagnostic studies such as ASO titer (for acute PSGN), C3 complement (for lupus), total serum albumin, cholesterol, and albumin/globulin ratio (for nephrotic syndrome and cirrhosis) may be obtained. RBC casts in the urine indicate glomerulonephritis. WBC casts indicate infection as an etiology, whereas hyaline casts suggest dehydration or acute tubular necrosis.[63]

BOX 172-3. Acute Renal Failure Etiologies in Children

Prerenal

Decreased Intravascular Volume or Dehydration

Burns or hemorrhage
Third spacing
Sepsis

Decreased Cardiac Output

Cardiac shock

Decreased Renal Arterial Blood Flow

Intrarenal

Glomerular Disease

Poststreptococcal and other glomerulonephritis
Pyelonephritis

Systemic Causes

Hemolytic-uremic syndrome
Henoch-Schönlein purpura or other vasculitides
Systemic lupus erythematosus
Sepsis or other causes of prolonged decreased perfusion

Toxins

Heavy metal poisonings such as lead, gold
Myoglobin or hemoglobin deposits
Antibiotics such as aminoglycosides
Anticonvulsants such as phenytoin
Contrast dyes

Postrenal

Obstructive

Nephrolithiasis or tumor
Posturethral valves
Intra-abdominal tumor obstructing urinary flow
Infection

Renal Vein Thrombosis

Ultrasonography is the test of choice for the preliminary evaluation of obstructive causes of renal failure. A noncontrast CT urogram can also readily identify the site of obstruction and avoids the use of nephrotoxic contrast material. A voiding cystourethrogram shows extrinsic pressure on the bladder by posterior urethral valves.

Differential Considerations

Significant dehydration can result in temporary decreased urine output and a slight rise in BUN and creatinine. After hydration and repletion of intravascular volume, urine output should improve and the elevated BUN and creatinine should resolve. Processes that can result in retention of fluids with associated renal failure include liver disease and decreased cardiac output.

Management

The initial management of a child with acute renal failure depends on the clinical evaluation. If hypovolemia resulting from dehydration or blood loss is thought to be the cause of the renal failure, immediate rehydration is necessary. A 20 mL/kg bolus of crystalloid should be given to prevent possible progression to acute tubular necrosis. If there is no urinary response after two boluses of crystalloid, diuretics may be useful in the euvolemic patient. Furosemide 1 mg/kg/dose every 2 to 6 hours IV may be tried if there is no evidence of obstruction. Bumetanide 0.015 to 0.1 mg/kg/dose every 6 to 24 hours IV (maximum 10 mg per 24 hours) can be useful if furosemide has no effect. Mannitol 0.75 g/kg/dose every 6 hours IV may also be helpful but is contraindicated if there is evidence of obstruction.

If a child is considered euvolemic and has no urine output despite diuretic therapy, renal-dose dopamine should be initiated (2 to 5 μg/kg/min). Consultation with a nephrologist is necessary.[62]

If hypertension with encephalopathy develops, a controlled 10% to 20% reduction in blood pressure should be achieved using nitroprusside or other IV blood pressure agents. Oral medications such as nifedipine or captopril are useful but are associated with a risk of the blood pressure dropping precipitously. Overaggressive reduction in blood pressure can result in hypoperfusion of central target organs such as the brain, heart, and kidneys that have become accustomed to higher perfusion pressures. Further discussion of hypertensive emergencies and treatment can be found in Chapter 83.

Hyperkalemia can result in cardiac dysrhythmias. Potassium levels higher than 6.5 mEq/L may cause changes on the electrocardiogram (ECG) such as peaked T waves and, if significant, widened QRS complexes. Hyperkalemia with resultant ECG changes should be treated with calcium chloride 20 to 30 mg/kg/dose (0.2 to 0.3 mL/kg/dose) IV over 10 to 15 minutes (maximum 500 mg or 5 mL/dose). Calcium alters the cardiac cells' action potentials, thereby decreasing the risk of arrhythmias. Calcium may be repeated in 5 minutes.

Sodium bicarbonate 1 to 2 mEq/kg/dose IV every 4 hours can also be administered. The resultant alkalosis helps move the potassium intracellularly by exchanging H^+ for K^+. Continued therapy with sodium bicarbonate should be administered in conjunction with pediatric nephrology as there is a risk of increasing volume load with repetitive dosages of sodium. Potassium binding agents such as sodium polystyrene sulfonate (Kayexalate) are administered orally or rectally and exchange sodium for potassium at a 1:1 ratio.

Glucose (50% dextrose in water) 0.5 to 1 g/kg should be given along with regular insulin (1 U for every 4 g of glucose administered). The insulin temporarily shifts the potassium intracellularly.

Nebulized albuterol can be also be used to shift potassium temporarily into the cells and lower serum K^+ by 1 to 1.5 mEq/L over 30 minutes.[64] Severe cases and those associated with renal failure should be immediately referred to a pediatric nephrologist for emergent dialysis.[62]

Acute renal failure may lead to seizures caused either by hypertensive encephalopathy or a metabolic derangement—most commonly hyponatremia resulting from dilution of the sodium by free water. Intractable hyponatremic seizures may rarely necessitate the use of hypertonic saline (3% normal saline). The amount of hypertonic saline to be administered may be calculated using the following formula:

Determine the amount of sodium milliequivalents needed to reach a level of at least 125 mEq/L: 0.6 × (body weight in kg) × (125 mEq/L measured sodium). There are 513 mEq/L of sodium in hypertonic saline.

Determine the volume of hypertonic saline needed to deliver the required amount of sodium:

Required sodium/513 mEq/L = volume of hypertonic saline to be infused. One half of this volume is administered in the first hour and the second half administered in the second hour if the patient remains symptomatic.

Normal saline (0.9%) is relatively hypertonic compared with serum and therefore may also be helpful in correcting the hyponatremia. Water restriction along with the administration of saline is usually only a temporary treatment because many of these hyponatremic patients ultimately require dialysis.

Sodium bicarbonate can also correct a persistent metabolic acidosis and maintain pH 7.1 or greater and a serum bicarbonate level of 15 mEq/L. The base deficit can determine the amount of bicarbonate needed: base deficit = 0.6 × (body weight in kg) × (desired bicarbonate level − the observed level), all divided by 2. Half the replacement is given in the first 3 hours with the remainder given over the next 24 hours.

Hemodialysis or peritoneal dialysis may be indicated for refractory fluid overload associated with hypertension, congestive heart failure, pulmonary edema, severe hyperkalemia, hypo- or hypernatremia, metabolic acidosis, myoglobinuria resulting from burn or crush injuries, or HUS with hemoglobinuria or encephalopathy.[62]

Table 172-2. Blood Pressure Limits in Children

Age (years)	Systolic (Upper Limit)	Diastolic (Upper Limit)
0-2	110	65
3-6	120	70
7-10	130	75
11-15	140	80

From Daniels SR: Consultation with the specialist. The diagnosis of hypertension in children: An update. *Pediatr Rev* 18:131, 1997.

Disposition

All children with acute renal failure should be admitted to the hospital. Any child with signs of congestive heart failure, pulmonary edema, significant hyperkalemia, or acidosis should be admitted to a monitored bed.

Hypertension

Perspective

Hypertension is defined as a systolic or diastolic blood pressure higher than 2 standard deviations above the mean for the age and sex of the patient (Table 172-2). This diagnosis requires three or more accurately measured blood pressures over the course of several weeks. A correct cuff size should be chosen (i.e., air bladder should cover 80% to 100% of the circumference and two thirds of the length of the upper arm).[58] It is recommended that all children receive yearly blood pressure measurements starting at the age of 3 years.[58] A child who is in pain or agitated may have falsely elevated blood pressure readings.

Principles of Disease

Hypertension occurs throughout childhood in both males and females. It probably occurs more often in black children than in white children, just as in the adult population. Predisposing factors include obesity, physical inactivity, and a strong family history.

Just as in adulthood, primary or essential hypertension is unrelated to a second systemic disease. Children diagnosed with primary hypertension are more likely to become adults with hypertension.[58] Secondary hypertension results from endocrinologic, cardiac, neurologic, or other factors such as certain drugs or poisons (Box 172-4). Children with significant hypertension usually have an underlying renal (glomerulonephritis) or renovascular cause.

BOX 172-4. Etiology of Hypertension in Children

Primary (or Essential)

Secondary

Renal

Glomerulonephritis
Henoch-Schönlein purpura
Pyelonephritis
Obstruction or reflux
Polycystic kidney disease
Diabetic nephropathy
Trauma
Renal transplant or hemodialysis
Tuberous sclerosis
Systemic lupus nephritis

Endocrine

Pheochromocytoma
Cushing's syndrome
Congenital adrenal hyperplasia
Corticosteroid treatment
Hyperthyroidism
Neuroblastoma
Ovarian tumor

Cardiac

Congestive heart failure
Coarctation of the aorta

Vascular

Hemolytic-uremic syndrome
Kawasaki syndrome
Renal artery thrombosis or stenosis

Neurology

Central nervous system tumor or infection
Central nervous system trauma or abuse
Increased intracranial pressure
Guillain-Barré syndrome

Oncology

Neuroblastoma
Wilms' tumor
Pheochromocytoma
Adrenal carcinoma

Drugs

Corticosteroids
Cocaine
Sympathomimetics
Oral contraceptives
Phencyclidine
Beta-blocker or clonidine withdrawal
Lead, mercury

Others

Iatrogenic fluid overload
Volume overload from end-stage renal disease

Clinical Features

There are a variety of clinical presentations of hypertension in children. First, asymptomatic or mildly symptomatic hypertension may show up in routine vital signs measured in children evaluated in the emergency department for unrelated illnesses. When asked, these children may complain of headaches, abdominal pain, irritability, or nose bleeds. Although the relationship between hypertension and epistaxis has not been substantiated in the literature, patients may present with nasal bleeding. Sometimes personality changes and difficulties in school are noted.

Urgent hypertension results in severe elevations in systolic or diastolic blood pressures (younger than 10 years of age: systolic blood pressure 160 mm Hg or higher, diastolic blood pressure 105 mm Hg or higher; older than 10 years of age: systolic blood pressure 170 mm Hg or higher, diastolic blood pressure 110 mm Hg or higher) but without signs of end-organ damage.

BOX 172-5. Diagnostic Evaluation in Hypertensive Children

Hypertensive Emergency (i.e., Evidence of End-Organ Damage)?

1. History of medications or drugs, or family history of cardiovascular disorders
2. Symptoms of headache or chest pain
3. Physical examination focused on acute neurological changes, funduscopic changes, pulmonary edema
4. Urinalysis for significant protein
5. Chest radiograph for cardiomegaly or congestive heart failure
6. Electrocardiogram for ventricular hypertrophy

Primary or Secondary Cause? Laboratory and Radiologic Tests to Consider

1. Urinalysis and urine culture
2. Urine catecholamines
3. Complete blood count with platelet count
4. Blood smear
5. Sodium, potassium, chloride, carbon dioxide, calcium, phosphorus, magnesium, uric acid
6. Blood urea nitrogen, creatinine
7. Serum C3 complement, antistreptolysin O titer, antinuclear antibody
8. Plasma renin level
9. Computed tomography urogram or intravenous pyelogram
10. Voiding cystourethrogram
11. Renal ultrasound or scan
12. Renal arteriogram

Hypertensive emergencies have clinical signs of end-organ damage. A severe elevation in blood pressure is associated with acute neurologic changes or encephalopathy, pulmonary edema, myocardial ischemia, or proteinuria. The ECG may show signs of ischemia or ventricular hypertrophy. Chest radiography may reveal cardiomegaly or pulmonary edema. Hypertensive emergencies require prompt recognition and treatment. However, overaggressive treatment of long-standing hypertension can produce relative hypotension and lead to worsening neurologic sequelae.

Hypertensive encephalopathy symptoms include headache, vomiting, altered mental status, visual disturbances (including blurry vision and diplopia), and seizures or stroke. Papilledema, decreased retinal venous pulsations, and cranial nerve palsies may be found on examination. The diagnosis is confirmed when the symptoms and signs improve rapidly after the blood pressure is lowered. Headache alone without any other associated symptoms or signs is not generally considered a hypertensive emergency.

Diagnostic Strategies

In addition to a thorough history and physical examination, laboratory and radiologic studies performed in the emergency department can often determine both the cause of the hypertension and whether a hypertensive emergency exists (Box 172-5).

Differential Considerations

Any situation that causes undue agitation or pain in a child can cause a transient rise in blood pressure. Therefore, the diagnosis of hypertension in a child should be based only on carefully measured blood pressures in a nonagitated child over several weeks. Secondary hypertension is more likely in symptomatic younger children, especially those without a strong family history.

Other diagnoses with presentations similar to that of hypertensive encephalopathy include meningitis, brain tumor, intracerebral hemorrhage, stroke, and uremia. These conditions, however, generally produce only a mild increase in the systolic blood pressure[65]; CT or lumbar puncture can also help identify these other diagnoses.

Management

The management of hypertensive emergencies is also discussed in Chapter 83. When a child with severe hypertension is seen in the emergency department, questions should focus on a history of hypertension, UTIs, hematuria, edema, or umbilical artery catheterization. A history of joint pain or swelling, palpitations, weight loss, flushing of the skin, drug ingestion, or family history is important.

A physical examination emphasizing the central nervous system and cardiopulmonary system is indicated. Examination of the fundus may reveal papilledema or hemorrhages. Signs of congestive heart failure or a difference in the upper and lower extremity blood pressures should be noted. A renal cause of the hypertension may be revealed by the presence of peripheral edema or palpable kidneys. An abdominal or flank bruit suggests renovascular hypertension. Initial laboratory tests should include a CBC, electrolytes, BUN, creatinine, urinalysis, urine culture, chest radiograph, and ECG.

A child with findings consistent with a hypertensive emergency (e.g., acute end-organ damage as found by physical examination, laboratory, or radiologic results) should have intravenous access and be monitored with continuous blood pressure readings; an arterial catheter is preferable. The goal of therapy is to reduce the mean arterial blood pressure by 10% to 20% over several minutes to hours, depending on the nature of the emergency. Headache and vomiting require blood pressure control over several hours, whereas intracranial bleeding or herniation requires reduction over several minutes. β-Blockers are contraindicated in patients with decreased cardiac output and clinical signs of congestive heart failure. Oral nifedipine is contraindicated in a patient with signs of end-organ damage, such as intracerebral bleeding, because of the inability to control the amount of blood pressure reduction. To avoid overaggressive treatment and resultant relative hypotension, medications that can be controlled by intravenous infusions are preferred (Table 172-3).

A hypertensive urgency is severe hypertension without evidence of end-organ damage. These patients should be started or restarted on antihypertensives to

Table 172-3. Medications Used in Hypertensive Emergencies

Medication	Dose	Time to Repeat Dose	Duration of Effect	Side Effects
Nitroprusside	0.3-0.5 µg/kg/min IV (max 10 µg/kg/min)	30-60 min	During infusion	Headache, abdominal pain, chest pain, gastrointestinal upset, seizures, thiocyanate and cyanide toxicity**
Hydralazine*	0.1-0.2 mg/kg IV (max 20 mg) slowly over 15 min	10-20 min	4-12 hr	Tachycardia, skin flushing, headache, vomiting, diarrhea, hypotension
Labetalol†,‡	May bolus 0.2-1 mg/kg IV (max 20 mg), then 0.4-1 mg/kg/hr IV (max 3 mg/kg/hr)	10 min	6 hr, but variable	Gastrointestinal upset, headache, sedation
Esmolol§,‖,¶	Load 100-500 µg/kg IV over 1-2 min, then maintenance 25-100 µg/kg/min	10 min	During infusion	Similar to labetalol
Phentolamine	0.1 mg/kg/dose IV (max 5 mg)	30 min	30-60 min	Tachycardia, abdominal pain

*Use with caution in renal patients.
†Avoid in asthma, pulmonary edema, and heart block.
‡Avoid in second and third trimesters of pregnancy.
§If inadequate response, readminister loading dose or increase maintenance dose by 25-50 µg/kg/min every 5-10 minutes.
‖Usual maintenance range 50-500 µg/kg/min.
¶Morphine may increase esmolol levels.
**Avoid in pregnancy.
Note: Diazoxide no longer recommended because of potential for acute drop in blood pressure.

prevent end-organ sequelae. Angiotensin-converting enzyme inhibitors or calcium channel blockers are useful as first-line therapy and are usually well tolerated. The child may be observed for a few hours after administration of the medication to evaluate effectiveness or complications. With no evidence of acute end-organ damage, the child can be safely discharged home, assuming good follow-up can be ensured.

Children with mildly elevated blood pressures (5 to 10 mm Hg above normal) unrelated to the emergency department visit require repeated blood pressure measurements before treatment for hypertension is begun. If the blood pressure is moderately elevated and the patient is asymptomatic, the patient may be discharged home for outpatient workup of the hypertension and follow-up with the patient's primary care physician for monitoring of blood pressure values. Thiazide diuretics or β-blockers may be started at low doses.

Disposition

A child with evidence of a hypertensive emergency (i.e., acute end-organ damage) must be admitted to a monitored bed for evaluation and treatment. A child with significantly elevated blood pressure, but without evidence of end-organ damage, can be discharged home assuming good follow-up can be ensured.

Henoch-Schönlein Purpura

Perspective

Henoch-Schönlein purpura is an immunoglobulin A–mediated systemic vasculitis involving the small blood vessels supplying the skin, gastrointestinal tract, and joints.[66] The peak incidence of HSP is between 4 and 7 years of age, with an overall occurrence rate of 13.5 episodes per 100,000 children annually.

Principles of Disease

Immune complex deposition results in a systemic vasculitis, with up to 33% of patients experiencing recurrences.[67] Approximately 50% of affected children have a history of previous upper respiratory tract infection, and as many as 75% have group A beta-hemolytic streptococcus cultured from the oropharynx. Other theorized predisposing factors include exposure to cold weather, certain foods, drugs, and insect bites. Varicella-zoster virus, *Mycoplasma* species, parvovirus, *Campylobacter enteritis,* parvovirus B19, and Epstein-Barr virus have also been implicated.

Clinical Features

The hallmark of HSP is a palpable, purpuric, or petechial rash most prominent on the lower extremities, starting around the lateral malleoli and extending to the buttocks. The cutaneous manifestations are the initial presenting complaint in 50% of patients. Arthralgia or arthritis occurs in 65% to 85% of patients[68] and usually involves the knee and ankle joints. Gastrointestinal complaints are present in up to 65% of patients, with the most common symptom being periumbilical, dull pain resulting from bleeding into the intestinal wall. The abdominal pain typically occurs concurrent with or immediately after the rash; however, in up to 15% of patients, abdominal pain can be the initial complaint.[69] Between 25% and 50% of children develop a self-limiting glomerulonephritis manifested by hematuria. Less than 1% of these patients develop chronic renal insufficiency. Children presenting with acute renal failure, nephritic syndrome, or hypertension are more likely to have unfavorable outcomes such as chronic renal failure.[70] Testicular involvement occurs in up to 35% of patients; they may present with severe scrotal edema that resembles acute testicular torsion.

Diagnostic Strategies

There are no specific tests to confirm HSP, and the diagnosis can be difficult if the classical rash is absent at the time of presentation. Screening tests such as urinalysis, BUN and creatinine, CBC, and coagulation studies may be needed to rule out other pathologic diseases. Typical ultrasound findings in patients with abdominal pain are intraluminal hematomas and duodenal wall thickening.[71] Intussusception may also complicate the disease.

Differential Considerations

Differential diagnoses include meningococcemia, Rocky Mountain spotted fever, intussusception, trauma, appendicitis, thrombotic thrombocytopenic purpura, juvenile rheumatoid arthritis, bacterial endocarditis, systemic lupus erythematosus, kidney stones, and primary renal disease.

Management

Treatment of HSP remains controversial because most cases resolve spontaneously and do not require therapy. NSAIDs can be used to treat joint pain, but close attention must be paid to renal function. Corticosteroids have been used to treat severe renal or gastrointestinal involvement. Prednisone or methylprednisolone pulse therapy has shown some benefit, but an acute, surgical process must be excluded before steroid initiation.[71] Therapy for patients with severe renal involvement also includes intravenous immunoglobulins, although promising results have also been seen in patients with severe abdominal pain.[72] Other treatment options for patients with severe HSP nephropathy include early treatment with oral immunosuppressants[73] and possibly the use of methylprednisolone and urokinase pulse therapy.[74] A nephrologist should be consulted for patients with renal involvement and good follow-up ensured.

Disposition

Patients with only skin manifestations of HSP can usually be discharged home with symptomatic therapy for the joint pain and malaise. NSAIDs or acetaminophen is usually sufficient, but close follow-up should be ensured. Patients with abdominal pain or renal involvement should be admitted for further evaluation and treatment.

Hemolytic-Uremic Syndrome

Perspective

HUS continues to be one of the most common causes of acute renal failure in children.[75] It most commonly involves infants and children, with a mean age at presentation of 3 years, but is rare after 5 years of age. There is no sex predilection and outbreaks can be sporadic or epidemic, especially when related to the most common offending agent, verotoxin produced by *E. coli* serotype O157:H7. Transmission is through person-to-person contact and also exposure to contaminated food, such as unpasteurized dairy products or beef.[76] Other causes of HUS include *Shigella* organisms, *S. pneumoniae*, *Aeromonas*, human immunodeficiency virus, and drugs; there are also hereditary, familial, and idiopathic forms.

Principles of Disease

Renal compromise is the result of injury to the renal vascular endothelium induced by viral or bacterial agents or the toxins released. Microangiopathic hemolytic anemia then results from injury to the RBCs by fibrin strands along the narrowed blood vessels. Platelets, complement, and fibrin are also deposited in the glomerular lumen and lead to a decrease in the glomerular filtration rate and renal failure.

Clinical Features

Patients present with watery diarrhea, crampy abdominal pain, and occasionally fever. From 2 to 3 days after onset of symptoms, patients develop increased abdominal pain and bloody stools, with up to 89% of patients developing bloody stools by day 5.[77] Toxic megacolon, ischemic colitis, intussusception, perforation, or delayed colonic stricture may occur. After the prodromal gastroenteritis, patients develop sudden onset of hemolytic anemia, thrombocytopenia, and acute renal insufficiency, with possible progression to renal failure. In a meta-analysis published in 2003, death or end-stage renal disease occurred in 12% of cases of diarrhea-associated HUS and 25% of survivors demonstrated long-term renal sequelae.[78] Pancreatic insufficiency resulting in insulin-dependent diabetes mellitus has also been reported. There are reports of HUS occurring in association with UTI as well.[79]

Central nervous system irritability may develop; it results in seizures in 40% of patients. Hypertension occurs in up to 50% of patients and may contribute to the development of encephalopathy. HUS recurrences have been associated with a 30% mortality rate.

Diagnostic Strategies

Leukocyte counts and C-reactive protein levels were found to be significantly higher in patients with verotoxin-producing *E. coli* O157:H7.[76] The peripheral blood smear shows microangiopathic changes such as teardrop cells, helmet cells, microspherocytes, and burr cells. The WBCs may be elevated and the platelet count may be less than 50,000/mm^3. The hemoglobin can be as low as 5 g/dL secondary to the rapid hemolysis that occurs.

Differential Considerations

The differential diagnosis of HUS includes thrombocytopenic thrombotic purpura, ulcerative colitis, intussusception, and other causes of acquired hemolytic anemia.

Management

Supportive therapy and early peritoneal dialysis account for the reduction in current mortality rates to less than 5%. Patients should be rehydrated; however, it is important not to overload these children with fluids. Hyperkalemia is common and should be treated with sodium bicarbonate, calcium gluconate or chloride, dextrose and insulin, and Kayexalate. Patients with severe hyperkalemia, hyperphosphatemia, and severe metabolic acidosis require dialysis.

Packed RBCs (5 mL/kg over 4 hours) are typically administered if the hemoglobin falls below 6 g/dL. Platelet transfusions are required only if there is active bleeding or before an invasive procedure. Hypertension is responsive to calcium channel blockers, labetalol, captopril, or nitroprusside in refractory cases. Seizures typically respond to benzodiazepines and phenytoin; however, if they are secondary to hyponatremia, treatment with 3% saline (4 mL/kg) may be indicated. Treatment for the colitis itself is also supportive because antimotility agents may lead to toxic megacolon. Antibiotics may enhance the release of verotoxin from the bacteria and therefore should be avoided. Hyperglycemia, ketonemia, and acidosis secondary to pancreatic islet cell necrosis are treated with insulin therapy.

Idiopathic HUS may be treated with plasmapheresis, especially if there is neurologic involvement. If this is unsuccessful, renal transplantation may be required. Unfortunately, idiopathic HUS can also recur in the transplanted kidney.

Disposition

Patients with HUS require admission, and a pediatric nephrologist and urologist should be consulted. Early dialysis and supportive therapy result in up to 90% of patients with acute renal failure regaining their baseline renal function.

KEY CONCEPTS

- *Priapism*: In low-flow priapism, cavernosal aspiration and irrigation have been effective when performed within the first 48 hours, and preferably within a few hours, of symptom onset. Phentolamine, phenylephrine, ephedrine, or 1:1,000,000 epinephrine is often added to the irrigation solution when performing corporal aspiration.
- *Phimosis and paraphimosis*: If there is vascular compromise of the glans penis, a dorsal split procedure may be necessary.
- *Testicular torsion*: Delay in diagnosis and treatment can result in loss of spermatogenesis and in severe cases a necrotic, gangrenous testis. Testicular salvage rates are time dependent, with a 96% success rate if detorsion is performed in less than 4 hours after symptom onset; if there is a greater than 24-hour delay in time to treatment, the success rate decreases to less than 10%.
- *Varicoceles*: Left sided varicoceles account for 85% to 95% of cases; intra-abdominal pathology should be suspected in cases of right-sided varicoceles because these are usually caused by inferior vena cava thrombosis or compression of the IVC by tumors.
- *Urinary tract infections*: In children younger than 2 years, a urinalysis alone is inadequate for ruling out UTIs because this study yields false-negative results in as many as 10% to 50% of patients.

REFERENCES

1. Hakim LS, et al: Evolving concepts in the diagnosis and treatment of arterial high flow priapism. *J Urol* 155:541, 1996.
2. Mulhall JP, Honig SC: Priapism: Diagnosis and management. *Acad Emerg Med* 3:810, 1996.
3. Powars D, Johnson C: Priapism. *Hematol Oncol Clin North Am* 10:1363, 1996.
4. Van Howe R: Cost-effective treatment of phimosis. *Pediatrics* 102:1, 1998.
5. Pontari MA: Phimosis and paraphimosis. In Seidman EJ, Hanno PM (eds): *Current Urologic Therapy*. Philadelphia, WB Saunders, 1994.
6. Dewan PA, Tieu HC: Phimosis: Is circumcision necessary? *J Paediatr Child Health* 32:285, 1996.
7. Chu C, Chen K, Diau G: Topical steroid treatment of phimosis in boys. *J Urol* 162:861, 1999.
8. Ashfield JE, et al: Treatment of phimosis with topical steroids in 194 children. *J Urol* 169:1106, 2003.
9. Kumar V, Javle P: Modified puncture technique for reduction of paraphimosis. *Ann R Coll Surg Engl* 3:126, 2001.
10. Turner CD, Kim HL, Cromie WJ: Dorsal band traction for reduction of paraphimosis. *Urology* 54:917, 1999.
11. Orden B, et al: Balanitis caused by group A beta-hemolytic streptococci. *Pediatr Infect Dis J* 15:920, 1996.
12. Persad R, et al: Clinical presentation and pathophysiology of meatal stenosis following circumcision. *Br J Urol* 75:91, 1995.
13. Langer J, Coplen D: Circumcision and pediatric disorders of the penis. *Pediatr Clin North Am* 45:801, 1998.
14. Kanegaye J: Penile zipper injury: A simple and less threatening approach using mineral oil. *Pediatr Emerg Care* 9:90, 1993.
15. Herberner TE: Ultrasound in the assessment of the acute scrotum. *J Clin Ultrasound* 24:405, 1996.
16. Paltiel HJ: Acute scrotal symptoms in boys with an indeterminate clinical presentation: Comparison of color Doppler sonography and scintigraphy. *Radiology* 207:223, 1998.
17. Knight PJ, Vassy LE: The diagnosis and treatment of the acute scrotum in children and adolescents. *Ann Surg* 200:664, 1984.
18. Kadish H, Bolte R: A retrospective review of pediatric patients with epididymitis, testicular torsion, and torsion of testicular appendages. *Pediatrics* 102:73, 1998.
19. Rabii R, Rais H, Hafiani M: Torsion of an undescended testis. Apropos of a case. *Ann Urol* 32:49, 1998.
20. Baker LA, et al: An analysis of clinical outcomes using color Doppler testicular ultrasound for testicular torsion. *Pediatrics* 105:604, 2000.
21. Nussbaum B, et al: Color Doppler sonography and scintigraphy of the testis: A prospective, comparative analysis in children with acute scrotal pain. *Pediatr Emerg Care* 18:67, 2002.
22. Coley BD, et al: Acute testicular torsion: Comparison of unenhanced power Doppler US, color Doppler US, and radionuclide imaging. *Radiology* 199:441, 1996.
23. Granados EA, Caicado P, Garat JM: Testicular torsion after 12 hours. III. *Arch Esp Urol* 51:978, 1998.
24. Cornel EB, Karthaus HF: Manual derotation of the twisted spermatic cord. *Br J Urol* 83:672, 1999.
25. Niedzielski J, Paduch D, Raczynski P: Assessment of adolescent varicocele. *Pediatr Surg Int* 12:410, 1997.
26. Kass E, Reitelman C: Adolescent varicocele. *Urol Clin North Am* 22:154, 1995.
27. Pillai S, Besner G: Pediatric testicular problems. *Pediatr Clin North Am* 45:813, 1998.
28. Bomalaski A, Mills J, Argueso L: Iliac vein compression syndrome: An unusual cause of varicocele. *J Vasc Surg* 18:1065, 1993.

29. Ulker V, Garibyan H, Kurth KH: Comparison of inguinal and laparoscopic approaches in the treatment of varicocele. *Int Urol Nephrol* 29:71, 1997.
30. Gahukamble DE, Khamage AS: Early versus delayed repair of reduced incarcerated inguinal hernias in the pediatric population. *J Pediatr Surg* 31:1218, 1996.
31. Shaw KN, Gorelick MH: Urinary tract infection in the pediatric patient. *Pediatr Clin North Am* 46:1111, 1999.
32. Jakobsson B, Esbjorner E, Hansson S: Minimum incidence and diagnostic rate of first urinary tract infection. *Pediatrics* 104:222, 1999.
33. American Academy of Pediatrics. Committee on Quality Improvement. Subcommittee on Urinary Tract Infection: Practice parameter: The diagnosis, treatment, and evaluation of the initial urinary tract infection in febrile infants and young children. *Pediatrics* 103:843, 1999.
34. Rushton H: Urinary tract infections in children—Epidemiology, evaluation and management. *Pediatr Clin North Am* 44:1133, 1997.
35. Munir V, Barnett P, South M: Does the use of volumetric bladder ultrasound improve the success rate of suprapubic aspiration of urine? *Pediatr Emerg Care* 18:346, 2002.
36. Doley A, Nelligan M: Is a negative dipstick urinalysis good enough to exclude urinary tract infection in pediatric emergency department patients? *Emerg Med* 15:77, 2003.
37. Bachur R, Harper MB: Reliability of the urinalysis for predicting urinary tract infections in young febrile children. *Arch Pediatr Adolesc Med* 155:60, 2001.
38. Pitetti RD, Choi S: Utility of blood cultures in febrile children with UTI. *Am J Emerg Med* 20:271, 2002.
39. Crain EF, Gershel JC: Urinary tract infections in febrile infants younger than 8 weeks of age. *Pediatrics* 83:363, 1990.
40. Hoberman A, et al: Oral versus intravenous therapy for urinary tract infections in young febrile children. *Pediatrics* 104:79, 1999.
41. McLoughlin TG, Joseph MM: Antibiotic resistance patterns of uropathogens in pediatric emergency department patients. *Acad Emerg Med* 10:347, 2003.
42. Michael M, et al: Short compared with standard duration of antibiotic treatment for urinary tract infection: A systematic review of randomized controlled trials. *Arch Dis Child* 87:118, 2002.
43. Dick PT, Feldman W: Routine diagnostic imaging for childhood urinary tract infections: A systematic review. *J Pediatr* 128:15, 1996.
44. Talan DA, Stamm EW, Hooton TM: Comparison of ciprofloxacin (7 days) and trimethoprim-sulfamethoxazole (14 days) for acute uncomplicated pyelonephritis in women. *JAMA* 283:1583, 2000.
45. Nelson DS, Gurr MB, Schunk JE: Management of febrile children with urinary tract infections. *Am J Emerg Med* 16:643, 1998.
46. Nairn SJ, Sugarman JM: Adequacy of follow-up in children diagnosed with urinary tract infections in a pediatric emergency department. *Pediatr Emerg Care* 11:156, 1995.
47. Feld LG, et al: Hematuria—An integrated medical and surgical approach. *Pediatr Clin North Am* 44:1191, 1997.
48. Feld LG, Meyers KE, Kaplan BS: Limited evaluation for microscopic hematuria in pediatrics. *Pediatrics* 102:965, 1998.
49. Demirkesen O, et al: Extracorporeal shockwave lithotripsy in the pediatric population. *J Endourol* 13:147, 1999.
50. Coward RJM, et al: Epidemiology of pediatric renal stone disease in the UK. *Arch Dis Child* 88:962, 2003.
51. Slavkovic A, et al: Extracorporeal shock wave lithotripsy for cystine urolithiasis in children: Outcome and complications. *Int Urol Nephrol* 34:457, 2002-2003.
52. Pinto E, Guignard JP: Renal masses in the neonate. *Biol Neonate* 68:175, 1995.
53. Schamberger RC: Pediatric renal tumors. *Semin Surg Oncol* 16:105, 1999.
54. Maxson WT: Benign proteinuria of childhood and adolescence: A survey. *Clin Pediatr* 2:662, 1963.
55. Loghman-Adham M: Evaluating proteinuria in children. *Am Fam Physician* 58:1145, 1998.
56. Mahan JD, Turman MA, Mentser MI: Evaluation of hematuria, proteinuria, and hypertension in adolescents. *Pediatr Clin North Am* 44:1573, 1997.
57. Matsell DG, Wyatt RJ, Gaber LW: Terminal complement complexes in acute poststreptococcal glomerulonephritis. *Pediatr Nephrol* 8:671, 1994.
58. Daniels SR: Consultation with the specialist. The diagnosis of hypertension in children: An update. *Pediatr Rev* 18:131, 1997.
59. Simckes AM, Spitzer A: Poststreptococcal acute glomerulonephritis. *Pediatr Rev* 16:278, 1995.
60. Louis CU, Morgenstern BZ, Butani L: Thrombotic complications in childhood-onset idiopathic membranous nephropathy. *Pediatr Nephrol* 18:1298, 2003.
61. Ulinski T, et al: Acute renal failure after treatment with non-steroidal anti-inflammatory drugs. *Eur J Pediatr* 163:148, 2004.
62. Belsha CW, Kohaut EC, Warady BA: Dialytic management of childhood acute renal failure: A survey of North American pediatric nephrologists. *Pediatr Nephrol* 9:361, 1995.
63. Stewart CL, Barnett R: Acute renal failure in infants, children and adults. *Crit Care Clin* 13:575, 1997.
64. Kemper MJ, Harps E, Muller-Wiefel DE: Hyperkalemia: Therapeutic options in acute and chronic renal failure. *Clin Nephrol* 46:67, 1996.
65. Proulx F, et al: Convulsions and hypertension in children: Differentiating cause from effect. *Crit Care Med* 21:1541, 1993.
66. Robson WL, Leung AK: Henoch-Schoenlein purpura. *Adv Pediatr* 41:163, 1994.
67. Walker W, et al: Miscellaneous intestinal inflammatory disease. In Walker WA, et al (eds): *Pediatric Gastrointestinal Disease*. Philadelphia, BC Decker, 1991.
68. Szer I: Henoch-Schoenlein purpura. *Curr Opin Rheumatol* 6:25, 1994.
69. Sharieff G, Francis K, Kupperman N: Atypical presentation of Henoch-Schoenlein purpura in two children. *Am J Emerg Med* 15:375, 1997.
70. Ulinski T, et al: Acute renal failure after treatment with non-steroidal anti-inflammatory drugs. *Eur J Pediatr* 163:148, 2004.
71. Wang L, et al: Successful treatment of mesenteric vasculitis caused by Henoch-Schönlein purpura with methylprednisolone pulse therapy. *Clin Rheumatol* 22:140, 2003.
72. Rostoker G, et al: High dose immunoglobulin therapy for severe IGA nephropathy and Henoch-Schönlein purpura. *Ann Intern Med* 120:476, 1994.
73. Tanaka H, et al: Early treatment with oral immunosuppressants in severe proteinuric purpura nephritis. *Pediatr Nephrol* 18:347, 2003
74. Kawasaki Y, et al: Efficacy of methylprednisolone and urokinase pulse therapy for severe Henoch-Schönlein nephritis. *Pediatrics* 111:785, 2003.
75. Flynn J: Causes, management approaches, and outcome of acute renal failure in children. *Curr Opin Pediatr* 10:184, 1998.
76. Kawamura N, Yamazaki T, Tamai H: Risk factors for the development of *Escherichia coli* O157:H7 associated with hemolytic uremic syndrome. *Pediatr Int* 41:218, 1999.
77. Cohen MB: *Escherichia coli* O157:H7 infection: A frequent cause of bloody diarrhea and the hemolytic-uremic syndrome. *Adv Pediatr* 43:171, 1996.
78. Garg AX, et al: Long term renal prognosis of diarrhea-associated hemolytic uremic syndrome. *JAMA* 290:1360, 2003.
79. Tarr P, et al: Hemolytic-uremic syndrome in a six-year-old girl after a urinary tract infection with Shiga toxin–producing *Escherichia coli* O103:H2. *N Engl J Med* 335:635, 1996.

CHAPTER 173

Neurologic Disorders

David H. Rubin, Dina Halpern Kornblau, Edward E. Conway, Jr., and Stuart M. Caplen

PERSPECTIVE

Many neurologic complaints, such as seizure, vertigo, ataxia, and headache appear in both adults and children. However, associated signs and symptoms and differential diagnoses in children are quite different than in the adult population. Finally, bacterial meningitis, once a predominantly pediatric disease, is now mainly a disease of adults and yet it remains imperative to recognize subtle signs and symptoms of this disease in infants and young children.

ACUTE BACTERIAL MENINGITIS

Perspective

Despite advances in medical care, acute bacterial meningitis (ABM) remains a potentially life-threatening emergency. The nationwide mortality rate among treated cases is 20% to 30% in neonates and adults and 2% in infants and children.[1] With the recommendation in 1991 that all infants, starting at 2 months of age, receive the conjugated vaccine against *Haemophilus influenzae* type b organisms, the incidence of bacterial meningitis caused by this organism has been reduced in children by more than 90%.[1,2] In fact, data show that the median age of meningitis in 1986 was 15 months and in 1995 was 25 years. Even with the best care, however, 10% to 30% of survivors of meningitis of all types demonstrate persistent, functionally important disabilities.[3,4] These include hearing deficits, seizures, learning and behavioral problems, and intelligence deficits. More than 90% of cases documented in the pediatric age group occur before 5 years of age.[1-3]

Neonates

Group B streptococcus accounts for more than half the cases of neonatal meningitis, whereas *Escherichia coli* and other coliforms are responsible for one fourth of cases.[5] The incidence of early-onset group B streptococcal disease has declined as a result of intrapartum prophylaxis. However, late-onset disease (after 7 days of life) has not.[6] *Staphylococcus epidermidis, Staphylococcus aureus, Streptococcus pneumoniae, Neisseria meningitidis,* group D streptococci, *Ureaplasma urealyticum, Haemophilus influenzae* type b, and nontypeable strains are less commonly seen in neonates. *Listeria monocytogenes* infection is rarely seen but is important because of its prevalence within some immigrant groups, its association with unpasteurized dairy products, and its resistance to cephalosporins.[5,6]

Infants and Children

Beyond the neonatal period, in the United States, *S. pneumoniae* and *N. meningitidis* account for 90% of the documented cases of ABM. Unusual organisms include *Salmonella* species, *Campylobacter* species, *L. monocytogenes,* group G streptococcus, *Francisella tularensis,* group B β-hemolytic streptococcus, and several anaerobic organisms.[1,2]

Principles of Disease

Host factors influence the degree of susceptibility to meningitis. Newborn infants younger than 1 month of age, particularly those born prematurely, are at greatest risk for ABM owing to their immunologic immaturity. Other groups predisposed to ABM include males, American Indians, African Americans, malnourished individuals, indigent urban dwellers, daycare center attendants, and people with immunodeficiency, including sickle hemoglobinopathies, acquired immunodeficiency syndrome, asplenia, renal disease, hepatic disease, diabetes mellitus, dysgammaglobulinemia, and immunosuppressive treatment including corticosteroids.

Bacterial meningitis is thought to develop through the interconnection of (1) infection of the respiratory tract, (2) development of bacteremia, (3) invasion of the meninges, and (4) inflammation of the meninges and brain.[6] Invasion of the meninges by bacterial pathogens is facilitated by mechanical disturbances. These include recent neurosurgical procedures such as ventriculoperitoneal shunt and lumbar puncture and skull fracture with a persistent cerebrospinal fluid (CSF) leak. Congenital or developmental central nervous system (CNS) abnormalities also predispose to bacterial seeding of the CNS. These include neurenteric fistula, intracranial cysts, and epidermoid or dermoid tumors, often with an associated congenital dermal sinus track.[7]

For ABM to occur, organisms must gain entrance into the subarachnoid space. On rare occasions, this occurs as a direct extension from a contiguous focus, such as sinusitis, mastoiditis, or otitis media. In the majority of cases, the bacterial organism gains access to the bloodstream and hematogenously seeds through inflamed capillaries within the choroid plexus. Most cases of ABM follow a progression of events. After exposure and nasopharyngeal colonization, there is an invasion of the blood. The organism can be recovered from the bloodstream in up to 90% of patients with CSF culture-proven bacterial meningitis.

If bacteria gain entrance into the subarachnoid space, they replicate. Bacterial cell wall constituents are liberated into the CSF. Host inflammatory mediators and cytokines, including interleukin-1, tumor necrosis factor, and platelet-activating factor, are produced and secreted by CNS macrophages and endothelial cells. As a result of an inflammatory response, vascular and parenchymatous cerebral changes occur. These include vasculitis, microthrombi formation, occlusion of venous sinuses, reduced blood flow, increased permeability of the blood-brain barrier, increased intracranial pressure, diffuse cerebral edema, and intracerebral hemorrhage.[8]

Clinical Features

In three fourths of children ultimately diagnosed with ABM, the clinical presentation is subacute, taking place over 2 to 5 days. At onset, affected children typically exhibit a variety of symptoms such as fever, malaise, decreased interest in surroundings, irritability, alteration in sleeping pattern, anorexia, nausea, vomiting, or diarrhea. These symptoms are nonspecific, occurring with equal frequency in children who are suffering from trivial and self-limited illnesses.[9] If examined early in the course, physical signs may be lacking. There is an absence of toxic appearance. Although the child may not look well to the parent, the physician may not otherwise be able to identify other signs of serious bacterial infection (SBI).

Children with this insidious presentation have a better prognosis than patients with ABM who present with a rapid progression of signs and symptoms. One fourth of children with ABM have an acute illness with manifestation such as vomiting, fever, and lethargy in less than 24 hours. In such patients, the diagnosis is rarely missed.[10] Those with fulminant illness exhibit a higher risk for death as well as for both immediate and long-term complications.[11]

In addition to the invasiveness of the offending organism, the other variable with the greatest impact on clinical expression is the age of the patient. As a rule, the younger and smaller the infant, the more nonspecific and ambiguous the symptoms and signs of ABM.[1,3,5]

The cutaneous expression of ABM may prove helpful and can suggest specific organisms. Petechial and purpuric eruptions may suggest meningococcemia but can also be seen in cases of pneumococcal disease and *H. influenzae* meningitis. Herpes simplex virus (HSV) infections in the neonate are suggested by blisters or erosions in or around the eye, mouth, or skin. These lesions may also be seen in patients with bullous impetigo, candidal infections, varicella, listeria, and syphilis.[6]

Neonatal Period (<1 Month of Age)

The clinical findings of ABM in the neonate include altered vital signs, behavior changes, neurologic aberrations, dermatologic findings, and gastrointestinal changes (Table 173-1). Temperature instability is the most common triggering event that leads to the consideration of SBI, including meningitis. In the first 30 days of life, patients who present to an emergency department with a temperature of 38° C (100.4° F) or higher are found to have SBI and ABM in 4% to 15% and 1% to 2% of cases, respectively.[11,12] The absence of fever does not eliminate the possibility of serious bacterial infection, as more than half of neonates with meningitis are afebrile or exhibit hypothermia. Other vital sign changes include tachycardia, bradycardia, tachypnea, and apnea. Apnea greater than 20 seconds may signify either seizure activity or a nonspecific medullary respiratory center dysfunction.

Neonates have a limited behavioral repertoire. However, a changed behavioral pattern can reflect early meningeal involvement. Restlessness, listlessness, increased or decreased sleeping time, and irritability may be clues. Irritability in a neonate without meningeal invasion is generally alleviated by human contact. An infant who is more irritable with cuddling should suggest the diagnosis of ABM. Neurologic manifestations of ABM in the neonate include high-pitched cry, incessant cry, absent cry, or moan. A vacant stare, hypertonicity, trembling chin, or bicycle motion of the extremities suggests a seizure. Focal or generalized tonic-clonic activity, although possible, is less commonly seen. Nuchal rigidity occurs in fewer than 25% of cases of neonatal ABM. A bulging fontanelle and diastasis of the sutures, both hallmarks of an increased intracranial pressure (ICP), are present in approximately 15% of neonatal ABM.

Table 173-1. Clinical Findings of Bacterial Meningitis

Feature	Newborn	Infant/Child
General	Apnea Tachypnea Hypothermia Hyperthermia Bradycardia	Fever Shaking chills Myalgia Neck, backache Tachycardia
Behavioral	Restlessness Paradoxical irritability Lethargy	Malaise Irritability Lethargy
Neurologic	High-pitched cry Nystagmus Vacant stare Seizure Opisthotonos Altered tone Nuchal rigidity Bulging fontanelle	Altered mentation Focal neurologic signs Hearing deficit Seizure Gait disturbance Photophobia Nuchal rigidity Kernig, Brudzinski sign
Dermatologic	Cyanosis Petechiae Purpura Delayed refill time Livedo reticularis	Cyanosis Petechiae Purpura Delayed refill time
Gastrointestinal	Altered feeding Diarrhea Vomiting Abdominal distention Jaundice	Anorexia Nausea Vomiting

Skin rashes are infrequent manifestations of neonatal meningitis.[13] One clue may be generalized pallor accompanied by indistinctly outlined truncal patches of blue discoloration (livedo reticularis). Difficulty feeding and unusual stooling patterns are nonspecific gastrointestinal complaints. Nonprojectile vomiting may appear in the course of meningitis and becomes projectile only after ICP has increased. Increased stool volume, irritability during defecation, abdominal distention, hepatomegaly, and jaundice can develop with meningitis.

One Month to 12 Months

Febrile patients in this age group who appear toxic are at high probability for invasive bacterial illness, including ABM. In young infants (<3 months of age), symptoms are similar to those of the neonate, but as the infant grows older, the social repertoire and motor capability expands, allowing for greater opportunity to assess for alteration in behavior, or signs and symptoms of bacterial meningitis. Nuchal rigidity, although not commonly present, is highly predictive for ABM in this age group. The absence of nuchal rigidity does not preclude the possibility of CNS infection; however, other signs are often present, such as poor tone, decreased interactiveness, inconsolability, alteration in gaze and focus, and a weak cry.

One Year to 5 Years

The cardinal features in this age group are fever, headache, vomiting, and neckache. Obtundation or lethargy are also common symptoms of meningitis but are nonspecific. Neck stiffness with difficulty flexing the neck is reliably seen after the first year of life, during the acute phase of meningitis. A patient may, rarely, exhibit torticollis.[14] One can attempt to elicit nuchal rigidity by forced flexion of the neck with the child in the supine position. However, this method is less reliable than attempting neck flexion with the child seated with the leg outstretched. Both of these maneuvers involve passive motion that many children voluntarily resist. More reliable methods that result in fewer false-negative and false-positive results involve active neck motion on the part of the child. In a toddler, a distracting object can be used to attract eye contact, and the active range of neck motion can be determined. Additionally, the neck stiffness that accompanies ABM may be displayed both in the prone and supine positions when the child's shoulders are placed at the edge of the examining table and minimal support of the occiput or forehead is given manually. A positive Kernig sign (flexion of the hip 90 degrees with subsequent pain on extension of the leg) and Brudzinski sign (involuntary flexion of the hips and knees following passive flexion of the neck while supine) are less reliable. Positive Kernig sign and Brudzinski sign are seen in approximately 43% and 66%, respectively, of children with ABM.[15]

Older than 5 Years

Headache, fever, stiff neck, and alteration of sensorium are common presenting signs and symptoms in children older than 5 years, as they are in the adult patient with ABM.

Diagnostic Strategies

Lumbar Puncture

Indications

Lumbar puncture is indicated in any child in whom bacterial meningitis is suspected. Patients to consider include those with classic signs and symptoms such as fever, stiff neck, and photophobia, but in infants and children classic signs are often absent. In a study by Walsh-Kelly, nuchal rigidity was present in only 27% of infants younger than 6 months of age with bacterial meningitis. By 12 months of age, 71% showed nuchal rigidity, which rose to greater than 95% by 19 months of age.[16] Therefore, the emergency physician must consider the constellation of presenting signs and symptoms and perform a lumbar puncture if meningitis is suspected.

Nuchal Signs. A lumbar puncture should be performed in ill children who have nuchal rigidity or a positive Kernig sign or Brudzinski sign and who have suspected meningitis. These three signs of meningeal irritation can also be seen in patients with parameningeal disease states other than ABM, so caution must be exercised in these cases.

Suspected Sepsis in Young Infants. Bacterial infections must be considered most strongly in the differential diagnosis of an infant younger than 3 months of age who is ill.[12] Current practice advocates that the possibility of SBI must be pursued with an ill young infant. No distinguishing features differentiate sepsis from meningitis in this age group. Because 50% of neonates with acute meningitis are bacteremic at the time of the initial evaluation, and because 25% of bacteremic neonates subsequently develop an intracranial infection, blood cultures and lumbar punctures should be undertaken concomitantly.[17,18] In infants older than 1 month of age but younger than 3 months of age, history and physical examination, even if augmented with selective laboratory investigations (excluding lumbar puncture), may fail to distinguish those infants with a serious bacterial infection such as ABM. Thus, a lumbar puncture should be performed as part of the sepsis evaluation.[19,20]

Toxic Appearance. A lumbar puncture should also be considered in any case in which the physician's global assessment suggests the child is toxic. Such observations include a blunted social response to overtures, poor perfusion, altered motor tone, and abnormal cry. Febrile pediatric patients of all ages who appear toxic have an increased incidence of SBI infection, including ABM.[11] Focal infections have been implicated as a source of dissemination of organisms into the CNS. Establishing an apparent infectious source for a particular presentation does not preclude the possibility of a more serious suppurative focus that may be intracranial.

If the patient exhibits clinical manifestations that are more severe than anticipated for an extracranial focus of infection, a lumbar puncture should be performed.

When obvious clues to the source of an apparent infectious process exist and an initial lumbar puncture is negative for an increasingly ill child, additional information can be obtained by repeating the lumbar puncture. The CSF composition may change from normal cellularity to marked pleocytosis within as little as 30 minutes.[21] A later reexamination of the CSF may be invaluable in establishing the nature of an occult intracranial infection.

Febrile Illness after Intimate Contact. All children who have prolonged and close physical involvement with patients who develop a serious bacteremic illness should have prompt medical evaluation. It is best to maintain a lower threshold for lumbar puncture when assessing febrile intimate contacts of patients with meningococcal or *Haemophilus* disease.[22]

Febrile Seizures. It is critical to exclude an intracranial infection when presented with a child whose febrile illness has been accompanied by a seizure. Lumbar puncture should be considered in patients who have characteristics that increase their risk of ABM. The historical features are age younger than 1 year, exposure to another child with meningitis or serious bacterial infection, and a physician visit within 48 hours before the seizure with fever. Generally, patients with complex features of the febrile seizure are at increased risk for meningitis. However, children with simple febrile seizures but who exhibit any physical findings that place them at risk for intracranial infection, including lethargy, decreased motor tone, positive doll's eye sign, inability to fix and follow, decreased response to painful stimuli, nuchal rigidity, full fontanelle, petechiae, or poor skin perfusion, should receive a lumbar puncture. Children 6 months to 5 years of age with a simple febrile seizure and who appear well (alert, active, playful) are extremely unlikely to have meningitis.[23]

Fever and Petechiae. Trivial to life-threatening infectious disease can cause fever and petechiae. There is no current optimal strategy for evaluating febrile children with petechial eruptions. Well-appearing febrile children with localized petechiae, especially above the nipple line, and with no purpura are unlikely to experience invasive bacterial disease. Patients at highest risk of invasive bacterial disease are more likely to appear ill, have generalized petechiae and purpura, or have signs of meningeal irritation.[24] In the high-risk group, unless contraindicated by apparent coagulopathy, lumbar puncture should be performed to exclude concurrent meningitis.[25]

Sepsis Suspected in an Abnormal Host. Immunocompromised pediatric patients are at risk for developing both opportunistic infections and invasive illness from pathogens common to all children. Immunologically incompetent children may not exhibit the typical manifestation of intracranial infections, including nuchal rigidity.[26] However, the impaired host who simply has a change in mental status should be suspected of having meningitis. CSF parameters in these patients are less sensitive indicators of the presence of bacterial meningitis compared with normal host response to a bacterial invasion of the meninges. A lumbar puncture nonetheless should be performed in the process of excluding sepsis in a compromised host.

Penetration of Dura. Fracture through the paranasal sinuses or anterior or middle cranial fossa and penetrating nasal injury or instrumentation may lead to dural tears. These defects are potential portals of entry for microorganisms into the CNS. CNS infection is generally seen within 2 weeks of the initial injury but may be delayed for years. Persistent CSF otorrhea or rhinorrhea may be encountered but is not a clinical prerequisite for posttraumatic meningitis. When patients with a recent or remote history significant for craniofacial trauma develop any constellation of symptoms suggestive of meningitis, lumbar puncture should be performed after a computed tomography (CT) scan.

Acute Hearing Loss. Hearing loss has been identified in up to one third of patients with ABM. Hearing impairment may be identified in the acute phase or become apparent only in the postmeningitic period. Its occurrence early in the course of the disease is usually overshadowed by dramatic symptoms. Of significance, hearing loss may precede the onset of systemic complaints and herald the appearance of meningitis. This is especially true for patients with an inner ear fistula or basilar skull fracture. Acute hearing loss should be an indication for lumbar puncture in traumatized patients who may have directly inoculated organisms into the labyrinth or basilar subarachnoid space. Lumbar puncture should also be promptly considered for patients who have subtle signs and symptoms suggestive of meningitis combined with acute hearing loss.

Contraindications

Herniation of the temporal lobes through the tentorium or herniation of the cerebellar tonsils through the foramen magnum rarely occurs in meningitis patients with increased ICP. Most children with ABM have some mental status changes, but rapid onset and progression to deep coma (Glasgow Coma Scale score <8) usually reflects increased intracranial pressure and lumbar puncture is contraindicated.[27] Focal neurologic signs suggestive of an abscess are further contraindications to lumbar puncture in children.

When not contraindicated, emergency lumbar puncture with CSF examination should be performed to confirm a presumptive diagnosis of ABM (Box 173-1).

BOX 173-1. Indications for Lumbar Puncture in Suspected Acute Bacterial Meningitis

- Signs or symptoms of meningitis or toxic appearance
- Suspected neonatal sepsis
- Febrile infant <2 months old
- Sepsis suspected in an abnormal host
- Consider lumbar puncture in suspected acute bacterial meningitis
  - Documented bacteremia
  - Febrile illness after intimate contact with person with meningitis or serious bacterial infection
  - Febrile seizure
  - Fever and petechiae

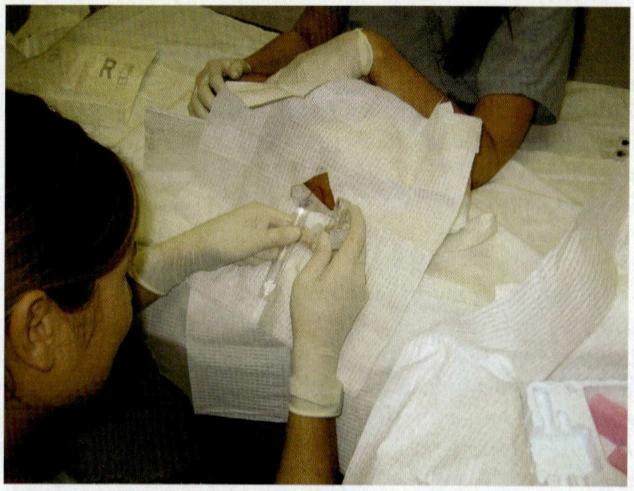

Figure 173-1. Lumbar puncture performed on a neonate in the lateral decubitus position with spine flexed and knees drawn upward toward the chest. (Courtesy of Marianne Gausche-Hill, MD.)

Patients with suspected bacterial meningitis should have the procedure completed in the lateral decubitus position with spine flexed and knees drawn upward toward the chest, with shoulders and back perpendicular to the table (Figure 173-1). Opening pressure should be obtained if possible in this position. In circumstances in which opening pressure measurement cannot be obtained, an alternative position is sitting with the thighs flexed toward the abdomen.

In the stable, monitored patient, the potential complications should not dissuade the physician from sampling the CSF. Lumbar pain can be eliminated in all pediatric patients with the use of an anesthetic agent. Prevention of post-lumbar puncture cephalgia is enhanced by using smaller gauge needles, restricting the sample fluid volume to 3 mL, and reinserting the stylet before removing the needle. The small risk of introducing bacterial skin flora is reduced with proper aseptic technique. The risk of creating meningitis by performing a lumbar puncture in the course of a bacteremic illness is a theoretical concern but does not occur. The information obtained from the lumbar puncture outweighs this hypothetical risk.

Standard Cerebrospinal Fluid Interpretation

A standard CSF examination includes bacterial culture and Gram stain from tube 1, protein and glucose assessment from tube 2, and blood cell count from tube 3. In all cases of culture-proven bacterial meningitis, up to 0% of patients have normal glucose and protein levels, few white blood cells, and a negative Gram stain smear.[15] Patients who have received antibiotics prior to their first lumbar puncture deserve special mention. Although the CSF can be sterilized after the administration of antibiotics in the emergency department, especially in cases of pneumococcal and meningococcal disease, the CSF profile is often unaffected for more than 12 to 24 hours after therapy.[6]

Table 173-2. Reported Values for Cerebrospinal Fluid Cellularity

	Total White Blood Cells/mm³		
Age	***Mean***	***Range***	***Threshold Exceeded***
Preterm	7	0-44	>9
Term newborn	8	0-32	>22
0-4 weeks	11	0-50	>35
4-8 weeks	7	0-50	>10
>8 weeks	2	0-8	>6

Glucose

The CSF glucose concentration must be interpreted in relation to a concomitant serum glucose value. The normal steady-state CSF serum glucose ratio is approximately 0.6. Hypoglycorrhachia, as defined as a ratio below 0.4, is characteristically found in cases of ABM with common pathogens and with *Mycobacterium tuberculosa*. Hypoglycorrhachia may also be associated with viral meningitis, although CSF glucose in these cases is typically normal.

Protein

The normal CSF protein range is 40 to 170 mg/dL in newborns and 15 to 45 mg/dL in children. Normal to modestly elevated protein concentration occurs in the course of viral meningitis. Higher levels of protein are encountered with ABM. In the face of a traumatic lumbar puncture, each 800 to 1000 red blood cells elevate the protein level by 1 mg/dL.

Cellularity

A representative cellularity profile is presented in Table 173-2. Unfortunately, these numbers have been largely derived from healthy or nonsystemically ill children.[28] The standard panic values that have been quoted are often greater than 2 standard deviations above the mean or are figures that are seen in only 5% to 10% of studied populations. Cellularity that exceeds these typical threshold values can be seen with conditions that indirectly influence the CNS; however, these cases should be considered as possible ABM and treated accordingly. These conditions include generalized seizure, shigellosis, and parameningeal focus of infections such as otitis media, sinusitis, and mastoiditis.[29] Patients with suspected sepsis or with distant foci of infection from the CNS such as pneumonia may also have increased cellularity. Classically in ABM, the total white blood cell count ranges from 1000 to 20,000.[15] A white blood cell count of greater than 2000 is present in more than one third of cases of ABM.[30] Significant pleocytosis can also accompany aseptic meningitis.

It is important to note that the practice of "correcting" for white blood cells in bloody CSF samples may have little scientific support. Underestimation of the white blood cell count in cases of culture-positive meningitis may be seen. Furthermore, consideration should be given to other illnesses, such as herpes simplex virus encephalitis, in which an increased number of red blood cells may be seen in the CSF.[6]

In the first month of life, up to 60% of the cells in the normal CSF are polymorphonuclear leukocytes (PMNs). Beyond 1 month in the normal state, not more than 3 PMNs/mm^3 should be seen. Shortly after invasion of the meninges, white blood cells can be sampled from the lumbar space. Traditional teaching suggests that a rise in PMNs is characteristic of ABM. However, PMNs and bands may be present in patients with viral meningitis as well.[31]

Gram Stain

The probability of visualizing bacteria on a stain depends on the number of bacterial organisms present at the time of sampling. One fourth of the smears are positive with 10^3 or more colony forming units (CFU) per milliliter, 60% of the smears are positive with 10^3 to 10^5 CFU/mL, and 97% are positive with 10^6 CFU/mL. A positive Gram stain necessitates immediate antibiotic therapy, even in the absence of increased white blood cells and protein levels or decreased glucose level in the CSF.

Other Cerebrospinal Fluid Tests

Antigen Detection

Commercial antigen detection kits are available for detecting the common pathogens causing ABM. Microbial antigens in CSF are detected by coagglutination, latex agglutination, countercurrent immunoelectrophoresis, enzyme-linked immunosorbent assay, and centrifugation-augmented solid-phase immunoassay. Because antigens remain measurable after antibiotic treatment, antigen detection proves to be most effective in cases of partially treated meningitis or in patients in whom the CSF Gram stain and culture are negative and ABM is strongly suspected. In any meningitic state, either untreated or pretreated, the CSF antigen detection kits are most sensitive when more than 500 white blood cells are present in the CSF.[32] The antigens are typically present at high levels in the CSF for several days, even after parenteral antibiotics have been initiated. A positive CSF assay result provides reliable bacteriologic diagnosis. A negative antigen test result cannot exclude the diagnosis of ABM.

Cytokines

Assayed concentrations of C-reactive protein, various interleukins, tumor necrosis factor, and prostaglandins are elevated with ABM.[33] These assays require sophisticated techniques and expensive equipment and take 5 hours to complete. For these reasons, the assays are of little utility for emergency physicians.

Polymerase Chain Reaction Testing

The diagnosis of HSV and enterovirus can be determined by polymerase chain reaction testing. Polymerase chain reaction assays for pneumococcus are still in the experimental phase.[6]

Other Laboratory Testing Instruments

The performance of other diagnostic tests in addition to CSF analysis should be guided by the clinical situation.

Blood cultures are of value in the patient with ABM. A pretreatment blood culture will identify the organism recovered from the CSF in 86% to 92% of cases. Cultures of body surfaces and orifices (e.g., nose and throat) are not helpful in identifying the causative pathogen. Positive cultures from urine, stool, and pleural spaces substantiate systemic bacterial disease but do not ensure the presence of an intracranial infection with the same organism.

Determination of serum electrolytes and serum glucose may be a benefit, as there can be changes in body water content and electrolytes. The serum sodium level may be below 135 mEq/L in more than half of ABM patients at the time of presentation.[34] The patient's blood glucose level should be estimated rapidly with a glucose oxidase tape, because hypoglycemia secondary to poor intake, vomiting, and metabolic derangements is a common complication. The estimated value should be confirmed with a serum sample submitted for electrolyte determinations.

There are no hematologic profiles that can consistently distinguish pediatric patients with ABM, yet a complete blood count is warranted because the total white blood cell count and platelet counts may aid prognostic risk assessment. Either thrombocytopenia or neutropenia at admission may be an ominous feature.

At the time of establishing the diagnosis of ABM in a moderately ill patient, the arterial blood gas determination can be performed on selected patients who are suspected to be hypoventilating, hypoxic, or have signs of metabolic acidosis.

A Gram-stained smear of a petechial or purpuric lesion may reveal an offending organism causing systemic invasion.[35] Serum C-reactive protein, erythrocyte sedimentation rate, and measurements of the various cytokines can be used to support the diagnosis of systemic bacterial infection. However, these tests are nonspecific and cannot be used to include or exclude a diagnosis of ABM. Elevated pretreatment values may be followed to determine the most effective length of therapy for ABM.

A urine specimen should be submitted for analysis. If the patient is pretreated with antibiotic agents, urine microbial antigen detection should be performed. Urine antigen detection may be positive in up to 87% of pretreated cases of ABM. Midstream clean-catch voided specimen or urine acquired by catheterization should be submitted. Urine from a bag specimen that is potentially contaminated by fecal material may yield false-positive results as a result of cross-reactivity with *E. coli* organisms.[36]

Radiology

Computed tomography of the head should be performed when the clinical findings suggest subdural empyema, cavernous sinus thrombosis, lateral sinus thrombosis, cerebral hemorrhage, brain tumor, brain abscess, or a parameningeal focus of infection. CT of the head without contrast should be performed on an emergency basis when the patient exhibits signs and symptoms of elevated ICP. There should be concern for

BOX 173-2. Differential Diagnosis of Acute Bacterial Meningitis

Infectious	Metabolic
Septicemia	Hypoglycemia
Rickettsemia	Ketoacidosis
Encephalitis	Hyponatremia
Subdural empyema	Hypernatremia
Spinal epidural abscess	Uremia
Intracranial epidural abscess	Urea cycle defect
Viral meningitis	**Miscellaneous**
Fungal meningitis	Intussusception
Tuberculous meningitis	Intoxication
Myocarditis	Toxic exposure
Shigellosis	Seizure disorder
Traumatic	Brain tumor
Shaken-impact syndrome	Arteriovenous malformation
Closed head injury	Ruptured dermoid cyst

raised ICP if the patient has cranial nerve palsy, absence of retinal venous pulsations, altered pupillary responses, papilledema, focal seizure, hemiparesis, ataxia, obtundation, persistent vomiting, decorticate or decerebrate posturing, or bradycardia unassociated with hypoxemia.[15] Patients with a ventriculoperitoneal shunt are a unique subset of patients, and if they demonstrate fever or signs of increased ICP, they should also undergo CT prior to tapping of the shunt for CSF. A decision to image the head or other body parts (such as chest) must not delay antibiotic administration.

Differential Considerations

Any of the manifestations of ABM can be expressed in a single patient. The most common expression is a combination of thermal instability, altered behavior, blunted mental status, and neck stiffness. The differential diagnosis for this constellation includes infectious, metabolic, traumatic, and miscellaneous conditions (Box 173-2).

Many conditions cause a child to appear ill. Any infectious agent can cause a child to appear ill, particularly in the first months of life. Infants with infectious disease are predisposed to exhibit altered affect, including significant changes in mental status, strongly suggesting an intracranial pathologic condition. Beyond infancy, children may appear toxic from any focal infection or with extensions from a primary focus leading to systemic invasion.[10] In addition to infection, a change in mental status may be seen with endocrinopathy, hypoglycemia, electrolyte imbalance, metabolic disease, uremia, seizure, unintentional trauma, abusive head injury, intussusception, and exposure to toxins.

Nuchal rigidity provokes strong consideration for ABM. However, neck stiffness associated with altered mentation or neurologic deficit can occur with spontaneous intracranial hemorrhage, hemorrhage into brain tumor, epidural abscess, or brain abscess. Other causes of stiff neck include retropharyngeal abscess, peritonsillar abscess, and torticollis.

Viral Meningitis

In the first few years of life, the signs and symptoms of bacterial and viral meningitis can be indistinguishable.[37] Beyond 1 year of age, the majority of children with viral meningitis have a relatively mild illness compared with children with ABM. Fever and retro-orbital or frontal headache are frequent symptoms of both diseases. Gastrointestinal symptoms such as anorexia, nausea, and diarrhea are more common with viral meningitis. There may be generalized myalgia, and patients often complain of neck ache or neck stiffness. However, reduction of active neck flexion is uncommon.

Modest elevation of PMNs in CSF specimens coupled with normal glucose level, normal to slightly elevated protein concentrations, and a negative Gram stain is anticipated with viral meningitis. These laboratory findings can confirm a clinical suspicion of viral meningitis. However, atypical findings such hypoglycorrhachia or significant pleocytosis can occur in 20% of encounters. This blurs the distinction between the two states and may alter management. Decision rules have been proposed to distinguish the two forms of meningitis but may be practically limited if they cannot identify every case of ABM.

Management

Management priorities for ABM include airway protection, oxygenation, and volume resuscitation with monitored preservation of organ function. If the capillary refilling time is delayed more than 2 seconds or the patient is hypotensive, the patient should be treated for shock. A bolus infusion of 20 mL/kg of normal saline or lactated Ringer's solution should be provided while an indwelling urinary catheter is inserted. Up to 40 mL/kg should be provided as bolus infusions. If there is a failure to stabilize vital signs after an infusion of 40 mL/kg of crystalloid solution and to maintain a 0.5 mL/kg/hr or greater urine flow, pressors should be given. In the patient without shock, an hourly infusion rate should be established that provides the normal maintenance of fluids. Fluid restriction, previously advocated, may be deleterious to the patient's survival and neurologic recovery.

Beyond support of cardiopulmonary and hemodynamic status, initial management of ABM includes prevention of hypoglycemia, control of seizures, and therapeutic agents to maintain cerebral blood flow.

Antibiotic Therapy

Intuitively, it makes biologic sense to advocate expeditious antibiotic administration for the patient suspected to have ABM. In reality, there are no studies to show that a duration of any given time frame arbitrarily chosen to constitute an "excessive delay" affects morbidity or mortality; however, most experts agree that antibiotics should be administered within 1 to 2 hours of presentation for patients with suspected ABM. The timing of antibiotic administration in a patient with CNS syndrome compatible with ABM should be driven by the specifics of the clinical scenario. A conservative approach for children with suspected ABM is to treat with empiric antibiotics and admit the patient to the hospital for observation. Strategies to stratify patients into low- and high-risk categories to restrict hospitalization and antibiotic therapy to children with suspected bacterial meningitis have been proposed. The following four categories are offered.

Nontoxic, Low-Risk. In a non-toxic, non-pretreated patient with a clinical picture of viral meningitis, if the CSF indices confirm a clinical suspicion of viral meningitis (negative Gram stain, few white blood cells in the CSF, and normal CSF protein and glucose levels), antibiotics can be withheld in consultation with the patient's primary care physician or a neurologist. Another option is to discharge the patient and schedule a repeat lumbar puncture within 12 hours after antibiotic therapy. These strategies are not without risk, as it is often difficult to distinguish viral meningitis from other infections such as Rocky Mountain spotted fever or ABM. If chemical parameters or cytologic assessment resemble ABM, the physician should begin empiric antibiotics and admit for observation.

Nontoxic, High-Risk. A nontoxic patient with high-risk historical features (such as pretreatment with antibiotics, exposure to an invasive organism [*H. influenzae* or *Neisseria meningitidis*], or age younger than 1 year) should cause increased physician concern for ABM. These patients should be the recipient of a blood culture and lumbar puncture. If the spinal fluid is cloudy, the physician should administer antibiotics rather than withhold them pending complete CSF analysis. In symptomatic patients exposed to a person with meningococcemia, the patient should be fully cultured, given empiric antibiotics, and admitted for observation until the results of all cultures are known, as the absence of meningitis does not imply that the patient does not have meningococcal disease.

Critical, Stable. For the patient with classic signs of ABM but who has a protected airway, adequate ventilation, normal perfusion, and no evidence of coagulopathy and is assessed as critical but stable, the emergency physician should perform a blood culture with phlebotomy and a second culture with introduction of an intravenous catheter, urinalysis and culture, blood chemistries, and a complete blood cell count, after which a lumbar puncture is performed. Antibiotics should be administered immediately after lumbar puncture and prior to the results of the CSF or other studies from the laboratory.

Critical, Unstable. A patient with a CNS syndrome, abnormal vital signs for age, an unprotected airway, active seizure, focal neurologic deficit, or coagulopathy is critical and unstable. The risk for an adverse outcome as a result of diagnostic lumbar puncture is magnified, especially if it is carried out before the patient is stabilized. Patients who clinically have increased ICP may experience fatal cerebral herniation (even after a normal CT scan) after a lumbar puncture.[27] One should acquire two blood culture samples and blood and urine for antigen detection. Antibiotics should be administered and the lumbar puncture deferred.

Table 173-3. Empiric Antibiotics for Acute Bacterial Meningitis

Age	Antibiotic	First IV Dose (mg/kg)
0-4 weeks	Ampicillin *plus*	50-100
	Gentamicin *or*	2.5
	Cefotaxime	50
4 weeks-2 months	Ampicillin *plus*	100
	Cefotaxime *or*	50
	Ceftriaxone *or*	100
	Chloramphenicol	25
>2 months	Cefotaxime *or*	50
	Ceftriaxone *and*	100
	Vancomycin	15

Emergency department antimicrobial treatment decisions are empirically based. The choice of antimicrobial agents should be based on the knowledge of the prevalent organisms responsible for intracranial infections and the regional patterns of their anti-microbial susceptibility. The initial regimen chosen for treatment should be broad enough to affect the various pathogens for the age group being treated (Table 173-3).

In the newborn, no single antibiotic has bactericidal activity against all the possible organisms commonly encountered. The most widely used combination therapy is ampicillin with an aminoglycoside or ampicillin plus cefotaxime, which is equally effective. For an infant older than 1 month of age and younger than 3 months of age, in the absence of evidence that suggests the presence of unusual organisms, conventional therapy is ampicillin and a third-generation cephalosporin. Beyond 3 months of age, monotherapy with a third-generation cephalosporin provides adequate coverage, except in cases in which there are resistant strains of *S. pneumoniae.* When gram-positive cocci are identified on the CSF Gram stain, the combination of a broad-spectrum cephalosporin and vancomycin is now routinely recommended.[38]

Steroid Therapy

The role of dexamethasone therapy for ABM has long been the focus of clinical interest. Consensus opinion suggests that for infants beyond 8 weeks old, dexamethasone can mitigate some neurologic sequelae, particularly hearing loss in cases of ABM caused by *H. influenzae.* The beneficial effect, if any, of dexamethasone on morbidity and mortality caused by other bacteria is less well defined.[1]

Provision of dexamethasone is not without risk. The most commonly reported deleterious effect of dexamethasone is gastrointestinal bleeding. The anti-inflammatory effects of dexamethasone have led to a false sense of clinical improvement, overshadowing the failure of the chosen antibiotic to eradicate an invasive organism. Reduced penetration of vancomycin with dexamethasone therapy has been demonstrated.[39] As we potentially approach a universal distribution of cephalosporin-resistant and penicillin-resistant *S. pneumoniae,* reducing the penetrating effect of vancomycin may cause undo harm. In summary, it is best to adhere to the latest recommendations of the American Academy of Pediatrics and limit the use of dexamethasone for the presumptive treatment of *H. influenzae* meningitis (a rare disease in the United States). Logistically, 0.15 mg/kg dexamethasone can be administered only after the completion of the Gram stain interpretation or on finding a positive test result for *H. influenzae* antigens.

For optimal management, close observation is mandated for the newly diagnosed and treated patient with ABM. Vital signs, systemic perfusion, and level of consciousness can rapidly change. Complications from the disease state such as shock or seizure, or complications from our interventions such as anaphylaxis or post-lumbar puncture herniation of cerebral contents, can be addressed only if the patient undergoes continuous monitoring.

Acyclovir

The issue of empiric treatment of a neonate or young infant (younger than 3 months of age) with acyclovir is controversial because identification of infected infants is challenging. Acyclovir should be administered in an ill or febrile infant with a history of maternal HSV infection, presence of vesicles on the skin, seizure, or focal neurologic findings. Acyclovir should be considered in cases of atypical presentations of sepsis or meningitis.[6] The dose of acyclovir is 20 mg/kg every 8 hours intravenously for 21 days in full-term immunocompetent infants. Polymerase chain reaction should be performed for HSV in these cases.

Disposition

A child newly diagnosed with ABM is best managed by experienced physicians and nurses who are capable of addressing critical care needs. When available, the best resource is a hospital that can provide pediatric intensive care. If transfer of the patient to another hospital is necessitated by the lack of appropriate inpatient pediatric care, the composition, expertise, and equipment of the interfacility transport team are important. It is best when the logistics are worked on in advance of the actual patient encounter.

SEIZURES

Perspective

A seizure is a paroxysmal event characterized by a change in behavior of the patient; it is caused by abnormal and excessive activity of a group of cortical neurons. The clinical appearance of the seizure depends on the location and extent of brain involved. Epilepsy is commonly defined as the occurrence of two or more unprovoked seizures. Provoked seizures, such as in the setting of acute head trauma or meningitis, do not constitute epilepsy. Epilepsy is most common in children and the elderly. In children, the highest incidence is in the first year of life. Although familial factors clearly play a role in the development of epilepsy, the exact role of genetic factors remains poorly understood.

Principles of Disease

Pathophysiology

The young, immature nervous system is more susceptible to seizures. Early in development, excitatory activity, which can lead to sustained firing, predominate, and inhibitory systems are undeveloped.[40] This is known as the period of vulnerability. A decrease in synaptic connections and alterations in the synthesis of neurotransmitters may also play a role.

Seizures and Brain Damage

It is well known that children with epilepsy are at a significant risk for cognitive impairment and behavioral abnormalities. Distinguishing the relative contribution of the effect of the seizures themselves from the underlying CNS pathologic condition and the effect of anticonvulsants is difficult. A single prolonged seizure has been convincingly shown to damage the brain, particularly the temporal lobes and hippocampus. Additionally, there is a growing body of evidence pointing to the lasting effect of repetitive, brief seizures in early childhood.[41] Repeated seizures in young experimental animals produce subtle but long lasting developmental effects on brain growth, behavioral milestones, and seizure thresholds.[42]

Clinical Features

Classification of Seizure Type

One of the first priorities in evaluating a child with a seizure is to determine the seizure type and, if possible, the seizure syndrome. Seizures are classified into two main types: partial and generalized (Box 173-3).[85,86]

Classification of Epilepsy: Epileptic Syndromes

An epileptic syndrome is characterized by a constellation of specific signs, symptoms, seizure types, prognoses, and electroencephalographic (EEG) findings. Determination of the epileptic syndrome provides information on prognosis and guides management decisions.

There are several well-described epileptic syndromes of infancy and childhood. Several of these syndromes are reviewed here (Box 173-4).

Infantile Spasms

Infantile spasms manifest during the first year of life and consist of rapid, jackknife flexor or extensor spasms that appear in clusters. An initial misdiagnosis of colic is common because these infants tend to cry and draw up their legs during the attack. The triad of infantile spasms, arrested psychomotor development, and a characteristic EEG pattern called *hypsarrhythmia* is known as West syndrome.[43] Hypsarrhythmia is an

BOX 173-3. Classification of Seizures[85,86]

Partial (focal, local) seizures
- Simple partial seizures (consciousness maintained)
  - With motor signs
  - With autonomic symptoms and signs
  - With somatosensory or special sensory symptoms
- Complex partial seizures (consciousness impaired)
  - Partial seizures evolving to secondary generalized tonic-clonic seizures

Generalized seizures (convulsive and nonconvulsive)
- Absence seizures (consciousness impaired, clonic, tonic, tonic or autonomic component)
  - Atypical absence (marked change in tone, not rapid in onset or cessation)
  - Myoclonic seizures
  - Clonic seizures
  - Tonic seizures
  - Tonic-clonic seizures
  - Atonic seizures

Unclassified epileptic seizures (includes all seizures that cannot be classified because of inadequate or incomplete data)

BOX 173-4. Modified Classification of Epileptic Syndromes[86]

I. Idiopathic epileptic syndromes (focal or generalized)
   A. Benign neonatal convulsions
   B. Benign childhood epilepsy
      1. Central midtemporal spikes (benign rolandic epilepsy of childhood)
      2. Occipital spikes
   C. Childhood/juvenile absence epilepsy
   D. Juvenile myoclonic epilepsy
   E. Idiopathic epilepsy—otherwise unspecified
II. Symptomatic epilepsy syndromes (focal or generalized)
   A. West syndrome (infantile spasms)
   B. Lennox-Gastaut syndrome
   C. Early myoclonic encephalopathy
   D. Epilepsia partialis continua
   E. Acquired epileptic aphasia (Landau-Kleffner syndrome)
   F. Temporal lobe epilepsy
   G. Frontal lobe epilepsy
   H. Posttraumatic epilepsy
   I. Other symptomatic epilepsy, not otherwise specified
III. Other epilepsy syndromes of uncertain or mixed classification
   A. Neonatal seizures
   B. Febrile seizures
   C. Reflex epilepsy
   D. Other unspecified

EEG pattern of extremely high-voltage slow waves, irregularly interspersed with spikes and sharp waves.

Approximately two thirds of children with infantile spasms have an underlying CNS disorder such as a congenital brain malformation or tuberous sclerosis; the remaining cases are cryptogenic in origin. The outcome is poor. Only half will attain remission of seizures and 90% to 95% of the children become mentally retarded.[44] The prognosis is substantially improved if development was normal before the onset of the spasms. In the United States, first-line treatment is adrenocorticotropic hormone. Vigabatrin has shown much promise, particularly in the treatment of infantile spasms associated with tuberous sclerosis, but is not approved for use yet in the United States.[45]

Lennox-Gastaut Syndrome

Lennox-Gastaut syndrome is characterized by mental retardation, multiple seizure types, and a classic EEG pattern of slow (less than 3 per second) spike and wave. The age of onset is between 1 and 8 years, and the syndrome can evolve from infantile spasms.[46] The patient usually has frequent seizures of multiple types, including atonic, atypical absence, myoclonic, tonic-clonic, and partial seizures. Adequate seizure control may be difficult. Traditionally, valproic acid has been the first-line treatment. However, in the last several years, several new anticonvulsants have shown promise in the treatment of Lennox-Gastaut syndrome. These include lamotrigine, topiramate, and felbamate.[47] Unfortunately, the prognosis remains poor.

Childhood and Juvenile Absence Epilepsy

This disorder begins most commonly between 4 and 12 years of age and is characterized by frequently recurrent absence seizures usually manifested by staring spells or periods of inattentiveness. Bursts of three per second spike-and-waves on the EEG during an absence spell is indicative of this syndrome. Generalized convulsive seizures occur in up to 50% of patients. Hyperventilation can trigger absence spells and can be used to diagnose absence epilepsy. Treatment is with ethosuximide or valproic acid, although lamotrigine is now being more commonly used in children. The prognosis is excellent and children usually outgrow this pattern by adolescence.[48]

Benign Rolandic Epilepsy of Childhood

Benign rolandic epilepsy is a partial epilepsy occurring between the ages of 3 and 13 years. Classically, the seizure occurs while sleeping and involves the face, with twisting of the mouth and anarthria. The seizure can secondarily generalize. There is a typical EEG pattern of central temporal (rolandic region) spikes during sleep. The prognosis is excellent; the seizures, as well as the EEG abnormalities, cease by 16 years of age. Carbamazepine, phenytoin, and valproic acid are all equally efficacious. However, there is considerable controversy as to whether brief seizures in this benign epilepsy syndrome warrant treatment at all.[49]

Febrile Seizures

Febrile seizures are defined as seizures in the presence of fever without CNS infection or other cause. Febrile seizures affect 5% of children before their fifth birthday. To satisfy the criteria for simple, or benign, febrile seizures, the seizure must be generalized, last less than 15 minutes, and occur in a child between 6 months and 5 years of age who is neurologically and developmentally normal.[50] Complex febrile seizures are diagnosed when multiple seizures occur during the same illness, seizures are prolonged (longer than 15 minutes), or there is a focal component to the seizure.

Febrile seizures typically occur early in the course of the febrile illness, while the temperature is rising, although it should be noted that almost half of children with a febrile seizure have a documented temperature of less than 39° C.

Overall, one third of children with a simple febrile seizure have a recurrence. Of these, one half will have a third event. The recurrence rate is inversely proportional to age, such that if the onset of febrile seizures is prior to the first birthday the recurrence risk is 50%; after 3 years of age, it is 12%.

Children with simple febrile seizures have an approximately 2% to 3% chance of developing epilepsy (compared with a 1% rate of epilepsy in the general population). Treatment with long-term anticonvulsants may reduce the risk of recurrence while on medication, but it does not affect the later risk of epilepsy.[51] Therefore, in most cases of simple febrile seizures, the risks of long-term anticonvulsant therapy outweigh its benefits. Acetaminophen or ibuprofen can be used to try to prevent fever spikes when the child develops fever or shows signs of the beginning of viral illness, but the seizure can occur before the parent is aware that the child has a fever. Published studies do not show a reduction in recurrence risk with the use of acetaminophen or ibuprofen.[52,53]

Use of pharmacologic agents to prevent recurrences is controversial. Rectal diazepam during the first 24 hours of the febrile illness is safe and effective in preventing a recurrence of a febrile seizure as well as effective in terminating prolonged or repetitive febrile seizures.[54] Limitations of its use are that the child may experience lethargy, ataxia, or dizziness while on the medications, making evaluation of mental status and behavior challenging, and the medication will not prevent afebrile seizure disorder in the future. Long-term anticonvulsant therapy is rarely warranted.

Neonatal Seizures

The frequency of seizures manifesting in the first month of life is greater than at any other time in childhood.[55] However, seizures in the newborn period may be difficult to recognize. There may be only subtle changes such as apnea, sustained eye deviation, chewing, or limb bicycling movements. Focal clonic movements are usually associated with an underlying structural lesion.

Although neonatal seizures have many causes, relatively few causes account for the majority of cases. These include hypoxic-ischemic encephalopathy, intracranial infection, congenital brain malformation, cerebrovascular events, and metabolic disturbances, particularly hypoglycemia and hypocalcemia. Although inborn errors of metabolism are rare, early treatment can be lifesaving. Pyridoxine deficiency presents with intractable seizures, unresponsive to anticonvulsants. A dose of 50 to 100 mg of pyridoxine, given intravenously or intramuscularly, will immediately stop the seizure and normalize the EEG.

Neonatal seizures have a high rate of morbidity and mortality. Overall, the rate of mental retardation and cerebral palsy in survivors of neonatal seizures is between 15% and 45%. The ultimate prognosis depends on the cause of the seizure.[56]

Status Epilepticus

Status epilepticus is a true neurologic emergency; it is associated with high rates of morbidity and mortality that increase with the duration of the seizure. Status epilepticus is somewhat arbitrarily defined as 30 minutes or longer of continuous seizure activity or sequential seizures without full recovery of consciousness between seizures. For the practitioner, any seizure lasting more than 5 minutes warrants intervention.[57] Status epilepticus occurs significantly more frequently in children, especially in those younger than 1 year of age; up to 70% of children with epilepsy onset before 1 year of age will experience at least one episode of status epilepticus. The incidence of morbidity and mortality due to status epilepticus in children appears to be lower than that in adults.[57,58]

Status epilepticus can be divided into two general types: convulsive and nonconvulsive. Although the diagnosis of convulsive status is usually obvious, the duration of the seizures is often underestimated because the intensity of the jerking tends to diminish with time; small-amplitude twitching or nystagmoid eye movements may become almost undetectable. The importance of careful observation cannot be overstated.

The hallmark of nonconvulsive status epilepticus is altered mental status. Patients demonstrate slow mentation, confusion, unresponsiveness, gross abnormal motor movements, twitches, lip smacking, mimicry, or automatisms. An EEG can confirm the diagnosis and should always be obtained if nonconvulsive status epilepticus is suspected.

In children, febrile illness is by far the most common precipitant of status epilepticus. Medication change, idiopathic epilepsy, metabolic derangements, and congenital abnormalities are the next most common. In contrast, the most common precipitants of status epilepticus in adults are cerebrovascular events, medication change, anoxia, drug or alcohol ingestion, and metabolic derangements.

Complications in patients with prolonged status epilepticus can involve any and all organ systems (Box 173-5). The overall mortality rate in pediatric status epilepticus cases is approximately 4%, in contrast to 10% to 25% in adult patients. However, the morbidity rate can be as high as 30%.[57,58]

Etiology of Seizures and Differential Considerations

When the emergency physician is confronted with a child with a suspected seizure, the first task is to determine whether the event was really a seizure. Not all paroxysmal events are seizures (Box 173-6).

Syncope is one of the most common systemic disturbances mistaken for epilepsy. It is characterized by the sudden impairment of consciousness (usually brief)

BOX 173-5. Complications of Status Epilepticus

Hypertension
Hypotension
Dysrhythmia
Congestive heart failure
Apnea
Aspiration pneumonia
Neurogenic pulmonary edema
Hyperglycemia
Hypoglycemia
Lactic acidosis
Electrolyte imbalance
Rhabdomyolysis
Uremia
Autonomic dysfunction
Hyperpyrexia
Cerebrospinal fluid pleocytosis

BOX 173-6. Episodic Disorders that May Mimic Seizures

- Newborns
  - Jitteriness
  - Benign neonatal sleep myoclonus
- Breath-holding spells
- Gastroesophageal reflux (Sandifer's syndrome)
- Migraine
- Syncope
- Sleep disorders
  - Sleep myoclonus
  - Narcolepsy
  - Nightmares
  - Night terrors
  - Somnambulism
- Tics
- Infantile shuddering attacks
- Paroxysmal choreoathetosis or dystonia
- Benign paroxysmal vertigo of childhood
- Psychologic
  - Pseudoseizures
  - Panic attack

with loss of motor tone. It results from the reversible cerebral anoxia precipitated by cardiogenic or noncardiogenic causes. If the anoxia is marked, the episode may be accompanied by tonic or clonic posturing. The patient usually complains of light-headedness before fainting and appears pale and sweaty. Postictal confusion does not occur.

Prolonged QT syndrome is one example of cardiogenic syncope. In most children, however, a cause of the syncope is never found. A complete history, physical examination, and electrocardiogram should be sufficient unless the history or physical examination suggest a specific cause.

Breath-holding spells are relatively common, occurring in 4% to 5% of children, primarily between 6 and 18 months of age. Breath-holding spells are triggered by pain or emotional upset that leads to crying. During expiration, the breath is held and the child becomes cyanotic or pale; this can progress to loss of consciousness. The infant is initially limp but then may develop a brief period of clonic movements or opisthotonos. The average attack lasts approximately 40 seconds.[59]

Migraine headaches can mimic seizures, particularly when accompanied by an aura, motor dysfunction, clouding of consciousness, nausea, or vomiting.

Disorders of sleep are distinguished by excessive daytime sleepiness or by disordered nighttime sleep. *Narcolepsy* is characterized by daytime sleep attacks, sleep paralysis, hypnagogic hallucinations (vivid hallucinations while falling asleep), and cataplexy (sudden loss of motor tone). These events can be mistaken for atonic or absence seizures. *Nocturnal enuresis* may raise the concern of a nighttime seizure with incontinence. It should be noted that nocturnal incontinence is seen in 5% to 17% of children; it usually occurs within the first few hours of sleep. *Night terrors* (pavor nocturnus) occur when the child suddenly appears to awaken and cries out. The child is usually unresponsive and inconsolable, and the event concludes with the child returning to sleep. *Sleepwalking (somnambulism)* and *sleep talking (somniloquy)* occur at least once in 15% of elementary school-age children.

Movement disorders can mimic seizures. *Tics* are rapid, repetitive, brief, involuntary movements that occur intermittently and in flurries. Those seen most commonly are eye blinking and head shaking. Patients do not lose consciousness. *Shudder attacks* are uncommon but easily mistaken for seizures. They have been described as resembling the chill one feels when cold water runs down the back. *Paroxysmal choreoathetosis* is an abnormal motor movement that may be spontaneous or triggered by the child's movement.

Children with behavioral or psychiatric disturbances can manifest behaviors that are episodic and unpredictable and appear epileptic. *Panic attacks* may be mistaken for complex partial seizures. The patient has a sudden sensation of intense fear accompanied by shortness of breath, dizziness, palpitations, sweating, choking, chest discomfort, and fear of dying. *Pseudoseizures,* also called *psychogenic seizures,* are involuntary events that mimic seizures; they can be as disabling as epileptic seizures. Many children with pseudoseizures also have epilepsy. Prolonged EEG monitoring may be necessary to differentiate an epileptic seizure from a pseudoseizure.

Hyperventilation syndrome most commonly occurs in adolescent girls with anxiety disorders. Common complaints include dyspnea, chest pain, tachycardia, light-headedness, circumoral numbness, and carpopedal spasm. Infants with gastrointestinal reflux may develop *Sandifer's syndrome,* characterized by episodes of abnormal posturing, arching of the back, retrocollis, and torticollis.

Etiology of Seizures in Children

Once the diagnosis of seizure is made, the next step is to classify the seizure and determine the cause. Seizures can be divided into three main categories:

BOX 173-7. Etiology of Acute and Remote Symptomatic Seizures

Acute Symptomatic Seizures

Febrile Seizures

Infectious
- Meningitis
- Encephalitis
- Brain abscess
- Shigella

Traumatic
- Cerebral contusion
- Hematoma: subdural, epidural, subarachnoid, intraparenchymal
- Impact seizure

Toxic
- Drug intoxication (see Box 173-5)
- Drug withdrawal

Metabolic
- Hypoglycemia
- Electrolyte disorder (sodium, calcium, magnesium)
- Hepatic or renal disorder
- Hyperosmolar states
- Inborn errors of metabolism (e.g., aminoacidurias)

Neoplastic
- Primary CNS tumor
- Metastatic CNS tumor

Vascular
- Arteriovenous malformation
- Subarachnoid hemorrhage
- Intraparenchymal hemorrhage
- Cerebral venous thrombosis
- Hypertensive encephalopathy

Miscellaneous
- Eclampsia
- Dialysis
- Post-immunization
- Hypoxia
- Hypoxic-ischemic encephalopathy
- Neurocutaneous disorder
- Neurodegenerative disease
- Ventriculoperitoneal shunt malfunction

Remote Symptomatic Seizures

Posttraumatic epilepsy
Cerebral dysgenesis
Neurocutaneous disorders (e.g., neurofibromatosis, tuberous sclerosis, Sturge-Weber syndrome)
Perinatal asphyxia
Intrauterine infection (i.e., TORCH)
Past history of stroke, meningitis, or any other disease that can cause brain damage

CNS, central nervous system; TORCH, toxoplasmosis, rubella, cytomegalovirus, and herpes simplex; may be modified to include syphil as STORCH.

acute symptomatic, remote symptomatic, and idiopathic seizures (Box 173-7).

Acute symptomatic seizures are provoked by an acute event. Fever is the most common cause of acute symptomatic seizure in children. Remote symptomatic seizures are due to an old, or remote, CNS lesion. Examples of this include head trauma (nonacute), congenital brain malformation, or any other chronic brain injury. *Idiopathic seizures* have no definable cause.

Acute Symptomatic Seizures

Central nervous system infection is a significantly more common cause of acute seizures in children than in adults.[60] Meningitis should always be considered in any person with seizures and fever. A child who has a normal mental status both before and after the seizure is unlikely to have meningitis.

Hypoglycemia (defined as a blood glucose concentration of less than 60 mg/dL in adults and children and less than 40 mg/dL in infants) can cause acute seizures. Hyponatremia (Na^+ <125 mEq/L) and hypernatremia (Na^+ >150 mEq/L) are both associated with seizures. Hyponatremia is the leading cause of nonfebrile seizures in children younger than 2 years of age. Common causes include increased water intake (especially improperly diluted formula). Hypernatremia is most commonly caused by dehydration.

Hypocalcemia and hypomagnesemia can lead to muscle spasms, paresthesias, hyperactive reflexes, weakness, tetany, and seizures. Hypocalcemia is a relatively common cause of neonatal seizures.

Posttraumatic seizures occur in as many as 15% of children after head injury. *Impact seizures* occur within 1 to 2 hours of the trauma; these in and of themselves are not associated with severe injury or with the later development of epilepsy. *Early posttraumatic seizures* occur within the first week of injury and may arise from cerebral edema, intracranial hemorrhage, laceration, or contusion. The occurrence of early posttraumatic seizures does not necessarily forecast the development of epilepsy. Phenytoin is effective in preventing early posttraumatic seizures but does not influence the development of late-onset epilepsy.[61]

Brain tumors cause a wide variety of symptoms, depending on their location and the type of tumor. In children, tumors are usually infratentorial and are therefore an unusual cause of seizures. Cerebral metastases are similarly rare in children.

Vascular malformations such as cerebral arteriovenous malformations occur in children. Subarachnoid hemorrhage is rare in pediatric patients, but seizures may be the presenting sign in 10% of patients. Ischemic stroke can manifest with a focal seizure. Congenital heart disease, sickle cell anemia, and homocystinuria are major risk factors for ischemic stroke in children.

Numerous drugs are known to cause seizures either at therapeutic dosages or from deliberate overdose. Although most drug-induced seizures are self-limited and do not result in permanent sequelae, as many as 15% of drug-related seizures manifest as status epilepticus.[62] Cyclic antidepressants, cocaine and other stimulants, antihistamines, theophylline, and isoniazid are

BOX 173-8. Drugs that May Cause Seizures

Anesthetic Agents
Etomidate
Enflurane
Methohexital
Lidocaine

Antibiotics
Penicillin
β-Lactams
Quinolones
Isoniazid
Metronidazole

Anticholinergics
Phenothiazines
Butyrophenones
Tricyclic antidepressants

Anticholinesterases
Organophosphates
Physostigmine

Anticonvulsants
Carbamazepine
Phenytoin

Antidepressants
Amitriptyline
Imipramine
Nortriptyline
Fluoxetine
Monoamine oxidase inhibitors

Antidysrhythmics
Mexiletine
Tocainide
Procainamide

Antihistamine
Diphenhydramine

Antipsychotics
Phenothiazines
Chlorpromazine
Thioridazine
Butyrophenones
Haloperidol

Antitumor Agents
Chlorambucil
Cyclosporin
β-Blockers
Propranolol
Metoprolol
Sotalol

Camphor
Carbon Monoxide
Cyanide
Contrast Agents
Ionic agents
Newer low-osmolality agents

Ethanol
Severe intoxication or withdrawal

Flumazenil
Hypoglycemic Agents
Insulin
Oral hypoglycemics

Lead
Narcotics
Fentanyl
Meperidine

Nicotine
Oxygen
Hyperbaric oxygen therapy

Sympathomimetics
Cocaine
Amphetamines
Phenylpropanolamine
Ketamine
Phencyclidine

Theophylline

the most common causes of drug-induced seizures (Box 173-8).

Seizures can occur during drug withdrawal, usually within 48 hours of drug cessation. Ethanol withdrawal may be seen in adolescent patients. Benzodiazepines and barbiturates produce an abstinence syndrome similar to ethanol withdrawal except that the onset of withdrawal symptoms and signs occurs later with these drugs than with alcohol. Flumazenil, a benzodiazepine receptor antagonist, has caused seizures by precipitating benzodiazepine withdrawal.

A hypertensive crisis can provoke seizures; conversely, status epilepticus can induce hypertension.[63] Reflex seizures are precipitated by a specific, identifiable stimulus. Some of the stimuli that induce seizure activity are light, eye closing, thinking, reading, startle, music, immersion in hot water, eating, and vestibular stimulation. Television and video games can induce seizures in photosensitive children.[64] Rarely, patients with ventriculoperitoneal shunt malfunctions present with seizures.[65]

Diagnostic Strategies

The initial diagnostic evaluation has several objectives. The first is to determine whether the event in question was actually a seizure. The second is to determine whether the seizure was an acute symptomatic seizure and, if so, to determine a specific underlying cause. If the seizure was not caused by an acute precipitant, the next objective is to determine, if possible, whether the seizure was a manifestation of epilepsy. If the patient arrives in the emergency department actively convulsing, attention must be immediately directed toward airway management and stopping the seizure.

A complete history is the cornerstone for establishing the diagnosis of a seizure and epilepsy. Effort should be extended to obtaining a description from an eyewitness. An adequate history should provide a clear picture of the clinical features of the episode, including the events just before and after it:

Events that led up to the attack: What was the patient doing at the time? Did the patient complain of anything such as dizziness, a bad smell, or flashing lights? Was the patient confused? Did the attack start abruptly?

The attack: Did the patient get stiff or limp? Did the patient shake? Was there a loss of consciousness? Was involvement on one side of the body different from involvement on the other side? Did the eyes or head turn in one direction? Was there incontinence? The observer should be asked to demonstrate the movements.

Events directly after the attack: Was the patient lethargic or confused? Did the patient complain of anything? Did the patient remember the event?

Possible precipitants of seizures, such as fever, illness, head injury, drug use, and any ingestion, should be detailed. Risk factors for epilepsy including a history of meningitis, head injury or febrile seizures, congenital abnormalities, developmental delay, or a family history of epilepsy should be sought. Any prior history of abnormal movements, staring spells, or myoclonic jerks should be obtained.

The occurrence of postictal confusion, headache, or fatigue can help differentiate a seizure from a nonepileptic event.[66] The movements in patients with partial seizures are usually simple and purposeless; they are not directed attacks or complex actions.

The general physical examination should be directed at signs of systemic disease that can cause seizure. Particular attention should be paid to signs of meningitis, head trauma, drug use, dehydration, hypertension, and heart disease. Skin lesions such as café au lait spots or hypopigmented nevi may point to a neurocutaneous disorder. An abnormal head circumference may point to hydrocephalus or abnormal brain growth. Attention to the presence of injury (e.g., oropharyngeal trauma, shoulder dislocation) is necessary to assist in securing the diagnosis of seizure and directing therapy to the injuries.

A careful neurologic examination must be performed. There is no one abnormality in the child with a seizure. The examination is directed toward signs of increased ICP (eye movement abnormality, pupil asymmetry, papilledema), focal findings, and developmental delay. The gait should be tested on all children who can walk.

Laboratory

Routine laboratory studies, including blood chemistry profile, liver function testing, complete blood cell count (CBC), and a toxicology screening test are not recommended in children who are neurologically normal after a seizure. Although hypoglycemia and electrolyte abnormalities can cause seizures, abnormalities sufficient to cause seizures are almost always associated with persistent abnormal mental status. In a study of 308 children who arrived at an emergency department with seizure, there were no significant abnormalities in serum electrolytes, calcium, glucose, or magnesium.[67] Uncomplicated simple febrile seizures usually do not require routine laboratory studies.

A lumbar puncture is mandated in the patient with an abnormal mental status or other signs of meningitis, regardless of whether fever is present. Most patients have an altered mental status in the postictal period. Therefore, if the concern for meningitis is low, the practitioner may opt to observe the patient over the next 30 to 60 minutes and if the patient's condition returns to baseline, a lumbar puncture can be avoided. In general, a child with a normal neurologic examination who had a brief seizure in the setting of fever can be assumed to have a simple febrile seizure. According to the American Academy of Pediatrics recommendations, lumbar puncture is not necessary in children older than 18 months with a first simple febrile seizure. However, lumbar puncture should be considered in the child younger than 12 months, as signs of meningitis can be subtle in this age group.[68]

A prolonged seizure, or seizure lasting 30 minutes or longer, can cause a mild elevation of white blood cells in the CSF, presumably from a transient disruption of the blood-brain barrier.[69]

Radiography/Imaging

There is considerable disagreement as to the need for neuroimaging in patients who come to the emergency department after a first seizure. Any child with an abnormal neurologic examination should undergo imaging acutely, as should most children with focal seizures or secondarily generalized seizures.[70] Children with generalized unprovoked seizures and normal examination findings do not usually require acute imaging. At follow-up evaluation, further information, such as an EEG with a focal abnormality, may warrant imaging, and neuroimaging can be done at that time.

If imaging is indicated in the acute period, either CT or magnetic resonance imaging (MRI) can be used. MRI provides superior anatomic detail, but the examination often requires sedation, and the patient cannot be closely monitored. CT provides rapid imaging and is highly sensitive for detecting acute blood and fractures; it therefore is the examination of choice in the unstable patient or in one suspected of having head trauma.

Special Procedures

The EEG reflects the activity of a large population of neurons, primarily that of cortical pyramidal neurons. The EEG produces distinctive patterns in epilepsy. In generalized epilepsy, changes in the EEG are evident over the entire brain at seizure onset. In partial epilepsy, changes in the EEG are restricted to a focal area, although the area of disturbance may spread.

Electroencephalography rarely needs to be performed in the acute setting unless there is the concern about nonconvulsive status or ongoing status in a patient who has been chemically paralyzed and intubated. The EEG assesses the underlying background activity of the brain and provides evidence of epileptiform activity. Distinctive patterns occur in specific epilepsy syndromes.

Epileptiform discharges correlate highly with susceptibility to seizures. Unfortunately, 10% to 40% of patients with known epilepsy do not show epileptiform abnormalities on routine EEG.[71] Techniques such as sleep deprivation, hyperventilation, and photic stimulation enhance the sensitivity of the EEG. Ideally, all EEGs should be performed with the patient awake, drowsy, and asleep. Occasionally, prolonged video-EEG monitoring may be necessary to record the EEG during the event in question.

Management

The vast majority of seizures are self-limited and without sequelae. For brief events, the only intervention required is to protect the patient from self-harm (Box 173-9). Patients who present to the emergency

BOX 173-9. Summary Approach to a Child with a Seizure

If the child is actively convulsing on presentation:
- Ensure adequate oxygenation and cardiorespiratory function
- Stop the seizure
- Prevent seizure recurrence
- Identify precipitating factors (e.g., hypoglycemia, electrolyte imbalance, low anticonvulsant levels, fever, trauma, CNS infection) and treat accordingly
- Further evaluate and treat the cause of status epilepticus

If the child presents after the event is over:
- Determine whether event was truly a seizure
- Determine seizure type
- Identify precipitating factors (e.g., hypoglycemia, electrolyte imbalance, low anticonvulsant levels, fever, trauma, CNS infection) and treat accordingly
- Determine further workup necessary to identify cause of seizure
- Determine whether anticonvulsant therapy is appropriate at this time

CNS, central nervous system.

department actively convulsing should be assumed to be in status epilepticus and treated accordingly.

Status Epilepticus

Airway Management

Status epilepticus represents a true medical emergency. The patient should be positioned to maximize ventilation and to prevent physical injury. The cervical spine must be protected if trauma cannot be excluded. Oxygen should be administered via nasal cannula or face mask, and a large suction catheter should be available to suction the patient's secretions. In the younger patient, the tongue may obstruct the airway. In this case, placement of a nasopharyngeal airway will keep the tongue forward and improve the patient's respiratory status. No attempts should be made to place anything in the patient's mouth.

If the airway cannot otherwise be maintained, there is respiratory failure, or there is clinical evidence of increased ICP, the patient should be intubated using rapid sequence intubation. Respiratory failure can occur during the administration of anticonvulsants. Use of a short-acting neuromuscular blocking agent such as succinylcholine or possibly rocuronium is recommended so that clinical signs of seizure activity will only be masked by the paralyzing agent for a short period of time.

Monitoring and Diagnostic Studies

Monitoring should include cardiovascular (heart rate, blood pressure) and pulmonary (respiratory rate, pulse oximetry) function. Hyperthermia should be treated with antipyretics and cooling blankets if necessary. Meticulous attention should be paid to avoiding hypoxia.

An intravenous line should be placed and blood samples drawn. Assuming the cause of the seizure is unknown, blood should be obtained for determination of serum electrolytes, glucose, sodium, calcium, magnesium, renal function, toxicology, antiepileptic levels (if indicated), and CBC. A rapid blood glucose level should be determined. If the glucose level is below normal, intravenous glucose should be given immediately. If necessary, an intraosseous line can be used to administer all medications, including anticonvulsants.

Administration of Antiepileptic Medication

The main principle of treatment of status epilepticus is to stop the seizure as rapidly as possible and prevent recurrence. The three most commonly used agents to treat convulsive status epilepticus are benzodiazepines, phenytoin, and barbiturates (Table 173-4).[72-73] More than half of patients with status epilepticus respond to therapy with a single antiepileptic drug. The average time to terminate status epilepticus is 15 to 30 minutes.

Benzodiazepines, particularly diazepam and lorazepam, are usually the initial drugs used in the treatment of status epilepticus. They diffuse quickly into the CNS, rapidly terminating seizure activity 75% to 90% of the time.[74] Both diazepam and lorazepam are equally effective in terminating status epilepticus, but lorazepam has a substantially longer duration of antiseizure effect (12 to 24 hours versus 15 to 30 minutes). The recommended pediatric intravenous dose of lorazepam is 0.1 mg/kg (maximum, 8 mg) at a rate of 1 to 2 mg/min. The recommended intravenous dose of diazepam is 0.2 to 0.5 mg/kg (maximum 10 mg) at a rate of 2 mg/min. Hypotension, respiratory depression, and impaired consciousness can occur in the course of benzodiazepine treatment.

One advantage of diazepam is that it can be administered rectally if intravenous access cannot be obtained; lorazepam is poorly absorbed rectally. If

Table 173-4. Antiepileptic Drug Therapy for Status Epilepticus

Drug	Initial Dose (mg/kg)	Rate	Repeat Dose	Time to Stop Seizure	Comments
A. Lorazepam	0.05-0.1 mg/kg IV/IO (max 8 mg)	2 mg/min	q 15 min (twice)	2-3 min	Watch for respiratory depression
or					
Diazepam	0.3-0.5 mg/kg IV/IO/PR (max 10 mg)	2 mg/min	q 15 min (twice)	1-3 min	
B. Fosphenytoin	20 mg PE/kg IV	150 mg PE/min	5-10 mg PE/kg	10-30 min	Monitor for hypotension, arrhythmia
or					
Phenytoin	20 mg/kg IV	1 mg/kg/min	5-10 mg/kg		No glucose in line (phenytoin only)
C. Phenobarbital	20 mg/kg IV	100 mg/min	5-10 mg/kg	20-30 min	Be prepared to intubate Avoid neuromuscular blockade if possible Monitor for hypotension
D. Midazolam Drip	0.2 mg/kg bolus	0.75-10 µg/k/min			Monitor EEG to burst suppression or suppression of epileptiform discharges
or					
Propofol	1-2 mg/kg bolus	2-10 mg/k/hr			
or					
Pentobarbital	10-15 mg/kg over 1 hour	0.5-1 mg/k/hr			

EEG, electroencephalogram; PE, phenytoin equivalents (see text).

Diastat, a rectal preparation of diazepam, is not available, the intravenous preparation can be inserted 4 to 6 cm into the rectum through a lubricated feeding tube. The appropriate rectal dosage is 0.5 mg/kg (maximum, 20 mg). Multiple doses of benzodiazepine may be required to stop the seizure; if so, the patient must be monitored carefully for respiratory depression. There have been recent reports on the use of buccal and intranasal midazolam in patients with status epilepticus, but this drug is not yet widely used.[75]

A long-term anticonvulsant agent should be given to prevent seizure recurrence. The first-line treatment is usually phenytoin or fosphenytoin. Fosphenytoin is a water-soluble phosphate ester of phenytoin (prodrug) that is rapidly converted in plasma to phenytoin. Unlike phenytoin, fosphenytoin can be administered intramuscularly, can be administered with common intravenous solutions, and is substantially less cardiotoxic and less sclerosing to the vasculature. Additionally, it can be given three times as rapidly as phenytoin. Fosphenytoin produces similar plasma concentrations to phenytoin in the same time period (10-30 minutes).

Phenytoin (or fosphenytoin) effectively terminates seizure activity in 40% to 90% of patients with generalized convulsive status epilepticus. The lower success rate is seen in patients with anoxic, metabolic, or toxic disturbances. The standard loading dose is 18 to 20 mg/kg at a rate of 1 mg/kg/min, not exceeding 50 mg/min. A dose of 20 mg/kg will therefore take a minimum of 20 minutes to be completed. The loading dosage of fosphenytoin is 20 PE (phenytoin equivalents)/kg at 150 mg/min. Cardiovascular status, including blood pressure and electrocardiogram, should be monitored carefully with either medication. If hypotension results, the rate of infusion should be decreased. If seizure activity continues, a second dose of lorazepam (0.1 mg/kg) and/or fosphenytoin/phenytoin (5-10 mg PE/kg or mg/kg) should be given.

If the seizure still has not stopped, phenobarbital, 20 mg/kg, should be loaded at a rate of 1 mg/kg/min (maximum of 100 mg/min). An additional dose of 5 to 10 mg/min can be given every 15 minutes if necessary, up to 40 mg/min. Significant side effects include depressed consciousness, apnea, and hypotension. These complications are more pronounced in the presence of benzodiazepines.

An intravenous preparation of valproic acid is now available. Its use in the treatment of status epilepticus is not fully defined as of yet.

In infants younger than 1 year, phenobarbital is usually the first-line medication because phenytoin is erratically absorbed in infants, and it is difficult to maintain appropriate levels. The loading dose is 20 mg/kg; additional dosages of 5 to 10 mg/kg can be used as needed. If the seizure continues, phenytoin or fosphenytoin is then used.

When status epilepticus is refractory to these medications, several treatments can be applied. In general, the patient is placed on a continuous intravenous infusion of medication while undergoing EEG monitoring. The dosage is titrated until suppression of electroencephalographic spikes or a burst suppression pattern is obtained. The infusion is maintained for 12 to 24 hours and then tapered. If seizure activity recurs, the infusion is restarted. Low-dose dopamine and/or dobutamine may be needed to treat hypotension.

Midazolam is a safe and effective benzodiazepine that has been shown to be extremely effective in terminating status epilepticus refractory to conventional agents. A bolus of 0.2 mg/kg is administered by slow intravenous injection, followed by infusion of 0.75 to 10 μg/kg/min.[76] The dose is increased every 15 minutes to effectiveness. The drug's short elimination half-life, rapid onset, and water solubility add to its safety profile. Tachyphylaxis may occur, requiring high doses.

Propofol has also shown to be highly effective in the treatment of refractory status epilepticus. An initial intravenous bolus dose of 1 to 2 mg/kg is followed by 2 to 10 mg/kg/hr.[77]

Pentobarbital, with an initial dose of 10 to 15 mg/kg intravenously over 1 hour, followed by 0.5 to 1.0 mg/kg/hr, is also effective. However, severe hypotension requiring inotropic support, cardiovascular toxicity, and postinfusion weakness are common complications, making this medication a less attractive choice. One potential benefit is the as-yet unproven possibility that barbiturates have cerebral protective effect. This awaits further elucidation. Another alternative is to use increasingly high phenobarbital dosing to maintain the patient in a barbiturate coma.

Nonconvulsive status epilepticus is more difficult to recognize and usually requires EEG for diagnosis. The hallmark of these entities is a change in mental status. Confusion, depression of consciousness, and emotional and behavioral changes are usually present. Acute treatment is with benzodiazepines. Valproic acid is a very effective anticonvulsant for this disorder and is now available in parenteral form. The typical loading dose is 20 mg/kg intravenously.[78] Valproic acid can also be administered by nasogastric tube or per rectum.

Identification and Treatment of Precipitators of Seizures

Once the seizure has been stopped, attention must be directed to the cause of the seizure. A child with normal neurologic examination findings who has had a brief seizure in the setting of fever can be assumed to have a simple febrile seizure. As noted earlier, according to the American Academy of Pediatrics recommendations, any further workup or treatment is solely directed at the cause of the underlying infection.[68]

Treatment of toxic metabolic seizures involves supportive care and treatment of the underlying disorder. Hypoglycemia must be identified immediately and treated aggressively as outlined previously. Severe hyponatremia resulting in seizures can be treated with the administration of an IV bolus of 3% saline. Hypocalcemia can be treated with 10% IV calcium gluconate.

Most toxic ingestions that cause seizures do not have an antidote. Isoniazid is one exception. The administration of intravenous pyridoxine can stop the seizures.

BOX 173-10. Advice to Parents about Simple Febrile Seizures[53]

- Febrile seizures occur in 2% to 5% of all children between the ages of 6 months and 5 years.
- These seizures may appear frightening to observers but are generally harmless.
- Simple febrile seizures often occur in the first 24 hours of the febrile illness and only occur once. If the seizure recurs, your child should be re-evaluated.
- A febrile seizure may be manifested by body stiffening, twitching of the face and/or arms and legs, eye rolling, jerking of the arms and legs, staring, or loss of consciousness.
- Febrile seizures generally last less than a minute but can last up to 15 minutes.
- Your child may appear not to be breathing and the skin color may become darker, if so, call 9-1-1 or emergency personnel and lay the child on the floor on his/her back and DO NOT place your fingers in the child's mouth.
- Febrile seizures do not cause brain damage or paralysis.
- A child who has febrile seizures has only a slightly increased risk of developing a seizure disorder compared with a child who never had a febrile seizure.
- Febrile seizures tend to run in families.
- Febrile seizures can recur with subsequent febrile illnesses. Medicines are generally not given to prevent simple febrile seizures.
- Using medicines such as acetaminophen or ibuprofen for fevers has not been shown to prevent febrile seizures.

Disposition

Decision to Hospitalize

In general, hospitalization is unnecessary for patients after a first unprovoked seizure, providing their neurologic examination findings are normal and good follow-up monitoring is possible. EEG and imaging studies can be done on an outpatient basis, as necessary.

Children with simple febrile seizures can almost always be sent home. The child should be treated with antipyretics for the duration of the febrile illness. Parents should be instructed on first aid, on when to call for emergency medical services, on beginning antipyretics at the start of any future febrile illness, and on follow-up with a primary care physician. Warden and colleagues[53] outlined advice on febrile seizures to be given to families in the emergency department (Box 173-10).

Children who have had a prolonged seizure, abnormal neurologic examination findings (or findings that are different from baseline), or a persistent alteration of mental status should be admitted. In addition, if adequate follow-up evaluation cannot be arranged, if there is concern that the patient will be lost to follow-up evaluation, or if there is extreme parental anxiety, the child should be admitted to the hospital. Children with acute symptomatic seizures will usually need to be admitted based on the underlying disorder.

Decision to Start Anticonvulsant Therapy

The decision to start anticonvulsant prophylaxis must take into account many variables. In particular, the decision must balance the risk of recurrent seizure (chance of recurrence and risk of injury during or as a result of seizure) with the risk of long-term medication use.

Risk of Recurrence of Seizures

Children with a first unprovoked seizure have a one-third rate of recurrence; 75% of these will have a third seizure and 75% of these will have a fourth.[79,80] Most recurrences occur within the first year; 90% occur within 2 years.[81] Children with Todd's paralysis and those with an abnormal EEG, a family history of epilepsy, or remote symptomatic seizures have a higher risk of recurrence than children without these risk factors. Children who have a seizure while asleep have twice the risk of recurrence as children who have their seizure while awake. Children whose first unprovoked seizure occurred while awake and who have a normal EEG have only a 21% 5-year recurrence risk.[81] These risk factors can guide the decision as to whether to place a child on long-term anticonvulsant medication. Overall, the general consensus is to not treat patients after a first unprovoked seizure.

Unlike a single, self-limited seizure, the occurrence of status epilepticus carries a high morbidity and mortality rate. Pediatric patients with prolonged status epilepticus (lasting for more than 1 hour) may experience significant sequelae, including epilepsy, mental retardation, and neurologic defects.

In addition, children who have poorly controlled epilepsy show progressive decline in IQ (intelligence quotient), and there is an increased incidence of psychiatric disorders in children with epilepsy.[82] Therefore, children with prolonged and/or repeated seizures warrant treatment.

Patients with acute symptomatic seizures may go on to develop epilepsy. The rate of epilepsy is dependent on the extent of injury, if any, during the acute event. For example, the risk of epilepsy after neonatal hypocalcemic seizures is negligible. On the other hand, head trauma with cerebral hemorrhage and contusion carries a high risk of epilepsy. In the acute period, a patient with acute symptomatic seizures who has a high risk of recurrence (e.g., head trauma or meningitis) should be treated prophylactically with anticonvulsants. When the patient is stable, the decision to continue or discontinue treatment is made. Clinical examination, neuroimaging, and EEG will guide the decision. There is no evidence that early treatment with anticonvulsant medications alters the later risk of epilepsy.[83]

Risks of Anticonvulsant Therapy

Side effects of anticonvulsant medications are common and include sedation, dizziness, blurred vision, ataxia, and gastrointestinal disturbance. These are usually dose related and can be significantly reduced by starting at a low dose and slowly increasing over several weeks.

Idiosyncratic reactions include hepatotoxicity, agranulocytosis, aplastic anemia, rash, Stevens-Johnson syndrome, and serum sickness. Anticonvulsants can interact with one another as well as with other medications. Erythromycin, isoniazid, and cimetidine are among the more common medications that alter drug levels. Many anticonvulsants are hepatically metabolized; dosage adjustment must be made in the patient with hepatic failure. Many of the newer anticonvulsant agents do not have drug interactions.

In several studies, the adverse effects of long-term anticonvulsant medications are often significant enough to outweigh the benefits of preventing a seizure recurrence after a single unprovoked seizure.

Choosing an Anticonvulsant

The choice of medication is dictated by the seizure type or syndrome and the side effect profile. The dose of a single medication is progressively increased until seizures are controlled or toxicity results. If monotherapy is unsuccessful, a second drug is slowly added or substituted. Drug levels must be monitored with the older anticonvulsant agents, particularly phenytoin (because of wide individual variation of metabolism and nonlinear elimination kinetics) and carbamazepine (which induces hepatic enzymes that are responsible for its own biotransformation). Many of the newer anticonvulsants do not require monitoring of drug levels.

Phenytoin, phenobarbital, valproic acid, and carbamazepine are all excellent medications for generalized and partial seizures. Long-term effects of phenytoin, namely hirsutism, gum hyperplasia, and facial coarsening make it a poor long-term choice in children. Side effects of phenobarbital include behavioral changes (hyperactivity, irritability), sleep disturbances, and lower IQ. For this reason, phenobarbital is rarely used in children older than 2 years. On the other hand, it is often used in infants because of its consistent absorption and excellent safety profile. Valproic acid has a relatively high incidence of hepatotoxicity, particularly in children younger than 2 years. Therefore, carbamazepine is the usual first drug of choice in patients with partial epilepsy. Carbamazepine is now available in a sustained-release preparation. Oxcarbazepine, a prodrug of carbamazepine, is also available.

Valproic acid is commonly the first-line treatment in the patient with primary generalized epilepsy. In particular, myoclonic and absence seizures, with or without generalized tonic-clonic seizures, are usually treated with valproic acid as first-line treatment. Carbamazepine will worsen absence and myoclonic seizures. Ethosuximide is effective for absence seizures; it is not effective for convulsive seizures.

In the last decade, several new anticonvulsants have been approved by the Food and Drug Administration (Table 173-5). These include gabapentin, felbamate, lamotrigine, topiramate, tiagabine, oxcarbazepine, and

Table 173-5. Summary of Commonly Used Anticonvulsants in Children

	Seizure Type	Average Daily Maintenance (mg/kg/d)	Therapeutic Level (μg/mL)	Dose-Related Side Effects (not including sedation and dizziness)	Idiosyncratic Effects
Phenytoin (Dilantin)	Partial, GTC	4-7	10-20	Ataxia, nystagmus, vertigo, hirsutism, gum hyperplasia	Stevens-Johnson syndrome
Carbamazepine (Tegretol)	Partial, GTC	15-30	6-12	Ataxia, nystagmus, vertigo	SIADH, aplastic anemia, Stevens-Johnson syndrome, hepatotoxicity
Valproic acid (Depakene/ Depakote)	Absence, myoclonic, atonic, GTC	15-60	40-120	Thrombocytopenia, weight gain, tremor, platelet dysfunction	Hepatotoxicity, pancreatitis, aplastic anemia, Stevens-Johnson syndrome
Phenobarbital	Partial, GTC	3-6	15-40	Hyperactivity, decreased IQ	
Diazepam (Diastat)	Clusters, status epilepticus	0.5 mg/k/dose PRN rectally	Level not routinely sent	Respiratory depression	
Clonazepam (Klonopin)	Myoclonic, atonic	0.1-0.2	Level not routinely sent	Increased secretions	
Ethosuximide	Absence	20-40	40-100	Nausea, gastrointestinal distress	
Gabapentin	Partial	900-3600 mg/day	Level not routinely sent	Cognitive abnormalities, exacerbation of preexisting hyperactivity	
Lamotrigine	Partial, Lennox-Gastaut	2-10	Level not routinely sent	Dizziness, diplopia, ataxia	Stevens-Johnson syndrome (especially if used with valproic acid)
Levitaractam	Partial	20-40	Level not routinely sent	Agitation, somnolence	
Topiramate	Partial, GTC, Lennox-Gastaut	5-9	Level not routinely sent	Kidney stones, psychomotor slowing	Hepatotoxicity

GTC, generalized tonic clonic seizure; PRN, as needed; SIADH, syndrome of inappropriate antidiuretic hormone secretion.

levetiracetam. These drugs are being used increasingly in the pediatric population both as second-line add-on therapy and, increasingly, as first-line therapy. Vigabatrin is used widely in Europe, but it is not currently approved for use in the United States. Lamotrigine has a similar anticonvulsant spectrum to valproic acid and is being used increasingly as first-line therapy.

Rectal diazepam (Diastat) is prescribed to prevent future episodes of status epilepticus or seizure clusters. It is given while a seizure is occurring to prevent status epilepticus.

Decision to Withdraw Anticonvulsant Therapy

Many practitioners consider withdrawal of anticonvulsants if the patient has remained seizure free for more than 2 years.[84] Several known risk factors increase the likelihood of recurrence. These include an age of onset greater than 12 years, a positive family history of epilepsy, a history of atypical febrile seizures, remote symptomatic epilepsy, and the presence of slowing on the EEG. A child with none of these risk factors has only a 12% risk of recurrence after having been seizure free for 2 years or more.

There is no consensus as to the length of time of withdrawal; medication tapers lasting anywhere from several weeks to several months have been used.

HEADACHES IN CHILDREN

Perspective

Headache is a common problem in children and adolescents. Even though the majority of patients have benign causes of headaches, which can usually be diagnosed by a careful history and physical examination, radiologic evaluation using CT or MRI or both may be necessary in selected cases. Proper diagnosis, treatment, and close monitoring of these patients are extremely important to ensure that no serious cause for the headache has been overlooked.

Studies of schoolchildren have indicated that 40% of children will experience a headache by 7 years of age and 75% will experience a headache by the time they are 15 years of age and also that migraine (one of the most common causes of headache in childhood) occurs in 1% of children by 7 years of age and 5% of children by 15 years of age. Studies in the United States have found that the highest incidence (246 per 100,000 person-years) of migraine headache occurs in boys 10 to 14 years old.[87]

Principles of Disease

There are several pathophysiologic theories to explain the mechanisms of headache. The *vascular theory* proposes that headaches are produced by dilation of intracranial or extracranial arteries. The change in vessel diameter triggers pain. Vasoconstrictive drugs, such as ergots, can relieve migraine pain. The *neuronal theory* proposes that headaches are due to a primary dysfunction of the brain; a wave of spreading neuronal depression is accompanied by decreased cerebral blood flow. Serotonin (5-hydroxytryptamine or 5-HT) may be a key mediator in this cascade of events. Serotonin agonists have been shown to relieve migraine pain. The *trigeminovascular theory* is an integrated hypothesis that combines elements of both theories. The trigeminal nerve makes synaptic connections with cerebral blood vessels, and the headache is an expression of the nerve-blood vessel interaction.[88]

Clinical Features

Headaches can be classified into five temporal patterns: acute, acute recurrent, chronic progressive, chronic nonprogressive, and mixed. An acute headache is new in onset and different from previous headaches; it can herald a broad range of conditions ranging from a viral illness to a subarachnoid hemorrhage. Acute recurrent headaches can be expressed as periodic events, which are separated by pain-free intervals. Chronic progressive headaches occur over weeks to months. They can signify serious medical disorders such as brain tumors or arteriovenous malformations. Chronic nonprogressive headaches usually occur for years and are classified as primary headaches (as opposed to secondary, symptomatic headaches). Mixed headaches are a combination of acute recurrent headaches (migraine) superimposed on a pattern of daily chronic nonprogressive headaches.[89,90]

The primary goal of the emergency physician is to differentiate symptomatic headaches from primary headaches such as migraine or tension headaches. The history is critical in evaluating children's complaints of headache and is the most important factor in determining the correct diagnosis. Both the patient and family should be asked about specific characteristics related to the headache. Rothner has created a "headache database" from which clinicians can formulate a diagnosis (Box 173-11).[90]

In addition to the important questions in Box 173-11, the clinician must focus on a detailed history of the neurologic system for any related symptoms (e.g., lethargy, ataxia, seizures, weakness, visual disturbances) and a general review of other organ systems. Warning signs of symptomatic headaches include new onset, occurrence with straining or athletics, association with neurologic symptoms, change in headache pattern, nocturnal awakening, and bioccipital headaches. Additional information related to the past medical history (e.g., history of recent head trauma, neurologic or psychiatric disorders, hospital admissions, and medications) is also important.

The physical examination, including vital signs, must be performed in a careful manner with particular attention to those findings unique to children. The child's height, weight, and head circumference should be compared to standard percentiles and the child's prior growth history; a change in the rate or direction of growth may indicate the presence of an intracerebral mass or hydrocephalus. Blood pressure should also be carefully measured with attention to age-appropriate cuff size and percentiles for age. A child's head should

BOX 173-11. Headache Database[90]

- Do you have more than one type of headache?
- How did the headache begin?
- Was there associated trauma or infection?
- How long has the headache been present?
- Are the symptoms worsening or staying the same?
- How often do the symptoms occur and how often do they last?
- Do the headaches occur at any special time or circumstance?
- Are the headaches preceded by warning signs?
- Where does it hurt?
- What is the quality of the pain? Is there pounding or sharp sensation?
- Do you have any associated symptoms during the headache? Abdominal pain? Is there any nausea or vomiting?
- Do you stop what you are doing during the headache?
- Do you have any other medical problems?
- Are you taking other medications?
- Are there activities that make the headache worse?
- Does any medication make the headache better?
- Does anyone in your family have headaches?
- What do you think is causing your headache?

BOX 173-12. Differential Diagnosis of Headache[89]

Aneurysm/arteriovenous malformation
Congenital malformation (e.g., Dandy-Walker syndrome)
Hydrocephalus
Hematoma—subdural, epidural (acute), intraparenchymal
Hypertension
Infectious: viral illness, abscess, meningitis, encephalitis
Metabolic
Neoplasm
Pseudotumor cerebri
Subarachnoid hemorrhage; berry aneurysm rupture
Toxic (medication, cocaine abuse, analgesia rebound)
Trauma

also be auscultated for bruits associated with arteriovenous malformations, and a skin examination should be performed for stigmata of neurocutaneous disorders such as neurofibromatosis. The neurologic examination should include particular attention to the child's mental status, language, and level of consciousness as well as a detailed neurologic examination (including cranial nerves, gait, cerebellar, sensory, and motor function, and deep tendon reflexes) and an ophthalmologic examination (including pupillary reactivity, visual acuity, extraocular movements, and a funduscopic examination). Observation of the interaction between the patient and family may also provide clues to potential family problems, depression, or anxiety.

Headache Syndromes and Differential Considerations

The list of differential considerations for headache is extensive (Box 173-12).[89]

Acute Headache

The acute headache is a common problem in children and adolescents and accompanies many infectious processes. In the absence of other signs of CNS involvement (such as nuchal rigidity or alteration in level of consciousness), headaches in febrile children are usually not evidence of CNS infection. In fact, nonspecific viral illnesses represent the majority of diagnoses in the child presenting to the emergency department with an acute headache.

The most common cause of subarachnoid hemorrhage in young adults is a ruptured cerebral aneurysm. In younger children, rupture of an arteriovenous malformation that is near the subarachnoid space may cause subarachnoid and intraparenchymal hemorrhage. A common site of bleeding is the anterior cerebral artery with resulting pressure on the third cranial nerve. Varying degrees of ptosis, lateral deviation of the eye, and pupillary dilation may be seen with this type of aneurysm.

If subarachnoid hemorrhage is suspected, CT of the head (non–contrast-enhanced) should be performed as soon as possible. If the CT scan does not show subarachnoid blood, a lumbar puncture must be performed, as a head CT scan is normal 5% to 10% of the time, especially if only a small amount of bleeding has occurred. The first and last samples taken in the lumbar puncture are examined for cells to eliminate the possibility of a traumatic tap (in a traumatic tap, the number of red blood cells would be expected to decrease by the last tube) and the presence or absence of xanthochromia.

Localized acute headaches are commonly due to sinusitis, otitis media, dental disorders, or head trauma. Dental disorders are usually accompanied by localized pain in the teeth, gums, or jaw. Temporomandibular joint dysfunction is usually seen with unilateral pain in the ear, jaw, or mouth. Headache associated with trauma must always be carefully evaluated for the possibility of subdural or epidural hematomas, fractures, and leptomeningeal cyst—a "growing" skull fracture in a child 3 years of age or younger with a history of recent trauma. Ophthalmologic problems such as astigmatism, refractory errors, eye strain, and squint are also occasionally responsible for headaches in children.

Chronic-Progressive Headache

The chronic-progressive headache category is composed of disorders that cause progressive severe headaches in children. The development of increased ICP, which can be caused by brain tumors, pseudotumor cerebri, hydrocephalus, brain abscess, and intracranial bleeding, is a major problem in this category. Headaches that awaken the child or are present when first awakening are a classic symptom of increased ICP. Impaired venous outflow in the supine position leads to excess fluid (blood, CSF, or edema) inside the skull, leading to increased pressure. Nocturnal or morning emesis may also suggest increased ICP. The physical examination may show symptoms of increased ICP (papilledema, brisk reflexes, cranial nerve deficits, upgoing toes, decreased level of consciousness) as well as focal symptoms related to the location of the lesion (e.g., hemiparesis, ataxia, visual field deficits).

Headaches may be the first symptom of a brain tumor and occur with increasing frequency with age. In a recent study, 18% of 0- to 5-year-olds, 52% of 6- to 10-year-olds, and 68% of 11- to 20-year-olds who had brain tumors presented with headaches. Only 38% of primary brain tumors were diagnosed within the first month after the onset of symptoms.[91] More than 50% of these children had at least three associated symptoms, such as nausea, vomiting, visual effects, problems with walking, weakness, and changes in personality, school performance, or speech. The most common neurologic findings were papilledema, abnormal eye movements, ataxia, abnormal tendon reflexes, and abnormal visual examination findings.[92,93]

Clinical findings of pseudotumor cerebri (idiopathic intracranial hypertension) are secondary to the increased ICP and include papilledema, sixth cranial nerve palsy, and visual field obstruction. This condition is more common in females and in younger compared with older age groups and is associated with obesity; use of outdated tetracycline; presence of otitis media or head trauma; use of vitamin A, steroids, birth control pills, or tetracycline; presence of menstrual irregularities or diseases that produce obstruction of the CSF pathways; and obstruction of the major venous sinuses. By definition, neuroimaging findings are normal. The lumbar puncture usually demonstrates elevated pressure, often over 20 cm H_2O and normal CSF protein and glucose levels. Neuroimaging should precede a lumbar puncture when increased ICP is suspected. Treatment can include diuretics and repeated lumbar puncture to remove CSF.[89] Hydrocephalus may be related to a previous episode of meningitis, subarachnoid hemorrhage, or head injury or may be congenital.

Brain abscess can result from meningitis, head trauma, chronic otitis media and sinusitis, or septic embolization in children with congenital heart disease. Focal neurologic signs as well as fever and headache may be present in these patients, but the patient may look surprisingly well. Before a lumbar puncture is performed and the opening pressure is measured, CT of the head with and without contrast enhancement should be performed to determine whether there is a mass lesion. The abscess can be missed without contrast enhancement. CSF findings usually include 10 to 200 leukocytes/mm^3, slightly elevated protein level, and normal glucose level. The CSF smear and culture usually do not reveal any organisms.

Subdural hematoma is associated with head trauma. Symptoms include those associated with increased ICP; seizures and other focal neurologic deficits may also be present. The diagnosis is confirmed by neuroimaging. Postconcussive headaches are common. These headaches can be severe and associated with dizziness and vomiting. Chronic progressive headache can also be a symptom of systemic diseases such as hypertension, collagen vascular disease, hypothyroidism, Lyme disease, mononucleosis, or inborn errors of metabolism.

BOX 173-13. 1998 Revised Criteria for Pediatric Migraine without an Aura*

A. Five or more attacks fulfilling features B through D below
B. Headache attack lasting *1-48 hours (adults 2-72 hours)*
C. Headache has at least two of the following features:
   1. Either *bilateral* or unilateral (frontal/temporal) location *(adults: unilateral)*
   2. Pulsating quality
   3. Moderate to severe intensity
   4. Aggravated by routine physical activities
D. At least one of the following accompanies headache:
   1. Nausea and/or vomiting
   2. Photophobia *and/or* phonophobia *(adults: both photo- and phonophobia)*

*Differences between pediatric and adult are italicized: shorter duration, bilateral representation, either photo- or phonophobia.

Migraine Headache

The diagnosis of migraine is based on symptoms of recurrent headaches separated by pain-free intervals. A revised classification of migraine syndromes has been made for pediatric migraine (Box 173-13).[94,95]

Migraine headaches are primarily classified into migraine with or without an aura. *Migraine without an aura,* also known as *common migraine,* is the most common type of pediatric and adolescent migraine and includes the following criteria: more than five attacks that last 2 to 72 hours (untreated), plus a minimum of two of the following criteria—unilateral location, pulsing quality, moderate to severe intensity, and aggravated by routine physical activities—and accompanied by at least nausea and/or vomiting and photophobia and phonophobia.

The main features that differentiate the pediatric from the adult migraine headache are a shorter duration (1-48 hours), unilateral or bilateral pain, and the presence of either photophobia or phonophobia. In children, malaise, irritability, and dizziness commonly occur before the onset of the headache.

Migraine with an aura, previously known as *classic migraine,* is diagnosed when at least two episodes occur with the following criteria: (1) reversible symptoms arising from focal cerebral or brainstem dysfunction, (2) gradual development of the headache over more than 4 minutes or several symptoms that occur in succession, (3) aura with a duration of less than 60 minutes, and (4) the appearance of a headache either before, simultaneously with, or within 60 minutes of the aura. In children, auras are most commonly visual, but sensory, motor, and psychic auras do occur.[94]

Hemiplegic migraine is characterized by the sudden onset of hemiparesis or hemisensory loss followed by headache in the contralateral hemisphere. This type of migraine is seen more frequently in children than adults. Even though symptoms usually last for hours or days, affected individuals are rarely left with permanent deficits. *Ophthalmoplegic migraine* is characterized by severe unilateral eye pain and headache, followed by ipsilateral third nerve palsy of varying degree. Less commonly, the fourth and sixth cranial nerves may be affected. *Basilar artery migraine*, also common in children, manifests with a combination of visual symptoms (e.g., transient bilateral blindness, blurred vision) and visual hallucinations, vertigo, ataxia, loss of consciousness, and drop attacks. An *acute confusional state* consists of a change in personality, orientation, or behavior. The *Alice in Wonderland syndrome* includes distortions in body images and shapes. Objects either appear much larger (macropsia) or smaller (micropsia) before, during, or after a headache.

Migraine variants are common. *Abdominal migraine* is characterized by recurrent abdominal pain, nausea, vomiting, and recurrent headaches. Benign paroxysmal vertigo occurs with the sudden onset of vertigo, pallor, and nystagmus. Paroxysmal torticollis is defined as recurrent episodes of head tilt associated with headache, nausea, and vomiting. It should be noted that this is a diagnosis of exclusion. A child with a head tilt, vomiting, and headache must first be evaluated for a posterior fossa lesion. *Ocular migraine* is characterized by transient monocular visual blurring to blindness with bright flashes of light.

Epilepsy and migraine headache are distinct clinical syndromes, yet they share several characteristics such as aura, vertigo, nausea, pallor, loss of consciousness, drowsy postictal state, confusion, and transient focal neurologic deficits. The incidence of seizures is higher in migraine patients than in the general population. The differentiation of these two clinical entities may be difficult in certain cases. Headache as the sole manifestation of a seizure is uncommon; however, headaches may frequently follow tonic, tonic-clonic, and brief complex-partial seizures. Bifrontal throbbing headaches may also follow episodes of status epilepticus. Further neurologic evaluation including EEG may occasionally be necessary to try to distinguish these two syndromes.

Chronic Nonprogressive Headache

Chronic nonprogressive headache is commonly seen in the adolescent population. Included in this category of headache are muscle contraction headache, depressive equivalents, and conversion headaches. The International Headache Society classification of headaches refers to these types of headaches as *tension headaches*. The symptoms of this type of headache include bilateral or frontal headache; nonthrobbing, pressing, or bandlike tightness of mild to moderate intensity; and the absence of nausea, vomiting, and an aura. These headaches are further classified as either episodic (10 episodes to fewer than 15/month lasting 30 minutes to 7 days) or chronic (more than 15 episodes/month for greater than 6 months).

Cluster Headache

Cluster headache is a distinctive headache syndrome more commonly seen in male subjects. The syndrome is rarely seen in those younger than 10 years of age. Cluster headache is characterized by one to several attacks recurring each 24 hours, over several weeks to months, with headache-free periods between the cluster headaches. The headache-free periods may last from months to years. The pain is throbbing, severe, and unilateral; occurs over the same orbitotemporal region; and is associated with ipsilateral scleral injection, lacrimation, nasal stuffiness, and, less often, partial Horner's syndrome. The pain lasts 30 minutes to several hours and can occur at any time of day or night.

Diagnostic Strategies

The diagnosis of a specific headache syndrome is usually determined by the history and physical examination. The primary concern of the emergency physician is to eliminate the possibility of an intracranial lesion or serious extracranial pathologic condition. Skull radiographs and EEG are of limited value in the routine emergency department evaluation of children with chronic headaches.

Radiology

Computed tomography of the head and MRI are excellent imaging instruments to evaluate patients with headaches.[89,96] MRI is particularly useful in detecting abnormalities in the sella turcica, temporal lobes, posterior fossa, and cervicomedullary junction. MRI is also advantageous because of its superior ability in detecting arteriovenous malformations and low-grade tumors. In general, an MRI provides superior anatomic detail compared to CT scan. However, a patient cannot be closely monitored during MRI. Therefore, CT is the method of choice in the potentially unstable patient and in the detection of acute bleeding. Indications for the use of neuroimaging are described in Box 173-14.[92]

Laboratory and Special Procedures

Lumbar puncture is occasionally helpful in the evaluation of patients with headache. If the possibility of mass lesion exists (history of early morning headaches and vomiting or focal neurologic findings on physical examination), radiologic imaging should precede the lumbar puncture. The lumbar puncture is a necessary procedure to determine the presence of an infectious process, hemorrhage, or pseudotumor cerebri.

In a patient with suspected chronic progressive headaches, the headaches may be a symptom of a systemic disease. Laboratory tests that may be considered include CBC, urinalysis, erythrocyte sedimentation rate, antinuclear antibody, liver function studies, thyroid function studies, serum lipids, serum magnesium, lactate, and pyruvate concentrations, and a Lyme disease titer.

BOX 173-14. Indications for Radiologic Imaging in Patients with Headache[92]

Strongly Indicated If . . .
- Abnormal neurologic examination findings
- Signs and symptoms of elevated intracranial pressure
- Meningeal signs plus focal neurologic findings or altered mental status
- Progressive and/or new neurologic signs
- Significant head trauma
- Severe nocturnal headaches that awaken the patient from sleep or are present upon awakening
- Severe (worst headache of life) headaches of increasing frequency and duration
- Presence of ventriculoperitoneal shunt
- Chronic progressive headache

Consider If . . .
- Headache or vomiting upon awakening
- Unvarying location of headache, especially occipital
- Persistent headache plus no family history of migraine
- Neurocutaneous syndrome
- Age <3 years (limited verbal skills)

Management

Treatment of primary childhood headaches requires attention to initial pharmacologic management as well as reassurance, removal of potential triggering factors, and initiation of a behavioral management program. A headache diary is important to help the patient identify potential triggers and the effects of medications. Common triggers include reduction in sleep, perimenstrual stress, missed meals, and foods such as caffeine, chocolate, processed meats, alcohol, hard cheeses, red wine, monosodium glutamate, yeast extracts, nuts, figs, aspartame, and sauerkraut. Children with primary headaches are not admitted for care unless the diagnosis is uncertain and a serious cause of secondary headache is being considered.

Migraine

Treatment of migraine headache includes analgesics, vasoconstrictors, sedatives, antiemetics, and other modalities. The patient should be placed in a quiet and safe environment. Simple analgesics and rest are the first line of treatment for patients with migraine as well as nonmigraine headache. These medications include acetaminophen (10-15 mg/kg/dose, 650-1000 mg for 12 years and older), and the nonsteroidal anti-inflammatory drugs (aspirin, 10-15 mg/kg/dose, 650-1000 mg for 12 years and older; ibuprofen, 5-10 mg/kg/dose, 400 mg for 12 years and older; or naproxen, 2.5-5.0 mg/kg/dose, 250-300 mg for 12 years of age and older maximum dose: 1250 mg/day).

For severe migraine episodes, more potent analgesics may be needed. These include ketorolac tromethamine (Toradol), a nonsteroidal anti-inflammatory, which can be used parenterally when vomiting is present (0.5 mg/kg every 6 hours IV/IM; maximum dose 30 mg), codeine (0.5-1.0 mg/kg/dose every 4 to 6 hours orally, maximum dose 60 mg), or oxycodone (0.05-0.15 mg/kg/dose every 4 to 6 hours orally, maximum dose 5 mg every 6 hours). Combination medications, such as Fiorinal (butalbital, aspirin, and caffeine), Fioricet (butalbital, acetaminophen, and caffeine), and Midrin (isometheptene, acetaminophen, dichloralphenazone) are also effective. The dose is 1 to 2 capsules in children older than 12 years of age. Caution should be used in prescribing these medications. In addition to producing an analgesic effect, these medications may produce alterations of emotional state, sedation, and psychological dependence.

In the adolescent population, vasoconstrictor drugs are used rarely; however, this class of medications is more commonly used in the adult population. Antiemetic agents such as promethazine (0.25-0.5 mg/kg/dose IM or PR every 4 to 6 hours as needed; adults, 12.5-25 mg every 4 to 6 hours as needed), metoclopramide (0.1-0.2 mg/kg/dose every 2 to 6 hours as needed), and prochlorperazine (>10 kg or >2 years of age, PO or PR 0.4 mg/kg/24 hr divided, three to four times per day, or IM 0.1 to 0.15 mg/kg/dose, three to four times per day. Dystonic reactions with these agents are more common in children and must be used with caution in this population.

Sumatriptan is a selective 5-HT_1 receptor agonist that can mediate cerebral vasoconstriction and block inflammatory response and can be administered orally, intranasally, or subcutaneously. Although not approved for the pediatric population, they should be considered in the adolescent population after failure to respond to conventional therapy.[92] In a recent pediatric study, there was a 78% response rate within 60 minutes using a single subcutaneous administration of 0.06 mg/kg.[97] Nasal sumatriptan (5-20 mg; repeat in 2 hours; maximum dose 40 mg/day) has been shown to be effective in the adolescent population,[98] along with oral preparations of 25 to 50 mg (repeat in 2 hours; maximum dose 200 mg/day). Sumatriptan should be avoided in people with cardiac disorders or hypertension and in patients who have received an ergot alkaloid in the preceding 24 hours. Other new 5-HT_1 agents such as zolmitriptan (Zomig) (at doses of 2.5 mg and 5 mg) compare favorably with sumatriptan. Cluster headaches, which are brief and may not respond to oral therapy, can be treated with inhalation of oxygen 4 to 5 L/minute, Cafergot, or sumatriptan.[90]

The use of pharmacologic agents for the prophylactic treatment of migraine headache in children requires careful observation and follow-up evaluation by the child's primary care physician. The indications to use these medications include more than two to three headaches per week and interference with lifestyle, particularly missed schooldays or inability to participate in social activities. Owing to the high spontaneous remission rate of childhood migraine, the placebo effect of many medications is very high. Controlled studies are extremely limited. Medications that have been used include propanolol (initiated slowly; 2 to 4 mg/kg/day divided three times a day, contraindicated in asthma patients), amitriptyline (initiated slowly; 25 mg at bedtime for adolescents, obtain a baseline electrocardiogram), calcium channel blockers, anticonvulsants (particularly valproic acid), cyproheptadine, and naproxen sodium. Cyproheptadine, valproic acid, and naproxen are available in liquid form, which is valuable in the pediatric population. Methysergide should be avoided in children owing to serious side effects, including retroperitoneal fibrosis. Amitriptyline may be useful for adolescents with a diagnosis of migraine and muscle contraction headaches and in depressed children with headaches.

PEDIATRIC ATAXIA

Perspective

Ataxia comes from the Greek word *ataktos* meaning "lacking order," and describes a pathologic abnormality of organization or modulation of movement.[99]

Pathophysiology

Ataxia can be caused by congenital abnormalities or can be acquired. Congenital ataxia is associated with CNS abnormalities. Acquired ataxia can be acute, episodic, or chronic. The chronic ataxias are usually caused by inherited metabolic or genetic disorders. Most commonly, ataxia is caused by cerebellar dysfunction. Lesions in the corticospinal tract or dorsal columns of the spinal cord may also be causative.

Clinical Features

Most children with ataxia are seen in the first few days after onset, usually because of a refusal to walk, unsteadiness of arm movements, or the sudden development of a wide-based "drunken" gait. History should include recent infection, injury, inadvertent drug ingestion, or other family members with the same problem. Mental state is usually normal in cases of postinfectious ataxia. If it is abnormal, consider ingestion, acute disseminated encephalomyelitis, or stroke. Nystagmus is common if the cerebellum is affected. Papilledema or cranial nerve palsies suggest hydrocephalus or a lesion.[99]

Differential Considerations

(Box 173-15)

BOX 173-15. Causes of Childhood Ataxia[99]

- Acute cerebellar ataxia
- Acute postinfectious demyelinating encephalomyelitis
- Brainstem encephalitis
- Drug ingestion
- Guillain-Barré syndrome
- Metabolic disorders
  - Amino acidopathies
  - Mitochondrial disorders
  - Organic acidopathies
  - Urea cycle disorders
- Migraine headaches
- Multiple sclerosis
- Neoplasm
- Opsoclonus-myoclonus syndrome
- Recurrent and chronic genetic ataxias
- Seizures
- Stroke

In children, 40% of ataxia cases are caused by acute cerebellar ataxia. Boys are more commonly affected, with the highest incidence at ages 2 to 4 years. Seventy percent of patients have a history of recent illness with multiple causative agents, but varicella virus is the most common, with up to 26% of cases. Coxsackievirus and echovirus are also found. The disease is thought to be due to an autoimmune phenomenon, which causes cerebellar demyelination.[100] Symptoms are maximal at onset, with the extremities affected more than the trunk. They range from unsteadiness and wide-based gait to an inability to walk. Mental status is normal, and nystagmus is common. Fever and seizures are uncommon.[1]

Acute postinfectious demyelinating encephalomyelitis can also cause ataxia and occurs in the recovery phase of a viral illness or vaccination. It is distinguished from acute cerebellar ataxia by alteration in consciousness and multifocal neurologic deficits as well as fever and the occurrence frequently of seizures.[99]

Brainstem encephalitis can involve the cerebellum, causing ataxia in association with focal neurologic abnormalities and respiratory irregularities. Etiologic agents include Epstein-Barr virus, *Listeria monocytogenes,* and enteroviruses.[99]

Up to 32% of cases of acute childhood ataxia are due to drug ingestion, most commonly after ingestion of anticonvulsants, benzodiazepines, alcohol, and antihistamines and less commonly after exposure to organic chemicals and heavy metals. Ataxia is usually accompanied by lethargy, confusion, and inappropriate speech or behavior. Nystagmus may be present.[99]

About 45% to 60% of all childhood brain tumors arise in the brainstem or cerebellum and can manifest with slowly progressive ataxia. Acute decompensation can occur with the development of hydrocephalus or hemorrhage into the lesion.[99]

Head injuries with cerebellar contusion or hemorrhage can cause ataxia. In patients with neck injuries, ataxia can be caused by vertebral artery dissection. Posterior circulation strokes are rare in children but should be considered after neck trauma due to vertebral artery dissection as a cause of ataxia.[101]

The opsoclonus-myoclonus syndrome consists of ataxia, rapid chaotic multidirectional eye movements, and myoclonic jerks of the extremities, head, trunk, and face. Most commonly, this is seen as presenting manifestation of neuroblastoma or ganglioneuroblastoma in which the ataxia is thought to be due to a paraneoplastic autoimmune phenomenon involving cross-reactivity of tumor and cerebellar antigens.[99]

Ataxia can be seen in patients with basilar migraine and can be associated with vertigo, hemiparesis, cranial nerve dysfunction, nausea, vomiting, or headache.[99]

Loss of sensory input to the cerebellum can cause a sensory ataxia. There is a positive Romberg sign, decreased deep tendon reflexes, and impaired proprioception and vibration sense. Fifteen percent of patients with Guillain-Barré syndrome have sensory ataxia. In the Miller-Fisher variant of Guillain-Barré syndrome, the triad of ataxia, areflexia, and ophthalmoplegia of vertical gaze can be seen.[99]

Ataxia can transiently be present in the ictal or postictal phase of seizures.[99]

Inborn errors of metabolism can manifest with ataxia, which can develop acutely or intermittently, depending on dietary intake or the presence of other illness. It should be considered when ataxia is accompanied by lethargy, encephalopathy, vomiting, diarrhea, or unusual body odor. Defects in urea acid cycle enzymes called aminoacidurias as well as defects in pyruvate and lactate metabolism can cause symptoms. Other hereditary diseases such as Niemann-Pick, Tay-Sachs, and Wilson's disease can also cause ataxia.[99]

Repeated attacks of ataxia can be the presenting symptom of multiple sclerosis.

A discussion of all the genetic disorders that can cause ataxia is too vast to be included here, but the two most common genetic disorders are Friedreich's ataxia and ataxia telangiectasia.

Friedreich's ataxia is an autosomal recessive condition characterized by progressive gait and limb disturbance. It is caused by mutation in the gene encoding a mitochondrial protein, frataxin, which results in loss of gene function. These patients develop dysarthria, lower limb areflexia, and proprioceptive sensory loss and high arched feet (pes cavus). Most patients are unable to walk by 30 years of age. The most common cause of death is cardiomyopathy causing intractable congestive heart failure as well as respiratory compromise from severe kyphoscoliosis.[102]

Ataxia telangiectasia is a recessive disorder caused by gene mutation that manifests as a truncal ataxia in infancy that leaves most patients wheelchair bound by age 12. Oculocutaneous telangiectasias usually appear by age 3 to 5. These patients also develop dysarthria, nystagmus, dystonic posturing, myoclonic jerks, and accelerated aging. They have deficient IgA and decreased IgE and IgM levels. They suffer from frequent sinus and pulmonary infections, as well as a 50 to 100 times greater chance of developing leukemia and lymphoma. The mean age of death from this disorder is 20 years.[102]

Diagnosis

The key to making the diagnosis is taking a complete history and performing a thorough physical examination. In particular, testing cerebellar function by looking for dysmetria and dysdiadochokinesia is helpful.[103] Urine and serum toxicology are the most likely laboratory tests to prove diagnostic. CT and MRI are usually normal in patients with postinfectious ataxia, but demyelination, tumor, hydrocephalus, or traumatic injuries may be identified. CSF may show mild pleocytosis or lymphocytosis in cases of acute postinfectious ataxia and is normal in most other cases. EEG is recommended for patients with altered consciousness and fluctuating clinical signs. Epileptiform discharges or slowing is seen in 66% of children with acute cerebellar ataxia. EEG can also diagnose nonconvulsive or convulsive seizures. The EEG is normal in the opsoclonus-myoclonus syndrome. Electromyography may be helpful if sensory ataxia is suspected and may help diagnose Guillain-Barré syndrome. Urinary catecholamines can be tested to diagnose neuroblastoma. Newborn errors of metabolism testing include a CBC; liver function tests; blood ammonia, lactate, pyruvate, and ketone levels; and acid-base status. Other tests include plasma and urinary amino acid assays, urine organic acids, serum biotinidase level, CSF pyruvate, and lactate assays. Genetic or other specialized testing may also be required. In the absence of developmental delay or positive family histories, however, these investigations for inborn errors of metabolism are unlikely to be helpful.[99]

Management

Children with ataxia usually require admission for a complete evaluation. Consultation with a pediatric neurologist should be sought for patients in whom the cause of the ataxia is not evident on emergency department evaluation.

Most children with acute cerebellar ataxia recover completely. Improvement is seen within a week and complete recovery in 3 months for 50% of children. Sixty-six to 90% recover completely. Some have persistent gait disturbances, ataxia, and delayed speech development. There is no evidence that immuno suppressive therapies improve outcome. Recovery is slower from acute postinfectious demyelinating encephalopathy. Corticosteroids may hasten recovery. Relapse can occur in up to 10% of children. Most children recover fully but some are left with significant permanent sequelae. Brainstem encephalitis should be treated with broad-spectrum antibiotics covering *Listeria monocytogenes* as well as using acyclovir for varicella and other viruses until an organism is discovered. Guillain-Barré patients will need to be admitted and may require intravenous immunoglobulins and plasmapheresis to reduce circulating antibodies.

PEDIATRIC VERTIGO

Perspective

Vertigo is defined as an illusion of movement, a sensation that the external world is revolving around an individual (objective vertigo) or that the individual is revolving in space (subjective vertigo). Vertigo does occur in the pediatric age group but is not common and has many potential causes.

Pathophysiology

Disease processes that affect the balance of the vestibular, visual, and proprioceptive systems can cause vertigo by affecting the neural activity of the vestibular nucleus. Diseases of the ear, the eighth cranial nerve, the neck, the brainstem, or, rarely, the eye can all lead to vertiginous symptoms. Vertigo is characterized as central or peripheral depending on whether the cause is in the central nervous system or not.

Clinical Features

Vertigo often manifests with dizziness. There may be a history of sudden falls, grasping for support, or unwillingness to move. History should include ear symptoms such as otalgia, hearing loss, or tinnitus. Other important historical features that should be asked about include headache, loss of consciousness, head trauma or barotrauma, and family history of migraine and seizure disorders.

Diagnostic Strategies

To determine the causes of vertigo, patients can be divided into those who have hearing loss and those who have normal hearing. Further characterization as to whether there is conductive or sensorineural hearing loss, the presence of trauma, and whether the cause is from the central nervous system or the peripheral nervous system from the labyrinth or eighth cranial nerve will help in diagnosis (Figure 173-2).

Differential Considerations

Although not as common in the pediatric age group as in adults, vertigo has many potential causes (Box 173-16).[104] It is usually helpful to separate those conditions that cause vertigo with and without associated hearing loss.

Benign paroxysmal vertigo of childhood is an episodic vertigo lasting seconds to minutes with occasional vomiting, which usually stops spontaneously for months to years. The most frequent cause of benign paroxysmal vertigo of childhood in children is a migraine headache,[105] with vertigo occurring as the aura of an episode.[106]

Patients with basilar artery migraines also present with vertigo, hemiparesis, ataxia, palsies of the third, sixth, or seventh cranial nerve, drop attacks, and blindness in various combinations followed by migraine headache. Children with benign paroxysmal vertigo of childhood or basilar migraines usually have a family history of migraine headaches.[107]

Benign positional vertigo is rare in children, and the earliest age at which it has been reported is 11 years.[107] It is believed to be due to an otolith that has moved out of its normal position in the utricle and can occur spontaneously as well as after trauma.

Ménière's disease, a syndrome with a combination of vertigo, fluctuating hearing loss, and tinnitus, is responsible for 1.5% to 4% of cases of pediatric vertigo.[108,109]

Vestibular neuronitis manifests with vertigo without hearing loss. A viral infection is thought to be the cause. Sixty percent of patients have a preceding cold. It manifests with severe vertigo that resolves in a few days, after which the child will have vertigo only with rapid head movements, which persists for weeks or months until central compensation occurs.[110]

Labyrinthitis is an inflammatory process involving the inner ear membranous labyrinth. It manifests with vertigo, hearing loss, and tinnitus. Viruses such as cytomegalovirus, rubella, and rubeola are etiologic agents. Bacterial labyrinthitis can also occur, usually associated with meningitis.[104]

Lyme disease and syphilis each cause vertigo if the inner ear is affected.[104]

Neurofibromatosis can manifest with vertigo if the patient develops neurofibromatosis of the superior vestibular nerve. Café au lait spots should be looked for. Other genetic syndromes are also associated with vertigo (see Box 173-16).[104]

Ototoxic drugs such as aminoglycosides and chemotherapeutic drugs can be a cause of vertigo, usually in association with hearing loss (Box 173-17).[104]

Cerebellar and brainstem lesions on occasion also manifest with vertigo. Cranial nerve deficits associated with vertigo may indicate a lesion or tumor.[110]

BOX 173-16. Causes of Pediatric Vertigo[104]

Central vertigo
Atrioventricular malformations
Brain abscess
Chiari malformations
Demyelinating disorders
Encephalitis
Meningitis
Migraine headaches
Neoplasm
Seizures
Trauma

Peripheral vertigo
Alport syndrome
Benign paroxysmal torticollis
Benign paroxysmal vertigo of childhood
Benign positional vertigo
Cholesteatoma
Diabetes mellitus
Down syndrome
Labyrinthine dysplasia/aplasia
Labyrinthine concussion
Labyrinthitis
Lyme disease
Otitis media suppurative and serous
Ototoxins
Ocular disorders
Pendred syndrome
Perilymphatic fistula
Radiation
Stenosis of the internal auditory canal
Syphilitic inner ear disease
Thyroid disease
Trauma
Usher syndrome
Vestibular neuronitis
Waardenburg syndrome

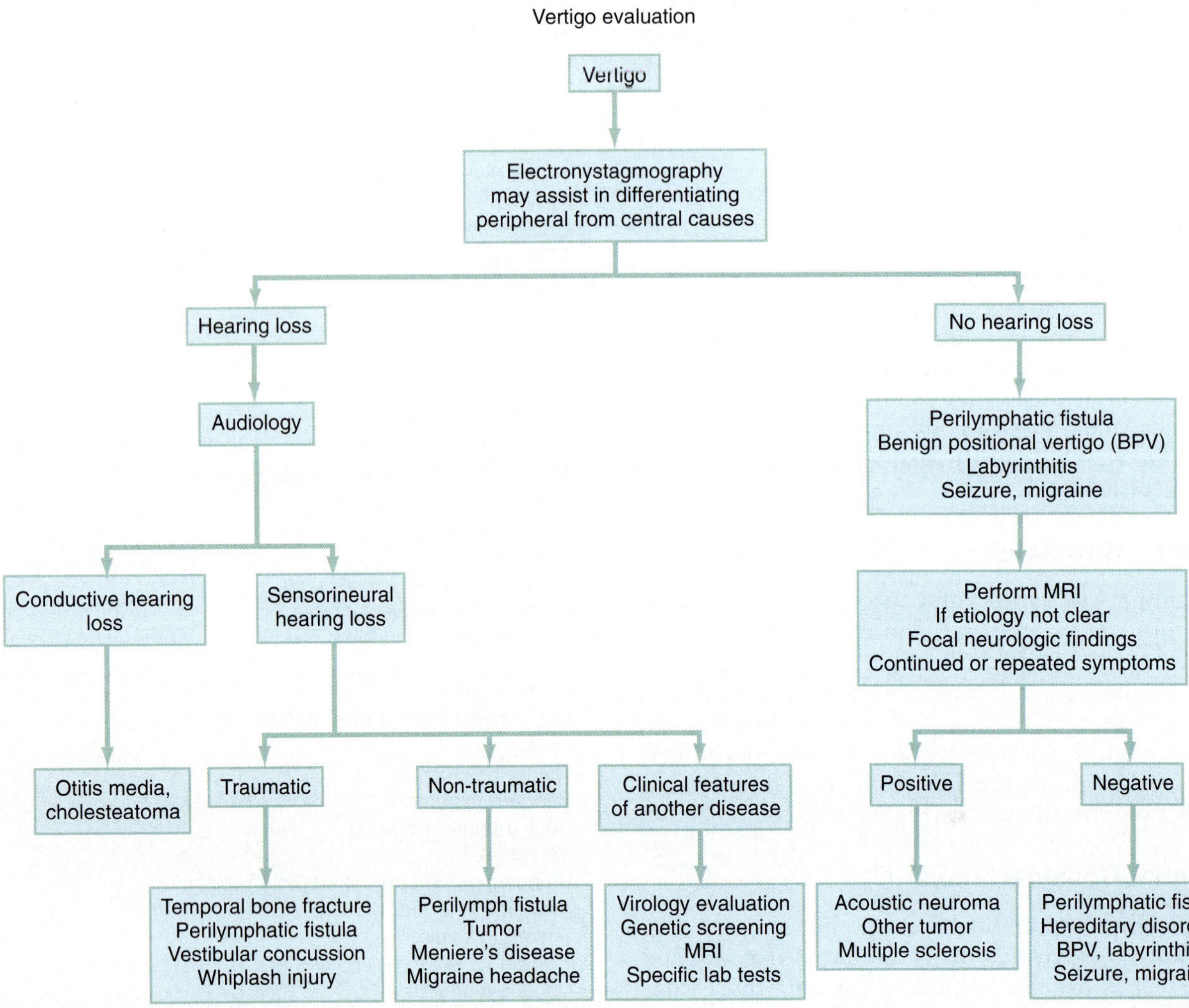

Figure 173-2. Vertigo evaluation. (Adapted from Rudolph C, Rudolph A [eds]: *Rudolph's Pediatrics,* 21st ed. New York, McGraw-Hill, 2003, pp 1246–1247.)

BOX 173-17. Causes of Vertigo Categorized by Conditions that Cause Hearing Loss

Hearing Loss

Conductive

Otitis media with effusion
Chronic suppurative otitis media or cholesteatoma should be considered

Sensorineural

Perilymphatic fistula
Tumor
Ménière's disease
Migraine headache
Genetic syndromes
Temporal bone fracture
Vestibular concussion

No Hearing Loss

Acute Vertigo

Perilymphatic fistula
Benign positional vertigo
Seizure
Labyrinthitis

Recurrent or Chronic Vertigo

Acoustic neuroma
Multiple sclerosis

Multiple sclerosis can have vertigo as one of the symptoms, and vertigo is the presenting symptom in 5% to 12% of cases.[110]

Endocrine disorders such as thyroid disease or diabetes mellitus have rarely been reported to cause vertigo.[110]

In posttraumatic vertigo, disturbances of cochlear and vestibular functions are the most common cause of late-onset vertigo from head injury in children. If labyrinthine damage is caused by trauma (labyrinthine concussion), vertigo, gait unsteadiness, and swaying toward the affected side is present with nausea and vomiting. Symptoms subside over a period of 4 to 6 weeks. Signs of vestibular dysfunction may be present many years after the injury. Positional nystagmus with the quick component toward the uninvolved side is usually present. Vestibular concussions can cause vertigo without hearing loss following blows to the parietal-occipital or temporal-parietal regions. It normally is continuous for several days followed by improvement but may reoccur intermittently with certain head positions. It is thought that a displaced otolith is responsible.[111]

Whiplash injuries of the neck can also cause vertigo, with up to 50% of patients having hearing loss or tinnitus. Posttraumatic migraine and seizures can also cause vertigo and occur in 5% to 7% of patients with closed head injuries.[111]

Perilymphatic fistula manifests with a sudden onset of sensorineural hearing loss. It is frequently associated with congenital cranial deformities and congenital abnormalities of the ear. However, barotrauma (flying, extreme coughing, retching, or straining) or direct trauma can also cause it. There is leakage of fluid from the oval or round window into the middle ear. Having the patient perform a Valsalva maneuver may stimulate vertigo. Hennebert's sign, which consists of nystagmus and vertigo after negative pressure is induced in the ear by a pneumatic otoscope, may be present.[107] Treatment is usually surgical repair.

Ocular disorders such as convergence insufficiency, strabismus, and amblyopia have been reported to cause a sensation of vertigo, and treatment of these disorders will eliminate the vertigo in children.[112]

Diagnostic Strategies

For most patients, the final diagnosis for the cause of the patient's vertigo may not be able to be made in the emergency department. A complete physical examination including otologic and neurologic evaluation is important. Looking for nystagmus and cerebellar testing is especially critical. Having the child hop as well as stand from a seated position on the floor with eyes open and closed may reveal vestibular dysfunction. Looking for physical signs of other disease processes such as café au lait spots in neurofibromatosis may aid in diagnosis. If a Valsalva maneuver or Hennebert maneuver initiates vertigo, the cause is probably a perilymphatic fistula. Vertical nystagmus is always from a central cause. Peripheral causes of nystagmus tend to extinguish or diminish after rapidly repeated stimulation whereas central nystagmus does not. Helpful laboratory tests in the vertiginous patient include glucose and electrolytes assessment, thyroid function tests, and viral titers or serologies (Lyme, syphilis), as the physical examination dictates.[104,107] The Hallpike-Dix positioning maneuver may help to diagnose benign positional vertigo.[110] A CT or MRI scan is indicated only in cases of central vertigo.

Management

Management of the vertiginous patient depends on the cause, which may not be evident in the emergency department.[113] For acute symptomatic relief, vestibular suppressants such as meclizine or diazepam may be helpful. Otoliths causing inappropriate stimulation may be restored to their proper place by Epley's maneuver.[107,114] Vestibular rehabilitation exercises that encourage patients to move their head while viewing a stimulus may assist in vestibular adaptation and reduce symptomatology.[107] Follow-up examination, testing, and treatment by a neurologist or an otolaryngologist for vertiginous patients is recommended. Very symptomatic children may need to be admitted to the hospital.

SYNCOPE

Perspective

Syncope is defined as a sudden, reversible, typically brief loss of consciousness and muscle tone (between 20 and 60 seconds) that usually reverses without intervention. The exact incidence of syncopal episodes is not known, but 15% to 25% of children and adolescents experience one episode by young adulthood.[115] The peak incidence occurs between 15 and 19 years of age, and females are affected more frequently than males. The presentation of these events can be quite frightening to the patient and those who witness them (parents, teachers, peers, coaches). Gordon and coworkers found that in a group of pediatric patients presenting to the emergency department, a mean of six diagnostic tests were performed per patient, 40% of these patients were admitted to the hospital, and total charges averaged $3000 per patient, yet significant pathologic conditions were found in less than 10% of the patients.[116]

Principles

The causes of syncope can be divided into autonomic, cardiac, and noncardiac. The most common cause of syncope is reflex syncope (also called autonomic, vasovagal, neurocardiogenic, or vasodepressor syncope or fainting). Venous pooling and decreased preload associated with prolonged standing is normally compensated for by reflex tachycardia and increased sympathetic tone. Patients who are prone to syncope have either a cardioinhibitory response causing bradycardia, a vasodepressor response causing hypotension, or, most commonly, a combination of both. Patients with cardiac syncope have decreased CBF resulting from poor cardiac filling or contractility, elevated afterload, or cardiac arrhythmias.

Clinical Features

Patients can have syncope during intercurrent illnesses, mild dehydration, or menses or after vigorous exertion. Those with situational syncope generally have typical triggers such as emotion, pain, hyperventilation, shower, cough, swallowing, urination, or defecation. Prior to the event, they may experience dizziness, lightheadedness, weakness, nausea, chest discomfort, palpitations, blurred vision, headache, tremulousness, and anxiety. After the event, loss of consciousness is brief (usually less than 20 seconds) and the patients are described as ashen appearing, with sweating and cool extremities.[117] Other examples of neurally mediated syncope include postural orthostatic tachycardia syndrome, chronic fatigue syndrome, and pandysautonomia.[118] Patients with postural orthostatic tachycardia syndrome and pandysautonomia have orthostatic palpitations rather than straightforward syncope, do not appear healthy between events, and complain of fatigue and exercise intolerance. Patients with pandysautonomia also have thermoregulatory, sweating, and bowel dysfunction.[118] Although cardiac causes of syncope are rare, they can be life threatening and should be suspected when the episode occurred during exercise or physical activity. Noncardiac causes include seizures. Helpful features to differentiate seizures form syncope include the following: seizures usually occur in a supine rather than an upright position, convulsions occur before rather than after the loss of consciousness, and a warm, flushed or cyanotic-appearing skin is present rather than pale and sweaty skin.

Diagnosis

Evaluation of the patient involves a description of the event, prior episodes, and past personal and family history. A detailed description of the event and particular note of any presyncopal symptoms such as sweating, nausea, pallor, visual changes, or a rapid change in position can suggest vasovagal syncope. A good physical examination with orthostatic heart rate and blood pressure obtained in supine, sitting, and standing positions and a detailed neurologic examination are essential. A baseline electrocardiogram should be obtained to rule out structural heart disease or an arrhythmia. If the history, physical examination, and electrocardiogram are typical for a neurally mediated event, further testing is not usually required. Family history of sudden death, early infarction or arrhythmia, prior personal history of fatigue and a known arrhythmia or heart defect, syncope preceded by chest pain or palpitations, syncope occurring during exercise, syncope without a prodrome, recurrent syncope (more than two or three episodes), or an event with neurologic sequela warrants additional testing.[119]

Differential Considerations

Cardiac causes of syncope may be life threatening. These include patients with an underlying structural abnormality of the heart, such as cardiomyopathies (hypertrophic, dilated, and restrictive), postoperative congenital heart anatomic changes (Mustard, Fontan), congenital coronary abnormalities, myocarditis, aortic stenosis, and pulmonary hypertension. Other cardiac abnormalities include those classified as electrical disorders and include long QT syndrome, Wolff-Parkinson-White syndrome, atrioventricular block, idiopathic ventricular fibrillation, and Brugada syndrome. Patients with an underlying cardiac abnormality warrant further investigation, which may include a 24- to 48-hour Holter monitor, echocardiogram, and/or exercise stress testing. Tilt-table testing can be used after diseases such as myocarditis, hypertrophic cardiomyopathy, and long-QT syndrome have been ruled out, because tilt-table testing on this subgroup can have fatal consequences.

Common noncardiac causes of syncope include neurologic disorders (seizures, migraines, tumor, and vertigo), breath-holding spells, electrolyte abnormalities (hypoglycemia), hyperventilation (hypocapnia), endocrinopathies, toxins (carbon monoxide), and drugs of abuse.

Management and Disposition

Syncope is a common pediatric problem and usually has a benign, neurally mediated cause. The management of patients with neurocardiogenic syncope is primarily that of education, involving avoidance of potential triggering events (hot crowded environments, volume depletion) and recognition of the early signs and symptoms so the patient can abort the syncopal episode (assume the supine position, ingest fluids, leg-crossing). The patient and the family must be reassured that these events are not life threatening. A simple approach is to encourage liberal fluid intake and to increase dietary salt intake. There is, however, a subgroup of patients with recurrent syncope or recurrent dizziness who require a trial of medication. There have been no large pediatric randomized studies of these medications, which include β-blockers, fludrocortisone, selective serotonin reuptake inhibitors, and α-agonists.[119]

KEY CONCEPTS

- Signs and symptoms of bacterial meningitis vary by age and can include nonspecific signs, such as irritability and lethargy in infants and young children.
- In suspected cases of bacterial meningitis, the first dose of parenteral therapy should be initiated promptly in the emergency department.
- A careful and detailed history is instrumental in determining whether an event was a seizure. If the event was a seizure, the history should delineate what type of seizure occurred (partial or generalized) and whether the patient fits into a known epilepsy syndrome.
- Status epilepticus is a neurologic emergency that carries a high rate of morbidity and mortality. Initial efforts should be directed at stopping the seizure and preventing seizure recurrence.
- The possibility of acute symptomatic, or provoked, seizures should always be considered, particularly because many of them are treatable.
- In patients with a febrile seizure, emergency physicians should address issues about first aid, use of antipyretics, recurrence risk, risk of epilepsy, and follow-up with a primary care physician and with the families.
- The majority of headaches in children have nonserious causes that can usually be diagnosed by a careful history and physical examination.
- Radiologic evaluation using CT or MRI, or both, may be necessary to rule out secondary causes of headache such as intracranial hemorrhage, subarachnoid hemorrhage, brain abscess, or brain tumor.
- Syncope, ataxia, and vertigo are common pediatric problems. Although most causes of these entities are benign, there are a few life-threatening conditions that should be considered in their evaluation.
- Most children with ataxia require admission to the hospital for evaluation and diagnosis.

REFERENCES

1. Saez-Lorens X, McCracken GH: Bacterial meningitis in children. *Lancet* 361:2139, 2003.
2. Centers for Disease Control and Prevention: Progress toward the elimination of *Haemophilus influenzae* type b disease among infants and children. United States 1998-2000. *MMWR* 51:234, 2002.
3. Kaplan SL: Clinical manifestations, diagnosis, and prognostic factors of bacterial meningitis. *Infect Dis Clin North Am* 13:579, 1999.
4. Grimwood K, et al: Adverse outcomes of bacterial meningitis in school-age survivors. *Pediatrics* 95:646, 1995.
5. Sadow KB, Durr R, Teach SJ: Bacterial infections in infants 60 days and younger: Epidemiology, resistance, and implications for treatment. *Arch Pediatr Adolesc Med* 153:611, 1999.
6. Peters ML: Suspected meningitis in the emergency department: Diagnosis and management. *Clin Ped Emerg Med* 4:186, 2003.
7. Kriss TC, Kriss VM, Warf BC: Recurrent meningitis: The search for the dermoid or epidermoid tumor. *Pediatr Infect Dis J* 14:697, 1995.
8. Leib SL, Tauber MG: Pathogenesis of bacterial meningitis. *Infect Dis Clin North Am* 13:527, 1999.
9. Morley CJ, Thornton AJ, Fowler MA: Symptoms and signs in infants less than 6 months of age correlated with the severity of their illness. *Pediatrics* 88:1119, 1991.
10. Bonadio WA: Assessing patient clinical appearance in the evaluation of the febrile child. *Am J Emerg Med* 13:321, 1995.
11. Singer JI, Vest J, Prints A: Occult bacteremia and septicemia in the febrile child younger than 2 years. *Emerg Med Clin North Am* 13:381, 1995.
12. Baker MD, Bell LM: Unpredictability of serious bacterial infection in febrile infants from birth to one month of age. *Arch Pediatr Adolesc Med* 153:508, 1999.
13. Arango CA, Rathore MH: Neonatal meningococcal meningitis: Case reports and review of literature. *Pediatr Infect Dis J* 15:1104, 1996.
14. McIntosh D, et al: Torticollis and bacterial meningitis. *Pediatr Infect Dis J* 12:160, 1993.
15. Lipton JD, Schafermeyer RW: Central nervous system infections: The usual and the unusual. *Emerg Med Clin North Am* 13:417, 1995.
16. Walsh-Kelly C, et al: Clinical predictors of bacterial versus aseptic meningitis in childhood. *Ann Emerg Med* 21(8):910, 1992.
17. Kellogg JA, et al: Frequency of low level bacteremia in infants from birth to 2 months of age. *Pediatr Infect Dis J* 16:381, 1997.
18. Schelonka RL, et al: Volume of blood required to detect common neonatal pathogens. *J Pediatr* 129:275, 1996.
19. Baker MD, Avner JR, Bell LM: Failure of infant observation scales in detecting serious illness in febrile, 4- to 8-week-old infants. *Pediatrics* 85:1040, 1990.
20. Jaskiewicz JA, et al: Febrile infants at low risk for serious bacterial infection: An appraisal of the Rochester criteria and implications for management. *Pediatrics* 94:390, 1994.
21. Korones DN, Shapiro ED: Occult pneumococcal bacteremia. What happens to the child who appears well at reevaluation. *Pediatr Infect Dis J* 13:382, 1994.
22. Shapiro ED: Prophylaxis for contacts of patients with meningococcal or *Haemophilus influenzae* type b disease. *Pediatr Inf Dis J* 1:132, 1982.
23. Green SM, et al: Can seizures be the sole manifestation of meningitis in febrile children? *Pediatrics* 92:527, 1993.
24. Mandl KD, Stack KM, Fleisher GR: Incidence of bacteremia in infants and children with fever and petechiae. *J Pediatr* 131:398, 1997.
25. Cnota JF, Barton LL, Rhee KH: Purpura fulminans associated with *Streptococcus pneumoniae* infection in a child. *Pediatr Emerg Care* 15:187, 1999.
26. Callaham M: Fulminant bacterial meningitis without meningeal signs. *Ann Emerg Med* 18:90, 1989.
27. Shetty AK, et al: Fatal cerebral herniation after lumbar puncture in a patient with normal CT scan. *Pediatrics* 103:1284, 1999.
28. Bonadio WA: The cerebrospinal fluid: Physiologic aspects and alterations associated with bacterial meningitis. *Pediatr Infect Dis J* 11:423, 1992.
29. Carraccio C, Blot NY, Kay Fisher MC: Cerebrospinal fluid analysis in systemically ill children without central nervous system disease. *Pediatrics* 96:48, 1995.
30. Spanos A, et al: Differential diagnosis of acute meningitis. *JAMA* 262:2700, 1989.
31. Baker RC, Lenane AM: The predictive value of cerebrospinal fluid differential cytology in meningitis. *Pediatr Infect Dis J* 8:329, 1989.
32. Werner V, Kruger RL: Value of bacterial antigen test in the absence of CSF leukocytosis. *Lab Med* 22:787, 1991.
33. Azuma H, et al: Clinical significance of cytokine measurement for detection of meningitis. *J Pediatr* 131:463, 1997.
34. Kumar V, Singhi P, Singhi S: Changes in body water compartment in children with acute meningitis. *Pediatr Infect Dis J* 13:299, 1994.
35. VanDeuren M: Rapid diagnosis of acute meningococcal infections by needle aspiration. *Br Med J* 306:1229, 1993.
36. Boyer D, Gordon RC, Baker T: Lack of clinical usefulness of a positive latex agglutination test for *Neisseria meningitidis* and *Escherichia coli* antigens in the urine. *Pediatr Infect Dis J* 12:779, 1993.
37. Rorabaug ML, et al: Aseptic meningitis in infants younger than 2 years of age: Acute illness and neurologic complications. *Pediatrics* 92:206, 1993.
38. *2003 Report of the Committee on Infectious Diseases of the American Academy of Pediatrics.* Elk Grove Village, Ill, American Academy of Pediatrics, 2003.
39. Chandy JC: Treatment failure with the use of a third-generation cephalosporin for penicillin-resistant pneumococcal meningitis: Case report and review. *Clin Infect Dis* 18:188, 1994.
40. Volpe JV: Neonatal seizures. In Volpe JV: *Neurology of the Newborn,* Philadelphia, WB Saunders, 1995.
41. Homes GL: Do seizures cause brain damage? *Epilepsia* 32:514, 1991.
42. Theodore W, Wasterlain CG: Do early seizures beget epilepsy? *Neurology* 53:898, 1999.
43. Pellock JM: Treatment of seizures and epilepsy in children and adolescents. *Neurology* 51:S8, 1998.
44. Holden KR, Clarke SL, Griesemer DA: Long term outcomes of conventional therapy for infantile spasms. *Seizure* 6:201, 1997.
45. Mackay M, Weiss S, Snead OC 3rd: Treatment of infantile spasms: An evidence-based approach. *Int Rev Neurobiol* 49:157, 2002.
46. Pellock JM: Treatment of seizures and epilepsy in children and adolescents. *Neurology* 51:S8, 1998.
47. Hancock E, Cross H: Treatment of Lennox-Gastaut syndrome. *Cochrane Database Syst Rev* (3)CD003277, 2003.
48. Pellock JM: Treatment of seizures and epilepsy in children and adolescents. *Neurology* 51:S8, 1998.
49. Peters JM, Camfield CS, Camfield PR: Population study of benign rolandic epilepsy: Is treatment needed? *Neurology* 57:537, 2001.
50. Baumann RJ, Duffner PK: Treatment of children with simple febrile seizures: The AAP practice parameter. *Pediat Neurol* 23:11, 2000.
51. Shinnar S, Glauser TA: Febrile seizures. *J Child Neurol* 17S:S44, 2002.

52. van Stuijvenberg M, et al: Randomized controlled trial of ibuprofen syrup administered during febrile illnesses to prevent febrile seizure recurrences. *Pediatrics* 102(5):51, 1998.
53. Warden CR, et al: Evaluation and management of febrile seizures in the prehospital and emergency department settings. *Ann Emerg Med* 41:215, 2003.
54. Dreifuss FE, et al: A comparison of rectal diazepam gel and placebo for acute repetitive seizures. *N Engl J Med* 338:1869, 1998.
55. Volpe JV: Neonatal seizures. In Volpe JV: *Neurology of the Newborn.* Philadelphia, WB Saunders, 1995.
56. Appleton RC, Martland TP, Scott R, Whitehouse W: The treatment of convulsive status epilepticus in children. The Status Epilepticus Working Party. *Arch Dis Childh* 83:415, 2000.
57. DeLorenzo RJ, et al: Epidemiology of status epilepticus. *J Clin Neurophys* 12:36, 1995.
58. Maytal J, et al: Low morbidity and mortality of status epilepticus in children. *Pediatrics* 83:233, 1989.
59. Dimario FJ: Breath-holding spells in childhood. *Am J Dis Child* 146:125, 1992.
60. DeLorenzo RJ, et al: Status epilepticus in children, adults, and the elderly. *Epilepsia* 33:S15, 1992.
61. The Brain Trauma Foundation, The American Association of Neurological Surgeons, The Joint Section on Neurotrauma and Critical Care: Role of antiseizure prophylaxis following head injury. *J Neurotrauma* 17:549, 2001.
62. Garcia PA, Alldredge BK: Drug induced seizures. *Neurol Clin* 12:85, 1994.
63. Proulx F, et al: Convulsions and hypertension in children: Differentiating cause from effect. *Crit Care Med* 21:1541, 1993.
64. Ritaccio AL: Reflex seizures. *Neurol Clin* 12:57, 1994.
65. Hack C, et al: Seizures in relation to shunt dysfunction in children with meningomyelocele. *J Pediatr* 116:57, 1990.
66. Ettinger AB, et al: Postictal symptoms help distinguish patients with epileptic seizures from those with nonepileptic seizures. *Seizure* 8:149, 1999.
67. Nypaver MM, et al: Emergency department laboratory evaluation of children with seizures: Dogma or dilemma? *Pediatr Emerg Care* 8:13, 1992.
68. Baumann RJ, Duffner PK: Treatment of children with simple febrile seizures: The AAP practice parameter. American Academy of Pediatrics. *Pediatr Neurol* 23:11, 2000.
69. Woody RC, Yamanchi T: Cerebrospinal fluid cell counts in childhood. *Pediatr Infect Dis J* 7:298, 1988.
70. Otsubo H, et al: Neuroimaging for investigation of seizures in children. *Pediatr Neurosurg* 18:105, 1992.
71. Pedley TA, Scheuer ML, Walczak TS: Epilepsy. In Rowland LP (ed): *Merritt's Textbook of Neurology,* 9th ed. Baltimore, Williams and Wilkins, 1995.
72. America's Working Group on Status Epilepticus: Treatment of convulsive status epilepticus. *JAMA* 270:854, 1993.
73. Hanhan UA, Fiallos MR, Orlowski JP: Status epilepticus. *Pediatr Clin North Am* 48:683, 2001.
74. Trieman DM: The role of benzodiazepines in the management of status epilepticus. *Neurology* 40:32, 1990.
75. Kondall JL, Reynolds M, et al: Intranasal midazolam in patients with status epilepticus. *Ann Emerg Med* 29:415, 1997.
76. Lowenstein DH, Alldredge BK: Status epilepticus. *N Engl J Med* 338:970, 1998.
77. Stecker MM, et al: Treatment of refractory status epilepticus with propofol: Clinical and pharmacokinetic findings. *Epilepsia* 39:18, 1998.
78. Hovinger CA, et al: Use of intravenous valproate in three pediatric patients with nonconvulsive or convulsive status epilepticus. *Ann Pharm* 33:579, 1999.
79. Hauser WA, et al: Risk of recurrent seizures after two unprovoked seizures. *N Engl J Med* 338:429, 1998.
80. Shinnar S, et al: The risk of seizure recurrence after a first unprovoked afebrile seizure in childhood: An extended follow-up. *Pediatrics* 98:216, 1996.
81. Shinnar S, et al: Sleep state and the risk of seizure recurrence following a first unprovoked seizure in childhood. *Neurology* 43:701, 1993.
82. Holmes GL: Do seizures cause brain damage? [review] *Epilepsia* 32:S14, 1991.
83. Musicco M, Beghi E, Solari A: Treatment of first tonic-clonic seizure does not improve the prognosis of epilepsy. First Seizure Trial Group (FIRST Group). *Neurology* 49:991, 1997.
84. Shinnar S, et al: Discontinuing antiepileptic drugs in children with epilepsy: A prospective study. *Ann Neurol* 35:534, 1994.
85. Commission on Classification and Terminology of the International League Against Epilepsy: Proposal for revised clinical and electroencephalographic classification of epileptic seizures. *Epilepsia* 22:489, 1981.
86. Commission on Classification and Terminology of the International League Against Epilepsy: Proposal for revised classification of epilepsies and epileptic syndromes. *Epilepsia* 30:389, 1989.
87. Stang PE, et al: Incidence of migraine headache: A population based study in Olmstead County, Minnesota. *Neurology* 42:1657, 1992.
88. May A, Goadsby PJ: The trigeminovascular system in humans: Pathophysiologic implications for primary headache syndromes of the neural influences on the cerebral circulation. *J Cerebr Blood Flow Metab* 19:115, 1999.
89. Lewis DW, Rothner DA: Headache in children and adolescents. In Johnson RT, Griffin JW, McArthur JC (eds): *Current Therapy in Neurological Diseases,* 6th ed. Philadelphia, Mosby, 2002.
90. Rothner DA: Headaches. In Swaiman KF, Ashwal S (eds): *Pediatric Neurology Principles and Practice.* St. Louis, Mosby, 1999.
91. Flores LE, et al: Delay in the diagnosis of pediatric brain tumors. *Am J Dis Child* 140:684, 1986.
92. Qureshi F, Lewis D: Managing headache in the pediatric emergency department. *Clin Ped Emerg Med* 4:159, 2003.
93. The Childhood Brain Tumor Consortium: The epidemiology of headache among children with brain tumor: Headache in children with brain tumors. *J Neurooncol* 10:31, 1991.
94. Headache Classification Committee of the International Headache Society: Classification and diagnostic criteria for headache disorders, cranial neuralgia, and facial pain. *Cephalgia* 8(supp 7):1, 1998.
95. Winner P, et al: Multicenter prospective evaluation of proposed pediatric migraine revisions to the HIS criteria. *Headache* 37:545, 1997.
96. Lewis DW, et al: Practice parameter: Evaluation of children and adolescents with recurrent headache. *Neurology* 59:490, 2002.
97. Linder SL: Subcutaneous sumatriptan in the clinical setting: The first 50 consecutive patients with acute migraine in a pediatric neurology office practice. *Headache* 36:419, 1996.
98. Winner P, et al: A randomized, double blind, placebo controlled study of sumatriptan nasal spray in the acute treatment of acute migraine in adolescents. *Pediatrics* 106:989, 2000.
99. Ryan M, Engle E: Acute ataxia in childhood. *J Child Neurol* 18:309, 2003.
100. Adams C, et al: Autoantibodies in childhood post-varicella acute cerebellar ataxia. *Can J Neurol Sci* 27:316, 2000.

101. Garg B, et al: Strokes in children due to vertebral artery trauma. *Neurology* 43:2555, 1993.
102. Paulson H, Ammache Z: Ataxia and hereditary disorders. *Neurol Clin* 19:759, 2001.
103. Avery M, First L (eds): *Pediatric Medicine*, 2nd ed. Baltimore, Williams & Wilkins, 1993, pp 785-787.
104. Rudolph C, Rudolph A (eds): *Rudolph's Pediatrics*, 21st ed. New York, McGraw Hill, 2003, pp 1246-1247.
105. Weisleder P, Fife TD: Dizziness and headache: A common association in children and adolescents. *J Child Neurol* 16:727, 2001.
106. Balkany TJ, Finkel RS: The dizzy child. *Ear Hearing* 7:138, 1986.
107. Tusa R, et al: Dizziness in childhood. *J Child Neurol* 9:261, 1994.
108. Akagi H, et al: Menieres disease in children. *J Pediatr Otorhinolaryngol* 6:259, 2001.
109. Meyerhoff W, et al: Ménière's disease in children. *Laryngoscope* 88:1504, 1978.
110. Eviatar L: Dizziness in children. Otolaryngol Clin North Am 27:557, 1994.
111. Eviatar L, et al: Post-traumatic vertigo in children: A diagnostic approach. *Pediatr Neurol* 2:61, 1995.
112. Anoh-Tanon MJ, et al: Vertigo is an underestimated symptom of ocular disorders: Dizzy children do not always need an MRI. *Pediatr Neurol* 23:49, 2000.
113. Golz A, et al: Evaluation of balance disturbances in children with middle ear effusion. *Int J Pediatr Otorhinolaryngol* 43:21, 1998.
114. Tusa R: Vertigo. *Neurol Clin* 19:23, 2001.
115. Driscoll DJ, Jacobsen SJ, Porter CJ, Wollan PC: Syncope in children and adolescents. *J Am Coll Cardiol* 29:1039, 1997.
116. Josnsrude CL: Current approach to pediatric syncope. *Pediatr Cardiol* 21:522, 2000.
117. Grubb BP, Kosinski D: Neurocardiogenic syncope and related syndromes of orthostatic intolerance. *Cardiol Rev* 5:121, 1997.
118. Tane RE, Walsh EP: Syncope in the pediatric patient. *Cardiol Clin* 15:277, 1997.
119. Massin MM: Neurocardiogenic syncope in children. *Pediatr Drugs* 5:327, 2003.

CHAPTER 174
Musculoskeletal Disorders

Kemedy K. McQuillen

PERSPECTIVE

Each year approximately 15 million children visit the emergency department because of unintentional injury. Trauma to the musculoskeletal system accounts for half of these visits.[1]

As a result of the physiologic and anatomic differences between children and adults, pediatric patients are susceptible to problems that do not affect the adult population. An understanding of these differences helps the emergency physician appropriately diagnose and treat musculoskeletal complaints in children. This chapter reviews the general principles and physiology of the pediatric musculoskeletal system, highlights the more common pediatric fractures, and describes musculoskeletal problems specific to the pediatric population.

PRINCIPLES OF DISEASE

Anatomy and Physiology

Several factors distinguish the pediatric musculoskeletal system from that of an adult. The most striking difference is the presence of a physis or growth plate. The physis is made up of proliferating cartilage cells between the metaphysis and epiphysis. Because it is composed of cartilage, the growth plate is the weakest part of the bone and is more likely to separate before the adjacent tendon or ligament tears. For this reason, sprains are less frequent in the pediatric population than in the adult population, and physeal injuries are common.

Another factor that influences pediatric musculoskeletal injuries is the presence of a thick, physiologically active periosteum that is easily stripped from the bony cortex. When injuries occur, the periosteum is often torn on the convex side while remaining intact on the concave side. As such, the periosteum reduces the amount of fracture displacement and, when it remains intact, aids the emergency physician and orthopedist in fracture reduction. The great bone-forming potential of the periosteum also facilitates the healing process: callus formation is vigorous and nonunion almost never occurs.

Growing bone is more porous, more pliable, and less dense than adult bone. These characteristics result in less strength, thus making children more susceptible to fractures. However, although it takes less force to cause deformation, pediatric bone is more likely to buckle when compressed or bow when bent. Finally, because the bones are still growing, there is greater remodeling potential with metaphyseal fractures. Growth can compensate for postreduction imperfections in both apposition and alignment, with deformities occurring in the plane of motion having the greatest potential for remodeling.

Fracture Patterns

As with adults, description of pediatric fractures includes the bony location (diaphysis, metaphysis,

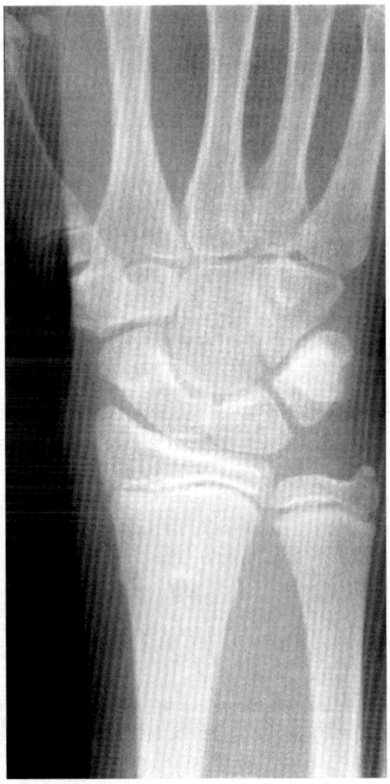

Figure 174-1. Buckle fracture of the distal end of the radius. Treatment is three to six weeks of immobilization.

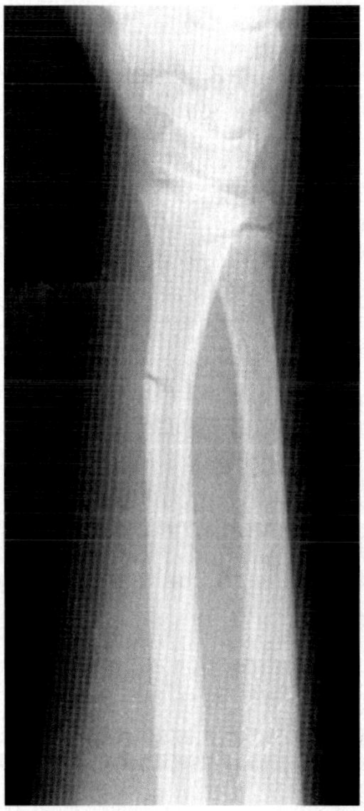

Figure 174-2. Greenstick fracture of the radius. This fracture may need to be completed to achieve an anatomic reduction.

physis, or epiphysis), configuration, relationship of fracture fragments to one another (angulation and displacement), and relationship of fracture fragments to adjacent tissue (open or closed). The inherent differences between pediatric and adult bone result in fracture configurations that are not found in the adult population. Pediatric fractures can be classified as follows:

- *Plastic deformation*: bone is bowed with no obvious cortical disruption.
- *Torus fracture* (buckle fracture): buckling of bone without cortical disruption; it tends to occur because of compression failure of the bone at the metaphyseal/diaphyseal junction (Figure 174-1). These fractures may be immobilized with a splint or cast or, if they involve the distal end of the radius, a Futura splint[2] or Prelude[3] backslab. The Futura splint and Prelude backslab can be removed by the family in 3 to 4 weeks or primary care provider, thereby obviating the need for orthopedic follow-up.
- *Greenstick fracture*: bone and one cortex are disrupted; the periosteum on the fracture's compression side remains intact (Figure 174-2).
- *Complete fracture*: the fracture propagates completely through the bone; included are transverse (Figure 174-3), spiral (Figure 174-4), and oblique fracture lines and comminuted (Figure 174-5) and butterfly fragments.

The presence of a relatively weak, cartilaginous physis in growing bone makes physeal injury common in the skeletally immature. Although injuries to the physis can occur at any age, they are more common during rapid skeletal growth. The Salter-Harris classification system is the most frequently used tool to

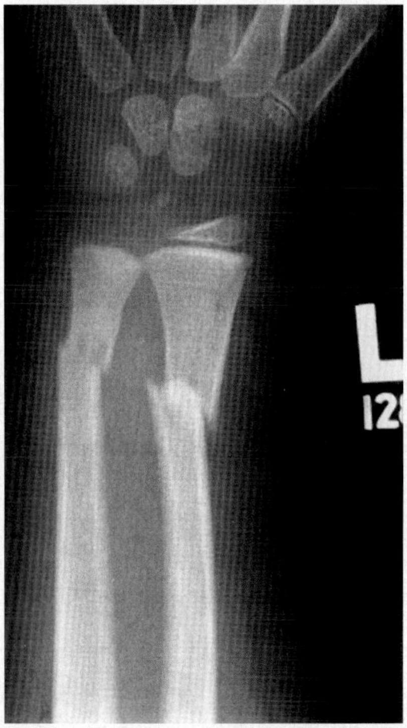

Figure 174-3. Transverse fractures of the radius and ulna.

describe physeal injuries. This classification system is based on the extent of involvement of the physis, epiphysis, and joint (Table 174-1). Type I and II Salter-Harris injuries (Figures 174-6 and 174-7) do not involve the germinal layer of the growth plate; therefore, the risk for growth arrest is small. In general, the higher the Salter-Harris classification, the greater the damage to

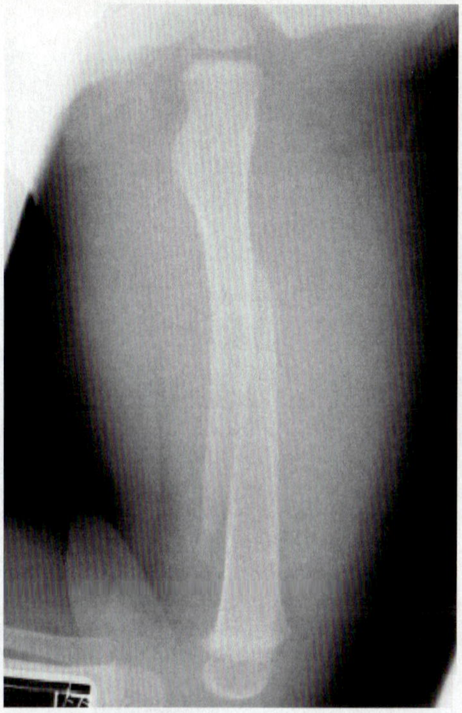

Figure 174-4. Spiral fracture of the femur.

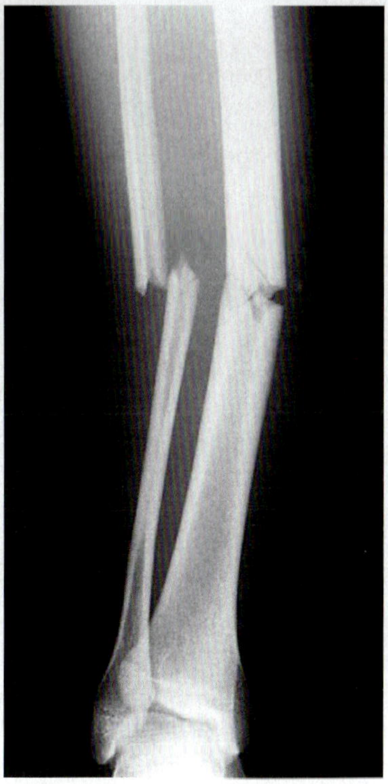

Figure 174-5. Comminuted fractures of the tibia and fibula.

Table 174-1. Salter-Harris Fracture Classification

Type I: Fracture extends through the physis (see Figure 174-6)	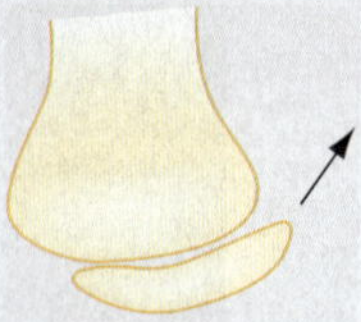
Type II: Fracture extends from the physis into the metaphysis (away from the joint space) (see Figure 174-7)	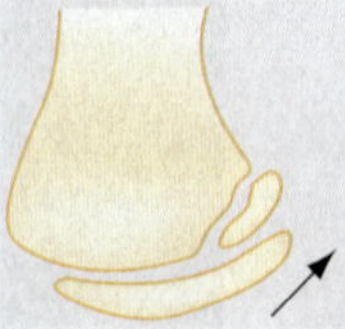
Type III: Fracture extends from the physis into the epiphysis (toward the joint space) (see Figure 174-8)	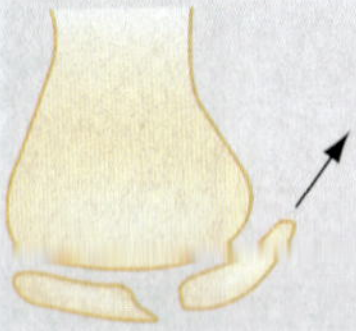
Type IV: Fracture extends from the physis into the metaphysis and epiphysis (see Figure 174-9)	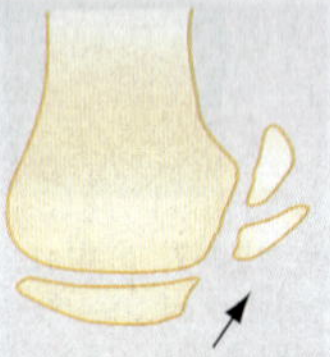
Type V: Crush injury of the physis (see Figure 174-10)	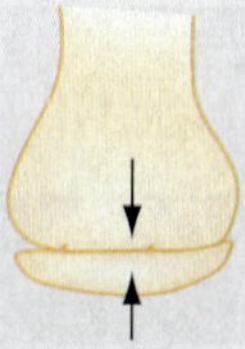

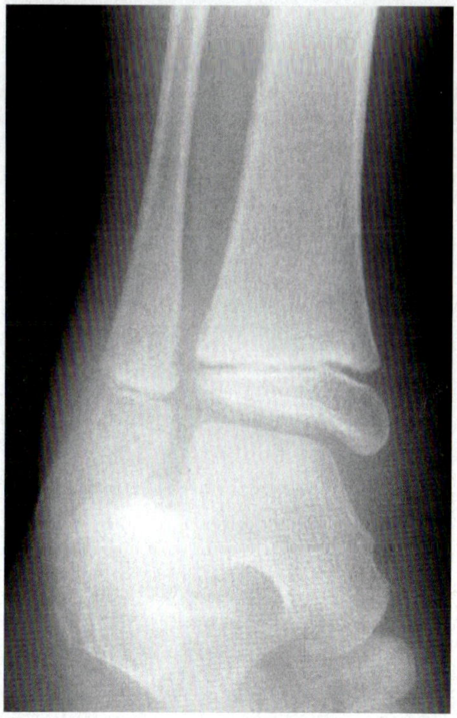

Figure 174-6. Salter-Harris type I fracture of the fibula. The only finding on examination was point tenderness over the distal end of the fibula. Radiographic findings include soft tissue swelling over the growth plate with minimal physeal widening.

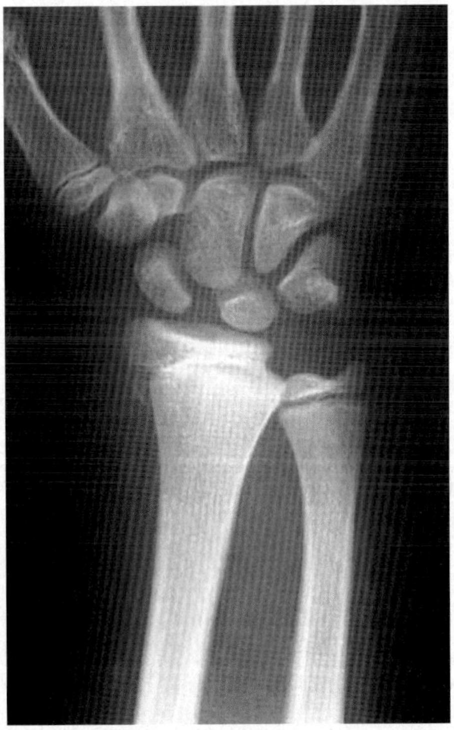

Figure 174-7. Salter-Harris type II fracture of the radius. The triangular piece of the metaphysis is referred to as the Thurston-Holland segment.

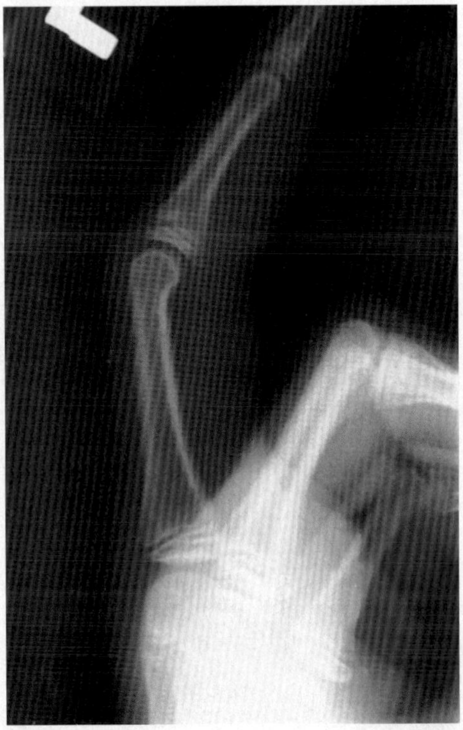

Figure 174-8. Salter-Harris type III fracture of the middle phalanx.

the growth plate and the greater the likelihood of growth arrest or limb length abnormalities (Figures 174-8 to 174-10). Type II fractures are the most common Salter-Harris injury and account for approximately three fourths of all growth plate injuries.

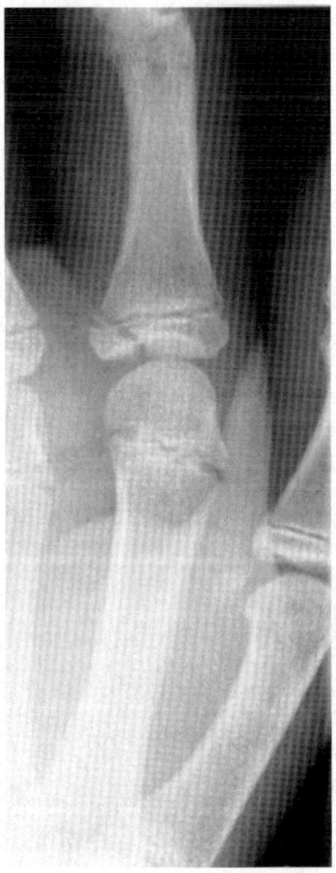

Figure 174-9. Salter-Harris type IV fracture of the proximal phalanx.

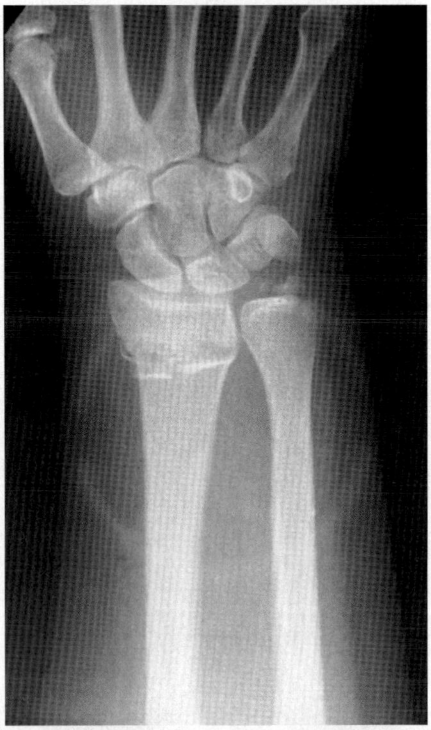

Figure 174-10. Salter-Harris type V fracture of the distal end of the radius. The crush injury has obliterated the physis.

SPECIFIC DISORDERS

Clavicle Fracture

Clavicle fractures are the most common childhood fracture.[4] Midshaft fractures account for approximately 85% of all clavicle fractures, whereas distal and proxi-

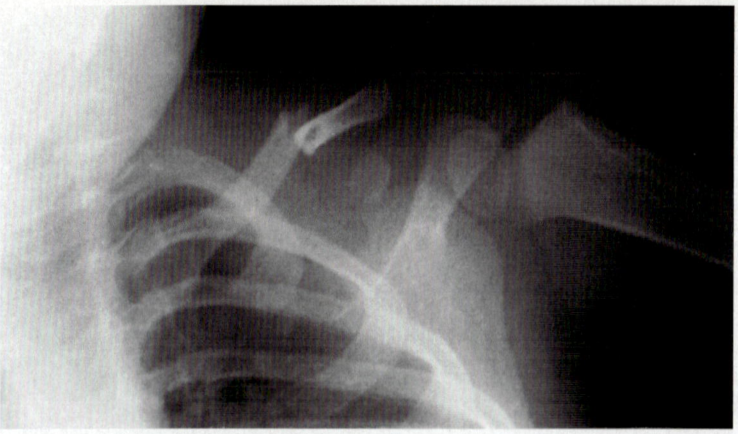

Figure 174-11. Fracture of the middle third of the clavicle.

mal fractures account for approximately 10% and 5%, respectively. The usual mechanism of injury is a fall on the shoulder or, less commonly, direct trauma to the bone itself. The child typically supports the affected side with the other hand and tilts the head toward the side of the fracture. Physical examination reveals point tenderness at the fracture site with or without an obvious bony deformity. With a minimally displaced fracture, shoulder motion may be tolerated. Otherwise, range of motion of the shoulder is limited by pain. Although complications are rare, the proximity of the clavicle to the great vessels and brachial plexus calls for a thorough neurovascular evaluation. The proximity to the pleural cap may also result in pneumothorax.

An anteroposterior (AP) radiograph of the clavicle (Figure 174-11) confirms the diagnosis. If clinical suspicion is high and the AP view does not reveal a fracture, a 30-degree cephalic view can be helpful. Specialized imaging studies are rarely needed, although computed tomography (CT) and duplex ultrasonography may be considered for proximal, posteriorly displaced fractures.[5]

Clavicle fractures do not require anatomic reduction for healing or function; therefore, treatment is directed at maintaining comfort with splinting, ice, and analgesics. Distal clavicular fractures in adolescents, however, may require surgical management. Figure-of-eight splinting helps bring the clavicle out to length, relieves muscle spasm, and minimizes motion at the fracture site. Previously the treatment of choice, the figure-of-eight splint has fallen out of favor with some physicians because of the risk for brachial plexus palsy with long-term use. Alternatively, a sling with or without a swath can be used to provide comfort by supporting the upper extremity and relieving the suspensory forces usually maintained by the clavicle. Most clavicle fractures heal without any problems, except for the development of bony callus at the fractures site; the younger the patient, the greater the potential for remodeling of this deformity.[6] As the fracture stabilizes and the comfort level improves, range-of-motion exercises can be started and gradually progressed. Younger children generally require shorter periods of immobilization (2 to 4 weeks) than do adolescents and adults (4 to 8 weeks).

Clavicle fractures can also occur during childbirth and represent more than 90% of obstetric fractures. They occur equally in males and females and on the right and left sides. Symptomatic neonatal clavicle fractures in the immediate postnatal period are characterized by "pseudoparalysis" of the affected arm; asymptomatic fractures may not be noticed until 10 days of age when the bony callus becomes apparent. The diagnosis is made with radiographs.

Supracondylar Fractures of the Humerus

Supracondylar fractures are the most common fracture around the elbow in the pediatric population. Most are sustained in children younger than 8 years. Until that age, the tensile strength of the ligaments and joint capsule is greater than that of the bone itself; the weaker bone therefore yields to the stronger ligament complex around the joint.[7]

Supracondylar fractures are classified as flexion or extension according to mechanism of injury. The extension type of fracture constitutes 95% of all supracondylar fractures and typically results from a hyperextension injury to the elbow when a child falls onto an outstretched arm. In this injury the olecranon forcefully abuts the olecranon fossa, and the forces are concentrated in the supracondylar area. This mechanism results in failure of the anterior cortex and displacement of the distal fragment posteriorly in relation to the proximal fragment. With extension-type supracondylar fractures, the degree of displacement and continuity of the cortex are further defined by the Gartland classification (Table 174-2).[8] In the less common flexion type of supracondylar fracture, the elbow is flexed when it hits the ground, and energy is transferred from the posterior aspect of the proximal end of the ulna to the distal end of the humerus. This mechanism results in a supracondylar fracture with anterior displacement of the distal fragment and failure of the cortex posteriorly.

Children with supracondylar humerus fractures can be seen with anything from mild swelling and elbow pain to a grossly displaced humerus. Gentle palpation is useful in determining the site of injury; however,

Table 174-2. Gartland Classification for Extension-Type Supracondylar Fractures

Type I	Nondisplaced fracture
Type II	Displaced fracture with intact posterior cortex
Type III	Displaced fracture with no cortical contact
	A: Posteromedial rotation of the distal fragment
	B: Posterolateral rotation of the distal fragment

Modified from Gartland JJ: Management of supracondylar fractures of the humerus in children. *Surg Gynecol Obstet* 109:145, 1959.

Table 174-3. Neurologic Examination of the Distal Upper Extremity

Nerve	Motor Findings	Sensory Findings
Radial	Wrist extension	Thumb and first finger web space
Ulnar	Wrist flexion and adduction	Little finger
	Finger spread	Ulnar aspect of palm of hand
Median	Wrist flexion and abduction	Thumb, index, and middle fingers
	Thumb opposition	Radial aspect of palm of hand
Anterior interosseous	Distal phalanx flexion (thumb/first finger)	None

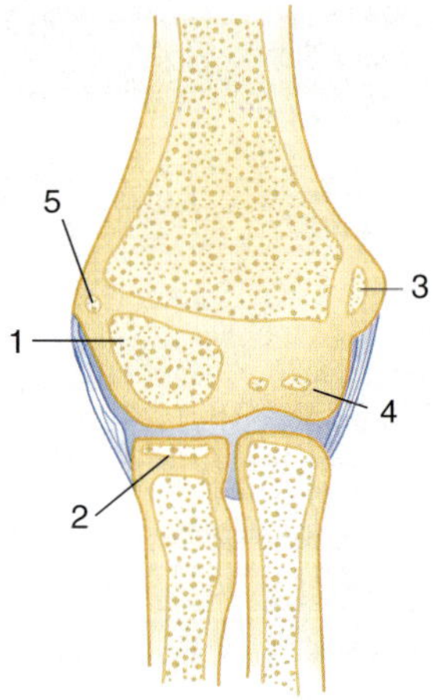

Figure 174-12. Ossification centers of the elbow. 1, Capitellum; 2, radial head; 3, medial epicondyle; 4, trochlea; 5, lateral epicondyle. (From Connolly JF: *DePalma's Management of Fractures and Dislocations.* Philadelphia, WB Saunders, 1981.)

Table 174-4. Sequence of Ossification around the Elbow (CRITOE)

Ossification Center	Age of Appearance
*C*apitellum	6-12 months
*R*adial head	4-5 years
Medial (*I*nternal) epicondyle	5-7 years
*T*rochlea	8-10 years
*O*lecranon	8-9 years
Lateral (*E*xternal) epicondyle	9-13 years

manipulation should be avoided because movement may cause further neurovascular damage. Children with extension-type supracondylar fractures hold the affected arm in extension with an S-shaped configuration of the elbow and have a prominence at the olecranon. Children with flexion-type supracondylar fractures hold the arm in flexion and have an empty space where the olecranon should be. In all cases it is important to carefully assess distal neurovascular status. Motor and sensory function should be evaluated by assessing the radial, ulnar, and median nerves (Table 174-3). Two-point discrimination on the fingers provides a sensitive means of assessing sensory status: an abnormal value (>6 mm) indicates a deficit. Vascular assessment should include evaluation of the pulse at the wrist and capillary refill of the hand. Patients should have ongoing assessment for the development of compartment syndrome of the forearm. If there is pain on flexion or extension of the fingers, forearm tenderness, or pain that is disproportionate to the injury, compartment pressures should be measured immediately. Unrecognized ischemic injury can result in Volkmann's ischemic contracture.

Radiographic evaluation of any elbow injury should include an AP view of the extended elbow and a lateral view of the flexed elbow. If these views do not show a fracture but clinical suspicion is high, oblique views are helpful. Even with proper radiographs, diagnosis of a pediatric elbow fracture can be difficult. The elbow is largely cartilaginous during early childhood, and the six secondary centers of ossification around the elbow can camouflage or be mistaken for fractures (Figure 174-12). These ossification centers can be remembered by the mnemonic CRITOE—*c*apitellum, *r*adius, *i*nternal (medial) epicondyle, *t*rochlea, *o*lecranon, and *e*xternal (lateral) epicondyle. The approximate age at which these sites ossify may be estimated at 1, 3, 5, 7, 9, and 11 years, respectively (Table 174-4).

Bony relationships are helpful when evaluating a radiograph for the presence of a supracondylar fracture (Figure 174-13). In a true lateral view, the anterior humeral line should bisect the capitellum. If the capitellum falls posterior to this line, an extension-type supracondylar fracture is likely. In all views, the proximal end of the radius and radial neck should point to the capitellum. Baumann's angle is also helpful in diagnosing subtle supracondylar fractures (Figure 174-14). This angle is formed by drawing a line that follows the growth plate of the capitellum and transecting it with a line that runs perpendicular to the axis of the humerus. The angle should be approximately 75 degrees. Baumann's angle should be the same in both elbows, and differences between elbows can be used to detect subtle supracondylar fractures. Postreduction alterations in Baumann's angle reliably predict the final carrying angle.[9]

Fat pads also provide a means for detecting occult supracondylar fractures. A lateral radiograph with the elbow flexed at 90 degrees may show an anterior fat pad protruding from the coronoid fossa. This finding is normal unless the pad is bulging or in the shape of a

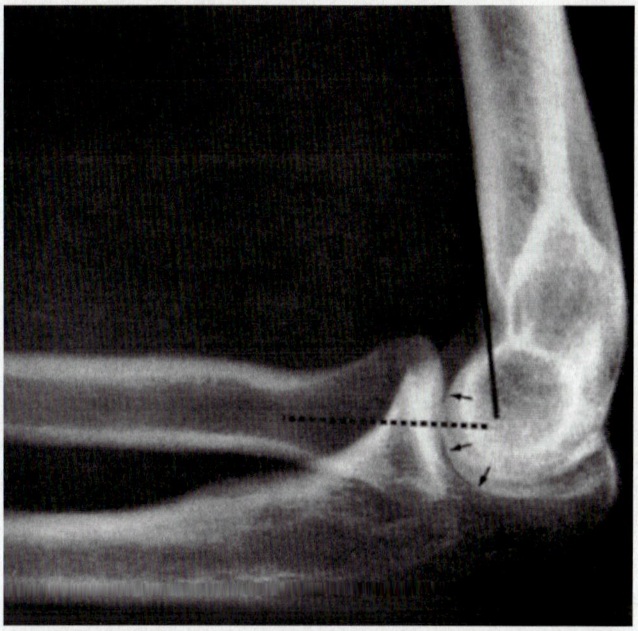

Figure 174-13. Lateral radiograph demonstrating the bony relationships in a normal elbow. The anterior humeral line *(solid)* and proximal radial line *(dashed)* bisect the capitellum. (From Weissman BN, Sledge CB: *Orthopedic Radiology.* Philadelphia, WB Saunders, 1986.)

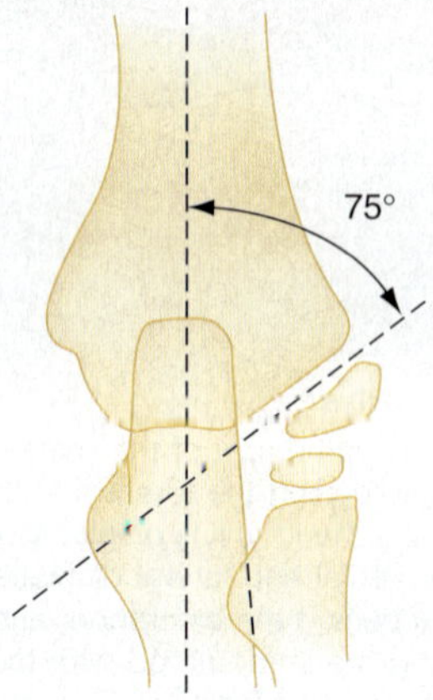

Figure 174-14. Baumann's angle in a normal elbow on an anteroposterior radiograph. (From Worlock P: Supracondylar fractures of the humerus: Assessment of cubitus varus by the Baumann angle. *J Bone Joint Surg Br* 68:755, 1986.)

ship's sail. This "sail sign" may indicate fluid in the joint, although alone it may not be a reliable predictor of a fracture. The posterior fat pad, however, sits snugly within the olecranon fossa and should never be seen unless there is a fracture around the elbow. In this case, blood pushes the fat pad laterally and thus makes it visible on a lateral radiograph of the elbow. Therefore, visualization of a posterior fat pad suggests the presence of an occult fracture around the elbow and, if the fracture is not seen, warrants oblique views of the elbow (Figure 174-15), splinting, and follow-up.

Plain radiographs are usually sufficient for diagnosing supracondylar fractures; however, if the diagnosis remains in question after AP, lateral, and oblique radiographs are obtained, ultrasound may be useful in

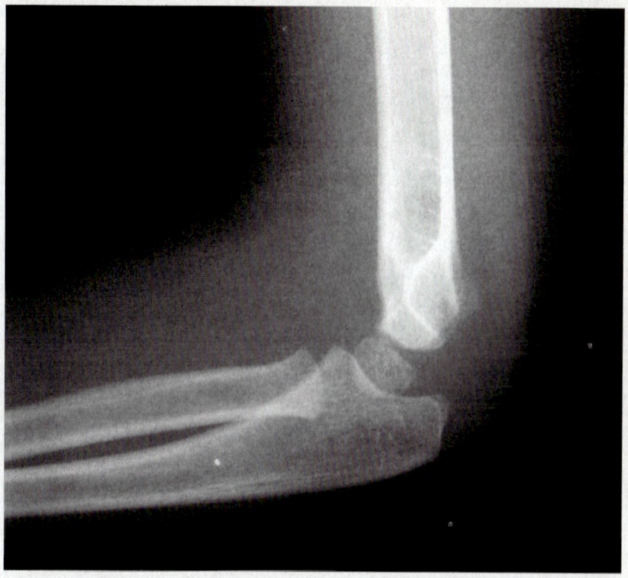

Figure 174-15. Lateral radiograph of a supracondylar fracture with an anterior fat pad "sail sign" and a posterior fat pad.

infants,[10] and magnetic resonance imaging (MRI) may be useful in older children.[11] With strong clinical suspicion, some orthopedic surgeons bypass MRI in favor of an intraoperative arthrogram.[12]

Emergency department treatment of supracondylar humeral fractures is determined by displacement and neurovascular status. A pale, pulseless cold hand mandates emergency consultation with an orthopedic surgeon. If an orthopedic surgeon is unavailable and the vascular supply has not been restored, reduction should be attempted (Figure 174-16). If necessary, reduction can be performed by a single operator: with the patient supine, the shoulder held in 90 degrees of forward flexion, and the elbow slightly flexed, both hands are placed on the arm proximal to the fracture and both thumbs are placed on the posterior aspect of the fracture fragment. Then, while directing the thumbs distally, the fragment is lifted onto the distal metaphysis. The return of blood supply is marked by the hand becoming warm and pink. If perfusion does not improve, another reduction may be attempted, with care taken to not entrap the brachial artery and median nerve. Multiple attempts at reduction increase the likelihood of neurovascular injury and swelling; therefore, no more than two reductions should be attempted. A supracondylar fracture with a pulseless hand that is warm and pink does not need to be reduced and should be splinted as it lies so that vascular status is not further compromised. The elbow should be splinted in relative extension because too much flexion in conjunction with swelling may obstruct the brachial artery and contribute to limb ischemia.

Gartland type I fractures can be splinted in the emergency department with the arm maintained in flexion and neutral rotation. Hospital admission is not required, but referral to an orthopedic surgeon the next day is recommended. These fractures are generally treated with 3 to 4 weeks of immobilization. Gartland

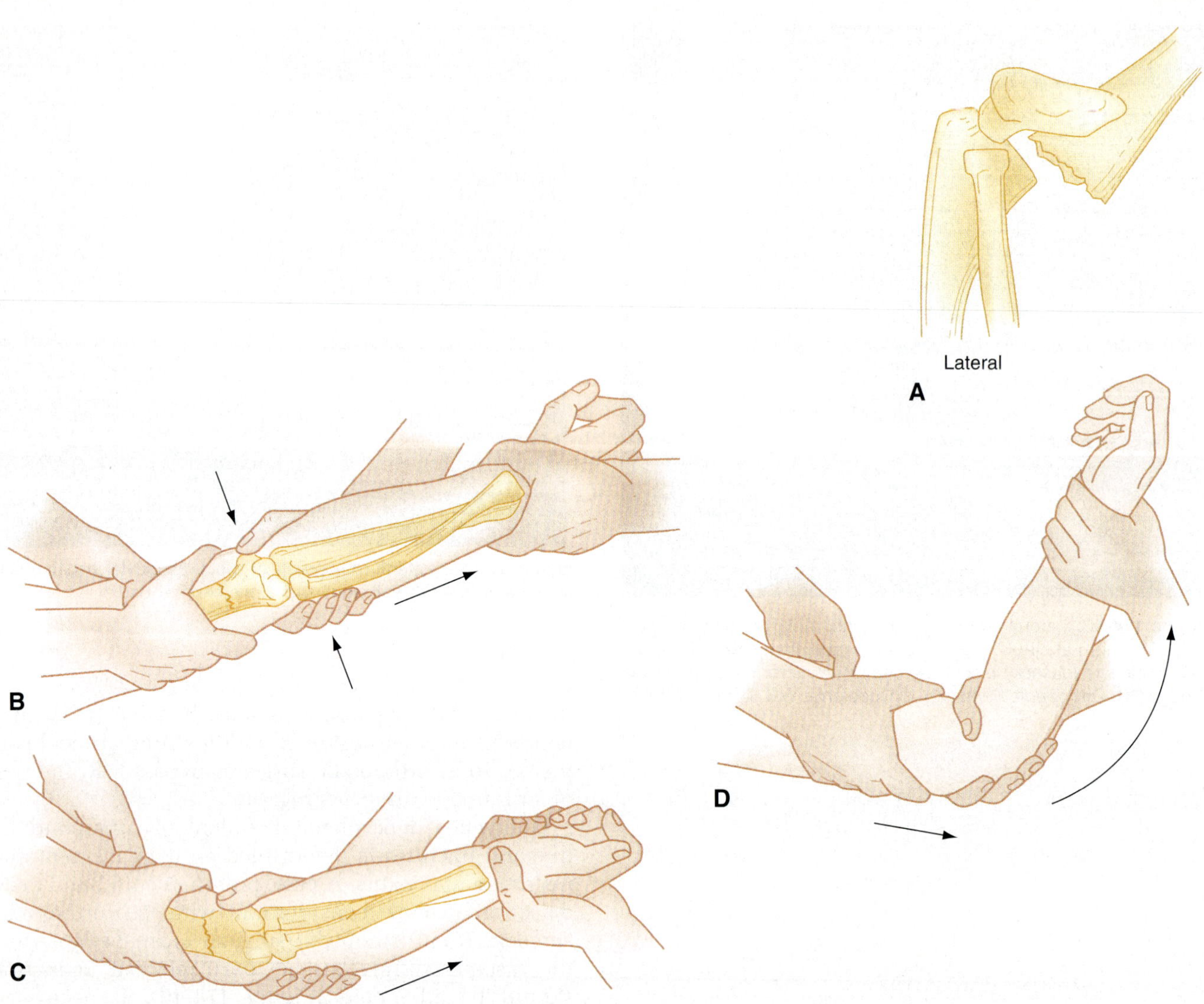

Figure 174-16. Steps in reduction of (**A**) a displaced supracondylar fracture. **B**, The assistant fixes the arm of the patient while the physician grasps the patient's wrist and applies steady traction in line with the long axis of the arm while keeping the forearm in the neutral, thumb-up position. **C**, If the distal fragment is displaced laterally, it is pushed inward with the physician's other hand. If it is displaced medially, it is pushed outward. Throughout manipulation, traction is maintained. **D**, After length is restored and the medial and lateral displacement corrected, the physician's thumb is placed over the anterior surface of the proximal fragment with the fingers behind the olecranon, and the elbow is gently flexed. The arm is then immobilized with the forearm pronated, and laterally displaced fractures are immobilized with the forearm supinated. (From Geiderman JM, Magnusson AR: In Rosen P, Barkin R [eds]: *Humerus and Elbow in Emergency Medicine: Concepts and Clinical Practice,* 4th ed. St Louis, CV Mosby, 1998.)

type III fractures require immediate orthopedic consultation and should be treated by either closed reduction and percutaneous pinning or open reduction and internal fixation in the operating room. Treatment of a partly displaced type II fracture is controversial. Some surgeons reduce and pin it in the operating room, whereas others perform closed reduction and keep it immobilized in a cast. However, treatment of displaced supracondylar fractures by closed reduction and casting is associated with higher complication rates than treatment by closed reduction and pinning is[13]; therefore, most are treated with pins and casting for 3 to 4 weeks.

The primary complications of supracondylar fractures are related to neurovascular injury. Type III fractures are at greatest risk, with neurovascular compromise occurring in as many as 49% of patients.[9] The median nerve is involved in half the cases and is associated with posterolateral displacement, and the radial nerve is involved in almost a third of patients and is associated with posteromedial displacement. Brachial artery injuries occur in approximately 40% of patients and are found with either type of displacement. Fortunately, the brachial artery has many branches around the elbow, and flow to the forearm and hand can be maintained even when the brachial artery is injured. Despite the frequency of neurovascular deficits immediately after the accident, most nerve palsies are caused by stretching or contusion and resolve spontaneously. The typical course for nerve injuries is complete resolution. Although motor function usually returns within 12 weeks, sensory function may not return for 6 months or longer.[14] If there is no clinical or electromyographic evidence of nerve recovery after 5 months, exploration and neurolysis are indicated.[15] Volkmann's ischemic contracture and

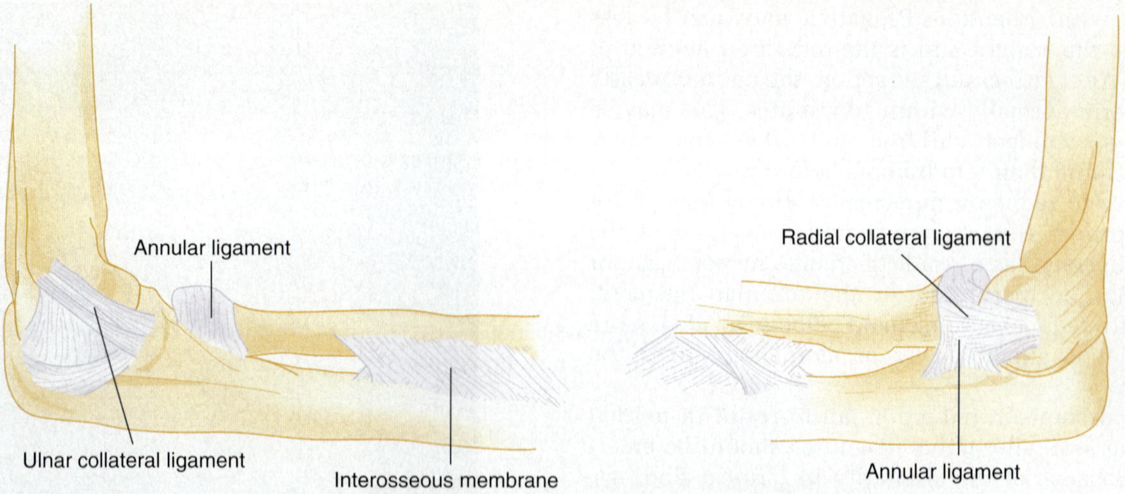

Figure 174-17. Nursemaid's elbow. In a nursemaid's elbow injury, as an axial force is applied, the annular ligament around the radial head is dislodged. The ligament is then partially dislocated into the radiocapitellar joint when the arm is released. (From Simon R, Kownigsknecht S: *Emergency Orthopaedics: The Extremities,* 2nd ed. E Norwalk, Conn, Appleton & Lange, 1987.)

permanent limb disability are the end result of untreated vascular injury. It is extremely rare and easily prevented by close observation and evaluation for the development of compartment syndrome. A few supracondylar fractures heal with a "gunstock" deformity; however, the combination of varus, hyperextension, and medial rotation of the limb is not a functional problem and, except in severe cases, requires no treatment. Severe cases can be corrected by humeral osteotomy.

Monteggia Fracture-Dislocation

Monteggia fracture-dislocation are characterized by a fracture of the proximal third of the ulna plus dislocation of the radial head. They can be very subtle, with only a minor greenstick fracture or bowing of the ulna. Isolated ulna fractures are rare in children; therefore, in all such fractures, AP and lateral radiographs of the elbow should be taken to rule out dislocation of the radial head.

Monteggia fracture-dislocations require urgent referral to an orthopedic surgeon for closed reduction of the radial head dislocation and repair of the ulna fracture. Complications include permanent radial head dislocation, valgus deformity of the arm, loss of pronation, and late radial nerve palsy.

Nursemaid's Elbow

Radial head subluxation, or nursemaid's elbow, is the most common upper extremity injury in children younger than 6 years who are taken to a pediatric emergency department.[16] It typically occurs when axial traction is placed on an extended and pronated arm, as when a child is pulled up or swung by the arms. It may also occur when a child falls onto an outstretched arm, sustains minor direct trauma to the elbow, or simply twists the arm. In infants, radial head subluxation can occur when an extended arm is caught beneath the infant's body while being rolled over. Pathologically, subluxation occurs when the annular ligament becomes loosened from the head of the radius and slips into the radiocapitellar joint, where it becomes entrapped (Figure 174-17).

Nursemaid's elbow is an injury that occurs in children a few months old to 5 years of age and has a peak incidence between 2 and 3 years of age.[17] It has been reported in children younger than 6 months[17] and has been seen in children as old as 9 years. It has a slight predilection for girls.

Children often have a consistent history followed by an acute onset of arm pain that may or may not be localized to the elbow. The affected arm is held still against the body, with the elbow slightly flexed and the arm pronated. Physical examination is significant for a lack of swelling, erythema, ecchymosis, or deformity. There may be mild tenderness on palpation of the radial head. Pain is elicited with supination, pronation, and elbow flexion.

The diagnosis of nursemaid's elbow is made clinically, and radiographs are not necessary. If, however, significant point tenderness, swelling, or ecchymosis is present or if the history suggests another injury, such as a supracondylar fracture, radiographs should be obtained. Though not commonly used as a diagnostic procedure, ultrasound may demonstrate a widened space between the radial head and capitulum.[18]

Radial head subluxation is an orthopedic injury that is easily reduced without sequelae. Classically, the affected elbow is gripped with the practitioner's thumb over the radial head, and with the other hand, the practitioner flexes and supinates the patient's arm. As the radial head relocates, the practitioner feels it click or clunk under the thumb. Hyperpronation of the forearm is also effective in reducing radial head subluxation. As is done in the flexion-supination maneuver, the practitioner holds the affected elbow with the thumb over the radial head, but then flexion-supination is replaced with hyperpronation of the forearm. Success rates range from 80%[17] to 92%[19] with supination and 93%[20]

to 98%[21] with pronation. Pronation may also be less painful to the patient and is the reduction method of choice.[21] After successful reduction, the child typically uses the arm normally within 10 minutes. This may be delayed in younger children and when the injury occurred more than 4 to 6 hours before reduction.

Inability to reduce a nursemaid's elbow may result from improper reduction technique, swelling of the annular ligament as a result of edema, hemorrhage, or hematoma, or disruption of the annular ligament. Failure to reduce a nursemaid' elbow is also more likely if it is attempted 12 or more hours after the injury.

If two attempts at reduction fail to result in normal use of the arm, alternative diagnoses should be entertained. Because of the similarity in clinical findings, children should be assessed for fractures of the clavicle and elbow. If no other pathology is found and the child is still not using the arm, a posterior splint should be applied with the elbow kept at 90 degrees and the forearm in supination. Follow-up evaluation with an orthopedic surgeon should be arranged for the next day.

Recurrence rates of radial head subluxation range from 5% to 39%, depending on the referral population studied.[17,19,21] With recurrent subluxations, immobilization in a posterior splint with the elbow maintained at 90 degrees and the forearm supinated may be warranted. The need for open reduction or repair of the annular ligament is exceedingly rare.

Toddler's Fracture

Toddler's fractures are oblique nondisplaced fractures caused by low-energy torsional forces applied to the very porous bone of infants and young children. Previously, it referred only to tibial fractures in children between 9 and 36 months of age, but the term is now applied more loosely. The mechanism of injury can be as mild as a child twisting on the leg while walking or a fall from an insignificant height. In some instances, there may be an unknown mechanism of injury. The child will have a limp or refuse to walk on the affected leg. Some children will revert to crawling and can crawl without pain. Examination may show mild swelling of the leg and point tenderness. Gentle twisting of the lower part of the leg may elicit pain.

AP and lateral radiographs may reveal a spiral or oblique fracture extending downward and medially through the distal third of the tibia (Figure 174-18). An internal oblique radiograph is helpful if there is no evidence of fracture on the AP or lateral views. If all views are negative, consideration should be given to fractures elsewhere in the limb. If no fracture is apparent, the child should be splinted for comfort and radiographs repeated in 10 days, at which time periosteal new bone or sclerosis of the fracture edges will make the fracture visible. If these radiographs are negative and the child is still limping, further evaluation should be undertaken to rule out osteomyelitis and malignancy. Bone scans are often helpful in assessing a limping toddler and are more sensitive for fractures than plain radiographs are. Treatment of a toddler's fracture consists of a below-knee walking cast for approximately 3 weeks.

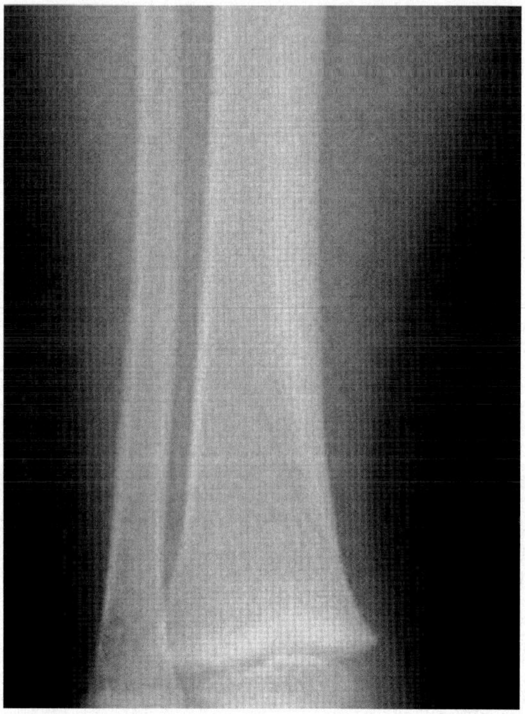

Figure 174-18. Toddler's fracture.

The presence of a spiral fracture without an appropriate history may raise concern of child abuse. Midshaft fractures, which are more common in abused children, tibial fractures in nonambulating children, or other unexplained or frequent injuries should prompt further evaluation.

Skeletal Aspects of Child Abuse

Perspective

Fractures are the second most common manifestation of child abuse, second only to soft tissue injury, and are present in up to 70% of physically abused children. Fractures associated with child abuse occur in the very young: 50% in children younger than 12 months[22] and 94% in children younger than 3 years.[23] With child abuse, a timely and accurate diagnosis is imperative because children who are returned to an abusive home face a 35% chance of repeated abuse and a 10% chance of death.

No fracture is pathognomonic for abuse, but certain fracture patterns are more worrisome than others. Any fracture in a child younger than 1 year, fractures of different ages, and bilateral or multiple fractures indicate a need for thorough assessment for intentional injury. Injuries that are especially concerning include complex skull fractures, rib fractures, metaphyseal fractures, and vertebral fractures or subluxations. Midshaft humeral and scapular fractures are nearly always associated with abuse, as are approximately 70% of femoral fractures in children younger than 1 year.

Specific Disorders/Injuries

Diaphyseal Fractures

Although multiple fractures of different ages are strongly suggestive of child abuse, the most common manifestation of child abuse is an isolated diaphyseal fracture, which occurs four times as often as classic metaphyseal fractures. The humerus, femur, and tibia are the most frequently fractured long bones; the radius and ulna are the most infrequently fractured. With the exception of supracondylar fractures, all fractures of the humerus in children younger than 3 years are strongly suggestive of abuse.[24]

Metaphyseal Fractures

Though less common than diaphyseal fractures, metaphyseal fractures are more specific for child abuse. Metaphyseal fractures most commonly affect the tibia, femur, and proximal end of the humerus. Corner fractures and bucket handle fractures, which may be the same fracture viewed in two different projections, result from violent shaking or forceful pulling or twisting of an infant's limb. The diagnosis is made by careful evaluation of high-quality plain radiographs. However, the tight adherence of the periosteum at the metaphysis precludes an active periosteal response, thus making these fractures difficult to diagnose even in the healing stages. Bone scans, though sometimes helpful, are difficult to interpret because of the normally increased radionuclide uptake in the metaphyseal area.

Rib Fractures

Rib fractures are present in 5% to 27% of cases of child abuse, with 90% occurring in children younger than 2 years. The young pediatric rib cage is very compliant, and it takes considerable force to break a rib. Because of the force involved, rib fractures are seldom seen in unintentional injury and are never seen after cardiopulmonary resuscitation.[25] In a child younger than 3 years, the positive predictive value of a rib fracture as an indicator of intentional trauma approaches 100%.[26] Posterior rib fractures are most common and result from maximal mechanical stress as the rib is levered over the transverse process of the vertebral body when infants are grasped and shaken. The ribs fail mechanically at the head or neck. Abuse-related rib fractures tend to be multiple and symmetrical and may be difficult to diagnose acutely by standard radiographs. Radiographs repeated at 7 to 10 days after the injury are advised if the initial films are negative but suspicion is high. Radiographic findings include callus formation or widening of the rib neck as a result of apposition of new bone subperiosteally. Bone scans can be helpful in detecting fractures in the acute setting.

Skull Fractures

Skull fractures are the second most frequent orthopedic injury in abuse and occur more commonly in abuse than in unintentional trauma.[22] Eighty percent occur in infants younger than 1 year, and although complex skull fractures are more suspicious for abuse, linear skull fractures are the most common type. Standard skull radiographs may not be adequate for diagnosis and are reported to miss more than 25% of head injuries. Children who meet high-risk criteria (the presence of rib fractures, multiple fractures or facial injury, or age younger than 6 months) should undergo CT or MRI to assess for occult head injury.[27]

Periosteal New Bone Formation

Periosteal new bone formation, which is one of the most common findings in cases of abuse, reflects separation of the periosteum from the bone and may be the only finding of orthopedic trauma related to child abuse. It may be present with or without a fracture. It results from shaking, from acceleration-deceleration forces applied to an unsupported limb, or from forceful gripping.

Diagnostic Strategies

Radiography

Conventional skeletal radiography is the screening examination of choice in cases of suspected physical abuse. Unsuspected fractures are found in 22% of physically abused children and are more common in the very young. A complete skeletal survey is recommended for all physically abused children younger than 2 years and for all infants younger than 1 year with evidence of abuse or neglect. Complete skeletal surveys are rarely indicated in children older than 5 years, and in children between 2 and 5 years old, the need for a skeletal survey is determined on a case-by-case basis. A skeletal survey consists of an AP view of the extremities (including the hands and feet), frontal and lateral views of the thoracolumbar spine, including the ribs, and an AP and lateral skull series. In cases in which abuse is strongly suspected but radiographs are negative, bone scanning serves as an adjunct and is complementary to the skeletal survey in detecting injury. It is sensitive for subtle rib, spine, and diaphyseal trauma, especially in the acute setting, but because findings can persist for years, it is not reliable in determining the age of the fracture.

Differential Considerations

Although most cases of intentional injury are easily diagnosed with a thorough history and physical examination, certain conditions can be confused with child abuse. Metaphyseal cupping and spurring and periosteal new bone formation are two normal variants that radiographically are almost identical to what is seen in cases of child abuse. These findings occur in more than 40% of normal infants. They appear between 2 and 3 months of age and may persist until 8 months of age. These findings can be differentiated from child abuse by subtle radiographic clues: normal-variant infantile metaphyseal spurs are in continuity with normal bone and cortex, and physiologic periostitis is bilateral, confined to the diaphysis, and smooth and lamellar in appearance. Physiologic periostitis also tends to be more obvious on the medial aspect of the bone and most commonly involves the femur, although it also is seen in the humerus and tibia. Radiographic differentiation between normal variants and trauma-related injury is extremely difficult, and the clinical findings must be taken into account.

Osteogenesis imperfecta (OI), a heritable disorder of connective tissue, is an alternative cause of multiple fractures with minimal trauma. In the United States, the estimated incidence is 1 in 20,000 persons. This estimate includes children in whom the condition is diagnosed within 1 year of birth but does not include milder forms of the disease that are not diagnosed until later in life. As such, the incidence of OI could be significantly higher. Most types of OI have been linked to mutations in type I collagen genes that interfere with either the synthesis or the construction of collagen subunits. Clinical features include bone fragility, ligament laxity, defective dentinogenesis, short stature, scoliosis, middle ear deafness, blue sclera and tympanic membranes, and misshapen skulls. On radiographs, the bones are diffusely osteopenic with thin cortices and attenuated trabecular patterns. The long bones have narrow diaphyses, and bowing and fractures are common (Figure 174-19).

There are four types of OI, and depending on the type, the severity of disease ranges from intrauterine demise to an infant with multiple fractures to an almost symptom-free adult (Table 174-5). The diagnosis of OI is made on the basis of the history, physical examination, and radiographic findings. Confirmation is by skin biopsy and culture of dermal fibroblasts for evaluation of type I collagen. However, because the molecular basis for the entire spectrum of disease has not been established, up to 10% of cases of OI would be missed with skin biopsy alone.[28] Emergency department management of children with OI includes appropriate orthopedic referral for fractures and primary care referral for hearing evaluation.

In addition to musculoskeletal complaints, children with OI are predisposed to abdominal pain and neurologic abnormalities. The abdominal pain is thought to be related to the trefoil-shaped pelvis and acetabular protrusion associated with OI. These structural abnormalities narrow the pelvic outlet and result in partial rectosigmoid obstruction and subsequent constipation or obstipation. Patients with this problem respond to an aggressive bowel program and disimpaction. Referral to a gastrointestinal specialist may be warranted.

Neurologic abnormalities associated with OI result from basilar impression. Basilar impression, or elevation of the floor of the posterior cranial fossa, is reported to occur in 25% of patients with OI.[29] It is seen most frequently in children with OI type IVB (71%),

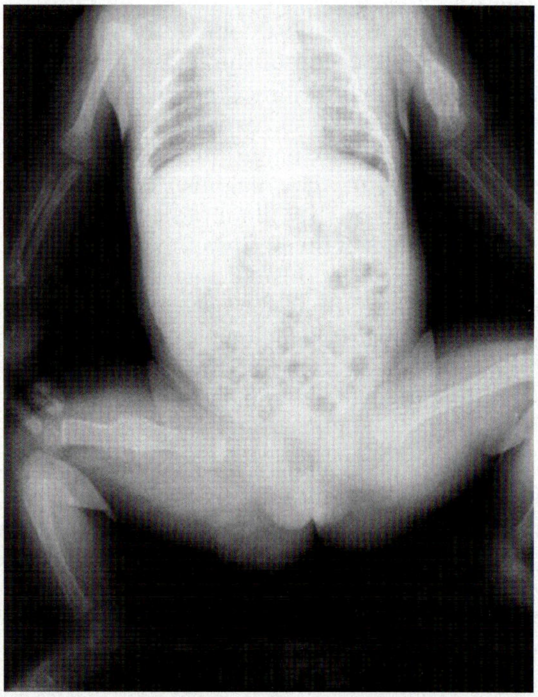

Figure 174-19. Radiograph of a child with osteogenesis imperfecta. Note the narrow diaphyses, osteopenia, and multiple fractures.

Table 174-5. Classification of Osteogenesis Imperfecta

Type	Inheritance	Bone Fragility	Sclerae*	Other
I	Autosomal dominant	Mild to moderate Onset of fractures after birth Most fractures in preschool years	Blue	Most common form of OI Presenile hearing loss Type A: normal teeth Type B: dentinogenesis imperfecta
II	Autosomal dominant—new mutation; autosomal recessive	Very severe Lethal in perinatal period	Dark blue	Subtypes A, B, and C based on radiographic findings
III	Autosomal dominant—new mutation; autosomal recessive	Moderate to severe Severe osteoporosis Fractures at birth with progressive deformity	Normal	Occasional deafness
IV	Autosomal dominant	Mild to moderately severe More severe than type I	Normal, gray or blue in infancy Normal by adolescence	Occasional deafness Type A: normal teeth Type B: dentinogenesis imperfecta

*Blue sclerae are normal in infants up to 4 months old.

and 50% of patients with this type of OI will have neurologic signs or symptoms of compression of the posterior fossa structures.[29] The signs (nystagmus, facial spasm, nerve paresis, pyramidal signs, and papilledema) may predate the symptoms (headache, neuralgia, imbalance, weakness, and incontinence). The most serious outcomes of basilar impression include brainstem compression, respiratory arrest, and sudden death. Any neurologic changes in a patient with OI mandate neurosurgical evaluation.

Several metabolic abnormalities can be associated with frequent fractures and radiographic abnormalities. *Rickets*, which results from vitamin D or calcium deficiency or hyperparathyroidism, can be manifested by diffuse osteopenia, fraying of the metaphysis, fractures, periosteal new bone formation, widening of the physis, and well-defined transverse stress fractures in the shafts of long bones. The diagnosis can be confirmed with laboratory testing. *Menkes' kinky-hair syndrome*, a rare X-linked recessive disorder involving inadequate copper absorption, is characterized by wormian skull bones, osteopenia, and metaphyseal fractures and spurring. These children have sparse, kinky hair, abnormal dentition, and developmental delay. Serum levels of copper and ceruloplasmin are low and confirm the diagnosis. *Hypervitaminosis A*, though a rare cause of fractures, does result in a thick periosteal reaction of tubular bones, most frequently the ulna and metatarsals, and widening of the cranial sutures. The epiphyses and metaphyses are normal. The diagnosis is based on the history and vitamin A levels.

Congenital syphilis can also mimic nonaccidental injury. Skeletal findings of congenital syphilis are frequently diffuse and symmetrical and involve the long bones, skull, and small bones of the hands and feet. Radiographic findings include osteolytic defects, periosteal reaction, and metaphyseal lucencies parallel to the physis. The diagnosis is confirmed by serologic testing.

Developmental Dysplasia of the Hip

Perspective

Developmental dysplasia of the hip (DDH), formerly known as congenital dislocation of the hip, is abnormal formation of the hip joint that occurs between organogenesis and fetal maturity.[30] It encompasses a spectrum of disease ranging from subluxatable, or loose, hips to frankly dislocated hips.

In white neonates, the incidence of dysplasia is 1%, and the incidence of dislocated hips is 0.1%. It is more common in Native American populations and less common in African American, Korean, and Chinese populations. There appears to be a familial predilection for the development of DDH; one British study noted that more than 20% of children who required treatment of DDH had a positive family history.[30] DDH is more common in girls and most frequently unilateral (80%). With unilateral involvement, there is a slight predilection for the left side. Associated birth factors include oligohydramnios, breech presentation, torticollis, talipes equinovarus, metatarsus adductus, and being first born.[31] DDH has also been associated with congenital muscular torticollis.[32] Postnatally, swaddling infants with their hips and knees in extension predisposes to dislocation.

Principles of Disease

The etiology of DDH is not entirely clear. Three theories have been postulated: mechanical issues related to fetal position and environment, primary acetabular dysplasia, and ligamentous laxity that is enhanced by maternal relaxin hormone. Each theory has merit, and it is most likely a combination of factors that contribute to the development of DDH.

Clinical Features

DDH may be diagnosed at birth, or despite frequent and appropriate physical examinations, it may not be discovered until later in life. In one study, 6% of children with documented DDH had normal physical examinations at birth.[30] Conversely, in more than 50% of infants found to have unstable hips at birth, the hips become spontaneously stable within 3.5 days.[33]

The manifestations and physical findings of DDH are as diverse as the disease itself. This variability is due to differences in the severity of the dysplasia and the progressive changes that occur over time. Up to 4 to 6 months of age, the diagnosis of DDH is based on physical examination findings of leg length, skinfold, and range-of-motion asymmetry and abnormal findings on the Barlow provocative test and the Ortolani reduction maneuver. Skinfold asymmetry can be noted in the groin, below the buttock, and along the thighs. Although skinfold asymmetry is not specific for DDH, being present in approximately 30% of infants with normal hips, it is sensitive, and the diagnosis of DDH is very unlikely in infants with normal skinfold symmetry. Range of hip motion is also helpful in diagnosing DDH; any asymmetries in hip flexion, abduction, and external rotation should prompt further investigation. Although the general physical examination can be helpful in assessing hip stability, the physical diagnostic cornerstones for diagnosing DDH in young infants are the Ortolani reduction maneuver and the Barlow provocative test. The Ortolani reduction maneuver is performed in an attempt to reduce a dislocated hip back into normal position, and the Barlow provocative test detects a subluxatable or dislocatable hip (Box 174-1). Abnormal findings include the presence of a "clunk" with the Ortolani test and any abnormal movement between the femoral head and the acetabulum with the Barlow maneuver.

After about 4 to 6 months of age, soft tissue contractures develop, the Ortolani and Barlow tests yield less information in detecting unstable hips, and range-of-motion abnormalities become more apparent. Parents may notice limited or asymmetric leg movements or difficulty with diapering. On examination there is limited abduction, relative shortening of the femoral segment (Galeazzi's sign) (Figure 174-20), and skinfold asymmetry. In children with bilateral DDH, the diagnosis is even more difficult beyond the first few months

BOX 174-1. Ortolani and Barlow Maneuvers

Ortolani (Reduction) Maneuver

1. Stabilize the pelvis with one hand.
2. With the other hand, slightly abduct the infant's hip.
3. With the index and long fingers over the greater trochanter, pull up the thigh to gently reduce the hip.

Barlow (Provocative) Test

1. Stabilize the pelvis with one hand.
2. Place the thumb on the inner aspect of the thigh near the lesser trochanter.
3. Adduct the hip.
4. Exert downward pressure on the thigh with the thumb and push it into the table.

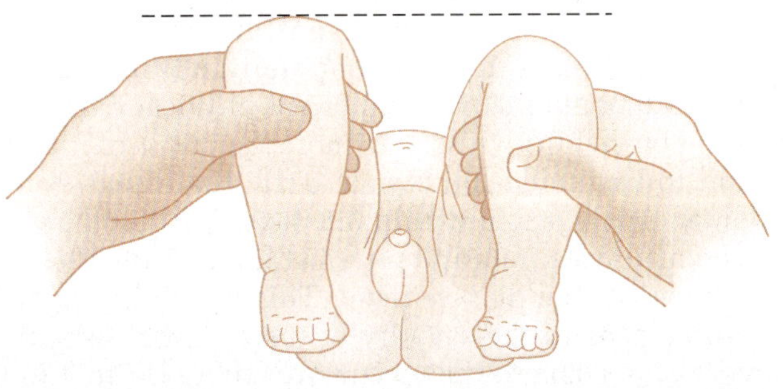

Figure 174-20. Galleazzi's sign. A positive Galeazzi test reveals asymmetry in the level of the patient's knees. (From Tolo VT, Wood B: *Pediatric Orthopedics in Primary Care.* Baltimore, Williams & Wilkins, 1983.)

of life because of the absence of asymmetry. After the development of contractures, physical findings in bilateral DDH include widening of the perineum, abduction less than 45 degrees, and the appearance of abnormally short thigh segments.

With the onset of walking, gait asymmetry or asymmetric in-toeing or out-toeing is a clue to the presence of DDH. Adduction and flexion contractures, a positive Galeazzi sign, hyperlordosis, and a waddling gait are common findings. Clinical observation reveals a Trendelenburg sign: while standing, the patient lifts one leg up at a time, and because the gluteal muscles are weakened on the affected side, the pelvis drops to the opposite side. With bilateral DDH, children have a wide-based waddling gait.

Diagnostic Strategies

Radiographs of infant hips are extremely difficult to interpret and may provide a false sense of security if they seem normal. Before the child is 3 to 6 months old, at which time the femoral head ossifies, an abnormal relationship between the upper end of the femur and the acetabulum may not be apparent. Additionally, in infants with unstable, but nondislocated hips, radiographs show the hip in position and its instability is not detected. Before femoral head ossification, a better diagnostic test is ultrasonography.[34] Because a large percentage of infants will have abnormal ultrasound findings in the first week of life, with many of these abnormalities resolving within a few weeks,[30] it is best to delay ultrasound in children with nondislocated, but possibly unstable hips until 4 to 6 weeks of age. Children with dislocated hips require immediate ultrasound. After approximately 6 weeks the ossific nucleus of the femoral head is detectable, and radiographs are more likely to reveal abnormalities and asymmetry. A standard AP pelvis radiograph with both legs extended in neutral abduction is then sufficient for diagnosis. Radiographic findings may include lateral displacement of Shenton's line and a widened acetabular angle; angles greater than 30 degrees are abnormal, and those greater than 40 degrees indicate dislocation.

Management

Treatment of DDH is most successful when begun early, and delay in detection may lead to a significantly worse prognosis. Patients with untreated abnormal hips that persist beyond the newborn period are at risk for osteoarthritis, pain, abnormal gait, leg length discrepancy, and decreased agility. For this reason, all children who are seen in the emergency department should have their hips examined until they are able to walk. Neonates who have a dislocated hip at birth should be referred to a pediatric orthopedist immediately. When a newborn has a loose, but nondislocated hip, referral can be made within 2 weeks. Children who are seen after the newborn period should be immediately referred to a pediatric orthopedic surgeon.

The essential, basic goals of treatment are concentric reduction of the hip. After concentric reduction, stability must be obtained so that when the leg is allowed to move, it does not sublux or dislocate. This position is maintained until all the dysplastic features of the bone and cartilage have resolved. The two most important complications are failure to achieve these goals and aseptic necrosis of the femoral head.

In the first 6 months of life, the Pavlik harness is the mainstay of treatment. It is a dynamic splint that allows movement while preventing hip extension or adduction. Other treatment options include the Craig and vonRosen splints.[35] If these modalities are unsuccessful, a hip spica cast is usually the next choice. Beyond 6 months of age, a hip spica cast or fixed orthosis is required. Surgical release of contracted muscles may be necessary in older infants and children, and open surgical reduction is required if complete closed reduction is not achieved. Femoral or pelvic osteotomy (or both) may be necessary to reduce and stabilize dislocated hips in children older than 2 or 3 years.[36] Beyond 4 years of age in bilateral cases and 8 years of age in unilateral cases, reduction should not be attempted. The risk of aseptic necrosis and the potential for a poor result are too high.[31]

Hip Pain in Children

Perspective

Hip pain in children is an extensive topic with myriad causes (Box 174-2). The extensive differential diagnosis precludes an in-depth review of the topic in this

BOX 174-2. Causes of Hip Pain in Children

Trauma
Hip or pelvis fractures
Overuse injuries

Infection
Septic arthritis
Osteomyelitis

Inflammation
Transient synovitis
Juvenile rheumatoid arthritis
Rheumatic fever

Neoplasm
Leukemia
Osteogenic or Ewing's sarcoma
Metastatic disease

Hematologic Disorders
Hemophilia
Sickle cell anemia

Miscellaneous
Legg-Calvé-Perthes disease
Slipped capital femoral epiphysis

chapter, but an overview of some of the more common causes of hip pain in children is presented.

Specific Disorders/Injuries

Transient Synovitis

Transient synovitis is the most common cause of hip pain in childhood.[37] It is a self-limited inflammatory condition caused by a nonpyogenic inflammatory response of the synovium. Although it has been reported in children as young as 3 months and occasionally occurs in adults,[38] its peak incidence is between 3 and 6 years of age. Transient synovitis of the hip affects boys more commonly than girls and has a slight predilection for the right side. Less than 5% of cases are bilateral. Approximately half the patients are initially seen acutely, usually within the first 3 days of the onset of symptoms, whereas the other half have a more insidious course, with symptoms occurring for weeks to months before medical evaluation.[39] Though most commonly affecting the hip, transient synovitis can also affect the knee.

The etiology of transient synovitis is unknown. Current theories imply an association with active or recent infection, trauma, or allergic hypersensitivity. At least half the children with transient synovitis have or recently have had an upper respiratory illness.[40] One study demonstrated a fourfold rise in viral titer in 45% of patients and elevated serum interferon levels, consistent with a concurrent viral infection, in 43% of patients with transient synovitis.[41] Trauma is commonly associated with transient synovitis, but no clear relationship has been demonstrated. Similarly, a causal association with an allergic reaction to an infectious agent has been suggested but not proved.

It is estimated that transient synovitis of the hip may occur in up to 3% of children. Hip or groin pain is the most common initial finding, but referred pain to the medial aspect of the thigh or knee is found in 10% to 30% of patients. Affected patients either walk with a limp or, with severe pain, refuse to walk at all. The leg is held in flexion with slight abduction and external rotation. On examination, passive movement is usually pain free; however, there may be pain and a slightly decreased range of motion with extreme internal rotation or abduction. Although most children with transient synovitis tend to otherwise be well, some will have a low-grade fever and malaise.

The diagnosis of transient synovitis is one of exclusion and relies on the history and physical examination in combination with limited laboratory testing and AP and "frog-leg" lateral radiographs of the pelvis. Laboratory tests are used to help differentiate children with transient synovitis from those with septic arthritis. In transient synovitis, laboratory values may be normal or may reveal mild elevations in the white blood cell count and erythrocyte sedimentation rate (ESR), both consistent with a nonspecific inflammatory process. One study showed that children with septic arthritis had a significantly higher mean ESR (44 mm/hr versus 19 mm/hr) and a higher mean white blood cell count (13.2×10^9/L versus 11.2×10^9/L) than children with transient synovitis did. The temperature of children with septic arthritis was also significantly higher (38.1° C versus 37.2° C). An ESR greater than 20 mm/hr, a temperature higher than 37.5° C, or both, identified 97% of all cases of septic arthritis of the hip. However, there was a wide overlap of values between the two groups, and with the same criteria, 50% of patients with transient synovitis would have unnecessarily undergone hip aspiration.[42] Another study that combined clinical and laboratory evaluation found four criteria to be more indicative of septic arthritis than transient synovitis: severe hip pain and spasm (present in 62% of patients with septic arthritis versus 12% of patients with transient synovitis), tenderness on palpation (present in 86% of patients with septic arthritis versus 17% of those with transient synovitis), a temperature of 38° C or higher (present in 81% of patients with septic arthritis versus 8% of those with transient synovitis), and an ESR of 20 mm/hr or greater (present in 90% of patients with septic arthritis versus 10.9% of those with transient synovitis). The same study found that the duration of symptoms, history of antecedent viral infection, and elevations in white blood cell count were not helpful in distinguishing between transient synovitis and septic arthritis.[43] An ESR higher than 50 mm/hr has been shown to herald serious disease and should be monitored closely.[44] Although radiographs of the hip and pelvis tend to be normal in transient synovitis, they are helpful in excluding other diseases. Radiographic findings consistent with transient synovitis include medial joint space widening, an accentuated pericapsular shadow, and Waldenström's sign, which is lateral displacement of the femoral epiphysis with surface flattening secondary to effusion. However, these findings are also apparent in Legg-Calvé-Perthes (LCP) disease and, if present, mandate close follow-up or further investigation with MRI. In unclear or atypical cases, ultrasonography, which is as accurate as CT or MRI in detecting effusions,[45-47] can be used to look for an intracapsular effusion or guide hip joint aspiration. Effusions are present in 60% to 70% of cases of transient synovitis; however, they are also present in septic arthritis, osteomyelitis, acute slipped capital femoral epiphysis (SCFE), LCP disease, rheumatoid and infectious arthritis, malignancy, and osteoid osteoma. As such, an effusion is neither sensitive nor specific for transient synovitis, and its presence should not, in and of itself, determine treatment. Nuclear scintigraphy in patients with transient synovitis is helpful in differentiating transient synovitis from osteomyelitis (with or without septic arthritis), LCP disease, and SCFE. Scintigraphy may demonstrate asymmetry in uptake in the capital femoral epiphysis, with decreased uptake early in the course of the disease and increased uptake later on. The early changes are also seen with very early LCP disease and suggest that some children with transient synovitis experience ischemia of the capital femoral epiphyses. This ischemia may be caused by an intracapsular effusion that tamponades vessels along the femoral neck. These ischemic findings have not yet been shown to have clinical significance.

Most cases of transient synovitis can be managed at home with close follow-up by the child's primary care provider. Generally, these children have a mild limp and, if treated with nonsteroidal anti-inflammatory drugs, often show improvement in symptoms. A complete blood count, ESR, and radiographs should be obtained. Patients with severe symptoms, fever, and an elevated ESR should be evaluated for septic arthritis. If there is any doubt about the diagnosis, immediate orthopedic consultation is necessary. Treatment of transient synovitis is twofold: (1) rest via non–weight bearing or, in cases of extreme pain, bed rest and (2) reduction of synovitis with anti-inflammatory medications. Temperatures should be monitored closely, and any fever should be reported to the physician. Children are allowed a gradual return to activity as the pain subsides, and full, unrestricted activity is permitted when the hip is completely pain free with no evidence of a limp. Although many children with transient synovitis have an effusion, aspiration of the joint is not routinely performed, and there is no strong evidence that aspiration shortens the clinical course or prevents osteonecrosis. Repeat examination is recommended for all children within 12 to 24 hours and then again after 10 to 14 days if the symptoms have not resolved.

The prognosis for children with transient synovitis is excellent. Up to 75% of patients have complete resolution of pain within 2 weeks and 88% within 4 weeks. The remainder may have less intense, but persistent pain for up to 8 weeks. Relapse is possible, though infrequent, and usually occurs within 6 months. In general, there are infrequent long-term sequelae of transient synovitis, including asymptomatic coxa magna (enlargement and deformity of the femoral head and neck caused by hypertrophy of cartilage secondary to inflammation) and mild degenerative cystic changes of the femoral neck. These changes persist for years and may be accompanied by radiographic degenerative change, but they do not tend to cause long-term functional disability. Additionally, a small number (2%) of cases of transient synovitis follow a clinical and radiographic course consistent with LCP disease. Whether this is due to ischemia of the capital femoral epiphyses during the early stages of synovitis or reflects an initial misdiagnosis is unclear. It is recommended that children with persistent symptoms undergo ultrasonography to evaluate for the presence of an effusion. Persistent joint effusion beyond 4 to 6 weeks is concerning for the subsequent development of LCP disease.[48] Some authors recommend routine 6-month follow-up radiographs for all children with transient synovitis,[39] whereas others reserve radiographs for children who remain symptomatic.[49]

Acute Septic Arthritis

Septic arthritis refers to microbial invasion and infection of the joint space. Bacterial pathogens are common in patients with acute septic arthritis, whereas fungal and mycobacterial pathogens tend to be associated with chronic septic arthritis. Acute septic arthritis occurs in all age groups but is more common in children: 70% of cases occur in children younger than 4 years, and the peak incidence is between 6 and 24 months. Boys are affected twice as frequently as girls. Predisposing factors include preceding viral infection, trauma, immunodeficiency, hemoglobinopathy, hemophilia with recurrent hemarthroses, diabetes, intravenous drug abuse, rheumatoid arthritis, and intra-articular injections or operations. Seventy-five percent of septic arthritis cases involve the joints of the lower extremity, with the knee being most commonly and the hip second most commonly involved. Other affected joints, in order of involvement, include the ankle, elbow, shoulder, and wrist. More than 90% of cases are monarticular.

Hematogenous seeding, local spread, or traumatic or surgical infection may cause septic arthritis. In children, it most commonly results from hematogenous spread as bacteria pass into the synovial space through the highly vascular synovial membrane. The synovial membrane lacks a limiting basement membrane, which facilitates bacterial translocation. The bacteria then bind to bone and cartilage and initiate an inflammatory response that breaks down the joint by two mechanisms: directly through the effects of proteolytic enzymes and indirectly through pressure necrosis caused by accumulation of purulent synovial fluid.

Contiguous spread of infection from osteomyelitis to the joint space occurs in approximately 10% of cases and is more common in newborns and young infants. In these children, blood vessels cross the physis and thereby connect the metaphysis and epiphysis and allow bacteria direct access into the joint space. Additionally, the joint capsules of the hip and shoulder overlie the bony metaphyses of the femur and humerus, thus facilitating direct extension of osteomyelitis into these joint spaces.

The most common bacterial causes of septic arthritis are listed in Table 174-6. Additional causative organ-

Table 174-6. Septic Arthritis Pathogens and Treatment

Age	Organism	Treatment
Birth to 2 months	Group B *Streptococcus* *Staphylococcus aureus* Gram-negative rods	Nafcillin, 50 mg/kg, and gentamicin, 2.5 mg/kg
2 months to 3 years	*Staphylococcus aureus* *Haemophilus influenzae* *Streptococcus pneumoniae*	Nafcillin, 50 mg/kg, and ceftriaxone, 50 mg/kg (consider vancomycin, 10 mg/kg)
3 years to 12 years	*Staphylococcus aureus* *Streptococcus pneumoniae* *Streptococcus pyogenes*	Nafcillin, 50 mg/kg, and ceftriaxone, 50 mg/kg (consider vancomycin, 10 mg/kg)
>12 years	*Staphylococcus aureus* *Streptococcus pneumoniae* *Neisseria gonorrhoeae*	Nafcillin, 50 mg/kg, and ceftriaxone, 50 mg/kg (consider vancomycin, 10 mg/kg)

isms include *Neisseria gonorrhoeae* in neonates and sexually active adolescents, *Pseudomonas aeruginosa* and *Candida* species in intravenous drug abusers, *Salmonella* species in children with sickle cell disease, and gram-negative bacteria in immunosuppressed children.

The clinical picture of septic arthritis varies with age. Clinically, infants tend to have fever, failure to feed, lethargy, pseudoparalysis of the extremity, and pain with diaper changes. In a recent study, however, neonates (younger than 1 month) were found to have less fever and fewer systemic signs of illness than older infants, thus making the diagnosis even more difficult.[49] Most older children have systemic symptoms of fever, malaise, poor appetite, and irritability, as well as localized symptoms of pain and limp or refusal to walk. With septic arthritis, the onset of symptoms is more acute than with osteomyelitis. Physical examination reveals local erythema, warmth, and swelling. If the hip is affected, it is often held in flexion, abduction, and external rotation. Range of motion is decreased because of pain and muscle spasm, and passive joint movement is painful. In infants, joint dislocation may be observed.

Laboratory studies helpful in diagnosing septic arthritis include a white blood cell count, ESR, C-reactive protein, blood cultures, and evaluation of joint fluid. Use of the white blood cell count and ESR is discussed in the section on transient synovitis. It should be noted that the ESR rises 24 hours or more after the onset of signs and symptoms of infection, so it may not be helpful during the first day of illness. C-reactive protein may be a better monitor of septic arthritis than the ESR is. It is a simpler test that requires only a finger stick sample of blood. It rises more quickly than the ESR does, is typically elevated at initial evaluation, and with appropriate therapy, will normalize within a week; in contrast, the ESR will not normalize for more than a month.[50]

Blood cultures should be included in the evaluation of a child with suspected septic arthritis. They are positive in 20% to 50% of cases[51] and, when positive, not only help direct antibiotic treatment but provide an organism for serum bactericidal testing as the children progress to oral antibiotics.

Evaluation of synovial fluid is the mainstay for diagnosing septic arthritis. If septic arthritis is being considered, joint aspiration should be performed without delay and the sample sent for Gram stain, aerobic and anaerobic cultures, cell count with differential, glucose determination, and a mucin clot test. The mucin clot test is a test of the integrity of hyaluronic acid, which tends to be degraded when bacteria are present. It is performed by placing two drops of 5% acetic acid into a mixture of 4 mL of water and 1 mL of synovial fluid while stirring with a glass rod. A normal result is a tight rope of mucin. The test is considered positive if the fluid's consistency changes to that of curdled milk as the clot flakes and shreds. Abnormal mucin clot test results are found with septic arthritis and rheumatic fever; however, with rheumatic fever, a fibrous band resembling a tethered rope forms on the glass stir rod. The synovial fluid in patients with septic arthritis tends to be turbid or grossly purulent with a white cell count greater than 40,000 cells/mm^3 and a predominance of polymorphonuclear cells. Synovial glucose may be low (synovial fluid/blood glucose less than 0.5) and protein and lactate elevated (Table 174-7). Because of the intrinsic immunoglobulins in the synovial fluid, culture of the fluid will be positive in only half the children with a clinical picture consistent with septic arthritis. Synovial fluid can be cultured on agar plates or blood culture media. Either way, the specimen requires immediate inoculation.

In septic arthritis, plain radiographs of the hip may be normal or, in the presence of a large joint effusion, may show periarticular soft tissue swelling, widening of the joint space, obliteration or displacement of the gluteal lines, and asymmetric fullness of the iliopsoas and obturator soft tissue planes. Late in the course of infection, subchondral bone erosions and narrowing of the joint space are seen. Ultrasonography is much more sensitive than plain radiography in detecting hip effusion and provides direct visualization of the fluid and needle during joint aspiration. Scintigraphy may also be useful in diagnosing septic arthritis; during the "blood pool" or delayed images of the joint, symmetrical uptake in periarticular tissue on both sides of the joint is seen. Scintigraphy is diagnostic of septic arthritis earlier than other imaging techniques are and is also a useful adjunct in identifying associated osteomyelitis or avascular necrosis of the femoral head. CT and MRI can confirm the presence of an effusion but do not dif-

Table 174-7. Synovial Fluid Findings in Different Types of Arthritis

	Character	WBC Count (/μL)	PMNs (%)	Mucin Clot	Other
Normal	Clear; yellow	<200	<10	Good	
Juvenile rheumatoid arthritis	Turbid	250-50,000	50-70	Fair to poor	50% with decreased complement
Reactive arthritis	Cloudy to turbid; may be clear	1000-150,000	50-70	Fair to poor	Increased complement
Lyme arthritis	Turbid	500-100,000	>50	Poor	
Septic arthritis	Turbid; white-gray	10,000-250,000	>75	Poor	Low glucose High lactate

PMN, polymorphonuclear leukocytes; WBC, white blood cell count.

ferentiate septic from nonseptic arthritis; however, they may be useful in complicated or atypical cases.[52]

Septic arthritis requires immediate admission, antibiotics, and surgical intervention. Surgical options range from needle aspiration to open surgical drainage, but no randomized controlled trials have compared these two treatment approaches. Some authors recommend surgical drainage in all infants and young children with septic arthritis because needle aspiration has been shown to be inferior in this population.[53] Indications for surgical drainage in children with septic arthritis include involvement of the hip joint, the presence of large amounts of pus or debris in the joint, loculated fluid, recurrence of joint fluid after four or five aspirations, and lack of clinical improvement within 3 days of the initiation of appropriate therapy.[54-57] In joints other than the hip, the need for surgical drainage is determined on a case-by-case basis.

Empirical antibiotic therapy for septic arthritis is directed against the most likely organisms based on patient age and comorbid conditions (see Table 174-6). Treatment may then be changed after culture and sensitivity results are known. To maximize culture results, antibiotics should not be given until a specimen of joint fluid is obtained. Initial treatment is parenteral to ensure adequate serum antibiotic concentrations. After the patient's clinical condition is stabilized, oral antibiotic therapy can be instituted. In general, doses two to three times those used for mild infections are sufficient. Response to therapy is measured by clinical improvement and acute phase reactants, including ESR and C-reactive protein.

The mortality rate associated with septic arthritis has fallen to less than 1%, but the morbidity remains significant. Sequelae include leg length discrepancy, persistent pain, limited range of motion and ambulation, and aseptic necrosis of the femoral head. Predictors of a poor outcome include infection of the hip and shoulder, adjacent osteomyelitis, a delay of 4 days or more before antibiotic and surgical intervention, and prolonged time to sterilization of synovial fluid.

Legg-Calvé-Perthes Disease

Idiopathic avascular necrosis of the proximal femoral epiphysis, also known as Legg-Calvé-Perthes disease, is named after the men who independently described it in the early 1900s. It usually occurs between the ages of 3 and 12 years, with the peak incidence between 5 and 7 years of age. LCP disease has been reported in teenagers as well as children as young as 2 years. Boys are affected three to five times more frequently than girls, and the disease is familial approximately 10% of the time. The disorder is bilateral in up to 20% of cases. LCP disease is associated with breech presentation, later-born children (particularly the third to sixth child), lower socioeconomic group,[58] higher parental age,[59] lower birth weight, attention-deficit/hyperactivity disorder,[60] delayed bone age,[61] short stature, smoking,[62] infection with human immunodeficiency virus,[63] and chronic renal disease.[64,65] The increased incidence of LCP disease in Japanese, Asians, Eskimos, and central Europeans and the decreased incidence in Native Australians, Native Americans, Polynesians, and African Americans suggest that racial factors may also play a role. Trauma is often related to the onset of symptoms of LCP disease, but a direct relationship between the two has not been clearly established.

Despite extensive research, the etiology of LCP disease remains unclear. Ponseti and colleagues[66] suggested that LCP disease is a local manifestation of a transient, generalized disorder of epiphyseal cartilage. Their histologic studies showed thickening and disorganization of the growth plate, which could block penetration of the blood vessels and render the femoral epiphysis avascular. Other etiologic theories involve abnormalities in the vascular anastomotic network around the femoral epiphysis, increased blood viscosity leading to infarction, and abnormalities in growth hormone.

Clinically, children with LCP disease initially have an insidious and stuttering onset of a limp. Associated pain, when present, is usually related to activity and relieved by rest. The pain tends to be localized to the groin or referred to the anteromedial aspect of the thigh or knee region. On examination, children have limited hip motion, particularly abduction and medial rotation. Early in the course of disease, the limited abduction is secondary to synovitis and muscle spasm. As the disease progresses, limitation of motion of the hip is due to deformity of the femoral head, and with time, the limited abduction may become permanent. Children with LCP disease have a positive Trendelenburg test (see the section "Developmental Dysplasia") accompanied by thigh, calf, and buttock atrophy related to disuse. With advanced disease and femoral head collapse, there may be limb length discrepancy.

The role of laboratory evaluation in the diagnosis of LCP disease is limited to ruling out other causes of hip pain (e.g., septic arthritis) when the diagnosis is in question or evaluating for hormonal, metabolic, or genetic causes in patients with bilateral hip involvement.

LCP disease is diagnosed and staged by plain radiographs taken in the AP and frog-leg lateral position. These radiographs show both the extent of epiphyseal involvement and the stage of the disease. Plain radiographs also supply prognostic information such as "head at risk" signs, lateral subluxation, and metaphyseal changes. These prognostic signs help guide treatment. In early LCP disease, radionuclide bone scanning may be diagnostic before the development of abnormalities on plain film. Bone scintigraphy has also been shown to provide accurate information concerning the extent of the necrotic process, as well as the degree of vascularization and therefore the stage of the disease. Scintigraphy, however, was not able to predict disease outcome.[67] When compared with plain radiographs and bone scan, MRI gives earlier and more reliable information about the extent of necrosis of the femoral head. MRI is also better than scintigraphy at showing revascularization. Despite the use of MRI in early LCP disease, its role in healed LCP disease is limited because it provides no further information regarding the configuration and structure of the femoral head than plain radiography does.[67] Arthrography is useful in delineating flattening of the femoral head, demonstrating the hinge abduction phenomenon with abduction of the leg, and in conjunction with plain films or CT, diagnosing osteochondritis dissecans after LCP disease.

There are four radiographic classification stages of LCP disease: initial, fragmentation, reossification, and healed. Radiographic findings in the initial stage include a femoral head that appears smaller than the opposite unaffected femoral head, widening of the medial joint space, a subchondral lucent zone (subchondral collapse—"crescent sign"), an irregular physeal plate, and a blurry and radiolucent metaphysis (Figure 174-21). In the fragmentation phase, the repair aspects of the disease become more prominent. The epiphysis begins to fragment, and there are areas of increased radiolucency as new bone forms, as well as areas of increased radiodensity. During the reossification stage, the repair process continues as normal bone density returns, radiodensities replace radiolucencies, and alterations in the shape of the femoral head and neck become apparent. The healed stage is the final radiographic stage of LCP disease, and radiographs of the proximal third of the femur taken during this stage of the illness will demonstrate any residual deformities.

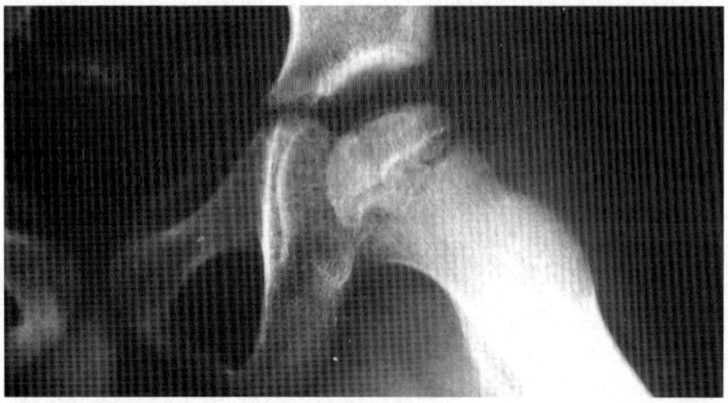

Figure 174-21. Crescent sign (subchondral lucent zone) in early Legg-Calvé-Perthes disease. (Courtesy Marianne Gausche-Hill, MD.)

Multiple prognostic classification systems of LCP disease have been devised. In general, a poor prognosis is associated with a greater degree of deformity of the femoral head and acetabulum at maturity, disease onset in children 6 to 8 years or older, female sex, and prolonged duration of disease.

When the diagnosis of LCP is suspected, orthopedic consultation is recommended. Goals in the treatment of LCP disease are to improve range of motion, prevent deformity, limit growth disturbance, and prevent degenerative joint disease. Treatment is not indicated in all children with LCP disease, but when indicated, it must be started in the initial or fragmentation phase of the disease. Treatment is recommended for patients who have a poor prognosis based on clinical and radiographic findings. The cornerstone for treatment of LCP is referred to as "containment": the femoral head is contained within the acetabulum to equalize pressure on the head and subject it to the molding action of the acetabulum to maintain the spherical nature of the femoral head. Containment can be achieved through nonoperative or operative methods, and optimal treatment is determined on a case-by-case basis.

Residual deformities resulting from LCP disease follow four patterns: coxa magna, premature physeal arrest, irregular head formation, and osteochondritis dissecans. Despite these deformities, most patients with childhood hip disease are capable of bony remodeling with subsequent improvement in femoral head deformities. During their early years, regardless of radiographic appearance, patients with LCP disease tend to do well.[68] The majority (70% to 90%) of patients with LCP disease are active and pain free and have good range of motion 20 to 40 years after the onset of symptoms. Only patients with flattened irregular femoral heads at the time of primary healing or premature physeal closure had clinical deterioration and increasing pain.[69] Later in life there is a marked reduction of function, with degenerative joint disease developing in the majority of patients by their 50s and 60s.[68] With noncontainment treatment, however, the outcome is not as good. Yrjonen found that at an average of 35 years of follow-up, 40% of patients had evidence of degenerative joint disease and 17% had either undergone total hip arthroplasty or had clinical symptoms that warranted total hip arthroplasty.[70]

Slipped Capital Femoral Epiphysis

SCFE refers to posterior and inferior slippage of the proximal femoral epiphysis on the metaphysis. The femoral head sits securely in the acetabulum, whereas the epiphysis separates from the femoral neck through the growth plate. The average annual incidence of SCFE is 2 per 100,000, with boys being affected more than twice as frequently as girls. The peak incidence occurs during the adolescent growth spurt: boys between 12 and 16 years of age (mean age, 13.5 years) and girls between 10 and 14 years of age (mean age, 11.5 years). The age at diagnosis decreases with increasing obesity. The majority of children with SCFE have delayed skeletal maturation, with bone age being as much as 20 months behind chronologic age. African American children are affected more frequently than white children. The literature reports SCFE to be bilateral in up to 80% of cases, although 30% to 40% of these cases are asymptomatic and discovered only on screening radiographs. In unilateral cases, the left hip is affected twice as often as the right.

SCFE is associated with endocrine disorders (hypothyroidism, panhypopituitarism, hypogonadism, and growth hormone administration), renal osteodystrophy, and radiation therapy. Most cases of SCFE, however, are idiopathic and associated with obesity. The etiology of idiopathic SCFE is unknown. It is likely to be multifactorial and related to biomechanical factors such as obesity and physeal architecture, as well as hormonal factors that weaken physeal strength. Obesity results in increased shear forces across a more vertically and posteriorly oriented growth plate that has been weakened by architectural irregularities and hormonal changes of puberty. The consequence is slippage of the epiphysis inferiorly and posteriorly in the direction of the weight-bearing force.

The traditional classification of SCFE was based on the duration of symptoms, with acute slippage defined as symptom duration of less than 3 weeks, chronic slippage defined as symptoms for 3 weeks or more, and acute-on-chronic slippage defined as symptoms for more than 3 weeks' duration with a recent, sudden exacerbation. Of late, this classification has been replaced by one based on stability: in stable SCFE, ambulation is possible (with or without crutches), whereas in unstable SCFE, ambulation is not possible (with or without crutches).[71] This classification system is preferred over the traditional classification because it does not rely on patient or parent recall for duration of symptoms and provides information regarding prognosis.

The signs and symptoms of SCFE vary with its stability. Children with stable SCFE have symptoms of intermittent limp and pain of several weeks' to months' duration. Stable SCFE is found in approximately 90% of all cases. The pain of SCFE may be localized to the hip but more commonly is poorly localized to the thigh, groin, or knee. Atypical manifestations of SCFE include weakness and easy fatigability of the affected limb and limping on exertion. With continued slippage, internal rotation, flexion, and abduction are lost, and parents and children may note progressive external rotation and shortening of the involved lower extremity with subsequent difficulty in daily activities such as tying shoes. On examination, children initially have a slight loss of internal rotation and experience pain only at the

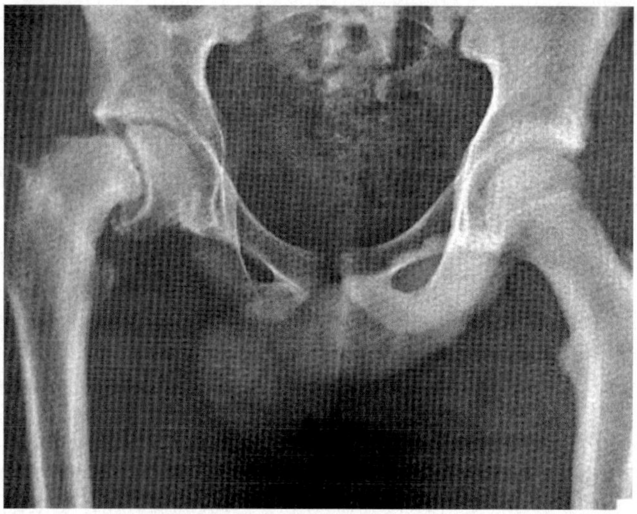

Figure 174-22. Anteroposterior radiograph of the pelvis with a unilateral slipped capital femoral epiphysis.

extremes of motion. Their gait is antalgic and muscle atrophy is minimal. As the slip becomes more severe, the gait becomes more antalgic, internal rotation is lost, abduction and flexion of the hip increase, thigh and gluteal muscle atrophy is more pronounced, and leg length discrepancy develops. A frequently seen sign associated with SCFE can be demonstrated during passive flexion of the affected hip: as flexion is increased from an extended position, the thigh abducts and externally rotates.

Unstable SCFE in children tends to initially come to attention after a sport-related injury or a fall with a twisting injury. They have an acute onset of extreme pain and, on examination, hold the hip in flexion, external rotation, and abduction. These children resist any type of movement of the affected leg, and if unstable SCFE is suspected, no passive movement should be attempted for fear of further displacing the epiphysis.

The diagnosis of SCFE is made with AP and lateral radiographs of both hips (Figure 174-22) With stable slippage, AP and frog-leg lateral pelvic radiographs should be obtained. When an unstable slip or a minimal slip is suspected, a cross-table radiograph replaces the frog-leg lateral view. Early in the course of SCFE the initial slippage is posterior; therefore, the AP view is normal or shows widening of the physis, and the slip is better seen on the lateral projection. Early findings on lateral radiographs include a minimal posterior step-off at the anterior physeal plate or widening of the growth plate. On AP radiographs, signs of slippage include Klein's line and the blanch sign of Steele. Klein's line is a line drawn along the superior margin of the femoral neck. With a normal hip, the line intersects or falls within the epiphysis, whereas in a hip with a slipped epiphysis, the line does not come in contact with the epiphysis. The blanch sign of Steele is a crescent-shaped area of increased density in the proximal portion of the femoral neck that is created by superimposition of the posteriorly displaced epiphysis on the femoral neck. The femoral metaphysis of the affected hip also appears to be more laterally displaced from the medial wall of the acetabulum. As the slip continues, the epiphysis continues to be displaced inferiorly and posteriorly relative to the metaphysis. Over time, remodeling smoothes away the superior and anterior portion of the femoral neck, and in an attempt to buttress the slippage, callus is formed at the inferior and posterior portions of the femoral neck. Unstable slips in children without previous symptoms will not have evidence of bone healing or remodeling.

Ultrasonography has been used in the diagnosis of SCFE but offers little, if any information over conventional radiography. CT and MRI can be used to confirm and quantitate epiphyseal displacement in patients who have symptoms but no radiographic findings suggestive of SCFE.

Slip severity is described in one of two ways. The simplest classification describes the amount of displacement of the femoral head on the femoral neck. In mild SCFE, the amount of displacement is less than a third, moderate SCFE has displacement between a third and a half, and severe SCFE is marked by the femoral head being displaced more than half the width of the femoral neck. A more accurate description of the magnitude of slippage is obtained by measuring the epiphyseal-shaft angle of Southwick. On a frog-leg lateral radiograph of the pelvis, a line is drawn between the anterior and posterior tips of the epiphysis at the physeal plate level. A second line is then drawn perpendicular to the epiphyseal line. Next, a line is drawn along the midshaft of the femur. The epiphyseal-shaft angle is formed by the intersection of the perpendicular and the femoral shaft lines. The magnitude of slip displacement is the angle of the involved hip minus the angle of the normal hip. If involvement is bilateral, 12 degrees is used as the control angle. Mild SCFE is less than 30 degrees, a moderate slip is between 30 and 50 degrees, and severe displacement is greater than 50 degrees.

When SCFE is diagnosed in the emergency department, the child should be made non–weight bearing, either with crutches or a wheelchair, and an immediate orthopedic consultation should be obtained. For a stable slip, definitive treatment is best if performed within a few days; however, hospital admission is prudent. With an unstable slip, some orthopedic surgeons recommend immediate fixation.

The goals of treatment are to prevent further slippage and achieve physeal stability. A stable slip can be fixed with internal fixation (pinning), bone graft epiphyseodesis, corrective osteotomy, or spica cast immobilization. Most orthopedic surgeons recommend internal fixation with a single central screw. Failure of this repair is very rare, and with new techniques that avoid opening the hip joint, it has become a procedure associated with minimal blood loss and wound complications and minimal need for hospitalization and rehabilitation. Postoperatively, non–weight bearing or touch-toe weight bearing for 4 to 6 weeks is followed by a gradual return to normal activity. Running and contact sports may be resumed once the physis is closed. With unstable SCFE, there is controversy regarding the timing of the surgery, the optimum number of fixative devices that should be used, whether reduction should be performed, and whether preliminary traction and bed rest should be used before surgery. Treatment is dependent on the degree of slippage and the preference and experience of the orthopedic surgeon.

The two most worrisome short-term complications of SCFE are avascular necrosis and chondrolysis; the risk for either process increases with the severity of the initial slippage.[72,73] Avascular necrosis has been reported to occur in 10% to 15% of children with SCFE. The risk is higher with unstable SCFE, greater degrees of slippage, attempts at reduction, and treatment with a spica cast. In children with stable slips treated by single-screw internal fixation without reduction, the rate of avascular necrosis is as low as 0% to 5%.[74]

Chondrolysis occurs in approximately 5% of SCFE patients, with an increased incidence in children with greater degrees of slippage. Chondrolysis can occur before and as a result of treatment. It should be suspected when pain and loss of motion are disproportionate to the severity of the slip. On radiographs, loss of articular cartilage may be seen. When SCFE is treated by spica cast immobilization, the rate of chondrolysis is reported to range from 19% to 67%.[73,75] Approximately 50% of cases of chondrolysis will resolve; however, it may progress to such severe pain and contractures that hip arthrodesis is needed.

Other complications of SCFE include nonunion, premature closure of the epiphyseal plate, and degenerative changes. Degenerative hip arthritis develops gradually over decades and has an earlier onset with more severe degrees of slippage.

Apophyseal Injuries

Perspective and Principles of Disease

The apophysis is a cartilaginous structure that serves as a site for insertion of tendons on the growing bone. It has its own growth plate, but it has a slower rate of growth than the nearby epiphyseal plate. Apophysitis is unique to patients with skeletal immaturity and involves inflammation of this actively growing bony prominence that is under great tensile stress. Common apophyseal injuries include medial epicondylitis, Osgood-Schlatter disease, and Sever's disease.

Apophysitis develops from a single episode of macrotrauma or from repetitive microtrauma to the secondary center of ossification, which causes multiple tiny avulsion fractures. This scenario sets up an inflammatory cycle that is perpetuated by continued activity and trauma to the apophysis.

Growth also contributes to the development of apophysitis. As the musculoskeletal system goes through a growth spurt, muscle development lags behind bony development. This difference in development leads to a muscle-tendon imbalance manifested as tight and inflexible muscle groups in which excessive stress is placed on the apophyseal centers where these muscles insert.

The true incidence of apophysitis is unknown. One study found an incidence of 18% in a population of

1000 patients seen at an urban general pediatric clinic over a 4.5-month period.[76] Another series, which looked at patient visits to a sports medicine clinic, found an incidence of 31%.[77] Children between 8 and 15 years of age are most frequently affected, with different apophyses being affected at different ages.

Specific Disorders/Injuries

Osgood-Schlatter Syndrome

In 1903 Osgood and Schlatter independently reported traumatically induced apophyseal injury to the tibial tubercle in adolescents.[78] This entity, Osgood-Schlatter syndrome, is the most common of the apophyseal disorders.[79] It is found most commonly in boys between 10 and 15 years old and in girls between 8 and 13 years old and is frequently bilateral. Boys are affected more often than girls, although this trend is changing as more girls are becoming increasingly involved in competitive sports. Bilateral involvement is found in 20% to 30% of patients.

Clinically, patients with Osgood-Schlatter syndrome have tenderness, pain, and swelling at the site of insertion of the patellar tendon on the tibial tubercle. The tibial tubercle may be prominent and the quadriceps tight. Pain is worsened with activities such as running or jumping by causing the quadriceps to contract and thereby stressing the tubercle. Extension of the knee against resistance causes pain, but resisted straight leg raises are painless. Osgood-Schlatter syndrome is a clinical diagnosis and radiographs are not generally indicated. However, if taken, lateral radiographs of the tibial tubercle may be normal or may show an enlarged, fragmented, and irregular tibial tuberosity with or without an overlying bony ossicle. Ultrasound, which has been proposed as a diagnostic tool by some authors, may reveal pretibial swelling, fragmentation of the ossification center, insertional thickening of the patellar tendon, or excessive fluid collection in the infrapatellar bursa.[80]

Treatment of Osgood-Schlatter syndrome is conservative and symptomatic. Initially, the pain can be effectively managed with ice, modification of activity, with or without nonsteroidal anti-inflammatory medications. After the acute inflammatory process has resolved, treatment focuses on strengthening and stretching of the quadriceps muscle. Mild pain during activity is not an absolute contraindication to participation; however, with more severe symptoms, the risk of avulsion of the tibial tubercle should be weighed against the benefits of competing. In rare instances, conservative therapy is insufficient and a 2- to 3-week trial of crutches is required. Steroid injections have been used in the past but are not currently recommended. Complete recovery without residual pain or weakness is the rule. Recovery usually occurs within weeks but, in some cases, may not be complete until the underlying growth plate is closed. However, if the patient reaches skeletal maturity and is still symptomatic, consideration should be given to surgical removal of the tibial tubercle or the bony ossicle overlying the tibial tubercle (or both).

Sever's Disease

Sever's disease, which was initially described in 1912,[81] is commonly manifested as posterior heel pain in an 8- to 13-year-old athlete. It is bilateral in 60% of cases. As with other apophyseal injuries, pain is exacerbated by activity. Sever's disease can be associated with growth, tight heel cords, or other biomechanical abnormalities. Frequently implicated sports are soccer and running.

Patients have pain at the insertion site of the Achilles tendon and plantar fascia on the calcaneus. Tenderness is elicited when the calcaneus is squeezed bilaterally. Dorsiflexion of the ankle is restricted. Radiographs may be normal or may show partial fragmentation and increased density of the calcaneal apophysis, although this finding can also be seen in normal feet.

As in Osgood-Schlatter syndrome, treatment of Sever's disease is conservative and symptomatic. Treatment consists of ice, massage, stretching of the plantar fascia and involved muscles (gastrocnemius-soleus complex and ankle invertors or evertors), nonsteroidal anti-inflammatory drugs, and shock-absorbing shoe inserts. Heel cups have also been found to be helpful, but they must be accompanied by stretching to avoid exacerbating the calf muscle contracture. Modification of activity may be necessary, and infrequently, a trial of crutches for 1 to 2 weeks is helpful. Plantar fasciitis can cause heel pain as well, but patients will experience tenderness along the plantar fascia, especially at the attachment of the fascia to the calcaneus. Treatment involves the use of anti-inflammatory agents, rest, and relaxation of the plantar fascia with heel support pads.

Elbow Apophysitis

Little Leaguer's elbow (medial epicondylitis), most commonly affecting the medial epicondyle, is an overuse phenomenon that results in inflammation at the site where the forearm flexor muscles originate. As its name suggests, it commonly affects baseball pitchers and is associated with overhead arm motion. It is also seen in other skeletally immature overhand athletes, including tennis players. Medial epicondylitis is caused by the excessive forces placed on the medial side of the elbow during the late cocking and acceleration phases of throwing.

Patients tend to be preadolescents with pain on the medial aspect of the elbow, diminished throwing effectiveness, and decreased throwing distance. Examination reveals localized tenderness and swelling over the medial epicondyle and pain with resisted flexion of the wrist. There may be a slight flexion contracture. Radiographs may be normal or may show fragmentation, sclerosis, and widening of the medial epicondylar apophysis. Treatment includes ice, nonsteroidal anti-inflammatory drugs, and modification of activity. Throwing is restricted until the symptoms have resolved. After resolution, the patient can begin a program of muscle stretching and strengthening and make a slow return to throwing. During recovery, alteration of the throwing style to reduce the degree of sidearm delivery is advisable. Recovery usually takes 4

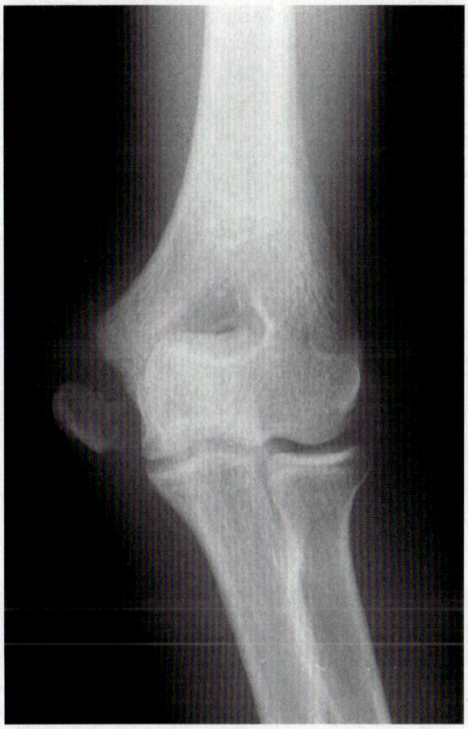

Figure 174-23. Avulsion injury of the elbow. This degree of displacement required surgical treatment.

to 6 weeks. If pain returns during resumption of pitching, rest should be reinstituted.

Apophysitis of the Hip

Apophyseal injuries of the hip involve sites around the hip where major abdominal and hip muscles either originate or insert: the anterior superior iliac spine, the anterior inferior iliac spine, the iliac crests, and the ischial tuberosities. Dancers and distance runners are most commonly affected. Patients with apophysitis of the hip have a dull pain located near the hip that is related to activity. Treatment includes strengthening and stretching of the abdominal and hip muscles and restriction of activity.

Avulsion Fractures

Apophysitis tends to have an insidious onset; therefore, any patient with a sudden onset of apophyseal pain after an acute traumatic event should be evaluated for an avulsion fracture. Such fractures occur when the muscular attachments to the apophyses are pulled off during strong active contractions against resistance. Examination will reveal localized tenderness and swelling. The diagnosis is usually readily apparent on plain films (Figure 174-23); however, bone scan and ultrasonography may play a role when the diagnosis is in question. Ultrasonography has the advantages of no radiation exposure, the ability to detect a fracture before the development of an ossification center, and the ability to provide a dynamic examination. Findings consistent with an avulsion fracture include a hypoechogenic zone, increased distance to the apophysis, dislocation of the apophysis, and mobility of the apophysis on dynamic examination.[82] Treatment of an avulsion fracture is based on the degree of separation. If the displacement is minimal (less than 2 cm with a hip avulsion and less than 5 mm with avulsion of the medial epicondyle[83]), immobilization for 4 to 6 weeks with subsequent slow resumption of activities is usually sufficient. With widely separated avulsion fractures, some authors recommend open reduction and fixation.[83]

KEY CONCEPTS

- Knowledge of the pediatric musculoskeletal system is imperative for appropriate evaluation and treatment of the skeletally immature.
- Child abuse must be suspected in children younger than 3 years with nonsupracondylar humerus fractures, femur fractures, rib fractures, and complex skull fractures.
- Children with displaced supracondylar fractures are at significant risk for neurovascular injury and should have frequent evaluations to assess for compartment syndrome.
- All children who are not yet walking should have a thorough hip evaluation with each visit to the emergency department.
- All patients with a gait disturbance need a thorough physical examination and directed laboratory and radiographic evaluation.
- Septic arthritis is a medical and surgical emergency that mandates immediate orthopedic consultation.
- Examine the hip of all patients with knee pain.

REFERENCES

1. Malek M, et al: The cost of medical care for injuries to children. *Ann Emerg Med* 20:997, 1991.
2. Davidson JS, et al: Simple treatment for torus fractures of the distal radius. *J Bone Joint Surg Br* 83:1173, 2001.
3. Solan MC, Rees R, Daly K: Current management of torus fractures of the distal radius. *Injury* 33:503, 2002.
4. Stanley D, Trowbridge EA, Norris SH: The mechanism of clavicle fractures: A clinical and biochemical analysis. *J Bone Joint Surg Br* 70:461, 1988.
5. Hanby CK, Pasque CB, Sullivan JA: Medial clavicle physis fracture with posterior displacement and vascular compromise: The value of three-dimensional computed tomography and duplex ultrasound. *Orthopedics* 26:81, 2003.
6. Rockwood CA Jr, Wilkins KE, Beaty JH: *Fractures in Children,* vol 3, 4th ed. New York, Lippincott-Raven, 1996.
7. Nork S, et al: The relationship between ligamentous laxity and the site of upper extremity fractures in children. *J Pediatr Orthop B* 8:90, 1999.
8. Gartland JJ: Management of supracondylar fractures of the humerus in children. *Surg Gynecol Obstet* 109:145, 1959.
9. Worlock P: Supracondylar fractures of the humerus: Assessment of cubitus varus by the Baumann angle. *J Bone Joint Surg Br* 68:755, 1986.
10. Skaggs D, Pershad J: Pediatric elbow trauma. *Pediatr Emerg Care* 13:425, 1997.
11. Williamson D, et al: Normal characteristics of the Baumann angle: An aid in the assessment of supracondylar fractures. *J Pediatr Orthop* 12:633, 1992.
12. Davidson RS, et al: Ultrasonographic evaluation of the elbow in infants and young children after suspected trauma. *J Bone Joint Surg Am* 76:1804, 1994.

13. Beltran J, et al: Pediatric elbow fractures: MRI evaluation. *Skeletal Radiol* 23:277, 1994.
14. Dormans JP, Squillante R, Sharf H: Acute neurovascular complications with supracondylar humerus fractures in children. *J Hand Surg [Am]* 20:1, 1995.
15. Culp RW, et al: Neural injuries associated with supracondylar fractures of the humerus in children. *J Bone Joint Surg Am* 72:1211, 1990.
16. Schutzman SA, Teach S: Upper extremity impairment in young children. *Ann Emerg Med* 26:474, 1995.
17. Schunk JE: Radial head subluxation: Epidemiology and treatment of 87 episodes. *Ann Emerg Med* 19:1019, 1990.
18. Kosuwon W, et al: Ultrasonography of pulled elbow. *J Bone Joint Surg Br* 75:421, 1993.
19. Quan L, Marcuse EK: The epidemiology and treatment of radial head subluxation. *Am J Dis Child* 139:1194, 1985.
20. McDonald J, Whitelaw C, Goldsmith LJ: Radial head subluxation: Comparing two methods of reduction. *Acad Emerg Med* 6:715, 1999.
21. Macias CG, Bothrer J, Wiebe R: A comparison of supination/flexion to hyperpronation in the reduction of radial head subluxation. *Pediatrics* 102:e10, 1998.
22. Leonidas J: Skeletal trauma in the child abuse syndrome. *Pediatr Ann* 12:875, 1983.
23. Herndon WA: Child abuse in a military population. *J Pediatr Orthop* 3:73, 1983.
24. Thomas SA, et al: Long bone fractures in young children: Distinguishing accidental injuries from child abuse. *Pediatrics* 88:471, 1991.
25. Feldman KW, Brewer DK: Child abuse, cardiopulmonary resuscitation and rib fractures. *Pediatrics* 73:339, 1984.
26. Barsness KA, et al: The positive predictive value of rib fractures as an indicator of nonaccidental trauma in children. *J Trauma* 54:1107, 2003.
27. Rubin DM, et al: Occult head injury in high-risk abused children. *Pediatrics* 111:1382, 2003.
28. Wallis GA, et al: Osteogenesis imperfecta type III: Mutations in the type I collagen genes COL1A1 and COL1A2 are not necessarily responsible. *J Med Genet* 30:492, 1993.
29. Sillence DO: Craniocervical abnormalities in osteogenesis imperfecta: Genetic and molecular correlation. *Pediatr Radiol* 24:427, 1994.
30. Marks DS, Clegg J, al-Chalabi AN: Routine ultrasound screening for neonatal hip instability: Can it abolish late-presenting congenital dislocation of the hip? *J Bone Joint Surg Br* 76:534, 1994.
31. Novaceck TF: Developmental dysplasia of the hip. *Pediatr Clin North Am* 43:829, 1996.
32. Tien YC, et al: Ultrasonographic study of the coexistence of muscular torticollis and dysplasia of the hip. *J Pediatr Orthop* 21:343, 2001.
33. Barlow TC: Early diagnosis and treatment of congenital dislocation of the hip. *J Bone Joint Surg Br* 44:292, 1962.
34. Boal DK, Schwenkter EP: The infant hip: Assessment with real-time ultrasound. *Radiology* 157:667, 1985.
35. Wilkinson AG: The efficacy of the Pavlik harness, the Craig splint and the von Rosen splint in the management of neonatal dysplasia of the hip. A comparative study. *J Bone Joint Surg Br* 84:716, 2002.
36. French LM, Dietz FR: Screening for developmental dysplasia of the hip. *Am Fam Physician* 60:177, 1999.
37. MacEwen GD, Dehse R: The limping child. *Pediatr Rev* 12:268, 1991.
38. Nyska M, et al: Benign synovitis of the hip in adults. *Br J Rheumatol* 32:820, 1993.
39. Haueisen DC, Weiner DS, Weiner SD: The characterization of "transient synovitis of the hip" in children. *J Pediatr Orthop* 6:11, 1986.
40. Koop S, Quanbeck D: Three common causes of childhood hip pain. *Pediatr Clin North Am* 43:1053, 1996.
41. Tolat V, et al: Evidence for viral aetiology of transient synovitis of the hip. *J Bone Joint Surg Br* 75:973, 1993.
42. Del Beccaro MA, et al: Septic arthritis versus transient synovitis of the hip: The value of screening laboratory tests. *Ann Emerg Med* 21:1418, 1992.
43. Taylor GR, Clark NM: Management of the irritable hip: A review of hospital admission policy. *Arch Dis Child* 71:59, 1994.
44. Huttenlocher A, Newman TB: Evaluation of the erythrocyte sedimentation rate in children presenting with limp, fever or abdominal pain. *Clin Pediatr (Phila)* 36:339, 1997.
45. Bickerstaff DR, et al: Ultrasound examination of the irritable hip. *J Bone Joint Surg Br* 72:549, 1990.
46. Egund N, et al: Computed tomography and ultrasonography for diagnosis of hip joint effusion in children. *Acta Orthop Scand* 57:211, 1986.
47. Galaski C, Royal S: The irritable hip: Scintigraphy is 192 children. *Acta Orthop Scand* 63:25, 1992.
48. Eggl H: Ultrasonography in the diagnosis of transient synovitis of the hip and Legg-Calvé-Perthes disease. *J Pediatr Orthop B* 8:177, 1999.
49. Hart JJ: Transient synovitis of the hip in children. *Am Fam Physician* 54:1587, 1996.
50. Klein DM, et al: Sensitivity of objective parameters in the diagnosis of pediatric septic hips. *Clin Orthop* 338:153, 1997.
51. Kallio MJT, et al: Serum C-reactive protein, erythrocyte sedimentation rate and white blood cell count in septic arthritis of children. *Pediatr Infect Dis J* 16:411, 1997.
52. Atkins BL, Bowler IEB: The diagnosis of large joint sepsis. A review. *J Hosp Infect* 40:263, 1998.
53. Brower AC: Septic arthritis. *Radiol Clin North Am* 34:193, 1996.
54. Syriopoulou V, Smith A: Osteomyelitis and septic arthritis. In Feigin R, Cherry J (eds): *Musculoskeletal Infections: Textbook of Pediatric Infectious Disease,* 3rd ed. Philadelphia, WB Saunders, 1992.
55. Dunkle LM: Toward optimum management of serious focal infections: The model of suppurative arthritis. *Pediatr Infect Dis J* 8:195, 1989.
56. Green NE, Edward K: Bone and joint infections in children. *Orthop Clin North Am* 18:555, 1987.
57. Nade S: Acute septic arthritis in infancy and childhood. *J Bone Joint Surg Am* 65:234, 1983.
58. Hall AJ, Barker DJ: Perthes's disease in Yorkshire. *J Bone Joint Surg Br* 71:229, 1989.
59. Hall AJ, et al: Perthes's disease of the hip in Liverpool. *Br Med J (Clin Res Ed)* 287:1757, 1983.
60. Loder RT, Schwartz EM, Hensinger RN: Behavioral characteristics of children with Legg-Calvé-Perthes disease. *J Pediatr Orthop* 13:598, 1993.
61. Cannon SR, Pozo JL, Catterall A: Elevated growth velocity in children with Perthes disease. *J Pediatr Orthop* 9:285, 1989.
62. Mata SG, et al: Legg-Calvé-Perthes disease and passive smoking. *J Pediatr Orthop* 20:326, 2000.
63. Gaughan DM, Mofenson LM, Hughes MD, et al: Osteonecrosis of the hip (Legg-Calvé-Perthes disease) in human immunodeficiency virus–infected children. *Pediatrics* 109:e74, 2002.
64. Burwell RG: Perthes disease: Growth and aetiology. *Arch Dis Child* 63:1408, 1988.
65. Boechat MI, et al: Avascular necrosis of the femoral head in children with chronic renal disease. *Radiology* 8:411, 2001.
66. Ponseti IV, et al: Legg-Calvé-Perthes disease: Histochemical and ultrastructural observations of the epiphyseal cartilage and physis. *J Bone Joint Surg Am* 65:797, 1983.
67. Kaniklides C: Diagnostic radiology in Legg-Calvé-Perthes disease. *Acta Radiol* 406:1, 1996.
68. Weinstein SL: Legg-Calvé-Perthes syndrome. In Morrisey RT, Weinstein SL (eds): *Lovell & Winter's Pediatric Orthopedics,* 4th ed. Philadelphia, Lippincott-Raven, 1996.

69. Weinstein SL: Legg-Calvé-Perthes disease: Results of long-term follow up. In Fitzgerald RH Jr (ed): *The Hip: Proceedings of the Thirteenth Open Scientific Meetings of the Hip Society.* St Louis, CV Mosby, 1985.
70. Yrjonen T: Prognosis in Perthes' disease after non-containment treatment: 106 hips followed for 28-47 years. *Acta Orthop Scand* 63:523, 1992.
71. Loder RT, et al: Acute slipped capital femoral epiphysis: The importance of physeal stability. *J Bone Joint Surg Am* 75:1134, 1993.
72. Rattey T, Piehl F, Wright JG: Acute slipped capital femoral epiphysis. Review of the outcomes and rate of avascular necrosis. *J Bone Joint Surg Am* 78:398, 1996.
73. Carney BT, Weinstein SL, Noble J: Long term follow up of slipped capital femoral epiphysis. *J Bone Joint Surg Am* 73:667, 1991.
74. Ward WT, et al: Fixation with a single screw for slipped capital femoral epiphysis. *J Bone Joint Surg Am* 74:799, 1992.
75. Meier MC, Meyer LC, Ferguson RL: Treatment of slipped capital femoral epiphysis with a spica cast. *J Bone Joint Surg Am* 74:1522, 1992.
76. de Inocencio J: Musculoskeletal pain in primary care pediatric care: Analysis of 1000 consecutive general pediatric clinic visits. *Pediatrics* 102:e63, 1998.
77. Micheli LJ, Fehlandt AF Jr: Overuse injuries to tendons and apophyses in children and adolescents. *Clin Sports Med* 11:713, 1992.
78. Osgood RB: Lesions of the tibial tubercle occurring during adolescence. *Boston Med J* 148:114, 1903.
79. Peck DM: Apophyseal injuries in the young athlete. *Am Fam Physician* 51:1891, 1995.
80. Blankstein A, et al: Ultrasonography as a diagnostic modality in Osgood-Schlatter disease. A clinical study and review of the literature. *Arch Orthop Trauma Surg* 121:536, 2001.
81. Sever JW: Apophysitis of the os calcis. *N Y Med J* 95:1025, 1912.
82. Lazovic D, et al: Ultrasound for the diagnosis of apophyseal injuries. *Knee Surg Sports Traumatol Arthrosc* 3:234, 1996.
83. Bennet JB, Tullos HS: Ligamentous and articular injuries in the athlete. In Morrey BF (ed): *The Elbow and Its Disorders.* Philadelphia, WB Saunders, 1985.

CHAPTER 175 Sudden Infant Death Syndrome and Apparent Life Threatening Events

Marianne Gausche-Hill

PERSPECTIVE

The National Institute of Child Health and Human Development defined the sudden infant death syndrome (SIDS) as the "sudden death of an infant less than 1 year of age which remains unexplained after a thorough case investigation, including performance of a complete autopsy, examination of the death scene, and review of the clinical history." Passed in 1974, the Sudden Infant Death Syndrome Act provided a needed focus on research and public information. It was not until 1992, however, that the American Academy of Pediatrics recommended that infants be placed to sleep in a nonprone position to reduce the risk of SIDS, and a Back to Sleep (BTS) campaign was initiated in 1994 by a joint effort of the U.S. Public Health Service, the American Academy of Pediatrics, the SIDS Alliance, and the Association of SIDS and Infant Mortality Programs. Since then, the frequency of prone sleeping has decreased from 70% to 20% and the SIDS rate has concomitantly decreased by greater than 40%.[1]

Epidemiology of Sudden Infant Death Syndrome

In 1994, SIDS declined from the second leading cause to the third leading cause of infant mortality. The 1995 data indicate that the SIDS rate declined 18.3% from 1994, demonstrating a continuing declining trend.[2] The overall incidence of SIDS in the United States was approximately 0.72 per 1000 live births in 1998, down from 1.5 per 1000 live births reported in the 1980s. Despite the dramatic decline in the incidence of SIDS, approximately 3000 infants still die each year of SIDS in the United States. SIDS remains the leading cause of postneonatal mortality in the United States, accounting for one third of all such deaths, and it is the third most common cause of infant deaths.[2,3] SIDS may occur at any time during the first 2 years of life, but it is rare (1%) in children younger than 1 month of age and in those older than 1 year (2%). Ninety-five percent of SIDS infants die before 6 to 8 months with a peak between 2 and 4 months of age.[4]

There is also epidemiologic variation among different racial and ethnic groups. In 1997, the rate was 1.53 per 1000 live births in the black population, 0.64 per 1000 in whites, 0.48 per 1000 in Hispanic Americans, 0.51 per 1000 among Asian Americans, and 5.93 per 1000 among Native Americans. The smaller proportionate decline in the postnatal SIDS mortality rate among black infants over the last decade has exacerbated the racial disparity.[5] In contrast, between 1985 and 1996, the decline in infant mortality rate and SIDS among Northwest American Indians and Alaskan Natives was of greater magnitude than the national decline in SIDS.[6]

Other epidemiologic risk factors include male sex and multiple births. Whereas triplets have an incidence as high as 8.3 per 1000, there does not appear to be an increased incidence among twin gestations. There also appears to be an increased incidence in the winter months, and 62% of SIDS cases occur during the colder season in California.[7]

Definitions

Because of the confusion that exists with the myriad of terms describing infants who present with cardiopulmonary distress, the 1986 National Institutes of Health Consensus Development Conference on Infantile Apnea and Home Monitoring delineated the following terms[8]:

Apnea is a cessation of airflow. The respiratory pause may be central or diaphragmatic (i.e., no respiratory effort), obstructive (usually caused by upper airway obstruction), or mixed. Short (<15 seconds) periods of central apnea can be normal at all ages.

Pathologic apnea is an abnormal respiratory pause that is prolonged (>20 seconds) or is associated with cyanosis, marked pallor, hypotonia, or bradycardia.

Apnea of prematurity is periodic breathing with pathologic apnea in a premature infant. Apnea of prematurity usually ceases by 37 weeks' gestation (menstrual dating) but occasionally persists past term.

Apnea of infancy is an unexplained episode of cessation of breathing for 20 seconds or longer or a shorter respiratory pause associated with bradycardia, cyanosis, pallor, or marked hypotonia. It generally refers to infants who are more than 37 weeks' gestational age at the onset of pathologic apnea. The term apnea of infancy should be reserved for those infants in whom no specific cause of an apparent life-threatening event (ALTE) can be defined.

Periodic breathing is a breathing pattern in which there are three or more respiratory pauses of greater than 3 seconds' duration with less than 20 seconds of respiration between the pauses. Periodic breathing may be a normal event.

Symptomatic premature infants are preterm infants who continue to have pathologic apnea at the time when they otherwise would be ready for discharge from the hospital.

An *apparent life-threatening event* is "an episode that is frightening to the observer and is characterized by some combination of apnea (central or occasionally obstructive), color change (usually cyanotic or pallid but occasionally erythematous or plethoric), marked change in muscle tone (usually limpness), choking, or gagging." Often the observer fears that the infant has died.[9] ALTE is a term used until a precise causative diagnosis can be established, but more than 50% of ALTEs never receive a definitive diagnosis despite an extensive workup. Previously used terms such as *near-miss SIDS* or *aborted crib death* should not be used because they imply an unproven, misleading association between an ALTE and SIDS.

Sudden infant death syndrome is "the sudden death of an infant under 1 year of age, which remains unexplained after a thorough case investigation, including performance of a complete autopsy, examination of the death scene, and review of the clinical history."

Breath-holding spells occur when infants perform a Valsalva maneuver in response to pain, fright, crying, coughing, or defecation. During the spell, minute ventilation decreases without any adverse effects. Breath-holding spells, however, if severe and prolonged, may result in cyanosis, unconsciousness, and seizures. Severe breath-holding spells are reported to occur in 5% of normal children before 6 years of age. Pallid breath-holding spells have been distinguished from cyanotic breath-holding spells. It is thought that pallid spells result from a primary central parasympathetic disturbance, leading to vagally mediated cardiac inhibition.[10] In contrast, cyanotic spells are hypothesized to have a more complex pathogenesis, involving the interaction of hyperventilation, Valsalva maneuvers, expiratory apnea, and intrinsic pulmonary mechanisms.[11]

BOX 175-1. Maternal Risk Factors for Sudden Infant Death Syndrome

Modifiable
Maternal smoking during pregnancy
Illicit drug use
Low socioeconomic status

Nonmodifiable
Maternal age <20 at first pregnancy
African American and American Indian descent
History of low parental education
Absence of prenatal care

PRINCIPLES OF DISEASE

Risk Factors for Sudden Infant Death Syndrome

In the 1980s, several risk factors were identified, such as low birth weight, preterm gestational age, cardiac dysrhythmias, young maternal age, maternal education, high parity, race, and poor socioeconomic status. Since then, many other predisposing factors have been proposed. Risk factors for SIDS may be divided into maternal, neonatal, and postnatal factors, and further differentiation may be made between modifiable and nonmodifiable risk factors (Box 175-1). Maternal smoking during pregnancy, age younger than 20 at the time of first pregnancy, short interpregnancy intervals, lack of prenatal care, illicit drug use (cocaine and narcotics), illness during pregnancy, being unmarried, and having a low socioeconomic status are characteristics that are prevalent in mothers of SIDS infants.[12]

Prenatal risk factors for SIDS (Box 175-2) include exposure to passive smoke, intrauterine growth retardation, multiple births, preterm birth, and low birth weight. The risk for SIDS is proportionately increased with decreasing gestational age and birth weight. Approximately 20% of all SIDS cases occur in the

BOX 175-2. Prenatal Risk Factors for Sudden Infant Death Syndrome (Nonmodifiable)

Exposure to passive smoking
Intrauterine growth retardation
Multiple births
Prematurity
Low infant birth weight (<2500 g)
Winter season

BOX 175-3. Postnatal Risk Factors

Modifiable

Exposure to environmental tobacco smoke
Excessively warm ambient temperature
Sheepskin or natural fiber bedding material (loose bedding)
Soft sleep surfaces
Bed sharing with adults

Nonmodifiable

? Infection
? Gastroesophageal reflux disease
? Cardiac arrhythmias

preterm population. Compared with age-matched control infants, infants born at less than 37 weeks and less than 33 weeks are 5 and 16 times, respectively, more likely to die of SIDS. A suboptimal intrauterine environment may lead to early spontaneous labor, which is associated with an increased risk of subsequent SIDS.[13]

The most important modifiable *postnatal risk factor* for SIDS (Box 175-3) is prone sleeping, with odds ratios ranging from 1.7 to 12.9. In the United States, there was a 40% decline in SIDS between 1992 and 1998, concurrent with a decrease in prone sleeping from 78% in 1992 to 17% in 1998.[1] Despite the association between the BTS campaign and the marked decline in SIDS, 20% of U.S. infants continue to sleep in the prone position, possibly because myths regarding the adverse effects of the supine sleeping position persist.[14] A study demonstrated that 25% of licensed child care centers were unaware of the association between SIDS and the prone position, and the proportion of SIDS in child care has not decreased despite a decline in the national SIDS rate.[15,16] In addition, many parents and health practitioners do not realize that the supine sleeping position is actually associated with other health benefits, such as decreased rates of nasal congestion, otitis media, and fever before the age of 1 month.[3]

Internationally, the supine sleeping position has led to a decline of nearly 50% in the incidence of SIDS in the United Kingdom, New Zealand, Australia, the Netherlands, Norway, Denmark, Ireland, and Tasmania. The original 1992 recommendation from the American Academy of Pediatrics identified any nonprone position (supine or side) as reducing the risk for SIDS. Since then, however, studies have demonstrated that side sleeping is associated with a higher risk for SIDS than the supine position.[1]

Other postnatal factors that are associated with SIDS include soft sleep surfaces and loose bedding, overheating, bed sharing, infection, gastroesophageal reflux (GER), poor postnatal weight gain, apnea, and cardiac arrhythmias. Polystyrene bead–filled pillows, soft pillows, quilts, comforters, sheepskin, and porous mattresses have been identified as a risk factor for SIDS, particularly when placed under the sleeping infant. An increased risk is associated with overheating with clothing and blankets as well as room temperature. Bed sharing may lead to suffocation of an infant by an overlying adult, and the risk of SIDS associated with co-sleeping is greater when the adult is under the influence of alcohol or other mind-altering drugs.[12] Thirty percent to 50% of SIDS infants have an infection, usually an upper respiratory tract infection, at the time of the acute event. Infection with respiratory syncytial virus is associated with apnea, particularly in premature infants, but no clear association exists between viral infections and SIDS.[12]

GER has been implicated in SIDS through an indirect mechanism.[17] The presence of gastric material in the lungs is found in 20% to 30% of SIDS autopsies, and there is continued controversy about whether aspiration is a contributory cause of death or merely an agonal phenomenon in SIDS. Physiologic GER may stimulate the laryngeal chemoreceptors when gastric contents are refluxed to the level of the pharynx. Although reflux may be innocuous, it may lead to SIDS in the young infant under conditions that promote depressed swallowing or arousal, such as prone sleeping, prematurity, sedatives, seizures, or upper respiratory tract infections.[10] Poor postnatal weight gain may also be associated with an increased risk of SIDS.[19] Mothers of SIDS victims are more likely to report apneic episodes (7.7% versus 3.0%) than control mothers, and there is an increased prevalence of SIDS in families who have members with obstructive sleep apnea.[20] A significant number of SIDS cases have been associated with a prolongation of the QT interval, but there is controversy over the study methods, and cardiac arrhythmias are thought to account for only a small number of SIDS cases.

Possible protective factors against SIDS have also been identified. A few retrospective studies have demonstrated a protective effect of breast-feeding; however, other analyses have failed to demonstrate the finding after adjustment for confounding variables. Thus, the Task Force on Infant Sleep Position and Sudden Infant Death Syndrome does not recommend breast-feeding as a strategy to reduce SIDS. Conversely, the use of pacifiers is associated with increased susceptibility to otitis media, an increased rate of dental malocclusion, and a shorter duration of breast-feeding. Thus, additional outcome studies are required before specific recommendations regarding pacifiers can be made.[21]

Factors that do not increase the risk of SIDS include maternal alcohol use, recent diphtheria-pertussis-tetanus or other vaccine administration, being a sibling of a SIDS victim, sickle cell disease, and bronchopulmonary dysplasia.

Pathophysiology and Etiology of Sudden Infant Death Syndrome

Autopsies of SIDS victims demonstrate the effects of chronic hypoxemia, but there are no specific findings that are pathognomonic of SIDS. Pathology typically reveals pulmonary artery smooth muscle hypertrophy, right ventricular hypertrophy, increased hematopoiesis in the liver, increased periadrenal brown fat, adrenal medullary hyperplasia, abnormalities in the carotid body, and brainstem gliosis.[12]

More than 70 theories have been proposed regarding the pathophysiology of SIDS. Delayed arousal response, autonomic dysfunction, suffocation, electrolyte abnormalities, mineral deficiencies, cardiac dysrhythmias, infection, anemia, hyperthyroidism, hyperthermia, upper airway obstruction, congenital anomalies, amino acid activation, and occult trauma are a few of the proposed theories.

A leading hypothesis states that SIDS may be due to a delayed or deficient arousal response, and in support of this theory, the brainstems of SIDS victims reveal hypoplasia and decreased neurotransmitter binding of the arcuate nucleus, a region that is involved in blood pressure responses, chemosensitivity, and hypercapnic ventilatory response. Prone sleeping may impair the arousal response, placing infants with a downregulated baroreceptor response at further disadvantage. Arousability is affected by gestational and postnatal age, and the arousal threshold is significantly elevated at 2 to 3 months, when the rate of SIDS is highest.[22] Prone sleep positions also cause a reduction in vasomotor tone with a lower resting blood pressure (79.6 versus 82.3 mm Hg), a higher peripheral skin temperature (33.7° C versus 33.3° C), and a faster heart rate. A combination of sleep-induced reduction in vasomotor control with a reduction in central venous return and cardiac distention may trigger a brainstem-mediated bradycardia. Decreased central venous return compromises pulmonary perfusion and causes worsening hypoxia.[23,24] Prone sleep positions may exacerbate the rebreathing of exhaled gases trapped in soft bedding material, leading to hypercarbia and worsening hypoxia.[25,26]

Although the exact mechanism of SIDS remains unclear, a theory that would bring together many of the preceding etiologies is the triple-risk theory. This model implies that lack of cardiorespiratory control and autonomic dysfunction are predisposing factors for SIDS. The circulatory effects of sleep, which involves the downregulation of the baroreceptor reflex, associated with a reduction in vasomotor control and decreased central venous return, cardiac output, and blood pressure may lead to the preterminal event progressive bradycardia (Figure 175-1). It is postulated that the prone sleeping position, overheating, co-sleeping, and the co-occurrence of an upper respiratory tract infection could exacerbate these effects.[27] As with neurocardiogenic syncope in the adult, poor central venous return and decreased cardiac distention lead to bradycardia, hypoxia from poor lung perfusion, and death.[28]

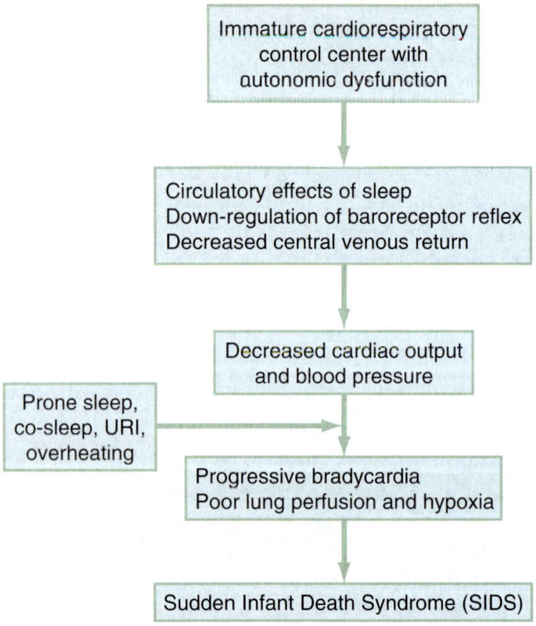

Figure 175-1. Triple-risk theory for the etiology of SIDS.

DIAGNOSIS OF SUDDEN INFANT DEATH SYNDROME

The diagnosis of SIDS is made at autopsy after postmortem evaluation fails to reveal a cause of death. If a suspected SIDS death has occurred, a thorough investigation of the death scene may identify contributing factors, such as accidental asphyxiation or hyperthermia. Any findings suggestive of child abuse should be reported, although fewer than 5% of SIDS victims are discovered to have died of child abuse. The estimated association between child abuse, including Munchausen's syndrome by proxy, and SIDS ranges between 2% and 40%. However, in families with recurrent unexpected deaths, the estimated association increases to 55%. Most investigations of the history, home circumstances, and postmortem examination are negative for child neglect or abuse. Child protection is rarely needed, but an investigation should be initiated if there is a recurrence of SIDS or an ALTE with a second baby.[29]

MANAGEMENT OF A SUDDEN INFANT DEATH SYNDROME CASE

In the management of a SIDS case, the death scene investigation should delineate the location and position of the infant, the room temperature, type of surface, presence of soft toys, pillows, bedding materials, and the general condition of the house.

Prehospital Considerations and Emergency Department Management

Prehospital care providers and emergency physicians may be involved in the resuscitation of infants who are apparent SIDS victims. In Los Angeles County, prehospital care personnel pronounced dead 26% of the pediatric coroner's cases in the field, of which 20% were SIDS deaths. If the infants are not pronounced dead in the field, they are brought to the emergency department for resuscitation. The decision to begin resuscitation and transport infants with signs of death in the field is a complex one. Often the scene is chaotic with personnel assessing and distraught family members pleading with prehospital providers to initiate care. Advantages of initiating transport include additional personnel in the emergency department to care for the child and family; physician involvement with care and declaration of death; and clergy and social services available for family support and grief counseling. As cardiopulmonary resuscitation is unsuccessful in the majority of cases, the physician must provide supportive care for the family. When the cause of death is unknown, appropriate samples (e.g., blood, urine) should be obtained. An autopsy should be performed in all SIDS deaths by a competent and experienced pathologist.

Psychosocial Considerations

The emergency physician and pediatrician must address psychosocial considerations in any SIDS case. The physician should be direct when informing parents that their child has died. The word "dead" or "died" should be used instead of confusing euphemisms such as "passed on." Parents universally experience intense guilt, and siblings may also have guilt over the loss of their brother or sister. Parents may further intensify the guilt by accusing one another of not taking adequate care of the infant. The police investigation may arouse suspicion in neighbors and friends and leave the parents and caretakers socially alienated. The overall toll of guilt and social alienation is enormous, and the effects are manifested in increased rates of miscarriage, divorce, and infertility after a SIDS death. The outcome of SIDS is dependent on the support provided for the family of the victim. Thus, the team approach, with the nurse, social worker, chaplain, emergency physician, and pediatrician together, may provide comfort and information to the grieving family. The parents may be given written information about local and national SIDS organizations (Box 175-4). The emergency physician and the pediatrician must recognize that they can play a pivotal role in helping the family to adjust to their loss, initiate the process of grieving, and educate the family about SIDS prevention.

In a review of 351 families who received counseling after an infant died unexpectedly, Smialek found the following interventions to be helpful: (1) openly accepting an individual's grief reactions, (2) allowing the family an opportunity to vocalize their feelings, (3) clarifying misconceptions, (4) allowing the family to hold or to be in the room alone with the dead infant, (5) providing a private place for the family to gather, and (6) providing an explanation for the cause of death and helping with funeral arrangements.[30]

BOX 175-4. Sudden Infant Death Syndrome Organizations

National SIDS Alliance
800-221-7437
American SIDS Institute
800-232-SIDS
CJ Foundation for SIDS
800-996-5002
The Compassionate Friends
630-990-0010
National SIDS Resource Center
703-822-8955

The American College of Emergency Physicians and the American Academy of Pediatrics jointly adopted a policy statement entitled "The death of a child in the emergency department." The published guidelines address critical issues, such as a family- and team-centered approach, providing support for families and communities, the importance of communication within the child's medical home, the identification of resources for use when a child dies, and postincident critical stress management.[31]

As an example of adopting a family- and team-centered approach, it is recommended that families be offered the option of being present during a resuscitation. Moreover, the family should be offered the decision whether or not to view the body. If they choose not to view the body, their decision should be respected, although viewing the body may help parents achieve closure and begin the grieving process. Different cultural and religious backgrounds influence a family's reactions, requests, and needs during the grieving process, and the emergency physician should be aware of the most common beliefs that are present in the community and be respectful of these backgrounds and traditions. Other strategies to improve the process of death notification may involve the inclusion of the victim's siblings and their peers in the immediate grieving process. The child's pediatrician should also be informed and included in the postincident phase because he or she can provide valuable support to the family in the days immediately after the death. A follow-up telephone call or letter from the emergency department may also facilitate the resolution of unanswered questions and help with the grief process. Finally, health care providers may also experience guilt, self-reproach, and sadness after a SIDS death, and it is important to arrange critical incident stress debriefing sessions in which health care providers may openly express and work through these emotions.

Team meetings may provide a forum for education, stress reduction, and supportive training on dealing with death in the emergency department.[31]

APPARENT LIFE-THREATENING EVENTS

Epidemiology

Estimates of the incidence of ALTEs in the United States range from 0.5% to 6%; however, the studies on which these estimates are based have methodologic flaws, and the true epidemiology is difficult to establish.[9] Most events occur at 2 to 3 months, but an ALTE can occur at any age. Approximately 1% to 3% of infants in the general population are reported to experience an ALTE. The average infant presenting after an ALTE is between 8 and 14 weeks of age, and 7% of these infants have a history of prematurity. Most studies also demonstrate a male predominance as high as 2 : 1.[9]

One of the most important questions yet to be answered is the degree to which ALTEs are associated with SIDS. Between 7% and 15% of children with ALTEs succumb to SIDS, and 6% of SIDS victims have had a previous ALTE.[32] Despite the significant decrease in SIDS rates since the initiation of the BTS program, the annual admission rate for ALTEs has remained unchanged, casting further doubt on the relationship between ALTE and SIDS.[33]

Pathophysiology and Etiology

The pathophysiology of an ALTE has not been clearly defined. Some studies demonstrate that ALTE infants experience autonomic dysfunction, whereby they respond with lower sympathetic stimulation and inhibited vagal withdrawal manifested as bradycardia, postural hypotension, and heart rate variability, particularly when stressed with carbon dioxide.[34-36] Polysomnographic studies in infants with ALTEs have demonstrated significantly more episodes of hypoxemia during sleep as well as increased inspiratory effort and thoracoabdominal asynchrony, which is thought to be due to compromised upper airway patency.[37] There may also be a relationship between anatomic causes of obstructive sleep apnea, intrapulmonary shunting, and upper and lower airway instability, such as tracheomalacia and esophageal atresia, and ALTEs.[38,39] Clinical investigation of first-degree relatives of ALTE infants with sleep-disordered breathing demonstrated smaller naso-oro-maxillomandibular traits compared with controls.[40]

Diagnosis

As an ALTE is only a description of a characteristic clinical presentation, determining the underlying cause is the greater challenge. However, a definitive diagnosis is not made in 50% of the cases.[41] The differential diagnosis for an ALTE is extensive (Box 175-5) and includes infection (sepsis, respiratory syncytial virus or other respiratory viruses, pertussis, or central nervous system infection), GER with or without obstructive apnea, congenital malformations (tracheomalacia, vascular rings, pulmonary slings), seizure disorder, cardiac dysrhythmias, congenital cardiac malformations, metabolic derangements (hypoglycemia), and child abuse.[41]

BOX 175-5. Etiologies of Apparent Life-Threatening Events

Cardiac
Dysrhythmias
Congenital heart disease

Child Abuse
Physical abuse
Munchausen syndrome by proxy

Gastrointestinal
Gastroesophageal reflux disease
Congenital malformations

Infectious
Meningitis or encephalitis
Pertussis
Respiratory syncytial virus
Sepsis

Metabolic
Hypoglycemia
Hypocalcemia
Hyponatremia
Inborn errors of metabolism

Neurologic
Seizure
Central nervous system tumor
Arnold-Chiari malformations
Subdural or epidural hematoma

Respiratory
Foreign body aspiration
Obstructive sleep apnea
Respiratory infection

Other
Breath-holding spells
Vasovagal syncope
Drug or toxin exposure

Injury associated with head trauma or child abuse may be difficult to distinguish in the absence of a reliable history. Intoxication, either accidental or intentional as in Munchausen's syndrome by proxy, can produce subsequent hypoventilation, hypoxia, cardiopulmonary arrest, and death. In a retrospective study of 196 infants who presented with an ALTE, the discharge diagnoses included seizure (25%), GER (18%), febrile convulsion (12%), bronchiolitis (9%), apnea (9%), pertussis (6%), choking (5%), upper respiratory tract infections (4%), cyanotic episode (2%), gastroenteritis (2%), asthma (1%), head injury (1%), feeding difficulties (1%), urinary tract infection (1%), and breath-holding (1%).[42]

Because GER is physiologic and occurs in most infants, establishing the diagnosis of GER does not prove that it is the cause of an ALTE. There has been emphasis on the causative role of laryngeal chemoreceptor stimulation. When isotonic fluids are infused into the larynx of human infants, there is a reflex arc that results in laryngeal adduction, apnea, bradycardia, and central pooling of blood. Mixed apnea from periodic breathing and obstructive apnea have been reported in children with ALTEs. An ALTE may be the first manifestation of an epileptic seizure, but the diagnosis is often difficult. A transient episode of apnea may be the only manifestation of a partial seizure, and the interictal electroencephalogram is characteristically normal. Seizures may be the causative etiology for up to 11% of ALTEs, and a normal interictal electroencephalogram does not exclude seizures as the precipitating factor.[43] QT prolongation has been associated with ALTE,[44] and an ALTE may also be a manifestation of child abuse, possibly of a smothering attempt, an intentional poisoning, or shaken baby syndrome.

Management

The infant who presents with a history of an ALTE may look well and act entirely normally at the time of the evaluation by the prehospital provider or the emergency physician. However, infants who are judged by prehospital personnel to have choked or turned blue or are showing other signs suggestive of a possible ALTE should be considered seriously ill and transported to the emergency department for evaluation.[42] Fifty percent of children who present to the emergency department after an ALTE have an entirely normal clinical examination, and the final diagnosis often correlates poorly with the prehospital presenting signs and symptoms, which often include cyanosis, breathing difficulties, abnormal movements, loss of consciousness, vomiting, pallor, and choking.[42]

In the emergency department, resuscitation must be the initial focus. Airway, breathing, and circulation should be stabilized. A complete history and physical examination should be performed. If possible, the physician should obtain a detailed description of the infant at the time of discovery (especially the color and muscle tone of the infant), the duration of the episode, the resuscitation measures used, and the infant's response to the resuscitation measures. Other questions that may be pertinent include the following: Was the infant awake or sleeping? Were there symptoms of airway obstruction? Does the infant have any history or symptoms suggestive of GER? Did the event occur after feeding? Did the episode occur after vigorous crying (suggestive of breath-holding)? Is there any family history of SIDS or apnea?

During the physical examination, the physician should note the presence of tachypnea, stridor, or wheezing. The skin should be examined for suspicious bruising (patterned bruises or truncal bruising suggestive of child abuse), the extremities for abnormalities (fractures, burns, healing wounds, or other signs of unusual injury), and the eyes for pupillary changes or retinal hemorrhages (shaken baby syndrome). A study demonstrated that a dilated funduscopic examination in 128 patients who presented with an ALTE detected retinal hemorrhages in 1.4% of the patients and helped detect child abuse in 2.3% of the patients. Thus, in addition to obtaining a detailed family and social history, it may be prudent to conduct a dilated funduscopic examination in children who present to the emergency department after an ALTE.[45]

BOX 175-6. Emergency Department Workup for the Infant Who Presents with an Apparent Life-Threatening Event

Laboratory Evaluation
Complete blood count
Serum glucose
Serum ammonia
Electrolytes, including calcium, magnesium, and phosphorus
Urinalysis
Blood, urine, and cerebral spinal fluid culture if younger than 1 month of age or consider if febrile
Toxicology screen
Electrocardiogram
Chest radiography

Other Imaging and Diagnostic Studies
Electroencephalogram
Computed tomography of the head
24-hour pH probe
Barium esophagram
Polysomnography for sleep disorders
Flexible and rigid laryngoscopy

There are no official evidence-based admission guidelines regarding the infant who presents with an ALTE. However, it is currently recommended that all infants younger than 1 year who present with color change, apnea, or change in muscle tone be hospitalized for observation and evaluation, as outlined in Box 175-6. Laboratory evaluation may include a complete blood count, serum glucose, electrolytes, serum ammonia (metabolic disease), cultures if younger than 1 month or febrile, and a toxicology screen. An electrocardiogram, chest radiograph, and computed tomography scan of the head without contrast may be performed in the emergency department. A skeletal survey may be obtained in selected cases. Once admitted, infants may also undergo an electroencephalogram, an evaluation for GER (24 hour pH probe and barium esophagram), polysomnography for sleep disorders, and possibly flexible and rigid laryngoscopy.

The outcome of an ALTE depends upon the underlying etiology. In a retrospective review of 196 ALTE patients, there were no deaths.[42] The follow-up revealed a high percentage of asthma and seizures as well as GER requiring Nissen fundoplication. Infants who survive an ALTE generally do well in follow-up. However, there are some rare complications. Pulmonary edema, aspiration pneumonia, and neurologic sequelae secondary to hypoxia may result.

Caffeine and Theophylline

Caffeine and theophylline have been shown to be useful in managing apnea of prematurity and in reducing periodic breathing in infants at risk for SIDS. A study of 300 patients with an ALTE or infants at increased epidemiologic risk of SIDS demonstrated that theophylline resulted in normal pneumograms in 94%

of the infants and improved the pneumogram in 100%. Theophylline is administered orally at a dose of 6 to 7.5 mg/kg/day, and serum levels should be maintained between 10 to 15 µg/mL. Theophylline levels should be checked periodically, and parents should be educated regarding potential side effects. The efficacy of the xanthine derivatives in preventing SIDS is unclear.

Home Monitoring

Monitoring devices measure chest wall movement and heart rate. Parents must learn about equipment maintenance, interpretation of alarms, and cardiopulmonary resuscitation. Technical support should be available to the parents 24 hours a day. Reports have shown a mortality rate of as high as 50% among infants receiving home monitoring. Technical errors and parental noncompliance are thought to contribute to the high mortality rate. Parents may misinterpret alarms when they sound, and the majority of alarms that parents felt required resuscitation were associated with normal electrocardiograms. Because of the lack of demonstrated efficacy and the frequency of false alarms, there is a great deal of controversy regarding the use of home monitoring.

The National Institutes of Health Consensus Development Conference on Infantile Apnea and Home Monitoring in 1986 defined several groups of infants as candidates for home monitoring[8]: (1) symptomatic premature infants who continued to exhibit apnea beyond term (40 weeks after conception), (2) term infants with unexplained apnea of infancy and a history of ALTE that required vigorous stimulation or resuscitation, (3) subsequent siblings of two or more SIDS victims, and (4) infants with bronchopulmonary dysplasia and infants with tracheostomies. The consensus panel also stated that normal asymptomatic infants who never experience ALTEs and who are not in other high-risk groups do not require monitoring, and for children who have had a less severe ALTE, monitoring should be determined on a case-by-case basis after considering with the family the potential benefits, uncertainties, and psychosocial burdens.[29]

Both pediatricians and emergency physicians are consulted about monitor alarms. The physician must be able to distinguish a false alarm from a true episode. Admission to the hospital for further care may be prudent if the event was associated with the infant changing color or requiring vigorous resuscitation.

FUTURE DIRECTIONS

Regarding SIDS, the American Academy of Pediatrics Task Force has made the following recommendations to parents[21]: (1) infants should be placed in the nonprone position for sleep, and the supine position is preferred; (2) infants should not be put to sleep on waterbeds, sofas, soft mattresses, or other soft surfaces; (3) soft materials should not be placed in the infant's sleeping environment; (4) bed sharing and co-sleeping may be hazardous and should be avoided; (5) overheating should be avoided; and (6) a certain amount of nonprone time while the infant is awake is recommended for developmental reasons and to prevent positional plagiocephaly. In order to achieve nationwide supine sleeping rates of at least 90% to 95%, health practitioners and parents must realize that supine sleeping is not associated with any adverse health outcomes or with diminished sleep. Moreover, outreach programs must tailor educational strategies to be acceptable to those of different cultural and ethnic backgrounds. Clearly, the BTS campaign should continue, and other potentially modifiable risk factors, such as maternal smoking, overheating, unsafe bedding, and bed sharing, should be addressed in educational efforts and public campaigns. Finally, it is crucial to define the contributions of genetic factors in autonomic dysfunction and neurotransmitter and receptor function in better characterizing the pathophysiology of SIDS.

KEY CONCEPTS

- *Epidemiology*: Despite the dramatic decline in the incidence of SIDS in the past several decades, SIDS remains the leading cause of postneonatal mortality in the United States, accounting for one third of all such deaths, and is the third most common cause of infant deaths.
- *Prevention*: Emergency physicians may play a key role in SIDS education and prevention. Parents must be taught the importance of the supine sleeping position, smoking cessation, and the elimination and avoidance of co-sleeping, overheating, and soft or loose bedding material.
- *Psychosocial considerations*: The team approach, with the nurse, social worker, chaplain, emergency physician, and pediatrician together, may help the family to adjust to their loss, initiate the process of grieving, and counsel the family about SIDS.
- *ALTE*: Although the infant who presents with a history of an ALTE may look well and act entirely normally at the time of the evaluation by the prehospital provider or the emergency physician, these infants and children require admission and monitoring as the final diagnosis and the presenting symptoms often correlate poorly. It is important to note that a definitive underlying etiology is not identified in 50% of the cases.

REFERENCES

1. Hunt CE, et al: Infant sleep position and associated health outcomes. *Arch Pediatr Adolesc Med* 157:469, 2003.
2. Contribution of selected metabolic diseases to early childhood deaths—Virginia, 1996-2001. *MMWR Morb Mortal Wkly Rep* 52:677, 2003.
3. Sudden infant death syndrome—United States, 1983-1994. *MMWR Morb Mortal Wkly Rep* 45:859, 1996.
4. Kum-Nji P, Mangrem CL, Wells P: Reducing the incidence of sudden infant death syndrome in the Delta region of the Mississippi: A three-pronged approach. *South Med J* 94:704, 2001.
5. Gibson E, Dembofsky C, Rubin S, Greenspan J: Infant sleep position 2 years into the "back to sleep" campaign. *Clin Pediatr (Phila)* 39:285, 2000.
6. Decrease in infant mortality and sudden infant death syndrome among Northwest American Indians and Alaskan

Natives—Pacific Northwest, 1985-1996. *MMWR Morb Mortal Wkly Rep* 48:181, 1999.
7. Adams EJ, et al: Changes in the epidemiology profile of sudden infant death syndrome as rates decline in California infants, 1990-1995. *Pediatrics* 102:1445-1451, 1998.
8. National Institutes of Health Consensus Development Conference on Infantile Apnea and Home Monitoring, Sept 29 to Oct 1, 1986. *Pediatrics* 79:292, 1987.
9. http://www.rain.org/~landon/ALTE (accessed September 19, 2003).
10. DiMario FJ, Bauer L, Baxter D: Respiratory sinus arrhythmia in children with severe cyanotic and pallid breath-holding spells. *J Child Neurol* 13:440, 1998.
11. Breningstall GN: Breath-holding spells. *Pediatr Neurol* 14:91, 1996.
12. Hauck F, Hunt C: Sudden infant death syndrome in 2000. *Curr Probl Pediatr* 30:237, 2000.
13. Smith G, Pell J, Dobbie R: Risk of sudden infant death syndrome and week of gestation of term birth. *Pediatrics* 111:1367, 2003.
14. Skadberg B, Morild I, Markestad T: Abandoning prone sleeping: Effect on the risk of sudden infant death syndrome. *J Pediatr* 132:340, 1998.
15. Moon R, Patel K, McDermott S: Sudden infant death in child care settings. *Pediatrics* 106:295, 2000.
16. Moon R, Billiter W: Infant sleep position policies in licensed child care centers after back to sleep campaign. *Pediatrics* 106:576, 2000.
17. Thach B: Sudden infant death syndrome: Can gastroesophageal reflux cause sudden infant death? *Am J Med* 108:144S, 2000.
18. Page M, Jeffrey H: The role of gastroesophageal reflux in the etiology of SIDS. *Early Hum Dev* 59:127, 2000.
19. Blair P, et al: Weight gain and sudden infant death syndrome: Changes in weight z scores may identify infants at greater risk. *Arch Dis Child* 82:462, 2000.
20. McNamara F, Sullivan C: Obstructive sleep apnea in infants: Relation to family history of sudden infant death syndrome, apparent life-threatening events, and obstructive sleep apnea. *J Pediatr* 136:318, 2000.
21. Task Force on Infant Sleep Position and Sudden Infant Death Syndrome: Changing concepts of sudden infant death syndrome: Implications for infant sleeping environment and sleep position. *Pediatrics* 105:650, 2000.
22. Horne R, et al: Effects of prematurity on arousal from sleep in the newborn infant. *Pediatr Res* 47:468, 2000.
23. Carolan P, Wheeler W, Ross J, Kemp J: Potential to prevent carbon dioxide rebreathing of commercial products marketed to reduce sudden infant death syndrome risk. *Pediatrics* 105:774, 2000.
24. Chong A, Murphy N, Matthews T: Effect of prone sleeping on circulatory control in infants. *Arch Dis Child* 82:253, 2000.
25. Franco P, et al: Auditory arousal thresholds are higher when infants sleep in the prone position. *J Pediatr* 132:240, 1998.
26. Kemp J, Livine M, White D, Arfken C: Softness and potential to cause rebreathing: Differences in bedding used by infants at high and low risk for sudden infant death syndrome. *J Pediatr* 132:234, 1998.
27. Chong A, Murphy N, Matthews T: Effect of prone sleeping on circulatory control in infants. *Arch Dis Child* 82:253, 2000.
28. Matthews T: Sudden infant death syndrome—A defect in circulatory control? *Child Care Health Dev* 28(Suppl 1):41, 2002.
29. Stanton A: Sudden unexpected death in infancy associated with maltreatment: Evidence from long-term follow-up of siblings. *Arch Dis Child* 88:699, 2003.
30. Smialek Z: Observations on immediate reactions of families to sudden infant death, *Pediatrics* 63:670, 1978.
31. Knazik S, et al: The death of a child in the emergency department. *Ann Emerg Med* 42:519, 2003.
32. McMurray S, Holinger L: Otolaryngologic manifestations in children presenting with apparent life-threatening events. *Otolaryngol Head Neck Surg* 116:575, 1997.
33. Mitchell E, Thompson J: Parental reported apnoea, admissions to the hospital and sudden infant death syndrome. *Acta Paediatr* 90:417, 2001.
34. Edner A, et al: Heart rate variability in infants with apparent life-threatening events. *Acta Paediatr* 89:1326, 2000.
35. Edner A, Ericson M, Milerad J, Katz-Salamon M: Abnormal heart rate response to hypercapnia in boys with an apparent life-threatening event. *Acta Paediatr* 91:1318, 2002.
36. Harrington C, Kirjavainen T, Teng A, Sullivan C: Altered autonomic function and reduced arousability in apparent life-threatening event infants with obstructive sleep apnea. *Am J Respir Crit Care Med* 165:1048, 2002.
37. Horemuzova E, Katz-Salamon M, Milerad J: Increased inspiratory effort in infants with a history of apparent life-threatening event. *Acta Paediatr* 91:280, 2002.
38. Cozzi DA, et al: Recurrent apparent life-threatening event relieved by glossopexy. *J Pediatr Surg* 31:1715, 1996.
39. Guilleminault C, Pelayo R, Leger D, Philip P: Apparent life-threatening events, facial dysmorphia and sleep-disordered breathing. *Eur J Pediatr* 159:444, 2000.
40. Guilleminault C, et al: Sleep-disordered breathing and upper-airway anomalies in first-degree relatives of ALTE children. *Pediatr Res* 50:14, 2001.
41. Davies F, Gupta R: Apparent life-threatening events in infants presenting to and emergency department. *Emerg Med J* 19:11, 2002.
42. Gray C, Davies F, Molyneux E: Apparent life-threatening events presenting to a pediatric emergency department. *Pediatr Emerg Care* 15:195, 1999.
43. Nunes M, Calcagnoto C, Costa da Costa J: Apparent life-threatening episodes as the first manifestation of epilepsy. *Clin Pediatr (Phila)* 42:19, 2003.
44. Goldhammer EI, et al: QT dispersion in infants with apparent life-threatening events syndrome. *Pediatr Cardiol* 23:605, 2002.
45. Pitetti R, et al: Prevalence of retinal hemorrhages and child abuse in children who present with an apparent life threatening event. *Pediatrics* 10:557, 2002.

CHAPTER 176

General Approach to the Pregnant Patient

Laurie J. Morrison

PERSPECTIVE

Epidemiology

There are remarkable trends in the epidemiology of fertility that may have an impact on the demographic and diagnostic profile of pregnant emergency department patients. The birth rates, fertility rates for all races, and the mean age of menarche in both the United States and Canada have fallen over the past decade. The age-specific fertility rate has declined in women younger than 30 years, and the rate of multiple births is rising.

The National Center for Health Statistics reported the number of U.S. live births for the year ending July 1, 1999, to be 3.96 million with a birth rate of 13.9 per 1000 population for all races.[1] In Canada during the year 2002-2003, the birth rate was 10.5 per 1000 population, with 331,522 births.[2] The 2003 report from the National Center for Health Statistics, Centers for Disease Control and Prevention reported that the birth rate for women in their early 20s, the principal child-bearing age, had fallen 9% from 1990 to 2001.[3,4] The overall birth rate for teens aged 15 to 19 dropped 3% per year from 1991 to 45.3 per 1000 teenagers in 2001.[3,4] The median age of menarche for adolescent American girls fell from 15.5 years in 1900 to 12.3 years in 2000 (Figure 176-1).[5] The Canadian general fertility rate has been declining since 1980, and Canada's growth rate is now only about three quarters of the growth rate in the United States.[6] Young American women have continued to have relatively high fertility rates, whereas fertility in young Canadian women has declined substantially in the last 20 years. In both countries there has been a relative decline in the last 6 years in the age-specific fertility rate for all age groups, except for women in their late 30s and early 40s. Fertility rates for women aged 35 to 39 have risen from 28.27 to 32.52 per 1000 women, whereas those for women 40 to 44 years of age have risen from 3.88 to 5.19 per 1000 women.[2]

From 1980 to 1997, the number of twin births in the United States rose 52% (from 68,339 to 104,137), and triplet and higher births rose 404% (from 1377 to 6737 births). At the same time, differences in twin birth rates between non-Hispanic white and African American mothers disappeared. Non-Hispanic white women were more than twice as likely as African American or Hispanic women to have a triplet birth.[7]

Statistical data concerning the pregnant patient demographics and frequency of use of the emergency department and the diagnostic profile are incomplete because most observational data sets group perinatal and pregnancy as "other medical diagnosis," which accounts for less than 2% of visits to the emergency department in the United States and Canada.[8] The diagnosis of pregnancy in the emergency department can be unexpected and not immediately apparent at the conclusion of the history and physical examination. A study of random pregnancy tests performed on female trauma patients revealed that 2% were pregnant.[9,10] Even when the chance of pregnancy was remote, female patients seeking treatment in the emergency department had a pregnancy rate of at least 10%.[10]

Pregnant patients may come to the emergency department with (1) symptoms related to an undiagnosed, normal pregnancy (abdominal discomfort, nausea, urinary frequency, breast swelling and tenderness, fatigue, or near syncope), (2) symptoms related to complications of pregnancy (see Chapter 177), or (3) symptoms of chronic medical illnesses that may be exacerbated by pregnancy (see Chapter 178). This chapter covers the following aspects of a normal pregnancy: physiologic changes, common initial symptoms, diagnostic tests, and considerations regarding treatment and referral.

Definitions

Gravidity refers to the number of pregnancies that the patient has had. This number includes all normal and abnormal pregnancies, including the current one.

Parity is the total number of times that the patient has given birth, regardless of outcome. Multiple births are counted individually for the purpose of calculating parity. Parity can be divided into four distinct categories; they are usually written on the chart parenthetically, adjacent to the parity level, and separated by hyphens. The four categories are identified by the letters T-P-A-L and refer to numbers of term infants, preterm infants, abortions, and children currently living (e.g., G10 P9 [6-1-2-7]).

Gestational age refers to the number of completed weeks of pregnancy from the last menstrual period.[9] A term infant is a child born between 38 and 42 completed weeks of gestation, a preterm infant is born before 38 completed weeks of gestation, and a postterm infant is born any time after 42 weeks' gestation.[11] The conceptus is considered an embryo from conception until after the 8th week, when it is termed a fetus. An abortus is a fetus or embryo removed or expelled from the uterus during the first half of gestation (20 weeks or earlier) and that weighs less than 500 g or measures

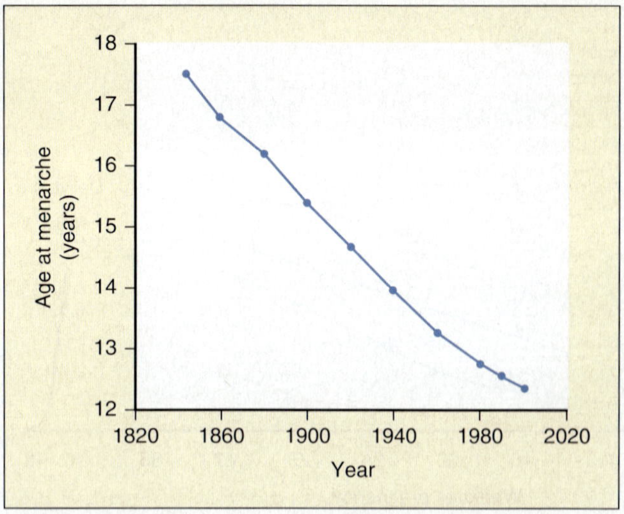

Figure 176-1. Age of menarche of European girls during the past 150 years. (Modified from Tanner JM: *Growth at Adolescence.* Oxford, Blackwell, 1962; Cunningham FG, et al: *Williams Obstetrics,* 19th ed. E Norwalk, Conn, Appleton & Lange, 1993; and MacDonald PC, et al: Recurrent secretion of progesterone in large amounts: An endocrine/metabolic disorder unique to young women? *Endocr Rev* 12:372, 1991.)

less than 25 cm.[11] Premature labor occurs before 37 weeks' gestation, and postmature labor occurs beyond 42 or 43 weeks' gestation.

PRINCIPLES OF DISEASE

Physiology of Pregnancy

Hormonal Role in Cyclic Ovulation and Fertilization

Near the end of each menstrual cycle, estradiol production in the ovary and corpus luteum is minimal. Most of the estrogen is in the form of estrone, produced by way of extraglandular aromatization of a plasma C19 steroid found in adipose tissue. At the midphase of each ovarian cycle, the rate of follicular development and ovarian estradiol secretion increases. Estradiol is essential for development, maturation, and ovulation of the follicle. After ovulation, the corpus luteum develops and produces progesterone in quantities exceeding the production of cortisol by the adrenal cortex. Progesterone is the "progestation steroid" essential to pregnancy.[11]

Fertilization occurs in the fallopian tube within minutes to hours after follicular ovulation. Implantation of the blastocyst in the endometrium occurs 6 days after fertilization. The life span of the corpus luteum is enhanced to maintain progesterone secretion. Human chorionic gonadotropin (hCG) originates in trophoblasts and augments corpus luteal production of progesterone until the trophoblastic production of progesterone is capable of maintaining pregnancy.[11]

The embryo-fetal-maternal biologic relationship results in maternal physiologic changes that permit embryonic-fetal development. The histocompatibility antigens are modified by trophoblasts to ensure maternal recognition and acceptance of the embryo-fetus. The fetus is protected from infection by the transplacental passage of selected antibodies. Nutrition and development are ensured by the placental transfer of nutrients in exchange for metabolic byproducts. Nutrition is preferentially transferred to the fetus at the expense of the maternal host.[11]

Maternal Adaptations to Pregnancy

Uterovaginal Structures

A nonpregnant uterus weighs 70 g and has a cavity capacity of 10 mL or less. At term, a normal pregnant uterus weighs approximately 1100 g and has a capacity of approximately 5 L, yet under specific circumstances it can accommodate 20 L or more. Uterine enlargement is asymmetric and is greatest in the fundus. In addition, placental attachment induces local myometrial hypertrophy that results in asymmetry.[11]

The cervix undergoes basal cell hyperplasia. The stratified squamous epithelium of the vagina and ectocervix is described as pink and glistening. The epithelium of the endocervix is columnar and appears reddish and velvety. The squamocolumnar junction is usually located at the external os of the cervix in a nonpregnant patient. In pregnancy, the columnar epithelium of the endocervix extends onto the ectocervix, is visualized as a reddish velvety lesion at the os, and is called pseudoerosion. It is hypothesized that the endocervical gland proliferation that occurs in pregnancy results in excessive glandular secretion of an alkaline solution that bathes the acidic ectocervix and encourages the growth of columnar epithelium onto the ectocervix. Excessive glandular secretion also results in a "mucosal plug" at the os. This plug prohibits ascending infection and is extruded just before labor.

The vaginal bacterium *Lactobacillus acidophilus* stimulates the metabolism of glycogen to lactic acid in the vaginal epithelium, which results in an acidic pH ranging from 3.5 to 6. It is thought that the acidic pH minimizes pathogenic bacterial overgrowth in the vagina.

Pregnancy-induced vaginal hyperemia and hypertrophy of the venous plexus result in a violaceous hue of the vaginal walls. In 1886 Chadwick described this color change at the vaginal introitus (Chadwick's sign). The color change begins as pale violet in the early months and progresses to a bluish and finally a dusky black tint near term.[12]

Cutaneous and Glandular Structures

In approximately 50% of pregnant women, striae gravidarum develop as a result of increased skin tension. The striae are reddish, depressed linear markings on the breasts, thighs, and abdominal wall that develop during the third trimester. The persistent striae in multiparous women are visualized as silver lines.[11] Increasing abdominal wall tension can also result in diastasis of the rectus muscles (diastasis recti).

Estrogen and progesterone are believed to have melanocyte-stimulating effects. Pregnancy-induced pigmentation changes include linea nigra, which is a

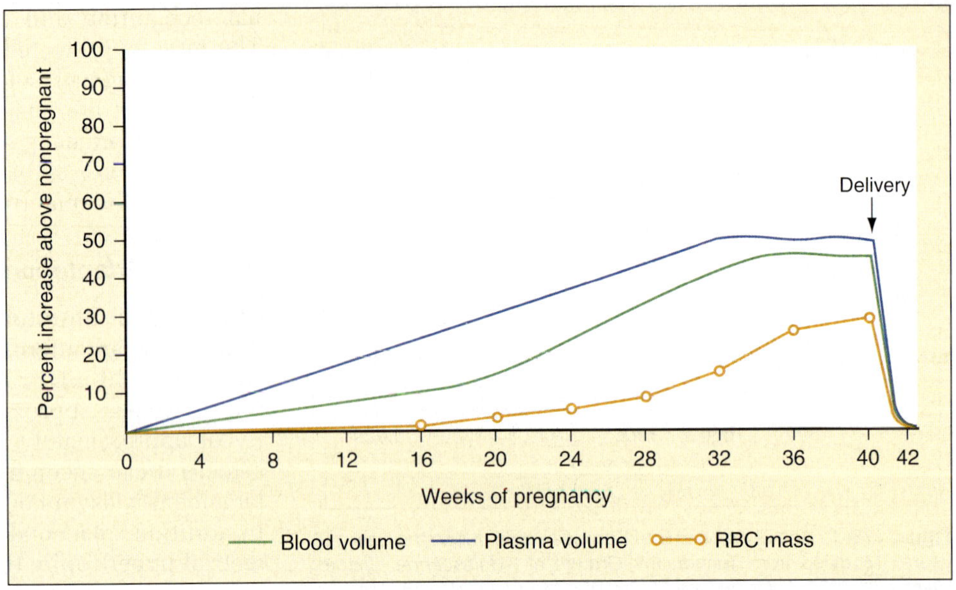

Figure 176-2. Changes in blood volume during pregnancy. (Modified from Scott DF: Anemia during pregnancy. *Obstet Gynecol Annu* 1:219, 1972.)

midline abdominal wall line, and chloasma or melasma gravidarum on the midface (the mask of pregnancy).

Vascular spiders, known as spider nevi, are seen in approximately two thirds of white and approximately 10% of African American pregnant women.[11] They are palpable, purpuric central lesions with tiny extensions resembling the legs of a spider. They preferentially occur in the face, neck, upper part of the chest, and arms. Palmar erythema is also more commonly seen in white women and is thought to be a result of increased estrogen. Changes in the breasts include initial tenderness and tingling, followed by an increase in size and nodularity. The latter changes result from hypertrophy of the mammary alveoli. The nipples enlarge and become more erect. The areolar area enlarges, and the glands of Montgomery (hypertrophic sebaceous glands) become more visible. Both the nipples and the areolae become more pigmented. During the second and third trimesters a thick yellow liquid, colostrum, can be expressed from the nipples.

Metabolism

The weight gain of pregnancy is attributed to the enlarging breasts and uterus, the amniotic sac and placenta, and the resultant increases in blood volume and extravascular fluid. In addition, the maternal host may accumulate reserves of water, fat, and protein. Weight gain is distributed throughout pregnancy and averages 1 kg in the first trimester and 5 kg in both the second and third trimesters.[13]

The average woman retains a minimum of 6.5 L of extra total body water during a normal pregnancy. The fetus, placenta, and amniotic fluid account for 3.5 L, and the remainder is attributable to the expanding maternal blood volume and the increase in size of the uterus and breasts.[11]

Water retention is due in part to a fall in plasma osmolality of 10 mOsm/kg. This fall in osmolality is the result of resetting of osmotic thresholds for thirst and secretion of vasopressin.[13] In addition, the enlarging uterus partially occludes the vena cava, more so in the supine position, and increases venous pressure distally, which results in pitting edema of the ankles and legs that may result in fluid shifts and accumulation of up to 1 L.

Pregnancy induces a state of peripheral resistance to insulin.[14] Biochemical evaluation for normal pregnancy reveals mild fasting hypoglycemia, postprandial hyperglycemia, hyperinsulinemia, and glucosuria.[15] Theoretically, this alteration in glucose metabolism ensures a persistent fetal glucose supply.[11] Pregnancy can result in clinical gestational diabetes or exacerbate existing diabetes.

Hematologic Indices

During pregnancy, plasma volume and erythrocyte production increase (450 mL, or 33%). The physiologic reasons for the increase in maternal blood volume are threefold: to minimize the effect of the erect and supine position on fetal and maternal circulation, to compensate for blood loss associated with parturition, and to meet the vascular needs of the enlarging uterus (Figure 176-2). Blood volumes are 45% above prepregnancy levels, and this same increase in blood volume is seen in patients with hydatidiform moles.[16]

Hemoglobin decreases slightly in pregnancy. The Centers for Disease Control and Prevention defined anemia in pregnancy as less than 11 g/dL during the first and third trimesters and less than 10.5 g/dL during the second trimester (Figure 176-3).[17] Total body iron stores in men are 4 g and in nonpregnant women vary between 2.0 and 2.5 g. For the most part, iron requirements, particularly during the latter half of pregnancy, exceed iron stores. The total iron requirement for pregnancy is 1 g: 200 mg for obligatory losses, 300 mg transferred to the fetus, and 500 mg for erythropoiesis. Iron supplementation during pregnancy is encouraged.[11]

Pregnancy has often been referred to as an "immunosuppressed state." Blood leukocyte counts during

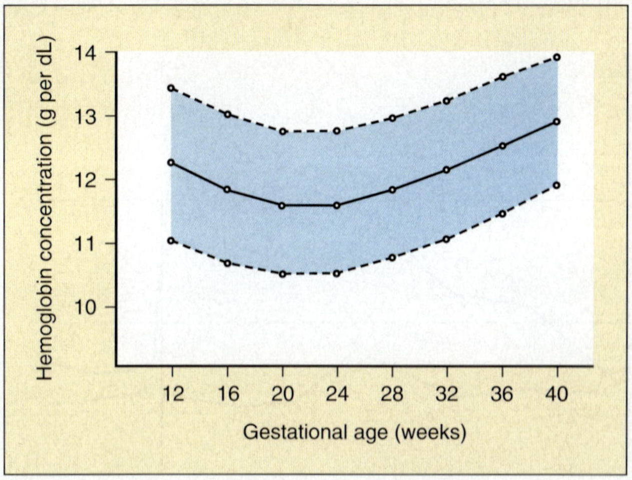

Figure 176-3. Mean hemoglobin concentrations *(solid circles)* and 5th and 95th percentiles *(open circles)* for healthy pregnant women taking iron supplements. (Modified from CDC criteria for anemia in children and childbearing-aged women. *MMWR Morb Mortal Wkly Rep* 38[22]:400, 1989.)

pregnancy normally vary from 5000/mL to 12,000/mL. However, polymorphonuclear leukocyte function is depressed, specifically with respect to chemotaxis and adherence, beginning in the second trimester and continuing throughout pregnancy. The reason remains unexplained.[18] It would appear that despite an increase in leukocyte numbers, the depressed function of polymorphonuclear leukocytes may predispose pregnant women to infection and may account for apparent improvement in some autoimmune diseases during pregnancy. Humoral antibody titers to viruses, including herpes simplex, measles, and influenza A, have been shown to decrease during pregnancy because of the expansion of plasma volume and subsequent hemodilutional effect of pregnancy.

The clotting times of whole blood remain unchanged. Pregnancy does induce increased levels of several coagulation factors, and the prothrombin time and partial thromboplastin time are both shortened. These changes are partially counteracted by the decrease in blood viscosity.

The platelet count decreases as pregnancy progresses.[19] Some believe it to be a result of pregnancy-induced platelet consumption.[20] An increase of 50% in plasma fibrinogen results in an elevated erythrocyte sedimentation rate.[21]

Some of the coagulation changes of pregnancy can be induced by the administration of contraceptive tablets containing estrogen and progestin.[11]

Cardiovascular System

As the diaphragm ascends during pregnancy, the heart is displaced upward and to the left and rotated on its long axis. In addition, normal pregnant women may have a benign form of pericardial effusion.[22] Thus, on a chest radiograph, the cardiac silhouette appears enlarged. The altered position of the heart results in a slight left axis deviation on the electrocardiogram. The resting heart rate increases 10 to 15 beats/min during pregnancy.[11]

Arterial blood pressure and vascular resistance decrease overall during normal pregnancy. Arterial blood pressure decreases during the second trimester and slowly rises during the third trimester. Cardiac output at rest in the lateral recumbent position steadily increases during pregnancy.[11] The changes in blood pressure and cardiac output during pregnancy reflect the physiologic balance of the decreasing blood pressure and vascular resistance concurrent with the increase in blood volume, maternal weight, and basal metabolic rate.

Arterial blood pressure is lowest in the lateral recumbent position and highest when sitting. Usually, blood pressure in the supine position is somewhere between these two levels. Some pregnant women become hypotensive in the supine position, a condition referred to as the supine hypotensive syndrome. In this position the enlarging pregnant uterus compresses the inferior vena cava, thereby decreasing venous return and cardiac output and resulting in arterial hypotension.[11] One study demonstrated significant lowering of arterial pressure distal to the level of uterine compression of the aorta in the supine position.[23] Thus, a supine pregnant woman with normal or hypotensive brachial pressure may have even lower uterine blood pressure. Accurate vital signs are best obtained with the patient in the left lateral decubitus position.

Venous pressure below the diaphragm increases throughout pregnancy (Figure 176-4). In the supine position, femoral venous pressure is initially 8 cm H_2O and rises to 24 cm before delivery. It has been shown with radiolabeled tracers that blood flow in the lower extremities is reduced in pregnancy unless the patient is in the lateral recumbent position. In the supine position, the enlarging uterus compresses the pelvic veins and inferior vena cava.[24,25] The resulting diminished blood flow and rise in femoral venous pressure may result in dependent edema, venous stasis, varicose veins in the legs and vulva, and hemorrhoids.

Respiratory System

An increased awareness of the need to breathe is present early in pregnancy.[26] A pregnant patient may report this sensation as dyspnea. During pregnancy, the diaphragm ascends 4 cm and the transverse diameter of the thorax increases by 2 cm. Tidal volume increases regardless of the ascension of the diaphragm as a result of increased diaphragmatic excursion. The increase in tidal volume lowers blood PCO_2 and paradoxically causes dyspnea.

Urinary System

By the second trimester the glomerular filtration rate (GFR) is increased by 50%.[27] This increase in GFR persists for the duration of the pregnancy. In the supine position, sodium and water excretion is reduced by 50%.[11] Nonetheless, pregnant women tend to accumulate dependent edema during the day and mobilize and excrete this fluid while asleep.

As a result of increased filtration, the plasma concentrations of creatinine and urea decrease during pregnancy. The increase in GFR and impaired tubular

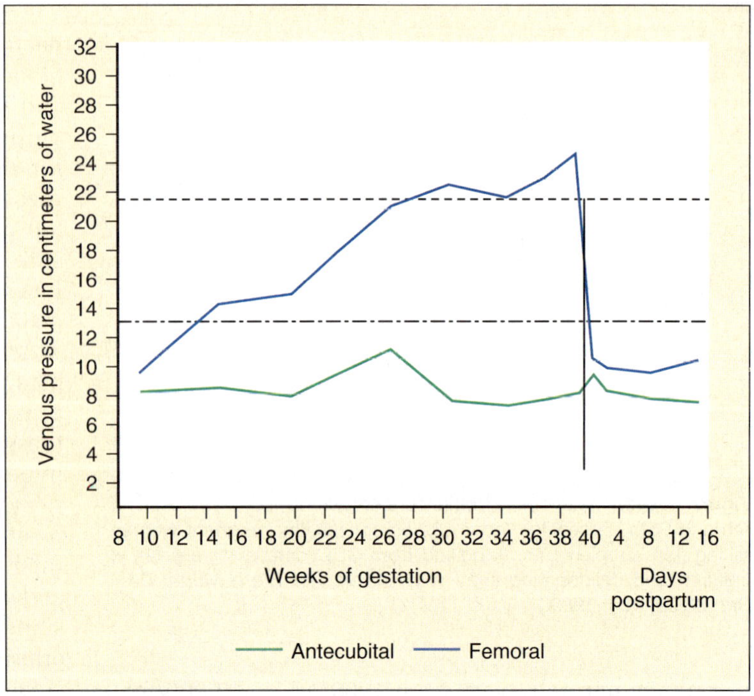

Figure 176-4. Serial changes in antecubital and femoral venous blood pressure throughout normal pregnancy and the early puerperium. These measurements were made on women in the supine position. (Modified from McLennan CE: Antecubital and femoral venous pressure in normal and toxemic pregnancy. *Am J Obstet Gynecol* 45:568, 1943.)

reabsorption of glucose result in glycosuria.[28] The presence of proteinuria and hematuria is usually pathologic. Active and vigorous labor may produce proteinuria in small amounts and hematuria as a result of trauma to the lower urinary tract.

The enlarging uterus rises out of the pelvis and compresses both ureters at the pelvic brim. The right ureter was preferentially compressed in 86% of pregnant women studied and may have been due to the engorged right ovarian vein complex compressing the right ureter.[29] Thus, a pregnant patient is at risk for hydronephrosis and hydroureter.

Gastrointestinal Tract

The gums become hyperemic and quite soft and may bleed with aggressive brushing. The epulis of pregnancy is a focal, highly vascular swelling of the gums that occurs spontaneously and resolves without treatment postpartum.

Gastric emptying and intestinal transit times are reduced during pregnancy as a result of mechanical and hormonal influences. The heartburn of pregnancy (pyrosis) occurs because of acid reflux in the lower part of the esophagus and is attributable to a hormonally mediated decrease in lower esophageal sphincter tone and an altered position of the stomach in response to the enlarging uterus. The latter results in higher intragastric pressure during pregnancy.[11]

Liver structure is unchanged during pregnancy; however, alkaline phosphatase activity is doubled. This increase may be attributable to placental alkaline phosphatase isoenzymes and high levels of circulating estrogen. Nonpregnant women taking estrogen can also have elevated levels of alkaline phosphatase.[30]

Contractility of the gallbladder is impaired, and a high residual volume is thought to be due to increased circulating progesterone.[11] Gallbladder stasis and increased cholesterol saturation may explain the increased prevalence of cholesterol stones in pregnancy.[31]

The cause of the cholestasis of pregnancy is unknown. The incidence is approximately 1 in 500 to 1000 pregnancies.[32,33] Cholestasis results in the accumulation of bile acids that undergo enterohepatic circulation and bacterial degradation to secondary bile acids. Pruritus gravidarum is a dermatologic manifestation of the retained bile acids.

Icterus gravidarum describes a mild form of jaundice resulting from the retention of conjugated bilirubin. The total bilirubin level may reach a maximum of 4.0 to 5.0 mg/dL.[11]

Pregnancy contributes to the development or exacerbation of existing hemorrhoids as a result of the associated increase in venous pressure distal to the uterus and concomitant constipation.

Endocrine System

The pituitary gland enlarges by 135% during pregnancy without compromise to the optic chiasma or visual fields. The level of serum prolactin rises during pregnancy, decreases postpartum, and increases in response to breast-feeding. The incidence of pituitary prolactinomas is not increased during pregnancy; however, tumor enlargement does occur.[11]

Normal pregnancy does not cause significant thyromegaly; therefore any goiter during pregnancy should be investigated. Thyroid regulation is altered in pregnancy, but maternal thyroid laboratory test results remain unchanged from nonpregnant levels. Fetal thyroid function is independent of and, for the most part, protected from the maternal thyroid status. However, a long-acting thyroid stimulator may cross the placenta in patients with Graves' disease and cause fetal thyrotoxicosis.

BOX 176-1. Summary of Risks during Pregnancy Attributed to Maternal Adaptation to Pregnancy

Physiologic
- Persistent colostrum secretion
- Angiomas or vascular spiders
- Excessive weight gain
- Iron deficiency anemia
- Increased risk of infection
- Gestational diabetes or exacerbation of existing diabetes mellitus
- Epulis
- Pruritus gravidarum
- Icterus gravidarum
- Inability to continue to use contact lenses

Mechanical or Positional
- Diastasis recti
- Striae gravidarum
- Lymphedema and dependent edema
- Venous stasis and increased risk of thromboembolism
- Supine hypotension syndrome
- Hydroureter and hydronephrosis
- Pyrosis
- Hemorrhoids
- Lordosis and kyphosis
- Meralgia paresthetica

Musculoskeletal System

Pregnant patients undergo postural changes to compensate for the anterior position of the enlarging uterus, and these changes result in pronounced lordosis and kyphosis. The weight of the enlarging breasts pulls the shoulders forward. The chin juts forward as a result of weak cervical spine flexors and shortened cervical spine extensors. The exaggerated lordosis and kyphosis shift the center of gravity over the lower extremities, and this realignment, in addition to the ligament laxity of pregnancy, may give rise to lower back discomfort, especially during the latter half of pregnancy.

In addition, in late pregnancy, anterior flexion of the neck and slumping of the shoulder girdle may result in traction on the ulnar and median nerves and is seen clinically as numbness, aching, and weakness in the upper extremities.[34]

Ophthalmologic System

An increase in corneal thickness is thought to be due to accumulation of fluid in pregnant women. Thus, it may be difficult for pregnant women to continue to use contact lenses. Moreover, Krukenberg spindles, or brownish red opacities in the posterior surface of the cornea, occur more often during pregnancy.[11]

Maternal adaptations to pregnancy, outlined in the previous section, are summarized in Box 176-1.

CLINICAL FEATURES

History

It is prudent practice to suspect pregnancy when assessing all female patients of childbearing age. Cyclic ovulation occurs on average for 38 years. Out of a possible 10,000 ovarian follicles, 500 achieve ovulation.[11] Thus, there are "500 opportunities for pregnancy which likely can be achieved by sexual intercourse on any one of 1500 days. Physicians of all specialties must be constantly vigilant and sensitive to the possibility that women of reproductive age may be pregnant irrespective of their presenting complaint."[11]

The reliability of the sexual and menstrual history has been notably poor. Ramouska and colleagues reported that 11.5% of women with abdominal pain or vaginal bleeding had positive pregnancy tests, in contrast to their perception that there was "no chance" that they were pregnant.[10,11] Missed diagnosis of pregnancy in adolescents was associated with failure to document a sexual or menstrual history. Adolescents rarely mentioned the possibility of pregnancy at triage (10%), and 10% denied being sexually active.[35]

Early signs and symptoms of pregnancy elicited during the history include cessation of menses, anorexia, nausea, easy fatigability, urinary frequency, breast swelling and tenderness, and the perception of fetal movement (quickening at 16 to 20 weeks).

Cessation of menses becomes suggestive of pregnancy when it occurs 10 days or more after the time that menstruation is expected. Intermittent, spontaneous vaginal bleeding or vaginal discharge is common during the first half of pregnancy, particularly in multiparous women. Most women without cervical lesions experience bleeding on or before the 40th day of pregnancy. This bleeding has been interpreted by some authors to be physiologic in origin and a result of implantation.[36] Nevertheless, any patient coming to the emergency department with vaginal bleeding during pregnancy should be considered at risk for a pathologic cause until proved otherwise.

It is possible to calculate the estimated date of conception in a regularly menstruating woman who has 28-day cycles and can give a reliable history. Nägele's rule is to add 7 days to the date of the first day of the last menstrual period and subtract 3 months.

Physical Examination

During the last half of pregnancy the physical examination should be done in the left lateral recumbent position to avoid supine hypotension syndrome.

The vital signs of a pregnant patient are essentially the same as those of a nonpregnant patient. The only changes are seen in the heart rate and blood pressure. The resting heart rate increases approximately 10 to 15 beats/min. Blood pressure in the brachial artery is highest in the sitting position, lowest when lying in the left lateral position, and intermediate in the supine position, except in pregnant women who have supine hypotension syndrome. Pathologic hypertension of pregnancy is defined as a sustained rise of 30 mm Hg systolic or 15 mm Hg diastolic over baseline values on at least two occasions, 6 hours or more apart.[11]

The fetal heart sound should be included as the fifth vital sign in the evaluation of a pregnant patient. It can be auscultated with a stethoscope at 17 weeks' gestation, on average, and by 19 weeks in nearly all pregnancies in nonobese women. With the use of Doppler ultrasonography, fetal cardiac activity can be detected as early as 8 weeks; however, it is more commonly heard by 10 weeks. It is possible to detect fetal heart activity at 48 days' gestation with echocardiography.

Auscultation of the pregnant abdomen reveals numerous findings that may be confusing. In addition to the fetal heart sound, it may be possible to identify sounds of fetal movement, the maternal pulse, maternal bowel sounds, and the fundic and uterine souffle. The fundic or umbilical cord souffle is created by blood rushing through the umbilical arteries. The whistling sound created is timed with the fetal pulse and present in 15% of pregnancies. The uterine souffle is a soft blowing sound timed with the maternal pulse and usually heard in the lower portion of the uterus. It is a function of blood flow through the dilated uterine vessels and can be heard in pregnancy and in women with uterine myomas or large tumors of the ovaries.[11]

Breast tenderness and fullness are common symptoms of pregnancy that can be appreciated on gentle physical examination. Objective breast changes include darkened areolae, more prominent glands of Montgomery around the nipple, engorged breasts with tiny bluish venules, and visible colostrum at the nipple with gentle massage of the breasts. This milky material may persist for months or even years, especially if the patient continues to breast-feed.

Increased skin pigmentation (melasma gravidarum) and abdominal striae occur not only in pregnancy but also in women who ingest estrogen-progestin contraceptives.

Braxton-Hicks contractions are painless contractions that occur spontaneously and irregularly early in pregnancy. They are also seen in patients with hematometra and those with uterine myomas. These contractions are not reliable for the diagnosis of pregnancy; however, they do not occur in ectopic pregnancy and thus their presence may be helpful in excluding the existence of an ectopic pregnancy.[11]

Uterine enlargement can be felt in nonobese women. At 6 to 8 weeks the uterus is about the size of an orange. At 12 weeks the top of the fundus should be at the level of the symphysis pubis, at 16 to 20 weeks at the level of the umbilicus, and at 36 to 38 weeks at the level of the xiphoid process of the sternum. Henceforth, the fetus descends into the pelvis, and fundal height may decrease accordingly.[37]

At approximately 6 to 8 weeks of pregnancy, Hegar's sign can be appreciated during an internal pelvic examination. Hegar's sign is softening of the lower uterine segment caused by hyperemia. In some cases the softening is sufficient to allow the examiner to easily distinguish the cervix from the fundus on palpation. It can be found in other conditions; however, it is not as easily palpated as it is in pregnancy (Figure 176-5).

The vaginal mucosa becomes hyperemic during pregnancy and with any other condition that causes congestion of the pelvic organs. In response, the color of the mucosa of the vaginal walls changes from pink to blue to violet and can be visualized at the vaginal introitus (Chadwick's sign).[12]

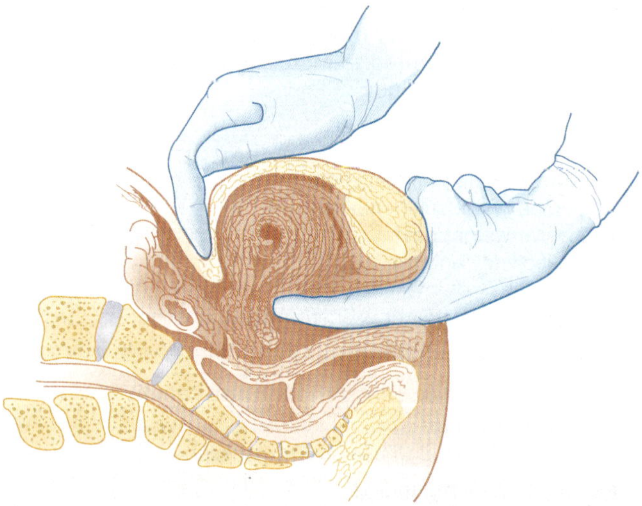

Figure 176-5. Hegar's sign. The softness and compressibility of the lower uterine segment can be so extreme that the fundus and cervix may even feel like separate organs. (Modified from Willson JR, et al: *Obstetrics and Gynecology,* 5th ed. St Louis, CV Mosby, 1975.)

At midpregnancy the fetus can be perceived by ballottement or palpated through the maternal abdominal wall in a nonobese patient. The fetus floats in a large volume of amniotic fluid. Thus, ballottement is perceived when pressure exerted on the uterus causes the fetus to sink and then rebound to its original position. Palpating the outline of the fetal body becomes easier near the end of pregnancy; however, subserosal myomas can simulate the fetal head and small parts, or both.[11]

DIAGNOSTIC STRATEGIES

Laboratory

Determination of urine or serum hCG is important in clinical management. Applications include diagnosis and monitoring of pregnancy and diagnosis and evaluation of the course of neoplastic trophoblastic disease or response to treatment (i.e., hydatidiform choriocarcinoma, gonadal teratoma, or a carcinoma with ectopic secretion of hCG).[38]

hCG assays are referenced to standard hCG preparations. Thus, the reference standard should always be noted when comparing results. One nanogram of hCG equals 9.3 mIU of the international reference standard provided by the World Health Organization (used in this text) and equals 5.0 mIU of the second international standard.[39]

Biologic assays for hCG are now only of historical interest. Since the 1960s, all hCG assays have been immunoassays. Enzyme-linked immunosorbent assay (ELISA) is the state-of-the-art pregnancy test. ELISA offers greater user convenience and has a sensitivity between 25 and 50 IU/L.

Over the years the pregnancy test has undergone a number of refinements. Antibodies are selected that act

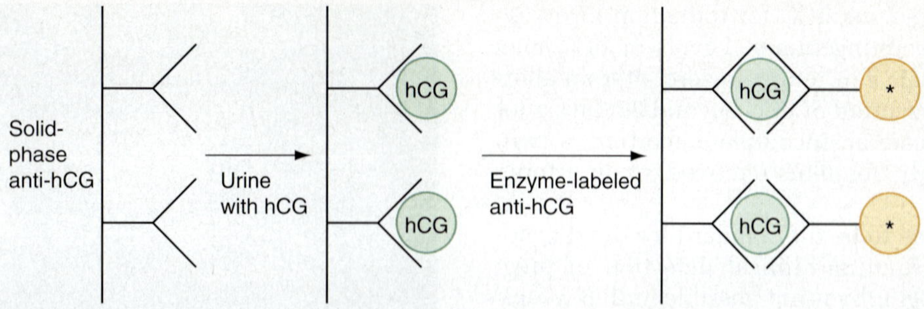

Figure 176-6. The principle of enzyme immunoassay (also sometimes known as "sandwich" or "immunometric" assays). hCG, human chorionic gonadotropin. (Modified from Chard T: Pregnancy tests: A review. *Hum Reprod* 7:701, 1992.)

against the purified β subunit of hCG, and this modification has resulted in improved sensitivity for low levels of hCG in the presence of luteinizing hormone. The development of monoclonal antibodies has improved specificity for the purified β subunit of hCG.

The fundamental process of ELISA involves an antibody adherent to a solid-faced support (usually plastic) that binds to a region of the hCG molecule. A second antibody chemically linked to an enzyme (for example, alkaline phosphatase) binds to another side of the trapped hCG molecule. The hCG molecule is sandwiched between the two antibodies. Excess enzyme-linked antibody is washed away, and a color developer is added and becomes blue when it comes in contact with the enzyme (Figure 176-6). The antibodies can be polyclonal or monoclonal. Many variations exist with respect to the solid-faced support and the method of developing the color reaction.

In July 1988 the first one-step pregnancy test became available. It was developed and patented by Unipath and is sold as Clearblue One Step. This test uses monoclonal antibodies specific for the β subunit of hCG. It includes a unique built-in control that shows a blue line when the test is complete and performed correctly.[40] This test appeals to consumers because it is rapid (takes less than 5 minutes), requires no manipulation by the user, offers hygienic sample handling, provides clear and easy-to-read results, and has a sensitivity between 25 and 50 mIU/mL.

The one-step test is an important development. Earlier studies revealed that results obtained by laypersons using more complicated home pregnancy tests were found to be less accurate than those performed by trained technologists. The incidence of false-negative results was 25%, and only a third of the lay users complied with the test instructions.

A well-designed ELISA applied to urine is not affected by drugs or a concurrent physiologic state. The only exception is exogenous hCG for induction of ovulation.[41]

Normal hCG levels in men and premenopausal women range from 0.02 to 0.8 IU/L. Postmenopausal women may have higher levels.[42] The blastocyst begins to secrete hCG 7 days after fertilization.[43] Thus, the hCG released can be detected as early as 6 to 8 days after conception.[44,45]

The initial doubling time is fast and has been attributed to the actual process of implantation. This is followed by a slower rate of doubling as trophoblast hCG and maternal circulatory hCG equilibrate (Figure 176-7).[45] hCG levels peak at 7 to 10 weeks of pregnancy with a mean value of 50,000 IU/L and a range of 20,000 to 200,000 IU/L.[46]

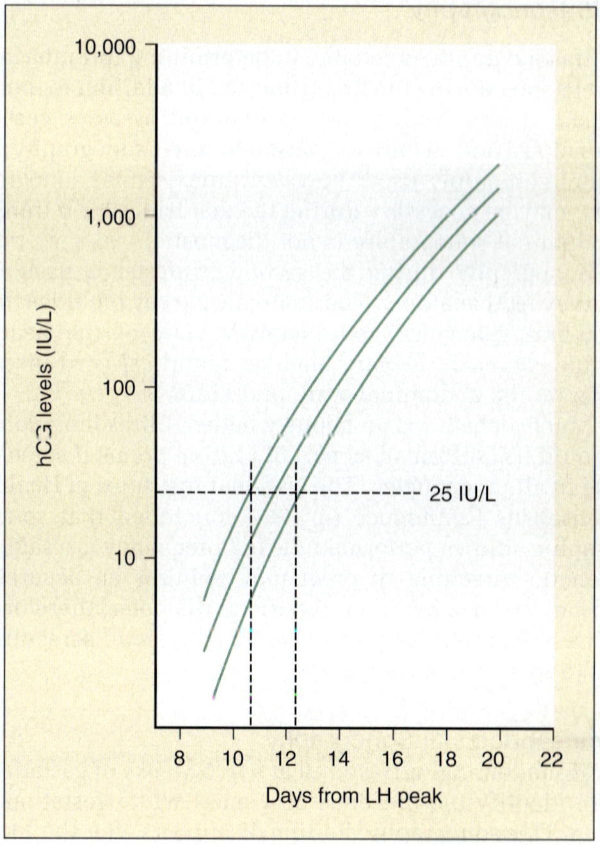

Figure 176-7. Levels of circulating human chorionic gonadotropin (hCG) in early pregnancy showing that an assay with a sensitivity of 25 IU/L would become positive in some subjects between 10 and 11 days after the peak in luteinizing hormone (LH) and in most subjects 12 to 13 days after the peak. (Modified from Chard T: Pregnancy tests: A review. *Hum Reprod* 7:701, 1992.)

hCG testing becomes positive in 98% of patients 7 days after implantation, which coincides with the time of the expected period. When a test with a sensitivity of 25 to 50 IU/L is used, a negative result 1 week from the expected time of the missed period essentially guarantees that a woman is not pregnant.[41]

The minimum number of false-positive results can be attributed to postmenopausal status, abortion in the first trimester, exogenous hCG for induction of ovulation, or an hCG-secreting tumor. Levels of hCG may take as long as 60 days to return to zero after an abortion.[47] Persistent elevation of hCG beyond 60 days after abortion may indicate an incomplete abortion, a twin pregnancy with only one fetus removed, or an ectopic pregnancy.[11]

hCG will continue to be the standard for the diagnosis of pregnancy. Routine clinical detection of pregnancy by ultrasonography is not possible until 6 weeks' gestation, when hCG is 1000 IU/L or more.[48-50]

Radiology

Ultrasonography

Ultrasonography is reliable in determining intrauterine pregnancy during the first trimester. In addition to diagnosis, it also locates the embryo and assesses gestational age and viability. Transabdominal sonography is more commonly used; however, transvaginal sonography may be necessary during the first trimester if transabdominal sonography is not diagnostic.

Sonography during the second trimester is used to survey fetal anatomy. The anatomic survey includes the cerebral ventricles, four-chamber view of the heart, spine, stomach, urinary bladder, umbilical cord insertion on the abdominal wall, and kidneys.[51]

Much debate exists about whether ultrasonography should be performed as part of routine prenatal screening in all pregnancies. The National Institutes of Health Consensus Conference in 1984 concluded that sonographic studies performed during pregnancy are safe.[52] Genetic screening of pregnancy requires an accurate gestational age based on biparietal diameter; therefore, ultrasonography as part of maternal genetic screening at 15 to 16 weeks is routine.

Transabdominal Sonography

Transabdominal ultrasound at 4 to 5 weeks of gestation can identify the presence of a small white gestational ring. This sonographic finding disappears after the 11th week of gestation.[11]

At 6 weeks the gestational sac can be visualized by transabdominal sonography (Figure 176-8). The sac is confirmed when two central uterine echoes are visualized within the hypertrophied endometrium. This diagnostic echo is called the double decidual sac sign. A healthy pregnancy can be determined by correlating the size of the sac with gestational age and quantitative hCG values.[53] At 8 weeks the fetal pole and fetal heart activity can be visualized reliably with transabdominal ultrasound in a normal pregnancy.

Transvaginal Sonography

Transvaginal sonography has greater resolution than transabdominal sonography and does not require a full bladder. Transvaginal ultrasound can identify an intrauterine gestational yolk sac at 5 weeks' gestation. This finding correlates with a quantitative hCG value of more than 1800 IU/L.[54] Fetal heart motion can be detected with transvaginal ultrasound at 6 weeks' gestation and correlates with an hCG level of 6770 IU/L and a crown-rump length of 2 mm.[11]

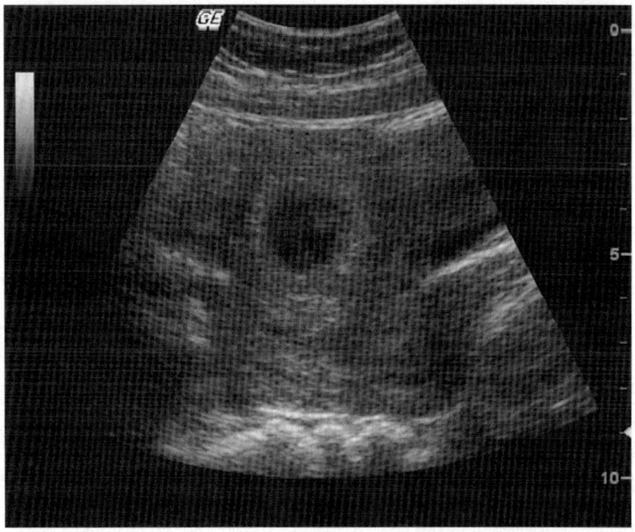

Figure 176-8. Transabdominal ultrasound showing a gestational sac with no fetal pole or yolk sac. (Courtesy of Andrew A. Common, MD.)

An intrauterine pregnancy can be diagnosed by sonographic findings in the following order of appearance: the double ring sign, the double gestational sac, the intrauterine fetal pole, and intrauterine fetal heart activity (Figure 176-9A to C). The gestational sac is eccentrically positioned within an asymmetrically thickened decidua. An ectopic pregnancy can be difficult to distinguish from a normal pregnancy and may be seen sonographically as a pseudosac or fluid collection centrally placed in the uterine cavity and surrounded by symmetrically thickened endometrium.[55]

Magnetic Resonance Imaging

No significant side effects have been documented to date with the magnetic field and radio waves used in magnetic resonance imaging. Gadolinium is the most common intravenous contrast agent, and allergic reactions with this agent are rare. The effects of strong magnetic fields on the fetus are unknown, and it is therefore recommended that pregnant women avoid magnetic resonance imaging.

Plain Radiographic Fetal Identification

The fetus can be reliably recognized by plain radiography after 16 weeks' gestation. Fetal foci of ossification can be identified as early as 14 weeks.[11]

Diagnostic Imaging Considerations in Pregnant Patients

The decision to perform imaging investigations of a pregnant patient must take into consideration the risk to the developing fetus of radiation, the inherent risk to the mother of the investigations, and the risk to the mother and fetus of missing the diagnosis because of reluctance to use available diagnostic imaging techniques. The adverse outcomes of intrauterine fetal exposure to the radiation used in radiography are

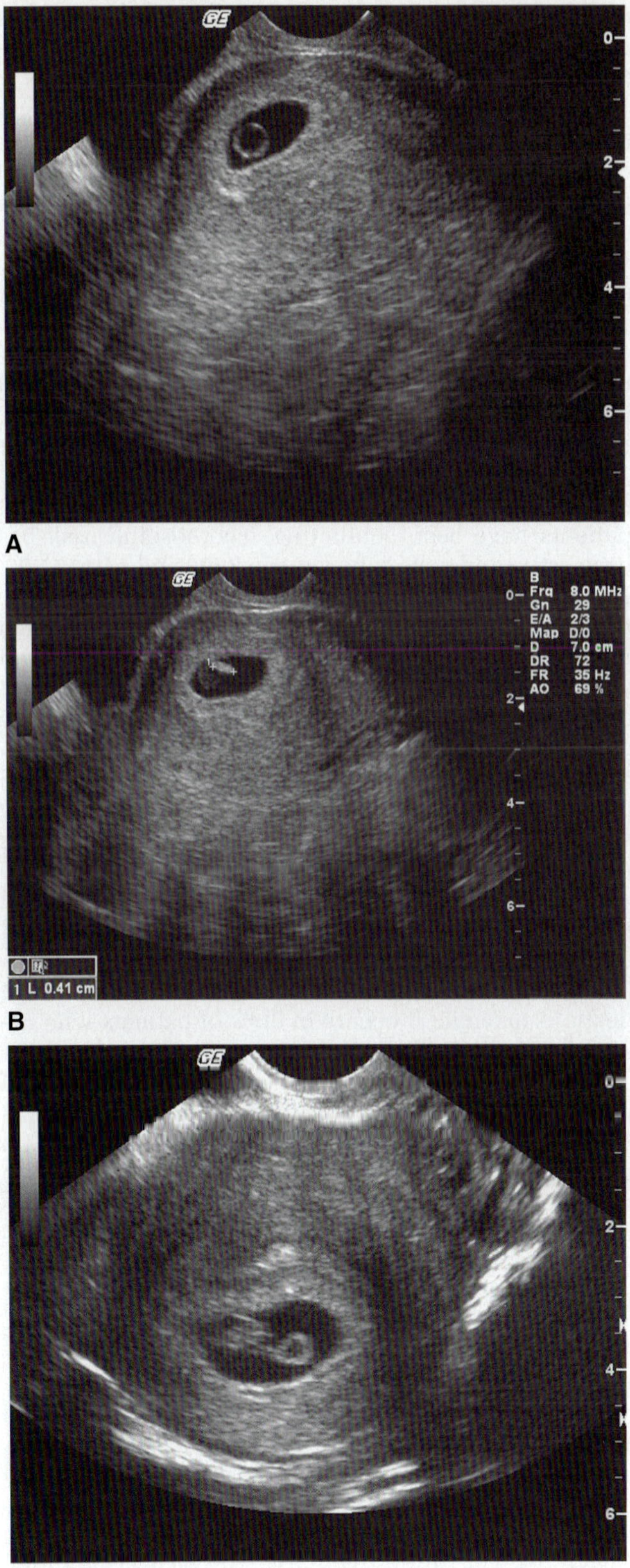

A

B

C

Figure 176-8. Transvaginal ultrasound images. **A**, Yolk sac. **B**, Fetal pole. **C**, Fetal pole, vitelline duct, and yolk sac. (Courtesy of Andrew A. Common, MD.)

minimal. Case-controlled studies report a slight, but statistically significant increase in the relative risk for childhood cancer.[56] Radiation is a dose-dependent teratogen.[57] The fetal central nervous system is most vulnerable to the teratogenic effects of radiation from 8 to 15 weeks after conception. The fetal dose of radiation is estimated from the ovarian or uterine dose. Pregnant women exposed to less than 5000 mrad have pregnancy outcomes similar to those of controls.[58] A study of childhood cancers in the offspring of female radiologists revealed a cancer frequency of 0.16% in children exposed to 1000 mrem of radiation in utero. This figure compares with a cancer frequency of 0.07% in children who were not exposed to radiation in utero.

Table 176-1. Fetal Radiation Exposure with Various Imaging Modalities

Procedure	Estimated Fetal Radiation Exposure (mrad)
Unilateral venography without an abdominal shield	305
Limited venography with an abdominal shield	<50
Pulmonary angiography via femoral access	405
Pulmonary angiography via brachial access with an abdominal shield	<50
Perfusion lung scan using ^{99m}Tc-MAA	
3 mCi	18
1-2 mCi	6-12
Ventilation lung scan using	
^{133}Xe	3-20
^{99m}Tc-DTPA	7-35
^{99m}Tc-SC	1-5
Ventilation-perfusion scan	<55

DTPA, diethylenetriaminepentaacetic acid; MAA, microaggregated albumin; SC, sulfur colloid.

Modified from Ginsberg JS, et al: Thrombotic complications in the obstetric patient. In Coleman RW, et al (eds): *Hemostasis and Thrombosis: Basic Principles and Clinical Practice*, 3rd ed. Philadelphia. JB Lippincott, 1994.

Table 176-1 outlines the estimated fetal radiation exposure associated with the more common diagnostic imaging modalities. Radiation exposure depends on the equipment and technique, and estimates listed may not be generalizable to every department.

A thoughtful, commonsense approach to the differential diagnosis will provide a sound basis for imaging investigations that will undoubtedly be in the best interests of the mother and the fetus. A commonsense approach will ensure that the risks of radiation exposure in the mother and fetus are balanced with the risk of missing the diagnosis and failing to act accordingly.

DIFFERENTIAL CONSIDERATIONS

The differential diagnosis of early pregnancy includes myomas, hematometra, adenomyosis, or an extrauterine mass or masses. Patients with these diagnoses excluding hematometra (a blood collection or retention in the uterus), typically have persistent regular menses. The enlarged uterus in these nonpregnant conditions is generally firmer and less elastic and boggy than it is in pregnancy.[11]

Spurious pregnancy is imaginary pregnancy or pseudocyesis (false phantom). It usually occurs in women nearing menopause or in women who have an overwhelming desire for pregnancy. The associated increase in abdominal girth is generally attributed to fat deposition, fluid accumulation, or intestinal gas. The menses may become unpredictable with respect to timing, duration, and amount of flow. This condition can be associated with changes in the breasts, including enlargement, galactorrhea, and increased areolar pigmentation. Patients may have morning sickness of psychogenic origin. The associated use of phenothiazines may cause amenorrhea, hyperprolactinemia, breast enlargement, and galactorrhea. Women with this condition may perceive fetal movements. Most commonly these movements can be attributed to muscular contractions of the abdominal wall and normal gastrointestinal peristalsis.[11]

The diagnosis is confirmed by the presence of a small uterus and a negative pregnancy test. The challenge in this condition is convincing the woman of the lack of pregnancy and dealing with the underlying reason for this delusion.

SPECIFIC DISORDERS

Perspective

In general, a pregnant patient should be treated and assessed in the same way as all other patients. However, the normal physiologic changes of pregnancy may mask or unmask underlying medical conditions. In addition, consideration should be given to the increased medical risks of pregnancy (e.g., deep vein thrombosis) and risk to the fetus when exposed to diagnostic imaging or surgical interventions.

Headache

The most common headache during pregnancy is a muscle contraction headache.[59] The patient has usually had a history of headaches before the pregnancy. The headaches begin on waking and increase in intensity during the day. The headache is described as a broad band, squeezing or constricting in quality, and localized to the vertex. The paracervical muscles are taut, and palpation usually reproduces or exacerbates the pain. During pregnancy these headaches are worsened by postural changes and psychosocial stress. Eighty percent of classic migraine sufferers have remission from attacks during pregnancy, particularly women with menstrual migraines.[60] Therefore, any headache other than a muscle contraction headache in a pregnant patient requires investigation.[61]

Brain tumors enlarge during pregnancy and shrink temporarily postpartum.[62] Most brain tumors become symptomatic during the second half of pregnancy, and they account for 10% of maternal deaths during pregnancy. Both pituitary gland and prolactin-secreting adenomas swell during pregnancy. Headache usually develops during the first trimester and precedes visual changes by approximately 1 month.[59] Occasionally, central venous thrombosis may occur during pregnancy and mimic eclampsia. The lack of proteinuria and hypertension points to the former diagnosis.[59] Central venous thrombosis is an unusual cause of postpartum headache that is associated with a mortality of 40%.[59]

Pseudotumor cerebri is benign intracranial hypertension in the absence of a mass lesion and hydrocephalus. Symptoms often include headache and papilledema. Other associated symptoms include decreased visual acuity, loss of color vision, defects in visual fields, and horizontal diplopia caused by abducens nerve palsy.[59] Pseudotumor cerebri associated with pregnancy usually occurs in obese women and begins during the third to fifth months of pregnancy. Symptoms resolve spontaneously after 1 to 3 months.[63]

Spontaneous subarachnoid hemorrhage accounts for 10% of maternal deaths. Reviews of the risk for subarachnoid hemorrhage in pregnant versus nonpregnant patients have been conflicting. The absolute risk has been estimated to be between 1 in 2000 and 1 in 10,000. The majority of intracranial bleeding is attributed to rupture of an arteriovenous malformation or a ruptured intracranial aneurysm. The overall risk for rupture of an arteriovenous malformation is identical in pregnant and nonpregnant patients without previous bleeding at 0.031 per patient-year.[64] Arteriovenous malformations usually bleed during the second trimester and during labor. Berry aneurysms initially bleed during the third trimester, and the incidence of bleeding increases as the pregnancy advances.

Nearly a third of cases of spontaneous subarachnoid hemorrhage are a result of bleeding disorders, bacterial endocarditis, metastatic tumor, and sickle cell disease. Cerebral hemorrhage is the most common cause of death in toxemia. It occurs in 60% of patients who die after becoming eclamptic.[59]

A new onset of headache during pregnancy should make the emergency physician wary. A thorough history and a detailed physical examination with emphasis on visual field and funduscopic examination can, in most cases, exclude the aforementioned serious disorders.

Chest Pain

The diagnosis of cardiac disease is complicated by the fact that the signs and symptoms of a normal pregnancy are suggestive of heart disease. Pregnancy is associated with easy fatigability, dyspnea, orthopnea, palpitations, syncope, peripheral edema, chest discomfort, and reflux. Symptomatic triggers for further cardiac evaluation include progressive orthopnea, dyspnea severe enough to limit activity, paroxysmal nocturnal dyspnea, syncope during or immediately after exertion, hemoptysis, and chest pain in an ischemic distribution at rest or associated with exertion, anxiety, or anger.[59]

Cardiovascular findings are altered in normal pregnancy. Peripheral edema is present in 80% of pregnant women. A third heart sound and systolic murmurs are common. Diastolic murmurs and systolic murmurs greater than II/VI deserve investigation. Other worrisome signs include cyanosis, clubbing, pulmonary rales, distended neck veins throughout the cardiac cycle associated with hepatomegaly and peripheral edema, persistent split S_2, and criteria of pulmonary hypertension (left parasternal lift and a loud P_2).[59]

The incidence of pulmonary embolism and deep vein thrombosis during pregnancy is unknown. In 1986 the National Institutes of Health held a consensus conference and concluded that the likelihood of venous thromboembolism during the puerperium after a normal pregnancy increased by a factor of 5 when compared with nonpregnant patients with similar demographics.[65] A pregnant patient is predisposed to deep vein thrombosis for the following reasons: (1) increased venous pressure, decreased distal venous flow, and significant venous stasis as a result of compression of the pelvic veins and inferior vena cava by the enlarging uterus; (2) the antepartum use of oral contraceptives before conception; and (3) the propensity for stasis in the workplace and at home as the pregnancy progresses.[11]

This increased risk for thromboembolism mandates thorough evaluation of a pregnant patient who complains of pleuritic chest pain, right-sided heart failure, and more subtle signs such as unexplained fever, dyspnea, or tachycardia.

Abdominal Pain

Displacement of the abdominal contents by the expanding uterus during pregnancy causes abdominal discomfort that may be associated with nausea, vomiting, gastroesophageal reflux, delayed gastric emptying, bowel irregularity, urinary frequency, and back and buttock pain. These symptoms may complicate the clinical assessment of a pregnant woman with abdominal pain. Delay or failure to diagnose and treat any underlying pathology may result in high maternal and fetal morbidity and mortality.

Obstetric causes of abdominal pain early in pregnancy include vascular congestion of the pelvic tissues, round ligament tension, ectopic pregnancy, and threatened abortion. Later in pregnancy, the obstetric differential diagnosis should include Braxton-Hicks contractions, toxemia, premature labor, abruptio placentae, or rupture of the uterus.[59] Nonobstetric causes include all diagnoses seen in a nonpregnant patient (e.g., cholecystitis, pyelonephritis, renal colic, ovarian torsion, salpingitis, corpus luteum cyst rupture or torsion, and degeneration of a uterine myoma). Common surgical diseases that may complicate pregnancy include appendicitis, cholecystitis, cholelithiasis, and intestinal obstruction.

The incidence of appendicitis in a pregnant patient is equal to that in a nonpregnant patient, but the perforation rate is higher. The state of pregnancy results in delays in diagnosis of appendicitis that contribute significantly to maternal and fetal morbidity and mortality.[66] Perinatal mortality in nonperforated appendicitis is 4.8%. It rises, however, to 27.8% with perforation at the time of surgery. The perforation rate is as high as 30% during the third trimester.[67]

The diagnosis is more difficult during the latter half of pregnancy, but it is challenging even in early pregnancy. Anorexia, nausea, and vomiting are symptomatic of appendicitis and may be misinterpreted as hyperemesis of pregnancy. As the uterus enlarges, the appendix moves upward and outward toward the right. As the appendix moves higher, the omentum is unable to surround the appendix and contain the infection if rupture occurs. Thus, appendiceal rupture in pregnant women results in generalized peritonitis.[11]

Musculoskeletal Pain

Hand symptoms are common during pregnancy. The median nerve is at risk for compression distally within the carpal tunnel. Approximately 25% of pregnant women complain of hand symptoms compatible with median nerve compression, but only 2.3% are actually found to have carpel tunnel syndrome.[68] Symptoms of carpal tunnel syndrome include burning, numbness, and tingling in the thenar aspect. The patient is often awakened from sleep with the onset of symptoms. In 80% of cases, the symptoms are bilateral. Because the symptoms usually resolve during the postpartum period, treatment is supportive. A sleep splint in slight flexion resolves the symptoms in 80% of patients.[69]

Postural changes in the cervical spine, the shoulder girdle, and the lumber spine result in pregnancy-related back pain. Lordosis is exaggerated and becomes progressively more symptomatic during pregnancy. Pain is localized to the sacroiliac joint and may radiate to one or both of the legs. The nature of the referred pain lacks the radicular quality of discogenic pain and does not extend beyond the knee.[59] Patients should avoid wearing high-heeled shoes because such shoes increase the lumbar lordosis and exacerbate the pain. Swimming and conditioning exercises are recommended.[59]

Meralgia paresthetica is a painful dysesthesia along the lateral aspect of the thigh caused by entrapment of the purely sensory lateral femoral cutaneous nerve as it passes beneath the inguinal ligament. It develops during the third trimester in obese pregnant women or in pregnant women with excessive and rapid weight gain. It resolves postpartum without treatment.[59]

Trauma

Trauma is the leading cause of death in young men and women. The American College of Obstetricians and Gynecologists reports that 1 in every 12 pregnancies is complicated by physical trauma.[70] Trauma is the leading cause of maternal death secondary to nonobstetric etiologies.[71] One study suggests that fetal mortality after trauma is significantly associated with higher injury severity scores (>28), lower final hemoglobin levels, higher numbers of transfusions, longer lengths of stay in the hospital, and a higher incidence of disseminated intravascular coagulation.[72] Other studies have not demonstrated a correlation between injury severity scores and maternal and fetal morbidity, and their authors advocate enhanced clinical vigilance for the unexpected when caring for obstetric trauma victims (see Chapter 35).[73]

Domestic Violence

Up to 35% of all emergency department visits by women are due to injuries or illnesses related to domestic violence. Domestic violence is conservatively estimated to occur in 10% to 20% of North American spousal relationships. Estimates of abuse during pregnancy vary widely from less than 1% to 37%. The wide variation in estimates is attributable to different study designs, definitions of abuse (Table 176-2), and sample population demographics.[74-83] Moreover, it is generally accepted that violence in the home is underreported and the prevalence is higher than studies estimate.

Violence may begin or increase during pregnancy.[83-87] Prevalence estimates in 1997 based on cross-sectional survey data obtained from interviews with 261 pregnant women suggest that 33.3% of women report abuse when asked. Of these, 26.7% were African Americans, 25.2% were of Hispanic origin, and 58.3% were white women.[88] Pregnant teenagers are at even greater risk for abuse from parents and partners.[89] Other significant demographic variables associated with abuse and pregnancy can be classified under the major headings of social instability, unhealthy lifestyle, and physical health problems.[87] Abused pregnant women are more commonly of lower educational levels, unmarried, unemployed, eating an unhealthy diet, abusing drugs and alcohol, and experiencing an unplanned pregnancy; they may also delay seeking prenatal care (Table 176-3).[87,90,91] Evidence of physical abuse is more common in the facial area in a nonpregnant patient,[83] whereas blunt abdominal trauma is the most common injury type in a pregnant patient.[84,87] Blunt abdominal trauma can result in miscarriage, abruptio placentae, fetal loss, premature labor, fetal fractures, low-birth-weight infants, and premature delivery. Other common injury sites in an abused pregnant patient are the breasts and genitals.

Not all abuse is physical abuse (see Table 176-2). Emotional abuse, including intimidation by the aggressor to maintain an abused women in the abusive relationship, has been well described.[92,93] Most abused women remain in the relationship, and few have any knowledge of the support services available to them.[87] Abused pregnant women often suffer from low self-esteem, despair, anxiety, fear, withdrawal, posttraumatic stress disorder, passivity, learned helplessness, and depression and have high rates of attempted suicide.[92-93]

Abused pregnant women may have vague physical symptoms, including headache, fatigue, insomnia, choking sensations, gastrointestinal complaints, pelvic pain, and backache. These symptoms may be manifestations of a deep depression or reactions to the adversity of the home environment.

Abused pregnant women do not believe that they have any control over the health of their fetus. They hold a strong belief that chance is the major determinant in fetal outcome. This perception and the associated behavior (e.g., cigarette smoking, alcohol and drug abuse) are unlikely to change unless the abused women leave the abusive situations. Only then will they be able to improve their sense of power and self-esteem and make changes in their behavior that are in the best interest of the fetus.[87]

Table 176-2. Proportion of Pregnant Women Attending a Prenatal Clinic Who Reported Abuse (N = 1014)*

No abuse	70.3%
Pushing, shoving, slapping	23.5%
Emotional (includes verbal abuse, being allowed no money, being kept away from family and friends)	21.2%
Kicking, biting, hitting with fist	13.2%
Damage to property or pets	12.0%
Throwing objects to intimidate	11.2%
Serious threat to life	5.8%
Choking, strangling	5.6%
Sexual abuse	5.3%
Using a knife, gun, or other weapon	3.7%

*Some women reported abuse in more than one category.
Modified from Webster J, et al: Domestic violence in pregnancy: A prevalence study. *Med J Aust* 161:468, 1994.

Table 176-3. Characteristics of Nonabused and Physically Abused Pregnant Women

Characteristic	Group: No (%) of Patients		
	Nonabused (n = 512)	*Abused (n = 36)*	*P Value**
Unmarried	69/503 (13.7)	35/36 (97.2)	≤.001
Failed to complete high school	41/488 (8.4)	25/33 (75.8)	≤.001
Born in Canada	275/496 (55.4)	21/35 (60.0)	NS
Unemployed or receiving social assistance	133/498 (26.7)	27/35 (77.1)	≤.001
Pregnancy unplanned	151/503 (30.0)	32/36 (88.9)	≤.001
Regularly smokes cigarettes	63/506 (12.5)	26/36 (72.2)	≤.001
Regularly drinks alcohol	83/430 (19.3)	23/33 (69.7)	≤.001
Uses illicit drugs	6/501 (1.2)	20/36 (55.6)	≤.001
Unhealthy diet	31/499 (6.2)	10/36 (27.8)	≤.001
Previous emotional problem	19/499 (3.8)	22/36 (61.1)	≤.001
Aware of abuse services	245/416 (58.9)	18/34 (52.9)	NS

*The χ^2 test was used to compare figures.
NS, not significant.
Modified from Stewart DE, Cecutti A: Physical abuse in pregnancy. *CMAJ* 149:1259, 1993.

Identification and appropriate follow-up are paramount in the emergency management of an abused pregnant patient. Most abused patients will not volunteer information regarding domestic violence unless specifically asked. They are more likely to disclose to another woman or medical personnel of either sex who offer protection, support, and access to help and who are very sympathetic.[84,87] Any physician's fear about offending an abused woman by pursuing direct questioning is unfounded.[87]

It is important to include queries about abuse in the history of a patient while separated from her partner. Direct questioning may take the form of the following: "How do you and your partner resolve disagreements?"; "Have you been hit or hurt by anyone in the last year?"[87]; "Are you concerned for your safety or the safety of your children?"; or "Many women come to the emergency department with similar problems and are victims of violence. Could this be what happened to you today?"[95]

During the history it is important to ask questions about the current pregnancy, the spousal relationship, the nature and location of injuries, the need for medical treatment in the past and present, the level of violence at home, the awareness of access to social and legal services, and the safety of children at home. With respect to the latter, it is well documented that spousal abuse is associated with child abuse.[75,92]

One should accept the patient's story in a nonjudgmental manner, but then communicate that such abuse is unacceptable and likely to escalate in the future. This should be followed by an offer to assist the patient in developing a safety plan, which should include community resources and information regarding protection, legal rights, and emergency shelters for her and her children.

If a pregnant patient is found to be at high risk and living in dangerous circumstances, it is prudent to arrange immediate shelter or hospital admission. All patients identified as victims of abuse should be referred to social services, community support groups, and if appropriate, substance abuse programs and referral for psychiatric and high-risk obstetric consultations.

Emergency department staff should receive education regarding the issues surrounding victims of violence and how to deal with a victim effectively, cooperatively, and expeditiously. In addition, it is important for the emergency department to develop strong links with battered women's services and to display posters and pamphlets about domestic violence and local resources.[87]

MANAGEMENT

Perspective

Assessment plus care of pregnant patients requires specialized equipment and access to specific ancillary tests. Basic equipment for the management of all obstetric and gynecologic emergencies includes a variety of specula and a Doppler ultrasonographic device for fetal heart readings. The specula should be available in at least four blade widths: extra narrow at 16 mm (e.g., Miltex Pedersen), narrow at 22 mm (e.g., Miltex Pedersen), regular at 25 mm (e.g., Pedersen), and wide at 35 mm (e.g., Graves). Speculum blades are available in three lengths: small at 7.7 cm, medium at 10.2 cm, and large at 17.8 cm. The medium-length Pedersen speculum provides adequate exposure for most women. Virginal or postmenopausal women may require a narrow or extra narrow speculum with a 10.2-cm-long blade. Obese patients or patients in whom the vaginal walls are loose and redundant may require the use of a Graves speculum.

Appropriate diagnostic imaging (transabdominal and transvaginal sonography, as well as color Doppler or impedance plethysmography) and laboratory testing (both quantitative and qualitative hCG testing) should be available at all times. If ready access to a high-risk obstetric unit is not available, prearranged agreements for transport to specialized centers for high-risk obstetric patients and neonates should be in place.

Health Promotion and Disease and Injury Prevention in Pregnancy

For some, the emergency department is where the diagnosis of pregnancy is first made and the time when the patient is introduced to both the emotional and physiologic realities of pregnancy. For others, it is simply the only source of prenatal care.

After complications of pregnancy and comorbid conditions have been excluded, pregnant patients should initially be counseled, appropriately referred, and encouraged to participate in regular prenatal care. The proportion of American women beginning prenatal care during the first trimester has consistently increased for 9 years to 82.8% in 1998. Statistics suggest that timely care rose 10% during the 1990s.[96,97]

Although the time for prenatal counseling is often limited in the emergency department, when it is performed it can provide the physician with an opportunity to have a positive impact on both fetal and maternal health. The following discussion is not inclusive of all prenatal issues; however, it does outline some of the most commonly identified risks and patient concerns, along with the appropriate advice that should be given.

Use of Seat Belts, Helmets, and Air Bags

The use of three-point seat belt restraints should be emphasized. There is no evidence that these restraints will increase the chance of fetal injury. The proper use of seat belts is a good predictor of a favorable maternal and fetal outcome in the case of vehicular trauma.[98] The lap belt should be snugly and comfortably placed low across the maternal pelvis, below the uterine corpus and fundus and across the thighs, with the shoulder belt positioned between the breasts and no excessive slack allowed anywhere in the belt.[99] The National Highway Traffic Safety Administration does not consider pregnancy to be an indication for the deactivation of air bags.[100] All patients should be encouraged to voluntarily or in compliance with the law wear helmets when riding a bicycle or a motorcycle. The latter modes of transportation are ill advised during pregnancy and certainly inappropriate during the third trimester.

Safe infant feeding should be reinforced. It is inappropriate and unsafe to breast-feed in a moving vehicle. Similarly, it is unsafe to remove the child from the restraining device to bottle-feed while in a moving vehicle.

Sexual Intercourse during Pregnancy

Sexual intercourse is considered harmless for a normal pregnant female. Most texts recommend abstinence during the last 4 weeks of pregnancy or when abortion or preterm labor is threatened.

Safety of Douching during Pregnancy

Certain guidelines must be adhered to for the proper use of douches during pregnancy. Hand-held bulb syringes are prohibited because of the risk of air embolism. The height of the douche bag should be limited to 2 ft or less above the level of the hips to prevent high fluid pressure. The nozzle should not be inserted more than 8 cm through the vulva.

Travel Restrictions during Pregnancy

Generally, travel is not prohibited during pregnancy. Airlines allow unrestricted travel until 35 to 37 weeks' gestation with normal pregnancies and no history of premature labor. Only short trips are allowed with more advanced pregnancy and require a doctor's letter of assurance that delivery is not imminent. It should be emphasized to a pregnant traveler that she should walk about at least every 2 hours to minimize the risk for thromboembolism. Cosmic radiation exposure for casual travelers is trivial. Pregnant airline employees or frequent flyers should consult a physician during pregnancy because their cosmic radiation from exposure in space is increased.[101]

Immunization during Pregnancy

The Advisory Committee on Immunization Practices posts guidelines for immunization during pregnancy on the U.S. Department of Health and Human Services, Centers for Disease Control and Prevention website. Immunization of pregnant women should be guided by risk-versus-benefit logic. Three guiding principles are important when considering vaccination during pregnancy: the risk of exposure is high, the infection could cause harm to the mother or infant, and the vaccine is unlikely to cause harm. Live virus vaccines are generally contraindicated during pregnancy because of the theoretical risk of transmission of the virus to the fetus. If a pregnant patient has received a live virus vaccine in the 3 months before the pregnancy, she should be referred for counseling on the potential risks to the fetus.[102] Comprehensive and specific guidelines for each vaccine are updated and posted on the website *http://www.cdc.gov/nip/publications/acip-list.htm.*

Importance of Regular Appropriate Exercise

Suitable regular exercise should be encouraged during pregnancy because it helps prevent venous stasis and thromboembolic disease, maintain regular bowel movements, improve posture and perineal muscle strength, and regulate weight gain. Sedentary lifestyles and work activities that are performed predominantly in the sitting position should be discouraged. The American College of Obstetrics and Gynecology recommends that healthy pregnant women without medical or obstetric complications adhere to the standard of exercise for nonpregnant patients recommended by the Centers for Disease Control and Prevention and the American College of Sports Medicine. The standard aimed at improving health and well-being includes an accumulation of 30 minutes or more of moderate activity daily. Pregnant patients with comorbidity require exercise also and should engage in regular exercise with close medical supervision.

Patients should be encouraged to strengthen the abdominal muscles; stretch the lower part of the back; balance pectoralis muscle strength with that of the trapezius, rhomboids, and latissimus dorsi; strengthen the cervical spine flexors; and perform regular pelvic tilt exercises in all positions to correct the postural imbalance of pregnancy and relieve discomfort.

Appropriate exercise includes low-impact and aquatic aerobics. High-impact activities should be avoided, especially during the latter half of pregnancy. Aggressive abdominal exercises are discouraged after 12 weeks' gestation because they may exacerbate the development of diastasis recti. Moderate regular abdominal strengthening exercises will minimize the lordosis of pregnancy. The Aerobics and Fitness Association of America recommends that exercise intensity during pregnancy be limited to an exercise heart rate range of 55% to 70% of the age-predicted maximum heart rate; class time should not exceed 1 hour and 15 minutes, including the time for stretch and relaxation exercises; and frequency should not exceed three times a week.

Diet, Vitamin Supplementation, and Weight Gain Recommendations

It is not recommended that pregnant patients take routine multivitamin supplementation; however, iron supplements may be recommended, especially during the latter half of pregnancy. It is also recommended that 1 mg of folic acid be taken daily, beginning 1 month before conception and continuing throughout the first trimester to reduce the risk for neural tube defects.

The American College of Obstetricians and Gynecologists recommends that the average weight gain for pregnant women be between 10 and 12 kg.[103] The normal physiologic consequences of pregnancy account for approximately 9 kg. The remainder is maternal fat storage.[104] The Centers for Disease Control and Prevention makes weight gain recommendations according to prepregnancy weight: underweight women, 13 kg; normal-weight women, 11 kg; and overweight women, 7 kg.[105]

Appropriate Management of Pregnant Patients with Substance Abuse Problems

The risks of smoking, illicit drug use, and excessive alcohol consumption during pregnancy are widely known by the lay public; however, despite warnings, some pregnant women continue to smoke and imbibe excessively. Cigarette smoking during pregnancy has declined steadily since 1989 to 12.9% in 1998. Nonetheless, tobacco use by pregnant teenagers continued to increase in 1998, particularly for African American teens.[106] The U.S. Department of Health and Human Services, Substance Abuse and Mental Health Services Administration concluded from their National Household Survey on Drug Abuse (1996 to 1997 database) that among women aged 15 to 44 who were currently pregnant, 2.5% used one or more illicit drugs in the past month, 1.3% engaged in "binge" alcohol use, and slightly less than 20% were past-month cigarette users. *Binge drinking* was defined as drinking five or more drinks on the same day at least once during the previous 30 days. When compared with a nonpregnant cohort, it would appear that women who abuse substances curtail their use during pregnancy and resume use postpartum. Substance abuse during pregnancy was more frequent in unmarried women without a high-school education. The prevalence decreased as the amount of adult education increased. The prevalence of drug abuse during the last month of pregnancy showed no difference between Hispanic and white pregnant females. Drug abuse while pregnant was significantly more common in African American than in Hispanic patients.[107]

KEY CONCEPTS

- The emergency physician should assume that a woman of childbearing age is pregnant because data show that 11.5% of women with abdominal pain or vaginal bleeding have positive pregnancy tests even when they have stated that there is "no chance" that they are pregnant.
- Accurate vital signs are best obtained with pregnant patients in the left lateral decubitus position. ELISA is the state-of-the-art urine pregnancy test. It offers excellent user convenience and has a sensitivity between 25 and 50 IU/L.
- The decision to perform diagnostic imaging investigations of a pregnant patient must take into consideration the risk to the developing fetus of radiation, the inherent risk to the mother of the investigations, and the risk to the mother and the fetus of missing the diagnosis because of reluctance to use available imaging techniques.
- In general, a pregnant patient should be treated and assessed in the same way as all other patients. However, the normal physiologic changes of pregnancy may mask or unmask underlying medical conditions.
- The emergency department encounter is an opportunity to reinforce or provide primary education and advice on health promotion and disease and injury prevention in pregnancy.

REFERENCES

1. National Center for Health Statistics: *Births, Marriages, Divorces, and Deaths for May 1991.* Hyattsville, Md, National Center for Health Statistics, 1991.
2. Statistics Canada, Catalogue No. 82F0075XCB.
3. Hamilton BE, Sutton PD, Ventura SJ: Revised birth and fertility rates for the 1990s and new rates for Hispanic populations, 2000 and 2001: United States. *Natl Vital Stat Rep* 51(12):1, 2003.
4. Minister of Industry, Science and Technology Statistics Canada: Births 1991, Ottawa, Ontario, Canada, 1993.
5. Chumlea WC, et al: Age at menarche and racial comparisons in US girls. *Pediatrics* 111:110, 2003.
6. Statistics Canada: Trends in Canadian and American fertility 1980 to 1999. *The Daily,* July 3, 2002.
7. Martin JA, Park MM: Trends in Twin and Triplet Births: 1980-97. *Natl Vital Stat Rep* 47(24):1, 1999.
8. Chan BTB, Schull MJ, Shultz SE: *Emergency Department Services in Ontario; Atlas Report (1993-2000).* Toronto, Ontario, Canada, Institute for Clinical and Evaluative Sciences, 2001.
9. Lippman S, et al: Detection of unknown early pregnancy: A matter of safety. *Postgrad Med* 83:129, 1988.
10. Ramoska EA, Sacchetti AD, Nepp M: Reliability of patient history in determining the possibility of pregnancy. *Ann Emerg Med* 18:48, 1989.
11. Cunningham FG, et al (eds): *Williams Obstetrics,* 19th ed. E Norwalk, Conn, Appleton & Lang, 1993.
12. Chadwick JR: Value of the bluish coloration of the vaginal entrance as a sign of pregnancy. *Trans Am Gynecol Soc* 11:399, 1886.
13. Lindheimer MD, et al: Water homeostasis and vasopressin release during rodent and human gestation. *Am J Kidney Dis* 9:270, 1987.
14. Freinkel N, Dooley SL, Metzger BE: Care of the pregnant woman with insulin-dependent diabetes mellitus. *N Engl J Med* 313:96, 1985.
15. Phelps RL, Metzger BE, Freinkel N: Carbohydrate metabolism in pregnancy. XVII. Diurnal profiles of plasma glucose, insulin, free fatty acids, triglycerides, cholesterol, and individual amino acids in late normal pregnancy. *Am J Obstet Gynecol* 140:730, 1981.
16. Pritchard JA: Changes in the blood volume during pregnancy and delivery. *Anesthesiology* 26:393, 1965.
17. CDC criteria for anemia in children and childbearing-aged women. *MMWR Morb Mortal Wkly Rep* 38(22):400, 1989.
18. Krause PJ, et al: Host defense during pregnancy: Neutrophil chemotaxis and adherence. *Am J Obstet Gynecol* 157:274, 1987.
19. Pitkin RM, Witte DL: Platelet and leukocyte counts in pregnancy. *JAMA* 242:2696, 1979.
20. Fay RA, Hughes AO, Farron NT: Platelets in pregnancy: Hyperdestruction in pregnancy. *Obstet Gynecol* 61:238, 1983.
21. Ozanne P, et al: Erythrocyte aggregation during normal pregnancy. *Am J Obstet Gynecol* 147:576, 1983.
22. Enein M, et al: Echocardiography of the pericardium in pregnancy. *Obstet Gynecol* 69:851, 1987.
23. Bieniarz J, et al: Aortocaval compression by the uterus in late pregnancy, III. Unreliability of the sphygmomanometric method in estimating uterine artery pressure. *Am J Obstet Gynecol* 102:1106, 1968.
24. Wright HP, et al: Changes in rate of flow of venous blood in the leg during pregnancy, measured with radioactive sodium. *Surg Gynecol Obstet* 90:481, 1950.
25. McLennan CE: Antecubital and femoral venous pressure in normal toxemic pregnancy. *Am J Obstet Gynecol* 45:568, 1943.
26. Milne JA, Howie AD, Pack AI: Dyspnoea during normal pregnancy. *Br J Obstet Gynaecol* 85:260, 1978.

27. Dunlop W: Serial changes in renal haemodynamics during normal human pregnancy. *Br J Obstet Gynaecol* 88:1, 1981.
28. Davison JM, Hytten FE: The effect of pregnancy on the renal handling of glucose. *Br J Obstet Gynaecol* 82:374, 1975.
29. Schulman A, Herlinger H: Urinary tract dilatation in pregnancy. *Br J Radiol* 48:638, 1975.
30. Song CS, Kappas A: The influence of estrogens, progestins, and pregnancy on the liver. *Vitam Horm* 26:147, 1968.
31. Cohen S: The sluggish gallbladder of pregnancy. *N Engl J Med* 302:397, 1980.
32. Fisk NM, Bye WB, Storey GN: Maternal features of obstetric cholestasis: 20 years experience at King George V Hospital. *Aust N Z J Obstet Gynaecol* 28:172, 1988.
33. Schorr-Lesnick B, et al: Liver diseases unique to pregnancy. *Am J Gastroenterol* 86:659, 1991.
34. Crisp WE, Defrancesco S: The hand syndrome of pregnancy. *Obstet Gynecol* 23:433, 1964.
35. Causey AL, et al: Pregnant adolescents in the emergency department: Diagnosed and not diagnosed. *Am J Emerg Med* 15:125, 1997.
36. Speert H, Guttmacher AF: Frequency and significance of bleeding in early pregnancy. *JAMA* 155:712, 1954.
37. Samuels P, Landon MI: Medical complication. In Gabbe S, et al (eds): *Obstetrics: Normal and Problem Pregnancies.* New York, Churchill Livingstone, 1986.
38. Iles RK, et al: Expression of beta human chorionic gonadotrophin by non-trophoblastic non-endocrine 'normal' and malignant epithelial cells. *Br J Cancer* 61:663, 1990.
39. Storring PL, Gaines-Das RE, Bangham DR: International Reference Preparation of Human Chorionic Gonadotrophin for Immunoassay: Potency estimates in various bioassay and protein binding assay systems; and International Reference Preparations of the alpha and beta subunits of human chorionic gonadotrophin for immunoassay. *J Endocrinol* 84:295, 1980.
40. O'Connor RE, et al: The comparative sensitivity and specificity of serum and urine HCG determinations in the ED. *Am J Emerg Med* 11:434, 1993.
41. Chard T: Pregnancy tests: A review. *Hum Reprod* 7:701, 1992.
42. Lee CL, et al: The purification and development of a radioimmunoassay for beta-core fragment of human chorionic gonadotrophin in urine: Application as a marker of gynaecological cancer in premenopausal and postmenopausal women. *J Endocrinol* 130:481, 1991.
43. Hay DL, Lopata A: Chorionic gonadotropin secretion by human embryos in vitro. *J Clin Endocrinol Metab* 67:1322, 1988.
44. Lenton EA, et al: Chorionic gonadotropin concentration in early human pregnancy: Comparison of specific and non-specific assays. *Fertil Steril* 35:40, 1981.
45. Lenton EA, et al: Normal and abnormal implantation in spontaneous in-vivo and in-vitro human pregnancies. *J Reprod Fertil* 92:555, 1991.
46. Rizkallah T, Gurpide E, Vande Wiele RL: Metabolism of HCG in man. *J Clin Endocrinol Metab* 29:92, 1969.
47. Steier JA, Bergsjo P, Myking OL: Human chorionic gonadotropin in maternal plasma after induced abortion, spontaneous abortion, and removed ectopic pregnancy. *Obstet Gynecol* 64:391, 1984.
48. Fossum GT, Davajan V, Kletzky OA: Early detection of pregnancy with transvaginal ultrasound. Fertil Steril 49:788, 1988.
49. Daya S, et al: Early pregnancy assessment with transvaginal ultrasound scanning. *CMAJ* 144:441, 1991.
50. Daya S, et al: Transvaginal ultrasound scanning in early pregnancy and correlation with human chorionic gonadotropin levels. *J Clin Ultrasound* 19:139, 1991.
51. American College of Obstetricians and Gynecologists: Ultrasonography in pregnancy. ACOG Technical Bulletin Number 187—December 1993. *Int J Gynaecol Obstet* 44:173, 1994.
52. National Institutes of Health: *Diagnostic Ultrasound Imaging in Pregnancy.* Bethesda, Md, U.S. Department of Health and Human Services, 1984.
53. Nyberg DA, et al: Early gestation: Correlation of HCG levels and sonographic identification. *AJR Am J Roentgenol* 144:951, 1985.
54. Nyberg DA, et al: Early pregnancy complications: Endovaginal sonographic findings correlated with human chorionic gonadotropin levels. *Radiology* 167:619, 1988.
55. Moore L, Wilson SR: Ultrasonography in obstetric and gynecologic emergencies. *Radiol Clin North Am* 32:1005, 1994.
56. Ginsberg JS, et al: Risks to the fetus of radiologic procedures used in the diagnosis of maternal venous thromboembolic disease. *Thromb Haemost* 61:189, 1989.
57. Ratnapalan S, Bona N, Koren G: Ionizing radiation during pregnancy. *Can Fam Physician* 49:873, 2003.
58. Bentur Y: Ionizing and nonionizing radiation in pregnancy. In Koren G (ed): *Maternal-Fetal Toxicology. A Clinician's Guide.* New York, Marcel Dekker, 2001.
59. Burrow G, Ferris T: *Medical Complications during Pregnancy,* 3rd ed. Philadelphia, WB Saunders, 1988.
60. Aube M: Migraine in pregnancy. *Neurology* 53(4 Suppl 1):S26, 1999.
61. Von Wald T, Walling AD: Headache during pregnancy. *Obstet Gynecol Surv* 57:179, 2002.
62. Bickerstaff ER, Small JM, Guest IA: The relapsing course of certain meningiomas in relation to pregnancy and menstruation. *J Neurochem* 21:89, 1958.
63. Digre KB, Varner MW, Corbett JJ: Pseudotumor cerebri and pregnancy. *Neurology* 34:721, 1984.
64. Grosset DG, et al: Stroke in pregnancy and the puerperium: What magnitude of risk? *J Neurol Neurosurg Psychiatry* 58:129, 1995.
65. National Institute of Health Consensus Development Conference: Prevention of venous thrombosis and pulmonary embolism. *JAMA* 256:744, 1986.
66. Cunningham FG, McCubbin JH: Appendicitis complicating pregnancy. *Obstet Gynecol* 45:415, 1975.
67. Weingold AB: Appendicitis in pregnancy. *Clin Obstet Gynecol* 26:801, 1983.
68. Voitk A, et al: Carpal tunnel syndrome in pregnancy. *CMAJ* 128:277, 1983.
69. Ekman-Ordeberg G, Salgeback S, Ordeberg G: Carpal tunnel syndrome in pregnancy. A prospective study. *Acta Obstet Gynecol Scand* 66:233, 1987.
70. American College of Obstetricians and Gynecologists: Trauma during pregnancy. ACOG Technical Bulletin 161, November 1991.
71. Moise KJ Jr, Belfort MA: Damage control for the obstetric patient. *Surg Clin North Am* 77:835, 1997.
72. Ali J, et al: Predictors of fetal mortality in pregnant trauma patients. *J Trauma* 42:782, 1997.
73. Schiff MA, Holt VL, Daling JR: Maternal and infant outcomes after injury during pregnancy in Washington State from 1989 to 1997. *J Trauma* 53:939, 2002.
74. Committee on Wife Assault: *Reports on Wife Assault.* Toronto, Ontario Medical Association, 1991.
75. Bland R, Orn H: Family violence and psychiatric disorder. *Can J Psychiatry* 31:129, 1986.
76. Nuttall SE, Greaves LJ, Lent B: Wife battering: An emerging problem in public health. *Can J Public Health* 76:297, 1985.
77. Flitcraft AH: Violence, values, and gender. *JAMA* 267: 3194, 1992.
78. Council on Scientific Affairs, American Medical Association: Violence against women. Relevance for medical practitioners. *JAMA* 267:3184, 1992.

79. Council on Ethical and Judicial Affairs, American Medical Association: Physicians and domestic violence. Ethical considerations. *JAMA* 267:3190, 1992.
80. Bain JE: Wife assault: Physicians cannot ignore it. *CMAJ* 144:283, 1991.
81. Lent B: Wife abuse in pregnancy: The role of the physician. *Perinatal Outreach Program of Southwestern Ontario Newsletter* 9(1), 1991.
82. Family and other intimate assaults—Atlanta, 1984. *MMWR Morb Mortal Wkly Rep* 39(31):525, 1990.
83. Helton AS, McFarlane J, Anderson ET: Battered and pregnant: A prevalence study. *Am J Public Health* 77:1337, 1987.
84. Webster J, Sweett S, Stolz TA: Domestic violence in pregnancy. A prevalence study. *Med J Aust* 161:466, 1994.
85. Berenson AB, et al: Drug abuse and other risk factors for physical abuse in pregnancy among white non-Hispanic, black, and Hispanic women. *Am J Obstet Gynecol* 164:1491, discussion 1496, 1991.
86. Amaro H, et al: Violence during pregnancy and substance use. *Am J Public Health* 80:575, 1990.
87. Stewart DE, Cecutti A: Physical abuse in pregnancy. *CMAJ* 149:1257, 1993.
88. Greenberg EM, McFarlane J, Watson MG: Vaginal bleeding and abuse: Assessing pregnant women in the emergency department. *MCN Am J Matern Child Nurs* 22:182, 1997.
89. Parker B, McFarlane J, Soeken K: Abuse during pregnancy: Effects on maternal complications and birth weight in adult and teenage women. *Obstet Gynecol* 84:323, 1994.
90. Gee V: *Perinatal Statistics in Western Australia: Ninth Annual Report of the Western Australian Midwives' Notification System, Perth 1991.* Perth, Health Services Statistics and Epidemiology, Branch Health Department of Western Australia, 1991.
91. Sampselle CM, et al: Prevalence of abuse among pregnant women choosing certified nurse-midwife or physician providers. *J Nurse Midwifery* 37:269, 1992.
92. Dickstein LJ: Spouse abuse and other domestic violence. *Psychiatr Clin North Am* 11:611, 1988.
93. Jaffe P, et al: Emotional and physical health problems of battered women. *Can J Psychiatry* 31:625, 1986.
94. Helton AS, Snodgrass FG: Battering during pregnancy: Intervention strategies. *Birth* 14:142, 1987.
95. Morrison LJ, Allan R, Grunfeld A: Improving the emergency department detection rate of domestic violence using direct questioning. *J Emerg Med* 19:117, 2000.
96. Notzon FC, et al: Maternal and child health statistics: Russian Federation and United States, selected years 1985-95. *Vital Health Stat 5* (10):i, 1, 1999.
97. National Center for Health Statistics website: http://www.cdc.gov/nchs.
98. Pearlman MD, et al: A comprehensive program to improve safety for pregnant women and fetuses in motor vehicle crashes: A preliminary report. *Am J Obstet Gynecol* 182:1554, 2000.
99. Van Hook JW: Trauma in pregnancy. *Clin Obstet Gynecol* 45:414, 2002.
100. National Conference on Medical Indications for Air Bag Disconnection. George Washington University Medical Center. Final Report, 1997. http://www.nhtsa.gov/airbags/air%20bag%conference%20final%20report.doc.
101. Barish RJ: In-flight radiation exposure during pregnancy. Obstet Gynecol 103:1326, 2004.
102. General recommendations on immunization: Recommendations of the Advisory Committee on Immunization Practices (ACIP). *MMWR Recomm Rep* 43(RR-1):1, 1994.
103. American College of Obstetricians and Gynecologists: *Standards for Obstetric-Gynecologic Services,* 7th ed. Washington, DC, American College of Obstetricians and Gynecologists, 1989.
104. Hytten F: Weight gain in pregnancy. In Hytten E, Chamberlain G (eds): *Clinical Physiology in Obstetrics.* Oxford, Blackwell, 1991.
105. U.S. Department of Health and Human Services, Centers for Disease Control and Prevention: 1996 Executive Summary entitled Pregnancy Nutrition Surveillance. Available at http://www.ars.usda.gov/dgac.
106. Centers for Disease Control and Prevention's National Center for Health Statistics: Births: Final data for 1998. 48(3 [PHS]):2000-1120, 1998.
107. National Household Survey on Drug Abuse: U.S. Department of Health and Human Services, Substance Abuse and Mental Health Services Administration. Available at http://www.samhsa.gov/oas/nhsda/1997main/nhsd1997mfweb-116.htm. 1997.

CHAPTER 177

Acute Complications of Pregnancy

Debra E. Houry and Jean T. Abbott

PERSPECTIVE

Acute complications of pregnancy can appear in all trimesters of pregnancy and can pose challenges in diagnosis and management. Recognition and management of life-threatening disorders of pregnancy, such as ectopic pregnancy in early pregnancy, pregnancy-induced hypertension in mid- and late pregnancy, and abruptio placentae in late pregnancy are relatively common and should be an integral part of the emergency physician's knowledge base. The emergency physician must consider the signs and symptoms, week of gestation, and stability of the patient when developing management strategies.

PROBLEMS IN EARLY PREGNANCY

Miscarriage

Perspective

Spontaneous miscarriage is common in pregnancy. Early pregnancy loss (positive human chorionic gonadotropin [hCG] finding but less than 6 weeks after last normal menstrual period) occurs in about one quarter of pregnancies, and another 10% or more of pregnancies are lost as miscarriages that are clinically recognized.[1,2] Thus, the overall embryonic and fetal loss rate after implantation ranges up to one third of detectable pregnancies. The risk of miscarriage rises with increasing maternal and paternal age, tobacco and alcohol use, increased parity, and history of vaginal bleeding; whereas the risk is only about 12% in females younger than 20 years old, it rises to about 30% in those older than 40 years of age.[2,3] About 80% of miscarriages occur during the first trimester; the rest occur before 20 weeks of gestation. Fetal demise after 20 weeks of gestation or when the fetus is more than 500 g is considered premature birth.

Threatened or actual miscarriage is commonly seen in the emergency department. Approximately 20% to 25% of clinically pregnant patients experience some bleeding. It is widely estimated that approximately 50% of all women who have bleeding during early pregnancy miscarry, although the risk is probably higher in the emergency department population.[3,4,5] Those with a history of bleeding who do not miscarry have otherwise fairly normal pregnancies, although they have about twice the risk of premature birth and low-birth-weight infants.[3,4]

Principles of Disease

Pathophysiology

The two major causes of miscarriage are uterine malformations and chromosomal abnormalities. In some cases, the ovum itself never develops (anembryonic gestation). In the majority of early miscarriages, fetal death precedes clinical miscarriage, often by several weeks. Indeed, although clinical symptoms of miscarriages are most common between 8 and 12 weeks of gestation, sonographic evidence in most cases demonstrates death before 8 weeks; if fetal viability can be demonstrated by heart activity at 8 weeks and a normal sonogram, the subsequent fetal loss rate is only 5% in asymptomatic patients and about 15% in symptomatic patients.[5]

Chromosomal abnormalities are associated with about 40% of miscarriages. Maternal factors that increase the risk of miscarriage include congenital anatomic defects, uterine scarring, leiomyomata, and cervical incompetence. Other conditions associated with increased miscarriage rates include toxins (alcohol, tobacco, cocaine), autoimmune factors, endocrine disorders including luteal phase defects, and occasional maternal infections.[2]

Terminology

Several stages of miscarriage are recognized. In *threatened miscarriage,* the patient has bleeding but a closed internal cervical os. The risk of miscarriage in this population is estimated at 35% to 50%, depending on patient demographics and severity of symptoms.[3,4] If the internal cervical os is open, the miscarriage is considered inevitable. If products of conception (POCs) are present at the cervical os or in the vaginal canal, the miscarriage is termed *incomplete. Completed* miscarriage occurs when the uterus has expelled all fetal and placental material, the cervix is closed, and the uterus is contracted. Establishing the diagnosis of completed miscarriage is difficult in the emergency department unless a gestational sac is visualized, because the cervix may close after an episode of heavy bleeding and clot passage without or after only partial expulsion of POCs. Unless an intact gestation is passed and recognized, completed miscarriage should be diagnosed only after a dilation and curettage (D&C) with pathologic confirmation of gestational products, a sonogram demonstrating an empty uterus with a prior known intrauterine pregnancy (IUP), or by reversion to a "negative" pregnancy test result, which may take up to several weeks.

Missed abortion is a relatively obsolete term referring to clinical failure of uterine growth over time. Because it is now known that fetal death occurs days or weeks before symptoms of miscarriage, ultrasonography or serial hormonal assays can provide more timely diagnosis of fetal death. The terms *anembryonic gestation* (when no fetus is seen) and *first-* or *second-trimester fetal death* (failure to see fetal heart activity in a fetus with at least a 5-mm crown-rump length) are more appropriate terms. Current technology facilitates recognition and timely treatment of early pregnancy failure.

Clinical Features

Patient history should include the estimated length of the gestation; time since last menstrual period; symptoms of pregnancy (and loss of pregnancy symptoms); degree of bleeding; duration of bleeding; presence of cramps, pain, or fever; and attempts by the patient to induce miscarriage. The severity of symptoms does not correlate well with the risk of miscarriage, although cramping and passage of clots are believed more likely to occur as the miscarriage becomes inevitable.[3]

The assessment of the patient who experiences first-trimester vaginal bleeding includes a careful abdominal examination to evaluate for tenderness or peritoneal irritation from a potential ectopic pregnancy as well as to determine uterine size (the uterus should not be palpable abdominally). Pelvic examination should be performed to evaluate whether the cervix is closed or open, to look for clots or fetal tissue, and to determine the degree of vaginal bleeding, as well as uterine size and tenderness. The cervix should be gently probed with a ring forceps (not a Q-tip) to determine whether the internal os (1.5 cm deep to the external os) is open or closed. This is unnecessary in the

Table 177-1. Landmarks for Gestational Age and hCG by Transvaginal Ultrasonography

Findings	Weeks from LMP	β-hCG (mIU/mL)
Gestational sac (25 mm)	5	1,000
"Discriminatory zone"	5-6	1,500-2,000
Yolk sac	6	2,500
Upper "discriminatory zone"	6-7	3,000
Fetal pole	7	5,000
Fetal heart motion	8	17,000

hCG, human chorionic gonadotropin; LMP, last menstrual period.
Adapted from Dart RG: Role of pelvic ultrasonography in evaluation of symptomatic first-trimester pregnancy. Ann Emerg Med 33(3):310-320, 1999.

BOX 177-1. Sonographic Criteria for Abnormal Pregnancy with Transvaginal Ultrasonography

- No gestational sac at β-hCG level of 3000 mIU/mL
- No yolk sac with gestational sac of 13 mm (or at 32 days since last menstrual period)
- 5-mm crown-rump length with no fetal heart tones
- No fetus with gestational sac of 25 mm mean diameter
- No fetal heart tones after 10–12 weeks' gestational age

β-hCG, human chorionic gonadotropin.
Adapted from Dart RG: Role of pelvic ultrasonography in evaluation of symptomatic first-trimester pregnancy. *Ann Emerg Med* 33:310, 1999.

patient who has a clearly open os or visible POCs but can be safely performed during the first trimester as long as the forceps are used gently and do not penetrate the cervix more than 2 or 3 cm. In the patient with second-trimester bleeding, probing should not be done, because the uterus is more vascular and the organized placenta may overlie the cervical os. Parous females normally have an open or lax external os, a finding of no significance. The adnexa may be enlarged, often unilaterally, either because the corpus luteum is cystic or because the pregnancy is ectopic. Significant adnexal or uterine tenderness should always raise the possibility of an ectopic pregnancy. Much less commonly, pelvic infection can cause uterine and adnexal tenderness during early pregnancy.

Any tissue that is passed should be suspended in saline or tap water (or viewed under low-power microscopy) to differentiate sloughing endometrium and organized clot from chorionic villi, which form fronds and appear feathery in the saline suspension. Except for the rare instance of heterotopic pregnancy (combined intrauterine and ectopic pregnancies), this reliably excludes ectopic pregnancy. Passage of tissue called the *endometrial cast* in ectopic pregnancy can easily be confused with intrauterine miscarriage if the physician does not confirm the absence of chorionic villi in the tissue.[6,7]

Diagnostic Strategies

A hemoglobin determination is useful to provide a baseline measurement and to evaluate the degree of bleeding in females whose bleeding persists. In addition, an Rh (*Rhesus*) type should be obtained. Ultrasonography is the primary means of evaluating the health of the fetus as well as its location (Table 177-1). Because historical and clinical estimation of gestational age are often inaccurate, ultrasonography is useful to provide an accurate measure of fetal age and viability. If fetal heart tones are identified, the risk of miscarriage is only about 5% in all women, and up to 15% in women with vaginal bleeding (Box 177-1).[5]

In the stable patient with threatened miscarriage, observation over time may be sufficient to determine when intervention is needed, as long as ectopic pregnancy has been excluded. Serial quantitative hCG levels are used to assess the health of the fetus if sonographic findings are indeterminate or if the gestational age is less than 6 to 7 weeks. The sonographic "discriminatory zone" is defined as the quantitative hCG level at which a normally developing IUP should reliably be seen. This is considered to be 6500 mIU/mL for transabdominal ultrasonography[8] and 3000 mIU/mL by transvaginal ultrasonography.[9] Ultrasonography can be performed or repeated when hCG levels rise to the level of 3000 mIU/mL. If hCG levels are flat or decline, or if sonographic criteria for fetal demise are demonstrated (see Box 177-1), the patient should be referred to a specialist for follow-up to be sure the miscarriage completes.

Differential Considerations

Of greatest concern is the possibility of ectopic pregnancy, which can masquerade as a threatened miscarriage in the early stages. Even in the patient with painless vaginal bleeding, the diagnosis of ectopic pregnancy must be considered. For this reason, early ultrasonography is imperative to locate the pregnancy in the patient who has bleeding or pain.

Other diagnoses should be considered. A small amount of bleeding occurs at the time of implantation of the blastocyst into the endometrium and occasionally at the time of the first missed menses. Molar pregnancy also is characterized by vaginal bleeding, usually during the late first trimester or the second trimester. This condition can be identified by ultrasonography. Cervical and vaginal lesions also can cause local bleeding and can usually be seen on vaginal inspection.

Management

After assessment of hemodynamic status and management of blood loss, a patient with a threatened miscarriage requires very little specific medical treatment. Anti-D immunoglobulin should be administered if the patient is Rh-negative (unless the father is known also to be Rh-negative). A 50-µg dose is used during the first trimester and a full 300-µg dose after the first trimester.[8] Ectopic pregnancy should always be considered, and ultrasonography employed urgently if risk factors for ectopic pregnancy are present or if the patient has pain. Although ectopic pregnancy can be associated with painless bleeding,[6,7] this occurs less frequently than bleeding associated with pain. Ultrasonography can be scheduled more routinely at a later time in patients without significant pain as long as the patient is aware that the potential for ectopic pregnancy exists until excluded by identifying an IUP. In the patient who is planning pregnancy termination, prompt referral should be encouraged and chorionic villi confirmed at the time of uterine evacuation.

Unless an IUP is diagnosed, the patient with threatened miscarriage should be given careful instructions to return if she has signs of hemodynamic instability, significant pain, or other symptoms that might indicate ectopic pregnancy (so-called ectopic precautions). In conjunction with gynecologic colleagues, an emergency department protocol is useful to determine when follow-up sonographic evaluation and serial hCG measurements should be obtained. In addition, recent studies have indicated that increased cancer antigen 125 (CA-125),[10] low progesterone levels,[11] and urinary hCG expression of certain molecular components[12] can also be predictors of early pregnancy loss, although they are not in widespread use.

Fifty percent or more of women with threatened miscarriage who are seen in emergency departments ultimately miscarry. Treatment to "prevent" miscarriage is not useful, because most fetuses can be shown to be nonviable 1 to 2 weeks before actual symptoms occur. In the vast majority of cases, spontaneous miscarriage is the body's natural method of expelling an abnormal or undeveloped (blighted) pregnancy. Thus a major goal of emergency department management should be patient education and support. Patients should be advised that moderate daily activities will not affect the pregnancy. Tampons, intercourse, and other activities that might induce uterine infection should be avoided as long as the patient is bleeding, and she should return immediately for fever, abdominal pain, or a significant increase in bleeding. Cramping from a known IUP can be safely treated with oral synthetic narcotics, if needed. If the patient passes tissue, it should be brought to a provider to examine for POCs, because differentiation of fetal parts or villi from decidual slough or casts is difficult.

Patient counseling is paramount with threatened miscarriage. Determination of fetal viability can be helpful in either reassuring the mother or preparing her for probable fetal loss. Miscarriages are associated with a significant grieving process, which is frequently more difficult because early pregnancy is unannounced and early fetal death is not publicly recognized. Because many women consider that small falls, injuries, or stress during the first trimester can precipitate miscarriage, patients should be reassured that they have done nothing to cause miscarriage. It is important to make them aware that miscarriage is common, that guilt is frequently felt but unfounded, and that grieving is normal.[13] A follow-up appointment should be scheduled after miscarriage to support the patient in resolving such issues.

Treatment of the patient with inevitable miscarriage includes either observation, dilation and evacuation, or D&C to remove the remaining intrauterine contents. When the miscarriage is incomplete, the uterus may be unable to contract adequately to limit bleeding from the implantation site. Bleeding may be brisk, and gentle removal of fetal tissue from the cervical os with ring forceps during the pelvic examination often slows bleeding considerably.

Management of patients with presumed completed spontaneous miscarriage is more complicated. If the patient brings tissue with her, this should be preliminarily inspected in the emergency department and then sent to the pathology department for evaluation. Unless an intact gestational sac or fetus is visualized, it is rarely clear clinically whether miscarriage is "complete." Recent studies have shown that in women with a history consistent with miscarriage who have minimal remaining intrauterine tissue as determined by ultrasonography, expectant management is safe, but only if ectopic pregnancy can be excluded.[14] If endometrial tissue is not seen with ultrasonography, bleeding is mild, and gestational age is less than 8 weeks, curettage is frequently unnecessary and the patient can be safely followed by a gynecologist for serial hormonal assays. Up to 80% of women with first-trimester miscarriage complete the miscarriage without intervention. The need for later visits and procedures may be decreased by uterine curettage, particularly if the fetal pole or a gestational sac is visible on the sonogram at the time of evaluation.[14] Medical management with misoprostol instead of D&C is also an option.[15] Consultation with an ob/gyn specialist is advised and if D&C is not performed. The patient should be instructed to return if uncontrolled bleeding, severe pain or cramping, fever, or tissue passage occurs. Follow-up is recommended in 1 to 2 weeks to ensure that the miscarriage is complete.

After miscarriage, the patient should be advised that fetal loss, even during the first trimester, can cause significant psychological stress. Follow-up in 1 to 2 weeks with a gynecologist should be provided. Some physicians prescribe antibiotics after D&C (usually doxycycline or metronidazole, as with pelvic inflammatory disease [PID]), particularly in patient populations at high risk for genital tract infections. Ergonovine or methylergonovine (0.2 mg PO twice daily) can be used to stimulate uterine involution. Anti-D immunoglobulin should be given if the patient is Rh negative. The patient should be advised to return if signs of infection (fever or uterine tenderness) occur, if bleeding resumes, or if further tissue is passed.

Ectopic Pregnancy

Perspective

Ectopic pregnancy, or pregnancy implanted outside the uterus, is an increasingly frequent problem that poses a major health risk to women during the childbearing years. It is the third leading cause of maternal death, responsible for 6% of maternal mortality.[16] The incidence of ectopic pregnancy has risen steadily over the past 35 years and now accounts for about 2% of all pregnancies. Although the incidence of ectopic pregnancy is highest in women aged 25 to 34, the rate is highest among older women and women belonging to minority groups. Simultaneous intrauterine and extrauterine gestations (heterotopic pregnancy) have historically been rare, occurring in about 1 in 4000 pregnancies; more recently, women who have undergone assisted reproduction techniques with embryo transfer have demonstrated a risk of one of the pregnancies being ectopic of 4% or greater.[17] In the emergency department, the incidence of ectopic pregnancy among women presenting with vaginal bleeding or pain in the first trimester is consistently about 10% in several series.[18,19]

Principles of Disease

Implantation of the fertilized ovum occurs about 8 to 9 days after ovulation. Risk factors for an abnormal site of implantation include prior tubal infection (50% of cases), anatomic abnormalities of the fallopian tubes, or abnormal endometrium (host factors). These result in failure of the embryo to implant in the endometrium. The risk of ectopic pregnancy increases approximately threefold after a patient has had PID. In recent studies, one fourth of patients with ectopic pregnancies have had tubal surgery, including tubal sterilization or removal of ectopic pregnancy.[20] If the patient is currently using an intrauterine device, increased risk can occur from complicating PID or from failure of the intrauterine device to prevent ectopic pregnancy as well as preventing endometrial implantation. All forms of contraception except intrauterine device use and tubal sterilization decrease the incidence of ectopic pregnancy. After an ectopic pregnancy, the risk of a subsequent ectopic pregnancy was 22% in one series of women trying to conceive again (Box 177-2).[21]

When abnormal implantation occurs in the fallopian tubes, on the ovaries, or in the cervix, the pregnancy grows at a less than normal rate, sometimes resulting in abnormally low or dropping hCG production. Leakage of blood occurs intermittently through the tubal wall or out the fimbrial ends, with spillage into the peritoneal cavity. Bleeding and other symptoms are usually intermittent. Three outcomes are possible: tubal abortion may occur into the peritoneal cavity or vagina, spontaneous involution of the pregnancy may occur, or rupture of the pregnancy with internal or vaginal bleeding may result. Implantation in the uterine horn (cornual pregnancy) is particularly dangerous, because the growing embryo can use the myometrial blood supply to grow larger (10 to 14 weeks' gestation) before rupture occurs.

BOX 177-2. Risk Factors for Ectopic Pregnancy

- Tubal surgery (for tubal sterilization or ectopic pregnancy)
- Pelvic inflammatory disease
- Smoking
- Advanced age
- Prior spontaneous abortion
- Medically induced abortion
- History of infertility
- Intrauterine device

Modified from Bouyer J, et al: Risk factors for ectopic pregnancy: A comprehensive analysis based on a large case-control, population-based study in France. *Am J Epidemiol* 157:185, 2003.

Clinical Features

The classic clinical picture of ectopic pregnancy is a history of delayed menses followed by abdominal pain and vaginal bleeding in a patient with known risk factors. Unfortunately, this history is neither sensitive nor specific. Risk factors for ectopic pregnancy are absent in almost half of patients. Fifteen to 20% of patients with symptomatic ectopic pregnancy have not missed a menstrual period, and occasionally the patient has no history of vaginal bleeding. Abdominal pain is most commonly severe, peritoneal in nature, and constant. Shoulder pain implies free fluid in the peritoneal cavity and is very suggestive of an ectopic pregnancy with significant hemorrhage. The pain of ectopic pregnancy can, however, be crampy, intermittent, or even absent.[6,7]

The physical examination findings in ectopic pregnancy are likewise variable. Vaginal bleeding, uterine or adnexal tenderness, or both in the patient with a positive pregnancy test result should always trigger consideration for ectopic pregnancy. Tachycardia is not always present, even with significant hemoperitoneum; hemoglobin is usually normal and hypotension may be seen.[7,22] The presence of peritoneal signs, cervical motion tenderness, or lateral or bilateral abdominal or pelvic tenderness indicates increased likelihood of an ectopic pregnancy. If significant peritoneal irritation is present, pain can preclude accurate bimanual examination. Adnexal masses are felt in only 10% to 20% of patients with ectopic pregnancy.[6,7] Vaginal bleeding is often mild. Heavy bleeding with clots or tissue usually suggests a threatened or incomplete miscarriage, although the patient with an ectopic pregnancy who has dropping hormonal levels may experience endometrial sloughing, which can be mistaken for passage of fetal tissue. Passed tissue should be examined, as with cases of miscarriage, in tap water or saline (or under low-power microscopy). Unless fetal parts or chorionic villi are seen, ectopic pregnancy should not be excluded in the patient with bleeding or passage of "tissue."

Diagnostic Strategies

Because both the history and the physical examination of the patient with ectopic pregnancy are insensitive and nonspecific, ancillary studies are required to locate the pregnancy in any emergency department patient who has abdominal pain or vaginal bleeding and a positive pregnancy test result. Recent technologic advances have allowed accurate detection or exclusion of ectopic pregnancy in the assessment of the woman with first-trimester vaginal bleeding or pelvic pain.

Ultrasonography and hormonal assays are the most commonly used ancillary tests. In addition, laparoscopy can be the most efficient diagnostic tool in some instances.

Ultrasonography

Ultrasonography is the primary method used to locate early gestation, establish gestational age, and assess fetal viability. Transabdominal ultrasonography is most useful for identifying IUPs with fetal heart activity, excluding ectopic pregnancy except in patients at high risk for heterotopic pregnancy due to infertility procedures.[9] Transvaginal ultrasonography is more sensitive, recognizes IUP earlier than transabdominal ultrasonography, and is diagnostic in up to 80% of stable patients presenting to the emergency department in the first trimester.[18,19] Correlation of sonographic results with quantitative hCG measurements can add to the predictive value. The risk of ectopic pregnancy and the chances of an indeterminate sonogram increase with lower hCG levels. With low hCG levels, the ability of ultrasonography to detect both normal and abnormal pregnancies declines. With hCG less than 1000 mIU/mL, the risk of ectopic pregnancy increases fourfold; ultrasonography is still diagnostic in a significant minority of patients (one third of patients with ectopic pregnancy), although the accuracy of sonographic findings may decrease.[19,23] Normal pregnancy is unlikely if no gestational sac is seen by transvaginal ultrasonography with an hCG level greater than 3000 mIU/mL, but the differential diagnosis includes both miscarriage and ectopic pregnancy.[23] Unfortunately, levels about 1500 mIU/mL develop in only about half of patients with ectopic pregnancies (see Table 177-1).[4,24]

Indeterminate sonograms, which demonstrate neither an IUP nor extrauterine findings suggestive of ectopic pregnancy (Box 177-3), occur in about 20% of emergency department evaluations of women with first-trimester bleeding or pain. Ectopic pregnancy is more likely among this subgroup with indeterminate sonograms if the hCG level is less than 1000 mIU/mL and when the uterus is empty. Endometrial debris and fluid in the uterus do not exclude ectopic pregnancy, however.[25]

BOX 177-3. Sonographic Findings in the Patient with Suspected Ectopic Pregnancy

Diagnostic of Intrauterine Pregnancy (IUP)
- "Double" gestational sac
- Intrauterine fetal pole or yolk sac
- Intrauterine fetal heart activity

Diagnostic of Ectopic Gestation
- Ectopic fetal heart activity
- Ectopic fetal pole

Suggestive of Ectopic Gestation
- Moderate or large cul-de-sac fluid without IUP
- Adnexal mass* without IUP

Indeterminate
- Empty uterus
- Nonspecific fluid collections
- Echogenic material
- Abnormal sac
- Single gestational sac

*Complex mass most suggestive of ectopic pregnancy, but cyst can also be seen with ectopic pregnancy.

Adapted from Dart RG: Role of pelvic ultrasonography in evaluation of symptomatic first-trimester pregnancy. *Ann Emerg Med* 33:310, 1999.

Hormonal Assays

The quantitative hCG levels have two primary uses in emergency department evaluation: serial levels can be used in the stable patient who can be followed as an outpatient, and a single level can be correlated with sonographic results for improved interpretation. hCG levels normally double every 1.8 to 3 days for the first 6 to 7 weeks of pregnancy, beginning 8 to 9 days after ovulation. An initial quantitative level can be measured at the time of the emergency department visit, particularly if the sonogram is indeterminate or the gestational age is estimated as less than 6 weeks. A repeat level should be measured 48 to 72 hours later. Levels that fall or double slowly are associated with abnormal pregnancy, either intrauterine or ectopic. However, normally rising hCG levels can be seen during early ectopic pregnancy, with falling levels of hCG seen initially in only half of ectopic pregnancies.[26]

A single low hCG level is also predictive of failed pregnancy. In one series, 25% of symptomatic first-trimester patients with hCG levels less than 1500 mIU/mL had an ectopic pregnancy; only 16% were diagnosed with a normal IUP.[4] Single quantitative hCG levels can also be useful in conjunction with ultrasonography; normal IUPs should be visible transvaginally at 3000 mIU/mL hCG (see Table 177-1). A benign course for ectopic pregnancy cannot be assumed with low hCG levels; ruptured ectopic pregnancies requiring surgery have been reported with very low or absent levels of hCG.[27]

Serum progesterone levels have been studied as an additional or alternative marker to determine which patients need further evaluation and follow-up for possible ectopic pregnancy. Progesterone rises earlier than hCG in normal pregnancy and plateaus with levels greater than 20 ng/mL, so measuring serial levels over time is not necessary. Levels less than 5 ng/mL exclude viable IUP (with rare exceptions) and could be useful when hCG levels are low, ultrasonography is indeterminate, and the clinician is considering D&E or laparoscopy. The ability of a progesterone level to differentiate ectopic pregnancy from a failed IUP is limited, however, and it is not a standard tool for evaluation at present.[28,29]

Other assays such as serum creatine kinase and interleukin levels and tumor necrosis factor α determinations have recently been studied to determine their utility in diagnosing ectopic pregnancy.[30] These levels are generally increased in patients with ectopic pregnancies but are not sufficiently discriminative to be of clinical value in the emergency diagnosis of ectopic pregnancy.

Other Ancillary Studies

Culdocentesis is not commonly used in stable patients with suspected ectopic pregnancy if ultrasonography is available. Culdocentesis is less sensitive and specific than ultrasonography for detecting hemoperitoneum, and several series report a nondiagnostic (i.e., dry) tap in about one quarter of patients.[31] Culdocentesis could be considered, however, to verify hemoperitoneum in the unstable patient who cannot tolerate the time required for ultrasonography or when emergency transfer is being considered for gynecologic consultation and definitive care.

Dilation and evacuation can be used in patients without a viable IUP or ectopic pregnancy on ultrasonography to differentiate intrauterine miscarriage from ectopic pregnancy. Identification of chorionic villi in endometrial samples is seen in about 70% of patients and excludes ectopic pregnancy (except in infertility patients). Identification of chorionic villi can be made even in 50% of women with an empty uterus on ultrasonography and limits the need for laparoscopy to exclude ectopic pregnancy in this population.[32]

Although invasive, laparoscopy is extremely accurate as a diagnostic (and therapeutic) procedure for possible ectopic pregnancy. It is the diagnostic treatment of choice in the unstable first-trimester patient with frank peritoneal signs and is also indicated in patients with significant peritoneal fluid or an ectopic gestation in the pelvic cavity. Medical alternatives for management of ectopic pregnancy have resulted in decreased indications in stable patients.[33,34]

Differential Considerations

The spectrum of clinical presentations in ectopic pregnancy is wide, so the differential diagnosis includes essentially all first-trimester complications. Threatened miscarriage, the most common alternative diagnosis, can be recognized by sonographic evidence of an IUP, either healthy or failed. Hypovolemia may be seen, particularly in incomplete miscarriage, but hypotension without significant vaginal hemorrhage is highly suggestive of ectopic pregnancy. Identification of fetal parts or chorionic villi in tissue expelled or obtained during D&C is useful to confirm a complication of IUP, although this is not sufficient to exclude ectopic pregnancy in the patient who has received infertility treatment and has an increased risk of heterotopic gestation.

A ruptured corpus luteum cyst should also be considered in the patient who has first-trimester bleeding associated with peritoneal pain or irritation. The corpus luteum normally supports the pregnancy during the first 7 to 8 weeks. Rupture causes pelvic pain and peritoneal irritation. Ultrasonography is helpful if it reveals an IUP (except in patients with in vitro fertilization). During early gestation, when ultrasonography is nondiagnostic, free fluid is usually visible by ultrasonography and serial observation may be required. If the patient is unstable (especially if an IUP cannot be identified by ultrasonography), laparoscopy or, rarely, laparotomy may be required to differentiate between the two conditions.

Management

Classically, approximately 20% of women with ectopic pregnancies manifest signs and symptoms warranting immediate intervention.[24] These included patients with significant hypovolemia, large amounts of peritoneal fluid, or an open cervical os. For patients with significant signs of hypovolemia, rapid volume resuscitation should be instituted with intravenous fluids and blood products as necessary, and a baseline hemoglobin level and type and crossmatch should be obtained. A D&C or evacuation procedure with examination of endometrial contents for products of conception can be performed urgently in the unstable patient with an open cervical os.

If the patient remains unstable, immediate surgery or rapid culdocentesis (to confirm intraperitoneal bleeding) followed by surgical exploration is the best method of management. Laparoscopy may be indicated for patients who stabilize with treatment, for those who are hemodynamically stable but exhibit significant peritoneal signs, and for those in whom ultrasonography is diagnostic or suggestive of ectopic pregnancy. All patients with ectopic pregnancy who are Rh-negative should be given Rh immunoglobulin 50 μg intramuscularly, unless the father is known to be Rh-negative.

The majority of patients who seek treatment for bleeding or pain during the first trimester of pregnancy are stable. In such patients, the goal should be to exclude ectopic pregnancy in a timely fashion. In the patient with significant pain by history or examination, or significant risk factors for ectopic pregnancy, ultrasonography should be performed before discharge. If the results are indeterminate, a quantitative hCG may be helpful in determining the patient's risk for ectopic pregnancy.

In low-risk patients with only minor symptoms or bleeding, ectopic pregnancy is still a possibility. Two general outpatient approaches can be considered. In most institutions, ultrasonography is the initial screening tool (Figure 177-1), by the emergency medical team or by radiology personnel. If an IUP is not seen, quantitative hCG levels help stratify patients by risk. Cost, availability, and convenience will drive the ordering of ancillary studies in different institutions. In all cases, if the patient is discharged, careful instructions are given for symptoms that would require her earlier return (ectopic precautions).

An alternative strategy using hCG first has also been used. However, waiting times for the serum assay can increase length of stay in the emergency department. In addition, ultrasonography is usually diagnostic of IUP or ectopic pregnancy, even if the hCG level is less than 1000 mIU/mL.[18,23] In most hands, the initial sonogram provides more rapid and accurate information at the time of an emergency department visit.

A significant minority of patients has indeterminate sonographic results and hCG levels less than 1500 mIU/mL. When the hCG levels never rise to the discriminatory zone, the differential diagnosis includes intrauterine fetal demise and ectopic pregnancy. Early D&C with identification of POCs can be useful to the

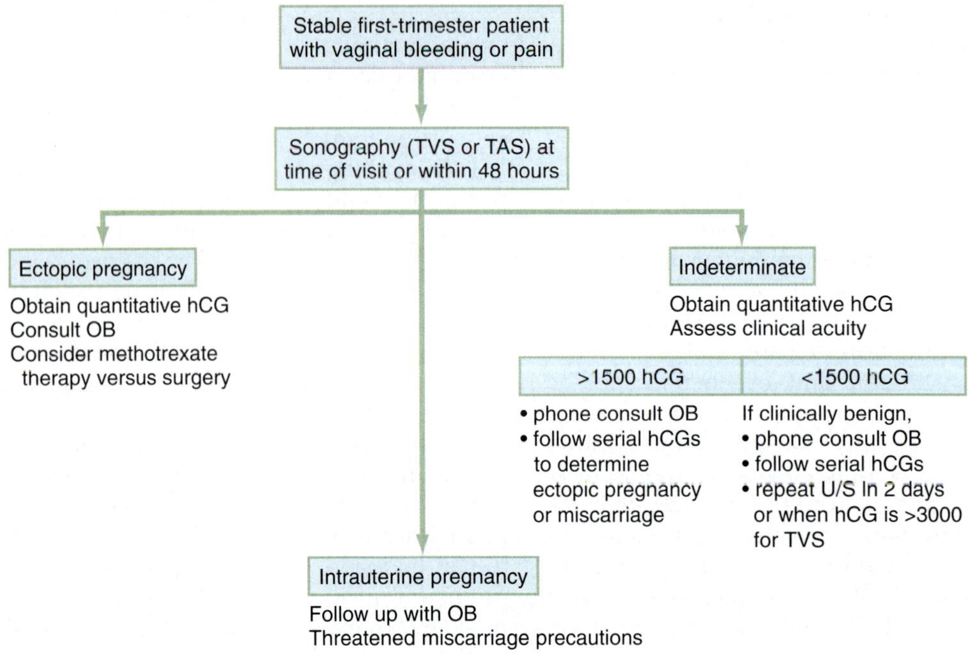

Figure 177-1. Management of vaginal bleeding or pain in the stable first-trimester pregnant patient. hCG, human chorionic gonadotropin; OB, obstetrics specialist; TAS, transabdominal ultrasonography; TVS, transvaginal sonography.

patient with nonrising hCG levels to detect chorionic villi and confirm a failed IUP or to strongly suggest ectopic pregnancy.[32] Alternatively, hCG levels can be followed until they reach zero, particularly if initial levels are low.

Although laparotomy may be required for emergency patients who have ectopic pregnancies, an increasing number of surgeries are being performed through the laparoscope. Salpingostomy is preferred to salpingectomy if the patient is stable and the procedure is technically feasible. Overall, the advent of transvaginal ultrasonography has resulted in a decreased number of surgeries and a trend toward nonoperative management.[35]

Nonoperative management has become standard in many areas for the stable patient with minimal symptoms.[36] Methotrexate is the drug most commonly used to treat early ectopic pregnancy. It causes destruction of rapidly dividing fetal cells and involution of the pregnancy. Medical treatment is most often used for patients with a tubal mass less than 4 cm in diameter and no sonographic evidence of rupture.[36] Medical therapies are associated with an 85% success rate.[37] Pelvic pain is common (60%) in patients receiving methotrexate, even when used successfully.[38] Indications of methotrexate failure and need for rescue surgery include decreasing hemoglobin levels, significant pelvic fluid, or unstable vital signs. All patients receiving methotrexate require close follow-up until the hCG level reaches zero, which may take 2 to 3 months.

Molar Pregnancy

Gestational trophoblastic disease (molar pregnancy) comprises a spectrum of diseases characterized by disordered proliferation of chorionic villi. In the absence of fetal tissue, the pregnancy is termed a *complete hydatidiform mole*. More rarely, if fetal tissue is present and trophoblastic hyperplasia is focal, it is called an *incomplete mole*. In approximately 15% of molar pregnancies, neoplastic gestational disease develops, with persistence of molar tissue after the pregnancy has been evacuated.[39] Metastatic disease can develop, requiring chemotherapy and intensive oncologic management.

Early molar pregnancy is usually not clinically apparent. Although patients sometimes seek treatment for apparent persistent hyperemesis gravidarum from high circulating levels of hCG, bleeding or intermittent bloody discharge or failure to hear fetal heart tones during the second trimester is the usual initial clue to diagnosis. If spontaneous abortion occurs with molar pregnancy, it is usually during the second trimester (before 20 weeks), and the patient or physician may note passage of grapelike hydatid vesicles. Uterine size is larger than expected by date (by more than 4 weeks) in approximately 30% to 40% of patients. Theca lutein cysts may be present on the ovaries as a result of excessive hormonal stimulation, and torsion of affected ovaries can be seen.

The diagnosis of hydatidiform mole is based on the characteristic sonographic appearance of hydropic vesicles within the uterus ("snowstorm" appearance). Alternatively, cystic changes are seen in partial molar pregnancies. In some cases, partial molar pregnancy is detected only on pathologic examination of abortion specimens.[40] Complications of molar pregnancy include preeclampsia or eclampsia (which can develop before 24 weeks of gestation), pulmonary embolization of trophoblastic cells, hyperemesis gravidarum, and significant uterine bleeding, either acute or chronic. Ultrasonography usually provides the diagnosis of complete molar pregnancy, either in the second-trimester patient who has "threatened miscarriage" or during sonographic assessment for fetal well-being and size. However, when ultrasonography is performed prior to

10 weeks' gestation, diagnosis of complete mole is only 58% sensitive and diagnosis of partial mole is made in 17% of cases.[40] Up to two thirds of molar pregnancies are diagnosed by pathologic specimens after miscarriage.[40]

COMPLICATIONS OF LATE PREGNANCY

Vaginal Bleeding in Later Pregnancy

Perspective

Bleeding during the second half of pregnancy occurs in about 4% of pregnancies. Only 20% of miscarriages occur after the first trimester, and the most important differential diagnoses after 12 to 14 weeks' gestation are abruptio placentae and placenta previa. Often the cause is not determined, although occult marginal placental separations (which can be recognized only by placental inspection at delivery) are held to be a common source of bleeding from above the cervix. Other causes of late vaginal bleeding include early labor, various cervical and vaginal lesions, lower genital tract infections, and hemorrhoids.

Bleeding during the second trimester before the fetus is potentially viable (14 to 24 weeks) is not benign. One third of fetuses are ultimately lost when maternal bleeding occurs. Management is supportive and expectant, because fetal rescue is impossible at this level of fetal immaturity. In the third trimester, vaginal bleeding is still associated with significant morbidity in about one third of women, but the treatment includes consideration of urgent delivery.[41]

Abruptio Placentae

Principles of Disease

Abruptio placentae, or separation of the placenta from the uterine wall, is believed to account for about 30% of episodes of bleeding during the second half of pregnancy. In addition, small subclinical or marginal separations may go undetected until the placenta is examined at delivery and probably account for many of the other self-limited episodes of bleeding for which no diagnosis is made. In cases of nontraumatic abruptio placentae, apparently spontaneous hemorrhage into the decidua basalis occurs, causing separation and compression of the adjacent placenta. Small amounts of bleeding may be asymptomatic and remain undetected until delivery. In other instances, the hematoma expands and extends the dissection; bleeding may be concealed or may be clinically apparent if dissection occurs along the uterine wall and through the cervix. Placental separation can be acute or can be an indolent problem throughout late pregnancy.

Abruptio placentae is most clearly associated with maternal hypertension and preeclampsia; it is also more common with increasing maternal age and parity, a history of smoking, thrombophilia, prior miscarriage, prior abruptio placentae, and cocaine use.[41,42] Placental separation can also be associated with blunt trauma to the abdomen. In such instances, the cause appears to be shearing of a nonelastic placenta from the easily distorted elastic uterine wall at the time of traumatic impact. Women who reported physical violence during pregnancy were twice as likely to have an abruption than women who did not report any violence.[43]

Clinical Features

Vaginal bleeding occurs in 80% of patients with abruptio placentae. Blood is characteristically dark and the amount is often insignificant, although the mother may have hemodynamic evidence of significant blood loss. Uterine tenderness or pain is seen in about two thirds of women; uterine irritability or contractions are seen in one third. With significant placental separation, fetal distress occurs and the maternal coagulation cascade may be triggered, causing disseminated intravascular coagulation.[41]

There is a wide spectrum of severity of symptoms and risk in placental separation. Assessment is generally based on clinical features, coagulation parameters, and signs of fetal distress. Slight vaginal bleeding, little or no uterine irritability, absence of signs of fetal distress, and normal coagulation characterize mild abruption. As the separation becomes more extensive, it is associated with more vaginal bleeding (or hidden maternal blood loss), increased uterine irritability with or without tetanic contractions, dropping fibrinogen levels, and evidence of fetal distress and maternal tachycardia. In cases of severe abruptio placentae (15% of cases), the uterus is tetanically contracted and very painful, maternal hypotension results from visible or concealed uterine blood loss, fibrinogen levels are less than 150 mg/dL, and fetal death can occur. Ultrasonography is insensitive in the diagnosis of abruptio placentae, often because the echogenicity of fresh blood is so similar to that of the placenta itself. Symptomatic or even fetus-threatening abruption can occur in the presence of a negative sonogram.[41,42]

Fetal distress and death occur in about 15% of patients with abruptio placenta, due to interruption of placental blood and oxygen flow. Risk of fetal death increases in proportion to both the percentage of placental surface involved and the rapidity of separation. Fetal distress may result from the loss of placental blood flow, from associated maternal hemorrhage (into the uterine cavity or externally), from increased uterine tone, or from resultant disseminated intravascular coagulation. Maternal death can result, usually from coagulopathy or exsanguination. Fetomaternal transfusion occurs in a significant minority of patients. Placental separation also predisposes the mother to amniotic fluid embolism.

Differential Considerations

The main alternative diagnosis in the woman with late-pregnancy bleeding is placenta previa, which is usually associated with painless, bright red bleeding and must be excluded with ultrasonography. Lower genital tract or rectal lesions and bloody show (blood-tinged cervical mucous plug) are also considerations.

In the patient with abdominal pain but no vaginal bleeding, abruptio placentae with concealed hemorrhage must be distinguished from other causes of abdominal pain in later pregnancy: complications of preeclampsia, pyelonephritis, various liver diseases, gallbladder disease, appendicitis, and ovarian torsion. Uterine irritability caused by abruptio placentae can also be confused with early labor; in one series almost one quarter of patients were misdiagnosed as having premature labor until fetal distress occurred. If the patient has acute catastrophic hypotension, amniotic fluid embolus (with or without abruptio placenta) and uterine rupture must be considered.[41]

Placenta Previa

Principles of Disease

Placenta previa, or implantation of the placenta over the cervical os, is the other major cause of bleeding episodes during the second half of pregnancy. The risk of placenta previa is increased with maternal age, multiparity, smoking, and prior cesarean section.[44] Bleeding occurs when marginal placental vessels implanted in the lower uterine segment are torn, either as the lower uterine wall elongates or with cervical dilation near the time of delivery. Early bleeding episodes tend to be self-limited unless separation of the placental margin is aggravated by iatrogenic cervical probing or onset of labor.

Clinical Features

Painless, fresh vaginal bleeding is the most common symptom of placenta previa. In about 20% of cases, some degree of uterine irritability is present, but this is usually minor. Vaginal examination usually reveals bright blood from the cervical os. Digital or instrumental probing of the cervix should never be done during the second half of pregnancy, because it can precipitate severe hemorrhage in the patient with an asymptomatic or minimally symptomatic placenta previa. In the emergency department, speculum examination of the vagina and cervix should be performed only in those settings where obstetric consultation is not readily available. It should be limited to an atraumatic partial speculum insertion to identify whether the bleeding is coming from the cervical os (and a presumed placenta previa), hemorrhoids, or a vaginal lesion that might not require urgent management.

Most cases of placenta previa identified during the midtrimester resolve by the time of delivery as the lower uterine segment elongates and the placenta no longer overlaps the cervical os. Central or total previa (which occurs in about 20% of cases) can, however, cause severe hemorrhage, with risk of exsanguination for the fetus and mother.

Diagnostic Strategies

Ultrasonography is the diagnostic procedure of choice for localizing the placenta and diagnosing placenta previa. Accuracy is excellent; visualization of the placenta as well as the internal cervical os is required. The bladder should be emptied prior to examination for suspected placenta previa to avoid overdiagnosis of placenta previa. Transvaginal ultrasonography is safe and even more accurate for visualizing the relationships between the placenta and the internal os.[45]

Management

Patients who experience vaginal bleeding during late pregnancy should have immediate obstetric consultation and arrangements for safe transfer to an appropriate obstetric facility. Emergency department management consists of maternal stabilization, with establishment of two large-bore intravenous lines and fluid resuscitation, as well as continuous fetal monitoring if available. A baseline hemoglobin level should be obtained, and blood should be sent for type and crossmatch; baseline coagulation studies including platelet count, prothrombin time, and partial thromboplastin time should be done; and fibrinogen level and presence of fibrin split products should be determined. Normal fibrinogen level in pregnancy is 400 to 450 mg/dL; values below 300 mg/dL indicate significant consumption of coagulation factors.

Blood loss requiring transfusions can occur in patients with placenta previa or abruptio placentae. Fresh frozen plasma or fresh whole blood may be needed because of the coagulopathy associated with significant abruptio placentae. Fetomaternal hemorrhage can occur with abruption. If the Rh-negative patient has not yet received her routine Rh immunoglobin prophylaxis at 28 weeks, 300 μg of Rh immune globulin should be administered within 72 hours (unless the father is known to be Rh-negative).[46] Transfer to the obstetric unit should be expedited if the patient is stable, or after initiation of resuscitation if she is unstable. If transfer to another hospital is required, a high-risk transfer team should be used if bleeding is significant or if the fetus is in distress. Although the bleeding source may not be identified or may be relatively benign, assessment is best accomplished by obstetricians who are accustomed to evaluating late-pregnancy complications and who can perform emergent cesarean section if needed.

In the obstetrics unit, fetal monitoring is continued. Ultrasonography is used primarily to locate the placenta and diagnose placenta previa; it may not be reliable in confirming the diagnosis of abruption placentae. Occasionally, subplacental hemorrhages of abruptio placentae can be seen and changes in size of the collection can be monitored. If evidence of placenta previa is absent or equivocal, vaginal examination is performed in the delivery suite, where emergency cesarean section can be performed if uncontrolled bleeding is encountered.

Patients who have significant abruptio placentae may require early delivery (either vaginal or surgical, depending on fetal status). If placenta previa is diagnosed or if abruptio placentae is considered mild, the patient is admitted for close monitoring. The goal is to support the patient, ideally until fetal maturity is demonstrated and a successful delivery can be accomplished.

Pregnancy-Induced Hypertension (Preeclampsia and Eclampsia)

Perspective

Hypertension is observed in approximately 6% to 8% of pregnancies and is generally divided into several categories.[47] Gestational hypertension occurs during pregnancy, resolves during the postpartum period, and is recognized by a new blood pressure reading of 140/90 mm Hg or higher. Preeclampsia is gestational hypertension with proteinuria (>300 mg/24 hours) and eclampsia is the occurrence of seizures in the patient with signs of preeclampsia. Progression of preeclampsia to eclampsia is unpredictable and can occur rapidly. Pregnancy-aggravated hypertension is chronic hypertension with superimposed preeclampsia or eclampsia. Chronic or coincidental hypertension is present before pregnancy or persists more than 6 weeks postpartum.[47,48]

Approximately 2% to 7% of pregnancies are complicated by pregnancy-induced hypertension. The incidence of actual eclampsia has progressively declined but is still one of the top three causes of maternal mortality.[16] The risk of pregnancy-induced hypertension is greatest in women younger than 20 years old; primigravidas; those with twin or molar pregnancies; those with hypercholesterolemia, pregestational diabetes, or obesity; and those with a family history of pregnancy-induced hypertension.[48]

Principles of Disease

Gestational hypertension/preeclampsia is a vasospastic disease of unknown cause unique to pregnant women. Vasospasm, ischemia, and thrombosis associated with preeclamptic changes cause injury to maternal organs, placental infarction and abruption, and fetal death from hypoxia and prematurity. The cause of eclampsia is not known, but recent research has centered on vascular responsiveness to endogenous vasopressors in the preeclamptic woman. Vascular responsiveness is normally depressed during pregnancy, which is a high output, low-resistance state. Gestational hypertension is characterized by an even greater elevation in cardiac output, followed by an abnormally high peripheral resistance as the disease develops clinical manifestations. In patients with preeclampsia, the cardiac output eventually drops as peripheral resistance rises.[49] The causes of these changes is not known, but they are associated with a relative increase in various substances, including those prostaglandins associated with vasoconstriction, and a generalized intravascular inflammatory reaction that results in vascular injury.[50] One study found that women with preeclampsia have significantly decreased prostacyclin production many months before the clinical onset of preeclampsia.[51]

The vasospastic effects of gestational hypertension/preeclampsia are protean. Intravascular volume is lower than in normal pregnancy; central venous pressures are normal, and capillary wedge pressures are variable. Liver effects are believed to be due to hepatocellular necrosis and edema resulting from vasospasm. Renal injury causes proteinuria and may result in decreased glomerular filtration. Microangiopathic hemolysis may result from vasospasm, causing thrombocytopenia. Central nervous system effects include microvascular thrombosis and hemorrhage, as well as focal edema and hyperemia.[48]

Clinical Features

Signs and Symptoms

The patient with gestational hypertension has mild systolic or diastolic blood pressure elevation, no proteinuria, and no evidence of organ damage. Mental status assessment, testing of reflexes, abdominal examination, liver function studies, and coagulation studies should all yield normal results. Preeclampsia is associated with kidney changes, and, in severe cases, other end-organ symptoms. Edema is often difficult to assess, because pregnancy is normally associated with excess extracellular fluid and dependent edema, and is no longer used as a criterion for recognizing preeclampsia. Proteinuria (>300 mg/24 hours) is variable at any given time and may not be detectable in a random urine specimen.[47]

In cases of severe preeclampsia, diastolic blood pressure can exceed 110 mm Hg, proteinuria is more severe, and there is evidence of vasospastic effects in various end organs. Central nervous system effects commonly include headache or visual disturbances. Thrombocytopenia may be present, liver function test findings may be elevated, and the liver is often tender. Renal dysfunction may be indicated by oliguria and elevated creatinine levels in addition to proteinuria.

Complications

The HELLP syndrome is a particularly severe form of preeclampsia that develops in 5% to 10% of women who have preeclamptic symptoms and is characterized by *h*emolysis, *e*levated *l*iver enzymes, and *l*ow *p*latelet count (fewer than 100,000/mm^3). Prothrombin time, partial thromboplastin time, and fibrinogen level are all normal, and blood studies reveal microangiopathic hemolytic anemia. Other complications of preeclampsia include spontaneous hepatic and splenic hemorrhage and abruptio placentae.

The most dangerous complication is eclampsia, which is the occurrence of seizures or coma in the setting of signs and symptoms of preeclampsia. Warning signs for development of frank eclampsia include headache, nausea and vomiting, visual disturbances, and mean arterial pressure greater than 160 mm Hg.[52] Elevated lactate dehydrogenase, aspartate aminotransferase, and uric acid concentrations are also predictive of increased morbidity for the patient with severe preeclampsia.[53] Particularly in early eclampsia before 32 weeks' gestation, seizures may develop abruptly and hypertension may not be associated with edema or proteinuria.[54] One third of eclamptic seizures occur after delivery, usually during the first 48 hours but occasionally as long as 28 days after delivery.[55] After 48 hours postpartum and without predelivery signs of preeclampsia, other diagnoses such as intracranial hemorrhage should be considered. Maternal complications of eclampsia include permanent central nervous system damage from recurrent seizures or intracranial bleeding, renal insufficiency, and death.

The maternal mortality rate from eclampsia has been reduced with modern management and is currently less than 1%. Perinatal mortality has also decreased, although it remains 4% to 8%.[48] Causes of neonatal death include placental infarcts, intrauterine growth retardation, and abruptio placenta. In addition, fetal hypoxia from maternal seizures and the complications of premature delivery mandated by the maternal condition contribute significantly to fetal mortality and morbidity.

Diagnostic Strategies

The patient who has severe preeclampsia should have an intravenous line and fetal monitoring initiated in a quiet but closely observed area. Blood testing should include complete blood cell count, renal function studies, liver function tests, platelet count, and coagulation profile. A baseline magnesium level should also be obtained. In the patient with actual seizures, serum glucose should be tested. If a history of preeclampsia is not obtained or the symptoms are refractory to magnesium sulfate therapy, a computed tomography (CT) scan of the head should be performed to exclude cerebral venous thrombosis or an intracranial bleed, either of which can occur in pregnancy (with or without pregnancy-induced hypertension) and may require specific treatment. CT scan abnormalities can be seen in half of patients with eclampsia. Patchy hemorrhage and microinfarcts of the cortex are characteristic, and may be due to loss of cerebral autoregulation in patients with severe pregnancy-related hypertension. Diffuse cerebral edema and increased intracranial pressure can also be seen.[56]

Differential Considerations

Peripheral edema is common in normal pregnancy, and it may be difficult to differentiate normal edema from that of early preeclampsia. Differentiation of gestational hypertension from preexistent hypertension is often impossible in an emergency department population if no record of normal blood pressure is available. Seizures during pregnancy may be due to epilepsy, as well as to other intracranial catastrophes such as thrombosis or hemorrhage.

Management

Prehospital

Eclampsia should always be considered in the patient with a seizure who is visibly pregnant (i.e., >20 weeks). Likewise, the pregnant patient who has trauma (e.g., in a single-vehicle motor vehicle crash) without obvious cause should be suspected of eclampsia. Moderate or severe preeclampsia associated with edema and hyperactive reflexes requires no prehospital treatment other than prophylactic venous access. If the patient has seizures, routine seizure management and protection of the patient's airway should be initiated. In some regions, magnesium sulfate is available to prehospital providers and can be given according to preset protocols, as described later. Diazepam can be administered as an anticonvulsant, although studies have suggested that it is not as effective as magnesium.[48,56]

Emergency Department

In the patient who has mild preeclampsia, appropriate management includes documentation of blood pressure and reflexes, weight, and testing to ensure normal end-organ function. Accurate determination of gestational age by ultrasonography is needed to allow optimal management if symptoms progress. Limitation of physical activities (including bed rest) is the only demonstrated means of reducing blood pressure and allowing the pregnancy to be sustained longer. Definitive treatment is delivery of the fetus. Arrangement for close follow-up is mandatory.

Hospitalization is usually required for patients with sustained hypertension above 140/90 mm Hg and signs of severe preeclampsia. Baseline laboratory studies to identify end-organ effects in the liver, kidney, and hematologic systems should be obtained. Both diuresis and antihypertensive therapy have been remarkably unsuccessful in improving fetal outcome or prolonging pregnancy. Admission does, however, allow the obstetrician to accurately assess fetal age and well-being, maternal organ function, and the effect of bed rest on blood pressure before deciding the optimal timing of delivery.[47]

Fulminant or severe preeclampsia, with marked blood pressure elevation (>160/110 mm Hg), associated with epigastric or liver tenderness, visual disturbance, or severe headache, is managed in the same way as eclampsia (Box 177-4). The goal is prevention of seizures and permanent damage to maternal organs. Magnesium sulfate is given for seizure prophylaxis.

BOX 177-4. Management of Eclampsia and Severe Preeclampsia

- Control seizures with magnesium sulfate.
- Control hypertension after seizure control if diastolic blood pressure > 105 mm Hg.
- Draw initial laboratory studies to assess organ injury:
  - Complete blood count and platelet count
  - Liver function tests
  - BUN, creatinine
- Monitor urine output: maintain at <25 mL/hr.
- Limit intravenous fluid administration unless significant losses occur.
- Avoid diuretics and hyperosmotic agents.
- Perform a CT scan of head if consciousness is decreased or seizures persist, lateralizing signs are present, or there are other concerns.
- Initiate steps to delivery.

BUN, blood urea nitrogen; CT, computed tomography.
Modified from Pritchard J, et al: The Parkland Memorial Hospital protocol for treatment of eclampsia: Evaluation of 245 cases. *Am J Obstet Gynecol* 161:261, 1989.

Seizures and coma are the hallmarks of eclampsia, the ultimate consequence of preeclampsia. As in all seizure patients, hypoglycemia, drug overdose, and other causes of seizures should be excluded with appropriate tests. Eclamptic seizures are controlled in almost all patients by adequate doses of magnesium sulfate, although the mechanism of action remains elusive; it is thought that membrane stabilizer and vasodilator properties are probably active in reducing cerebral ischemia. Magnesium has little antihypertensive effect but is the most effective anticonvulsant, preventing recurrent seizures while maintaining uterine and fetal blood flow. The goal of magnesium sulfate therapy is to terminate ongoing seizures and prevent further seizures. A loading of dose of 6 g IV magnesium, followed by 2 g IV/ hour, is recommended. Magnesium administration should be accompanied by clinical observation for loss of reflexes (which occurs at about 10 mg/dL) or respiratory depression (which occurs at levels over 12 mg/dL, although actual serum magnesium levels are rarely monitored). The infusion should be stopped if signs of hypermagnesemia are seen; such patients may require assisted ventilation. Calcium gluconate, 1 g given slowly into a secure vein, will reverse the adverse effects of hypermagnesemia.[48]

Despite ongoing controversy, the familiarity, physiologic advantages to the fetus, wide margin of safety, and high success rate in controlling seizures make magnesium sulfate the first-line drug in patients with eclampsia. Several recent reports highlight an international consensus that magnesium sulfate is more effective than nimodipine, phenytoin, or diazepam for prophylaxis against or treatment of eclamptic seizures.[48,57] If seizures persist after the recommended doses of magnesium sulfate have been administered, further therapy should be given in conjunction with obstetric consultation and a careful search for other causes of seizures (e.g., hypoglycemia, intracranial bleed) should be instituted.

Although magnesium sulfate is not a direct antihypertensive, the hypertension associated with eclampsia is often controlled adequately by stopping the seizures. Rapid lowering of blood pressure can result in uterine hypoperfusion, so specific antihypertensive treatment is initiated only if the diastolic blood pressure remains above 105 mm Hg after control of seizures. Many patients do not require specific antihypertensive treatment after treatment with magnesium sulfate. The antihypertensive used most often by obstetricians is hydralazine. The dose is 5 mg/IV, with repeated doses of 5 to 10 mg IV every 20 minutes as needed to keep the diastolic blood pressure below 105 mm Hg. Nimodipine and labetalol have also been reported to be safe and effective, although they are less widely used.[48,57] Other antihypertensive agents are not well studied in this population, where there are specific risks to uncontrolled lowering of blood pressure and loss of uteroplacental blood flow.

Although total body water in the eclamptic patient is excessive, intravascular volume is contracted and the eclamptic patient is very sensitive to further volume changes. Hypovolemia results in decreased uterine perfusion. Thus, diuretics and hyperosmotic agents should be avoided in patients with eclampsia. Although intravascular volume expansion in the face of volume contraction, increased systemic resistance, and vasospasm would seem reasonable, invasive monitoring has demonstrated that vasospasm is not reversed with intravenous fluid administration. Rather, excessive intravenous fluids increase extravascular fluid stores that are difficult to mobilize postpartum, resulting in a higher incidence of pulmonary edema in patients treated aggressively with fluid therapy. Invasive pulmonary artery pressure monitoring may be required for accurate fluid management in the eclamptic patient.

Amniotic Fluid Embolus

Perspective

Amniotic fluid embolus (AFE) is the release of amniotic fluid into the maternal circulation during intense uterine contractions or uterine manipulation, or at areas of placental separation from the uterine decidua basalis (abruptio placentae), triggering a rapidly fatal anaphylactoid-type maternal response. Although AFE most commonly occurs during labor, in which circumstance the maternal mortality rate is 25% or higher, it can also occur after induced abortions and miscarriage and spontaneously during the second and third trimesters. AFE can also occur after amniocentesis or in association with abruptio placentae after abdominal trauma. Although it is a rare syndrome, AFE is responsible for 13% to 30% of maternal deaths and is the fifth leading cause of direct maternal death.[58]

Clinical Features

Amniotic fluid embolus should be suspected during the second or third trimester of pregnancy, particularly in the setting of uterine manipulation or contraction, when a patient experiences sudden hypotension, hypoxia, and coagulopathy. The embolization of amniotic fluid and the particulate matter suspended in it triggers a profound immunologic response when it enters the maternal circulation. Half of the cases of mortality occur during the first 2 hours when vasospasm, release of vasoactive substances, and mechanical plugging of vessels, particularly in the maternal pulmonary vascular tree, trigger abrupt cardiopulmonary collapse.[58] In survivors, disseminated intravascular coagulation, acute respiratory distress syndrome, and left ventricular dysfunction develop. An initial seizure is seen in about 10% of patients. Bleeding diathesis may be the initial sign in some women.

Diagnostic Strategies

When AFE is suggested, a complete blood cell count, coagulation studies, arterial blood gases, and chest radiograph should be obtained. Urinary output should be monitored after urinary catheter placement. The diagnosis is usually made with certainty only at autopsy, with the finding of fetal hairs, squamous cells, and debris in the maternal circulation. Because squamous epithelial cells can be seen normally in the maternal pulmonary circulation, the typical clinical syndrome is also required for diagnosis.[58]

Differential Considerations

Catastrophic pulmonary embolus, drug-induced anaphylaxis, and septic shock must be considered in the differential diagnosis. Seizure occurs in patients with eclampsia, but in that condition hypertension, rather than cardiovascular collapse, should be observed. Coagulopathy may be seen in patients with preeclampsia (HELLP syndrome), abruptio placentae, or other chronic coagulopathies seen in the nonpregnant patient.

Management

Amniotic fluid embolus is uncommon, so treatment is mainly anecdotal and based on animal studies. The most helpful modalities appear to be high-flow oxygen, support of ventilation and oxygenation with intubation, aggressive fluid resuscitation, inotropic cardiovascular support, and anticipation and management of consumptive coagulopathy. A few reports have indicated that plasma exchange may be helpful to remove triggering cytokines.[59] Adequate management usually requires invasive hemodynamic monitoring in an intensive care unit.

Rh (Anti-D) Immunization in Pregnancy

Rh immunization occurs when an Rh-negative woman is exposed to Rh-positive fetal blood. Small numbers of fetal cells enter the maternal circulation spontaneously throughout pregnancy, but the maternal immune system is only triggered by significant loads of fetal cells, which can occur during the third trimester and at delivery. Sensitization occurs in up to 15% of Rh-negative women carrying Rh-positive fetuses. To prevent this, anti-D immunoglobulin (RhoGAM) is routinely administered to Rh-negative mothers (if the father is Rh-positive or his status is unknown) at about the 28th week of gestation to protect the mother from spontaneous sensitization, which occurs during the third trimester. Transplacental hemorrhage can also occur during uterine manipulation, threatened miscarriage (even without fetal loss), spontaneous miscarriage, surgery for ectopic pregnancy, and amniocentesis, although the risk is not clear. Anti-D immunoglobulin (RhoGAM) should be administered when these events occur. A dose of 50 μg can be used if the patient is at less than 12 weeks' gestation, although many pharmacies only carry the 300-μg dose, which can also be given. After 12 weeks, a 300-μg dose should be given. The half-life of immunoglobulin is 24 days, and it needs to be administered within 72 hours of a sensitization event to prevent antibody development.[60]

The Kleihauer-Betke test of maternal blood has been used to detect fetal cells in the maternal circulation. Unfortunately, the test is difficult to perform, not immediately available in most emergency laboratories, and only sensitive enough to detect 5 mL of fetal cells in the maternal circulation. Because only 0.1 mL of fetal cells is required to sensitize the mother, routine immunoglobulin administration has been recommended in situations likely to result in sensitization. Patients with third-trimester bleeding are not at increased risk of sensitization compared with patients with normal pregnancy; RhoGAM should be administered only if the patient did not receive her prophylactic dose at 28 weeks.[46] In instances of significant blunt trauma to the uterus, the Kleihauer-Betke test should be ordered to detect the rare large fetal transfusions that may require specific fetal blood therapy or administration of additional immunoglobulin to the mother. The standard dose (300 μg) is sufficient to prevent maternal immunization for fetal transfusions of up to 15 mL of red blood cells or 30 mL of whole blood.[60]

MEDICAL AND SURGICAL PROBLEMS IN THE PREGNANT PATIENT

Perspective

Clinicians must be aware of a variety of illnesses, both related and unrelated to pregnancy, that may have altered symptomatology, risk, and treatment in the pregnant patient (Tables 177-2 and 177-3).

Abdominal Pain

Gynecologic Problems

Several gynecologic diseases must be considered in evaluating the pregnant patient who has abdominal pain. These include threatened miscarriage and ectopic pregnancy, which were discussed in the first part of this chapter. A patient with either complication of pregnancy can complain of nonspecific abdominal pain, either in the midline or laterally, and may show intermittent or constant symptoms. A careful history can be helpful in differentiating gradual progression of inflammatory or infectious diseases (such as ovarian cyst expansion or, rarely, PID) from sudden peritonitis caused by spillage of blood or cyst fluid into the peritoneal cavity, or from the colicky pain of renal stones or the ischemic pain of ovarian torsion. In addition, examination of the abdomen, back, and pelvis helps localize the pain to areas and specific organs, thus narrowing the differential diagnosis and guiding the selection of ancillary studies.

Appendicitis

Perspective

Appendicitis is the most common surgical emergency in pregnant patients. The incidence of appendicitis in pregnant patients is the same as in nonpregnant patients, but delays in diagnosis contribute to an increased rate of perforation, which results in significant fetal mortality and maternal morbidity. During the first half of pregnancy, diagnostic findings are usually similar to those in the nonpregnant woman, but the clinical picture becomes less classic during the second half of pregnancy.

Table 177-2. Differential Diagnosis of Abdominal Pain in Pregnancy

Diagnosis	Gestational Age	Comments
Gynecologic		
Miscarriage	<20 weeks, 80% <12 weeks	Ultrasonography to confirm location
Septic abortion	<20 weeks	Fever, uterine tenderness
Ectopic pregnancy	<14 weeks	Must always consider in first trimester until intrauterine pregnancy confirmed
Corpus luteum cyst	<12 weeks	Sudden focal peritoneal pain; no fever
Ovarian torsion	Especially <24 weeks	Ischemic pain
Pelvic Inflammatory disease	<12 weeks	Very rare
Chorioamnionitis	>16 weeks	Tender uterus, fever; amniocentesis reveals white blood cells
Abruptio placentae	>16 weeks	Focal uterine tenderness, fetal distress, variable bleeding
Preeclampsia	>20 weeks	Hypertension, proteinuria, edema, right upper quadrant pain
Nongynecologic		
Appendicitis	Throughout	Guarding may be less prominent; location changes
Cholecystitis	Throughout	Confirm with ultrasonography
Hepatitis	Throughout	Confirm with liver function tests
Pyelonephritis	Throughout	Flank pain, fever, positive catheterized urinalysis

Table 177-3. Differential Diagnosis of Common Symptoms in Pregnancy

Diagnosis	Gestational Age	Comments
Vaginal Bleeding		
Miscarriage	<20 weeks	Usually no fetal heart activity at 8 weeks; decreasing hCG
Ectopic pregnancy	<14 weeks	Evaluate with ultrasonography
Molar pregnancy	12-24 weeks	No fetal heart tones, characteristic sonogram
Cervical lesions	Throughout	Perineal and vaginal inspection
Vaginitis/cervicitis	Throughout	White blood cells on wet mount, with culture
Placenta previa	>16 weeks	Ultrasonography to localize placenta
Abruptio placentae	>16 weeks	Ultrasonography to exclude previa; fetal distress, tenderness
Seizure		
Eclampsia	>24 weeks	Blood pressure >140/90 mm Hg; usually history of PIH, edema, proteinuria
Amniotic fluid embolus	>12 weeks	Hypotension, respiratory distress, DIC
Epilepsy	Throughout	History; lack of PIH findings
Dyspnea		
Pulmonary embolus	Especially 6 weeks prepartum and postpartum	Usual diagnostic studies
Dyspnea of pregnancy	>24 weeks	Exclude other causes
Pulmonary infection	Throughout	Examination; roentgenography
Amniotic fluid embolus	>12 weeks	Uterine manipulation, bleeding diathesis, hypotension
Jaundice		
Cholestasis of pregnancy	>24 weeks	Well patient; itching and jaundice
Hepatitis	Throughout	Abnormal liver function tests
Acute fatty liver	>24 weeks	Rapid liver failure; coma, seizures, hypoglycemia
Bleeding Diathesis		
Eclampsia	>24 weeks	Blood pressure > 140/90 mm Hg; proteinuria, edema, HELLP syndrome
Amniotic fluid embolus	>12 weeks	Respiratory distress, cardiovascular collapse
Abruptio placentae	>20 weeks	Uterine tenderness; vaginal bleeding; fetal distress

DIC, disseminated intravascular coagulation; hCG, human chorionic gonadotropin; HELLP, hemolysis, elevated liver enzymes, low platelets; PIH, pregnancy-induced hypertension.

Principles of Disease

During pregnancy, the appendix is usually displaced counterclockwise out of the right lower quadrant after the third month of gestation. Displacement of the abdominal wall away from the abdominal viscera results in difficulty palpating organs and loss of signs of parietal peritoneal irritation. By the last trimester, the appendix is located deep in the right upper quadrant, superior to the iliac crest (Figure 177-2). However, one recent study questioned this finding, and found that only 23% of pregnant patients had the location move from the right lower quadrant, even in the third trimester.[61] The physiologic increase in white blood cell count and erythrocyte sedimentation rate in pregnancy also must be considered when evaluating the patient with possible appendicitis.

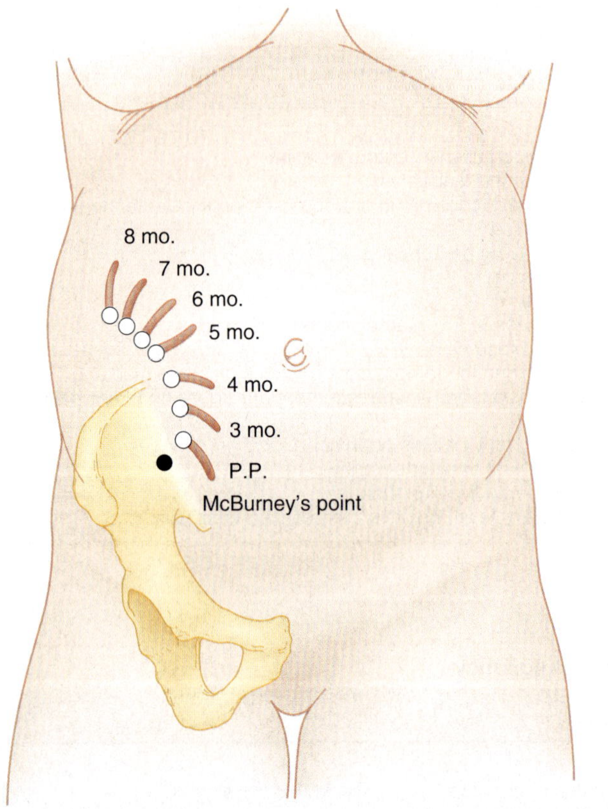

Figure 177-2. Locations of the appendix during succeeding months of pregnancy. In planning an operation, it is better to make the abdominal incision over the point of maximal tenderness unless there is great disparity between that point and the theoretical location of the appendix. P.P., post partum. (From Gabbe: Normal and problem pregnancies, as modified from Baer JL: *JAMA* 98:1359, 1932.)

Clinical Features

The gastrointestinal symptoms of appendicitis, such as anorexia, nausea, and vomiting, mimic those of pregnancy, particularly during the first trimester, making such symptoms relatively nonspecific. Right-sided abdominal pain is the most constant finding, although this is less reliable later in pregnancy. Peritoneal signs are likewise most common during the first trimester. Lack of fever, leukocytosis, or tachycardia has been reported.[62] The cause of these differences in clinical findings in pregnant patients with appendicitis may be a blunted inflammatory response from elevated maternal levels of pregnancy-related steroids. Pyuria without bacteruria is seen in about 20% of patients.

Because of confounding factors, the misdiagnosis rate for appendicitis is 30% to 35% overall in pregnancy, with a 40% to 50% rate of removal of normal appendix during the third trimester.[62,63] In contrast to the relative safety of performing an exploratory laparotomy or laparoscopy during pregnancy, the risk of fetal loss from failure to diagnose appendicitis and perforation is considerable, so clinical vigilance is required in the absence of classic signs. In later pregnancy, when peritoneal signs are often absent and the uterus obscures normal physical findings, diagnosis is frequently delayed and the perforation rate may approach 25%.

Differential Considerations

Pyelonephritis, cholecystitis, and pregnancy-related diseases such as ectopic pregnancy, broad ligament pain, corpus luteum cyst leakage, and ovarian torsion must be considered in the patient who has right-sided abdominal pain. Pyelonephritis is the most common condition that is confused with appendicitis. During its migration, the appendix takes up a position very near the kidney, resulting in a high incidence of pyuria and flank pain (see Figure 177-2). In cases of appendicitis, unless there is coincident urinary tract infection, the urine is free of bacteria, a feature distinguishing it from pyelonephritis. Salpingitis, another common misdiagnosis, is very rare in pregnancy, although it can occur before 12 weeks of gestation.

Diagnostic Strategies

Leukocytosis is common in pregnant patients with appendicitis, although it is rarely high enough to distinguish it from the physiologic leukocytosis of pregnancy. Pyuria in a catheterized urine specimen suggests pyelonephritis, but it is also seen in 20% of patients with appendicitis.[62] Bacteruria is uncommon. Ultrasonography, using graded-compression techniques, has been reported to be more than 90% accurate in diagnosing appendicitis in pregnant patients. Castro[64] has reported the utility of helical CT in diagnosis, with fetal radiation exposures of only 300 mrad, using rectal contrast and a limited study. Otherwise, laparoscopy or laparotomy is the diagnostic procedure of choice in the pregnant patient suspected of having appendicitis. Early exploration is to be encouraged even more in pregnant than in nonpregnant patients because of the variability of clinical signs and the increased fetal risk if diagnosis is delayed.

Management

The pregnant patient with suspected appendicitis should be admitted to the hospital after appropriate consultation with surgeons and obstetricians. Ultrasonography or CT scan should be considered as diagnostic options. The patient should be kept on nothing by mouth (NPO) status, with intravenous fluid hydration to maintain intravascular volume. Although prompt surgery is required if the diagnosis is clear, in unclear cases a period of inpatient observation may allow clarification of signs and symptoms.

Gallbladder Disease

Perspective

Cholelithiasis is present in about 5% of pregnant women and is the second most common nonobstetric surgical condition in pregnant patients. The natural history of asymptomatic cholelithiasis is believed to be similar to that in nonpregnant women, with less than half of patients with gallstones developing symptoms.[65]

Principles of Disease

Changes in gallbladder kinetics are believed to be due to high pregnancy-related steroid levels. Progesterone decreases smooth muscle tone and induces cholestasis, causing an increased risk of stone formation.

Clinical Features

The signs and symptoms of acute cholecystitis during pregnancy are the same as those in nonpregnant women. Epigastric or right upper quadrant pain and tenderness and nausea predominate. Leukocytosis must be evaluated with care because of the increased white blood cell count seen normally in pregnancy. Likewise, a slightly elevated amylase level can be normal during pregnancy, and alkaline phosphatase, which is produced by the placenta, may be twice the nonpregnant level. A history of self-limited pain episodes associated with food intake is useful in suggesting the diagnosis.

Diagnostic Strategies

Ultrasonography is a reliable means of recognizing stones within the gallbladder, although it may not differentiate symptomatic from asymptomatic stones. In the patient with right upper quadrant pain, simultaneous sonographic evaluation of the liver is useful although technically difficult, particularly during the third trimester, when subcapsular liver hematomas and other intrinsic hepatocellular disease can occur but may be hidden under the ribs.

Differential Considerations

Pyelonephritis should be considered in the patient with right upper quadrant pain with or without fever. During the third trimester, appendicitis can also be associated with right upper quadrant pain. Hepatitis occurs in pregnancy; liver distention and inflammation associated with pregnancy-induced hypertension can also cause right upper quadrant pain. In addition, spontaneous intrahepatic bleeding can occur in late pregnancy, mimicking cholecystitis. Because of the potential for other serious diseases, diagnostic studies should always be performed to verify a clinical diagnosis of cholecystitis in pregnancy.

Management

The patient who has fever, leukocytosis, prolonged pain, or evidence of complicated cholecystitis should be admitted for inpatient management. Some patients can be managed conservatively with intravenous hydration, bed rest, fluids, analgesics, and antibiotics for prolonged or complicated cholecystitis. Discharge should be considered only in patients with uncomplicated and sonographically proven cholelithiasis who do not meet admission criteria after consultation with an obstetrician. Early follow-up should be arranged and the patient should be given careful instructions to return if she experiences fever, vomiting, or persistent pain. In one study, one third of pregnant women with biliary colic failed conservative treatment but were treated safely, often using newer laparoscopic techniques.[66]

Liver Disorders

Perspective

Pregnancy is associated with several unique liver abnormalities, in addition to more usual hepatic diseases. Clinicians should recognize the symptoms of liver disease during pregnancy as well as the hepatic diseases unique to pregnant women. Liver metabolism increases during pregnancy, but hepatic blood flow is unchanged and little change occurs in liver function. Bilirubin, transaminases, and prothrombin times are unchanged from the nonpregnant state. Alkaline phosphate levels may be up to double the nonpregnant values, and amylase levels may also be slightly elevated.[67]

Hepatitis

Hepatitis is the most common cause of liver disease in pregnancy, accounting for 40% of jaundice in pregnancy. Management and treatment are unchanged from that for nonpregnant patients. Maintaining adequate nutrition is a priority. Vertical transmission of hepatitis B can occur if the disease is not recognized and prophylaxis should be administered to the newborn.

Acute Fatty Liver of Pregnancy

Acute fatty liver of pregnancy is a disorder of the third trimester that can result in hepatic failure, complicated labor, and fetal mortality. The disease is rare, occurring most often in primiparous patients and patients with twin gestations.

Principles of Disease. The cause of acute fatty liver of pregnancy is unknown, although the liver abnormalities and clinical picture are similar to those of Reye's syndrome. Microscopically, fatty infiltration of the hepatocytes with edema and vacuolization can be seen, but there is no necrosis or inflammation. Liver function returns to normal after delivery if the patient can be supported through the acute phase. Although often seen in patients with preeclampsia and having some of the same characteristic abnormalities, the linkage between the two is not well established.[68]

Clinical Features. Nausea and vomiting or liver dysfunction during the third trimester should trigger consideration of a diagnosis of acute fatty liver. Additionally, symptoms of anorexia, fatigue, and headache occur initially, and the liver is usually tender. The disease may progress to coagulopathy, jaundice, seizures, and hepatic coma. The diagnosis is often delayed.[68]

Diagnostic Strategies. Typically, leukocytosis is present, the platelet count is low, prothrombin time and partial thromboplastin time are elevated, and fibrin split products are present. Hypoglycemia may occur. Serum transaminase levels are elevated, although rarely above 500 U/L, and should be measured in all patients who have systemic gastrointestinal symptoms during the third trimester. In contrast to Reye's syndrome, the serum ammonia level is only mildly elevated. Hyperuricemia is usually present. Bilirubin is elevated late in the course of the disease. The CT scan is usually normal, as is the sonogram. Liver biopsy is used to make the diagnosis.[69]

Differential Considerations

Liver tenderness and coagulopathy most often suggest preeclampsia during the third trimester.[69] Jaundice and aminotransferase level rises are unusual in cases of liver disease associated with pregnancy-induced hypertension, and rapid progression of hepatic failure, hypoglycemia, and coagulopathy is unlikely in cases of preeclampsia. The patient with viral hepatitis is likely to have more marked elevations in transaminase levels. Drug-induced hepatic failure should be excluded by history and toxicologic screen for acetaminophen or other toxins if appropriate. Cholecystitis may also be characterized by right upper quadrant pain but is not associated with coagulopathy or progressive liver failure.

Management

The patient with acute fatty liver of pregnancy requires immediate stabilization if experiencing seizure or coma. Hypoglycemia may occur, and coagulation parameters should be assessed. Fluid resuscitation and replacement of clotting factors may be required, and the patient should be admitted to an obstetric service capable of managing this serious disease. The diagnosis is usually made with liver biopsy if the disease has not progressed to severe coagulopathy. Rapid delivery is usually advisable when the diagnosis has been established. Fresh frozen plasma, platelet transfusions, and glucose may be needed to sustain the patient until delivery can be accomplished. After delivery, infants of mothers with acute fatty liver of pregnancy are at risk for postpartum hypoglycemia and liver dysfunction, and therefore should be monitored closely.[69]

Intrahepatic Cholestasis of Pregnancy

Intrahepatic cholestasis of pregnancy, also termed *idiopathic jaundice of pregnancy* or *pruritus gravidarum*, is a syndrome that occurs during the third trimester of pregnancy. It is the second most common cause of jaundice in pregnancy, after hepatitis. Histologically, the disease is characterized by cholestasis and dilated canaliculi in the biliary tree. The liver itself is normal. It is more common with increasing maternal age and with multiple gestations.[70]

Clinical Features. Generalized pruritus and mild jaundice are the hallmarks of intrahepatic cholestasis of pregnancy. Although insomnia and fatigue occasionally accompany the pruritus, the patient appears nontoxic, without fever, vomiting, diarrhea, or significant malaise. The bilirubin level is rarely above 5 mg/dL, the alkaline phosphatase level can be elevated 7-fold to 10-fold, and transaminase levels are in the normal range. Resolution occurs when the woman delivers. Women with intrahepatic cholestasis of pregnancy are at increased risk for preterm delivery and meconium passage.[70]

Differential Considerations and Management. Exclusion of more serious entities, such as viral hepatitis, acute fatty liver, drug-induced cholestasis, or complicated cholecystitis, is required. Outpatient management is appropriate, provided the diagnosis is clear and the patient has close obstetric follow-up. Symptomatic treatment with antihistamines, ursodeoxycholic acid, bile salts, guar gum, and other medications has been tried with variable success.[71]

Hyperemesis Gravidarum

Nausea and vomiting are common in pregnancy, particularly from 6 to 20 weeks of gestation. *Hyperemesis gravidarum* is defined as nausea and vomiting that causes starvation metabolism, weight loss, dehydration, and prolonged ketosis. It occurs in a small minority of pregnant patients. Wernicke's encephalopathy can complicate hyperemesis.[72] The cause of hyperemesis gravidarum is not clear; associations have been made with increasing estradiol and hCG levels, as well as with maternal cytokines.[73,74] One study also reported an increased infection rate with *Helicobacter pylori* in patients with hyperemesis gravidarum.[75] Initial management involves rehydration with intravenous fluids, antiemetics, and demonstration of ability to take oral hydration. Patients may require enteral nutrition. Most standard antiemetics are in Food and Drug Administration category C and are used successfully to treat hyperemesis gravidarum. A short course of oral prednisolone has been reported to be therapeutic for intractable hyperemesis.[76] Bilirubin and alkaline phosphatase levels can be mildly elevated but should return to normal levels after delivery.

Thromboembolic Disease in Pregnancy

Principles of Disease

Thromboembolic disease accounts for almost 20% of obstetric mortality, making it the leading cause of death in pregnancy.[16] Pregnancy is a hypercoagulable state, with increased coagulation factors and stasis as pregnancy progresses and significant vascular trauma at the time of delivery. The risk of venous thrombosis increases during pregnancy to five to six times that of nonpregnant women. The risk is increased throughout pregnancy but is highest during the puerperium. Women who smoke, have varicose veins, or have a prior superficial venous thrombosis, as well as women who deliver prematurely or have postpartum hemorrhage, are at higher risk.[77]

Clinical Features

Clinical signs of pain, tenderness, and swelling are poor predictors of deep vein thrombosis in pregnancy (as in nonpregnancy). The clinical diagnosis of pulmonary embolus is likewise difficult. Although tachypnea, dyspnea, and pleuritic pain are commonly associated with pulmonary embolus, the symptoms are nonspecific and in pregnancy may be associated with such diverse diseases as hepatic inflammation, pyelonephritis, and diaphragmatic impingement from the pregnancy.

Diagnostic Strategies

An arterial blood gas analysis should be undertaken, although arterial blood gases in pregnancy normally show a respiratory alkalosis from progesterone-induced respiratory stimulation, and the alveolar-arterial (A-a) oxygen difference is normal (the pregnant normal A-a gradient can be as high as 20 mm Hg) in the majority of patients with pulmonary embolus.[78] A chest radiograph (shielding the pelvis and uterus) should be obtained to exclude other disease processes. The diaphragm is normally symmetrically elevated during late pregnancy.

Noninvasive impedance plethysmography and Doppler ultrasonography are useful in the diagnosis of deep vein thrombosis of the femoral or popliteal veins in pregnancy, and these studies provide the least risk to the patient. Abnormal flow study results can be found in the normal patient studied in the supine position during late pregnancy, so positive results should be confirmed with the patient positioned on her left side. An unequivocally abnormal flow study finding is sufficient reason to treat the pregnant patient in most cases. However, normal leg study results can be seen with isolated iliac vein disease, which is common in pregnancy. If thromboembolic disease is suspected, further indirect Doppler testing or CT may be required.[79] The risk of treatment usually outweighs the risk of definitive studies when the diagnosis is still in doubt.

Technetium-labeled ventilation-perfusion scans expose the fetus to less than 50 mrad of radiation, making them safe. One recent study found that only 2% of pregnant women had high-probability scans; no adverse events occurred during follow-up in 104 women who were not heparinized and had normal or nondiagnostic scans.[80] Labeled fibrinogen studies are contraindicated in pregnancy. The average fetal radiation dose in helical CT scans is less than that from ventilation-perfusion scans, making it a potentially attractive alternative, although studies of its accuracy in pregnancy have not yet been done.[81] A pulmonary angiogram may be required if the diagnosis of pulmonary embolus is unclear after less invasive studies.

Management

Warfarin (Coumadin) is contraindicated during pregnancy because of its association with a high risk of abortion or fetal malformation, and continued risk to the fetus during the second and third trimesters. Heparinoids are used to treat thromboembolic disease during pregnancy. Unfractionated heparin carries a poorly understood risk of fetal osteoporosis, thrombocytopenia, prematurity, or miscarriage, but the alternatives carry greater risk. In general, acute anticoagulation with intravenous heparin is followed by subcutaneous heparin twice daily, usually continued for 3 to 6 months postpartum in patients who have deep vein thrombosis or pulmonary embolus during pregnancy. Reports of the efficacy and safety of low-molecular-weight heparin in pregnancy are beginning to appear, but it is not yet the standard of care.[82] Low-molecular-weight heparin has several advantages over unfractionated heparin in pregnancy: fixed dosages, less frequent dosing, and decreased risk of osteoporosis and thrombocytopenia. In patients with a history of deep vein thrombosis or pulmonary embolus, prophylaxis for subsequent gestations is usually recommended.[83]

Genitourinary Infections

Urinary Tract Infection

Principles of Disease

Although the risk of asymptomatic bacteruria (9%) does not increase in pregnancy, it appears that pregnancy predisposes the patient to develop symptomatic lower or upper tract genitourinary infections.[84] Mechanical pressure on the bladder and ureters, poor emptying of the bladder with voiding, and progesterone-induced smooth muscle relaxation that inhibits ureteral peristalsis appear to contribute to increased risk of infection during pregnancy.

Identification of patients with asymptomatic bacteruria by prenatal screening in early pregnancy identifies about 95% of individuals at risk for subsequent bacteruria during the pregnancy. Because up to 30% of women who have asymptomatic bacteruria will develop pyelonephritis if untreated, treatment of bacteruria is cost effective and important.[85]

Clinical Features and Diagnostic Strategies

The pregnant patient who comes to the emergency department with lower urinary tract symptoms (dysuria, frequency, and urgency) or upper tract symptoms (fever, malaise, or back pain) should have a pelvic examination and evaluation of an uncontaminated urine specimen (preferably catheterized). There is a predominance of right-sided symptoms during pregnancy, probably the result of increased mechanical forces on the right ureter, but left-sided flank pain or bilateral symptoms may be caused by pyelonephritis. Rarely, urinalysis may yield normal results or cultures may produce negative findings, either because of failure to report lower colony counts or because of complete obstruction of the involved ureter.

The major risk of asymptomatic and lower urinary tract infection is spread to the renal parenchyma. Acute pyelonephritis carries considerable morbidity in pregnancy, including maternal sepsis, permanent renal injury, and premature labor.[85] The risk of prematurity can be minimized by effective treatment and continued monitoring for recurrence. The development of premature labor in the woman who has pyelonephritis is ominous and can be prevented only by aggressive recognition and treatment earlier in pregnancy.

Differential Considerations

Vaginitis, herpes genitalis, chlamydial infection of the urethra, or ovarian torsion can masquerade as urinary tract symptoms. A history of external dysuria (burning at the perineum with urination) suggests herpes or vaginitis. A pelvic examination should be performed to obtain cervical cultures and to identify perineal or vaginal causes of dysuria. Appendicitis, cholecystitis, pancreatitis, and liver diseases in pregnancy must be considered in the differential diagnosis of upper urinary tract infection. Back pain may also be a sign of premature labor. Careful evaluation of an uncontaminated catheterized urine specimen is essential to making the correct diagnosis.

Management

Patients with asymptomatic bacteruria or lower urinary tract signs and symptoms should be treated with 7 to 10 days of an antibiotic that is active against usual urinary pathogens and is safe in pregnancy.[86] The most common choices are a cephalosporin, nitrofurantoin, or a sulfonamide (except during the third trimester). Single-dose therapy for these infections during pregnancy has been proposed but may not be appropriate in an emergency department population with questionable follow-up and a relatively high incidence of occult upper urinary tract infection.

Patients with fever, back pain, and evidence of acute pyelonephritis in pregnancy are usually admitted for intravenous antibiotic administration, although outpatient parenteral therapy can be effective and safe in selected patients.[87] In such cases, intravenous hydration, obstetric consultation, and urine cultures should be initiated. At least one parenteral dose of antibiotics should be given, with antibiotic coverage guided by known organism susceptibilities in a given hospital. Because the resistance of *Escherichia coli* to ampicillin is considerable in most regions, cephalosporins or a combination of a penicillin and an aminoglycoside (which must be carefully monitored because of variable clearance by infected kidneys) is the usual intravenous medication administered. Cultures must be performed to ensure that the original choice of antibiotic was correct, and the patient must have a repeat culture and be followed closely after treatment.

Vaginitis

Bacterial Vaginosis

Bacterial vaginosis (formally known as *Gardnerella* vaginitis or *Haemophilus vaginalis* vaginitis) is an overgrowth of multiple endogenous vaginal bacteria, producing in some cases discharge and excess vaginal odor. Prevalence rates for bacterial vaginosis in pregnancy are estimated at 15% to 20%. Bacterial vaginosis is associated with an increased risk of amnionitis, premature rupture of membranes, fetal prematurity, and postpartum infection after vaginal delivery. Therapy during the second trimester is recommended even when the patient is asymptomatic to prevent the sequelae of premature rupture of membranes. Management includes a 7-day course of metronidazole or a 7-day course of clindamycin. Intravaginal treatment is not recommended in pregnant patients.[86]

Candida albicans Vaginitis

The incidence of vulvovaginal candidiasis is increased during pregnancy by high levels of estrogen and other steroids. It is not increased in the pregnant patient who has recently been on antibiotics[88] and there is no association of *Candida* colonization with low birth weight or preterm delivery.[89] Treatment with vaginal azoles for 7 days during pregnancy is considered safe, with an estimated 85% to 100% cure rate.[86] Recurrent disease may require longer treatment or treatment of a potential *Candida* reservoir in the patient's partner.

Trichomoniasis

Trichomoniasis is a sexually transmitted vaginitis caused by a protozoan parasite, *Trichomonas vaginalis.* Of patients who have trichomoniasis, 50% are asymptomatic. The recommended treatment is metronidazole, a one-time dose of 2 g, for symptomatic patients only.[86] The organism is rarely aggressive during pregnancy but is associated with adverse pregnancy outcomes if untreated.

Sexually Transmitted Diseases in Pregnancy

Sexually transmitted diseases are treated in pregnant patients according to the latest Centers for Disease Control and Prevention guidelines, which should be referenced for the latest treatment guidelines. In general, the tetracyclines and quinolones are contraindicated in pregnant patients. Treatment of genital tract infections may be important in preventing preterm labor and the morbidity of prematurity.

Chlamydia trachomatis Infection

Chlamydia trachomatis infection is the most common sexually transmitted disease, both in the United States and worldwide. Its prevalence is currently three to five times that of *Neisseria gonorrhoeae* infection.[86] Clinical diagnosis is difficult during pregnancy because cervical mucus is usually cloudy and contains white blood cells. Routine *Chlamydia* screening during pregnancy is important to prevent complications of preterm labor and postpartum endometritis, both of which are more common in patients who have chlamydial cervical infections.[90] Chlamydial conjunctivitis has become epidemic among infants born to mothers with chlamydial cervical infections. In addition, neonatal pneumonia caused by *Chlamydia* is common. Recommended treatment during pregnancy or breast-feeding is a 7-day course of erythromycin base or amoxicillin. Azithromycin (single 1-g dose) is an acceptable alternate treatment.[86]

Herpes Simplex Infection

Herpes simplex virus infections pose a significant risk in pregnancy to both the mother and the newborn. Women who have genital herpes during the third trimester have an increased risk of transmission (30-50%) compared with woman with herpes simplex virus infection in the first trimester (1%). The virus can be transmitted prenatally via intrauterine infection and via vaginal delivery, particularly when herpetic lesions are present. Infections in the neonate often are disseminated or involve the central nervous system, causing significant morbidity and mortality. In the emergency department, culturing of new suspected herpetic lesions of the cervix, vagina, or perineum identifies patients at risk for perinatal complications. Although the risk of oral acyclovir use in pregnancy is not well known, it is recommended for first-episode genital herpes. Suppressive acyclovir therapy can reduce the need for cesarean section in women whose first clinical episode of genital herpes simplex virus occurred during pregnancy but may not eliminate the need for cesarean sections in women with recurrent herpes simplex virus.[86] Treatment should be undertaken with obstetric consultation and careful patient monitoring.

Neisseria gonorrhoeae Infection

Gonococcal infection of the cervix occurs during pregnancy in 1% of women. Symptoms are similar to those in nonpregnant women. Salpingitis is rare but may develop during the first trimester from upper genital extension of cervical infection. Some practitioners believe that the incidence of the disseminated infection is increased in pregnant patients because of elevated progesterone levels and increased vascularity in the area of the cervix. Diagnosis and treatment of gonococcal infections are unchanged by pregnancy, and treatment includes cephalosporins or spectinomycin.[86] Treatment for possible coexistent chlamydial infection is recommended for pregnant and nonpregnant women. The major complications of third-trimester gonococcal infection are neonatal gonococcal ophthalmia and sepsis.[86]

Upper Genital Tract Infection

Pelvic Inflammatory Disease

Pelvic inflammatory disease is very rare in pregnancy and does not occur after the first trimester. Differential diagnosis includes ectopic pregnancy, septic abortion, and appendicitis, all of which are more common. In the patient with suspected infection, smears or cultures for *Chlamydia* and gonorrhea should be obtained. Given the risk of endometrial infection in pregnancy and the need to consider other diagnoses, pregnant patients who have suspected PID require hospital admission and intravenous antibiotics.[86]

Chorioamnionitis

After 16 weeks of pregnancy the chorioamniotic membranes adhere to the cervical os and may become infected. Chorioamnionitis is diagnosed by the findings of fever and uterine tenderness in a patient past 16 weeks of pregnancy. The diagnosis is confirmed by amniocentesis. Urgent obstetric consultation should be obtained, and hospital admission for intravenous antibiotics is required.

KEY CONCEPTS

- The emergency physician must determine the type of miscarriage (incomplete, complete, inevitable, and threatened) because management priorities for these patients are different.
- The history and the physical examination of the patient with ectopic pregnancy are insensitive and nonspecific; therefore, ancillary studies are required to locate the pregnancy in any emergency department patient who has abdominal pain or vaginal bleeding and a positive pregnancy test result.
- The major conditions associated with vaginal bleeding in the second half of pregnancy include abruptio placentae and placenta previa. Patient history, physical examination, and results of ultrasonography must be used together by the emergency physician to distinguish these conditions.
- Appendicitis is the most common surgical emergency in pregnancy and the presentation of these patients may not be classic, leading to a misdiagnosis rate of 30% to 35% overall in pregnant patients.
- The treatment of eclampsia includes magnesium sulfate for seizures, reduction of blood pressure, and delivery of the fetus.

REFERENCES

1. Wang X, et al: Conception, early pregnancy loss, and time to clinical pregnancy. *Fertil Steril* 79:577, 2003.
2. Garcia-Enguidanos A, et al: Risk factors in miscarriage. *Eur J Obstet Gynecol* 102:111, 2002.
3. Chung TK, et al: Threatened abortion: Prediction of viability based on signs and symptoms. *Aust N Z J Obstet Gynaecol* 39:443, 1999.
4. Kohn MA, et al: Beta-human chorionic gonadotropin levels and the likelihood of ectopic pregnancy in emergency department patients with abdominal pain or vaginal bleeding. *Acad Emerg Med* 10:119, 2003.
5. Frates MC, et al: Pregnancy outcome after a first trimester sonogram demonstrating fetal cardiac activity. *J Ultrasound Med* 12:383, 1993.
6. Abbott JT, et al: Ectopic pregnancy: Ten common pitfalls in diagnosis. *Am J Emerg Med* 8:515, 1990.
7. Dart RG, et al: Predictive value of history and physical examination in patients with suspected ectopic pregnancy. *Ann Emerg Med* 33:283, 1999.
8. Ory SJ: New options for diagnosis and treatment of ectopic pregnancy. *JAMA* 267:534, 1992.
9. Dart RG : Role of pelvic ultrasound in evaluation of symptomatic first trimester pregnancy. *Ann Emerg Med* 33:310, 1999.
10. Azogui G, et al: CA-125 is elevated in viable pregnancies destined to be miscarried: A prospective longitudinal study. *Fertil Steril* 65:1059, 1996.
11. Perkins SL, et al: Comparison of serum progesterone as an indicator of pregnancy nonviability in spontaneously pregnant emergency room and infertility clinic populations, *Fertil Steril* 73:499, 2000.
12. O'Connor JF, et al: Differential urinary gonadotropin profiles in early pregnancy and early pregnancy loss. *Prenat Diagn* 18:1232, 1998.
13. Zaccardi R, et al: Loss and grief reactions after spontaneous miscarriage in the emergency department. *Ann Emerg Med* 22:5, 1993.
14. Luise C, et al: Outcome of expectant management of spontaneous first trimester miscarriage. *BMJ* 324: 873, 2003.
15. Wood SL, et al: Medical management of missed abortion: A randomized clinical trial. *Obstet Gynecol* 99:563, 2002.
16. Chang J: Pregnancy-related mortality surveillance—United States, 1991-1999. *MMWR Surveill Summ* 52:1, 2003.
17. Braude P, Rowell P: Assisted conception. III—Problems with assisted conception. *BMJ* 327:920, 2003.
18. Kaplan BC, et al: Ectopic pregnancy: Prospective study with improved diagnostic accuracy. *Ann Emerg Med* 28:10, 1996.
19. Barnhart KT, et al: Diagnostic accuracy of ultrasound above and below the β-hCG discriminatory zone. *Obstet Gynecol* 94:583, 1999.
20. Bouyer J, et al: Risk factors for ectopic pregnancy: A comprehensive analysis based on a large case-control, population-based study in France. *Am J Epidemiol* 157:185, 2003.
21. Bouyer J, et al: Sites of ectopic pregnancy: A 10 year population-based study of 1800 cases. *Hum Reprod* 17:3224, 2002.
22. Snyder HS: Lack of tachycardic response to hypotension with ruptured ectopic pregnancy. *Am J Emerg Med* 8:23, 1990.
23. Dart R: Normal intrauterine pregnancy is unlikely in emergency department patients with either menstrual days >38 or B-hCG >3,000 but without a gestational sac on ultrasonography. *Acad Emerg Med* 4:967, 1997.
24. Barnhart K, et al: Prompt diagnosis of ectopic pregnancy in an emergency department setting. *Obstet Gynecol* 84:1010, 1994.

25. Dart RG: Subclassification of indeterminate pelvic ultrasonography: Prospective evaluation of the risk of ectopic pregnancy. *Ann Emerg Med* 39:382, 2002.
26. Barnhart KT, et al: Presumed diagnosis of ectopic pregnancy. *Obstet Gynecol* 100:505, 2002.
27. Kalinski MA, et al: Hemorrhagic shock from a ruptured ectopic pregnancy in a patient with a negative urine pregnancy test result. *Ann Emerg Med* 40:102, 2002.
28. Stovall TG, Ling FW: Ectopic pregnancy: Diagnostic and therapeutic algorithms minimizing surgical intervention. *J Reprod Med* 38:807, 1993.
29. Dart R, et al: Progesterone as a predictor of ectopic pregnancy when ultrasound is indeterminate. *Am J Emerg Med* 20:575, 2002.
30. Soriano D, et al: Serum concentrations of interleukin-2R, IL-6, IL-8, and tumor necrosis factor alpha in patients with ectopic pregnancy. *Fertil Steril* 79:975, 2003.
31. Chen PC, et al: Sonographic detection of echogenic fluid and correlation with culdocentesis in the evaluation of ectopic pregnancy. *AJR* 170:1299, 1998.
32. Dart R, et al: Utility of a dilatation and evacuation procedure in patients with symptoms suggestive of ectopic pregnancy and indeterminate transvaginal ultrasonography. *Acad Emerg Med* 6:1024, 1999.
33. Shalev E, et al: Transvaginal sonography as the ultimate diagnostic tool for the management of ectopic pregnancy: Experience with 840 cases. *Fertil Steril* 69:62, 1998.
34. Kontoravdis A, et al: The diagnostic value of laparoscopy in 2365 patients with acute and chronic pelvic pain. *Int J Obstet Gynecol* 52:243, 1996.
35. Atri M, et al: Effect of transvaginal sonography on the use of invasive procedures for evaluating patients with a clinical diagnosis of ectopic pregnancy. *J Clin Ultrasound* 31:1, 2003.
36. Carson SA, Buster JE: Ectopic pregnancy. *N Engl J Med* 329:1174, 1993.
37. Potter M, et al: Predictors of success with methotrexate treatment of tubal ectopic pregnancy at Grady Memorial Hospital. *Am J Obstet Gynecol* 188:1192, 2003.
38. Heard K, et al: Rupture of ectopic pregnancy after medical therapy with methotrexate: A case series. *J Emerg Med* 16:857, 1998.
39. Mungan T, et al: Hydatidiform mole: Clinical analysis of 310 patients. *Int J Obstet Gynecol* 52:233, 1996.
40. Sebire NJ, et al: The diagnostic implications of routine ultrasound examination on histologically confirmed early molar pregnancies. *Ultrasound Obstet Gynecol* 18:662, 2001.
41. Obstetrical Hemorrhage. In Cunningham G, et al (eds): *Williams Obstetrics*, 21st ed. New York, McGraw Hill, 2001, pp 619-670.
42. Toivonen S, et al: Reproductive risk factors, Doppler findings, and outcome of affected births in placental abruption: A population-based analysis. *Am J Perinatol* 19:451, 2002.
43. Rachana C, et al: Prevalence and complications of physical violence during pregnancy. *Eur J Obstet Gynecol* 103:26, 2002.
44. Miller DA, et al: Clinical risk factors for placenta previa-placenta accreta. *Am J Obstet Gynecol* 177:210, 1997.
45. Mustafa SA, et al: Transvaginal ultrasonography in predicting placenta previa at delivery: A longitudinal study. *Ultrasound Obstet Gynecol* 20:356, 2002.
46. Balderston KD, et al: Is the incidence of fetal-to-maternal hemorrhage increased in patients with third-trimester bleeding? *Am J Obstet Gynecol* 188:1615, 2003.
47. Sibai BM: Diagnosis and management of gestational hypertension and preeclampsia. *Obstet Gynecol* 102:181, 2003.
48. Hypertensive Disorders in Pregnancy. In Cunningham G, et al (eds): *Williams Obstetrics*, 21st ed. New York, McGraw Hill, 2001, pp 567-618.
49. Bosio PM, et al. Maternal central hemodynamics in hypertensive disorders of pregnancy. *Obstet Gynecol* 94:978, 1999.
50. Redman CWG, et al: Preeclampsia: An excessive maternal inflammatory response to pregnancy. *Am J Obstet Gynecol* 180:499, 1999.
51. Mills JL, et al: Prostacyclin and thromboxane changes predating clinical onset of preeclampsia. *JAMA* 282:356, 1999.
52. Witlin AG, et al: Risk factors for abruptio placentae and eclampsia: Analysis of 445 consecutively managed women with severe preeclampsia and eclampsia. *Am J Obstet Gynecol* 180:1322, 1999.
53. Martin JN, et al: Early risk assessment of severe preeclampsia: Admission battery of symptoms and laboratory tests to predict likelihood of subsequent significant maternal morbidity. *Am J Obstet Gynecol* 180:1407, 1999.
54. Mattar F, et al: Eclampsia: Risk factors for maternal morbidity. *Am J Obstet Gynecol* 182:307, 2000.
55. Chames MC, et al: Late post-partum eclampsia: A preventable disease? *Am J Obstet Gynecol* 186:1174, 2002.
56. Thomas SV: Neurological aspects of eclampsia. *J Neurol Sci* 155:37, 1998.
57. Belfort MA, et al: Comparison of magnesium sulfate and nimodipine for the prevention of eclampsia. *N Engl J Med* 348:304, 2003.
58. Gilbert WM, et al: Amniotic fluid embolism: Decreased mortality in a population-based study. *Obstet Gynecol* 93:973, 1999.
59. Tuffnell DJ: Amniotic fluid embolism. *Curr Opin Obstet Gynecol* 15:119, 2003.
60. Moise KJ: Management of rhesus alloimmunization in pregnancy. *Obstet Gynecol* 100:600, 2002.
61. Hodjati H, et al: Location of the appendix in the gravid patient: A re-evaluation of the established concept. *Int J Gynecol Obstet* 81:245, 2003.
62. Mourad J, et al. Appendicitis in pregnancy: New information that contradicts long-held clinical beliefs. *Am J Obstet Gynecol* 185:259, 2000.
63. Hee P, Viktrup L: The diagnosis of appendicitis during pregnancy and maternal and fetal outcome after appendectomy. *Int J Gynaecol Obstet* 65:129, 1999.
64. Castro MA, et al: The use of helical computed tomography in pregnancy for the diagnosis of acute appendicitis. *Am J Obstet Gynecol* 184:954, 2001.
65. Indar AA, et al: Acute cholecystitis. *BMJ* 325:639, 2002.
66. Glasgow RE, et al. Changing management of gallstone disease during pregnancy. *Surg Endosc* 12:241, 1998.
67. Stone K: Acute abdominal emergencies associated with pregnancy. *Clin Obstet Gynecol* 45:553, 2002.
68. Castro MA, et al: Reversible peripartum liver failure: A new perspective on the diagnosis, treatment, and cause of acute fatty liver of pregnancy, based on 28 consecutive cases. *Am J Obstet Gynecol* 181:389, 1999.
69. Usta IM, et al: Acute fatty liver of pregnancy: An experience in the diagnosis and management of fourteen cases. *Am J Obstet Gynecol* 171:1342, 1994.
70. Mullally BA, et al: Intrahepatic cholestasis of pregnancy. *Obstet Gynecol Surg* 57:47, 2001.
71. Burrows RF, et al: Interventions for treating cholestasis in pregnancy. *Cochrane Database Syst Rev* 4:CD000493, 2001.
72. Spruill SC, et al: Hyperemesis gravidarum complicated by Wernicke's encephalopathy. *Obstet Gynecol* 99:875, 2002.
73. Lagiou P, et al: Nausea and vomiting in pregnancy in relation to prolactin, estrogens, and progesterone. *Obstet Gynecol* 101:639, 2003.
74. Kaplan PB: Maternal serum cytokine levels in women with hyperemesis gravidarum in the first trimester of pregnancy. *Fertil Steril* 79:498, 2003.
75. Frigo P, et al: Hyperemesis gravidarum associated with *Helicobacter pylori* seropositivity. *Obstet Gynecol* 91:615, 1998.

76. Nelson-Piercy C, et al: Randomised, double-blind, placebo-controlled trial of corticosteroids for the treatment of hyperemesis gravidarum. *Br J Obstet Gynecol* 108:9, 2001.
77. Danilenko-Dixon DR, et al: Risk factors for deep vein thrombosis and pulmonary embolism during pregnancy or post partum. *Am J Obstet Gynecol* 184:104, 2001.
78. Powrie RO, et al: Alveolar-arterial oxygen gradient in acute pulmonary embolism in pregnancy. *Am J Obstet Gynecol* 178:394, 1998.
79. Anand SS, et al: Does this patient have deep vein thrombosis? *JAMA* 279:1094, 1998.
80. Chan WS, et al: Suspected pulmonary embolism in pregnancy. *Arch Intern Med* 162:1170, 2002.
81. Winer-Muram HT, et al: Pulmonary embolism in pregnant patients: Fetal radiation dose with helical CT. *Radiology* 224:487, 2002.
82. Jacobsen AF, et al: Low molecular weight heparin (dalteparin) for the treatment of venous thromboembolism in pregnancy. *Br J Obstet Gynecol* 110:139, 2003.
83. Ginsberg JS, et al: Management of venous thromboembolism during pregnancy. *J Thromb Haemost* 1:1435, 2003.
84. Uncu Y, et al: Should asymptomatic bacteriuria be screened in pregnancy? *Clin Exp Obstet Gynecol* 29:281, 2002.
85. Smaill F: Antibiotics for asymptomatic bacteriuria in pregnancy. *Cochrane Database Syst Rev* 2:CD000490, 2001.
86. Sexually transmitted diseases treatment guidelines 2002. Centers for Disease Control and Prevention. *MMWR Recomm Rep* 2002 51(RR-6):1, 2002.
87. Millar LK, et al: Outpatient treatment of pyelonephritis in pregnancy: A randomized controlled trial. *Obstet Gynecol* 86:560, 1995.
88. Glover DD, et al: Longitudinal investigation of candida vaginitis in pregnancy: Role of superimposed antibiotic use. *Obstet Gynecol* 91:115, 1998.
89. Cotch MF, Hillier SL, Gibbs RS, Eschenbach DA: Epidemiology and outcomes associated with moderate to heavy Candida colonization during pregnancy. Vaginal Infections and Prematurity Study Group. *Am J Obstet Gynecol* 178:374, 1998.
90. Rastogi S, et al: Effect of treatment for *Chlamydia trachomatis* during pregnancy. *Int J Gynaecol Obstet* 80:129, 2003.

CHAPTER 178

Chronic Medical Illness During Pregnancy

Edward J. Newton and Kirsten K. Calder

PERSPECTIVE

This chapter concentrates on selected chronic medical conditions in the pregnant patient that may deteriorate precipitously, placing both the mother and the fetus at risk. Many pregnant patients have limited access to prenatal care or choose not to avail themselves of such care. Consequently, the initial intervention for a serious medical condition often takes place in the emergency department. Recognition of risk factors for chronic disease is an important aspect of the screening of these patients.

PRINCIPLES OF DISEASE

Medical illness can complicate pregnancy in a variety of ways. The physiologic adjustments of pregnancy, such as anemia or increased cardiac output, may exceed the patient's previous compensatory mechanisms, resulting in initial symptom onset or rapid decompensation during pregnancy. Certain chronic medical conditions also pose a serious threat to the mother's health or result in a poor fetal outcome. Finally, some medical illnesses result in a difficult delivery or the need for special resuscitation measures in the neonate, and the emergency physician must be prepared for these events.

Although the incidence of purely obstetric causes of morbidity and mortality has progressively decreased, the incidence of pregnancy in chronically ill patients has increased because of improved survival of patients with diseases such as diabetes, epilepsy, renal failure, and various cancers. Also, the demographics of pregnancy are changing in that maternal age at the time of first pregnancy is increasing.[1] Advances in assisted reproduction, including in vitro fertilization and oocyte donation, has made it possible for older women—including those who are postmenopausal—to become pregnant. Older pregnant women experience an increased rate of antepartum and intrapartum complications, including gestational diabetes and hypertension[1,2] and are at higher risk for certain complications such as coronary artery disease.

SPECIFIC DISORDERS

Asthma

Asthma is the most common pulmonary problem in pregnancy, affecting up to 4% of gestations,[3] and the prevalence appears to be increasing. The overall effect of pregnancy on asthma is that one third of patients will experience a worsening of the disease, one third will have improvement, and one third will have no change. The effect of asthma on the fetus is controversial, but recent studies reveal an increased risk of complications including preeclampsia, gestational diabetes mellitus, prematurity, intrauterine growth retardation, meconium-stained amniotic fluid, and congenital malformations.[4-6]

Several changes in respiratory physiology during normal pregnancy affect the management of asthma in this context. Both the tidal volume and the minute ventilation rise, increasing by up to 50% by term. This increase in minute ventilation, or "hyperventilation of pregnancy," lowers the resting PCO_2 by an average of 10 mm Hg to a PCO_2 of 32 mm Hg. In response to chronic hyperventilation, there is a compensatory increase in the renal excretion of bicarbonate, with serum levels averaging 19 mEq/mL. The net result is a slight respiratory alkalosis, with a serum pH ranging from 7.40 to 7.45. It is important to keep these "normal" values in mind when gauging the severity of an asthma exacerbation in the pregnant patient.

The treatment strategy in the care of the pregnant asthmatic patient is to control the disease and to prevent episodes of status asthmaticus, thereby avoiding fetal hypoxia. Acute asthma exacerbations pose a significant maternal and fetal risk, and the pregnant patient should be managed as aggressively as the non-pregnant patient. In fact, patients whose asthma is well controlled generally have normal pregnancies and the risks from inadequately treated disease far outweigh the risks of therapy.[4,7]

Therapy for acute exacerbations as well as maintenance disease control is largely unchanged in pregnancy, although there are a few medications to avoid, if possible (Tables 178-1 and 178-2).[3,8,9] As in the non-pregnant patient, inhaled β-agonists are the first-line agents for both chronic use and treatment of an acute asthma exacerbation. Although safe from a teratogenic perspective, these medications are powerful tocolytics and will usually halt active labor. Selective agonists are preferred, since nonselective agents such as epinephrine theoretically decrease uteroplacental blood flow via α-mediated effects. Ipratropium bromide, an anticholinergic bronchodilator, can also be used in conjunction with β-agonists.

Corticosteroids remain a core component of treatment for asthma in the pregnant patient. In fact, current data support the chronic use of inhaled corticosteroids in most asthmatic patients whose disease is of at least moderate severity.[8] Other agents including the methylxanthines and newer agents including nedocromil, salmeterol, montelukast, or zafirlukast are acceptable and can be continued throughout pregnancy if a high level of control has been achieved. Conversely, zileuton has been shown to be teratogenic in animals and should be avoided during pregnancy.[9]

Magnesium sulfate recently has received a great deal of attention in the acute treatment of refractory asthma exacerbations because it has a wide safety profile and potent bronchodilator properties. Very little literature exists concerning its use in the pregnant asthmatic patient, although large doses have been used for the treatment of eclampsia for many years and it appears to be safe and may be effective for treating asthma.[10] Caution should be exercised when using magnesium during labor because it relaxes uterine smooth muscle.

Perhaps the most important tenet of treatment to recognize is that if the mother is hypoxic, the fetus is hypoxic as well. The fetus is more sensitive to hypoxia than the mother, and normal maternal oxygen saturation does not preclude fetal distress. Supplemental oxygen should be administered to all pregnant patients with an acute asthma exacerbation.

Hypertension

Chronic Hypertension and Hypertensive Emergencies

Chronic hypertension is defined as elevated blood pressure that is present before the onset of pregnancy or that begins prior to the 20th week of gestation. It affects 1% to 5% of pregnancies and represents a significant source of maternal and fetal mortality and morbidity (see Table 178-1).[11,12] The emergency physician might be required to provide therapy for hypertensive emergencies in patients with chronic hypertension and to differentiate between the various hypertensive disorders of pregnancy (Table 178-3). Although treatment of mild disease during pregnancy is not indicated,[12] patients with more severe blood pressure elevations probably need maintenance medical therapy (see Table 178-1). This is best done by the patient's primary care practitioner in conjunction with her obstetrician.

In the treatment of hypertension in pregnancy, the emergency physician must balance the goal of reducing maternal blood pressure with the requirements to maintain cardiac output and minimize adverse effects for both mother and fetus. Precipitous and marked decreases in blood pressure may significantly diminish uteroplacental blood flow. Nearly all of the major classes of antihypertensive agents are acceptable in the pregnant patient, with the exception of angiotensin enzyme inhibitors and angiotensin II receptor blockers. β-Blockers may have adverse fetal effects when given early in pregnancy but are considered safe later in gestation.[13] Hydralazine, labetalol, and sodium nitroprusside (Table 178-4) are the agents most commonly used for hypertensive emergencies associated with eclampsia and are also appropriate for such emergencies in the patient with chronic hypertension.

Diagnosis of preeclampsia in the pregnant patient with chronic hypertension is challenging but necessary. Patients with chronic hypertension are more likely to develop preeclampsia, a situation that results in increased morbidity and mortality as compared with either process in isolation. Coexistence of the two disorders should be suspected in the following settings: (1) new onset of proteinuria prior to 20 weeks' gestation in a patient with known hypertension, and (2) pregnant patients with hypertension and proteinuria prior to 20 weeks' gestation who develop an acute increase in proteinuria or blood pressure, thrombocytopenia, or increased transaminases.[11]

Pulmonary Hypertension

Primary (idiopathic) pulmonary hypertension, Eisenmenger's syndrome (pulmonary hypertension associ-

Table 178-1. Gestational Effects and Treatment of Medical Illnesses During Pregnancy

Medical Illness	Gestational Concerns	Treatment
Asthma	Fetal—IUGR, PTD, hypoxia, meconium-stained amniotic fluid, fetal loss Maternal—preeclampsia, gestational hypertension, gestational diabetes, hyperemesis gravidarum, need for labor induction	Treatment of acute exacerbations is the same as for the nonpregnant patient. Fetal monitoring for exacerbations during the third trimester is recommended even in absence of maternal hypoxia. Maintenance therapy also unchanged with the following precautions: **Corticosteroids:** inhaled agents preferred to limit side effects but oral route may be necessary with severe, persistent disease; patients on long-term steroids require "stress dose" hydrocortisone during labor and delivery **Methylxanthines:** safe but debatable benefit; use only in refractory disease; reduced clearance during pregnancy may result in maternal toxicity and fetal tachycardia **Leukotriene receptor antagonists:** avoid zileuton
Acute coronary syndrome	Fetal—perinatal death, PTD Maternal—uterine hemorrhage and abruption (related to use of antiplatelet, antithrombotic, and fibrinolytic agents)	Standard medical therapy is the same as for the nonpregnant patient, although antiplatelet, antithrombotic, and fibrinolytic agents should be avoided when delivery is imminent. Avoid maternal hypotension when using nitrates—may result in fetal distress. Avoid β-blockers in the first trimester (teratogenic). Coordinate definitive care (fibrinolytics versus PCI) with cardiology
Valvular heart disease	Fetal—perinatal death, PTD Maternal—decompensated heart failure, thromboembolism, death	Subcutaneous heparin therapy indicated for patients with prosthetic valves and atrial fibrillation. Avoid warfarin. **Mitral stenosis:** diuresis and β-blockade; valvuloplasty or open cardiac surgery for severe symptomatic disease; consider pregnancy termination in patients with atrial fibrillation or severe stenosis **Mitral and aortic regurgitation:** diuresis in patients with pulmonary congestion; surgical therapy for acute regurgitant lesions; consider pregnancy termination in patients with symptomatic disease **Aortic stenosis:** avoid hypotension and the supine hypotensive syndrome—position left lateral decubitus; vigorous fluid replacement during delivery; valvuloplasty or open cardiac surgery for severe symptomatic disease
Hypertension	Fetal—perinatal death, IUGR, PTD Maternal—progression of target end-organ damage, superimposed preeclampsia, abruption	Fetal cyanide poisoning might develop after several hours of sodium nitroprusside—avoid prolonged infusions. The most commonly used agents include methyldopa, labetalol, and hydralazine. Avoid β-blockers in the first trimester (teratogenic). Avoid ACEIs and ARBs.
Iron deficiency anemia	Fetal—low birth weight, PTD, low fetal iron stores, fetal loss (with severe anemia) Maternal—preeclampsia, high-output heart failure (rare); effects on maternal mortality unclear	Oral iron supplementation is indicated to improve maternal iron stores. Several over-the-counter preparations are available. There is a delay from onset of therapy to increase in serum hemoglobin. Parenteral iron replacement is safe and effective, although rarely required. Transfusion is rarely required but may be necessary with severe, symptomatic anemia.
Sickle cell anemia	Fetal—fetal loss, IUGR, PTD and premature rupture of membranes Maternal—↑ need for cesarean section, preeclampsia, infection, heart failure, pulmonary infarction, ↑ incidence of painful crises; maternal mortality low with treatment; false-positive Apt and Kleihauer-Betke tests 2° to persistent hemoglobin F	Management of pain crises and infections is the same as for the nonpregnant patient with rest, hydration, narcotic analgesia, supplemental oxygen, and antibiotics as indicated. Narcotic analgesics should not be withheld but the need for neonatal respiratory support should be anticipated if delivery is imminent. Prophylactic transfusion is not indicated. Fetal monitoring and assessment of fetal well-being are indicated for viable pregnancies. Chronic maintenance care includes pneumococcal vaccination, supplement folate and usually iron. Hydroxyurea has been discouraged during pregnancy, but few adverse fetal effects have been reported in humans.
Epilepsy	Fetal—various congenital malformations associated with AEMs; fetal hypoxia and bradycardia; fetal loss Maternal—variable changes in seizure frequency; alterations in AEM levels; increased seizure frequency secondary to voluntary medication noncompliance; abruption, anemia, hyperemesis gravidarum, preeclampsia, need for labor induction and cesarean section, premature rupture of membranes	Management of status epilepticus is the same as for the nonpregnant patient. Maintenance therapy should be coordinated by the patient's neurologist (or primary care practitioner) and obstetrician—in general, a single AEM given at the lowest effective dose is recommended. Patients with pregravid seizure control with AEM monotherapy should continue their current regimen. There is limited experience with newer AEMs, but these are likely to have a more favorable side effect profile. Folate supplementation is mandatory for patients taking older AEMs. Administer oral vitamin K to the mother during the last month of pregnancy and parenteral vitamin K to the newborn.

Continued

Table 178-1. Gestational Effects and Treatment of Medical Illnesses During Pregnancy—cont'd

Medical Illness	Gestational Concerns	Treatment
Myasthenia gravis (MG)	Fetal—transient neonatal myasthenia syndrome Maternal—variable changes in disease severity; arrest of labor; disease exacerbation in the postpartum period	Management is the same as for the nonpregnant patient. Ventilatory support is the most important aspect of therapy; note that patients with myasthenia gravis are relatively resistant to depolarizing paralytic agents—higher doses may be required. Pyridostigmine therapy can be continued. Patients on maintenance corticosteroids require "stress dose" hydrocortisone during labor and delivery. Plasmapheresis is safe during pregnancy.
Diabetes mellitus—insulin-dependent, non–insulin-dependent, and gestational	Fetal—congenital malformations; macrosomia; IUGR: fetal loss; neonatal hypoglycemia, jaundice, hypomagnesemia, and hypocalcemia Maternal—preeclampsia, "brittle" diabetes, ↑ need for cesarean section; mothers with GDM have ↑ risk for development of postpartum diabetes	Every attempt should be made to maintain maternal serum glucose of 100 mg/dL. Note that insulin requirements decrease during the immediate postpartum period and the mother may not need insulin for 24 to 48 hours after delivery. Insulin therapy—using either intermittent dosing or continuous subcutaneous infusion—is standard of care for patients with both IDDM and NIDDM. Management of DKA is the same as for the nonpregnant patient with the addition of an assessment of fetal well-being and continuous fetal heart monitoring. GDM often manageable with diet alone but may require insulin therapy when fasting plasma glucose remains >105 mg/dL.
Hyperthyroidism	Fetal—PTD, low birth weight, fetal thyroid dysfunction, fetal loss Maternal—preeclampsia, heart failure	Management of thyroid storm is the same as for the nonpregnant patient and includes a search for the underlying precipitant. Therapy for hyperthyroidism in the absence of thyroid storm: **Reversal of sympathetic effects:** propanolol in standard doses is useful until thyroid hormone synthesis has been blocked by thioamides **Thioamides:** both propylthiouracil and methimazole at the lowest effective dose are acceptable **Surgical therapy:** thyroidectomy useful in refractory cases **Other:** avoid iodide if possible; hydrocortisone decreases peripheral conversion of T_4 to the more active T_3 and can be used during pregnancy. Radioactive iodine is absolutely contraindicated.
Hypothyroidism	Fetal—congenital malformations, low birth weight, fetal loss, fetal thyroid dysfunction and goiter Maternal—preeclampsia, abruption, postpartum hemorrhage, ↑ need for cesarean section	Maintenance therapy includes levothyroxine 0.15 mg/day. Appropriate treatment prevents adverse obstetric and fetal outcomes. Myxedema coma is rare but when present treatment is the same as for the nonpregnant patient.
Tuberculosis	Fetal—fetal loss, low birth weight, PTD; fetal and neonatal tuberculosis Maternal—preeclampsia; potential for delayed diagnosis and treatment out of concern for the fetus	**PPD positive/chest radiograph negative:** 6- to 9-month course of isoniazid (starting after the first trimester) for patients with recent conversion (<2 years); patients who have been PPD positive >2 years may defer treatment until after delivery but should still be offered a course of isoniazid since it is safe in pregnancy **Active tuberculosis:** 9-month course (starting immediately) of isoniazid plus rifampin or ethambutol **Multidrug-resistant tuberculosis:** warrants aggressive therapy without regard to potential teratogenicity Pyridoxine is mandatory for all patients receiving isoniazid.
HIV/AIDS	Fetal—HIV infection, PTD, fetal loss; neonatal drug withdrawal if the mother uses intravenous drugs Maternal—postpartum endometritis, uterine bleeding (in the setting of thrombocytopenia)	**Antiretroviral therapy:** 1. Highly active retroviral therapy (HAART) should be offered to all pregnant patients with HIV and viral load > 1000. The HAART regimen should include zidovudine (AZT) to prevent vertical transmission of the virus. 2. There are specific HAART drug-related concerns during pregnancy—decisions regarding therapy are best made by appropriate specialists. 3. ART monotherapy is not recommended except in those patients with a low viral load who do not wish to take HAART. In these cases, AZT is appropriate reduce disease transmission. Cesarean section is recommended with viral load > 100. Opportunistic infections require standard therapies despite the potential fetal effects.
Syphilis	Fetal—congenital syphilis, fetal loss, PTD, IUGR, nonimmune hydrops	Primary, secondary, early latent (<1 year): benzathine penicillin G (BPG), 2.4 million units IM × one dose Late latent (>1 year or unknown duration): BPG, 2.4 million units IM weekly × three doses Neurosyphilis: aqueous penicillin G, 2-4 million units IV q 4 hours × 10-14 days or procaine penicillin G, 2.4 million units IM and probenecid 500 mg PO q 6 hours × 10-14 days

ACEI, angiotensin-converting enzyme inhibitor; AEM, antiepileptic medicine; AIDS, acquired immunodeficiency syndrome; ARB, angiotensin II receptor blocker; DKA, diabetic ketoacidosis; GDM, gestational diabetes mellitus; HIV, human immunodeficiency virus; IDDM, insulin-dependent diabetes mellitus; IUGR, intrauterine growth retardation; NIDDM, non–insulin-dependent diabetes; PCI, percutaneous coronary intervention; PTD, preterm delivery.

Table 178-2. Drugs Used in the Treatment of Asthma During Pregnancy

Pharmacologic class	Examples	Comments	Dosages
Inhaled β-agonists	Albuterol	First-line therapy	Continuous nebulization or 2 puffs q4-6 hours
	Metaproterenol		2 puffs q4-6 hours
Injectable β-agonists	Epinephrine	Decreases uteroplacental blood flow	0.3 mL SC of 1:1000 conc.
	Terbutaline	May inhibit labor	0.25 mL SC
Inhaled corticosteroids	Beclomethasone	Not for use in mild asthma Preferred steroid for maintenance therapy	2-4 puffs qid
Systemic corticosteroids		Indications for use in acute exacerbations:	
Oral	Prednisone	inadequate response to β-agonists, steroid dependence	Maintenance therapy variable; consider alternate-day regimens 60 mg PO q6h for exacerbations
Intravenous	Prednisolone		125 mg IV q6h
Anticholinergics	Ipratropium bromide	Limited efficacy, ↓ clearance in third trimester; follow serum levels	2 puffs q6h
Methylxanthines	Theophylline	Use only in refractory disease	400-1200 mg/day
	Aminophylline	Not for routine use in the emergency department; ↓ aminophylline clearance in pregnancy may result in maternal toxicity	4-5 mg/kg IV, then 0.5 mg/kg/hr IV
Leukotriene modifiers	Montelukast	Limited data on their efficacy in acute asthma exacerbations or pregnancy	10 mg PO qhs
	Zafirlukast		20 mg PO BID
Smooth muscle relaxants	Magnesium sulfate	Limited data on its efficacy in pregnancy	2-3 g IV; may repeat q4h

Table 178-3. Hypertensive Disorders of Pregnancy

	Chronic Hypertension	Gestational Hypertension	Preeclampsia
Definition	1. Hypertension* that antedates pregnancy 2. Hypertension diagnosed prior to 20 weeks of gestation	Hypertension diagnosed after 20 weeks gestation in the absence of preeclampsia; considered transient if hypertension resolves by 12 weeks postpartum or chronic if it persists beyond that period	Hypertension[+] that begins after 20 weeks of gestation occurring in association with other clinical findings (see below)
Findings			
Time of onset	< 20 weeks gestation	Usually third trimester	≥ 20 weeks gestation
Severity	Mild to severe	Mild	Mild to severe
Proteinuria	Absent	Absent	Usually present
Hyperuricemia	Rare	Absent	Usually present
Thrombocytopenia	Absent	Absent	Present in severe disease
Liver dysfunction	Absent	Absent	Present in severe disease

*Defined as blood pressure > 140 mm Hg systolic or > 90 mm Hg diastolic.
[+]Defined as blood pressure > 140 mm Hg systolic or > 90 mm Hg diastolic in a previously normotensive female or increases in systolic and diastolic pressures of 30 mm Hg and 15 mm Hg respectively.
Adapted with permission from Sibai BM: Drug therapy: Treatment of hypertension in pregnant women. *N Engl J Med* 335:257-265, 1996.

Table 178-4. Antihypertensive Agents for Hypertensive Emergencies

Antihypertensive Agents	Dose	Comment
Hydralazine	5 to 10 mg IV Repeat every 20 minutes until target blood pressure is achieved	Consider another agent if inadequate response despite administration of 20 mg
Labetalol	20 mg IV Can double the dose every 10 minutes until target blood pressure is achieved	Consider another agent if inadequate response despite administration of 220 mg Standard contraindications apply
Sodium nitroprusside	Infusion rates vary—start at 0.1 μg/kg/min	Avoid prolonged infusions—fetal cyanide toxicity is possible after several hours

ated with intracardiac left-to-right shunts), and secondary vascular pulmonary hypertension (i.e., secondary to connective tissue disease) have extremely high mortality in association with pregnancy, ranging from 30% to 52%. The majority of deaths are a result of heart failure.[14] Unfortunately, mortality is unaffected by peripartum management in most cases, although some patients benefit from selective pulmonary artery vasodilators such as prostacyclin and inhaled nitric oxide.[14] The primary goals of the emergency physician are to ensure high right ventricular filling pressures by diligently maintaining adequate volume status and to obtain early consultation with obstetrics and cardiology specialists. Patients with early gestations should be referred for elective pregnancy termination.

Cardiac Disorders

Acute Coronary Syndromes

Coronary artery disease is rare in pregnant women, and acute myocardial infarction (MI) is reported to occur in fewer than 1 in 10,000 pregnant patients; however, MI in this setting requires special considerations in management and carries a worse prognosis with a maternal mortality rate of 21% overall and 35% during the peripartum period.[15] Normal physiologic changes of pregnancy such as increased cardiac output and reduced oxygen-carrying capacity secondary to physiologic anemia have the potential to exceed the threshold for angina if a fixed coronary artery stenosis is present. Pregnancy-specific abnormalities such as hypercoagulability and preeclampsia might contribute to acute coronary thrombosis as well. The risk of MI in a patient with significant coronary atherosclerosis increases with the duration of the gestation and peaks during labor, which is associated with further increases in cardiac output as well as increased systolic and diastolic blood pressures.

A significant percentage of pregnant women with MI have normal coronary arteries—29% overall and 75% of those with postpartum MI. Other pathophysiologic mechanisms besides atherosclerosis that cause MI in the pregnant patient include coronary artery dissection, coronary artery aneurysm, and vasospasm; the relative significance of these lesions varies according to the gestational period. Atherosclerotic disease causes the majority of MIs in the antepartum period and coronary artery dissection is responsible for most postpartum events.[15] Pulmonary embolus, reflux esophagitis, biliary colic, chest pain from mitral valve prolapse, and aortic dissection are all more common than myocardial ischemia during pregnancy and need to be considered in the differential diagnosis. It is also important to consider cocaine use in the pregnant patient presenting with chest pain. Unfortunately, some women continue to use illicit drugs during their pregnancy, and it is possible that pregnancy enhances cocaine-induced cardiovascular toxicity.[16]

The diagnosis of angina is primarily clinical. Because normal pregnancy is often associated with electrocardiographic changes such as left axis deviation, minor ST wave depression, and T wave inversion,[17] treadmill evaluation may be necessary. Echocardiography is useful in correlating suspicious electrocardiographic findings with wall motion abnormalities. The enzymatic diagnosis of MI is unchanged except during and after delivery, when troponin is preferred over creatinine kinase and myoglobin, which are both elevated above baseline during this time period.[18] Angiography is generally avoided because the large dose of radiation poses a risk to the fetus, but it can be used in certain clinical situations.

Treatment of acute MI during pregnancy is similar in most respects to treatment of the nonpregnant patient. Survival of the mother is the primary concern, and therapy to improve maternal outcome should not be withheld. Standard treatment includes aspirin, nitroglycerin, β-blockers, and antithrombotic agents. However, there are potential adverse effects of such therapy on the mother and fetus (see Table 178-1). Heparin has long been considered the antithrombotic agent of choice in pregnant patients, but newer lower molecular weight agents, specifically dalteparin and enoxaparin, appear to be efficacious and safe.[19,20] Heparin might be preferable for patients in the late third trimester, since there is a more predictable response to protamine sulfate should labor begin. The use of magnesium sulfate has not been studied in pregnant patients with MI but would presumably be safe, considering its long history of use in eclampsia, and it may improve survival in patients with acute MI complicated by hypomagnesemia.

Experience with thrombolytic therapy in pregnancy is limited and is more extensive with disorders other than MI (i.e., pulmonary embolus). Although such therapy may reduce maternal and fetal mortality, pregnancy is considered a relative contraindication to its use. A comprehensive review of cases in which thrombolytic agents were used during pregnancy reveals significant hemorrhagic complications in 8.1% of cases.[21] Reported effects have included maternal hemorrhage, maternal death, placental abruption, preterm delivery, fetal death, and fetal intracranial hemorrhage, although the causal relationship in many of these cases is unclear. The majority of patients had favorable maternal and fetal outcomes, but most were being treated for indications other than MI.[15,21] Because thrombolytic therapy precludes major surgery in the days immediately after administration, the emergency physician must carefully consider whether to use these agents in pregnant women who are close to term, especially if the need for cesarean delivery is anticipated.

Cardiac surgery, including coronary artery bypass grafting, during pregnancy is associated with a maternal mortality rate of 2.2% and fetal mortality rate of 9.5%.[22] Emergency angioplasty with stent placement has been reported with good maternal and fetal outcomes.[23]

In the setting of peripartum MI, labor should be conducted with continuous monitoring of both the mother's hemodynamic status and fetal well-being. There are benefits and risks of both vaginal and operative delivery. Cesarean section avoids prolonged exertion by the mother but subjects the patient to general anesthesia and other typical postoperative complications. Therefore, assisted vaginal delivery (i.e., vacuum) is preferred unless there is an obstetric reason for cesarean section.[15] Resolution of angina may occur during the postpartum period as physiologic demands lessen, but its occurrence during pregnancy merits a complete investigation.

Valvular Heart Disease

Maternal valvular heart disease can be congenital or acquired and is one of the leading causes of nonobstetric death.[24] Acquired valvular disease is mainly the result of rheumatic fever and endocarditis. In the United States, most cases of significant congenital heart disease are identified and corrected surgically before puberty. Still, in many patients valvular heart disease remains undiagnosed until cardiac decompensation occurs. Asymptomatic or mildly symptomatic valvular disease is generally considered low risk, and most of these patients tolerate pregnancy without any ill effects. On the other hand, advanced aortic stenosis, aortic and mitral lesions associated with moderate to severe ventricular dysfunction or pulmonary hypertension, and prosthetic valves can result in significant maternal mortality and require directed therapy.[25] All patients with suspected valvular disease should undergo echocardiography.

Mitral Stenosis

Mitral stenosis is the most important lesion to detect in early pregnancy because maternal mortality is appreciable. The increased resting heart rate seen in normal pregnancy shortens left ventricular diastolic filling time and consequently results in reduced stroke volume. The demand for increased cardiac output during pregnancy creates a vicious cycle in which further acceleration of heart rate occurs. This tachycardia, combined with the expanded plasma volume of pregnancy, ultimately produces high left atrial pressures, pulmonary vascular congestion, and the symptoms and physical findings typical of left ventricular failure. Atrial fibrillation is common and is associated with a maternal mortality rate of 15% during pregnancy.[24] Treatment is aimed at reducing plasma volume and slowing the heart rate (see Table 178-1). Emergency commissurotomy can be performed at any time during the pregnancy if the mother's status deteriorates, and this procedure is tolerated relatively well by the fetus.[24] Treadmill testing is useful in predicting how well the patient will tolerate pregnancy and labor. Delivery should be conducted under epidural anesthesia with the use of forceps to decrease straining.

Aortic and Mitral Regurgitation

In most cases, regurgitant valvular lesions are well tolerated during pregnancy and may even improve as the reduced systemic vascular resistance of pregnancy allows more forward and less regurgitant flow. Consequently, if the mother is relatively asymptomatic before becoming pregnant, it is likely that she will do well during pregnancy. However, in the setting of ventricular dilation or atrial fibrillation, it is recommended that the mother terminate the pregnancy because of the high risk of congestive heart failure or systemic embolization. Acute aortic insufficiency resulting from acute bacterial endocarditis is an indication for immediate surgical repair at any stage of pregnancy.[24]

Aortic Stenosis

Symptomatic aortic stenosis during pregnancy usually occurs in the setting of a congenital bicuspid valve and is uncommon.[25] Older reports note a high rate of maternal mortality with severe aortic stenosis (up to 17%); however, more recent series have reported uniformly successful outcome of pregnancy with aortic stenosis.[26] It is particularly important to avoid the supine hypotensive syndrome with aortic stenosis, because sudden death can occur. Invasive hemodynamic monitoring and vigorous replacement of fluids are indicated during delivery.

Hematologic Disorders

Anemia

By far the most common medical complication of pregnancy is anemia. Up to 50% of all pregnancies manifest some type of anemia.[27] The physiologic adaptations to pregnancy include expansion of plasma volume in excess of the increase in red blood cell (RBC) mass, resulting in the dilutional, physiologic anemia of pregnancy. Any type of anemia can complicate pregnancy, but the three types most commonly involved are iron deficiency, macrocytic, and sickle cell anemia.

Iron Deficiency Anemia

Iron deficiency anemia is common, occurring in approximately 20% of pregnancies in industrialized countries.[28] Without iron supplementation, this number doubles.[29] Apart from chronically low or marginal iron stores in many women, diversion of maternal iron to the fetus for development of its own RBCs and iron stores and increased maternal demand for iron exacerbate the deficiency during pregnancy. Any episodes of blood loss during pregnancy tax an already stressed hematopoietic system and need to be taken very seriously.

Maternal anemia has relatively little impact on perinatal mortality until a hemoglobin level of 6.0 g/mL is reached.[24] Less severe anemia (hemoglobin < 11.0 g/mL) is associated with an increase in preterm delivery and low birth weight. Iron supplementation (see Table 178-1) is indicated to improve maternal iron stores but has not been proven to improve either of these fetal outcome measures, and pregnant women with mild, dilutional anemia generally have uncomplicated pregnancies.[28,29] Iron deficiency anemia secondary to malnutrition or disease is more worrisome.[29] Pregnant patients are subject to other causes of iron deficiency anemia, such as chronic blood loss from the gastrointestinal or genitourinary tracts, and these possibilities need to be considered.

The diagnosis of iron deficiency anemia is most accurately made by analysis of bone marrow, because all other methods have limitations. Serum ferritin levels less than 10 g/L, transferrin saturation less than 16%, and reticulocyte counts less than 1% are characteristic of iron deficiency anemia. Serum ferritin is the preferred test, but values can be affected by inflammation and by the dilutional effect of increased plasma volume characteristic of pregnancy. It is recommended that serum ferritin levels be determined during the first trimester if possible to minimize the dilutional effect.[28] Although RBC indices classically reveal a microcytic and hypochromic anemia, these indices are found in only 11% of pregnant patients with iron deficiency anemia and are not a reliable screening tool.[24]

Megaloblastic Anemia

Megaloblastic anemia is most commonly caused by dietary deficiency of vitamin B_{12} or folate, although in pregnancy folate deficiency is responsible for almost all cases. It is estimated that 1% to 4% of pregnancies in the United States are complicated by megaloblastic anemia, although 9% to 30% of pregnant women show depletion of folate stores and the megaloblastic bone marrow changes that precede anemia.[24] Patients with multiple gestations have an eightfold increased risk of developing folate deficiency and megaloblastic anemia. Other patients at higher risk include those with malnutrition, hyperemesis gravidarum, malabsorption syndromes, anticonvulsant therapy, alcoholism, and chronic hemolysis. Iron deficiency and megaloblastic anemias often coexist, making the peripheral blood smear difficult to interpret. Effects on the fetus depend on the degree of anemia and include neural tube defects, preterm delivery and intrauterine growth retardation.[30] Consequently, oral folate supplementation with 1 mg/day is routinely prescribed. Treatment response is usually brisk and transfusion is rarely required.

Sickle Cell Anemia

Sickle cell disease (SCD) is one of the major sources of maternal and fetal complications in the United States. The sickle cell trait has a prevalence of 8% in African Americans.[31] The details of the pathophysiology and genetics of SCD are discussed in Chapter 119, but it is useful to review the most common phenotypes that affect pregnancy. The sickle gene can be homozygous (hemoglobin SS or SCD), and this form of the disease is responsible for most pregnancy complications. The sickle gene can also be heterozygous with normal hemoglobin A (sickle cell trait or hemoglobin SA), in which case symptoms are rare except under extreme environmental conditions. The hemoglobin S can also be heterozygous with a large number of abnormal hemoglobins such as hemoglobin C, several variants of thalassemia, and other rare hemoglobin variants, and each variant has its own complication profile. Of these, the most relevant in terms of pregnancy complications is hemoglobin SC.

Patients with SCD are subject to many chronic medical problems secondary to a variety of pathophysiologic mechanisms, including sickling of RBCs, anemia, immunosuppression caused by autosplenectomy, and the need for repeated transfusion. The mortality rate is 20% in the first decade of life, but many patients now live longer than 40 years and fertility is generally unaffected, so it is likely that the emergency physician will encounter pregnant patients with the disease. The incidence of serious medical complications of pregnancy in patients with SCD ranges from 50% to 80% and includes preeclampsia, antepartum and postpartum infections, more frequent pain crises, heart failure, and pulmonary infarction.[31,32] Despite these complications, the maternal mortality rate is less than 1% with current treatment.

Sickle cell disease also results in adverse effects on the fetus (see Table 178-1). Placental infarction is common, with small-for-gestational-age and low-birth-weight infants resulting from placental insufficiency. In addition, the need for emergency cesarean section for fetal distress is increased.[33] A high rate of fetal loss has been noted in the past, although a recent study found no increase in the rate of perinatal death.[32] An incidental complication is that the Apt test and Kleihauer-Betke test to distinguish fetal from maternal blood will yield false-positive results because of the compensatory persistence of hemoglobin F in the mother.

Treatment of SCD in pregnant patients is similar to treatment in nonpregnant patients (see Table 178-1). Folate supplementation is standard even in the nonpregnant state because of the increased turnover of RBCs. Supplemental iron is controversial because of the fear of iron overload. Because iron stores tend to be low in pregnant patients, even those with SCD, most specialists provide iron supplements. Transfusion is reserved for patients with symptomatic anemia, cardiovascular instability, or acute chest syndrome, preoperatively for anticipated blood loss, and for a hematocrit less than 18%.[31] Hydroxyurea has not been used extensively in pregnancy because of fears of fetal toxicity, but there have not been any adverse effects among the few cases reported.

Neurologic Disorders

Epilepsy

Epilepsy is the most common neurologic complication of pregnancy, occurring in 0.8% of all gestations.[34] Epilepsy refers to a broad spectrum of seizure disorders that range from relatively benign and infrequent seizures to a disabling condition with daily, poorly controlled generalized convulsions; therefore, care must be individualized. Management of epilepsy during pregnancy must balance the risk of increased frequency and duration of seizures to both the mother and the fetus against the teratogenic risks of antiepileptic medications (AEMs).

The effect of pregnancy on epilepsy is variable. Most (50-83%) epileptic patients experience no change in their seizure frequency, whereas 20% to 33% experience more frequent seizures, and 7% to 25% experience improvement in their seizure disorders.[35] Deterioration may be due to alterations in the volume of distribution or metabolism of AEMs, resulting in subtherapeutic levels or a voluntary noncompliance with medications to avoid teratogenic effects on the fetus. In addition, pregnancy-associated increased levels of estrogen, decreased levels of γ-aminobutyric acid, respiratory alkalosis, and fatigue have all been implicated as potential causes of increasing seizure frequency.[36]

All of the older, commonly used AEMs have measurable teratogenic effects. A twofold to threefold increase exists in the incidence of serious congenital malformations in offspring of epileptic mothers taking AEMs.[37] The "fetal anticonvulsant syndrome" has been described and consists of neural tube defects, cleft palate, major limb defects, microcephaly, mental deficiency, and cardiac anomalies. Controversy exists as to whether infants of epileptic patients not taking AEMs have an increased incidence of congenital malformations compared with the general population. A recent study comparing these infants with infants born to mothers without epilepsy found a similar incidence of malformations.[37]

Care should be provided by specialists in high-risk obstetrics and neurology disciplines; however, emergency physicians may be forced to confront this problem in several clinical scenarios—the pregnant patient with a first-time seizure or status epilepticus and the patient with epilepsy who is found to be pregnant.

New-Onset Seizure

Pregnant patients may seek treatment for idiopathic new-onset seizures; however, drug toxicity or withdrawal, head injury, meningitis, stroke, and eclampsia should be considered as possible causes. The most important of these is eclampsia. Eclampsia generally occurs in the setting of progressive preeclampsia, although the diagnosis may be difficult. Preeclampsia consists of the triad of hypertension, peripheral edema, and proteinuria. Patients in the immediate postictal phase often manifest hypertension resulting from massive sympathetic discharge, and even those with normal pregnancies may have mild edema of the lower extremities. Consequently, urinalysis should be performed to search for proteinuria, which may be the only differentiating factor in the initial assessment of these patients. After a period of observation, blood pressure in the noneclamptic patient will revert to normal or low. If the patient remains hypertensive or manifests other signs of eclampsia, magnesium sulfate and other agents are indicated to prevent further seizures and to control blood pressure. In patients who do not manifest signs of eclampsia, investigation of the cause of the seizure should proceed as with the nonpregnant patient (see Chapter 100).

Status Epilepticus

Pregnant patients with known epilepsy may arrive in the emergency department in status epilepticus. Any of the causes of seizures, including eclampsia, may result in status epilepticus. Despite this, status epilepticus in pregnancy is relatively rare and only anecdotal reports are available to guide therapy.[38] The risk of status epilepticus to both the mother and the fetus clearly outweighs the potential for adverse teratogenic effects, and standard resuscitative measures as well as drug therapy are indicated. Continuous fetal monitoring should be instituted as soon as possible and the mother positioned to avoid the supine hypotensive syndrome.

Pregnant Epileptic Patient

Patients with epilepsy coming to the emergency department for unrelated reasons may be found to be pregnant. Although no immediate change in their therapeutic regimen needs to be made, these patients should be advised of the potential risk of AEMs in pregnancy and be referred to appropriate specialists. Unintentional pregnancy is seen even in patients taking oral contraceptives, because AEMs can cause increased clearance of these medications, thereby reducing their efficacy.[39]

There are many obstetric complications related to prolonged seizure activity and long-term treatment with an AEM for patients with such ictal events is indicated (see Table 178-1). Many patients who have nonconvulsive seizure disorders or who have been free of seizures for a sufficient period can be taken off AEMs, but this decision should be deferred to the patient's primary physician or neurologist. Because diphenylhydantoin, carbamazepine, valproate, and possibly other AEMs interfere with folate metabolism, oral supplementation with at least 0.4 mg/day is recommended for all women of child-bearing age taking AEMs.[35] Higher doses are recommended for women using AEMs known to cause neural tube defects. Many AEMs, including carbamazepine, diphenylhydantoin, and phenobarbital, cause neonatal vitamin K deficiency, resulting in a high rate of infant mortality (>30%) as well as coagulopathy in up to 50% of neonates, with serious bleeding episodes in 7%.[35,40] Consequently, the mother should receive oral vitamin K (10 mg) during the last month of gestation, and vitamin K 1 mg intramuscularly or intravenously should be given to the newborn.[35]

Experience with the newer AEMs, such as gabapentin, felbamate, lamotrigine, topiramate, and tiagabine, in pregnant patients is limited, but these agents are likely to have a more desirable side effect profile and have less interference with folate metabolism.[41]

Multiple Sclerosis

Multiple sclerosis (MS) affects 250,000 Americans and is twice as common in women as men. The peak age of onset is from 20 to 35 years of age, which overlaps peak childbearing years. The disease is characterized by intermittent episodes of central nervous system demyelination with consequent neurologic impairment that follows a relapsing-remitting course. Progressive neurologic deficits and permanent disability develop in certain patients.

The impact of pregnancy on the course of MS has been closely studied in various cohorts of women, and a pattern has emerged. Like other autoimmune diseases, the frequency and severity of exacerbations of MS improve because of the immunosuppressant effects of pregnancy. During the 3 months after delivery, the rate of relapse increases and then returns to the prepregnancy baseline.[42] The long-term effects of pregnancy on the disease course may be beneficial. Several studies have found that patients who had at least one pregnancy after the onset of MS had a significantly longer interval until wheelchair dependence than patients who did not have a pregnancy (18.6 years versus 12.5 years)[43] and were less likely to develop progressive disease.[44] Studies involving a shorter period of follow-up do not reveal such a benefit. Children of parents with MS have an increased susceptibility to develop MS themselves, reflecting at least a partial genetic component to the disease. Labor may be complicated by uncoordinated voluntary motor activity in pushing, but generally pregnancies in these patients progress without undue complications.

Spinal Cord Injury

Because spinal cord injury (SCI) occurs mainly in young persons and usually does not impair fertility, there is a relatively large population of paraplegic and quadriplegic patients who become pregnant. Although many of these pregnancies are uneventful, these patients are at risk for certain complications.

The incidence of urinary tract infection is relatively high, and these infections often progress to pyelonephritis during pregnancy with the resultant increased risk of fetal loss, prematurity, and maternal sepsis. The increased coagulability of pregnancy combined with chronic immobilization results in an increased incidence of venous thrombosis and pulmonary embolus.[45]

A unique problem in the patient with SCI is the detection of the onset of labor, which may be painless and precipitous. Patients with spinal cord lesions below T12 have an intact uterine nerve supply and will experience labor pains; however, with lesions above T10, labor may be imperceptible or experienced as only mild abdominal discomfort. In 85% of patients with lesions above T5 to T6, labor is heralded by an explosive autonomic dysreflexia.[46,47] This manifests as severe paroxysmal hypertension, pulsatile headache, tachycardia, blotching of the skin, diaphoresis, piloerection, mydriasis, and nasal congestion. Because the response is not specific to labor and may be precipitated by distention of bowel or bladder, other causes must be pursued as well. Pregnant patients with SCI who have these symptoms should be assessed for cervical dilation and have uterine contractions monitored. Emergency department treatment is directed at restoring normal blood pressure with nitroprusside, nitroglycerin, or hydralazine. Definitive therapy is with regional anesthesia. Both spinal and epidural anesthesia obliterate and prevent this response and should be used as soon as possible during labor for all women with SCI.[47] Because of the difficulty in detecting labor, pregnant patients with SCI are often admitted for observation at 35 weeks' gestation.

Myasthenia Gravis

Myasthenia gravis is a rare disorder in which autoimmune destruction of the postsynaptic cholinergic receptor results in profound muscle fatigability. Treatment with cholinesterase inhibitors can supply additional acetylcholine to achieve virtually normal muscle contractility but must be titrated to avoid precipitating a cholinergic crisis. Adjustments in medication dosing are frequently required to preserve this balance.

The effect of pregnancy on myasthenia gravis is unpredictable in the individual patient, but overall approximately one fifth to one third experience exacerbation of disease with the remainder having improvement or no change in disease severity.[48,49] Improvement during the last two trimesters of pregnancy is likely due to the relative immunosuppressant effect seen during that time.[49]

Several important pregnancy complications are associated with myasthenia gravis. Because of weight gain, anemia, and other physiologic adjustments of pregnancy that may result in fatigue, the distinction between normal pregnancy symptoms and myasthenia may be difficult. Although uterine contractile force is unaffected by myasthenia gravis, labor may be prolonged because of fatigue of abdominal muscles during active pushing. Arrest of labor can occur, requiring the use of high forceps or other extraction methods.[50] Ten to 20% of neonates born to mothers with myasthenia develop a transient neonatal myasthenic syndrome that may be life-threatening.[48,49] The onset of neonatal myasthenia may be delayed as much as 1 week and consists of poor feeding and suck, diminished reflexes, hypotonia, and respiratory failure. As with adults, the symptoms respond to cholinesterase inhibitors, but treatment should be done in an intensive care unit setting, and these neonates should be observed for at least 1 week. The duration of the syndrome depends on the clearance of maternal antibodies, and medication must be continually adjusted. Finally, maternal myasthenia gravis can exacerbate precipitously during the postpartum period as the protective immunosuppressant effect of pregnancy dissipates.

Treatment in the emergency setting is no different than treatment for nonpregnant patients and might include ventilatory support, pyridostigmine, corticosteroids, and plasmapheresis (see Table 178-1). Continuous pulse oximetry and arterial blood gas determination will guide respiratory therapy. For patients presenting with weakness, a "Tensilon challenge test" or its equivalent can distinguish myasthenic from cholinergic crisis but should only be attempted after appropriate ventilatory assistance is provided. Use of immunosuppressive medications may be associated with a higher incidence of congenital malformations, although azathioprine appears to be safe. Epidural anesthesia is recommended for labor and delivery; sedatives and other agents that increase fatigue should be avoided during this time.[49]

Renal Disorders

Several alterations in renal hemodynamics occur during pregnancy. Both the glomerular filtration rate and effective renal plasma flow increase by 30% to 50% compared with the nonpregnant state.[51] Because no substantial alterations are present in the production of creatinine or urea nitrogen, levels of these solutes decrease from average nonpregnant values of 0.7 and 12.0 mg/dL to 0.5 and 9.0 mg/dL, respectively. Thus, blood urea nitrogen and creatinine levels considered normal in nonpregnant women (creatinine > 0.8 mg/dL and blood urea nitrogen > 13 mg/dL) indicate underlying renal impairment and warrant further investigation.

In the past, chronic renal parenchymal disease of any severity was considered a virtual contraindication to pregnancy, but this view has changed with recent studies that show good pregnancy outcomes and preserved renal function in the majority of patients with mild to moderate insufficiency. On the other hand, patients with severe renal dysfunction have a much higher risk of further decline in renal function as well as poor fetal outcome.[51,52] Other variables that have been shown to adversely affect pregnancy outcome are prepregnancy hypertension and a history of long-term hemodialysis. Conception is uncommon in women on long-term dialysis and is extremely risky for both the mother and the fetus. Pregnancy termination is usually advised. Typically, less than 50% of these pregnancies result in a viable infant, although recent advances in maternal and neonatal care may improve the success rate.[53]

Pregnant women with preexisting renal disease or hypertension are more susceptible to preeclampsia. Because worsening of the underlying renal disease is manifested by hypertension and proteinuria, differentiation from preeclampsia can be difficult. It is always best to treat the patient for presumed preeclampsia, but measurement of serum magnesium levels is indicated prior to use of magnesium sulfate.

Pregnant women with chronic renal failure require aggressive and timely management to optimize their chances for a successful gestation without causing further deterioration in renal function. Baseline renal function studies are done early in pregnancy and then reassessed every 4 to 6 weeks. Evidence of renal function deterioration or the development or exacerbation of hypertension warrants admission for specialized inpatient care. Failure to reverse these parameters is usually an indication to terminate the pregnancy.

Metabolic and Endocrine Disorders

Diabetes

Diabetes is one of the most common chronic disorders that complicate pregnancy, affecting 3% to 5% of all pregnancies.[54] Three types of diabetes are involved in pregnancy: type I or insulin-dependent diabetes mellitus (IDDM), type II or non–insulin-dependent diabetes mellitus (NIDDM), and gestational diabetes mellitus (GDM) in which glucose tolerance becomes abnormal during pregnancy but returns to normal after delivery. Although pregnant patients with NIDDM tend to have less severe disease than those with IDDM, maternal and fetal complications relate more to the duration of diabetes as well as the presence of vascular complications or severe renal insufficiency rather than to the type of diabetes. All pregnant patients with diabetes are considered "brittle" and demand close follow-up by appropriate specialists.

Maternal Complications

The physiology of glucose regulation during pregnancy is complex. During the first trimester, under the influence of elevated progesterone and estrogen levels, the sensitivity to insulin increases. When combined with emesis, increased use of glucose by the placenta and fetus, and a decrease in hepatic glucose production, hypoglycemia occurs more easily. Consequently, patients with IDDM are at risk for hypoglycemic coma during early pregnancy and insulin dosage should be decreased. During later gestation, however, there is progressive insulin resistance that peaks during the third trimester.[54,55] Pregnancy also predisposes to ketosis and this effect is exacerbated in the setting of emesis.

The effects of pregnancy on underlying diabetes vary depending on the organ system. The data are limited, but pregnancy termination is generally advised for diabetic patients with coronary artery disease because of the cardiovascular demands of pregnancy and the high mortality of acute MI during pregnancy.[54,56] Patients with diabetic nephropathy are at increased risk for severe preeclampsia and often experience a transient increase in proteinuria with resolution after delivery. Those patients with severe renal dysfunction are more likely to experience permanent effects. Retinopathy does not appear to be permanently affected by pregnancy, but it may worsen during pregnancy, especially in patients with hypertension and in the setting of overaggressive correction of hyperglycemia.[54,56,57] Autonomic neuropathy does not accelerate during pregnancy, but the combination of hyperemesis gravidarum and gastroparesis often causes problems. Frequent vomiting results in dehydration and inadequate intake of food that can result in hypoglycemic episodes if the insulin dosage is not adjusted accordingly.

Diabetic ketoacidosis occurs in 1% to 3% of insulin-requiring diabetic patients during pregnancy and may represent the initial presentation of diabetes. Diabetic ketoacidosis is most commonly seen in those patients with IDDM but also complicates pregnancies in women with NIDDM and GDM.[55] Common precipitating events include hyperemesis, use of β-mimetic medications for tocolysis, use of corticosteroids, infection, and noncompliance or errors in insulin dosage.[55] The serum pH may be deceptively normal in a pregnant patient with diabetic ketoacidosis, because the initial pH tends to be higher in pregnancy due to physiologic hyperventilation. Loss of gastric acid through vomiting will also counteract the metabolic acidosis of diabetic ketoacidosis. Serum glucose may be only moderately elevated because the fetus continues to secrete insulin and use glucose.[24] Maternal mortality is rare in appropriately treated diabetic ketoacidosis. Fetal mortality rates are decreasing with advances in diabetic and obstetric care but still remain relatively high, ranging from 9% to 50%.[55,56]

Fetal Complications

Diabetes has many deleterious effects on the fetus (see Table 178-1). Both hyperglycemia and hypoglycemia appear to be teratogenic during early pregnancy. The rate of congenital malformations in patients with prepregnancy diabetes is increased threefold to fourfold over the nondiabetic population.[58] The poorly controlled diabetic patient is also more likely to have either macrosomic or low-birth-weight infants. Glucose crosses the placenta and prolonged fetal exposure to maternal hyperglycemia induces fetal pancreatic hyperplasia and high insulin production. Elevated insulin levels in turn promote fetal growth, resulting in macrosomia. Consequently, the incidence of fetopelvic disproportion, shoulder dystocia, and asphyxia during delivery is high in diabetic pregnancies.[24,54] Conversely, preeclampsia and placental infarction secondary to vascular disease may result in impaired fetal development. After delivery, continued high insulin secretion in the absence of a maternal glucose supply results in neonatal hypoglycemia in 25% of cases.[59] The incidence of respiratory distress syndrome is increased in infants of diabetic mothers with inadequate glycemic control because surfactant production is decreased. Macrosomic infants have an increased risk of intrauterine fetal demise during the last weeks of gestation but lack of fetal lung maturity may prevent early elective delivery.[54]

Management

Treatment of NIDDM and IDDM requires individualized and carefully adjusted insulin administration (see Table 178-1). Treatment of diabetic ketoacidosis does not differ from treatment given in the nonpregnant state except that fetal viability and well-being should be assessed. The timing of delivery is a balance between the delayed fetal lung maturity and the condition of the fetus or mother. Generally, elective delivery for poorly controlled diabetic patients is timed to occur about 2 weeks early to avoid fetal growth into the macrosomic range. Patients undergoing elective delivery prior to 39 weeks' gestation require amniocentesis to assess fetal lung maturity. For patients with term gestations, fetal size is estimated by ultrasonography and a nonstress test is performed to determine the fetus's ability to tolerate labor.[54]

Gestational Diabetes

Gestational diabetes is more common than IDDM or NIDDM and has little impact on the fetus if detected and treated early in the pregnancy; however, untreated GDM carries a fourfold increase in fetal mortality.[59] The implication of GDM is greater for the mother in that 17% to 63% will develop diabetes within the following decade.[60,61] Patients at increased risk include those with obesity, poor insulin secretion, and onset early in pregnancy.[60]

The issue of screening for GDM is controversial. Some sources recommend universal screening while the American Diabetes Association advocates selective screening of patients at increased risk for GDM. This group includes patients older than 25 years of age; certain high-risk ethnic groups; and patients with obesity, known first-degree relatives with diabetes, a personal history of diabetes or glucose intolerance, and a personal history of poor pregnancy outcome.[54] A positive screening test is an indication for a formal 3-hour glucose tolerance test. Treatment is initially aimed at dietary control, followed by insulin administration if dietary control is unsuccessful (see Table 178-1). Practitioners have avoided oral medications in the past but studies show that glyburide is safe and effective for GDM.[54,62]

Thyroid Disorders

Thyroid function remains essentially unchanged during pregnancy despite an increase in thyroglobulin levels. Human chorionic gonadotropin stimulates the thyroid gland and is structurally similar to thyroid-stimulating hormone; high circulating levels of human chorionic gonadotropin during the first trimester may cause a temporary and clinically insignificant increase in free thyroxine (T_4). However, free triiodothyronine (T_3), T_4, and thyroid-stimulating hormone levels usually remain within normal range.[63,64] Negligible amounts of maternal thyroid hormone, thyroid-stimulating hormone, or exogenous thyroxine cross the placenta; however, thyroid-releasing hormone from the hypothalamus and thyroid-stimulating immunoglobulin G do cross the placenta and can also cause fetal hyperthyroidism.[63]

Hyperthyroidism

The peak incidence of autoimmune disease and thyroid disease is in women of childbearing age, and 0.2% of pregnancies are complicated by hyperthyroidism.[63] Because the symptoms of hyperthyroidism resemble the physiologic changes expected during pregnancy in many respects, the diagnosis may not be immediately evident. Symptoms such as dyspnea, heat intolerance, hyperemesis, tachycardia, palpitations, systolic flow murmurs, increased appetite, and fatigue are common to both conditions, making clinical diagnosis difficult. In cases of suspected hyperthyroidism, thyroid function studies are indicated and will confirm the presence of disease.

The most common cause of hyperthyroidism is Graves' disease, in which autoimmune thyroid-stimulating immunoglobulin G results in increased production and release of thyroid hormone. Patients with Graves' disease have other characteristic findings in addition to the more nonspecific signs and symptoms of sympathetic stimulation. These include a diffusely enlarged, soft, mildly tender thyroid gland; exophthalmos; and dermopathy. Thyroid storm is the most serious manifestation of disease. It may be precipitated by stressors such as infection and delivery and manifests with fever, dysrhythmias, congestive heart failure, psychosis, and circulatory collapse. As with other autoimmune conditions, transient improvement during pregnancy is common, with rebound and clinical deterioration occurring after delivery.[64]

There are several obstetric concerns for both mother and fetus in the setting of untreated hyperthyroidism (see Table 178-1).[63] In addition, Graves' disease places the fetus at risk for autoimmune-mediated thyroid dysfunction. One to 2% of neonates of mothers with Graves' disease have transient hyperthyroidism lasting 3 to 12 weeks because of the transfer of maternal thyroid-stimulating immunoglobulin G across the placenta. The condition gradually clears as maternal antibodies are metabolized. These infants may have goiter, congestive heart failure, premature craniosynostosis, frontal bossing, low birth weight, pulmonary hypertension, and hypertrophic cardiomyopathy. The mortality rate from severe neonatal hyperthyroidism approaches 25%, so the condition must be recognized promptly and treated aggressively.[65]

Treatment of hyperthyroidism (see Table 178-1) occurs in two stages. The first priority is the reversal and stabilization of the end-organ and hemodynamic effects of sympathetic stimulation, followed by reduction in the production of thyroid hormone. Most patients respond to pharmacologic manipulation, although thyroidectomy may be considered in severe cases. Use of ^{131}I radionuclide to ablate the maternal thyroid is absolutely contraindicated because it will also destroy the fetal thyroid gland.

Propylthiouracil is typically preferred over methimazole because of a more rapid onset of effect, although either drug can be used. Both drugs cross the placenta and can cause fetal hypothyroidism.[63] Consequently, neonatal thyroid function must be assessed periodically. Both drugs also enter breast milk, but they are still considered safe for breast-feeding.[63] Iodides transiently block the release of stored T_4 from the thyroid gland and inhibit organification of iodide. However, the fetal thyroid is extremely sensitive to iodide, which may result in neonatal goiter and hypothyroidism. Therefore, iodide use should be reserved for severe cases and should not be continued beyond 7 to 10 days during pregnancy.

Postpartum Thyroiditis

Postpartum thyroiditis is a common but relatively benign condition that develops in 5% to 9% of parturients within 9 months of delivery. Patients typically experience transient hyperthyroidism followed by transient hypothyroidism.[64] Pharmacologic treatment may be required; however, the need for medication seems to be confined to those patients with hypothyroidism.[63,64] Up to 30% of patients with postpartum hypothyroidism may have permanent thyroid failure several years later, and this percentage may be even higher in subsequent years.[64]

Hypothyroidism

Overt hypothyroidism is often associated with infertility, so most cases seen during pregnancy are less severe or subclinical forms. Subclinical hypothyroidism may become overt during pregnancy, because physiologic adjustments result in a greater requirement for thyroid hormone production. In addition, iodine deficiency may be exacerbated by pregnancy, because renal losses of iodine increase as the glomerular filtration rate increases and as the fetus diverts iodine for its own thyroid hormone synthesis. The resulting lack of thyroid hormone results in increased thyroid-stimulating hormone level and goiter formation.

Symptoms are identical to those in the nonpregnant state and include coarse hair, dry skin, fatigue, weight gain, cold intolerance, constipation, irritability, and paresthesias. Myxedema coma is extremely rare but must be considered with other causes of coma in a pregnant patient.

As with hyperthyroidism, there is an increased incidence of adverse maternal and fetal effects (see Table 178-1).[63,66,67] Treatment consists of the replacement of thyroid hormone at a dosage of 0.15 mg/day orally, which is slightly higher than the recommended dosage in nonpregnant patients.[63] The fetus produces its own thyroid hormone after 12 weeks' gestation and is consequently euthyroid at birth.

Congenital hypothyroidism, associated with cretinism and severe mental retardation, occurs in 1 in 4000 births. It is most often the result of sporadic thyroid dysgenesis or various genetic disorders rather than maternal thyroid dysfunction.[68] Diagnosis is often difficult, since clinical signs and symptoms may be masked by maternal thyroid hormone.[63] Congenital hypothyroidism is amenable to in utero diagnosis and treatment, and screening for congenital hypothyroidism is mandated in most developed countries.

Systemic Infections

Tuberculosis

The effect of tuberculosis on pregnancy is unclear. Some studies reveal a significant increase in gestational complications (see Table 178-1), but these outcomes are likely significantly influenced by the site of disease and specifics of treatment. Complications are more likely in patients with inadequate or delayed treatment, delayed diagnosis, and extrapulmonary (extranodal) tuberculosis.[69-71] A recent study found no significant increase in gestational complications in 111 pregnant patients with properly treated tuberculosis.[72] On the other hand, exposure to undiagnosed and untreated active disease places the infant at significant risk for acquiring tuberculosis during the first year of life, with significant mortality. In addition, the fetus can become infected via the placenta or aspiration of infected amniotic fluid, but congenital tuberculosis is rare if the mother has received appropriate therapy.[71]

Current recommendations are to administer a tuberculin skin test early in pregnancy to all patients at high risk for disease and to obtain a chest radiograph if the purified protein derivative (PPD) skin test is positive or if the patient's signs and symptoms suggest tuberculosis. Definitive treatment varies depending upon the duration of PPD positivity and whether the patient has active disease (see Table 178-1).[73] Isoniazid, ethambutol, and rifampin in their usual doses have not been shown to be teratogenic to human fetuses and are acceptable during pregnancy. On the other hand, streptomycin causes fetal ototoxicity when given at any time during gestation, and little is known about the safety of pyrazinamide during pregnancy.[71] These agents as well as the other less commonly used medications should be avoided in pregnancy except in the case of multidrug-resistant disease. Bacille Calmette-Guérin vaccine is recommended for infants with a negative tuberculin skin test who are at high risk for infection by virtue of prolonged exposure to individuals who are untreated or noncompliant with treatment.[71]

Human Immunodeficiency Virus and Acquired Immunodeficiency Syndrome

The human immunodeficiency virus (HIV) is one of the leading health problems in pregnancy. In 2002, 26% of cases of acquired immunodeficiency syndrome (AIDS) in the United States were in women, with the vast majority (80%) in their childbearing years.[74] Estimates of the seroprevalence of HIV in pregnant women vary on a regional basis. In some African countries, these figures range from less than 1% to 24%.[75,76] In the United States, the nationwide prevalence ranges from 1.5 to 1.7 per 1000 women but is as high as 2% in some inner city populations.[77,78] Vertical transmission of HIV in the United States declined by 67% from 1992 through 1997, a decline that coincides with the implementation of routine voluntary testing and zidovudine (AZT) prophylaxis for HIV-positive pregnant women.[79] However, vertical transmission remains a global concern; it is estimated that perinatal infection occurs in 10% to 60% of deliveries if the mother is untreated.[80]

The mechanism of vertical transmission is unknown, but the majority of cases are thought to occur during delivery through exposure to maternal blood and secretions; other infants are likely infected in utero or via breast-feeding. Various factors influence the rate of transmission, the most important of which is maternal viral load; others include vaginal delivery, intravenous drug use, and prolonged rupture of membranes.[80] In countries in which alternative nutritional sources are available, breast-feeding should be avoided because it doubles the risk of fetal infection. Antepartum AZT therapy that is continued through delivery decreased the rate of vertical transmission from 25.5% to 8.3% in one study and decreased the rate to 4.25% in a smaller, more recent investigation.[81,82] Because of this beneficial effect, voluntary screening should be offered to all pregnant women, and all pregnant patients presenting to the emergency department should be referred to anonymous testing centers or specialty clinics if their HIV status is unknown. Although long-term data are not available, AZT has not been found to cause any specific congenital abnormalities; however, it is associated with reversible neonatal anemia.[83] Other infections, such as with cytomegalovirus, syphilis, and hepatitis B and C, can also be vertically transmitted concurrently with HIV.

The incidence of prematurity, stillbirth, and low birth weight is higher with symptomatic maternal HIV infection. Seropositive mothers have an increased risk of postpartum endometritis, but asymptomatic patients generally have good pregnancy outcomes.[84-86]

Commonly used serologic tests for HIV yield positive results in virtually all of these neonates because of transfer of maternal antibodies. These findings may remain positive for up to 18 months and are not an accurate indicator of neonatal infection; in fact, the vast majority of infants are seronegative after these antibodies clear. In addition, some children in whom HIV has been directly isolated using culture or detection of viral RNA have been clear of the virus in subsequent testing.[87] Only a fraction of exposed infants develop HIV infection, but of these, approximately 20% develop AIDS during the first year of life.[88] Common initial symptoms are generalized lymphadenopathy, hepatosplenomegaly, and thrush. Infants with AIDS typically present with recurrent bacterial infections, *Pneumocystis* pneumonia, encephalopathy, and lymphoid interstitial pneumonia.[88,89] Isolation of virus within the first week of life is associated with the onset of early, severe disease.[89] The rapidity of disease progression in the infant is also directly proportional to the severity of the mother's HIV illness as manifested by the viral load and CD4 count. Early antiretroviral treatment during infancy has been shown to reduce the likelihood of death as well as the development of AIDS.[90]

The effect of pregnancy on the course of HIV in the mother is unclear. CD4 lymphocyte counts transiently decrease in normal pregnancy but then normalize postpartum. Counts remain depressed in the HIV-infected patient.[91] It seems intuitive that the incidence of opportunistic infections would increase, but this does not occur, at least in women with mild to moderate HIV disease.[92,93]

Treatment of the pregnant patient with HIV includes appropriate antiretroviral treatment (see Table 178-1)[80] as well as standard therapy for opportunistic infections when they occur. Use of highly active antiretroviral treatment (HAART) has become commonplace in nonpregnant patients and limits the emergence of resistant organisms within an individual. There is limited experience using HAART during pregnancy, but recent studies suggest that there is no increase in serious adverse effects. Protease inhibitors have been linked to an increase in prematurity and low birth weight, but there is disagreement about this association.[83,94] The risk of perinatal HIV transmission increases with the degree of maternal viral load, even in the setting of prophylactic AZT therapy.[80,95] Consequently, pregnant patients with HIV infection should be offered the more effective HAART regimen, particularly if the viral load is greater than 1000 copies.[80]

Syphilis

Fortunately, the incidence of syphilis in the United States in 2000 was the lowest it has been since 1941.[96] Likewise, the incidence of congenital syphilis has been declining but the disease remains a concern among those patients without access to prenatal care.[97]

Syphilis causes numerous gestational complications (see Table 178-1), but its most significant sequela is congenital syphilis. This syndrome is characterized by clinical abnormalities such as hepatosplenomegaly, osteochondritis, jaundice, lymphadenopathy, rhinitis, Hutchinson's teeth, and anemia. Perinatal mortality for cases occurring from 1992 to 1998 was 6.4%.[98] If untreated, vertical transmission rates are high at approximately 50% but can be reduced to negligible levels (2%) with appropriate penicillin therapy.[99] Screening for all pregnant patients is indicated at the first prenatal visit and at 32 to 36 weeks for high-risk patients.[99] Either Venereal Disease Research Laboratory or rapid plasma reagin testing can be used to detect nontreponemal antibody. Pregnancy may cause false-positive results for nontreponemal studies, so confirmation using specific treponemal tests is indicated for a positive Venereal Disease Research Laboratory test or rapid plasma reagin finding. Patients with latent syphilis and those whose titers fail to respond to therapy should undergo cerebrospinal fluid analysis to screen for tertiary syphilis.[100]

Treatment is identical to that given to nonpregnant patients using benzathine penicillin G (see Table 178-1).[100] Penicillin-allergic patients should undergo skin testing and desensitization if the skin test result is positive because erythromycin, although adequate for the mother, is not reliably effective in preventing congenital syphilis.

Hepatitis

Hepatitis B

The prevalence of hepatitis B virus infection among pregnant women varies depending on the population studied. In U.S. urban areas, 0.14% to 5.79% of pregnant women are positive for HbsAg, with Asians having the highest seroprevalence.[101] The rate of vertical transmission depends on the acuity of maternal infection and when during the gestation it occurs. Perinatal transmission approaches 90% in mothers who are seropositive for HBsAg and HBeAg and is more likely if the mother has acute infection during the third trimester or first few months postpartum, or if she is a chronic carrier.[102,103] Infection earlier in pregnancy does not result in high rates of perinatal transmission because maternal antibody to HBsAg has time to clear the virus from both mother and fetus. Of babies who develop hepatitis B virus infection, 60% to 90% become chronic carriers as adults and are at risk for complications such as cirrhosis and hepatocellular carcinoma.[102]

Routine screening for hepatitis B virus during early pregnancy is recommended because treatment with hepatitis B immunoglobulin and hepatitis B vaccine is very effective in reducing the rate of vertical transmission.[103] Infant immunization and treatment with hepatitis B immunoglobulin is 85% to 95% effective in preventing perinatal disease transmission, and vaccination is recommended for all infants in the United States. The treatment schedule varies depending on maternal seropositivity. Infants of HBsAg-positive mothers should receive hepatitis B immunoglobulin and the first dose of vaccine within 12 hours of birth. Pregnancy is not a contraindication to either therapy, and all pregnant patients who are exposed to hepatitis B virus should also receive hepatitis B immunoglobulin and vaccine.[103]

Hepatitis C

As with hepatitis B virus, the prevalence of hepatitis C infection among pregnant women varies depending on the population; overall, 1% of pregnant women has hepatitis C but the prevalence is as high as 4.3% in some urban areas.[104,105] Vertical transmission of hepatitis C is much less common than hepatitis B virus but can occur. The rate of perinatal transmission is increased by the presence of viremia, coinfection with HIV, and a history of intravenous drug use. Overall, vertical transmission occurs in 1.7% of mothers with anti-hepatitis C antibodies, but this increases to 4% to 7% in viremic mothers and is greater than 8% in intravenous drug use patients. The rate increases sixfold for those with HIV.[105] No available vaccine exists to prevent hepatitis C, although testing of potentially infected neonates is advised to identify those at risk for chronic hepatitis.

Inflammatory Disorders

Rheumatic diseases or collagen vascular diseases are characterized by sterile inflammation in multiple anatomic sites. The most common rheumatic diseases encountered in pregnancy are systemic lupus erythematosus (SLE), rheumatoid arthritis (RA), scleroderma, and juvenile rheumatoid arthritis. Patients with collagen vascular disease may have preexisting cardiovascular or renal compromise and may not tolerate the increased intravascular volume that occurs during pregnancy. The following discussion focuses on SLE, which is the rheumatic disease responsible for the majority of gestational complications. Most of the treatment guidelines for SLE are relevant to other rheumatologic disorders as well.

Systemic Lupus Erythematosus

Systemic lupus erythematosus primarily affects women of reproductive age, and fertility is usually unaffected. The disease course during pregnancy is a matter of controversy but it seems that flare-ups are common.[106] The gestational effects of SLE are variable, depending on the severity of underlying disease. Although many patients do well, lupus pregnancies are associated with an increased rate of complications, including preeclampsia, preterm delivery, intrauterine growth retardation, and fetal loss.[106,107] The risk of preeclampsia is increased in patients with preexisting renal disease and antiphospholipid antibodies.[106] Increasing proteinuria warrants a careful evaluation to distinguish between lupus glomerulonephritis and preeclampsia. The presence of RBC casts in the urine sediment, increasing titers of anti-DNA antibody, decreasing levels of C3 and C4, disease activity in other organs, and a positive response to prednisone point to lupus nephritis.[106]

Numerous other organ systems in addition to the kidneys are involved in SLE, and differentiation from pregnancy-related changes may be difficult. Thrombocytopenia occurs in normal pregnancies and is also common in patients with SLE, although the clinical significance varies from patient to patient. Anemia is a frequent complication of lupus and magnifies the normal dilutional anemia of pregnancy; this anemia can compromise the fetus even if the mother is relatively asymptomatic.

Various musculoskeletal and cutaneous symptoms associated with pregnancy, such as arthralgias and facial and palmar erythema can also resemble active SLE. In addition, preexisting lupus rashes become more erythematous because of the increased cutaneous blood flow during pregnancy. Arthritis occurs in approximately 90% of SLE patients, and many develop inflammatory effusions late in pregnancy.

Neurologic disease in SLE may manifest as psychosis, seizures, chorea, or peripheral neuropathy. The incidence of these complications is low during pregnancy, although the occurrence of seizures in late pregnancy in patients with coexistent hypertension and renal insufficiency poses a diagnostic dilemma between the neurologic effects of SLE and eclampsia.

Other Rheumatologic Diseases

Rheumatoid arthritis is characterized by chronic, destructive, symmetric joint inflammation. Less common manifestations include the development of subcutaneous nodules, neuropathy, pleuropericarditis, and vasculitis. Systemic symptoms, including weight loss, lymphadenopathy, and fatigue, are common. Approximately two thirds of patients with RA experience an amelioration of symptoms during pregnancy, although often an exacerbation follows delivery.[108] RA appears to have little effect on pregnancy outcome. Patients with other rheumatologic diseases including Sjögren's syndrome, scleroderma, CREST syndrome (calcinosis, Raynaud's phenomenon, esophageal dysmotility, sclerodactyly, and telangiectasia), and polymyositis may have symptomatic improvement during pregnancy.

Treatment

The rheumatologic diseases are very similar with respect to the therapeutic approach. Corticosteroids form the basis of treatment for most disease complications and exacerbations. Prednisone and methylprednisolone do not readily cross the placenta and are considered relatively safe to use during pregnancy, even at high dosages. Although animal studies suggest an increased incidence of cleft palate, no teratogenic effects have been documented in humans. Steroid use during pregnancy predisposes the patient to GDM and hypertension, and these patients require close follow-up.[106,109]

Aspirin can be effective in treating thrombocytopenia in pregnant SLE patients and is often used as the mainstay of therapy in nonpregnant RA patients. Nonsteroidal anti-inflammatory drugs are also a mainstay of therapy in many patients with rheumatic diseases. There are numerous potential adverse effects of aspirin and nonsteroidal anti-inflammatory drugs on gestation, including premature closure of the fetal ductus arteriosus, increased maternal bleeding secondary to platelet dysfunction, and prolongation of gestation and labor. On the other hand, aspirin has gestational benefits as well, since it reduces the incidence of perinatal death and preeclampsia in high-risk patients, including those with renal disease.[110] Use of these agents during the last weeks of pregnancy should be avoided to minimize the risks of maternal and fetal hemorrhage and premature ductus closure.[106]

Acute flares often require institution of cytotoxic drugs. Cyclophosphamide and methotrexate are contraindicated during the first trimester and should be used only in extreme circumstances because of their teratogenicity and abortifacient properties. Azathioprine has a better documented safety profile because of its use in renal transplant patients and is the cytotoxic agent of choice during pregnancy. Although the drug and its metabolites cross the placenta, there is not a significant increase in congenital malformations. Cyclosporin A is an acceptable alternative to azathioprine.[106]

Other agents used in the treatment of SLE or RA include chloroquine, injectable gold complexes, D-penicillamine, and sulfasalazine. These drugs cross the placenta, and reports of congenital malformations have been associated with their use. On the other hand, hydroxychloroquine appears safe, and its use may allow for a decrease in corticosteroid dosage.[106,111]

KEY CONCEPTS

- The physiologic demands of pregnancy may cause previously occult medical conditions to become apparent.
- The physiologic adjustments of pregnancy alter the normal ranges for certain laboratory values. The adjusted values need to be considered in interpreting results.
- The possibility of pregnancy must be considered in the differential diagnosis of certain conditions, including new-onset seizures or status epilepticus (eclampsia), glucose intolerance (GDM), persistent vomiting (hyperemesis gravidarum), and thyroid disorders.
- The immunosuppressive effects of pregnancy may cause temporary improvement in inflammatory and autoimmune conditions. This beneficial effect is lost in the postpartum period, resulting in exacerbations of asthma, thyroid disorders, and myasthenia gravis. Medication requirements can change drastically during pregnancy and the postpartum period.
- Certain medical conditions in the mother result in neonatal complications requiring special resuscitative measures.

REFERENCES

1. Berkowitz GS, et al: Delayed childbearing and the outcome of pregnancy. *N Engl J Med* 322:659, 1990.
2. Paulson RJ, et al: Pregnancy in the sixth decade of life: Obstetric outcomes in women of advanced reproductive age. *JAMA* 288:2320, 2002.
3. Blaiss MS: Management of rhinitis and asthma in pregnancy. *Ann Allergy Asthma Immunol* 90:S16, 2003.
4. Schatz M: Asthma and pregnancy. *Lancet* 353:1202, 1999.
5. Beckmann CA: The effects of asthma on pregnancy and perinatal outcomes. *J Asthma* 40:171, 2003.
6. Wen SW, et al: Adverse outcomes in pregnancies of asthmatic women: Results from a Canadian population. *Ann Epidemiol* 11:7, 2001
7. Schatz M, et al: Perinatal outcomes in the pregnancies of asthmatic women: A prospective controlled analysis. *Am J Respir Crit Care Med* 151:1170, 1995
8. Luskin AT: An overview of the recommendations of the Working Group on Asthma and Pregnancy. *J Allergy Clin Immunol* 103:S350, 1999.
9. The use of newer asthma and allergy medications during pregnancy. The American College of Obstetricians and Gynecologists (ACOG) and The American College of Allergy, Asthma and Immunology (ACAAI). *Ann Allergy Asthma Immunol* 84:475, 2000.
10. How HY, et al: Bronchodilating effect of IV magnesium sulfate in pregnant asthmatic patients [abstract]. *Ann Emerg Med* 20:952, 1990.
11. Report of the National High Blood Pressure Education Program Working Group on High Blood Pressure in Pregnancy. *Am J Obstet Gynecol* 183:S1, 2000.
12. Livingston JC, Sibai BM: Chronic hypertension in pregnancy. *Obstet Gynecol Clin North* Am 28:447, 2001.
13. The sixth report of the Joint National Committee on prevention, detection, evaluation, and treatment of high blood pressure. *Arch Intern Med* 157:2413, 1997.
14. Weiss BM, Hess OM: Pulmonary vascular disease and pregnancy: Current controversies, management strategies, and perspectives. *Eur Heart J* 21:104, 2000.
15. Roth A, Elkayam U: Acute myocardial infarction associated with pregnancy. *Ann Intern Med* 125:751, 1996.
16. Woods JR Jr, et al: Pregnancy enhances cocaine's actions on the heart and within the peripheral circulation. *Am J Obstet Gynecol* 170:1027, 1994.
17. Gei AF, Hankins GDV: Cardiac disease and pregnancy. *Obstet Gynecol Clin North Am* 28:465, 2001.
18. Shivvers SA, et al: Maternal cardiac troponin I levels during normal labor and delivery. *Am J Obstet Gynecol* 180:122, 1999.
19. Laurent P, et al: Low molecular weight heparins: A guide to their optimum use in pregnancy. *Drugs* 62:463, 2002.
20. Greer IA: Exploring the role of low-molecular-weight heparins in pregnancy. *Semin Thromb Hemost* 28:25, 2002.
21. Turrentine MA, et al: Use of thrombolytics for the treatment of thromboembolic disease during pregnancy. *Obstet Gynecol Surv* 50:534, 1995.
22. Bernal JM, Miralles PJ: Cardiac surgery with cardiopulmonary bypass during pregnancy. *Obstet Gynecol Surv* 41:1, 1986.
23. Craig S, Ilton M: Treatment of acute myocardial infarction in pregnancy with coronary artery balloon angioplasty and stenting. *Aust N Z J Obstet Gynecol* 39:194, 1999.
24. Cherry SH, Merkatz IR (eds): *Complications of Pregnancy: Medical, Surgical, Gynecologic, Psychosocial and Perinatal,* 4th ed. Baltimore, Williams & Wilkins, 1991.
25. ACC/AHA guidelines for the management of patients with valvular heart disease: A report of the American College of Cardiology/American Heart Association Task Force on practice guidelines. *JACC* 32:1486, 1998.
26. Lao TT, et al: Congenital aortic stenosis and pregnancy: A reappraisal. *Am J Obstet Gynecol* 169:540, 1993.
27. Meeks GR, et al: Iron deficiency anemia. In Kitay D (ed): *Hematologic Problems in Pregnancy.* Oradell, NJ, Medical Economics, 1987, pp 26-48.
28. Haram K, et al: Iron supplementation in pregnancy-evidence and controversies. *Acta Obstet Gynecol Scand* 80:683, 2001.
29. Scholl TO, Reilly T: Anemia, iron, and pregnancy outcome. *J Nutr* 130:S443, 2000.
30. Scholl TO, Johnson WG: Folic acid: Influence on the outcome of pregnancy. *Am J Clin Nutr* 71(Suppl):S1295, 2000.
31. Hassan M, et al: HCV in sickle cell disease. *J National Med Assoc,* 95:864-867, 872-874, 2004.
32. Sun PM, et al: Sickle cell disease in pregnancy: Twenty years of experience at Grady Memorial Hospital, Atlanta, Georgia. *Am J Obstet Gynecol* 184:1127, 2001.
33. Seoud MA, et al: Outcomes of pregnancies complicated by sickle cell and sickle-C hemoglobinopathies. *Am J Perinatol* 11:187, 1994.
34. Schupf N, Ottman R: Likelihood of pregnancy in individuals with idiopathic/cryptogenic epilepsy: Social and biologic influences. *Epilepsia* 35:750, 1994.
35. Pennell PB: Pregnancy in the woman with epilepsy: Maternal and fetal outcomes. *Semin Neurol* 22:299, 2002.
36. Devinsky O, Yerby MS: Women with epilepsy. *Neurol Clin North Am* 12:479, 1994.
37. Holmes LB, et al: The teratogenicity of anticonvulsant drugs. *N Engl J Med* 344:1132, 2001.
38. Mendez-Quijada J, et al: Status epilepticus in pregnancy: A case report. *J Reprod Med* 35:289, 1990.
39. Mattson RH, Cramer JA: Epilepsy, sex hormones, and antiepileptic drugs. *Epilepsia* 26:40S, 1985.
40. Krumholz A: Epilepsy in pregnancy. In Goldstein PJ, Stern BJ (eds): *Neurologic Disorders in Pregnancy,* 2nd ed. Mount Kisco, NY, Futura, 1992, pp 25-51.
41. Palmieri C, Canger R: Teratogenic potential of the newer antiepileptic drugs: What is known and how should this influence prescribing? *CNS Drugs* 16:755, 2002.
42. Confavreux C, et al: Rate of pregnancy-related relapse in multiple sclerosis. *N Engl J Med* 339:285, 1998.
43. Damek DM, Shuster EA: Pregnancy and multiple sclerosis. *Mayo Clin Proc* 72:977, 1997.
44. Runmarker B, Anderson O: Pregnancy is associated with a lower risk of onset and a better prognosis in multiple sclerosis. *Brain* 118:253, 1995.
45. Westgren N, Levi R: Motherhood after traumatic spinal cord injury. *Paraplegia* 32:517, 1994.
46. Hughes SJ, et al: Management of the pregnant woman with spinal cord injuries. *Br J Obstet Gynaecol* 98:513, 1991.
47. American College of Obstetricians and Gynecologists: ACOG Committee Opinion: Number 275, September 2002. Obstetric management of patients with spinal cord injuries. *Obstet Gynecol* 100:625, 2002.
48. Batocchi AP, et al: Course and treatment of myasthenia gravis during pregnancy. *Neurology* 52:447, 1999.
49. Djelmis J, et al: Myasthenia gravis in pregnancy: Report on 69 cases. *Eur J Obstet Gynecol* 104:21, 2002.
50. Fox MW: Selected neurologic complications of pregnancy. *Mayo Clin Proc* 65:1595, 1990.
51. Henders CL, Lucas MJ: Renal disease in pregnancy. *Obstet Gynecol Clin North Am* 28:593, 2001.
52. Abe S: An overview of pregnancy in women with underlying renal disease. *Am J Kidney Dis* 17:116, 1991.
53. Chao A-S, et al: Pregnancy in women who undergo long-term dialysis. *Am J Obstet Gynecol* 187:152, 2002.
54. Gabbe SG, Graves CR: Management of diabetes mellitus complicating pregnancy. *Obstet Gynecol* 102:857, 2003.

55. Kamalakannan D, et al: Diabetic ketoacidosis in pregnancy. *Postgrad Med J* 79:454, 2003.
56. Lucas MJ: Diabetes complicating pregnancy. *Obstet Gynecol Clin North Am* 28:513, 2001.
57. ACOG technical bulletin, Diabetes and pregnancy. Number 200—December 1994. Committee on Technical Bulletins of the American College of Obstetricians and Gynecologists. *Int J Gynaecol Obstet* 48:33, 1995.
58. Sheffield JS, et al: Maternal diabetes mellitus and infant malformations. *Obstet Gynecol* 100:925, 2002.
59. Reece EA, Homko C: Diabetes-related complications of pregnancy. *J Natl Med Assoc* 85:537, 1993.
60. Kjos SL, Buchanan TA: Current concepts: Gestational diabetes mellitus. *N Engl J Med* 341:1749, 1999.
61. Damm P, et al: Predictive factors for the development of diabetes in women with previous gestational diabetes mellitus. *Am J Obstet Gynecol* 167:607, 1992.
62. Langer O: Oral hypoglycemic agents in pregnancy: Their time has come. *J Matern Fetal Neonat Med* 12:376, 2002.
63. American College of Obstetricians and Gynecologists: ACOG Practice Bulletin. Clinical management guidelines for obstetrician-gynecologists. Number 37, August 2002. Thyroid disease in pregnancy. *Obstet Gynecol* 100:387, 2002.
64. Lazarus JH: Thyroid dysfunction: Reproduction and postpartum thyroiditis. *Semin Reprod Med* 20:381, 2002.
65. Mestman J: Hyperthyroidism in pregnancy. *Clin Obstet Gynecol* 40:45, 1997.
66. Leung AS, et al: Perinatal outcome in hypothyroid pregnancies. *Obstet Gynecol* 81:349, 1993.
67. Wasserstrum N, Anania CA: Perinatal consequences of maternal hypothyroidism in early pregnancy and inadequate replacement. *Clin Endocrinol (Oxf)* 42:353, 1995.
68. Smallridge RC, Ladenson PW: Hypothyroidism in pregnancy: Consequences to neonatal health. *J Clin Endocrinol Metab* 86:2349, 2001.
69. Jana N, et al: Perinatal outcome in pregnancies complicated by pulmonary tuberculosis. *Int J Gynaecol Obstet* 44:119, 1994.
70. Jana N, et al: Obstetrical outcomes among women with extrapulmonary tuberculosis. *N Engl J Med* 341:645, 1999.
71. Ormerod P: Tuberculosis in pregnancy and the puerperium. *Thorax* 56:494, 2001.
72. Tripathy SN, Tripathy SN: Tuberculosis and pregnancy. *Int J Obstet Gynecol* 80:247, 2003.
73. ACOG technical bulletin. Pulmonary disease in pregnancy. Number 224—June 1996. American College of Obstetricians and Gynecologists. *Int J Obstet Gynaecol* 54:187, 1996.
74. Centers for Disease Control. HIV/AIDS Surveillance Report, No. 14, 2002.
75. Kigadye RM, et al: Sentinel surveillance for HIV-1 among pregnant women in a developing country: 3 years' experience and a comparison with a population serosurvey. *AIDS* 7:849, 1993.
76. Hinderaker SG, et al: Low HIV-seroprevalence in pregnant women in a rural area in Tanzania. *Acta Obstet Gynecol Scand* 80:1152, 2001.
77. Landesman S, et al: Serosurvey of human immunodeficiency virus infection in parturients. *JAMA* 258:2701, 1987.
78. Davis SF, et al: Trends in HIV prevalence among childbearing women in the United States, 1989-1994. *J Acquir Immune Defic Syndr Hum Retrovirol* 19:158, 1998.
79. Lindegren ML, et al: Trends in perinatal transmission of HIV/AIDS in the United States. *JAMA* 282:531, 1999.
80. Minkoff H: Human immunodeficiency virus infection in pregnancy. *Obstet Gynecol* 101:797, 2003.
81. Connor EM, et al: Reduction of maternal-infant transmission of human immunodeficiency virus type-1 with zidovudine treatment. *N Engl J Med* 331:1173, 1994.
82. Carneiro M, et al: Vertical HIV-1 transmission: Prophylaxis and paediatric follow-up. *Placenta* 22(Suppl A):S13, 2001.
83. European Cooperative Study: Exposure to antiretroviral therapy in utero or early life: The health of uninfected children born to HIV-infected women. *J Acquir Immune Defic Syndr* 32:380, 2003.
84. Kumar RM, et al: Impact of maternal HIV-1 infection on perinatal outcome. *Int J Gynaecol Obstet* 49:137, 1995.
85. Temmerman M, et al: Maternal human immunodeficiency virus-1 infection and pregnancy outcome. *Obstet Gynecol* 83:495, 1994.
86. De Santis M, et al: Drug addiction in pregnancy: The HIV infection. *Fetal Diagn Ther* 9:125, 1994.
87. Jehuda-Cohen C: A new look at HIV transmission from seropositive mothers to their infants: The facts beyond serology. *Isr J Med Sci* 30:364, 1994.
88. Natural history of vertically-acquired human immunodeficiency virus-1 infection. The European Collaborative Study. *Pediatrics* 94:815, 1994.
89. Mayaux M-J, et al: Neonatal characteristics in rapidly progressive perinatally acquired HIV-1 disease. *JAMA* 275:606, 1996.
90. Abrams EJ, et al: Maternal health factors and early pediatric antiretroviral therapy influence the rate of perinatal HIV-1 disease progression in children. *AIDS* 17:867, 2003.
91. Biggar RJ, et al: Immunosuppression in pregnant women infected with human immunodeficiency virus. *Am J Obstet Gynecol* 161:1239, 1989.
92. Melvin AJ, et al: Effect of pregnancy and zidovudine therapy on viral load in HIV-infected women. *J Acquir Immun Defic Syndr Hum Retrovirol* 14:232, 1997.
93. Hocke C, et al: Prospective cohort study of the effect of pregnancy on the progression of human immunodeficiency virus infection. The Group d'Epidemiologie Clinique du SIDA en Aquitaine. *Obstet Gynecol* 86:886, 1995.
94. Tuomala RE, et al: Antiretroviral therapy during pregnancy and the risk of an adverse outcome. *N Engl J Med* 346:1863, 2002.
95. Mofenson LM, et al: Risk factors for perinatal transmission of human immunodeficiency virus type 1 in women treated with zidovudine. Pediatric AIDS Clinical Trials Group Study 185 Team. *N Engl J Med* 341:385, 1999.
96. Centers for Disease Control and Prevention: Primary and secondary syphilis—United States 2000-2001. *MMWR* 51:971, 2002.
97. Centers for Disease Control and Prevention: Congenital syphilis—United States, 2000. *MMWR* 50:573, 2001.
98. Gust DA, et al: Mortality associated with congenital syphilis in the United States, 1992-1998. *Pediatrics* 109:E79, 2002.
99. Wendel GD, et al: Treatment of syphilis in pregnancy and prevention of congenital syphilis. *CID* 35(Suppl 2):S200, 2002.
100. Genç M, Ledger WJ: Syphilis in pregnancy. *Sex Transm Infect* 76:73, 2000.
101. Euler GL, et al: Hepatitis B surface antigen prevalence among pregnant women in urban areas: Implications for testing, reporting, and preventing perinatal transmission. *Pediatrics* 111:1192, 2003.
102. Levy M, Koren G: Hepatitis B vaccine in pregnancy: Maternal and fetal safety. *Am J Perinatol* 8:227, 1991.
103. Hepatitis in pregnancy. ACOG Technical Bulletin Number 174—November 1992. *Int J Obstet Gynaecol* 42:189, 1993.
104. Silverman NS, et al: Hepatitis C virus in pregnancy: Seroprevalence and risk factors for infection. *Am J Obstet Gynecol* 169:583, 1993.

105. Roberts EA, Yeung L: Maternal-infant transmission of hepatitis C virus infection. *Hepatology* 36(Suppl 1):S106, 2002.
106. Mok CC, Wong RWS: Pregnancy in systemic lupus erythematosus. *Postgrad Med J* 77:157, 2001.
107. Yasmeen S, et al: Pregnancy outcomes in women with systemic lupus erythematosus. *J Matern Fetal Med* 10:91, 2001.
108. Nelson JL, et al: Maternal-fetal disparity in HLA class II alloantigens and the pregnancy-induced amelioration of rheumatoid arthritis. *N Engl J Med* 329:466, 1995.
109. Rayburn WF: Glucocorticoid therapy for rheumatic diseases: Maternal, fetal and breast-feeding considerations. *Am J Reprod Immunol* 28:138, 1992.
110. Coomarasamy A, et al: Aspirin for prevention of preeclampsia in women with historical risk factors: A systematic review. *Obstet Gynecol* 101:1319, 2003.
111. Levy RA, et al: Hydroxychloroquine (HCQ) in lupus pregnancy: Double-blind and placebo-controlled study. *Lupus* 10:401, 2001.

CHAPTER 179

Drug Therapy and Substance Abuse

Rania Habal and Diane Sauter

PERSPECTIVE

The placenta previously was believed to act as a barrier, excluding toxins from the fetal circulation and protecting the fetus from environmental and pharmacologic exposures. In 1961, when an epidemic of amelia, a rare malformation characterized by an absence of limbs, was linked to the use of thalidomide during pregnancy, the vulnerability of the fetus to medications came into focus. Thalidomide was a sedative-hypnotic agent introduced in 1956. It immediately became popular in the treatment of nausea and vomiting during the first trimester of pregnancy, but in the years that followed, it was established that thalidomide was the agent responsible for the amelia/phocomelia epidemic. By the time thalidomide was withdrawn from the market, an estimated 5850 children were affected worldwide.[1] Similarly, it took an epidemic of debilitating congenital anomalies and deaths in the children of fishermen in Minimata, Japan, to recognize the teratogenicity of environmental pollutants.[2,3] Minimata disease was due to the ingestion of fish contaminated by methylmercury, an industrial byproduct that was dumped into Minimata Harbor early in the 20th century. These two events sparked the development of numerous control agencies to oversee the safety of drugs in pregnancy and numerous environmental protection laws.

Thalidomide's legacy continues to haunt physicians worldwide. Many physicians are reluctant to prescribe medications to pregnant women or to nursing mothers. The fact is, however, only a few medications have been identified as teratogens, and medication use during pregnancy is extremely common. In a worldwide survey of more than 14,000 patients, the World Health Organization reported that more than 86% of women used at least one prescription drug while pregnant. In a similar survey in the United States, more than 80% of pregnant women reported using medications during pregnancy, with 30% using more than four drugs.[4,5] The contribution of these substances to the incidence of birth defects is thought to be low, accounting for 1% to 3% of all live birth defects.[5,6]

The emergency physician (1) must be able to discuss the risks and benefits of drug prescribing with a pregnant patient so that an informed decision may be made; (2) must be familiar with the acute and chronic untoward effects of drugs of abuse on the mother, the pregnancy, and the fetus; and (3) must understand the psychology of addiction and provide help in a nonjudgmental manner. Early intervention and referral to a maternal drug rehabilitation program and other social programs may hold the key to a successful and healthy pregnancy and delivery.

PRINCIPLES OF DISEASE

Major birth defects affect 3% to 5% of all live births. Most are of unknown etiology, but 1% to 3% of these are thought to be due to pharmaceutical substances.[5,6] Defects include major anatomic and physiologic abnormalities. A teratogen is any chemical, pharmacologic, environmental, or mechanical agent that can cause deviant or disruptive development of the conceptus. Included in this definition are physical malformations, growth retardation, fetal demise, and functional impairment.[7] Although serious effects on the mother are identified immediately, a drug's teratogenic effect may not be apparent for years.[8] Typically, there is variability in the expression of teratogenicity among animal species and among humans.[8] Malformations may range from subtle neurobehavioral effects to devastating physical deformities and physiologic effects, including death. Why one pregnancy would be affected and not another remains to be elucidated. Highly teratogenic

BOX 179-1. Drugs and Agents Considered Human Teratogens

Angiotensin-converting enzyme inhibitors
Methotrexate, aminopterin
Androgens
Busulfan
Chlorobiphenyls
Cocaine
Coumarin derivatives
Diethylstilbestrol
Ethanol (in large doses)
Isotretinoin
Lithium
Methyl mercury
Paramethadione, trimethadione
Phenytoin
Tetracycline
Thalidomide
Valproic acid

Modified from Shepard TH: *Catalog of Teratogenic Agents,* 10th ed. Baltimore, Johns Hopkins University Press, 2001.

BOX 179-2. Food and Drug Administration Classification: Teratogenic Risk of Drugs

Class A: Controlled studies have shown no risk. Adequate, well-controlled studies in pregnant women have failed to show risk to fetus.

Class B: No evidence exists of risk for humans. Animal studies show risk or are negative, but no human studies have been done.

Class C: Use may engender risk for fetus. Human studies are lacking, and animal studies may be positive or lacking. Potential for benefit may outweigh potential for harm.

Class D: Positive evidence of risk is based on studies or postmarketing data. Potential for benefit may outweigh potential for harm.

Class X: Drugs are contraindicated in pregnancy based on human or animal studies or postmarketing reports that indicate benefit is clearly outweighed by risk.

medications seem to be few in number, estimated at less than 30 drugs (Box 179-1).[8,9]

When examining the effects of substances on the outcome of pregnancy, it is important to keep in mind that the process of establishing the risk and safety of drugs in pregnancy is tedious and often flawed. For ethical reasons, few controlled prospective human studies analyzing the risk-benefit relationship for any given exposure are available. As a result, much current knowledge has been derived from case reports, case-controlled studies, or cohort studies, which are inherently weak in establishing a causal relationship.[9-11] Knowledge extrapolated from animal models, although valuable in determining risk initially, is not always applicable to humans.[9-11]

During the 9 months of gestation, the mother and fetus are exposed to a variety of chemicals. In evaluating data on the relationship between an exposure during pregnancy and a particular outcome, a multitude of confounding factors make the determination of a causal link difficult. The genetic background of the fetus, timing and duration of the exposure, environmental factors, occurrence of multiple exposures, presence of nutritional deficits, and illicit drug use all contribute to the outcome of pregnancy.[7-10] Additionally, in the presence of disease, the outcome of pregnancy may be related to the medical condition and not the medication itself, and separating the risks of an anomaly from the expected background risk may be difficult.[7-10]

The study of teratogenicity is hindered further by several additional factors. First, the history of drug or environmental exposure is often obtained in retrospect, after 9 months of pregnancy and the delivery of an abnormal infant. By that time, significant recall bias may have been introduced, which may depend on the outcome of the birth.[10] Second, because many pregnancies are spontaneously aborted before maternal knowledge that conception has occurred, the cited prevalence of drug-induced birth defects may not be accurate.[9-11] Finally, as in the case of diethylstilbestrol, teratogenicity may not be apparent for years after birth. Large population studies are needed to understand the connection between the outcome of a pregnancy and an associated in utero exposure.[12]

Classification of Teratogenic Risk

To aid physicians in determining the teratogenic potential of a particular medication, the U.S. Food and Drug Administration has published a classification system that assigns risk based on currently available human and animal studies and case reports. Drugs are assigned one of five letters—A, B, C, D, and X—depending on the strength of evidence for their safety or teratogenicity (Box 179-2). This classification system has been criticized as oversimplistic and perhaps inaccurate because it relies on data that are generally of poor quality. Some clinicians believe that the classification system conveys the incorrect impression that there is a gradation of reproductive risk from exposure across categories (i.e., that risk increases from A to B to C to D to X) and that the drugs within a given category present similar reproductive risks.[13] The Food and Drug Administration has acknowledged these problems and is working to change the present regulations.

Drug Transfer Across the Placenta

The degree to which the fetus is affected by a given pharmaceutical agent and the nature of that effect depend on multiple factors. The transport of maternal substrates to the fetus and of waste products from the fetus to the mother is established during week 5 of gestation.[14,15] Drug transfer across the placenta occurs most commonly by simple passive diffusion or by protein transport. A thin layer of trophoblastic cells is all that separates maternal from fetal circulation. The degree to which a drug gains access to fetal circulation depends on molecular size, ionic state, lipid solubility, and extent of protein binding. Drugs with a molecular weight of less than 5000 D readily diffuse. Anionic forms diffuse through the lipid layer more readily than ionized forms. Free drug diffuses more readily than a drug that is bound to plasma proteins. Because fetal pH is slightly more alkalotic than maternal pH, weak organic acids (e.g., salicylate) may become ion trapped in the fetal circulation, increasing fetal exposure.[14]

Drugs may affect the fetus through a variety of mechanisms. Some drugs may alter the availability of substrates, such as vitamins, glucose, oxygen, and amino acids, needed for normal nutrition and growth.[14] Others may directly affect cellular growth and differentiation. The age of the fetus is crucial in determining the impact of any given exposure. During the time of organogenesis (days 21 to 56 of fetal life), the fetus is much more vulnerable to toxic insults. The major body organs are formed during this period, and exposure to a teratogen at this time may result in major anatomic defects. The central nervous system (CNS) develops over a longer period (10 to 17 weeks) so that later exposures may affect neurologic development and subsequent function. Exposure after the period of organogenesis may affect the growth and development of the fetus but does not have an impact on organogenesis.[14,15]

Drug Transfer During Lactation

For the most part, drugs and substances that are ingested or injected by the mother diffuse passively into milk, then back into the maternal circulation for excretion. The amount of drug diffusing into milk depends on many factors. Lipid-soluble and nonionic substances diffuse more readily, and highly protein-bound substances diffuse less readily. Whether a substance is concentrated in maternal milk or not, the neonate generally is able to detoxify it with no adverse effects, and only a few drugs pose a danger to a breast-feeding infant. The interruption of breast-feeding should not be advocated except in the rare situations of known drug toxicity to the infant.[16,17] Table 179-1 summarizes medications and their effects in pregnancy and lactation.

DRUG THERAPY DURING PREGNANCY

Analgesic Agents

Acetaminophen

Acetaminophen or paracetamol is widely used during pregnancy, and no significant increase in the incidence of congenital malformations has been identified. As a result, acetaminophen currently is considered safe for short-term use and at therapeutic doses at any time during pregnancy.[15,18,19] Acute and chronic overdoses of acetaminophen have been associated, however, with a fatal outcome.[20] Acetaminophen is safe during lactation because only a little is excreted into breast milk, and the small amount that does get through is tolerated by the neonate's sulfhydration pathway.[18]

Nonsteroidal Anti-Inflammatory Drugs and Salicylate

Nonsteroidal anti-inflammatory drugs (NSAIDs) interfere with the enzyme cyclooxygenase, which converts arachidonic acid to cyclic endoperoxides, prostacyclin, and thromboxane. In addition to its role in inflammation, thromboxane A_2 regulates platelet adhesiveness. The progress of normal labor and delivery depends to some extent on prostaglandin. Interference with prostaglandin delays the onset of labor and increases its duration. The normal maintenance of a patent ductus arteriosus in utero is also a prostaglandin-dependent phenomenon. Increased pulmonary pressures that follow the premature closure of the ductus provoke hypertrophy of the small pulmonary vessels, which may interfere with the rapid reduction of pulmonary vascular resistance necessary for the fetus to establish normal pulmonary circulation after birth.[15,21,22]

Salicylate is the most thoroughly studied of the class of NSAIDs and is generally not recommended as an analgesic for use in pregnancy. Salicylate is readily absorbed, and although the extent of protein binding limits the free fraction available for diffusion across the placenta, salicylate that is unbound readily diffuses. Salicylate levels peak in the fetus within 60 to 90 minutes of maternal administration. Because early in pregnancy the fetus has a higher pH than the mother, the fetus may ion trap salicylate, perhaps resulting in a greater fetal risk for salicylate toxicity or congenital anomalies. Although salicylates were shown to be teratogenic in animal models, two meta-analyses in humans failed to show a teratogenic effect to salicylates, although there was a trend toward a slightly increased incidence of gastroschisis when used in the first trimester.[21,22] Low-dose aspirin had no effect on perinatal mortality and was not associated with an increased risk for miscarriage.[22] Low-dose aspirin therapy (60 to 90 mg/day) late in pregnancy also has been found to be effective in treating certain inflammatory conditions associated with pregnancy (antiphospholipid antibody syndrome and lupus) without the production of adverse effects in either the mother or the neonate.[23] Chronic use of low-dose aspirin in patients with pregnancy-induced hypertension may increase the risk of abruption, however.[24]

Aspirin has been associated with an increased risk of perinatal bleeding, increased of postmaturity, significant prolongation of labor, and a decrease in birth weight.[15] The increased risk of bleeding may extend to the neonate because platelet dysfunction and reduced factor XII activity have been noted.[15,22] Additional effects of salicylates on neonates include derangements of intracellular glucose metabolism through effects on the Krebs cycle, resulting in an increased risk of hypoglycemia and in some reports fetal death.[25,26] For all these reasons, salicylates are not recommended for analgesia in pregnant women. Aspirin is poorly excreted in breast milk and is safe for short-term use during lactation.[15] High-dose salicylate schedules may result in severe metabolic acidosis in newborns.[27]

Table 179-1. Summary of Medication Safety in Pregnancy and Laction

Medication Class	Pregnancy	Lactation
Analgesic agents		
Acetaminophen or paracetamol	Safe	Safe
Nonsteroidal anti-inflammatory drugs (NSAIDs)		
Salicylate	Not recommended	Safe for short-term use
Other NSAIDs	Not recommended	Safe
Opiates/opioids	Safe	Safe
Morphine	Caution at time of delivery due to respiratory depression in newborn	
Meperidine		
Oxycodone		
Antibiotics		
Penicillin	Safe	Safe
Dicloxacillin		May interfere with culture results in neonates
Ampicillin		
Penicillin derivatives		
Cephalosporins	Safe	Safe
		May interfere with culture results in neonates
Chloramphenicol	Safe until term. *Do not* use at term, as it can cause "gray baby syndrome"	Unknown safety
Macrolides	Safe. *Do not* use estolate salt of erythromycin, as it can cause hepatotoxicity in pregnant patient	Safe
Erythromycin		Azithromycin preferred over erythromycin
Azithromycin		
Clarithromycin		
Clindamycin		
Sulfonamides	Not recommended near term, as can cause kernicterus	Safe
		Except in premature infants or infants with G6PD deficiency or hyperbilirubinemia
Aminoglycosides	Not recommended	Safe
Tetracycline	Not recommended	Not recommended
Fluoroquinolones	Not recommended	Safe
Metronidazole	Not recommended	Not recommended
Antifungals		
Nystatin	Safe	Safe
Clotrimazole and ketoconazole	Safe	Safe
Fluconazole	Not recommended	Not recommended
Antituberculous agents		
INH	Safe	Safe
Rifampin	Safe	Safe
Ethambutol	Safe	Safe
Antiviral agents		
Acyclovir	Safe	Safe
Anticoagulants		
Warfarin	Not recommended	Safe
	Causes fetal warfarin syndrome	
Heparin	Safe	Safe
Low-molecular-weight heparin	Safe	Safe
Anticonvulsants		
Phenytoin	Not recommended	Safe
	Causes fetal hydantoin syndrome in 5–10%, but may be used in selected cases	
Carbamazepine	Not recommended	Safe
Valproic acid	Not recommended	Safe
	Class D	
Phenobarbital	Not recommended	Not recommended
	Class D	
Ethosuximide	Not recommended	Safe
	Class C	
Primidone	Not recommended	Not recommended
	Class D	
Trimethadione	Not recommended	Not recommended
	Class D	
	Fetal loss 85%	
Benzodiazepines	Safe	Not recommended
	Class C	May cause apnea in newborn
Newer drugs		
Felbamate	Safe	Unknown
Levetiracetam	Safe	Unknown
Gabapentin	Safe	Unknown
Lamotrigine	Not recommended	Unknown
Antidycrhythmics		
Digoxin	Safe	Safe
Disopyramide	Safe	Safe
Quinidine	Safe	Safe
Procainamide	Safe	Unknown
Lidocaine	Safe, except with high doses	Safe

Table 179-1. Summary of Medication Safety in Pregnancy and Laction—cont'd

Medication Class	Pregnancy	Lactation
Amiodarone	Not recommended Class D, may use with refractory cases.	Not recommended
Adenosine	Safe	Safe
Antihypertensives		
Angiotensin-converting enzyme inhibitors	Not recommended Class D	Safe (captopril and enalapril only)
Angiotensin II receptor antagonists	Not recommended	Unknown
β-Blockers	Safe	Safe
Labetalol		Monitor neonate for adverse events
Atenolol	Caution in first trimester with atenolol	
Metoprolol		
Propranolol		
Calcium channel blockers	Safe	Safe
Diltiazem	Safe	Safe
Verapamil	Caution for dehydration and electrolyte abnormalities	
Nifedipine		
Diuretics	Safe	Safe
Bendroflumethiazide	Caution: can cause hypotension	
Chlorthalidone	Labetolol preferred	
Hydrochlorothiazide		
Hydralazine	Safe (first-line therapy for hypertension) Class C	Safe
Methyldopa	Safe Class C Second-line agent to labetalol	Unknown Unknown
Clonidine		
Nitroprusside		
Medications used in the treatment of asthma, allergies, and upper respiratory infection		
β-Adrenergics	Safe	Safe
Albuterol		
Metaproterenol		
Terbutaline		
Ipratropium	Safe	Safe
Cromolyn sodium	Safe Little data available	Unknown
Corticosteroids	Safe	Safe
Prednisone		
Theophylline	Safe	Safe
Aminophylline		
Leukotriene antagonists	Safe	Safe
Zileutron	Not recommended Caution: may cause mutagenic effects	Not recommended
Antihistamines	Safe	Not recommended
Chlorpheniramine	Safe	Not recommended
Diphenhydramine	Safe	Not recommended
Dimenhydramine	Safe	Not recommended
Doxylamine	Safe	Not recommended
Hydroxyzine	Safe	Not recommended
Meclizine	Not recommended in first trimester	Not recommended
Loratadine		Not recommended
Decongestants	Safe	
Pseudoephedrine	Not recommended	Not recommended
Phenylpropanolamine		Not recommended
Drugs used for nausea and vomiting of pregnancy		
Dopamine antagonists	Safe	Unknown
Phenothiazines		
Promethazine		
Chlorpromazine		
Perphenazine		
Metoclopramide		
5-HT_3 Antagonists	Safe	Safe
Ondansetron		
Medications used in the treatment of diabetes		
Insulin	Safe	Safe
Sulfonylurea	Not recommended	Not recommended
Glyburide	Not recommended	Caution: nursing infants should be monitored
Glipizide	Not recommended	Caution: nursing infants should be monitored
Metformin	Not recommended	Not recommended
Acarbose	Safe	Safe No studies have been done
Rosiglitazone	Not recommended	Not recommended
Pioglitazone	Not recommended	Not recommended
Antacids		
Ranitidine	Safe	Safe

G6PD, glucose-6-phosphate dehydrogenase.

With the exception of indomethacin, the nonsalicylate NSAIDs have been less well studied during pregnancy and lactation, but they seem to be safe in breast-feeding.[15] Indomethacin is commonly used as a tocolytic agent but has been associated with premature closure of the ductus arteriosus, neonatal pulmonary hypertension, periventricular hemorrhages, and oligohydramnios and fetal nephrotoxicity.[15,27a] In a cohort study, the use of NSAIDs during pregnancy was associated with an increased risk of miscarriage, but not of congenital anomaly, preterm birth, or low birth weight.[28]

Opiates

Morphine, meperidine, and oxycodone are considered safe analgesic agents for use at any time during pregnancy.[15] The use of codeine has been associated with the development of certain congenital defects, but it is unclear whether this association is statistically significant.[15] The use of opiates during labor may result in respiratory and CNS depression in the newborn. Chronic use of opiates during pregnancy may result in neonatal addiction and withdrawal.[15] Because opiates are poorly concentrated in milk, opiate analgesia may be used safely during breast-feeding.[15] Meperidine is associated with an increased incidence of neurobehavioral abnormalities in nursing infants compared with morphine.[15,29]

Antibiotics

Penicillin and Derivatives

Penicillin, dicloxacillin, ampicillin, and other penicillin derivatives (including procaine and benzathine penicillin) are considered safe for use in pregnancy. They have been used extensively since the 1940s and are thought to be the safest antibiotics available for pregnant patients.[30,31] Oral probenecid also is considered safe.[31] Penicillins are considered safe during breast-feeding, but their use may interfere with culture results if a neonatal fever workup is required.[15] Other side effects include allergic responses and the occurrence of loose stools in the infant.

Cephalosporins

Most cephalosporins are considered safe during pregnancy and breast-feeding, although there are no controlled studies examining their safety.[15,30,31] Some cephalosporins are excreted into breast milk and may have the same implications for the infant as described for penicillin.[15]

Chloramphenicol

No relationship has been found between the use of chloramphenicol and congenital anomalies. Although it is considered safe throughout most of pregnancy, chloramphenicol should be used with caution at term. It has been associated with the development of cardiovascular collapse (the "gray baby" syndrome) in a neonate.[15,30,31] The safety of chloramphenicol during breast-feeding is unknown.

Macrolides

Erythromycin, azithromycin, clarithromycin, and clindamycin are considered to be safe for use in pregnancy and compatible with breast-feeding, although there are no well-controlled studies examining their effects on the fetus. The estolate salt of erythromycin has been associated with the development of hepatotoxicity in pregnant women[15,30,31] and should be avoided. Erythromycin seems to be safe in breast-feeding despite the fact that it is highly concentrated in breast milk. Occasional reports have linked it to pyloric stenosis.[16] Azithromycin is poorly concentrated in breast milk and may be the preferred agent in lactating mothers.[16,17]

Sulfonamides

The primary use of sulfonamides during pregnancy is in the treatment of uncomplicated urinary tract infection. The sulfonamides readily cross the placenta to the fetus during all stages of gestation. Fetal levels may reach 90% of maternal plasma concentrations. Sulfonamides are contraindicated in pregnancy near term because they compete with bilirubin for protein-binding sites, leaving large amounts of free bilirubin to diffuse, be deposited in the infant's brain, and cause kernicterus.[15,30,31] Sulfonamides are excreted into breast milk in low concentrations and are generally tolerated by a healthy neonate. They should be avoided, however, in ill or premature infants and in infants with hyperbilirubinemia or glucose-6-phosphate dehydrogenase deficiency.[15,16]

Aminoglycosides

Aminoglycosides readily cross the placenta. Their use in pregnancy has been linked to fetal ototoxicity, especially when high doses are used. The pattern of abnormalities is not consistent, however. Gentamicin is selectively taken up by the fetal kidney and may cause nephrotoxicity in the fetus.[15,30,31] Gentamicin is secreted in small amounts in breast milk and is poorly absorbed from the gastrointestinal tract. It seems to be compatible with lactation.[15,30,31]

Tetracycline

Tetracycline should be avoided during pregnancy. It is associated with the development of fatty liver in pregnant women[15,30,31] and readily crosses the placenta and reaches the fetus, where it chelates calcium, causing abnormalities in bone growth and staining of decidual teeth. Tetracycline also has been associated with fetal genitourinary anomalies, inguinal hernias, and limb abnormalities.[15,30,31] Because tetracycline binds to breast milk calcium, only a little reaches the nursing infant, and it may be used for short periods (≤10 days) during breast-feeding.[16] Prolonged use of tetracycline is associated with stained teeth.[16]

Doxycycline does not bind to calcium and is associated less with stained teeth than tetracycline. Doxycycline is present in greater quantities in breast milk. Although doxycycline is not contraindicated when prescribed for short periods, its long-term use is not advocated.[15,16,30,31]

Fluoroquinolones

Fluoroquinolones have been linked to numerous toxic effects on bone and cartilage growth in infants and should be avoided during pregnancy, particularly the first trimester.[15,30,31] Because of these effects, some clinicians avoid prescribing them during lactation. The American Academy of Pediatrics considers fluoroquinolones compatible with breast-feeding, however, because breast-fed infant plasma levels are low.[16]

Metronidazole

Human data on the use of metronidazole during pregnancy are mixed,[15,30,31] and it is best avoided during the entire pregnancy. Metronidazole possesses a mutagenic effect and was found to be carcinogenic in mice.[15,30,31] In view of its mutagenic effects and because it is highly concentrated in breast milk and poorly metabolized by infants 6 months old and younger, it is not recommended during breast-feeding.[16]

Antifungals

Nystatin has a long safety profile during pregnancy and lactation. It is poorly absorbed from skin, mucous membranes, and gastrointestinal tract.[15,30,31] Clotrimazole, miconazole, and ketoconazole seem to be safe during pregnancy and lactation, although ketoconazole is teratogenic in rats. As a result of the long-standing safety record of nystatin, the other agents are considered second-line treatment of fungal infections in pregnancy.[15,30,31]

Fluconazole is associated with a slight increase in craniofacial, bone, and joint abnormalities when high doses are used.[15,30,31] These anomalies were not noted when lower doses were used or with single-dose therapy. No data are available concerning use of fluconazole during lactation,[15,16] and it should be used with caution.

Antituberculous Agents

Untreated tuberculosis places the mother and fetus at greater risk than the use of antituberculous medications. Isoniazid crosses the placenta, but it does not seem to affect the fetus and is considered safe in pregnancy.[15,30,31] It also is considered safe during breast-feeding.[16] Rifampin crosses the placenta and occasionally has been implicated in case reports of congenital anomalies. There are, however, no controlled studies documenting these effects, and it is recommended as first-line therapy along with isoniazid in pregnant women with tuberculosis.[15,30,31] Rifampin is considered compatible with breast-feeding.[16] Ethambutol crosses the placenta, but has not been associated with any congenital defect.[15,30,31] It is considered safe for use in pregnancy and during breast-feeding.[16]

Antiviral Agents

Acyclovir is a purine analogue, commonly used in the treatment of herpesvirus infections. During pregnancy, acyclovir is indicated for life-threatening maternal herpes simplex virus infections, such as disseminated disease and herpes encephalitis, and varicella pneumonia, which carries a maternal mortality of 44% if untreated.[32] The Centers for Disease Control and Prevention also recommend treatment of the first episode of genital herpes during pregnancy with oral acyclovir.[33] In humans, acyclovir seems to cross the placenta readily and reach higher concentrations in fetal circulation than in maternal circulation. There are no reports of teratogenicity or adverse effects in the fetuses or newborns of mothers using acyclovir.[15,31,34] Acyclovir is concentrated in milk, where levels may be higher than in plasma. Because there are no reported adverse outcomes in infants of mothers taking acyclovir or infants treated with acyclovir for disseminated herpes, it is considered safe in breast-feeding.[15,16]

Anticoagulants

During the normal course of pregnancy, plasma concentrations of several procoagulants are increased, whereas fibrinolysis and the inhibition of coagulation are suppressed.[35,36] These changes result in hypercoagulability and an increased risk for thromboembolic phenomena during pregnancy. Pulmonary embolism has emerged as the leading cause of maternal mortality during pregnancy.[35]

The management of venous thrombosis and pulmonary embolism during pregnancy is problematic. The use of warfarin (Coumadin) derivatives is contraindicated because of a known risk of congenital anomalies with its use in pregnancy. As a result, when anticoagulation is indicated during pregnancy, heparin is considered the agent of choice.[15] Whenever possible, the diagnosis of venous thrombosis should be confirmed with a ventilation-perfusion lung scan, venography, or less invasive venous Doppler flow studies before the initiation of therapy.[35]

Warfarin is a known human teratogen and affects 4% to 5% of exposed fetuses. The risk from exposure is greatest during 6 to 9 weeks of gestation and seems to be dose dependent.[15,35,36] The fetal warfarin syndrome is associated with multiple abnormalities, such as hypoplasia of the nasal bones, midline dysplasia including agenesis of the corpus callosum, optic atrophy and blindness, mental retardation, seizures, and stippling of the bones with scoliosis and shortening of limbs.[15,35,36] Additionally, exposed infants are at an increased risk of prematurity, abortion, and stillbirths.[15,35,36] The type of anomaly seen depends on the timing and duration of warfarin ingestion. Warfarin-induced CNS malformations may occur at any time during pregnancy.[15,35,36] Abnormalities in the axial skeleton are more prominent when warfarin is ingested during the early stages of pregnancy. Because warfarin is so highly protein bound, only a little is secreted into milk, and use by breast-feeding mothers is acceptable.[16] Caution should be used in breast-feeding premature infants because they may be at increased risk for intraventricular hemorrhage.[16,35]

Unfractionated heparin is a highly charged heterogeneous molecule with a molecular weight between 5000 and 35,000 D. It does not cross the placenta and does not present a direct risk to the fetus. Early reports on the use of heparin for the prevention or treatment of venous thromboembolism during pregnancy concluded that the risks to the fetus from prematurity, stillbirth, and hemorrhage might affect one third of infants. More recently, the increased risks previously associated with heparin were determined to be related to underlying maternal medical problems rather than heparin.[15,35,36] When anticoagulation during pregnancy is required, heparin is considered the agent of choice.[15] Its use sometimes is associated with maternal osteopenia and immune-mediated thrombocytopenia. Patients need careful monitoring for these adverse effects. The risk of maternal hemorrhage at delivery is significant. Because of its high molecular weight, heparin is not excreted in breast milk and is compatible with breast-feeding.[15,16] Additionally, it is quickly destroyed in the stomach when ingested.

Low-molecular-weight heparin may be used during pregnancy and in the postnatal period for therapeutic or prophylactic anticoagulation.[37] All currently available low-molecular-weight heparin products have been used safely during pregnancy. Data are limited, however, because of their relatively recent introduction.[16,35]

Although pregnancy remains a contraindication for the use of thrombolytic therapy, these agents have been used successfully in pregnant women in cases of life-threatening pulmonary embolus or myocardial infarction. Alteplase, which has a high molecular weight, most likely does not cross the placenta. To date, no teratogenic effects have been reported in humans. Maternal hemorrhagic complications have been noted when alteplase was used during the intrapartum period but not at any other time.[15,38] Although no specific recommendations exist, alteplase most likely would be safe for use in nursing mothers because it has a short half-life.[16]

Anticonvulsants

The occurrence of generalized seizures during pregnancy has been associated with an increased risk of spontaneous abortion, hypoxic injury to the fetus, and impaired neuropsychologic functioning.[39] Anticonvulsants are known teratogens, however, and 30% of neonates exposed to commonly used anticonvulsants exhibit congenital anomalies. The risks for birth defects increase with the duration of exposure and with the number of agents used.[39-43] Despite the risks, most practitioners believe that it is important to control seizures during pregnancy. Monotherapy seems to be the most appropriate option and is recommended at the lowest effective anticonvulsant dose. Dividing the daily dose to decrease peak plasma levels should be considered. The physiologic changes that accompany pregnancy result in lower maternal serum levels of most anticonvulsant medications. Adjustment of the dosage upward often is required to maintain adequate seizure control.[15]

Phenytoin

Phenytoin is a human teratogen and readily crosses the placenta. The parent compound and all metabolites have been identified in fetal tissues. Of chronically exposed fetuses, 5% to 10% develop the fetal hydantoin syndrome.[15] This syndrome is characterized by various degrees of ossification abnormalities of the extremities and digits, craniofacial abnormalities including cleft lip and palate, impaired growth, delayed neurologic development, and cardiovascular anomalies.[15,40,41] The last-mentioned include atrial septal defects, ventricular septal defects, coarctation of the aorta, and endocardial cushion defects.[15,40] Phenytoin also has been associated with hemorrhagic disease of the newborn, presumably because it competitively inhibits placental transport of vitamin K. This inhibition results in a decrease in fetal levels of the vitamin K–dependent clotting factors, resulting in severe and potentially lethal hemorrhage during the first day of life.[15,39] To avoid this rare complication, some clinicians have advocated the use of vitamin K during the last month of pregnancy. Evidence does not support its use, however.[39] Phenytoin also has been linked to a variety of tumors in infants. Phenytoin use is considered safe in breast-feeding.[16]

Carbamazepine

Carbamazepine use during pregnancy is associated with a syndrome similar to fetal hydantoin syndrome, which is thought to be secondary to a toxic, teratogenic metabolite and not the parent compound itself.[15,42] In one study, carbamazepine was associated with a twofold increase in major congenital abnormalities compared with nonexposed fetuses.[40] These abnormalities include craniofacial defects, fingernail hypoplasia, and developmental delay.[15,42] In addition, in utero exposure to carbamazepine is associated with low birth weights and a 1% to 2% risk of neural tube defects.[40] Carbamazepine also has been reported to induce hemorrhagic disease of the newborn.[39] The use of carbamazepine is considered compatible with breast-feeding.[16]

Valproic Acid

Valproic acid, a class D medication that should not be used in pregnancy, is an eight-carbon, branched-chain carboxyl acid that has been approved since 1978 for the treatment of absence seizures.[43] It is teratogenic in laboratory animals and in humans. It readily crosses the placenta and concentrates in the fetus. The concentration of valproic acid in the fetus is related to decreased albumin levels and increased levels of free fatty acids in the mother that occupy binding sites on maternal albumin; this increases the fraction of valproic acid available to equilibrate across placental membranes. Many authors have described a syndrome of defects associated with the use of valproic acid. The characteristics of the syndrome include multiple minor facial anomalies, low birth weight, delayed neurologic development, congenital heart defects, neural tube defects, hypospadias, strabismus, nystagmus, tracheomalacia, afibrinogenemia, and hyperglycemia.[15,39,40,43] Several mechanisms have been proposed to explain the teratogenic effects of valproic acid, including inhibition of intestinal folic acid absorption; inhibition of liver microsomal epoxide hydrolase, resulting in fetal exposure to reactive epoxides; and interference with glutathione, lipid metabolism, or embryonic pH.[15,39,40,43] Valproic acid is present in breast milk in low levels and is considered safe during breast-feeding.[16]

Phenobarbital

Phenobarbital is considered a class D medication in pregnancy. It is associated with a slightly increased risk of congenital abnormalities, including congenital heart disease and cleft lip or palate and some minor malformations associated with the fetal hydantoin syndrome.[15,39,40] It is occasionally associated with hemorrhagic disease in the newborn and may result in neonatal withdrawal.[15] Breast-fed infants of mothers taking phenobarbital have developed toxicity characterized primarily by sedation. These infants must be monitored closely for sedation while breast-fed and after breast-feeding for symptoms of withdrawal.[16]

Ethosuximide

Ethosuximide is indicated primarily for the treatment of petit mal or absence seizures. It is considered a class C agent in pregnancy. Its use has been loosely associated with congenital cardiac abnormalities, orofacial clefting, and hydrocephalus.[15] Ethosuximide also may induce hemorrhagic disease of the newborn resulting from interference with the vitamin K–dependent clotting factors. The use of ethosuximide is considered compatible with breast-feeding.[16]

Primidone

Primidone is considered a class D agent in pregnancy and lactation. It is used in the treatment of partial and generalized tonic-clonic seizures. It is metabolized to phenobarbital, and its use in pregnancy has been associated with the same problems associated with phenobarbital. Dysmorphic features similar to the features seen with hydantoin, congenital cardiac disease, orofacial clefting, and microcephaly have been described with the use of primidone.[15] This drug also may interfere with the vitamin K–dependent clotting factors and induce hemorrhagic disease of the newborn. Neonatal withdrawal may occur after birth. Similar to phenobarbital, primidone should be used with caution during breast-feeding, with attention given to the development of sedation and withdrawal after breast-feeding is stopped.[15,16]

Trimethadione

Trimethadione is used primarily in the treatment of petit mal and absence seizures. It is considered a class D medication in pregnancy and lactation. Fetal loss is reported to be 85%,[15] and in fetuses that survive, a congenital syndrome, including epicanthal folds, V-shaped eyebrows, low-set ears, irregular teeth, microcephaly, mental retardation, and orofacial clefting, may be seen in 70%. Trimethadione is contraindicated in pregnancy.[15]

Benzodiazepines

Data on the fetal effects of benzodiazepines have been inconsistent. Some case reports and case-controlled studies have shown a significantly increased risk of oral clefts, whereas others have failed to show any increased risk for fetal anomalies.[15,44] Different benzodiazepines may have different effects and risks. Whatever the risks, they seem to be small.[44] Neonates exposed to benzodiazepines may exhibit signs of toxicity, including apnea, cyanosis, unresponsiveness, hypotonia, poor feeding, and withdrawal symptoms characterized by irritability and tremulousness.[15]

Clonazepam is a benzodiazepine used largely for refractory myoclonic seizures. It is considered a class C medication for use in pregnancy and lactation. There is no conclusive evidence of human teratogenicity associated with its use, although there is an increased risk of congenital cardiac effects.[15] Because of the reported risk of apnea, it is recommended that neonates exposed to benzodiazepines through breast-feeding be monitored closely.[15,16]

Newer Drugs

No adequate studies of human teratogenicity have been published regarding felbamate, levetiracetam, gabapentin, and lamotrigine, but all except lamotrigine seem to be safe during pregnancy. Lamotrigine seems to have an increased incidence of birth defects.[15] Safety in lactation is unknown.[15]

Cardiovascular Preparations

Antidysrhythmics

Digoxin, disopyramide, and quinidine all are considered safe for use during pregnancy and lactation.[45] Of the three agents, digoxin and quinidine have the longest records of safe use during pregnancy and are first-line agents for the treatment of significant maternal dysrhythmias.[38]

Procainamide also is well tolerated and should be considered a first-line treatment of wide-complex tachydysrhythmias during pregnancy.[46] The use of procainamide in nursing mothers is controversial because procainamide and its metabolite *N*-acetylprocainamide have been found in breast milk.[15,16]

Lidocaine is a weak base. It crosses the placenta rapidly and becomes ion trapped in the fetus. There is no evidence of a link between lidocaine and any fetal malformations.[31,45,46] High doses used near term are associated with neonatal CNS depression, apnea, hypotonia, seizures, and bradycardia.[31,38] For this reason, the lowest effective dose should be used in the mother.[31] Care also should be taken not to inject lidocaine into a major blood vessel.[31] Lidocaine is considered compatible with breast-feeding.[16]

Few studies have addressed the use of the newer class IC agents. Encainide and flecainide have been used safely to terminate maternal and fetal tachycardia.[15,45,46] Flecainide also is considered compatible with breast-feeding.[15,16]

Amiodarone, a class D agent, is used for refractory ventricular and supraventricular arrhythmias and is now recommended as first-line therapy for ventricular tachycardias. It contains large amounts of iodine and may result in congenital goiter. Neonatal hyperthyroidism and hypothyroidism have been reported.[15] Additionally, amiodarone use during pregnancy has been linked to many congenital abnormalities, including growth retardation, structural cardiac abnormalities, corneal deposits, and developmental delay.[15,45,46] Its use during pregnancy should be limited to cases of refractory disease. The effects of maternal use of amiodarone on breast-fed infants are unknown. Because of its high iodine content, its excretion into milk, and its long elimination half-life, amiodarone should not be used in nursing mothers.[15]

Adenosine

Adenosine is a naturally occurring compound that is metabolized quickly in the body. It has been used safely throughout pregnancy and is the drug of choice in terminating maternal supraventricular tachycardia despite the absence of large-scale studies.[15,45-47]

Antihypertensives

Angiotensin-Converting Enzyme Inhibitors

The angiotensin-converting enzyme (ACE) inhibitors are categorized as category D drugs for use in pregnancy. ACE inhibitors are embryocidal in animals and increase the rate of stillbirths in some species. Although they seem to be safe in humans during the first trimester of pregnancy, many adverse fetal effects have been noted with their use during the second and third trimesters, precluding their use.[48] In the fetus, renal perfusion is generally low and depends on high levels of angiotensin. Because ACE inhibitors decrease levels of angiotensin II, they interfere with glomerular flow and renal perfusion, interfering with normal renal development.[15] Reported adverse neonatal effects include oligohydramnios, anuria, renal agenesis resulting in death, increased risk of stillbirth, intrauterine growth retardation (IUGR), fetal skull abnormalities, pulmonary hypoplasia, respiratory distress syndrome, and fetal and neonatal hypotension.[15,48,49] Captopril and enalapril are considered compatible with breast-feeding.[15,16]

Angiotensin II Receptor Antagonists

Angiotensin II receptor antagonists have been reported to result in fetal abnormalities similar to the abnormalities seen with ACE inhibitors, including renal agenesis, neonatal anuria, oligohydramnios, IUGR, persistent patent ductus arteriosus, abnormal ossification, and death.[15] Angiotensin II receptor antagonists should be avoided during pregnancy.[15] Their safety in lactation is unknown.

β-Blockers

All β-adrenergic blocking agents cross the placenta. The steady-state maternal-to-fetal ratio depends on the relative lipid solubility of the individual agent. The greatest experience with β-blockers has been with women requiring treatment during the last trimester of pregnancy, at which time they seem to be safe. Long-term in utero exposure and first-trimester exposure have not been studied.[15,31]

Labetalol, atenolol, and metoprolol are considered safe for use in pregnancy and lactation.[50] Atenolol seems to cause fetal harm when used in the first trimester, however, and IUGR and persistent β blockade in the newborn when used for prolonged periods in the third trimester. It seems to be safe in the third trimester when prescribed for short periods. Similarly, propranolol is associated with fetal and neonatal adverse effects, especially when dosages exceeding 160 mg/day are used. These adverse effects include IUGR, hypoglycemia, bradycardia, respiratory depression at birth, and hyperbilirubinemia.[15,31] β-Blockers are reportedly safe in breast-feeding, but close monitoring of the infant for adverse effects is recommended.[15,16]

Calcium Channel Blockers

The calcium channel blockers are considered safe for use during pregnancy. Diltiazem, verapamil, and nifedipine have been used frequently during the first trimester of pregnancy without any increase in the risk of congenital anomalies.[15,31,51] Fetal distress secondary to maternal hypotension has been reported with the use of sublingual nifedipine. These agents also are considered safe for use during breast-feeding.[15,16]

Diuretics

Thiazide diuretics have been used successfully for the treatment of hypertension in pregnancy but may result in electrolyte abnormalities in neonates when given near term.[31] An increase in perinatal mortality and congenital defects possibly caused by volume depletion has been reported.[31] First-trimester use has been associated with an increase in congenital anomalies.[15] Bendroflumethiazide, chlorthalidone, and hydrochlorothiazide are considered safe during breast-feeding.[16]

Hydralazine

Hydralazine previously was considered the drug of choice for the parenteral treatment of acute severe hypertension during pregnancy. Hydralazine is associated with higher rates of maternal hypotension, however, which may affect perinatal outcome.[15,31] It also is associated with a lupus-like syndrome.[15,31] Because other agents, in particular labetalol, are safer and just as effective, hydralazine is no longer recommended as a first-line agent in the treatment of hypertensive emergencies in pregnant women.[15,31,52] Hydralazine is safe in lactation.[15,16]

Methyldopa

Methyldopa is considered safe in pregnancy. Many clinicians use it as first-line therapy to treat hypertension during pregnancy.[50] Methyldopa is compatible with breast-feeding.[31]

Clonidine

Clonidine is categorized as a class C medication for use during pregnancy. It has been used during all three trimesters with few adverse effects on the pregnancy. Transient neonatal hypertension has been reported in neonates with in utero exposure to clonidine.[15,31] Its effects on breast-feeding neonates are unknown.

Nitroprusside

The use of nitroprusside for the treatment of hypertensive emergencies in pregnancy has all of the advantages and disadvantages seen in nonpregnant patients. Advantages include its rapid onset, rapid metabolism, and rapid excretion. Disadvantages of nitroprusside include the need for constant monitoring and cumbersome administration. During prolonged administration of high doses, nitroprusside may result in cyanide toxicity. It readily crosses the placenta and reaches fetal levels of cyanide that are twice maternal levels. Standard doses do not seem to subject the fetus to major risk of toxicity, but with the availability of safer alternatives, notably labetalol, nitroprusside is considered a second-line agent.[15,16,31] When used, monitoring plasma and red blood cell cyanide and maternal pH are recommended. Nitroprusside is considered a category C medication. No data are available on its use during breast-feeding.[15,16]

Asthma, Allergy, and Upper Respiratory Infection Medications

β-Adrenergics

Pregnant women with asthma are at risk of neonatal death, preterm birth, low-birth-weight infants, preeclampsia, and small-for-gestational-age infants. Asthmatic mothers also may have a higher rate of chorioamnionitis, hypertensive disorders of pregnancy, cesarean section, and prolonged hospital stay than control mothers.[53,54] Better asthma control has been associated with an improved outcome.[53] Albuterol, metaproterenol, and terbutaline seem to be safe in pregnancy; none have been linked to congenital anomalies.[15] β-Adrenergic agents have been used during the last trimester to treat premature labor. Adverse reactions are related to the drugs' cardiovascular and metabolic effects, which are transient and generally well tolerated by the fetus. Transient hyperglycemia followed by insulin secretion may occur, resulting in neonatal hypoglycemia.[15] The concentration of albuterol in breast milk has not been studied, but similar to other β-mimetics, it seems compatible with breast-feeding.[16]

Ipratropium

Ipratropium has not been found to be teratogenic in numerous animal models. Although human data are few, ipratropium seems to be safe for use during pregnancy and lactation.[15,16]

Cromolyn Sodium

Cromolyn sodium is considered safe for use in pregnancy, but adequate data are not available.[15,31]

Corticosteroids

Corticosteroids are commonly used during pregnancy for the treatment of various disorders, including autoimmune diseases, hyperemesis gravidarum, and asthma. Inhaled corticosteroids are mainstay therapy for the prevention of asthma exacerbations during pregnancy. They are not considered human teratogens, although in a meta-analysis, pooled data from case-control studies showed a small but significant increase in oral clefts associated with first-trimester use.[15,55,56] Additionally, there seems to be an increased risk for IUGR and preeclampsia when corticosteroids are used during the third trimester.[15] Other authors also have raised concerns about the development of congenital adrenal hyperplasia in newborns. Prednisone is considered safe during breast-feeding.[15,16]

Theophylline

Theophylline is considered a useful bronchodilator in the management of asthma and chronic obstructive pulmonary disease during pregnancy. There are no reports of congenital abnormalities in the offspring of mothers taking theophylline. Aminophylline may reduce the frequency of respiratory distress syndrome in premature newborns.[15]

Leukotriene Antagonists

There are no reports of teratogenicity for montelukast and zafirlukast, and they may be continued during pregnancy.[53] Zileuton seems to be mutagenic in animal studies and should be avoided in pregnancy and lactation.[53]

Antihistamines

Antihistamines have been used in different capacities during pregnancy—as antihistamines in the treatment of allergic reactions and as antiemetics in the treatment of nausea and vomiting of pregnancy. Antihistamines have been linked to the development of retrolental fibroplasia in premature infants when given during the last 2 weeks of pregnancy.[15] A meta-analysis reviewing 24 studies and involving more than 200,000 patients confirmed the safety of antihistamines, including chlorpheniramine, diphenhydramine, dimenhydramine, doxylamine, hydroxyzine, and meclizine, during pregnancy.[57] An interaction between diphenhydramine and temazepam has been reported in animal experiments, and at least one human pregnancy resulted in stillbirth.[15] The mechanism of this adverse interaction is unknown.

Because little information on the use of newer generation antihistamines, such as cetirizine and loratadine, during pregnancy is available, their use in the first trimester is not recommended. They may be acceptable alternatives in severe allergies if the first-generation antihistamines are not tolerated.[15] First-generation antihistamines are not recommended during breast-feeding because they may inhibit lactation. Additionally, neonates receiving antihistamines appear to develop serious adverse CNS effects, including seizures, especially when premature.[15,16]

Decongestants

Pseudoephedrine is a known animal teratogen; however, no human teratogenicity has been reported.[15] The American Academy of Pediatrics considers pseudoephedrine compatible with breast-feeding.[31] Two cases of amelia have been associated with the use of oxymetazoline, a topical sympathomimetic vasoconstrictor and decongestant.[58] Phenylpropanolamine use may be associated with placental vasoconstriction and in utero hypoxemia.[15] A statistically significant association between first-trimester use of this medication and eye and ear abnormalities has been reported.[15] Use of most decongestants is not recommended during pregnancy or lactation.[16]

Drugs Used for Nausea and Vomiting of Pregnancy

Dopamine Antagonists

Phenothiazines, such as promethazine, chlorpromazine, perphenazine, and metoclopramide, are commonly used in the treatment of nausea and vomiting of pregnancy. Although some investigators have reported a teratogenic effect from these substances, most studies show no association between phenothiazine use and congenital malformations.[15,57]

5-HT$_3$ Antagonists

Ondansetron, a serotonin 5-HT$_3$ receptor antagonist, has been shown to be safe in pregnant rats and in a small randomized study in humans.[15,57] It is not clear, however, whether ondansetron offers any additional antiemetic activity compared with promethazine.[57]

Diabetes Medications

Insulin has been used safely during pregnancy and lactation for many years and is the drug of choice for glucose control in pregnancy. Sulfonylurea drugs traditionally have not been used during pregnancy. They are regarded as possibly teratogenic and less effective than insulin in the control of gestational diabetes. Sulfonylurea drugs also have been associated with neonatal hypoglycemia when used at term.[15] In reality, there is little information about their use in pregnant women. In a randomized study, glyburide proved to be as effective and safe during pregnancy as insulin.[59] Glyburide and glipizide are highly protein-bound, second-generation sulfonylureas. Although glyburide and glipizide are not likely to pass into breast milk, nursing infants should be monitored.

Metformin has not been associated with fetal malformations in animals, but there are no controlled studies analyzing its effect in humans.[15] Metformin has been associated with serious adverse effects in adults, including severe life-threatening metabolic acidosis and hepatotoxicity. Because of its potential for serious effects in adults, metformin is not recommended for use in lactating mothers.[60]

Human experience with acarbose, an oral α-glucosidase inhibitor that decreases the rate of digestion of carbohydrates, is limited, but it was not associated with birth anomalies in animals.[15] Acarbose is a large molecule and is not likely to be excreted into breast milk and is probably safe in lactation, although no controlled studies have been done.[60] Similarly, experience with rosiglitazone and pioglitazone, or insulin sensitizers, is limited in humans, and these agents are not recommended for use in pregnant or lactating women.[15]

Antacids

Ranitidine has not been shown to be teratogenic and seems to be safe for long-term use during pregnancy and lactation.[15,16]

SUBSTANCE ABUSE IN PREGNANCY

Perspective

Substance abuse during pregnancy is common. In a nationwide survey conducted in 2002, the National Household Survey on Drug Abuse (NHSDA) found that among pregnant women aged 15 to 44 years, more than 3% reported using illicit drugs in the month before their interview, and 9% used alcohol.[61] Alcohol and cigarettes are the most commonly abused substances during pregnancy, and marijuana is the most commonly used illicit drug.[61] Although the rates of drug use during pregnancy were significantly lower than the rates for nonpregnant women of the same age,[61] the true prevalence is likely to be higher because pregnant women consistently underreport drug use. Other methods to establish prevalence also have limitations. Urine toxicologic screening can test only for recent drug use, and meconium and hair analysis are tedious and time-consuming.[62]

Principles of Disease

The effects of drugs and alcohol on a pregnant woman may be classified into three categories, each character-

BOX 179-3. Maternal Complications of Drug and Alcohol Use

Respiratory complications: infections, noncardiogenic pulmonary edema, acute respiratory distress syndrome, pneumothorax, pneumomediastinum, hyperactive airway disease, pulmonary granulomatosis, pulmonary infarction, ventilatory failure
Cardiovascular complications: hypertension, hypotension, ventricular dysrhythmias, myocardial infarction, endocarditis, congestive heart failure, cardiogenic pulmonary edema, myocarditis, aortic dissection, deep vein thrombosis, vasculitis
Neurologic complications: seizures, hemorrhagic and ischemic cerebrovascular accidents, subarachnoid hemorrhage, septic emboli to the brain, cerebral abscesses, ischemic spinal cord injury, neuropathies, psychosis, coma
Infectious complications: human immunodeficiency virus and all of its complications, hepatitis, endocarditis, pneumonia, skin abscesses, sexually transmitted disease, septic emboli
Renal and gastrointestinal complications: acute tubular necrosis, ischemia, pigment nephropathy, gastritis, peptic ulcer disease, bowel ischemia, bowel perforation, pancreatitis, hepatitis, cirrhosis
Metabolic complications: anorexia, malnutrition, vitamin deficiencies, rhabdomyolysis

BOX 179-4. Obstetric and Fetal Complications of Drug and Alcohol Abuse

Placenta previa
Abruptio placentae
Premature rupture of membranes
Spontaneous abortion
Intrauterine growth retardation
Fetal demise
Premature delivery
Neonatal and developmental effects
Birth defects

ized by a special set of problems and complications: effects on the mother (Box 179-3); effects on the course of pregnancy and delivery; and effects on the fetus, newborn, and developing child (Box 179-4). Reports on drug use in pregnancy often have limitations that must be considered. Many studies do not control for confounding variables, such as inadequate nutrition, housing, and lack of prenatal care, all of which can affect the pregnancy. Additionally, many drug users use multiple substances simultaneously, making it difficult to differentiate each drug's contribution to the outcome of pregnancy.[63] In the NHSDA survey, 20% of women who reported using marijuana also used another illicit substance. A large proportion also smoked cigarettes and drank alcohol.[61] Concomitant use of multiple drugs has been shown to increase the risk of adverse effects on the fetus. Infants exposed to multiple drugs have the highest prenatal morbidity of all groups, the highest incidence of cesarean section, the highest incidence of prematurity, the highest incidence of poor growth, and an increased incidence of IUGR and fetal distress.[64]

BOX 179-5. Alcohol-Related Birth Defects

Central Nervous System
Cognitive impairment
Sensory impairment
Language impairment
Delayed motor development and poor coordination
Seizure disorder
Hyperactivity, attention deficit disorder
Abnormal myelination
Microcephaly
Corpus callosum agenesis

Craniofacial Abnormalities
Midface hypoplasia
Flat philtrum
Low nasal bridge
Thin upper lip
Microphthalmia, strabismus, ptosis
Short palpebral fissures

Cardiovascular
Ventricular and atrial septal defects
Tetralogy of Fallot
Great vessel abnormalities

Urogenital
Hydronephrosis, renal dysplasia, hypospadias

Gastrointestinal
Absent abdominal wall

Specific Disorders

Alcohol

Alcohol is the oldest and the most common recreational substance used during pregnancy. Its effects on the mother and newborn evolve in a dose-dependent fashion. Social drinking (<one drink per day) carries minimal risks to mother and fetus. Consumption of more than 5 oz of absolute alcohol per day is associated with a 40% risk of fetal malformation.[65,66] Persistent heavy drinking during pregnancy (>2 oz of absolute alcohol per day) may result in an increased risk of spontaneous abortion[67] and other, less clearly defined links, such as low birth weights and preterm labor. The most notable effects of chronic alcohol use affect the development of the fetus, especially the CNS, the face, and the cranium.

Fetal Alcohol Syndrome

The spectrum of anomalies related to alcohol use ranges from minor behavioral abnormalities to a syndrome of structural, cognitive, and behavioral deficits termed the *fetal alcohol syndrome* (Box 179-5). Fetal alcohol syndrome affects 2 out of 1000 live births and is the most common cause of preventable mental retardation in the United States. In its full expression, fetal alcohol syndrome is characterized by IUGR, craniofacial anomalies, and CNS defects. Craniofacial abnormalities include midface hypoplasia, flat or absent philtrum, low nasal bridge, short palpebral fissures, low-set ears, and a thin upper lip. CNS defects include microcephaly, agenesis of the corpus callosum, seizure disorder, and abnormal myelination.[68,69] These abnormalities may be manifested by various neurodevelopmental disorders, including mental retardation, cognitive impairment, sensory impairment, language impairment, poor coordination, and attention deficit disorder with hyperactivity.[70]

The mechanisms underlying the wide range of adverse cellular and biochemical effects of gestational alcohol use are multifactorial. Ethanol, which readily crosses the placenta and dissolves in the amniotic fluid, induces oxidative stress on fetal tissues, causing mitochondrial and cell membrane damage.[71] Ethanol and its metabolite, acetaldehyde, disrupt cellular differentiation and growth, limit DNA and protein synthesis, and inhibit cell migration. Ethanol and acetaldehyde also decrease the transfer of amino acids, glucose, folic acid, zinc, and other nutrients across the placental barrier, indirectly affecting fetal growth through intrauterine nutrient deprivation. Other mechanisms implicated in the development of fetal abnormalities relate to alcohol's effects on the activity of prostacyclin and thromboxane, which result in placental vessel constriction.[72] Elevated levels of erythropoietin, often seen in cord blood of alcohol-exposed newborns, is evidence of a state of chronic fetal hypoxia.[72]

Marijuana

Marijuana, or cannabis, which contains tetrahydrocannabinol, is the most commonly used illicit drug during pregnancy.[61,73] Tetrahydrocannabinol diffuses slowly across the placenta, despite its high lipid solubility. Cord blood concentrations are 2.5 to 6 times lower than in the maternal blood. The mechanism of this concentration gradient is not well understood given the highly lipophilic nature of the compound. It may be due to high maternal plasma protein binding or a placental filtering mechanism.[15] Tetrahydrocannabinol and its metabolites can be detected in neonatal urine and meconium.[62,74] Other noted side effects of tetrahydrocannabinol include the inhibition of DNA, RNA, and protein synthesis, and a transitory impairment of cellular immunity and macrophage function.[75]

Despite its widespread use during pregnancy, it is not clear that marijuana is associated with long-term consequences for the neonate. Data regarding the effects of marijuana are inconsistent. Some studies report an increased incidence of meconium staining, dysfunctional labor, placental abruption, preterm delivery, low birth weight, IUGR, and postnatal growth retardation.[15,73,74,76] Other studies failed to find a clear link between marijuana use and any of the reported complications. A meta-analysis did not find that cannabis, in the amounts typically consumed by pregnant women, causes low birth weight.[77] Heavier use (greater than four marijuana cigarettes per week) may affect the birth weight in a dose-dependent fashion.[77]

Studies on the long-term neurologic development of neonates and infants prenatally exposed to marijuana also have shown conflicting results. Neonates may exhibit tremors, exaggerated startle reflexes, abnormalities in sleep patterns, and a decrease in habituation to visual stimuli.[15,74,76,78] Long-term follow-up of these children shows no significant effects on cognitive function or language development.[78]

Phencyclidine

Phencyclidine (PCP) was introduced in 1957 as a dissociative anesthetic similar to ketamine. Its medical use soon fell out of favor because patients became agitated and delusional during the postoperative recovery period. It is now manufactured and used illegally as a hallucinogen and sold under various street names, such as *angel dust, peace pill,* and *superweed,* among others. PCP usually is smoked in combination with marijuana, but may be snorted, taken orally, or injected intravenously.[79]

Little is known regarding the effects of gestational PCP use on the outcome of pregnancy and offspring. PCP has been shown to cross the placenta readily and accumulate at higher concentrations in fetal tissue than maternal blood.[15,80] PCP also has been noted to inhibit *N*-methyl-D-aspartate receptor function in the brain.[81] Because *N*-methyl-D-aspartate may be critical in the differentiation and the survival of neuronal cells during fetal growth, PCP theoretically may have devastating effects on fetal CNS development. To date, however, no significant long-term consequences to the fetus have been established. Studies on the effects of PCP on birth weight, length, and head circumference have had inconsistent results.

Neonates born to mothers intoxicated with PCP at delivery may exhibit behaviors and physical signs similar to those of adults acutely intoxicated with it. The most characteristic of these features are sudden outbursts of agitation with rapid changes in levels of alertness, increased lability and poor consolability, poor attention span, hypertonia, depressed neonatal reflexes, and jitteriness. These signs are self-limited and may be controlled easily with supportive care.[15,82,83]

Cocaine

Cocaine is an alkaloid derived from the leaves of *Erythroxylon coca,* a shrub that is indigenous to South and Central America. Its mind-altering properties and local anesthetic properties have been known for centuries, but it was not until modern times that its potential for abuse and its devastating effects have been recognized.[84] Cocaine blocks the reuptake of catecholamines, most notably dopamine, norepinephrine, and serotonin. This results in the perpetuation of adrenergic stimulation. It may be snorted, injected, or smoked in its freebase form (crack).[84] After an intravenous injection, 80% of the cocaine dose is rapidly metabolized and inactivated by liver and plasma cholinesterases. The remainder is demethylated in the liver, producing norcocaine, which is even more vasoactive than the parent compound. Factors that decrease the activity of pseudocholinesterases and factors that increase hepatic *N*-demethylation result in increased toxicity of cocaine.[84] Pregnancy stimulates hepatic *N*-demethylation and increases the toxicity of cocaine.[84,85] The toxicity and lethality of cocaine, which are largely due to its vasoconstrictive effects, may be increased by repeated use and by the concomitant use of ethanol; this results in the formation of cocaethylene, which has been implicated in the occurrence of sudden death in cocaine users.[84]

Cocaine and its metabolites readily pass through the placenta; achieve variable concentrations in the fetus; and have been detected in the urine, meconium, and hair of neonates.[15,62] A dose-dependent inverse relationship seems to exist between maternal plasma cocaine levels and placental blood flow, paralleling uterine artery vasoconstriction and uterine vascular resistance.[86,87] These changes are accompanied by a simultaneous increase in the maternal and fetal blood pressure and heart rate and a decrease in fetal blood oxygen content and other nutrient substances. Chronic decreases in placental blood flow result in chronic fetal hypoxemia, which is associated with adverse effects on fetal growth.[86,87]

The earliest reports on the complications of cocaine use during pregnancy greatly exaggerated and dramatized its effects on the mother, the pregnancy, and the neonate. The original cocaine literature was replete with reports linking its use to an increased risk of spontaneous abortion, premature labor and delivery, low birth weight, IUGR, precipitous delivery, placental abruption, embryonic and fetal demise, meconium staining of amniotic fluid, low Apgar scores, and stillbirths. In addition, many reports linked prenatal cocaine use to numerous structural anomalies in the neonate. These early reports did not control for confounding variables, however, such as polysubstance abuse and socioeconomic variables. More recent, rigorously designed studies have failed to reproduce many of the previously reported complications, such as an increase in the risk for spontaneous abortion, premature labor, or premature delivery.[15,88] Similarly, newer studies did not find an increase in the incidence of sudden infant death syndrome, unless the infants weighed less than 2500 g.[89] The only consistently observed obstetric effect of cocaine use during pregnancy is a slightly increased incidence of placental abruption,[15,90] and the only consistent fetal effect is a slightly reduced birth weight.[15,91] More recent studies have failed to show any reproducible or specific teratogenic effects of cocaine.

During the crack epidemic, a "crack baby" syndrome was described. Increased irritability, nervousness, tremors, hyperactivity, abnormal muscle tone and movements, and an aggressive suck characterized these neonates, and the symptoms persisted for a few days to weeks after birth.[92] More recent data, albeit incomplete, are showing a trend toward a self-limited nature of these symptoms within a supportive environment.

Amphetamines

Amphetamines enhance the release and block the reuptake of catecholamines from the CNS, resulting in many adrenergic effects similar to those caused by cocaine.[93] Methamphetamine is one of the most potent amphetamines sold on the streets. Other amphetamines, such as 3,4-methylenedioxyamphetamine (MDMA), have a predominantly serotoninergic effect. In low doses, MDMA has mild sympathetic effects but heightens pleasure and sexuality. At high doses, it has side effects similar to its parent compound.[93]

Little is known about the effect of amphetamines on the course and outcome of pregnancy. Clinical studies are limited by sample size and several confounding factors, such as polysubstance use and lack of prenatal care. Experience with designer amphetamines, such as MDMA, is even more limited. The most frequently reported effects of amphetamines on pregnancy are an increased risk of placental abruption, prematurity, preterm delivery, and sudden infant death syndrome.[15,94] Data from different studies present conflicting results, however. Amphetamine use is associated with an increased risk of congenital malformations compared with cocaine use.[95,96] Cleft lip and palate have been described in children of amphetamine-using women with some regularity, and similar effects have been reproduced in animal studies, confirming the teratogenicity of amphetamines. Prenatal exposure also has been implicated in the development of cardiac and CNS anomalies.[96] In addition, amphetamine use during pregnancy results in low-birth-weight infants, a finding most probably the result of vasoconstrictive effects on the fetomaternal circulation.[94] Amphetamine-exposed infants exhibit a high incidence of irritability, hypertonia, tremors, abnormal sleep patterns, abnormal feeding, vomiting, tachycardia, and tachypnea. These symptoms are self-limited and usually resolve without specific therapy when the drug has been eliminated.[94]

Opiates and Opioids

Opiates and opioids are highly addictive substances; opiates are derived from the poppy plant, *Papaver somniferum*, and opioids are synthesized in the laboratory. They readily diffuse across the placenta. Peak fetal levels are noted within 1 hour of the intravenous injection of morphine. Heroin, morphine, methadone, and their metabolites may be detected in amniotic fluid, meconium, and neonatal urine. These drugs may be detectable in amniotic fluid long after cord blood levels fall to zero, suggesting that fetal exposure to a dose of opiates or opioids is prolonged.[97,98]

The emergency department presentations of acute heroin use are attributable to CNS depression and range from drowsiness to frank coma with respiratory and cardiovascular collapse. In addition, the intravenous use of drugs is associated with cellulitis, bacteremia, endocarditis, sepsis, hepatitis, acquired immunodeficiency syndrome (AIDS), and other sexually transmitted diseases,[64] which may greatly affect the pregnancy and its outcome. When interpreting research data, it is important to keep in mind these confounding medical factors. In addition, social factors, such as lack of prenatal care, poor nutrition, and polydrug use, are amplified in this patient population.[63]

Pregnancy-related complications of opioid and opiate use include premature labor, premature rupture of membranes, chorioamnionitis, meconium staining, preeclampsia, placental abruption, fetal wastage, and fetal death. Whether these complications are due to a direct effect of the drug or to a combination of confounding factors remains to be determined.[15,98,99] Fetal effects include IUGR, low birth weight, and premature birth. These effects have been observed in illicit heroin use and, to a lesser extent, in methadone-maintained pregnancies.[15,99]

The effects of opioid and opiate intoxication on the neonate do not differ from the effects seen in adults. At birth, an acutely intoxicated neonate may be unresponsive, bradypneic, apneic, or cyanotic. Severe hypoxia also may lead to cardiorespiratory arrest requiring resuscitation. The chronic exposure of the fetus to these substances leads to dependence. Neonates born to opioid- or opiate-addicted mothers are themselves addicted to the same substances. At birth, the neonate's withdrawal from narcotics leads to one of the most dramatic complications of opioid or opiate dependence, termed the *neonatal abstinence syndrome.* This syndrome, which occurs in 60% to 80% of infants born to narcotic-dependent mothers, develops within 48 to 72 hours after birth, but may be delayed 2 weeks. The neonatal abstinence syndrome is characterized by signs of CNS hyperactivity, autonomic instability, and respiratory and gastrointestinal abnormalities. Affected neonates develop irritability, tremulousness, hypertonia, mottling of the skin, diaphoresis, piloerection, tachycardia, tachypnea, respiratory distress, wheezing, vomiting and diarrhea, volume depletion, and aspiration.[98-100] Myoclonic jerks are common, and in 7% of neonates these progress to generalized convulsions.[98-100] Infants born at term are more susceptible to the neonatal abstinence syndrome than premature infants, owing to differences in the maturation level of the CNS and differences in total amount of drug exposure.[101] Methadone-dependent neonates have more frequent and more severe symptoms than heroin-exposed neonates.[98] Despite these complications, methadone continues to be recommended during pregnancy because it offers an opportunity for providing comprehensive medical care and stabilization of the nutritional and social environment.[98]

Summary

The assessment and management of drug-dependent pregnant women pose additional challenges to the emergency physician. It is important to obtain an understanding of the psychology and physiology of addiction, and remain objective and nonjudgmental toward these patients. Acutely intoxicated and critically ill patients should be managed in a conventional manner. When medically stable, the most important part of the therapeutic management of drug-dependent pregnant patients is the referral to a drug maintenance program. Drug maintenance programs, such as methadone maintenance, provide a stable nutritional and social environment; decrease the risk of infectious complications in the mother and the fetus; and reduce the problems of cyclic intrauterine fetal withdrawal, chronic fetal hypoxia, and intrauterine death.[102]

KEY CONCEPTS

- Chemically induced birth defects are believed to be responsible for approximately 1% to 3% of anomalous births.
- The age of the fetus is crucial in determining the impact of any given exposure; during the time of organogenesis (days 21 to 56 of fetal life), when major body organs are formed, exposure to a teratogen may result in major anatomic defects.
- Certain medications, such as anticonvulsants, warfarin derivatives, NSAIDs, sulfonamides, fluoroquinolones, ACE inhibitors, and oral hypoglycemic agents, are known teratogens or cause potential toxic effects in the newborn and should be avoided, if possible, during pregnancy.
- Fetal alcohol syndrome affects 2 out of every 1000 live births in the United States and results in a wide variety of anatomic abnormalities (craniofacial and CNS defects) and neurodevelopmental disorders (mental retardation, poor coordination, and attention deficit disorder with hyperactivity).
- Neonatal abstinence syndrome occurs in 60% to 80% of infants born to narcotic-dependent mothers and is characterized by signs of CNS hyperactivity, autonomic instability, and respiratory and gastrointestinal abnormalities.
- The most important part of the therapeutic management of drug-dependent pregnant patients is the referral to a drug maintenance program.

REFERENCES

1. Rogers JM, Kavlock RJ: Developmental toxicology. In Klaasen CD (ed): *Casarrett and Doull's Toxicology: The Basic Science of Poisons,* 6th ed. New York, McGraw-Hill, 2001.
2. Goyer RA: Toxic effects of metals. In Klaasen CD (ed): *Casarrett and Doull's Toxicology: The Basic Science of Poisons,* 6th ed. New York, McGraw-Hill, 2001.
3. Wax PM: Toxicologic plagues and disasters in history. In Goldfrank LR, et al (eds): *Goldfrank's Toxicologic Emergencies,* 7th ed. New York, McGraw-Hill, 2002.
4. Mitchell AA, Cottler LB, Shapiro S: Effect of questionnaire design on recall of drug exposure in pregnancy. *Am J Epidemiol* 123:670, 1986.
5. Mitchell AA, Hernandez-Diaz S, Louik C, Werler MM: Medication use in pregnancy: 1976-2000. *Pharmacoepidemiol Drug Saf* 10:S146, 2001.
6. Botto LR, Mastroiacovo P: Surveillance for birth defects and genetic diseases. In Khoury MJ, Burke W, Thomson EJ (eds): *Genetics and Public Health in the 21st Century Using Genetic Information to Improve Health and Prevent Disease.* Oxford, Oxford University Press, 2000.
7. Schardein J: Principles of teratogenesis. In Schardein JL (ed): *Chemically Induced Birth Defects.* New York, Marcel Dekker, 1993.

8. Mitchell AA: Systematic identification of drugs that cause birth defects—a new opportunity. *N Engl J Med* 349:2556, 2003.
9. Shepard TH: *Catalog of Teratogenic Agents,* 10th ed. Baltimore, Johns Hopkins University Press, 2001.
10. Koren G, et al: Drug therapy: Drugs in pregnancy. *N Engl J Med* 338:1128, 1998.
11. Rubin P: Fortnightly review: Drug treatment during pregnancy. *BMJ* 28:1503, 1998.
12. Saunders EJ, Saunders JA: Drug therapy in pregnancy: The lessons of diethylstilbestrol, thalidomide, and bendectin. *Health Care Women Int* 11:423, 1990.
13. Doering PL, Boothby LA, Cheok M: Review of pregnancy labeling of prescription drugs: Is the current system adequate to inform of risks? *Am J Obstet Gynecol* 187:333, 2002.
14. Garland M: Pharmacology of drug transfer across the placenta. *Obstet Gynecol Clin North Am* 25:21, 1998.
15. Briggs GG, et al: *Drugs in Pregnancy and Lactation,* 6th ed. Baltimore, Lippincott Williams & Wilkins, 2002.
16. The American Academy of Pediatrics Committee on Drugs: The transfer of drugs and other chemicals into human milk. *Pediatrics* 108:776, 2001.
17. Hale T: *Medications and Mother's Milk,* 9th ed. Amarillo, Tex, Pharmasoft Publishing, 2000.
18. Thulstrup AM, et al: Fetal growth and adverse birth outcomes in women receiving prescriptions for acetaminophen during pregnancy. *Am J Perinatol* 16:321, 1999.
19. McElhatton PR, et al: Paracetamol poisoning in pregnancy: An analysis of the outcomes of cases referred to the teratology information service of the National Poisons Information Service. *Hum Exp Toxicol* 9:147, 1990.
20. Riggs BS, et al: Acute acetaminophen overdose during pregnancy. *Obstet Gynecol* 74:247, 1989.
21. Sørensen HT: Aspirin in early pregnancy is not associated with an increased risk of congenital anomalies—meta-analysis. *Evidence-based Obstet Gynecol* 5, 2003.
22. Kozer E, et al: Aspirin consumption during the first trimester of pregnancy and congenital anomalies: A meta-analysis. *Am J Obstet Gynecol* 187:1623, 2002.
23. Sibai BM, et al: Low-dose aspirin in pregnancy. *Obstet Gynecol* 74:551, 1989.
24. Sibai BM, et al: Prevention of eclampsia with low-dose aspirin in healthy, nulliparous women. *N Engl J Med* 329: 1213, 1993.
25. Peterson RG: Consequences associated with non-narcotic analgesics in the fetus and newborn. *Fed Proc* 44:2309, 1985.
26. Rejent TA, Baik BA: Fatal in utero salicylism. *J Forens Sci* 30:942, 1985.
27. Clark JH, Wilson WG: A 16-day-old breastfed infant with metabolic acidosis caused by salicylate. *Clin Pediatr (Phila)* 20:53, 1981.
27a. Macones GA, Marder SJ, Clothier B, Stamilio DM: The controversy surrounding indomethacin for tocolysis. *Am J Obstet Gynecol* 184:264, 2001.
28. Nielsen GL, Sørensen HT, Larsen H, Pedersen L: Risk of adverse birth outcome and miscarriage in pregnant users of non-steroidal anti-inflammatory drugs: Population-based observational study and case-control study. *BMJ* 322:266, 2001.
29. Wittels B, Scott DT, Sinatra RS: Exogenous opioids in human breast milk and acute neonatal neurobehavior: A preliminary study. *Anesthesiology* 73:864, 1990.
30. Dasche JS, Gilstrap LC III: Antibiotic use in pregnancy. *Obstet Gynecol Clin North Am* 24:617, 1997.
31. Ives TJ, Tepper RS: Drug use in pregnancy and lactation. *Pharmacother Prim Care Physician* 17:623, 1990.
32. Broussard RG, Payne DK, George RB: Treatment with acyclovir of varicella pneumonia in pregnancy. *Chest* 99: 1045, 1991.
33. 1998 guidelines for treatment of sexually transmitted diseases. Centers for Disease Control and Prevention. *MMWR Recomm Rep* 47(RR-1):1, 1998.
34. Acyclovir pregnancy registry and valacyclovir pregnancy registry: Final study report. 1 June 1984 through 30 April 1999. London, Glaxo-Wellcome, 1999.
35. Brown HL, Bobrowski RA: Anticoagulation. *Clin Obstet Gynecol* 41:545, 1998.
36. Greer IA: Prevention and management of venous thromboembolism in pregnancy. *Clin Chest Med* 24:123, 2003.
37. Sanson BJ, et al: Safety of low-molecular-weight heparin in pregnancy: A systematic review. *Thromb Haemost* 81:668, 1999.
38. Roth A, Elkayam U: Acute myocardial infarction associated with pregnancy. *Ann Intern Med* 125:751, 1996.
39. Malone FD, D'Alton ME: Drugs in pregnancy: Anticonvulsants. *Semin Perinatol* 21:114, 1997.
40. Holmes LB, et al: The teratogenicity of anticonvulsant drugs. *N Engl J Med* 344:1132, 2001.
41. Buehler BA, et al: Prenatal prediction of risk of the fetal hydantoin syndrome. *N Engl J Med* 322:1567, 1990.
42. Jones KL, et al: Pattern of malformations in the children of women treated with carbamazepine during pregnancy. *N Engl J Med* 320:1661, 1989.
43. Cortariu C, Zaidman JL: Developmental toxicity of valproic acid. *Life Sci* 48:1341, 1991.
44. Dolovich LR, et al: Benzodiazepine use in pregnancy and major malformations or oral cleft: Meta-analysis of cohort and case-controlled studies. *BMJ* 317:839, 1998.
45. Joglar JA, Page RL: Treatment of cardiac arrhythmias during pregnancy: Safety considerations. *Drug Saf* 20:85, 1999.
46. Page RL: Treatment of arrhythmias during pregnancy. *Am Heart J* 130:871, 1995.
47. Elkayam U, Goodwin TM: Adenosine therapy for supraventricular tachycardia during pregnancy. *Am J Cardiol* 75:521, 1995.
48. Shotan A, Widerhorn J, Hurst A, Elkayam U: Risks of angiotensin-converting enzyme inhibition during pregnancy: Experimental and clinical evidence, potential mechanisms, and recommendations for use. *Am J Med* 96:451, 1994.
49. Mastrobattista JM: Angiotensin-converting enzyme inhibitors in pregnancy. *Semin Perinatol* 21:124, 1997.
50. Rey E, et al: Report of the Canadian Hypertension Society consensus conference: 3. Pharmacologic treatment of hypertensive disorders in pregnancy. *Can Med Assoc J* 157:1245, 1997.
51. Magee LA, et al: The safety of calcium channel blockers in human pregnancy: A prospective, multicenter, cohort study. *Am J Obstet Gynecol* 174:823, 1996.
52. Seely EW: Hypertension in pregnancy: A potential window into long-term cardiovascular risk in women. *J Clin Endocrinol Metab* 84:1858, 1999.
53. Schatz M: Asthma and pregnancy. *Lancet* 353:1202, 1999.
54. Liu S, et al: Maternal asthma and pregnancy outcomes: A retrospective cohort study. *Am J Obstet Gynecol* 184:90, 2001.
55. Czeizel C, Rockenbauer M: Population-based case control study of teratogenic potential of corticosteroids. *Teratology* 56:335, 1998.
56. Magee LA, Mazzotta P, Koren G: Evidence-based view of safety and effectiveness of pharmacologic therapy for nausea and vomiting of pregnancy (NVP). *Am J Obstet Gynecol* 186:5, 2002.
57. Seto A, Einarson T, Koren G: Pregnancy outcome following first trimester exposure to antihistamines: Meta-analysis. *Am J Perinatol* 14:119, 1997.
58. van den Anker JN, et al: Severe limb deformities: Analysis of a cluster of five cases born during a period of 45 days. *Am J Med Genet* 45:659, 1993.

59. Langer L, et al: A comparison of glyburide and insulin in women with gestational diabetes mellitus. *N Engl J Med* 343:1134, 2000.
60. Everett JA: Use of oral antidiabetic agents during breastfeeding. *J Hum Lact* 13:319, 1997.
61. Substance Abuse and Mental Health Services Administration. Results from the 2002 National Survey on Drug Use and Health: National Findings (Office of Applied Studies, NHSDA Series H-22, DHHS Publication No. SMA 03-3836). Rockville, Md, Substance Abuse and Mental Health Services Administration, 2003.
62. Ostrea EM: Testing for exposure of illicit drugs and other agents in the neonate: A review of laboratory methods and the role of meconium analysis. *Curr Probl Pediatr* 29:41, 1999.
63. LaGasse LL, et al: Interpreting research on prenatal substance exposure in the context of multiple confounding factors. *Clin Perinatol* 26:39, 1999.
64. Cisek JE: Substance users. In Goldfrank LR, et al (eds): *Goldfrank's Toxicologic Emergencies,* 7th ed. New York, McGraw-Hill, 2002, pp 1666-1676.
65. Larsson G, et al: Prospective study of children exposed to variable amounts of alcohol in utero. *Arch Dis Child* 60:316, 1985.
66. Yip L: Ethanol. In Goldfrank LR, et al (eds): *Goldfrank's Toxicologic Emergencies,* 7th ed. New York, McGraw-Hill, 2002, pp 980-1003.
67. Abel EL: Maternal alcohol consumption and spontaneous abortion. *Alcohol Alcohol* 32:211, 1997.
68. Jones KL, et al: Pattern of malformation in offspring of chronic alcoholic mothers. *Lancet* 1:1267, 1973.
69. Clarren SK, Smith DW: The fetal alcohol syndrome. *N Engl J Med* 298:1063, 1978.
70. Day NL, et al: Prenatal exposure to alcohol: Effect on infant growth and morphologic characteristics. *Pediatrics* 84:536, 1989.
71. Henderson GI, et al: Ethanol, oxidative stress, reactive aldehydes and the fetus. *Front Biosci* 4:D541, 1999.
72. Shibley IA Jr, Pennington SN: Metabolic and mitotic changes associated with the fetal alcohol syndrome. *Alcohol Alcohol* 32:423, 1997.
73. Day N, Richardson G: Prenatal marijuana use: Epidemiology, methodologic issues, and infant outcome. *Clin Perinatol* 18:77, 1991.
74. Bishai R, Koren GG: Maternal and obstetric effects of prenatal drug exposure. *Clin Perinatol* 26:75, 1999.
75. Tang JL, et al: Marijuana and immunity: Tetrahydrocannabinol-mediated inhibition of growth and phagocytic activity of the murine macrophage cell line, P388D1. *Int J Immunopharmacol* 14:253, 1992.
76. Lee MJ: Marijuana and tobacco use in pregnancy. *Obstet Gynecol Clin North Am* 25:65, 1998.
77. English DR, et al: Maternal cannabis use and birth weight: A meta-analysis. *Addiction* 92:1553, 1997.
78. Dahl RE, et al: A longitudinal study of prenatal marijuana use. *Arch Pediatr Adolesc Med* 149:145, 1995.
79. Olmedo R: Phencyclidine and ketamine. In Goldfrank LR, et al (eds): *Goldfrank's Toxicologic Emergencies,* 7th ed. New York, McGraw-Hill, 2002, pp 1034-1045.
80. Nicholas JM, et al: Phencyclidine: Its transfer across the placenta as well as into breast milk. *Am J Obstet Gynecol* 15:143, 1982.
81. Deutsch SI, et al: Neurodevelopmental consequences of early exposure of phencyclidine and related drugs. *Clin Neuropharmacol* 21:320, 1998.
82. Rahbar F, et al: Impact of intrauterine exposure to phencyclidine (PCP) and cocaine on neonates. *J Natl Med Assoc* 85:349, 1993.
83. Golden NL, et al: Neonatal manifestations of maternal phencyclidine exposure. *J Perinat Med* 15:185, 1987.
84. Hollander JE, Hoffman RS: Cocaine. In Goldfrank LR, et al (eds): *Goldfrank's Toxicologic Emergencies,* 7th ed. New York, McGraw-Hill, 2002, pp 1004-1019.
85. Woods JR Jr, Plessinger MA: Pregnancy increases cardiovascular toxicity to cocaine. *Am J Obstet Gynecol* 162:529, 1990.
86. Plessinger MA, Woods JR Jr: Maternal, placental, and fetal pathophysiology of cocaine exposure during pregnancy. *Clin Obstet Gynecol* 36:267, 1993.
87. Woods JR Jr, et al: Effect of cocaine on uterine blood flow and fetal oxygenation. *JAMA* 257:957, 1987.
88. Lutiger B, et al: Relationship between gestational cocaine use and pregnancy outcome: A meta-analysis. *Teratology* 44:405, 1991.
89. Fares I, et al: Intrauterine cocaine exposure and the risk for sudden infant death syndrome: A meta-analysis. *J Perinatol* 17:179, 1997.
90. Hulse GK, et al: Assessing the relationship between maternal cocaine use and abruptio placentae. *Addiction* 92:1547, 1997.
91. Hulse GK, et al: Maternal cocaine use and low birth weight newborns: A meta-analysis. *Addiction* 92:1561, 1997.
92. Madden JD, et al: Maternal cocaine abuse and effect on the newborn. *Pediatrics* 77:209, 1986.
93. Chiang WK: Amphetamines. In Goldfrank LR, et al (eds): *Goldfrank's Toxicologic Emergencies,* 7th ed. New York, McGraw-Hill, 2002, 1020-1033.
94. Oro AS, Dixon SD: Perinatal cocaine and methamphetamine exposure: Maternal and neonatal correlates. *J Pediatr* 111:571, 1987.
95. Little BB, et al: Methamphetamine abuse during pregnancy: Outcome and fetal effects. *Obstet Gynecol* 72:541, 1988.
96. Thomas DB: Cleft palate: Mortality and morbidity in infants of substance abusing mothers. *J Pediatr Child Health* 31:457, 1995.
97. Szeto HH: Kinetics of drug transfer to the fetus. *Clin Obstet Gynecol* 36:246, 1993.
98. Kaltenbach K, et al: Opioid dependence during pregnancy: Effects and management. *Obstet Gynecol Clin North Am* 25:139, 1998.
99. Glantz JC, Woods JR: Cocaine, heroin, phencyclidine: Obstetric perspectives. *Clin Obstet Gynecol* 36:279, 1993.
100. Wright ML, Robinson MJ: Neonatal abstinence syndrome. *Arch Dis Child Fetal Neonatal Educ* 73:F122, 1997.
101. Doberczak TM, et al: Neonatal opiate abstinence syndrome in term and preterm infants. *J Pediatr* 118:933, 1992.
102. Joseph H, et al: Methadone maintenance treatment (MMT): A review of historical and clinical issues. *Mt Sinai J Med* 67:347, 2000.

CHAPTER 180

Labor and Delivery and Their Complications

Sean Henderson and William K. Mallon

PERSPECTIVE

Emergency department births are rare. In general, the emergency physician quickly triages patients in labor and transfers them to the obstetric service for management when possible, maintaining a continuum of care with their primary providers. Because some births are precipitous, or obstetric resources may not be immediately available, the emergency physician must possess the basic skills for intrapartum management of normal and abnormal deliveries. Because some deliveries occur in the home or prehospital setting, postpartum care occasionally is required in the emergency department.[1-3]

Limitations of the Emergency Department

The emergency department is a suboptimal location for the management of a complicated delivery.[4] The obstetric suite has greater resources; experienced personnel; and technology such as tocodynamometry, ultrasonography, fetal scalp electrodes, intrauterine pressure monitors, vacuum extractors, and forceps to optimize maternal and fetal outcomes. The obstetrician also has the prenatal care database. Information contained therein includes accurate gestational dates, presence of multiple gestations, estimated fetal weights, detailed maternal pelvimetry, placental anatomy, amniocentesis results, maternal blood type and Rh, and prior documented obstetric complications. This database allows the obstetrician to anticipate complications of labor and delivery. It is difficult, if not impossible, to compile or obtain these data in the emergency department while preparing for imminent delivery.[5] Finally, in some situations, cesarean section is the best way to ensure successful maternal and fetal outcomes. This surgical option is not available in the emergency department except in dire perimortem circumstances. These are compelling arguments against emergency department delivery when an obstetrician and obstetric suite are available.

Epidemiology of Emergency Delivery

Perinatal infant mortality rates for normal pregnancies with good prenatal care and delivery by an obstetrician are 0.04%.[6] Extensive epidemiologic data regarding emergency department deliveries are lacking. These deliveries should be considered high risk, however. A perinatal mortality rate of 8% to 10% for deliveries in the emergency department has been reported.[6] Maternal morbidity also may be increased relative to the general obstetric population.

There are multiple causes of the "high-risk" emergency department delivery profile. The emergency department often is selected by an obstetric population with unexpected complications. Antepartum hemorrhage, premature rupture of membranes (PROM), eclampsia, premature labor, abruptio placentae, precipitous delivery, malpresentation, and umbilical cord emergencies are overrepresented in the emergency department population.

Psychosocial factors further skew the epidemiology of emergency department deliveries. Women without adequate prenatal care often deliver in the emergency department. Pregnant women who have drug or alcohol problems or are victims of domestic violence represent a disproportionate number of patients who deliver in the emergency department.[6] Women who are unaware or in denial of their pregnancies (usually young and obese) also tend to end up in the emergency department when labor begins.[7-10] Illegal aliens who wish their children to be born in the United States also contribute to the emergency department obstetric population. For each of these groups, all of whom are compromised by psychosocial factors, inadequate prenatal care makes the subsequent delivery high risk.

Patient Transfer Considerations

Because of the high risk associated with emergency department delivery, laboring patients should be transported to a facility that has obstetric and neonatal resources. The management of a premature infant may require highly specialized intensive care that is unavailable at many community hospitals. The desire to transfer a woman with an impending high-risk delivery to such a facility must be tempered, however, by clinical and medicolegal judgment.[11,12]

Medicolegal Considerations

Transfer, with resultant en route delivery, can be disastrous for the mother and fetus. Such a transfer violates federal law. The Consolidated Omnibus Reconciliation Budget Act (COBRA) of 1989 was based on an "inappropriate" obstetric transfer.[13] Federal law has identified labor as a condition unsuitable for transfer because of its unstable nature. Although the intent of this legislation is to protect women from medical and financial "dumping," COBRA also may force emergency physicians to perform difficult high-risk deliveries that might have better outcomes if transferred.

BOX 180-1. Levels of Nursery Care

Level 1 Nurseries

These nurseries care for infants presumed healthy. In such units, screening and surveillance are primary responsibilities.

"Rooming-in" units are encouraged, with emphasis on support of breast-feeding and assessment of parenting skills.

Level 2 Nurseries

These nurseries care for infants >30 weeks' gestation and >1200 g who require special attention short of circulatory or ventilator support and major surgical procedures. Because they address the greatest diversity of neonatal disorders, these nurseries present perhaps the greatest challenge to health care providers. A high percentage of the problems in such nurseries relates to obstetric complications (e.g., birth trauma, fetal distress, obstetric anesthesia).

Level 3 Nurseries

These nurseries are staffed and equipped to care for all newborn infants who are critically ill, regardless of the level of support required. They are regional institutions serving as referral centers for other nurseries and for this reason are often linked with transport services.

Perinatal Centers

A perinatal center provides services to high-risk mothers and to infants requiring level 3 nursery care. Ample data show a higher neonatal survival rate for high-risk pregnancies cared for in such centers.

Nursery Requirements

For many emergency department deliveries, labor will have progressed to a point where tocolysis is contraindicated and delivery is imminent. Generally, this is the point when the mother feels the urge to push or the head is crowning. Whenever possible, a neonatologist or pediatrician should attend high-risk preterm (<36 weeks' gestation) deliveries, and preparations for neonatal resuscitation and high-level nursery care should be initiated (Box 180-1).[14]

NORMAL DELIVERY

Normal labor and delivery proceed to a good outcome without physician intervention in most cases. The mother and fetus are extremely vulnerable during labor and delivery, however, and medical attendance decreases morbidity and mortality. Although the epidemiology and high complication rate associated with emergency department births demand caution, most are normal deliveries. Knowledge of normal labor and delivery mechanics aids safe vaginal delivery and facilitates the identification of complications.

Whenever a woman in the third trimester of pregnancy seeks treatment in the emergency department, the possibility that she is in labor must be considered. A wide array of nonspecific symptoms may herald the onset of stage 1 labor. Abdominal pain, back pain, cramping, nausea, vomiting, urinary urgency, stress incontinence, and anxiety all can be symptoms of labor. After 24 weeks' gestation, any medical assessment should include the mother and the fetus because fetal viability becomes established near that time. In addition, given the generally high-risk nature of this patient population and the abundance of bodily fluids that the health care provider and newborn are exposed to during delivery, serologic testing for infectious disease may be warranted. With the development of rapid bedside testing technology, human immunodeficiency virus (HIV) and hepatitis screening before delivery is indicated in a significant group of patients presenting with active labor.

False Labor

Braxton Hicks contractions, or false labor, must be differentiated from true labor. During the third trimester, the uterus develops into a contractile organ. After 30 weeks' gestation, the previously small and uncoordinated contractions of the uterus become more synchronous and may be perceived by the mother. Although usually painless, the patient may indicate that her uterus or lower abdomen has become firm. By definition, this muscular activity is not associated with cervical dilation.

Examination should reveal a minimally dilated cervix and intact membranes. Care not to rupture the membranes is important to avoid inducing labor prematurely. Braxton Hicks contractions do not increase in frequency or duration the way the contractions of true labor do. If the diagnosis remains in doubt, external electrical monitoring of uterine activity excludes true labor. Any discomfort associated with false labor usually is relieved with mild sedation and analgesia.

True Labor

True labor is characterized by cyclic uterine contractions of increasing frequency, duration, and strength, culminating in delivery of the fetus and placenta. In contrast to Braxton Hicks contractions, true labor causes cervical dilation to begin, marking the first stage of labor.

Bloody Show

Early in pregnancy, the cervix becomes increasingly vascular and develops edema, giving the cervix a boggy texture. The vascularity of the cervix also increases, giving rise to Chadwick's sign (a blue-violet coloration). At the onset of labor, the cervical mucous plug is expelled, resulting in what is called a *bloody show*. The bleeding associated with the process is slight, and usually only a few dark red spots are noticed. The dark color is due to its venous origin, and it is admixed with the mucous components of the cervical plug. The significance of a bloody show is that it is a fairly reliable indicator of the onset of labor (stage 1). Bloody show is not a contraindication to vaginal examination for determination of cervical effacement and dilation. If bleed-

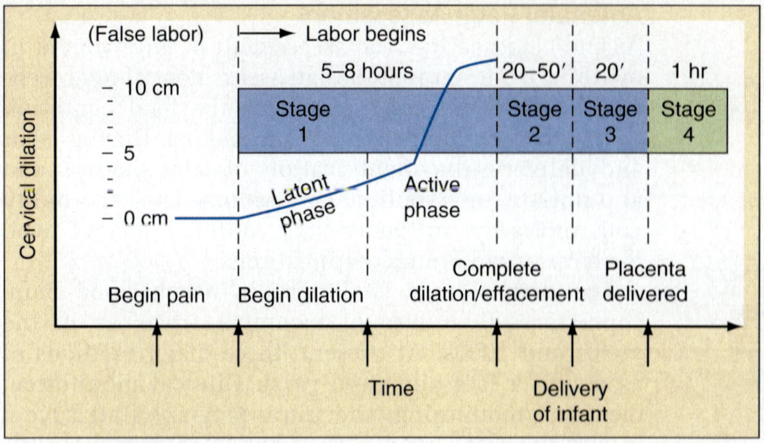

Figure 180-1. Stages of labor and delivery. Stage 1, cervical stage; stage 2, fetal expulsion; stage 3, placental expulsion (20 minutes); stage 4, uterine contraction (1 hour postpartum).

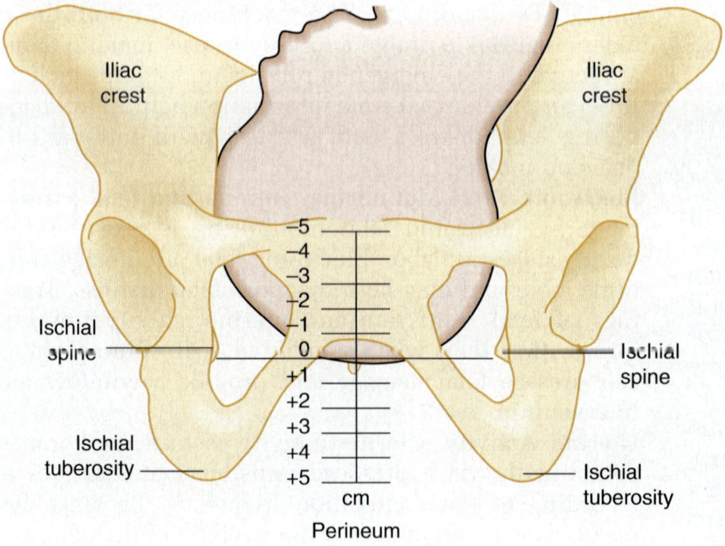

Figure 180-2. Fetal stations. The level of the ischial spines is considered "0" station. The silhouette of the infant's head is shown approaching station +1. (Courtesy of Ross Laboratories, Columbus, Ohio.)

ing continues or is of a larger volume, more serious causes should be suspected, such as placenta previa and placental abruption, which are contraindications for a vaginal examination.

Stages of Labor

First Stage of Labor

The first stage of labor is the cervical stage and ends when the cervix is fully dilated and paper thin (fully effaced). Stage 1 is divided into a latent phase, with slow cervical dilation, and an active phase, with more rapid dilation. In multiparous women, the active phase can progress rapidly into stage 2 of labor (delivery of the fetus). Most women who deliver in the emergency department arrive while in the active phase of stage 1 or in early stage 2 labor (Figure 180-1).[6]

The duration of the first stage of labor averages 8 hours in nulliparous women and 5 hours in multiparous women. During this time, frequent assessment of fetal well-being is important. For low-risk pregnancies, fetal heart tones should be auscultated approximately every 30 minutes. For higher risk pregnancies, continuous external electrical monitoring may help identify fetal distress, allowing appropriate intervention.

The accurate determination of the stage of labor depends on examination of the cervix. A sterile approach using sterile gloves, a sterile speculum, and povidone-iodine (Betadine) solution is indicated to prevent ascending infection, such as chorioamnionitis. The cervix should be evaluated for the following:

1. *Effacement* refers to the thickness of the thinning cervical canal relative to the uneffaced cervix. A paper-thin cervix is 100% effaced.
2. *Dilation* indicates the width of the cervical opening in centimeters. Complete, or maximum, dilation is 10 cm.
3. *Position* describes the relationship of the fetal presenting part to the birth canal. The most common position of the head is occiput anterior.
4. *Station* indicates the relationship of the presenting fetal part to the ischial spines (Figure 180-2).
5. *Presentation* specifies the anatomic part of the fetus leading through the birth canal.

In 95% of all labors, the presenting part is the occiput or vertex. On palpation, both are smooth surfaces with 360 degrees of firm bony contours and palpable suture lines. Palpation of the suture lines and the fontanelles

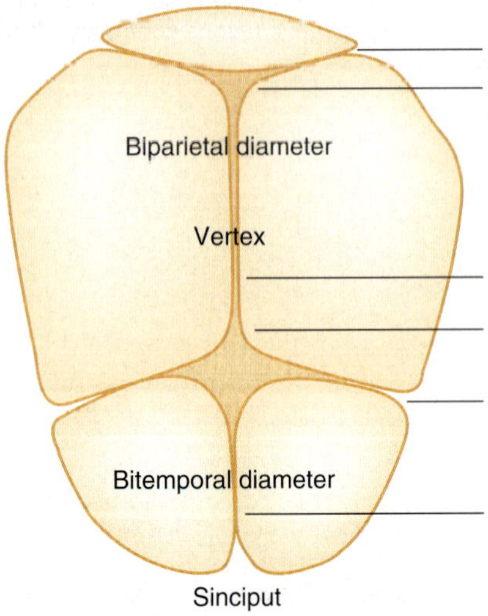

Figure 180-3. Bony landmarks of the fetal skull. (Modified from Willson JR, et al: *Obstetrics and Gynecology,* 9th ed. St. Louis, Mosby, 1991.)

where they join allows the examiner to determine in which direction the fetus is facing. Three sutures radiate from the posterior fontanelle, and four radiate from the anterior fontanelle (Figure 180-3). The lateral margins should be examined carefully for fingers or facial parts that indicate compound or brow presentations.

Leopold's maneuvers may confirm the lie of the fetus (Figure 180-4). After labor has begun, particularly during the active phase of stage 1, Leopold's maneuvers are difficult to use. The firm contractions of the uterus prevent the identification of fetal "small parts." The third and fourth maneuvers are "negative" because of engagement of the head within the birth canal. Other modalities of assessing the lie may be necessary, such as emergency department ultrasonography, if presentation remains in question.[15]

Maternal examination also provides a rough guide to gestational age. At 20 weeks' gestation, the uterine fundus reaches the umbilicus. Approximately 1 cm of fundal height is added per week of gestation until 36 weeks. At that time, the fundal height decreases as the fetus "drops" into the pelvis (Figure 180-5). These estimates help to establish prematurity rapidly.

Second Stage of Labor

The second stage of labor is characterized by full dilation of the cervix, accompanied by the urge to bear down and push with each uterine contraction. The fetal station advances to +3, with crowning of the presenting part as expulsion begins. Stage 2 uterine contractions may last 1 to 2 minutes and recur after a resting phase of less than 1 minute. The median duration of this stage is 50 minutes in nulliparous women and 20 minutes in multiparous women. More rapid progression through stage 2 should be anticipated for low-birth-weight premature infants.

Antenatal Fetal Assessment

As indicated earlier, the assessment of any woman in the third trimester includes an assessment of fetal well-being. After 24 weeks' gestation, the fetal condition begins to affect clinical decision making. During labor and delivery, the identification of fetal distress and appropriate intervention can reduce fetal morbidity and mortality in genetically normal infants who develop intrapartum complications.

The diagnosis of fetal distress has become more sophisticated because of technical advances in the 1980s and 1990s. At present, three major methods of assessing a fetus in utero exist. Clinical monitoring, electrical monitoring, and ultrasonography all have a role in the assessment of the fetus.[16,17] External electrical monitoring and ultrasonography merit consideration for use in the care of women laboring in the emergency department. The machinery for both these technologies is portable and easy to use, making them attractive to the emergency physician.[18,19] Both modalities can provide real-time information helpful for diagnosing fetal distress and assisting with intrapartum decision making.

Electronic Fetal Monitoring. Intrapartum fetal assessment by electronic fetal monitoring is most useful during stage 1 of labor. Electronic fetal monitoring confirms labor and may help diagnose fetal distress. Tracings of fetal heart rate and uterine activity provide information that, when combined with clinical data, can presage fetal damage and provide a window for intervention.

Uterine Activity. Uterine activity is measured transabdominally via a pressure transducer and creates a recording of the contraction frequency. Because the measurements are indirect, the strength of the contractions correlates poorly with the tracing. The tracings are position and placement sensitive. Documentation of organized cyclic uterine contractions confirms the onset of labor and rules out Braxton Hicks contractions that are too disorganized to register in this fashion. Premature onset of labor also can be diagnosed, and the efficacy of tocolysis can be documented using external electrical monitoring.

Fetal Cardiac Activity. Fetal heart rate tracings have several components that can be assessed: baseline heart rate, variability, accelerations, decelerations, and diagnostic patterns. Baseline heart rate, by definition, is maintained for 15 minutes in the absence of a uterine contraction (i.e., between contractions) and is the most important aspect of fetal heart rate monitoring.

Variability can be instantaneous (beat-to-beat) or long-term over intervals of 1 minute or more. Both types of variability are indicators of fetal well-being. Accelerations of heart rate are an important component of long-term variability. Accelerations occur during fetal movement and reflect an alert, mobile fetus. Brief periods of umbilical cord compression also can cause accelerations by decreasing the venous return and reflexively generating fetal tachycardia. Decreased variability corresponds to an inactive, unresponsive fetus. Fetal acidemia, hypoxemia, and a wide array of drugs

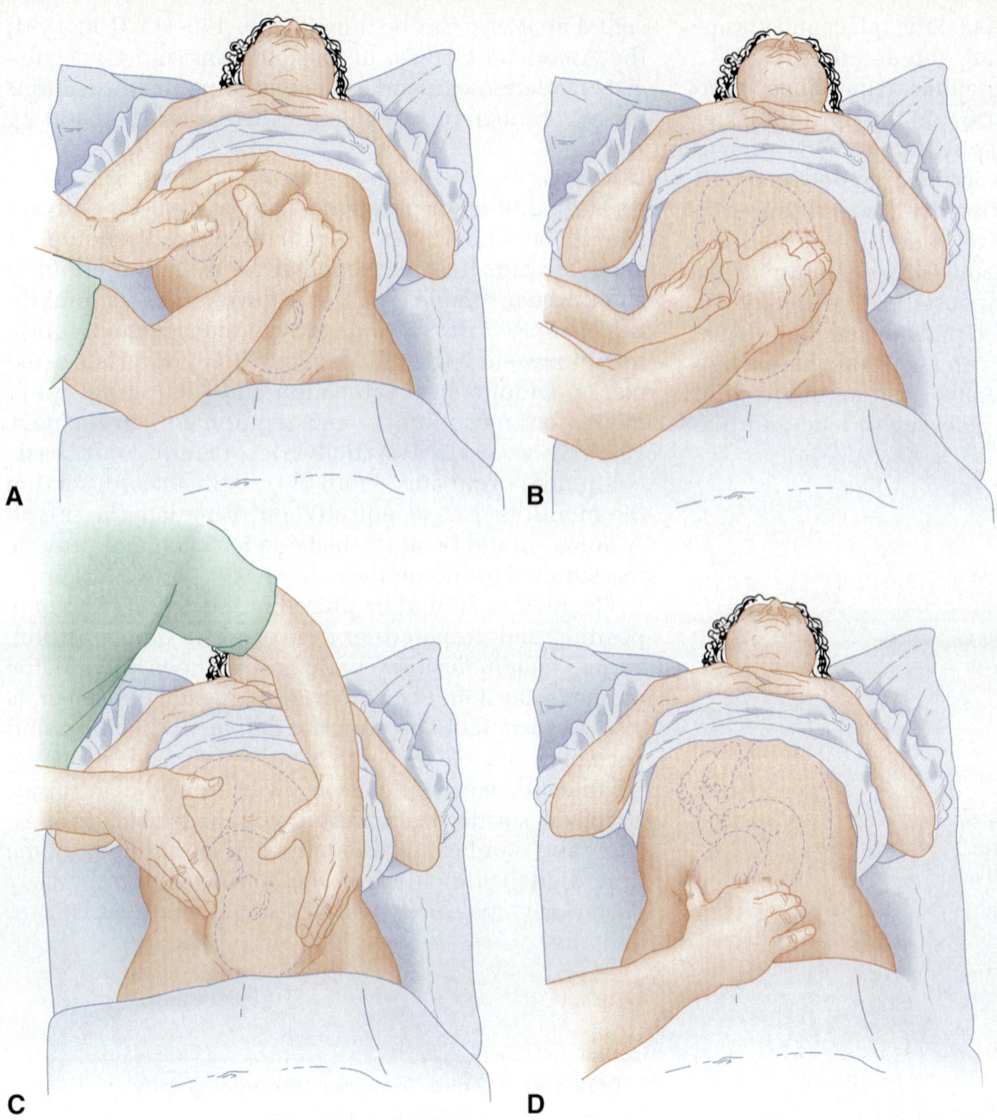

Figure 180-4. Leopold's maneuvers. **A,** The first Leopold maneuver reveals what fetal part occupies the fundus. **B,** The second Leopold maneuver reveals the position of the fetal back. **C,** The third Leopold maneuver reveals what fetal part lies over the pelvic inlet. **D,** The fourth Leopold maneuver reveals the position of the cephalic prominence. (Modified from Willson JR, et al: *Obstetrics and Gynecology,* 9th ed. St. Louis, Mosby, 1991.)

can cause decreased variability. Analgesics, sedative-hypnotics, phenothiazines, and alcohol all have been reported to cause decreased variability.

Decelerations in the fetal heart rate are more complicated, and their interpretation must be integrated with the clinical situation. There are three types of deceleration: variable, early, and late (Figure 180-6). These terms refer to the timing of the deceleration relative to the uterine contraction.

Variable and early decelerations are common. Present on more than 50% of all tracings, these heart rate changes can represent physiologic reflexes associated with head compression in the birth canal or intermittent cord compression. Variable decelerations that are persistent and repetitive usually indicate repeated episodes of umbilical cord compression. The resultant hypoxia and acidosis may cause fetal distress. Attempts to shift maternal and fetal weight off the umbilical cord by changing position are indicated. If these variable decelerations continue, the situation calls for efforts to hasten the delivery or, if obstetric backup becomes available, to perform an emergency cesarean section.

Late decelerations are more serious and most often indicate uteroplacental insufficiency. The tracing contours are generally smooth, with the heart rate nadir occurring well after maximal uterine contraction. The lag, slope, and magnitude of late decelerations correlate with increasing fetal hypoxia. Late decelerations are particularly ominous in association with poor variability, nonreactivity, and baseline bradycardia. Immediate delivery to prevent further hypoxia is indicated when these findings are present.

The need for newborn resuscitation should be anticipated and preparation for critical care established for these deliveries. Overall, 30% of infants with late decelerations have good outcomes. The remaining 70% have suboptimal outcomes related to either the underlying pathologic condition or hypoxia.

Finally, some diagnostic fetal heart rate tracings are important. For the emergency physician, the most important of these is the sinusoidal tracing. Tracings of this type have low baseline heart rates and little beat-to-beat variability. The sinusoidal tracing is an ominous finding that is often premorbid. The differential diagnosis includes erythroblastosis fetalis, placental abruption, fetal hemorrhage (trauma), and amnionitis.

Ultrasonography. Ultrasonographic techniques have wide application to obstetric care. In the third trimester or during labor, ultrasonography can provide crucial information pertaining to the impending delivery.[18] Of immediate interest are fetal viability, lie, and presentation. Ultrasonography also reveals multiple gestations, allowing time for preparation and early communication with other specialists (from obstetrics, neonatology, and anesthesia).[15] When a technician and radiologist are available, gestational age can be established, a biophysical profile can be generated, the amniotic fluid index can be measured, and a survey of fetal and placental anatomy can be done (Table 180-1).[19-21] In 1991, the American College of Obstetricians and Gynecologists made recommendations regarding the indications for ultrasonography in the third trimester (Box 180-2).

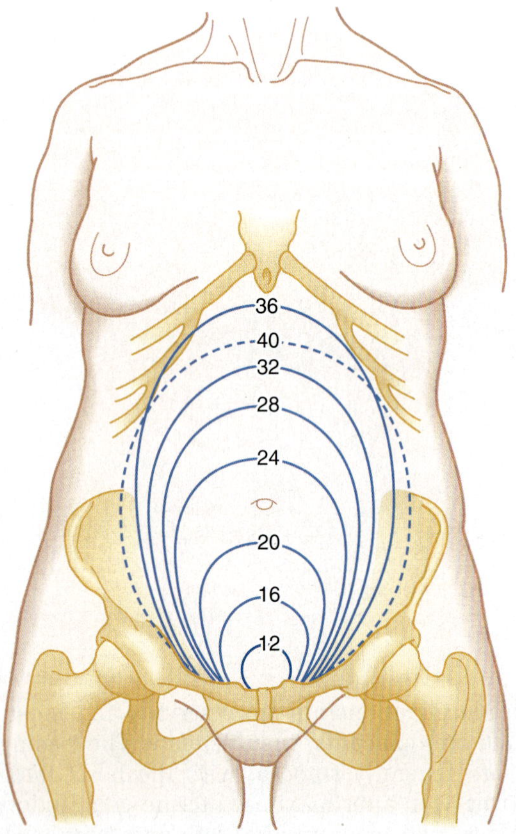

Figure 180-5. Height of fundus by weeks of normal gestation with a single fetus. *Dotted line* indicates height after lightening. (Modified from Barkaukas V, et al: *Health and Physical Assessment*. St. Louis, Mosby, 1994.)

Delivery

As stage 2 of labor progresses, preparation for delivery should be under way. A radiant warmer should be available and heated. Neonatal resuscitation adjuncts should be available, such as a towel, scissors, umbilical clamps, bulb suction, airway management equipment (oxygen, bag/mask device with appropriate-sized masks, endotracheal intubation and suctioning equipment for meconium), and equipment to achieve vascular access. Most deliveries require only basic equipment to cut and clamp the umbilical cord, suction the mouth and nose, and dry and stimulate the infant. A nurse should be at the bedside to coach and provide reassurance to the mother.

The mother should be placed in the dorsal lithotomy position and prepared for delivery. The Sims position, or left lateral position with knees drawn toward the mother's chest and back to the emergency physician, is also an acceptable position for delivery. The vulva and perineum are cleared and gently scrubbed, directing all mucoid debris and feces away from the introitus. A repeat sterile examination to assess labor progression and confirm presentation is performed. Some firm digital stretching of the perineum, particularly posteriorly, may prevent tears and lacerations later in delivery.

BOX 180-2. Third-Trimester Ultrasonography: Possible Indications

- Determine number of fetuses
- Establish fetal presentation
- Identify fetal heart motion
- Locate placenta
- Measure amniotic fluid
- Determine gestational age
- Survey fetal anatomy
- Diagnose cord prolapse
- Diagnose third-trimester bleeding
- Rule out abruption

Table 180-1. Biophysical Profile: 30 Minutes of Ultrasonographic Observation

Element Assessed	Normal Score = 2	Abnormal = 0
Fetal heart rate reactivity	2 accelerations > 15 beats/min for >15 sec	<2 accelerations
Amniotic fluid index	1 pocket > 1 cm in orthogonal planes	No large pockets
Fetal muscle tone	1 episode of active flexion-extension with full return to flexed posture	<1 episode or slow, incomplete actions
Body movements	3 discrete moves	≤2
Breathing motions	1 episode of fetal breathing of at least 60 sec duration during 30 min of observation	No breathing activity *or* The absence of 1 episode of fetal breathing of at least 60 sec duration during 30 min of observation

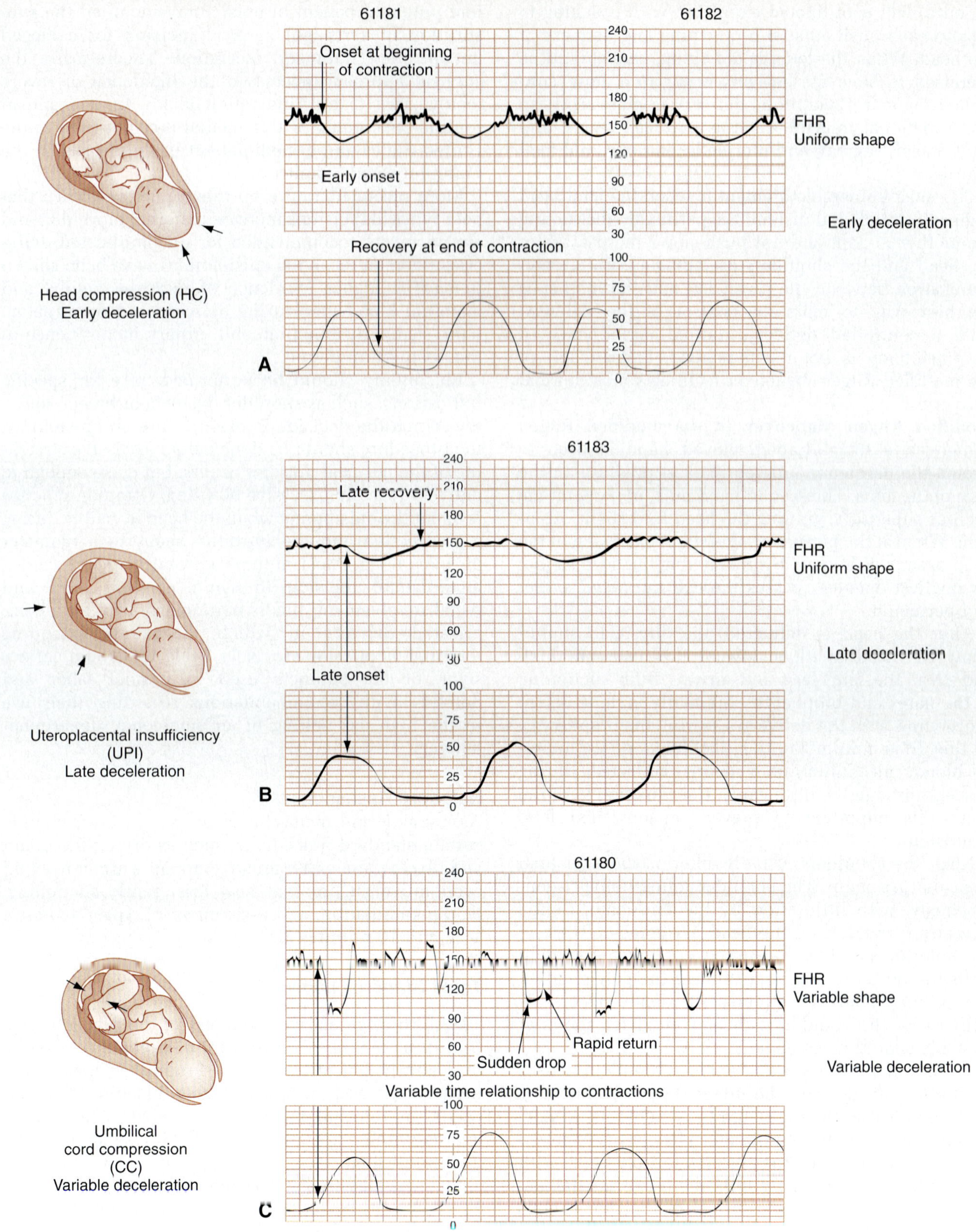

Figure 180-6. Deceleration patterns of the fetal heart rate (FHR). **A,** Early deceleration caused by head compression. **B,** Late deceleration caused by uteroplacental insufficiency. **C,** Variable deceleration caused by cord compression. (Modified from Lowdermilk DL, et al: *Maternity and Women's Health Care,* 6th ed. St. Louis, Mosby, 1997.)

Controlled, coordinated expulsion with coaching to sustain each push aids with crowning and delivery of the head. When the fetus is crowning, care should be exercised to have the delivery occur in a slow, controlled manner. Precipitous delivery is more likely to cause maternal injuries, such as perineal, rectal, urethral, labial, vaginal, and uterine lacerations, and fetal injuries.[22,23]

The most vulnerable moment is when the fetal head begins to stretch and distend the perineum. Instructing the mother to pant and not push slows the passage of the head and the shoulders as indicated. Calm communication between the physician and the mother is the best way to maintain control of the delivery. With a controlled delivery, routine performance of an episiotomy is not recommended. Instead, use of the modified Ritgen maneuver facilitates most normal deliveries.[23]

Modified Ritgen Maneuver. In the modified Ritgen maneuver, a towel-draped, gloved hand is used to stretch the perineum and gently exert pressure on the chin of the fetus. The second hand puts pressure on the occiput superiorly, guiding the head into slight extension. When at the perineum, this slight extension of the head promotes delivery by positioning the head so that its smallest diameter passes through the pelvic outlet and perineum.

After the head is delivered, the physician should allow the head to rotate toward the maternal thigh and clear the fetal face and airway. Bulb suctioning of the nares and oropharynx optimally is done before proceeding with the delivery. Clearing the oropharynx at this time minimizes the likelihood of aspiration of blood, meconium, and debris collected during descent through the birth canal. Coordination with the mother is important to prevent uncontrolled fetal expulsion.

Next, the shoulders, usually anterior shoulder first, clear the perineum. The shoulders often deliver spontaneously, with little effort by the physician. Gentle downward traction on the head promotes delivery of the anterior shoulder. A subsequent upward motion pulls the posterior shoulder through the pelvic outlet, minimizing maternal trauma. If delay occurs in delivery of the shoulders, the potential for shoulder dystocia should be considered.

As the infant clears the perineum, attention focuses on the umbilical cord. The infant should be kept low or at the level of the perineum to promote blood flow into the infant from the placenta. The cord is clamped and cut. Clamps should be placed 4 to 5 cm apart, with the proximal clamp 10 cm from the infant's abdomen. An adequate umbilical stump is important for venous access if the child requires resuscitation.

The infant is now clear of the mother and can be wrapped in towels and moved to the warmer. Gentle drying with a towel usually provides adequate respiratory stimulation. If not, flicking the soles of the feet and rubbing the back are other modalities. Spanking the newborn should not be performed.

Episiotomy. Previously the need for episiotomy in normal deliveries was an area of controversy. The original potential benefit of episiotomy included the substitution of a straight surgical incision for a ragged uncontrolled traumatic laceration. Theoretically the surgical approach decreased the incidence of severe rectovaginal tears. This rationale led to widespread routine episiotomy, with a medial incision used in the United States and a mediolateral incision used in the Commonwealth countries.

More recent literature on this topic has shown that both types of incisions increase maternal morbidity and are no longer recommended for uncomplicated deliveries. Women receiving episiotomies have been shown to have a higher incidence of perineal trauma and maternal blood loss during delivery and more pelvic pain, sexual dysfunction, and urinary incontinence in the postpartum period.[24]

Episiotomy should be performed only for specific indications, such as shoulder dystocia or breech delivery. When the decision is made to use an episiotomy, the procedure should be done before excessive stretching of the perineal muscles occurs, but close enough to delivery to avoid excessive bleeding. Common practice is to cut the episiotomy when the head is visible during a contraction and the introitus opens to a diameter of 3 or 4 cm. Most authors currently recommend a mediolateral incision to avoid perineal tears and rectal involvement; this is particularly true for a complicated delivery in which lacerations extending the surgical incision are likely. Table 180-2 summarizes some of the adjuncts used in normal labor and delivery with recommendations regarding their use in the high-risk setting of an emergency department delivery.

Newborn Assessment

Assessment and management of the newborn include certain standard procedures, such as drying the infant and placing him or her under a radiant warmer to avoid evaporative and radiant heat loss, gentle suctioning, tactile stimulation, and assignment of Apgar scores at 1, 5, and 10 minutes after birth.

Third Stage of Labor

The third stage of labor, delivery of the placenta, is a time of patient observation with frequent checks of the tone and height of the uterine fundus. As long as the uterus remains firm and excessive bleeding does not occur, no uterine massage is needed. Attempts to express the placenta before it separates are contraindicated.

Signs of placental separation include the following:

1. The uterus becomes more firm and globular.
2. There is a sudden gush of blood.
3. As the placenta passes into the vagina, its bulk displaces the uterus upward in the abdomen.
4. The umbilical cord begins to protrude 5 to 10 cm further out of the vagina, indicating placental dissociation.

These signs usually occur within 5 to 10 minutes of the delivery of the infant but may be delayed 20 minutes. Beyond 25 minutes, the possibility of abnormal adher-

Table 180-2. Risk-Benefit Analysis of Routine Adjuncts to Normal Labor and Delivery

Practice or Procedure	Risk	Benefit	Utility in the ED
NPO status and IV hydration	Fluid overload, osmolar and acid-base disturbances	Venous access, decreased risk of aspiration	Yes
Enemas	Time-consuming	Reduced pain caused by constipation	Minimal to none
Pubic shaving	Infections and irritation	None	None
Nitrous oxide analgesia	Incomplete pain control	Self-administered, minimal fetal side effects, noninvasive	Yes
Narcotic analgesia	Neonatal depression	Excellent pain control	As needed
Regional anesthesia (paracervical or pudendal block)	Technically difficult, incomplete pain control	Excellent pain control when technically successful	Variable (operator-dependent)
Electronic fetal monitoring	Increased incidence of surgical intervention	Early diagnosis of fetal distress	Variable (operator-dependent)
Ultrasonography	None	Rapid augmentation of database	Yes (operator-dependent)
Amniotomy	Augmented labor, prolapsed umbilical cord	None	No
Episiotomy	Poor maternal outcomes	None for uncomplicated delivery	No
Ritgen maneuver	None	Decreased birth trauma	Yes

NPO, nothing by mouth; IV, intravenous.

ence of the placenta to the uterus increases. Exploration of the uterus is preferable to umbilical traction as a method of placental delivery (see section on postpartum hemorrhage).

In a normal delivery, the placenta is expelled spontaneously with only slight assistance. Examination of the placenta and umbilical cord is an essential part of the delivery process. A segment of the umbilical cord should be kept available as a source of cord blood. Abnormalities of the cord should be noted at this time. Normally a three-vessel structure, the umbilical cord is filled with a connective tissue known as *Wharton's jelly* and is approximately 50 to 60 cm long and 12 mm in diameter. Normal architecture places the two umbilical arteries on either side of the single umbilical vein.

A two-vessel cord (one umbilical artery) occurs in 1 of 500 deliveries, caused by aplasia or atrophy. Approximately 30% of these infants have congenital defects, and the entity is more common in African Americans. An association also exists between fetal structural anomalies and placental vascular occlusion or thrombosis.[25]

The placenta should be examined for abnormalities. Clots adherent to the uterine aspect may indicate placental abruption. Infarcted areas of placenta may be seen. Accessory lobes (succenturiate placenta if completely separate) and abnormal cord insertion are common abnormalities. The umbilical cord and placenta routinely should be held for pathologic review.[26] The discovery of an incomplete placenta or membranes should alert the emergency physician to the possibility of postpartum complications and should be noted.

Fourth Stage of Labor

The fourth stage of labor denotes the first hour after delivery of the placenta and is a critical period. Postpartum hemorrhage is most likely to occur during this hour. Careful examination and repair of any lacerations should occur at this time. The cervix and vaginal fornices must be visually inspected to avoid missing deep lacerations as a result of delivery.

Oxytocin should be infused to promote contraction of the uterus and control hemorrhage. The uterus should be evaluated frequently for tone and massaged transabdominally if any sign of relaxation exists. Oxytocin should not be given before delivery of the placenta because this may result in the trapping of placental fragments or an undetected twin.

SPECIFIC DISORDERS

Third-Trimester Complications Associated with Delivery

Obstetric problems in the third trimester often result in the initiation of labor. Premature labor, PROM, and third-trimester bleeding are relatively common complications encountered by the emergency physician. The fundamental question to be addressed in this clinical setting is to determine whether the fetus would fare better in utero or delivered.

Premature Labor

Premature, or preterm, labor and fetal immaturity are the leading causes of neonatal mortality. *Preterm labor* is defined as uterine contractions with cervical changes before 37 weeks' gestation. Women with premature labor are a heterogeneous group. Many underlying conditions result in preterm labor, which occurs in 8% to 10% of all pregnancies. Some factors linked to this problem include demographics, reproductive history, uterine anomalies, iatrogenic complications, infections, and lifestyle or psychosocial stressors (Box 180-3).[27] The unexpected nature of premature labor often results in an emergency department visit. When delivery is not imminent, the patient can be moved to the obstetrics unit for further care.

BOX 180-3. Factors Linked to Preterm Labor

Demographic and Psychosocial
Extremes of age (>40 yr, teenagers)
Lower socioeconomic status
Tobacco use
Cocaine abuse
Prolonged standing (occupation)
Psychosocial stressors

Reproductive and Gynecologic
Prior preterm delivery
Diethylstilbestrol exposure
Multiple gestations
Anatomic endometrial cavity anomalies
Cervical incompetence
Low pregnancy weight gain
First-trimester vaginal bleeding
Placental abruption or previa

Surgical
Prior reproductive organ surgery
Prior paraendometrial surgery other than genitourinary (appendectomy)

Infections
Urinary tract infections
Nonuterine infections
Genital tract infections (bacterial vaginosis)

Clinical Features

The diagnosis of preterm labor requires the identification of uterine activity and cervical changes before 37 weeks' gestation. Early maternal signs and symptoms include an increase or change in vaginal discharge, pain resulting from uterine contractions (sometimes perceived as low back pain), pelvic pressure, vaginal bleeding (usually bloody show), and fluid leak.

Diagnostic Strategies

If uterine contractions and cervical changes are present and the estimated fetal weight on ultrasonography is less than 2500 g, the diagnosis of premature labor is likely. The differentiation of false labor (Braxton Hicks contractions) from true labor is best done by electrical monitoring. Ultrasonography also may aid in the diagnosis because fetal breathing movements make the diagnosis of false labor unlikely. The initial evaluation of a woman with possible preterm labor should include urinalysis, complete blood count, and pelvic ultrasonography. If delivery is not imminent, these studies can be performed in the emergency department or obstetrics area, whichever would provide the best monitoring. When possible, these patients should be transferred to a perinatal center with an associated intensive care unit.

If fetal assessment reveals intrauterine demise or major congenital anomalies, or if the mother is critically ill because of eclampsia or another diagnosis that mandates the termination of pregnancy, preterm labor should not be treated. When pregnancy is contraindicated or the fetus nonviable, termination of preterm labor by fetal expulsion is beneficial.[27]

BOX 180-4. Commonly Used Tocolytic Agents

Magnesium sulfate 4-6 g bolus over 30 min
 2-4 g/hr infusion
Terbutaline 2.5 mg PO q2-4 h
 0.25-0.50 mg SC
 0.010-0.080 mg/min IV
Ritodrine 10-20 mg PO q4h
 0.050-0.350 mg/min IV
Isoxsuprine 20 mg PO q4h

PO, orally; SC, subcutaneously; IV, intravenously.

Management

A viable fetus and healthy mother are indications for medical management directed toward the prolongation of gestation. An important exception is the combination of preterm labor and PROM. When patients with PROM, fetal disorders, and maternal contraindications are excluded, only one fourth of all women in premature labor are candidates for medical management.[28]

The treatment of preterm labor includes multiple modalities. Tocolytics to interrupt labor and fetal maturation therapy combined with bed rest and hydration are used in hopes of prolonging pregnancy (Box 180-4). These patients optimally should be transferred to an appropriate center before delivery whenever possible because medical management fails in more than 25% of preterm patients in whom it is attempted.[29] Attempts to transfer these women to perinatal centers should occur when transfer without delivery en route is possible.

Tocolysis. The two classically used tocolytics were intravenous magnesium sulfate and the β-mimetic drugs. Other medications that have been shown to be as or more effective include prostaglandin synthetase inhibitors (nonsteroidal anti-inflammatory drugs) and calcium channel blockers.[30,31] When indicated and in coordination with an obstetric consultant, tocolytics initiated in the emergency department may arrest premature labor and prevent imminent delivery. Allowing labor to continue may result in precipitous delivery of an immature, critically ill neonate.[32]

Magnesium Sulfate. Magnesium sulfate competitively inhibits calcium uptake into smooth muscle and allows relaxation. Magnesium also may produce respiratory and neurologic depression in the dosages used, and women treated with magnesium require monitoring. Cardiac dysrhythmias also have been reported.[33] These effects can be reversed rapidly by the administration of calcium-containing solutions (i.e., 1 g of 10% calcium gluconate solution). Because women with premature labor are at risk for ascending infections, early treatment with antibiotics often is indicated during magnesium therapy.[34]

β-Mimetics. β-Mimetics (ritodrine and terbutaline) cause smooth muscle relaxation by activating enzymes that bind calcium to the sarcoplasmic reticulum. This effect is mediated by β_2-receptors that increase cyclic adenosine monophosphate concentrations in the myometrium. The dosage of the β-mimetic is titrated to biologic effect. Only treatment success or side effects limit their administration. The dosage needed to eliminate uterine activity is unpredictable and varies. β-Mimetics freely cross the placenta and cause fetal tachycardia.

Pulmonary edema is the main adverse effect of high-dose β-mimetics. This complication is more likely to occur in mothers with preexisting cardiac disease, multiple gestations, and maternal infection. This form of pulmonary edema is high-output failure and tends to occur when there is sustained maternal tachycardia greater than 120 beats/min. β-Mimetics should be gradually titrated according to uterine activity and maternal heart rate. Eventually, tachyphylaxis and receptor downregulation decrease the effectiveness of these drugs over 24 to 48 hours.[29]

β_1-Related side effects can be problematic in diabetic mothers. β_1 Stimulation can lead to diabetic ketoacidosis and the usual cascade of metabolic and electrolyte abnormalities.[35] Surveillance of the urine for glucose and ketones is recommended. Fetal heart stimulation can result in increased cerebral perfusion pressures. A premature infant's central nervous system vasculature is frail and may not tolerate these changes. β-Mimetics are associated with an increased incidence of fetal intraventricular hemorrhage.[36]

The prostaglandin synthetase inhibitors, specifically indomethacin and sulindac, have been shown to be superior to magnesium and the β-mimetics in multiple trials. Maternal side effects include a prolonged bleeding time. In the fetus, pulmonary hypertension, patent ductus arteriosus constriction, necrotizing enterocololitis, and intraventricular hemorrhage all have been reported.[31,37]

Calcium channel blockers also have been used as tocolytics with success. Nifedipine or nicardipine may be given. Onset is more rapid than magnesium, and the maternal and fetal side effect profiles are good.[30,31]

Aggressive titratable tocolytics are best for the initial 24 to 48 hours. After uterine contractions have been stopped, the patient usually can be maintained on oral agents, although the benefits of maintenance tocolysis, studied to date primarily with β-mimetics and magnesium, have yet to be shown.[31] The contraindications to tocolytics are important to review before initiating these therapies (Box 180-5). Any patient receiving tocolytics should be externally monitored (electrically) for signs of fetal distress.

BOX 180-5. Contraindications to Tocolysis

Absolute
Acute vaginal bleeding
Fetal distress (not tachycardia alone)
Lethal fetal anomaly
Chorioamnionitis
Preeclampsia or eclampsia
Sepsis
Disseminated intravascular coagulopathy

Relative
Chronic hypertension
Cardiopulmonary disease
Stable placenta previa
Cervical dilation > 5 cm
Placental abruption

Premature Rupture of Membranes

Clinical Features

PROM, also known as *amniorrhexis*, is defined as rupture of the amniotic and chorionic membranes before the onset of labor. Three percent of all gestations are affected by PROM.[38] During pregnancy, the chorionic and amniotic membranes protect the fetus from infection and provide an environment that allows fetal growth and movement. The amniotic fluid is constantly exchanged by fetal swallowing and urination and umbilical cord transfer. The fetal airway also contains a secreted fluid that allows for fetal breathing movements, promoting fetal respiratory development. This fluid is produced at 5 mL/kg/hr at term gestation and is resorbed rapidly by the pulmonary lymphatics, blood vessels, and upper airway at birth.

The word *premature* in PROM refers to rupture before labor, not to fetal prematurity. In 10% to 15% of PROM cases, the fetus is at or near term, and PROM may result in normal labor. When PROM is associated with fetal prematurity, there is significant fetal morbidity and mortality. PROM is the inciting event in one third of all preterm deliveries.

After the membranes rupture, the period from latency to the onset of labor varies. Longer latent periods are common earlier in pregnancy, and the latency shortens as gestational age increases. At term, labor is a desirable result of PROM, but with fetal immaturity labor is problematic because delivery would result in fetal complications, such as hyaline membrane disease.

Diagnostic Strategies

The diagnosis of PROM usually can be established by history, physical examination, and rapid bedside testing.[39] The patient usually describes a spontaneous gush of watery fluid followed by a low-level persistent seepage. In most cases, the patient suggests the diagnosis and usually is correct. Urinary incontinence or excess vaginal or cervical secretions occasionally are confused with PROM.

Examination of women with potential PROM should be performed under sterile conditions to prevent ascending infection. Direct digital examination of the cervix should be avoided. The incidence of infection has been shown to be proportional to the number of examinations. A moist perineum and watery fluid pooling in the vaginal vault, with the characteristic odor of amniotic fluid, confirm the diagnosis. Nitrazine paper testing reveals a pH of 7.1 to 7.3 typical of amniotic fluid (normal vaginal pH in pregnancy is 3.5 to 6.0). Table 180-3 summarizes the bedside testing modalities available to confirm the diagnosis of PROM. Visualization of the cervix for prolapsed cord or abnormal fetal

Table 180-3. Bedside Testing for Premature Rupture of Membranes

Method	Result
Nitrazine	Amniotic fluid pH 7.1 to 7.3 turns nitrazine paper yellow; >7.3 is blue
Ferning	Amniotic fluid crystallizes
Smear combustion	Amniotic fluid, when flamed, turns white and crystallizes
	Vaginal secretions caramelize and turn brown

presentation (prolapse of a small part) should be done during the uterine evaluation for effacement and dilation. Cultures for group B streptococci, *Chlamydia,* and gonorrhea should be obtained.

Management

When the diagnosis of PROM is established, management depends on several factors: gestational age and maturity of fetus, presence of active labor, presence or absence of infection, and degree of fetal well-being or distress.[40] Obstetric consultation and admission are indicated. Further emergency department management may be for clarification of these factors or for delivery, if imminent.

Gestational age may be well known by menstrual history and previous ultrasonographic scans. In the absence of such data, immediate ultrasonography provides an estimated gestational age quickly. Fetal maturity is a more complex determination. Beyond 36 weeks' gestation, fetal pulmonary maturity is likely. If the gestational age is less than 36 weeks, testing the amniotic fluid for the lecithin-to-sphingomyelin ratio or for phosphatidylglycerol can establish maturity. Fluid pooling in the posterior vaginal vault can be used for this purpose.

In the immature fetus, administration of corticosteroids can accelerate pulmonary maturation. The benefit of this strategy has been shown with preterm labor; however, this therapy is less well documented for PROM. In PROM, treatment with steroids seems to decrease the incidence and severity of hyaline membrane disease, but it may increase the risk of maternal infectious complications. Rupture of the membranes also stimulates fetal lung maturation, making it more difficult to establish a treatment benefit in PROM compared with preterm labor. When gestational age is less than 26 weeks, the latent interval to delivery is often 1 week. Tocolytics are an obvious choice, but to date their use is controversial. When tocolytics are used, the goal is to temporize, allowing time for therapy to take effect. These treatment decisions should be coordinated with the receiving obstetrician.

All patients with PROM should be assessed for intra-amniotic infection. Infectious complications should be diagnosed and treated before the mother develops overt clinical signs of infection.[41] The signs and symptoms of chorioamnionitis are late manifestations of advanced infection and include fever, tachycardia, leukocytosis, uterine tenderness, and purulent vaginal discharge for the mother and tachycardia with or without loss of variability for the fetus.[42]

BOX 180-6. Chorioamnionitis Evaluation

Fluid in Vaginal Vault
Phosphatidylglycerol

Cervical Cultures
Escherichia coli and other gram-negative bacteria
Neisseria gonorrhoeae

Vaginal Cultures
Chlamydia spp.
Mycoplasma hominis
Group B streptococci

Amniocentesis Studies
Gram stain (group B streptococci)
Culture
Glucose
Lecithin-to-sphingomyelin ratio

Maternal Signs and Symptoms
Premature rupture of membranes
Uterine tenderness
Fever
Tachycardia
Malodorous vaginal discharge
Leukocytosis

Fetal Signs and Symptoms
Decreased activity
Abnormal biophysical profile (ultrasonographic examination)
Fetal tachycardia
Decreased variability of fetal heart rate

Chorioamnionitis

Box 180-6 summarizes the findings and evaluation of chorioamnionitis. Prophylactic antibiotic treatment has been controversial. It seems that early treatment, however, even before evidence of infection occurs, decreases neonatal morbidity and delays delivery, allowing fetal maturation.[42,43]

Third-Trimester Bleeding

Two entities, placenta previa and abruptio placentae, merit special consideration when they occur in the context of active labor.

Placenta Previa

Clinical Features. The classic symptom of placenta previa is painless, bright red vaginal bleeding in the third trimester. The uterus remains soft, and fetal lie is often abnormal; breech, oblique, or transverse lie is common. The initial bleeding is often self-limited and not lethal. This bleeding usually occurs as cervical effacement exposes the placenta. The earlier in the effacement process the bleeding begins, the lower the placenta lies. Although labor and cervical effacement usually provoke the bleeding, other precipitants, such as sexual intercourse or minor trauma, may be identified. Instrumentation, digital examination of the cervix, and speculum examination can provoke severe, exsanguinating hemorrhage.[44]

If obstetric evaluation cannot be obtained, a partial speculum insertion to identify blood loss at the os may be done. Transvaginal ultrasonography also can be used with care to diagnose placenta previa. Ideally a "double setup," in which preparations for immediate cesarean section are made before the examination, protects the patient if any hemorrhage occurs. If possible, the vaginal examination should be performed in the delivery suite with the obstetrician in attendance.

For the fetus, the greatest risk is due to preterm delivery. Placenta previa can occur at 20 weeks' gestation. One third of cases of placenta previa occur at less than 30 weeks' gestation. In addition to prematurity, the fetus is at risk because of an increased incidence of congenital abnormalities and intrauterine growth retardation that are associated with placenta previa.

Diagnostic Strategies. A vaginal examination is contraindicated. The diagnosis is best pursued by ultrasonography, which usually yields the diagnosis quickly; however, the emergency physician must keep the limitations of ultrasonography in mind. Obesity, a posteriorly located placenta, and ultrasonographic shadows of the fetal head all can result in false-negative scans. A distended bladder pushing the lower uterine segment into a horizontal plane also can result in false-positive results. Transvaginal probes also have been used when transabdominal ultrasonography is unsuccessful. Although described as relatively safe, some potential to provoke hemorrhage is present owing to placement of the ultrasonographic probe.[45]

Management. In all cases of placenta previa, admission and obstetric consultation are indicated. Cesarean section is the preferred method of delivery. The decision to perform cesarean section depends on fetal maturity, the presence or absence of labor, and placental position. When placenta previa is diagnosed early in pregnancy, the condition may resolve. Placental migration away from a low uterine insertion is well described during the second trimester. Because prematurity is the main determinant of fetal outcome, conservative expectant management is indicated.[46] If delivery by cesarean section is anticipated, steroids can be administered to accelerate fetal lung development. Tocolysis is controversial. If tocolytics are used, magnesium sulfate is superior to β-mimetics because it does not produce increases in heart rate or decreases in maternal blood pressure. These vital sign changes are particularly problematic in a patient who also may be hemorrhaging because they mimic volume loss.[47] Vaginal delivery should be considered only with a dead or nonviable fetus in cases of placenta previa. A previable fetus (<20 weeks) also may be delivered vaginally.

Abruptio Placentae

Clinical Features. Placental abruption ranges in severity from trivial to lethal. Areas of clotted blood may be incidentally found attached to the retroplacental surfaces in otherwise normal deliveries. The associated bleeding can be overt or concealed in 20% to 30% of cases. The diagnosis of abruption must be considered even in the absence of bleeding. The amount of bleeding does not correlate with the size of the abruption. Abruption is the most common cause of intrapartum fetal death and accounts for 15% of all perinatal mortality. A significant number of abruption survivors experience neurologic morbidity as well.[48]

The clinical picture of placental abruption can be distinguished from that of placenta previa by the presence of abdominal pain in abruption. The patient's pain is caused by uterine contractions, which tend to be of high frequency and low amplitude. The bleeding is venous and darker than that of previa, although color is rarely of diagnostic value. The picture is often subtle and has been described as "deceptively variable." Intermittent pain, concealed hemorrhage, and difficulty with ultrasonographic diagnosis are common problems.[49,50]

Diagnostic Strategies. Misdiagnosis of abruption as false labor (Braxton Hicks contractions) or as nonobstetric pain can be disastrous. Uterine irritability may be perceived as back pain and be misdiagnosed as a musculoskeletal problem. Every woman with premature labor should have the diagnosis of placental abruption considered. Fresh placental hemorrhage has an echogenicity similar to normal placental tissue; a negative ultrasonographic result does not rule out life-threatening abruption. Ultimately, ultrasonographic establishment of the diagnosis is less important than the effect of the abruption on mother and fetus. If the diagnosis cannot be excluded, obstetric consultation is mandatory.

Electronic fetal monitoring for fetal distress is essential because abruption can progress, especially when trauma is the cause. Fetal distress can develop suddenly, requiring immediate cesarean section. Monitoring has become the preferred means of diagnosing clinically significant abruption. D-dimer testing may have a role in identification of abruptio placentae, but it is controversial.[51] Because disseminated intravascular coagulation (DIC) is associated with abruptio placentae, a platelet count, fibrin split product level, and fibrin levels also are indicated.

Management. Fetal status and the presence or absence of labor are the most important factors in management. Most women with significant placental abruption spontaneously go into labor. Cesarean section improves fetal survival and is being used more liberally. Vaginal delivery can be used for minor (grade I) abruptions without evidence of fetal distress. In severe abruptions with documented intrauterine fetal demise, vaginal delivery is preferred because no fetal benefit can be obtained by surgical delivery.

Placental abruption causes more maternal complications than other causes of third-trimester bleeding. Uncontrolled hemorrhage from DIC extending into the postpartum period can be life-threatening.[52] Severe maternal hypovolemia also is associated with renal failure. Although prerenal decreases in glomerular filtration rate caused by volume losses or inadequate volume resuscitation are part of the cause, additional mechanisms seem to provoke acute tubular necrosis. As noted, maternal hypertension is an important predisposing factor for abruption. When abruption with hypovolemia occurs in conjunction with pregnancy induced hypertension, the risk of renal failure and acute tubular necrosis is high.

Circumvallate Placenta

Circumvallate placenta occurs when the membranous chorion has an abnormal insertion at the periphery of the placenta, giving rise to a cuplike fold at the placental periphery. The precise cause of this abnormality is unknown, but a familial tendency suggests a genetic factor. This defect is uncommon, but when it occurs, it often causes second-trimester and third-trimester bleeding. It is usually painless and mimics placenta previa. Ultrasonography shows no evidence of previa, however, suggesting the diagnosis. When hemorrhage produces fetal distress, immediate cesarean section is indicated.[53]

Vasa Previa

When insertion of the umbilical cord on the placenta is velamentous and the unsupported vessels present in advance of the fetus, vasa previa exists. As labor progresses, these vessels can tear with resultant hemorrhage. Ruptured vasa previa is rare but becomes much more common with multiple gestations, often complicating twin and triplet deliveries.

In vasa previa, the umbilical vessels are essentially part of the amniotic membrane. Rupture of membranes followed by intrapartum hemorrhage strongly suggests the diagnosis. Because the circulatory volume of the fetus is small, even a small amount of bleeding has dire consequences for the fetus. Fifty percent of fetal mortality in vasa previa is a result of exsanguination at delivery. Emergency cesarean section is required for fetal salvage. When vascular rupture occurs, the prognosis is poor. Color flow Doppler studies may facilitate diagnosis.[54]

The presence of fetal blood can be established by the alum-precipitated toxoid test for alkali stability. The alum-precipitated toxoid test determines whether the blood in the vaginal vault is fetal or maternal. Maternal blood is alkali unstable, and the cells lyse, turning the serum yellow when alkali is added. Failure of the blood to lyse with alkali establishes a fetal source. Alternatively, a Wright's stain of the blood reveals the nucleated red blood cells present in cord blood. When a viable delivery occurs after vasa previa, fetal transfusion should be considered during the resuscitation phase.

Vertical Transmission of Human Immunodeficiency Virus

Emergency deliveries may involve women who are known to be HIV positive and women who are infected but have never been tested. The latter group generally includes vulnerable pregnant women with little or no prenatal care who are prone to emergency department delivery. In both situations, antiretroviral therapy at emergency department presentation—even while labor progresses—can decrease vertical HIV transmission.

In November 2002, the U.S. Food and Drug Administration approved the OraQuick Rapid HIV-1 Antibody Test (OraSure Technologies, Bethlehem, Pa).[55] Point-of-care testing for HIV with a median turnaround time of 45 minutes realistically allows the emergency physician to initiate intrapartum and neonatal antiretroviral therapy when the test is positive. As usual, serologic confirmation is recommended, but emergent interventions can proceed based on the bedside result.[56] Since 1994, it has been known that immediate treatment during labor can decrease significantly vertical transmission to the newborn.[57,58]

A positive HIV test in some cases may allow for a change in the method of delivery. Cesarean section decreases the rate of HIV transmission compared with vaginal delivery methods. In a 1999 meta-analysis from the United States and Europe, vertical HIV transmission was decreased by cesarean section with an odds ratio of 0.43 (95% confidence interval: 0.33, 0.56). The protective effect of surgical delivery over other delivery methods persisted even when the data were stratified for receipt of antiretroviral therapy.[59]

Ideally, decisions regarding the mode of delivery and the need for antiretroviral therapy can be made before the rupture of membranes. It seems that transmission increases after that time and continues as the fetus traverses the birth canal.[60] When antiretroviral therapy and elective cesarean section are employed, the likelihood of vertical transmission is reduced by 87% compared with women receiving neither intervention.[59]

This relatively new diagnostic and therapeutic burden on the emergency physician faced with an emergency department delivery is difficult and has real-time pressure associated with it. The data indicate that antiretroviral treatment and the mode of delivery make labor a true emergency for an HIV-positive patient. For the emergency physician, mobilizing an on-call obstetric consultant to perform a prompt cesarean section of a patient the consultant does not know and who comes with occupational and medicolegal risk is not easy. Currently the main obstacle to this type of care is the availability of point-of-care HIV testing. Since the late 1990s, the results supporting this approach have become increasingly robust and seem to justify the efforts.[61,62]

Complicated Delivery

Perspective

Deliveries complicated by dystocia, malpresentation, or multiple gestations are life-threatening emergencies. The emergency physician cannot "solve" these obstetric problems with cesarean section and may face the prospect of an extremely high-risk vaginal delivery. Abnormal delivery increases the risk of fetal and maternal complications.

Aggressive attempts to obtain obstetric, neonatal, and anesthesia support are warranted. If the delivery proceeds in the emergency department, preparations for maternal and neonatal resuscitation should be made. The potential for two critically ill patients is real, although the fetus is proportionally at greater risk.

Table 180-4. Drug and Labor Interactions

Drug	Effect on Labor
Barbiturates	In anesthetic doses can stop labor
Alcohol	Decreases oxytocin release, smooth muscle relaxant
Cocaine	Increased prematurity, placental infarction
Caffeine or aminophylline	Increased duration of labor
Narcotics	Increased latent phase, slow dilation (minimal effect once in active labor)
Atropine, scopolamine	Lower uterine segment relaxation, decreased frequency of contractions
Halothane	Strong inhibition of labor
IV nitroglycerin	Profound uterine relaxation

IV, intravenous.

Table 180-5. Relative Incidence of Malpresentations

Malpresentation	Incidence
Breech presentation	1/25 live births
Shoulder dystocia	1/300 live births
Face presentation	1/550 live births
Brow presentation	1/1400 live births

BOX 180-7. Breech Presentations

Frank Breech
60-65% of all breech presentations
Hips flexed, knees extended
Buttocks act as good dilating wedge
Incidence of cord prolapse approximately 6.4%

Complete Breech
Least common, occurs in approximately 5% of all breech presentations
Hips and knees flexed
Buttocks act as good dilating wedge
Incidence of cord prolapse is 5-6%

Incomplete Breech
25-35% of all breech presentations
Incomplete hip flexion, single or double footling
Poor wedge
Increased incidence of prolapsed cord (15-18%)

Principles of Disease

Knowledge of abnormal labor and its anatomy and physiology are important for the emergency physician facing a complicated delivery. Intrapartum management skills may allow the emergency physician to proceed with delivery, averting disaster.

Dystocia and Malpresentation

Dystocia, or abnormal labor progression, accounts for one third of all cesarean sections and half of primary cesarean sections. Because rapid surgical resolution is unavailable to the emergency physician, intrapartum management skills are important. The delay in delivery associated with dystocia is a major ally to the emergency physician because obstetric assistance often becomes available.

Dystocia can be divided into three etiologic categories. Labor fails to progress when there are problems related to the pelvic architecture (the passage), when there are fetal size or presentation problems (the passenger), and when uterine expulsive forces are inadequate. Table 180-4 summarizes important labor-drug interactions that may be involved. Although it is useful to consider these causes independently, dystocia usually is caused by a combination of factors. Presentation problems are particularly important because they become apparent during stage 2 of labor and require immediate action.

There are physician-related factors in the diagnosis of dystocia. An obstetrician may be content to reach a diagnosis of dystocia because surgical options are available. True fetopelvic disproportion is much less common than dystocia, however. The diagnosis of dystocia has been challenged as the reason for many unnecessary cesarean sections. For the emergency physician faced with delivery, the rarity of true fetopelvic disproportion means that vaginal delivery would be possible in most cases. Fetal malpresentation and shoulder dystocia are relatively common delivery complications (Table 180-5). It is likely that the incidence of these problems is higher in the emergency department obstetric population.

As the fetus enters the birth canal, the body diameters usually are minimized to facilitate passage. In shoulder dystocia and malpresentation, such as breech, face, or brow, the fetal orientation within the birth canal creates a mechanical obstruction to delivery. Labor arrest and fetal asphyxia are common results. For the obstetrician, vaginal delivery may be abandoned in favor of cesarean section to improve maternal and fetal outcomes. When delivery is imminent, however, intrapartum management skills are critical to successful delivery. An understanding of the mechanical problems associated with these deliveries helps the emergency physician choose from a variety of maneuvers that can resolve these life-threatening obstetric emergencies.

Breech Delivery

Perspective. Breech is the most common malpresentation, occurring in approximately 4% of all deliveries. Three types of breech presentation exist: frank, incomplete, and complete (Figure 180-7 and Box 180-7). The main mechanical problem with breech presentations is that the buttocks do not provide a sufficient wedge to dilate the cervix completely. The relatively large aftercoming head becomes trapped within the birth canal. Cord prolapse can occur because the breech does not completely occlude the cervical opening.

The terminology for breech deliveries is complicated. By convention, the presentation (frank, incomplete, and complete) is followed by the relationship of the

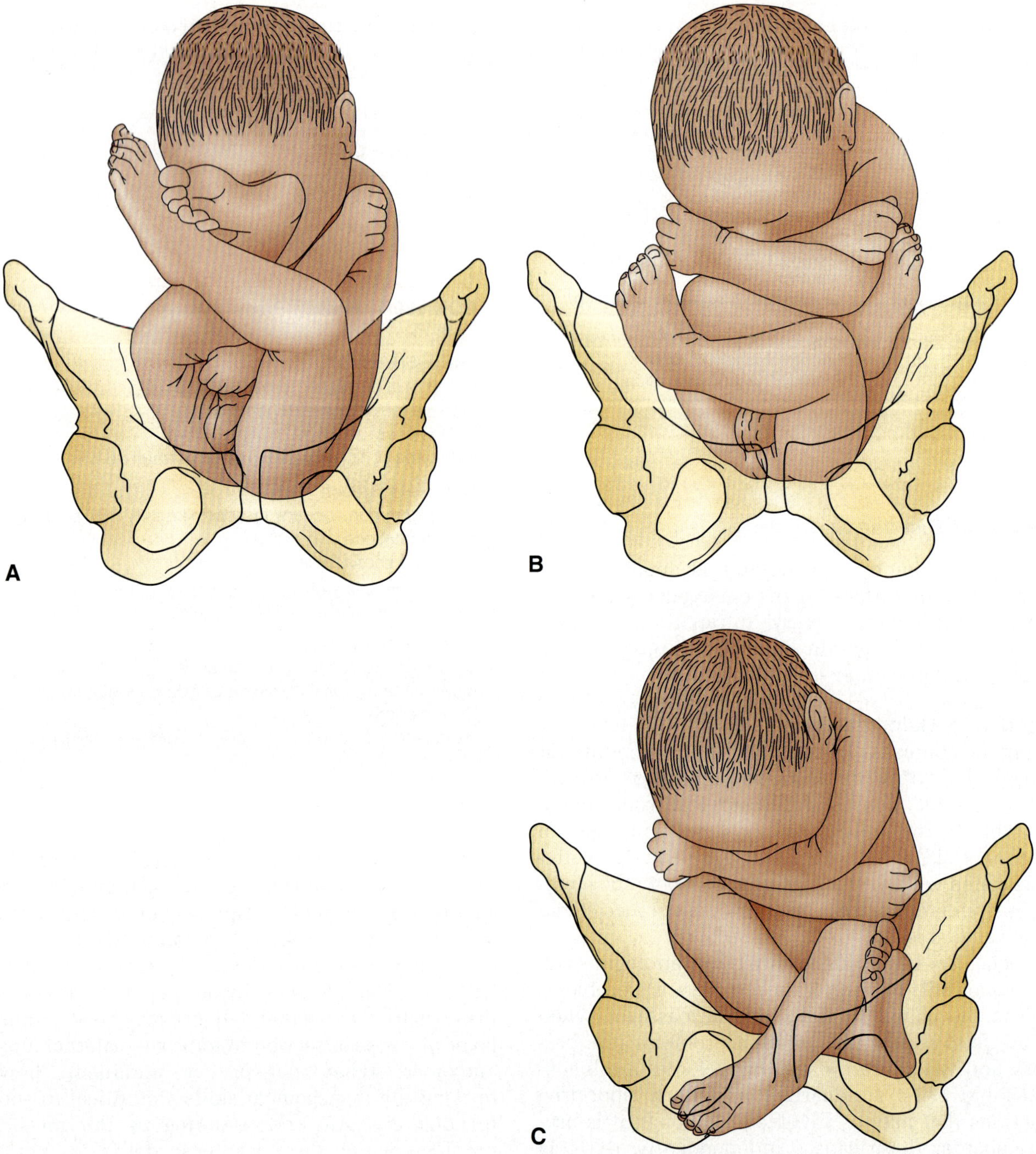

Figure 180-7. Breech presentations. **A,** Frank breech presentation. **B,** Complete breech presentation. **C,** Incomplete breech presentation. (Modified from Cunningham FG, et al: *Williams Obstetrics,* 19th ed. Norwalk, Conn, Appleton & Lange, 1993.)

fetus to the birth canal, using the fetal sacrum as a reference point. The mode of delivery used also has specific terminology. *Spontaneous breech delivery* refers to vaginal delivery without manual aid, almost always of a small premature infant. *Assisted breech delivery* and *partial breech extraction* are terms that apply when delivery is manually assisted after the umbilicus clears the perineum. The head may be delivered by intrapartum maneuvers or forceps. Complete breech extraction consists of the application of traction to the lower extremities or groin before delivery of the buttocks. This approach is never indicated for a singleton breech because it increases the chances of head entrapment. Confusion arises because the word *complete* as used here describes the mode of delivery, not the presentation.

Slightly less than 4% of deliveries are breech; the incidence is increased in premature or congenitally abnormal fetuses. Of term infants who die during the neonatal period, 50% are products of breech deliveries. Despite the association of low birth weight and anomalies with breech presentation, more than two thirds of breech fetuses weigh more than 2500 g, and in 50% no predisposing factor can be identified. These normal, full-term infants are at the greatest risk for complications related to delivery.

Overall, one third of breech fetal deaths are believed to be preventable. Asphyxia is often due to umbilical cord prolapse or entrapment of the aftercoming head. Fetal head and neck trauma can occur if inappropriate delivery techniques are used. Planned cesarean section for these patients means they usually are deleted from the pool of potential emergency department deliveries. Since the 1990s, however, obstetricians have been attempting to decrease cesarean rates. As part of this process, some centers have proposed a trial of labor and vaginal delivery for selected full-term infants with frank breech presentations.[63] The potential for the emergency physician to encounter a breech presentation may be increasing.

Diagnostic Strategies. Before labor, Leopold's maneuvers facilitate the diagnosis of breech presentation. Leopold's first maneuver identifies a firm round mass (the head) in the upper portion of the uterus. The third maneuver reveals the softer breech at the pelvic inlet. For the emergency physician, active labor often limits the use of Leopold's maneuvers, and vaginal examination is required. Sterile technique is indicated if ruptured membranes are suspected. If the membranes are intact, caution not to rupture them should be exercised because intact membranes improve the fetal dilating wedge.

The differentiation of a vertex presentation from a breech by tactile vaginal examination is not always simple. Any time a fontanelle is not identified on examination, a breech presentation should be suspected. During the vaginal examination, it is helpful to remember that the face and the skull have a complete circle of bone, whereas the anus is flanked by bone on only two sides.

If time allows, immediate ultrasonographic studies or plain radiographs are indicated for all breech presentations to obtain information on the position of the fetal arms and neck. If the fetus has a hyperextended neck, vaginal delivery is associated with a 70% incidence of spinal cord injuries. If possible, labor should be delayed to allow cesarean section.[64] Likewise, if the arms are over the head, they increase the dystocia when the head enters the birth canal. For term infants, labor arrest and asphyxia or brachial plexus injuries are common outcomes of vaginal delivery. If ultrasonography reveals anencephaly or massive hydrocephaly, vaginal breech delivery should be allowed to continue because cesarean section is undesirable.

Management. Premature infants in the breech position often deliver spontaneously without difficulty. As the infant comes to term, dystocia becomes increasingly common. When committed to a vaginal delivery, knowledge of breech dystocia mechanics may allow atraumatic delivery. The key goals are to maximize the size of the passage and to minimize the dystocia of the aftercoming head. Box 180-8 summarizes the actions associated with successful vaginal breech delivery.

The Mauriceau maneuver is the use of the fetal oral aperture to flex the fetal neck and draw in the chin. Because fetal neck extension is associated with cord injuries and worsening dystocia, this maneuver is crucial to successful vaginal delivery. While the Mauriceau maneuver is used, the fetal pelvis should be supported to avoid abdominal injuries. Generous episiotomy, or even episioproctotomy, may be necessary to facilitate the Mauriceau maneuver in a full-term infant. If the aftercoming head cannot be delivered quickly, the chances of good fetal outcome are poor.

BOX 180-8. Vaginal Breech Delivery

Actions to Do as Able

Monitoring fetal heart rate
Focused history
Diagnosis of breech lie
Cervical dilation and station determination
Ultrasonography or plain radiography
Evaluation for prolapsed cord if spontaneous rupture of membranes
Generous episiotomy
Knee flexion and sweep out legs
Pulling out a 10-15 cm loop of cord (room to work) after umbilicus clears perineum
Use of bony pelvis as means of holding infant
Keeping face and abdomen away from symphysis, and using rotation to deliver the most accessible arm
Mauriceau maneuver

Actions to Avoid

Inappropriate transfer with delivery en route
Misdiagnosis of cervical dilation
Iatrogenic rupture of membranes (cord prolapse)
Moving patients or leaving unmonitored
Traction on the fetus during delivery
Grasping fetus by the waist, causing abdominal organ injury
Arm entrapment over head
Neck hyperextension

Shoulder Dystocia

Perspective. Shoulder dystocia is the second most common malpresentation. In contrast to a breech presentation, which may be diagnosed antepartum, shoulder dystocia develops intrapartum. Maternal and fetal factors are associated with shoulder dystocia. Maternal factors include diabetes, obesity, and prolonged second stage of labor; fetal factors include macrosomia, postmaturity, and erythroblastosis fetalis. The combination of prenatal data, estimated fetal weight, and fetal biometry cannot reliably identify most deliveries complicated by shoulder dystocia. The unpredictable nature of shoulder dystocia increases its risk of being an emergency department problem. That shoulder dystocia responds well to a variety of intrapartum maneuvers means that delivery skill is an important determinant of fetal outcome.

Shoulder dystocia occurs in 1 in 300 deliveries in a general obstetric population. As with malpresentation, it has been suggested that the incidence may be higher in the emergency department. In diabetic mothers with infants weighing more than 4000 g, the incidence may be 23%; however, most shoulder dystocia occurs in deliveries of infants of average birth weight.[65]

The consequences of shoulder dystocia can be devastating. As with breech presentation, infant com-

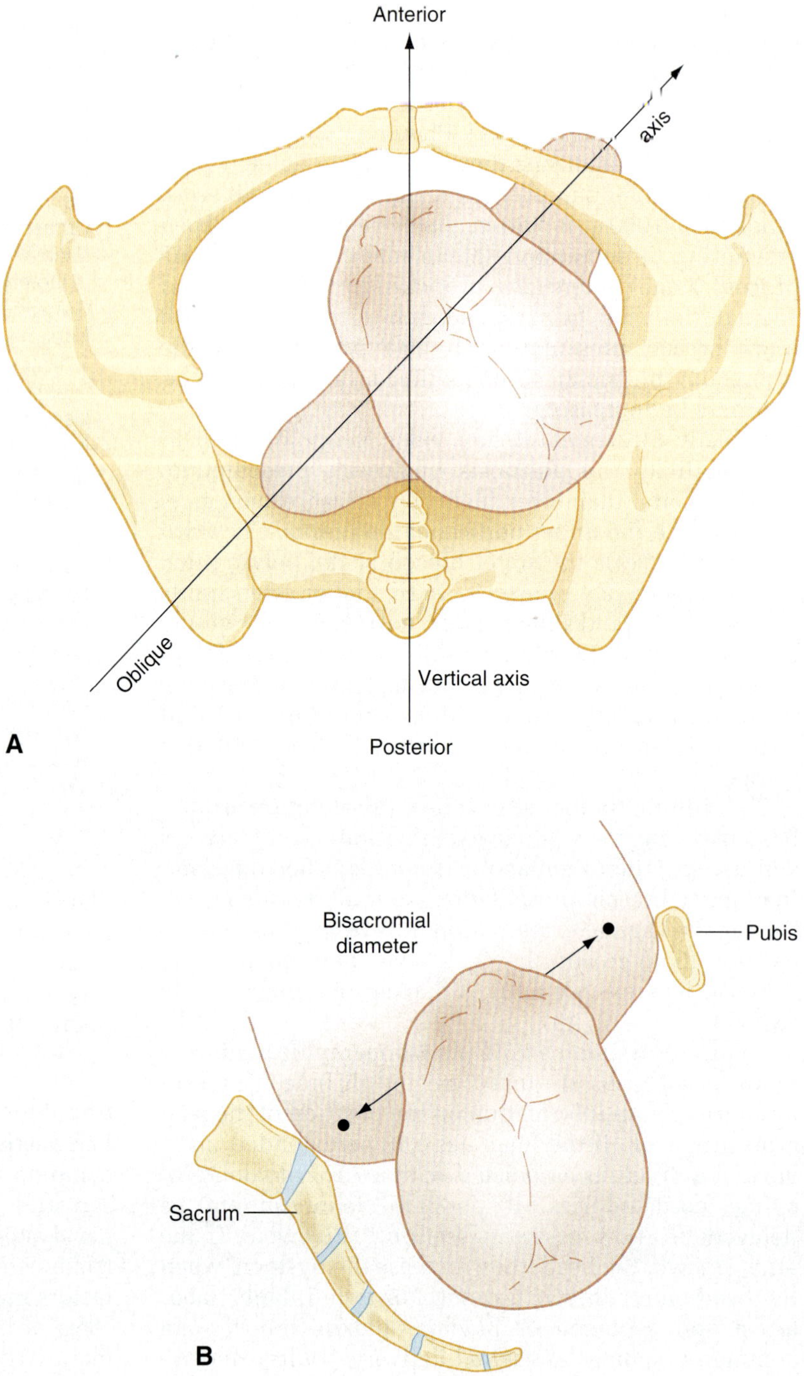

Figure 180-8. A, Normal delivery. As the fetal head rotates, the shoulders assume an oblique position and enter the pelvis one at a time. **B,** Shoulder dystocia. Both shoulders attempt to clear the pelvis simultaneously, forcing the bisacromial diameter into the opening.

plications are more common and severe than maternal complications. Asphyxia, traumatic brachial plexus injuries, and humeral and clavicular fractures contribute to a complication rate of 20%.[66] Maternal complications are related to traumatic delivery and include cervical, vaginal, perineal, and rectal tears.

Diagnostic Strategies. Shoulder dystocia is diagnosed clinically by an inability to deliver either shoulder. The fetal head may appear to retract toward the maternal perineum. This finding is known as the "turtle sign" and suggests the diagnosis. Traction on the head extends and abducts the shoulders, increasing the bisacromial diameter and worsening the dystocia. Figure 180-8 shows the normal and abnormal relationship of the shoulders to the birth canal and illustrates why the bisacromial diameter is an important element of fetal biometry.

Normally the shoulders negotiate the maternal pelvis in sequential fashion, anterior shoulder first. With shoulder dystocia, both shoulders attempt to clear the maternal pelvis simultaneously. In addition to the turtle sign, examination often reveals that the fetal shoulders are on a vertical axis (rather than oblique). These findings in combination with an arrested delivery with the fetal head on the perineum confirm the diagnosis of shoulder dystocia.[67]

Management. When shoulder dystocia becomes evident, knowledge of intrapartum delivery maneuvers can be lifesaving. Successful vaginal delivery is most likely when a directed sequential approach to each

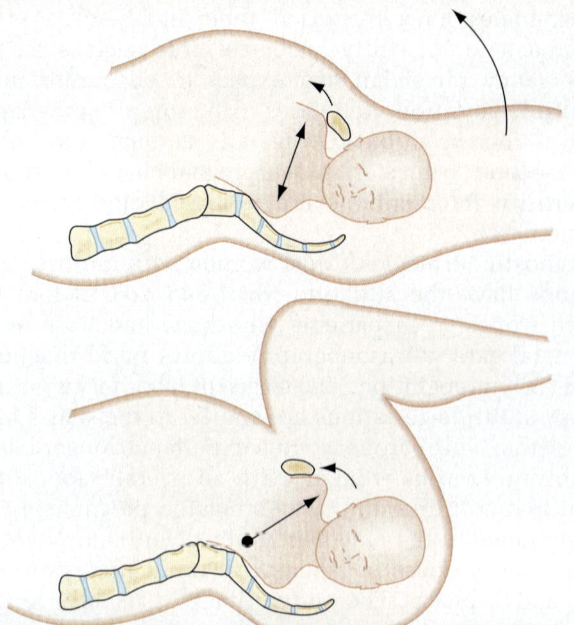

Figure 180-9. McRoberts' maneuver. A, Bisacromial diameter pinned behind pubic symphysis. B, Removing the maternal legs from the stirrups and putting the knees up to the chest fulcrums the pubic symphysis over the impacted anterior shoulder.

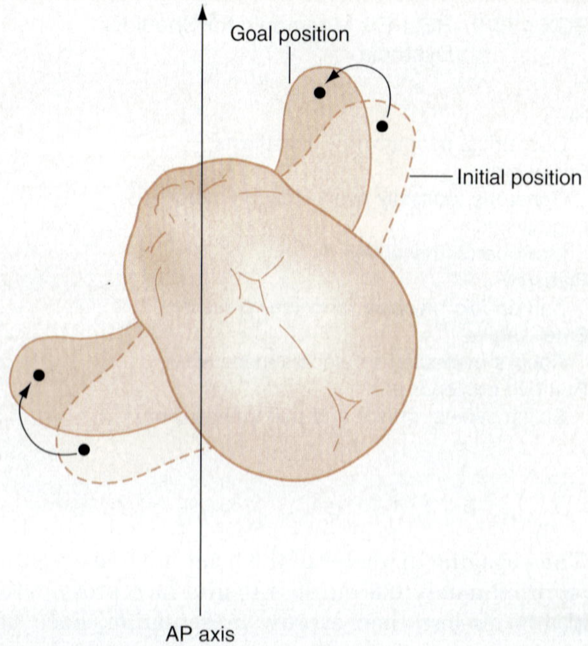

Figure 180-10. Rubin's maneuver decreases the bisacromial diameter. AP, anteroposterior.

maneuver is used. Rapid resolution of shoulder dystocia is important to avoid fetal asphyxia. Obstetric and neonatology assistance may improve the outcome, and aggressive attempts to obtain help in these areas are warranted.

Initial attempts to resolve shoulder dystocia involve increasing the anteroposterior diameter of the passage. Posteriorly, an episiotomy (or episioproctotomy) should be used to provide working room. The opening created increases access to the posterior shoulder. Anteriorly, room can be generated by draining the bladder with a Foley catheter.

The next step is to use the McRoberts' maneuver (Figure 180-9). Maternal leg flexion to a knee-chest position may disengage the anterior shoulder, allowing rapid vaginal delivery to follow. This maneuver "walks" the pubic symphysis over the anterior shoulder, helping the fetus to pass through the birth canal one shoulder at a time.

If the McRoberts' maneuver does not free the anterior shoulder, suprapubic pressure may accomplish the goal. Pressure may slip the anterior shoulder beneath the pubis or cause the posterior shoulder to retreat into the hollow of the sacrum. Digital pressure on the posterior shoulder (via the episiotomy) may help facilitate posterior shoulder retreat. Use of these intrapartum maneuvers resolves most cases of shoulder dystocia. If delivery is still impossible, more drastic interventions are warranted. Decreasing the bisacromial diameter may be possible by pushing the most accessible shoulder toward the fetal chest (Rubin's maneuver) (Figure 180-10). Often both shoulders assume the same attitude, decreasing the bisacromial diameter and allowing delivery. Attempts to manipulate the shoulders for Rubin's maneuver may be transabdominal, via the introitus (anterior shoulder), or via the episiotomy (posterior shoulder).

If the shoulders remain undeliverable, the next step is to "corkscrew" the shoulders through the aperture. Fetal rotation of 180 degrees is achieved by pushing the most accessible shoulder in toward the chest. The fetal axilla can be snared with a digit, or a hand can be slid in along the fetal spine to sweep the hips and generate rotation. Wood's corkscrew maneuver is difficult to perform but should be attempted before reaching for an arm. A slightly oblique anteroposterior position for the shoulders provides the largest passage through the pelvic outlet.

At this juncture, if the fetus remains trapped and several attempts have failed to yield delivery, consideration of episioproctotomy or delivery of an arm is appropriate. A hand is introduced along the posterior aspect of the posterior shoulder. This would be a tight fit, requiring tactile identification of fetal anatomy. The posterior arm is swept across the chest, bringing the fetal hand up to the chin. Attempts to splint the humerus may prevent fractures and brachial plexus injuries. The fetal hand is grasped and pulled out of the birth canal across the face, delivering the posterior shoulder. The mnemonic *HELPER* (Box 180-9) has been proposed to help keep these steps organized and to facilitate a sequential approach. These steps successfully deliver almost all cases of shoulder dystocia.

Face, Brow, and Compound Presentations

Face and brow presentations also yield a larger engaging aspect of the fetal head and predispose to labor arrest. Although these abnormal presentations can be diagnosed with ultrasonography or Leopold's maneuvers, most are discovered during labor via vaginal examination. Approximately half are discovered during the second stage of labor.

BOX 180-9. HELPER Mnemonic for Shoulder Dystocia

Help
  Obstetrics, neonatology, anesthesia
Episiotomy
  Generous, possibly even episioproctotomy
Legs flexed
  McRoberts' maneuver
Pressure
  Suprapubic pressure, shoulder pressure
Enter vagina
  Rubin's maneuver or Wood's maneuver
Remove posterior arm
  Splint, sweep, grasp, and pull to extension

The engaging diameter of the head in vertex position is approximately 0.8 cm less than a face presentation and 1.5 cm less than a brow presentation. Face presentations are described using the chin as a reference point. Mentum anterior deliveries are possible, and many mentum posterior lies spontaneously convert to mentum anterior. The obstetric adage "if a face presentation is progressing, leave it alone" arises from this frequent spontaneous conversion. Brow presentations also may convert to face presentations. Failure to do so would result in labor arrest in term-sized infants.

A persistent mentum posterior face and brow presentation cannot be delivered vaginally if the fetus is full term. The resultant labor arrest requires symphysiotomy or cesarean section. Prolongation of the second stage is the most common outcome of both of these malpresentations at term. For the emergency physician, this prolonged second stage may provide a window during which obstetric help may arrive.

Compound presentations are presentations in which a small part enters the birth canal with the head. Small and premature fetuses may proceed to vaginal delivery without incident.

Labor arrest and umbilical cord prolapse are accepted indications for cesarean section in the setting of face, brow, and compound presentations. Manipulation of a compound presentation, including attempts to reduce the hand or arm, increases the rate of cord prolapse. Manipulations, such as attempted reduction or traction, are contraindicated. Cord prolapse rates are 10% to 20% even without manipulation. Close monitoring and careful examination are indicated.

Multiple Gestations

Perspective. Twin gestations account for less than 1% of all deliveries. Even with obstetric care in a delivery suite, twins contribute disproportionately to perinatal mortality, representing more than 10% of the perinatal deaths.[68] Maternal and fetal complications increase with multiple gestations.

The management of triplets and higher multiples of gestation is similar to that of twins. Although multiple gestations are relatively rare in naturally conceived pregnancies, fertility drugs and artificially induced pregnancies have increased their incidence. As the approach to infertility becomes more aggressive, the emergency physician can expect to encounter more multiple-gestation deliveries. Heterotopic pregnancy also is increased, but this usually is diagnosed before the second trimester. Most pregnancies that follow infertility interventions are followed closely by the obstetrician.[69]

Diagnostic Strategies. Most women with multiple gestations have the situation identified well before the third trimester. In patients who have had little or no prenatal care, ultrasonography allows rapid diagnosis and early preparation. The stages of labor for twins and other multiple gestations are similar to the stages for a singleton. Nulliparous women experience longer labors than multiparous women, with an overall labor duration that is similar to that of singleton pregnancies. Of importance to the emergency physician is a relatively short latent phase of labor, with rapid progression to the active phase. The active phase is usually longer, however. The prolongation of the active phase is due to overdistention of the uterus and malpresentation and may allow time for obstetric assistance to arrive.

Vertex twin A and vertex twin B occur in approximately 40% of deliveries. In the remaining 60%, one or both of the twins has a malpresentation, especially twin B. Delivery problems with twin B cause most of the preventable perinatal mortality of twin gestation.[70]

Management. The presentation of the twins is an important determinant for the safety of vaginal delivery. Twins that are vertex-vertex can be delivered vaginally. If twin B is nonvertex, some obstetricians recommend cesarean section to prevent delivery-related complications for twin B. External cephalic version also may be attempted to convert twin B to a vertex lie and then proceed to vaginal delivery. Breech extraction is a third, more difficult, option. All obstetricians agree that if twin A is nonvertex, abdominal delivery is the preferred route. In such cases, efforts should be made to delay delivery until an operative approach can be used.[71,72] Proceeding vaginally can result in the "stuck twin" syndrome and poor outcome.

The interval between the delivery of twin A and twin B is variable. Although in most cases twin B delivers in minutes, prolonged interdelivery times with good fetal outcomes have been reported. When twin B does not follow rapidly, in utero assessment is important to document fetal well-being. If the membranes are intact and fetal monitoring is used, the delivery of twin B (especially nonvertex) should not be hastened. Repeat ultrasonographic evaluation may help confirm twin B's presentation and well-being during the interdelivery period.

After every emergency department delivery, particularly deliveries that are precipitous or that occur in the prehospital setting, the mother should be examined for the possibility of twins. Ongoing labor may be confused with postpartum cramping, only to have twin B and all of the potential complications surprise the clinician. This situation is particularly relevant for women with inadequate prenatal care and low-birth-weight infants.

Umbilical Cord–Related Emergencies

Perspective

Umbilical cord–related complications can occur in normal and abnormal deliveries. Immediate intervention is required to prevent fetal morbidity and mortality. The spectrum of cord-related emergencies includes prolapsed cord, nuchal loops of the umbilical cord, body coils, cord knots, and entangled cords in monoamniotic twins. Cord length is believed to be proportional to fetal activity in utero during the first and second trimesters. Excess cord length increases the potential for umbilical cord complications of all types. Because the umbilical cord supplies the fetus with all of its oxygen, interruption of cord circulation before establishment of fetal respiration is a life-threatening emergency. Fetal asphyxia caused by cord circulation compromise is potentially preventable with appropriate delivery interventions.

Umbilical Cord Prolapse

Clinical Features

Umbilical cord prolapse occurs when the umbilical cord precedes the fetal presenting part. Most instances of cord prolapse are unexpected and develop during the second stage of labor. Any time the presenting part does not fill the birth canal completely, the umbilical cord may prolapse, particularly if it is longer than normal. PROM also is associated with umbilical cord prolapse.[73]

Cord prolapse has a variable rate of association with different fetal presentations. Compound, shoulder, and breech presentations all yield gaps and a relatively poor dilating wedge. Table 180-6 summarizes the rates of umbilical cord prolapse with various fetal presentations. Overall, malpresentations account for 50% of cord prolapse cases, and prolapse may be the first indication of a malpresentation.[74] Previous series report the incidence of cord prolapse to range from 1 in 160 to 1 in 600 births, with an associated perinatal mortality of 8.6% to 49%.[75]

Diagnostic Strategies

Umbilical cord prolapse may be overt or occult, requiring a pelvic examination to reveal the umbilical cord lying beside the presenting part. The diagnosis also may be made with Doppler ultrasonography.[76] In most cases, the diagnosis is obvious, and the cord is encountered at the perineum or introitus.

Table 180-6. Conditions Associated with Umbilical Cord Prolapse

Presentation	Incidence (%)
Vertex	0.14
Breech	2.5-3.0
Frank breech	0.4
Complete breech	5
Incomplete breech	10
Shoulder	5-10
Compound	10-20
Face or brow	Rare

Management

Whenever a prolapsed cord occurs with a viable infant, cesarean section is the delivery method of choice. If surgical delivery is available, maneuvers to preserve umbilical circulation should be begun immediately and maintained. The mother should be placed in the knee-chest position with the bed in Trendelenburg as the presenting part is digitally elevated off the umbilical cord.[77] It is crucial that the mother be instructed *not* to push, to avoid further compression of the cord. Placement of a Foley catheter and instillation of 500 to 750 mL of saline into the bladder may help lift the fetus off the cord, particularly in the first stage of labor. Tocolysis with ritodrine has been described as another method of relieving pressure on the umbilical cord.

Preparation for an emergency ("crash") cesarean section should be under way. The time from prolapse to surgical intervention is an important factor in fetal outcome. Perinatal mortality rates of approximately 15% are reported for prolapsed cord deliveries; however, if cesarean section can be done within 10 minutes, the mortality rate decreases to 5%.[78] These numbers have implications for the availability of obstetric and surgical backup for the emergency department.

If surgical delivery cannot be done in a timely fashion, funic reduction (manual replacement of the cord into the uterus) and rapid vaginal delivery may be the only options available. The same maneuvers to decrease cord compression are used, and the umbilical cord is pushed gently retrograde above the presenting part. Manipulation and cord trauma should be kept to a minimum because the resultant vasospasm can cause fetal hypoxia. After funic reduction, the development of umbilical cord body coils or nuchal loops is common and should be expected.[79]

The emergency physician should prepare for resuscitation of a distressed newborn. If one is available, a neonatologist should attend the delivery. Delivery without delay is essential, and generous episiotomy should be used as needed to expedite the delivery.

Cord Entanglement

The umbilical cord can become tangled on itself, spontaneously knotting. Umbilical cord knots are related to intrauterine movements early in pregnancy. Approximately 4% to 5% of stillbirths are found to have knots that are believed to have resulted in fetal demise. Despite this association, cord knots can persist without associated problems as long as perfusion is maintained.

Loose umbilical cord knots pulled tight at delivery may cause fetal distress. As with cord prolapse, this situation must be resolved quickly to prevent fetal asphyxia. Rapid delivery and avoidance of further cord traction optimize fetal outcome. No specific interventions exist to deal with this problem.

Cord Fetal Entanglement

A long umbilical cord can become entangled with the fetus. Because the fetal limbs are short and flexed in most presentations, they are rarely involved. Loops around the neck and body do occur, however. Umbilical cord loops can be single or multiple, and there are reports of six nuchal loops. Cord fetal entanglement does not usually result in fetal distress. No evidence exists that these entanglements result in low Apgar scores, and only rarely do they cause problems during delivery.

During delivery, loose nuchal coils should be reduced at the perineum. Loose body coils usually disentangle spontaneously. The reduction process may be aided by slipping them over the extremities or forward over the head. Occasionally, loops are tight enough to impede delivery and cannot be reduced. The solution is to clamp and cut the cord and deliver the infant rapidly, establishing ventilation to prevent asphyxia. The high frequency of nuchal loops (one in five births) means that the emergency physician should expect to encounter this problem.

Maternal Complications of Labor and Delivery

Perspective

Maternal complications of labor and delivery include obstetric trauma, postpartum hemorrhage, uterine inversion and rupture, amniotic fluid embolism, coagulation disorders, and infections. Many of these problems can be managed nonsurgically in the emergency department. When severe, these complications threaten the reproductive future and the life of the mother. Treatment may require emergent surgical intervention.

Postpartum Hemorrhage

Clinical Features

Postpartum hemorrhage is the most common complication of labor and delivery. Defined as hemorrhage greater than 500 mL, it affects 5% to 8% of all deliveries, and it accounts for 25% of obstetric deaths.[80] Postpartum hemorrhage is divided into immediate and delayed categories. The immediate category includes blood loss that occurs within the first 24 hours, and the delayed category is hemorrhage 24 hours to 6 weeks after delivery. The clinical picture is as expected with any cause of blood loss. Shock states may occur rapidly with postpartum bleeding.

Differential Considerations

The differential diagnosis of postpartum hemorrhage is logical, and the emergency physician can identify most cases quickly. The differential diagnosis leads the emergency physician to the aspects of the examination that confirm the diagnosis.

Uterine Atony. The most common cause of serious immediate postpartum hemorrhage is laxity of the uterus after delivery. Postpartum bleeding from the placental implantation site normally is limited by myometrial constriction that occludes the surrounding vessels. If the uterus cannot or does not contract, ongoing hemorrhage will occur. Uterine atony causes 50% of the cases of postpartum hemorrhage. Predisposing factors include overdistention of the uterus, grand multiparity, prolonged labor, excessive manipulation of the uterus, and general anesthesia with halogenated compounds. Despite the myriad causes, uterine atony is a diagnosis of exclusion. Physical examination to rule out obstetric trauma and retained products of conception must be done before reaching the diagnosis. On examination, the uterus is palpable as a soft, boggy mass.

After other causes have been excluded, therapy to augment myometrial contraction should be instituted to prevent further hemorrhage. Two-handed uterine massage may stimulate uterine contraction. One hand exerts pressure transabdominally, while the other supports the uterus via the introitus. Oxytocics in conjunction with massage usually provide enough stimuli to control bleeding. Blood should be typed, crossmatched, and available for resuscitation should these measures fail.

Maternal Birth Trauma. Uncontrolled delivery, macrosomia, and malpresentation all may result in maternal birth-related trauma. Although genitourinary structures are most commonly involved, any of the birth canal–associated anatomy may be injured with resultant postpartum hemorrhage. Maternal birth trauma is the second most common cause of postpartum hemorrhage, accounting for 20% of the cases. Tears and lacerations may involve the perineum, rectum, cervix, vagina, vulva, and urethra. Blood vessels beneath the vulvar or vaginal epithelium also can be injured without frank hemorrhage, resulting in the formation of large, contained hematomas. These hematomas may go unrecognized for hours, gradually enlarging and eventually resulting in hemorrhagic shock. This type of hemorrhage should be suspected whenever there is evidence of ongoing blood loss and no identifiable obstetric site of bleeding (a firm uterus and negative examination for lacerations). Delayed postpartum hemorrhage at these sites also can occur and is often a diagnostic challenge.

Tears. Vaginal tears, especially posteriorly over the ischial spines, should be diagnosed early by postpartum exploration, rather than hours later when the mother is hemorrhaging. The vulva, including periurethral structures, should be examined. Although minor tears may be left, any laceration involving subcutaneous tissue should be repaired with absorbable suture.

Vulvar tears are relatively uncommon. The most common sites of tears are the vaginal, perineal, and rectal structures. Tears are classified as first, second, third, and fourth degree. First-degree tears involve the perineal skin and vaginal mucous membranes without involvement of the underlying fascia and muscle. Second-degree lacerations extend through the skin into the fascia and muscles of the perineal body but not into the rectal sphincter. Third-degree tears involve the skin, mucous membranes, perineal body, and anal sphincter. Fourth-degree involvement extends through the above and into the rectal mucosa. These lacerations also are associated with tears in the region of the urethra.

The repair of these tears and the repair of episiotomies are virtually identical. Commonly, repair of the episiotomy is delayed until the placenta is delivered, which allows an uninterrupted approach to potentially complicated repairs. The goal of these repairs is to restore anatomy and provide hemostasis with a minimum of suturing. Third-degree and fourth-degree tears should be repaired by the obstetrician in an operating room.

Retained Products of Conception. Approximately 10% of postpartum hemorrhage is due to retained placental tissue. Normally the plane of cleavage between the zona basalis and the zona spongiosa results in clean separation of the placenta from the uterus. When this occurs, the placental tissue delivers as a single unit, without evidence of fragmentation. Occasionally, accessory placental tissue exists as succenturiate placenta, but this also should cleave normally and deliver spontaneously.

Any placental defect or evidence of accessory placental tissue may signify a retained cotyledon. Retained fragments prevent myometrial constriction and result in hemorrhage. Inappropriate traction on the placenta during stage 3 of labor can result in tears with retained products of conception, which may cause immediate and delayed postpartum hemorrhage. The timing of the bleeding does not eliminate the possibility of this diagnosis.

Treatment requires removal of the remnant placental tissue. Digital uterine exploration with blunt dissection of the fragments from the myometrium allows myometrial contraction. Normal placental tissue cleaves away easily, allowing removal. Abnormally adherent tissue is not freed by this mechanism.

Placenta Accreta, Increta, and Percreta. Placenta accreta, increta, and percreta describe various degrees of abnormal placental attachment to the uterus. Abnormal attachment results in retained products of conception and postpartum hemorrhage. Placental villi may invade the myometrium at the site of implantation, firmly rooting the placenta and obliterating the normal cleavage plane. When the placenta adheres without the intervening decidua basalis, it is termed *placenta accreta*. In *placenta increta,* the villi extend into the myometrium. In *placenta percreta,* the villi extend full thickness through the myometrium.[81]

The incidence of these placental disorders is 1 in 2000 to 7000 deliveries. Placenta accreta occurs in 80% of the cases. Associated risk factors include multigravidity, prior cesarean sections, placenta previa, previous curettage, and uterine infections. These conditions may cause a defect in the development of the decidua basalis that results in a visible change in the ultrasonographic appearance of the placenta.[82,83]

Management

Uterine Exploration and Placental Removal. In the face of ongoing hemorrhage and retained products of conception, attempts to remove the placenta manually are indicated. The procedure entails risk of infection, perforation, and increased hemorrhage but may be the most expeditious way to control bleeding.[84] Before beginning, good vascular access should be established, and blood products should be available.

The umbilical cord is traced through the cervical os to the placenta, allowing the identification of a placental margin. The placental membranes are digitally perforated, and the placenta is gradually divided from the myometrium. The palmar surface of the hand should be directed toward the placenta, taking care to avoid uterine perforation. After placental removal, the uterus should be explored for retained cotyledons. Removal of any further fragments still present requires curettage of the uterine cavity by an obstetrician. Placenta accreta, percreta, and increta may be diagnosed in this way because these conditions are not digitally dissectible.

Hysterectomy may be required if the retained products of conception cannot be removed. When emptied, the uterus can be stimulated to contract. Uterine massage, oxytocin, and prostaglandins all may be used.

Uterine Packing. Uterine packing to decrease postpartum hemorrhage was widely used previously but now is uncommon. For the emergency physician, this technique may be used with resultant tamponade, preventing further blood loss. The procedure has limited morbidity and is straightforward. The physician introduces 15 to 20 yards of 4-inch gauze with a ring forceps and packs it into the uterus using a layering technique. A special "uterine packer" is available to help direct gauze high into the uterus but is not necessary.

Opponents of packing point out that an atonic uterus may accommodate a large volume of packing and blood without effective tamponade. Packing also may increase the risk of postpartum infection even when prophylactic antibiotics are given. As with all uterine manipulation and instrumentation, some risk of perforation also exists. Because dilation and curettage and hysterectomy sometimes are not available to the emergency physician, the importance of uterine packing as an option is increased. This approach is a temporizing measure.[85]

Pelvic Vessel Embolization. Pelvic bleeding postpartum can be difficult to control. Hysterectomy as a solution requires a surgeon and destroys the woman's reproductive capability. Radiographic embolization of the bleeding vessels by an invasive radiologist is another option. The procedure does not require an anesthesiologist, operating room, or obstetrician and may be more available on an emergent basis.[86]

A catheter is placed in the aorta and fluoroscopically guided to the bleeding sites that are imaged by radiopaque dye. The vessels are embolized with absorbable gelatin sponges placed via the catheter. If no definitive vessel is identified or the bleeding is diffuse, the iliac arteries can be embolized. Because recanalization usually occurs, future reproductive capability is preserved.[87]

Aortic Compression. Direct compression of the aorta against the anterior surface of the vertebral column decreases blood flow to the pelvis and lower extremities. Although not a permanent solution, this intervention is another reasonable temporizing measure that can be used while more definitive interventions are readied. Direct aortic compression also can be used to limit hemorrhage while uterine packing and embolization are carried out. The pressure required often is uncomfortable to the patient, but the need may justify the discomfort. Patient body habitus may limit the ability to compress the aorta effectively.[88]

Hysterectomy. Most postpartum hemorrhages are controllable with oxytocics and massage or uterine exploration for products of conception. Rarely, hemorrhage continues despite the interventions outlined. Life-threatening obstetric bleeding may require emergency hysterectomy. The desire to preserve the woman's reproductive capabilities must not be given priority if her life is in jeopardy.[89] A timely search for the refractory cause of hemorrhage is warranted because coagulopathies may complicate obstetric hemorrhage. DIC can occur as a consequence of placental abruption, eclampsia, amniotic fluid embolism, postpartum infections, and dilution of clotting factors caused by aggressive volume resuscitation. Retained products of conception and dead fetal tissue contain excess thromboplastin, which can initiate DIC. All women with severe postpartum hemorrhage should be evaluated for DIC. As with DIC from nonobstetric causes, clinical signs of bleeding are associated with hypofibrinogenemia, thrombocytopenia, and elevated levels of fibrin split products and D dimer.[90]

Uterine Inversion

Uterine inversion is a serious complication of delivery that occurs during stage 4 of labor. Inversion of the uterus is associated with immediate postpartum hemorrhage, which can be life-threatening. Uterine inversion is relatively uncommon, complicating 1 in 2000 to 2500 deliveries. Uterine inversion is classified according to its duration into acute, subacute, and chronic. Traction on the umbilical cord during stage 3 of labor can cause this problem, although it also may occur spontaneously. Risk factors include primiparity, fundal implantation of the placenta, fundal pressure during delivery, and oxytocin use.[91]

Clinical Features

Clinically the patient notes the sudden onset of severe abdominal pain. Abdominal examination reveals tenderness and an absence of the uterine corpus, which is visualized in the vaginal vault or bulging from the introitus. When the diagnosis is made, the appropriate mobilization of resources should begin simultaneously with efforts to reestablish the correct anatomic position of the uterus.

Management

The highest likelihood for successful repositioning of the inverted uterus is immediately after inversion occurs. If the placenta is still adherent, it should not be removed until after repositioning. Removing the placenta while the uterus is inverted is associated with excessive blood loss. The initial attempt to reposition the uterus should be to push the fundus upward via the introitus. Digital pressure should be directed toward the mother's umbilicus along the long axis of the uterus. Contraction of the cervical uterine segments can create a muscular ring, preventing repositioning. Cervical ring contraction takes some time to develop—hence the urgency of repositioning.

If initial attempts fail and a cervical ring develops, pharmacologic attempts to relax the uterus are indicated. Sedation and tocolytics can be used to facilitate uterine replacement. Terbutaline followed by magnesium sulfate have been used successfully to relax cervical rings. If obstetric and anesthesia backup become available, halogenated anesthetics are potent relaxers of cervical rings. When the uterus has been repositioned, the muscle relaxants should be halted, and oxytocin and prostaglandin therapy should be initiated. Firm manual pressure via the introitus should be maintained until uterine contraction begins, the cervical ring contracts, and the uterus can no longer invert.

Uterine Rupture

Criticism of the high rate of cesarean delivery in the United Stated has led to an advocacy of vaginal birth after cesarean (VBAC). Prior cesarean section is no longer an automatic indication for repeat cesarean delivery. The high success rate and relative safety of VBAC are countered partly by the risk of uterine rupture. Dehiscence of a surgical scar occurs in 0.3% to 1.7% of VBAC deliveries.[92] As more women have VBACs, emergency physicians can expect to encounter uterine rupture.

Clinical Features

Uterine rupture is an unpredictable event occurring late in pregnancy or as stage 1 of labor changes to the active phase. The severity of rupture ranges from simple scar dehiscence to complete fetal extrusion. Significant fetal mortality is associated with the event, and mortality increases with the degree of fetal expulsion through the rupture. Minimal fetal extrusion results in a perinatal mortality rate of less than 1%, whereas complete extrusion results in a 10% to 20% mortality rate. Maternal death is rare, but significant hemorrhage is common, complicating one third of cases. Maternal genitourinary injury also may occur in association with uterine rupture.

Diagnostic Strategies and Difficulties

The diagnosis of uterine rupture is sometimes difficult because pain is not always present. Risk for uterine rupture with VBAC generally cannot be predicted based on maternal characteristics except that women with a prior "classic" vertical incision and women who have had more than three cesarean sections are at increased risk. Intrapartum vaginal bleeding may signal the problem, but its absence by no means precludes rupture. Fetal distress with prolonged late decelerations may suggest a problem but does not confirm rupture. Emergency ultrasonography may reveal the problem, but good sensitivity data are lacking.

Management

If the diagnosis is suspected, delivery should be hastened to limit fetal hypoxia. Emergency cesarean section is the best method to speed delivery and repair the injury. The American College of Obstetricians and Gynecologists guidelines for uterine rupture identify a

30-minute window of opportunity that maximizes fetal outcome.[93] At surgery, the maternal condition dictates whether uterine repair or hysterectomy is indicated. In the absence of opportunity for emergency laparotomy, appropriate interventions remain speculative. Oxytocic agents (especially ergonovine) may enlarge the rupture and are contraindicated.

Amniotic Fluid Embolism

Amniotic fluid embolism is a rare and catastrophic complication of labor and delivery. Uterine trauma at or around the time of delivery, amniocentesis, and miscarriage also may result in amniotic fluid embolism. The diagnosis is usually clinically evident with sudden onset of dyspnea, tachycardia, and oxygen desaturation. DIC frequently follows, and maternal morbidity is high. Occasional postpartum bleeding may be the initial symptom of amniotic fluid embolism, accompanied by lesser degrees of respiratory failure. Central hemodynamic monitoring and inotropic support may be needed.[94,95]

Postpartum Endometritis

Perspective

Puerperal infections affect 2% to 8% of all pregnancies. Operative delivery, PROM (>24 hours), prolonged stage 2 of labor (>12 hours), and frequent or excessive pelvic examinations all have been linked to these ascending gynecologic infections. Of all puerperal deaths, 8% have infection and sepsis as a direct or contributing factor.[96] Causative organisms for these infections include gram-negative coliforms, *Bacteroides,* and streptococci. More rarely, *Chlamydia* and *Mycoplasma* species have been implicated. Infection occurs when these bacteria proliferate and invade the uterus or other tissues along the birth canal.

Clinical Features

Endometritis is the most common puerperal infection, usually developing on the second or third day postpartum. Typically the lochia has a foul odor, and the white blood cell count is elevated. Fever and abdominal pain indicate greater severity, often warranting inpatient care and intravenous antibiotics. A search for retained products of conception is indicated, particularly if bleeding is ongoing.

Management

Treatment in the emergency department is empiric and directed at the most likely organisms. Clindamycin in conjunction with an aminoglycoside is usually used, although second-generation and third-generation cephalosporins are acceptable alternatives.[97] Most patients require admission.

Postpartum Cardiomyopathy

Perspective

For unclear reasons, the postpartum period is associated with the relatively sudden onset of cardiomyopathy in healthy women without evidence of prior cardiac disease. Estimates indicate that postpartum cardiomyopathy (PPCM) occurs in 1 of 4000 pregnancies and is more common in African American women and multiparous women. Proposed etiologies include viral, immunologic, toxic, and genetic factors, but in most cases no specific cause is found.[98] Mortality rates for PPCM range from 18% to 56%.

Clinical Features

Symptom onset varies, as does the severity of the cardiomyopathy. Onset is usually days to weeks after delivery, and symptoms range from mild fatigue to acute pulmonary edema. PPCM is often unrecognized in its milder form, leading to the consensus that the condition may be more prevalent than reported. Dyspnea on exertion, orthopnea, and fatigue may be easily misinterpreted as normal in a mildly anemic woman who is breast-feeding a new infant at home. The emergency physician must not dismiss these symptoms because congestive heart failure and dysrhythmias may ensue.

Management

Treatment with diuretics, vasodilators, and oxygen relieves the symptoms in many cases. Angiotensin-converting enzyme inhibitors are contraindicated if PPCM occurs during the last month of pregnancy (owing to teratogenicity), but should be considered a mainstay of treatment postpartum. Amlodipine (a dihydropyridine calcium channel blocker) also may have a role in the treatment of PPCM.[99,100]

Cardiac function returns to normal in half of patients with PPCM during the following 6 months. Others have residual left ventricular dysfunction and a cardiac mortality of 85% over the next 5 years. The presence of cardiomyopathy after one pregnancy does not predict recurrence during subsequent pregnancies.[101] Most physicians recommend against future pregnancies, however, believing that there is some residual cardiac function impairment. If such a pregnancy cannot be avoided, it should be considered high risk and followed closely.

Postpartum Depression

Perspective

Postpartum depression affects 10% to 15% of mothers and is likely underdiagnosed. Although in many cases it is self-limiting and considered minor, the suicide of a young woman with a new infant is an enormous and possibly preventable tragedy. The condition has been recognized as having important consequences for the mother, infant, and family, even when self-limited.[102] Risk factors for postpartum depression include maternal attributes, such as low self-esteem, anxiety, and neuroticism; poor marital adjustment; adverse socioeconomic factors; and recent life stressors.

Clinical Features

Women with delivery problems and fetal complications may develop maternal despair. The method of delivery also may play a role in the development of postpartum depression. Studies reveal that women anticipating normal delivery who subsequently go on to emergent cesarean section are at increased risk.[103] Maternal self-blame for failure of labor to progress, fetal distress, or cephalopelvic disproportion may result in clinical depression. The loss of the "natural" birthing experience is a significant injury to the psyche of these women.[104]

When unrecognized, these women are at high risk for suicide and may come to the emergency department with overdoses or other manifestations of an attempt. Most women with postpartum depression do not have vegetative signs or symptoms. Early discharge from childbirth hospitalization does not seem to be a factor in postpartum depression.[105,106]

Management

Early identification and referral are the key components of therapy. Dismissal of postpartum fatigue as normal, without considering the diagnosis of postpartum depression, can be disastrous. As with other depressed patients in the emergency department, depression is rarely the chief complaint. Many of these women also fear that they will harm their infants and are ashamed of these emotions. Sensitivity to the possibility of depression is crucial to successful treatment. Suicide in a new mother is a real possibility that must be addressed in these patients.[107] Occasionally the patient requires inpatient psychiatric care with suicide precautions.

KEY CONCEPTS

- Emergency department deliveries should be considered high risk. A perinatal mortality rate of 8% to 10% for deliveries in the emergency department has been reported. To a large extent, the emergency department is selected by an obstetric population with unexpected complications. Antepartum hemorrhage, PROM, eclampsia, premature labor, abruptio placentae, precipitous delivery, malpresentation, and umbilical cord emergencies all are overrepresented in emergency department deliveries.
- Women with the urge to push or with the head of the infant crowning are at imminent risk of delivery, and their infants should be delivered in the emergency department. Otherwise, transfer of a woman with an impending high-risk delivery to a perinatal center must be tempered by clinical and medicolegal judgment.
- Most deliveries require only basic equipment to cut and clamp the umbilical cord and to dry and suction the infant. Given that most emergency department deliveries are high risk, however, the emergency physician must have the equipment and staff available to care for a newborn requiring further resuscitation.
- Maternal complications of labor and delivery include obstetric trauma, postpartum hemorrhage, uterine inversion and rupture, amniotic fluid embolism, coagulation disorders, and infections. Many of these problems can be managed nonsurgically in the emergency department.
- Deliveries complicated by dystocia, malpresentation, or multiple gestations are life-threatening emergencies. The emergency physician must develop strategies to treat each of these potential complications of delivery.

REFERENCES

1. Higgins SD: Emergency delivery: Prehospital care, emergency department delivery, perimortem salvage. *Emerg Med Clin North Am* 5:529, 1987.
2. Pons PT: Prehospital considerations in the pregnant patient. *Emerg Med Clin North Am* 12:1, 1994.
3. Moscovitz HC, et al: Care and outcome of out-of-hospital deliveries. *Acad Emerg Med* 7:757, 2000.
4. Anderson GV Jr, Anderson GV Sr: Umbilical cord prolapse in the emergency department. *J Emerg Med* 7:207, 1989.
5. Harper RG, et al: Unexpected, unattended deliveries. *N Y State J Med* 90:330, 1990.
6. Brunette DD: Prehospital and emergency department delivery: A review of eight years experience. *Ann Emerg Med* 18:1116, 1989.
7. Chasnoff JJ, et al: Cocaine use in pregnancy. *N Engl J Med* 313:666, 1985.
8. Amara H, et al: Violence during pregnancy and drug abuse. *Am J Public Health* 80:575, 1990.
9. Verenson A, et al: Perinatal morbidity associated with violence experienced by pregnant women. *Am J Obstet Gynecol* 170:1760, 1994.
10. Abbott J, et al: Domestic violence against women: Incidence and prevalence in an emergency department population. *JAMA* 273:1763, 1995.
11. Katz VL, Hansen AR: Complications in the emergency transport of pregnant women. *South Med J* 83:7, 1990.
12. Ayres RJ Jr: Legal considerations in prehospital care. *Emerg Med Clin North Am* 11:853, 1993.
13. Strobos J: Tightening the screw: Statutory and legal supervision of interhospital patient transfers. *Ann Emerg Med* 20:302, 1991.
14. Low RB, et al: Emergency transport of pregnant patients: The national experience. *J Emerg Med* 6:41, 1988.
15. Trott A: Diagnostic modalities in gynecologic and obstetric emergencies. *Emerg Med Clin North Am* 5:405, 1987.
16. Paul RH, et al: Clinical fetal monitoring: The evaluation and significance of intrapartum baseline fetal heart rate variability. *Am J Obstet Gynecol* 123:206, 1975.
17. Chang TS, Lepanto L: Ultrasound in the emergency setting. *Emerg Med Clin North Am* 10:1, 1982.
18. Howe RS, et al: Embryonic heart rate in human pregnancy. *J Ultrasound Med* 10:367, 1991.
19. Jehle D: Emergency department sonography by emergency physician. *Am J Emerg Med* 7:605, 1989.
20. Eden RD, et al: A modified biophysical profile for antenatal fetal surveillance. *Obstet Gynecol* 71:365, 1988.
21. Phelan JP, et al: Amniotic fluid volume assessment with the four-quadrant technique at 36-42 weeks gestation. *J Reprod Med* 32:540, 1987.
22. Shiono P, et al: Midline episiotomies: More harm than good? *Obstet Gynecol* 75:765, 1990.
23. Borgatta L, et al: Association of episiotomy and delivery position with deep perineal laceration during spontaneous delivery in nulliparous woman. *Am J Obstet Gynecol* 160:294, 1989.
24. Webb DA, Culhane J: Hospital variation in episiotomy use and the risk of perineal trauma during childbirth. *Birth* 29:132, 2002.
25. Macpherson T: Fact and fancy: What can we really tell from the placenta? *Arch Pathol Lab Med* 115:672, 1991.
26. Salatia CM, Vintzilcos AM: Why all placentas should be examined by a pathologist in 1990. *Am J Obstet Gynecol* 163:1282, 1990.
27. Gonik B, Creasy K: Preterm labor: Its diagnosis and management. *Am J Obstet Gynecol* 154:3, 1986.

28. Travis BE, McCullough M: Pharmacotherapy of preterm labor. *Pharmacotherapy* 13:28, 1993.
29. Canadian Preterm Labor Investigators Group: Treatment of preterm labor with the β-adrenergic agonist ritodrine. *N Engl J Med* 327:308, 1992.
30. Berkman ND, et al: Tocolytic treatment for the management of preterm labor: A review of the evidence. *Am J Obstet Gynecol* 188:1648, 2003.
31. Rodts-Palenik S, Morrison JC: Tocolysis: An update for the practitioner. *Obstet Gynecol Surv* 57:S9, 2002.
32. Beall MH, et al: A comparison of ritodrine, terbutaline, and magnesium sulfate for the suppression of preterm labor. *Am J Obstet Gynecol* 153:854, 1985.
33. Elliott JP: Magnesium sulfate as a tocolytic agent. *Am J Obstet Gynecol* 147:277, 1983.
34. Parsons MT, et al: Thermic effects of tocolytic agents: Decreased temperature with magnesium sulfate. *Obstet Gynecol* 69:88, 1987.
35. Spellacy WN, et al: The acute effects of ritodrine infusion on maternal metabolism measures of glucose, insulin, glucagon, triglycerides, cholesterol, placental lactogen, and chorionic gonadotropin. *Am J Obstet Gynecol* 131: 637, 1978.
36. Groome LF, et al: Neonatal periventricular-intraventricular hemorrhage after maternal β-sympathomimetic tocolysis. *Am J Obstet Gynecol* 167:873, 1992.
37. Sawdy RJ, Lye S, Fisk NM, Bennett PR: A double-blind randomized study of fetal side effects during and after the short-term maternal administration of indomethacin, sulindac, and nimesulide for the treatment of preterm labor. *Am J Obstet Gynecol* 188:1046, 2003.
38. Wenstrom KD, et al: Premature rupture of membranes. *Obstet Gynecol Clin North Am* 19:241, 1992.
39. Janetta O: A new simple test for detecting rupture of the fetal membranes. *Obstet Gynecol* 63:575, 1984.
40. Capeless EL, Mead PB: Management of preterm premature rupture of membranes: Lack of a national consensus. *Am J Obstet Gynecol* 157:11, 1987.
41. Johnston MM, et al: Antibiotic therapy in preterm, premature rupture of membranes: A randomized prospective double blind trial. *Am J Obstet Gynecol* 163:743, 1990.
42. Amon L, et al: Ampicillin prophylaxis in preterm premature rupture of the membranes: A prospective randomized study. *Am J Obstet Gynecol* 159:539, 1988.
43. Kenyon S, Boulvain M, Neilson J: Antibiotics for preterm rupture of membranes. *Cochrane Database Syst Rev* 2:CD001058, 2003.
44. Iyasu S, et al. The epidemiology of placenta previa in the United States. *Am J Obstet Gynecol* 168:1424, 1987.
45. Haines CJ, Stock A: The diagnosis of marginal placental abruption in placenta previa using transvaginal sonography. *Aust N Z J Obstet Gynaecol* 32:174, 1992.
46. Droste S, Keil K: Expectant management of placenta previa: Cost-benefit analysis of outpatient treatment. *Am J Obstet Gynecol* 170:1254, 1994.
47. Mover JR: Placenta previa: Antepartum conservative management, inpatient versus outpatient. *Am J Obstet Gynecol* 170:1683, 1994.
48. Fleming AD: Abruptio placentae. *Crit Care Clin* 7:865, 1991.
49. Lowe TW, Cunningham FG: Placental abruption. *Clin Obstet Gynecol* 33:406, 1990.
50. Nyberg DA, et al: Sonographic spectrum of placental abruption. *AJR Am J Roentgenol* 148:161, 1987.
51. Neiger R, et al: Plasma fibrin D-dimer in pregnancies complicated by partial placental abruption. *Tenn Med* 90:403, 1997.
52. Gilabert J, et al: Abruptio placentae and disseminated intravascular coagulation. *Acta Obstet Gynecol Scand* 64:35, 1985.
53. Bey M, et al: The sonographic diagnosis of circumvallate placenta. *Obstet Gynecol* 78:515, 1991.
54. Hata K, et al: An accurate diagnosis of vasa previa with transvaginal color Doppler ultrasonography. *Am J Obstet Gynecol* 171:265, 1994.
55. Approval of a new rapid test for HIV antibody. *MMWR Morb Mortal Wkly Rep* 51:1051, 2002.
56. Centers for Disease Control and Prevention (CDC): Rapid point-of-care testing for HIV-1 during labor and delivery—Chicago, Illinois, 2002. *MMWR Morb Mortal Wkly Rep* 52:866, 2003.
57. Conner EM, Sperling RS, Gelber R, et al: Reduction of maternal-infant transmission of HIV-1 with zidovudine treatment. *N Engl J Med* 331:1173, 1994.
58. Mofenson LM, Centers for Disease Control and Prevention, U.S. Public Health Service Task Force: U.S. Public Health Service Task Force recommendations for use of antiretroviral drugs in pregnant HIV-1 infected women for maternal health and interventions to reduce perinatal HIV-1 transmission in the United States. *MMWR Recomm Rep* 51(RR-18):1, quiz CE1, 2002.
59. The mode of delivery and the risk of vertical transmission of HIV-1—a meta-analysis of 15 prospective cohort studies. The International Perinatal HIV Group. *N Engl J Med* 340:977, 1999.
60. Landesman SH, et al: Obstetrical factors and the transmission of HIV-1 from mother to child. *N Engl J Med* 334:1617, 1996.
61. Moodley D, et al: A multicenter randomized controlled trial of nevaripine versus a combination of zidovudine and lamuvidine to reduce intrapartum transmission of HIV-1. *J Infect Dis* 187:725, 2003.
62. Simonds RJ, et al: Impact of zidovudine use on risk and risk factors for perinatal transmission of HIV. *AIDS* 12:301, 1998.
63. Collea JV, et al: The randomized management of term frank breech presentation: Vaginal delivery versus caesarean section. *Am J Obstet Gynecol* 129:186, 1978.
64. Seffah JD, Armah JO: Antenatal ultrasonography for breech delivery. *Int J Gynaecol Obstet* 68:7, 2000.
65. Carlan SJ, et al: Shoulder dystocia. *Am Fam Physician* 43:1307, 1991.
66. Nocon JJ, et al: Shoulder dystocia: An analysis of risks and obstetric maneuvers. *Am J Obstet Gynecol* 168:1732, 1993.
67. Morrison JC, et al: The diagnosis and management of dystocia of the shoulder. *Surg Gynecol Obstet* 175:515, 1992.
68. Vecciana M, et al: Labor and delivery management of the multiple gestation. *Obstet Gynecol Clin North Am* 22:235, 1995.
69. Malloy D, et al: Multiple-sited (heterotopic) pregnancy after in vitro fertilization and gamete intra-fallopian transfer. *Fertil Steril* 53:1068, 1990.
70. Adams DM, Chervenak FA: Intrapartum management of twin gestation. *Clin Obstet Gynecol* 33:52, 1990.
71. Greig PC, et al: The effect of presentation and mode of delivery on neonatal outcome in the second twin. *Am J Obstet Gynecol* 167:901, 1992.
72. Gocke SE, et al: Management of the nonvertex second twin: Primary caesarean section, external version, or primary breech extraction. *Am J Obstet Gynecol* 161:111, 1989.
73. Koonings PP, et al: Umbilical cord prolapse: A contemporary look. *J Reprod Med* 35:690, 1990.
74. Barnett WM: Umbilical cord prolapse: A true obstetrical emergency. *J Emerg Med* 7:149, 1989.
75. Critchlow CW, et al: Risk factors and infant outcomes associated with umbilical cord prolapse: A population based case-control study among births in Washington state. *Am J Obstet Gynecol* 170:613, 1994.

76. Johnson RL, et al: Duplex ultrasound diagnosis of umbilical cord prolapse. *J Clin Ultrasound* 15:282, 1987.
77. Katz Z, et al: Management of labor with umbilical cord prolapse: A five year study, *Obstet Gynecol* 72:278, 1988.
78. Migliorini GD, Pepperell RJ: Prolapse of the umbilical cord: A study of 69 cases. *Med J Aust* 2:522, 1977.
79. Barrett JM: Funic reduction for the management of umbilical cord prolapse. *Am J Obstet Gynecol* 165:654, 1991.
80. Druelinger L: Postpartum emergencies. *Emerg Med Clin North Am* 12:219, 1994.
81. Zahn CM, Yoemans ER: Postpartum hemorrhage, placenta accreta, uterine inversion, and puerperal hematomas. *Clin Obstet Gynecol* 33:422, 1990.
82. Shapiro JL, et al: Postpartum ultrasonographic findings associated with placenta accreta. *Am J Obstet Gynecol* 167:601, 1992.
83. Petrovic O, et al: Placenta accreta: Postpartum diagnosis and a potentially new mode of management using real time ultrasonography. *J Clin Ultrasound* 22:204, 1994.
84. Reed BD: Postpartum hemorrhage. *Am Fam Physician* 37:111, 1988.
85. Goldrath MH: Uterine tamponade for the control of acute uterine bleeding. *Am J Obstet Gynecol* 147:869, 1983.
86. Gilbert WM, et al: Angiographic embolization in the management of hemorrhagic complications of pregnancy. *Am J Obstet Gynecol* 166:493, 1992.
87. Mitty HA, et al: Obstetric hemorrhage: Prophylactic and emergency arterial catheterization and embolotherapy. *Radiology* 188:183, 1993.
88. Rilep DP, Burgess RW: External abdominal aortic compression: A study of a resuscitation maneuver for postpartum hemorrhage. *Anaesth Intensive Care* 22:571, 1994.
89. Stanco LM, et al: Emergency peripartum hysterectomy and associated risk factors. *Am J Obstet Gynecol* 168:879, 1993.
90. Gerbasi FR, et al: Increased intravascular coagulation associated with pregnancy. *Obstet Gynecol* 75:385, 1990.
91. Lago JD: Presentation of acute uterine inversion in the emergency department. *Am J Emerg Med* 9:239, 1991.
92. Leung AS, et al: Uterine rupture after previous caesarean delivery: Maternal and fetal consequences. *Am J Obstet Gynecol* 169:945, 1993.
93 American College of Obstetricians and Gynecologists: Vaginal birth after previous cesarean. *ACOG Practice Bulletin 5*. Washington DC, ACOG, 1999.
94. Davies S: Amniotic fluid embolism and isolated DIC. *Can J Anaesth* 47:481, 2000.
95. Green BT, Umana E: Amniotic fluid embolism. *South Med J* 93:721, 2000.
96. Hillier SL, et al: A case-control study of chorioamnionitis in prematurity. *N Engl J Med* 319:972, 1988.
97. Rusnik E, et al: Early postpartum endometritis: Randomized comparison of ampicillin/sulbactam versus ampicillin, gentamicin and clindamycin. *J Reprod Med* 39:467, 1994.
98. Rizeq MN, et al: Incidence of myocarditis in peripartum cardiomyopathy. *Am J Cardiol* 74:474, 1994.
99. Pearson GD, et al: Peripartum cardiomyopathy: NHLBI and the Office of Rare Disease (NIH) workshop recommendations and review. *JAMA* 283:1183, 2000.
100. Packer M, et al: For the PRAISE study group: Effect of amlodipine on morbidity and mortality in severe chronic heart failure. *N Engl J Med* 335:1107, 1996.
101. Witlin AG, et al: Peripartum cardiomyopathy: An ominous diagnosis. *Am J Obstet Gynecol* 176:182, 1997.
102. Jermain DM: Treatment of postpartum depression. *Am Pharm* NS35:33, 1995.
103. Boyce PM, Todd AI: Increased risk of postnatal depression after emergency caesarean section. *Med J Aust* 157:172, 1992.
104. Wolman W, et al: Postpartum depression and companionship in the clinical birth environment: A randomized, controlled study. *Am J Obstet Gynecol* 168:1388, 1993.
105. Atkinson LS, Baxley EG: Postpartum fatigue. *Am Fam Physician* 50:113, 1994.
106. Thompson JF, et al: Early discharge and postnatal depression: A prospective cohort study. *Med J Aust* 172:532, 2000.
107. O'Hara MW, et al: Prospective study of postpartum depression: Prevalence, course, and predictive factors. *J Abnorm Psychol* 93:158, 1984.

Section III **THE GERIATRIC PATIENT**

CHAPTER 181 The Elder Patient

Diane M. Birnbaumer

There are no diseases of the aged, but simply diseases among the aged.

Leonard Larson, 1960

PERSPECTIVE

The population of the United States is becoming proportionately more elderly, with the proportion of people older than age 65 increasing at twice the rate of younger people. In 2000, 12.4% of the population were older than age 65, and by 2030, one in five people may be older than age 65.[1] The fastest growing subset of the U.S. population is people age 85 and older. This group is also the fastest growing population seen in the emergency department. About 35% of total health care dollars are spent on patients older than age 65.[2]

These changing demographics have affected the practice of emergency medicine. Currently, elders account for 15% to 19% of emergency department visits, and 46% of these patients are admitted. This

Table 181-1. **Physiologic Changes of Aging and Potential Effects**

Physiologic Change	Potential Effect
Nervous System	
Decreased efficiency of blood-brain barrier	Increased risk of meningitis Potential for exaggerated medication responses
Decreased response to changes in temperature	Impaired thermoregulation
Alteration of autonomic system function	Variations in blood pressure; risk of orthostatic hypotension Reduced erectile function Urinary incontinence
Alterations in neurotransmitters	Slowing of complex mental functioning
Skin/Mucosa	
Atrophy of all skin layers	Decreased insulation Increased risk of skin injury Increased risk of infection
Sweat glands decreased in number or activity	Potential for hyperthermia
Musculoskeletal System	
Progressive bone loss	Increased risk of fractures
Atrophy of fibrocartilaginous and synovial tissues	Joint instability and pain Impaired balance and mobility
Decrease in lean body mass	Alteration in pharmacokinetics
Increase in proportion of adipose tissue	Alteration in pharmacokinetics
Immune System	
Decrease in cell-mediated immunity	Increased susceptibility to neoplasms Tendency to reactivate latent diseases
Decreased antibody titers	Increased risk of infection
Cardiovascular System	
Decreased inotropic response	Less efficient response to myocardial wall stress
Decreased chronotropic response	Decreased maximal heart rate
Increased peripheral vascular resistance	Increased blood pressure
Decreased ventricular filling	Changes in organ perfusion
Pulmonary System	
Decreased vital capacity	
Decreased lung/airway compliance	Increased airway resistance
Decreased chemoreceptor response to hypercapnia/hypoxemia	Potential for rapid decompensation
Decreased ventilatory drive	Decreased Pa_{O_2} and increased Pa_{CO_2}
Decreased diffusion capacity	Decreased Pa_{O_2}
Hepatic Function	
Decrease in hepatic cell mass	Reduced ability to regenerate
Decrease in hepatic blood flow	Alteration in pharmacokinetics
Alterations in microsomal enzyme activity	Alteration in pharmacokinetics
Renal System	
Decrease in renal cell mass	Decreased drug elimination
Thickening of basement membrane	Decreased drug elimination
Reduced hydroxylation of vitamin D	Risk of hypocalcemia, osteoporosis
Decrease in total body water	Alteration in pharmacokinetics
Decreased thirst response	Risk of dehydration/electrolyte abnormalities
Decreased renal vasopressin response	Risk of dehydration/electrolyte abnormalities
Gastrointestinal System	
Decrease in gastric mucosa	Increased risk of gastric ulcer
Decrease in bicarbonate secretion	Increased risk of gastric ulcer
Decrease in blood flow to gastrointestinal system	Increased risk of perforation
Decreased epithelial cell regeneration	Longer healing times

group accounts for nearly 43% of all emergency department admissions and 47% of all critical care admissions.[3] In general, elderly patients presenting to the emergency department are more likely to have an emergent condition than younger patients and spend a longer time being evaluated in the emergency department.[4] As this patient population increases, their presence will continue to have a direct clinical impact on the emergency department.

PRINCIPLES OF DISEASE

Physiologic Changes of Aging

Physiologic changes of aging affect virtually every organ system and can have many effects on the health and functional status of elders (Table 181-1). Heart disease is the leading cause of hospitalization and death in elders.[2] Increased peripheral vascular resistance with aging leads to an increased risk of hypertension. Decreased inotropic and chronotropic functioning of the heart compromises the patient's ability to respond to physiologic stressors. Atherosclerosis is common and contributes not only to the rate of heart disease, but also to the risk of vascular conditions (e.g., stroke, mesenteric ischemia, peripheral vascular disease, aortic dissection, abdominal aortic aneurysms).

Elders are at higher risk for infections. Decreases in antibody titers make this population more prone to infection in general. *Immunosenescence* of cell-mediated immunity predisposes patients to reactivation of latent diseases (particularly tuberculosis) and may be associated with increased susceptibility to neoplasms. Cancer is the second most common cause of hospitalization and death in older patients.[2]

Fractures are the fifth leading cause of hospitalization, reflecting the high rate of osteoporosis among elders, particularly women. Arthritis is the most prevalent outpatient disease in elders because of the wear on the cartilaginous joints, particularly of the knees, hips, and hands.[2] Arthritis greatly affects quality of life, with patients reporting fair or poor health approximately three times more often than patients without arthritis.[5]

Although the physiology of aging often affects a patient's functional status, laboratory values usually are within the normal range. Abnormal laboratory values in elders should be evaluated as abnormal findings and should *not* be attributed to "normal effects of aging."

Pharmacologic Considerations

Polypharmacy, drug interactions, and misuse and abuse of medications in elders are crucial health care issues. Elders currently consume more than 30% of the prescription drugs in the United States, and this figure is projected to increase to 50% by 2020. More than 40% of elders use 5 or more drugs weekly, and 12% use 10 or more.[6]

Although multiple medications may be necessary to treat the medical problems that occur with aging, significant adverse health effects may result. Underlying medical problems, multiple physicians, changing pharmacokinetics of aging, and treating side effects of one medication with another drug all contribute to this problem. Studies have shown that 12% to 30% of admitted elders have adverse drug reactions or interactions as a primary or major contributing factor to their admission,[7] and 25% of these drug reactions or interactions are serious or life-threatening.[8]

Pharmacokinetics may change with age. Altered gastrointestinal motility and blood flow, decreased lean body mass, increased proportion of adipose tissue, decreased creatinine clearance, and decreased hepatic blood flow all may alter the absorption, distribution, and clearance of medications. Despite these changes, the bioavailability of most medications is not significantly altered in elders. Medication interactions and side effects pose significant problems, however, particularly because so many elders take multiple medications. Emergency physicians unwittingly may contribute to this problem by adding a new medication at discharge that may have an adverse drug interaction with a patient's preexisting medications. In addition, the altered pharmacokinetics in elders necessitates caution when medications are administered in the emergency department, particularly sedative-hypnotics and narcotics. A good rule of thumb is "start low and go slow."

The medications most often implicated in adverse reactions in elders in the ambulatory setting are cardiovascular medications, followed by diuretics, nonopioid analgesics, hypoglycemics, and anticoagulants.[9] Caution should be used when prescribing any of these classes of drugs because they can contribute to morbidity and mortality in this group. If possible, some drugs should be avoided completely.

Narcotics and sedative-hypnotic drugs lead to decreased cognition and an increased risk of falls and accidents. Diuretics may cause dehydration or electrolyte imbalance and should be prescribed with caution. Nonsteroidal anti-inflammatory drugs (NSAIDs) may have serious and potentially lethal side effects, particularly in elders. The toxicity of NSAIDs includes azotemia, worsened hypertension, and congestive heart failure as a result of sodium retention; gastrointestinal toxicity ranges from bleeding to perforation.[10,11] The data support using extreme caution when prescribing NSAIDs. These complications can be seen in patients taking widely available over-the-counter formulations of these drugs. Recent evidence shows a significant increase in cardiovascular risk with the use of COX-2 inhibitors, which must be taken into consideration when prescribing these agents.

With these concerns about medications in elders, the issue of pain management is difficult. Although a "first, do no harm" philosophy is laudable, treatment of pain is one of the most important remedies physicians have to offer their patients. Three major considerations influence the choice of medication for elderly patients. First, chronic pain (e.g., arthritis pain) may need to be treated differently from an acute painful condition (e.g., wrist fracture). Second, the patient's underlying medical problems, social situation, and baseline functional status need to be considered. Third, starting with low doses and titrating upward to effect is the safest way to use these medications.

Overall, *acetaminophen* has the highest safety profile in elders and often is the drug of choice for chronic painful conditions (e.g., degenerative joint disease). Care must be taken to avoid inadvertent excessive dosing, but acetaminophen is safe and should be considered first-line management for chronic pain and acute conditions causing mild to moderate pain.

NSAIDs effectively ease pain, but these agents have a ceiling analgesic effect; increasing the dose increases the risk of side effects without increasing the analgesic benefit. These agents should be used as second-line agents after acetaminophen in chronic or acute painful conditions, and low doses should be used.

Narcotics may be necessary for acutely painful conditions and chronic conditions refractory to acetaminophen or NSAIDs. The common side effect of constipation from these agents can be problematic, and older patients need to be instructed to exercise regularly, eat high-fiber foods or supplements, and keep well hydrated. Because these agents may decrease cognition in elders, starting with low doses and titrating upward as needed is particularly important.

Psychosocial Issues

The problems of drug dependence and alcohol abuse should be considered when treating elders. Alcohol dependence is a factor in 14% of elders who come to the emergency department and is more prevalent than suspected.[12,13] These patients often present with gastrointestinal complaints or after falls or other trauma. Iatrogenic dependence on prescription drugs, particularly sedative-hypnotics, also is more prevalent than suspected. The routine use of sedative-hypnotics in elders should be avoided, and duration of their use when necessary should be limited. Dependence on these drugs may cause decreased cognition, and withdrawal from these agents can be life-threatening.

Psychiatric disease in elders often manifests in atypical fashion. *Depression,* a common problem, may manifest as agitation, anxiety, and somatic complaints, in addition to the typical depressive symptoms.[14-16] Depression often follows chronic illness, loss of physical mobility, diminished cognitive function, bereavement from the death of a spouse or long-time friend, and financial pressures, all of which are common features of old age.[15,16] Social isolation and loss of independence produce a sense of helplessness and hopelessness that may result in suicidal ideation or action. Certain types of depression, such as "late-life delusional depression" and involutional depression, occur exclusively in old age. In addition, depression may be caused by medication side effects or reversible physiologic conditions (e.g., thyroid disease, malnutrition). Elders often respond to pharmacologic treatment of depression but are prone to develop adverse effects from tricyclic antidepressants; selective serotonin reuptake inhibitors seem to be safer.[17] A phenomenon known as *sundown syndrome* occurs in elderly demented patients, who become highly agitated and disoriented after dark when visual sensory input is diminished and the environment becomes unfamiliar.[18]

EVALUATION AND CLINICAL FEATURES

The evaluation of elders can be frustrating and difficult. Elders living independently have an average of 3 medical problems, which increases to 10 for elders living in care facilities. Underlying illnesses complicate the evaluation. Studies have shown that many emergency physicians are uncomfortable evaluating elders because managing an elderly patient with a specific complaint is significantly more difficult than managing the same problem in a younger patient. Use of ancillary services can be increased 50% in elders, most likely because of vague or atypical presentations and complicated medical backgrounds.

History

Obtaining a medical history from an elderly patient requires meticulous and painstaking work. Cognitive and physical deficits must be recognized, and the emergency physician often needs to be creative and thorough.

Cognitive deficits may compromise an elder's recall and result in an inaccurate medical history. Enlisting family members, consulting with the patient's primary care physician, and reviewing past medical records may be necessary. Particular attention should be paid to past medical and surgical problems and to the patient's current medications, including over-the-counter and herbal preparations.

Physical deficits also may impede the history taking process. Sequelae from previous strokes (e.g., aphasia) are usually obvious. In addition, elders often have difficulty hearing, which impairs communication and can lead to dangerous misunderstandings. Because elders tend to lose the ability to hear high-pitched sound earlier than other ranges, physicians should lower the pitch of their voice and speak loudly to ensure that the patient can hear questions, always bearing in mind the patient's privacy. Because hearing loss can be embarrassing for the patient, the physician should address the issue with sensitivity to allow for adequate communication while maintaining the patient's dignity.

Physical Examination

Because of the physiologic changes that occur with aging, elders may have vague complaints that could be the only indication of a life-threatening medical or surgical problem. The physical examination of an elder should be more thorough than that of a younger patient with a similar complaint. The physician also must be aware that the physical examination may be misleadingly benign in an elder, despite the presence of a potentially lethal illness. In addition to physiologic changes that may affect the physical examination, medications may alter the response of elders to physiologic stressors. Antihypertensives in particular may alter the patient's ability to mount tachycardia in response to hypovolemia or sepsis (β-blockers) or may predispose the patient to hypotension.

Fever or lack of fever in elders is significant. Of elders with a serious infection, 30% present with a blunted or absent fever response.[19] The temperature measurement must be accurate; oral temperatures may be spuriously low in elders, so rectal temperatures should be taken when fever is uncertain in a patient with a possible infectious disease. When fever is present, elders are much more likely to have a serious (nonviral) infection than younger patients.[20] Of febrile elders presenting to an emergency department, 89% prove to have an infectious disease. About one third are respiratory tract infections; one fifth, urinary tract infections; and nearly 20%, bacteremia or sepsis.[20] Fever in an elder must be taken seriously, with appropriate ancillary testing and a low threshold for admission. A lack of fever does not exclude infection, and emergency physicians should consider radiographic and laboratory tests in elders with vague complaints.

DIAGNOSTIC STRATEGIES

More diagnostic tests tend to be performed in elders presenting to the emergency department than in their younger counterparts.[4] Increased use of resources is often necessary because the accuracy of diagnosis needs to be higher in elders because they have less reserve. Because elders may present with only vague complaints despite having significant medical or surgical problems, this increased use of resources seems warranted.

SPECIFIC DISORDERS

Myocardial Infarction

The incidence of atypical presentation of myocardial infarction increases with increasing age.[21,22] In patients older than age 85, atypical presentation of myocardial infarction may be typical, and a lack of chest pain may be the rule. Studies show, however, that only 2% to 6% of elders with myocardial infarction have an asymptomatic presentation.[22] A painless myocardial infarction is more common with increasing age and occurs in women more often than men. Sudden onset of dyspnea may be the presenting complaint in 35% to 59% of elders with myocardial infarction. Other presenting complaints include syncope, flulike symptoms, nausea, vomiting, confusion, and weakness. The prognosis for myocardial infarction in elders who present atypically is the same as for elders who present typically; atypical presentations are not more benign.

Infections

Elderly patients are more prone to infectious diseases than younger patients, with greater morbidity and higher mortality from these diseases. Common infections occur regularly, but aging causes this patient population to be more susceptible to unusual organisms. Although immunosenescence is a contributing factor, predisposing illnesses and institutionalization are more significant causes of this increased risk of infection. Hospitalization carries the risk of acquiring nosocomial infections. Instrumentation and catheterization, also significant risk factors for acquiring infectious diseases, should be kept to a minimum, and early ambulation and discharge should be a goal.

Evaluating infections may be difficult because 48% of elders with proven bacterial infections do not have a fever.[20] In addition, the sensitivity of an elevated white blood cell count and elevated band count is poor, about 44% and 32%, respectively.[19] The absence of these findings does not eliminate the presence of sepsis.

Table 181-2. Differential Diagnoses of Abdominal Pain in Elderly Patients

Disorder	Incidence (%)
Cholecystitis/biliary colic	12-41
Nonspecific abdominal pain	9.6-23
Appendicitis	2.5-15.2
Obstruction	7.3-14
Hernia	4-9.6
Perforation	2.3-7
Pancreatitis	2-7.3
Diverticular disease	3.4-7

Several infections, particularly pneumonia, urinary tract infections, and sepsis, occur more often in elders.[23,24] *Pneumonia* is one of the 10 leading causes of hospitalization and death in elders.[2] With decreased vital capacity, lung and airway compliance, ventilatory drive, and ciliary function, the infection takes hold more easily in these patients. Pneumonia likely results from decreased cough response, decreased ciliary function, and increased esophageal reflux with microaspiration. Pneumococcus is still a common cause of pneumonia, but gram-negative organisms also are common, as are mixed infections. Reactivation of *tuberculosis* also must be considered in this age group.

Urinary tract infections have a high incidence in the elderly. The incidence of bacteriuria is 20% in men older than age 70 and 20% in women ages 65 to 70, increasing to 23% to 50% in women older than age 80. Laxity of the pelvic floor and urinary incontinence are significant risk factors in women; prostate enlargement is the most common cause in men. The incidence of urinary tract infections increases dramatically in patients with chronic indwelling catheters.

Abdominal Pain

Abdominal pain may be the most difficult presenting complaint to evaluate in elderly patients. Despite this difficulty, most patients have a specific diagnosis made in the emergency department. Two thirds of elders with abdominal pain are admitted, and nearly one fifth go directly to the operating room from the emergency department.

The differential diagnoses (Table 181-2) of abdominal pain in elders differ significantly from those in younger patients, particularly in regard to the number of serious and potentially life-threatening causes. More than 60% of the causes of abdominal pain in elders are surgical in nature, a rate nearly double that of younger patients. In addition, these surgical causes have a 10-fold higher risk of mortality compared with younger patients.[25]

Because of the physiologic changes of aging, even life-threatening causes of abdominal pain may present with few or no alarming findings, and elders may complain of vague abdominal pain despite the occurrence of a catastrophic process. The complication rates of typically benign processes in younger patients are dramatically higher in older patients. With aging, the abdominal musculature decreases, and patients are less able to manifest guarding and rebound. In addition, the omentum shrinks and is less able to contain intra-abdominal processes. Atherosclerotic disease, with its resultant decrease in blood flow, causes increased perforation rates in diseases such as cholecystitis and appendicitis. This increased rate of vascular disease also contributes to higher rates of vascular causes of abdominal pain, such as mesenteric ischemia and leaking or ruptured abdominal aortic aneurysms. The high prevalence of gallstones in elders leads to an increased risk of cholecystitis.

Because of vague presentation and high rate of serious disease, evaluating an elderly patient with abdominal pain often requires an extensive battery of laboratory and radiographic tests. Elderly patients with potentially catastrophic intra-abdominal processes may not present with a fever or an elevated white blood cell count,[26,27] so adjunctive tests, such as ultrasonography, computed tomography, radionuclide studies, and occasionally angiography, may be important. Because many elderly patients with abdominal pain have a serious disease, the patient should be considered for admission and close observation if the diagnosis is still unclear after a workup. If the patient is not admitted, a prolonged period of emergency department observation or re-evaluation within 12 hours is prudent.

Major Trauma

Major trauma in elders (see also Chapter 37) is relatively uncommon, constituting 8% to 15% of cases in major trauma databases; however, elder trauma patients experience higher mortality and poorer functional recovery for a given trauma score compared with younger patients.[28-30] In any elderly trauma patient, the circumstances leading to the injury need to be determined. Motor vehicle crashes, particularly crashes involving a single vehicle, may result from transient loss of consciousness from dysrhythmias, syncope, medication side effects, transient ischemic attacks, strokes, or myocardial infarctions. These serious medical problems require simultaneous diagnosis and treatment in the setting of trauma and at times may take priority over the trauma assessment.

The presence of comorbid illness and the limited physiologic reserve in the cardiopulmonary and renal systems often complicate the trauma resuscitation in this age group. More aggressive ventilatory support and early use of invasive hemodynamic monitoring are indicated to guide volume resuscitation.[31] Shock is poorly tolerated in elders because hemodynamic compensation is limited, and end-organ failure occurs earlier.

Certain injuries are more common and more severe in elders.[32] A subdural hematoma may occur after relatively trivial head trauma, and chronic subdural hematoma may present as progressive dementia with only subtle "hard" neurologic findings. Increasing ankylosis of the spine, osteoarthritis, and decreased bone density as a result of osteoporosis make the geriatric cervical spine more susceptible to fracture. Preexisting pulmonary pathology and a brittle thoracic wall account for the greater severity of pulmonary contusions and the higher incidence of rib fractures and resultant complications (e.g., atelectasis, pneumonia). Skeletal fractures are more common and lacerations of atrophic skin are more difficult to repair and more prone to infection. This thin skin also is prone to decubitus breakdown in patients who are immobile, even for short periods (e.g., spinal immobilization on a backboard).

PREVENTIVE CARE

Immunizations

Pneumonia, influenza, accidents, and adverse events are among the top seven causes of death in elders.[2] These conditions account for 15% of admissions and are potentially preventable. Annually, 36,000 adults die of complications from influenza and pneumococcal infections, and most of these deaths occur in elders. Immunization could reduce the incidence of clinical and serologic influenza by half in this patient population. The Centers for Disease Control and Prevention (CDC) has set a goal of an 80% immunization rate for patients in high-risk groups, including elders. Studies have shown that the actual vaccination rate falls significantly below this goal; in patients 65 years old, 66% and 62% were vaccinated for influenza and pneumococcus, with the lowest rates among nonwhite ethnic groups and people of lower socioeconomic means.[33] To combat this problem, the CDC has recommended that potential vaccination sites be extended to include walk-in clinics and emergency departments. Data suggest that half of elders who had not been hospitalized or seen their primary care physician in the previous 3 years had made at least one visit to an emergency department, and many are willing to be vaccinated in the emergency department.[34]

Despite this information, controversy exists regarding vaccination of elders in the emergency department. In one study, half of all emergency physicians surveyed were reluctant to give vaccinations in the emergency department, citing time constraints and their concern over delivering primary care in the emergency department. In this same study, 89% of emergency physicians rarely or never administer influenza vaccine, and 94% rarely or never give pneumococcal vaccine.[34] In addressing the feasibility of vaccinating elders in the emergency department, another study found that 50% to 60% of eligible elders want to be and are able to be vaccinated during an emergency department visit.[35] Considering the low threshold we have in the emergency department for administering another vaccine, the tetanus vaccine, it seems feasible that influenza and pneumococcal vaccination programs could be set up relatively easily in the emergency department and could save lives.

Falls

In combination with vaccinations, education about accident prevention in the home could have a considerable impact on the overall morbidity and mortality in elders; falls and adverse events are the seventh leading cause of death in elders.[8] A primary care or social service provider more appropriately supplies this instruction; however, the emergency department may be an additional resource for providing educational services to elders on a case-by-case basis, particularly in reference to any specific incident that led to the need for emergency care. Studies suggest that the leading cause of falls in elders is related to the use of pharmacologic agents, often prescription drugs.[36] Reviewing the patient's medications, looking for agents that might cause decreased cognition or dehydration, and addressing the need for these agents with the patient and the primary care provider could decrease significantly the risk for falls and resultant morbidity and mortality. In addition, informing the patient's primary care provider that the patient has fallen may facilitate education by the primary physician.

KEY CONCEPTS

- Evaluation of elders often requires patience and diligence, including accessing other resources.
- Polypharmacy and side effects of prescription and nonprescription drugs often occur in elderly patients and should be considered in their evaluation.
- Physiologic changes that occur with aging may make evaluation of elders difficult and must be taken into account. A more in-depth evaluation, including ancillary testing, than one would perform for a younger patient with the same complaint is often indicated.
- Elderly patients may have a blunted fever response to infection and a less elevated white blood cell count.
- Myocardial infarction frequently presents atypically in elderly patients.
- Abdominal pain in an elderly patient often is caused by a surgical condition and may require an extensive workup in the emergency department, including radiographic studies.
- Elderly trauma patients have a higher morbidity and mortality than their younger counterparts because of exacerbation of underlying medical problems.

REFERENCES

1. U.S. Bureau of the Census: *The 65 Years and Over Population: 2000. Census 2000 Brief.* Washington, DC, U.S. Government Printing Office, 2000.
2. Desai MM, Zhang P: Surveillance for morbidity and mortality among older adults—United States, 1995-1996. *MMWR Morb Mortal Wkly Rep* 48:7, 1999.
3. Strange GR, Chen EH: Use of emergency department by elder patients: A five-year follow-up study. *Acad Emerg Med* 5:1157, 1998.
4. Aminzadeh F, Dalziel WB: Older adults in the emergency department: A systematic review of patterns of use, adverse outcomes, and effectiveness of interventions. *Ann Emerg Med* 39:238, 2002.
5. Health-related quality of life among adults with arthritis—behavioral risk factor surveillance system, 11 states, 1996-1998. *MMWR Morb Mortal Wkly Rep* 29:366, 2000.
6. Kaufman DW, et al: Recent patterns of medication use in the ambulatory adult population of the United States: The Slone Survey. *JAMA* 287:337, 2002.
7. Willcox SM, Himmelstein DU, Woolhandler S: Inappropriate drug prescribing for the community dwelling elderly. *JAMA* 272:292, 1994.
8. McDonnell PJ, Jacobs MR: Hospital admissions resulting from preventable adverse drug reactions. *Ann Pharmacother* 36:1331, 2002.
9. Gurwitz JH, et al: Incidence and preventability of adverse drug events among older persons in the ambulatory setting. *JAMA* 239:1107, 2003.
10. Jones RH, Tail CL: Gastrointestinal side effects of NSAIDs in the community. *Br J Clin Pract* 49:67, 1995.
11. Buffum M, Buffum C: Nonsteroidal anti-inflammatory drugs in the elderly. *Pain Manag Nurs* 1:40, 2000.
12. Ganry O, et al: Prevalence of alcohol problems among elderly patients in a university hospital. *Addiction* 95:107, 2000.
13. Friedmann PD, et al: The effect of alcohol abuse on the health status of older adults seen in the emergency department. *Am J Drug Alcohol Abuse* 25:529, 1999.
14. Casey DA: Depression in the elderly. *South Med J* 87:559, 1994.
15. Muller-Spahn F, Kock C: Clinical presentation of depression in the elderly. *Gerontology* 40:10, 1994.
16. Jorm AF: The epidemiology of depressive states in the elderly: Implications for recognition, intervention, and prevention. *Social Psychiatry Psychiatr Epidemiol* 30:53, 1995.
17. Naranjo CA, et al: Recent advances in geriatric psychopharmacology. *Drugs Aging* 7:184, 1995.
18. Little JT, et al: Sundown syndrome in severely demented patients with probable Alzheimer's disease. *J Geriatr Psychiatry Neurol* 8:103, 1995.
19. Norman DC: Fever in the elderly. *Clin Infect Dis* 31:148, 2000.
20. Marco CA, et al: Fever in geriatric emergency patients: Clinical features associated with serious illness. *Ann Emerg Med* 26:18, 1995.
21. Tresch DD, et al: Comparison of elderly and younger patients with out-of-hospital chest pain: Clinical characteristics, acute myocardial infarction, therapy, and outcomes. *Arch Intern Med* 156:1089, 1996.
22. Gregoratos G: Clinical manifestations of acute myocardial infarction in older patients. *Am J Geriatr Cardiol* 10:345, 2001.
23. Beck-Sague C, Benerjee S, Jarvis WR: Infectious diseases and mortality among US nursing home residents. *Am J Public Health* 83:1739, 1993.
24. Michielsen W, et al: Bacterial surveillance cultures in a geriatric ward. *Age Ageing* 22:221, 1993.
25. Marco CA, et al: Abdominal pain in geriatric emergency patients: Variable associated with adverse outcomes. *Acad Emerg Med* 5:1163, 1998.
26. Potts FE IV, Vukov LF: Utility of fever and leukocytosis in acute surgical abdomens in octogenarians and beyond. *J Gerontol A Biol Sci Med Sci* 54:M55, 1999.
27. Parker JS, Vukov LF, Wollan PC: Abdominal pain in the elderly: Use of temperature and laboratory testing to screen for surgical disease. *Fam Med* 28:193, 1996.
28. Knudson MM, et al: Mortality factors in geriatric blunt trauma patients. *Arch Surg* 129:448, 1994.
29. Schiller WR, Knox R, Chleborad W: A five-year experience with severe injuries in elderly patients. *Accid Anal Prev* 27:167, 1995.
30. Zietlow SP, et al: Multisystem geriatric trauma. *J Trauma* 37:985, 1994.
31. DeMaria EJ: Evaluation and treatment of the elderly trauma victim. *Clin Geriatr Med* 9:461, 1993.
32. Lonner JH, Koval KJ: Polytrauma in the elderly. *Clin Orthop* 318:136, 1995.

33. Centers for Disease Control and Prevention (CDC): Public health and aging: Influenza vaccination coverage among adults aged > or =50 years and pneumonococcal vaccination coverage among adults aged > or =65 years—United States, 2002. *MMWR Morb Mortal Wkly Rep* 52:987, 2003.
34. Wrenn K, Zeldin M, Miller O: Influenza and pneumococcal vaccination in the emergency department: Is it feasible? *J Gen Intern Med* 9:245, 1994.
35. Rodriguez RM, Baraff L: Emergency department immunization of the elderly with pneumococcal and influenza vaccines. *Ann Emerg Med* 22:1729, 1993.
36. Ensrud KE, et al: Central nervous system-active medications and risk for falls in older women. *J Am Geriatr Soc* 10:1629, 2002.

Section IV **THE PATIENT WITH COMPROMISED IMMUNE FUNCTION**

CHAPTER 182

The Immunocompromised Patient

Michael J. Burns and Mark I. Langdorf

PERSPECTIVE

Infections in immunocompromised patients are more common and severe, progress more rapidly, are more often fatal, and are caused by a wider variety of organisms than in individuals with intact immunity.[1,2] This chapter presents an approach to the immunocompromised patient that focuses on presentation, diagnosis, and emergency therapy (Table 182-1).

PRINCIPLES OF DISEASE

A brief description of the human immune system aids in understanding the defects that predispose immunocompromised patients to disease. Defense mechanisms consist of surface barriers, such as skin, enzymes, and mucus, as well as innate (natural) and acquired (adaptive) responses. Fundamentally, innate responses occur to the same extent regardless of how often the body encounters the infectious agent, whereas acquired responses improve on repeated exposure.[3] Innate immunity is activated immediately upon exposure to an infecting agent, rapidly controlling replication and allowing the requisite 3 to 5 days for the adaptive component to clone sufficient T and B cells to respond more specifically.[4]

Non–Microbe-Specific Immunity

Physical Barriers

The first line of defense against microorganisms consists of physical barriers, including skin, gastrointestinal and respiratory mucosa, and gastric acid. Cutaneous acidity, maintained by bacterial metabolism of sebaceous lipids, inhibits dermal bacterial growth. Only with disruption of this barrier, through trauma, burns, or inflammation, can bacteria gain entry. Mucous membranes are continually bathed in secretions that contain antimicrobial properties, including lysozyme, which lyses bacterial cell walls, and immunoglobulin G (IgG) and secretory IgA, which block attachment of organisms to host cells.[5]

In the respiratory tract, mucociliary transport and the cough reflex combine to remove particulate matter and microbes, but this mechanism is impaired with smoking and ineffective cough, as in the debilitated or elderly patient. Mechanical ventilation or tracheostomy introduces large numbers of microbes that often overwhelm natural clearance.[6]

Gastric acid and pancreatic enzymes have antibacterial properties that prevent overgrowth in the upper gastrointestinal tract. Normal peristalsis and mucosal shedding help maintain normal gut flora. Alterations in these factors increase susceptibility to infection. For example, broad-spectrum antibiotics alter normal flora, permitting overgrowth of pathogens such as *Candida* species, multiantibiotic-resistant bacteria, and *Clostridium difficile*, which can result in pseudomembranous colitis.

Acute-Phase Response

The metabolic changes that occur during systemic infection and inflammation constitute the acute-phase response. The liver is central to this process and manifests a stress response by decreasing albumin synthesis while increasing production of proteins that enhance the number and function of phagocytes and assist in complement activation. One of these proteins is *C-reactive protein* (CRP), sometimes measured clinically as a nonspecific indicator of infection or inflammation. Muscle proteolysis is also part of this response and may result in the weight loss characteristic of chronic inflammatory or infectious states.

Invading microorganisms activate the acute-phase response, which is not microbe specific. The response delivers humoral and cellular immune components to sites of inflammation and initiates antigen-antibody responses. Cytokines, platelet-activating factor, and hormone-like proteins, including interferons, are

Table 182-1. Incidence of Compromised Immune Function in Groups of Emergency Department Patients

Condition	Incidence (%)
Old age	10-20
Diabetes	5
Alcoholism	10-20
Drug abuse	5-10
Cancer	5
Transplantation	<1
Malnutrition	2-3
HIV/AIDS	1-10
Immunosuppressive drugs	2-4
Burns	<1
Renal or hepatic failure	2-3
Autoimmune disorders	<1

AIDS, acquired immunodeficiency syndrome; HIV, human immunodeficiency virus.

secreted from various immune cells and play important roles in mediating this response. Three cytokines stimulate hematopoiesis of their specific cell lines. *Erythropoietin* has clinical usefulness for treating anemia, as in chronic renal failure. *Granulocyte colony-stimulating factor* (G-CSF) is used to reduce the depth and duration of neutropenia during chemotherapy in cancer patients, and *interleukin 11* stimulates platelet production to combat chemotherapy-induced thrombocytopenia.[7]

Clinically, these cytokines result in migration and adhesion of polymorphonuclear leukocytes and monocytes to sites of bacterial invasion. These cells release granules of substances that vasodilate and increase vascular permeability, leading to edema, warmth, and redness, but also allow both phagocytic cells and humoral components to concentrate at the site of infection.

Both erythrocyte sedimentation rate (ESR) and CRP levels rise with inflammation and infection. The CRP rises within a few hours, and the ESR rises over several days. The ESR reflects binding of fibrinogen to red blood cells, increasing red cell mass and thus rate of fall in serum. Depletion of fibrinogen, as in liver disease or consumptive coagulopathy, may make the ESR paradoxically low, even in the presence of inflammation.

Reticuloendothelial System

The reticuloendothelial system, composed of tissue macrophages and their blood-borne counterparts, monocytes, removes particulate matter including microbes from the lymph and blood. The tissue component is concentrated in the lymph nodes, spleen, liver, marrow, and lung and has particular affinity for encapsulated bacteria such as pneumococci, meningococci, and *Haemophilus influenzae*. The vital importance of this non–microbe-specific system is demonstrated by the overwhelming sepsis from encapsulated organisms in patients who are functionally or surgically asplenic.

Adaptive (Microbe-Specific) Immunity

Humoral Immunity

Antibodies

Antibodies are produced by B lymphocytes, and each B cell produces a single microbe-specific antibody type. Stimulation by an antigen (or microbe) causes proliferation of this particular B cell so that large quantities of a specific circulating antibody can be produced. Furthermore, B cells are active in presenting antigens to T lymphocytes, which promotes cell-mediated immunity. Disorders of B cells and their antibodies also produce disease when inappropriate types and quantities of antibodies, especially to self, are produced, resulting in autoimmune processes characteristic of collagen vascular disease. Impairing immunity further, antibodies in systemic lupus erythematosus (SLE) may be directed against neutrophils, resulting in moderate to severe neutropenia and monocytosis. Susceptibility to infection in SLE patients is proportional to the degree of neutropenia.[8]

Immunoglobulins. Five distinct classes of immunoglobulin antibodies exist. *IgM* is the first immunoglobulin to appear in response to a new antigen. Although it has less affinity at binding antigens than IgG, IgM provides some recognition of antigens and begins B cell proliferation before the subsequent development of IgG.[9] Clinically, IgM is detectable earlier in serum than IgG and serves as a marker for a patient's early response to acute infection. *IgD* has no particular relevance to emergency care.

Secretory IgA is the predominant immunoglobulin present in gastrointestinal fluids, nasal and oral secretions, tears, and other mucous fluids. IgA inhibits cell adherence of viral, bacterial, and protozoan pathogens and therefore prevents invasion by organisms through the respiratory or gastrointestinal tract.[10,11] High concentrations of IgA are secreted in colostrum and may be responsible for the lower incidence of infection in breast-fed versus formula-fed babies. IgA also binds dietary proteins, and because it does not activate complement, IgA may shield the body from antigenic responses to common food proteins.

IgE, which is expressed in high concentration on the surface of mast cells and basophils, is responsible for immediate-type hypersensitivity responses. When these cells come in contact with antigens, degranulation of mediators occurs, resulting in the clinically deleterious effects of urticaria, anaphylaxis, and asthma.

IgG accounts for 75% of the total immunoglobulin mass and is more widely distributed through tissues than other types. It crosses the placenta and provides fetal immunity during the first 6 months of life. Congenital or cellular deficiencies of IgG lead to infection with encapsulated organisms because the predominant subtype (IgG2) has affinity for the dense polysaccharides of bacterial cell capsules, such as those of *Streptococcus pneumoniae* and *H. influenzae*.

Complement

Another crucial component of the humoral response is the complement cascade. This complex interaction of

30 proteins is important in producing inflammation and leukocytosis and in recruiting leukocytes to sites of infection by production of chemoattractants. Complement also neutralizes viruses, enhances opsonization of bacteria, and produces bacterial cell wall and membrane lysis.

Both IgG and IgM, when in contact with an antigen, activate the classical pathway, whereas molecules with repeating chemical structures (e.g., bacterial cell walls and capsules) activate the cascade through the alternative pathway. Components of C3, the merging point of the classical and alternative paths, provide opsonization and modulate the response of lymphocytes (cell-mediated immunity). Opsonization is important in defense against infection with *S. pneumoniae*, *Streptococcus pyogenes*, *H. influenzae*, and *Staphylococcus aureus*. The terminal leg of the cascade, C5 through C9, forms the membrane attack complex, which inserts into cell walls and membranes and leads to cell death.

Individuals with inherited complement deficiencies are predisposed to frequent and recurrent infections with *S. pneumoniae*, *H. influenzae*, and especially *Neisseria meningitidis*.[12] The risk of meningococcal infection is increased several thousandfold and most often develops in persons deficient in late complement components (C5 to C8). Paradoxically, the disease is usually milder with complement deficiency, and mortality is likewise reduced 5-fold to 10-fold compared with normal individuals.[13] This suggests that the host response may be, in part, responsible for the severity of disease in normal individuals, although attenuated in complement deficiency, but the true cause of this paradox remains unclear. Patients older than 10 years with meningococcemia should be tested for inherited complement deficiencies because they may benefit from immunization with capsular polysaccharide.

Acquired deficiencies of complement function may develop in persons with rheumatologic diseases, especially SLE. Approximately 40% of patients with SLE have an inhibitor of C5a-derived chemotaxis in their serum that results in enhanced susceptibility to infection.[14]

Cell-Mediated Immunity

Cell-mediated immunity (CMI) generally includes immune responses that are mediated by T lymphocytes, natural killer (NK) cells, and mononuclear phagocytes. CMI is vitally important in the control of infections caused by microbes that survive and replicate intracellularly, including virtually all viruses, some bacteria (obligate and facultative intracellular types) and fungi, and protozoan pathogens. Current understanding involves regulation by CMI cells of all aspects of the immune response.

It has been estimated that T and B cells have the capacity to recognize 10^{15} distinct antigens.[3] The concept of vaccination is based on deliberate exposure to a harmless version of a pathogen, which generates memory B lymphocytes but not clinical infection. The immune system is then primed to mount a secondary immune response with strong and immediate protection if the real pathogen is encountered in the future. However, mutation of microbes (antigenic drift) defeats this memory process, as exemplified by the yearly influenza pandemics that continue to kill thousands around the globe.

Only 5% of lymphocytes are in circulating blood. Most mature and are active in the marrow, thymus, spleen, and lymph nodes. The latter two sites expose T cells to circulating antigen from invading microbes.[8] Specialized antigen-presenting cells in the lymphoid system sequester antigen and antigen-antibody complexes and present them to T cells. Presentation involves internalization and processing of the antigen, followed by formation of peptides that bind to a cell surface molecule called the *major histocompatibility complex* (MHC). Only with this specific presentation can a T lymphocyte become activated against a particular antigen.

Two major types of T lymphocytes are CD4 (helper cell) and CD8 (suppressor cell), corresponding to type II and type I of MHC, respectively. CD4 lymphocytes provide help for other cells in the immune system, including enhanced B cell antibody production and production of cytokines. CD8 lymphocytes are generally cytotoxic and are thought to mediate the eradication of virally infected target cells and certain tumors. Infected cell death occurs when CD8 cells extrude granules with proteolytic enzymes that perforate the membrane. A decline in the number of CD4 cells, with predominance of CD8 cells, is responsible for the increased susceptibility to infection in patients with acquired immunodeficiency syndrome (AIDS).[5] Despite the cytotoxicity of CD8 cells, immunity is reduced without adequate numbers of CD4 cells.

Patients with defects in CMI are at increased risk for disseminated infection with intracellular bacteria, such as *Mycobacterium tuberculosis*, *Listeria monocytogenes*, and *Salmonella* species. The deoxyribonucleic acid (DNA) viral infections, such as cytomegalovirus, herpes simplex, and varicella-zoster, also affect these patients more severely, as do fungal infections with *Candida*, *Cryptococcus*, *Mucor*, *Aspergillus*, and *Pneumocystis*. Finally, even some protozoa are pathogenic without intact CMI, as infections with *Toxoplasma gondii* demonstrate.[15,16] Some infections are seen only below a certain CD4 cell count. *Pneumocystis* pneumonia is seen almost exclusively in patients with counts less than 200 cells/mm^3, whereas almost all patients with toxoplasmosis or cryptococcal meningitis have counts less than 100.

Natural killer cells, another kind of lymphocyte effector cell in CMI, are also important in defense against intracellular infections, particularly herpesviruses. These cells recognize the absence of self MHC but, unlike CD8 cells, do not require the presence of foreign MHC to kill other cells. Beneficially, infection with certain viruses can mask cells' ability to express MHC on their surface, leading to attack by NK cells. However, NK cells also have deleterious effects by rejecting bone marrow transplants because the donor marrow lacks the proper proteins to be recognized as self.

Granulocytic Phagocytes

Granulocytic phagocytes are the cellular effectors of microbe killing, engulfing them and enzymatically lysing their cell membranes or walls. Two major types are polymorphonuclear leukocytes (also called neutrophils) and macrophages (the tissue version of circulating monocytes). Macrophages have surface receptors that recognize nonvertebrate carbohydrates such as mannose, which form the cell wall of some microorganisms. Hence they can identify and attack "invaders" rather than "self."

Eosinophils and basophils, also types of granulocytes, are derived from common progenitor cells in bone marrow. They are less involved in the ingestion of organisms.[5] *Eosinophils* mediate the destruction of certain parasites through release of toxic proteins. Normally only 3% of total granulocytes, this cell type can reach 20% during times of high parasite load. *Basophils* (rare in circulation) and their tissue counterparts, mast cells, have high affinity for IgE and, when exposed to antigens, release granules with histamine, prostaglandins, and leukotrienes, which affect the allergic-inflammatory response with increased vascular permeability, bronchospasm, and vasodilation.[3]

Neutrophils constitute 90% of circulating granulocytes and spend only 6 to 8 hours of their average 4-day life in circulation (the remainder in tissues). Effective antibacterial activity depends on the ability of neutrophils to travel to sites of infection, a process known as *chemotaxis*. The neutrophils move by means of a cytoskeleton, which incorporates actin and myosin, stimulated by complement factors C3a and C5a. The locomotion of neutrophils along vascular endothelium is facilitated by adherence to cell surface proteins, such as interleukins and tumor necrosis factor α, whose production is enhanced in the acute-phase response.[5]

One half of all neutrophils that leave the bone marrow circulate in the plasma. The other half become marginated, adhering to endothelium, primarily in the lung, liver, and spleen. During periods of stress or with endogenous or exogenous catecholamines or corticosteroids, these neutrophils demarginate and enter the circulation. As long as the patient is not neutropenic, demargination causes an increased peripheral neutrophil count composed of mature cells, whereas with infection, an increased proportion of immature (band) forms is typically seen.

Neutrophils (and macrophages in tissue) bind to and ingest bacteria, a process called *phagocytosis*. This process is enhanced by proteins called *opsonins* that bind to bacterial surfaces. CRP, one of the acute-phase response proteins, fulfills this function for certain bacteria, including *S. pneumoniae*. IgG and complement protein C3b also opsonize bacteria, again illustrating the interdependence of the immune system. Actual killing takes place within granulocytes when cytoplasmic granules enzymatically produce potent oxidants.

Granulocytes further control bacterial proliferation at the site of infection by elaborating lactoferrin, which locally binds free iron necessary for bacterial replication.

In addition to phagocytosis, macrophages (located in the spleen, alveoli, liver, and lymph nodes) modulate the immune response by presenting antigens to lymphocytes and releasing cytokines and complement components. Activation of macrophages to ingest bacteria depends on interaction with interferon-γ, a cytokine manufactured by T cells.[5] Thus, the once clear demarcation between cellular and humoral immunity is breaking down as more is understood about the immune system. In reality, the two systems are interdependent for their activation and modulation.

SPECIFIC IMMUNOCOMPROMISED STATES

Solid-Organ Transplants

See Chapter 183.

Cancer

Patients with cancer frequently have multiple immune defects that predispose them to infection, such as neutropenia and impaired T cell and B cell function, which are induced by cancer chemotherapy or by the disease process itself. Other factors leading to infection include defects in physical barriers (skin and mucous membranes), splenic dysfunction or splenectomy, use of long-term intravascular catheters, frequent use of complex invasive diagnostic and therapeutic procedures, toxic effects of radiation therapy, and frequent colonization with antimicrobial-resistant pathogens. Advances in the treatment of cancer (e.g., allogeneic bone marrow and autologous stem cell transplantation, platelet transfusion, granulocyte colony-stimulating factor, implanted central venous catheters) have increased survival during episodes of profound immunosuppression, allowing patients to receive more intense cytotoxic cancer chemotherapy regimens. This has resulted in long survival of patients with neoplastic diseases that were formerly rapidly fatal.[17]

Neutropenia

Principles of Disease

Neutropenia is defined as a neutrophil count of less than 500 cells/mm^3, including band forms, or less than 1000 cells/mm^3 and expected to fall to less than 500.[18,19] It usually results from cytotoxic chemotherapy or radiation therapy but is occasionally caused by the disease process itself, especially in hematologic malignancies. In addition, cancer chemotherapeutic agents and radiation therapy can cause functional defects in granulocytes. Neutropenia, as well as the functional defects induced by cancer therapy, predisposes cancer patients to the development of certain bacterial and fungal infections (Box 182-1).

The incidence and severity of infection in cancer patients with neutropenia are inversely proportional to the absolute neutrophil count and directly proportional to the duration of neutropenia. Although the incidence of infection begins to rise as the neutrophil count falls below 500/mm^3, most severe infections and almost all

BOX 182-1. The Immunocompromised Patient: Factors Predisposing to Infection and the Most Common Pathogens

Neutropenia

Bacteria

Gram-negative bacilli
- *Escherichia coli*
- *Klebsiella pneumoniae*
- *Pseudomonas aeruginosa*
- *Enterobacter* sp.
- *Serratia* sp.
- *Citrobacter* sp.
- *Proteus* sp.
- *Stenotrophomonas maltophilia*

Gram-positive cocci
- *Staphylococcus epidermidis*
- *Staphylococcus aureus*
- *Viridans* streptococci
- Less common: *Enterococcus* sp.

Gram-positive rods
- *Corynebacterium* sp.
- Less common: *Bacillus* sp.

Fungi

Candida sp.
Aspergillus sp.
Less common: *Mucor* sp., *Rhizopus* sp., *Trichosporon beigelii*, *Fusarium* sp., *Pseudallescheria boydii*

Cellular Immune Dysfunction

Bacteria

Listeria monocytogenes
Salmonella sp.
Mycobacterium tuberculosis
Mycobacterium avium-intracellulare
Legionella sp.
Nocardia sp.

Fungi

Cryptococcus neoformans
Histoplasma capsulatum
Coccidioides immitis
Candida sp.
Aspergillus sp.
Pneumocystis jiroveci (formerly *carinii*)

Viruses

Herpes simplex
Varicella-zoster
Cytomegalovirus
Epstein-Barr
Less common: Measles, adenovirus

Parasites

Toxoplasma gondii
Cryptosporidium sp.
Stronglyoides stercoralis

Humoral Immune Dysfunction (Antibody Deficiency)

Bacteria

Streptococcus pneumoniae
Haemophilus influenzae
Neisseria meningitidis
S. aureus

Splenectomy/Functional Asplenia

Bacteria

S. pneumoniae
H. influenzae
N. meningitidis
Capnocytophaga canimorsus
Bordetella holmesii

Parasites

Babesia sp.

Complement Deficiency

Bacteria

N. meningitidis
S. pneumoniae
H. influenzae

bacteremias occur when the neutrophil count is less than 100.[20] Fever in the neutropenic patient is defined as a single temperature of 38.3° C (101° F) or higher or a temperature of 38.0° C (100.4° F) or higher over 1 to 2 hours.[19] In neutropenic patients the temperature should be taken orally or tympanically, not rectally. Even though fever can be suppressed or lessened by immunosuppressive agents such as corticosteroids and nonsteroidal anti-inflammatory drugs, most cancer patients with infection manifest fever despite the use of these agents.[21] Although it is uncommon, immunocompromised patients can have serious local or systemic infections without fever, which may occur with unexplained tachypnea or tachycardia, mental status changes, metabolic acidosis, increased volume requirements, rapid changes in serum glucose or sodium, or acute abdominal pain. Because cancer patients with severe neutropenia or a history of splenectomy can develop the rapid onset of life-threatening infections, urgent evaluation and prompt initiation of antimicrobial therapy in the emergency department are essential.

The most common sites of infection in neutropenic patients are the lung (25%); mouth and pharynx (25%); gastrointestinal tract (15%); skin, soft tissue, and intravascular catheters (15%); perineum and anorectal area (10%); urinary tract (5%); and nose and sinuses (5%).[22] Pneumonia and anorectal infection are more likely to be associated with bacteremia. Bacteremia may occur without a source being discovered despite intensive investigation. Historically, the most important bacteria causing infections in these patients have been three gram-negative bacilli—*Escherichia coli*, *Klebsiella pneumoniae*, and *Pseudomonas aeruginosa*—and four gram-positive cocci—*Staphylococcus epidermidis*, viridans group streptococci, *Enterococcus* species, and *S. aureus*. Many centers treating large numbers of cancer patients have seen a decrease in the gram-negative bacilli just listed and an increase in infections caused by other gram-negative bacilli, such as *Enterobacter*, *Citrobacter*, and *Serratia* species, which are capable of rapidly developing resistance to cephalosporins and extended spectrum penicillins.

Over the past 20 years, infection with gram-positive organisms (e.g., coagulase-negative staphylococci, *S. aureus*, viridans streptococci, and *Enterococcus* species) has increased and has now become the leading cause of bacterial infection (50% to 70% at some centers) in febrile neutropenic cancer patients in the United States, Canada, and Western Europe, whereas gram-negative organisms still predominate in developing countries.[23,24] Most of these gram-positive infections do not result in immediately life-threatening infections compared with the rapid lethality of many gram-negative infections. In the past 15 years, life-threatening bloodstream infections caused by viridans streptococci (especially *Streptococcus mitis*) have become common in many cancer centers and are often resistant or respond poorly to penicillins and cephalosporins. These infections may present with a toxic shock–like syndrome, rash, pneumonia, or acute respiratory distress syndrome. Risk factors include aggressive cytoreduction therapy for acute leukemia or allogeneic bone marrow transplantation (especially after high-dose cytosine arabinoside treatment), profound neutropenia, severe oral mucositis, prophylactic use of trimethoprim-sulfamethoxazole (TMP-SMX) or fluoroquinolones, use of antacids or H_2 receptor antagonists, and childhood.[25,26]

Anaerobes are uncommon but may be important in certain mixed infections (e.g., mouth, abdominal, perianal).

Aspergillus and *Candida* species are the most common fungi producing infection in cancer patients with fever and neutropenia.[22,27,28] They are most likely to develop in neutropenic patients who have been treated with broad-spectrum antimicrobials and whose fever has persisted for more than 7 days. *Aspergillus* species usually produce necrotizing infections in the lung or sinuses. Pulmonary aspergillosis often arises with pleuritic pain, hemoptysis, and localized wheezing. The chest radiograph demonstrates pleural effusion or focal infiltrates; computed tomography (CT) is more sensitive in detecting pulmonary infiltrates compatible with aspergillosis and may demonstrate a distinct halo of low attenuation surrounding a pulmonary infiltrate. This pattern is highly suggestive of invasive aspergillosis, although mucormycosis and other disorders occasionally produce a similar picture. Invasive aspergillosis originating in the paranasal sinuses may extend to the surrounding bone and brain. It may begin as a black eschar on the nose or palate and is easily misdiagnosed as dried blood. Patients presenting with head or facial pain or swelling, or proptosis, should be rapidly evaluated for invasive aspergillosis and mucormycosis. *Candida* species produce infections of the skin, oral cavity, and esophagus as well as fungemia.

Less common fungi producing infection in these patients include *Mucor* and *Rhizopus* species (necrotizing pneumonia and sinusitis), *Trichosporon* species (pneumonia, fungemia), and *Pseudallescheria boydii* (soft tissue infection). Other than *Candida* species, these fungi are rarely found in blood cultures. Specific diagnosis requires biopsy of involved tissue demonstrating invasion by organisms.

Clinical Features

Although infection is the most common cause of fever in the cancer patient with neutropenia, noninfectious causes of fever need to be considered, such as drug toxicity, drug allergy, transfusion reactions, and pulmonary emboli.[17] Fever is frequently the only sign of infection because these patients are unable to mount a full inflammatory response at a site of infection.[22] Usual symptoms and signs of infection may not be present, especially when the neutrophil count is less than 100/mm^3. When pneumonia develops, purulent sputum may be absent, and the initial chest radiograph may not show an infiltrate. Pyuria may be absent in the presence of urinary tract infection. Areas of cellulitis may have diminished or absent induration and redness and no purulent drainage. Tenderness may be the only finding in perineal and anal infections. The neutropenic patient with a documented infectious cause of fever may be difficult to distinguish from the patient with fever not caused by infection. The performance of a procedure before the onset of fever, the presence of chills, "toxic appearance" as perceived by the physician, and lack of localized findings on examination are not helpful in determining whether the patient is bacteremic.[29] Only 20% of febrile neutropenic patients have a clinical focus of infection identified at presentation, and only 30% of patients have positive blood cultures. Characteristic clinical findings may be associated with infection with specific pathogens, as shown in Table 182-2.

Table 182-2. Characteristic Clinical Findings in Neutropenia That May Be Associated with Infection with Specific Pathogens

Characteristic Clinical Findings	Suspect Pathogens
Ulcerative lesions in the mouth	Viridans streptococci, herpes simplex, *Candida*, anaerobes
Necrotizing skin lesions	*Pseudomonas aeruginosa, Aeromonas hydrophila, Aspergillus, Mucor*
Nontender subcutaneous nodules	*Nocardia, Cryptococcus*
Nontender pink skin papules	*Candida*
Black eschar of nose or palate	*Aspergillus, Mucor*
Generalized macular red rash	Viridans streptococci
Right lower quadrant abdominal pain, tenderness, distention, bloody diarrhea	Typhlitis (neutropenic enterocolitis) caused by *Pseudomonas aeruginosa, Escherichia coli, Clostridium septicum*
Perineal pain and tenderness without inflammation or abscess	Gram-negative bacilli, anaerobes
Redness or pain at vascular catheter sites	Coagulase-negative staphylococci, *Corynebacterium, Bacillus* species

Diagnostic Strategies

The emergency evaluation of the cancer patient with fever and neutropenia should include a meticulous search for subtle symptoms and signs of inflammation at the sites most often infected: oral cavity and pharynx, lower esophagus, lung, skin, perineum including anus, bone marrow aspiration sites, vascular catheter sites, and tissue around the nails.[20] In nearly two thirds of patients, the initial evaluation does not identify a focus of infection.[21] Two sets of blood cultures should be obtained. If the patient has a central venous catheter, cultures of blood should be obtained from each lumen of a multilumen catheter and from at least one peripheral site. Specimens for culture should also be obtained from any site of inflammation, including inflamed or draining catheter exit sites. Complete blood count, electrolytes, transaminases, blood urea nitrogen, and creatinine should be obtained to plan supportive management and to monitor occurrence of drug toxicity.

Urine culture should be obtained if symptoms or signs of a urinary tract infection are present, if a urinary catheter is in place, or if the urinalysis is abnormal. Examination of the cerebrospinal fluid is not recommended as a routine procedure but should be done if subtle symptoms or signs of meningitis (low-grade headache, confusion) are present.

A chest radiograph should be obtained even when symptoms or signs of pneumonia are absent. Radiographic evaluation of the sinuses should be performed if facial pain or swelling is present. Other imaging techniques such as ultrasonography, CT, magnetic resonance imaging, and radionuclide studies are indicated in selected cases. For example, pneumonia is detected by high-resolution CT of the chest in more than one half of febrile neutropenic patients with normal findings on chest radiographs.[30]

A stool culture for bacterial pathogens should be obtained if diarrhea is present. *Cryptosporidium parvum*, a protozoan, may cause profuse, watery diarrhea; acid-fast staining or immunofluorescence testing of stool is required to detect it. *C. difficile* colitis may cause diarrhea and occasionally produces abdominal pain in the absence of diarrhea. *C. difficile* toxin assay of the stool is necessary for diagnosis.

Management

Antibiotic Therapy. Broad-spectrum antimicrobial therapy should be initiated promptly in the febrile neutropenic patient if the neutrophil count is less than 500/mm^3 or if the neutrophil count is 500 to 1000/mm^3 and is expected to drop.[19] Moreover, even afebrile neutropenic patients who have signs and symptoms (e.g., abdominal pain and tenderness) compatible with an infection should be treated promptly with antibiotics (Table 182-3).

Many antibiotic regimens appear effective in controlled trials, and none have proved to be superior. Use of a single antimicrobial agent is preferred in most patients, as it is less expensive, less toxic, and there is no conclusive evidence of a benefit from multiple drugs.[31,32] Factors that must be considered when choosing an antimicrobial agent for a particular patient include renal and hepatic function, drug allergies, suspected site of infection, organism suspected, and cost. In addition, antimicrobial resistance for a certain organism can vary even from hospital to hospital in the same geographic area. Thus, choosing an appropriate empirical antimicrobial regimen requires knowledge of the local causes of infection and local antimicrobial resistance patterns. In the absence of a written hospital protocol, immediate telephone consultation with an oncologist or an infectious disease specialist may be of great assistance in deciding on the best initial empirical therapy at a particular institution.

Monotherapy with intravenous cefepime, ceftazidime, imipenem, or meropenem is recommended by most authorities, with an aminoglycoside (gentamicin, tobramycin, or amikacin) added for the more seriously ill patient.[19,22,33,34] Monotherapy, without an aminoglycoside, may be advantageous in the patient with mild to moderate renal dysfunction or for patients taking nephrotoxic drugs such as cisplatin, cyclosporine, or amphotericin B. Ceftazidime-resistant gram-negative bacilli have become common pathogens at some centers. In addition, ceftazidime is the least active against gram-positive organisms, compared with cefepime, cefotaxime, or ceftriaxone. Cefepime, a broad-spectrum cephalosporin with excellent activity against both gram-positive and gram-negative organisms, including *P. aeruginosa*, is now the preferred agent at many centers. The carbapenems (imipenem, meropenem) provide excellent activity against gram-negative organisms (including *P. aeruginosa*), gram-positive organisms (with the exception of *Enterococcus* species and methicillin-resistant staphylococci), as well as anaerobic bacteria. Alternative regimens include piperacillin-tazobactam alone or with an aminoglycoside or single daily doses of an aminoglycoside plus ceftriaxone.

For patients who are allergic to β-lactam antibiotics (e.g., penicillins, cephalosporins, imipenem, meropenem), aztreonam can be used for coverage of gram-negative bacilli, including *P. aeruginosa*. Because aztreonam is not active against gram-positive or anaerobic bacteria, it should be combined with an antimicrobial such as vancomycin. If anaerobes are suspected (i.e., oral, abdominal, or perianal infection) in the β-lactam–allergic patient or in the patient receiving cephalosporin monotherapy, an antianaerobic drug such as clindamycin or metronidazole should be administered. Empirical treatment with intravenous fluoroquinolones is not recommended in the febrile neutropenic cancer patient because of frequent prophylactic use of these agents in the cancer patient and because of rapid emergence of resistance in gram-negative bacilli.[19]

When a focus of infection is identified at the initial evaluation, the choice of empirical therapy should cover the most likely pathogens causing infections at the site. For example, patients with pneumonia may need coverage for *Legionella* (fluoroquinolone, azithromycin, doxycycline, or erythromycin), *Pneumocystis* (TMP-SMX), or fungi (amphotericin B) in addition to standard antibacterial coverage. Agents

Table 182-3. Selected Antimicrobial Agents Useful in the Immunocompromised Patient

	Dosage		
Drug	***Adult***	***Child***	**Precautions/Comments**
Aminoglycosides			
Gentamicin	2 mg/kg loading dose, then 5 mg/kg/day IV q8-12h, *or* 5-7 mg/kg IV once daily	Same as adult	Decrease maintenance dose in elderly or with renal dysfunction
Tobramycin	Same as gentamicin	Same as adult	
Amikacin	10 mg/kg/day loading dose, then 15 mg/kg/day IV q12h or once daily	Same as adult	
Extended-Spectrum Penicillins/β-Lactamase Inhibitors			
Ticarcillin/clavulanate	3.1 g IV q4-6h	200-300 mg/kg/day IV q6h	For *Pseudomonas aeruginosa* administer with aminoglycoside
Piperacillin/tazobactam	3.375 g IV q6h	240-400 mg/kg/day IV q6h	
Cephalosporins			
Ceftazidime	1-2 g IV q6-8h	150 mg/kg/day IV q8h	Both active against *P. aeruginosa,* but cefepime more active than ceftazidime against gram-positive organisms and some resistant gram-negative bacilli
Cefepime	1-2 g IV q8h	150 mg/kg/day IV q8h	
Carbapenems			
Imipenem/cilastatin	0.5-1 g IV q6h	60-100 mg/kg/day IV q6h	Adjust dose in elderly or with renal dysfunction
Meropenem	0.5-1 g IV q8h	60-120 mg/kg/day IV qh8	Seizures associated with imipenem Cross-allergenic with penicillin Broad-spectrum against gram-positive and gram-negative organisms, including *P. aeruginosa* and anaerobes
Other			
Aztreonam	1-2 g IV q8h	120 mg/kg/day IV q6h	Active against gram-negative bacilli including *P. aeruginosa* Not active against gram-positive organisms Safe in penicillin-allergic patient
Vancomycin	1 g IV q12h	40 mg/kg/day IV q6-12h	Infuse over 2 hours (flushing, hypotension with rapid infusion)
Amphotericin B	0.5-1.5 mg/kg/day IV once daily	Same as adult	Refer to infectious disease or pharmacology text
Acyclovir			Infuse over 1 hour
Herpes simplex, mucocutaneous*	5 mg/kg IV q8h *or* 400 mg PO three times a day	250 mg/m² IV q8h, *or* 15 mg/kg/day PO q4h	
Herpes zoster			
Not severe†	800 mg PO five times a day	20 mg/kg PO four times a day	
Severe	10 mg/kg IV q8h	500 mg/m² IV q8h	Elderly: 7.5 mg/kg IV q8h
Primary varicella	10 mg/kg IV q8h	500 mg/m² IV q8h	

*Alternative for herpes simplex: famciclovir 250 mg three times a day, or valacyclovir 1 g two times a day PO.
†Alternative for herpes zoster: famciclovir 500 mg three times a day, or valacyclovir 1 g three times a day PO q8-12h.

effective against anaerobes (clindamycin, metronidazole, imipenem, meropenem, piperacillin-tazobactam) should be considered for patients with perianal or oral infection and those with abdominal pain, who may have appendicitis, diverticulitis, or typhlitis (neutropenic enterocolitis). Acyclovir should be considered for patients with ulcerative or vesicular lesions who may have herpes simplex virus or varicella-zoster virus infections. Ganciclovir may be required to treat cytomegalovirus infection, which is rare in febrile neutropenic cancer patients. Foscarnet may be needed for acyclovir-resistant herpes simplex or ganciclovir-resistant cytomegalovirus infections.

Routine empirical use of vancomycin for the febrile neutropenic cancer patient is not recommended.[25,35] There is great concern about the development of vancomycin-resistant organisms.[36] Randomized clinical trials have shown no survival advantage to including vancomycin in the initial therapy for all neutropenic patients, even those with indwelling catheters. Because most infections with gram-positive bacteria are indolent, vancomycin therapy can be safely delayed for 24 to 48 hours in most patients until a vancomycin-requiring gram-positive infection has been identified. Indications for initial empirical vancomycin therapy include serious catheter-related infections, known colonization with penicillin-resistant pneumococci or methicillin-resistant *S. aureus*, positive blood culture for gram-positive organism before final identification and susceptibility testing, shock, severe mucositis, and fluoroquinolone use as prophylaxis as well as at institutions where methicillin-resistant *S. aureus*, vancomycin-susceptible enterococci, and *S. mitis* are frequent pathogens.

Amphotericin B (and its lipid formulations) is the drug of choice for treatment of invasive fungal infections in patients with neutropenia.[19,35,37] Up to one third of febrile neutropenic patients not responding to a week of antibiotics have systemic fungal infections, usually *Candida* or *Aspergillus*. New antifungal agents, such as voriconazole, itraconazole, and caspofungin, may be indicated in selected cases, but empirical use of fluconazole is not recommended because of lack of activity against *Aspergillus* and some *Candida* species.

Cell Stimulation Therapy. To treat neutropenia, some centers now routinely use human recombinant hematopoietic or colony-stimulating growth factors (G-CSF—*filgrastim*, *pegfilgrastim*; GM-CSF—*sargramostim*) to stimulate the proliferation and maturation of bone marrow progenitor cells and increase the number and function of these committed cell populations. They are safe and well tolerated but are very expensive. Although treatment with these agents after chemotherapy may shorten the hospital stay and the duration of fever, controlled trials show no good evidence that they prolong survival or affect the frequency of severe infections. Use of these agents should be limited to high-risk neutropenic patients, such as those with severe sepsis, multiorgan failure, or recurrent febrile neutropenia and elderly patients.[19,38]

Inpatient versus Outpatient Management. Febrile neutropenic cancer patients can be classified into high-risk and low-risk groups.[19,39] Factors associated with *high-risk patients* include (1) status as inpatient when fever and neutropenia develop, (2) presence of comorbid medical conditions, (3) uncontrolled cancer, and (4) neutropenia expected to last more than 10 days. These patients should always be treated in the hospital with intravenous antibiotics. *Low-risk patients* generally have an excellent outcome with therapy and (1) are clinically stable outpatients with solid tumors, (2) have no coexisting medical conditions or significant focal infection (e.g., pneumonia, cellulitis), (3) are clinically well with cancer that is not progressing, and (4) have an expected duration of neutropenia of 10 days or less. Randomized controlled clinical trials have shown that low-risk patients with fever and neutropenia may be treated with oral antibiotics, such as ciprofloxacin plus amoxicillin-clavulanate, in the hospital.[40-42] An evolving concept is outpatient management of low-risk patients, both children and adults. Hospitalization exposes low-risk patients to potential iatrogenic complications and antimicrobial-resistant nosocomial pathogens, and outpatient treatment allows an improved quality of life for patients and their families. Some low-risk patients may be hospitalized initially, stabilized over 48 to 72 hours, and then discharged home to continue parenteral or oral antibiotics, or the entire febrile episode might be treated at home using parenteral or oral antibiotics. Outpatient treatment should not be attempted without consultation with the patient's oncologist. Patients sent home from the emergency department need adequate instruction and must have support from family and friends as well as easy access and 24-hour transportation to a hospital in case of emergency.[43-45]

Non-neutropenic Conditions

Perspective

Evaluation of the non-neutropenic cancer patient who presents to the emergency department should focus on the presenting symptoms and the presence or absence of fever. Prompt initiation of antimicrobial therapy in the patient with fever is not always indicated. If fever is unexplained, it is often best to observe the patient and perform serial examinations and cultures. Indications for antibiotics in these patients include signs of sepsis, mental status changes, abdominal pain, or identification of a focal site of infection.[46]

Impaired Cell-Mediated Immunity

The T cell defects resulting from impaired CMI in cancer patients usually result from cancer chemotherapy or corticosteroid treatment. The cancer itself impairs CMI in patients with Hodgkin's disease, non-Hodgkin's lymphoma, and hairy cell leukemia. The patient becomes susceptible to infection with intracellular pathogens, including bacteria, fungi, parasites, and viruses.

Bacterial Infections. *L. monocytogenes* is one of the more common bacterial organisms producing infection in cancer patients with impaired CMI.[47-49] *Listeria* infection is also seen in patients with organ transplants, diabetes, cirrhosis, and AIDS and those receiving high-dose corticosteroids. Fever is the most common presenting symptom, and no early characteristics distinguish *Listeria* infection from bacteremias caused by other organisms. Meningitis, which may be accompanied by cerebritis or brain abscess, is the most common focus of infection in these patients and may arise with personality changes or focal neurologic signs. Cerebrospinal fluid examination frequently does not reveal the organism on Gram stain, but protein is elevated and pleocytosis is present. Treatment should be with ampicillin, usually with gentamicin added for synergy. TMP-SMX is the alternative drug for patients with penicillin allergy. Cephalosporins, such as ceftriaxone and cefotaxime, are not active against *Listeria*.

Infections caused by *Salmonella* species are common in patients with impaired CMI, including cancer, and usually present with fever with or without enteritis.[50] Other organ systems may also be involved. Treatment depends on local sensitivity patterns but may include ampicillin, TMP-SMX, a third-generation cephalosporin, or a fluoroquinolone.

Patients with solid tumors, lymphoma, and leukemia (especially hairy cell leukemia) are at increased risk for pneumonia from *Legionella* species, with the highest risk in cancer patients receiving high-dose corticosteroids.[51,52] Non-*pneumophila* species of *Legionella* (e.g., *micdadei*, *bozemanii*) are particularly common in these patients.[53] Clinical and radiographic manifestations of *Legionella* infection in the immunocompromised patient often differ from those in the immunocompetent host. For example, pleuritic chest pain may be a prominent symptom in the former and may mimic pulmonary embolism. These patients can have fever without any other symptoms of pneumonia despite the presence of radiographic pulmonary infiltrates. In addition, the chest radiograph may reveal an expanding pulmonary nodule or cavitation of a nodule or infiltrate rather than the usually lower lobe alveolar filling defects. Hyponatremia (serum sodium less than 130 mEq/L) is particularly common. Although gastrointestinal and neurologic symptoms and elevated serum transaminase levels are common in patients with *Legionella* infections, prospective studies have shown that these are not more common in patients with *Legionella* than in those with other causes of pneumonia. The treatment of choice for immunocompromised patients with *Legionella* is a fluoroquinolone or azithromycin (alternatively, doxycycline or erythromycin, each combined with rifampin).

Nocardiosis is an uncommon but often severe bacterial infection that occurs in cancer patients and others with defective CMI.[54,55] Pneumonia with nodular infiltrates is the most common manifestation, but *Nocardia* may also produce cellulitis, subcutaneous abscesses, meningitis, and brain abscess. Diagnosis requires biopsy, tissue stains, and culture.

Mycobacterial Infections. Tuberculosis and other mycobacterial diseases may produce severe disease in patients with defective CMI and may present as fever of undetermined origin, pneumonia, lymphadenopathy, or skin lesions.[56,57] It is easily mistaken for signs caused by the patient's underlying disease or treatment. Disseminated nontuberculous mycobacterial infections are more common in patients with hairy cell leukemia or chronic myelogenous leukemia. Fever, cough, and weight loss are usual symptoms.

Fungal Infections. Infection with *Cryptococcus neoformans* is common in patients with Hodgkin's and non-Hodgkin's lymphoma, chronic myelogenous leukemia, and chronic lymphocytic leukemia, especially those taking high-dose corticosteroids.[58] Meningitis is the most common manifestation, often arising with low-grade fever and subacute headache.

Impaired CMI in cancer patients may result in reactivation of *Histoplasma capsulatum* and *Coccidioides immitis* with resultant disseminated disease. Infections with *Candida* species are also common in cancer patients with defective CMI, but disseminated disease is less likely than in patients with neutropenia. Invasive aspergillosis may develop in cancer patients receiving high-dose corticosteroids, but not as commonly as in those with organ transplants or prolonged neutropenia. *Pneumocystis jirovecii* (formerly *carinii*) pneumonia is most common in patients with AIDS, leukemia, and lymphoma and in patients with solid tumors taking high doses of corticosteroids.

Parasitic Infections. Reactivation of central nervous system infection with the protozoan *T. gondii* occurs most often in cancer patients with lymphoma and leukemia. *Strongyloides stercoralis* is the only helminthic organism producing severe infection in patients with deficient CMI, almost exclusively in those receiving high-dose corticosteroids.[59] Larvae of the parasite disseminate from intestine to the lung and other organs. Wheezing, cough, dyspnea, and hemoptysis are common symptoms. Chest radiographs may show focal or diffuse infiltrates. Dissemination is often accompanied by bacterial infections, usually caused by enteric gram-negative bacilli carried by the parasites from the intestinal tract. Diagnosis includes examination of sputum and stool for parasites. The treatment of choice is thiabendazole or ivermectin.

Viral Infections. The most common viruses producing serious infections in cancer patients with defective CMI are varicella-zoster, herpes simplex, and cytomegalovirus.[60] Visceral dissemination is common in primary varicella in nonimmune children and adults. When an immunocompromised child or adult is exposed to varicella, varicella-zoster immune globulin can be given within 72 hours of exposure to ameliorate the disease. Herpes zoster infection is common in cancer patients, particularly those with Hodgkin's and non-Hodgkin's lymphoma and leukemia. Disease usually remains localized to the primary dermatome, but dissemination occurs in approximately 11% of cancer patients. Dissemination is usually limited to the skin, but visceral involvement (lung, liver) occasionally occurs. Skin lesions in primary varicella or zoster often become hemorrhagic in these patients. Reactivation of herpes simplex virus is common in these patients, resulting in severe mucocutaneous infection in oral or genital areas. Spread may occur to the esophagus, lungs, or other organs. Herpetic lesions in cancer patients tend to be larger and deeper than in the immunocompetent patient. Acyclovir given intravenously is the treatment of choice for varicella-zoster and herpes simplex infections in immunocompromised patients, but some authorities recommend oral famciclovir or valacyclovir for stable patients to avoid hospitalization.

Cytomegalovirus infection may occur in cancer patients treated with corticosteroids. Measles virus, although uncommon, may produce severe infection in cancer patients with defective CMI. Fever, rash, pneumonia, and encephalitis are common manifestations. Immune serum globulin may be given after exposure to ameliorate disease. Common community respiratory viruses, such as respiratory syncytial virus, influenza, and adenovirus, may produce severe or fatal pneumonia in immunocompromised patients with cancer.[60]

Humoral Immune (B Cell) Defects

Hypogammaglobulinemia is common in patients with chronic lymphocytic leukemia and myeloma. Low immunoglobulin levels predispose these patients to infections with encapsulated bacteria, such as *S. pneumoniae*, *H. influenzae*, and *N. meningitidis*.[61,62] Pneumonia is the most common manifestation, but sepsis, otitis media, cellulitis, and urinary tract infection may occur. After receiving cytotoxic agents and corticosteroids for treatment, these patients become susceptible to infections associated with impaired CMI as well as bacterial infections caused by *S. aureus* and gram-negative bacilli. Regular infusions of intravenous immunoglobulin may decrease the incidence of infection in these patients but may not result in improvement in quality or duration of life and are probably not cost effective. They should receive pneumococcal vaccine, but many do not respond.

Disruption of Natural Barriers

Disruption of natural anatomic barriers (e.g., mucous membranes, skin) by ulcerating tumors, chemotherapy, radiation, diagnostic and therapeutic procedures, and catheters can lead to infection by gram-positive and gram-negative organisms, including anaerobes.[63] Oral mucositis, a debilitating and intensely painful condition associated with radiation therapy and high-dose chemotherapy, frequently results in serious local and systemic infections, including life-threatening sepsis with viridans streptococci.[64] Cancers may cause partial or total obstruction of body lumens and cavities. Stenosis of a lumen may result from radiation. Bronchial obstruction by tumor can lead to pneumonia. Obstruction of the urinary tract may result in infection. Gastrointestinal tract obstruction can lead to perforation and peritonitis.

Opportunistic Infections Mimicking Neoplasm

In patients with cancer, infectious agents can produce laboratory, radiologic, or physical findings that resemble those caused by the spread of tumor. For example, mass lesions in the brain caused by *Nocardia* or *Toxoplasma* can be mistaken for cancer metastases. *Aspergillus*, *Mucor*, *Rhizopus*, and related fungi invade blood vessel walls and produce thrombosis, which may result in Budd-Chiari syndrome (hepatic vein obstruction), nephrotic syndrome, or oculomotor palsy that may be incorrectly attributed to the spread of tumor. Renal vein thrombosis can be caused by infection with gram-negative bacilli. *Candida* fungus balls may develop in one or both ureters, producing a picture of postrenal obstructive uropathy. *Histoplasma*, *Pneumocystis*, *Legionella*, *Aspergillus*, *Nocardia*, and other organisms can produce pulmonary nodules in patients with cancer and be mistaken for pulmonary metastases.

Pulmonary Infections in the Immunocompromised Patient

In neutropenic cancer patients, pneumonia is commonly caused by gram-negative bacilli early in neutropenia and fungal organisms such as *Aspergillus* late. In those with impaired CMI, cytomegalovirus, *Pneumocystis*, *Legionella*, *Nocardia*, mycobacteria, and fungal infections predominate. Pneumococcal pneumonia is most common in patients with impaired humoral immunity. Patients with primary lung cancer or with pulmonary metastases from other cancers develop postobstructive pneumonia, lung abscess, and empyema related to *S. aureus*, gram-negative bacilli, and anaerobes. Mimics of pneumonia in the immunocompromised host include pulmonary emboli and infarction, congestive heart failure, metastatic or primary carcinoma, lymphangitic spread of carcinoma, alveolar hemorrhage, leukoagglutinin reactions, and radiation- and drug-induced pneumonitis. An acute presentation of "pneumonia" suggests bacterial pneumonia, pulmonary emboli, congestive heart failure, or pulmonary hemorrhage. Subacute presentation suggests a fungal, nocardial, mycobacterial, or viral etiology.[65,66]

Diabetes

Diabetic patients have increased susceptibility to infection because of defects in immune function, provision of substrate for fungal and bacterial growth, vascular insufficiency related to microangiopathy and atherosclerosis, and sensory neuropathy that leads to wound neglect.[67-69]

All steps of neutrophil and monocyte/macrophage function are impaired in diabetic patients, including adherence to bacteria, chemotaxis, phagocytosis, and intracellular killing. These defects are exacerbated by hyperglycemia and improved by tight glucose control. Although decreased lymphocyte proliferative responses to phytohemagglutinin and certain pathogens have been described, cellular immunity appears to be normal or only minimally affected by diabetes. Humoral immunity is normal in diabetics.

Infections seen with increased frequency in diabetic patients include rhinocerebral mucormycosis, malignant (or necrotizing) otitis externa, pneumonia caused by *S. aureus* and gram-negative bacilli, tuberculosis, emphysematous cholecystitis, urinary tract infections including emphysematous cystitis and pyelonephritis, necrotizing fasciitis involving the perineum and lower extremities (usually polymicrobial), and foot infections with osteomyelitis. Diabetics are not more likely to develop pneumococcal pneumonia but are more likely to become bacteremic and have a higher mortality rate.

Alcoholism and Cirrhosis

Alcohol consumption predisposes to infection through direct suppression of the immune system, alterations in blood flow, depression of mental status, and delay in seeking medical care.[70]

Numerous immunologic abnormalities are present in patients with alcoholic cirrhosis.[71] There is deficient hepatic clearance and killing of bacteria by reticuloendothelial cells, as well as splenic hypofunction. Complement deficiency occurs because the liver is the primary site of C3 synthesis. Neutrophils show defective chemotaxis.[72] Cellular immune deficiency occurs and is exacerbated by malnutrition. Bactericidal activity of IgM antibody against gram-negative pathogens such as *E. coli* and *H. influenzae* is decreased.

Acute ethanol intoxication is associated with granulocytopenia and diminished leukocyte mobilization and is reversible with abstinence. Ethanol intoxication interferes with most respiratory tract defense mechanisms, resulting in alterations of normal flora, impaired mechanical and cellular clearance because of a suppressed cough reflex, decreased ciliary motility, and resultant aspiration. These effects are often compounded by malnutrition, cigarette smoking, and chronic lung disease. Alcoholics exhibit an increased incidence of oropharyngeal colonization by gram-negative bacteria (35% to 59% of ambulatory alcoholic patients) compared with control subjects (14% to 18%). Alcoholics are also more likely to aspirate because of loss of reflex glottic closure associated with acute intoxication, withdrawal seizures, and encephalopathy.

Infections occurring with increased frequency in patients with alcoholism and cirrhosis include spontaneous bacteremia and sepsis caused by *E. coli*, *K. pneumoniae*, *Salmonella*, streptococci, *Vibrio vulnificus*, and *Aeromonas*; spontaneous bacterial peritonitis, usually caused by *E. coli*, *K. pneumoniae*, *S. pneumoniae*, or enterococci; pneumonia related to pneumococci, gram-negative bacilli (*E. coli*, *K. pneumoniae*, *H. influenzae*), and anaerobes; tuberculosis; meningitis caused by *S. pneumoniae* and *L. monocytogenes*; and skin and soft tissue infections with *S. aureus*, streptococci, and gram-negative bacilli. Nasopharyngeal and cutaneous diphtheria also occurs.[73]

Renal Failure

Infections cause up to 20% of all deaths among patients with chronic renal failure and are the second most common cause of mortality after coronary artery disease.[74,75] Disruption of cutaneous barriers at vascular access sites and peritoneal dialysis catheter sites as well as numerous immune system defects are mainly responsible for the increased incidence of infection. Uremic pruritus with excoriation, epidermal and sweat gland atrophy, dryness, and vesicular eruptions also compromise the cutaneous barrier. Reduced renal clearance of unknown toxins, nutritional deficiencies, and administration of immunosuppressive medications lead to aberrant immune regulation early in the course of renal failure. Neutrophils show reduced mobility, chemotaxis, adherence, phagocytosis, and intracellular bactericidal activity, and leukopenia is commonly present.

CMI is severely impaired, with decreased activation and proliferation of T lymphocytes and reduced NK cell activity, which cannot be reversed by hemodialysis. Furthermore, humoral immunity is adversely affected, resulting in deficient production of certain IgG subclass antibodies. Poor response to vaccines is common but can be improved by reinforced vaccination schedules, increased vaccine dosage, and adjunct immunomodulators.[76]

Additional predisposing factors to infection in uremic patients include low serum albumin, iron overload, increased intracellular calcium, circulating low-molecular-weight uremic toxins, metabolic acidosis, circulating inhibitors to chemotactic factors, decreased production of endogenous pyrogens, and invasive vascular procedures for dialysis access.

Skin and soft tissue infections, especially those caused by *S. aureus*, are a major cause of infectious morbidity and mortality and are particularly severe in diabetics and in those with peripheral vascular disease or peripheral neuropathy. Vascular access site infections are frequent, usually caused by *S. aureus* but occasionally gram-negative bacilli and enterococci. Bacteremia may lead to hematogenous osteomyelitis, usually involving the ribs or thoracic vertebrae, as well as endocarditis, meningitis, epidural abscess, and septic arthritis. Although the incidence of pneumonia is not increased overall in renal failure, it is often more severe, and there is an increased incidence of *Legionella* pneumonia. Tuberculosis as well as fungal infections caused by *Candida* species, *Cryptococcus*, *Histoplasma*, and *Coccidioides* occur with increased frequency. In addition, *C. difficile* colitis occurs more frequently and is more severe in patients with chronic renal failure. Infections of the urinary tract are more prevalent, with urinary bladder catheterization the most frequent predisposing factor. There is a poor correlation between the presence of pyuria and urinary tract infection in these patients. *Candida* infection of the urinary tract may develop in patients with chronic renal failure treated with broad-spectrum antibiotics.

Up to two thirds of patients receiving chronic ambulatory peritoneal dialysis have peritonitis in their first year, and one third may be forced to discontinue dialysis because of recurrent infections. *S. aureus* and *S. epidermidis* predominate, followed by streptococci, gram-negative bacilli, and *Candida* species.

Splenectomy and Functional Asplenia

The spleen is the most important organ in the reticuloendothelial system and is the primary site for IgM synthesis, the first early immune response of the body. Opsonin production in the spleen facilitates phagocytosis of bacteria by intracellular macrophages. Patients without a spleen also have decreased production of neutrophils, NK cells, and immunomodulating cytokines.[77]

The spleen is the principal site of clearance of pneumococci from the blood. Splenectomy or functional asplenia predisposes to overwhelming pneumococcal infection and fulminant infection with other encapsulated organisms (*H. influenzae*, *N. meningitidis*, and *Capnocytophaga canimorsus* after dog bites) and gram-negative bacilli (*E. coli*, *P. aeruginosa*). Asplenic persons who become infected with *Babesia microti*, a malaria-like protozoan transmitted by tick bite in the United States, develop severe and often fatal hemolysis. Ehrlichiosis, another tick-borne infection, is severe and sometimes fatal in asplenic patients. In addition, the gram-negative coccobacillus *Bordetella holmesii* produces a non–life-threatening acute febrile illness with bacteremia in patients with asplenia. Pneumococcal sepsis represents 50% to 90% of cases. Most healthy adults who die after fulminating pneumococcal sepsis have had a splenectomy or have a congenitally small or abnormal spleen.[78-81]

Children younger than 2 years are at the greatest risk for overwhelming pneumococcal sepsis. The risk is highest in the first few years after splenectomy but persists throughout life. Persons undergoing splenectomy for a hematologic disorder or lymphoma are at much higher risk for overwhelming postsplenectomy infection than those undergoing splenectomy for trauma. This is probably because of the occurrence of splenic implants (splenosis) or accessory spleens in traumatized patients. Patients with autosplenectomy from sickle cell anemia are at high risk for overwhelming bacterial infections as well. Patients may present with sepsis syndrome or with meningitis or pneumonia.

Splenectomy may be performed in several types of cancer, including Hodgkin's lymphoma, chronic lymphocytic leukemia, chronic myelogenous leukemia, and hairy cell leukemia. Infections in the early postoperative period (30 to 60 days) are common and include pneumonia, wound infections, urinary tract infections, sepsis, and intra-abdominal abscesses. Later, serious infections from pneumococci, meningococci, and *H. influenzae* increase, similar to those in patients without cancer who have had splenectomy or functional asplenia.

Functional hyposplenism occurs in a variety of conditions besides sickle cell disease, including hereditary spherocytosis, hemoglobin SC disease, ulcerative colitis, celiac disease, sarcoidosis, amyloidosis, rheumatoid arthritis, and SLE. The presence of anatomic or functional hyposplenism may be recognized by finding Howell-Jolly bodies in red blood cells on a peripheral blood smear.

When overwhelming postsplenectomy infection occurs, often no obvious source of infection is found. Initial influenza-like symptoms, such as fever, rigors, malaise, myalgias, headache, and vomiting, are followed by rapid progression to septic shock with disseminated intravascular coagulation, purpura, and multiorgan dysfunction. The mortality rate is high. In addition, meningitis without overwhelming infection or shock is a common presentation of pneumococcal infection in asplenic patients.[82] When fever develops in a person at risk for this disorder, treatment with an antimicrobial agent effective against *S. pneumoniae* should be initiated without delay.

Use of pneumococcal vaccine in patients at risk is especially important now that antimicrobial-resistant *S. pneumoniae* have become prevalent. Asplenic persons should be immunized against pneumococcus, *Hemophilus influenzae* type B, influenza virus, and possibly meningococcus. Persons with functional hyposplenism related to serious underlying diseases often respond poorly to pneumococcal vaccine. Prophylaxis with oral penicillin or amoxicillin should be taken for 2 to 5 years after splenectomy, up to age 21. These patients should have standby antibiotics at home and should be provided with information and a medical alert bracelet. Fatal pneumococcal infection has occurred in patients immunized with pneumococcal vaccine who are also taking penicillin.

An emergency department–based pneumococcal vaccine program, if implemented, could reduce mortality in high-risk patients while remaining cost effective.[83]

IMMUNOSUPPRESSIVE THERAPY

Corticosteroids

High doses of corticosteroids alter the distribution and function of neutrophils, monocytes, and lymphocytes, resulting in profound effects on the immune system. Corticosteroids suppress inflammation and enhance susceptibility to infection by impairing the mobilization and function of neutrophils and mononuclear cells at sites of primary lodgment of microorganisms in tissues. Corticosteroids produce decreased chemotaxis of neutrophils and monocytes and inhibit phagocytosis and intracellular killing of microorganisms. Corticosteroids also severely impair CMI, probably a result of inhibition of the migration of lymphocytes to the site of antigen challenge, inhibition of lymphokine production, and consequent inhibition of lymphocyte proliferation. Moreover, patients receiving high-dose corticosteroids have infection risks related to anatomic abnormalities of the underlying disease, treatment with other immunosuppressive agents, cancer chemotherapeutic agents, radiation, and implantation of foreign bodies.[84-86]

Acute administration of corticosteroids produces marked alterations in circulating leukocyte numbers. Basophils, eosinophils, and monocytes decrease, whereas neutrophils are increased. These changes occur within 4 to 6 hours and abate by 24 to 48 hours after a single steroid dose. There is a redistribution of lymphocytes, predominately T cells, out of the circulation, resulting in lymphocytopenia. Acute or chronic corticosteroid therapy has little effect on serum immunoglobulin levels.

The most common infections occurring in patients receiving high-dose corticosteroids are those caused by pyogenic bacteria (*S. aureus*, streptococci, and gram-negative bacilli). Despite the profound depression of CMI that occurs in patients taking corticosteroids, these patients generally have few infections commonly recognized as associated with defective CMI. The most common are tuberculosis and severe or disseminated infections caused by varicella-zoster and herpes simplex viruses. Patients receiving moderate doses of corticosteroids for asthma and other disorders are at increased risk for lethal primary varicella infection.[87] Other infections seen with corticosteroid use include those caused by *Listeria*, *Salmonella*, *Legionella*, *Nocardia*, invasive fungi, *Pneumocystis*, *Cryptosporidium*, and *Strongyloides*. Patients with neurologic diseases have much higher rates of infectious complications than patients with intestinal, hepatic, or renal disease. The infectious complications related to corticosteroid use increase with doses of prednisone equivalents of greater than 20 mg/day in adults, with total doses of more than 700 mg, and with treatment longer than 30 days. The risk of adrenal suppression can be decreased by using prednisone doses less than 7.5 mg/day, giving doses early in the day, avoiding split doses, and using alternate-day dosing.

Because corticosteroids have a profound impact to decrease leukocyte accumulation at inflammatory sites, the whole cascade of responses leading to local manifestations of infection is slowed. These effects result in late presentation of serious infections because of diminished clinical signs of inflammation. The ability of parietal cavities to localize sepsis is reduced. In addition, prolonged administration of corticosteroids results in delayed wound healing. For example, skin sutures should be left in place 50% to 100% longer than in normal patients. Short-term treatment has little effect on wound healing.[88]

The diagnosis of peritonitis resulting from perforation of colonic diverticula, appendicitis, peptic ulcer, or another primary intra-abdominal condition is a particularly difficult problem in the patient taking corticosteroids.[89] Peritonitis caused by perforation of colonic diverticula in patients taking high-dose corticosteroids is not uncommon. These patients have abdominal discomfort but may have few abdominal findings. Fever and tachycardia may be absent or mild, and clinical signs of peritoneal irritation are blunted. Delays in diagnosis are common, leading to greater morbidity and mortality. Patients taking high-dose corticosteroids who have abdominal discomfort need rapid and aggressive investigation for life-threatening abdominal disease. Plain upright or lateral decubitus radiographs of the abdomen should be obtained immediately. These may reveal free intraperitoneal air even though the patient has minimal signs of peritoneal irritation. A CT scan of the abdomen and pelvis may be needed emergently in these patients. Broad-spectrum antimicrobials to cover for gram-negative enteric bacilli and anaerobes should be administered without delay.

Patients receiving high-dose or long-term treatment with corticosteroids may have a host of other complications unrelated to the effects on the immune system. These include iatrogenic Cushing's syndrome, peptic ulcer disease, benign intracranial hypertension (pseudotumor cerebri), glaucoma, posterior subcapsular cataract, pancreatitis, avascular necrosis of bone (especially the femoral and humoral heads), psychosis, poor wound healing, hyperglycemia, diabetic ketoacidosis, hyperosmolar nonketotic diabetic coma, myopathy, and osteoporosis, resulting in vertebral compression fractures and other spontaneous fractures. In addition, adrenocortical insufficiency may occur on withdrawal of therapy.

Other Immunosuppressive Medications

Commonly used immunosuppressive drugs include cyclosporine, tacrolimus, sirolimus, mycophenolate, azathioprine, and methotrexate. They may be used to treat a wide variety of conditions, including autoimmune diseases (e.g., rheumatoid arthritis and psoriasis), nephrotic syndrome, inflammatory bowel disease, and prevention and treatment of organ transplant rejection.[90] These drugs depress immune function, especially CMI, and patients may present to the emergency department with an infectious complication. In addition, they have a narrow therapeutic window, wide-ranging toxic side effects, and have many significant drug-drug and drug-food interactions. Patients may present to the emergency department for evaluation of symptoms caused by an adverse drug reaction. Before prescribing any new medications or discontinuing or changing the dose of current medications, the physician needs to check carefully for drug interactions. It may be very helpful to notify the patient's physician when these patients come to the emergency department. For a more detailed discussion of the toxic effects of these agents, refer to Chapter 183.

Infliximab and etanercept are tumor necrosis factor inhibitors that have become available for treatment of rheumatoid arthritis and are also being used for psoriasis and Crohn's disease. Serious infections have been reported after treatment with these agents, especially tuberculosis, frequently disseminated and extrapulmonary at presentation, but also bacterial sepsis.[91]

KEY CONCEPTS

- Patients with variable degrees of immunocompromise are common in emergency department practice.
- Infections in immunocompromised patients are more difficult to diagnose and cause increased morbidity and mortality. Early use of broad-spectrum antibiotics is indicated after appropriate cultures of all potential sites of infection, including intravascular catheters.
- Fever in cancer patients receiving chemotherapy indicates infection until proved otherwise, most often caused by gram-positive and gram-negative bacteria but also by a wide variety of fungal, viral, mycobacterial, and protozoal organisms.
- Diabetics, alcoholics, and patients with renal failure, cirrhosis, and collagen vascular diseases all have varying degrees of immunosuppression.
- Patients with functional or surgical asplenia are at high risk for overwhelming sepsis from encapsulated bacteria.
- High doses of corticosteroids cause profound dysfunction (or profound alteration in the function) of neutrophils and mononuclear cells, and impair cell-mediated immunity, resulting in a marked increase in infections caused by pyogenic bacteria, varicella-zoster and herpes simplex viruses, tuberculosis, and a wide variety of other bacteria, fungi, and parasites.

REFERENCES

1. Swenson KK, et al: Recognition and evaluation of oncology-related symptoms in the emergency department. *Ann Emerg Med* 26:12, 1995.
2. Conces DJ: Opportunistic pneumonia. *Curr Probl Diagn Radiol* 22:3, 1993.
3. Delves PJ, Roitt IM: The immune system. First of two parts. *N Engl J Med* 343:37, 2000.
4. Medzhitov R, Janeway C Jr: Innate immunity. *N Engl J Med* 343:338, 2000.
5. Rubin JT, Lotze T: Immune function and dysfunction: A primer for the radiologist. *Radiol Clin North Am* 30:507, 1992.
6. Newhouse M, Sanchis J, Biennenstock J: Lung defense mechanisms. *N Engl J Med* 295:990, 1976.
7. Delves PJ, Roitt IM: The immune system. Second of two parts. *N Engl J Med* 343:108, 2000.
8. Gin-Shaw S, Moore GP: Selected white cell disorders. *Emerg Med Clin North Am* 11:507, 1993.
9. Buckley RH, Dees SC, O'Fallon WM: Serum immunoglobulins. I. Levels in normal children and in uncomplicated childhood allergy. *Pediatrics* 41:600, 1968.
10. Heyworth MF: Immunology of *Giardia* and *Cryptosporidium* infections. *J Infect Dis* 166:465, 1992.
11. Bessen D, Fischetti VA: Passive acquired mucosal immunity to group A streptococci by secretory immunoglobulin A. *J Exp Med* 167:1945, 1988.
12. Figueroa JE, Densen P: Infectious diseases associated with complement deficiencies. *Clin Microbiol Rev* 4:359, 1991.

13. Ross SC, Densen P: Complement deficiency states and infection: Epidemiology, pathogenesis and consequences of neisserial and other infections in an immune deficiency. *Medicine (Baltimore)* 63:243, 1984.
14. Perez HD, Lipton M, Goldstein IM: A specific inhibitor of complement (C5a)-derived chemotactic activity in serum from patients with systemic lupus erythematosus. *J Clin Invest* 78:29, 1978.
15. Klastersky J: Infections in cancer patients with suppressed cellular immunity. *Recent Results Cancer Res* 132:147, 1993.
16. Francis P, Walsh TJ: Current approaches to the management of fungal infections in cancer patients. *Oncology* 6:81, 1992.
17. Rolston KV, Bodey GP: Infections in patients with cancer. In Kufe DW, et al (eds): *Holland-Frei Cancer Medicine 6*. Hamilton, Ontario, BC Decker, 2003, pp 2633-2658.
18. Alexander SW, Pizzo PA: Current considerations in the management of fever and neutropenia. *Curr Clin Top Infect Dis* 19:160, 1999.
19. Hughes WT, et al: Infectious Diseases Society of America 2002 guidelines for the use of antimicrobial agents in neutropenic patients with cancer. *Clin Infect Dis* 34:730, 2002.
20. Schimpff SC, Scott DA, Wade JC: Infections in cancer patients: Some controversial issues. *Support Care Cancer* 2:94, 1994.
21. Pizzo PA: Fever in immunocompromised patients. *N Engl J Med* 341:893, 1999.
22. Giamarellou H, Antoniadou A: Infectious complications of febrile leukopenia. *Infect Dis Clin North Am* 15:457, 2001.
23. Zinner SH: Changing epidemiology of infections in patients with neutropenia and cancer: Emphasis on gram-positive and resistant bacteria. *Clin Infect Dis* 29:490, 1999.
24. Wisplinghoff H, Seifert H, Wenzel RP, Edmond MB: Current trends in the epidemiology of nosocomial bloodstream infections in patients with hematological malignancies and solid neoplasms in hospitals in the United States. *Clin Infect Dis* 36:1103, 2003.
25. Haslam DB: Managing the child with fever and neutropenia in an era of increasing microbial resistance. *J Pediatr* 140:5, 2002.
26. Tunkel AR, Sepkowitz KA: Infections caused by viridans streptococci in patients with neutropenia. *Clin Infect Dis* 34:1524, 2002.
27. Patterson TF, et al: Invasive aspergillosis. Disease spectrum, treatment practices, and outcomes. *Medicine (Baltimore)* 79:250, 2000.
28. Stevens DA, et al: Practice guidelines for diseases caused by *Aspergillus*. Infectious Diseases Society of America. *Clin Infect Dis* 30:696, 2000.
29. Pizzo PA, Robichaud KJ, Wesley R, Commers JR: Fever in the pediatric and young adult patient with cancer: A prospective study of 1001 episodes. *Medicine (Baltimore)* 61:153, 1982.
30. Heussel CP, et al: Pneumonia in febrile neutropenic patients and in bone marrow and blood stem cell transplant recipients: Use of high resolution computed tomography. *J Clin Oncol* 17:796, 1999.
31. Furno P, Bucaneve G, Del Favero A: Monotherapy or aminoglycoside-containing combinations for empirical antibiotic treatment of febrile neutropenic patients: A meta-analysis. *Lancet Infect Dis* 2:231, 2002.
32. Paul M, Soares-Weiser K, Leibovici L: Beta lactam monotherapy versus beta lactam-aminoglycoside therapy for fever with neutropenia: Systematic review and meta-analysis. *BMJ* 326:1111, 2003.
33. Raad II, et al: Treatment of febrile neutropenic patients with cancer who require hospitalization: A prospective randomized study comparing imipenem and cefepime. *Cancer* 98:1039, 2003.
34. Choice of antibacterial drugs. *Treat Guidel Med Lett* 2:13, 2004.
35. Pizzo PA: Empirical therapy and prevention of infection in the immunocompromised host. In Mandell GL, Bennett JE, Dolin R (eds): *Principles and Practice of Infectious Diseases*. Philadelphia, Churchill Livingstone, 2000, pp 3102-3112.
36. Recommendations for preventing the spread of vancomycin resistance. Recommendations of the Hospital Infection Control Practices Advisory Committee (HICPAC). *MMWR Recomm Rep* 44(RR-12):1, 1995.
37. Gotzsche PC, Johansen HK: Routine versus selective antifungal administration for control of fungal infections in patients with cancer. *Cochrane Database Syst Rev* (2):CD000026, 2002.
38. Ozer H, et al: 2000 update of recommendations for the use of hematopoietic colony-stimulating factors: Evidence-based, clinical practice guidelines (American Society of Clinical Oncology Growth Factors Expert Panel). *J Clin Oncol* 18:3558, 2000.
39. Koh A, Pizzo PA: Empirical oral antibiotic therapy for low risk febrile cancer patients with neutropenia. *Cancer Invest* 20:420, 2002.
40. Freifeld A, et al: A double-blind comparison of empirical oral and intravenous antibiotic therapy for low-risk febrile patients with neutropenia during cancer chemotherapy. *N Engl J Med* 341:305, 1999.
41. Kern WV, et al: Oral versus intravenous empirical antimicrobial therapy for fever in patients with granulocytopenia who are receiving cancer chemotherapy. *N Engl J Med* 341:312, 1999.
42. Innes HE, et al: Oral antibiotics with early hospital discharge compared with inpatient intravenous antibiotics for low-risk febrile neutropenia in patients with cancer: A prospective randomized controlled single centre study. *Br J Cancer* 89:43, 2003.
43. Mullen CA: Ciprofloxacin in treatment of fever and neutropenia in pediatric cancer patients. *Pediatr Infect Dis J* 22:1138, 2003.
44. National Comprehensive Cancer Network: NCCN practice guidelines for fever and neutropenia. *Oncology* 13:197, 1999.
45. Uzun O, Anaissie EJ: Outpatient therapy for febrile neutropenia: Who, when, and how? *J Antimicrob Chemother* 43:317, 1999.
46. Freifeld AG, Walsh TJ, Pizzo PA: Infections in the cancer patient. In DeVita VT, Hellman S, Rosenberg SA (eds): *Cancer: Principles and Practice of Oncology*, 5th ed. Philadelphia, Lippincott-Raven, 1997, pp 2659-2704.
47. Gellin BG, Broome CV: Listeriosis. *JAMA* 261:1313, 1989.
48. Khardori N, et al: Spectrum and outcome of microbiologically documented *Listeria monocytogenes* infection in cancer patients. *Cancer* 64:1968, 1989.
49. Lorber B: Listeriosis. *Clin Infect Dis* 24:1, 1997.
50. Cohen JI, Bartlett JA, Corey GR: Extraintestinal manifestations of *Salmonella* infections. *Medicine (Baltimore)* 66:349, 1987.
51. Edelstein PH: Legionnaires' disease. *Clin Infect Dis* 16:741, 1993.
52. Stout JE, Yu VL: Legionellosis. *N Engl J Med* 337:682, 1997.
53. Fang GD, Yu VL, Vickers RM: Disease due to the Legionellaceae (other than *Legionella pneumophila*): Historical, microbiological, clinical and epidemiological review. *Medicine (Baltimore)* 68:116, 1989.
54. Berkey P, Bodey GP: Nocardial infection in patients with neoplastic disease. *Rev Infect Dis* 11:407, 1989.
55. Lerner PI: Nocardiosis. *Clin Infect Dis* 22:891, 1996.
56. Kaplan MH, Armstrong D, Rosen P: Tuberculosis complicating neoplastic disease: A review of 201 cases. *Cancer* 33:850, 1974.
57. Akiyama H, Maruyama T, Uetake T: Systemic infection due to atypical mycobacteria in patients with chronic myelogenous leukemia. *Rev Infect Dis* 13:815, 1991.

58. Kaplan MH, Rosen P, Armstrong D: Cryptococcosis in a cancer hospital: Clinical and pathological correlates in forty-six patients. *Cancer* 39:2265, 1977.
59. Siddiqui AA, Berk SL: Diagnosis of *Strongyloides stercoralis* infection. *Clin Infect Dis* 33:1040, 2001.
60. Whimbey E, Englund JA, Couch RB: Community respiratory virus infections in immunocompromised patients with cancer. *Am J Med* 102:10, 1997.
61. Paradisi F, Giampaolo C, Cinelli R: Infections in multiple myeloma. *Infect Dis Clin North Am* 15:373, 2001.
62. Tsiodras S, Samonis G, Keating MJ, Kontoyiannis DP: Infection and immunity in chronic lymphocytic leukemia. *Mayo Clin Proc* 77:1039, 2000.
63. Glauser M: Alterations of host defenses: The key to the multifaceted spectrum of infections in immunocompromised patients. *Recent Results Cancer Res* 121:321, 1991.
64. Wilkes JD: Prevention and treatment of oral mucositis following cancer chemotherapy. *Semin Oncol* 25:538, 1998.
65. Cunha B: Pneumonias in the compromised host. *Infect Dis Clin North Am* 15:591, 2001.
66. Rolston KV: The spectrum of pulmonary infections in cancer patients. *Curr Opin Oncol* 13:218, 2001.
67. Geerlings SE, Hoepelman AI: Immune dysfunction in patients with diabetes mellitus. *FEMS Immunol Med Microbiol* 26:259, 1999.
68. Calvet HM, Yoshikawa TT: Infections in diabetes. *Infect Dis Clin North Am* 15:407, 2001.
69. Delamaire M, et al: Impaired leucocyte functions in diabetic patients. *Diabet Med* 14:29, 1997.
70. MacGregor RR, Louria DB: Alcohol and infection. *Curr Clin Top Infect Dis* 17:291, 1997.
71. Nelson S, Kolls JK: Alcohol, host defence and society. *Nat Rev Immunol* 2:205, 2002.
72. Engelish G, Wright DG, Hartshorn KL: Acquired disorders of phagocyte function complicating medical and surgical illnesses. *Clin Infect Dis* 33:2040, 2001.
73. Johnson DH, Cunha BA: Infections in cirrhosis. *Infect Dis Clin North Am* 15:363, 2001.
74. Minnaganti VR, Cunha BA: Infections associated with uremia and dialysis. *Infect Dis Clin North Am* 15:385, 2001.
75. Bloembergen WE, Port FK: Epidemiological perspectives on infections in chronic dialysis patients. *Adv Ren Replace Ther* 3:201, 1996.
76. Johnson DW, Fleming SJ: The use of vaccines in renal failure. *Clin Pharmacokinet* 22:434, 1992.
77. Sumaraju V, Smith LG, Smith SM: Infectious complications in asplenic hosts. *Infect Dis Clin North Am* 15:551, 2001.
78. Brigden ML: Detection, education and management of the asplenic or hyposplenic patient. *Am Fam Physician* 63:499, 2001.
79. Davidson RN, Wall RA: Prevention and management of infections in patients without a spleen. *Clin Microbiol Infect* 7:657, 2001.
80. Lutwick LI: Life threatening infections in the asplenic or hyposplenic individual. *Curr Clin Top Infect Dis* 22:78, 2002.
81. Shepard CW, et al: *Bordetella holmesii* bacteremia: A newly recognized clinical entity among asplenic patients. *Clin Infect Dis* 38:799, 2004.
82. Schutze GE, et al: Invasive pneumococcal infections in children with asplenia. *Pediatr Infect Dis J* 21:278, 2002.
83. Stack SJ, Martin DR, Plouffe JF: An emergency department-based pneumococcal vaccination program could save money and lives. *Ann Emerg Med* 33:299, 1999.
84. Stuck AE, Minder CE, Frey FJ: Risk of infectious complications in patients taking glucocorticosteroids. *Rev Infect Dis* 11:954, 1989.
85. Lionakis MS, Kontoyiannis D: Glucocorticoids and invasive fungal infections. *Lancet* 362:1828, 2003.
86. Klein NC, Go H, Cunha BA: Infections associated with steroid use. *Infect Dis Clin North Am* 15:423, 2001.
87. Dowell SF, Bresee JS: Severe varicella associated with steroid use. *Pediatrics* 92:223, 1993.
88. Nohr C: Host defenses. In Meakins JL (ed): *Surgical Infections: Diagnosis and Treatment.* New York, Scientific American, 1994, pp 21-28.
89. Nathans A, et al: Peritonitis and other intra-abdominal infections. In Howard RJ, Simmons RL (eds): *Surgical Infectious Diseases*, 3rd ed. Norwalk, Conn, Appleton & Lange, 1995, pp 959-1009.
90. Smith JM, Nemeth TL, McDonald RA: Current immunosuppressive agents: Efficacy, side effects, and utilization. *Pediatr Clin North Am* 50:1283, 2003.
91. Keane J, et al: Tuberculosis associated with infliximab, a tumor necrosis α-neutralizing agent. *N Engl J Med* 345:1098, 2001.

Section V **THE PATIENT WITH AN ORGAN TRANSPLANT**

CHAPTER 183

The Solid-Organ Transplant Patient

Matthew T. Keadey and Douglas W. Lowery III

PERSPECTIVE

The successful rehabilitation of patients with end-stage renal, pulmonary, hepatic, and cardiac failure through organ transplantation is one of the great achievements of modern biomedical science. Because 1-year survival rates for all solid-organ transplants exceed 80% and many patients survive much longer, increasing numbers of transplant patients with complications are being seen in the emergency department.

PRINCIPLES OF DISEASE

Transplanted organs are devoid of their native innervations and have surgical anastomoses to a variety of structures, including arteries, veins, heart chambers, bronchi, ureters, intestines, and even the bladder, depending on the allograft. Pain is therefore an unreliable sign of underlying disease. Furthermore, the normal inflammatory responses that signal the development of disease are suppressed in these patients, and the immunologic defenses against infection and malignancy are impaired. Subtle symptoms and signs may be the harbingers of serious or even life-threatening complications of organ transplantation, and each complaint merits careful investigation. Even in the most advanced stages of severe disease, patients may have few specific complaints and physical findings. Consideration of the anatomic relationships relevant to the allograft may assist in anticipating leakages or blockages of vital connections. Familiarity with the physiologic capacity of the allograft aids in interpreting chief complaints in the context of possible organ failure.

Transplant organ complications can generally be placed into one of three categories: rejection, infection, and drug toxicity. In any transplant recipient presenting to the emergency department, each category must be considered in the differential diagnosis. Often the exact etiology is not determined until the patient has been admitted to the hospital. In addition, complications can be further categorized by time since transplantation. This information can help the clinician focus investigative efforts and tailor treatment regimens.

Infection

Lifelong immunosuppression is necessary for all recipients of solid-organ transplants except those with transplants from identical twins. Because of this, infection is the primary cause of death after transplantation. Two thirds of transplant patients have at least one significant infection, most commonly during the surgical recovery period.[1,2]

Signs of infection in this population of patients are often blunted by an impaired inflammatory response. Even the most benign-appearing skin lesion, pulmonary nodule, or nonspecific complaint may indicate serious disease. Aggressive management usually translates into increased survival of patients and graft function.[1]

There are three primary sources of infection in transplant recipients: before transplantation, community acquired after transplantation, and nosocomial. The timing of infection can be separated into three time periods: within the first month after transplantation, between 1 and 6 months after transplantation, and more than 6 months after transplantation. These distinctions are useful in predicting the etiologic agents of the infection (Box 183-1).

First Month after Transplantation

Infections occurring in the first month after transplantation are likely to be related to the technical procedure, catheters, and intubation. In addition, the typical causes of postoperative fever must always be considered in the workup. Nosocomial pathogens are prominent, and management is similar to that for any immunosuppressed patient recently discharged from the hospital.[2]

BOX 183-1. Infectious Pathogens in Transplant Patients

Exposure before Transplantation
Tuberculosis
Histoplasmosis
Coccidioidomycosis
Blastomycosis
Strongyloides stercoralis
Hepatitis B and C
Human immunodeficiency virus (HIV)
Cytomegalovirus (CMV)
Epstein-Barr virus (EBV)
Varicella-zoster virus
Herpes simplex virus

Community-Acquired Exposure after Transplantation
Influenza
Primary varicella
Salmonellosis
Tuberculosis and fungal infections (see above)
Legionellosis
Nocardiosis
Cryptococcosis
CMV
EBV

Nosocomial Exposure
Aspergillosis
Legionellosis
Pseudomonas aeruginosa and other gram-negative bacilli

Modified from Gorbach S (ed): *Infectious Diseases*, Philadelphia, WB Saunders, 1992.

One to Six Months after Transplantation

Infections occurring from 1 to 6 months after transplantation are divided into two general types: viral infection with immunomodulating viruses and the resulting opportunistic infections. Immunomodulating viruses include cytomegalovirus (CMV), hepatitis B and C viruses, and Epstein-Barr virus (EBV); opportunistic infections include *Pneumocystis*, *Listeria*, and fungal species.

CMV is the most important and prevalent immunomodulating virus 1 to 6 months after transplantation.[1] CMV infection may produce disease in multiple systems, including the gastrointestinal tract, kidneys, retina, skin, and central nervous system. However, pneumonitis is particularly common and may arise insidiously. CMV infection may be primary or due to reactivation from latent viral particles found in lymphocytes. Typically, signs of CMV infection occur at a median of 40 days after transplantation. Survival from CMV infection has improved with earlier diagnosis by aggressive use of bronchoscopy and treatment with ganciclovir and CMV-specific immunoglobulin. Despite treatment, however, CMV infection is often fatal.[3,4]

In addition, active CMV infection can trigger or exacerbate organ rejection. CMV has been linked to a particular form of glomerulopathy in renal allograft recipients as well as acute hepatic dysfunction and the disappearing bile duct syndrome of chronic hepatic allograft dysfunction.[5,6] Furthermore, both acute cardiac dysfunction and accelerated coronary artery atherosclerosis of chronic heart transplant rejection have been linked to CMV.[7,8]

EBV infection causes clinical effects similar to those caused by CMV. EBV contributes to the net state of immunosuppression and can cause a mononucleosis-like syndrome associated with lymphadenopathy, weakness, and low-grade fevers. Because CMV and EBV often coexist, it is unknown whether EBV causes or triggers graft rejection independently. EBV has also been implicated in B cell lymphoproliferative syndrome, histologically similar to polymorphic B cell lymphoma.[9]

Six Months after Transplantation

Six months or more after transplantation, patients with functioning solid-organ allografts receiving immunosuppressive therapy are divided into three groups relative to infection susceptibility: healthy transplant, chronic viral infection, and chronic rejection.

Healthy Transplant

Healthy transplant patients have no chronic viral infection and a functioning allograft. They have a mildly increased susceptibility to normal, community-acquired infections, such as influenza, urinary tract infection, and pneumococcal pneumonia.

Chronic Viral Infection

Chronic viral infections are typically from CMV, EBV, or hepatitis B or C. Progressive disease may develop as a result of the combination of viral infection and long-term immunosuppressive therapy (e.g., CMV retinitis). Patients are also susceptible to progressive liver disease from hepatitis B or C and the malignancies of hepatocellular carcinoma and B cell lymphoproliferative disorder, which are associated with hepatitis B virus and EBV infection, respectively.[1,2]

Primary varicella infection leads to rapid dissemination with pneumonia, pancreatitis, hepatitis, encephalitis, and disseminated intravascular coagulation. Patients who are varicella-zoster virus (VZV) seronegative need high doses of intravenous (IV) varicella-zoster immune globulin as soon as possible after any exposure to chickenpox or zoster. This therapy can be lifesaving, provided it is administered early in the course before dissemination occurs.[1,2]

Reactivation of latent VZV infection, manifested as cutaneous herpes zoster, affects at least 10% of solid-organ transplant recipients. Fortunately, VZV is usually confined to a single dermatome and does not disseminate. Hospitalization for IV acyclovir therapy should be considered because this has been shown to speed healing but does not change the incidence of painful neuralgia. However, facial zoster specifically involving the cornea and disseminated infections found in more than one dermatome are indications for admission.[1]

Herpes simplex virus (HSV) reactivation is common after solid-organ transplantation and can manifest as oral or anogenital lesions, more often ulcers than vesicles. Some transplant centers have patients take oral acyclovir for 3 to 6 months after transplantation, whereas others choose to treat HSV immediately at the first sign of recurrence.[10] Typically, these patients can be treated as outpatients if they can tolerate oral medications and their pain is controlled.

Chronic Rejection

Patients with chronic rejection require ongoing aggressive immunosuppressive treatment to protect the allograft. These patients are at highest risk for life-threatening opportunistic infections with fungi (e.g., *Cryptococcus*, *Coccidioides*, *Blastomyces*, *Histoplasma*), bacteria (e.g., *Listeria*, *Nocardia*), and parasites (e.g., *Pneumocystis*, *Toxoplasma*, *Strongyloides*).

Fungal infections are distinct to geographic regions, and patients typically present with subacute respiratory complaints associated with fever and focal, disseminated, or miliary infiltrates on chest radiographs. Invasive candidiasis and aspergillosis are also problems in the chronically immunosuppressed group. Primary infections in the lungs, gastrointestinal tract, or nasal sinuses lead to fungemia and seeding of IV lines and wounds. Treatment is with antifungal agents such as amphotericin B, paying special attention to potential renal toxicity.

Diverticulitis is the principal bacterial gastrointestinal infection observed in transplant recipients. Because of chronic steroid therapy, inflammation is suppressed, leading to an increased incidence of perforation before diagnosis. Patients complain of an insidious onset of pain, change in bowel habits, and sometimes fever, but they typically lack peritoneal signs. Transplant patients also have increased susceptibility to invasion of the mucosa with salmonellae (nontyphoidal) and *Listeria*. Both organisms can be present as acute diarrheal syndromes that progress to bacteremia or meningitis.[1,2]

Pulmonary infection with *Nocardia asteroides* may occur in transplant patients. Primary infection is subacute, with cough, fever, pleurisy, purulent sputum, and subsequent metastatic infection of the brain and skin. Seizures or subcutaneous nodules may be the presenting complaint with primary *Nocardia* infection.

Pneumocystis carinii pneumonia (PCP) is often found in combination with CMV infection because CMV inhibits alveolar macrophage function. (Figure 183-1) Fortunately, its incidence is reduced with prophylactic low-dose trimethoprim-sulfamethoxazole (TMP-SMX). Without prophylaxis, infection develops 1 to 6 months after transplantation and arises subacutely with fever, nonproductive cough, progressive dyspnea over several days, and an interstitial infiltrate on chest radiographs. Differentiation from CMV pneumonia is impossible without bronchoscopic confirmation. Treatment of PCP includes IV TMP-SXM and steroids, depending on the degree of hypoxia.

Disseminated toxoplasmosis is a particular problem in heart transplant patients. Toxoplasmosis can lie dormant in the tissues, especially the heart, and can be reactivated during immunosuppression, resulting in myocarditis, brain abscesses, or diffuse encephalitis.

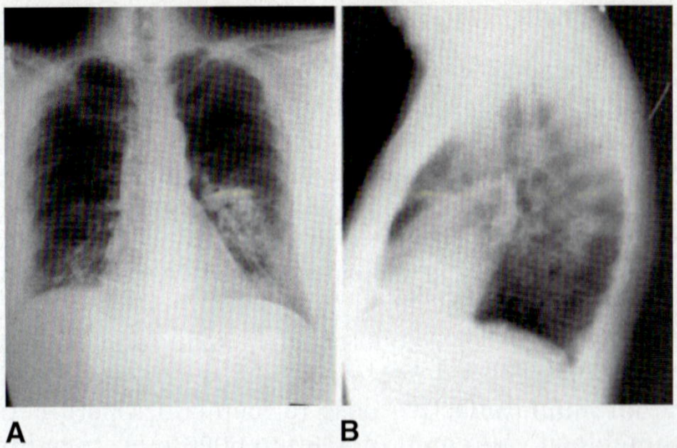

Figure 183-1. **A** and **B,** Bilateral perihilar and lower lobe alveolar infiltrates in a cardiac transplantation recipient from *Pneumocystis carinii*. (From Tewari S, Maurer J: Pulmonary considerations of organ transplantation. In Ginnes LG, Cosimi AB, Morris PJ [eds]: *Transplantation*. Malden, Mass, Blackwell Science, 1999, p 617.)

Treatment of toxoplasmosis is with a combination IV sulfadiazine and pyrimethamine daily, typically for more than 4 weeks.

Strongyloides stercoralis, an intestinal nematode that normally causes few or no symptoms, can become an invasive pathogen. Normally, cell-mediated immunity keeps the parasite in check, but during immunosuppression a *hyperinfection syndrome* can develop causing a necrotizing hemorrhagic enterocolitis. The exaggeration of the normal life cycle of the parasite has a major impact on the gastrointestinal tract and lungs (hemorrhagic pneumonia). Disseminated strongyloidiasis occurs when the larvae migrate from the gastrointestinal tract into all portions of the body. Both dissemination and hyperinfection are associated with frequent gram-negative bacteremia and meningitis secondary to impairment of the blood-gut barrier.

Mycobacterial disease can arise as an opportunistic reactivation or as a primary infection. Even disseminated disease can be clinically silent, with invasion of the bowel, skin, and gastrointestinal tract being common. Pulmonary disease can be absent, miliary, or cavitary (Figure 183-2). Treatment is a significant problem because typical agents used to treat mycobacteria can cause graft dysfunction.[1,2]

Rejection

Rejection typically occurs in three phases: hyperacute, acute, and chronic. Not only does the course of rejection vary from patient to patient, but also each individual typically has a lifelong course of waxing and waning immuno responses to the allograft, mandating ongoing surveillance of the status of the graft.

Hyperacute rejection has become rare with careful donor-recipient matching. It typically occurs in the immediate perioperative or postoperative period. *Acute rejection* occurs within the first months after transplantation. It usually arises with constitutional symptoms and signs of transplant organ insufficiency. Expeditious laboratory assessment, including possible allograft biopsy, can confirm the diagnosis of rejection,

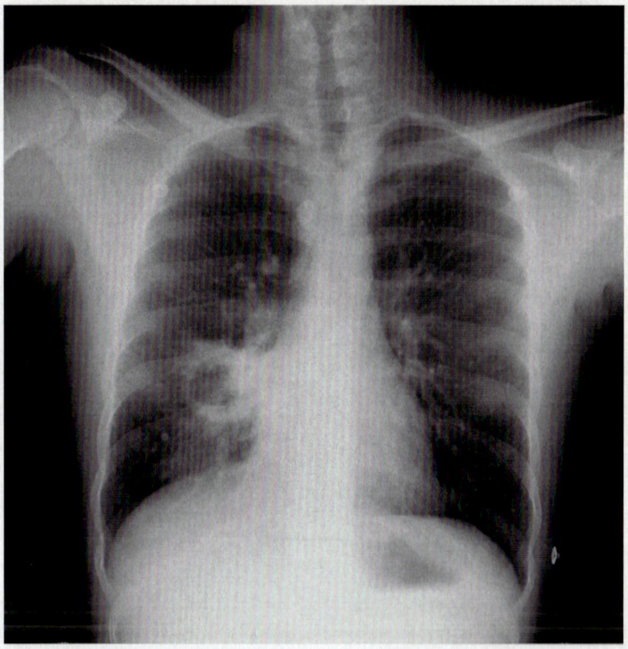

Figure 183-2. 22-year-old male with a kidney transplant who presents with fever and a cough. Diagnosed with reactivated tuberculosis by sputum analysis.

and the appropriate adjustment can be made in the patient's immunosuppressant regimen. Acute rejection can occur at any time if immunosuppressants are stopped. *Chronic rejection* has a time course of years and results in gradual failure of the transplanted organ.[11]

Drug Toxicity and Immunosuppression

Pharmacology of Immunosuppression

The single greatest advancement in the treatment of patients with transplanted organs has been the advent of effective immunosuppressants, used to prevent and abort transplant rejection. Immunosuppressive therapy is the cornerstone for success in organ transplantation and requires correctly timed drug combinations to establish a delicate balance between immunosuppression, rejection, and susceptibility to infection. Multiple agents are used and patients commonly take more than one immunosuppressant agent. An example of a three-drug protocol is:

- A calcineurin inhibitor (cyclosporin or tacrolimus)
- A purine synthesis inhibitor (azathioprine or mycophenolate mofetil)
- A corticosteroid

Recognizing the side effects, toxicities, and potential drug interactions of immunosuppressant medications is an important component in the care of any transplant patient.

Cyclosporine

A variety of new immunosuppression strategies are being tested, but the mainstay of transplant immunosuppression has been cyclosporine, and its introduction in 1980 revolutionized transplant survival.[12,13]

Table 183-1. Drug Interactions with Cyclosporine

Agent	Pharmokinetic Action	Effect
Carbamazepine Nafcillin Phenobarbital Phenytoin Rifampin	Induce cytochrome P450 enzymes	Decreased half-life and immunosuppressive effect
Colchicine Diltiazem Fluconazole Fluoroquinolones Ketoconazole Macrolide antibiotics Oral contraceptives Verapamil	Inhibit cytochrome P450 enzymes	Increased half-life and potential drug toxicity or immunosuppression
Aminoglycosides Amphotericin B Cimetidine Nonsteroidals Sulfur	Interact at a glomerular or tubular level	Increased nephrotoxicity

Cyclosporine inhibits both cellular and humoral immunity by binding to cyclophilins, which block cytokine transcription and production and thereby inhibit lymphocyte signal transduction. It is classified as a calcineurin inhibitor. The result is a potent immunosuppression of helper-inducer T cells without affecting the suppressor T cell subset.[12,14] The helper-inducer T cells enhance antibody recognition and production by B cells.

Cyclosporine has significant risks. It exhibits dose-related nephrotoxicity, which is additive to that of other nephrotoxic drugs typically used after transplantation, such as amphotericin B, aminoglycosides, and high-dose TMP-SMX. Cyclosporine causes renal tubular injury and direct renal artery vasospasm in a dose-dependent fashion.[12] Up to one third of patients are reported to have some degree of nephrotoxicity. The drug-induced renal arterial vasospasm leads to arterial hypertension in many recipients. Hypertension must be treated aggressively using standard regimens to preserve renal function and prevent atherosclerosis. Cyclosporine may also worsen hyperlipidemias common in cardiac patients.[15] Therefore, monitoring blood levels and renal function is routine during therapy.

Cyclosporine causes hyperuricemia and gout in transplant patients. The nephrotoxic effects of cyclosporine make the management of gouty attacks in a transplant patient very difficult.[16]

Cyclosporine levels are altered by many common posttransplantation medications (Table 183-1). Drugs that inhibit cytochrome P-450 metabolism, such as erythromycin and ketoconazole, produce elevated cyclosporine levels and enhanced toxicity.[17] Treatment with rifampin can increase metabolism, which triggers episodes of organ rejection. Cyclosporine also causes hepatotoxicity, hyperkalemia, hirsutism, tremor, and gingival hyperplasia.[12]

Azathioprine

Azathioprine is an antimetabolite derivative of 6-mercaptopurine. Long an important component of immunosuppressive therapy for solid-organ transplant recipients, azathioprine functions by inhibiting both deoxyribonucleic acid (DNA) and ribonucleic acid (RNA) synthesis, resulting in suppression of lymphocyte proliferation. It is usually used in combination with other agents.

Azathioprine is a bone marrow toxin, and patients exhibit dose-related neutropenia. The drug is given at the minimum effective dose to maintain a peripheral white blood cell count of 4000 to 6000/mm^3. Azathioprine has also caused hepatic dysfunction and gastrointestinal disturbances.[18]

Corticosteroids

Corticosteroids have been used for immunosuppression since the 1960s. Glucocorticoids have a wide range of effects on the immune system, specifically the T lymphocytes. Because of the significant long-term toxic effects associated with chronic glucocorticoid administration, every effort is made to minimize the dosage of glucocorticoids. *Combination therapy*, in which two or more immunosuppressants are administered simultaneously, has decreased the reliance on long-term, high-dose glucocorticoid administration for allograft survival.[19]

Long-term corticosteroid therapy causes osteoporosis, cataracts, gastrointestinal bleeding, glucose intolerance, steroid skeletal myopathy, bone disease, and adrenal suppression (Figure183-3).[20] Acute administration may lead to glucose and electrolyte abnormalities as well as altered mental status. Acute withdraw or severe illness may lead to an addisonian crisis.

Mycophenolate Mofetil

Mycophenolate mofetil (MMF) is a newer agent used to prevent and suppress organ rejection after solid-organ transplantation.[20] MMF is an antimetabolite with more potent and selective inhibition of lymphocytic proliferation. It appears to reduce the incidence of acute rejection but with no significant change in the long-term survival of transplant recipients or their allografts.[14]

MMF has the advantage of a low side effect profile. The mostly mild effects resulting from its gastrointestinal and hematologic toxicity include abdominal pain, nausea, diarrhea, gastroenteritis, leukopenia, and thrombocytopenia. Because magnesium and aluminum antacids interfere with the absorption of MMF, care should be exercised when treating the gastrointestinal symptoms.[21]

Antilymphocyte Monoclonal Antibody Preparations

OKT3 and antithymocyte globulin are used in short courses to reverse allograft rejection.[20,22] OKT3 is a mouse-derived monoclonal antibody to T cells. When

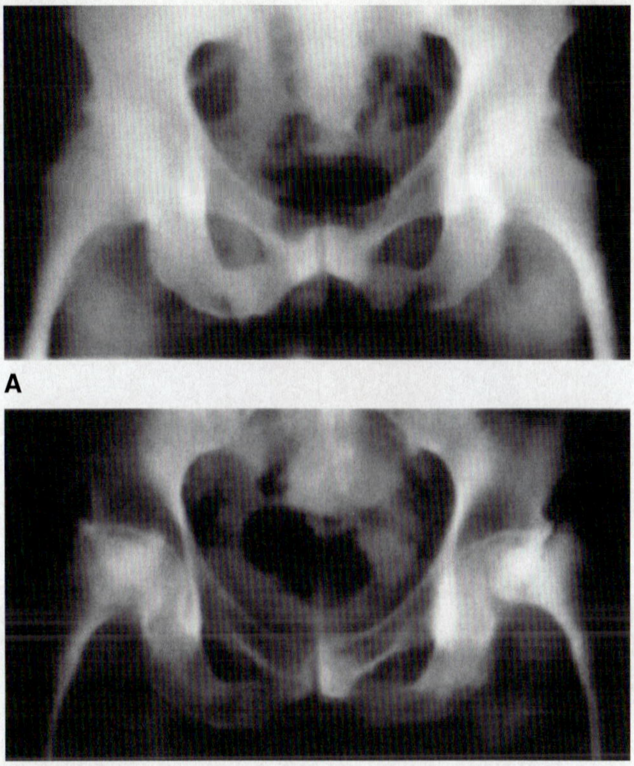

A

B

Figure 183-3. Radiographic appearance of a 24-year-old renal transplant patient with early (**A**) and late (**B**) findings consistent with avascular necrosis from chronic steroid use. (From Walker RG: Steroids and transplantation. In Ginnes LG, Cosimi AB, Morris PJ [eds]: *Transplantation*. Malden, Mass, Blackwell Science, 1999, p 121.)

used against acute rejection, it is administered intravenously for 10 to 14 days, usually in the hospital initially because chills, fever, hypotension, and headache often occur. Pulmonary edema may also develop in overhydrated, oliguric patients. OKT3 is effective in more than 90% of first rejections. Patients can develop antibodies against these agents, which limits the duration of therapy and availability for repeated use.[14]

OKT3 toxicity is common because of T cell activation and lymphokine release caused by these agents. When receiving these agents, patients are at increased risk for infection with opportunistic pathogens, particularly CMV. An increased risk of lymphoproliferative disease also exists.[20,22]

Tacrolimus

Tacrolimus is a macrolide compound that binds to lymphocyte proteins and inhibits cytokine synthesis. Used as either primary or rescue therapy for allograft rejection, tacrolimus has been shown to be effective for rejection in all types of solid-organ transplants.[23,24]

As with cyclosporine, tacrolimus causes nephrotoxicity as well as neurotoxicity. Hyperglycemia and hyperkalemia are also seen. Tacrolimus can also cause anorexia, diarrhea, dyspepsia, and nausea. Macrolide antibiotics should not be prescribed to patients taking tacrolimus because they may induce acute toxicity.[23]

SPECIFIC DISORDERS

Clinical Features

The pertinent clinical features of organ transplant complications are as extensive as the elements of the history and physical examination. Allograft rejection symptoms are usually vague and nonspecific. Complications of the organ itself, such as abscess or obstruction, often result in localized symptoms and dysfunction of the transplanted organ. The clinical features of infectious complications depend on the nature of the pathogenic organism, location of the infection, and level of active immunosuppression. Traumatic transplant organ injury is uncommon, and care should center on the diagnosis and management of the more common traumatic conditions. However, careful attention must be paid to maintaining the appropriate level of immunosuppression and watching for the typical transplant-related complications.[25] Still, every complaint and finding in the organ transplant recipient must be examined in the most suspicious light to avoid missing catastrophic illness.

Diagnostic Strategies

Transplant patients should undergo careful and often extensive laboratory and radiographic evaluation to rule out the myriad infectious etiologies as well as to assess the functioning of the allograft and survey for signs of drug toxicity. Laboratory assessments should include organ-specific measures of function as well as a careful search for evidence of infection. If infection is suspected, appropriate cultures and serologies should be obtained. Radiologic interventions focus on sources of infection and the relevant anatomy of the patient's allograft.

MANAGEMENT

Heart Transplant

General Approach

Human heart transplantation was first performed in 1967. Currently, more than 2000 procedures are done annually in the United States. The 5-year survival rates for adults and children are now 70% and 80%, respectively.[26] Typically, the recipient heart is removed and replaced by the donor heart (orthotopic transplant) (Figure 183-4A and B), but occasionally the recipient heart is left in place with the donor heart anastomosed to the native vessels (heterotopic transplant).

Patients are usually discharged from the hospital within 2 to 3 weeks to home. In the Stanford experience, 37% of heart transplant patients made at least one emergency department visit in the ensuing 3 years (range, one to six visits). The most common complaints are fever (37%), shortness of breath (13%), gastrointestinal (nausea, vomiting, diarrhea) (10%), and chest pain (9%). Sixty percent of these patients are admitted,

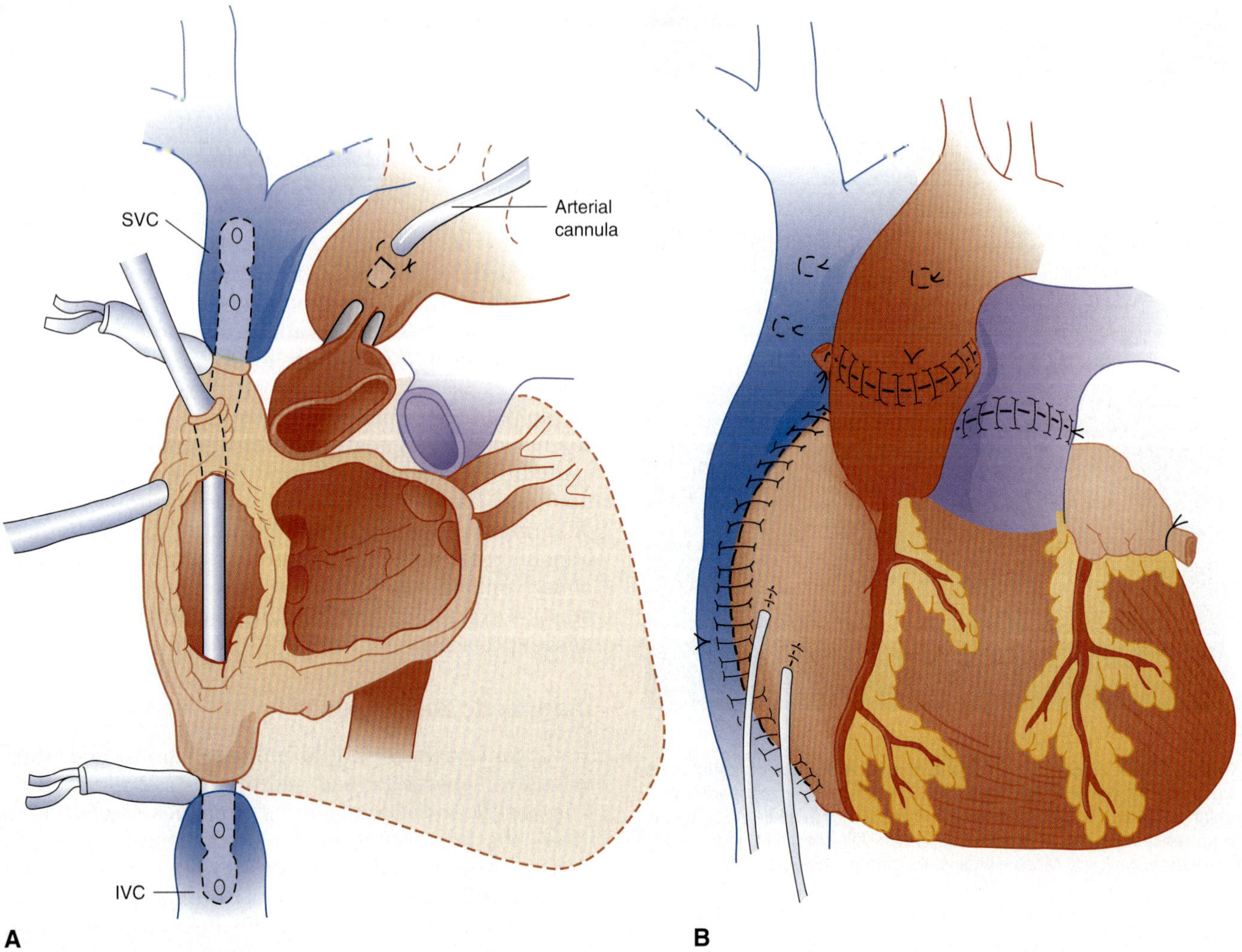

Figure 183-4. A and **B,** Typical anastomoses of an orthotopic heart transplant. (From Hunt SA, Schroeder JS, Berry GJ: Cardiac transplantation, mechanical ventricular support, and endomyocardial biopsy. In Furster VL, et al: *Hurst's The Heart*. New York, McGraw Hill, 2001, pp 729-730.)

compared with an overall emergency department admission rate of 15%, reflecting an appropriately high concern for rejection or localized or systemic infection. The most common emergency department diagnoses are sepsis (18%), rejection (11%), and pneumonia (8%).[15] In trauma, the diagnosis of myocardial contusion may be made in these patients by usual means, notwithstanding the lack of a "gold standard." Treatment for the transplanted heart should be no different from that for native hearts. Baseline tachycardia is expected because of denervation of the vagus. Tamponade is possible because of scarring, which may contain pericardial fluid or blood under pressure. Blind pericardiocentesis is discouraged.[25]

Infection and rejection are the leading causes of mortality in the first year. Any heart transplant patient presenting to the emergency department with congestive heart failure (CHF), fever (>38° C), shortness of breath, hypoxia, hypotension, poorly controlled hypertension, or new dysrhythmia should be admitted. Chest pain is rarely related to cardiac ischemia because the denervated heart is incapable of producing angina.[27] Accelerated atherosclerosis of the graft vessels is the hallmark of chronic rejection, but the ischemia is manifest as CHF, ventricular dysrhythmias, hypotension, syncope, or sudden death.[28,29] A CMV infection appears to be a risk factor for accelerated atherosclerosis.[8,17,30]

Drug Toxicity

Lifelong immunosuppression is required in these patients. Most centers use a three-drug regimen of cyclosporine, prednisone, and azathioprine. Each drug has a potential for toxicity, and the combination of cyclosporine and prednisone worsens the hyperlipidemias common in many of these patients.[15,31]

Rarely, cyclosporine toxicity can result in a neurotoxic syndrome of seizures, confusion, cortical blindness, and quadriplegia, even progressing to coma. Seizure management is with standard anticonvulsants.[32-34]

Rejection

Acute rejection occurs in 75% to 85% of patients within the first 3 months. Its manifestations may be subtle with cyclosporine included in the immunosup-

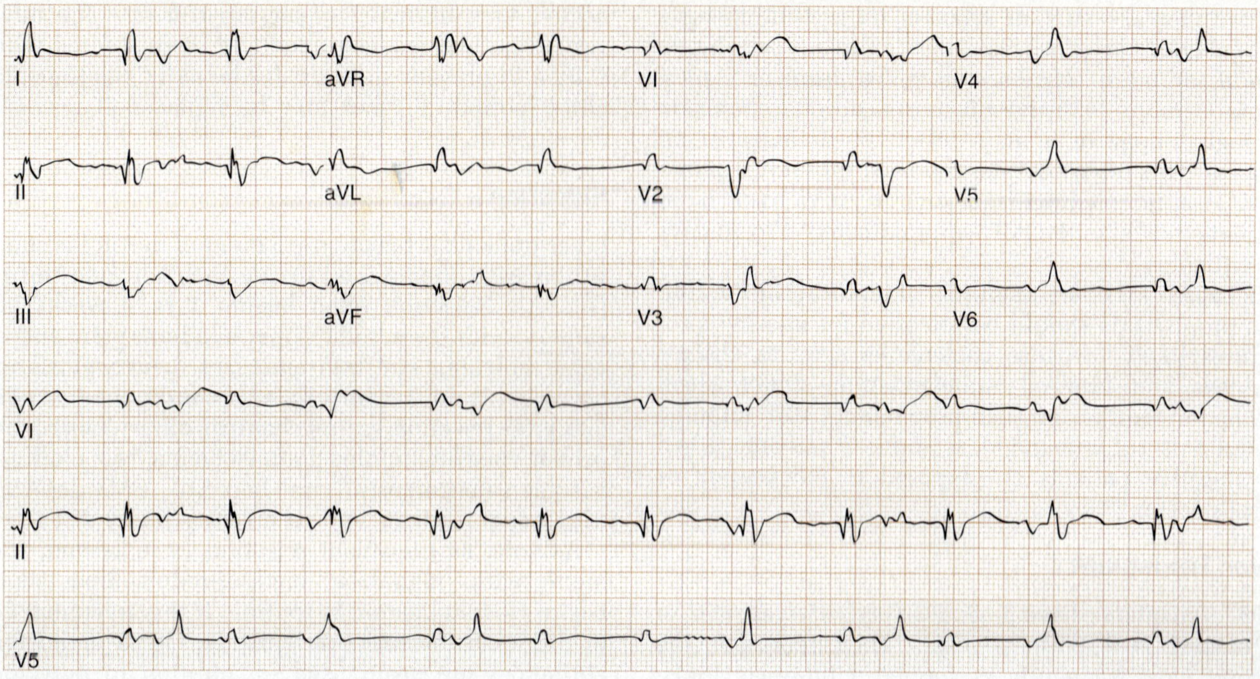

Figure 183-5. A 68-year-old male status postheterotopic heart transplant; native heart rate of 55 and donor heart rate of 75 beats per minute.

pressive regimen. Previously, rejection was obvious, with decreased QRS voltage, a new S_3 heart sound, new-onset CHF, or atrial dysrhythmias. Currently, these features are present only during episodes of severe rejection, and the diagnosis of rejection is made by endomyocardial biopsy showing lymphocyte infiltration or myocyte necrosis.[1,15] Because most episodes of early or mild rejection are asymptomatic, frequent biopsies are performed to monitor the success of the immunosuppressive regimen.[35,36]

Acute rejection is treated with increased doses of corticosteroids (methylprednisolone, 500 to 1000 mg/day) and cyclosporine or with OKT3 or antithymocyte globulin. Immunosuppression is continued lifelong, with endocardial biopsies at least every 3 months.[36,37]

The transplanted heart maintains a rate of 100 to 110 beats/min without vagal parasympathetic tone. The electrocardiogram typically demonstrates two P waves (Figure 183-5). One wave is from the native sinus node in the posterior right atrium, which is left in place with its vena caval connections during surgery. The second P wave is from the donor sinoatrial node, which should conduct to the ventricles as usual with a normal PR interval. The heart rate can increase with exercise or stress through the effects of endogenous catecholamines, up to 70% of maximum for age. Exogenous pressor drugs work well in the transplanted heart. Upregulation of β-adrenergic receptors appears to occur in the graft, with a slightly enhanced response to norepinephrine and isoproterenol.[32,37-39] Antihypertensive agents can be used to treat hypertension, even of crisis proportions, as in the nontransplant patient. Atropine is ineffective at increasing the sinus node rate or relieving atrioventricular block.

Infection

Infection in heart transplant patients has many causes. One fourth of deaths after transplantation result from infection. The most vulnerable period is the first 3 months, when immunosuppression is maximal. Although one third of patients have a major infection develop in the first year, life-threatening infection after 1 year is rare.[1,17]

In the first month, nosocomial infection predominates, with the usual gram-positive and gram-negative bacteria. After the first 3 months, patients experience an overall 20% per year rate of infection. The most common skin infection is herpes zoster; high-dose acyclovir limits cutaneous and visceral dissemination, even when begun more than 3 days after the onset of rash. Nausea, vomiting, or diarrhea should prompt a search for CMV by culture and serologic testing.[2,15,35]

All heart transplant patients with fever should be presumed to have a new infection. An aggressive diagnostic workup, including blood and urine cultures, computed tomography (CT) scan, lumbar puncture, and bronchoscopy, should begin in the emergency department. In addition, complete blood count, glucose, serum chemistries, blood urea nitrogen and creatinine, chest radiograph, and electrocardiogram are recommended. In one series of 131 emergency department visits by such patients, 23 patients were admitted with a diagnosis of "rule out sepsis" and 12 (52%) had an infecting organism identified.[15]

Any new headache with or without visual changes may be the first symptom of meningitis or brain abscess, and a CT scan of the head and a lumbar puncture should be obtained. Fever, lethargy, headache, altered mental status, or seizures are presenting signs of *Listeria*, cryptococcal meningitis, *Toxoplasma gondii*, or brain abscesses from *Nocardia* or *Aspergillus*. A more definitive diagnosis can often be made through biopsy of a mass lesion or drainage of an abscess. This often obviates the need for lumbar puncture. Aseptic meningitis occurs in 10% to 14% of patients treated with OKT3 approximately 6 to 10 days after therapy.[1,17]

Because of the attendant risk of endocarditis, antibiotic prophylaxis should be provided for invasive procedures likely to cause bacteremia, such as abscess drainage and urethral catheterization. Endotracheal intubation requires no such prophylaxis. VZV immune globulin is recommended as soon as possible when seronegative patients are exposed to chickenpox or herpes zoster.[2,15]

Liver Transplant

Liver transplants have 1- and 3-year survival rates of 86% and 76%, respectively.[26] They represent the second most frequently performed solid-organ transplant procedure. Complications are common, and loss of function of the graft organ is rapidly life threatening. Postoperative complications include intra-abdominal hemorrhage, vascular thrombosis, and biliary leaks or obstructions.[18]

Anatomic Considerations

The typical liver transplant is connected to its host by five anastomoses (Figure 183-6). The vessels are connected first, allowing organ reperfusion. The biliary system is then reconstructed and often stented with a T tube to prevent stenosis. In the early posttransplantation period, T tubes may be replaced if restenosis develops.

Rejection

Liver transplant rejection is common despite immunosuppressive therapy, occurring in up to one third of patients. Rejection often begins 1 to 2 weeks after surgery, with fever, right upper quadrant pain, and elevated bilirubin and transaminases. Leukocytosis may occur but is nonspecific. Related conditions that simulate graft rejection are mechanical biliary obstruction, primary nonfunctioning graft, ischemia from clotting of vascular anastomoses, viral hepatitis, CMV infection, drug hepatotoxicity, and recurrent primary disease.[40,41]

As soon as transplant rejection is suspected, treatment with high-dose methylprednisolone should begin. Hospitalization is routine. If this treatment fails to diminish the rejection episode, OKT3 monoclonal antibodies are again used in addition to polyclonal antilymphocyte globulin.[40]

Infection

The risk of infection is highest in the postoperative recovery period. After the first postoperative month, opportunistic infections replace the common postsurgical complications. Viral (CMV, HSV), fungal (*Aspergillus*, *Candida*, *Cryptococcus*), protozoan (*Pneumocystis*, *Toxoplasma*), and unusual bacterial (*Nocardia*,

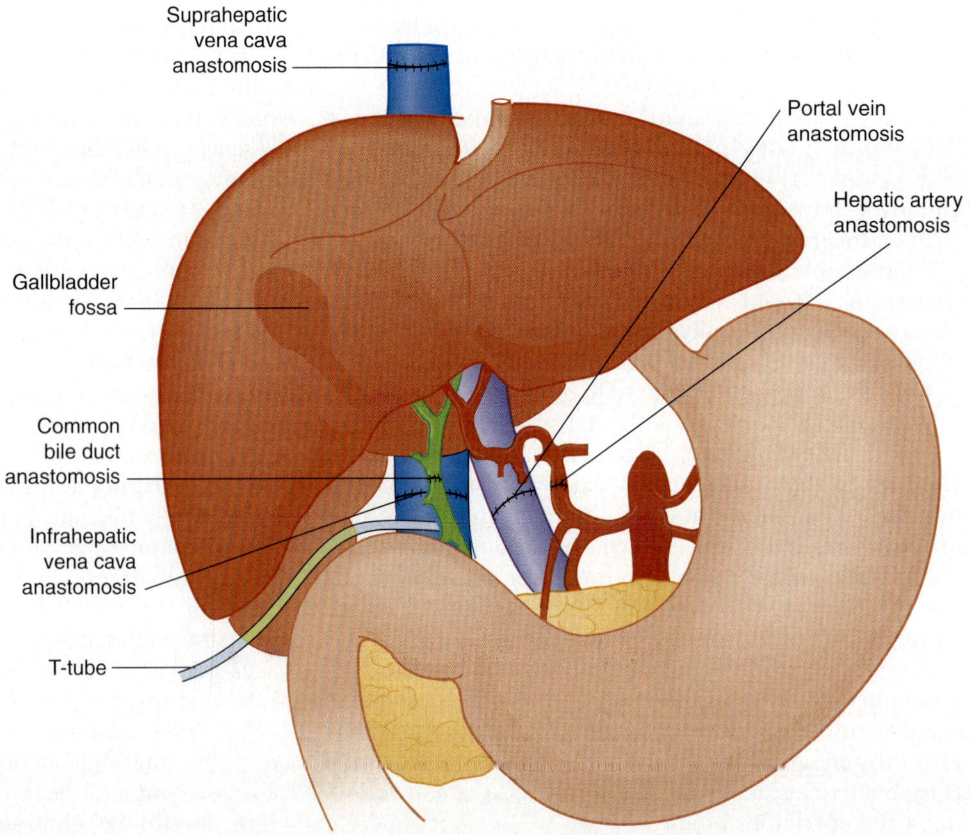

Figure 183-6. Typical anastomoses of an orthotopic liver transplant. (From Powelson JA, Cosimis AB, Liver transplantation. In Ginnes LG, Cosimi AB, Morris PJ [eds]: *Transplantation*. Malden, Mass, Blackwell Science, 1999, p 352.)

Legionella, Listeria) infections occur. In addition, liver transplant patients are at risk for cholangitis because a biliary stent is left in place for many weeks and colonization by staphylococcal species, enterococci, and gram-negative organisms is common. Subsequent injury to the graft during diagnostic biopsy or cholangiography can cause clinical cholangitis or liver abscess. Because immunosuppressive therapy must be continued indefinitely, these patients remain at risk for opportunistic infection for the rest of their lives.[40,42,43]

Kidney (Renal) Transplant

With survival rates of 96% at 1 year and 91% at 3 years, renal transplants have proved highly successful. They are the most common solid-organ transplants in the United States.[26] Injury of the transplanted kidney is rare, despite its location in the retroperitoneal area of the anterior pelvis, where it may be at risk from direct blows as well as seatbelt injuries.[25]

Infection

The classic example of bacterial infection in transplanted organs is pyelonephritis in renal allografts. It often occurs in the first month after surgery during high-dose immunosuppression. This timing presents an increased risk of sepsis. Responsible organisms are the usual gram-positive organisms associated with wound infections and gram-negative organisms from the gut. Pyelonephritis occurs in 35% of patients during the first 4 months but can be prevented with prophylactic antibiotics. All patients with a transplant who have pyelonephritis are admitted to the hospital for aggressive antibacterial therapy.[44,45]

Hepatitis C virus infection is the most common cause of hepatitis in renal transplant patients. It may be transferred to the recipient by blood transfusion or through the donor organ because pretransplantation antibody testing is a poor predictor of latent hepatitis C virus infection. Liver disease develops in approximately 50% of seropositive patients, occurring approximately 4 months after transplantation. Most patients develop chronic hepatitis, with accompanying immune defects and susceptibility to sepsis and spontaneous bacterial peritonitis. No specific effective treatment is available for hepatitis C virus infection. Pretransplantation screening with newer techniques is the only current avenue of prevention.[1,44]

Rejection

Early kidney transplant rejection is mediated through attack by T lymphocytes against antigenic donor tissues, including cytotoxic CD8 and CD4 cells, but B lymphocytes, natural killer cells, and macrophages also infiltrate the foreign tissues. The B lymphocytes manufacture specific antibodies, which results in microvascular lesions impairing perfusion.

Chronic transplant rejection occurs after several years of adequate function and is a result of nephrosclerosis. This process involves proliferation of the vascular intima of renal vessels with a marked decrease in the lumen size. Systemic hypertension ensues as the graft fails from ischemia and tubular and glomerular atrophy.[46]

With cadaveric kidney transplants, histocompatibility differences are almost universal and routinely require long-term immunosuppressive therapy. Immunosuppression is accomplished with a combination of azathioprine, prednisone, and cyclosporine. Azathioprine inhibits both DNA and RNA synthesis, which inhibits lymphoid cell proliferation by halting mitosis while making existing cells unable to respond to antigen exposure with messenger RNA production. Prednisone is begun at a high dose immediately after transplantation but tapered rapidly to minimize interference with wound healing and reduce wound infection. On diagnosis of acute rejection, high-dose methylprednisolone (500 to 1000 mg) is begun daily and continued for 3 days. After 6 to 12 months, many patients only need lower doses (10 to 20 mg/day).[44-47]

Clinically, renal graft rejection arises as fever, swelling and tenderness over the allograft, and decreased urine output. Early therapy can save the graft. A subtle rise in serum creatinine should prompt great concern. Renal ultrasonography should be performed to rule out obstruction, abscess, and perirenal collections of blood, pus, or lymph. Early consultation with the nephrologist is prudent.

Lung Transplant

The lung may be transplanted alone or in combination with the heart, with 1-year survival rates of 76% and 56%, respectively.[26] Lung transplants are usually done unilaterally, except for cystic fibrosis. Inequity of lung sounds is to be expected. There is no published experience with lung injury after transplantation. Comparison of chest radiography with preinjury studies is critical in the evaluation of trauma. Chest tube placement on the transplanted side may be difficult because of adhesions and loculations.[25]

Rejection

Although still rare, lung transplantation is increasing in frequency; more than 800 are performed annually in the United States. Most patients develop early rejection, and 25% to 40% have chronic rejection. An episode of acute rejection can occur as early as a few days after transplantation or as late as several years. Clinically, the patient presents with cough, dyspnea, and fever. Rales and rhonchi are heard on lung examination, with deterioration in oxygenation and pulmonary function. Early rejection is often accompanied by infiltrates on the chest radiograph. When rejection occurs more than a month after transplantation, 75% of radiographs are normal or unchanged. The diagnosis of rejection is made by transbronchial biopsy showing lymphocytic infiltration.[17,48]

Suspected episodes of acute rejection are treated with high-dose methylprednisolone (500 to 1000 mg/day). This is successful in reversing most episodes, but OKT3 can be used in refractory cases.[49]

Chronic lung transplant rejection is a leading cause of late morbidity and mortality. Antecedent acute rejection and CMV pneumonia are risk factors. Pathologically, vascular sclerosis and progressive limitation to airflow result from obliterative bronchiolitis. Rejection can occur several years after transplantation, but the mean time to onset is 8 to 12 months. Clinically, this rejection mimics an upper respiratory infection or bronchitis. If dyspnea is a component of the presenting complaint, a search for transplant rejection should be initiated.[48-51]

Chronic rejection is treated with high-dose methylprednisolone (500 to 1000 mg/day), with the first dose begun in the emergency department. Antilymphocyte antibodies are used as well, but relapse of the rejection episode is common.

Infection

Transplanted lungs are highly susceptible to pneumonia because they are colonized by bacteria during the ventilator stage of the brain-dead donor. After transplantation, diminished mucociliary clearance, decreased cough reflex (because the transplanted lung is denervated), and defective function of alveolar macrophages are present. The most common infections are caused by gram-negative bacteria, especially *Pseudomonas* and *Staphylococcus aureus*. Antibiotic therapy should be aggressively directed toward any pathogenic bacteria cultured from the tracheobronchial tree. On long-term follow-up, most pneumonias are gram negative, but community-acquired infections occur as well. *Pneumocystis* pneumonia is uncommon because of routine prophylaxis with TMP-SMX.[1,49]

CMV pneumonia is the most common opportunistic pulmonary infection after lung transplantation. Patients are at highest risk between 3 weeks and 4 months. Clinically, CMV infection closely resembles transplant rejection; tissue biopsy and viral culture are required to differentiate the two entities. Treatment with ganciclovir is effective. Colonization by *Candida* is common, but not invasive disease. *Aspergillus* provides the most significant fungal threat to the transplanted lung. Reactivation of tuberculosis is rare.[49,50]

Pancreas Transplant

The pancreas may be transplanted singly or in combination with a kidney, typically secondary to diabetes. Pancreatic transplants have a high complication rate, with 1-year graft survival rates as low as 72%.[26] Because the exocrine functions of the allograft pancreas are usually drained into the bladder, genitourinary complaints are also common. Duodenocystostomy fistula may form in the early posttransplantation period. The clinical findings are abdominal pain, tenderness, hyperamylasemia, leukocytosis, and elevated serum creatinine. Other types of pancreatic transplant complications include urinary tract infections, hematuria, reflux pancreatitis, rejection, and pancreatic graft thrombosis.[52-54]

Anatomic considerations are important when these patients suffer major trauma because pancreas transplants are placed in the pelvis overlying the iliac vessels. Because exocrine secretions are drained into the bladder for excretion, patients have a chronic non–anion gap acidosis through loss of bicarbonate into the bladder. This condition should not be confused with lactic acidosis. These trauma patients should not require exogenous insulin unless the graft is injured. Positive amylase on peritoneal lavage (CT is recommended if the patient is stable) can result from either native organ or graft trauma or from a ruptured bladder. CT scanning should be done with rectal contrast in addition to IV and oral contrast to better define the native and transplanted pelvic organs.[25]

Islet cell transplantation is under investigation as a means to treat diabetes mellitus.[55] This procedure is in its infancy, but, if successful, it may negate the need for future pancreas transplants and the resultant complications.

DISPOSITION

Patients with solid-organ transplants presenting to the emergency department have a much higher than average rate of hospitalization.[25,43] Because of the insidious nature of the diseases affecting this immunosuppressed population, a thorough approach to evaluation is warranted in all patients. If organ rejection, infection, or drug toxicity is evident, local transplantation specialists should be consulted. Physicians without significant transplant experience should notify the patient's transplant center to obtain consultation and coordinate follow-up care. Patients who are discharged require careful instructions and close follow-up.

KEY CONCEPTS

- The possibility of organ rejection, infection, or drug toxicity should be considered in all organ transplant patients who present to the emergency department.
- The symptoms and signs of significant medical problems are often subtle in transplant patients.
- A patient's inability to take oral immunosuppressants for even a single day should be considered an emergency condition.
- When infectious disease is evident, every effort should be made to administer the appropriate antibiotics as soon as possible. Unusual infectious etiologies should be considered.
- When prescribing care in the emergency department, the physician must be careful to avoid drug interactions and toxicity.

REFERENCES

1. Dummer JS, Ho M: Infections in solid organ transplant recipients. In Mandell GL, Bennett JE, Dolin R (eds): *Mandell, Douglas, and Bennett's Principles and Practice of Infectious Disease*, 5th ed. Philadelphia, Churchill Livingstone, 2000, pp 3148-3156.
2. Rubin RH, Fishman JA: Infection in the organ transplant recipient. In Ginns LC, Cosimi AB, Morris PJ (eds): *Transplantation*. Malden, Mass, Blackwell Science, 1999, pp 747-769.
3. Sweny P: Infection in solid organ transplantation. *Curr Opin Infect Dis* 6:412, 1993.

4. Sweny P, Burroughs AK: Infections in solid organ transplantation. *Curr Opin Infect Dis* 7:436, 1994.
5. Richardson WP, et al: Glomerulopathy associated with cytomegalovirus viremia in renal allografts. *N Engl J Med* 305:57, 1981.
6. O'Grady JG, et al: Cytomegalovirus infection and donor/recipient HLA antigens: Interdependent cofactors in pathogenesis of vanishing bile duct syndrome after liver transplantation. *Lancet* 2:302, 1988.
7. Rubin RH: The indirect effects of cytomegalovirus infection on the outcome of organ transplantation. *JAMA* 261:3561, 1989.
8. Grattan MT, et al: Cytomegalovirus infection is associated with cardiac allograft rejection and atherosclerosis. *JAMA* 262:3561, 1989.
9. Benkerron M, Durandy A, Fischer A: Therapy for transplant-related lymphoproliferative disease. *Hematol Oncol Clin North Am* 7:467, 1993.
10. Pettersson E, et al: Prophylactic oral acyclovir after renal transplantation. *Transplantation* 39:279, 1985.
11. Dallman MJ: Immunobiology of graft rejection. In Ginns LC, Cosimi AB, Morris PJ (eds): *Transplantation*. Malden, Mass, Blackwell Science, 1999, pp 23-36.
12. Keown PA: Molecular and clinical therapeutics of cyclosporine in transplantation. In Ginns LC, Cosimi AB, Morris PJ (eds): *Transplantation*. Malden, Mass, Blackwell Science, 1999, pp 101-112.
13. Harlan DM, Kirk AD: The future of organ and tissue transplantation: Can T-cell costimulatory pathway modifiers revolutionize the prevention of graft rejection? *JAMA* 282:1076, 1999.
14. Halloran PF: Immunosuppressive agents in clinical trails in transplantation. *Am J Med Sci* 313:283, 1997.
15. Sternbach GL, et al: Emergency department presentation and care of heart and heart/lung transplant recipients. *Ann Emerg Med* 21:1140, 1992.
16. Pratt PW, Ball GV: Gout: Clinical and laboratory features. In Klippel JH (ed): *Primer on the Rheumatic Diseases*. Atlanta, Arthritis Foundation, 1997, pp 209-218.
17. Petri WA: Infections in heart transplant recipients. *Clin Infect Dis* 18:141, 1994.
18. Freeman L, Awad SH: Evaluation and management of solid organ transplant patients in the emergency department. *Emerg Med Rep* 25(2):11, 2004.
19. Walker RG: Steroids and transplantation. In Ginns LC, Cosimi AB, Morris PJ (eds): *Transplantation*. Malden, Mass, Blackwell Science, 1999, pp 115-123.
20. Bungardner GL, Roberts JP: New immunosuppressive agents. *Gastroenterol Clin North Am* 22:421, 1993.
21. Rayhill SC, Sollinger HW: Mycophenolate mofetil: Experimental and clinical experience. In Ginns LC, Cosimi AB, Morris PH (eds): *Transplantation*. Malden, Mass, Blackwell Science, 1999, pp 147-162.
22. Parlevliet KJ, Schellekens PT: Monoclonal antibodies in renal transplantation: A review. *Transplant Int* 5:234, 1992, pp 127-136.
23. Klintmalm GB: Tacrolimus. In Ginns LC, Cosimi AB, Morris PJ (eds): *Transplantation*. Malden, Mass, Blackwell Science, 1999.
24. Gerber D, Bonham C, Thomson A: Immunosuppressive agents: Recent developments in molecular action and clinical application. *Transplant Proc* 30:1573, 1998.
25. Barone GW, et al: Trauma management in solid organ transplant recipients. *J Emerg Med* 15:169, 1997.
26. Scientific Registry of Transplant Recipients website. Accessed at *www.ustransplant.org*, April 17, 2004.
27. Gao SZ, et al: Acute myocardial infarction in cardiac-transplant recipients. *Am J Cardiol* 664:1092, 1989.
28. Hosenpud JD: Coronary artery disease after heart transplantation and its relation to cytomegalovirus. *Am Heart J* 138:S469, 1999.
29. Weis M, von Scheidt W: Cardiac allograft vasculopathy: A review. *Circulation* 96:2069, 1997.
30. Wagoner LE: Management of the cardiac transplant recipient: Roles of the transplant cardiologist and primary care physician. *Am J Med Sci* 314:173, 1997.
31. Hunt SA, Schroeder JS: Managing patients after cardiac transplantation. *Hosp Pract* 24:83, 1989.
32. Cooper DK, et al: Does central nervous system toxicity occur in transplant patients with hypocholesterolemia receiving cyclosporine? *J Heart Transplant* 8:221, 1989.
33. Rubin AM: Transient cortical blindness and occipital seizures with cyclosporine toxicity. *Transplantation* 47: 572, 1989.
34. Velu T, Debusscher L, Stryckmans PA: Cyclosporine-associated fatal convulsions. *Lancet* 1:219, 1985.
35. Cainelli F, Vento S: Infections and solid organ transplantation rejection: A cause and effect relationship? *Lancet Infect Dis* 2:543, 2002.
36. Taylor AJ, Bergin JD: Cardiac transplantation for the cardiologist not trained in transplantation. *Am Heart J* 129:578, 1995.
37. Miniati DN, Robbins RC, Reitz BA: Heart and heart-lung transplantation. In Braunwald E (ed): *Heart Disease: A Textbook of Cardiovascular Medicine*, 6th ed. Philadelphia, WB Saunders, 2001, pp 615-630.
38. Borow KM, et al: Cardiac and peripheral vascular responses to adrenoceptor stimulation and blockage after cardiac transplantation. *J Am Coll Cardiol* 14:1229, 1989.
39. Yusuf S, et al: Increased sensitivity of the denervated transplanted human heart to isoprenaline both before and after beta-adrenergic blockade. *Circulation* 75:696, 1987.
40. Powelson JA, Cosimi AB: Liver transplantation. In Ginns LC, Cosimi AB, Morris PJ (eds): *Transplantation*. Malden, Mass, Blackwell Science, 1999, pp 324-366.
41. Jain A, et al: Immunosuppressive therapy. *Surg Clin North Am* 79: 59, 1999.
42. Munoz SJ, et al: Long-term care of the liver transplant recipient. *Clin Liver Dis* 4:691, 2000.
43. Savitsky EA, Uner AB, Votey SR: Evaluation of orthotopic liver transplant recipients presenting to the emergency department. *Ann Emerg Med* 31:507, 1998.
44. Patel R: Infections in recipients of kidney transplants. *Infect Dis Clin North Am* 15:901, 2001.
45. Rubin RH: Infectious disease complications of renal transplantation. *Kidney Int* 44:221, 1991.
46. Ponticelli C: Renal transplantation strengths and shortcomings. *J Nephrol* 14(Suppl 14):S1, 2001.
47. Lo A, Alloway RR: Strategies to reduce toxicities and improve outcomes in renal transplant recipients. *Pharmacotherapy* 22:316, 2002.
48. Glover FL, et al: The past, present, and future of lung transplantation. *Am J Surg* 173:523, 1997.
49. Ginns LC, Wain JC: Lung transplantation. In Ginns LC, Cosimi AB, Morris PJ (eds): *Transplantation*. Malden, Mass, Blackwell Science, 1999, pp 490-550.
50. Midthun DE, et al: Medical management and complications in the lung transplant recipient. *Mayo Clin Proc* 72:175, 1997.
51. Scott JP, et al: Posttransplantation physiologic features of the lung and obliterative bronchiolitis. *Mayo Clin Proc* 72:170, 1997.
52. Hickey DP, et al: Urological complications of pancreatic transplantation. *J Urol* 157:2042, 1997.
53. Stegall MD, et al: Pancreas transplantation for the prevention of diabetic nephropathy. *Mayo Clin Proc* 75:49, 2000.
54. Allen RM: Pancreas transplantation. In Forsythe JLR (ed): *Transplantation Surgery*. London, WB Saunders, 1997.
55. Markmann JF, et al: Insulin dependence following isolated islet transplantation and single infusions. *Ann Surg* 237:741, 2003, pp 741-749.

CHAPTER 184

Alcohol-Related Disease

David B. McMicken and John T. Finnell

PERSPECTIVE

Epidemiology

The disastrous effects and widespread incidence of alcoholism are well known to the emergency physician. Motor vehicle accidents, drowning, suicides, homicides, divorce, violent crime, child abuse, unemployment, and disruption of the family are often either directly or indirectly associated with excessive alcohol consumption. The tragic effects of alcohol not only affect the individual drinker but also have far-reaching implications for the family, community, and workplace. The prevalence of alcoholism or inappropriate drinking among emergency department patients ranges from 8% to 40%. The 5-year mortality rate among alcohol-intoxicated emergency department patients was 2.4 times that of a comparison group in one study.[1]

A simple, rapid, and respectful screening test for alcoholism is the four *CAGE* questions. Have you ever felt:

the need to ***C***ut down on your drinking?
Annoyed by criticism of your drinking?
Guilty about your drinking?
the need to drink an ***E***ye opener in the morning?

Positive answers to two or more of these questions are sufficient to identify individuals who require more intensive evaluation.[2] Also, a positive answer to the question "Have you ever had a drinking problem?" plus evidence of alcohol consumption in the previous 24 hours provides greater than 90% sensitivity and specificity as a screening tool for identifying alcoholism.

Alcohol is the most common recreational drug taken by Americans, and per capita consumption is increasing. Alcoholism permeates all levels of society and is the leading cause of mortality and morbidity in the United States, with a cost to the nation estimated to be greater than $130 billion annually. An estimated 18 million alcoholics reside in the United States. More than 100,000 alcohol-related deaths occur each year, and alcohol is the third leading cause of preventable death in the United States.[3]

Definition and Natural History

A precise definition of alcoholism is difficult. A proposed definition encompassing the features of alcoholism is "a primary chronic disease with genetic, psychosocial, and environmental factors influencing its development and manifestations." The disease is often progressive and fatal. It is characterized by impaired control over drinking, preoccupation with and use of alcohol despite adverse consequences, and distortions in thinking, most notably denial. Each of these symptoms may be periodic or continuous.[4] When drinking adversely affects an individual's physical health, ability to function in society, or interpersonal relationships, alcoholism is present. Certainly, the patient who has a dependence on ethanol can be labeled "alcoholic."

The cause of alcoholism is not completely understood but appears to be a complex interaction between biologic and environmental factors. Data show that a genetic variability of enzymes for alcohol metabolism may be a risk factor. The validity of genetic factors is supported by family, twin, and adoption studies.[5]

The natural history of alcoholism is variable, and it may appear in any patient despite age or social status. The age of onset of alcoholism continues to decrease. Up to 6% of high school seniors drink daily, and it is not unusual to see children younger than 16 years of age who have already graduated from an alcohol detoxification program.[6] Many individuals also begin drinking heavily after age 60.

The fourth edition of the *Diagnostic and Statistical Manual of Mental Disorders* (*DSM-IV*) has two categories for substance disorders, which include alcohol abuse. It lists criteria for substance abuse and substance dependence.[7] The chronic *substance abuse* of alcohol eventually leads to *acquired tolerance*, a condition in which larger and larger doses of alcohol are required for the same effect. An *inborn tolerance* also exists. A wide variance in the behavioral abnormalities is manifested, independent of the patient's drinking experience.

Continued alcohol abuse progresses to *substance dependence*, defined in DSM-IV as a maladaptive pattern of substance use leading to clinically significant impairment, as manifested by three or more of the following occurring in the same 12-month period:

1. Physiologic dependence, as evidenced by tolerance or withdrawal
2. Alcohol taken in larger amounts or over a longer period than was intended
3. Persistent desire or unsuccessful efforts to control alcohol consumption
4. Great amount of time spent in activities necessary to obtain alcohol or recover from its effects
5. Important social, occupational, or recreational activities forsaken for sustained alcohol use
6. Continued alcohol use despite knowledge of having a persistent or recurrent physical or psychological problem that is likely to have been caused or exacerbated by alcohol

PRINCIPLES OF DISEASE: METABOLISM OF ALCOHOL

Ethanol is rapidly absorbed from the stomach and small intestine. It is distributed uniformly to all organ systems, including the placenta if present. Most alcohol is metabolized in the liver. The oxidation of alcohol is a complex process involving three enzyme systems, all contained in the hepatocyte. The pharmacokinetic properties of alcohol metabolism are well known. The class I alcohol dehydrogenase (ADH) isoenzymes, ADH1, ADH2, and ADH3, oxidize ethanol. ADH2 and ADH3 have polymorphic properties with distinct kinetic properties. At the ADH3 locus, two alleles account for pharmacokinetic differences of 2.5-fold in maximum velocity of ethanol oxidation.[8]

$$\text{Ethanol} \xrightarrow[\text{NAD} \longrightarrow \text{NADH}]{\text{Alcohol dehydrogenase}}$$

$$\text{Acetaldehyde} \xrightarrow[\text{NAD} \longrightarrow \text{NADH}]{\text{Alcohol dehydrogenase}}$$

$$\text{Acetyl coenzyme A} \xrightarrow[\text{Cycle}]{\text{Citric acid}} CO_2 + H_2O$$

An alternative pathway, the *microsomal ethanol-oxidizing system* (MEOS), can be induced by chronic alcohol exposure. Many effects of alcoholism are produced by the toxic byproducts (hydrogen, acetaldehyde), the acceleration of metabolism of other drugs, and activation of hepatotoxic compounds by these metabolic pathways.

Although the liver is the major site of ethanol metabolism, other tissues contribute to its metabolism. ADH is found in the gastric mucosa, but the gastric metabolism of alcohol is decreased in women. This increased bioavailability of ethanol or decreased first-pass metabolism may explain the enhanced vulnerability of women to acute and chronic complications of alcoholism.

Studies have shown two alcohol elimination curves. The alcohol elimination rate approximates zero-order kinetics (constant rate) for lower ethanol levels and first-order kinetics (amount of drug removed over time is proportional to the concentration of the drug) for higher levels, especially in chronic alcoholics. The MEOS pathway may account for the increased elimination rate of ethanol.

The absorption and elimination rates of alcohol vary by individual and depend on many factors: diet, gender, body weight and habitus, speed of consumption, gastric motility, presence of food in the stomach, smoking history, age, whether the person is a chronic alcohol consumer with enzyme induction and high activity MEOS, advanced cirrhosis, presence of ascites, and the state of nourishment.[9] There is enormous variation among patients in the rate of disappearance of ethanol from the blood, ranging from 9 to 36 mg/dL/hr in published data.

Table 184-1. Physiologic Effects and Blood Alcohol Levels

Blood Alcohol Concentration (mg/dL)	Effects*
20-50	Diminished fine motor control
50-100	Impaired judgment; impaired coordination
100-150	Difficulty with gait and balance
150-250	Lethargy; difficulty sitting upright without assistance
300	Coma in the novice drinker
400	Respiratory depression

*These effects are for the occasional drinker. Chronic drinkers can function at much higher alcohol concentrations because of tolerance. On the other hand, patients may become comatose with low levels of alcohol in mixed alcohol-drug overdose.

Although the clearance rate may be as high as 36 mg/dL/hr in some chronic drinkers, 20 mg/dL/hr is a reasonable rate to assume in any intoxicated emergency department patient. This holds true for adults, adolescents, and children. In the unusual circumstance that an accurate prediction of the rate of clearance is required, a second measurement should be obtained several hours after the initial value.[10]

Physiologic effects vary directly with the blood alcohol (Table 184-1). Diminished fine motor control and impaired judgment appear with alcohol concentrations as low as 20 mg/dL (0.02 mg%), but wide individual variability exists. Chronic alcoholics can exhibit impressive tolerance. The *blood alcohol concentration* (BAC) of a person cannot be accurately determined without quantitative testing. More than 50% of the adult population are obviously intoxicated with a level of 150 mg/dL (0.15 mg%). As the ethanol level rises, the patient's level of consciousness declines, eventually ending in coma. Death is caused by aspiration or respiratory depression.

In most states, the legal level of intoxication is 80 to 100 mg/dL (0.08 to 0.1 mg%). Many states now allow administrative driver's license revocation at BACs as low as 20 mg/dL (0.02 mg%).

Expired breath alcohol or saliva testing can be used to obtain a reliable approximation of BAC in a cooperative patient. This value can be used as a rapid screen for alcohol intoxication.[11]

DIFFERENTIAL CONSIDERATIONS

Acute alcohol intoxication is a diagnosis of exclusion. Before assuming that a patient's behavior is caused only by alcohol, other conditions must be considered. Hypoglycemia, hypoxia, carbon dioxide narcosis, mixed alcohol-drug overdose, ethylene glycol or methanol poisoning, hepatic encephalopathy, psychosis, severe vertigo, and psychomotor seizures can manifest in a manner similar to ethanol intoxication. The possibility of occult head trauma and the presence of associated metabolic disorders need to be recognized after alcohol intoxication has been established. Adequate history from paramedics and family, repeated physical examinations by the same physician, and diagnostic adjuncts can help resolve this dilemma.

MANAGEMENT

Ethanol is similar to general anesthetics that act on the lipid moiety of cell membranes. Because there are no specialized receptors for alcohol, a specific antagonist does not exist.

Comatose or stuporous patients need to have their airway and breathing evaluated. The airway is protected as necessary, including endotracheal intubation. Gastric lavage and activated charcoal are of little value in ethanol overdose because of the rapid absorption of alcohol but may be appropriate in a suspected mixed drug-alcohol overdose.

Thiamine (100 mg intravenously [IV]) to prevent or treat Wernicke's syndrome, glucose (dextrose, 25 to 50 g IV) for hypoglycemia, and naloxone (0.8 mg IV) for possible opioid ingestion are considered in comatose patients. Whenever possible, hypoglycemia should be documented before the administration of empirical glucose. With the airway maintained and respirations supported, the patient's liver eventually metabolizes the alcohol, and the patient should recover.

Glucose (dextrose, 25 g IV) produces a dramatic response in alcohol-induced hypoglycemic patients. Unlike hypoglycemia of other causes, alcohol-induced hypoglycemia may be unresponsive to glucagon because of depleted liver glycogen stores. The possibility of precipitating Wernicke's encephalopathy by administering glucose before thiamine has little scientific merit. Although Wernicke's encephalopathy is a medical emergency, alcohol-induced hypoglycemia is a much more common condition with serious and permanent morbidity if left untreated. Therefore, thiamine can be given in a timely fashion, but glucose therapy should never be delayed.[12]

Intoxicated patients require evaluation and treatment in the emergency department regardless of their obstreperousness. Inappropriate discharge and failure to diagnose are two common areas of liability when treating the alcohol-dependent patient. The theoretical liability for detention by reasonable restraint is less than the potential liability for injury sustained by the alcohol-dependent patient or an innocent bystander after premature discharge. Discharge (after excluding significant abnormal laboratory values or suspected head injury) can be considered if a concerned, sober adult is willing to take responsibility for and remain with the patient for the next 24 to 48 hours.

ALCOHOL WITHDRAWAL SYNDROME

Principles of Disease

The neurophysiology of alcohol withdrawal is complex and not fully understood. Chronic alcohol consumption has a depressant effect on the central nervous system (CNS). The hallmark of alcohol withdrawal is CNS excitation with increased cerebrospinal fluid (CSF), plasma, and urinary catecholamine levels.

Chronic alcohol consumption affects central adrenergic α-receptors, glutamate, central adrenergic β-receptors, the inhibitory neurotransmitter γ-aminobutyric acid (GABA), and dopamine turnover. The effectiveness of lofexidine and clonidine (α_2-adrenergic agonists), propranolol and atenolol (β-blockers), haloperidol (dopamine blocker), and benzodiazepines and propofol (GABA transmission blockers) in suppressing the signs and symptoms of alcohol withdrawal supports this concept.[13,14]

Differential Considerations

Alcohol withdrawal syndrome can initially be confused with acute schizophrenia, encephalitis, drug-induced psychosis, thyrotoxicosis, anticholinergic poisoning, and withdrawal from other sedative-hypnotic-type drugs. It may be difficult to differentiate between alcohol withdrawal and alcohol-induced hypoglycemia.

Acute schizophrenia usually has its onset in adolescence or early adulthood. Manifestations include multiple bizarre delusions and a flat affect with the patient otherwise oriented. The patient in alcohol withdrawal is usually older (20s or 30s), hyperactive, and often disoriented.

Encephalitis can produce headache, confusion, fever, and seizures. Thyrotoxicosis is more common in women, and its features include irritability, insomnia, tremor, weight loss despite a good appetite, palpitations, and frequent stools. Physical examination may reveal lid lag, tachycardia, and a bruit over the thyroid. No relationship exists between the onset of encephalitis or thyrotoxicosis and alcohol consumption.

Anticholinergic poisoning can occur with several different drugs or plant ingestion. The classic clinical picture is a patient with dry mouth, dry eyes, dry skin, hypoactive bowel sounds, urinary retention, and delirium. Amphetamine and cocaine intoxications produce anorexia, insomnia, and physical signs of CNS sympathetic overactivity.

In opioid withdrawal, patients complain of abdominal pain and diarrhea, the mental status is usually normal, the patient is afebrile, and seizures are uncommon (with the exception of meperidine). In contrast, patients with major alcohol withdrawal are usually disoriented and febrile and may have seizures.

Signs of alcohol withdrawal usually begin 6 to 24 hours after a decrease in the patient's usual intake of alcohol. If patients manifest withdrawal 3 days or more after their last drink, drugs with a longer half-life should be considered. The barbiturate and benzodiazepine withdrawal syndromes usually progress more slowly, with a higher frequency of seizures later (7 days versus 2 days), and status epilepticus is more common than with alcohol withdrawal.

Clinical Features

Isbell's classic study in 1955 confirmed the relationship between alcohol and the withdrawal syndrome.[15] He documented that the severity of signs and symptoms depends on both the dose and the duration of ethanol consumption. The withdrawal syndrome may occur any time after the blood alcohol level starts to fall. Therefore, only a reduction, not the abrupt cessation, of ethanol intake may result in withdrawal.

The withdrawal syndrome usually develops 6 to 24 hours after the reduction of ethanol intake and lasts from 2 to 7 days. The alcohol withdrawal state ranges from mild withdrawal with insomnia and irritability to major withdrawal with diaphoresis, fever, disorientation, and hallucinations.

Minor alcohol withdrawal occurs as early as 6 hours and usually peaks at 24 to 36 hours after cessation of or significant decrease in alcohol intake. It is characterized by mild autonomic hyperactivity: nausea, anorexia, coarse tremor, tachycardia, hypertension, hyperreflexia, sleep disturbances (e.g., insomnia, vivid dreams), and anxiety.[16]

Major alcohol withdrawal occurs after more than 24 hours and usually peaks at 50 hours but occasionally takes up to 5 days to manifest after the decline or termination of drinking. The syndrome is characterized by pronounced anxiety, insomnia, irritability, tremor, anorexia, tachycardia, hyperreflexia, hypertension, fever, decreased seizure threshold, auditory and visual hallucinations, and finally delirium.[17]

Delirium tremens is the extreme end of the spectrum and consists of gross tremor, profound confusion, fever, incontinence, frightening visual hallucinations, and mydriasis. It seldom appears before the third postabstinence day. Only 5% of patients hospitalized for alcohol withdrawal develop delirium tremens. Other causes of delirium to be considered in the alcoholic patient include sepsis, meningitis, hypoxia, hypoglycemia, hepatic failure, and intracranial bleeding. True delirium tremens is rare and is not synonymous with alcohol withdrawal. Seizures can occur in major withdrawal or delirium tremens.

Management

Prehospital Care

The alcohol-dependent patient in withdrawal may also have a mixed alcohol-drug ingestion, occult head trauma, or cervical spine injury. Patients who are unable to sit without assistance or have an altered mental status require IV access. Thiamine (100 mg), naloxone (0.8 mg), and glucose (dextrose, 25 g) may be given in an IV bolus. Although rapid blood glucose testing is preferable, it is acceptable to give glucose for altered mental status if this testing is not readily available. The airway must be maintained and respirations supported. Emergency medical service personnel should monitor the patient's vital signs and neurologic status. The cervical spine should be immobilized if trauma is suspected. It is usually best to withhold additional treatment until the patient can be evaluated in the emergency department. Emergency medical service personnel should be alert for other medical disorders that accompany alcoholism, such as pneumonia, sepsis, gastrointestinal bleeding, pancreatitis, hepatic failure, hypoglycemia, and intracranial hemorrhage.

Hospital Care

Initial Assessment

Family, friends, bystanders, or paramedics may give more reliable historical data than the patient. Accurate vital signs are essential. This may require a rectal temperature. Hyperthermia, hypothermia, tachypnea, or tachycardia may suggest serious disorders that often accompany the alcohol-dependent patient. These disorders should be considered during this first assessment.

A rapid, thorough examination should be done with attention to the level of consciousness, signs of hepatic failure, or coagulopathy. Signs of trauma are sought, such as subcutaneous emphysema, ecchymosis, subconjunctival hemorrhage, Battle's sign, or fractures. The neurologic examination should search for focal findings, including central facial nerve palsy, hemiparesis, asymmetry of reflexes, or asymmetry of pupillary response.

Treatment Plan

The alcohol withdrawal syndrome must be promptly recognized and treated. Treatment is necessary (1) to provide relief from anxiety and hallucinations, (2) to halt progression to major withdrawal and withdrawal seizures, (3) to allow detection of a treatable primary psychiatric illness, (4) to prepare the patient for long-term alcohol abstinence with the lowest risk of new drug dependence, and (5) to calm the patient and allow adequate examination for the detection of medical illnesses that typically accompany alcoholism, such as gastritis, dehydration, pancreatitis, pneumonia, electrolyte disorders, and hepatitis.

Detention by reasonable restraint is an option to prevent potential injury patients may inflict on themselves or the hospital staff. Appropriate restraints are preferable to allowing decision-incapacitated patients to sign an "against medical advice" (AMA) form and be discharged.

Pharmacologic Intervention

Patients suffering from alcohol withdrawal should receive pharmacologic intervention along with supportive care. More than 150 different drugs and drug combinations have been reported in the literature for the treatment of alcohol withdrawal. The ideal drug for alcohol withdrawal would have a rapid onset, a wide margin of safety, a metabolism not dependent on liver function, and limited abuse potential. Although no one drug class fits all these requirements, benzodiazepines are clearly the mainstay of treatment.

Benzodiazepines. The benzodiazepines have superior anticonvulsant activity, have the least respiratory and cardiac depressive effect of all the CNS depressants, and can be given parenterally in the uncooperative patient. By interacting with receptors linked to the GABA-associated chloride ion channel, benzodiazepines substitute for the withdrawal of the GABA-potentiating effect of alcohol and abate withdrawal signs and symptoms.[18]

Numerous benzodiazepines, including alprazolam (Xanax), chlordiazepoxide (Librium), clorazepate

(Tranxene), diazepam (Valium), lorazepam (Ativan), midazolam (Versed), and oxazepam (Serax), have been studied. No evidence of clear superiority of any one benzodiazepine exists. Lorazepam has good bioavailability with oral, intramuscular (IM), and IV routes. It is rapidly and completely absorbed from IM sites in agitated patients with no IV access. Lorazepam's half-life is intermediate (7 to 14 hours), and it reaches a steady state in 36 to 48 hours without active metabolites. Excessive sedation, confusion, and ataxia are potential complications of all benzodiazepines with prolonged half-lives. Lorazepam is metabolized (conjugated) in the liver, yielding inactive products. Although lorazepam's half-life increases in patients with cirrhosis or liver failure, it is much less than the increase with chlordiazepoxide. Lorazepam's elimination is only minimally altered in patients with renal failure and in elderly persons.

Lorazepam may be given IV in a dose of 2 to 4 mg, depending on the severity of the withdrawal. Dosing can be repeated at 10- to 30-minute intervals for patients in severe withdrawal. An IM dose of 0.07 mg/kg can be used. The oral schedule for moderate withdrawal is 6 mg/day in three divided doses, tapering the amount by 1 to 2 mg/day over 4 to 6 days. If lorazepam is unavailable, diazepam can be given, with 5 mg IV every 5 to 10 minutes in major withdrawal until the patient is calm. When patients are admitted to the hospital, symptom-triggered dosing of benzodiazepines has been shown to be superior to a fixed dose schedule.[19]

The dosage of benzodiazepines required for alcohol withdrawal is highly variable. Practically, the dose is titrated to the patient's agitation. Massive IV drug doses have been required in patients with delirium tremens, including a recorded 2640 mg of diazepam and 35 mg of haloperidol over 48 hours, 75 mg of midazolam in 1 hour, and 2850 mg of midazolam over 5 days.[20]

Butyrophenones. Haloperidol, a dopamine antagonist, can be considered in patients with major alcohol withdrawal or delirium tremens not responding to IV benzodiazepines. Haloperidol is more potent than chlorpromazine, has lower anticholinergic properties, and has less propensity to cause cardiovascular side effects or lower the seizure threshold. Haloperidol has little effect on myocardial function or respiratory drive, and its safety and efficacy by the IV, IM, or oral route in the emergency department have been established. Haloperidol has no anticonvulsant properties.

Haloperidol and lorazepam in combination are safe and may be synergistic. Safe use in extremely high doses in patients with serious underlying medical illness has been documented in several studies: 240 mg of haloperidol and 480 mg of lorazepam given over 24 hours in a patient and 485 mg of haloperidol over 8 hours in another patient without significant adverse effects. Some advocate an aggressive protocol with escalating doses of the combination of haloperidol and lorazepam.[21]

β-Blockers. Alcohol withdrawal has been associated with increased noradrenergic activity. Benzodiazepines do not possess any direct antiadrenergic effects. Propranolol and atenolol have been studied in alcohol withdrawal. In one study, vital signs and clinical (tremor) and behavioral (agitation, anxiety) signs in patients taking atenolol and oxazepam resolved more rapidly than in patients taking placebo and oxazepam. Over 4 to 5 days of treatment the atenolol group required substantially smaller doses of oxazepam on each treatment day.

β-Blockers can be considered as an adjunctive therapy in mild to moderate alcohol withdrawal. Relative contraindications include insulin-dependent diabetes, hypotension, lung disease with bronchospasm, congestive heart failure, and second-degree or third-degree heart block.

α-Agonists. The α-adrenergic agonist clonidine has proved effective in opiate withdrawal. Clonidine is not a controlled substance and has little or no addictive or abuse potential. It improves vital signs and the subjective complaints of alcohol withdrawal. Clonidine appears to be most effective in attenuating blood pressure changes versus other withdrawal symptoms. Theoretically, clonidine avoids the potential for oversedation and the dependence on benzodiazepines and may be helpful with mixed alcohol-apioid withdrawal. It is ineffective in preventing seizures. Clonidine may be considered in patients with mild alcohol withdrawal with no history of alcohol-related seizures who are candidates for an outpatient program or who have coincident opiate addiction.

Anticonvulsants. Carbamazepine, gabapentin, and valproate have been tried in outpatient treatment of mild to moderate alcohol withdrawal with some success.[22,23]

Emergency Department and Outpatient Approaches

Rapid, aggressive control of alcohol withdrawal is crucial. The cornerstone of treatment is a benzodiazepine. Lorazepam may be preferable because of its previously discussed qualities.

An initial test dose of 1 to 2 mg of lorazepam or 5 mg of diazepam IV can be given to the patient in the emergency department. The doses can be repeated with observation of the patient for 2 to 6 hours guiding the emergency physician concerning the dose required for outpatient treatment. Patients remain under observation or are admitted until the manifestations of withdrawal do not progress after the effects of the benzodiazepine have dissipated.[18]

Outpatient treatment consists of lorazepam, 1 to 2 mg three times a day in a tapering dose for 3 to 6 days; chlordiazepoxide, 25 to 100 mg three times a day, in a tapering dose for 3 to 6 days; or diazepam, 30 mg once a day tapered over 5 days depending on the severity of symptoms. Adequate diet, abstinence, and participation in a rehabilitation program in the community are also desirable. Any patient requiring 300 mg of chlordiazepoxide or 60 mg of diazepam per day to control withdrawal should be considered for admission. Patients with major alcohol withdrawal (disorientation, hallucinations, diaphoresis, or fever) are admitted. Doses approximately equivalent to 100 mg of chlordiazepoxide are 20 mg of diazepam and 5 mg of lorazepam.[18]

Haloperidol (5 mg IV) or propofol (100 mg IV) can be considered in major withdrawal or delirium tremens not responding adequately to benzodiazepines. In stable admitted patients, β-blockers may be considered as an adjunct to benzodiazepine therapy if no contraindications are present. Combination therapy is reasonable in alcohol withdrawal; benefits include reduction of the risks associated with prolonged and heavy sedation, faster symptom resolution, and quicker recovery.

Benzodiazepines should be used only for the minimum time required to avoid their abuse, addiction, and withdrawal in the alcoholic. The previous suggestions are only guidelines, and therapy must be individualized.

Adjunctive Therapy

Patients being treated for major alcohol withdrawal should receive thiamine (100 mg IV) and magnesium (2 g IV). Although magnesium sulfate does not decrease the severity of withdrawal symptoms, the incidence of delirium, or seizures, it carries no significant risk or cost. In the nonacute setting, oral magnesium supplementation in chronic alcoholics improves liver function tests, electrolyte balance, and muscle strength.[24] Multivitamin preparations may be considered for chronic malnutrition. Although their clinical benefit is not proved, they carry no significant risk or cost.[14]

If present, volume depletion can be corrected with normal saline. Reversal of electrolyte and metabolic disorders (hypomagnesemia, hypophosphatemia, hypokalemia, and acidosis) is discussed in the following section. Although treatment of electrolyte disorders and acidosis benefits the patient, it does little to abate the withdrawal syndrome.

Phenothiazines are contraindicated because they can produce hypotension, lower seizure threshold, disturb central temperature regulation, and cause extrapyramidal effects in the dosages required to calm patients in alcohol withdrawal.

ALCOHOL-RELATED SEIZURES

With the various medical problems related to alcohol abuse, the differential diagnosis and management of seizures remain among the most challenging and controversial (Box 184-1). A patient arriving at the emergency department with seizures should be questioned about alcohol intake. From 20% to 40% of seizure patients presenting to an emergency department have their seizures related to alcohol abuse.[25] Alcohol is a causative factor in 15% to 24% of patients with status epilepticus.[26]

The primary consideration in the initial care of these patients is the recognition and treatment of life-threatening causes of seizures, such as CNS infection, hypoglycemia, or intracranial hematoma.

BOX 184-1. Differential Diagnosis of Alcohol Related Seizures

- Withdrawal (alcohol or drugs)
- Exacerbation of idiopathic or posttraumatic seizures
- Acute intoxication (amphetamines, anticholinergics, cocaine, isoniazid, organophosphates, phenothiazines, tricyclic antidepressants, salicylates, lithium)
- Metabolic (hypoglycemia, hyponatremia, hypernatremia, hypocalcemia, hepatic failure)
- Infectious (meningitis, encephalitis, brain abscess)
- Trauma (intracranial hemorrhage)
- Cerebrovascular accident
- Sleep deprivation
- Noncompliance with anticonvulsants

Alcohol may act in one of several ways to produce seizures in patients with or without underlying foci: (1) by its partial or absolute withdrawal after a period of chronic inebriation, (2) by an acute alcohol-related metabolic brain disorder (e.g., hypoglycemia, hyponatremia), (3) by creating a situation leading to cerebral trauma, or (4) by precipitating seizures in patients with idiopathic or posttraumatic epilepsy. Moreover, alcoholics are more susceptible to other causes of seizures, including cerebral infarction, subarachnoid hemorrhage, neurosyphilis, acquired immunodeficiency syndrome (AIDS), brain abscess, and meningitis.[27]

Alcohol Withdrawal Seizures

Alcohol withdrawal is one of the most common causes of adult-onset seizures. Descriptions of alcohol withdrawal seizures (AWSs) were based on data collected on 241 alcohol abusers with seizures or alcohol-related illness complicated by seizures initially described by Victor and Brausch.[28] These patients with AWSs were confirmed alcoholics of many years with the onset of seizures in adulthood. The seizures occurred 6 to 48 hours after the cessation of drinking. Ninety percent had one to six generalized tonic-clonic seizures, which occurred abruptly without warning. Sixty percent experienced multiple seizures, usually two to four within a 6-hour period. However, more recent data suggest a much lower repeat seizure rate of 13% to 24%.[29]

The incidence of partial (focal) seizures, common with posttraumatic epilepsy, is increased by alcohol withdrawal. However, partial seizures still should be considered indicative of a mass lesion until proved otherwise.

The term *alcohol withdrawal seizure* is reserved for seizures with the characteristics described by Victor and Brausch.[28] The term *alcohol-related seizure* (ARS) is used to refer to all seizures in the aggregate associated with alcohol use, including this subset of AWSs.

Management

Historically, up to one third of patients with AWSs progressed to delirium tremens because of inadequate treatment. Currently, this proportion has decreased to less than 5% with early, aggressive benzodiazepine therapy.

An IV line of normal saline with magnesium, similar to the alcohol withdrawal regimen, should be established. If the patient has an altered mental status, thiamine, dextrose, and naloxone should be considered. Again, empirical glucose bolus dosing should not be used if a prompt, accurate determination of blood glucose is possible.

Although fever may suggest meningitis, it may be found in intracranial hemorrhage, brain abscess, alcohol withdrawal, toxic ingestions, and infections outside the CNS. Temperature can rise as a result of tonic-clonic seizure. If meningitis is suspected but a possibility of increased intracranial pressure exists, the patient can have specimens drawn for blood cultures and be started empirically on antibiotics. A lumbar puncture (LP) may be delayed until a space-occupying lesion is ruled out with computed tomography (CT) scanning, but antibiotics cannot be delayed if meningitis is a possibility.

Contraindications of LP include intracranial mass, papilledema, localizing neurologic findings, coagulopathy, and local infection in the area of the LP. If an LP is performed relatively soon after a single IV dose of antibiotics (1 to 2 hours), subsequent CSF cultures are likely to remain positive in most adult patients. In addition, the CSF leukocyte count, protein level, and glucose concentration are not significantly affected. Delay in administering antibiotics in meningitis adversely affects patients' morbidity and mortality. LP should be considered in febrile alcoholics with delirium, with the previous precautions. Interestingly, occult CNS infections in febrile alcoholics with an altered mental status are uncommon.[30]

Patients Presenting with a Normal Neurologic Examination

New-Onset Alcohol-Related Seizures

Patients with new-onset ARSs must be thoroughly evaluated. This includes alcoholics who claim to have had seizures in the past but for whom no documentation of previous seizures or of an appropriate workup is available. Metabolic disorders, toxic ingestion, infection, and structural abnormalities are ruled out by history, repeated physical examinations, laboratory testing including electrolytes and glucose, and CT scan, as necessary. An electroencephalogram scheduled during follow-up may be considered (but its value is limited) in the patient whose seizures have not been explained.[31]

If the initial assessment is normal, patients who remain seizure free and symptom free with no sign of withdrawal after 4 to 6 hours of observation may be discharged. Optimal outpatient treatment includes clear guidelines for follow-up and re-evaluation and the help of a concerned family member or friend (who is not a drinking partner). Ideally, this individual should remain with the patient for 1 to 2 days. These criteria may be difficult to meet, and the physician must use discretion in deciding to admit for observation when the patient is at risk for serious injury. The ideal disposition is participation in a detoxification-rehabilitation program.

It may be unclear whether the patient has had a pure AWS or the new onset of epilepsy in the setting of alcohol ingestion. At this point, such a patient probably does not require further treatment. The literature provides little useful information about the natural history, including the risk of subsequent seizures, in patients presenting with an unprovoked seizure.[32] Beginning anticonvulsants in a patient after a new-onset single seizure is controversial, and the final decision about treatment should be individualized and made after consultation with a neurologist or the patient's primary care provider. The patient with a first-time ARS who has a history consistent with AWS and a negative workup can be treated as presented in the next section.

Seizures in the Alert Patient with a History of Seizures during Prior Withdrawal

Alcoholic patients with the manifestations of alcohol withdrawal who have not had a recent seizure but relate a history of AWSs are seen frequently in the emergency department. The risk of seizure increases 10-fold in this subset of patients.

Benzodiazepines alone are sufficient to prevent AWSs.[29] Many of these patients are sporadically taking one or more anticonvulsants. It is difficult, if not impossible, to decide in the emergency department whether these anticonvulsants were given for idiopathic epilepsy, posttraumatic epilepsy, or AWSs. To prevent AWSs effectively, detoxification with benzodiazepines should be initiated early because most AWSs occur within the first 24 hours after alcohol withdrawal. Treatment should be started with the understanding the patient will be observed for 4 to 6 hours and referred to a detoxification-rehabilitation program (if available).

An initial dose of 2 mg of lorazepam or 10 mg of diazepam can be given orally or 1 to 2 mg of lorazepam or 5 mg of diazepam given IV to the patient in the emergency department. This dose may be repeated depending on the patient's response. The patient is observed for 4 to 6 hours, which guides the dose required for outpatient treatment.

Prescribing anticonvulsants, such as benzodiazepines (other than a short 3- to 6-day course for alcohol withdrawal) and phenytoin, to the outpatient alcoholic may increase the potential for addiction and paradoxically may increase the number of acute seizures. The poorly compliant alcoholic patient may do better without outpatient anticonvulsants for a concurrent seizure disorder. Therefore, the ideal disposition is admission to a detoxification-rehabilitation unit.

Alert Patient with a Seizure before or after Presentation

The alcoholic patient with a documented history of ARSs who experiences a single seizure or a short burst of seizures should be treated with lorazepam, 2 mg IV. These patients usually require observation with careful monitoring of neurologic status for at least 6 hours before discharge.

Patients with an Abnormal Neurologic Presentation

New-Onset Partial Seizures

Partial (focal) seizures are reported to account for up to 24% of ARSs. Conversely, studies have shown that 17% to 21% of patients with partial ARSs have structural lesions (hematomas, tumors, or vascular abnormalities).[33] These primary causes of partial ARS, such as prior head trauma, may be missed in the history taking. As a result, an urgent CT scan is indicated to evaluate new-onset partial seizures.

The patient with a documented history of a focal ARS who has been previously evaluated does not require an emergency CT scan provided a return to baseline occurs promptly. A patient with a focal ARS associated with normal neuroimaging can be managed with supportive care, observation for 4 to 6 hours, and benzodiazepines for withdrawal signs or symptoms. Appropriate follow-up should be arranged.

Status Epilepticus

When multiple seizures are interrupted only by brief periods of incomplete recovery or major motor convulsions are continuous for more than 30 minutes, status epilepticus is present. Although fewer than 8% of ARS patients go into status epilepticus, alcohol is implicated in 15% to 24% of status epilepticus cases.[34] Status epilepticus may also be the first presentation of ARSs.

The most common cause of status epilepticus is discontinuation or erratic compliance with an anticonvulsant drug regimen, followed by ARS. However, status epilepticus may arise for a variety of reasons and is often multifactorial. Thus, it is essential to screen for all possible factors underlying repeated or prolonged seizures, even when a probable cause is thought to be readily apparent.

After airway management and the initiation of two IV lines, IV lorazepam is given, along with thiamine, dextrose, and naloxone. Although lorazepam and diazepam are both effective in terminating seizures in status epilepticus, lorazepam is preferable because its anticonvulsant effect lasts several hours, whereas diazepam's anticonvulsant effects last only 20 to 30 minutes. Because of this, lorazepam is associated with fewer recurrent seizures and fewer repeated doses are required compared with diazepam.[35,36]

Lorazepam 4 mg can be given at 2 mg/min diluted in an equal volume of solution and repeated in 10 minutes if seizures persist. Diazepam is given at a rate of 5 mg/min, up to 20 mg. Intravenous benzodiazepines are associated with the complications of respiratory depression and hypotension.

If seizures persist after lorazepam or diazepam, a loading dose of phenytoin (Dilantin), 18 mg/kg, or fosphenytoin (Cerebyx), 15 to 20 phenytoin equivalents mg/kg, is administered in the second IV line. Additional doses of 5 mg/kg of phenytoin, to a maximum of 30 mg/kg or 1500 mg/24 hours, can be given if status is not terminated.

Most of the cardiac abnormalities associated with phenytoin infusion are caused by its solvent, propylene glycol. Caution is advised in patients who have preexisting heart disease. Using a 20-gauge line proximal to the forearm to avoid purple glove syndrome and keeping the phenytoin rate less than 50 mg/min helps to minimize the problem of hypotension and bradycardia. Fosphenytoin does not contain propylene glycol and is safe and well tolerated at IV rates of 100 to 150 mg/min. Rapid achievement of therapeutic free phenytoin levels without significant side effects has been documented using fosphenytoin in patients with status epilepticus.[37] The cost of fosphenytoin is approximately 20 times greater than that of phenytoin. Interestingly, emergency department studies comparing phenytoin and fosphenytoin (not involving status epilepticus) found no advantage of fosphenytoin over phenytoin.[38-40]

Phenobarbital at a maximum rate of 50 mg/min to 100 mg/min IV, with a loading dose of 20 mg/kg, was recommended in the past for a patient who does not respond to phenytoin and lorazepam or diazepam. (By this time, the admitting physician should be involved with the patient's care). Phenobarbital can be used in patients with cardiac disease or phenytoin allergy. The cardiorespiratory depressant effects of phenobarbital and lorazepam are additive. Experts have suggested skipping phenobarbital and considering pentobarbital, propofol, midazolam, or valproic acid instead at this stage.[41-43]

It is often difficult to rule out a CNS infection in alcoholics with status epilepticus because of concomitant hyperthermia, serum leukocytosis, and CSF pleocytosis. If CSF infection is a possibility, an LP should be considered.

Obtundation

The obtunded or stuporous patient with a history of seizure activity poses a diagnostic challenge. The patient's decreased level of consciousness (LOC) may be the result of a postictal state, occult head trauma, unrecognized metabolic disorder, or poisoning. The first task is to determine the possibility of hypoglycemia (diagnosed and reversed at the bedside in seconds to minutes) or a neurosurgical lesion—intracranial mass (with morbidity and mortality directly related to the time of surgical intervention).

Patients with focal neurologic findings on physical examination, new-onset seizures, partial (focal) seizures, or evidence of acute head trauma should be considered for an urgent CT scan. If the LOC is consistently improving, the patient is unlikely to have an immediate life-threatening problem. An unimproved or deteriorating LOC requires a CT scan.

No History of Seizures, No Current Seizure

In the alcoholic patient in withdrawal who lacks a history of seizures, benzodiazepines generally have sufficient anticonvulsant activity to prevent withdrawal seizures.

Phenytoin-Anticonvulsant Conundrum

Phenytoin has no significant benefit over placebo in preventing recurrence of AWSs.[25,44] Considering the risks of phenytoin and no demonstrated benefit in the setting of AWS, it is not indicated for the treatment of an AWS. The sudden withdrawal of phenytoin may potentiate the convulsive effects of alcohol withdrawal. Withdrawal seizures may occur in epileptic patients withdrawn from phenytoin. In patients with status epilepticus, alcohol and noncompliance with anticonvulsant regimens may be synergistic.

Alcoholic patients with preexisting seizure disorders pose a dilemma when they are supposed to be taking antiepileptic drugs but their blood levels suggest noncompliance. This is especially problematic when their epileptic attacks are uncommon and appear to occur exclusively in the context of alcohol withdrawal. Some of these patients may have AWSs and may have been misdiagnosed. Others may have a seizure disorder that appears to be confined to the setting of alcohol withdrawal. Such patients have demonstrated that they cannot maintain compliance with their treatment.

A patient currently taking phenytoin for an antecedent seizure disorder who presents with a seizure while intoxicated falls into a different category. Such an episode could be an isolated event in a usually compliant patient without a history of chronic alcohol abuse. In this patient a seizure in the setting of a subtherapeutic phenytoin level may represent the consequences of noncompliance with phenytoin versus AWS.

OTHER CLINICAL FEATURES AND MANAGEMENT

Cardiovascular Effects

Acute and chronic ethanol consumption can affect the mechanical function of the heart, produce dysrhythmias, and exacerbate coronary artery disease (CAD). It may alter myocardial function by direct toxic effects, associated hypertension, or indirectly by altering specific electrolytes. Acute intoxication has minimal effects on patients who are not chronic alcoholics and do not have preexisting CAD. Acute intoxication can decrease cardiac output in both alcoholic and nonalcoholic patients with preexisting cardiac disease.[45]

Several studies have linked moderate alcohol consumption (up to two drinks per day in men and one in women) to a protective effect from CAD. As much as 50% of the relative risk reduction of CAD can be explained by increased levels of high-density lipoprotein (HDL) and its subfractions HDL-2 and HDL-3. Genetic variations in the ADH allele may account for these changes. Low to moderate alcohol consumption is found to decrease platelet aggregation, raise plasma levels of endogenous tissue plasminogen activator,[46] and lower insulin resistance. Experimental data suggest that alcohol may have antioxidant properties, produce effects on smooth muscles through interactions with nitric oxide, and alter plasma total homocysteine levels.[47,48]

Studies suggest that moderate alcohol consumption, through a reduced risk of CAD, may also protect individuals from congestive heart failure (Box 184-2).[49] All of these beneficial effects are lost in heavy drinkers, in whom chronic alcoholism is associated with hypertension and congestive cardiomyopathy.

The typical patient with alcoholic cardiomyopathy is a man older than 30 with a greater than 10-year history of chronic alcohol intake. The signs and symptoms are no different from those of low-output congestive heart failure of other causes: dyspnea, palpitations, weakness and fatigue, jugular venous distention, poor R wave progression, nonspecific electrocardiographic abnormalities, and biventricular enlargement on a chest radiograph. Echocardiography shows four-chamber enlargement with decreased left and right ventricular contractile function. Up to one third of chronic alcoholic patients have left ventricular dysfunction demonstrated by a radionuclide ventriculogram, usually coexisting with skeletal muscle disease. Women appear to be more sensitive to the toxic effects of alcohol on striated muscle and are at greater risk for cardiomyopathy and myopathy. The diagnosis is made by obtaining a history of prolonged alcohol use and excluding hypertensive, coronary, valvular, and congenital disease.

Heavy alcohol consumption (more than 2 ounces a day) has a detrimental effect on those with preexisting CAD. It can reduce exercise tolerance, induce coronary vasoconstriction, and raise heart rate and blood pressure.[50] Additive cardiovascular effects of ethanol and nicotine contribute to dysrhythmias and sudden death in patients with CAD. In one study, nearly half the patients with alcohol withdrawal had prolongation of the QT interval. Prolonged QT can precipitate a dysrhythmia, resulting in sudden death.[51] There is an increased incidence of sudden death among heavy drinkers regardless of concomitant CAD or smoking.

Supraventricular (usually atrial fibrillation) and ventricular (usually transitory ventricular tachycardia) dysrhythmias, the "holiday heart," have been documented in alcoholic patients who have been drinking heavily. One study reported that alcohol contributes to or causes new-onset atrial fibrillation in approximately two thirds of patients younger than 65. Alcohol also affects cardiac function indirectly by lowering potassium and magnesium levels. Data from the Framingham Heart Study indicate that patients with lower levels of potassium and magnesium have higher rates of dysrhythmias.[52]

Left ventricular ejection fractions improve with either abstinence or sustained decrease of alcohol consumption starting at 1 year and continue to improve over at least 4 years. Tachydysrhythmias as a result of episodic drinking commonly revert to sinus rhythm with abstinence and do not require immediate intervention if the patient is hemodynamically stable. Nevertheless, correction of electrolyte abnormalities is prudent.

Pulmonary Effects

Alcohol reduces the mobilization of alveolar macrophages and their bactericidal capacity. Their impairment is greatest in alcoholics with hepatic cirrhosis. These effects, along with aspiration, decreased airway

BOX 184-2. Risks and Benefits of Light, Moderate, and Heavy Drinking

Light/Moderate Drinking			
Risks		***Benefits***	
Established	Heavy drinking	Probable	Decreased risk of coronary heart disease Decreased risk of ischemic stroke Decreased risk of gallstones
Unresolved	Breast cancer Fetal damage	Possible	Decreased risk of diabetes Decreased risk of peripheral vascular disease
Unlikely	Bowel cancer Hemorrhagic stroke High blood pressure		
Heavy Drinking			
Risks		***Benefits***	
Noncardiovascular	Liver cirrhosis Pancreatitis Certain cancers Accidents Homicides Suicides Fetal damage Degenerative central nervous system disorders	None	
Cardiovascular	High blood pressure Arrhythmia Hemorrhagic stroke Cardiomyopathy		

From Klatsky A: Drink to your health. *Sci Am* February, 2003. Copyright © Scientific American, Inc.

sensitivity, concomitant smoking, and malnutrition, probably account for the increased incidence of pneumonia, particularly lobar pneumonia, among alcoholic patients.[53]

At least 80% of alcoholics are smokers, making it difficult to distinguish between alcohol-induced and tobacco-induced injury to the lungs. Most studies have failed to show an independent effect of alcohol on pulmonary function. The high prevalence of respiratory disease in alcoholics is largely caused by smoking. Chronic alcohol abuse has been shown to increase the risk of developing adult respiratory distress syndrome in the intensive care unit setting.[54]

Alcohol ingestion has been shown to induce bronchospasm in some asthmatics and to increase ventricular ectopy and sleep apnea in patients with chronic obstructive pulmonary disease. Alcoholic patients with hepatic cirrhosis can have hypoxemia develop as a result of precapillary shunting in their lungs. Hyperventilation and a respiratory alkalosis are also seen with hepatic cirrhosis. Low to moderate alcohol consumption (one or two drinks per day) has been shown to decrease the risk of pulmonary embolus and deep venous thrombosis in elderly patients.[55]

Gastrointestinal and Hepatic Effects

Esophagus and Stomach

Alcoholic patients have a higher incidence of esophagitis, gastric cancer, and esophageal carcinoma than the general population. Acute alcohol ingestion also decreases lower esophageal sphincter pressure, delays gastric emptying, and disrupts the normal gastric mucosal barrier. Vomiting is common among drinkers. Forceful or persistent emesis can lead to a Mallory-Weiss tear or Boerhaave's syndrome.

Gastrointestinal Bleeding

Alcohol has a close association with gastrointestinal bleeding. Causes include Mallory-Weiss tears, esophagitis, esophageal varices, acute and chronic gastritis, thrombocytopenia, portal hypertensive gastropathy, qualitative and quantitative platelet disorders, and prolonged clotting times. Alcohol may exacerbate gastric mucosal damage when combined with nonsteroidal anti-inflammatory drugs (NSAIDs), but ethanol itself is not a risk factor for peptic ulcer disease. An inverse relationship exists between consumption of alcohol, particularly wine, and active *Helicobacter pylori* infection. Peptic ulcer disease is the most common cause of bleeding in alcoholic patients with upper gastrointestinal hemorrhage as well as those who do not drink.[56]

Liver

The liver is the primary site of ethanol metabolism. Hepatic damage has been recognized for centuries as the hallmark of chronic alcohol abuse. The production of cytokines such as tumor necrosis factor α is one of the earliest events in many types of liver injury. This cascade may trigger the production of other cytokines that together enlist inflammatory cells, kill hepatocytes, and initiate healing through fibrogenesis. There is no one test that can be used to diagnose alcoholic liver disease (ALD) reliably. However, the ratio of aspartate transaminase (AST) to alanine transaminase (ALT) may provide a hint that alcohol is likely the cause of liver injury.[57] ALD is the most common liver disorder in the western world and, along with hepatitis C, is a leading cause of liver transplantation.

Fatty Infiltration

The earliest, mildest, and most common liver change seen in alcoholism is the accumulation of macrovesicular fat in the hepatocytes, predominantly involving triglycerides. Alcoholic fatty liver is usually asymptomatic, associated with mild elevations of AST and ALT, and subsides with abstinence. It is usually detected by the finding of hepatomegaly on physical examination or abnormalities on ultrasonography or CT but is confirmed only by liver biopsy. Fatty liver is usually a reversible disorder if the patient can refrain from drinking.[58]

Alcoholic Hepatitis

Alcoholic hepatitis is a more serious complication than fatty infiltration and develops in up to 35% of heavy drinkers.[59] These individuals usually have right upper quadrant pain, a tender enlarged liver, fever, jaundice, leukocytosis, and altered liver function tests. AST levels are usually less than 300 IU/L, and ALT levels are typically less than one half the AST level. Alcoholic hepatitis can have a range of clinical manifestations, from mildly symptomatic hepatomegaly to fulminant hepatic failure. The severity of the disease can be estimated in the emergency department by a prolonged prothrombin time/international normalized ratio (INR).[60]

Symptomatic patients with alcoholic hepatitis require admission. Emergency department evaluation includes complete blood count, electrolytes, blood urea nitrogen, glucose, prothrombin time/INR, liver function tests, and urinalysis. If the patient has an abnormal prothrombin time/INR and is actively bleeding, fresh frozen plasma should be started in the emergency department. Steroids are indicated in severe cases (encephalopathy, coagulopathy).[61] Steroids are not indicated in patients with gastrointestinal bleeding or concurrent infection. Up to 80% of patients who continue to drink after having alcoholic hepatitis eventually develop cirrhosis.

Alcoholic Cirrhosis

Cirrhosis is the disruption of the normal architecture of the liver by scarring and regenerating nodules of parenchyma. Alcoholism is the most common cause of cirrhosis in the United States and is responsible for approximately 50% of all cirrhotic deaths.

Alcoholic cirrhosis usually requires 10 to 15 years of chronic drinking, often punctuated by one or more episodes of acute hepatic decompensation. The clinical outcome is determined by the development of complications of portal hypertension and by hepatic dysfunction. We are just beginning to understand the pathogenesis of alcoholic cirrhosis in animal models. Why hepatic damage develops in some alcoholic patients and not in others exposed to identical amounts of alcohol remains a mystery. The disorder was originally described as "nutritional cirrhosis," but it has been shown that alcohol, independent of malnutrition, produces liver damage. Alteration of the normal hepatic architecture by fibrosis and nodule formation may eventually lead to portal hypertension. Portal hypertension may in turn be complicated by ascites and esophageal varices. Alcoholic cirrhosis is the most common cause of hepatic encephalopathy.[58]

Hepatitis C antibodies are found in one third to one half of alcoholics with ALD. Patients with ALD and hepatitis C have histologically more severe disease, shorter survival, and increased rates (by a factor of 10) of cirrhosis and liver cancer.[62]

No specific therapy of proven benefit exists for ALD other than abstinence, proper diet, and management of the subsequent hepatic decompensation (i.e., ascites and encephalopathy). A 60% decrease in mortality has been associated with decreasing the amount of alcohol consumed over 1 year.[63] Liver biopsy is the only way to identify precisely which type of ALD is present. Biopsy is contraindicated in patients with coagulopathy that has not been corrected. Although cirrhosis is irreversible, its progression may be halted with abstinence.

Pancreas and Intestines

The association of ethanol with pancreatitis is well established, but the exact pathogenesis still eludes investigators. Hypotheses include reflux of duodenal contents and bile into the pancreatic duct, obstruction by a plug of pancreatic juice rich in proteins, and a direct toxic effect of ethanol. Ethanol abuse is associated with both acute and chronic pancreatitis.

The diagnosis of alcoholic pancreatitis can be difficult because asymptomatic alcoholics may have an elevated amylase level. In addition, up to 30% of patients with acute alcoholic pancreatitis have an amylase value within normal limits. Serum lipase rises after amylase and remains elevated longer. It appears to be a more reliable indicator of alcoholic pancreatitis, especially when more than three times normal.[64] Alcohol is only one of several causes of acute pancreatitis; other causes include biliary tract disease, hypercalcemia, hypertriglyceridemia, penetrating peptic ulcer, abdominal trauma, and reactions to various drugs. Alcohol is the leading cause of chronic pancreatitis.

Diarrhea and impaired intestinal absorption are common problems of the chronic alcoholic. Alcohol increases small intestine transit time and decreases brush border enzyme activity. Thiamine, vitamin B_{12}, amino acids, folic acid, and glucose have all been shown to have impaired absorption in alcoholics. Dietary deficiencies in folic acid and protein, pancreatic insufficiency, abnormal biliary secretion, and direct toxic effects of ethanol on the gastrointestinal tract all contribute to malabsorption. Abstinence and adequate nutrition reverse the diarrhea and much of the malabsorption.[58]

Neurologic Effects

Altered Mental Status and Coma

Alcohol is often associated with an altered level of consciousness. Coma or an altered mental state may be caused by acute intoxication, mixed alcohol-drug overdose, postictal states, head trauma, hypoglycemia, shock from gastrointestinal bleeding or sepsis, hypothermia, hyperthermia, hepatic encephalopathy, methanol–isopropyl alcohol–ethylene glycol poisoning, or Wernicke-Korsakoff syndrome.

A potential pitfall for the clinician is ascribing the cause of the patient's altered mental state to acute intoxication without considering the aforementioned conditions. These potentially catastrophic diagnoses are usually revealed by a thorough history and physical examination, a blood alcohol level (coma is rare in patients with blood alcohol levels less than 200 mg/dL), and close observation (an intoxicated patient's LOC should constantly improve over time). Patients with a less than classical presentation or course should receive appropriate laboratory analysis and a head CT scan.

Neuropathy

A symmetrical sensorimotor polyneuropathy is common after chronic alcohol abuse. It usually manifests itself in the lower extremities. Its causes are thought to be a combination of nutritional deficiency with thiamine or B_{12} deficit and a direct neurotoxic effect of alcohol. Burning pain and paresthesia are common presenting complaints. Findings on physical examination include loss of light touch, decreased pinprick, and reduced lower extremity deep tendon reflexes. Distal muscle weakness is a late finding. The neuropathy may lead to nonhealing ulcers on the feet.

"Saturday night palsy" or "honeymooner's syndrome," an entity caused by radial nerve compression, consists of wristdrop. The patient usually has spent the night with the arm drooped over the back of a chair, bench, or a companion, compressing the radial nerve against the humerus and producing a neurapraxia.

Treatment of alcoholic neuropathy is abstinence, adequate diet, and thiamine. Complete recovery is rare. With radial nerve neurapraxia, function usually returns after a few weeks to months.

Wernicke-Korsakoff Syndrome

The classical description of Wernicke's encephalopathy includes (1) oculomotor disturbances (usually nystagmus and ocular palsies), (2) abnormal mentation (usually confusion), and (3) ataxia resulting in part from thiamine deficiency. Currently, Wernicke's encephalopathy, a medical emergency with a mortality rate of 10% to 20%, remains a clinical diagnosis and is poorly recognized because the complete triad is found in as few as 12% of patients.[14] Alternatively, contemporary criteria require two of these signs: (1) dietary deficiencies, (2) oculomotor abnormalities, (3) cerebellar dysfunction, and (4) either an altered mental state or mild memory impairment.[65] The diagnosis should be entertained in any alcoholic or malnourished patient presenting with ocular abnormalities, ataxia, altered mental status, hypothermia, or coma.

Genetic and environmental factors may also play a part in the pathogenesis in this disorder. An inborn enzymatic error, a thiamine-dependent enzyme, transketolase, is deficient or less responsive in some patients with the Wernicke-Korsakoff syndrome. This may explain why the disorder develops in only a few alcoholics. Persons with transketolase deficiency are asymptomatic until they are stressed by thiamine deficiency. Protracted vomiting, inadequate diet, and malabsorption all contribute to thiamine deficiency in the alcoholic.[66]

Korsakoff's psychosis or amnesic state, also called alcohol-induced persisting amnestic disorder, is a disorder with primarily recent memory impairment, inability to learn new information or recall previously learned information, apathy, and confabulation. Although common, confabulation is not essential for the diagnosis. Age older than 40 years and many years of heavy alcohol use are risk factors. The onset may be abrupt or insidious.

In addition to chronic alcoholism, thiamine deficiency should be considered in other chronically ill patients (e.g., AIDS, hyperemesis gravidarum, thyrotoxicosis) and those undergoing dialysis or long-term furosemide therapy for congestive heart failure and disseminated cancer.[12,67]

Alcoholics with altered mental status should receive thiamine (100 mg IV) and either a rapid blood glucose determination or empirical dextrose (25 g IV). Naloxone (0.08 mg IV) should be considered if warranted by the clinical picture. Treatment for Wernicke-Korsakoff syndrome consists of abstinence, adequate diet, and thiamine. The ophthalmoplegia and nystagmus usually have a good response to thiamine (hours to days). The ataxia and mental changes may take days to weeks to improve and usually have a poorer prognosis. Less than 25% of patients show any real recovery, 50% show some recovery, and the remainder show no response despite adequate thiamine replacement. Because magnesium is a cofactor for this enzyme system, serum levels should be corrected.

Patients with Wernicke's syndrome require admission and aggressive thiamine and magnesium repletion. Recovery is variable in the Korsakoff or alcohol amnesic state.

Cerebrovascular Accident

As with CAD, many studies have shown that drinking light to moderate amounts of alcohol may decrease the risk of ischemic stroke. Conversely, several studies have linked heavy drinking to an increased risk of intracranial hemorrhage and ischemic brain injury. Chronic alcohol consumption is believed to increase the risk of hemorrhage through alcohol-induced hypertension, impaired hemostasis, decreased circulating levels of clotting factors, excessive fibrinolysis, and disseminated intravascular coagulation. In addition, cardiac dysrhythmias or cardiomyopathy may precipitate thromboembolic phenomena.[68] Fifty percent of middle-aged patients (45 to 55 years) with no apparent cause for their cerebrovascular accidents suffer from alcoholism.[7]

Myopathy

Several studies have reported elevated creatine kinase values in patients who had been on drinking sprees. Although these patients were asymptomatic, many had muscular tenderness on examination. In these patients, cardiomyopathy often coexists. Both acute and chronic forms of this myopathy are recognized. Many chronic alcoholics have mild proximal muscle weakness and muscle atrophy on examination.

Type II muscle fiber atrophy is found in chronic alcoholic myopathy. The role of ethanol, toxic metabolites, hypokalemia, hypocalcemia, hypomagnesemia, hyponatremia, malnutrition, unrecognized compression or crush injury, and other factors in the pathogenesis of atrophy remains to be determined.[69]

Movement Disorders

Alcohol withdrawal is associated with tremor, ataxia, and myoclonus. Acute alcohol consumption ameliorates essential tremor and myoclonus. Persistent tremor is occasionally seen in chronic alcoholism. This alcoholic tremor may persist up to 1 year after abstinence. Although the pathophysiology is poorly understood, studies have confirmed that essential tremor and alcoholic tremor are distinct entities.[70]

Alcoholic Cerebellar Degeneration

Characterized by ataxia of the extremities, cerebellar ataxia of alcoholism results in a wide-based stance and uncoordinated gait. Lower extremity involvement predominates, although the arms may rarely be involved. Pathologic changes consist of degeneration of elements in the cerebellum, especially the Purkinje cells. The diagnosis is based on history, physical examination, and magnetic resonance imaging or CT (which show severe cerebellar atrophy). Treatment consists of abstinence, adequate nutrition, and thiamine.[71]

Infections

Alcohol is an immunosuppressive drug. Animal and human studies have implicated acute and chronic ethanol ingestion in causing decreased serum bactericidal activity, impaired mononuclear phagocyte function, diminished cell-mediated immune functions, reduced delayed hypersensitivity reaction, and defective polymorphonuclear neutrophils. Neutropenia may be found in up to 8% of hospitalized alcoholics.[72]

Alcohol ingestion prevents the normal delivery (chemotaxis) of polymorphonuclear neutrophils to sites of bacterial infection. Chronic alcohol exposure depresses the development and expression of cell-mediated immunity. This depression may contribute to the high incidence of tuberculosis and head, neck, and upper gastrointestinal cancers in alcoholics. Alcohol's suppression of macrophage function reduces the reticuloendothelial system's ability to clear particles. This may contribute to spontaneous bacteremia, spontaneous peritonitis, and pneumonia. Primary antibody response to new antigens is also depressed. Malnutrition and liver failure also contribute to an immunocompromised state in the alcoholic.

The most common infection seen in alcoholism is pneumonia. Associated risk factors for pneumonia in alcoholics include smoking, decreased ciliary function, decreased surfactant production, depressed cough reflex, malnutrition, and poor oral hygiene. Although alcoholic patients may contract a variety of bacterial pneumonias, *Streptococcus pneumoniae* is still the most common organism. Periods of alcoholic stupor with incomplete glottic closure and subsequent aspiration can lead to aspiration pneumonia. *Klebsiella pneumoniae*, classically associated with alcoholism, is currently more common in patients with cytotoxic chemotherapy, hematologic malignancy, and transplantation than the chronic alcoholic. In addition, these infections now tend to be nosocomial rather than community acquired.[72]

Alcoholism is also associated with a higher incidence of *tuberculosis*—55 times higher than that of the general population in one study. Alcoholism itself does not seem to influence the long-term relapse rates in tuberculous patients if they have closely supervised therapy of adequate duration. Homeless alcoholic patients are believed to constitute an important reservoir of tuberculosis in the United States. Spontaneous bacterial peritonitis occurs in cirrhotic patients with ascites and has a high mortality rate (50% to 90%). A common presentation consists of fever, abdominal pain, and peritonitis. *Escherichia coli*, *K. pneumoniae*, and *S. pneumoniae* are the most common bacteria cultured from the ascitic fluid. Patients with ascites and fever should have a diagnostic paracentesis as part of their evaluation.

Hepatitis C appears to be related to concomitant IV drug use rather than the direct effect of alcohol abuse. Alcoholism is associated with a high prevalence of unsafe sexual behavior and human immunodeficiency virus (HIV) seropositivity.[73] New evidence suggests a potential for greater immunologic changes in HIV-1–positive patients who also consume alcohol.[74]

The most serious impairment of the various host defenses occurs in patients with alcoholic cirrhosis and liver failure. Chronic alcoholics with cirrhosis have been reported to develop spontaneous bacteremia and to have a higher incidence of bacterial endocarditis. Alcoholism and cirrhosis increase the mortality rate in pneumococcal meningitis.

Fever in the chronic alcoholic may result from a vast array of causes. The most common infection remains pneumonia. Occult urinary tract infections are more common than expected. The most common noninfectious causes of fever are alcohol withdrawal and alcoholic hepatitis. A leukocytosis is associated with both, often making the differentiation from infection difficult. Both infectious and noninfectious causes may coexist, as well as multiple sources of infection. Most febrile alcoholics without an identifiable source are best served by hospitalization.

After the appropriate cultures and Gram stain, treatment for spontaneous bacterial peritonitis consists of a third-generation cephalosporin such as cefotaxime. Inoculating 10 mL of ascitic fluid into blood culture bottles at the bedside increases the percentage of positive cultures.[75]

Endocrine Effects

Male hypogonadism and feminism have long been recognized in chronic alcoholics. Alcohol's effects on both the testes and the hypothalamus decrease testosterone production in men.[76] Alcohol may cause impotence by CNS sedation, secondary depression, or decreased testosterone production. Decreased testosterone, increased estrogen (in patients with liver disease), and increased prolactin can lead to decreased libido, feminization, and gynecomastia in male alcoholics and to abnormalities in lactation and menstruation in women. In female alcoholics, increased levels of testosterone and estrogen are found. Estrogen replacement therapy may increase hormonal levels threefold and thus increase the risk of cholelithiasis and breast cancer.[77]

It is difficult to distinguish between obesity, alcoholism, and Cushing's syndrome because facial fullness, weakness, fatigue, and easy bruising related to thinning of the skin can be present in all three conditions. An alcohol-induced pseudo-Cushing's syndrome has also been described that resolves with abstention.[76]

Metabolic Effects

Carbohydrates

Alcohol-induced hypoglycemia is relatively uncommon, occurring in 1% to 4% of intoxicated emergency department patients. It is more frequently seen in chronic alcoholics.[78] Coma, seizures, hemiparesis, and a variety of other neurologic signs have been described in patients presenting with alcohol-induced hypoglycemia. Starvation, depletion of liver glycogen stores, decreased plasma cortisol levels, impaired release of growth hormone, and inhibition of gluconeogenesis may contribute to this phenomenon.

Hyperglycemia and diabetes may be found in chronic alcoholism. However, studies in men exploring the association between light to moderate alcohol use and risk for type 2 diabetes suggest that an inverse relationship may exist.[79] Alcohol abuse can lead to chronic pancreatitis, resulting in underproduction of insulin by the damaged pancreatic cells. Alcohol also impairs peripheral glucose utilization, causing a relative insulin resistance (similar to type 2 diabetes). In diabetic patients, alcohol can induce hypoglycemia and may also mask the signs of hypoglycemia. This effect has been found to be more prominent in the fasting state.[80]

Ethanol can be found as an active ingredient in hundreds of prescription and nonprescription drugs. Concentrations of 60% or greater can be found in some oral preparations, which pose a potential threat to the pediatric patient by producing profound intoxication or alcohol-induced hypoglycemia. Children seem particularly susceptible because of relatively decreased glycogen stores and delayed diagnosis. Hypoglycemia can also be seen with aspirin intoxication, prior gastric bypass surgery, hypothermia, or overwhelming sepsis.

Lipids

A reversible hypertriglyceridemia occurs in many chronic alcoholics. Ethanol increases hepatic synthesis of triglycerides. Abstention is necessary to reduce elevated triglyceride levels. Except for its relationship to fatty infiltration of the liver, the clinical significance of this hyperlipidemia is unknown.[81]

Uric Acid

Hyperuricemia is common with heavy drinkers. Alcohol increases urate levels by inhibiting renal clearance of urate and increasing urate synthesis by enhancing the turnover of adenine nucleotides. Although alcohol use can exacerbate primary gout, it is unlikely that alcohol itself can induce secondary gout.

Electrolytes

Ethanol has numerous effects on electrolytes and mineral metabolism as summarized in Table 184-2. Hyponatremia and hypokalemia are common findings in active drinkers. Vomiting, diarrhea, magnesium depletion, malnutrition, and metabolic alkalosis contribute to these abnormalities.

Alcoholism may be the most common cause of severe magnesium deficiency in adult outpatients. Thirty percent of alcoholics are magnesium deficient as a result of malabsorption, malnutrition, diarrhea, vomiting, and increased urinary losses. Correcting the magnesium level has been shown to improve liver enzyme levels and to correct other electrolytes.[12,24]

Hypocalcemia is a common finding in alcoholic patients with magnesium depletion. The mechanism is related to diminished parathyroid hormone secretion, decreased tissue responsiveness to parathyroid hormone, decreased vitamin D metabolism, and decreased calcium release from bone independent of parathyroid hormone. Correction of magnesium depletion is necessary to restore calcium to normal levels. Hypoalbuminemia, pancreatitis, or vitamin D deficiency may also contribute to low serum calcium or low total body stores of calcium in the alcoholic patient.[82]

Hypophosphatemia is found in 30% to 50% of admitted patients with alcoholism. Phosphorus depletion results from malnutrition, vomiting, respiratory alkalosis, diarrhea, enhanced release of calcitonin, phosphate-binding antacids, and urinary loss (related to vitamin D deficiency and secondary hyperparathyroidism). Hypophosphatemic patients are often found to have low magnesium levels.[83] Rehydration, carbohydrate repletion, and parenteral alimentation further exacerbate phosphorus depletion. Glucose bolus and

Table 184-2. Effect of Ethanol on Mineral Metabolism

Mineral	Cause of Depletion	Additional Effect of Compartment Shifts	Consequences
Magnesium	Alcohol Diarrhea Poor intake Phosphate depletion Hyperaldosteronism	↓ Hyperventilation ↓ Free fatty acids	Pseudohypoparathyroidism Myopathy Potassium depletion Phosphate depletion ECG abnormalities Seizures
Phosphorus	Poor intake Diarrhea Metabolic alkalosis Hypomagnesemia	↓ Metabolic alkalosis ↓ Respiratory alkalosis ↓ Glucose (refeeding) ↑ Hypoparathyroidism (secondary to hypomagnesemia) ↑ Rhabdomyolysis	Rhabdomyolysis Platelet dysfunction WBC dysfunction CNS dysfunction Cardiac failure Renal tubular acidosis
Calcium	Poor intake Steatorrhea Hypovitaminosis K	↓ Hypoparathyroidism (secondary to hypomagnesemia) ↓ Rhabdomyolysis ↓ Hypovitaminosis D ↓ Hyperphosphatemia ↓ Pancreatitis ↓ Hypoalbuminemia ↑ Recovery from rhabdomyolysis	Tetany Seizures
Potassium	Poor intake Metabolic alkalosis Hyperaldosteronism Diarrhea	↓ Glucose (refeeding) ↓ Hyperventilation ↑ Rhabdomyolysis	Weakness Paralysis Myopathy Sudden death

↓, out of plasma; ↑, into plasma.
CNS, central nervous system; ECG, electrocardiographic; WBC, white blood cell.
From Kaysen G, Noth R: The effects of alcohol on blood pressure and electrolytes. *Med Clin North Am* 68:239, 1984.

infusion have been shown to produce a significant fall in serum inorganic phosphate levels. Severe hypophosphatemia (less than 1 mg/dL) has been associated with acute respiratory failure; myocardial depression; dysfunction of erythrocytes, leukocytes, and platelets; CNS irritability; and rhabdomyolysis.

Although chronic alcoholics requiring admission often have potassium, magnesium, and phosphate depletion, empirical treatment with potassium and phosphate is discouraged. Serum levels and renal function should be determined. Unintended hyperkalemia and hyperphosphatemia can produce significant morbidity, and phosphate infusion exacerbates hypocalcemia if present. Because most magnesium is intracellular, a normal serum magnesium level does not necessarily mean that total body magnesium levels are normal. If the serum level is normal, total body levels may be either normal or low. As long as renal function is adequate, empirical magnesium treatment can be considered. Abstinence and a proper diet resolve electrolyte and nutritional deficiencies in the ambulatory alcoholic patient who is healthy enough to be treated as an outpatient.

Correcting these problems is usually the responsibility of the admitting physician. Therapy may be initiated in the emergency department. In most cases, oral supplementation is sufficient. In more severe cases, to correct both hypokalemia and hypophosphatemia, 20 mEq of potassium phosphate per liter of IV solution can be given. Two grams (16.2 mEq) of magnesium sulfate (maximum 30 to 40 g/day) may be given IV at a rate not to exceed 150 mg/min (equivalent to 1.5 mL of 10% solution).

Alcoholic Ketoacidosis

Alcoholic ketoacidosis most frequently occurs in severe chronic alcoholics who have had a recent binge followed 1 to 3 days later by protracted vomiting, decreased food intake, dehydration, and abstinence. Nausea, vomiting, and abdominal pain are common presenting complaints.[84]

These patients have tachypnea, dehydration, ketonuria, and little or no glucosuria. Serum glucose levels are usually less than 200 mg/dL. Normal blood pH may be found despite ketonemia because of coexisting respiratory alkalosis and metabolic alkalosis.

The exact mechanism responsible for this increase in ketone bodies is unclear. Acute starvation superimposed on chronic malnutrition, as well as release of an alcohol-induced block in ketogenesis allowing marked ketosis, may explain the disorder. An increased ratio of reduced (NADH) to unreduced nicotinamide adenine dinucleotide (NAD) in the alcoholic predisposes to the accumulation of β-hydroxybutyrate and the inhibition of gluconeogenesis. The common occurrence of hypoglycemia in alcoholic ketoacidosis adds further weight to this hypothesis.

The alcoholic patient with metabolic acidosis presents an interesting challenge. Most of these patients have an increased anion gap acidosis. In addition, a very high osmolal gap (>25 mOsm/kg) has been found to be very specific (88%) for methanol or ethylene glycol ingestion.[85] Quick examination of a urine specimen in the emergency department can be helpful in determining the cause of the acidosis: glucosuria may suggest diabetes; crystalluria can be seen in ethylene

Table 184-3. Origins of Hematologic Disorders in Acute and Chronic Alcoholism

	Direct Effect of Alcohol	Nutritional Deficiency	Liver Involvement or Sequelae
RBC disorders			+
Hypervolemia			
Decreased production			
Vacuolization of precursors	+		
Megaloblastic anemia		+	
Sideroblastic anemia		+	
Iron deficiency anemia			+
Increased destruction			
RBC abnormalities			+
Hypersplenism			+
Hypophosphatemia			+
WBC disorders			
Morphologic changes			
Hypersegmentation		+	
Megaloblastic changes		+	
Decreased production			
Granulocytopenia	+	+	+
Lymphopenia	+		
Altered function			
Granulocytes	+		
Lymphocytes	+		
Disorders of hemostasis			
Coagulation factors			
Vitamin K–dependent factors		+	+
Other factors			+
Platelets			
Quantitative			
Thrombocytopenia	+	+	+
Thrombocytosis			
Qualitative	+		

RBC, red blood cell; WBC, white blood cell.
From Hamilton GC, Jurisic MA: *Top Emerg Med* 6:75, 1984.

glycol poisoning; low specific gravity, proteinuria, and casts can be seen in renal failure; leukocytes and bacteria are present with urosepsis; and significant ketones in an otherwise normal urine may indicate starvation or alcoholic ketosis.

Treatment of alcoholic ketosis consists of volume replacement by normal saline, glucose, thiamine, and correction of hypokalemia. This can be accomplished with 5% dextrose in normal saline and either 30 mEq of potassium chloride or 30 mEq of oral potassium. Bicarbonate is seldom necessary for the uncomplicated case but may be considered in the rare patient who has a pH less than 7.1. If no serious complicating illness is present, the ketosis is reversed in 12 to 24 hours with this treatment.

Clinical improvement may be detected within hours of therapy. Nevertheless, most patients with alcoholic ketoacidosis need 1 or 2 days of inpatient treatment to correct fluid, electrolyte, and nutritional balance.[3]

Hematologic Effects

The alcoholic presents the clinician with a myriad of hematologic abnormalities. The direct toxic effect of ethanol and its metabolites, secondary nutritional deficiency, and hepatic disease, individually or in combination, affect red blood cells (RBCs), white blood cells (WBCs), platelets, hemostasis, and the immune system (Table 184-3).[86]

Anemia

A common effect of alcohol on the hematopoietic system is anemia. Several different mechanisms are responsible for anemia in the alcoholic.

Megaloblastic anemia resulting from folate deficiency is the most common type of anemia in alcoholics. The mean corpuscular volume (MCV) is typically increased but may be normal when iron deficiency coexists. Malnutrition, inability of the cirrhotic liver to store folate, excessive urinary loss, and malabsorption decrease folate stores. Alcohol accelerates the development of megaloblastic anemia in individuals with depleted folate (MCV > 100 fL) stores by an unknown mechanism.

Macrocytosis is the most common hematologic manifestation of the chronic alcoholic. It may be caused by folate deficiency, reticulocytosis (the younger reticulocytes are larger), liver disease (producing an abnormal lipid coating of RBC membrane), or vitamin B_{12} deficiency. The most common cause is the idiopathic macrocytosis of alcoholism.

Iron deficiency anemia is common among alcoholic patients and usually is a result of blood loss from the gastrointestinal tract. Alcoholics are subject to chronic inflammatory diseases such as endocarditis, tuberculosis, empyema, lung abscess, malignancy, and hepatic disease. These chronic inflammatory illnesses can produce the anemia of chronic disease, a mild micro cytic or normocytic anemia in which the serum iron is low, the total serum iron-binding capacity is low or low-normal, and serum ferritin is increased. With iron deficiency anemia the serum iron is decreased, the total serum iron-binding capacity is elevated, and serum ferritin is decreased.

Ethanol also has a direct toxic effect on erythropoiesis. Bone marrow biopsies reveal vacuolization of erythroid precursors, resulting in decreased reticulocytosis and a reversible sideroblastic anemia. Sideroblastic anemia, usually in the presence of malnutrition with pyridoxine deficiency and folate deficiency, occurs in 25% to 30% of anemic alcoholics.

Hemolytic Syndromes and Erythrocyte Abnormalities

A variety of hemolytic syndromes have been associated with alcoholism. Zieve's syndrome is a transient hemolytic anemia with hyperlipidemia and fatty infiltration of the liver. Acquired stomatocytosis, a condition characterized by abnormally shaped RBCs that are susceptible to hemolysis and acanthocytosis (spur cell anemia), has been associated with alcohol abuse. Zieve's syndrome and stomatocytosis may be reversed with abstinence. Spur cells are RBCs with spicules. Spur cell hemolytic anemia is frequently linked to alcoholics with cirrhosis. With jaundice and splenomegaly, spur cell hemolytic anemia is usually fatal. When severe hemolysis is present, remission is rare.[87]

These syndromes are associated with liver disease, which alters the lipid composition of the RBC membrane, and congestive splenomegaly, which produces hemolysis. Severe hypophosphatemia (<1 mg/dL) can also result in hemolysis. The pathogenesis of these syndromes, specificity for alcoholism, and relationship to membrane injury or hemolytic anemia are uncertain at present.[86]

Leukocyte Abnormalities

Leukopenia is often seen in the alcoholic patient and has several possible causes. Sepsis, folate deficiency, and hypersplenism all lead to a decreased WBC count. Alcohol has a direct toxic effect on WBC production in the bone marrow. Granulocyte mobilization (chemotaxis) and adherence are also impaired, resulting in a decreased inflammatory response.

Platelet Disorders

Thrombocytopenia can occur with folate deficiency, sepsis, disseminated intravascular coagulation, or splenic sequestration. The direct toxic effects of alcohol decrease measured survival time and impair production of platelets in the bone marrow. Qualitative platelet function is also impaired. Binge drinking is associated with a reactive thrombocytosis potentially responsible for acute stroke and sudden death.[88]

Hemostasis

Alcoholic patients have several potential causes for developing a bleeding diathesis. Thrombocytopenia, qualitative platelet disorders, deficient production of hepatic clotting factors, gastrointestinal variceal formation, and vitamin K deficiency may occur in these patients. A complete blood count, peripheral smear, platelet count, reticulocyte count, thrombin time, prothrombin time/INR, and partial thromboplastin time are required to evaluate episodes of significant bleeding. Bleeding associated with coagulation abnormalities may require immediate intervention. Fresh frozen plasma can be given for immediate correction of coagulation factor depletion; vitamin K (10 mg IV) takes 6 to 10 hours to reverse the vitamin K–dependent factors II, VII, IX, and X. Because of poor diet and impaired hepatobiliary function, alcoholics may have insufficient vitamin K storage and thus benefit from vitamin K delivery. However, alcoholic patients with profound liver failure are unable to produce precoagulation factors II, VII, IX, X, and IV; vitamin K therapy in this case is futile. Platelet transfusions should be started in the emergency department for adult patients with active bleeding whose platelet count is less than 50,000/mm^3.

Oncologic Effects

Chronic alcohol use is associated with an increased incidence of upper alimentary and respiratory tract cancers. The direct or indirect mechanism (e.g., tumor promoter) producing this relationship remains to be explained. Ethanol may promote carcinogen activation by its effect on the cytochrome P-450 system through (1) nutritional deficiencies (particularly vitamin A) that accompany prolonged heavy drinking, (2) contaminants such as nitrosamines and hydrocarbons, or (3) increased permeability of mucous membranes to other carcinogens.[89] Smoking certainly has its own role as a cause of neoplasia and is difficult to isolate in these studies. Alcohol may act synergistically with tobacco and malnutrition to produce oropharyngeal cancer. The type of alcohol is increasingly shown to influence cancer risk. In one study, wine did not increase the risk of upper digestive tract tumors but rather lowered it compared with beer or whiskey, possibly because of the anticarcinogenic properties found in wine versus beer and other alcohols.[90]

In general, alcohol increases the risk of cancer of the mouth, pharynx, larynx, and esophagus. Chronic hepatitis B infection may sensitize the liver to alcohol, producing hepatocellular carcinoma. Evidence also supports a relationship between invasive breast cancer and alcohol consumption. Women who consume two to five drinks per day have a relative risk of 1.41 compared with nondrinkers.[91] Moderate alcohol consumption has been shown to lead to an increased risk of colorectal and prostate cancer.[92] The association is less clear between alcohol consumption and lung or pancreatic cancer.

Hypothermia

Acute alcohol ingestion is one of the most common precipitating factors for accidental hypothermia and exacerbates hypothermia of other causes. Several studies have implicated acute ethanol ingestion in 33% to 73% of patients presenting with a core temperature less than 35° C.[93] Alcohol use predisposes to hypothermia by depression of hypothalamic thermoregulation, peripheral vasodilation producing heat loss, CNS depression, sepsis, inability to shiver, hypoglycemia, and increased risk of environmental exposure. Hypothermia may be the presentation of Wernicke's syndrome, possibly caused by lesions of the posterior hypothalamus, hypoglycemia, or sepsis. Intoxicated patients also may have slower rewarming rates.

Psychiatric Effects

Forty-five percent of alcohol-dependent adults are diagnosed with one or more additional psychiatric conditions during their lifetime. Of alcoholic men admitted to a psychiatric ward, approximately 40% had a psychiatric disorder unrelated to substance abuse. In particular, antisocial personality disorder, schizophrenia, mood disorders, and anxiety disorders are found in this group. Up to 17% of all alcoholics eventually die by suicide.[94,95]

Depression and antisocial personality are the two most common psychiatric disorders that correlate with alcoholism, with a prevalence of 30% to 60% in most studies. Chronic alcohol use can produce an imbalance in the serotoninergic system. This imbalance may lead to increased anxiety, aggression, and depression. Interestingly, aggressive behavior is linked more strongly to depression than to alcohol dependence.[96] Secondary depression may be caused by alcoholism, or the primary affective disorder may be present with secondary alcoholism. Mild depressive symptoms are also common in alcohol withdrawal. Antisocial individuals are at high risk for alcoholism and drug dependence, although an unstable, unhappy childhood environment appears to be more important to the development of sociopathy than alcohol. Alcoholism, major depression, and antisocial personality all predispose to suicide attempts, and interaction among the three is particularly dangerous.

Problem drinking is found in up to 50% of patients hospitalized for schizophrenia. In one urban aftercare program for schizophrenic patients, alcohol use was found to be strongly associated with poor medication compliance, psychosocial problems, hostility, cognitive disorganization, poor medical health, and higher rates of rehospitalization.[97]

As many as 50% of alcoholic women exhibit symptoms of other psychiatric disorders. Although many patients turn to alcohol because of a primary psychiatric illness, alcohol can produce anxiety, hallucinations, paranoia, and depression and has been associated with a nearly twofold increased risk of suicide.[95]

An alcoholic patient who presents to the emergency department with an apparent psychiatric disorder poses a diagnostic dilemma. Does the patient have a primary affective disorder with secondary alcoholism, or is the patient manifesting anxiety or depressive behavior because of alcoholism? In general, alcoholic patients with psychiatric disorders are best treated with medications that are specific for their psychiatric condition.[98]

Many alcoholics with mild depression have spontaneous resolution of symptoms with abstinence. Nevertheless, depression meeting DSM-IV criteria is best treated with antidepressants.[99] If abstinence can be achieved, underlying psychiatric disorders are more easily diagnosed and treated.

ALCOHOL-DRUG INTERACTIONS

Alcohol ingestion is associated with a vast number of drug interactions (Table 184-4). These may occur through several mechanisms: (1) altered absorption, (2) enhanced metabolism and activated toxic metabolites through the hepatic MEOS pathway, (3) additive or synergistic effects, (4) disulfiram-ethanol-like reactions, and (5) congeners, compounds found in alcoholic beverages. In general, chronic alcoholism is associated with an increased rate of drug clearance resulting from enhanced metabolism and enzyme induction (cytochrome P-450 system). Conversely, acute alcohol intoxication reduces clearance for other drugs, increasing their serum concentration because of competition for a partially shared detoxification pathway.[100]

Altered Absorption

Propranolol may delay gastric emptying and thus prolong gastric contact. Other compounds, such as erythromycin and metoclopramide, may increase gastric emptying.

Enhanced Metabolism and Toxic Metabolites

Most alcohol is metabolized by ADH. A small percentage of alcohol is metabolized by the MEOS–cytochrome P-450 system, which is also responsible for the metabolism of various drugs. The MEOS metabolic pathway is enhanced in chronic alcoholics. Therefore, the induction of MEOS is associated with the acceleration of the degradation of these other drugs. For example, the half-lives of warfarin, phenytoin, and isoniazid are 50% shorter in abstaining alcoholics than in nondrinkers. Barbiturates, diazepam, propranolol, and rifampin may have increased rates of clearance when taken by chronic alcoholics. This effect can persist for days to weeks after the cessation of drinking.[58,100]

Acetaminophen is the most widely used analgesic in the United States and is often recommended to alcoholic patients instead of NSAIDs to prevent gastritis. Chronic alcohol ingestion may enhance acetaminophen hepatotoxicity by accelerating the biotransformation to toxic byproducts. A few case reports exist of severe or lethal acetaminophen toxicity in alcoholics taking therapeutic doses of the analgesic. Greatly elevated AST levels (3000 to 48,000 in one series), increased ALT levels, and greatly elevated prothrombin/INR times may help to distinguish acetaminophen hepatotoxicity from alcoholic hepatitis.[101] Increased vulnerability seems to occur immediately after cessation of

Table 184-4. Effects and Mechanisms of Alcohol-Drug Interactions

Clinical Effect	Mechanism	Drugs Involved	Comments
Increased blood alcohol levels	Inhibition of gastric ADH	Cimetidine Ranitidine Aspirin	Debatable role
Increased blood alcohol levels	Increased rate of gastric emptying	Cisapride Erythromycin	
Liver damage	Increased hepatotoxicity (chronic or "heavy" alcohol use)	Acetaminophen Isoniazid Phenylbutazone	"Heavy" drinkers can experience severe consequences even with therapeutic doses.
	Decreased metabolism of drug (acute alcohol use)	Narcotics Barbiturates Benzodiazepines Chloral hydrate Warfarin	"Binge" drinkers may develop toxicity from standard doses.
May require higher dosages	Induction of enzymes	Benzodiazepines Phenytoin Propranolol Warfarin	Chronic alcoholics
Increased bleeding time		Aspirin NSAIDs	
Sedation Psychomotor impairment		Antihistamines Barbiturates Benzodiazepines Narcotics Tricyclic antidepressants	
	Disulfiram-like reactions	Oral hypoglycemics Antibiotics: metronidazole Sulfonamides Griseofulvin Cefoperazone Nitroglycerin	
Hypoglycemia Hypotension		Long-acting oral hypoglycemics Aldomet Hydralazine Nitroglycerin	

ADH, alcohol dehydrogenase; NSAIDs, nonsteroidal anti-inflammatory drugs.
Data from Fraser AG: Pharmacokinetic interactions between alcohol and other drugs. *Clin Pharmacokinet* 33:79, 1997; and Adams WL: Interactions between alcohol and other drugs. *Int J Addict* 30:1903, 1995.

drinking. A synergistic effect apparently occurs with alcohol, fasting, and acetaminophen use in combination with depleted glutathione stores. Other studies have failed to demonstrate increased hepatotoxicity after acetaminophen overdose in heavy drinkers versus nondrinkers.[102]

Additive or Synergistic Effects

Alcohol has long been known to have additive or even synergistic effects with several drugs. Acute intoxication decreases the rate of drug metabolism, which is at least partially explained by competition for the same enzymatic process in the liver. For example, ethanol has additive sedative effects when taken with first-generation antihistamines, barbiturates, cyclic antidepressants, benzodiazepines, phenothiazines, propoxyphene, propofol, and narcotics. Alcohol may also increase the activity of methyldopa and nitroglycerin. Alcohol can increase tetracycline levels by 30%. Selective serotonin reuptake inhibitors do not appear to affect alcohol kinetics or psychomotor performance.

When cocaine and ethanol are taken concomitantly, a third drug is formed. Cocaethylene is a neurologically active compound, significantly more toxic than cocaine to the heart, liver, and brain, that is more addicting and more lethal than cocaine alone. Cocaethylene produces a higher incidence of confusion, lower mean Glasgow Coma Scale (GCS) scores, and a higher incidence of violent trauma and more often requires endotracheal intubation.[103] Hemodynamically, these patients demonstrate an elevated heart rate (1.5 to 5 times normal) and blood pressure greater than with either drug alone. Sudden death is increased 18- to 25-fold over that associated with use of cocaine alone. Plasma levels of cocaine in this combined group were higher than in those who used cocaine alone.[104]

Gastrointestinal Bleeding

Ethanol increases aspirin-induced prolongation of bleeding time and reduces the metabolism of warfarin, leading to increased anticoagulant effects. There is an increased risk of upper gastrointestinal bleeding when alcohol is combined with NSAIDs. This may be the most dangerous additive or synergistic effect of alcohol.[105]

Disulfiram and Similar Reactions

Most patients pretreated with disulfiram (Antabuse) who then consume even small amounts of alcohol experience an extremely unpleasant reaction. These patients develop a hypersensitivity to ethanol and experience a direct response within 15 minutes and lasting 30 minutes to several hours. The reaction consists of skin flushing on the head that spreads to the trunk, along with nausea, vomiting, headache, chest and abdominal discomfort, diaphoresis, vertigo, palpitations, and confusion. A severe reaction may produce hypotension, seizures, and dysrhythmias. Disulfiram-ethanol reaction is thought to occur by either the accumulation of acetaldehyde secondary to inhibition of the aldehyde dehydrogenase enzyme, which may be deficient in some Asians, or another unknown toxic factor. This incapacitating reaction has been used to discourage chronic alcohol ingestion.

A similar but milder disulfiram-ethanol-like reaction has been described when alcohol combines with several different drugs. The reaction may occur days to weeks after the last dose of medication. Four cephalosporins (cefamandole, cefoperazone, cefotetan, moxalactam), metronidazole, chloramphenicol, griseofulvin, nitrofurantoin sulfonamides, all sulfonylureas, and chloral hydrate have been reported to produce this reaction when combined with alcohol ingestion. Life-threatening toxic reactions between griseofulvin and small amounts of ingested alcohol have been reported.[106]

Treatment for disulfiram reaction is symptomatic and includes IV fluids, dopamine for persistent severe hypotension, observation, an antiemetic, and cardiac monitoring.

Congeners

Congeners are compounds in alcoholic beverages other than ethanol and water. Some beers and wines contain tyramine. Hypertensive crisis may occur in patients treated with monoamine oxidase inhibitors who drink these alcoholic beverages.

Oral Hypoglycemics

Oral hypoglycemic agents and alcohol can interact through multiple mechanisms, producing unpredictable glucose levels. Profound hypoglycemia can occur when alcohol and oral hypoglycemic agents are combined. Patients taking metformin may have an increased risk for developing lactic acidosis when combined with heavy drinking. A disulfiram-ethanol-like reaction has been described with many hypoglycemic agents.[100]

THE ADOLESCENT PATIENT

Injury is the most common cause of adolescent morbidity and mortality. Alcohol is often associated with these injuries.[107] Adolescent drinking is associated with a myriad of negative consequences including suicides, driving under the influence and resultant fatalities, unsafe or increased sexual activity, sexual assault, and acquaintance or date rape. Seventy-eight percent of high school students have tried alcohol, and 30% admit to binge drinking at least once a month.[108]

The age of drinking onset may be an indicator for increased risk of alcohol-related injury. Adolescents who began drinking regularly before age 14 years were at least three times more likely to be diagnosed with alcohol dependence than those who began drinking at age 21. In addition, adolescents who began drinking before age 21 were significantly more likely during their lives to have been injured while under the influence of alcohol.[109]

Adolescent drinkers account for nearly 20% of all alcohol consumption, spending an estimated $22.5 billion in 1999.[110]

THE ELDERLY PATIENT

Active problem drinking is found in 14% of elderly (older than 65) emergency department patients. Fifty percent of older people drink some alcohol, and 2% to 4% meet criteria for alcohol abuse or dependence. Common screening tests (e.g., CAGE) tend to be less sensitive in this age group. Alcohol may exacerbate underlying disease by masking anginal chest pain, worsening hypertension, and inducing dysrhythmias.[111] However, elderly persons consuming low to moderate levels of alcohol may have a decreased risk for developing dementia and heart failure.[112] More than 75% of people age 65 or older use more than one prescribed medication. Aging alters gastrointestinal absorption, lowers volume of distribution, diminishes homeostatic responses, and reduces renal and hepatic function.[100] Elderly persons may also demonstrate increased end-organ sensitivity, particularly involving the CNS, with concomitant drug use. Therefore, elderly patients are at increased risk for alcohol and drug interactions.

Elderly patients also are more likely to have neuropsychiatric complications of alcoholism. Sleep problems, anxiety, depression, and dementia are often observed. Alcohol has been involved in one third of suicides in elderly persons. Older subjects have also been shown to perform less well on tests of perception and attention than younger subjects at all blood alcohol levels. This may result in an increased risk of fractures from falling and osteoporosis.

Overall, prognosis is age related with respect to cirrhosis. One study reported a 1-year mortality rate of 50% in those older than 60 versus 7% for those younger than 60.[58]

PREGNANCY

More than 2000 scientific reports have confirmed alcohol's teratogenic effects. According to the National Institute on Drug Abuse, almost 19% of all children born in the United States have been exposed to alcohol during gestation.[113] Pregnant women who reported any use of alcohol, binge drinking, or frequent drinking were more likely to be older than 30 years, employed, and unmarried.[114]

Fetal alcohol syndrome is characterized by a triad of CNS defects, including mild to moderate mental retardation; dysmorphology, involving mostly facial structures; and growth deficiencies, usually consisting of short stature and microcephaly.[115] Fetal alcohol syndrome is now considered the most common identifiable source of mental retardation. Children exposed to alcohol prenatally may exhibit increased activity levels, cognitive and attention deficits, perseverative behavior, and language and motor problems. Unfortunately, these developmental and cognitive handicaps persist into adulthood.[116]

Ethanol rapidly diffuses across the placenta and is distributed to all fetal tissue with a predilection for gray matter. Although infants of mothers who drink heavily have the poorest outcome, children of mothers who consume only two or three alcoholic drinks a day also display abnormalities. Even in the absence of growth retardation or congenital abnormalities, children born to women who consume excessive alcohol during pregnancy appear to be at increased risk for attention deficit disorders. These findings are referred to as *fetal alcohol effects.*

No known safe amount of alcohol consumption during pregnancy exists. The American Academy of Pediatrics recommends abstinence from alcohol for women who are pregnant or who are planning a pregnancy.[117]

TRAUMA

Alcohol and trauma are inextricably linked. Independently, the tragic effects of both are numerous; in combination, they are staggering. Injury is the leading cause of death between the ages of 1 and 44. It accounts for more than 140,000 deaths per year, and for each death, two patients have permanent disabling injuries. In the United States, alcohol is the major risk factor for virtually all categories of intentional and unintentional injury. These include motor vehicle accidents, including pedestrians and cyclists; burns; drownings; suicides; crimes, including assault, sexual assault, and murder; and all forms of domestic violence, including spousal battering and sexual abuse. Besides increasing the frequency and severity of injury, alcohol significantly complicates the management of the trauma victim.[3] Alcohol intoxication may alter the initial assessment of injury severity, resulting in an increased need for invasive diagnostic and therapeutic procedures (e.g., intubation, diagnostic peritoneal lavage, ultrasound, CT scan, intracranial pressure monitoring).[118]

Alcohol may diminish the patient's capacity to respond to hemorrhagic shock by altering hemodynamic effects and acid-base balance. Volume depletion as a result of the diuretic effect of alcohol or vomiting can impair the reserve of the intoxicated trauma patient. Peripheral vasodilation caused by alcohol may contribute to hypotension and hypothermia. Although these effects may be minimal, they underscore the need for early and adequate fluid resuscitation in these patients. Intoxicated patients with severe non-neurologic trauma may have lower blood pressures and carbon dioxide levels (indicative of a compensatory hyperventilation) on hospital arrival than sober patients. More important, a poorly understood cardiac depressant effect also increases the depth of shock and volume requirements for resuscitation. Alcohol-induced skin vasodilation may be accompanied by an increase in skeletal muscle, mesenteric and renal bed constriction, and left ventricular stroke work. Thus, the overall effect on systemic vascular resistance and blood pressure may be balanced.[119]

Intoxication renders the signs and symptoms of intra-abdominal and retroperitoneal injury less reliable than usual. If the risk of an intra-abdominal injury exists, further evaluation (e.g., ultrasonography, CT) should be considered.

Alcohol intoxication predisposes to abdominal wall laxity and thus less protection from blunt trauma.[119] These patients are also likely to have full stomachs, increasing the risk of gastric injury after trauma and predisposing to vomiting and aspiration, especially during airway management. The fatty liver changes of alcoholism can result in hepatomegaly. Portal hypertension in alcoholics may produce splenomegaly. These organs can become more vulnerable to the effects of trauma because of their enlarged size, protrusion beneath the protection of the ribs, and increased intracapsular pressure. One study compared intoxicated patients with isolated blunt splenic injury with a control group matched for age, abbreviated injury severity score, initial hematocrit, and grade of splenic injury. The intoxicated group had significantly greater blood transfusion requirements in the first 24 hours and underwent splenectomy more often.[120]

Alcohol intoxication contributes to CNS injury in many ways. It is associated with aggressive behavior, impaired reflexes and coordination, and inappropriate avoidance responses. A higher degree of trauma to the spinal cord and much worse neurologic and functional recovery occur in patients who are intoxicated during trauma compared with sober patients.[121] Experimental evidence suggests that alcohol acts synergistically with mechanical injury of the spinal cord to amplify the trauma response by increasing edema formation within the contused tissue.[122]

No consensus exists on the indications for an emergency CT scan in patients with "minor head injury" (loss of consciousness, posttraumatic amnesia, GCS score of 13 to 15, normal neurologic examination). One disturbing prospective study found that GCS plus 1 hour of observation were unable to predict positive head CT scans in ethanol-intoxicated patients with minor head trauma. Patients with signs of head trauma and focal or generalized seizures need an urgent CT scan. CT scans of the head should be performed for any patient with deteriorating mental status, focal neurologic findings, new-onset seizures even without obvious signs of history of trauma, failure to improve over time, or mental status changes out of proportion to the degree of intoxication.[123]

ADMISSION GUIDELINES AND DISPOSITION

Optimal outpatient therapy for chronic alcoholics includes concerned family or friends to ensure that the patients take their medications properly, appear at their follow-up appointments, abstain from alcohol, and maintain an adequate diet. Alcoholic patients who undergo outpatient treatment need close supervision; therefore, a follow-up appointment within 24 to 48 hours should be considered.

Most alcoholics suffer from a combination of medical, psychiatric, and social problems. Hospitalization is often necessary to diagnose and treat these multiple problems. Moreover, with alcoholics who are no longer able to care for themselves, hospitalization is often dictated for this reason alone. Unfortunately, many managed care and Medicaid plans limit or do not cover inpatient detoxification. In attempting to choose medical versus psychiatric admission, a medical illness usually takes priority.

Acute Intoxication

Acute intoxication alone seldom requires admission. However, combined alcohol-drug overdose or associated medical, psychiatric, or social problems may require hospitalization. *Acute alcohol intoxication is a diagnosis of exclusion.*

Alcohol levels that may be tolerated by an adult can be lethal in children. It is prudent to admit children with acute intoxication unless close psychosocial follow-up can be ensured. Children presenting with hypoglycemia or medical complications should be admitted. Child abuse or neglect should be considered.

Alcohol Withdrawal

Patients with signs of major withdrawal (fever, hallucinations, confusion, extreme agitation) require admission. Patients with mild alcohol withdrawal should be observed in the emergency department. After 4 to 6 hours of observation and treatment, the alert, oriented patient whose vital signs, physical examination, and appropriate laboratory analysis are within normal limits may be released. Nevertheless, the patient requires treatment for the underlying disease of alcoholism and should be advised or referred accordingly.

Seizures

Patients experiencing their first ARS are usually admitted. Admission allows initiation of drug therapy, diagnostic evaluation, and continuous monitoring of the patient's status. However, the alcoholic patient with a first time ARS may be discharged to a suitable social situation when (1) the patient's alcohol withdrawal is mild and easily controlled either by supportive care or with low-dose benzodiazepines; (2) the diagnostic workup, including a head CT scan, is unremarkable; (3) the patient has had less than two seizures; and (4) the patient has been observed to be alert and oriented, with normal vital signs, physical examination, and laboratory studies, during the 6 hours since the last seizure, and appropriate outpatient follow-up can be ensured.

Patients with a documented history of ARS can be discharged if, along with these criteria, they have had no more than two ARSs over a 6-hour period with a lucid interval between seizures and are observed to be seizure free and at baseline mental and physical status for at least 6 hours after their last ARS. Three to six brief, self-limited seizures may occur with AWS. Nevertheless, admission for patients with two or more seizures is advised because of the potential for deterioration to status epilepticus. This is especially appropriate in the malnourished, immunocompromised, homeless, or noncompliant alcoholic patient.

Patients with partial seizures or focal neurologic findings on physical examination require admission unless these findings have been previously documented. Patients with seizures associated with head trauma or with mixed alcohol-drug withdrawal are admitted. Status epilepticus or recurrent seizures during observation in the emergency department indicate a lack of seizure control also requiring hospitalization.

Psychiatric and Social Problems

Alcoholic patients requiring admission with acute intoxication, ARS, alcohol withdrawal, or medical or surgical disorders are usually best managed on acute care floors and should not be initially admitted to a general psychiatric service. Some psychiatric and social conditions in the alcoholic can still be better handled on a general psychiatric unit: psychosis, exacerbation of schizophrenia, depression with suicidal tendencies, any patient who is a danger to self or others, or alcoholic hallucinosis with an otherwise clear sensorium.

Patients who are no longer able to care for themselves may also require admission. Although these patients' ultimate destination is a rehabilitation center or a board-and-care program, hospitalization may be necessary to rule out medical or psychiatric illness and to treat impending withdrawal symptoms. Patients who wish to stop drinking are usually admitted to a detoxification unit to treat impending withdrawal. Data and interest are increasing for outpatient drug therapy in alcohol dependence. The U.S. Food and Drug Administration has approved disulfiram and naltrexone for treatment of alcohol dependence.[1] Naltrexone, ondansetron, acamprosate, or acamprosate plus naltrexone have had mixed results facilitating abstinence.[124,125] Most communities have either an Alcoholics Anonymous (AA) chapter or a treatment center for anyone who desires help with alcohol. In small communities, clergy or social workers can usually arrange rehabilitation.

Alcohol kills—it kills the alcoholic and it kills unintended victims by the acts of inebriated persons. Whatever medical, psychological, or social problem brings the alcoholic to the emergency department, the underlying problem is alcoholism and the ultimate goal is abstinence. This disease surely progresses if alcoholism is not first recognized and the patient is given the opportunity to participate in a rehabilitation program.[126] It is up to the emergency physician to intervene on behalf of the patient and the public.

KEY CONCEPTS

- Moderate alcohol consumption is defined as one to two drinks per day in men and one in women.
- Benzodiazepines are the mainstay of treatment for alcohol withdrawal and alcohol withdrawal seizures.
- Inappropriate alcohol consumption or alcohol dependence should be considered in emergency department patients in almost any clinical situation, including trauma, potential drug-alcohol reactions, pneumonia, cardiomyopathy, new-onset atrial fibrillation, hepatitis, gastrointestinal bleeding, pancreatitis, altered mental status, depression, suicide, magnesium deficiency, and anemia.
- Minor alcohol withdrawal occurs as early as 6 hours and usually peaks at 24 to 36 hours after the cessation of or significant decrease in alcohol intake.
- Major alcohol withdrawal occurs after more than 24 hours and usually peaks at 50 hours (but occasionally takes up to 5 days) after the decline or termination of drinking.
- Delirium tremens is the extreme end of the alcohol withdrawal spectrum and consists of gross tremor, profound confusion, fever, incontinence, frightening visual hallucinations, and mydriasis.
- Not all alcohol-related seizures are alcohol withdrawal seizures.

REFERENCES

1. Swift RM: Drug therapy for alcohol dependence. *N Engl J Med* 340:1482, 1999.
2. Kitchens JM: Does this patient have an alcohol problem? *JAMA* 272:1782, 1994.
3. National Institute on Alcohol Abuse and Alcoholism: *Seventh Special Report to Congress on Alcohol and Health*. Rockville, Md, Department of Health and Human Services, 1990.
4. Morse RM, et al: The definition of alcoholism. *JAMA* 268:1012, 1992.
5. Liu IC, Blacker DL, Xu R, et al: Genetic and enviromental contributions to the development of alcohol dependence in male twins. *Arch Gen Psychiatry* 61:897, 2004.
6. Werner MJ, Adger H: Early identification, screening, and brief intervention for adolescent alcohol use. *Arch Pediatr Adolesc Med* 14:1241, 1995.
7. American Psychiatric Association: *Diagnostic and Statistical Manual of Mental Disorders*, 4th ed. Washington, DC, American Psychiatric Association, 1994.
8. Hines LM, et al: Genetic variation in alcohol dehydrogenase and the beneficial effect of moderate alcohol consumption on myocardial infarction. *N Engl J Med* 344:549, 2001.
9. Jones AW: Disappearance rate of ethanol from the blood of human subjects: Implications in forensic toxicology. *J Forensic Sci* 38:104, 1993.
10. Brennan DF, et al: Ethanol elimination rates in an ED population. *Am J Emerg Med* 13:276, 1995.
11. Christopher TA, Zeccardi JA: Evaluation of the QED saliva alcohol test: A new, rapid, accurate device for measuring ethanol in saliva. *Ann Emerg Med* 21:1135, 1992.
12. Krishel S, SaFranek D, Clark RF: Intravenous vitamins for alcoholics in the emergency department: A review. *J Emerg Med* 16:419, 1998.
13. Coomes TR, et al: Successful use of propofol in refractory delirium tremens. *Ann Emerg Med* 30:285, 1997.
14. Davis KM, Wu JV: Role of glutaminergic and GABAergic systems in alcoholism. *J Biomed Sci* 8:7, 2001.
15. Isbell H, et al: An experimental study of the etiology of "rum fits" and delirium tremens. *Q J Study Alcohol* 16:1, 1955.
16. Turner RC, et al: Alcohol withdrawal syndromes: A review of pathophysiology, clinical presentation and treatment. *J Gen Intern Med* 4:432, 1989.
17. Berk WA, Todd K: Relationship of abstinence to the presentation and peak intensity of signs and alcohol withdrawal. *Ann Emerg Med* 22:339, 1993.
18. Mayo-Smith MF: Pharmacological management of alcohol withdrawal. *JAMA* 278:144, 1997.
19. Dappan JB, et al: Symptom-triggered versus fixed schedule doses of benzodiazepines for alcohol withdrawal. *Arch Intern Med* 162:1117, 2002.
20. Nolop KB, Natow A: Unprecedented sedative requirements during delirium tremens. *Crit Care Med* 13:246, 1985.
21. Adams F, Fernandez F, Anderson BS: Emergency pharmacotherapy of delirium in the critically ill cancer patient. *Psychosomatics* 27:33, 1986.
22. Voris J, et al: Gabapentin for the treatment of ethanol withdrawal. *Subst Abus* 24:129, 2003.
23. Malcolm R, et al: Update on anticonvulsants for the treatment of alcohol withdrawal. *Am J Addict* 10(Suppl):16, 2001
24. Gullestad L, et al: Oral magnesium supplementation improves metabolic variables and muscle strength in alcoholics. *Alcohol Clin Exp Res* 16:986, 1992.
25. Rathlev NK, et al: The lack of efficacy of phenytoin in the prevention of recurrent alcohol-related seizures. *Ann Emerg Med* 23:513, 1994.
26. Lowenstein DH, Alldredge BK: Status epilepticus at an urban public hospital in the 1980s. *Neurology* 43:483, 1993.
27. Brust JC: Acute neurologic complications of drug and alcohol abuse. *Neurol Clin* 16:503, 1998.
28. Victor M, Brausch C: The role of abstinence in the genesis of alcoholic epilepsy. *Epilepsia* 8:1, 1967.
29. D'Onofrio GD, et al: Lorazepam for the prevention of recurrent seizures related to alcohol. *N Engl* J Med 340:5, 1999.
30. Wrenn KD, Larron S: The febrile alcoholic in the emergency department. *Am J Emerg Med* 9:57, 1991.
31. Sand T, et al Clinical utility of EEG in alcohol-related seizures. *Acta Neurol Scand* 105:18, 2002.
32. Scheuer M, Pedley T: Current concepts: The evaluation and treatment of seizures. *N Engl J Med* 323:1468, 1990.
33. Earnest MP, et al: Intracranial lesions shown by CT scans in 259 cases of first alcohol-related seizures. *Neurology* 38:1561, 1988.
34. Lowenstein DH: Status epilepticus: An overview of the clinical problem. *Epilepsia* 40:53, 1999.
35. Treatment of convulsive status epilepticus: Recommendations of the Epilepsy Foundation of America's Working Group on Status Epilepticus. *JAMA* 270:854, 1993.
36. Cock HR, Schapira AHV: A comparison of lorazepam and diazepam as initial therapy in convulsive status epilepticus. *Q J Med* 95:225, 2002.
37. Runge JW, et al: Intravenous fosphenytoin for emergent seizure control. *Ann Emerg Med* 25:139, 1995.
38. Coplin WM, et al: Randomized evaluation of adverse events and length of stay with routine ED use of phenytoin or fosphenytoin. *Neurol Res* 24:842, 2002.

39. Johnson J, et al: Inappropriate fosphenytoin use in the ED. *Am J Emerg Med* 19:293, 2001.
40. Rudis MI, et al: Cost-effectiveness of oral phenytoin, intravenous phenytoin, and intravenous fosphenytoin in the ED. *Ann Emerg Med* 43:386, 2004.
41. Shorvon S: The management of status epilepticus. *J Neurol Neurosurg Psychiatry* 70(Suppl II):ii22, 2001.
42. Smith BJ: Treatment of status epilepticus. *Neurol Clin* 19:153, 2001.
43. Yu KT, et al: Safety and efficacy of intravenous valproate in pediatric status epilepticus and acute repetitive seizures. *Epilepsia* 44:724, 2003.
44. Chance J: Emergency department treatment of alcohol withdrawal seizures with phenytoin. Ann Emerg Med 20:520, 1991.
45. Segal LD, et al: Alcohol and the heart. *Med Clin North Am* 68:147, 1984.
46. Ridker PM, et al: Association of moderate alcohol consumption and plasma concentration of endogenous tissue-type plasminogen activator. *JAMA* 272:929, 1994.
47. Fagrell B, et al: The effects of light to moderate drinking on cardiovascular diseases. *J Intern Med* 246:331, 1999.
48. Agrawal DP: Cardioprotective effects of light-moderate consumption of alcohol: A review of putative mechanisms. *Alcohol Alcohol* 2002;7:409, 2002.
49. Walsh CR, et al: Alcohol consumption and risk for congestive heart failure in the Framingham Heart Study. *Ann Intern Med* 136:181, 2002.
50. Mukamal KJ, et al: Prior alcohol consumption and mortality following acute myocardial infarction. *JAMA* 285:1965, 2001.
51. Otero-Anton E, et al: Prolongation of the QTc interval during alcohol withdrawal syndrome. *Acta Cardiol* 52:285, 1997.
52. Tsuji H, et al: The associations of levels of serum potassium and magnesium with ventricular premature complexes (the Framingham Heart Study). *Am J Cardiol* 74:232, 1994.
53. Thomsen JL: Diseases of the airways and lungs in forensic autopsy material of alcoholics. *Med Sci Law* 37:23, 1997.
54. Moss M, et al: The role of chronic alcohol abuse in the development of acute respiratory distress syndrome in adults. *JAMA* 275:50, 1996.
55. Pahor M, et al: Alcohol consumption and risk of deep venous thrombosis and pulmonary embolism in older persons. *J Am Geriatr Soc* 44:1030, 1996.
56. Brenner H, et al: Inverse graded relation between alcohol consumption and active infection with *Helicobacter pylori*. *Am J Epidemiol* 149:571, 1999.
57. Diehl AM: Liver disease in alcohol abusers: Clinical perspective. *Alcohol* 27:7, 2002.
58. Lieber CS: Hepatic and other medical disorders of alcoholism: From pathogenesis to treatment. *J Stud Alcohol* 59:9, 1998.
59. Purohit V, Russo D: Cellular and molecular mechanisms of alcoholic hepatitis: Introduction and summary of the symposium. *Alcohol* 27:3, 2002.
60. Alcoholic liver: The ACG's recommendations. *J Crit Illness* 14:204, 1999.
61. Mathurin P, et al: Corticosteroids improve short-term survival in patients with severe alcohol hepatitis. *J Hepatol* 36:480, 2002.
62. Khan KN, Yatsuhashi H: Effect of alcohol consumption on the progression of hepatitis C virus infection and risk of hepatocellular carcinoma in Japanese patients. *Alcohol* 35:286, 2000.
63. Sigal SH, Lieber CS: Treating the most severe manifestations of alcoholic liver disease. *J Crit Illness* 11:155, 1996.
64. Gumaste V, Dave P, Serery G: Serum lipase: A better test to diagnose acute alcoholic pancreatitis. *Am J Med* 92:239, 1992.
65. Harper C: The neuropathology of alcohol-specific brain damage, or does alcohol damage the brain? *J Neuropathol Exp Neurol* 57:101, 1998.
66. Reuler JB, Girard DE, Cooney TG: Wernicke's encephalopathy. *N Engl J Med* 312:1035, 1985.
67. Roberts JR: Thiamine deficiency in the non-alcoholic patient. *Emerg Med News* 8, 1996.
68. Brust JC: Acute neurologic complications of drug and alcohol abuse. *Neurol Clin* 16:503, 1998.
69. Haller RG, Knochel JP: Skeletal muscle disease in alcoholism. *Med Clin North Am* 68:91, 1984.
70. Cardoso F, Jankovic J: Movement disorders. *Neurol Clin* 11:625, 1993.
71. Charness ME, Simon RP, Greenberg DA: Ethanol and the nervous system. *N Engl J Med* 321:442, 1989.
72. Cook RT: Alcohol abuse, alcoholism, and damage to the immune system: A review. *Alcohol Clin Exp Res* 22:1927, 1998.
73. Avins AL, et al: HIV infection and risk behaviors among heterosexuals in alcohol treatment programs. *JAMA* 271:515, 1994.
74. Szabo G: Consequences of alcohol consumption on host defense. *Alcohol Alcohol* 34:830, 1999.
75. Runyon BA, et al: Short-course versus long course antibiotic treatment of spontaneous bacterial peritonitis. *Hepatology* 100:1737, 1990.
76. Noth RH, Walter RM: The effects of alcohol on the endocrine system. *Med Clin North Am* 68:133, 1984.
77. Ginsburg ES, et al: Effects of alcohol ingestion on estrogens in postmenopausal women. *JAMA* 276:1747, 1996.
78. Sucov A, Woolard R: Ethanol-associated hypoglycemia is uncommon. *Acad Emerg Med* 2:185, 1995.
79. Ajani UA, Hennekens CH, Spelsberg A, Manson JE: Alcohol consumption and risk of type 2 diabetes mellitus among US male physicians. *Arch Intern Med* 160:1025, 2000.
80. Bell DS: Alcohol and the NIDDM patient. *Diabetes Care* 19:509, 1996.
81. Baraona E, Lieber CS: Alcohol and lipids. *Recent Dev Alcohol* 14:97, 1998.
82. Vamvakas S, et al: Alcohol abuse: Potential role in electrolyte disturbances and kidney diseases. *Clin Nephrol* 49:205, 1998.
83. Elisaf MS, Siamopoulos KC: Mechanisms of hypophosphataemia in alcoholic patients. *Int J Clin Pract* 51:501, 1997.
84. Fulop MF: Alcoholic ketoacidosis. *Endocrinol Metab Clin North Am* 22:209, 1993.
85. Almaghamsi AM, Yeung CK: Osmolal gap in alcoholic ketoacidosis. *Clin Nephrol* 48:52, 1997.
86. Lindenbaum J: Hematologic complications of alcohol abuse. *Semin Liver Dis* 7:169, 1987.
87. Zieve L: Jaundice, hyperlipemia and hemolytic anemia: A heretofore unrecognized syndrome associated with alcoholic fatty liver and cirrhosis. *Ann Intern Med* 48:471, 1958.
88. Renaud SC, Ruf JC: Effects of alcohol on platelet functions. *Clin Chim Acta* 246:77, 1996.
89. Devita VT Jr: *Cancer: Principles and Practice of Oncology*, 4th ed. Philadelphia, JB Lippincott, 1993.
90. Gronbaek M, et al: Population based cohort study of the association between alcohol intake and cancer of the upper digestive tract. *BMJ* 317:844, 1998.
91. Smith-Warner SA, et al: Alcohol and breast cancer in women: A pooled analysis of cohort studies. *JAMA* 279:535, 1998.
92. Sesso HD, Paffenbarger RS Jr, Lee IM: Alcohol consumption and risk of prostate cancer: The Harvard Alumni Health Study. *Int J Epidemiol* 30:749, 2001.
93. Kortelainen ML: Drugs and alcohol in hypothermia and hyperthermia related deaths: A retrospective study. *J Forensic Sci* 32:1704, 1987.

94. O'Connor PG, Schottenfeld RS: Patients with alcohol problems. *N Engl J Med* 338:592, 1998.
95. Bourgeois JA, et al: Comorbid affective disorders and personality traits in alcohol abuse in patients at an Air Force Medical Center. *Mil Med* 164:103, 1999.
96. Bacaner N, et al: The relationship among depressive and alcoholic symptoms and aggressive behavior in adult male emergency department patients. *Acad Emerg Med* 9:120, 2002.
97. Drake RE, Osher FC, Wallach MA: Alcohol use and abuse in schizophrenia: A prospective community study. *J Nerv Ment Dis* 177:408, 1989.
98. Swift RM: Drug therapy for alcohol dependence. *N Engl J Med* 340:1482, 1999.
99. Mason BJ, et al: A double-blind, placebo controlled trial of desipramine for primary alcohol dependence stratified on the presence or absence of major depression. *JAMA* 275:761, 1996.
100. Fraser AG: Pharmacokinetic interactions between alcohol and other drugs. *Clin Pharmacokinet* 33:79, 1997.
101. Wootton FT, Lee WM: Acetaminophen hepatotoxicity in the alcoholic. *South Med J* 83:1047, 1990.
102. Makin A, Wiiliams R: Paracetamol hepatotoxicity and alcohol consumption in deliberate and accidental overdose. *Q J Med* 93:341, 2000.
103. Andrews P: Cocaethylene toxicity. *J Addict Dis* 16:75, 1997.
104. Vanek VW, et al: Concurrent use of cocaine and alcohol by patients treated in the emergency department. *Ann Emerg Med* 28:508, 1999
105. Henry D, Dobson A, Turner C: Variability in the risk of major gastrointestinal complications from nonaspirin nonsteroidal anti-inflammatory drugs. *Gastroenterology* 105:1078, 1993
106. Fett DL, Vukov LF: An unusual case of severe griseofulvin-alcohol interaction. *Ann Emerg Med* 24:95, 1994.
107. Maio RF, et al: Adolescent injury in the emergency department: Opportunity for alcohol interventions? *Ann Emerg Med* 35:252, 2000.
108. Foster SE, Vaughan RD, Foster WH, Califano JA Jr: Alcohol consumption and expenditures for underage drinking and adult excessive drinking. *JAMA* 289:989, 2003.
109. Hingson RW, Heeren T, Jamanka A, Howland J: Age of drinking onset and unintentional injury involvement after drinking. *JAMA* 284:1527, 2000.
110. Garfield CF, Chung PJ, Rathouz PJ: Alcohol advertising in magazines and adolescent readership. *JAMA* 289:2424, 2003.
111. Adams WL: Potential for adverse drug-alcohol interactions among retirement community residents. *J Am Geriatr Soc* 43:1021, 1995.
112. Ruitenberg A, et al: Alcohol consumption and risk of dementia: The Rotterdam Study. *Lancet* 359:281, 2002.
113. Young NK: Effects of alcohol and other drugs on children. *J Psychoactive Drugs* 29:23, 1997.
114. From the Centers for Disease Control and Prevention. Alcohol use among women of childbearing age—United States, 1991-1999. *JAMA* 287:2069, 2002.
115. Gottlieb MI: Alcohol and pregnancy: A potential for disaster. *Emerg Med* 26:73, 1994.
116. O'Connor MJ, et al: Psychiatric illness in a clinical sample of children with prenatal alcohol exposure. *Am J Drug Alcohol Abuse* 28:743, 2002.
117. American Academy of Pediatrics, Committee on Substance Abuse, Committee on Children with Disabilities: Fetal alcohol syndrome and fetal alcohol effects. *Pediatrics* 91:1004, 1993.
118. Jurkovich GJ, et al: Effects of alcohol intoxication on the initial assessment of trauma patients. *Ann Emerg Med* 21:704, 1992.
119. Marx J: Alcohol and trauma. *Emerg Med Clin North Am* 8:929, 1990.
120. Rappaport W, et al: The effect of alcohol in isolated blunt splenic trauma. *J Trauma* 30:1518, 1990.
121. Kiwerski J, Krasuski M, Wozniak E: Sequelae of injuries of thoracic vertebrae with spinal cord trauma in persons under the influence of alcohol. *Pol Tyg Lek* 44:910, 1989.
122. Brodner R, Gilder JV, Collins WJ: Experimental spinal cord trauma: Potentiation by alcohol. *J Trauma* 21:124, 1981.
123. Stein S, O'Malley K, Ross S: Is routine computed tomography scanning too expensive for mild head injury? *Ann Emerg Med* 20:1290, 1991.
124. Krystal JH, et al: Naltrexone in the treatment of alcohol dependency. *N Engl J Med* 345:1734, 2001.
125. Kenna, GA, McGeavy HE, Swift RM: Pharmacotherapy, pharmacogenomics and the future of alcohol dependence treatment, part 2. *Am J Health Syst Pharm* 61:2380, 2004.
126. Davidson P, et al: Intoxicated ED patients: A five year follow-up of morbidity and mortality. *Ann Emerg Med* 30:593, 1997.

CHAPTER 185

Substance Abuse

Stephen A. Colucciello and Christian Tomaszewski

PERSPECTIVE

The use and abuse of psychoactive substances are not unique to our country or century. People utilized hallucinogenic plants to achieve altered states of consciousness in prehistoric times, and psychoactive substances have been used in all eras and cultures ever since. As Osler remarked, "The desire to take medicine is, perhaps, the great feature which distinguishes man from other animals."[1] The human cost of substance abuse is high, and deaths secondary to psychoactive substances nearly doubled during the 1980s.[2]

EPIDEMIOLOGY

A variety of stereotypes come to mind when compiling the profile of a substance abuser. These stereotypes pose dangerous traps for the clinician. Physicians are likely to ignore the possibility of drug intoxication in the well-dressed businessman or in those at the extremes of age. Children may ingest psychoactive substances they find on coffee tables or floors after parties or passively inhale smoke in rooms where drugs are used. Some parents deliberately give psychoactive substances to their children in an attempt to calm or abuse them.

Recently, increasing numbers of teens have been ingesting dextromethorphan-containing over-the-counter products such as Coricidin HBP Cough & Cold tablets.[3] These are known on the streets as Triple-C, Red Devils, Red C, Red Box, or skittles. Other dextromethorphan compounds that include cough medicines, such as NyQuil or Robitussin DM, provide the sought-after high known as the "robo-buzz." Teens abusing such over-the-counter preparations may present to the emergency department with anticholinergic syndromes and demonstrate tachycardia, hypertension, mydriasis, somnolence, or agitation.[4]

The elderly also abuse substances, and geriatric patients may suffer new-onset psychosis as a result of cocaine or drug withdrawal when hospitalized. Drug use is frequent among pregnant women, resulting in both maternal and fetal morbidity. Up to 7% of women delivering babies have urine toxicology screens positive for illicit drugs.[5] Manifestations of abuse may be acute, as in abruptio placentae or premature birth, or insidious, producing growth retardation and birth defects.

Some of the best data regarding the direct impact of drug abuse on emergency departments come from the Drug Alert Warning Network (DAWN), sponsored by the Substance Abuse and Mental Health Services Administration Office of Applied Studies. DAWN collects data from hospital emergency departments and medical examiners that include drug-related emergency department visits or deaths. The inclusion criteria involve patients who abuse illegal drugs or use legal substances for a nonmedical purpose.

According to DAWN statistics, drug-related emergency department visits increased from 323,100 in 1978 to an all-time high of 518,521 in 1994. Most of this increase was due to heroin, with its more pronounced addiction problems. By 1996, drug-related emergency department visits decreased by 6% from 518,500 to 487,600. However, in 1996, cocaine-related episodes reached their highest level since the DAWN survey began in 1978. Although reported cocaine exposures have decreased over the last 5 years, deaths and major medical morbidity have increased significantly.[6,7]

According to DAWN, in 2002, there were 670,307 drug abuse related emergency department episodes in the United States, equivalent to a rate of 261 emergency department episodes per 100,000 population.[8] Other important findings in this report included the following:

- Eight of 10 emergency department drug mentions (81%) come from only seven categories: alcohol-in-combination, cocaine, heroin, marijuana, benzodiazepines, antidepressants, and analgesics. In 2002, alcohol-in-combination was a factor in 31% of emergency department drug episodes (207,395 mentions), cocaine in 30% (199,198), marijuana in 18% (119,472), and heroin in 14% (93,519). Collectively, the benzodiazepines, antidepressants, and analgesics constituted 359,266 emergency department mentions in 2002, or nearly 30% of total emergency department drug mentions.
- Of the most common illicit drugs, only amphetamines showed a significant increase in emergency department mentions (17%, from 18,555 to 21,644), but amphetamines and methamphetamine, when considered together, were statistically unchanged from 2001 to 2002.
- Among the less frequently mentioned major substances of abuse, only two drugs increased significantly from 2001 to 2002: inhalants (187%, from 522 to 1496) and PCP (25%, from 6102 to 7648). Mentions of LSD decreased significantly (−68%, from 2821 to 891). MDMA ("ecstasy") (4026), γ-hydroxybutyrate (GHB; 3330), miscellaneous hallucinogens (1428), and ketamine (260) were statistically unchanged from 2001 to 2002.
- Trends in emergency department mentions of the club drugs MDMA (ecstasy) (4026) and GHB (3330) appear to have leveled off, with GHB mentions lower in 2002 than in 2000 (from 4969). Estimates for flunitrazepam (Rohypnol) continued to be too imprecise for publication.

Cocaine continues to be the most frequently mentioned illicit drug, followed by marijuana/hashish, heroin/morphine, and amphetamines (Figure 185-1).

Drug problems are more prevalent among the disadvantaged minority and lower socioeconomic groups. As a result, these groups bear the brunt of drug-related problems, such as incarceration, acquired immunodeficiency syndrome, and tuberculosis.

CLINICAL FINDINGS

History

A complete drug history should be obtained from patients reporting drug reactions, acute anxiety or other psychiatric problems, and acute cardiopulmonary or neurologic symptoms. This information should include use of legal and illegal substances, prescription and over-the-counter medications, vitamins, herbals, tonics, and potions. The possibility of suicidal ingestions should be considered, and the physician should specifically ask if the patient is suicidal when appropriate. The physician who is neutral and nonjudgmental in approach is more likely to obtain accurate information.

Patients should be questioned as to what they thought they took, and when. Prehospital care providers, family members, and friends may be able to provide additional information. Patients who are brought from the scene of a club, "rave," or circuit party with altered mental status may be under the influence of a "club drug" such as MDMA (ecstasy), GHB, flunitrazepam (Rohypnol), or ketamine. Other club drugs

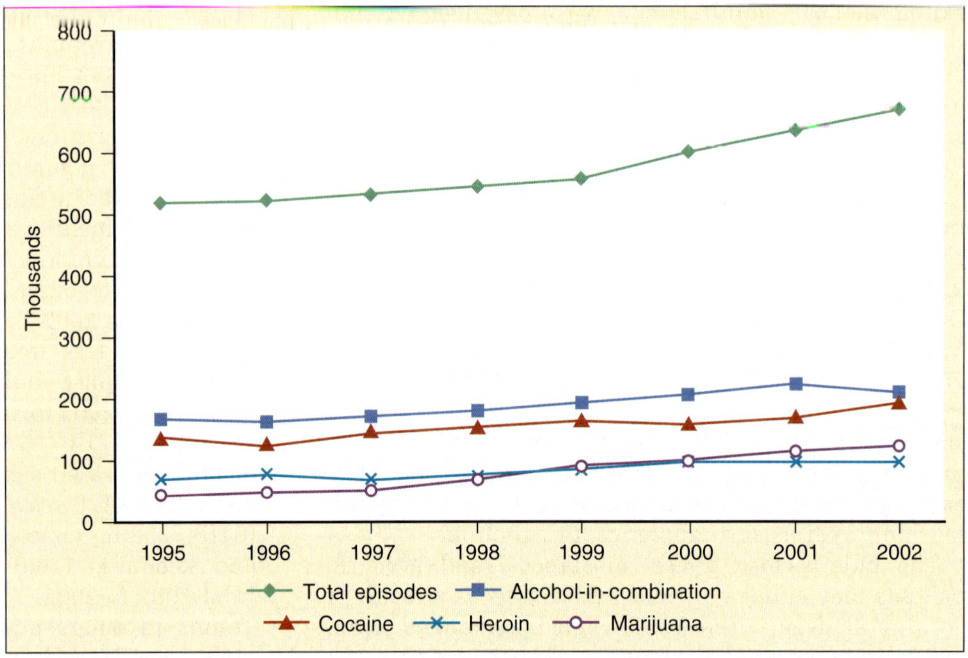

Figure 185-1. Emergency department drug-related episodes and alcohol-in-combination, cocaine, heroin, and marijuana mentions. 1995 through 2002. (From Emergency Department Trends From the Drug Abuse Warning Network, Final Estimates 1995-2002. Rockville, Md, Department of Health and Human Services Substance Abuse and Mental Health Services Administration Office of Applied Studies, 2003.)

such as "verve" and "jolt" are sold on the Internet as precursor molecules to GHB, known as γ-butyrolactone (GBL). These dangerous drugs are especially appealing to teens.[9]

Knowledge of drug interactions assists in the diagnosis and care of substance abuse victims. A careful medication history for all legal and illegal drugs, including ethanol, may pinpoint the source of an adverse reaction. For example, a variety of agents can heighten the effects of cocaine. Some abusers co-ingest small amounts of organophosphates to decrease pseudocholinesterase activity and prolong the effects of cocaine.[10] The co-ingestion of ethanol and cocaine results in an active metabolite, cocaethylene, which also extends cocaine's effects. Serotonin syndrome, manifested by muscle rigidity, hyperthermia, diarrhea, and seizures, may result when sympathomimetic drugs are taken concurrently with selective serotonin reuptake inhibitors such as fluoxetine. Amphetamines elevate serotonin either directly or by reversible inhibition of monoamine oxidase (MAO). In fact, a selective serotonin reuptake inhibitor can result in flashbacks in prior users. MAO inhibitors can provoke hypertensive crisis in patients taking sympathomimetics. Interactions between agents commonly prescribed for patients with human immunodeficiency virus and recreational drugs may be associated with serious clinical consequences, as protease inhibitors and nonnucleoside reverse transcriptase inhibitors can inhibit or induce the cytochrome P450 system.[11]

Illicit drug laboratories are not known for their quality control, and many drugs are combined or "cut" with other substances to increase profits. Up to 50% of street samples lack the alleged drug. Some additives may be innocuous, such as local anesthetics or sugars, but others, such as strychnine, may be lethal. Some drugs, such as phencyclidine (PCP), are deliberately sold as a different drug, such as lysergic acid diethylamide (LSD). Drug combinations and unanticipated additives or substitutions often produce a clinical picture discordant with what the patient claims to have taken.

Some physicians believe that the RAFFT score is useful in detecting substance abuse in adolescents and that any positive response to the following questions warrants further evaluation[12]:

Relax: Do you drink/use drugs to relax, feel better about yourself, or fit in?

Alone: Do you ever drink/use drugs while you are by yourself, alone?

Friends: Do any of your closest friends drink/use drugs?

Family: Does a close family member have a problem with alcohol or drugs?

Trouble: Have you ever gotten into trouble from drinking or using drugs?

Physical Examination

Documentation of vital signs is essential. The presence of fever has profound implications, yet temperatures are frequently neglected in violent or agitated patients. Because rapid mouth breathing, dry mucous membranes, and agitation all produce unreliable oral temperatures, a rectal temperature best confirms suspected hyperthermia. Patients should be undressed and completely examined, with particular attention paid to the skin, eyes, and nervous system.

Physical examination includes evaluation for specific toxidromes. Adrenergic and cholinergic findings are especially significant. The presence of diaphoresis, mydriasis, or hyperactive bowel sounds suggests sympathetic overload. This contrasts with the anticholinergic syndrome of dry skin and mouth and absent bowel sounds. The neurologic examination should incorporate a mental status evaluation, addressing both level of consciousness and appropriateness of affect. The skin provides important clues to the existence or sequelae of substance abuse, such as residue of drugs on the hand or face or track marks from intravenous drug use.

DIFFERENTIAL DIAGNOSIS

It is clinically dangerous to assume that abnormal behavior or altered mental status in the unkempt young patient is due to drug intoxication. Many serious illnesses can manifest as an "OD," including sepsis, meningitis, head trauma, poisoning, intracranial hemorrhage, and drug withdrawal. Hypoglycemia and other metabolic and endocrine derangements are important considerations.

COMPLICATIONS

Illicit drugs produce a wide variety of complications involving all major organ systems. They are responsible for up to 5% of intensive care admissions, generating 10% of costs.[13] Neurologic complications are especially prominent. In some series, almost 10% of strokes occur secondary to drug abuse.[14] Vascular insults include cerebral infarction, cerebral and cerebellar hemorrhage, and subarachnoid bleed, usually secondary to cocaine and other sympathomimetics, PCP, or heroin. Seizures are frequently associated with substance abuse, and although single generalized tonic-clonic seizures are more common, status epilepticus can occur. Although sympathomimetics, such as cocaine and amphetamines, are responsible for the majority of seizures, heroin and PCP play a significant role.

The dangers of substance abuse extend far beyond the toxic effects of a particular drug. Associated hazards include the risk of human immunodeficiency virus infection, not only secondary to intravenous injection, but also as a result of a promiscuous lifestyle associated with the drug culture. In one study, human immunodeficiency virus seroprevalence was 12.7% among injection drug users and 7.5% among crack smokers. Almost 20% of cocaine abusers have a positive purified protein derivative (tuberculosis) test result in some locales. Sexually transmitted disease is common, especially in the sex-for-drugs culture of crack cocaine. Syphilis in particular is endemic among crack abusers.

The lungs are target organs for impurities in intravenous drugs, and pyrogens become trapped in this massive filter. Acutely, this can produce "cotton fever," characterized by high fever, tachycardia, and tachypnea 10 to 20 minutes after injection. This benign self-limited illness contrasts with the long-term restrictive and obstructive lung diseases that accompany the prolonged intravenous abuse of methylphenidate. Right-sided endocarditis is a frequent sequela of chronic intravenous drug abuse, and the nonspecific flulike symptoms that accompany this disease can easily mislead the clinician. In addition to endocarditis and acquired immunodeficiency syndrome, intravenous drug abusers develop septic pulmonary emboli, cellulitis, botulism, tetanus, and other infectious complications. They may develop unusual sites of osteomyelitis or septic arthritis involving the lumbar spine, sternoclavicular, or sacroiliac joints.

Psychiatric complications are frequent and include anxiety, depression, suicidal ideation, mood swings, paranoia, and panic attacks. Paranoia and depression and associated suicide attempts are common among stimulant abusers, and hallucinations of parasites under the skin are common in those addicted to amphetamines. Sympathomimetics are strongly associated with aggressive behavior and street crime. Traumatic injuries are endemic among substance abusers, and arise from both assault and motor vehicle crashes. At times, trauma can be occult, and the unwary physician may overlook a stab wound in a patient whose clinical picture is predominated by drug-induced agitation.

DIAGNOSTIC ADJUNCTS

All patients with acute alterations in mental status require either a bedside glucose test-strip measurement or the empiric administration of 50% dextrose solution. The complete blood cell count is of little value, except to follow serial hemoglobins if occult trauma or hemolysis is suspected. Patients who are unstable hemodynamically or with altered mental status need assessment of electrolytes, blood urea nitrogen level, and creatinine level. Arterial blood gas may be useful in assessing acid-base status, as well as measuring oxygenation and ventilation. Rhabdomyolysis, most likely seen with sympathomimetic abuse, is best detected by measurement of serum creatinine kinase. Rhabdomyolysis is usually defined as creatinine kinase levels more than 5 to 10 times normal. Dipstick urinalysis is insensitive for this condition, but may screen positive for hemoglobin without accompanying red blood cells. The electrocardiogram will occasionally diagnose a myocardial infarction in patients with drug-related chest pain but has limited sensitivity and specificity.

The use of qualitative toxicology screens is controversial. Although unsuspected drugs may be detected, this knowledge rarely affects patient management.[15,16] Emergency physicians are often confused as to which drugs are screened for on their own hospital's toxicology panel. Qualitative toxicology screens are less important than the patient history and clinical status, but quantitative levels of suspected substances, such as acetaminophen or acetylsalicylic acid, may be valuable in certain circumstances. A new generation of rapid bedside urine toxicology screens may provide timely information, but their use requires further study. One paper evaluated the test characteristics of four point-of-care toxicology assays for drugs of abuse: Triage Panel for Drugs of Abuse plus TCA, QuickScreen Pro-Multi Drug Screening Tests, Syva Rapid Test d.a.u. 5 and d.a.u. 2, and Rapid Drug Screen.[17] In this study, Triage was the most dependable and reproducible on-site drug-screening device.

MANAGEMENT

Agitation

Few antidotes exist for psychoactive drug intoxication and, with a few notable exceptions, treatment is symptomatic and supportive. Violent or agitated patients require sedation. Benzodiazepines such as lorazepam (Ativan) can sedate patients with sympathomimetic symptoms, whether owing to drug intoxication or withdrawal. For other patients, butyrophenones, such as haloperidol (Haldol) are safe and rapidly effective. In the past, droperidol (Inapsine) was used with success; however, a "black-box" warning from the Food and Drug Administration (FDA) requiring continuous electrocardiographic monitoring before, during, and after use has removed it from most emergency department formularies. Most authorities advise against phenothiazines in the drug-intoxicated patient because of their strong anticholinergic effects and potential to produce hypotension and lower the seizure threshold.

Body Packers and Stuffers

Patients may present with ingested drugs that are not yet absorbed from the gastrointestinal tract. The body *stuffer* swallows loosely packaged drugs, or the raw drug itself, in an attempt to conceal contraband on arrest. The body *packer* (a "mule") delivers professionally packaged drugs in their intestines, usually on a flight from another country. In many cases, these packets can be visualized radiographically.

There is considerable debate with regard to the best approach to body packers. In asymptomatic cases, the patient's right to refuse care usually supersedes local laws for forcible removal of such evidence. Patients who are significantly confused from drug effects (or comatose) are incapable of refusing lifesaving interventions.

Referral

After acute medical issues have been managed, substance abusers should be asked whether they would like help in overcoming their addiction. Studies show that intervention may be most successful in abusers of heroin, nonprescribed methadone, and benzodiazepines. Users of crack cocaine appear to be more resistant to treatment.[18]

SELECTED SUBSTANCES OF ABUSE

The remainder of the chapter reviews selected substances of abuse. Other commonly abused drugs are discussed in the following chapters: hallucinogens (see Chapter 154), cocaine (see Chapter 152), jimson weed (see Chapter 148), and γ-hydroxybutyrate (see Chapter 163).

SOLVENTS (see Chapter 153)

Epidemiology

In the United States, abuse of petroleum vapors was first reported in the 1940s. Today, hydrocarbons are frequently abused by adolescents with adjustment disorders, rebellion, and polysubstance abuse. Solvent abuse occurs in up to 13% of teenagers in some areas and is most common among minority populations, especially Hispanics and Native Americans.[19,20] There have been numerous deaths from volatile hydrocarbons, most of which occur between the ages of 14 and 16 years.

Hydrocarbons are ubiquitous in both home and industry and can be found in solvents, typewriter correction fluid, paints, lacquers, glues, aerosols, refrigerants, and various propellants (Table 185-1). Trichloroethylene and other chlorinated hydrocarbons are used as solvents and degreasers in many household products. The most commonly abused hydrocarbons include chlorinated agents, such as trichloroethane, trichloroethylene and related compounds, and the aromatic petroleum distillates toluene and gasoline. Gasoline remains the cheapest high available to indigent youths and accounts for 83% of hydrocarbon abuse in children younger than 9 years.[21]

Hydrocarbon abuse generally occurs through inhalation; however, ingestion and even intravenous abuse have been reported. Inhalation involves a variety of techniques. "Sniffers" inhale fumes from an open container, and "huffers" spray liquid onto a cloth, which then covers their mouth and nose. "Baggers" pour the liquid into a bag and then place it over their face. Because of the high concentrations and potential for asphyxia, the risk of sudden death is greatest among baggers.[20] "Fire breathing" is the practice by which butane is inhaled and then set aflame during exhalation for an inspiring visual effect.

Pathophysiology

Inhaled hydrocarbons rapidly cross the alveoli into the bloodstream and are quickly distributed throughout the body. They are strongly lipophilic and traverse the blood-brain barrier within minutes. Hydrocarbons initially produce central nervous system (CNS) stimulation or disinhibition, similar to alcohol intoxication, and increased levels lead to a general anesthetic effect and respiratory depression. As a result, solvent abusers are at risk of cerebral hypoxia.

Toluene abuse produces a mixed metabolic acidosis with associated electrolyte disturbance. Chronic abusers develop a distal renal tubular acidosis characterized by bicarbonate wasting, profound hypokalemia, hypophosphatemia, and a urine pH greater than 5.5.[22] Although the renal tubular acidosis produces a narrow anion gap acidosis (hyperchloremia), a concomitant wide gap acidosis may also occur, as a result of acid

Table 185-1. Volatile Substances of Abuse and Their Sources

Class	Example	Source	Special Concerns
Aliphatic hydrocarbons	Butane/isobutane	Lighter fluid	Thermal injury
	Propane	Bottled gas	
	n-Hexane	Paints/thinners, rubber cement	Polyneuropathy
	Gasoline	Fuel	Possible lead poisoning/thermal injury
Halogenated hydrocarbons	Freons	Refrigerants, propellants	Frostbite of lips
	Trichloroethane	Cleaning solvent	
	Trichloroethylene	Typing correction fluid, PVC cement	
	Tetrachloroethylene	Dry cleaning fluid	
	Methylene chloride	Paint stripper	Carbon monoxide poisoning
	Carbon tetrachloride	Solvent, refrigerant	Hepatorenal failure
Aromatic hydrocarbons	Toluene	Solvent, adhesives Paints/thinners	RTA, hypokalemia
	Benzene	Chemical/plastic industry	Hemotoxicity
	Xylene	Solvent, paints/thinners	
Alkyl nitrites	Amyl nitrite	Cyanide antidote kit	Methemoglobinemia
	Propyl, isopropyl	Room odorizer	Methemoglobinemia
	Butyl, isobutyl	"Head" shop	Methemoglobinemia
Oxygenated compounds	Acetone	Nail polish remover	
	Dimethyl ether	Aerosol, propellants	
	Ethyl acetate	Balsa wood cement	
	Nitrous oxide	Aerosol propellant	

PVC, polyvinyl chloride; RTA, renal tubular acidosis.
Data from Flanagan RI, et al: *Drug Safety* 5:359, 1990; and Linden CH: *Emerg Med Clin North Am* 8:559, 1990.

metabolites.[23] In severe overdoses, rhabdomyolysis may occur secondary to electrolyte disorders, muscle compression, or direct muscle toxicity.

Animal studies demonstrate that hydrocarbon inhalation, especially the chlorinated hydrocarbons, produces "cardiac sensitization," in which the heart becomes irritable and overly responsive to endogenous catecholamines. This sensitization predisposes patients to ventricular tachycardia and fibrillation. Such dysrhythmias are presumed responsible for the many cases of sudden death among solvent abusers. Exertion after hydrocarbon inhalation seems to precipitate many of these arrests.[24] Most inhaled hydrocarbons are pulmonary irritants and produce bronchial and laryngeal spasm. Patients with acute-on-chronic exposure are most likely to experience respiratory distress and can develop wheezing, pulmonary edema, or respiratory failure.[25]

Many hydrocarbons exist in complex mixtures that include other toxins, such as carbon tetrachloride, methanol, or methylene chloride. Carbon tetrachloride may lead to hepatic and renal failure, whereas methanol produces inebriation, ataxia, abdominal pain, and "snowstorm" blindness. Methylene chloride, a chlorinated hydrocarbon, is slowly metabolized in the liver to carbon monoxide. In addition to the initial solvent narcosis, sustained carbon monoxide levels produce headache, nausea, vomiting, chest pain, or loss of consciousness. Aromatic hydrocarbons are metabolized in the liver, whereas aliphatic hydrocarbons, and alkyl halides, are eliminated by the lungs and, to some extent, excreted by the kidneys.

Hydrocarbons lead to a variety of dermal insults. Because they are skin and mucous membrane irritants, many users develop contact dermatitis.

Clinical Findings

The diagnosis of solvent abuse may be hindered by the patient's reluctance to admit to this activity. Because solvent abuse often occurs in groups, the patient's friends might provide the necessary history. Physical examination provides important clues, such as the characteristic odor on the breath or clothes. Conjunctival injection, and even corneal damage, is common due to the solvent's irritant effect. Telltale flecks of paint around the nose and mouth or on the hands distinguish paint sniffers and huffers (see Chapter 156, Figure 156-1). Severe frostbite of the lips occurs in patients who abuse Freon gas (chlorofluorocarbons), and swelling may lead to airway compromise (Figure 185-2).[26] Some patients report wheezing, whereas others exhibit tachycardia and cardiac dysrhythmias. Alterations in mental status are common and range from excitation and euphoria to delusions, irritability, lethargy, and coma. Visual and auditory hallucinations may also be present.

Toluene abuse causes three clinical syndromes in which either gastrointestinal complaints, neuropsychiatric symptoms, or muscular weakness may predominate.[27] The weakness from hypokalemia may be so profound as to result in quadriparesis and respiratory failure.[28,29] Gastrointestinal symptoms include abdominal pain, nausea, and vomiting; the neuropsychiatric presentation involves altered mental status, headache, loss of consciousness, and ataxia.

Complications

High doses of toluene may result in seizures and stroke-like syndromes, and some patients die from massive cerebral edema.[30] Chronic hydrocarbon abuse leads to a variety of often permanent neurologic abnormalities

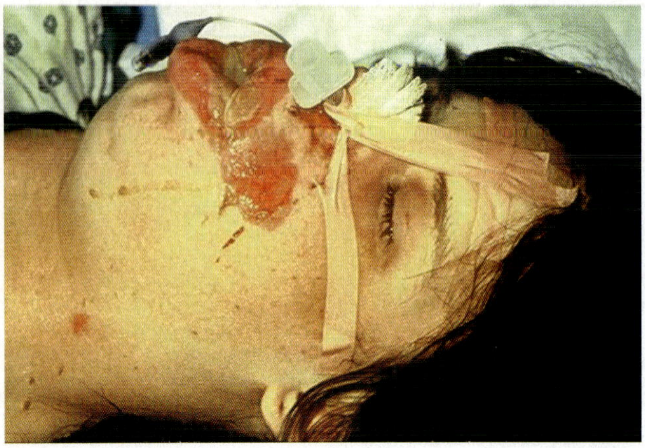

Figure 185-2. Freon abuser. (Copyright Stephen Colucciello.)

that include cognitive, cerebellar, cranial nerve, and peripheral nerve dysfunction.[31] Pendular nystagmus and memory loss are characteristic, and persistent abuse results in progressive irreversible encephalopathy as well as cerebellar ataxia. In such cases, magnetic resonance imaging demonstrates diffuse cerebral and cerebellar atrophy with loss of differentiation between gray and white matter, which correlates with the degree of dementia.[32]

Multiorgan failure occurs with massive overdose. Renal and hepatic failure develops with heavy, chronic abuse, particularly in the case of chlorinated agents. Urinary calculi, proteinuria, and hematuria ensue during chronic abuse.[33] Hydrocarbons may cause fatal asthma or lead to diffuse pulmonary injury and acute respiratory distress syndrome. Myocarditis and myocardiopathy have also been reported with long-term abuse. An overlapping syndrome of lead poisoning can occur from sniffing old gasoline containing organoleads.[34] Other signs of lead poisoning, such as anemia and basophilic stippling, provide clues to this diagnosis.

One of the most dramatic complications of hydrocarbon abuse is accidental self-immolation.

Ancillary Data

Symptomatic patients should be placed on a cardiac monitor and pulse oximeter. A chest radiograph is necessary for those with respiratory distress to detect noncardiogenic pulmonary edema. In the case of symptomatic toluene abuse, analysis of electrolytes, phosphorus, and calcium may reveal significant abnormalities. Hypokalemia may be profound, less than 1.5 mEq/L. Hypercalcemia, which is often present during metabolic acidosis, may drop precipitously after treatment, producing tetany. An arterial blood gas analysis will assist in determining acid-base status. Measurement of carbon monoxide is important if there is concomitant exposure to methylene chloride. Chronic abusers of chlorinated hydrocarbons should have liver function tests performed, particularly if there is icterus or right upper quadrant tenderness. Urinalysis is helpful in patients who have abused toluene, as measurement of urinary pH will assist in the diagnosis of renal tubular acidosis. Symptomatic toluene abusers should have their creatinine kinase level measured to detect rhabdomyolysis. Laboratory screening for the presence of hydrocarbons is not necessary in acute management. Testing may be helpful under special circumstances, such as the need to document an industrial exposure or in the investigation of a fatality.[35]

Differential Considerations

Patients who abuse hydrocarbons can present with psychosis, bizarre behavior, or visual hallucinations—symptoms compatible with a host of different medical conditions. Profound muscle weakness seen with toluene abuse can occur with other disorders characterized by hypophosphatemia or hypokalemia. Toluene-induced weakness is distinguished from Guillain-Barré syndrome in that reflexes are maintained and motor strength returns with electrolyte replacement.[27] Chronic abuse can result in cognitive and brainstem abnormalities common to many degenerative diseases. Peripheral neuropathy of the stocking-glove type may occur, and the differential diagnosis must include heavy metal toxicity, vitamin deficiency, and alcoholism.

Many nonvolatile gases are also inhaled for their psychoactive effect. Nitrous oxide, or laughing gas, is an analgesic commonly abused by medical and dental personnel. The public can obtain nitrous oxide in canisters sold as propellants for whipped cream ("whippets"). Helium, used professionally by mixed-gas divers, is used recreationally to raise the pitch of the voice. The greatest danger posed by both helium and nitrous oxide is anoxic death from asphyxia. In addition, long-term abuse of nitrous oxide can result in manifestations of vitamin B12 deficiency, including peripheral neuropathy.[36]

Management (Box 185-1)

Hydrocarbon toxicity is treated supportively. Early in the course of management, any hydrocarbons present on the skin should be washed off to prevent absorption. In the prehospital setting, medics should provide supplemental O_2. They should calm the patient to avoid any exertional stress, which could precipitate dysrhythmias. Cardiac dysrhythmias can be treated with routine protocols, including defibrillation if necessary. Although there are concerns regarding the administration of catecholamines in patients with sensitized hearts, the withholding of epinephrine for cardiac arrest cannot be justified.

Hypotension is a rare complication of hydrocarbon toxicity and may respond to bolus infusions of crystalloid fluid. Bronchospasm should be treated with inhaled β-1 agonists, such as albuterol, but epinephrine should be avoided because of the potential for myocardial sensitivity and dysrhythmias. Toluene abusers with acidosis require aggressive fluid therapy and replacement of potassium and phosphorus, based on laboratory evaluation. Although renal abnormalities and acidosis resolve in hours to days with simple hydration, some authorities use sodium bicarbonate to treat profound acidosis. If rhabdomyolysis occurs, vigorous hydration is the mainstay in the treatment of

BOX 185-1. Acute Clinical Features and Treatment of Hydrocarbon Abuse

Clinical Findings

Acute

Irritation of the mucous membranes
Conjunctival infection
Reactive airway disease
Hallucinations
Seizures
Dysrhythmias, including ventricular fibrillation
Sudden death
Weakness/electrolyte disorders

Chronic

Hepatic failure
Encephalopathy
Cerebellar ataxia
Renal tubular acidosis
Hypokalemia
Hypophosphatemia
Peripheral neuropathy

Ancillary Data

Traces or odor of paint and solvent on bands and face
Liver function tests in chronic chlorinated hydrocarbon exposure
Electrolytes in symptomatic patients
Calcium and phosphorus level in symptomatic toluene exposure
Creatinine kinase level if rhabdomyolysis is suspected
Carboxyhemoglobin after methylene chloride exposure

Management

Oxygen
Hydration
Correction of electrolyte abnormalities (potassium, phosphorus, calcium)
Careful use of dopamine or norepinephrine for hypotension resistant to fluids
Nebulized albuterol for bronchospasm
Defibrillation, as necessary

rhabdomyolysis. In severe cases, sodium bicarbonate and mannitol may prevent myoglobin from precipitating in the tubules.

Disposition

The CNS effects of acute hydrocarbon toxicity are usually short lived, and patients with mild alterations of mental status may be monitored and discharged after resolution of symptoms. Symptomatic patients require admission. Indications for intensive care monitoring include severe weakness, electrolyte abnormalities, acidosis, rhabdomyolysis, persistent dysrhythmias, respiratory distress, seizures, or coma.

NITRITES

Epidemiology

Nitrites have become increasingly recognized as drugs of abuse since the 1960s. Initially, nitrites were available only by prescription. Amyl nitrite "poppers" were previously used in the treatment of angina and should be found in the cyanide antidote kit. Today, nitrites such as butyl nitrite ("Locker Room") and isobutyl nitrite ("rush") are sold without a prescription. Head shops that offer other drug paraphernalia openly market these products as stimulants.

Volatile nitrites are inhaled in the belief that their vasodilating properties enhance sexual arousal. Juvenile drug abusers, college-age males, and male homosexuals are prominent among nitrite abusers. Commercially available nitrites possess names with aggressive sexual overtones, including bang, bolt, bullet, climax, flash, highball, locker room, poppers, rush, snappers, liquid gold, and thrust.[37]

Pathophysiology

Volatile nitrites are rapidly absorbed through the lung and have a variety of toxic effects. They are potent vasodilators that may cause syncope and headache. Fortunately, these vascular effects are short-lived and resolve before or soon after emergency department presentation. Nitrites produce significant hemolysis in patients with glucose-6-phosphate dehydrogenase (G6PD) deficiency, owing to the drug's membrane oxidant effect. Rare cases of hemolysis have occurred in patients with normal G6PD levels.[38,39] Damage to the cell membrane leads to denaturation, precipitation of protein, and development of Heinz bodies within the red blood cell.

The most significant effect of nitrites is the development of methemoglobinemia. Nitrites oxidize hemoglobin to methemoglobin through transformation of the ferrous ion (Fe^{2+}) to the ferric ion (Fe^{3+}). Methemoglobin is incapable of binding oxygen and shifts the hemoglobin dissociation curve to the left, further impairing tissue delivery. Methemoglobinemia produces varying levels of central and peripheral cyanosis. In the normal person, small amounts of endogenous methemoglobin are reduced to hemoglobin by methemoglobin reductase, utilizing G6PD as a cofactor. As methemoglobin levels increase, the metabolic pathways are overwhelmed. Although it is suggested that the natural half-life of methemoglobin is approximately 1 hour, longer half-lives have been reported.[40] The combination of methemoglobinemia and hemolytic anemia produced by nitrites leads to dangerous tissue hypoxia.

Clinical Findings

The most dramatic presentation of volatile nitrite intoxication is central cyanosis unresponsive to oxygen. Patients present with dusky blue lips and varying degrees of cyanosis of the head, trunk, and extremities. They are frequently tachycardic and may be agitated or confused. In patients without anemia, cyanosis occurs with methemoglobin levels greater than 15%. Patients with severe anemia may never develop cyanosis, despite significant levels of methemoglobin.

Neurologic complaints are common and include transient headaches, euphoria, aggression, confusion, or lethargy. Initially, speech may be incomprehensible, and the patient's gait ataxic. Headache, dizziness, weakness, and hypotension generally occur with levels greater than 30%. Symptoms of severe hypoxia such as lethargy, dysrhythmias, respiratory distress, and seizures appear at levels greater than 60%. In these rare cases, the patient may present with unstable vital signs secondary to cardiac ischemia.[40] Secondary to the nitrite's irritant effect, the sclera may be injected, and contact dermatitis appears on the face, nose, lips, and hands. Because these flammable substances can be ignited by cigarettes or lighters, volatile nitrites are also responsible for serious facial burns.

Complications

Severe, untreated methemoglobinemia leads to progressive acidosis, respiratory distress, and cardiovascular collapse. Occasionally, nitrite abuse can lead to death. Massive hemolysis has also been reported, even in the absence of an intrinsic red blood cell defect.[41]

Ancillary Data

Arterial blood appears darker than normal and is often described as being "chocolate brown" in color. Whereas normal venous blood turns red when oxygen is bubbled through it, blood with significant methemoglobin remains dusky. Pulse oximetry gives a false reading owing to absorptive interference from methemoglobinemia. When methemoglobin levels exceed 30%, the pulse oximeter tends toward a mean of 85% saturation, regardless of true O_2 saturation.[42] Oxygen saturation must be measured on a co-oximeter, rather than calculated by the arterial blood gas analyzer. A measured saturation lower than the calculated level implies a dyshemoglobinemia from methemoglobin, carboxyhemoglobin, or sulfhemoglobin.

The co-oximeter best determines actual methemoglobin levels. This spectrophotometrically obtained value is usually expressed as a percentage (methemoglobin ÷ total hemoglobin × 100%). Symptomatic patients require cardiac monitoring, and those with chest pain or altered mental status need an electrocardiogram. A complete blood cell count and peripheral smear will diagnose hemolysis. Measurement of nitrite levels is generally unavailable and, more important, not useful.

Differential Considerations

The emergency physician should consider a number of different causes when faced with a patient with cyanosis (see Chapter 30). These include pulmonary disorders, abnormalities of ventilation or perfusion, low cardiac output, and dyshemoglobins. Most cyanotic patients improve with oxygen, whereas patients with methemoglobinemia do not. Other agents that can cause methemoglobinemia include dapsone, lidocaine, aniline dyes, sulfonamides, phenacetin, and the quinolones. Other abnormal hemoglobins, such as sulfhemoglobin, also produce cyanosis unresponsive to oxygen. However, these abnormal hemoglobins do not respond to treatment with methylene blue. In the infant, congenital hemoglobinopathies, lack of methemoglobin reductase, and heart disease must be considered in the differential diagnosis.

BOX 185-2. Clinical Features and Treatment of Nitrite Abuse

Clinical Findings
Tachypnea
Tachycardia
Cyanosis unresponsive to oxygen
Headache
Nausea
Weakness
Mucosal irritation
Transient euphoria or combativeness
Syncope
Hypotension

Ancillary Data
Methemoglobin level
Arterial blood gas
Oxygen saturation gap (calculated – measured)
Chocolate-brown blood
Cyanosis unresponsive to oxygen
Peripheral smear for hemolysis (pulse oximetry is unreliable)

Management
High-flow oxygen
Intravenous fluids for hypotension
Intravenous methylene blue (1%) at 1 mg/kg over 5 min, may repeat in 1 hour if no response, do not exceed 7 mg/kg/day
Consider hyperbaric oxygen or transfusion for recalcitrant cases

Management (Box 185-2)

Symptomatic patients require oxygen, and those with cyanosis benefit from a nonrebreather mask set at a high flow rate. Hypotension should be treated with a rapid infusion of crystalloids. Although recreational nitrites are almost universally inhaled, in the rare case of ingestion, activated charcoal may be helpful. Patients who are asymptomatic or with methemoglobin levels below 25% to 30% rarely require treatment, as endogenous nicotinamide adenine dinucleotide methemoglobin reductase will convert the methemoglobin to hemoglobin within several hours.

Methylene blue is the treatment of choice for patients who are symptomatic or have levels above 30%. This substance acts as a cofactor that accelerates the reduction of methemoglobin.[43] One to 2 mg/kg of 1% methylene blue is given intravenously over 5 minutes and repeated in 1 hour if needed. No more than 7 mg/kg should be given in a 24-hour period, as larger doses may paradoxically *increase* methemoglobinemia owing to the oxidant effects of methylene blue.[44] High doses of methylene blue can also result in hemolysis. Methylene blue may be ineffective in patients with methemoglobin reductase deficiency, G6PD deficiency, or ongoing absorption of an ingested nitrite. Although the undiagnosed G6PD-deficient patient is theoretically at risk for hemolytic anemia induced by methylene blue, as a practical matter, such hemolysis is extremely rare.

In cases of life-threatening methemoglobinemia (levels ≥70%) unresponsive to adequate doses of methylene blue, alternate treatments must be used. Hyperbaric oxygen has been used to good effect, supplying all the dissolved oxygen necessary for life.[45] As a last resort, exchange transfusion may benefit recalcitrant cases. Anemic patients in particular may profit from transfusion.

Disposition

Symptomatic patients require admission and serial methemoglobin determinations. Ingested nitrites can cause recurrent or persistent methemoglobinemia and, as a result, even mildly symptomatic patients should be hospitalized. Asymptomatic patients without cyanosis can be safely discharged after a period of observation. This includes those who required only a single dose of methylene blue and have remained asymptomatic for several hours. Serial measurements of methemoglobin are prudent in such cases.

PHENCYCLIDINE

Epidemiology

In the first half of 1999, slightly more than 2000 emergency department visits involved PCP. The number of PCP cases, which began to decline in 1996, has leveled off. PCP was developed in 1957 as a non-narcotic general anesthetic chemically similar to ketamine. PCP [1-(1-phenylcyclohexyl] piperidine hydrochloride is still commercially available as an animal tranquilizer but was removed from human medical practice because of the high incidence of adverse effects that occurred on emergence from anesthesia. Phencyclidine was popularized in Haight-Ashbury during the late 1960s and was often sold as a substitute for LSD. Currently, the drug is most often used by adolescents, particularly inner-city black males, and its popularity waxes and wanes in proportion to the availability of other, more desirable sympathomimetics, such as crack cocaine; it has been termed a drug of "downward mobility."[40] PCP can be ingested or injected, but it is most often smoked by "dusting" the chemical on tobacco or marijuana cigarettes. Alternatively, cigarettes can be "doped" by dipping them in liquid PCP. PCP is often contaminated with benzene, toluene, isopropanol, phenol, benzocaine, ketamine, or ephedrine.[47] Drugs such as LSD or cocaine are often sold as PCP and vice versa. Phencyclidine may be absorbed percutaneously and cause intoxication in law enforcement personnel, manufacturers, and dealers. Children become symptomatic by ingesting butts of PCP or through passive inhalation of the smoke.

There are a large number of street names for PCP, including angel dust, crystal joint, super grass, peace pill, hog, and rocket fuel. The practice of combining PCP with crack cocaine is known as space basing.

Pathophysiology

Although its mechanism is debated, PCP probably blocks acetylcholine at postsynaptic sites and inhibits reuptake of catecholamines.[48] It produces a rapid effect when smoked, and symptoms occur within 2 to 5 minutes. Users remain intoxicated for 4 to 6 hours and may not return to normal for 24 to 48 hours. Effects are prolonged in large overdoses, particularly if ingested, and some patients remain symptomatic for days to weeks. Because PCP is fat soluble, it accumulates in adipose tissue and the brain, resulting in recurrent and fluctuating symptoms.[46] The drug is metabolized in the liver and subsequently excreted into the urine. PCP is a weak base with a pKa of 8.5 to 9.6 and accumulates in the stomach regardless of whether it is smoked, injected, or absorbed through the skin. Hypoglycemia occurs in up to 22% of PCP users.[49]

Clinical Findings

Dramatic and fluctuating behavioral effects characterize PCP intoxication. Patients present with altered mental status and violent, agitated behavior. They may be calm or catatonic one minute, and raging and uncontrollable the next. PCP intoxication occurs in three stages: (1) mild psychiatric signs and symptoms; (2) progressive stupor with an intact response to deep pain; and (3) deep coma with loss of pain response.[50] The acute brain syndrome associated with PCP is characterized by disorientation, confusion, and memory loss, as well as violent behavior. Neurologic effects include dystonias, ataxia, jerky movements, and oculogyric crisis.[49] Some patients display general rigidity and athetoid movements, and children in particular may have bizarre staring spells. Public nudity is a frequent associated behavior.

Patients are frequently hypertensive with mild tachycardia and often demonstrate a mixture of cholinergic, anticholinergic, and adrenergic signs. Cholinergic findings include diaphoresis, myosis, bronchospasm, and salivation. Anticholinergic and adrenergic findings include mydriasis and urinary retention. The eyes provide important clues to PCP intoxication. Horizontal nystagmus is extremely common, but nystagmus can be vertical, rotary, or mixed.[49] A blank, open-eyed stare with roving gaze and dilated pupils is common and has been referred to as "Groucho eyes."

Complications

Large ingestions produce a variety of severe complications, most of which are trauma related. Delusions of invulnerability have led to many deaths during PCP intoxication. The dissociative effect prevents the patient from experiencing pain, and the loss of impulse control may lead patients to mutilate themselves or attack armed police officers. Disseminated intravascular coagulation and liver failure occur in conjunction with life-threatening hyperthermia. Neurologic complications are frequent, most notably seizures and coma. Prolonged coma, which occurs in up to 10% of patients, is associated with increased morbidity. Subarachnoid hemorrhage has also been reported. Respiratory problems include stridor, aspiration pneumonia, and apnea.[49]

Rhabdomyolysis induced by PCP occurs through a wide variety of mechanisms that include profound voluntary exertion, fighting against restraints, and myoclonic or dystonic muscle contractions. Rhabdomyolysis can progress to acute renal failure, particularly in the presence of hyperthermia or dehydration.[illegible]

Ancillary Data

Symptomatic patients require immediate glucose testing. Because rhabdomyolysis is one of the most serious complications of PCP use, the creatinine kinase level should be measured, and elevated levels followed in a serial manner. Leukocytosis is frequent, but not a prognostic indicator. However, serial hemoglobins or hematocrits may assist in the detection of occult trauma. Liver function tests, electrolytes, blood urea nitrogen, and creatinine influence management in the critically ill.

A qualitative urine drug screen can be used to confirm the diagnosis of PCP intoxication. However, quantitative serum and urinary levels of PCP do not correlate with clinical effects and are not useful in management. Chronic users excrete PCP metabolites in the urine for 1 to 2 weeks, but because PCP is excreted only in acid urine, patients with profoundly alkalotic urine may test falsely negative for PCP.

Differential Considerations

The behavioral effects of PCP can be difficult to distinguish from those of other mind-altering substances, such as hallucinogens, sympathomimetics, and particularly cocaine. However, the diaphoresis characteristic of cocaine is usually absent with PCP. Hyperthermia seen with PCP intoxication has a broad differential diagnosis, including sepsis, neuroleptic malignant syndrome, serotonin syndrome, and other drug-related causes. PCP intoxication must be distinguished from acute psychosis, thyroid storm, pheochromocytoma, and hypoglycemia. Head trauma, hypoxia, electrolyte disorders, and CNS infections may all be confused with drug intoxication; a rapid bedside toxicology screen may be helpful. Nystagmus, fluctuating mental status, and mixed autonomic findings provide additional clues to toxicity.

BOX 185-3. Clinical Features and Treatment of Phencyclidine

Clinical Findings
- Violent, agitated, bizarre behavior
- Fluctuating mental status
- Catatonia, staring spells
- Psychosis
- Nystagmus
- Hypertension
- Tachycardia
- Hyperthermia
- Seizures
- Rhabdomyolysis
- Dystonia
- Mydriasis or myosis
- Stupor or coma

Ancillary Data
- Stat glucose
- Creatinine kinase
- Urine toxicologic screen (only if diagnosis unclear)

Management
- Physical or chemical restraints
- Benzodiazepines for agitation, seizures
- Butyrophenones for agitation, psychosis
- Multiple dose charcoal
- Aggressive cooling
- Intravenous nitroprusside or phentolamine for hypertension

Management (Box 185-3)

Neither hemodialysis nor hemoperfusion is indicated owing to the large volume of distribution and significant protein binding. Because there is no specific antidote for PCP, treatment is supportive.

Sedation

Agitated patients with loss of impulse control present a real and immediate danger to emergency department personnel. Verbal "talk-down" therapy is not effective with PCP-intoxicated patients, and combative patients should be restrained. Sedation should also be used, as patients may suffer muscle damage and rhabdomyolysis if they struggle against restraints. Reports of incredible strength in such patients are part of emergency department legend, and restraints must be unbreakable. Strong leather or specially designed polymers are most effective, as cloth restraints may tear. The physician must *not* remove the restraints at the first sign of tranquility, because brief periods of relative calm are shattered by periods of raging psychosis.

Intravenous benzodiazepines, or butyrophenones, such as haloperidol or droperidol, are effective means of controlling agitation. Haloperidol (Haldol) is extremely effective in managing patients with PCP intoxication[49]; it decreases delusions, hallucinations, disorganized thinking, and assaultive behavior. Some patients may require up to 100 mg/day of haloperidol, and the addition of ascorbic acid may be more effective than either drug alone.[52] Benzodiazepines are also beneficial in the agitated patient and are particularly useful in controlling seizures. Benzodiazepines are safest when administered intravenously and titrated to effect. Seizures that are refractory to high doses of benzodiazepines may respond to phenobarbital.

Treatment of Complications

Hyperthermia may be treated in a variety of ways, including immersion in an ice-water bath, or combining tepid mist and cooling fans. Benzodiazepines are a useful adjunct to prevent shivering and provide sedation.

Rhabdomyolysis may lead to acute renal failure, and adequate hydration is essential. Intravenous crystalloids should be administered to produce a urine output of at least 2 mL/kg per hour. Mannitol and bicarbonate therapy, occasionally used in the treatment of rhabdomyolysis from other causes, have not been studied in PCP intoxication.

Hypertensive crises respond to a nitroprusside drip or intravenous phentolamine, 2.5 to 5 mg every 5 minutes titrated to effect. Dosages above 20 mg should rarely be needed (see Chapter 83).

Drug Elimination

The elimination of PCP may be enhanced by multiple doses of activated charcoal, even if the drug was smoked or injected.[46] Because PCP accumulates in the stomach, continuous nasogastric suction has been proposed; however, no data exist regarding the efficacy of this approach. Multiple doses of activated charcoal are preferred, as it avoids the acid-base disturbances associated with continuous suction.

Acidification of the urine through systemic administration of acid has been recommended to achieve ion trapping and enhance urinary PCP excretion. However, only a small percentage of PCP is excreted unchanged in the urine, and the induction of metabolic acidosis carries significant risks by increasing the chance of myoglobinuric renal failure. For these reasons, forced acid diuresis is not recommended for patients with PCP intoxication. Anecdotal reports suggest a benefit for verapamil, but no clinical trials substantiate these case reports. In fact, animal studies indicate that verapamil may actually increase PCP toxicity.[53]

Disposition

Patients with hyperthermia, hypertension, seizures, or altered mental status require hospitalization and often intensive care. Patients with any signs of severe poisoning may have a prolonged course and will require admission. Because of PCP's fluctuating symptomatology, patients who appear calm and cooperative must be observed for several hours before discharge, to ensure that symptoms do not return.

KETAMINE

Ketamine is best known to emergency physicians for its role in conscious sedation. However, it is becoming an increasingly important drug of abuse in the club scene and can be injected, swallowed, snorted, or smoked. One recent emergency department review found that common presenting symptoms included anxiety, chest pain, and palpitations. Tachycardia was the most common physical examination finding, but nystagmus was actually rare. The most frequent complications of ketamine abuse in this series included agitation and rhabdomyolysis.[54] Symptoms were transient, and most patients were discharged from the emergency department within 5 hours of presentation. Patients intoxicated with ketamine may benefit from benzodiazepines or haloperidol.[55]

AMPHETAMINES AND AMPHETAMINE-LIKE DRUGS

(see Chapter 152)

Historical Perspective

Plants containing psychoactive amphetamines were ingested before recorded history. Alexander the Great sent the amphetamine-containing weed, khat, to one of his generals as a cure for depression. Amphetamines became popular in America after their widespread use as a stimulant during World War II. Hallucinogenic amphetamines were first used clinically in psychotherapy in the 1970s, and during the 1980s abuse was widespread among college students. "Designer" chemical variant formulations of amphetamines have flourished over the last decade.

Epidemiology

Amphetamines occur in a variety of forms and are cheaply and easily manufactured in illicit labs as tablets, capsules, powders, gelatin, or impregnated in pieces of paper. "Ice," which is the pure hydrochloride salt of methamphetamine, is marketed in crystalline form for smoking, insufflation, or injection. Methcathinone is a synthetic amphetamine derived from the evergreen shrub khat. Street names for methamphetamine include speed, crank, and go; the names ice and crystal are reserved for its crystalline form. The hallucinogenic amphetamines are methoxylated or methylene dioxylated analogues of amphetamines and mescaline (Table 185-2) and include MDMA (3,4-methylenedioxymethamphetamine), MDM (methylenedioxymethamphetamine), MDEA (3,4-methylenedioxymethamphetamine), 2-CB (4-bromo-2,5-methoxyphenyl-ethylamine), DOM (dimethoxyamphetamine), and bromo-DOB (bromodimethoxyamphetamine). There are more than 50 types of hallucinogenic amphetamines, and many have not been classified. Most hallucinogenic amphetamines are ingested, but some are insufflated nasally or injected. Hallucinogenic amphetamines carry a wide variety of colorful street names: MDMA (Adam, ecstasy, Eve, essence), MDEA (Eve), MDA (harmony, love, speed for lovers), DOM (STP—serenity, tranquility, and peace), DOB (LSD-25 and golden eagle).

Natural sources of amphetamine-like substances have been increasingly touted as legal highs. Chewing the East African herb khat (*Catha edulis*) releases several amphetamine-like substances. *Ma huang*, a Chinese herbal medicine derived from the *Ephedra* plant, contains large amounts of ephedrine and is abused for its ability to stimulate the CNS and cause euphoria. Ephedra-containing nutritional supplements are sold over the counter with names such as herbal ecstasy, blasting caps, cloud 9, diet fuel capsules, diet prep, and ener-trim.

Although amphetamine use is widespread, in certain subcultures, abuse is endemic. College students ingest amphetamines hoping to remain alert while "cram-

Table 185-2. Commonly Abused Amphetamines and Their Derivatives

Street Name	Common Name	Special Features
Speed, uppers	Amphetamine and dexamphetamine	
	Methamphetamine hydrochloride	
Crank, speed	Mixed isomers	
Ice, crank, crystal	D-Isomer	Smokable
	Propylhexedrine	
Khat	Cathionine	*Catha edulis* plant
Serenity, Tranquility, Peace	Designer amphetamines	
	4-Methyl-2,5-dimethoxy-amphetamine (DOM, STP)	Hallucinations
Golden eagle, LSD-25, tile, MOA	4-Bromo-2,5-dimethoxy-amphetamine (DOB)	Hallucinations
	Para-methoxy-amphetamine (PMA)	Hallucinations
Love drug, love pill	3,4-Methylenedioxy-amphetamine (MDA)	Hallucinations
Adam, ecstasy	3,4-Methylenedioxymethamphetamine (MDMA)	Euphoria
Eve	3,4-Methylenedioxyethamphetamine (MDEA)	Euphoria
Cat	Methcathinone	Euphoria, hallucinations

Data from Jerrard DA: *J Emerg Med* 8:733, 1990; and Shield TO: Amphetamines. In Haddad LM, Winchester JF (eds): *Clinical Management of Poisoning and Drug Overdose*. Philadelphia, WB Saunders, 1990.

ming." Abuse is prominent among certain motorcycle gangs of the Southwest. Smokable forms of amphetamines, such as crank, are found most commonly in Hawaii and the West Coast. Hallucinogenic amphetamines are often ingested at parties called "raves," where young people gather in a large warehouse, listen to loud music, and dance all night. At these parties, multiple drugs are ingested, yielding a mixed clinical picture. MDMA is particularly popular in colleges, and at one institute 39% of the students interviewed admitted to its use.[56]

Pathophysiology

Amphetamines belong to the phenylethylamine family. They release catecholamines and block their reuptake, resulting in stimulation of both α- and β-adrenergic receptors. At high doses, serotonin may be released. Substitution of various positions of the phenylethylamine molecule produces a variety of physiologic effects, ranging from CNS stimulation and cardiovascular excitation to hallucinogenic properties. The "toxic" dose for amphetamines ranges from 1 to 5 mg for DOB to 150 mg for MDMA.[21]

Hallucinogenic amphetamines stimulate both the dopaminergic and the serotonergic system. Amphetamines and related compounds can produce central hyperthermia, probably secondary to activation of CNS dopamine receptors. Peripherally induced hyperthermia occurs with muscle rigidity or severe exertion, as in all-night dancing. The combination of MAO inhibitors and hallucinogenic amphetamines results in a particularly dangerous reaction. The amphetamines release norepinephrine and serotonin, and the MAO inhibitor prevents their degradation. This may result in a serotonin syndrome characterized by life-threatening hypertension, hyperthermia, and hypertonicity.[57]

Amphetamines have large volumes of distribution and are eliminated primarily by hepatic transformation. A number of amphetamines have significant renal elimination. Clinical intoxication with amphetamines can last as long as 24 hours.

Clinical Findings

The neurologic abnormalities seen with amphetamine use include hallucinations, agitation, and twitching. Methamphetamine use is particularly associated with delusions of parasitosis. Known as *formication*, this sensation of ants or bugs crawling under the skin causes patients to pick at themselves and even engage in self-mutilation. Hallucinogenic amphetamines provoke panic attacks and cause auditory or visual hallucinations. Large ingestions may lead to a florid psychosis. Fever, tachycardia, hypertension, diaphoresis, pallor, and piloerection arise from sympathetic stimulation. Teens who overdose on ecstasy typically present to the emergency department on a weekend night with increased temperature and altered mental status. This presentation is sardonically known as "Saturday Night Fever" in some emergency departments. Patients can attain body temperatures of 42.9° C (109° F) and still survive with aggressive management.

Ocular manifestations include nystagmus, mydriasis, blurred vision, and intraretinal hemorrhages.[58] Muscles may become extremely rigid, and patients may exhibit clenching, tremulousness, and hyperreflexia. Myoclonus, muscle spasms, and bruxism are common. Cardiovascular toxicity results in tachycardia, palpitations, and dysrhythmias; respiratory rates are usually increased. Nausea, vomiting, and diarrhea may occur.

Complications

The severely intoxicated patient presents with a constellation of rigid body, dilated pupils, high temperature, and seizures, leading to rhabdomyolysis and possible acute renal failure. Delirium and even coma may ensue; ischemic stroke, intracranial hemorrhage, and cerebral edema have been reported.[59,60] Peripheral vasospasm can lead to ischemia and gangrene, ultimately requiring amputation of the limb. Amphetamines have both acute and chronic effects on the heart. Severe cases are characterized by hypotension and cardiovascular collapse. Myocardial infarction and fatal dysrhythmias occur after either inhalation or ingestion of amphetamines.

Deaths from sympathetic amines result from ingestions of as little as 200 mg. The time course of amphetamine mortality is biphasic. Early deaths occur secondary to cardiac dysrhythmias, seizures, and CNS depression; late deaths (24-48 hours) result from the complications of malignant hyperthermia, such as rhabdomyolysis, renal failure, disseminated intravascular coagulation, metabolic acidosis, and cardiovascular collapse.[61] In addition, some early deaths are due to intracranial hemorrhage from abuse of ephedrine, often sold on the street as speed. Jaundice and hepatomegaly occur with hepatotoxicity. Some researchers suggest that a history of hallucinogenic amphetamine misuse should be sought in young people presenting with any of these findings.

Chronic amphetamine abuse can produce necrotizing vasculitis, which involves multiple organ systems. Cardiomyopathy has also been reported. In addition to their direct toxicity, amphetamines and hallucinogenic amphetamines may be contaminated during distribution or manufacture. Two cases of lead poisoning characterized by hepatitis, nephritis, and encephalopathy have been associated with methamphetamine abuse.[62]

Diagnostic Adjuncts

Patients with moderate to severe symptoms require laboratory assessment. Measurement of electrolytes detects hyperkalemia and acidosis, whereas arterial blood gas analysis assists in the management of the dyspneic or acidotic patient. Complete blood cell count, creatinine kinase level, renal function, urinalysis, and coagulation studies are indicated in patients at risk for disseminated intravascular coagulation and rhabdomyolysis, such as those with hyperthermia or muscle rigidity. Hyponatremia is common in abuse of ecstasy (MDMA).[63] Liver function tests are necessary in the very ill or jaundiced. If respiratory distress is present, a chest radiograph will detect pulmonary edema or acute respiratory distress syndrome. Computed tomography of the head is valuable when there are persistent alterations of mental status, seizures, or neurologic deficit. Although amphetamines and their analogues can be detected by thin-layer chromatography or gas liquid chromatography, blood levels do not correlate with toxicity. Clinical diagnosis is usually sufficient, but qualitative analysis may be helpful if the patient does not volunteer a history of ingestion.

Differential Considerations

The differential diagnosis of amphetamine overdose is extremely broad. Patients may present with a host of complaints, including altered mental status, stroke, seizures, hypertensive crisis, chest pain, and peripheral ischemia. The existence of generalized sympathetic stimulation is an important clue to amphetamine toxicity. Hyperpyrexia and confusion may be caused by sepsis, but such patients often have an identifiable infectious source. Thyroid storm and pheochromocytoma can mimic amphetamine overdose, as can the serotonin and neuroleptic malignant syndromes. Cocaine intoxication is often clinically indistinguishable from other sympathomimetic toxicity, except that amphetamine effects are more prolonged.

BOX 185-4. Clinical Features and Treatment of Amphetamine Abuse

Clinical Findings
Tachycardia
Hypertension
Hyperthermia
Diaphoresis
Hallucinations
Myocardial ischemia
Hemorrhagic cerebral infarct
Pneumomediastinum
Pneumonitis
Rhabdomyolysis
Renal failure
Hyperkalemia
Metabolic acidosis
Seizures
Dysrhythmias
Cardiomyopathy

Ancillary Data
ECG (for chest pain)
Chest radiography (for chest symptoms)
Creatinine kinase
CT scan of brain for persistent altered mental status, neurologic deficit, or seizures

Management
Oxygen
Intravenous fluids for hypotension
Benzodiazepines or butyrophenones for agitation or seizures
Dopamine or norepinephrine for unresponsive hypotension
Phentolamine or nitroprusside for hypertension
Lidocaine for ventricular dysrhythmias
Nitroglycerin for myocardial ischemic pain
Aggressive cooling and possibly paralysis for hyperthermia
Fluids, mannitol, or bicarbonate for rhabdomyolysis

ECG, electrocardiogram; CT, computed tomography.

Management (Box 185-4)

Cardiovascular Complications

Severe hypertension requires aggressive treatment with a titratable intravenous drug, such as nitroprusside or phentolamine. The use of β-blockers should be avoided, as their administration may result in unopposed α effects, causing coronary and peripheral arterial vasoconstriction. The use of intravenous or intra-arterial nitroprusside may be effective for severe vascular spasm. Few studies have addressed the management of amphetamine-induced dysrhythmias. In cases of supraventricular tachycardia, a titratable agent such as intravenous diltiazem may be safe. Standard cardiac protocols are indicated in cases of life-threatening ventricular dysrhythmias.

Agitation and Seizures

Agitation and seizures should be managed aggressively. If uncontrolled, they may lead to rhabdomyolysis and life-threatening hyperthermia. While benzodiazepines best manage these symptoms, the physician must be prepared to secure the airway if oversedation occurs. Haloperidol appears to be a reasonable alternative. Although there is the theoretical concern that haloperidol may lower the seizure threshold, this has not been identified as a problem in a large series of patients treated for amphetamine toxicity.[64] Patients with seizures unresponsive to high doses of benzodiazepines and barbiturates usually require intubation and paralysis. In such cases, continuous electroencephalographic monitoring should be used to detect electrical status epilepticus and guide subsequent drug administration.

Hyperthermia

Patients with hyperthermia require aggressive external cooling to prevent neuronal damage. Although sedation with benzodiazepines usually aids cooling, paralysis is occasionally necessary for refractory agitation and seizures. There is little evidence that dantrolene influences the outcome of hyperthermia caused by sympathomimetic drugs. However, it may be considered for hyperthermia unresponsive to other cooling measures.[65]

Rhabdomyolysis

Rhabdomyolysis should be treated with intravenous crystalloid fluid to ensure a urine output of at least 2 mL/kg per hour. The benefits of bicarbonate and mannitol loading in this setting remain unclear, and these drugs should probably be reserved for severe cases unresponsive to fluid loading.

Decontamination and Drug Elimination

If the drug is ingested, activated charcoal can assist in decontamination. Gastrointestinal decontamination (whole bowel irrigation) should be used in any suspected case of body packing. Urine acidification is contraindicated because of the increased danger of renal failure and the lack of proven efficacy.

Disposition

In the absence of complications, patients can be discharged once they become asymptomatic. Extended observation is necessary in the case of ingestions to ensure that delayed effects do not occur, especially if the drug was swallowed in packaged form. Patients with chest pain after amphetamine use represent an understudied group. A reasonable policy is monitoring and institution of a cardiac ischemia workup for any patient who manifests prolonged chest pain (20-30 minutes or longer) that sounds cardiac or occurs in a patient with multiple cardiac risk factors.

KEY CONCEPTS

- For the majority of patients with toxin-induced violent behavior, butyrophenones, such as haloperidol (Haldol), are safe and rapidly effective sedating agents. In patients with suspected sympathomimetic (e.g., cocaine, amphetamines) intoxication, benzodiazepines such as lorazepam (Ativan) should be utilized.
- Toluene abuse causes three clinical syndromes in which either gastrointestinal complaints, neuropsychiatric symptoms, or muscular weakness may predominate. Profound weakness, and even transient quadriparesis secondary to hypokalemia and hypophosphatemia, is the most dramatic presentation.
- The most significant effect of nitrites is the development of methemoglobinemia. Methylene blue is the treatment of choice for patients who are symptomatic or have levels above 30%.
- Dramatic and fluctuating behavioral effects characterize PCP intoxication. These are difficult to distinguish from the behaviors associated with other mind-altering substances, such as hallucinogens, sympathomimetics, and particularly cocaine. Notably, the diaphoresis characteristic of cocaine is usually absent with PCP.
- The severe hypertension that may ensue requires aggressive treatment with a titratable intravenous drug, such as nitroprusside or phentolamine. The use of β-blockers should be avoided, as their administration can result in unopposed α effects, causing coronary and peripheral arterial vasoconstriction.

REFERENCES

1. Osler W: Recent advances in medicine. *Science* 17:170, 1891.
2. Wysowski DK, et al: Mortality attributable to misuse of psychoactive drugs, 1979-88. *Public Health Rep* 108:565, 1993.
3. Banerji S, Anderson IB: Abuse of Coricidin HBP cough & cold tablets: Episodes recorded by a poison center. *Am J Health Syst Pharm* 58:1811, 2001.
4. Kirages TJ, Sule HP, Mycyl MB: Severe manifestations of Coricidin intoxication. *Am J Emerg Med* 21:473, 2003.
5. Vaughn AJ, et al: Community wide estimation of illicit drug use and delivering limit: Prevalence, demographics and associated risk factors. *Obstet Gynecol* 82:92, 1993.
6. Litovitz TL, Schmitz BF, Bailey KM: 1989 Annual Report of the American Association of Poison Control Centers National Data Collection System. *Am J Emerg Med* 8:394, 1990.
7. AAPCC: 1994 Annual Report of the American Association of Poison Control Centers toxic exposure surveillance system. *Am J Emerg Med* 13:551, 1995.
8. Department of Health and Human Services: Emergency Department Trends From the Drug Abuse Warning Network, Final Estimates 1995-2002. Rockville, Md, DHHS Substance Abuse and Mental Health Services Administration Office of Applied Studies, 2003.
9. Winickoff JP, Houck CS, Rothman EL, Bauchner H: Verve and Jolt: Deadly new Internet drugs. *Pediatrics* 106:829, 2000.
10. Hoffman RS, et al: Decreased plasma cholinesterase activity enhances cocaine toxicity in mice. *J Pharmacol Exp Ther* 263:698, 1992.
11. Antoniou T, Tseng AL: Interactions between recreational drugs and antiretroviral agents. *Ann Pharmacother* 36:1598, 2002.

12. Bastiaaens L, Francis G, Lewis K: The RAFFT as a screening tool for adolescent substance use disorders. *Am J Addict* 9:10, 2000.
13. Baldwin WA, et al: Substance abuse related admissions to adult intensive care., *Chest* 103:101, 1993.
14. Sloan MA, et al: Occurrence of stroke associated with use/abuse of drugs. *Neurology* 41:1358, 1991.
15. Brett AS: Implications of discordance between clinical impression and toxicology analysis in drug overdose. *Arch Intern Med* 148:437, 1988.
16. Mahoney JD, et al: Qualitative serum toxic screening in the management of suspected drug overdose. *Am J Emerg Med* 8:16, 1990.
17. Peace MR, Tarnai LD, Poklis A: Performance evaluation of four on-site drug-testing devices for detection of drugs of abuse in urine. *J Anal Toxicol* 24:589, 2000.
18. Gossop M, Marsden J, Stewart D, Kidd T: The National Treatment Outcome Research Study (NTORS): 4-5 year follow-up results. *Addiction* 98:291, 2003.
19. Esmail A, et al: Deaths from volatile substance abuse in those under 18 years: Results from a national epidemiological study. *Arch Dis Child* 69:356, 1993.
20. Linden CH: Volatile substances of abuse. *Emerg Med Clin North Am* 8:559, 1990.
21. Spiller HA, Krenzelok EP: Epidemiology of inhalant abuse reported to two regional poison centers. *J Toxicol Clin Toxicol* 35:167, 1997.
22. Battle DC, Sabatini S, Kurtzman NA: On the mechanism of toluene induced renal tubular acidosis. *Nephron* 49:210, 1988.
23. Carlisle EJ, et al: Glue-sniffing and distal renal tubular acidosis: Sticking to the facts. *J Am Soc Nephrol* 1:1019, 1991.
24. Carlton RF: Fluorocarbon toxicity: Aerosol deaths and anaesthetic reactions. *Ann Clin Lab Sci* 6:411, 1976.
25. Cronk SL, Barkley DE, Farrell MF: Respiratory arrest after solvent abuse. *Br Med J Clin Res Ed* 290:897, 1985.
26. Wegener EE, Barraza KR, Das SK: Severe frostbite caused by freon gas. *South Med J* 84:1143, 1991.
27. Streicher H, et al: Syndromes of toluene sniffing in adults. *Ann Intern Med* 94:758, 1981.
28. Kao KC, et al: Hypokalemic muscular paralysis causing acute respiratory failure due to rhabdomyolysis with renal tubular acidosis in a chronic glue sniffer. *J Toxicol Clin Toxicol* 38:679, 2000.
29. Patel R, Benjamin J Jr: Renal disease associated with toluene inhalation. *J Toxicol Clin Toxicol* 24:213, 1986.
30. D'Costa DF, Gunasekera MP: Fatal cerebral oedema following trichloroethane abuse. *J R Soc Med* 83:533, 1990.
31. Hormes JT, Felley CM, Rosenberg NL: Neurologic sequelae of chronic solvent vapor abuse. *Neurology* 36:698, 1986.
32. Rosenberg NL, et al: Toluene abuse causes diffuse central nervous system white matter changes. *Ann Neurol* 23:611, 1988.
33. Kaneko T, et al: Urinary calculi associated with solvent abuse. *J Urol* 147:1365, 1992.
34. Edminster SC, Bayer MJ: Recreational gasoline sniffing: Acute gasoline intoxication and latent organolead poisoning. Case reports and literature review. *J Emerg Med* 3:365, 1985.
35. Ramsey J, Flanagan R: The role of the laboratory in the investigation of solvent abuse. *Hum Toxicol* 1:299, 1982.
36. Brodsky JB, Cohen EN: Adverse effects of nitrous oxide. *Med Toxicol* 1:362, 1986.
37. Sarvessvaran ER, Fysh R, Bowen DA: Amyl nitrite related deaths. *Med Sci Law* 32:267, 1992.
38. Beaupre SR, Schiffman FJ: Rush hemolysis, a "bite cell" hemolytic anemia associated with volatile liquid nitrite use. *Arch Fam Med* 3:545, 1994.
39. Brandes JC, Bufill JA, Pisciotta AV: Amyl nitrite-induced hemolytic anemia. *Am J Med* 86:252, 1989.
40. Bradberry SM, et al: Fatal methemoglobinemia due to inhalation of isobutyl nitrite. *J Toxicol Clin Toxicol* 32:179, 1994.
41. Bogart L, Bonsignore J, Carvalho A: Massive hemolysis following inhalation of volatile nitrites. *Am J Hematol* 22:327, 1986.
42. Barker SJ, Tremper KK, Hyatt J: Effects of methemoglobinemia on pulse oximetry and mixed venous oximetry. *Anesthesiology* 70:112, 1989.
43. Bodansky O: Mechanism of action of methylene blue in treatment of methemoglobinemia. *JAMA* 142:923, 1950.
44. Whitwan JG, Taylor AR, White JM: Potential hazard of methylene blue. *Anesthesia* 34:181, 1979.
45. Tomaszewski C, Thom SR: Use of hyperbaric oxygen in toxicology. *Emerg Med Clin North Am* 12:437, 1994.
46. Baldridge EB, Bessen HA: Phencyclidine. *Emerg Med Clin North Am* 8:541, 1990.
47. Shesser R, Jotte R, Olshaker J: The contribution of impurities to the acute morbidity of illegal drug use. *Am J Emerg Med* 9:336, 1991.
48. Smith RC, Heltzer HY, Arora RC: Effects of phencyclidine on catecholamine and serotonin uptake. *Biochem Pharmacol* 26:1435, 1979.
49. McCarron MM, et al: Acute phencyclidine intoxication: Clinical patterns, complications and treatment. *Ann Emerg Med* 10:290, 1981.
50. Milhorn HT Jr: Diagnosis and management of phencyclidine intoxication. *Am Fam Phys* 43:1293, 1991.
51. Patel R, Connor G: A review of 30 cases of rhabdomyolysis-associated acute renal failure among phencyclidine users. *J Toxicol Clin Toxicol* 23:547, 1985.
52. Castellani S, et al: Phencyclidine intoxication: Assessment of possible antidotes. *J Toxicol Clin Toxicol (B)* 19:313, 1982.
53. McCann DJ, Smith CM, Winter JC: A caution against use of verapamil in phencyclidine intoxication. *Am J Psychiatry* 43:679, 1986.
54. Weiner AL, Vieira L, Mckay CA, Bayer MJ: Ketamine abusers presenting to the emergency department: A case series. *J Emerg Med* 18:447, 2000.
55. Giannini AJ, Underwood NA, Condon M: Acute ketamine intoxication treated by haloperidol: A preliminary study. *Am J Ther* 7:389, 2000.
56. Peroutka SJ: Incidence of recreational use of 3,4-methylenedimethoxymethamphetamine (MDA, "ecstasy") on an undergraduate campus. *N Engl J Med* 317:1542, 1987.
57. Smilkstein MJ, et al: MAO/MDMA interaction: Agony after ecstasy. *Clin Toxicol* 25:149, 1987.
58. Wallace RT, et al: Sudden retinal manifestations of intranasal cocaine and methamphetamine abuse. *Am J Ophthalmol* 114:158, 1992.
59. Woods JD, Henry JA: Hyperpyrexia induced by 3,4-methylenedioxyamphetamine ("Eve") [letter]. *Lancet* 340:305, 1992.
60. Rothrock JF, Rubinstein R, Lyden PD: Ischemic stroke associated with methamphetamine inhalation. *Neurology* 38:589, 1988.
61. Screaton GR, et al: Hyperpyrexia and rhabdomyolysis after MDMA ("ecstasy") abuse. *Lancet* 339:677, 1992.
62. Allcott JV III, Barnhart RA, Mooney LA: Acute lead poisoning in two users of illicit methamphetamine. *JAMA* 258:510, 1987.
63. Gowing LR, Henry-Edwards SM, Irvine RJ, Ali RL: The health effects of ecstasy: A literature review. *Drug Alcohol Rev* 21:53, 2002.
64. Derlet RW, Albertson TE, Rice P: Antagonism of cocaine, amphetamine, and methamphetamine toxicity. *Pharmacol Biochem Behav* 36:745, 1990.
65. Singarajah C, Lavies NG: An overdose of ecstasy: A role for dantrolene. *Anesthesia* 47:686, 1992.

CHAPTER 186

Evaluation of the Developmentally and Physically Disabled Patient

Maria Stephan

THE DEVELOPMENTALLY DISABLED PATIENT

Perspective

The Americans with Disabilities Act defines a disability as an impairment that limits a major life activity.[1] Developmental disability is a chronic or physical impairment that results in the delay or failure to achieve normal developmental milestones.[2] These impairments usually occur before age 22 and cause significant functional impairments in areas such as independent living, self-care, receptive and expressive language, learning, and economic self-sufficiency.[3] Autism, cerebral palsy, and syndromes with chromosomal deviations are types of developmental disabilities. Tables 186-1 and 186-2 list the characteristics of persons with certain syndromes or metabolic abnormalities associated with developmental disabilities who may present to the emergency department. People with a developmental disability may be either cognitively or physically disabled or both. Developmental disabilities are often associated with mental retardation, defined as having an IQ of 70 or below and at least two impairments in adaptive functioning.[4] Approximately 1% to 2.5% of the population suffers from mental retardation.[5]

There has been a change in social and political attitudes toward persons with developmental disabilities. In 1992, the American Association of Mental Retardation revised its official definition from one that viewed mental retardation as an individual trait to thinking of it as an expression of the interaction between a person with limited intellectual functioning and the environment. Therefore, the diagnosis of mental retardation relies on the assessment of adaptive behavior and not just on IQ. The etiology of mental retardation is multifactorial. It may result from gene and chromosomal abnormalities, both prenatal and postnatal infections, metabolic disorders, hypoxic-ischemic injury, malnutrition, and other unknown influences.

The primary difficulty posed by these individuals in the emergency department is obtaining an adequate history and physical examination. Sometimes maladaptive behavior is encountered in patients with developmental disabilities, making the examination difficult. Generally, more reliance is placed on the caregiver's report, as comprehensive medical records may not be available. Careful observation of nonverbal communication such as facial expression, gesturing, and posture can be helpful. When presenting for evaluation of an acute illness, most disabled patients receive more tests than nondisabled patients. Certain procedures, such as suturing, casting, or pelvic examinations, may require premedication with benzodiazepines or conscious sedation.[6]

Whenever possible, patients should be involved in making decisions about their health care. However, disabled patients may be unable to make informed decisions on their behalf, and documentation of guardianship is usually necessary before or during their care. Appointed guardians have limits to their decision-making power. They cannot write a living will (advance directive) for a patient and are expected to obtain medical consultation about important decisions such as surgery. Any ethical decisions, such as do not resuscitate orders, may have to be reviewed by a probate court.

Specific Medical Problems of the Disabled

Seizure Disorders

Mental retardation, multiple seizure types, and central nervous system (CNS)-related complications with medical therapy are a common clinical scenario for the emergency physician. Thirty percent of all developmentally delayed patients have a seizure disorder, and the incidence of seizures in patients with cerebral palsy (CP) approaches 50%.[7,8] Patients with developmental disabilities and epilepsy account for 18% of patients with known causes for seizures and 5% of new cases of epilepsy annually. The risk for seizure disorders increases with decreasing IQ. Seizures may have an atypical appearance with subtle signs such as eye deviation, brief changes in level of consciousness or behavior, falls, or incontinence. First-time seizures should be thoroughly evaluated and not assumed to be secondary to the developmental disability.[9] Two thirds of patients with severe disabilities have incomplete seizure control and patients frequently require polytherapy with both broad-spectrum and partial-onset antiepileptic drugs (AEDs).[10] Children with mental retardation average 3 AED exposures in contrast to 1.9 exposures in children with normal cognition.[11] Complications of polytherapy with AEDs include CNS toxicity, with delirium, hallucinations, and myoclonus. Valproic acid is frequently effective for treating seizures in patients with developmental disabilities. Phenytoin is also effective for treating tonic-clonic and partial-onset seizures. Only 25% of patients with symptomatic generalized epilepsy enter complete seizure remission.[12] Newer AEDs that may be effective for patients with developmental disabilities and uncontrolled epilepsy are topiramate, lamotrigine, levetiracetam, and zonisamide.

Vagal nerve stimulation therapy is a newer nonpharmacologic therapy useful for reducing seizures in patients with developmental disabilities with intractable seizures. It requires the implantation of a pacemaker-like device that stimulates the left vagus nerve intermittently and on demand. The continuous cyclic stimulation every 3 to 5 minutes produces a prolonged effect on the brain and results in a median reduction in seizure frequency of 30% to 40%.[13] Complete seizure control is rarely achieved. Side effects include hoarseness, throat pain, coughing, paresthesia, and dyspnea and can usually be resolved with adjustment of the stimulation settings.

Cerebrospinal Fluid Shunts

Advances in medical and surgical care have improved the lives of many patients with developmental disabilities. Those with hydrocephalus may have cerebrospinal fluid (CSF) shunts placed to prevent increased intracranial pressure (ICP) caused by tumors, congenital anomalies, hemorrhage, postinfectious obstruction, and other sources. As with any indwelling catheter or appliance, these may be associated with malfunction, infections, and other complications. Many of these CSF shunts are placed in children. Differentiating between shunt complications and common pediatric illnesses may be difficult. More than half of all shunt procedures performed each year are for shunt revision or removal, caused by malfunction or infection.[14]

Shunt malfunction is the most common complication of these devices. Approximately 30% to 40% of shunt procedures eventually result in a malfunction, and 67% of patients experience a shunt malfunction in their lifetime.[15] Obstruction of the shunt catheters accounts for most shunt malfunctions; however, infection, disconnection of shunt components, catheter migration, inadequate drainage, and overdrainage can also cause malfunction.

The signs of shunt malfunction are numerous: swelling or erythema around the shunt tract, bulging or full fontanelle, increase in head circumference with splitting sutures, headache, irritability, increased seizures, vomiting, papilledema, lethargy, ataxia, neck or back pain, blurred vision, sun-setting eyes, behavioral changes, or "just not acting right."[16,17] Seizures are associated with shunt malfunction but not as the sole presenting symptom. Parents have been shown to be as accurate as physicians at diagnosing shunt malfunction before diagnostic testing.[18]

The second most common complication of CSF shunts is infection. The incidence of shunt related infections has been reported to be between 2% and 30% per shunt procedure with a lower incidence in more recent studies.[17] Children younger than 1 year have a higher rate of shunt infection. Half of all shunt infections occur in the first 2 weeks after a shunt procedure, 70% to 80% occur within 2 months, and 80% to 90% within 4 months.[17,19] The most common pathogens identified are coagulase-negative staphylococcal species, *Staphylococcus epidermidis* and *Staphylococcus aureus*, and gram-negative rods.[17,19] Other pathogens that cause meningitis, such as pneumococcus and *Haemophilus influenzae*, have also been isolated in shunt infections.[19] Shunt infections may appear as erythema, swelling, cellulitis, or wound infection overlying the shunt tract.[17,19] Most children with shunt infections present with vague, nonspecific signs and symptoms. Although fever is present in most infections, the classical signs of meningeal irritation are much less common.[17] Any CSF that is obtained should be sent for culture, Gram stain, protein, glucose, and cell count. Elevated white blood cell count, neutrophils, and protein in the CSF are suspicious for infection.[15,17] Bacteria seen on Gram stain are indicative of shunt infection. Patients with ventriculoatrial shunts tend to be bacteremic and may develop sepsis, endocarditis, glomerulonephritis, hypocomplementemia, and thromboembolic events.[17,19]

Overdrainage of CSF can lead to the slit ventricle syndrome. When too much CSF is drained, the ventricle collapses, the ventricular wall or choroid plexus blocks the fenestrations in the proximal catheter, and ICP begins to rise.[19,20] The patient complains of symptoms similar to those of a shunt malfunction until the ICP rises to a level that reexpands the ventricle, after which symptoms resolve. Some patients are sensitive to position; the slight increase in ICP when lying down is enough to relieve the overdrainage, and the lower ICP when standing is sufficient to cause overdrainage.[20] Computed tomography (CT) of these patients reveals small- to normal-sized ventricles.

Radiographic studies used to evaluate shunts include plain radiographs, commonly known as a shunt series, head CT, ultrasonography, and radionucleotide clearance study. They aid in detection of disconnections, kinks, and migration of the shunt catheters and assess ventricular size (CT) or flow through the proximal and distal catheters (radionucleotide clearance study).[15]

Evaluation of shunt function can be difficult and fraught with many pitfalls. Pumping the shunt reservoir has been taught as a way to assess shunt function; however, it has poor sensitivity and must be carefully interpreted.[17,19]

Medical treatment of patients with signs of increased ICP includes hyperventilation and diuretics, such as acetazolamide and mannitol.[17] If cerebral herniation is imminent and unresponsive to medical management, a ventricular puncture through the burr hole can be performed.[15,17,19] When possible, it is preferable to have a neurosurgeon perform this procedure.

Migration of the distal catheter has been reported through intact abdominal wall, into the mediastinum, into the thoracic cavity, and through abdominal and pelvic organs.[15] Migration into the thoracic cavity can cause symptomatic hydrothorax. Abdominal pseudocysts develop in 0.8% to 10% of patients.[19] Other rare abdominal complications attributed to CSF shunts include intussusception, intractable hiccups, omental cyst torsion, and volvulus around the catheter.[15]

Table 186-1. Potential Disorders, Listed by Organ System, of Selected Syndromes Associated with Developmental

Organ System	Myotonic (Muscular) Dystropy	Duchenne Dystrophy	Down Syndrome (Trisomy 21)
Cardiac	Disturbance of conduction system	Arrhythmias, Cardiomyopathy	A-V canal VSD PDA
Pulmonary	Respiratory muscle weakness Fibrosis Pneumonia	Respiratory muscle weakness Pneumonia	Pulmonary vascular disease
Gastrointestinal	Reduced esophageal motility Fecal impaction Intestinal pseudo-obstruction	Constipation	Duodenal atresia Tracheoesophageal fistula
Eye/ear	Cataracts Retinal degeneration	—	Brushfield spots Refractive error Lens opacities
Hematologic/immunologic	—	—	Leukemia Transient myeloproliferative syndrome
Central nervous system	Mental retardation Apathy Dementia	Mental retardation	Mental retardation
Endocrine	Hyperinsulinemia	—	Goiter Hyperthyroidism
Skin	Frontal baldness	Pressure sores	—
Peripheral nerve	Neuropathy	—	—
Liver/kidney	Elevated transaminase levels Gallstones	—	—
Bones	Multiple malformations	Fractures	Atlanto-axial instability
Potential emergency department presentation	Chest pain Palpitations Respiratory distress Abdominal pain	Chest pain Abdominal pain Fractures	Cyanosis Chest pain Congestive heart failure

ASD, atrial septal defect; A-V, atrioventricular; PDA, patent ductus arteriosus; UTI, urinary tract infection; VSD, ventricular septal defect.

Failure to Thrive

Adults with developmental disabilities often present with multiple nonspecific symptoms that represent a decline in overall functioning. Possible etiologies may include medical illness, changes in sensory perception, undiagnosed pain syndromes, medication side effects, response to environmental changes, or neuropsychiatric conditions. Patients may have oromotor control problems that may lead to difficulty with sucking, chewing, or swallowing. Some patients with CP have been reported to have an oral aversion, avoiding having anything placed in their mouths.[21] The presence of dysphagia, combined with the fact that spasticity and dyskinesia are high energy-requiring states, causes many children with CP to be malnourished. Some infants and young children require supplemental feedings with gastrostomy tubes. Reasonable evaluation in the emergency department may include screening tests such as a complete blood count, renal function studies, urinalysis, electrolytes, or electrocardiogram. Further evaluation is best done with the assistance of a neurologist or psychiatrist who has experience in caring for persons with developmental disabilities. Neuropsychiatric testing, CNS imaging, electroencephalography, and lumbar puncture are the most common additional tests obtained.[8]

Gastrostomy Tubes

Neurologic diseases constitute the most frequent indication for a gastrostomy tube (GT). GTs allow enteral feeding in patients with swallowing dysfunction, severe gastroesophageal reflux, esophageal atresia, esophageal burns or strictures, craniofacial abnormalities, chronic malabsorption, and severe failure to thrive. A low-profile balloon tip, mushroom tip, and the collapsible wing tip replace the GT when the stoma matures in 3 weeks to 3 months. Common complications encountered include wound infection, hemorrhage, mucosal injury, obstruction of the tube, dislodgement of the tube, detachment of the stomach from the abdominal wall, peritonitis, aspiration, granulation tissue formation, leakage around the tube, bowel obstruction, and fistula formation.[22]

Disabilities

Turner's (XO) Syndrome	Marfan's Syndrome	Osteogenesis Imperfecta	Fetal Alcohol Syndrome
Bicuspid aortic valves Dilation of aortic root Coarctation of aorta Aortic stenosis, mitral valve prolapse, anomalous pulmonary venous return	Aortic root dilation Aortic regurgitation Mitral valve prolapse Endocarditis	Cor pulmonale in adults	VSD ASD Tetralogy of Fallot Aortic coarctation
—	Pneumothorax	Pneumonia	—
Inflammatory bowel disease Gastrointestinal bleed Delayed gastric emptying	—	—	—
Anterior segment dysgenesis Bilateral otitis	Blue sclera Lens dislocation Iridodonesis	Otosclerosis Early deafness Blue sclera	Microphthalmia
—	—	—	—
Mental retardation to normal cognitive function	Normal cognitive function	Hydrocephalus Brainstem compression Basilar invagination	Mental retardation Hyperactivity in childhood
Goiter Autoimmune thyroid disease Short stature	—	—	—
Neck webbing Pigmented nevi	—	Thin, translucent	Webbed neck
—	—	—	—
Horseshoe kidney Double collecting system Ureteropelvic junction obstruction Hypertension	—	—	Renal anomalies
Scoliosis	Tall stature Long arm span Joint laxity	Thin cortices Multiple fractures Pectus excavatum or carinatum	Microcephaly Joint anomalies Maxillary hypoplasia
Chest pain Gastrointestinal bleed Hypertension UTI	Chest pain Endocarditis	Fractures Headache Congestive heart failure	Aspiration UTI Seizures

If the GT is nonfunctioning, removal and replacement may be necessary. New tubes may be misplaced, most often into the peritoneal cavity. The ease of replacement of a transabdominal feeding tube depends on the surgical procedure performed and the length of time since placement of the original feeding tube. Nonoperative tube replacement techniques are safe only through an established tract between the skin and bowel. If the approach is unclear, a Foley catheter is often a reasonable temporary replacement. The Foley catheter size depends on the size of the child or adult. Catheter replacement should not be attempted in the immediate postoperative period.[22]

Musculoskeletal Disorders

Atlantoaxial Instability

Approximately one in seven persons with trisomy 21 (Down syndrome) has increased ligamentous laxity of the upper cervical spine.[23,24] Complaints of neck or shoulder pain, torticollis, upper extremity weakness, gait changes, changes in bowel or bladder function, and reflex abnormalities may be related to spinal cord compression caused by excess movement of C1 and C2 vertebrae. Evaluation of these patients should include cervical spine radiographs, including flexion and extension views. Atlantoaxial instability is characterized by a space of 5 mm or greater between the posterior segment of the anterior arch of C1 and the anterior portion of the odontoid process of C2. Patients with trisomy 21 undergoing a procedure requiring general anesthesia (i.e., risk of neck manipulation for intubation) should be evaluated beforehand for atlantoaxial instability.

Cerebral Palsy

Patients with CP develop joint contractures. Hip subluxation and dislocation are common in nonambulatory patients including patients with meningomyelocele. Hip subluxation and dislocation may cause pain and commonly interfere with proper wheelchair seating. Foot and hand deformities are also common in patients with CP and may require surgical intervention.[21]

Table 186-2. Selected Metabolic Disorders Associated with Developmental Disabilities: Evaluation, Treatment, and Potential Disorders Listed by Organ System

	Urea Cycle Defects	Organic Acidemias	Carbohydrate Metabolism Defects
Categories	Carbamyl-phosphate deficiency (CPS) Ornithine transcarbamylase (OTC) Citrullinemia Argininemia	Multiple acyl-CoA dehydrogenase deficiency	Galactosemia Glycogen storage diseases
Laboratory Evaluation	Ammonia, glucose, electrolytes, blood gas	Ammonia, blood gas Glucose, electrolytes Lactate, pyruvate, amino acids	Urinary reducing substances (galactosemia) Glucose, electrolytes, lactic acid
Treatment	Sodium benzoate Arginine administration Sodium phenylacetate D10W	Bicarbonate Glucose	Glucose No galactose-containing foods
Potential Disorders by Organ System			
Cardiac			A-V canal VSD PDA
Pulmonary		Apnea	Pulmonary vascular disease
Gastrointestinal	Vomiting Hepatomegaly Failure to thrive	Poor feeding, vomiting	Jaundice Hepatomegaly Diarrhea, vomiting Milk intolerance, failure to thrive
Eye/ear			Cataracts
Hematologic/immunologic			Hemolysis *E. coli* sepsis Galactosemia
Central nervous system	Mental retardation Obtundation Seizures, headache Personality changes Ataxia, neurodegeneration Progressive spastic diplegia	Obtundation Seizures Irritability Increased intracranial pressure	Mental retardation Irritability Seizures Pseudotumor cerebri
Skin		Peeling skin	
Renal		Unusual odor in urine	Galactosuria
Potential Emergency Department Presentation	Altered mental status Seizures, vomiting Shock Neonatal catastrophe	Altered mental status Seizures, vomiting Liver failure Neonatal catastrophe	Vomiting, diarrhea Failure to thrive Hyperbilirubinemia, cataracts Altered mental status

A-V, atrioventricular; D10W, 10% dextrose in water; PDA, patent ductus arteriosus; VSD, ventricular septal defect.

Scoliosis is common in children with CP. The incidence of scoliosis is much higher in the nonambulatory patient than in the ambulatory patient. Factors that lead to scoliosis include asymmetric muscle imbalance, posture, and other structural factors. Surgical treatment is indicated when scoliosis continues to progress, or when the degree of curvature is severe (generally over 40 degrees).[21]

Fractures

Patients living in institutions are known to be at increased risk for fractures.[25] These individuals may be predisposed to injury because of impulsive or aggressive behavior, poor frustration tolerance, or impaired judgment. In addition, many of these individuals have seizure disorders that result in falls or movements that lead to injury. Medications used to control seizure activity may cause osteomalacia, resulting in pathologic fractures. Physical impairments may include severe contractures and osteoporosis, placing the individual at high risk for fractures.[26] Health care staff have been reported to witness only 27% of fractures in these patients.[25] Most fractures are diagnosed by subtle findings of erythema or swelling or by a change in the patient's behavior. Patients who are less functional (e.g., nonambulatory) are at greater risk for fractures. Therefore, any patient with erythema, swelling, or a change in ability to function should be examined for possible fractures. Also, the possibility of abuse or neglect should be considered whenever these patients present to the emergency department.

Cardiovascular Disorders

The reported incidence of congenital cardiac defects in newborns with developmental disabilities ranges from 30% in infants with fetal alcohol syndrome to 50% or greater in those with trisomy 21.[23,24] The most common abnormalities are ventricular or atrial septal defects and mitral valve prolapse. It is important to remember the need for appropriate endocarditis prophylaxis in such patients.

Psychiatric Disorders

Coexisting psychiatric disorders are estimated to be three to four times more common in persons with developmental disabilities than in the general population. Although any type of mental illness can occur, affective disorders and attention-deficit hyperactivity disorders are the most common.[7] Overall, 30% to 40% of patients with mental retardation have emotional disorders compared with 10% in the general population. Patients with developmental disabilities are especially vulnerable to behavioral side effects of AEDs (28% versus 6% in the normal population).[11] Schizophrenia and psychotic illness are uncommon. Diagnosis is difficult and usually requires input from the caregiver, family, and primary care physician.

Pulmonary Disorders

Poor nutritional status, impairment of airway clearance by muscular weakness or poor coordination, and decreased pulmonary reserve (resulting from obesity or chest wall or spine deformity) increase the risk of significant morbidity and mortality from respiratory infections. Other conditions that have adverse effects on the airway and lung include drooling, feeding problems, gastroesophageal reflux, aspiration, spasticity, and scoliosis. Chronic aspiration may result in chemical pneumonitis with permanent lung damage.

Gastrointestinal Disorders

Gastroesophageal Reflux Disease

The prevalence of gastroesophageal reflux disease (GERD) in developmentally disabled institutionalized patients with an IQ less than 50 is high.[27] Anticonvulsant drugs, constipation, CP, scoliosis, feeding gastrostomy, tube feeding, and inactivity have all been described as predisposing factors in this group.[27] Symptoms of GERD include persistent vomiting, hematemesis, rumination, regurgitation, food refusal, pneumonia, and failure to thrive. If the diagnosis is not clear, endoscopy and 24-hour pH probe testing should be performed. Medical therapy with proton pump inhibitors is efficacious with minimal side effects.[28]

Hepatitis

The prevalence of hepatitis B virus in individuals with developmental delay is much higher than in the general population (ranging up to 13.5%).[29] The prevalence of hepatitis B surface antigen is particularly high in patients with Down syndrome.[29,30] This increase in hepatitis has been ascribed to behavioral issues such as aggressive behavior, dribbling or spitting, taking objects in the mouth and sharing food, and unhygienic toilet habits. In this high-risk population, vaccination for hepatitis B is recommended. The prevalence of hepatitis C in developmentally delayed individuals is the same as in the general population.[29]

Fecal Impaction

Constipation and fecal impaction are common in developmentally disabled patients. Difficulties in swallowing, poor diet and fluid intake, inability to appreciate the sense to defecate, and constipating medication may all lead to constipation. High impaction may present as diarrhea from passage of feces and fluid around a partially obstructing mass. In these cases, rectal examination may show little stool in the rectal vault. A plain abdominal radiograph is valuable in the diagnosis of this disorder. Management consists of bowel retraining regimens and stool softeners. It may include rectal stimulation, stimulant laxative suppositories, stool softeners, disposable enema, and a low-bulk diet. Digital disimpaction may be necessary.

Dental Disorders

The oral health of patients with developmental disabilities is dependent largely on their caregiver's knowledge, attitudes, and practices about looking after teeth and going to the dentist. Surveys of the dental health of adults in this group have consistently identified multiple problems. Poor oral and denture hygiene, a high prevalence of gingival disease and untreated dental caries, a high proportion of missing and filled teeth, heavy tooth wear as a result of bruxism, increased traumatic injuries to the teeth and mouth, defects of tooth enamel, and delayed eruption have all been reported.[31]

Orofacial muscle tone abnormalities lead to malocclusions. Tooth enamel defects are common and may lead to caries. Motor problems and oral sensitivity may make brushing difficult. Mouth breathing and some medications used to treat spasticity, such as sedatives, may decrease the amount of saliva and thus increase the propensity for developing dental caries.[31]

Skin

Nonambulatory patients are at significant risk for developing decubitus ulcers. It is important to evaluate the skin thoroughly and treat early signs of breakdown aggressively. Caregivers should be instructed on appropriate pressure relief. It is also important to evaluate the skin around orthoses. If there is a reddened area under an orthosis that does not disappear within 20 minutes of removal of the orthosis, it needs to be adjusted or replaced.

Poor oromotor control combined with decreased sensation and poor head control may cause drooling, which may result in skin irritation and breakdown. It may also cause social embarrassment and decreased social integration. Medications that may be tried include scopolamine patches, glycopyrrolate, cetirizine, or other antihistamines.[21]

Cerebral Palsy

CP is a nonprogressive disorder of posture and movement, often associated with epilepsy and abnormalities of speech, vision, and intellect resulting from a defect or lesion of the developing brain. The prognosis for normal intellect is often excellent. CP is a common disorder with an estimated prevalence of 1 to 2 per 1000 population.[32] The United Cerebral Palsy Association estimates that there are approximately 500,000 adults with CP in the United States.[33]

Congenital CP is present at birth but may not be detected for months. Risk factors include complicated labor and delivery including hypoxia, prematurity, multiple births, infections during pregnancy, and fetal stroke.

Motor involvement may take several forms: spastic, athetoid, ataxia, and mixed forms.[21,33] Spastic CP affects 70% to 80% of patients. The muscles are stiff and permanently contracted. It may affect one limb or multiple extremities. Patients with spastic hemiplegia have decreased spontaneous movements on the affected side. Spasticity is responsible for the equinovarus deformity of the foot. The affected child often walks on tiptoes because of the increased tone. Ankle clonus, a positive Babinski sign, increased deep tendon reflexes, and weakness of the hand and foot dorsiflexors may be present. Approximately 30% of patients with spastic hemiplegia have a seizure within the first 2 years of life and 25% have cognitive abnormalities including mental retardation. Spastic diplegia consists of bilateral spasticity of the legs with brisk reflexes, ankle clonus, a bilateral Babinski sign, and scissoring posture. Severe spastic diplegia is characterized by disuse atrophy and impaired growth of the lower extremities and by disproportionate growth with normal development of the upper torso. Spastic quadriplegia is the most severe form of CP. Marked motor impairment of all extremities and the high association with mental retardation and seizures are seen. Swallowing difficulties are common secondary to supranuclear bulbar palsies, often leading to aspiration pneumonia. Neurologic examination reveals increased tone and spasticity in all extremities, often with flexion contractures in the elbows and knees.

Athetoid (dyskinetic) CP is characterized by uncontrolled, slow, writhing movements of the muscles. This type of CP is seen in 10% to 20% of CP patients. Ataxic CP affects the sense of balance and depth perception. A wide-based gait, poor gait coordination, and intention tremor may be observed. This type affects approximately 5% to 10% of CP patients.[21]

Several management tools for spasticity have been introduced, including pharmacologic agents and surgical procedures. Baclofen, a γ-aminobutyric acid agonist administered intrathecally by an indwelling implanted pump, has been shown to reduce spasticity, improve muscle extensibility, improve joint range of motion, and decrease requirement for corrective orthopedic surgery.[34] Intrathecal baclofen binds to receptors in the spinal cord, causing inhibition of spinal reflexes. The most common side effects are drowsiness, dizziness, nausea, hypotension, and headache, but they are much less common than with oral dosing. Unfortunately, life-threatening complications can occur. Overdose can occur with incorrect pump filling or programming and may result in respiratory depression and reversible coma. Withdrawal may cause increased spasticity, severe hyperthermia, and rhabdomyolysis followed by multisystem failure and death.[34] Early symptoms of withdrawal include itching, dysphoria, irritability, a dramatic increase in spasticity, tachycardia, fever, and changes in blood pressure.

Selective dorsal rhizotomy is a neurosurgical procedure in which a percentage of the dorsal rootlets of the lumbar spinal nerves is sectioned, resulting in a dramatic and permanent reduction in lower limb spasticity. This essentially causes irreversible denervation atrophy. Selective dorsal rhizotomy has been shown to improve range of motion and gait in young children with spastic diplegia CP.[35] The risks of surgery include hypotonia, weakness, sensory changes, and bladder dysfunction. Use of intramuscular botulinum toxin A has resulted in a reduction of muscle tone with some reestablishment of a functional balance between spastic flexors of the elbow, wrist, and fingers and the weakened extensors. The toxin blocks neuromuscular transmission by inhibiting the release of acetylcholine. The single most reported benefit is a reduction in elbow flexion posturing when walking rapidly, which has more to do with cosmesis than function.[36]

A number of medications have been found to decrease spasticity, including diazepam, tizanidine, dantrolene, and clonidine. Trihexyphenidyl (Artane) has been found to improve upper extremity function, expressive language, and drooling in children with dystonic CP.[21]

THE PHYSICALLY DISABLED PATIENT

Hearing Impaired

The size of the deaf community in the United States is unclear, and estimates range from 100,000 to more than 1 million.[37] The population of Americans with some degree of hearing loss is estimated as 20 million. Hearing loss is the sixth most common chronic condition in the United States. Hearing loss is an impairment that affects communication. The categories of "deaf" and "hearing impaired" are not discrete divisions. They represent a continuum of inability to hear, analogous to that of visual impairment. Of those with congenital or prevocal deafness, a few learn to communicate verbally with appropriate hearing aids and training.[38]

A deaf person is not simply deaf. Deaf persons have a range of classifications for themselves. People who describe themselves as "deaf" simply have the physical condition of not being able to hear and understand speech. People describing themselves as "Deaf" are those who embrace the condition and belong to a culture of others like themselves with a similar background, language, value system, and personal experiences.[38] Deaf people have poorer health and appear to use health care services differently from hearing people.[39,40] They report suboptimal communication with health care providers, including a reliance on speech reading and written communication.[41] This has caused feelings of frustration, mistrust, and avoidance of health care institutions and health care providers.[40,41] Successful communication strategies in an encounter with a patient depend on characteristics of the individual involved and the environment in which the communication occurs. People with hearing loss often have good suggestions on how to best communicate with them, and it is important to enlist their help.

After assessing the degree of deafness, communication guidelines include (1) gaining the patient's attention (i.e., if the patient is turned away from you, touch the edge of the bed), (2) using available assistive devices (hearing aids), (3) decreasing background noise, and (4) communicating clearly (avoid gum chewing, do not cover your mouth, keep explanations simple, establish eye contact, and do not shout).

Communication between the physician and a hearing-impaired patient may take several forms. Writing is the method most frequently used with patients who are completely deaf.[42] Although prelingually deaf adults have normal cognitive abilities compared with hearing individuals, their ability to read and write English is often impaired.

American Sign Language (ASL), the second method normally used, is the third most commonly used language in the United States after English and Spanish. It has its own vocabulary, syntax, sign number, and grammar and is not simply spoken English encoded for visual perception (i.e., words spelled with the fingers). The Americans with Disabilities Act requires that a sign language interpreter be provided at medical encounters whenever requested by a deaf person. Qualified interpreters provide simultaneous translation of everything that is said. It is important to emphasize that under federal regulations a physician can choose among various types of auxiliary aids and services "as long as it will result in effective communication." There is no statute, regulation, or judicial decision mandating that a physician provide an ASL interpreter for all hearing-impaired patients under all circumstances.[43] However, effective communication must be provided in each case and the results should be documented.

Lipreading is another method of communication. It is a skill most congenitally deaf persons do not acquire adequately for communication in most of their daily interactions. The average profoundly deaf lipreader understands approximately one third of what is said to him or her under optimal conditions.[44] People who lose their hearing over time can better supplement the loss with lipreading. They already know the spoken language, and their lipreading skills improve gradually as their hearing becomes less reliable.

The fourth method of communication is through the text teletype writer (TTY). A TTY is a small battery-operated keyboard with a display panel for the typed message. Some prefer this to ASL, which is often condensed and abbreviated in conveying details. The TTY may be more useful for the explanation of medical procedures and unfamiliar medical terminology and therefore may decrease confusion. The technology can also be used to communicate with another TTY by telephone. Hearing persons trying to call a deaf patient using this device use a statewide relay service. The service types into the TTY whatever a person says into the receiver at one end of the line and reads what the deaf person types into the TTY at the other end. Electronic mail may become another useful method for follow-up conversations.

Social services may be a valuable resource to help the deaf patient. Deaf patients may require extra help in obtaining medicines or medical supplies, in understanding their disease and its treatment, and in organizing subsequent appointments and interpreter services.

Visually Impaired

Legal blindness is defined as "visual acuity of 20/200 or worse in the better eye with correction, or a visual field which subtends to an angle of not greater than 20 degrees" (Federal Regulations: PL 94-142, 1975).[45] Studies have found blindness second only to cancer in the degree of dread with which it is regarded by the American public. Partially sighted persons are those whose visual acuity falls between 20/70 and 20/200 in the better eye corrected.[46]

Although there is no one "right" way to interact with the blind or partially sighted patient, following a few basic guidelines can make the interaction a more positive and rewarding experience. The patient should be addressed directly when the physician enters the room, and all actions should be clearly explained before they happen. It is useful to repeat what is happening as a procedure is conducted, including warnings about potential discomfort. The patient's name should be used when requesting a specific response because blind patients do not have the visual cues that a person is speaking directly to them. When a patient must be moved from the examining room to another area of the emergency department, an explanation of why the move is necessary (e.g., to obtain a radiograph) and orientation to the new situation can be helpful. Appropriate communication strategies, such as Braille or large-print educational materials, are helpful. The Optacon (Telesensory Systems) is a device that allows printed material to be optically scanned and translated into a tactile array, enabling the blind to have access to the printed material.[45,46] Most important, active advocacy by the physician is necessary to promote effective communication, assessment, and therapy.

Spinal Cord Injury

The prevalence of spinal cord injury (SCI) continues to be significant (0.9 cases per 1000), accounting for 10,000 new cases per year in the United States.[47,48] Cervical SCI occurs in at least 1.5% to 3% of major trauma victims, the majority of whom are young men between the ages of 15 and 35 years.[49,50] Patients with SCI can present a significant diagnostic challenge. Not only are they predisposed to certain complications from their injury, but also findings of common medical and surgical problems may be masked, resulting in high morbidity and mortality.

Knowledge of the anatomic level of injury is necessary to interpret the patient's complaint and physical examination. A complete lesion eliminates motor function and sensation distal to the injury. In the cervical region, spinal cord roots exit above the similarly numbered vertebrae down to C7. The C8 nerve root exits below the seventh cervical vertebra, and all subsequent nerve roots exit below the identically numbered vertebrae. Because the spinal cord ends at the L1 or L2 interspace, anatomic disruption below this level may cause the cauda equina syndrome. Incomplete lesions include the central cord syndrome, Brown-Séquard syndrome, anterior cord syndrome, posterior cord syndrome, and unclassified neurologic symptoms. These lesions give rise to typical patterns of motor function or sensation loss below the level of cord injury.[51] The complications of SCI may represent the wide range of problems found in physically disabled patients.

Autonomic Dysreflexia

Autonomic dysreflexia (AD) syndrome can occur at any time after spinal shock has subsided in SCI patients.[52] It represents a cluster of symptoms that result in an exaggerated sympathetic response to noxious stimuli. It occurs in more than 80% of patients with cord lesion above T8 and can result in subarachnoid hemorrhage and stroke.[53,54] Recognition of the clinical features is extremely important because, although it is usually managed successfully, failure to do so can have dire consequences, including death. On rare occasions, the condition is also seen in paraplegic patients with lesions below T6, but in this situation the reaction is usually somewhat milder. AD is more common in patients with complete lesions than in those with incomplete lesions, and the reaction seems to be less severe in the latter group.[53]

The pathophysiologic origin of AD is a disrupted feedback system between the sympathetic and parasympathetic branches of the autonomic nervous system. These spinal reflex mechanisms remain intact despite the patient's injury. A noxious stimulus below the level of the lesion produces an afferent impulse that generates a generalized sympathetic response, which in turn results in vasoconstriction below the neurologic lesion.[53] With lesions at or above the T6 level, the splanchnic vascular bed becomes involved, which provides the critical mass of blood vessels required to cause elevation of the blood pressure. The patient with AD may develop severe headache, shortness of breath, nausea, or blurred vision. Bradycardia, sweating piloerection, and flushing above the spinal lesion and pallor below the lesion may also be noted. Sweating and piloerection below the lesions have also been reported. The triad of bitemporal throbbing headache, head and neck sweating, and systolic hypertension is reported in 72% of patients.[55] Atypical presentations of AD include chest pain, urinary retention, increased spasticity without the usual hypertension-induced anxiety, sweating, headache, and bradycardia.[48] Any noxious stimulus occurring below the level of the injury to the spinal cord can trigger an episode of AD. Stimulation of the lower urinary tract accounts for most episodes of AD, and bladder distention appears to be the precipitant in 75% to 85% of cases.[53] The distention can result from a blocked or kinked catheter or insufficient frequency of intermittent catheterization. Urinary tract infection, kidney stones, tight-fitting clothes, gallstones, and appendicitis are other common precipitants.

Initial treatment includes raising the head of the bed and blood pressure monitoring. The patient should be carefully examined to identify the etiology of AD, with specific attention to potential urinary retention or fecal impaction. Gentle and careful rectal examination is necessary, as digital insertion risks stimulation of a spastic anal sphincter that may exacerbate the crisis.[56] If the hypertension persists or symptoms worsen, nifedipine has been recommended. Hydralazine and nitroprusside are alternatives.[54,56] Sustained observation or admission is necessary if the patient requires antihypertensive therapy.

Orthostatic Hypotension

Orthostatic hypotension (OH) is defined as an acute or progressive decline in the mean blood pressure of more than 10 to 15 mm Hg in the erect position.[57] It may arise as light-headedness or loss of consciousness seen during transfers from a lying to sitting or upright position. OH is common in SCI patients, especially those with cervical spine injuries.

Positional hypotension results from venous pooling in the splanchnic bed and lower extremities secondary to deficient vasomotor tone. In addition, quadriplegics have lower resting levels of epinephrine and norepinephrine, and there is no significant increased release of catecholamines when a quadriplegic changes position from lying to sitting. Blood pressure levels can decrease as much as 50% when changing from a lying to upright position in these individuals. Tachycardia may be found as a compensatory mechanism but is usually insufficient.

The treatment of OH is usually nonpharmacologic. If this condition appears as a new finding, an etiology must be sought. Urosepsis and bowel obstruction can masquerade as OH and should be considered. New-onset OH usually responds well to intravenous fluids. In recurrent OH, treatment is directed toward decreasing venous pooling. This can be accomplished by sequential repositioning in a gradual manner from a supine to upright position. This conditioning gradually increases tolerance and may be aided by use of an abdominal binder to decrease visceral and abdominal vasculature. Sympathomimetic and other vasoactive agents such as ephedrine and pseudoephedrine have been used, but some studies have found them ineffective.[58]

Thromboembolic Disease

The incidence of thromboembolism with acute SCI ranges from 4% to 100%, depending on the detection method used.[59] Pulmonary embolism is reported in up to 5% of patients and is a leading cause of death among SCI patients.[49,60] Deep venous thrombosis occurs in 12% to 20% of patients in the first 2 weeks after injury, with an increased frequency in quadriplegics. Most patients have preventive treatment initiated during the first 90 days after injury.[61] Prophylactic therapies include "minidose" heparin, low-molecular-weight heparin, external calf compression with or without aspirin, and range-of-motion exercises.[49]

Unilateral leg swelling may be the only sign of deep venous thrombosis in a patient with SCI. Attenuated sensory input makes a high index of suspicion essential in evaluation of these patients. Unexplained fever, cough, and shortness of breath may be the only clues to PE.[49,62] Leg manipulation, upright posture, and range-of-motion exercises should be avoided as these actions may result in dislodgement and embolization of the thrombus.

Gastrointestinal Problems

Acute Abdomen

Acute abdominal processes reportedly account for 10% of deaths in SCI patients. Peptic ulcers and superior mesenteric artery syndrome are particularly common in SCI patients. Peptic ulcers occur in 5% to 25% of SCI patients, usually within 6 weeks after injury. Long-term administration of anti-inflammatory agents has been associated with more than double the rate of gastric erosion and ulcer.[63] Superior mesenteric artery syndrome is obstruction of the third portion of the duodenum by vascular compression of the superior mesenteric artery against the aorta. It results from loss of areolar tissue around the duodenum in chronic SCI, usually from concomitant weight loss.[64] Distention, abdominal discomfort, postprandial emesis, and weight loss are the usual presenting symptoms. Other etiologies of a surgical abdomen must also be considered in SCI patients with such symptoms.[65,66]

The presentation of an acute abdomen in SCI patients depends on the level of injury and subsequent ability to sense abdominal pain. With cord lesions at or below T12, abdominal visceral sensation is intact. Therefore, abdominal emergencies arise with the same degree of localization and quality of pain as in patients without cord lesions.[51,66] However, patients with spinal cord lesions above T12 have altered symptoms because the sensory nerves of the overlying dermatomes innervate the parietal peritoneum. A poorly localized, dull or heavy sensation is often reported as the earliest symptom of the acute abdomen in these patients. Referred pain has been reported as a "burning" sensation of the skin area of the dermatome supplying the irritated viscera. Pain may be referred because the thoracic sympathetic, splanchnic, hypogastric, or pelvic nerves to the dorsal root ganglion and then to the spinal cord convey visceral sensation.[67]

The early symptoms of intra-abdominal pathology are often subtle: anorexia, unexplained fatigue, and changes in micturition. These may be associated with fever, tachycardia, cardiac dysrhythmias, diaphoresis, and restlessness. In one study of acute appendicitis in SCI patients, 81% of patients had fever, 77% presented with abdominal distention, and 23% had a palpable mass.[65] Interestingly, the mean duration from the onset of symptoms to presentation was 4 days. Abdominal guarding and rigidity do not develop in the patient with a high cord lesion, but spasticity suggests an acute abdomen.

Fecal Impaction

Constipation and fecal impaction are the most common gastrointestinal complications in patients with chronic SCI. Normal bowel function is controlled by the vagus nerve, which supplies parasympathetic innervation to the esophagus, stomach, small intestine, and ascending and transverse colons. The pelvic nerve supplies the descending and rectosigmoid colon. Sympathetic control, which acts to diminish peristalsis and secretion, travels by splanchnic nerves that arise from T4 to L3 and synapse in the celiac and mesenteric ganglia.[51] Fecal impaction results from the interruption of impulses of the pelvic parasympathetic outflow, which leaves the distal transverse and descending colon without organized peristalsis. Autonomic nervous system imbalance and release of the external anal sphincter from central control are responsible for the majority of gastrointestinal complications in the SCI patient.

A sense of fullness, epigastric discomfort, or fever with AD may be the presenting symptoms. High impaction may result in diarrhea from passage of feces and fluid around a partially obstructing mass. In these cases, rectal examination may show little stool in the rectal vault. A plain radiograph is valuable in the diagnosis of this disorder.[68]

Management consists of bowel retraining regimens and stool softeners. This may include rectal stimulation, stimulant laxative stool suppositories, stool softeners, disposable enema (i.e., Fleet), and a low-bulk diet. A high enema may be necessary to manage an acute impaction. Digital disimpaction may be necessary, but the potential for stimulating an autonomic dysfunction response must be anticipated.

Respiratory Problems

Pneumonia

Long-term respiratory complications are a major source of morbidity and mortality in SCI patients. Pneumonia remains the major cause of death.[48,49] Pneumonia is relatively uncommon in the first year after injury, but its frequency increases over time. Pneumonia in patients with SCI is associated with a reduction in high volume and expiratory force resulting in chronic hypoventilation, mild hypercarbia, and ineffective cough, predisposing the individual to aspiration, atelectasis, and pneumonia. The impairment of abdominal, intercostal, and diaphragmatic muscles associated with progressively higher lesions in the spinal cord results in a higher incidence of aspiration and pneumonia among quadriplegics.[68,69]

Reflex Airway Closure

Reflex airway closure is a near-asphyxiation event that occurs in response to aspiration of inert substances such as water, saline, barium, nasogastric feeding solutions, or gastric contents with pH above 3.0. These substances cause acute bronchospasm from an intrinsic pulmonary reflex reaction.[51] The patient usually presents with acute dyspnea immediately after the episode of aspiration. Occasionally, the patient is in no distress but complains of aspirating a liquid. The chest radiograph is usually without infiltrate. Residual pulmonary infiltrate suggests a previous chemical pneumonitis or foreign body aspiration.

If the patient is in distress, tracheal suctioning and intubation may be necessary. Otherwise, an aerosolized β_2 agonist, such as albuterol, may be administered to a stable patient. If the patient clears, observation for 6 hours is suggested to monitor the stability of respiratory status. Discharge instructions should outline the risks of recurrent aspiration and require the patient to return for respiratory distress.

Acute Tracheostomy Obstruction

Elective removal of the tracheostomy tube usually results in spontaneous closure of the stoma in 2 to 5 days.[51] However, the tracheostomy may be kept open with a prosthetic "tracheostomy button" to maintain long-term access to the airway. This is most desirable in high quadriplegics with poor respiratory reserve who are in danger of acute respiratory decompensation. If respiratory distress occurs with a functioning tracheostomy, suctioning should be performed to remove any plugging. If this is unsuccessful, the tracheostomy tube should be replaced under oxygen supplementation.

Decubitus Ulcer and Infection

Pressure ulcers develop in 15% of SCI patients after the first year.[48] The pathophysiology of these ulcers is primarily unrelieved pressure and compression of the subcutaneous tissue against bone prominences. The most common sites of occurrence are the ischium, trochanter, sacrum, and heel. Poor nutritional status predisposes an SCI patient to the development of ulcers. The development sequence of decubitus ulcer consists of hyperemia followed by ischemia and necrosis. Necrosis extends over time and ultimately ulcerates through the skin. A small skin defect may be found to tract extensively under the skin. Up to 88% of patients with decubitus ulcers may have concomitant infections. Common causative organisms are *Enterobacter*, *Pseudomonas* spp, and *Streptococcus faecalis*.[68,70]

When superficial hyperemia is recognized as impending ischemia, adequate pressure relief can prevent decubitus ulcers. Effective padding and repositioning every 2 hours are effective treatment. The treatment of ulcers is dependent on their depth. Shallow ulcers can be managed with debridement of necrotic tissue until bleeding tissue is encountered. Debridement of necrotic tissue, followed by packing, is essential. Clean ulcers can be loosely packed with saline wet-to-dry dressings. Moderately contaminated ulcers should be dressed with silver sulfadiazine cream. Systemic antibiotics are not helpful unless there is cellulitis, osteomyelitis, or sepsis. Deep decubitus ulcers extend to superficial muscle of deep connective tissue. Ulcers that penetrate to the bone or muscle should be seen by a plastic surgeon for debridement and surgical correction by either a myocutaneous flap or skin graft.

Urinary Tract Problems

Progressive Renal Dysfunction

Life expectancies for these patients remain substantially below normal. SCI mortality rates are up to 21 times higher than corresponding rates for persons without spinal injuries.[71] Urinary tract morbidity is the second leading cause of death in the SCI patient.[71] SCI produces profound alterations in lower urinary tract function. Incontinence, elevated intravesical pressure, reflux, stones, and neurologic obstruction, commonly found in the spinal cord–injured population, increase the risk of urinary infection. Abnormal renal function tests are found in only 11% of SCI patients after 5 years, but the rate increases to 26% at 20 years. The percentage of abnormal tests is lower in patients treated with intermittent catheterization than in those who have a suprapubic catheter placed.[48]

Neurogenic Bladder

Micturition is normally initiated by conscious relaxation of the external sphincter, which is the only structure in the urinary tract under volitional control. This relaxation leads to a decrease in sympathetic tone causing relaxation of the internal sphincter and detrusor disinhibition. Decreased sympathetic tone, in turn, leads to increased parasympathetic tone, causing detrusor contraction and thus expulsion of urine. Maintenance of low intravesicular storage pressure is critical for urinary tract function. Intravesicular storage pressures higher than 35 to 40 cm H_2O are likely to cause renal deterioration.[72,73] Vesicoureteric reflux is caused by either abnormally high pressure within the bladder or a structural abnormality in the ureterovesical junction or bladder wall.

Most individuals with lesions between C1 and L1 have reflex dyssynergistic bladder-increased detrusor tone, with lack of coordination between the detrusor and sphincter muscles. The sphincters do not relax during detrusor contraction, which leads to high intravesical pressure and reflux.[74] The consequences of ureteral obstruction include hydronephrosis, pyelonephrosis, and renal stones.

Neurogenic bladder management usually consists of reflex emptying, clean intermittent catheterization, or placement of an indwelling catheter or external collecting device (condom catheter), in addition to the use of cholinergic and anticholinergic agents. Other procedures that may be undertaken to enhance bladder function include sphincterotomy to decrease intravesical pressure and ensure emptying, suprapubic catheter placement, urinary diversion procedures, and placement of an artificial urinary sphincter.

Urinary Retention

Urinary retention in SCI patients is most often due to obstruction, either mechanical or pharmacologic. Mechanical causes include stones, clots, sediment, and displacement of the catheter.[51] Pharmacologic urinary retention is usually the result of a single anticholinergic agent or the additive effects of multiple agents such as oxybiotin, tricyclic antidepressants, and over-the-counter cold preparations. The patient with urinary retention should be assessed for any associated anticholinergic symptoms.

If a catheter is present, the balloon is deflated and removed. If no catheter is present, gentle insertion of either a straight or Foley catheter should be attempted. On insertion, a "give" of the catheter as it passes through the bladder neck is the usual finding in sphincter spasm. If a catheter cannot be passed, suprapubic aspiration of bladder contents may be necessary along with urologic consultation. Treatment of pharmacologic retention requires discontinuation of the medication. Bladder irrigation with sterile normal saline may also decrease the likelihood of recurrent urinary obstruction but is usually reserved for hospitalized patients.

Urinary Tract Infection

The significance of pyuria in patients with SCI and indwelling or intermittent catheters is often problematic. Complete bladder emptying is considered to be the most effective barrier to urinary tract infection (UTI). In patients with neurogenic bladders, high residual urine volumes favor bacterial growth and inhibit the antibacterial activity of the bladder mucosa. Consequences of UTI are structural damage and dysfunction of the urinary tract. In addition, UTIs are responsible for most bacteremic episodes in the SCI population.[71,73]

With the development of a neurogenic bladder, the classic symptoms of UTI are not observed. Presenting symptoms include increased spasticity, dysreflexia, cloudy or odoriferous urine, and a change in residual volumes. Findings of fever or chills suggest sepsis or tissue invasion. Patients who void on their own, or who are intermittently straight catheterized, should have sterile urine. The line between bacterial colonization and infection is often difficult to determine in the neurologically impaired patient. Marked pyuria appears to be correlated with the presence of catheters, infection with gram-negative organisms, and bacterial tissue invasion. Infectious bacteruria can be distinguished from colonization on the basis of significant pyuria (>50 leukocytes per high-power field) or detection of combined leukocyte esterase and nitrite positivity on dipstick urinalysis.[71,74] Urine culture and sensitivities are indicated for all patients who undergo treatment, but the decision to treat should be based on the patient's symptoms. Common pathogens in SCI patients include *Escherichia coli*, coagulase negative *Streptococcus*, *Klebsiella pneumoniae*, and *Pseudomonas aeruginosa*. Initial treatment should consist of ciprofloxacin or norfloxacin for 7 to 10 days, with adjustments made on the basis of urine cultures and sensitivity.[71,75] Symptomatic patients with indwelling catheters can be treated as outpatients with ciprofloxacin or norfloxacin. If sepsis is suspected or cannot be ruled out, the patient requires hospitalization.

Neurologic Problems

Posttraumatic Syrinx

Posttraumatic syrinx (cystic myelopathy) is defined as any fluid-filled cystic cavity in the spinal cord, other than enlargement of the central canal, occurring after trauma to the spinal cord. The cystic cavity does not communicate with the fourth ventricle, central canal, or subarachnoid space. The annual incidence is approximately 3% of all SCI patients and is more common in quadriplegics. It may occur up to 30 years after the original injury. Posttraumatic syrinx begins at the original site of cord injury and extends cephalad in 80% and caudad in 20% of patients. Extension is predominantly in larger cysts, which can range up to 35 cm long. The etiology of cystic myelopathy is unknown. One theory is that cavitation in the cord develops after hematomyelia or necrosis of a myelomalacic core that results from the original injury.[51,76]

Syrinx development is suggested by new onset of pain, numbness, sensory change, or weakness that may be exacerbated by laughing, coughing, sneezing, or straining. The pain can be dull, aching, and constant in the neck or behind the ear and at the same time burning and intermittent in the upper limbs. It is generally located at or above the site of the original spinal injury but may be referred to the abdomen or lower extremity. The diagnosis is made by magnetic resonance imaging (MRI) of the spinal cord. The treatment is neurosurgical removal of the syrinx fluid with instillation of a shunt to prevent its reaccumulation.

Orthopedic Problems

Long bone fractures of the lower extremities occur in SCI patients, with an annual incidence from 0.3% to 2.5%. As SCI patients age, they experience an increased fracture rate, which may be the result of years of immobility-related bone loss. In any case of extremity swelling in an SCI patient, fracture should be considered in the differential diagnosis. Signs and symptoms may be minimal, even if the femur is involved.

Multiple Sclerosis

Multiple sclerosis (MS) is an autoimmune disease of the CNS that reportedly affects 350,000 persons in the United States with an annual incidence of about 12,000.[77] MS typically arises between the ages of 18 and 45. MS occurs more commonly in individuals of western European ancestry and is uncommon in certain ethnic and racial groups, such as Eskimos, Native American Indians, and Africans.[2] Susceptibility is also associated with particular genetic factors, such as human leukocyte antigen HLA-DR2.[77,78]

The histopathologic lesion in MS is the plaque, which is a localized area of demyelination in the white matter tracts of the CNS. Myelin destruction is probably mediated by the combined actions of infiltrating T lymphocytes and macrophages. The inflammatory cells may also be the source of cytokines that lead to oligodendral death and axonal degeneration. These white matter plaques, visible by MRI, have a predilection for the periventricular areas of the cerebrum, brainstem, spinal cord, and optic nerves. The initial trigger for the disease process has yet to be identified but may be quite diverse. One hypothesis has considered the role of immune dysregulation in the development of an autoimmune response against CNS myelin antigens.[77,79] Mechanistically, this may involve an infectious trigger (e.g., virus, bacteria) that generates antigen exposure followed by an initially appropriate neutralizing immune response.[77,78]

MS can be classified into a variety of subtypes. Most patients initially present with neurologic attacks followed by remissions. This type of MS is referred to as relapsing-remitting (RR) MS and affects 85% of patients. Primary progressive MS occurs in about 10% of the MS population and involves a steady, almost imperceptible myelopathy from the onset not associated with relapses. In this form of the disease there is a much lower level of inflammatory markers and an equal distribution in men and women. The secondary progressive (SP) subtype of MS is characterized by a steady, insidious progressive deterioration of neurologic function, with or without ongoing relapses. SP MS most commonly produces disability with myelopathy, including a decline in ambulation, spasticity, and bladder and bowel dysfunction.[77-79]

The spectrum of clinical signs and symptoms of MS is very diverse. The initial symptom of MS is often blurred or double vision, red-green color distortion, or even blindness in one eye. Optic neuritis is one of the most common findings. It occurs in up to 64% of MS patients at some time during their illness.[80] Patients typically complain of loss of central vision with pain on movement of the globe. Visual loss is usually unilateral, and other causes must be considered. Management of intraocular disease should include an ophthalmology consultation. No treatment has proved effective in optic neuritis, including steroids.

Vertigo, vomiting, and nystagmus are present in 30% of patients and are due to lesions near the vestibular complex. Diplopia may stem from involvement of the third, fourth, or sixth cranial nerve or internuclear ophthalmoplegia. This lesion involves the medial longitudinal fasciculus running between the sixth and third nerve nucleus. Although common in MS, internuclear ophthalmoplegia can be seen in vascular disease, brainstem tumors, or Wernicke's encephalopathy. Lesions in the cerebellum produce ataxia, intention tremor, or affect fine movements of hands, feet, or speech.[79] Approximately half of all persons with MS experience cognitive impairments such as difficulties with concentration, attention, memory, and judgment, but such symptoms are usually mild and are frequently overlooked.[77]

Abnormalities of the spinal cord may produce dysautonomias involving the vesicourethral and gastrointestinal tracts and sexual function. Bladder dysfunction is common and occurs in association with motor dysfunction of the lower extremities. Morbidity and mortality in more than half of patients with MS are secondary to hydronephrosis, pyelonephrosis, and septicemia from urologic dysfunction. Severe constipation and sexual dysfunction are present in patients with advanced MS. Fever, acute illness, and stress may acutely worsen symptoms in MS patients. Evaluation of the underlying cause of fever or illness is warranted. As the acute illness is treated, resolution of the underlying symptoms should occur.

To diagnose MS, the patient must have either two or more discrete episodes at least 1 month apart or a slow or stepwise progression of symptoms over at least 6 months.[80] In addition, the patient should be between 10 and 50 years at onset with evidence of two or more lesions of the CNS demonstrated by clinical examination or MRI findings that should predominantly involve the white matter. Finally, CSF abnormalities (the presence of oligoclonal immunoglobulin G [IgG] bands, elevated IgG synthesis rate, and elevated IgG index) should be present. MRI scanning is abnormal in 85% to 95% of patients. Multiple discrete lesions are noted in the supratentorial white matter, especially the paraventricular area. With gadolinium enhancement, MRI distinguishes active from inactive lesions. CT scanning is useful to exclude structural lesions of the CNS.[79,80]

Magnetic resonance spectroscopy (MRS) is a new tool being used to investigate MS. Unlike MRI, which provides an anatomic picture of lesions, MRS yields information about the biochemistry of the brain in MS. Evoked potential tests, which measure the speed of the brain's response to visual, auditory, and sensory stimuli, can sometimes detect lesions the scanners miss. Like imaging technologies, evoked potentials are helpful but not conclusive because they cannot identify the cause of lesions.[79]

Some patients may experience atypical symptoms. Spasticity and tonic muscle spasms are due to spinal cord lesions. Spasticity may be relieved by physical therapy or diazepam use. Painful spasms may respond to anticonvulsants such as phenytoin or carbamazepine. Patients confined to wheelchairs are at high risk for carpal tunnel syndrome, sciatic neuropathy, or peripheral neuropathy.

The differential diagnosis of MS includes virtually any disease of the CNS that may cause focal deficits. These include stroke or transient ischemic attack, migraine headache, brain or spinal tumor, subdural hematoma, spinal degenerative disease, transverse myelitis, systemic lupus erythematosus and other vasculitides, Lyme disease, syphilis, human immunodeficiency virus infection, and adrenomyeloleukodystrophy.

MS is a chronic disease characterized by periods of relapses and remission. The development of new symptoms does not change the prognosis or treatment. However, the emergency physician should not assume that each new neurologic symptom is due to MS. Careful history and examination of each symptom must be undertaken to avoid misdiagnosis.

No treatment for MS has been found to be truly effective. Agents used in treatment have included corticosteroids, azathioprine, cyclophosphamide, cyclosporine, and interferon. Although corticosteroids have been the mainstay in treatment of MS, studies suggest they are not effective, and the effectiveness of high-dose parenteral methylprednisolone appears to be marginal.[81-83] However, interferon β1a and 1b, glatiramer acetate, and intravenous immunoglobulin have been shown to decrease the rate of relapse.

KEY CONCEPTS

- Understanding the specific medical disorders that are associated with each type of disability can facilitate the care of disabled patients.
- Complications in disabled patients may be associated with high-technology equipment (e.g., gastrostomy tubes, CSF shunts, tracheostomies, Foley catheters).
- The care of a patient with mental retardation can be enhanced by focusing on recent changes in the patient's behavior as explained by the caregiver; by observing nonverbal communications such as facial expression, gesturing, and posture; by erring on the side of performing ancillary tests or observing the patient in unclear cases; and by adequately premedicating the patient for necessary procedures.
- Patients with chronic spinal cord injury experience several unique problems including autonomic dysreflexia, orthostatic hypotension, superior mesenteric artery syndrome, and posttraumatic syrinx. An understanding of the presentation and treatment of these disorders improves the care these patients receive in the emergency department. The signs and symptoms of intra-abdominal catastrophes and orthopedic fractures can be subtle in patients with chronic SCI.
- The new onset of seizures in patients with developmental disabilities and new neurologic symptoms in patients with multiple sclerosis require evaluation and should not be simply ascribed to the underlying disease.

REFERENCES

1. Patel DR, Greydanus D: The pediatric athlete with disabilities. *Pediatr Clin North Am* 49:803, 2002.
2. Messinger-Rapport BJ, Rapport DJ: Primary care for the developmentally disabled adult. *J Gen Intern Med* 12:629, 1997.
3. AARP Disability Initiative: *Facts about Children with Developmental Disabilities and Their Families*. Washington, DC, American Association of Retired Persons, 1994.
4. Griswold KS, Goldstein MZ: Issues affecting the lives of older persons with developmental disabilities. *Psychiatr Serv* 50:315, 1999.
5. Murphy CC, et al: Epidemiology of mental retardation in children. *Ment Retard Dev Disabil Res Rev* 4:6, 1998.
6. Minihan P, et al: Managing the care of patients with mental retardation: A survey of physicians. *Ment Retard* 30:239, 1993.
7. Tyler C, Bourguet C: Primary care of adults with mental retardation. *J Fam Pract* 44:487, 1997.
8. Counsellman DL: Caring for adults with mental disabilities. Problems tend to be complex among this growing population. *Postgrad Med* 106:181, 1999.
9. Coulter DL: Epilepsy and mental retardation: An overview. *Am J Ment Retard* 98:1, 1993.
10. Sunder TR: Meeting the challenge of epilepsy in persons with multiple handicaps. *J Child Neurol* 12(Suppl 1): S38,1997.
11. Harbond MG: Significant anticonvulsant side effects in children and adolescents. *J Clin Neurosci* 7:210, 2000.
12. Sillanpaa M: Long term prognosis in seizures with onset in childhood. *N Engl J Med* 338:1916,1998.
13. Scherrman J, et al: Vagus nerve stimulation: Clinical experience in a large patient series. *J Clin Neurophysiol* 18:408, 2001.
14. Bondurant CP, Jimenez DF: Epidemiology of cerebrospinal fluid shunting. *Pediatr Neurosurg* 23:254, 1995.
15. Madsen MA: Emergency department management of ventriculoperitoneal cerebrospinal fluid shunts. *Ann Emerg Med* 15:1330, 1986.
16. Guertin SR: Cerebrospinal fluid shunts: Evaluation, complications, and crisis management. *Pediatr Clin North Am* 34:203, 1987.
17. Schwatrz G, Seamens C: Medical hardware inside software: CSF shunts and indwelling devices in children. *Pediatr Emerg Med Rep* 2:39, 1997.
18. Watkins L, et al: The diagnosis of blocked cerebrospinal fluid shunts: A prospective study of referral to a paediatric neurosurgical unit. *Childs Nerv Syst* 10:87, 1994.
19. Teoh D: Pediatric surgical emergencies. Tricks of the trade: Assessment of high tech gear in special needs children. *Clin Pediatr Emerg Med* 3:62, 2002.
20. Walker ML, et al: Diagnosis and treatment of the slit ventricle syndrome. *Neurosurg Clin North Am* 4:707, 1993.
21. Green L, et al: Primary care of children with cerebral palsy. *Clin Fam Med* 5:467, 2003.
22. Samuels L: Gastrostomy, gastroenterostomy, duodenostomy, and jejunostomy tubes. In Roberts J, Hedges J (eds): *Clinical Procedures in Emergency Medicine*, 3rd ed. Philadelphia, WB Saunders, 1998, pp 704-710.
23. Down Syndrome Medical Interest Group (DSMIG), Cohen WI: Healthcare guidelines for individuals with Down syndrome. *Downs Syndr Q* 1:1, 1996.
24. Martin BA: Primary care of adults with mental retardation living in the community. *Am Fam Physician* 56:485, 1997.
25. Peabody TD, Stasikelis PJ: Fractures in adults at an institution for the developmentally disabled. *Clin Orthop* 366:217, 1999.
26. Bohmer CJM, et al: The prevalence of gastroesophageal reflux disease in institutionalized disabled individuals. *Am J Gastroenterol* 94:804, 1999.
27. Bohmer CJ, et al: Gastroesophageal reflux disease in intellectually disabled individuals: How often, how serious, how manageable? *Am J Gastroenterol* 95:1868, 2000.
28. Vellinga A, et al: Hepatitis B and C in institutions for individuals with mental disability. *J Intellect Disabil Res* 43:445, 1999.
29. Nespoli L, et al: Immunologic features of Down's syndrome: A review. *J Intellect Disabil Res* 37:543, 1993.
30. Strum PF, et al: Femur fractures in institutionalized patients after hip spica immobilization. *J Pediatr Orthop* 13:246, 1993.
31. Cumella S, et al: Needs for oral care among people with intellectual disability not in contact with dental services. *J Intellect Disabil Res* 44:45, 2000.
32. Pschirrer ER, Yeomans ER: Does asphyxia cause cerebral palsy? *Semin Perinatol* 3:215, 2000.
33. Murphy KP: Medical problems in adults with cerebral palsy: Case examples. *Assist Technol* 11:97, 1999.
34. Gertzen PC, et al: Intrathecal baclofen infusion and subsequent orthopedic surgery in patients with spastic cerebral palsy. *J Neurosurg* 88:1009, 1998.
35. Wright FV, et al: Evaluation of selective dorsal rhizotomy for the reduction of spasticity in cerebral palsy: A randomized controlled trial. *Dev Med Child Neurol* 40:239, 1998.
36. Graham HK: Botulinum toxin A in cerebral palsy: Functional outcomes. *J Pediatr* 137:300, 2000.
37. Ralston E, et al: Physician's attitudes and beliefs about deaf patients. *J Am Board Fam Pract* 9:167, 1996.

38. Sneed S, Joss D: Deafness and hearing loss—A global health problem. *Work* 12:93, 1999.
39. Kurz RS, et al: The effects of hearing impairment on health services utilization. *Med Care* 29:878, 1991.
40. Steinberg A, et al: Deaf women: Experiences and perceptions of healthcare system access. *J Womens Health* 11:729, 2002.
41. Zazove P, et al: The health status and health care utilization of deaf and hard-of-hearing persons. *Arch Fam Med* 2:745, 1993.
42. Ebert D, Heckerling P: Communication with deaf patients. Knowledge, beliefs and practices of physicians. *JAMA* 273:227, 1995.
43. Jackson J: Health care providers' responsibilities toward hearing-impaired patients. *NJ Med* 100:22, 2003.
44. Lotke M: She won't look at me. *Ann Intern Med* 123:54, 1995.
45. Moller MA: Working with visually impaired children and their families. *Pediatr Clin North Am* 40:881, 1993.
46. Thompson L, Kaufman L: The visually impaired child. *Pediatr Clin North Am* 50:225, 2003.
47. Alexander JT, Haid RW: Upper cervical trauma outcome assessment. *Clin Neurosurg* 44:305, 1997.
48. McKinley WO, et al: Long term medical complications after traumatic spinal cord injury: A regional model systems analysis. *Arch Phys Med Rehabil* 80:1402, 1999.
49. Urdaneta F, Layon AJ: Respiratory complications in patients with traumatic cervical spine injuries: Case report and review of the literature. *J Clin Anesth* 15:398, 2003.
50. Chui WC, et al: Ligamentous injuries of the cervical spine in unreliable blunt trauma patients: Incidence, evaluation and outcome. *J Trauma* 50:457, 2001.
51. Herr R, Speed J: The patient with spinal cord injury. In Herr R, Cydulka R (eds): *Emergency Care of the Compromised Patient.* Philadelphia, JB Lippincott, 1994, pp 43-65.
52. Keely BR: Recognition and treatment of autonomic dysreflexia. *Crit Care Nurs* 17:170, 1998.
53. Blackmer J: Rehabilitation medicine 1. Autonomic dysreflexia. *CMAJ* 169:931, 2003.
54. Karlsson AK: Autonomic dysreflexia. *Spinal Cord* 37:383, 1991.
55. Kewalramani LS: Autonomic dysreflexia in traumatic myelopathy. *Am J Phys Med* 59:1, 1980.
56. McGuire TJ, Kumar VN: Autonomic dysreflexia in the spinal cord injured. What the physician should know about this medical emergency. *Postgrad Med* 80:81, 1986.
57. Blackmer J: Orthostatic hypotension in spinal cord injured patients. *J Spinal Cord Med* 20:212, 1997.
58. Schwartz JJ: Orthostatic hypotension II. Clinical diagnosis, testing and treatment. *Arch Intern Med* 144:1037, 1984.
59. Waring WP, Karonas RS: Acute spinal cord injuries and the incidence of clinically occurring thromboembolic disease. *Paraplegia* 29:8, 1991.
60. Merli G, et al: Etiology, incidence and prevention of deep venous thrombosis in acute spinal cord injury. *Arch Phys Med Rehabil* 74:199, 1993.
61. Sommer RM, et al: Clinical physiologic considerations and anesthetic management of patients with spinal cord injury. In Errico TJ, Bauer BA, Waugh T (eds): *Spinal Trauma.* Philadelphia, JB Lippincott, 1991, pp 435-453.
62. Powell M, et al: Duplex ultrasound screening for deep vein thrombosis in spinal cord injured patients at rehabilitation admission. *Arch Phys Med Rehabil* 80:1044, 1999.
63. Tunaka M, Uchiyami M, Itano H: Gastroduodenal disease in chronic spinal cord injuries. *Arch Surg* 114:185, 1979.
64. Ramos M: Recurrent superior mesenteric artery syndrome in a quadriplegic patient. *Arch Phys Med Rehabil* 56:86, 1975.
65. Strauther GR, et al: Appendicitis in patients with previous spinal cord injury. *Am J Surg* 178:403, 1999.
66. Neumoyer LA, et al: The acutely affected abdomen in paraplegic spinal cord injury patient. *Ann Surg* 21:561, 1990.
67. Juler GL, Eltarai IM: The acute abdomen in spinal cord injury patients. *Paraplegia* 23:118, 1985.
68. Viroslav J, Rosenblatt R, Tomazevic S: Respiratory management, survival and quality of life for high level traumatic tetraplegias. *Respir Care Clin North Am* 2:313, 1996.
69. Montgomerie JZ: Infections in patients with spinal cord injuries. *Clin Infect Dis* 25:1285, 1997.
70. Sugarman B, Brown D, Musher D: Fever and infection in spinal cord patients. *JAMA* 278:66, 1982.
71. Siroky M: Pathogenesis of bacteriuria and infection in the spinal cord injured patient. *Am J Med* 113(Suppl 1A):67S, 2002.
72. Lightner DJ: Contemporary urologic management of patients with spinal cord injury. *Mayo Clin Proc* 73:434, 1998.
73. Madersbacher HG: Neurologic bladder dysfunction. *Curr Opin Urol* 9:303, 1999.
74. Liptak GS, et al: Screening for urinary tract infection in children with neurogenic bladders. *Am J Phys Med Rehabil* 72:122, 1993.
75. Pedersen SS, et al: Peroral treatment with ciprofloxacin of patient with spinal cord lesion and bacteriuria caused by multiple resistant bacteria. *Paraplegia* 28:41, 1990.
76. Rossier AB, et al: Posttraumatic cervical syringomyelia. *Brain* 108:439, 1985.
77. Frohman EM: Multiple sclerosis. *Med Clin North Am* 87:867, 2003.
78. O'Connor P: Key issues in the diagnosis and treatment of multiple sclerosis. *Neurology* 59(6 Suppl 3):S1, 2002.
79. Pellagrino T: The patient with multiple sclerosis. In Herr R, Cydulka R (eds): *Emergency Care of the Compromised Patient.* Philadelphia, JB Lippincott, 1994, pp 91-99.
80. Rodriguez M: Multiple sclerosis: Basic concepts and hypothesis. *Mayo Clin Proc* 64:570, 1989.
81. Sharrack B, et al: The effect of oral and intravenous methylprednisolone treatment on subsequent relapse rate in multiple sclerosis. *J Neurol Sci* 173:73, 2000.
82. Goodin DS: The use of immunosuppressive agents in the treatment of multiple sclerosis: A critical review. *Neurology* 41:980, 1991.
83. Palace J: New and old treatments for multiple sclerosis. *Neurologia* 13:162, 1998.

CHAPTER 187

Pain Management

Paul M. Paris and Donald M. Yealy

PERSPECTIVE

The relief of acute pain is key in the modern practice of emergency medicine.[1] Why should pain relief assume such an importance to this specialty?

1. Pain is the most common complaint of emergency department patients, seen in one half to three quarters of all patients.[2,3]
2. One essential mission of all health care providers is the relief or prevention of suffering, and we have the tools readily available for this mission.
3. Patients judge physicians by how they treat pain. Satisfaction with emergency care often depends on the techniques and timeliness of analgesia as well as the discharge plans for pain relief.[4]
4. Many of the diagnostic and therapeutic procedures in the practice of emergency medicine cause pain if appropriate analgesia is not used. Pain during subsequent procedures may actually be increased if successful analgesia was not provided during previous procedures.[5]
5. Unrelieved pain is associated with a long list of potential negative physiologic outcomes, including, but not limited to,
   a. increased sympathetic outflow,
   b. increased peripheral vascular resistance,
   c. increased myocardial oxygen consumption,
   d. increased production of carbon dioxide,
   e. hypercoagulability,
   f. decreased gastric motility, and
   g. decreased immune function.
6. The Joint Commission on Accreditation of Healthcare Organizations (JCAHO) now requires hospitals to develop comprehensive programs for the measurement, treatment, documentation, and institution of quality improvement efforts related to acute pain management.[6]
7. Poorly treated acute pain can aid in the development of chronic pain syndromes.

Methods must be not only effective but also safe. Physicians often believe they practice safe analgesia because side effects seldom develop. In reality, physicians often prescribe a suboptimal drug in an inadequate dose at an excessive interval or via an inappropriate route.

Pain relief is best addressed with a plan that incorporates administration, nurses, and clinicians. Triage algorithms should consider pain as a medical emergency. The degree of pain and the overall acuity should determine the rapidity of care. Pain scales should be used, with frequent charting of the patient's subjective report of degree of pain in a fashion analogous to the recording of vital signs.

We provide an overview of the principles and practice of providing analgesia in emergency medicine. The definitions of important terms relating to analgesic practices are listed in Box 187-1.

ACUTE VERSUS CHRONIC PAIN

Acute pain is a symptom of noxious or tissue-damaging stimulation produced by a tissue injury or illness (Box 187-2). Acute pain usually is caused by an identifiable pathologic condition and serves the useful function of warning the individual that a potentially threatening illness or injury exists, thus motivating the patient to seek medical assistance. Acute pain also may force the patient to limit certain activities that could potentially exacerbate the underlying pathophysiology. Chronic pain is a complex disease that lasts for months to years and serves no useful function to the patient. It commonly has no readily identifiable or treatable cause. Patients with chronic pain commonly seek aid in the emergency department, presenting challenges to emergency physicians because there is no quick fix for their problems. They often have a multitude of problems that may include sleep and appetite disturbances, irritability, and somatic preoccupations. It is common for chronic pain patients to arouse animosity in the emergency department staff because of their demands and limited provider ability to "fix" things.

Although acute pain often last days to weeks, and chronic pain for more than 3 months, this distinction does not define the emergency department approach to these two syndromes. For example, pain from bony metastases, while often long in duration, is best categorized as persistent acute pain (because of the underlying tissue distortion). Similarly, sickle-cell vaso-occlusive events are frequent but best considered recurrent or persistent acute pain syndromes rather than chronic. Another approach to categorization is to distinguish malignant "chronic" (applied solely because of duration) pain from other forms of chronic pain. Irrespective of the specific classification scheme used, acute pain (including malignant) therapy requires analgesia and removal of the cause (if possible), whereas chronic nonmalignant pain therapy seeks adaptation, return to functioning, and psychosocial improvements primarily.

Patients with chronic pain syndromes visiting the emergency department can be classified into four categories (Box 187-3). Therapy for groups 2 and 3 should

BOX 187-1. Definitions of Terms Related to Analgesia

Analgesia—relief from pain
Anesthesia—a state with five conditions as follows:
1. Analgesia
2. Amnesia
3. Unconsciousness
4. Muscle relaxation
5. Physiologic stability

Local anesthesia—creating an area of insensibility to pain by the injection of a local anesthetic agent
Hypnotic—an agent that promotes the onset of sleep
Induction agent—a drug that promotes the quick, short-lived onset of unconsciousness, allowing endotracheal intubation to be performed (there should be unresponsiveness to command and loss of the ciliary reflex)
Nociceptor—a receptor that is sensitive and responsible for transmitting a noxious stimulus
Noxious stimulus—a stimulus that is damaging or potentially damaging and results in sensation of pain
Pain—an unpleasant sensory and emotional experience arising from actual or potential tissue damage or described in terms of such damage
Sedative—an agent that decreases activity, moderates excitability, and calms the patient
Conscious sedation—pharmacologically producing a state of profound sedation while maintaining all protective reflexes
Dissociative sedation—a chemically produced (e.g., ketamine) unique state with the following features:
1. Analgesia
2. Amnesia
3. Cooperation
4. Maintenance of all protective reflexes

Unconscious sedation—sedation associated with loss of protective reflexes
Rapid tranquilization—chemically sedating severely agitated or violent patients

BOX 187-2. Acute Versus Chronic Pain

Acute Pain	Chronic Pain
Is a symptom of injury or illness	Is the problem
Serves a biologic purpose	Has no biologic function
Causes anxiety	Causes depression
Is associated with identifiable pathology	May or may not be associated with identifiable pathology
Is present for less than 6 months	Is present for more than 6 months

Adapted from Stewart CE, MacMurdo D: Chronic pain. In Paris PM, Stewart RD (eds): *Pain Management in Emergency Medicine.* Norwalk, Conn, Appleton & Lange, 1988.

involve referral to a multidisciplinary pain evaluation and treatment center where a team of professionals can attempt to treat the multiple manifestations of these diseases. Patients with a significant change in the pattern of their chronic pain caused by cancer or a terminal illness should be evaluated for a new process to

BOX 187-3. Categories of Chronic Pain Patients

1. Patients with chronic pain caused by cancer or a terminal illness (e.g., acquired immunodeficiency syndrome)
2. Patients with well-known syndromes (e.g., tic douloureux)
3. Patients with no objectively confirmed cause for the complaints
4. Patients who are frankly malingering or feigning pain

account for the pain. Opioids should be used liberally to bring pain relief in patients with terminal illnesses.[7] The remainder of this chapter focuses on the treatment of acute pain.

PATHOPHYSIOLOGY OF ACUTE PAIN

Pain Conduction Pathways

The pain experience can be divided into four separate processes, namely receptor activation, information transmission, signal modulation, and perception.

Receptor Activation

The somatosensory system is responsible for sensation of pain as well as tactile, proprioceptive, and thermal sensations. Receptors responsible for transmitting information related to noxious stimuli are called *nociceptors*. These receptors are free nerve endings and are widespread throughout the skin and deeper tissues. They are capable of converting mechanical, thermal, or chemical stimulation into electrical activity. Strong mechanical pressure may result in a release of a variety of chemicals (potassium, prostaglandin, cyclic adenosine monophosphate, leukotrienes, bradykinins, serotonin, substance P, thromboxanes, platelet-activating factor) that sensitize receptors or actually result in conduction of nociceptive stimuli. Nociceptors in the viscera respond to different stimuli than those in the skin and soft tissues. Receptors are individually connected to a specific nerve fiber.

Information Transmission

Peripheral Nerve Fibers

All sensory neurons are composed of a cell body, which is located in the dorsal root ganglia, and a receptor located within a given dermatome. A variety of classification systems have been described to catalog nerve fibers, but the relatively simple system in Table 187-1 allows a basic understanding of the roles of different fibers.

Dorsal Horn

The dorsal horn is the gray matter in the posterior aspect of the spinal cord (Figure 187-1). It is the anatomic area of the spinal cord where pain integration, modification, and relay occur. The dorsal horn is structured in six layers called *laminae*. Each lamina receives specific types of nerve fibers, and the various laminae are connected by multiple interneurons. *Sub*

Table 187-1. Peripheral Nerve Fibers

Fiber	Sensation	Dorsal Horn Termination	Ascending Tract	Conduction Rate (M/sec)	Mean Diameter (µmol/L)	Myelin
A-α	Light touch	Deep	Ipsilateral dorsal column	100	15	Heavy
A-β				50	8	
A-δ	Sharp pricking	Superficial	Contralateral spinothalamic tract	15	3	Thin
C	Long-lasting burning	Superficial	Contralateral spinothalamic tract	1	1	None

Adapted from Paris PM, Uram M, Ginsburg MJ: Physiological mechanisms of pain. In Paris PM, Stewart RD (eds): *Pain Management in Emergency Medicine.* Norwalk, Conn, Appleton & Lange, 1988.

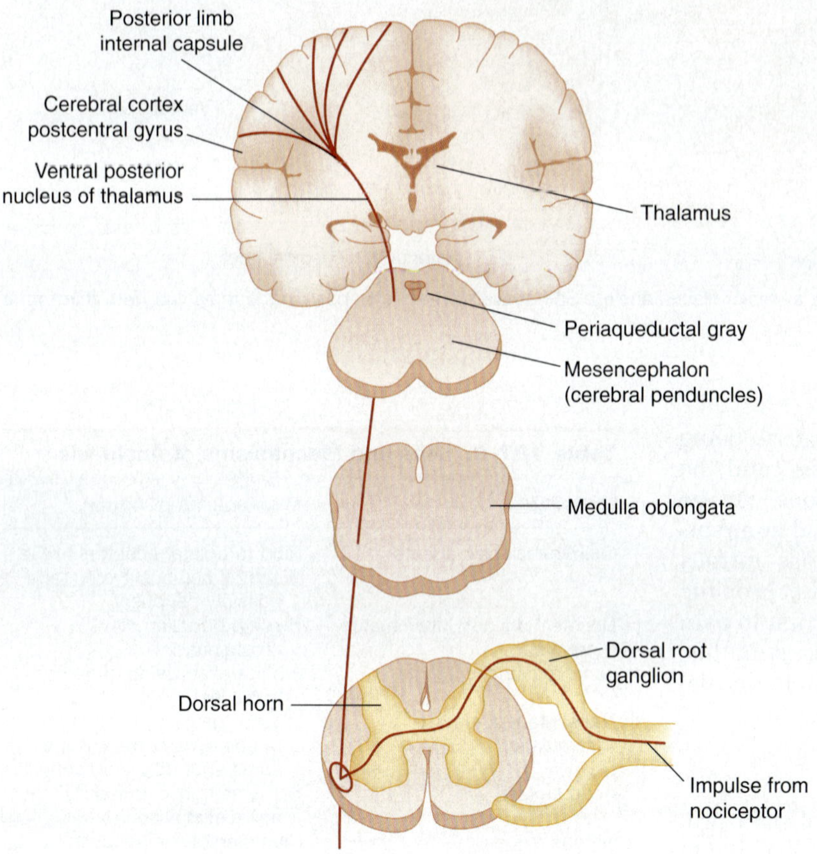

Figure 187-1. Diagram tracing the path of the major tract that carries pain stimuli to the brain, the lateral spinothalamic tract.

stantia gelatinosa is the term given to laminae II and III, and many of the A-δ and C fibers synapse at this level of the spinal cord.

Ascending Tracts Associated with Pain and Tactile Stimuli

Fibers carrying pain impulses exit the dorsal horn and ascend the spinal cord to the brain. The predominant pathways for pain conduction are the spinothalamic tract and the spinoreticular tract; both are located in the anterior lateral aspect of the spinal cord (Figure 187-2).

The spinoreticular tract ends in synapses in the reticular formation, with subsequent neurons going to the thalamus and then to the cerebral cortex.

Signal Modulation

It is now generally accepted that pain sensation can be modified—multiplied or divided—in the descending tracts that modulate sensory information that is transmitted from the periphery. The two primary pathways identified originate in the midbrain (periaqueductal gray matter and locus ceruleus) and medulla (nucleus raphe magnus and nucleus reticularis giganto-cellularis). The nociceptive modulation is transmitted to the spinal cord via the dorsolateral funiculus. Electrical stimulation of this pathway produces analgesia comparable to that produced with opioids. Several specific neurotransmitters are involved in these pathways, including serotonin and norepinephrine. It is believed that the activation of this system is responsible for the placebo effect.

Pain Perception and Reaction

The threshold for the perception of a painful stimulus (that is, "Is pain present?") is similar in everyone, whereas the threshold for pain tolerance varies widely. These thresholds can be lowered by certain chemicals (e.g., the mediators of inflammation). The discrete cognitive processes and pathways involved in the inter-

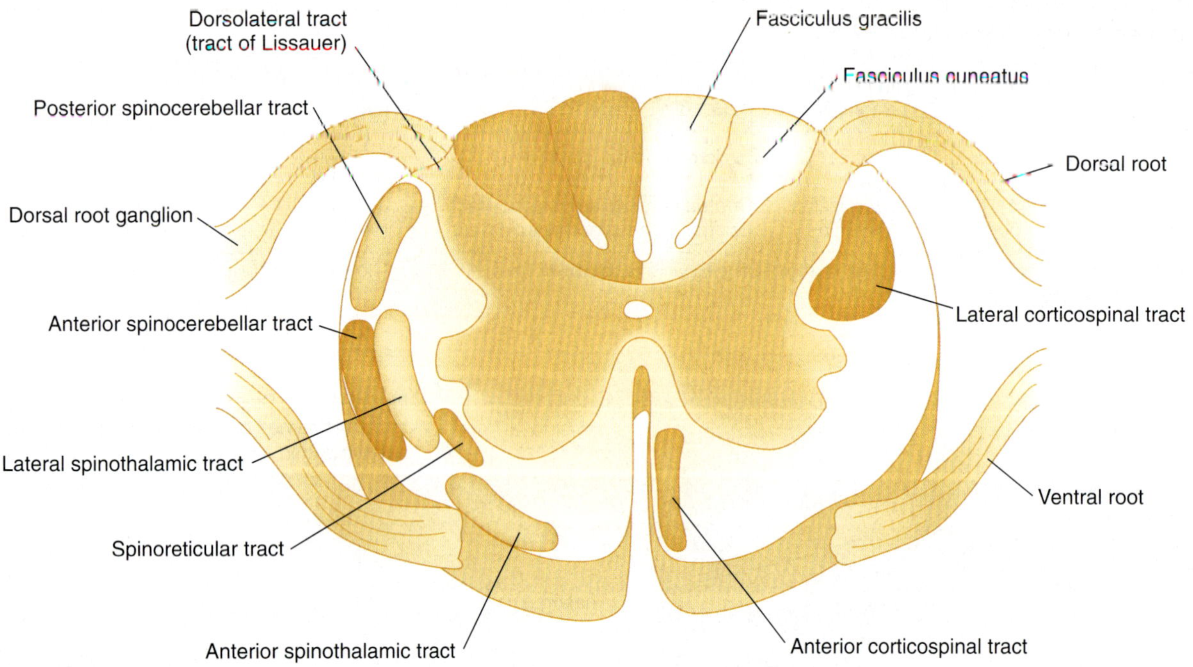

Figure 187-2. Cross-section of entire spinal cord with all major tracts labeled. Spinothalamic tract synapses in the thalamus, with third-order neurons ascending the somatosensory cortex.

pretation of painful stimuli remain a mystery, being affected by culture, personality, experiences, and the underlying emotional state. These reactions can be greatly influenced by both pharmacologic and nonpharmacologic interventions. For drugs such as nitrous oxide and low-dose opioids, much of the effect is on the cognitive interpretation and emotional reaction to pain rather than on the transmission of the pain stimulus. Noninvasive techniques (e.g., distraction and hypnosis) can limit pain perceptions and increase tolerance.

Sites of Analgesia

At each level in the physiologic process of pain production or transmission, interventions are available to alter the process (Table 187-2).

Table 187-2. Sites and Mechanisms of Analgesia

Modality	Mechanisms of Action
Opioid analgesic agents	Bind to opiate receptors in the central nervous system and possibly periphery
Nonsteroidal anti-inflammatory agents	Block production of prostaglandins
Local anesthetic agents	Block transmission of nerve impulses
Transcutaneous nerve stimulation	Closes "gate" in dorsal horn of spinal cord; may also be some endorphin component
Acupuncture	Same as transcutaneous nerve stimulation
Nitrous oxide	Blunts emotional reaction to pain; endogenous opioid system may play a role
Ketamine	Dissociates thalamocortical and limbic systems
Hypnosis	Causes cognitive reinterpretation of pain stimulus
Biofeedback	Decreases muscle tension
Music	Decreases anxiety and allows cognitive focus on stimuli other than pain
Placebo	Activates descending pain inhibitory paths; also possibly endorphins
Distraction	Allows cognitive focus on stimuli other than pain

MANAGEMENT PRINCIPLES

Pain Evaluation and Documentation

Pain is a complex experience—a composite of anatomic, chemical, and psychological factors that affect people differently. Unfortunately, no singular test or physiologic index exists to measure pain reliably.[8] Numerical rating scales, employing a verbal 0 to 10 "none to worst" report, have been validated in the emergency department setting.[9] Conversely, visual analogue scales, often consisting of a 10 cm straight line with anchors at either extreme (similar to verbal scales), are used in research because of beliefs regarding accuracy and reproducibility but offer little practical advantage over verbal reports in the daily practice of medicine (Table 187-3).[10]

The only accurate barometer in treating pain is the patient's report. Pain behavior is unique to each individual and is a product of many influences, including past experiences with pain, cultural background, and the psychosocial makeup of the patient. Changes in facial expressions or vital signs do not correlate reliably with a patient's subjective sensation of pain. Patients may be experiencing severe pain despite

Table 187-3. Techniques for Grading Pain Intensity Before and After Treatment*

Technique	How Pain Is Graded	Application
Five-point global scale	0 = None 1 = A little 2 = Some 3 = A lot 4 = Worst possible	Routine bedside evaluation
Verbal quantitative scale	0 . . . 5 . . . 10 None Worst Possible	Routine bedside evaluation
Visual analogue scale (10-cm line, slide-rule devices)	No Pain ———— Worst Possible Pain Place a mark on the line to show how much pain you are having.	Routine bedside evaluation When "hard copy" is desirable Can be used with children age 6 years and older
Behavioral and physiologic parameters	Restlessness, grimacing, vocalization, sweating, lacrimation, pupil dilation, tachycardia, hypertension, and discoordinate mechanical ventilation may all be signs of pain. (These signs have not been validated so should be used with caution.)	Unconsciousness, unresponsive, confused, critically ill patients
Observer-generated assessment of function	Can patient perform important functions associated with recovery (deep breathing, cough, spirometry, range of motion in joint, ambulation)? Yes/No	Adjunct to patient-generated subjective pain reports Should be used in all patients
Global satisfaction question	Are you satisfied with your pain relief? Yes/No	Clarification of confusing response; for unsophisticated patients
Observer-generated pediatric pain scales	Observe facial expressions, crying, cardiorespiratory responses; compare with children who are not in pain.	Neonate to age 3 years and some aged 3-6 years
Patient-generated pediatric pain scales		Over age 6 years and some aged 3-6 years
a. *Pictorial*	☺ ☹	
Faces	Point at (or circle, or color) the face that shows how you feel.	
Draw a picture of your pain	Estimate location, character, intensity from drawing.	
b. *Numeric*		
"Pieces of Hurt" (poker chips)	Poker chips represent pain that child can give to therapist.	
Hurt thermometer	Similar to visual analogue scale for adults.	

*Many problems can be mislabeled as pain. The reports of pain obtained using these techniques must be interpreted carefully. Pain should be assessed both at rest and during stimulation (deep breathing, coughing, ambulation).
Modified from Ready BL, Edwards WT: *Management of Acute Pain.* Seattle, I.A.S.P. Publications, 1992.

BOX 187-4. The Visual Analogue Pain Scale

No pain									Unbearable pain
1	2	3	4	5	6	7	8	9	10

smiles or even laughter. Simply stated, pain exists if the patient says it does. Including a pain scale as a routine part of vital signs is now mandated (by the JCAHO and other agencies) (Box 187-4).[b] This encourages clinicians to initially and frequently communicate with patients to assess their pain. It also allows charts to be used for continuous quality improvement efforts to improve pain control practices on a departmental level.

Oligoanalgesia

Physicians in a variety of specialties tend to underestimate the degree of patient pain and, more importantly, undertreat it.[11] Numerous studies confirm inadequate treatment of pain by both physicians and nurses in a variety of medical and surgical settings involving adults and children. Studies in emergency departments have demonstrated the same insensitivity and lack of success in treating the acute pain state.[12] Data from the National Hospital Ambulatory Medical Survey evaluated all isolated closed fractures of extremities and clavicle and showed that only 64% of patients received an analgesic and only 42% received an opioid.[13] As in other studies, children and elderly patients were less likely to receive analgesics than patients in other age groups. Unfortunately, recent studies show only modest improvements in emergency medicine based pain management.

A recent review suggests that the oligoanalgesia phenomena may emanate from "(1) a lack of educational emphasis on pain management practices in nursing and medical school curricula and postgraduate training programs; (2) inadequate or nonexistent clinical quality management programs that evaluate pain management; (3) a paucity of rigorous studies of populations with special needs that improve pain management in the emergency department, particularly in geriatric and pediatric patients; (4) clinicians' attitudes toward opioid analgesics that result in inappropriate diagnosis of drug-seeking behavior and inappropriate concern about addiction, even in patients who have obvious acutely painful conditions and request pain relief; (5) inappropriate concerns about the safety of opioids compared with nonsteroidal anti-inflammatory drugs that result in their underuse (opiophobia); (6) unappreciated cultural and sex differences in pain reporting by patients and interpretation of pain reporting by providers; and (7) bias and disbelief of pain reporting according to racial and ethnic stereotyping."[14]

Even when analgesia is administered in the emergency department, there frequently is a long delay. When opioids are used, they frequently are given in subtherapeutic doses. One study of trauma centers showed that of the 38% of patients who did receive an analgesic, the average time of administration of the first dose of analgesic was 109 minutes after arrival.[15]

One of the most common excuses for withholding analgesia in the emergency department is the fear of masking the diagnosis. This unproven historical belief, which originated before modern diagnostic approaches, including imaging, were developed, has no validity and has not been supported by any recent study. Patients can be made comfortable without impeding normal diagnostic approaches.

Inadequate treatment of acute pain does not seem to be limited to the United States. A study in Costa Rica showed that analgesic agents were given to only 11% of adults and 4% of children.[16] The most striking finding was that opioids were not used for any patients, including those who had severe pain.

A study from the United Kingdom looked at 172 children with limb trauma and discovered that only 49% received any analgesic, of which 70% received only paracetamol and 30% morphine. An Australian study of 176 patients with femoral neck fractures showed that only 49% received prehospital analgesia despite a protocol that would have encouraged analgesic use.

Priorities

Correcting the problems of inadequate treatment of a patient's pain requires a major effort by educational institutions in all specialties of medicine, surgery, and emergency medicine. For emergency medicine, the approach to analgesia in acute care medicine must emphasize the following:

1. Safety: Ongoing, untreated pain is harmful to the patient and must be mitigated. Conversely, analgesic agents can cause harm. Any analgesic procedure or agent must be administered with proper technique and monitoring to ensure safety.
2. Speed of onset: Triage protocols can decrease time to administration of analgesics. Nebulized fentanyl can also provide rapid analgesia.[17,18]
3. Ease of administration: Techniques used must be suited to the emergency department environment and to staff resources. For most patients, oral agents given early are ideal, whereas intravenous medications are needed for severe pain or when oral use cannot occur.

Table 187-4. Opioid Receptors and Their Actions

Receptor	Action
μ (MOP)	Supraspinal analgesia Euphoria Miosis Urinary retention Low addiction potential Respiratory depression Gastrointestinal actions Cardiovascular effects Addiction risk
κ (KOP)	Spinal analgesia Dysphoria* Psychotomimetic effects* Several subtypes proposed Low addiction potential
δ (DOP)	Primarily spinal analgesia. Binds enkephalin
ε	Identified in animals

OP, opioid peptide receptor.

Opioid Analgesic Agents

In the emergency department, opioid analgesic agents are the mainstay of therapy for most of the conditions that cause moderate to severe acute pain.

Mechanism of Action

The physiologic actions of opioids are primarily mediated through their binding to specific opiate receptors in the spinal cord and brain. Recently, peripheral opiate receptors have also been implicated in analgesia. Several different classes of opiate receptors exist, and the unique actions of various opioids are explained by the specific binding properties of the agent to the different receptors. The classification of opioid receptors is currently changing. The traditional classification system of using Greek letters, namely mu (μ), kappa (κ), delta (δ), and epsilon (ε) is changing (Table 187-4). The Greek symbols have been replaced by their Arabic alphabet equivalents, followed by OP for "opioid peptide receptor." Stimulation of opioid receptors inhibits pain conduction in nociceptive pathways by inhibiting the release of neurotransmitters. There is also inhibition of the postsynaptic membrane.

Common Therapeutic Mistakes

Opioids are often poorly used.[12] Common mistakes seem to result from a lack of understanding of the basic pharmacologic principles of this class of analgesics (Box 187-5).

Reluctance to Use Opioid Analgesic Agents

In 1680, Sydenham wrote "among the remedies it has pleased Almighty God to give to man to relieve his

BOX 187-5. Common Errors in the Use of Opioid Analgesic Agents that Limit Their Efficacy

Reluctance to use this class of agents
Wrong dose
Wrong route of administration
Wrong frequency
Wrong opioid
Inappropriate use of adjunctive agents
Excessive suspicion of drug-seeking behavior

BOX 187-6. Disadvantages of Intramuscular Opioid Administration

Pain on injection
Delayed onset of action
Inability to predict effect
Inability to easily titrate dosage
Diurnal variation in level achieved
Disease state may affect level achieved
Level dependent on muscle used
Hematomas may occur if coagulopathy exists
Poor technique may damage other structures

sufferings, none is so universal and so efficacious as opium."[19] Centuries later, this statement is still accurate, but a reluctance to use opioids continues to exist among clinicians. Physicians have an irrational fear of creating opioid addiction in patients or causing uncontrollable life-threatening side effects (e.g., respiratory depression). When comparing the occurrence and the severity of side effects, one can actually make a strong case that opioids are safer than nonsteroidal anti-inflammatory drugs (NSAIDs).

The iatrogenic creation of opioid addiction, a new addiction where one did not previously exist, is a relatively rare phenomenon. The results of the Boston Drug Collaborative Study showed that only 4 in 11,892 inpatients treated with opioid analgesic agents developed new opioid abuse.[20] The authors concluded iatrogenic development of addiction is rare in medical patients treated with opioid analgesic agents unless they have a prior history of addiction. Even as lay press addiction stories abound (recently surrounding oxycodone preparations), many experts believe this most often represents a change in addiction rather than creation of a "new" addict.

Suspicion of Drug-Seeking Behavior

Some patients feign pain to receive opioids. Suspected drug-seeking behavior should be well documented and the information relayed to other emergency physicians in a way that does not violate the Healthcare Insurance Portability and Accountability Act (HIPAA) or state or federal statutes. Patients should be given the benefit of the doubt until it is obvious the patient is trying to deceive the hospital staff. It is possible to maintain patient confidentiality and act in the best interest of the patient while maintaining files of suspected nontherapeutic drug seeking.[21] Such files must be stored in a secure fashion, such as a password-protected computerized system with limited access, and the process must be guided by the approval of a qualified individual or committee.

If one is suspicious, but uncertain, of opioid-seeking behavior, use of parenteral opioids can be limited to those in the agonist-antagonist class (e.g., nalbuphine [Nubain] or butorphanol [Stadol]). These drugs work well as analgesic agents without creating much of the euphoria that opioid abusers may seek. Another approach is to tell patients they will be receiving a potent opioid analgesic agent that has very few side effects except in persons addicted to opioids, in which case it precipitates withdrawal symptoms. If the clinician is fooled and administers a parenteral opioid, it represents one consequence of having a humane approach to the treatment of acute pain. When writing prescriptions for oral opioids, caution must be taken if there is a suspicion of opioid abuse. In these cases, the number of pills should be limited and the drug that is most notorious for abuse, Oxycontin, should be avoided.

Wrong Dosage

The most important factor in achieving adequate analgesia with a given opioid is titrating the dosage to achieve the desired degree of analgesia. A wide interpatient variability exists in the effective analgesic concentration. The "one amp" approach of treating all patients with 10 mg of morphine is ineffective and potentially dangerous in many patients.[19] The proper way to achieve the effective dosage for moderate to severe pain is to use a deliberate intravenous titration.

Wrong Route of Administration

The intramuscular route of administration of opioids—while common—has several disadvantages (Box 187-6). The intramuscular route does not allow timely titration. When using the intramuscular route, one must estimate the proper dose and then wait 20 to 60 minutes to observe for peak effect. If too small a dose is used, the patient must experience another painful injection and wait another 20 to 60 minutes to determine whether effective analgesia is achieved. If too large a dose is given, the patient is at risk of side effects. In short, IM opioids have little role in acute pain management in the emergency department—most patients are best managed with oral agents if mild to moderate pain exists and intravenous agents if pain is moderate to severe.

If an intravenous line cannot be established, the subcutaneous route is preferable to the intramuscular route because it is less painful. The rate of absorption for a subcutaneous injection is almost identical to one given by the intramuscular route.

Opioids can be delivered through the oral transmucosal or intranasal mucosal route.[22,23] The potent opioid buprenorphine can be given by sublingual route. Fentanyl is available in an impregnated, sweetened matrix called a Fentanyl Oralet (oral transmucosal fentanyl citrate). Nasal butorphanol and sufentanil also produce rapid clinical effects.

Wrong Frequency

Optimal use of opioids requires titrating the initial "loading" dose to desired relief of pain, then the administration of repeated doses at a frequent enough interval to prevent the return of significant discomfort.

The best way to determine the need to administer another dose of opioid is to use the patient's subjective impression. The dose of opioid to prevent pain is less than the dose to treat well-established pain. Patient-controlled analgesia is a technique that uses a computerized delivery system that allows patients to self-administer a prescribed dose of opioid at a predetermined frequency based on their own determination of need. A recent study using patient-controlled analgesia for sickle cell pain crisis in a pediatric emergency department showed that this technique could be used safely and result in quicker care with high patient satisfaction.[24]

Wrong Opioid

In general, most opioids are effective in achieving analgesia if given in the proper dose. The major exception to this rule is the use of oral codeine and propoxyphene.

At any dose, codeine is a weak analgesic. Although it sometimes suffices for mild to moderate pain, it is rarely successful for moderate to severe pain. Codeine has a high incidence of inducing nausea, vomiting, and constipation and can cause abdominal pain. Studies have not distinguished the analgesic superiority of acetaminophen plus codeine versus acetaminophen alone. Oxycodone and hydrocodone are excellent oral opioid analgesics. The long-acting oxycodone preparation Oxycontin has been abused so widely that its use in the practice of emergency medicine should be limited to management of patients with chronic pain of known cause (e.g., malignancy).

Propoxyphene (Darvon, Darvocet) has limited indications for use. Many studies have shown its analgesic efficacy to be no better or only marginally better than placebo. In toxic doses, it can cause early refractory seizures, respiratory arrest, and significant risk of death. In those patients who have had success with the use of propoxyphene for past episodes of pain, it may be a reasonable choice for mild to moderate pain.

Oral meperidine is similarly not recommended because of its unsatisfactory side effect profile, significant abuse potential, and lack of analgesic efficacy due to its significant hepatic first-pass metabolism.

The most commonly used parenteral opioids are morphine, hydromorphone, and meperidine (Table 187-5). Morphine has many advantages over meperidine, including a longer half-life, much less central nervous system (CNS) toxicity, a metabolism that is little affected by renal or hepatic disease, and no myocardial depression.[19] Hydromorphone has a longer half-life and effect than morphine, with similar actions otherwise.

Meperidine is contraindicated in patients on monoamine oxidase inhibitors. Rare but potentially fatal malignant hyperthermia may be induced by this combination. The historical rationale for using meperidine rather than morphine was based on a presumed lack of smooth muscle stimulation, notably biliary spasm. In reality, all opioid agonists have similar smooth muscle effect in equipotent doses. Because of the many

Table 187-5. Meperidine versus Morphine

	Meperidine	Morphine
Half-life	2½-3 hr	2½-3 hr
Parenteral potency	⅛ morphine	
Oral/parenteral potency	50%	15%
Respiratory depression	Moderate	Moderate
Abuse potential	High	High
Metabolism	Hepatic	Hepatic
Liver disease	Half-life prolonged	Half-life unaffected
Renal disease	Increased CNS toxicity	Unaffected (active metabolite accumulation)
Histamine release	Yes	Yes
Biliary tract spasm	Significant	Significant
Urinary tract spasm	Yes	Yes
Side effects	Similar to morphine but higher CNS toxicity	See text
Cardiovascular system	Increased pulse, decreased contractility, decreased peripheral vascular resistance	No change or increased pulse, no change in contractility, decreased peripheral vascular resistance
Allergic reactions	Extremely rare	Extremely rare
Constipation	Minimal	Moderate
Cough suppression	Minimal	Marked
Routes of administration	PO, IM, IV, SQ	PO, IM, IV, SQ
Dose-response curve	Very steep	Steep
Interaction with MAO inhibitors	Potentially lethal	Not reported

CNS, central nervous system; IM, intramuscularly; IV, intravenously; MAO, monoamine oxidase; PO, orally; SQ, subcutaneously.
Modified from Paris PM, Blenko JW: Narcotic agonist-antagonist analgesics. In Paris PM, Stewart RD (eds): *Pain Management in Emergency Medicine.* Norwalk, Conn, Appleton & Lange, 1988.

advantages of morphine, it is the preferred agent for most situations in emergency medicine that require parenteral analgesia. Meperidine has been removed from pain treatment guidelines and many hospital formularies.

Incorrect Use of Adjuvant Agents

Adjuvant analgesic agents have a primary indication other than pain relief but are often combined with analgesic agents to enhance pain relief. Some of the agents that have been used as adjuvant analgesics are antidepressants, neuroleptics, hydroxyzine, corticosteroids, benzodiazepines, anticonvulsants, and caffeine.

A historical practice for clinicians was to use less than the full analgesic dose of an opioid and to combine it with another agent in an attempt to potentiate the given dose of opioid and decrease side effects (e.g., nausea, vomiting, and respiratory depression). In general, this practice could add to the potential toxicity of other agents. The most commonly used adjunctive agents for this purpose are phenothiazines and hydroxyzine (Vistaril, Atarax). Use of adequate and appropriate dosages of opioids provides at least equal efficacy at less cost than the use of a lower dosage of opioid with an adjuvant agent.

Although many different phenothiazines have been used to potentiate the analgesic effect of opioids, most studies do not show any significant benefit of their use. Some authors believe that some phenothiazines (e.g., promethazine [Phenergan]) may be antianalgesic. Considering the side effects of phenothiazines and the absence of compelling evidence of efficacy, their use to potentiate opioids is not well founded.

Hydroxyzine is commonly used as an adjunct to opioids. This drug has been shown to potentiate opioid analgesia. The major disadvantage of hydroxyzine is that it is not approved for intravenous use and therefore is most commonly given as a potentially painful intramuscular injection. Hydroxyzine can potentiate the sedation and respiratory depression associated with opioids. When titrating the dose of an opioid intravenously, there is little need for the routine use of hydroxyzine.

In general, antinausea drugs are not used routinely when administering opioids, and nausea can be expected to abate when the pain is managed. Antinauseant medication should be reserved for cases of severe nausea and vomiting that persist after analgesia has been obtained.

Parenteral Opioids

The terminology and classification system used to describe opioid analgesic agents can be confusing. The commonly used word *narcotic* has legal implications and is imprecise because it includes many classes of drugs that are not opioids. The term *opiate* defines a naturally occurring or semisynthetic derivative of opium alkaloid. The term *opioid*, as used in this chapter, is the most correct, because it refers to all natural opiates, plus all synthetic drugs that bind opiate receptors and produce effects similar to those of the natural opiates (Table 187-6).

Morphine

Morphine is the opioid analgesic agent to which all other opioids are compared. When administered intra-

Table 187-6. Opioid Classification

Generic Name	Proprietary Name	Oral Dose	Parenteral Dose	Duration	Comments	Precaution
Naturally Occurring Alkaloids and Semisynthetic Opiates						
Natural						
Morphine sulfate		30-60 mg	10 mg	3-4 hr	Standard opioid for all comparisons. Duration may vary widely, especially in patients with severe pain, or elders.	Respiratory depression, hypotension, histamine release, sedation.
Codeine		30-100 mg	30-100 mg	4 hr	Excellent cough suppressant. Poor analgesic.	Much constipation, nausea and vomiting. Decreased with supine position. Abuse potential.
Semisynthetic						
Hydromorphone	Dilaudid	2-6 mg	1-2 mg	2-4 hr	Very soluble, allowing small volumes to be used for injection. Available as suppository.	Much euphoria.
Hydrocodone	Hycodan Vicodan Lorcet Vicoprofen	5-10 mg	Not available	3-4 hr	Excellent cough suppressant. Greater potency than codeine. Perhaps fewer side effects.	Greater abuse potential than codeine.
Oxycodone	Percodan Percocet Tylox	5-10 mg	15 mg	3 hr	Parenteral form not available in United States. Very effective analgesic.	Euphoria predisposes to abuse.

Continued

Table 187-6. Opioid Classification—cont'd

Generic Name	Proprietary Name	Oral Dose	Parenteral Dose	Duration	Comments	Precaution
Meperidine and Related Phenylpiperidines						
Meperidine	Demerol	250-300 mg	75-125 mg	2-3 hr	See Table 187-5 for comparison with morphine. No advantages and several disadvantages vs morphine.	CNS tachycardia. Caution if renal or hepatic failure. Avoid with MAO inhibitors.
Fentanyl	Sublimaze	Not available	100-200 µg	1-2 hr	No histamine release. Good for short periods. Transcutaneous and transmucosal absorption.	May produce truncal rigidity in higher doses
Alfentanil	Alfenta	Not available	1 µg/kg	1-1.5 hr	Minimal cardiovascular side effects. Less potent, with shorter half-life than fentanyl. Shortest half-life of all opioids. Administered by intravenous infusion during general anesthesia.	Muscular rigidity in high dose or if administered too quickly. Expensive.
Sufentanil	Sufenta	Not available	5-15 µg	1-1.5 hr	Minimal cardiovascular side effects. More potent, with shorter half-life than fentanyl.	Muscular rigidity in high dose or if administered too quickly. Expensive.
Remifentanil	Ultiva	Not available	0.5-1 µg/kg	6 min		Muscle rigidity and decreased blood pressure possible. Expensive.
Methadone and Related Drugs						
Methadone	Dolophine	10-20 mg	10 mg	4-6 hr	Analgesic half-life not the same as plasma half-life. Not much euphoria.	Long plasma half-life may produce cumulative toxicity.
Propoxyphene	Darvon-N	100 mg	Not available	3 hr	Very weak analgesic.	Overdoses are complicated and serious.
Nalorphine Type						
Pentazocine	Talwin	50-100 mg	30-60 mg	2-3 hr	Suppositories available.	Increased cardiac stroke work. High incidence of psychotomimetic effects.
Nalbuphine	Nubain	40 mg	5-15 mg	3-4 hr	Minimal if any hemodynamic effects. Ceiling on respiratory depression. Low abuse potential.	Can precipitate withdrawal if dependence on opioid agonist.
Butorphanol	Stadol	Not available	1-4 mg	4-7 hr	Nasal metered-dose available.	Cardiovascular effects similar to pentazocine. Can precipitate withdrawal.
Dezocine	Dalgan	Not available	5-20 mg		More potent analgesia than other agonists/antagonists.	Mild cardiovascular depression.
Buprenorphine	Buprenex		0.3-0.6 mg	5-6 hr	Partial agonist. Can be given sublingually. Long analgesic action.	Not completely antagonized by naloxone.

CNS, central nervous system; IV, intravenous; MAO, monoamine oxidase.
Adapted from Paris PM, Blenko JW: Opioid agonist-antagonist analgesics. In Paris PM, Stewart RD (eds): *Pain Management in Emergency Medicine.* Norwalk, Conn, Appleton & Lange, 1988.

venously, morphine reaches its peak of action in a few minutes and has a half-life of 1.5 to 2 hours in healthy young adults, and slightly longer in elderly patients. The clinical duration of action is variable but is in the range of 3 to 4 hours in most patients. It is common for repeat doses to be required earlier than the total duration interval, especially in patients with severe pain syndromes. Morphine is conjugated to an active and inactive metabolite in the liver, with renal excretion of the conjugate. The active metabolite is morphine-6-glucuronide; this substance has little analgesic activity but can cause profound sedation.

The cardiovascular effects of analgesic doses of morphine are relatively minimal. Morphine does not decrease cardiac contractility, but it does cause the release of histamine, which results in peripheral venous and arteriolar dilation. The property of increasing venous capacitance is what makes morphine so helpful in the treatment of cardiogenic pulmonary edema. In patients who are relatively hypovolemic, this effect can lead to a decrease in blood pressure. If hypotension does occur, patients should first be treated with fluid administration and supine positioning. Naloxone is not effective at blocking the decreased peripheral vascular resistance. On occasion, morphine can increase vagal tone, leading to a decrease in heart rate.

Like most other opioids, morphine releases histamine, which may result in urticaria and, rarely, an increase in bronchospasm in patients with reactive airways disease. True immunoglobulin-mediated allergies are rare for morphine and other opioids.

Like other opioids, morphine has significant effects on the gastrointestinal tract. Morphine increases antral tone and decreases gastric motility, thereby delaying stomach emptying. Because colonic peristalsis is slowed significantly, constipation commonly results from opioid use. Morphine, like the other pure agonist opioids, causes a significant increase in biliary pressure.[19] The increased intrabiliary pressure usually is not associated with symptoms.

Meperidine

Meperidine has several disadvantages compared with morphine (see Table 187-5). The duration of action of meperidine is only 2 to 3 hours, which is less than that of morphine. Perhaps the greatest disadvantage of meperidine is the CNS toxicity that is caused by a metabolite, normeperidine, which is a cerebral irritant. The adverse CNS actions that can be caused by normeperidine include anxiety, disorientation, tremors, seizures, hallucinations, and psychosis. Normeperidine is renally excreted and also has a longer half-life in elderly patients. Repeated doses of meperidine should be avoided when possible in patients with renal insufficiency and in elderly patients.

Of particular concern is the potentially lethal interaction of meperidine with monoamine oxidase inhibitors. Meperidine can also cause a serotonin syndrome in patients who are taking a selective serotonin reuptake inhibitor.[25] The majority of studies have not definitively shown a marked advantage for the use of meperidine in patients with biliary tract disease or pancreatitis. Meperidine has been removed from formularies, or its indication has been limited in many hospitals.

Fentanyl

Fentanyl (Sublimaze) is a synthetic opioid of the phenylpiperidine group that has some unique properties that make it a useful agent in emergency medicine. The most prominent properties of fentanyl are its short half-life, lack of histamine release, and lack of decrease in cardiac contractility. Fentanyl is lipid soluble, which allows it to cross the blood-brain barrier rapidly and thus have a rapid onset of action (<5 minutes). The half-life of fentanyl is 90 minutes, but the duration of action is often less because of redistribution, which makes it an ideal agent for brief procedures (e.g., dislocated joint relocation and incision and drainage of abscesses). Emergency department use of fentanyl is associated with a very low (1.1%) incidence of potentially serious complications.[26]

Because fentanyl and its derivatives are the only opioid analgesic agents that do not release histamine, they are ideal for treating pain in patients with bronchospastic lung disease. High or repeated doses of fentanyl may produce muscle rigidity. This side effect usually occurs with anesthetic doses (>15 μg/kg) and may be so severe that it interferes with respiration but is exceedingly rare with analgesic use. This rigidity can be treated with naloxone or (if severe) neuromuscular blockade plus intubation. Fentanyl does not directly decrease cardiac output, but it may blunt central sympathetic output, which can potentially decrease cardiac output in selected patients who depend on sympathetic drive. Combining fentanyl with nitrous oxide or benzodiazepines can also cause mild cardiovascular compromise.

Because fentanyl can be readily absorbed through the oral mucosa, it has been put into a candy matrix, oral transmucosal fentanyl citrate. This is particularly useful for treating children. The nebulized inhaled fentanyl has been described in the emergency department treatment of patients with abdominal pain.[18] Intranasal delivery of fentanyl in children with a variety of painful conditions also is an analgesic option.[17]

Alfentanil (Alfenta) and sufentanil (Sufenta) are fentanyl derivatives with even shorter durations of action. These agents are commonly used for anesthesia and procedural analgesia/sedation, though not commonly in the emergency department. Sufentanil can also be given by the intranasal and transmucosal routes.[23,27]

Remifentanil

Remifentanil is the first opioid from a new class of ultrashort-acting 4-anilidopiperidines.[28] It is rapidly hydrolyzed by nonspecific plasma and tissue esterases with a duration of action of less than 6 minutes. Like fentanyl, it does not release histamine and seems to be safe for use in patients with renal failure and chronic liver disease. In large doses, it has also been associated with muscle rigidity, like fentanyl, and several cases of bradycardia have been described. Despite not increasing histamine concentrations, a mild decrease in blood pressure may occur. Because of its very short duration of action, this drug may play an increasing role in procedural analgesia/sedation. It is supplied as a lyophilized powder only available for intravenous use. There has been little emergency department experience with this drug.

Hydromorphone

Hydromorphone (Dilaudid) has a few unique properties that make it useful for selected emergencies. It is a potent analgesic agent with excellent bioavailability

BOX 187-7. Properties of the Agonist-Antagonists

- Ceiling on respiratory depression
- Moderate to potent analgesia in therapeutic dose
- Less euphoria than agonists
- Less abuse potential than agonists
- Slower development of tolerance than agonists
- Milder withdrawal than agonists
- Precipitation of withdrawal in patients dependent on agonists
- Probably fewer side effects than agonists
- Extensive first-pass effect with oral administration (hepatic metabolism)
- Possible psychotomimetic effects
- Sedation most common side effect
- Pentazocine only agonist-antagonist subject to Controlled Substance Act
- Butorphanol available in nasal spray

Adapted from Paris PM, Blenko JW: Opioid agonist-antagonist analgesic. In Paris PM, Stewart RD (eds). *Pain Management in Emergency Medicine.* Norwalk, Conn, Appleton & Lange, 1988.

when given orally. Since it lasts longer than morphine and many other opioids after an intravenous dose (4-6 hours), it is an excellent choice in many severe pain syndromes, especially sickle cell vaso-occlusive events. It is also one of the few opioids commercially available as a rectal suppository.[19] Because hydromorphone has high solubility, large doses of the drug can be given in small quantities of fluid for subcutaneous or intramuscular injection.

Opioid Agonist-Antagonist Analgesic Agents

The agonist-antagonist group of opioids were synthesized in an attempt to provide analgesia with little or no respiratory depression and abuse. It is believed that the analgesia provided by these agents is caused by agonist action at the κ (KOP) receptors, whereas the ceiling on respiratory depression is caused by antagonism of the μ (MOP) receptors (Box 187-7, Table 187-6).

The primary advantages of these drugs are the ceiling on respiratory depression (not absence) and diminished abuse potential. Some practitioners have also suggested that a ceiling may exist on analgesia, but whether this has clinical significance is unclear.

Pentazocine

Pentazocine (Talwin) was first introduced in 1967. Today, because of its side effect profile, it has little use. The most significant side effect is a psychotomimetic reaction in up to 7% of patients taking this agent. This reaction may include visual or auditory hallucinations, disorientation, dysphoria, and feelings of depersonalization or panic. Another unique side effect of pentazocine is a fibrous myopathy that occurs after intramuscular injections. Abuse of pentazocine seems to occur less commonly than abuse of morphine or heroin but still is a problem. Winthrop Laboratories has now added 0.5 mg of naloxone to its tablets (Talwin Nx) to combat parenteral use of the oral form. Because naloxone is not absorbed through the gastrointestinal tract, the oral route for the drug remains effective. There are no emergency medicine indications for which pentazocine offers an advantage over other available opioids.

Nalbuphine

Nalbuphine (Nubain) has many potential uses as a parenteral analgesic. Its major advantages are a ceiling on respiratory depression and no demonstrated cardiovascular side effects. The half-life of the drug is 3.5 hours, and the effects of renal or hepatic disease on metabolism are not completely known. Psychotomimetic reactions occur but in fewer than 1% of patients, which is much less often than with pentazocine.[29] Abuse potential of nalbuphine seems to be low.

The usual therapeutic parenteral dose is 10 mg, but as with all other opioids, the dose must be individualized. Nalbuphine currently is not subject to regulation under the Controlled Substance Act. This fact may be a benefit in some emergency medical service systems[30] where opioids are currently not used because of the difficulties of maintaining distributions of controlled substances. When nalbuphine is used in a prehospital or hospital environment, patients subsequently may require higher doses of morphine or other pure μ-agonist opioids.

Butorphanol

Butorphanol (Stadol) is a synthetic opioid with properties similar to those of nalbuphine. One major difference, however, is that butorphanol increases systemic and pulmonary artery pressures. Because it increases cardiac afterload, butorphanol is not recommended in cases of myocardial infarction or states of decreased myocardial contractility.

The major advantage of this drug is its transmucosal absorption, with a transnasal preparation commercially available.[31] The latter allows rapid, easily self-titrated analgesia to patients. Each nasal spray delivers 1 mg. The most common side effect of butorphanol is sedation. Psychotomimetic reactions have been described but are rare. The usual therapeutic dose is 2 to 4 mg. The half-life is 3 hours; hepatic metabolism and renal excretion both contribute to drug elimination.

Dezocine

Dezocine is a newer agonist-antagonist opioid under investigation. Currently, it is not available in the United States. It may provide more potent analgesia than other members of the agonist-antagonist class of drugs.[32] Dezocine does cause some respiratory depression, but it has a ceiling effect like the other agonist-antagonist opioids. It may cause mild cardiovascular depression in selected patients.

Buprenorphine

Buprenorphine (Buprenex) is a semisynthetic opioid analgesic agent in the agonist-antagonist category, but it differs from the other drugs in that it acts as a partial agonist at the μ opiate receptor.[33] Opioid antagonists do not completely reverse the actions of buprenorphine. Buprenorphine is well absorbed orally and sublingually. Buprenorphine is gaining use in the treatment of opioid dependence. Little information has been published on analgesic uses of buprenorphine in emergency medicine.

Oral Opioids

Many oral opioids suffer from the first-pass effect of hepatic metabolism, requiring the dosage to be adjusted accordingly. If the proper dosage is used, then the oral route is excellent for moderate pain and a good follow-up to intravenous analgesics for severe pain. Oral opioids are appropriate for moderate pain and are often safer and more effective than nonopioid analgesic agents. Most emergency medicine conditions for which oral opioid analgesics are prescribed are fairly short-lived and require no more than 10 to 20 doses, with cancer and sickle cell vaso-occlusive pain as notable exceptions.

Codeine with acetaminophen or aspirin (Tylenol #4, Tylenol #3, Empirin with codeine, Bufferin with codeine) is a commonly used oral opioid. This group of preparations enjoyed great and undeserved popularity because of the relative lack of euphoria it produces and a belief that it has a lesser abuse potential. Codeine commonly produces nausea, often with vomiting. Even in higher doses, codeine is not a very effective analgesic agent, performing frequently no better than placebo. It has no legitimate role as an analgesic in modern emergency medicine practice. Patients under consideration for a codeine analgesic should simply be given acetaminophen or an NSAID. If the pain is believed to be too severe for an NSAID, a more potent opioid (e.g., oxycodone or hydrocodone) is indicated.

Propoxyphene (Darvon, Darvocet-N) was once one of the most commonly prescribed drugs in the United States. This drug is a poor analgesic agent, only marginally if at all better than placebo. Overdoses with this opioid can be toxic, with refractory seizures and respiratory depression leading to death. For these reasons, the use of propoxyphene compounds in emergency medicine should be rare.

Oxycodone (Percodan, Percocet, Tylox) is a potent, effective oral analgesic. The major drawback to this agent is that it causes significant euphoria in many patients, making it a popular drug of abuse. For moderate to severe acute pain, it is an excellent choice, but the quantity of pills prescribed should be limited to only a few days' supply for most emergency medicine indications. A long-acting oxycodone preparation (Oxycontin) has received much negative publicity because of its abuse potential. Although this agent has many indications for the treatment of chronic pain syndromes, it has few indications in the practice of emergency medicine.

Hydrocodone (Anexsia, Zydone, Vicodin, Hycodan, Lorcet, Vicoprofen), a semisynthetic derivative of codeine, has gained great popularity in the last decade. Drug manufacturers have promoted it as more potent than codeine with fewer gastrointestinal side effects. The few controlled studies that have compared hydrocodone to codeine also suggest that it is a more effective analgesic with fewer side effects. Hydrocodone may cause some euphoria and has become one of the most commonly abused oral opioids.[34]

Oral morphine has one sixth the potency of parenteral morphine, but it is still an excellent analgesic agent if given in the proper dose. It is a mainstay of therapy in patients with cancer pain. In addition to short-acting oral preparations, a long-acting oral preparations (MS Contin) is available in 15, 30, 60, and 100 mg tablets.

Oral meperidine has half the potency of the parenteral preparation, and it is generally not recommended because of the superiority of other oral agents. The risk of neurotoxicity may be higher when using meperidine orally.

Methadone (Dolophine) is widely used as a treatment for opioid addiction. It is able to suppress opioid withdrawal and causes little or no euphoria. The long plasma half-life (24-36 hours) allows it to suppress opioid withdrawal with a single daily oral dose, but its duration of action as an analgesic is only 4 to 5 hours. When methadone is used to treat pain, care must be taken to avoid the increasing sedation that can occur with multiple daily doses.

Tramadol

Tramadol (Ultram, Ultracet) is a unique centrally acting analgesic. The affinity of tramadol for the μ (MOP) receptor is 6000 times less than that of morphine; its analgesia persists in the presence of naloxone, leading to the conclusion that the opioid receptor binding activity accounts for only a fraction of its analgesic effect. Its other actions are caused by inhibition of reuptake of norepinephrine and serotonin. The major side effect to this agent is seizures, reported even in patients receiving therapeutic doses as well as occurring during sudden discontinuation of the drug. When administered with selective serotonin reuptake inhibitors, the risk of the serotonin syndrome is increased. This drug has a long history of widespread use in Europe; it is actually unrestricted in Germany and is the most popular analgesic agent in that country. Tramadol can be administered orally with 60% bioavailability and seems to have an excellent safety profile.[35]

Respiratory depression has not been reported in recommended dosages. Tramadol has very little potential for abuse or addiction. Tramadol should be considered a mild analgesic and not a good choice for moderate to severe pain. In a dental model, tramadol was found to have similar effect to 60 mg of codeine but was less effective than a codeine/NSAID combination or a full dose NSAID regimen.[36] An emergency department study of acute musculoskeletal pain showed tramadol to be less effective than any combination of hydrocodone plus acetaminophen.[37]

Opioid Use in Abdominal Pain

In his treatise on abdominal pain, Cope stated, "Though it may appear cruel, it is really kind to withhold morphine until one is certain whether surgical interference is necessary, i.e., until a reasonable diagnosis has been made." He added, "If morphine be administered, it is possible to die happy in the belief that he is on the road to recovery, and in some cases the medical attendant may for a time be induced to share the same delusive hope." This outdated philosophy was written before modern diagnostic techniques were developed and before the ability to accurately titrate the intravenous use of opioids. Now, several studies have concluded that the titrated use of low doses of opioids does not interfere with the diagnostic timing and accuracy.[38-40] Furthermore, many physicians have suggested that it actually improves the ability to make an accurate diagnosis by improving patient cooperation with examination. In the modern edition of the Cope text, the current author Silen stated that, "The cruel practice of withholding analgesics is to be condemned, but I suspect that it will take many generations to eliminate it because the rule has become so firmly ingrained in the minds of physicians."[41]

Several small studies have been conducted questioning the safety of administering opioid analgesics to children and adults with acute abdominal pain. Almost all of these studies have agreed that analgesic therapy provides relief of discomfort without compromising diagnosis or definitive therapy.[42,43]

When opioids are used in the treatment of abdominal pain, a few basic principles should be followed. The dosage of the opioid should be titrated to provide patient comfort but not to seek complete pain obliteration. While limiting the pain, the search for the cause and any change must be ongoing, often through repeat examinations, directed testing, surgical consultation, or close observation. Patients who have a resolution of pain should be observed for a few hours and be provided careful follow-up and discharge instructions if a nonemergency cause is found.

Nonopioid Analgesic Agents/ Nonsteroidal Anti-Inflammatory Drugs

Nonopioid analgesic agents are the most widely used analgesics in the practice of emergency medicine. The classification system for nonopioid analgesics is inexact. They have no anti-inflammatory activity, so they are not considered NSAIDs.

The mechanism of action of NSAIDs is thought to be inhibition of the cyclooxygenase enzyme and thereby interference with prostaglandin production. NSAIDs also inhibit production of leukotrienes. The pharmacologic actions and therapeutic advantage of giving NSAIDs are dependent on the degree to which selected prostaglandins and leukotrienes are inhibited. Prostaglandin inhibition accounts for the antipyretic and anti-inflammatory properties. A newer class of NSAID agents, cyclooxygenase 2 (COX-2) inhibitors, are now available. These agents offer similar analgesic and anti-inflammatory effects to those of nonselective (and usually cheaper) traditional NSAIDs, with a lower degree of gastric and renal side effects. The magnitude of the latter benefits is debated and likely small and seen in high-risk patients or with prolonged use. In the emergency department, they offer no particular advantage over traditional NSAIDs in treating acute pain or inflammatory syndromes.

The most commonly used of the nonopioid analgesic agents are aspirin, acetaminophen, and ibuprofen; however, more than 20 different NSAIDs are currently available in the United States. The most common emergency department indications for acetaminophen and NSAIDs include musculoskeletal pain, dysmenorrhea, and headache. They are also effective for pain associated with inflammation such as pericarditis and pleuritis.

The NSAIDs have become one of the mainstays of therapy in patients with renal colic. The inhibition of prostaglandin lessens renal capsule distention (through diminished renal blood flow) and ureteral peristalsis, causing less pain.[19] NSAIDs are also effective in providing some analgesia in patients with biliary colic.[44] Rather than decide between an NSAID and an opioid for colic syndromes, an optimal approach is to use both agents.

The Safety Myth

The widespread use of acetaminophen and NSAIDs is largely the result of the perceived safety of these drugs, especially less respiratory depression and abuse potential. Although these drugs lack the selected side effects of opioids, they are not problem free and can cause significant morbidity and even mortality. Even the safest of the nonnarcotic analgesic agents, acetaminophen, has serious side effects. Because NSAIDs are associated with numerous potentially serious side effects, they should be used only when considered to be particularly effective for a given type of pain and not automatically prescribed for all pain conditions because of the misperception that they are "safer than opioids."

Side Effects

As a group, and because of their wide use, NSAIDs are responsible for more serious drug-related side effects than any other class of analgesic drugs. The majority of these side effects occur in patients who are taking NSAIDs for chronic conditions. It is estimated that there are more than 100,000 hospital admissions and approximately 16,500 deaths each year from gastrointestinal bleeding related to NSAID use for osteoarthritis and rheumatoid arthritis.[45] One survey estimated that for every 100,000 people taking NSAIDs each year, there are 300 gastrointestinal-related deaths, 5 liver-related deaths, 4 renal-related deaths, and some number of congestive heart failure–related deaths.[46] The major side effects of NSAID analgesic agents are gastrointestinal bleeding, renal failure, anaphylaxis, and platelet dysfunction. Aspirin is not recommended as an antipyretic for children with viral syndromes because of its association with Reye's syndrome.

One of the little publicized theoretical concerns regarding NSAIDs is its potential inhibition of bone healing. Animal evidence suggests that prostaglandins promote bone formation and that NSAIDs might inhibit the process. Animal experiments have confirmed the inhibition of fracture healing, but human evidence is currently unconvincing.[47]

Routes of Administration

The NSAIDs can be administered by the oral, rectal, topical ophthalmic, and parenteral routes. Indomethacin (Indocin) suppositories are useful in treating patients unable to tolerate oral medications because of vomiting. Ketorolac tromethamine (Toradol) is the first NSAID analgesic agent available for intravenous and intramuscular use in the United States. It is not more effective in relieving pain than other NSAIDs at equipotent doses. A study comparing 60 mg of intramuscular ketorolac to 800 mg of oral ibuprofen showed no difference in the efficacy of analgesia for the treatment of acute musculoskeletal pain.[48] In general, ketorolac is best used only in cases in which a parenteral NSAID is required, such as renal colic.

Diclofenac ophthalmic solution has been shown to be effective in decreasing discomfort from corneal abrasions.[49]

Acetaminophen

Acetaminophen has analgesic and antipyretic properties due to actions on the CNS. It has been postulated that acetaminophen may act on the recently identified COX-3 enzyme in the brain.[50] The analgesic actions of acetaminophen are comparable to those of NSAIDs, and it may be that the combination of acetaminophen with an NSAID actually improves analgesia. Acetaminophen's lack of peripheral activity accounts for its absence of anti-inflammatory properties.

Acetaminophen is available in many formulations, including caplets, tablets, and liquid and rectal formulations. The recommended dose of acetaminophen for an adult is 325 to 1000 mg not to exceed 4000 mg/day. Acetaminophen is metabolized in the liver primarily through conjugation to sulfate or glucuronides. A minor pathway for the oxidative metabolism of acetaminophen produces the toxic metabolite *N*-acetyl-*p*-benzoquinoneimine (NAPQI). NABQI requires glutathione for detoxification and elimination. Hepatic toxicity can occur when glutathione pathways are overwhelmed by an increase in NAPQI or a decrease in glutathione. Hepatic toxicity is rare with ingestions less than 10 g in a 24-hour period unless underlying liver disease exists or concomitant alcohol abuse is ongoing. In the latter cases, therapeutic doses can cause clinical hepatotoxicity.[51] Acetaminophen toxicity is discussed in Chapter 146.

Ibuprofen

Ibuprofen is the most widely used drug in the NSAID class. It is now available over the counter in a variety of preparations, including tablets, liquid suspension, and suppository. Ibuprofen is rapidly absorbed in the upper gastrointestinal tract. It is an excellent analgesic and there is little reason to think other NSAIDs offer any particular analgesic advantage. Ibuprofen has minimal interaction with other medications.

COX-2 Specific Inhibitors

The NSAIDs produce analgesic, anti-inflammatory, and antipyretic effects primarily by altering production of leukotrienes (Figure 187-3). This is accomplished via inhibition of cyclooxygenase, which is present in two isoforms in humans (COX-1 and COX-2). Most traditional (or nonselective) NSAIDs block both of these isoforms, although at low doses COX-1 effects are more prominent. Each isoform is found in specific areas (Box 182-8). Another difference in these isoforms is in function and response to stimuli. COX-1 serves as a "clean up" or reparative agent in addition to anti-inflammatory and analgesic actions and is minimally increased after stimuli. COX-2 is normally present in lower levels but is inducible, and its levels are closely related to the response to stimuli, especially inflammation or injury.

Three agents, rofecoxib (Vioxx), celecoxib (Bextra), and valdecoxib (Celebrex), offer selective COX-2 inhibition and are approved for use in the United States. For practical purposes, these agents appear to share similar effect and side effect profiles, even though direct comparisons are lacking.

In September 2004, Merck announced a voluntary withdrawal of rofecoxib. Based on the APPROVe trial, there was a small but real increase for cardiovascular events, especially myocardial infarction and stroke in

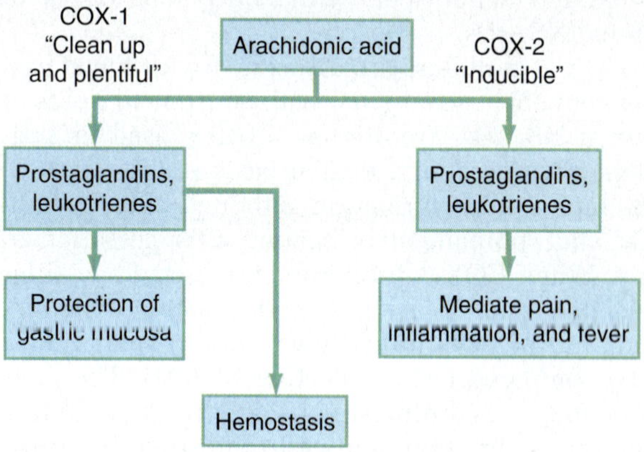

Figure 187-3. Mechanism of action of nonsteroidal anti-inflammatory drug.

BOX 187-8 Anatomic Distribution of COX-1 and COX-2

COX-1	COX-2
Synovium	Synovium
Stomach	Central nervous system
Platelets	Kidney (ascending limb of Henle, papillae)
Endothelial cells	Female reproductive tract
Kidney (arteries, arterioles, glomeruli, collecting ducts)	
Many other tissues	

patients who had been taking rofecoxib for 18 months. The FDA is currently investigating closely this entire class of drugs. Nonetheless, these data have little impact on emergency department prescribing practice, where COX-2 agents offer no real advantage over non-selective agents, given the short duration of usual therapy. Celecoxib can be started at 100 mg bid or 200 mg once daily.

The COX-2 inhibitors are eliminated primarily by the liver, with drug interactions similar to those seen with traditional NSAIDs (e.g., warfarin, lithium, angiotensin-converting enzyme inhibitors). Also, both agents (like traditional NSAIDs) can precipitate asthma, urticaria, and other allergic manifestations in patients with known aspirin hypersensitivity. Celecoxib is metabolized by the cytochrome P450 system and shares allergic potential with sulfonamides.

The major advantage of the COX-2 inhibitors is the ability to provide anti-inflammatory effects and moderate analgesia with less risk of gastrointestinal side effects compared with nonselective NSAIDs, albeit at a much higher cost per dose.[52] Although the Food and Drug Administration–approved indications for the COX-2 inhibitors are not identical, each appears effective in persistent inflammatory pain syndromes (osteoarthritis and rheumatoid arthritis) and other leukotriene-mediated pain syndromes (e.g., dysmenorrhea and postsurgical pain). Their role in other pain syndromes that are often either short-lived (e.g., sprain, renal and biliary colic) or non-leukotriene-mediated (e.g., headache or sickle cell vaso-occlusive crisis) is not well studied, although COX-2 inhibitors will likely afford similar relief seen with equipotent doses of traditional NSAIDs.

The COX-2 inhibitors are associated with fewer gastrointestinal effects compared with equipotent doses of traditional NSAIDs. Traditional NSAIDs used in anti-inflammatory doses on a regular basis produce a 10% to 20% rate of ulcer formation, although often asymptomatic and spontaneously healing after cessation of therapy. When COX-2 inhibitors are used for similar periods, the rate of *asymptomatic* gastric irritation, erosion, and ulcer is much lower (approximately 3% to 10%) compared to nonselective NSAIDs. The rates of symptomatic gastrointestinal side effects, including perforation, obstruction, and gastrointestinal bleeding, are also lower, but the difference is much smaller (2%-4% with traditional NSAIDs vs 0.5-2% with COX-2 inhibitors, depending on doses used and concomitant use of low-dose aspirin).[53]

The frequency of renal failure does not appear to be different between COX-2-inhibiting agents and traditional NSAIDs. COX-2 inhibitors also have limited effects on platelet function and bleeding time, although the benefit of this compared to traditional NSAID use in practice is not well defined.

Patients prescribed a COX-2 inhibitor should be counseled about potential side effects, including the smaller but still present risk of upper gastrointestinal bleed, and drug/disease interactions rather than assuming that risk is eliminated. In particular, higher doses of either selective or nonselective agents increase the risk of symptomatic gastric complications, as does use together with other irritative agents (e.g., low-dose aspirin or corticosteroids). COX-2 inhibitors are many times more expensive than their nonselective siblings, and infrequently offer an advantage to offset the additional cost.

General Guidelines for Nonopioid Analgesic Agents

Several general guidelines suggested by Kaplan may be useful when choosing a nonopioid analgesic agent[54]:

- Elderly patients are more likely to suffer adverse effects from NSAIDs than are younger patients.
- For most indications, there is little clinical evidence that any one of these agents is consistently more effective than another, but in some cases, the patient may respond to one nonopioid analgesic and not another.
- There is a 50-fold cost differential between some of the newer NSAIDs such as ketorolac, diclofenac, etodolac, ketoprofen, celecoxib, and rofecoxib, and the older NSAIDs, such as aspirin, acetaminophen, ibuprofen, and naproxen. In patients to whom cost is of concern, prices should be considered in selecting an agent.
- A number of dosages or regimens are available for NSAIDs: Piroxicam, oxaprozin, nabumetone, Naprelan (naproxen sodium), and rofecoxib can be administered once daily; regular naproxen, etodolac, sulindac, diflunisal, ketoprofen (Oruvail) extended release, and other selected salicylate derivatives can be administered twice daily. Sustained-release indomethacin and celecoxib can be administered once or twice daily.
- Most NSAIDs have potent anti-inflammatory actions. Those possessing no or only minimal anti-inflammatory action include acetaminophen and mefenamic acid.
- All NSAIDs have the potential for producing gastrointestinal distress. The least irritating NSAIDs appear to be nonacetylated salicylates, acetaminophen, ibuprofen, naproxen, and sulindac. The COX-2 NSAIDs offer little real safety benefit in short-term use (as is often prescribed in the emergency department). Hypersensitivity reactions can occur after initial administration or rechallenge with an NSAID. In aspirin-intolerant patients, it appears that acetaminophen has the lowest cross-reactivity.
- NSAIDs may interfere with the antihypertensive actions of numerous drugs.

Skeletal Muscle Relaxants

Skeletal muscle relaxants have been marketed as an adjunct to analgesics in the management of musculoskeletal pain with a "spasm" component, principally back pain. This practice has been based on a number of small, poorly designed studies, and there is currently no clear evidence that the addition of a skeletal muscle relaxant to an analgesic offers any superiority over the analgesic (in adequate doses) alone. In one small trial, 10 mg of cyclobenzaprine three times a day was compared in a double-blind fashion with ibuprofen 800 mg three times a day in 77 patients with acute myofascial strain secondary to minor trauma.[55] There was no difference in pain scores or satisfaction, but there was an increased incidence of side effects in the group receiving the cyclobenzaprine. A meta-analysis of "muscle relaxants" for low back pain concluded that in the 30 trials that met inclusion criteria, there was insufficient evidence to demonstrate with statistical likelihood that these agents are more effective than placebo for short-term relief. Evidence is strong, however, that they are associated with an increase in CNS side effects, particularly sedation.[56] Skeletal muscle relaxants should not be used in the management of acute musculoskeletal pain as a substitute for proper doses of effective analgesics. A benzodiazepine, offering sedation and anxiolysis, may be a reasonable adjunct in cases of particularly disabling or difficult pain.

Nitrous Oxide/Oxygen Mixtures

The analgesic and anesthetic properties of nitrous oxide were discovered more than 200 years ago. Combined with oxygen, a mixture of nitrous oxide and oxygen in a 50:50 ratio has been shown to be safe when self-administered by the patient. This technique is one of the original forms of patient-controlled analgesia. Nitrous oxide and oxygen administered by nasal mask have long been used by dentists. Experience in children would indicate that the nasal mask facilitates use in this group, but experience in emergency medicine with nitrous oxide has been greatest with self-administered hand-held masks in the ratio of 50:50.[57]

Basic Pharmacology and Physiology

In its pure form, nitrous oxide is a colorless gas that is heavier than air. It is nonflammable but supports combustion when mixed with oxygen. The most notable physical property important for its use as a medical gas is its ability to diffuse through membranes, although it is poorly soluble in blood. The actual mechanism of analgesia and anxiolysis has not been fully delineated.

In the two-tank, self-administered system, a fixed-ratio nitrous oxide/oxygen mixture is delivered to the patient through a demand valve activated when the patient inhales through a face mask or mouthpiece. A −3 to −5 cm H_2O pressure must be produced within the mask or mouthpiece to activate the flow of gas. This element provides the fail-safe and patient-controlled aspects of the system.

Physiologic effects of inhaling the gas mixture are slight with the low-dosage self-administered forms. No documented adverse hemodynamic effects have occurred with the self-administered forms of this agent. This safety has also been confirmed in the prehospital care setting.

The nitrous oxide to oxygen ratio must be adjusted for altitude because patients will not obtain adequate pain relief otherwise. At significant elevations (e.g., Denver, 5000 ft), nitrous oxide may need to be increased to 70%. This would mean, however, that oxygen concentration is only 30%, which can be a problem in patients who need a greater degree of oxygen supplementation.

In 10% to 15% of patients, nitrous oxide is ineffective.[57] It is much more potent as an anxiolytic than as an analgesic agent. As with all analgesic agents, its success should be determined by the patient's subjective feedback. When necessary, nitrous oxide should be supplemented with other analgesics.

Contraindications

Nitrous oxide-oxygen mixtures are relatively or absolutely contraindicated in the following patients:

- Those with altered consciousness or unable to follow instructions
- Patients with head injury
- Patients with decompression sickness

Patients with severe chronic obstructive pulmonary disease who retain CO_2 should be given nitrous oxide-oxygen mixtures carefully because the mixture contains 50% oxygen. Because nitrous oxide does diffuse into body cavities, it can worsen a pneumothorax or bowel obstruction. However, one swine experiment failed to show any hemodynamic compromise as a result of nitrous oxide administration in an experimental pneumothorax model.[58]

Side Effects

Minor side effects of the analgesic gas mixture have been reported in 5% to 50% of patients. Most common is light-headedness, with occasional patients complaining of paresthesias and nausea. Although the use of nitrous oxide for anesthesia has been associated for some years with nausea and vomiting, clinical experience and recent studies suggest that low-dosage forms do not cause a significant incidence of these complications. Side effects usually resolve within minutes of discontinuation.

Indications

Nitrous oxide/oxygen mixtures can be used in the emergency department or prehospital care setting to reduce anxiety in patients and to manage mild to moderate pain states. The gas mixture is particularly useful in the prehospital environment to provide safe and effective sedation and analgesia to injured patients, particularly those who are trapped or facing a long extrication or transport time. Patients in labor and those suffering burns, fractures, and other trauma also respond favorably to nitrous oxide. Even minor procedures (e.g., venipuncture) may be an indication for nitrous oxide if the patient is extremely apprehensive and has a significant aversion to needles.

Precautions

Nitrous oxide is a potent medication and should be dispensed with care and regard for patient and attendant safety. It should be used with a scavenging device to prevent trace concentrations in the environment being raised above National Institute of Occupational Safety and Health (NIOSH) standards. Roland and colleagues[59] showed a reduction in fertility among female dental assistants exposed to long periods of nitrous oxide at trace levels. Since that study, NIOSH has been very careful in recommending that scavenging devices be used routinely.[60] Scavenging devices are now available that collect exhaled air and remove it from the patient care areas. These devices can reduce nitrous oxide levels far below 1200 ppm, the level now considered standard for use with the agent in the emergency department.

Nitrous oxide levels in ambulances vary with the airflow within the patient compartment of the vehicle. If air conditioning or fans are operating and the ambulance is moving, trace levels of nitrous oxide are reduced to safe levels even without scavenging devices. Chronic use or abuse of nitrous oxide has been associated with B_{12} antagonism and secondary hematologic effects as well as development of a myelopathy.[61,62]

Concern regarding abuse by medical personnel familiar with nitrous oxide use exists, although no cases of repeated abuse have been reported in ambulance or emergency department settings. A strict protocol of accountability for its use must be in place in both settings. Such a protocol should balance security with ready availability so that clinicians will not be dissuaded from using the agent for pain relief in patients. A simple locking mechanism can be added to cylinders of the gas in the ambulance; in the emergency department, the delivery valve or mouthpiece can be locked in the drug box or opioid cupboard. After use of nitrous oxide, adults should not be allowed to drive a motor vehicle or operate machinery for at least 1 hour.

Nitrous oxide can be used carefully in conjunction with intravenous opioids, but the dosage of opioids should be lowered and the patient watched carefully. The problems of oversedation with analgesic therapy are not so great when the self-administered form of nitrous oxide is used. Some myocardial depression has been described with the combined use of nitrous oxide and opioids.

Local Anesthesia

Mechanism of Action

Peripheral nerves are responsible for transmitting pain information from the pain receptors to the spinal cord. Nerve fibers themselves vary in their anatomy and function. Each fiber consists of an axon surrounded by a covering called the Schwann cell. The Schwann cell can cover the axon in numerous ways. If several axons are covered by a single-layer projection of one Schwann cell, the nerve fiber is said to be *unmyelinated*. A *myelinated* axon is one that is covered by the projection of a Schwann cell that wraps itself many times around the axon. Hence, the myelinated fiber has a many-layered phospholipid cover called the *myelin sheath*.

Embedded in the phospholipid membrane are protein channels through which sodium and other ions can pass. An impulse is generated in the nerve fiber by a sudden influx of sodium ions through the protein channel, a process called *depolarization*. Repolarization follows, during which the resting transmembrane potential is reestablished through active transport mechanisms. Cutaneous pain receptors, when stimulated, cause sodium channels in the nerve endings to open, which depolarizes the nerve and causes the sensation of pain.

Local anesthetics are much more effective at penetrating unmyelinated or lightly myelinated fibers than heavily myelinated ones. This differential explains the fact that ordinarily local anesthetic agents provide sensory block without a motor block.

The effect of local anesthetic agents is the result of their ability to reversibly block the protein channel of the lipid membrane and therefore prevent the sudden influx of sodium ions into the axon (i.e., depolarization). Although other substances also can block the sodium channel, no substance does it as reliably, quickly, or effectively as local anesthetic agents, which do not have to be placed within the nerve because they penetrate the membrane on their own.

The sequence of events after injection of a local anesthetic begins when tissue buffers increase the pH of the agent, thus releasing some of its lipid-soluble base form. Its lipid solubility allows this nonionized moiety to penetrate the lipid membrane of the axon where it then ionizes and enters the sodium channel, thus blocking it. A receptor is likely associated with this process. In simple terms, the ionized form of the agent plugs up the channel. Such a mechanism does not explain the action of benzocaine, for example, which does not ionize. It may be that benzocaine-like drugs cause the channel to swell, thus blocking the passage of sodium ions.

Classes of Local Anesthetic Agents

Local anesthetic agents are chemical compounds that consist of an aromatic and an amine group separated by an intermediate chain. The class that has an ester link between the intermediate chain and aromatic portion are called amino esters; procaine, chloroprocaine, and tetracaine are the only ones in use today. Amides have an amide link and are more commonly used; lidocaine, mepivacaine, prilocaine, bupivacaine, and etidocaine are examples. Esters are unstable in solution and are metabolized in the body by the plasma enzyme cholinesterase. The amides, after absorption into the body, are destroyed by enzymes in the liver.[63]

Profiles

Each local anesthetic has a predictable effect when used in appropriate doses and by the appropriate route. The main considerations in the clinical use of these agents are potency, duration of anesthesia, and speed of onset (Table 187-7).

Potency

The ability of a local anesthetic drug to penetrate the lipid membrane of the axon determines its potency. Agents that have a high lipid solubility (e.g., tetracaine, etidocaine) are more potent than those with a low lipid solubility (e.g., procaine, mepivacaine).

Table 187-7. Characteristics of Common Local Anesthetic Agents

Agent	Trade Name(s)	Potency (Lipid Soluble)	Duration (min)	Onset	Comments
Procaine (ester)	Novocaine Neocaine	1	60-90	Slow	Solutions of 0.5%-2%; infiltration, blocks
Tetracaine (ester)	Pontocaine	8	180-600	Slow	Topical eye
Lidocaine (amide)	Xylocaine Dilocaine Ultracaine	3	90-200	Rapid	Most commonly used; 1½ times as toxic as procaine infiltration, blocks
Mepivacaine (amide)	Carbocaine	2.4	120-240	Very rapid	Slightly less potent than lidocaine; 75% as toxic as procaine infiltration, blocks, epidurals
Bupivacaine (amide)	Marcaine	8	180-600	Intermediate	Blocks; recent toxicity reported, now not used in emergency department for intravenous regional
Etidocaine (amide)	Duranest	6	180-600	Rapid	Twice as toxic as lidocaine blocks; epidurals

Modified from Paris PM, Weiss LD: Narcotic analgesics: The pure agonists. In Paris PM, Stewart RD (eds): *Pain Management in Emergency Medicine.* Norwalk, Conn, Appleton & Lange, 1988.

Duration of Anesthesia

Agents that bind well to protein in the sodium channel are longer acting and provide anesthesia of long duration. Tetracaine and bupivacaine have a high affinity for protein and provide long-lasting anesthesia, whereas procaine, poorly bound, does not.

Onset of Action

In most cases, it is helpful to have an anesthetic agent that acts quickly. The speed of onset of any local anesthetic agent is directly related to how quickly that agent, after injection, can diffuse through tissues to the nerve and through the nerve membrane to the axoplasm. After injection, the local anesthetic solution will be in two forms, ionized and nonionized. The percentage of the solution in the nonionized form is determined by the pKa of the agent (the pH at which 50% of the solution is nonionized and 50% is ionized). Because only the nonionized form of the agent will diffuse through membranes, solutions with a larger percentage of nonionized form at tissue pH have a more rapid onset of anesthesia. That is, local anesthetic agents with higher pKas take effect more slowly. At a tissue pH of 7.4, 5% of tetracaine (pKa 8.5) is in the nonionized form compared with 35% of lidocaine (pKa 7.9) solution. Low tissue pH (5 or 6) in surrounding infected tissue inhibits local anesthesia by direct infiltration in situations such as abscess incision and drainage, because the anesthetic is primarily in an ionized state.

Several other factors influence the clinical performance of local anesthetic agents. In the clinical dosages used, these agents (except cocaine) are vasodilators, which tend to shorten the duration of anesthesia. Injection of the solutions into vascular tissues not only shortens the duration of anesthesia but also increases systemic absorption and hence the chance of toxicity. For these reasons, a vasoconstrictor is sometimes added to local anesthetic solutions. Epinephrine, in a dose of 10 μg/mL (1:200,000), is the usual additive. Less bleeding occurs when this preparation is used.

Allergy

Patients sometimes provide a history of allergy to local anesthetic agents, but it is not an immunoglobulin-mediated true allergy. Allergy to ester agents has been reported and is most probably caused by the preservative methylparaben and its breakdown products. True allergy to the amide group is exceedingly rare. When allergy is reported, it is often caused by one of the preservatives used. Because the two groups do not cross-react, if a patient gives a history of allergy to an agent of one group, an agent from the other group can be used. A study of 236 patients with apparent adverse reactions to local anesthetics were tested using commercial preparations of unrelated local anesthetics. The study confirmed that no patient exhibited a systemic reaction.[64] In those patients who insist they are allergic to all "caine" anesthetic agents, and the allergy is believed to be legitimate (a very rare circumstance), diphenhydramine (Benadryl) can be used; 1 mL of a 50-mg/mL ampule can be diluted to 5 to 10 mL (1% to 0.5% solution) and can be used for local infiltration or nerve block. Diphenhydramine may cause direct tissue toxicity and should be avoided when possible in areas with poor collateral circulation (e.g., digits, penis, pinna, nose).[65]

Local and Systemic Toxicity

Many reactions to local anesthetic infiltration are autonomically mediated (e.g., vasodepressor syncope) attacks from the injection or from the inadvertent intravascular injection of an anesthetic solution containing epinephrine; however, both local and systemic toxicity can occur, even when these agents are injected locally.

Local Toxicity

Local anesthetic agents are directly toxic to tissue, depending on the concentration. The use of a vasoconstrictor in the anesthetic solution produces a reduction in blood flow that may theoretically increase

Table 187-8. Guidelines for Maximum Doses of Commonly Used Agents*

Agent	Without Epinephrine	With Epinephrine
Lidocaine HCl†	3-5 mg/kg	7 mg/kg
Mepivacaine HCl	8 mg/kg	7 mg/kg‡
Bupivacaine HCl§	1.5 mg/kg	3 mg/kg

*All maximum doses should be reduced 20% to 25% in very young, old, and very sick patients.
†A lidocaine level of 0.5 to 2.0 μg/mL may be reached for every 100 mg of lidocaine infiltrated for blocks.
‡Epinephrine adds to the potential cardiac toxicity of this drug.
§Not to be used for pudendal blocks or intravenous regional anesthesia. Not recommended for children younger than 12 years old.
Adapted from Stewart RD: Local anesthesia. In Paris PM, Stewart RD (eds): *Pain Management in Emergency Medicine.* Norwalk, Conn, Appleton & Lange, 1988.

BOX 187-9. Techniques that Can Be Used to Reduce the Pain of Injection

- Buffering of local anesthetic agents
- Countorirritation
- Changing size of needle used
- Slowing rate of injection
- Changing depth of injection
- Changing site of injection
- Use of topical anesthetics
- Warming solution
- Distraction techniques

the wound healing time and the vulnerability of the wound to infection, although this has never been demonstrated.

Although the evidence of direct local toxicity and the role of vasoconstriction in the healing of wounds are controversial, it is perhaps wise clinical practice to restrict the use of vasoconstrictors to well-vascularized areas and to ensure that wounds are well irrigated. Nerve blocks are preferable to local infiltration for wounds that are contaminated or old. Epinephrine-containing solutions have traditionally been taught to be contraindicated on digits, the penis, ears, or the nose. Recent literature, however, suggests that dilute epinephrine can be used safely on digits and possibly these other areas as well.[66,67] A comprehensive review of the use of epinephrine in digits has concluded that it was safe when diluted to 1:200,000 or less, but it should not be used in patients with vascular disease.[68]

Systemic Toxicity

All local anesthetics can produce systemic toxicity in high blood or CNS concentrations. Table 187-8 provides a rough guideline to safe doses that can be administered for local anesthesia. It must be remembered that these "safe doses" depend on the location and rate of administration. As little as 1 mL of local anesthetic injected into the vertebral artery during a stellate ganglion block can cause seizures, while much larger doses are well tolerated when used in infiltration. The more lipophilic agents (e.g., etidocaine, bupivacaine) are more cardiotoxic. Cardiac toxicity is also increased by the use of epinephrine.[63] Special care should be exercised in children and in performing certain blocks known to produce high blood levels (e.g., intercostal). In pediatric patients, total dose guidelines are important and the maximum dose must be calculated before administration.

Central Nervous System Toxicity. A wide variety of symptoms may be experienced by the patient with local anesthetic toxicity. These include light-headedness, headache, tingling of lips or tongue, drowsiness, ringing of ears, difficulty with concentration, abnormal body sensations, slurred speech, and twitches.[69] A very clear predicted relationship exists between the local anesthetic blood level and the CNS symptoms that are experienced. Increasing the intravenous dose of lidocaine from 1 mg/kg to 1.5 mg/kg increases the incidence of experiencing CNS subjective side effects from 10% to 80%. CNS toxicity may result in seizures. The clinical spectrum begins with drowsiness and progresses to confusion, convulsions, and coma. Direct intravascular injection of a large dose can provoke CNS symptoms, which usually begin with circumoral paresthesias, tinnitus, and light-headedness and progress to dysarthria, drowsiness, and tonic-clonic seizures. Longer-acting, more potent agents (e.g., bupivacaine and etidocaine) are more likely than lidocaine to cause CNS symptoms at lower blood levels.[69] Some classes of anticonvulsants (e.g., phenytoins [Dilantin]) are strikingly ineffective as prophylaxis or therapy for local anesthetic-induced seizures. The benzodiazepines work best for treating local anesthetic-induced seizures. Thiopental (pentothal), 50 to 100 mg IV, can also be used as an anticonvulsant.

Cardiovascular Effects. Local anesthetic agents have direct effects on cardiac automaticity, conductivity, contractility, and vascular tone. In animal experiments, the cardiac toxicity of bupivacaine is commonly seen before the CNS toxicity, and this toxicity is exacerbated by epinephrine.

Management of cardiovascular collapse caused by toxic levels of local anesthetic agents should follow standard advanced cardiac life support guidelines. Unless the overdose is massive, the toxicity should be relatively short-lived because of the redistribution of the lipophilic agents. Hypotension can be treated with fluids and α-adrenergic agents. Dysrhythmias that occur should be treated by standard algorithms.

Reducing the Pain of Injection

Counterirritation by scratching the skin or repetitive pinching of the skin during needle puncture or injection has been shown to reduce discomfort[70] (Box 187-9).

The addition of sodium bicarbonate to lidocaine immediately before injection significantly reduces patient discomfort.[71,72] A standard preload syringe of sodium bicarbonate (8.4% in 50 mL) can be used as a multidose vial and the bicarbonate added to a syringe containing lidocaine in a ratio of 1:10 (e.g., 1 mL bicarbonate to 10 mL lidocaine, or 0.5 mL to 5 mL). Buffered lidocaine can be kept in the emergency department and has been shown to stay effective for up to 1 week.[73] Slow injection of this combination can produce painless anesthesia. Bupivacaine (Marcaine) can also be buffered, but the ratio should be 1:50 (i.e., 0.1 mL bicarbonate to 5 mL bupivacaine). One study concluded that slow injection attenuates pain of infiltration to a greater degree than buffering of the solution.[74]

Injection of local anesthetic into the edges of the laceration has been shown to be less painful than injection through intact skin surrounding the wound.[75] On the other hand, subdermal injection requires more time to produce anesthesia, an effect not seen for at least 5 minutes. When time permits, warming the anesthetic or the application of a topical anesthetic agent can also greatly decrease the initial sensation associated with needle injection.[76,77]

Topical Anesthesia

Several agents are useful when applied to mucosal surfaces. Caution must be used, as 1% equals 10 mg/mL of the anesthetic. Therefore, a 5% solution has 50 mg/mL.

1. Cocaine: This agent is unique among local anesthetic agents because it is a potent vasoconstrictor and is therefore useful intranasally. A 4% (40 mg/mL) solution provides rapid and effective anesthesia for the treatment of epistaxis and other procedures on the nose. Higher concentrations are not necessary. Although the accurate dose is unknown, more than 200 mg should not be exceeded in adults. Cocaine should not be used in patients with known coronary artery disease because it may cause coronary artery vasoconstriction. It is also a component in TAC (tetracaine, epinephrine, and cocaine).
2. Lidocaine: This drug, used in 2% or 4% solution in a viscous matrix, can be useful in endoscopic procedures, including passing nasogastric tubes and gastric lavage tubes. It can be helpful in the cleansing of open abrasions and "road rash." Lidocaine jelly (2%) can be used for urethral anesthesia, but to be effective it must be injected into the urethra with a catheter-tip syringe and be in contact with the area for 5 to 20 minutes. Lidocaine spray (4%) has been demonstrated to decrease the discomfort of nasogastric tube insertion. Lidocaine spray (10%) is useful for upper airway anesthesia, including intranasal use. It is supplied in a metered-dose spray with a long delivery stem.
3. Tetracaine: This potent ester is used for surface anesthesia of the cornea (Pontocaine) and is a component of TAC solution.
4. Benzocaine: Almost insoluble in water, benzocaine is so poorly absorbed from mucous membranes that it is used commonly in intraoral preparations to dull the discomfort of needle puncture. It comes in various flavors.
5. TAC: The combination of tetracaine, adrenaline (epinephrine), and cocaine (TAC) was popular in the past, but has been largely replaced with LET and EMLA, which do not contain cocaine. Between 5 and 10 mL on sterile cotton is applied to the open wound, which is covered with gauze and held in place for 10 to 20 minutes. Complete anesthesia is evident in approximately 85% of cases of the scalp and face and a lower percentage of extremity wounds.[78] Application of the solution to the mucous membranes (eye, intranasal) can result in toxic blood levels of both tetracaine and cocaine; this complication has caused death.[79]
6. LET: A solution of lidocaine, epinephrine, and tetracaine (LET) has been studied in an attempt to find an effective topical anesthetic solution that avoids the potential complications of cocaine. The solution has been called LET, TLE, and LAT. The combination of tetracaine, lidocaine, and epinephrine is as effective and less expensive than TAC.[80-83] Since it requires 20 minutes for analgesia, one study showed success when the application was administered at the time of triage in children with a simple laceration.[84]
7. EMLA: EMLA is a *e*utectic *m*ixture of *l*ocal *a*nesthetic agents—namely, lidocaine and prilocaine—along with some other chemicals to allow the mixture to be kept in oil phase.[85] *Eutectic* refers to a property whereby combining the agents results in a melting point that is higher than that of either agent alone. The mixture is thickened to a cream that should be applied on the desired area with an occlusive dressing 30 to 60 minutes before the desired procedure is performed. Heating the EMLA for 20 minutes improves analgesia over 20 minutes without heat but is far less effective than a routine 60 minute application with or without heat.[86] After such application, local anesthesia is achieved for 1 to 5 hours. Possible indications for use of EMLA would be venipuncture, arterial puncture, lumbar puncture, or arthrocentesis when a 30- to 60-minute delay in performing the procedure is not an impediment. It may be particularly useful in children. The most significant side effect is the development of methemoglobinemia. Currently, EMLA is not recommended for use on mucous membranes or for skin wounds. In open wounds, EMLA has a theoretical disadvantage of decreasing local tissue defenses.[87] It has limited depth of penetration; hence, for many procedures, it is advantageous to inject an additional anesthetic.
8. Ethyl Chloride and Flori-Methane sprays: These sprays are occasionally used for limited skin incisions, e.g., small superficial abscess drainage. The agents evaporate quickly and supply a short lived (less than 1 minute) but effective local anesthetic. Any injection or incision should be made immediately after or even during the application of the agent.

The major advantage to the use of topical anesthesia is that it is well tolerated and nonthreatening, especially to children. Although its use in wounds is questioned because of animal work showing increased wound infection and problem with healing times, recent clinical experience refutes this claim.[87,88] It does demonstrate a benefit in starting intravenous lines, selected injection sites, and limited incisions.

Intravenous Regional Anesthesia (Bier Block)

The intravenous regional anesthesia procedure is an effective and rapid technique to anesthetize extremities for fracture reduction or repair of extensive wounds. The method involves the intravenous injection of a local anesthetic agent (lidocaine, prilocaine) into a previously exsanguinated limb. This procedure has been adapted for use in the emergency department in the form of a minidose of 100 mg of lidocaine. A safe alternative is to use the relatively nontoxic local anesthetic agent prilocaine.

Nonpharmacologic Interventions

Transcutaneous Electrical Nerve Stimulation

Physicians have attempted to treat pain with electricity since 46 AD, when Scribonus Largus used the electric eel to provide analgesia for headache, arthritis, and gout. Modern use of electric stimulation was greatly accelerated with the publication of the gate control theory by Melzack and Wall in 1965.[89] This theory suggests that the selective stimulation of large myelinated A fibers closes a spinal cord gate, thereby inhibiting pain transmission of small unmyelinated C fibers.

The basic components of a transcutaneous electric nerve stimulation system include a pulse generator, amplifier, and electrodes. Most transcutaneous electric nerve stimulation generators are capable of producing electric impulses with different waveforms, pulse widths, and frequencies. Some are also capable of modulating the patterns of stimulation. More simple and inexpensive disposable devices better suited to the practice of emergency medicine are also available.[90] While transcutaneous electric nerve stimulation has been successfully used in a variety of acute pain conditions such as fractured ribs and acute myofascial pain secondary to injury, it has not been well studied in emergency medicine.[91]

Hypnosis

Trance can be accomplished quickly in the emergency department. The induction of trance allows the patient to refocus attention away from pain and anxiety-producing stimuli to other images and feelings. Hypnosis can be used as an adjunct to pharmacologic interventions or, in some cases, as a substitute. Trance can often be induced after the clinician utters just a few sentences.[92]

When using nitrous oxide, patients are susceptible to suggestion. The clinician can enhance the efficacy of nitrous oxide administration by taking advantage of the trance and using the techniques of guided imagery and posthypnotic suggestion. Even when trance induction is not formally attempted, the verbal skills used in hypnosis can be valuable in most therapeutic encounters.

Psychological Techniques

One of the most neglected aspects of the treatment of pain is the attention to the psychological factors involved in reaction to a given painful stimulus and the use of proper communication techniques to ameliorate pain and suffering. Patients who present to the emergency department in pain are focused on the painful stimuli and the threatening, unfamiliar environment of the hospital. They are frightened by the loss of control and fear of what the pain represents. By recognizing these patient concerns and establishing a trusting physician-patient relationship, the physician can mitigate reactions to a given painful stimulus and lessen the suffering.

Attempts should be made to distract patients from the pain of their condition or procedures they must undergo. Providing patients with a portable stereo cassette player and their choice of music lessens their pain during laceration repair.[93]

Pain Management in Children

Several studies have shown that children are less likely than adults to receive analgesic agents for their painful conditions. Although safety should be a primary concern with any therapeutic intervention, when used properly most of the techniques described in this chapter can be adapted to use in children. Overall, the same general principles that apply to providing analgesia to adults apply to children. The major difference in providing analgesia to children is the difficulty of accurately assessing subjective sensation of pain, particularly in the very young. The most common indication for providing analgesia in children in an emergency department is for procedural analgesia and sedation. The same drugs used for analgesia in adults are safe in children in size- and age-adjusted doses.

The general approach to a child can be important in developing a trusting relationship with both child and parent. Techniques in communicating with children should take into account the unique developmental aspects of each age group. Words should be chosen carefully, with care taken to avoid threatening words. All equipment (e.g., syringes, scissors, and suture holders) should be kept out of sight of the child. Play therapy and a slow, friendly, nonthreatening manner can be invaluable. The decision to separate children from their parents must be individualized, but many authorities suggest avoiding the separation when possible. Parents can help distract the child and reinforce the suggestions of the medical team.

Children deserve even more attention than adults with regard to safe and effective analgesia because their early experiences will affect their lifelong outlook and trust in the medical profession. Recently, there has been much interest in providing children analgesia and sedation by less threatening routes of administration. Transmucosal fentanyl in the form of lollipops and transnasal butorphanol and transnasal midazolam are examples.

Pediatric Pharmacology

Most of the principles relating to the pharmacokinetics of drugs, including absorption, distribution, and elimination, are similar for children and adults.[94] In neonates and infants younger than 3 months old, clearance of opioids may be slow compared with older children. Opioids in this age group may also have a greater effect because of decreased protein binding, resulting in higher levels of free drug, and an immature blood-brain barrier that allows passage of a greater degree of opioid. These patients need to have lower dosages of local anesthetics because of decreased protein binding and decreased metabolism. For mild pain, acetaminophen can be very effective in doses of 15 mg/kg orally or 20 mg/kg rectally every 4 hours. Aspirin is also an excellent analgesic but should be avoided during febrile illnesses because of the possible relationship to Reye's syndrome. Tolectin, ibuprofen, and naproxen are officially approved for use in children and are probably equally efficacious for painful conditions.

Pain Management in the Elderly

Approximately 80% of elderly patients have at least one chronic ailment commonly associated with pain.[95] Many studies have attempted to determine whether people lose pain sensitivity with increasing age, but results have varied with different experimental models. Extra caution must be taken to avoid side effects when using analgesic agents in elderly patients. This group needs lower dosages of opioid analgesic agents. In addition, opioids seem to produce sedation and constipation more often. NSAIDs must also be used cautiously in this group because of the many potentially serious side effects (e.g., worsening renal function and gastrointestinal bleeding).

Prehospital Analgesia

Because the prehospital environment is less controlled, safety becomes of paramount importance during analgesic administration. The basic tenets of establishing rapport with the patient, providing reassurance, using gentle movement and handling, using proper splinting, and controlling the temperature are the groundwork on which pharmacologic support can be added.[96]

Unfortunately, despite protocols allowing for use of drugs such as nitrous oxide and opioids, moderate to severe pain is treated in only the minority of patients in the prehospital environment.[97] The study of lower extremity or hip fractures showed that only 18% of patients received an analgesic.[98] Another study of suspected extremity fractures showed that despite a protocol allowing the use of either morphine sulfate or nitrous oxide, among 1073 patients analgesia was administered to only 18 patients (1.8%). These studies have led the National Association of EMS Physicians to publish a position paper encouraging more liberal use of analgesics in the prehospital environment.[99]

Self-administered 50% nitrous oxide offers many advantages for use in the field. Opioids also should be used when indicated. For the pain of myocardial ischemia, morphine should be titrated. Nalbuphine also has been described as safe and effective in the field treatment of trauma patients.[30]

In disaster and war situations, ketamine has been described as a useful analgesic agent in the field. Fentanyl has been shown to be a safe analgesic agent in prehospital air medicine use.

KEY CONCEPTS

- Pain is best treated early; untreated or undertreated pain begets more pain. A corollary is not to allow previous relief to completely vanish before redosing (whether orally or parenterally).
- Analgesia and a search for the cause of pain should happen in tandem; withholding pain relief until diagnostic certainty exists is inhumane and may impede the evaluation.
- Pain scales should be used routinely, and continuous quality improvement programs should be based on adequacy of pain therapy.
- Unrelieved pain is associated with a long list of negative psychological and physiologic outcomes.
- Titrated opioid analgesics should be the mainstay of emergency department therapy of moderate to severe pain.
- For the majority of opioid indications in the emergency department, morphine is a suitable agent.
- The NSAIDs are effective in a wide variety of acute pain states but also have a wide variety of significant side effects that need to be considered when used for more than 1 or 2 days.
- COX-2 specific inhibitors are much more expensive than NSAIDs but do offer the advantage of less risk of gastrointestinal side effects, particularly in selected patients.
- Topical and local anesthetics can be used to prevent or ameliorate discomfort associated with the majority of the emergency department procedures.

REFERENCES

1. Ducharme J: Acute pain in pain control: state of the art. *Ann Emerg Med* 35:592, 2000.
2. Tanabe P, Buschmann M: A prospective study of ED pain management practices and the patient's perspective. *J Emerg Nurs* 25:171, 1999.
3. Berthier F, et al: Comparative study of methods measuring acute pain intensity in an ED. *Am J Emerg Med* 16:132, 1998.
4. Fosnocht DE, Swanson ER, Bossert P: Patient expectations for pain medication delivery. *Am J Emerg Med* 19:399, 2001.
5. Weisman SJ, Bernstein B, Schechter NL: Consequences of inadequate analgesia during painful procedures in children. *Arch Pediatr Adolesc Med* 152:147, 1998.
6. Bry PH, Dahl JL: The new JCAHO pain standards: Implications for pain management nurses. *Pain Mgmt Nurs* 1:3, 2000.
7. Hough SW, Portenoy RS: Medical management of cancer pain. In Warfield CA, Bajwa ZH (eds): *Principles & Practices of Pain Medicine*, 2nd ed. New York, McGraw Hill, 2004, pp 465-476.
8. Hobbs GJ, Hodgkinson V: Assessment, measurement, history, and examination. In Rowbotham DJ, Macintyre PE

(ed): *Clinical Pain Management: Acute Pain.* New York, Oxford University Press, 2003, pp 93-112.
9. Bijur PE, Latimer CT, Gallagher EJ: Validation of a verbally administered numerical rating scale of acute pain use in the emergency department. *Acad Emerg Med* 10:390, 2003.
10. Ready LB, Edwards WT: *Management of Acute Pain: A Practical Guide.* Seattle, IASP Publications, 1992.
11. Marquie L, et al: Pain rating by patients and physicians: Evidence of systemic miscalibration. *Pain* 102:289, 2003.
12. Ducharme J, Barbar C: A prospective blinded study on emergency pain assessment of therapy. *J Emerg Med* 15:571, 1995.
13. Brown JC, et al: Emergency department analgesia for fracture pain. *Ann Emerg Med* 42:197, 2003.
14. Rupp T, Delaney KA: Inadequate analgesia in emergency medicine. *Ann Emerg Med* 43:494, 2004.
15. Silka PA, Roth MM, Geiderman JM: Patterns of analgesic use in trauma patients in the ED. *Am J Emerg Med* 20:298, 2002.
16. Jantos TJ, et al: Analgesic practice for acute orthopedic trauma in Costa Rican emergency departments [abstract]. *Prehospital Disaster Med* 1:A43, 1994.
17. Borland ML, Jacobs I, Geelhoed G: Intranasal fentanyl reduces acute pain in children in the emergency department: A safety and efficacy study. *Emerg Med* 14:275, 2002.
18. Bartfield JM, Flint RD, McErlean M, Broderick J: Nebulized fentanyl for relief of abdominal pain. *Acad Emerg Med* 10:215, 2003.
19. Jaffe JH, Martin WR: Opioid analgesics and antagonists. In Gilman AG, et al (eds): *The Pharmacological Basis of Therapeutics,* 10th ed. New York, McGraw-Hill, 2001, pp 569-619.
20. Porter J, Jick H: Addiction rare in patients treated with narcotics. *N Engl J Med* 302:123, 1980.
21. Geiderman JM: Keeping lists and naming names: Habitual patient files for suspected nontherapeutic drug-seeking patients. *Ann of Emerg Med* 41:873, 2003.
22. Schutzman SA: Comparison of oral transmucosal fentanyl citrate and intramuscular meperidine, promethazine and chlorpromazine for conscious sedation for children undergoing laceration repair. *Ann Emerg Med* 28:385, 1996.
23. Portenoy RK, et al: Oral transmucosal fentanyl citrate (OTFC) for the treatment of breakthrough pain in cancer patients: A controlled dose, titration study. *J Pain* 79:303, 1999.
24. Melzer-Lange MD, et al: Patient controlled analgesia for sickle cell pain crisis in a pediatric emergency department. *Ped Emerg Care* 20:2, 2004.
25. Weiner AL: Meperidine as a potential cause of serotonin syndrome in the emergency department. *Acad Emerg Med* 6:156, 1999.
26. Chudnofsky CR, et al: The safety of fentanyl use in the emergency department. *Ann Emerg Med* 18:635, 1989.
27. Schutzman SA: Comparison of oral transmucosal fentanyl citrate and intramuscular meperidine, promethazine and chlorpromazine for conscious sedation for children undergoing laceration repair. *Ann Emerg Med* 28:385, 1996.
28. Vercauteren M, et al: Intranasal sufentanil for preoperative sedation. *Anaesthesia* 43:270, 1988.
29. Schmidt WK, et al: Nalbuphine. *Drug Alcohol Depend* 14:339, 1985.
30. Hyland-Mcguire P, Guly HR: Effects on patient care of introducing prehospital intravenous nalbuphine hydrochloride. *J Accident Emerg Med* 15:99, 1998.
31. Gillis JC, Benfield P, Goa KL: Transnasal butorphanol: A review of the pharmacodynamic and pharmacokinetic properties, and therapeutic potential in acute pain management. *Drugs* 38:225, 1989.
32. O'Briens JJ, Benfield P: Dezocine: A preliminary review of its pharmacodynamic and pharmacokinetic properties and therapeutic efficacy. *Drugs* 38:225, 1989.
33. Kosten TR, et al: Buprenorphine for cocaine and opiate dependence. *Psychopharmacol Bull* 28:15, 1992.
34. Mitka M. Abuse of prescription drugs. Is a patient ailing or addicted? *JAMA* 283:1126, 2000.
35. Lehmann KA: Tramadol for the management of acute pain. *Drugs* 47:19, 1994.
36. Moore PA: Pain management in dental practice: Tramadol vs. codeine combinations. *J Am Dent Assoc* 130:1075, 1999.
37. Turturro MA, Paris PM, Larkin GL: Tramadol versus hydrocodone-acetaminophen in acute musculoskeletal pain: A randomized, double blind clinical trial. *Ann Emerg Med* 32:139, 1998.
38. Mackway-Jones K: Analgesia and assessment of abdominal pain. J Accid Emerg Med 17:128, 2000.
39. Brewster GS, Herbert ME, Hoffman JR: Medical myth: Analgesia should not be given to patients with an acute abdomen because it obscures the diagnosis. *West J Med* 172:209, 2000.
40. Vermeulen B, et al: Acute appendicitis: Influence of early pain relief on the accuracy of clinical and US findings in the decision to operate: a randomized trial. *Radiology* 210:639, 1999.
41. Silen W: *Cope's Early Diagnosis of the Acute Abdomen,* 21st ed. New York, Oxford University Press, 2004.
42. Kim MK, Straite RT, Sato TT, Hennes HM: A randomized clinical trial of analgesia of children with abdominal pain. *Acad Emerg Med* 9:281, 2002.
43. Thomas SH, Silen W: Effect on diagnostic efficiency of analgesia for undifferentiated abdominal pain. *Br J Surg* 90:5, 2003.
44. Henderson SO, Swadron S, Newton E: Comparison of intravenous ketolorac and meperidine in the treatment of biliary colic. *J Emerg Med* 23:237, 2003.
45. Singh G: Recent considerations in nonsteroidal anti-inflammatory drug gastropathy. *Am J Med* 105:31S, 1998.
46. Hernadez-Diaz S: Epidemiologic assessment of the safety of conventional nonsteroidal anti-inflammatory drugs. *Am J Med* 110:20, 2001.
47. Do NSAIDs inhibit bone healing? In Moore A, Edwards J, Barden J, McQuay H (eds): *Bandolier's Little Book of Pain.* New York, Oxford University Press, 2003, pp 153-160.
48. Turturro MA, et al: Intramuscular ketorolac versus oral ibuprofen in acute musculoskeletal pain. *Ann Emerg Med* 26:117, 1995.
49. Szucs PA, et al: Safety and efficacy of diclofenac ophthalmic solution in the treatment of corneal abrasions. *Ann Emerg Med* 35:131, 2000.
50. Schwab JM, Schluesener HJ, Laufer S: COX-3: Just another COX or the solitary elusive target of paracetamol? *Lancet* 361:981, 2003.
51. Matin A, Williams R: Paracetamol hepatotoxicity and alcohol consumption in deliberate and accidental overdose. *Q J Med* 93:341, 2000.
52. Wolfe M, Lichtenstein D, Singh G: Gastrointestinal toxicity of nonsteroidal anti-inflammatory drugs. *N Engl J Med* 340: 1888, 1999.
53. Silverstein FE, et al: Gastrointestinal toxicity with celecoxib vs. nonsteroidal anti-inflammatory drugs for osteoarthritis and rheumatoid arthritis. *JAMA* 284:1247, 2000.
54. Kaplan R: Non-narcotic analgesia. In Paris PM, Grass J (eds): *Textbook of Acute Pain Management.* Philadelphia, WB Saunders, private communication.
55. Turturro MA, Frater CR, D'Amico FJ: Cyclobenzaprine with ibuprofen versus ibuprofen alone in acute myofascial strain: A randomized, double-blind clinical trial. *Ann Emerg Med* 41:818, 2003.
56. van Tulder MW, et al: Muscle relaxants for nonspecific low back pain: A systematic review within the framework of the Cochran collaboration. *Spine* 28:1978, 2003.

57. Annequin D, et al: Fixed 50% nitrous oxide oxygen mixture for painful procedures: A French survey. *Pediatrics* 105: 850, 2000.
58. Seaberg DC, Yealy DM, Ilkhanipour K: Effective nitrous analgesia on a pneumothorax. *Acad Emerg Med* 2:287, 1995.
59. Roland AS, et al: Reduced fertility among the women employed as dental assistants exposed to high levels of nitrous oxide. *N Engl J Med* 327:993, 1992.
60. US Department of Health and Human Services: Controlling exposures to nitrous oxide during anesthetic administration. *NIOSH Alert.* Washington, D.C., US Department of Health and Human Services, 1994.
61. Butzkueven H, King JO: Nitrous oxide myelopathy in an abuser of whipped cream bulbs. *J Clin Neurosci* 7:73, 2000.
62. Ogundipe O, et al: Sickle cell disease and nitrous oxide-induced neuropathy. *Clin Lab Haematol* 21:409, 1999.
63. Covino BG: Pharmacology of local anesthetic agents. *Br J Anaesth* 58:701, 1986.
64. Berkun Y, et al: Evaluation of adverse reactions to local anesthetics: Experience with 236 patients. *Ann Allergy Asthma Immunol* 91:342, 2003.
65. Green SM, Rothrock SG, Gorchynski J: Validation of diphenhydramine as a dermal local anesthetic. *Ann Emerg Med* 23:1284, 1994.
66. Sylaidis P, Logan A: Digital blocks with adrenaline: An old dogma refuted. *J Hand Surg [Br]* 1:17, 1998.
67. Wilhelmi BJ, et al: Epinephrine in digital blocks: Revisited. *Ann Plast Surg* 41:410, 1998.
68. Kenkler K: A comprehensive review of epinephrine in the finger: To do or not to do. *Plast Reconstr Surg* 108:114, 2001.
69. de Jong RH: *Local Anesthetics.* St Louis, Mosby, 1994.
70. Fosko SW, Gibney MD, Harrison B: Repetitive pinching of the skin during lidocaine infiltration reduces patient discomfort. *J Am Acad Dermatol* 39:74, 1998.
71. Bartfield JM, Ford DT, Homer PJ: Buffered versus plain lidocaine for digital nerve blocks. *Ann Emerg Med* 22:216, 1993.
72. Ong EL, Lim NL, Koay CK: Towards a pain-free venipuncture. *Anaesthesia* 55:260, 2000.
73. Fatovich DM, Jacobs IG: A randomized controlled trial of buffered lidocaine for local anesthetic infiltration in children and adults with simple lacerations. *J Emerg Med* 17:223, 1999.
74. Scarfone RJ, Jasani M, Gracely EJ: Pain of local anesthetics: Rate of administration and buffering. *Ann Emerg Med* 31:30, 1998.
75. Bartfield JM, Sokaris SJ, Raccio-Robak N: Local anesthesia for lacerations: Pain of infiltration inside vs. outside the wound. *Acad Emerg Med* 5:100, 1998.
76. Mader TJ, Playe SJ, Garb JL: Reducing the pain of local anesthetic infiltration: Warming and buffering have a synergistic effect. *Ann Emerg Med* 23:550, 1994.
77. Pryor GJ, Kilpatrick WR, Opp DR: Local anesthesia in minor lacerations: Topical TAC vs lidocaine. *Ann Emerg Med* 9:568, 1980.
78. Hegenbarth MA, et al: Comparison of topical tetracaine, adrenaline, and cocaine anesthesia with lidocaine infiltration for repair of lacerations in children. *Ann Emerg Med* 19:63, 1990.
79. Dailey RH: Fatality secondary to misuse of TAC solution. *Ann Emerg Med* 17:159, 1988.
80. Ernst AA, et al: Topical lidocaine adrenaline tetracaine (LAT gel) versus injectable buffered lidocaine for local anesthesia in laceration repair. *West J Med* 167:79, 1997.
81. Blackburn PA, et al: Comparison of tetracaine-adrenaline-cocaine (TAC) with topical lidocaine-epinephrine (TLE): Efficacy and cost. *Am J Emerg Med* 13:315, 1995.
82. Ernst AA, et al: LAT (lidocaine-adrenaline-tetracaine) versus TAC (tetracaine-adrenaline-cocaine) for topical anesthesia in face and scalp lacerations. *Am J Emerg Med* 13:151, 1995.
83. Schilling CG, et al: Tetracaine, epinephrine (adrenaline), and cocaine (TAC) versus lidocaine, epinephrine, and tetracaine (LET) for anesthesia of lacerations in children. *Ann Emerg Med* 25:203, 1995.
84. Priestley S, et al: Application of topical local anesthetic at triage reduces treatment time for children with lacerations: A randomized controlled trial. *Ann Emerg Med* 42:34, 2003.
85. Gagrag NM, Pennant JH, Watcha MF: Eutectic mixture of local anesthetics (EMLA cream). *Anesth Analg* 78:574, 1994.
86. Liu DR, Kirchner HL, Petrack EM: Does using heat with eutectic mixture of local anesthetic cream shorten analgesic onset time? A randomized, placebo-controlled trial. *Ann Emerg Med* 42:27, 2003.
87. Powell DM, et al: Damage to tissue defenses by EMLA cream. *J Emerg Med* 9:205, 1991.
88. Martin JR, et al: The effect of local anesthetics on bacterial proliferation: TAC versus lidocaine. *Ann Emerg Med* 19:987, 1990.
89. Melzack R, Wall PD: Pain mechanisms: A new theory. *Science* 150:971, 1965.
90. Merrill DC: Clinical evaluation of FasTENS, an inexpensive, disposable transcutaneous electrical nerve stimulator designed specifically for postoperative electroanalgesia. *Urology* 33:27, 1989.
91. Nash TP: Transcutaneous electrical nerve stimulation. In Rice ASC, Warfield CA, Justins D, Eccleston C (eds): *Clinical Pain Management: Practical Applications & Procedures.* London, Arnold, 2003, pp 343-354.
92. Bierman SF: Hypnosis in the emergency department. *Am J Emerg Med* 7:238, 1989.
93. Menegazzi JJ, et al: A randomized controlled trial of the use of music during laceration repair. *Ann Emerg Med* 20:348, 1991.
94. Berde CB, Sethna N, Koka BV: Pediatric pain management. In Warfield CA (ed): *Principles and Practice of Pain Management,* New York, McGraw-Hill, 1993, pp 325-346.
95. Nation EM, Warfield CA: Pain in the elderly. *Hosp Pract* 4:113, 1989.
96. Stewart RD: Pain control in prehospital care. In Paris PM, Stewart RD (eds): *Pain Management in Emergency Medicine.* Norwalk, Conn, Appleton & Lange, 1988, pp 313-322.
97. Turturro M: Pain, priorities and prehospital care. *Prehosp Emerg Care* 6:486, 2002.
98. McEachin CC, McDermott JT, Swor R: Few emergency medical services patients with lower-extremity fractures receive prehospital analgesia. *Prehosp Emerg Care* 6:406, 2002.
99. Alonso-Serra HM, Wesley K: National association of EMS physicians standards and clinical practices committee. *Prehosp Emerg Care* 7:482, 2003.

CHAPTER

188 Procedural Sedation and Analgesia

Carl R. Chudnofsky and Marie M. Lozon

Performing painful diagnostic and therapeutic procedures has become a routine aspect of emergency department care. Accordingly, the ability to safely provide adequate sedation and analgesia for patients of all ages has become a necessary skill for emergency physicians.[1,2]

Procedural sedation and analgesia (PSA) is the use of analgesic, dissociative, or sedative agents to prevent the pain, anxiety, and unpleasant memories associated with painful diagnostic and therapeutic procedures. All of the agents used for PSA have the potential for serious adverse effects, including respiratory depression and cardiovascular compromise (Table 188-1). This chapter presents an overview of sedation and analgesia for procedures. Recommendations are based on current medical evidence whenever possible. Where no evidence exists, practice guidelines and consensus opinions are provided.

TERMINOLOGY

The Sedation Continuum

The progression from mild sedation to general anesthesia represents a dynamic *continuum* that lacks distinct separation between stages (Figure 188-1). Low doses of sedative-hypnotic agents induce mild sedation, with little danger of adverse events. However, as more medication is administered, the patient will move along the sedation continuum, experiencing a progressive decline in level of consciousness with an attendant risk of adverse respiratory and cardiovascular events. If medication administration continues, the patient will ultimately reach a state of general anesthesia with loss of protective airway reflexes and ventilatory drive.[3]

The transition from one level of sedation to the next is often difficult to predict and will vary from patient to patient. Moreover, the sedation continuum is not drug-specific, in that varying states from mild sedation to general anesthesia can be achieved with virtually all nondissociative PSA agents (e.g., opioids, benzodiazepines, barbiturates, etomidate, propofol).[3]

Definitions

Prior to 2001, three levels of sedation were defined: *conscious sedation*, *deep sedation*, and *general anesthesia*.[4,5] According to guidelines published by the American Academy of Pediatrics in 1985, conscious sedation requires the patient to respond purposefully to verbal command or physical stimulus.[4] Despite this requirement, the term *conscious sedation* soon became the catchall for describing all levels of sedation, including deep sedation in which the patient is not easily aroused and during which there is a higher risk for loss of protective airway reflexes and spontaneous respiration. By the late 1990s, it became clear to most clinicians that the term *conscious sedation* was really an oxymoron, particularly in pediatrics, where the goal of sedation is often complete sleep and immobility.[6] Thus, although historically popular, the widely misinterpreted and misused term *conscious sedation* has been discarded.

In 2001 the Joint Commission on the Accreditation of Healthcare Organizations (JCAHO) adopted new sedation terminology and definitions that more closely reflect the current state of PSA.[7] These new terms—*minimal sedation*, *moderate sedation*, *deep sedation*, and *general anesthesia*—are defined in Box 188-1. The new definitions provide much clearer descriptions of the varying states and degrees of sedation and have been accepted by most specialty societies.[1,8,9] A fifth category of sedation, *dissociative sedation*, has been advocated to describe the level of sedation achieved with the use of ketamine.[10]

APPROACH TO SEDATION AND ANALGESIA FOR PROCEDURES

Preprocedure Patient Assessment

There have been no studies evaluating the relationship between PSA outcome and preprocedure patient evaluations. Nevertheless, an increased risk of adverse events may exist in select subsets of patients such as the elderly, those with abnormal facial or neck anatomy, and patients with underlying cardiopulmonary disease.[1,8] Consequently, most practice guidelines recommend (and the JCAHO requires) a history and focused physical examination prior to PSA.[7,8]

Important historical information includes the patient's age; comorbid illness and injuries; underlying medical problems; previous problems with PSA and general anesthesia; drug allergies and current medications; and tobacco, drug, and alcohol use. The physical examination should focus on vital signs, auscultation of the heart and lungs, and evaluation of the airway for a potentially difficult intubation or difficulty providing bag/mask ventilation (see Chapter 1). There is no literature to support the need for specific laboratory or radiologic testing prior to PSA. Diagnostic testing should be guided by the patient's underlying medical

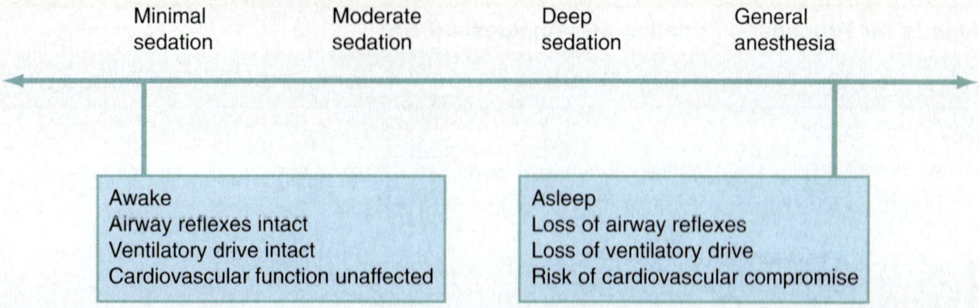

Figure 188-1. Schematic representation of the sedation continuum. As increasing doses of nondissociative agents are given, patients move along the sedation continuum, experiencing a progressive decline in their level of consciousness and an increased risk of adverse respiratory and cardiovascular events. If medication administration continues, the patient will ultimately reach a state of general anesthesia with loss of protective airway reflexes and ventilatory drive. The transition from one level of sedation to the next is often difficult to predict and varies from patient to patient.

BOX 188-1. Current PSA Terminology and Definitions

*Minimal sedation** (anxiolysis): A drug-induced state during which patients respond normally to verbal commands. Although cognitive function and coordination may be impaired, ventilatory and cardiovascular functions are unaffected.

*Moderate sedation** (formerly "conscious sedation"): A drug-induced depression of consciousness during which patients respond purposefully to verbal commands, either alone or accompanied by light tactile stimulation. Reflex withdrawal from a painful stimulus is not considered a purposeful response. No interventions are required to maintain a patent airway, and spontaneous ventilation is adequate. Cardiovascular function is usually maintained.

Deep sedation:* A drug-induced depression of consciousness during which patients cannot be easily aroused but respond purposefully following repeated or painful stimulation. The ability to independently maintain ventilatory function may be impaired. Patients may require assistance in maintaining a patent airway and spontaneous ventilation may be inadequate. Cardiovascular function is usually maintained.

General anesthesia:* A drug-induced loss of consciousness during which patients are not arousable, even by painful stimulation. The ability to independently maintain ventilatory function is often impaired. Patients often require assistance in maintaining a patent airway, and positive pressure ventilation may be required because of depressed spontaneous ventilation or drug-induced depression of neuromuscular function. Cardiovascular function may be impaired.

Dissociative Sedation†: A trancelike cataleptic state induced by the dissociative agent ketamine characterized by profound analgesia and amnesia, with retention of protective airway reflexes, spontaneous respirations, and cardiopulmonary stability.

*Joint Commission on Accreditation of Healthcare Organizations: *Accreditation Manual for Hospitals.* Oakbrook Terrace, Ill, Joint Commission on Accreditation of Healthcare Organizations, 2001.
†Green SM, Krauss B: The semantics of ketamine. *Ann Emerg Med* 36:480, 2000.

condition and the likelihood that the results will affect some aspect of PSA.[1,8]

Procedural sedation and analgesia should be avoided or delayed in patients with hemodynamic instability or respiratory distress. These patients require stabilization (e.g., fluid resuscitation, endotracheal intubation) before PSA. Similarly, patients with severe ischemic heart disease or chronic obstructive pulmonary disease may benefit from anesthesia consultation and definitive care in the operating room. Certain procedures, although possible in the emergency department, may be more efficiently and safely performed in the operating room, including procedures expected to last more than 1 hour. PSA should be performed with caution or not at all in patients who suffered an adverse event with prior PSA or general anesthesia. Likewise, extreme caution and the judicious use of sedating agents are indicated in patients who may be difficult to manually ventilate or intubate.

The need for preprocedure fasting has been controversial. At question is whether nonfasted patients undergoing PSA are at increased risk for vomiting and aspiration, similar to nonfasted patients undergoing general anesthesia. While this question has not been definitively answered, years of experience and recent data suggest the answer is "no."

It is well known that loss of protective airway reflexes and manipulation of the airway during intubation and extubation increases the risk of aspiration in patients undergoing general anesthesia. In contrast, most patients undergoing PSA do not require airway manipulation, and the combination of vomiting and loss of protective airway reflexes is an extremely rare occurrence.[1]

Agrawal and his colleagues[11] evaluated 905 children undergoing PSA in a pediatric emergency department. They found no difference in adverse events between the 509 children who did not meet current American Academy of Pediatrics fasting guidelines and the 396 children who did. In a study of "sedation disasters," Cote and colleagues[12] failed to identify a single case of aspiration in any nonoperating room setting during a 27-year study period. These studies suggest that fasting prior to PSA is unnecessary. Indeed, the American

Table 188-1. Agents for Procedural Sedation and Analgesia (PSA)

Agent	Class	Route	Usual Total Dose*	Onset	Duration†
Fentanyl (Sublimaze)	Opioid	IV	2-3 μg/kg	1-2 min	20-30 min
		TM	10-15 μg/kg	15-30 min	60-120 min
Midazolam (Versed)	Benzodiazepine	IV	0.02-0.1 mg/kg (adult) 0.05-0.15 mg/kg (child)	1-2 min	30 min
		IM	0.05-0.15 mg/kg	10-15 min	60-120 min
		PO	0.5-0.75 mg/kg	15-30 min	60-90 min
		PR	0.5-0.75 mg/kg	10-30 min	60-90 min
		IN	0.2-0.5 mg/kg	10-15 min	45-60 min
Methohexital (Brevital)	Barbiturate	IV	0.75-1.0 mg/kg	<1 min	5-10 min
		PR	20-30 mg/kg	7-8 min	20-60 min
Ketamine (Ketalar)	Phencyclidine derivative	IV	1-2 mg/kg	1 min	15 min
		IM	4-5 mg/kg	5 min	15-30 min
		PO	5-10 mg/kg	30-45 min	2-4 hrs
		PR	5-10 mg/kg	5-10 min	15-30 min
		IN	3-6 mg/kg	5-10 min	—
Propofol (Diprivan)	Alkylphenol derivative	IV	1.0 mg/kg	<1 min	8-10 min
		Infusion	25-125 μg/kg/min		
Etomidate	Imidazole derivative	IV	0.1-0.2 mg/kg	<1 min	5-8 min
		PO	50 mg (adult dose)	10-20 min	30-60 min
		PR	4.5 mg/kg	4 min	40-60 min
Nitrous oxide	Anesthetic gas	Inhalation	30-50%	1-2 min	5 min

CNS, central nervous system; COPD, chronic obstructive pulmonary disease; IM, intramuscular; IN, intranasal; IV, intravenous; PO, oral; PR, rectal;
*Response to dosage is highly individualized and the drug must be carefully titrated.
Doses provided are usual total doses. See Box 188-2 for drug administration strategies.
†Duration may vary with dose.

College of Emergency Physicians' current policy on emergency department PSA points out that recent oral intake is not a contraindication to PSA but should be considered in choosing the depth and target level of sedation.[1]

Circumstances permitting, the physician should discuss with the patient the indications, risks, benefits, and alternatives for PSA and document this discussion in the emergency department record. However, there is no literature to suggest that the use of an informed consent form separate from the general informed consent obtained at emergency department registration has an effect on patient satisfaction or on clinical outcome. Thus, unless mandated by institutional policy, there is no need to obtain separate written informed consent prior to PSA.

Serious Adverse Effects	Advantages	Comments
Respiratory depression Muscular/glottic rigidity	Rapid onset Short duration Easily titrated Favorable cardiovascular profile	Respiratory depression is more pronounced when coadministered with other respiratory depressants. Does not cause histamine release.
Respiratory depression	Rapid onset Short duration Easily titrated Low incidence of pain with injection and phlebitis Can administer via multiple routes	Prolonged sedation may occur in elderly patients. Respiratory depression is more pronounced in elderly patients, patients with COPD, and when coadministered with other respiratory depressants. Reduce dosage in patients with COPD and patients older than 60 years of age (see text for details).
Apnea/respiratory depression	Rapid onset	Risk of hypotension is increased in hypovolemic patients.
Hypotension	Short duration Airway reflexes maintained Predictable when given PR	Coughing, hiccups, and laryngospasm may occur. Does not provide analgesia. Not recommended to facilitate endotracheal intubation.
Hypertension Tachycardia	Rapid onset Short duration	Respiratory depression may occur with rapid IV bolus, exceptionally high doses, in the presence of CNS abnormalities, and in ill neonates.
Laryngospasm (rare) Increased intracranial and intraocular pressure Emergence phenomena Emesis	No respiratory depression Airway reflexes maintained Can administer via multiple routes Predictable when given IM Effective bronchial dilator	Laryngospasm may occur in infants younger than 3 months of age and in patients with concurrent respiratory infections. In children, administer with atropine (0.1 mg/kg; min 0.1 mg, max 0.5 mg) or glycopyrrolate (0.005 mg/kg; max 0.25 mg) in the same syringe. Contraindications include children younger than 3 months of age, active pulmonary infection, cardiovascular disease (angina, heart failure, aneurysm, uncontrolled hypertension), traumatic brain injury, CNS mass lesions, hydrocephalus, glaucoma, and acute globe injury.
Respiratory depression	Rapid onset	Procedures lasting >8-10 min will require repeat boluses or a constant infusion.
Hypotension	Short duration	Safety has not been documented for extended emergency department administration.
Injection pain	Cerebral protective Antiemetic effects	To prevent injection pain, administer IV lidocaine, 0.5 mg/kg with a rubber tourniquet in place, 30 to 120 sec before propofol.
Respiratory depression Myoclonus	Rapid onset Short duration	Data are still somewhat limited, but appears to be safe and effective for emergency department PSA; further studies needed to better define its uses and safety profile.
Emesis Injection pain Adrenal suppression	Minimal cardiovascular effects Cerebral protective	Adrenal suppression is not clinically relevant with one-time administration.
Diffusion hypoxia	Rapid onset	Indicated for constant low-intensity pain or nonpainful anxiety-provoking procedures.
Expansion of gas-filled structures	Short duration Minimal cardiovascular and respiratory effects	For cooperative/older patients, administer via a demand-valve. For uncooperative/younger patients, administer via continuous-flow technique.
Emesis		The continuous-flow technique requires two physicians and is associated with a greater incidence of emesis (10%). Contraindications include pneumothorax, bowel obstruction, middle ear effusion, severe COPD, traumatic brain injury, indwelling balloon-tipped catheters, and patients who are intoxicated or cannot follow directions.

TM, transmucosal.

Personnel

Personnel providing PSA should have an understanding of the pharmacology of the agents being administered, the ability to monitor the patient's response to the medications given, and the skills necessary to recognize and manage all potential complications.

The optimal number of personnel required to perform emergency department PSA has not been established. However, current practice guidelines recommend that in addition to the physician performing the procedure, a support person (e.g., nurse, respiratory therapist) capable of recognizing the complications of PSA be present to closely monitor the patient.[1,2,8,9] During moderate sedation, this individual may assist with minor, interruptible tasks. However, during deep sedation, the support person monitoring the patient should have no other responsibilities that would interfere with the advance level of monitoring and documentation appropriate for this level of sedation.[8] Finally, since it is not always possible to predict the level of sedation that will be reached for an individual patient, advanced life support should be immediately available whenever PSA is being performed.

Supplies and Equipment

Although rare, PSA can result in allergic reactions, respiratory depression, or cardiopulmonary arrest. Consequently, equipment to manage the patient's airway and supplies to treat allergic reactions, oversedation, and cardiopulmonary arrest should be readily available. Equipment for patient monitoring is discussed separately in the next section.

The room in which the procedure is being performed should have suction capability and an oxygen source. An appropriately sized bag/mask device and oral and nasal airways should be ready at the bedside. Intubation supplies and a crash cart containing advanced life support drugs and defibrillator must be immediately available. When opioids or benzodiazepines are being employed, the opiate antagonist naloxone and the benzodiazepine antagonist flumazenil are readily available.

Except in rare circumstances, drugs used for PSA in adults should be administered intravenously. Hence, all adults undergoing emergency department PSA should have an intravenous line placed. The need for intravenous line placement in children will depend on the presence of comorbid conditions and the route of drug administration chosen by the physician. In addition, placement of an intravenous line should be considered in children when there is a high likelihood that multiple drug doses will be required.

The need for supplemental oxygen and its benefits during PSA have not been studied. Supplemental oxygen may prevent hypoxemia in some patients. However, patients receiving supplemental oxygen may have normal oxygen saturation despite significant ventilatory depression. Unfortunately, there are few scientific data to guide the clinician. Thus, for the present time, the use of supplemental oxygen should be in accordance with institutional protocols or at the discretion of the treating physician.

Monitoring

Close patient monitoring is paramount to providing safe PSA and involves assessing the patient's level of consciousness and respiratory status and measuring vital signs, including heart rate, respiratory rate, blood pressure, and oxygen saturation.

Monitoring the level and adequacy of sedation has often been difficult due to the lack of an objective, accurate, and simple method of measuring the depth of sedation. Recently, however, there has been increased interest in using Bispectral Index (BIS) monitoring as an accurate and simple way of assessing level of sedation during emergency department PSA.[10,11]

The BIS is a noninvasive monitoring system consisting of a sensor attached to the patient's forehead and a monitor that provides a reading between 0 (no brain activity) and 100 (fully awake). The BIS uses bispectral analysis of the electroencephalographic waveform and other features within the electroencephalogram to detect subtle changes in levels of sedation, loss of consciousness, and recall. The BIS has been validated as an objective measure of sedation depth in the operating room. No recent studies in the emergency department have found BIS monitoring reliably predictive for patients undergoing PSA who were sedated to the point of general anesthesia from those with lesser degrees of sedation. However, BIS monitoring did not discriminate as well between patients with mild-to-moderate sedation or moderate-to-deep sedation.[13]

Miner and his colleagues prospectively evaluated the correlation between BIS scores and respiratory depression, perception of pain, recall of the procedure, and satisfaction in 108 adult patients undergoing PSA. They found that patients with BIS scores > 70 had significantly less respiratory depression than patients with BIS scores of <70. In addition, patients with BIS scores of >85 had more pain, more recall, and were less satisfied compared with patients whose BIS scores were <85. The authors concluded that BIS scores between 70 and 85 represented the optimal level of sedation.[15]

There are still insufficient data to support the widespread use of BIS monitoring, but it may eventually have a role in emergency department PSA. It should be pointed out that BIS monitoring does not work for PSA with the dissociative agent ketamine.

It is well known that most of the drugs used for PSA can cause respiratory depression (see Table 188-1); hence, continuous assessment of respiratory status is imperative. A support person should be present to closely monitor the patient's level of consciousness, chest wall motion, and air movement. Pulse oximetry should be utilized to provide a noninvasive estimate of arterial oxygen saturation. However, its use should not be considered a substitute for clinical assessment. The use of pulse oximetry is particularly important in patients at increased risk of developing hypoxemia, such as when high doses of drugs or multiple drugs are used, or when treating patients with significant comorbidity. However, no studies have demonstrated that identifying a decrease in oxygen saturation alone has an impact on patient outcome. In fact, when the patient's level of consciousness or respiratory efforts can be adequately assessed, PSA has an extremely low risk of morbidity and mortality.[12] This is reflected in the current American College of Emergency Physicians clinical policy on PSA, which suggests that pulse oximetry may not be necessary when the patient's level of consciousness is minimally depressed and verbal communication can be continually monitored.[1] Despite this, pulse oximetry is widely available and noninvasive and should be used in most, if not all, cases of PSA.

Since PSA can cause hypoventilation, monitoring $ETCO_2$ has been suggested as an adjunct to pulse oximetry. Theoretically, increases in $ETCO_2$ should precede a fall in oxygen saturation; therefore, monitoring $ETCO_2$ may detect inadequate ventilation before hypoxemia occurs.[14] Unfortunately, data regarding $ETCO_2$ monitoring during emergency department PSA are sparse.[16]

At the present time, there is insufficient evidence to recommend $ETCO_2$ monitoring for all patients receiving PSA in the emergency department. If available, it should be considered when ventilatory efforts cannot be directly observed and when supplemental oxygen is being administered.[8]

Vital signs, including heart rate, respiratory rate, blood pressure, and oxygen saturation, should be monitored closely during the procedure. This is particularly true 5 to 20 minutes after the patient receives intravenous medications and during the immediate post-procedure period when patients are at greatest risk of complications. However, the optimal frequency at which vital signs should be recorded has not been studied. In many cases, the frequency of vital sign documentation is driven by institutional policies. When no such policies exist, a reasonable approach for patients undergoing minimal or moderate sedation would include documentation at baseline, after drug administration, on completion of the procedure, during early recovery, and at completion of recovery. During deep sedation, some experts advocate recording vital signs every 5 minutes,[8] but there is no proof that this practice improves outcomes.

There is no evidence that cardiac monitoring during PSA is of any benefit. However, in older patients or in those with a history of cardiovascular disease, hypertension, or dysrhythmia, the use of continuous electrocardiographic monitoring is prudent. In young patients without underlying cardiovascular disease, continuous electrocardiographic monitoring is likely unnecessary as long as continuous pulse oximetry (that allows visual monitoring of heart rate) is being utilized. Nevertheless, because it is inexpensive and readily available, continuous electrocardiographic monitoring is commonly recommended for all patients.[1,8]

Recovery

During the immediate post-procedure period, when all stimulation has stopped and pain and anxiety have been controlled, the patient is at increased risk for complications. Consequently, patients must be observed closely following completion of the procedure. Monitoring should continue until the patient is completely back to baseline function and ready for discharge. Drowsy patients should not be left unattended, particularly when they are in other areas of the hospital (e.g., radiology). If patients are transported out of the emergency department before they have completely returned to baseline function, a trained caregiver with appropriate monitoring equipment and resuscitation supplies must accompany them.

Discharge Criteria and Instructions

A normal mental status and baseline cognitive and motor function are prerequisites to discharge. The patient should understand and follow directions, speak clearly, and ambulate unassisted (infants should sit unassisted). Vital signs and respiratory status should be within normal limits, pain and discomfort should be addressed, and any nausea and vomiting should be resolved. Every effort should be made to send the patient home with a responsible adult. In one study that addressed time of discharge after emergency department PSA, Newman and associates[17] found that serious adverse effects rarely occurred after 25 minutes from the final medication administration. Those that did occur late were all preceded by a separate adverse effect during the expected peak drug effect (i.e., the late adverse effect was not the first adverse effect for that patient). The authors concluded that, when using similar medication regimens (midazolam/fentanyl, midazolam/morphine, midazolam/ketamine, lorazepam/diphenhydramine), discharge from the emergency department may be safe approximately 30 minutes after administration of the final sedation medication if no adverse effects have occurred.

The patient should be advised not to drive or participate in other dangerous activities (e.g., operate power tools, ride bicycles, use swing sets) for 24 hours. Children should be watched closely at home for at least 8 hours. Although the duration of action of most agents used for PSA is relatively short, some patients may experience subtle cognitive deficits or mild drowsiness for 8 or more hours. If the patient experiences nausea or vomiting, a clear liquid diet is indicated until these symptoms resolve. In general, nausea and vomiting are short lived, and most patients will advance to a normal diet very quickly. Standard discharge instructions for the presenting complaint (i.e., abscess, fracture, dislocation) and those signs and symptoms (e.g., confusion, difficulty breathing) that should prompt an immediate return or telephone call must also be provided.

PHARMACOLOGY

Agents for PSA, dosing recommendations, and adverse effects are provided in Table 188-1. Individual agents are discussed in detail here.

Route of Administration

For nondissociative agents, intravenous titration to the desired level of sedation and analgesia provides the safest, most rapid, and most predictable results. Drugs given by other routes (e.g., intramuscular, oral, intranasal, rectal) generally have a slower onset of action, are difficult or impossible to titrate, often provide unpredictable results, and may cause prolonged sedation. One exception to this rule is PSA in pediatric patients. In some children, the benefits of intravenous drug administration may be outweighed by the difficulty in obtaining intravenous access. In this situation, intramuscular, oral, nasal, or rectal administration can be used. In addition, the inhalation route using nitrous oxide may be an alternative for selected procedures. Use of these alternative routes requires dosing modification (see Table 188-1).

An intramuscular injection is a simple and economic method of parenteral administration that avoids the need for intravenous line placement. Disadvantages include pain with injection, particularly if multiple doses are required, and a delayed and often unpredictable onset with most agents. An exception to this is the dissociative agent ketamine, which provides consistent and predictable results when given intramuscularly.

Advantages of oral, nasal, and rectal administration are ease of delivery and patient acceptance; however, because of variability in gastrointestinal absorption, gastric emptying time, and gastrointestinal motility, patient response to orally administered agents is less predictable. In addition, oral administration may increase the risk of aspiration when the child is deeply sedated. Nasal and rectal administration avoids local gastrointestinal effects and therefore produces more predictable results.

Opioids

Parenteral opioids are commonly used as analgesics before performing painful procedures. For PSA, many clinicians prefer to combine an opioid with another agent, usually a benzodiazepine, to increase the amnesic and sedative effects. The most commonly used opioids are meperidine, morphine, and fentanyl. Fentanyl has become the opioid of choice for PSA in the emergency department because of its rapid onset and short duration of action, high potency (it is 1000 times more potent than meperidine), and favorable cardiovascular profile.

When given intravenously, fentanyl rapidly crosses the blood-brain barrier, producing analgesia in as little as 90 seconds. Serum fentanyl levels rapidly decline from peak concentrations because of extensive tissue uptake, producing a serum half-life of 90 minutes and duration of action of 30 to 40 minutes. The combination of potency and short half-life permits the administration of multiple small doses that can be titrated easily to the desired clinical effect.[18]

The typical dose of intravenous fentanyl for both children and adults is approximately 2 to 3 μg/kg. The ultimate dose depends on the patient's age and pain threshold, the procedure being performed, the concomitant use of other agents, and the presence of underlying medical problems. In children, oral transmucosal fentanyl citrate (OTFC) can be used when intravenous access is not feasible. The OTFC is a fentanyl-impregnated, sweetened matrix in lozenge form on a holder ("fentanyl lollipop"). Transmucosal delivery allows a rapid onset of action because direct absorption into the systemic circulation avoids first-pass metabolism by the liver. It has been shown to produce sedation and relieve pain 12 to 30 minutes after administration.[19] Despite a rapid onset, transmucosal delivery does not allow easy titration. The dose of OTFC is 10 to 15 μg/kg. Larger doses (15-20 μg/kg) have been shown to cause more nausea and vomiting without improving analgesia or sedation.[18]

Adverse effects reported with fentanyl use include respiratory depression, muscular and glottic rigidity, seizures, pruritus, and nausea and vomiting. Fentanyl has minimal effect on the cardiovascular system and when carefully titrated is seldom associated with hypotension or bradycardia.[18,19]

Fentanyl induces respiratory depression by reducing the responsiveness of the brainstem respiratory center to carbon dioxide. Maximal respiratory depression occurs 5 minutes after intravenous administration. The magnitude of respiratory compromise is dose-dependent and is intensified by the coadministration of other respiratory depressants, particularly midazolam.[20,21] Furthermore, delayed respiratory depression secondary to redistribution of fentanyl from peripheral tissues has been reported following high-dose (>50 μg/kg) fentanyl anesthesia. With slow, careful titration, clinically significant respiratory depression is rare. Similar results have been demonstrated in which patients received a combination of fentanyl and midazolam or fentanyl and diazepam to facilitate painful procedures in the emergency department.[18,20,21]

High-dose fentanyl general anesthesia may result in muscular and glottic rigidity ("board chest"). The resulting fall in chest wall compliance, glottic closure, or both may lead to difficulty in providing or an inability to provide adequate manual ventilation. Fortunately, rigidity has never been reported with the use of fentanyl in the emergency department. This is most likely because much smaller doses of fentanyl are used for PSA (2-3 μg/kg) compared to general anesthesia (50-100 μg/kg). In fact, rigidity does not begin to occur until 8.8 to 17 μg/kg have been given.[22] Although less well recognized, generalized rigidity significant enough to prevent ventilation may also occur with intravenous morphine and meperidine.[23] Regardless of the responsible agent, rigidity can be reversed with naloxone or succinylcholine.

Generalized seizure activity has also been reported during induction of anesthesia using high doses of fentanyl. Nevertheless, prospective studies of patients experiencing motor activity resembling seizures while undergoing fentanyl anesthesia fail to demonstrate a seizure focus on a simultaneous electroencephalogram.[24] It has been suggested that these patients may have been experiencing myoclonus produced by opioid depression of higher central nervous system (CNS) inhibitory centers or a pronounced form of muscular rigidity. In any event, seizures or seizure-like activity has never been reported with the use of fentanyl in the emergency department.

Mild facial pruritus is commonly associated with fentanyl administration; however, generalized pruritus, urticaria, or anaphylactoid reactions are seldom seen because fentanyl causes little or no histamine release compared with other commonly used opioids.[25] Similarly, fentanyl has been reported to induce less vomiting than other opioid analgesics.

Benzodiazepines

Benzodiazepines, including diazepam, lorazepam, and midazolam are commonly used to provide sedation in a variety of outpatient settings. However, when rapid, short-term sedation is required, midazolam is most commonly used.

As with other benzodiazepines, midazolam exhibits sedating, hypnotic, anxiolytic, amnesic, anticonvulsant, and muscle relaxant properties. Midazolam possesses a unique imidazole ring structure that imparts both water solubility and lipophilicity. When the pH is less than 4, the ring opens, making the drug water-soluble. This obviates the need for solvents and results in a lower incidence of injection pain and phlebitis as compared with non-water-soluble benzodiazepines such as diazepam and lorazepam. When the pH is greater than 4, the ring closes, increasing the drug's lipophilicity. This allows midazolam to rapidly cross the blood-brain barrier and produce sedation in 1 to 3 minutes. It also results in rapid redistribution of the drug from the brain to peripheral tissues, producing a serum half-life of 1.5 to 3 hours and duration of action of approximately 30 minutes. Because midazolam does not possess significant analgesic properties, it is commonly combined with fentanyl or another opioid when used to facilitate a painful procedure. Midazolam has been shown to be a safe and effective agent for PSA, both when used alone and in combination with fentanyl.[18,26]

The recommended total intravenous dose of midazolam for adults is 0.02 to 0.1 mg/kg. Like fentanyl, the final dose of midazolam depends on the patient's age and pain threshold, the procedure being performed, the concomitant use of other agents, and the presence of underlying medical problems. In elderly patients, the total dose should be reduced by approximately one half. In children, the intravenous dose is 0.05 to 0.15 mg/kg. When intravenous access is not possible or practical, midazolam administered orally, intranasally, or rectally has been shown to be safe and effective in facilitating laceration repair in preschool-age children.[27,28]

Midazolam causes central respiratory depression through decreased sensitivity to carbon dioxide. Ventilatory depression is dose dependent, peaking approximately 3 minutes after intravenous administration. Maximal depression may occur sooner with rapid administration.[20] The severity of respiratory compromise is increased in the presence of barbiturates, opioids, alcohol, or other CNS depressants. Respiratory depression is also more pronounced and sedation lasts longer in patients with chronic obstructive pulmonary disease and in the elderly.

Midazolam does not produce significant cardiovascular effects in sedative doses. Changes in heart rate, cardiac index, and pulmonary vascular resistance are minimal. Its predominant effect is a decrease in systemic vascular resistance, resulting in a slight reduction in blood pressure. This may be more pronounced with the coadministration of fentanyl.[21] When midazolam is carefully titrated, even when combined with fentanyl, clinically significant cardiovascular effects are rare. Other adverse effects such as pain with intravenous administration, local irritation, and thrombophlebitis are occasionally reported with midazolam, but they occur less frequently and are less severe than with diazepam. Headache, nausea, emesis, coughing, and hiccups occur infrequently. In children, there have been reports of paradoxical agitation following the use of midazolam.[27]

Barbiturates

Methohexital is an ultra-short-acting barbiturate that was once popular for both sedation and rapid sequence intubation in the emergency department but is less frequently prescribed as other agents have become available. Although data are somewhat limited, the use of methohexital in the emergency department appears to be safe and effective, particularly for orthopedic procedures and radiologic imaging.[30-32]

Methohexital has a rapid onset of action, producing an unconscious, sleep-like state in less than 1 minute. It also has a brief duration of action, with most patients awake in less than 10 minutes. Rapid onset and short duration of unconsciousness make methohexital an excellent agent for short procedures such as cardioversion, bone or joint reduction, and CT scans in children.[31] It should be noted that while methohexital causes profound amnesia, it does not provide significant analgesia. Consequently, some physicians coadminister small doses of an opioid for extremely painful procedures.

For PSA in both children and adults, a dose of 0.75 to 1 mg/kg IV produces a rapid onset of unconsciousness with minimal cardiorespiratory effects. In children, methohexital can be given rectally at a dose of 25 mg/kg.[30]

Depressed respiratory drive and apnea may be seen following administration of methohexital, but several studies of methohexital use in emergency department patients demonstrate that respiratory depression has a low incidence and is generally transient and mild. Most patients respond to supplemental oxygen and repositioning of the airway. A small percentage of patients may require a brief period of assisted ventilation, but no emergency department patients have required intubation or a change in disposition after receiving methohexital for procedural sedation.[30-32]

Methohexital has a direct myocardial depressant effect. This may cause a slight drop in blood pressure with a compensatory elevation in heart rate. Methohexital also causes venodilation, but systemic vascular resistance usually remains unchanged. Clinically, the effects on heart rate and blood pressure are variable, and in most cases, transient and insignificant.[30-32] However, methohexital does have the potential to cause significant hypotension and should be used with caution in patients with hemodynamic instability or occult blood loss.

Methohexital may also cause activation of respiratory reflexes, including coughing, hiccups, and rarely, laryngospasm. Coughing and hiccups are usually transient and of no serious consequence. Laryngospasm is rare and usually mild. It may be reduced or eliminated by removing any inciting stimulus. Heightened airway reflexes and failure of adequate jaw relaxation reduce the effectiveness of methohexital in facilitating endotracheal intubation.

Similarly, sodium pentothal was historically used for procedural sedation, but its use for this purpose has largely been abandoned with the availability of newer agents.

Ketamine

Ketamine hydrochloride is a derivative of the street drug phencyclidine. It causes dissociation between the thalamoneocortical and limbic systems, preventing the higher centers from perceiving visual, auditory, or painful stimuli.[33] This creates a dissociative "trance-like" state often accompanied by a blank stare and nystagmus. Muscle tone is maintained or increased and random movements of the extremities unrelated to painful stimuli may occur. In contrast to other agents used for PSA, when given to otherwise healthy patients at recommended doses, ketamine does not cause respiratory depression.[34] Muscular tone of the tongue and pharynx are preserved, and protective airway reflexes such as coughing, sneezing, and swallowing are maintained or slightly enhanced. In addition, ketamine causes bronchial smooth muscle relaxation and has been used successfully in combination with succinylcholine to facilitate intubation of patients with status asthmaticus and to treat bronchospasm in asthmatic patients requiring mechanical ventilation.[35]

Ketamine is both water soluble and lipophilic, which allows for painless parenteral administration and a rapid onset. Peak levels occur 1 minute after intravenous administration and 5 minutes after an intramuscular injection. The duration of action is 15 minutes for the intravenous route and 15 to 30 minutes when given intramuscularly. Complete recovery generally requires 1 to 2 hours.

The intravenous dose of ketamine to obtain the dissociative state is 1.5 to 2 mg/kg given at a rate of 0.5 mg/kg/min. For short procedures, particularly in children, the intramuscular route is simple and effective. A dose of 4 to 5 mg/kg IM is required to consistently achieve the dissociative state; larger doses offer no additional benefit.[36] However, intravenous administration is recommended for prolonged procedures in children to avoid repeated intramuscular injections. In this situation, an initial dose of 1 mg/kg is administered intravenously, followed by repeat doses of 0.05 to 0.1 mg/kg as needed.

Ketamine stimulates salivary and tracheobronchial secretions. In children, coadministration of atropine (0.01 mg/kg; minimum dose, 0.1 mg; maximum dose, 0.5 mg) or glycopyrrolate (0.005 mg/kg; maximum dose, 0.25 mg) is recommended and can be given in the same syringe.[33] The use of atropine appears to be unnecessary in adult emergency department patients.[37] Ketamine can also be given orally, transmucosally, nasally, and rectally. These routes produce longer induction and recovery times (see Table 188-1).

Ketamine inhibits reuptake of catecholamines, resulting in mild to moderate increases in heart rate, blood pressure, and cardiac output. The hypertensive response is more pronounced with rapid intravenous administration and is greater in adults than children.[33] Because of the resultant increase in oxygen consumption, this can be harmful in patients with cardiovascular disease, particularly coronary artery disease. The combination of a benzodiazepine (e.g., midazolam, diazepam) with ketamine will help attenuate unwanted hypertension and tachycardia, allowing safe sedation in many patients with ischemic heart disease. Despite this, when alternative agents are available, it would be prudent to avoid ketamine in these patients.

Although respiratory depression is extremely rare, it can occur with a rapid intravenous bolus, exceptionally high doses, in the presence of CNS abnormalities, or when administered to ill neonates. Laryngospasm, presumably from stimulation of hypersensitized laryngeal reflexes, has been reported in infants younger than 3 months of age and in patients with concurrent respiratory infections; thus, ketamine is contraindicated in these patients. In the largest emergency department study to date (1022 cases), Green and colleagues[38] noted transient laryngospasm in 0.4% of children who received ketamine for emergency department PSA. None of these patients required intubation or a change in disposition or suffered any other serious sequelae. Furthermore, in healthy children older than 3 months, pooled data of 11,589 administrations reveal only 2 cases (0.017%) of laryngospasm severe enough to necessitate intubation.[33]

Neuromuscular effects of ketamine include skeletal muscle hypertonicity and rigidity and random movement of the head or extremities unrelated to painful stimuli. These movements rarely interfere with performance of painful procedures but can make obtaining computed tomography scans difficult.[39] Brief myoclonic twitching, sometimes confused with seizures, may also be seen. However, these occurrences are not seizures and are not associated with electroencephalographic changes. In fact, ketamine may suppress epileptic activity. Ketamine does cause elevation of intraocular and intracranial pressure and is contraindicated in patients with open globe injuries or in patients with traumatic brain injury or other CNS abnormalities.

Emesis occurs in 0% to 9.0% of patients receiving ketamine.[33,38-40] In children, the incidence appears to be age related, with a higher risk in patients aged 5 years and older.[38] However, since vomiting almost always occurs during the late recovery phase when the patient is awake and alert, and since protective airway reflexes are maintained, significant aspiration following administration of ketamine is extremely rare.

Emergence phenomena manifested by hallucinations and nightmares occur in up to 30% of adults receiving ketamine. Risk factors include age greater than 16 years, female sex, rapid intravenous administration, and use of large doses.[38] Administration of a benzodiazepine can reduce or eliminate emergence reactions and is recommended for all adults receiving ketamine.

Emergence phenomena, particularly recovery agitation, can also occur in children. These reactions are generally mild and occur less often than in adults.[40] In Green's study of 1022 children, mild recovery agitation (whimpering or crying) was noted in 17.6% of patients, with more pronounced agitation in only 1.6%. The incidence was age-related, with agitation occurring in 12.1% of children aged 5 years or older, and 22.5% in those younger than 5 years.[38] Only 2 of 1022 children had reactions that treating physicians judged severe enough to require treatment, and both children responded promptly to small doses of midazolam.

Despite the fact that these reactions are generally very mild, children routinely receive a benzodiazepine when ketamine is used for PSA.[41-44] Recent studies suggest, however, that this practice is unnecessary and may even be harmful. In a study of 104 children receiving ketamine in a pediatric emergency department, Sherwin and associates[41] found that recovery agitation was common, but the magnitude was very low (median score of 5 mm on a 100-mm visual analogue scale). Moreover, the addition of midazolam did not alter the incidence or severity of these reactions. In another study, the use of midazolam actually resulted in more recovery agitation in children 10 years or older, and a higher incidence of oxygen desaturation in children younger than 10 years.[40] Based on current data, there is no evidence to support the prophylactic administration of benzodiazepines to children receiving ketamine. Rather, their use should be reserved to treat unpleasant reactions if they occur.

Propofol

Propofol is an ultrashort-acting sedative hypnotic derived from the alkylphenols. It is highly lipid soluble but is insoluble in aqueous solution. The onset of sedation is very rapid, occurring within one circulation time after intravenous injection. Plasma levels fall quickly, producing a very short duration of action, usually less than 10 minutes. Moreover, because propofol does not accumulate, sedation clears quickly and completely. This suggests that propofol may allow quick discharge from the emergency department.

Propofol produces dose-dependent levels of sedation ranging from minimal sedation to general anesthesia. When used for emergency department PSA, deep sedation is usually the goal. Because it has such a short duration of action, procedures lasting longer than 8 to 10 minutes will require a continuous intravenous infusion or repeat bolus doses.

Propofol possesses antiemetic properties and decreases intracranial pressure but does not provide analgesia. Hence, some clinicians administer an opioid, such as fentanyl or morphine, for painful procedures.[45,46] Adverse effects include respiratory depression, hypotension, and pain on injection.

Propofol causes dose-related apnea and respiratory depression. However, in emergency department studies to date, clinically significant respiratory depression is unusual.[47-50] In most cases, it is transient, with most patients requiring only jaw thrust or repositioning of the airway and, rarely, a brief period of assisted ventilation. The need for intubation after the use of propofol for emergency department PSA has not been reported.

Propofol commonly results in a drop in both systolic and diastolic blood pressure. However, when used for sedation in healthy adult and pediatric emergency department patients, the decline in blood pressure is usually transient, and treatment is rarely if ever required.[5,32,48-50] Nevertheless, propofol can cause significant hypotension, especially when given by rapid bolus and/or to patients with hypovolemia. Hence, it would be prudent to avoid propofol in hypovolemic patients and those at risk for occult blood loss.

Propofol causes pain with intravenous injection in up to 70% of patients. A meta-analysis of 56 studies (6624 patients) comparing various analgesic interventions with placebo concluded that intravenous lidocaine, 0.5 mg/kg, given with a rubber tourniquet in place 30 to 120 seconds before injection of propofol was the best way to prevent this pain.[51]

Etomidate

Etomidate is a nonbarbiturate, ethyl-carboxylated, imidazole derivative structurally unrelated to other sedative-hypnotic agents. It causes sedation and hypnosis by enhancing neurotransmission at GABA receptors located in the CNS. Etomidate is fast acting and its effects are short lived. After intravenous administration, onset of sedation occurs in less than 1 minute and clears in 10 to 15 minutes.

Etomidate can be more difficult to titrate than other sedative hypnotic agents (e.g., midazolam) and generally produces deep sedation. For emergency department PSA, etomidate is generally administered intravenously but can be given by other routes (see Table 188-1). The initial intravenous dose is usually 0.1 to 0.2 mg/kg given over 90 seconds. Additional doses of 0.05 to 0.1 mg/kg can be administered every 2 to 3 minutes until the desired level of sedation is achieved. Long procedures may require repeat boluses or a constant infusion.

Etomidate has little effect on the cardiovascular system and may be cerebral protective, making it an excellent agent for patients with the potential for hemodynamic instability (e.g., trauma patients, gastrointestinal hemorrhage) or increased intracranial pressure (e.g., patients with traumatic brain injury).[52] Adverse effects include respiratory depression, myoclonus, nausea and vomiting, pain on injection, and adrenal suppression.

A brief period of apnea may occur following administration of etomidate. It is more likely to happen with rapid administration (<80 seconds), when higher doses are used (>0.2 mg/kg), and in older patients (>55 years of age).[53,54] At typical PSA doses (0.1-0.2 mg/kg), respiratory depression is rare. When it does occur, it is generally transient and mild, although some patients may require a brief period of assisted ventilation.[55,56] No studies have reported the need to intubate a patient after the use of etomidate for emergency department PSA.

Myoclonus associated with etomidate is typically described as benign muscle contractions of variable regularity and symmetry.[57] While the precise mechanisms have yet to be described, myoclonus is most likely related to hyperexcitability of the brain neurons affecting muscle movement and control. In emergency department studies evaluating the use of etomidate for PSA, the incidence of myoclonus has ranged from 0% to 21%.[52,53,55] When myoclonus does occur, it is generally minor and short-lived, does not cause post-sedation muscle discomfort, and rarely interferes with the procedure.[55,56] However, myoclonus is occasionally described as severe and, as such, could potentially lead to respiratory compromise.[57] Thus, even though myoclonus-induced respiratory depression has not been reported with emergency department use, it is important for clinicians using etomidate to be aware of this possibility.

The risk of nausea and vomiting after administration of etomidate appears to be dose related and is generally not a problem with the typical doses used for emergency department PSA (0.1-0.2 mg/kg). In emergency department studies published to date, the incidence of nausea and vomiting ranges from 0% to 5%.[55,56] More importantly, there have been no documented cases of aspiration.

Pain on injection is also reported with etomidate and is most likely caused by the propylene glycol solvent. Using larger veins, flushing with saline, pretreating with fentanyl, or mixing 1 mL of lidocaine with each 10 mL of etomidate can reduce the discomfort.[54] Alternatively, a lipid-emulsion formulation is available that is associated with decreased injection pain.[53]

Etomidate suppresses adrenal function by inhibiting 11-beta-hydroxylase activities. This seems to be clinically relevant only for patients on long-term infusions. One-time administration has not been reported to cause inadequate stress responses or significant electrolyte abnormalities.[54] In one study of emergency department patients requiring rapid sequence intubation, Schenarts and colleagues[58] found that patients who received etomidate (0.3 mg/kg) had a lower 4-hour serum cortisol response to cosyntropin stimulation than patients who were induced with midazolam. However, cortisol levels in both groups remained within normal limits, and the difference between the groups resolved within 12 hours.

Nitrous Oxide

Nitrous oxide is a colorless, sweet-smelling gas that has been used since the 1950s for sedation and analgesia in a variety of inpatient and outpatient settings. It rapidly diffuses across biologic membranes, producing sedation and analgesia in as little as 1 to 2 minutes. Its duration of action is likewise very short, usually around 3 to 5 minutes. The drug is excreted unchanged by the lungs and it does not bind to hemoglobin. Consequently, it has little effect on organ systems other than the CNS.[59] Nitrous oxide is thought to exert its analgesic and sedative effects by binding opiate receptors in the CNS. Clinically, however, its sedative and anxiolytic effects are more evident than its analgesic properties. Therefore, for more painful procedures, some clinicians prefer to also administer a short-acting opioid such as fentanyl.

The usual dose of nitrous oxide for PSA ranges from 30% to 50%. Lower concentrations (30%) may be less effective for emergency department use, particularly in children younger than 6 years of age.[60] Higher concentrations (i.e., 65%-70%) are required at high altitudes. Nitrous oxide must be administered with at least 30% oxygen to avoid hypoxia (i.e., the maximum concentration of nitrous oxide is 70%). However, the use of a 70/30 nitrous/oxygen mix can result in deep sedation with loss of protective airway reflexes. In addition, nitrous oxide can diffuse into any air-filled space, possibly worsening conditions where there is an abnormal collection of air, such as bowel obstruction and pneumothorax. Other adverse effects include nausea, dizziness, voice change, euphoria, and laughter. Nitrous oxide is a known teratogen and mutagen and should not be used in pregnant patients or around pregnant staff members.

The use of nitrous oxide requires a well-ventilated room with a scavenger system to prevent inhalation by emergency department staff. A double-tank system is commonly used to deliver the nitrous oxide and O_2 mixture. The system relies on a mixing valve preset to deliver a fixed ratio of nitrous oxide to oxygen and will deliver gas only when O_2 is flowing. The double-tank system contains a fail-safe device that automatically stops the flow of nitrous oxide when the O_2 supply is depleted.

The safest method to administer nitrous oxide is via a self-administered demand-valve. The demand-valve requires that the patient generate a negative pressure of 3 to 5 cm H_2O within a handheld mask or mouthpiece for gas to flow. If patients become too somnolent, they will not be able to generate sufficient negative pressure or the mask will fall from their face; in either case, delivery of nitrous oxide will cease. This feature significantly reduces the risk of oversedation. Unfortunately, uncooperative patients and those too small to generate sufficient negative pressure will be unable to utilize a demand-valve. For these patients, a continuous-flow technique utilizing a mask strapped over the nose or nose and mouth can be used.[61] This technique requires an additional physician dedicated to continuous gas titration to avoid oversedation and is associated with a higher rate of emesis.[61,62] In addition, the mask may interfere with procedures involving the perioral and nasal areas of the face.

REVERSAL ("RESCUE") AGENTS

Naloxone

Naloxone is a pure opioid antagonist with a high affinity for μ-opiate receptors and less affinity for the κ- and λ-receptors. It is the most commonly used agent for reversal of opioid-induced sedation and respiratory depression. It has a rapid onset of action and a mean half-life of 64 minutes. However, the clinical effects of opioid reversal may last only 15 to 30 minutes. Naloxone can also be administered via the intramuscular, subcutaneous, or endotracheal routes but should optimally be given intravenously when used for reversal of PSA.

The dose of naloxone for adults is 0.1 to 2 mg IV; for complete reversal, at least 2 mg should be given. If the procedure has not been completed, but the patient becomes overly sedated or experiences respiratory depression, partial reversal can be achieved using incremental doses of 0.1 to 0.4 mg. Because large doses of naloxone are not associated with toxicity, dosing recommendations are similar for children. For partial reversal, smaller initial doses (e.g., 0.005-0.05 mg/kg) can be used.

When administered for reversal of PSA, naloxone is associated with very few adverse effects. Potential problems include acute opioid withdrawal in patients addicted to opioids and resedation in patients who have received a long-acting opioid (e.g., meperidine, morphine). Therefore, these patients should be observed for 90 to 120 minutes after administration of naloxone. Alternatively, nalmefene, a long-acting opioid antagonist, can be used. Resedation is usually not a problem for patients who have been given fentanyl in doses recommended for PSA. Nevertheless, these patients should be observed for a minimum of 1 hour after administration of naloxone. This is especially important for patients who have received large doses of fentanyl to ensure that redistribution of fentanyl within the body does not result in recurrence of sedation.

Flumazenil

Flumazenil is an imidazobenzodiazepine derivative that antagonizes the effects of benzodiazepines by competitively and reversibly binding to GABA-benzodiazepine receptors in the CNS. After an intravenous injection, the onset of reversal is usually evident within 1 to 2 minutes, with peak effect occurring after 6 to 10 minutes. The duration of action is dose related. A dose of 1.0 mg (maximum recommended dose for reversal of PSA) will sustain antagonism for approximately 48 minutes.[63]

Data regarding the use of flumazenil to reverse PSA in the emergency department is sparse. One study has demonstrated that a dose of 1.0 mg of flumazenil is safe and effective in reversing the sedating and psychomotor effects of midazolam without interfering with its amnesic effect or diminishing the analgesic effect of coadministered fentanyl.[64] However, its use does not obviate the need for close monitoring of the patient's respiratory status and aggressive intervention to assist breathing when needed.

Data regarding indications for flumazenil use in the context of PSA are lacking. Possible indications for its use may include hypoventilation unresponsive to stimulation or a brief period of bag/mask ventilation or deep sedation with loss of protective airway reflexes. Routine reversal is not recommended, and PSA should not be planned with reversal in mind.

To reverse sedation in adults, flumazenil should be administered intravenously in increments of 0.2 mg until the desired level of consciousness is achieved, or a maximum of 1.0 mg has been given. Incremental doses should be given 60 seconds apart with each dose administered over 15 seconds.

Serious potential adverse effects of flumazenil include seizures, benzodiazepine withdrawal, and resedation. Risk factors for seizures include (1) concurrent major sedative-hypnotic withdrawal, (2) recent therapy with repeated doses of parenteral benzodiazepines, (3) myoclonic jerking or seizure activity before administration of flumazenil, and (4) concurrent cyclic antidepressant poisoning. In addition, flumazenil may precipitate seizures in patients taking a benzodiazepine for control of an underlying seizure disorder.

Flumazenil can cause benzodiazepine withdrawal in patients who chronically take benzodiazepines. This may occur after only 2 weeks of benzodiazepine use.[63] Withdrawal is more likely to occur with high doses of flumazenil (>1.0 mg); therefore, the lowest possible dose of flumazenil required for adequate reversal should be used.

Resedation may be a problem if flumazenil is used to reverse a long-acting benzodiazepine, such as diazepam or lorazepam, or if it is administered to a patient who has received a large dose (>10 mg) of midazolam. In one recent study of emergency department patients requiring PSA for cardioversion, five of six patients (average weight 71 kg; range, 70-76 kg) who received midazolam (0.2 mg/kg) followed by flumazenil (0.5 mg bolus followed by 0.5 mg infusion over 1 hour) experienced resedation prior to discharge.[50] Hence, these patients should be observed for at least 2 hours after receiving flumazenil. Even when small doses of midazolam are used, it is advisable to observe patients for at least 60 minutes after administration of flumazenil. If resedation occurs, repeat doses of flumazenil can be administered at 20-minute intervals as needed. Repeat doses should be given in increments of 0.2 mg with a maximum of 1.0 mg every 20 minutes and no more than 3.0 mg within any 1 hour.

Drug Selection and Administration

When selecting a strategy for PSA, the clinician must consider the type of procedure being performed, specific procedural requirements, the length of the procedure and whether it may need to be repeated, and the ability to use topical, local, or regional anesthesia (Table 188-2). One must also take into account the patient's age, comorbid conditions, and past medical history. When more than one PSA strategy may be appropriate, the clinician is encouraged to choose the agents that they are most familiar with, as there are few scientific data comparing one PSA regimen to another. Once the agent or agents have been chosen, proper drug administration is the key to safe and effective use.

Procedures can be divided into three broad categories: (1) noninvasive, (2) low pain, high anxiety, and (3) high pain, high anxiety procedures (see Table 188-2). For noninvasive procedures in which complete immobilization is required (e.g., computed tomography), rectal methohexital is safe, effective, and easily administered. Alternatives include intravenous metho-

Table 188-2. Drug Selection Strategies

Procedure Type	Common Emergency Department Examples	Recommendation	Alternatives	Comments
Noninvasive	Radiologic imaging Echocardiography	Methohexital (PR)	Methohexital (IV) Etomidate (IV) Midazolam (IV)	IV access is often not required in these patients. Methohexital given rectally is likely safer than methohexital or etomidate given IV. Midazolam does not consistently render children motionless.
Low pain High anxiety	Simple laceration repair Lumbar puncture Simple foreign body removal Eye irrigation Slit lamp examination	Midazolam (IV, PO, IN, PR)	Ketamine (IM) Nitrous oxide	These procedures generally do not require more than moderate sedation, and analgesia can usually be provided using local or topical anesthesia.
High pain High anxiety	Abscess irrigation and drainage Fracture/joint reduction Burn debridement Chest tube placement Cardioversion Sexual assault examination	Midazolam and Fentanyl (IV) or Ketamine (IM/IV)	Propofol (IV) or Etomidate (IV) or Methohexital (IV) plus: Fentanyl (IV)	Evidence now exists to support the use of any of these agents. However, there are far more data supporting the safety and efficacy of midazolam/fentanyl and ketamine for emergency department use than the other regimens. In children, administer ketamine IV or IM with atropine or glycopyrrolate. In adults, administer ketamine IV preceded by midazolam IV.

IM, intramuscular; IN, intranasal; IV, intravenous; PO, oral; PR, rectal.

hexital, intravenous etomidate, or intravenous midazolam. These agents will provide adequate sedation, but intravenous access is seldom required for these procedures, and intravenous administration may increase the risk of adverse events. In addition, midazolam does not consistently render children motionless.

Low pain, high anxiety procedures such as laceration repair and lumbar puncture generally require only minimal to moderate sedation, whereas analgesia can usually be provided with topical or local anesthetics. For these procedures, midazolam provides safe and effective sedation and can be administered via multiple routes. Alternatives include intramuscular or intravenous ketamine or nitrous oxide (see Table 188-2).

Ketamine may work well, but complete dissociation is generally not necessary for procedures in this category. If available, nitrous oxide can also provide adequate sedation and seems to work particularly well for laceration repair. In a recent study of children 2 to 6 years of age requiring facial suturing, Luhmann and associates[61] found that a 50:50 mixture of nitrous oxide and oxygen delivered via a continuous-flow system (rather than via a demand-valve) was more effective in reducing stress and had fewer adverse effects and shorter recovery times than oral midazolam. However, the continuous-flow system required the presence of two physicians (one to administer the nitrous oxide and the other to perform the procedure) and was associated with a higher incidence of emesis (10%).

For procedures that cause high pain and high anxiety (e.g., fracture or joint reduction, abscess irrigation and drainage), the use of intravenous fentanyl/midazolam or intravenous ketamine (or intramuscular in children) are strongly supported by current literature. Alternatives include intravenous propofol, intravenous etomidate, or intravenous methohexital. While evidence to support the use of these agents is growing, there remain far more data substantiating the safety and efficacy of fentanyl/midazolam and ketamine for emergency department use (see Table188-2).

The combination of fentanyl and midazolam remains one of the most popular and most broadly recommended regimens to facilitate a wide variety of emergency department procedures. These agents have a rapid onset and short duration of action; they can be titrated to the desired level of sedation and analgesia (Box 188-2); and they have a long safety record with emergency department use. They should be used with caution in elderly patients and in patients with chronic obstructive pulmonary disease who have a higher incidence of respiratory depression and prolonged sedation.

Multiple studies have demonstrated the safety and efficacy of ketamine in pediatric patients.[33,34,38,39] As a result, it has become one of the most widely used agents for emergency department PSA in children. While data regarding the use of ketamine in adult emergency department patients is limited, a recent study has demonstrated a high success rate with minimal complications.[37] Ketamine should be avoided in children younger than 3 months of age, and in patients with uncontrolled hypertension, ischemic heart disease, and upper respiratory infections and those at risk for elevated intraocular or intracranial pressure.

Over the past several years, propofol has been gaining popularity and acceptance as a safe and effective agent for emergency department PSA in both children and adults. Propofol's popularity stems from its clinical properties, including an almost immediate

BOX 188-2. Drug Administration Strategies

Methohexital

- Adults: 1.0 mg/kg IV bolus with additional 0.5 mg/kg boluses as needed.
- Children: 1.0 mg/kg IV bolus with additional 0.5 mg/kg boluses as needed up to a maximum of 2.0 mg/kg or 25 mg/kg rectally*
- Methohexital should be given over 60 seconds to avoid apnea and respiratory depression.

Ketamine

- Adults: 1.5 to 2.0 mg/kg IV over 2 minutes with additional 0.5 mg/kg boluses as needed; administer midazolam 0.05 mg/kg approximately 1 minute prior to ketamine to attenuate cardiovascular stimulation and reduce or eliminate emergence phenomena.
- Children: 1.5 to 2.0 mg/kg IV over 2 minutes with additional 0.5 mg/kg boluses as needed, or 4 to 5 mg/kg IM; add atropine 0.01 mg/kg (minimum dose 0.1 mg; maximum dose, 0.5 mg) or glycopyrrolate (0.005 mg/kg to a maximum dose of 0.25 mg) to the same syringe to prevent excessive salivation.
- Ketamine should be given at a rate of 0.5 mg/kg/min or over 90 to 120 seconds to avoid respiratory depression.

Propofol†

- Adults: 1.0 mg/kg IV bolus with additional 0.5 mg/kg boluses as needed, or a constant infusion at 25 to 125 μg/kg/min titrated to effect.
- Children: 1.0 mg/kg IV bolus (maximum 40 mg) with additional 0.5 mg/kg boluses (maximum 20 mg per bolus) as needed, or a constant infusion at 25 to 125 μg/kg/min titrated to effect.
- Bolus doses of propofol should be given over 60 to 120 seconds to avoid apnea and respiratory depression.

Etomidate

- Adults: 0.1 mg/kg IV bolus with additional 0.05 to 0.1 mg/kg boluses as needed.
- Children: 0.1 mg/kg IV bolus with additional 0.05 to 0.1 mg/kg boluses as needed.
- Etomidate should be given over 90 to 120 seconds to avoid respiratory depression.

Nitrous oxide

- Adults: 50% nitrous oxide (50% oxygen) via demand-valve.
- Children: 30% to 50% nitrous oxide (70% to 50% oxygen) via demand-valve or continuous-flow using a nasal mask (continuous-flow technique requires the presence of two physicians).

Fentanyl and midazolam

- General Principles of Administration:
- The dose of each drug ultimately depends on the patient's age and pain threshold, the procedure being performed, the concomitant use of other drugs, and the presence of underlying medical problems.
- Strive to achieve a "balanced" effect of analgesia and sedation. For example, if the patient is very drowsy but experiencing pain, additional analgesia (fentanyl) is indicated. On the other hand, if the patient is too alert, then more sedation (midazolam) should be given.
- The drugs must be slowly and carefully titrated to the desired level of analgesia and sedation. Administer each dose over 1 minute and wait 2 to 3 minutes between doses to fully appreciate the effects of the previous dose and avoid overdosing.
- The endpoint of drug administration is a patient who is very drowsy and frequently falls asleep when not stimulated. There is a variable amount of ptosis present, nystagmus occurs, and the speech is slurred and often not understandable. However, airway reflexes are intact; the ability to swallow is preserved; and the patient is arousable to verbal or painful stimuli, although the response to pain is greatly tempered. At the height of pain, patients may grimace or express objections. This does not signify inadequate analgesia or sedation, but rather a lack of general anesthesia.
- If respiratory depression occurs, patients should be encouraged to take several deep breaths. In most cases, this is all that is required. Administration of a painful stimulus may also be helpful. If necessary, naloxone or flumazenil can be administered. A brief period of assisted ventilation using a bag/mask device may be performed until the patient resumes spontaneous respiration, eliminating the need for reversal agents.
- Adults: An initial dose of 1 to 1.5 μg/kg of fentanyl is given, and the effect is observed. This is followed by an initial dose of 1 to 2 mg of midazolam. All doses are administered over 1 minute. Additional fentanyl and midazolam are given in increments (50 μg per dose of fentanyl, 1 mg per dose of midazolam) at 2- to 3-minute intervals until the desired level of analgesia and sedation is achieved. In elderly patients or those with significant underlying cardiorespiratory disease, initial and incremental doses of both agents should be halved.
- Children: An initial dose of 1 μg/kg of fentanyl and 0.05 mg/kg of midazolam is administered as previously described. Subsequent doses of fentanyl are given in increments of 0.25 to 0.5 μg/kg, and additional midazolam is administered in doses of 0.02 to 0.03 mg/kg until the desired level of analgesia and sedation is achieved. The principles of slow careful titration, achievement of a balanced effect, and endpoints of drug administration are identical in adults and children.

*For rectal use of methohexital, add 5 mL of sterile water or saline to a 500 mg vial of methohexital and mix well; this provides a methohexital solution of 100 mg/mL. Administer the appropriate dose of methohexital using a small rubber feeding tube or plastic intravenous catheter with the needle removed; be sure to deliver methohexital into the rectum, not the colon, and squeeze or tape the buttocks together immediately after administration to avoid expulsion.
†To prevent injection pain with propofol, place a rubber tourniquet distal to the injection and administer 0.5 mg/kg of IV lidocaine 30 to 120 seconds before propofol. Be sure to remove the tourniquet prior to propofol administration.

onset of action after intravenous administration, uniformly successful sedation, extremely rapid recovery, and antiemetic effects. Propofol's acceptance as an appropriate agent for emergency department use has been driven by a number of recent studies demonstrating safe administration by emergency physicians.[32,45,46] However, before using propofol for the first time, it is advisable to spend some time observing propofol sedation by an experienced clinician, as there is a "learning curve" with respect to dosing and titration.

Based on current data, propofol appears best suited for brief intensely painful procedures (e.g., cardioversion, fracture reduction) or brief procedures that require complete immobilization (e.g., ocular examination). The safety of propofol for extended administration in the emergency department has not been documented.[65]

Since propofol typically induces deep sedation, close patient monitoring is mandatory. In the majority of the emergency department studies to date, two physicians were present; one to administer propofol and observe the patient, and another to perform the procedure.[32,46,48] However, there is no evidence that the presence of two physicians improves outcome. Tactics to decrease the risk of aspiration should also be employed, including avoidance of oversedation (and therefore the need for assisted ventilation) and adopting a more conservative approach to recent oral intake.[65]

Although etomidate enjoys widespread acceptance as an induction agent for emergency department RSI, limited data are available to support its safety and efficacy for PSA. In a prospective study of 60 patients, Ruth and associates[56] found that 98% of patients were successfully sedated with etomidate. There was a low incidence of adverse effects, including oxygen desaturation below 90% (5 patients), myoclonus (4 patients), vomiting (1 patient), pain on injection (1 patient), and a brief episode of bradycardia (1 patient). Several other studies have demonstrated similar results.[52,53,55] Intravenous methohexital is not easily titrated and may be associated with a slightly higher incidence of apnea and respiratory depression when compared with a combination of fentanyl and midazolam or ketamine.[30] The use of rectal methohexital has demonstrated use in sedating children for radiologic procedures.[31]

SPECIAL CONSIDERATIONS FOR PEDIATRIC PATIENTS

Although it is clear that children may find even the most routine emergency department procedures terrifying, they historically have received less pain control and anxiolysis than adult patients with similar conditions.[66,67]

Over the last several years, PSA agents previously restricted to use in the operating suite have been used with increasing frequency in pediatric ambulatory treatment settings. In response to reports of adverse outcomes (including deaths), the American Academy of Pediatrics Committee on Drugs has published guidelines for PSA.[5,9] These documents provide a useful, pediatric-focused adjunct to the Practice Guidelines set forth by the American College of Emergency Physicians.[1]

Approach to Sedation in Children

When planning a strategy for performing a painful procedure on a child in the emergency department, one must balance the desire to reduce pain and fear in the child with the level of safety and invasiveness inherent in some methods of PSA. In some cases, a calm and reassuring bedside manner combined with distraction techniques may be successful. For other procedures, the use of topical agents such as EMLA cream (eutectic mixture of local anesthetics), tetracaine/adrenaline/cocaine, and lidocaine/epinephrine/tetracaine solutions and gels, in conjunction with transmucosal anxiolytics, may provide adequate sedation and analgesia and obviate the need for placement of an intravenous line (see Table 188-2). Local anesthetics are potential cardiac depressants and can cause CNS depression or excitation, even if injected intradermally. Maximum recommended doses should be calculated in advance to avoid overdosing in small children.[5] Intravenous PSA is indicated when intravenous access is required for other reasons and when the clinician believes that the benefits of intravenous administration outweigh the potential problems (e.g., pain, technical difficulty) associated with intravenous line placement. In addition, intravenous administration should be considered when repeat doses of medications are likely to be needed (i.e., for prolonged procedures).

Guidelines for patient preparation, personnel requirements, monitoring, drug administration, recovery care, and discharge criteria for children receiving PSA are similar to those outlined for adults, but some special concerns should be highlighted. Dosages must be calculated precisely using the child's current weight, not the parent's estimate. Equipment to manage the airway and resuscitation supplies must be size appropriate, and the treating physician must be skilled in airway management and pediatric resuscitation.

Pharmacology

Agents used for PSA often have different pharmacokinetics in infants and children than in adults. The body's content of water, muscle, and fat vary significantly from birth to adulthood, and this, along with factors such as protein-binding capacity and the level of maturity of hepatic and renal function, can affect the half-life elimination of medications. While not universally true for all drugs, neonates have more prolonged clearance times than children older that 2 years, but after 2, the half-life is longer than in adults. As the child approaches the teen years, the pharmacokinetics approach adult patterns. Precise dosing according to weight and anticipation of age-dependent responses to these medications are essential for their safe use. The benefits of intravenous drug administration may be outweighed by the difficulty in obtaining intravenous access in some children. In this situation, alternative routes of administration (e.g., oral, nasal, rectal, intramuscular) can be used (see Table 188-1).

Opioids

As in adults, fentanyl has become the opioid of choice for PSA in children. When administered intravenously, it should be titrated slowly, keeping in mind that the potential for respiratory depression is enhanced when fentanyl is used in concert with other sedatives.[68,69] The metabolism of fentanyl in small infants (<3 months) is prolonged. Therefore, some authors recommend starting with one third of the usual dose in neonates and small infants to avoid respiratory compromise.[68]

The OTFC appears to be an attractive option for premedication for laceration repair in the emergency department. It has been most extensively studied as a preinduction agent in children and carries the same risk of respiratory depression as intravenous fentanyl[70]; therefore, standard PSA monitoring is required.

The indications for fentanyl use in children are similar to those for adults, namely relatively short, painful procedures such as abscess incision and drainage, fracture and joint reduction, burn debridement, and complex laceration repair. As with adults, combination with midazolam for additional sedation and amnesia is often preferred. A safe and efficacious method for titrating these medications is described in Box 188-2. Careful titration is also important in children, and the physician responsible for PSA should not allow the painful procedure to begin until the desired level of sedation and analgesia is achieved.

Benzodiazepines

Midazolam has become a popular agent for sedation in the pediatric age group because of its rapid onset of sedation, short duration of action, and minimal pain on injection compared with other benzodiazepines. In addition, midazolam is effective by almost any route of administration (e.g., intravenous, intramuscular, nasal, oral, rectal), making it ideal for sedating the child who does not require intravenous access (see Table 188-1).

Oral administration is simple but can take up to 30 minutes to achieve effective sedation. Nasal midazolam will provide adequate sedation more rapidly than oral administration, often within 10 minutes. However, in school-age children, it is not feasible to deliver intranasally the volume of the intravenous formulation required to achieve the desired level of sedation.

To facilitate painful procedures, intravenous midazolam is often combined with fentanyl; however, midazolam alone via a transmucosal route (i.e., intranasally or orally) can be quite useful for sedating the anxious or uncooperative child for a procedure that is brief and only mildly painful (e.g., administration of local or regional anesthesia for laceration repair, lumbar puncture). Often, with transmucosal midazolam and a topical anesthetic, a minor procedure can be completed with minimal discomfort. Although popular with many practitioners as a sedating agent for painless imaging studies, midazolam does not consistently render the child motionless, and additional medications may be needed to obtain an acceptable study.

Flumazenil has been shown to successfully antagonize the hypnotic effects of midazolam in pediatric cases of overdose and reversal of preoperative or intensive care unit sedation.[71,72] The most commonly used dose is 0.02 mg/kg with a maximum of 0.2 mg. Resedation can occur in children receiving flumazenil for benzodiazepine overdose and occasionally PSA; therefore, the patient should be observed for at least 1 hour if flumazenil has been given. Other serious adverse effects are rare, but when they do occur, they are similar to those in adults (i.e., seizures). Therefore, flumazenil should be avoided in children on chronic benzodiazepines or those taking medications that could lower the seizure threshold. Less serious effects include agitation and crying.

Paradoxical reactions to benzodiazepines including agitation, combativeness, and inconsolability are occasionally seen in young children. A recent report demonstrated that flumazenil brought about abatement of paradoxical reactions within a few minutes in children who had been given midazolam to facilitate endoscopy.[73]

Barbiturates

Pentobarbital, thiopental, and methohexital are the most commonly used barbiturates for sedation in children. They have been most extensively studied as induction agents for general anesthesia and as sedatives for healthy children undergoing prescheduled radiologic studies.[68] Because of its long duration of action, pentobarbital is less desirable for procedural sedation in the emergency department.

Thiopental is a short-acting barbiturate used extensively for anesthetic induction and rectally for sedation before imaging studies. When given intravenously at doses of 0.5 to 2.0 mg/kg, it produces deep sedation lasting 10 to 15 minutes. The potential for respiratory depression, hypotension, and a longer recovery period are greater than with methohexital.[68] Thiopental is safe in children with seizure disorders. As mentioned, rectal methohexital has demonstrated efficacy for sedating children undergoing imaging procedures.

Ketamine

Ketamine hydrochloride has analgesic, sedative, and amnesic properties and is an excellent agent for children who require analgesia and sedation for self-limited painful procedures. It is indicated for complex laceration repair, fracture reduction or pin placement, foreign body extraction, and abscess incision and drainage and for extremely agitated children who require an examination for sexual abuse.[33] Coadministration of an antisialagogue in the same syringe with ketamine is recommended. Some authors prefer glycopyrrolate (0.005 mg/kg to a maximum dose of 0.25 mg) to atropine because of its somewhat greater antisialagogic effect and its lack of penetration of the blood-brain barrier.

As discussed previously, emergence reactions are common in children who receive ketamine, but the severity of these reactions are generally very mild.[41] Midazolam does not alter the incidence or the severity of these reactions, and therefore it is no longer recommended.

An often overlooked but important aspect to ketamine use in children is a discussion with the parents of what to expect following drug administration. If unexpected, the trancelike appearance, nystagmus, and sudden purposeless movements can be disconcerting to many parents.

Propofol

The use of propofol for emergency department PSA has been described earlier. Children tend to require somewhat higher doses than adults to achieve the optimal level of sedation for a given procedure. An intermittent bolus of 0.5 to 1 mg/kg can be given, with repeated doses as necessary, or propofol can be continuously infused at 25 to 125 μg/kg/minute, maintaining heart rate and blood pressure within 20% of baseline. When injected, propofol is quite painful at the site, which is difficult for children. This can be relieved somewhat by selecting the largest vein possible and premixing the propofol with lidocaine, as described previously.[51]

Other Agents

Although historically very popular for sedating children for a wide variety of procedures, the use of chloral hydrate, a pure sedative hypnotic, offers no advantage to currently available agents. Moreover, its delayed onset (>40 minutes), prolonged recovery time, and residual sedation (often lasting up to 24 hours) make it unsatisfactory for emergency department use. Likewise, the combination of meperidine (Demerol), promethazine (Phenergan), and chlorpromazine (Thorazine), also known as DPT or the "lytic" cocktail, is not recommended. Unacceptable rates of sedation failure, prolonged sedation times, the risk of respiratory depression, and the possibility of dystonic reactions (from the combination of phenothiazines) argue against its use.[74,75]

REFERENCES

1. American College of Emergency Physicians: Clinical policy: Procedural sedation and analgesia in the emergency department. *Ann Emerg Med* 45:177, 2005.
2. Innes G, et al: Procedural sedation and analgesia in the emergency department. Canadian consensus guidelines. *J Emerg Med* 17:145, 1999.
3. Krauss B, Green SM: Sedation and analgesia for procedures in children. *N Engl J Med* 342:938, 2000.
4. American Academy of Pediatrics Committee on Drugs: Guidelines for the elective use of conscious sedation, deep sedation, and general anesthesia in pediatric patients. *Pediatrics* 76:317, 1985.
5. American Academy of Pediatrics Committee on Drugs: Guidelines for monitoring and management of pediatric patients during and after sedation for diagnostic and therapeutic procedures. *Pediatrics* 89:1110, 1992.
6. Green SM, Krauss B: Procedural sedation terminology: Moving beyond "conscious sedation." *Ann Emerg Med* 39:433, 2002.
7. Joint Commission on Accreditation of Healthcare Organizations: Accreditation manual for hospitals. Oakbrook Terrace, Ill, Joint Commission on Accreditation of Healthcare Organizations, 2001.
8. American Society of Anesthesiology: Practice guidelines for sedation and analgesia by non-anesthesiologists. *Anesthesiology* 96:1004, 2002.
9. American Academy of Pediatrics Committee on Drugs: Guidelines for monitoring and management of pediatric patients during and after sedation for diagnostic and therapeutic procedures: Addendum. *Pediatrics* 110:836, 2002.
10. Green SM, Krauss B: The semantics of ketamine. *Ann Emerg Med* 36:480, 2000.
11. Agrawal D, et al: Preprocedural fasting state and adverse events in children undergoing procedural sedation and analgesia in a pediatric emergency department. *Ann Emerg Med* 42:636, 2003.
12. Cote CJ, Karl HW, Notterman DA: Adverse sedation events in pediatrics: A critical incident analysis of contributing factors. *Pediatrics* 105:805, 2000.
13. Gill M, et al: A study of bispectral index monitor during procedural sedation and analgesia in the emergency department. *Ann Emerg Med* 41:234, 2003.
14. Agrawal D, et al: Bispectral index monitoring quantifies depth of sedation during emergency department procedural sedation and analgesia in children. *Ann Emerg Med* 43:247, 2004.
15. Miner JR, et al: Bispectral electroencephalographic analysis of patients undergoing procedural sedation in the emergency department. *Acad Emerg Med* 10:638, 2003.
16. Miner JR, Heegaard W, Plummer D: End-tidal carbon dioxide monitoring during procedural sedation. *Acad Emerg Med* 9:275, 2002.
17. Newman DH, et al: When is a patient safe for discharge after procedural sedation? The timing of adverse effect events in 1,367 pediatric procedural sedations. *Ann Emerg Med* 42:627, 2003.
18. Chudnofsky CR, et al: The safety of fentanyl use in the emergency department. *Ann Emerg Med* 18:6, 1989.
19. Schutzman SA, et al: Oral transmucosal fentanyl citrate for premedication of children undergoing laceration repair. *Ann Emerg Med* 24:1059, 1994.
20. Wright SW, et al: Comparison of midazolam and diazepam for conscious sedation in the emergency department. *Ann Emerg Med* 22:201, 1993.
21. Bailey PL, et al: Frequent hypoxemia and apnea after sedation with midazolam and fentanyl. *Anesthesiology* 73:826, 1990.
22. Hill AB, et al: Prevention of rigidity during fentanyl-oxygen induction of anesthesia. *Anesthesiology* 55:452, 1981.
23. Mostert JW, et al: Clinical comparison of fentanyl with meperidine muscle rigidity. *J Clin Pharmacol J New Drugs* 8:382, 1968.
24. Scott TC, Sarnquist FH: Seizure-like movements during a fentanyl infusion with absence of seizure activity in a simultaneous EEG recording. *Anesthesiology* 62:812, 1985.
25. Flacke JW, et al: Histamine release by four narcotics: A double-blind study in humans. *Anesth Analog* 66:723, 1987.
26. Ramoska EA, Linkenheimer R, Glasgow C: Midazolam use in the emergency department. *J Emerg Med* 9:247, 1991.
27. Shane SA, Fuchs SM, Khine H: Efficacy of rectal midazolam for the sedation of preschool children undergoing laceration repair. *Ann Emerg Med* 24:1065, 1994.
28. Connors K, Terndrup TE: Nasal versus oral midazolam for sedation of anxious children undergoing laceration repair. *Ann Emerg Med* 24:1074, 1994.
29. Reves JG, et al: Midazolam: Pharmacology and uses. *Anesthesiology* 62:310, 1985.
30. Austin T, et al: Safety and effectiveness of methohexital for procedural sedation in the emergency department. *J Emerg Med* 24:315, 2003.
31. Pomeranz ES, et al: Rectal methohexital sedation for CT imaging of pediatric patients in the ED. *Pediatrics* 105:1110, 2000.
32. Miner JR, et al: Randomized clinical trial of propofol versus methohexital for procedural sedation during fracture and dislocation reduction in the emergency department. *Acad Emerg Med* 10:931, 2003.

33. Green SM, Johnson NE: Ketamine sedation for pediatric procedures: Part 2, review and implications. *Ann Emerg Med* 19:1033, 1990.
34. Kim G, et al: Ventilatory response during dissociative sedation in children: A pilot study. *Acad Emerg Med* 10:140, 2003.
35. Hemmingsen C, Nielsen PK, Odorico J: Ketamine in the treatment of bronchospasm during mechanical ventilation. *Am J Emerg Med* 12:417, 1994.
36. Green SM, et al: What is the optimal dose of intramuscular ketamine for pediatric sedation? *Acad Emerg Med* 6:21, 1999.
37. Chudnofsky CR, et al: A combination of midazolam and ketamine for procedural sedation and analgesia in adult ED patients. *Acad Emerg Med* 7:228, 2000.
38. Green SM, et al: Intramuscular ketamine for pediatric sedation in the emergency department: Safety profile in 1,022 cases. *Ann Emerg Med* 31:688, 1998.
39. Green SM, Nakamura R, Johnson NE: Ketamine sedation for pediatric procedures: Part 1, A prospective series. *Ann Emerg Med* 1:1024, 1990.
40. Wathen JE, et al: Does midazolam alter the clinical effects on intravenous ketamine sedation in children? A double-blind, randomized, controlled, emergency department trial. *Ann Emerg Med* 36:579, 2000
41. Sherwin TS, et al: Does adjunctive midazolam reduce recovery agitation after ketamine sedation for pediatric procedures? A randomized, double blind, placebo-controlled, emergency department trial. *Ann Emerg Med* 35:229, 2000.
42. Hostetler MA, Davis CO: Prospective age-based comparison of behavioral reactions occurring after ketamine sedation in the ED. *Am J Emerg Med* 20:463, 2002.
43. Luhmann JD, et al: Sedation for peritonsilar abscess drainage in the pediatric emergency department. *Pediatr Emerg Care* 18:1, 2002.
44. Acworth JP, Purdie D, Clark RC: Intravenous ketamine plus midazolam is superior to intranasal midazolam for emergency paediatric procedural sedation. *Emerg Med J* 18:39, 2001.
45. Bassett KE, et al: Propofol for procedural sedation in children in the emergency department. *Ann Emerg Med* 42:773, 2003.
46. Godambe SA, et al: Comparison of propofol/fentanyl versus ketamine/midazolam for brief orthopedic procedural sedation in a pediatric emergency department. *Pediatrics* 112: 116, 2003.
47. Guenther E, et al: Propofol for sedation by emergency physicians for elective pediatric outpatient procedures. *Ann Emerg Med* 42:783, 2003.
48. Skokan EG, et al: Use of propofol sedation in a pediatric emergency department: A prospective study. *Clinical Pediatrics* 40:663, 2001.
49. Havel CJ Jr, Strait RT, Hennes H: A clinical trial of propofol vs. midazolam for procedural sedation in a pediatric emergency department. *Acad Emerg Med* 6:989, 1999.
50. Coll-Vincent B, et al: Sedation for cardioversion in the emergency department: Analysis of effectiveness in four protocols. *Ann Emerg Med* 42:767, 2003.
51. Picard P, Tramer MR: Prevention of pain on injection with propofol: A quantitative systematic review. *Anest Analg* [illegible], 2000.
52. Dickinson R, Singer AJ, Carrion W: Etomidate for pediatric sedation prior to fracture reduction. *Acad Emerg Med* 8:74, 2001.
53. Vinson DR, Bradbury DR: Etomidate for procedural sedation in emergency medicine. *Ann Emerg Med* 39:592, 2002
54. Dursteler BB, Wightman JM: Etomidate-facilitated hip reduction in the emergency department. *Am J Emerg Med* 18:204, 2000.
55. Burton JH, et al: Etomidate and midazolam for reduction of anterior shoulder dislocation: A randomized controlled trial. *Ann Emerg Med* 40:496, 2002.
56. Ruth WJ, Burton JH, Bock AJ: Intravenous etomidate for procedural sedation in emergency department patients. *Acad Emerg Med* 8:13, 2001.
57. Van Keulen SG, Burton JH: Myoclonus associated with etomidate for ED procedural sedation and analgesia. *Am J Emerg Med* 21:556, 2003.
58. Schenarts CL, Burton JH, Riker RR: Adrenocortical dysfunction following etomidate induction in emergency department patients. *Acad Emerg Med* 8:1, 2001.
59. Stewart RD: Nitrous oxide sedation/analgesia in emergency medicine. *Ann Emerg Med* 14:2, 1985.
60. Gamis AS, Knapp JF, Glenski JA: Nitrous oxide analgesia in a pediatric emergency department. *Ann Emerg Med* 18:177, 1989.
61. Luhmann JD, et al: A randomized clinical trial of continuous-flow nitrous oxide and midazolam for sedation of young children during laceration repair. *Ann Emerg Med* 37:20, 2001.
62. Krauss B: Continuous-flow nitrous oxide: Searching for the ideal procedural anxiolytic for toddlers. *Ann Emerg Med* 37:61, 2001.
63. Philip BK: *Flumazenil: A Review of the Literature.* New Jersey, Excerpta Medica, 1992.
64. Chudnofsky CR, et al: The safety and efficacy of flumazenil in reversing conscious sedation in the emergency department. *Acad Emerg Med* 4:944, 1997.
65. Green SM, Krauss B: Propofol in emergency medicine: Pushing the sedation frontier. *Ann Emerg Med* 42:792, 2003.
66. Hostetler MA, Szilagyi PG, Auinger P: Do children in the emergency department really receive less analgesia and sedation than adults [abstract]? *Acad Emerg Med* 7:549, 2000.
67. Strauss SG, Lynn AM, Spear RM: Progress in pain control for very young infants. *Contemp Pediatr* 12:80, 1995.
68. Cote CJ: Sedation for the pediatric patient. *Pediatr Clin North Am* 41:31, 1994.
69. Yaster M, Desphanpande KT: Management of pediatric pain with opioid analgesics. *J Pediatr* 113:421, 1988.
70. Friesen RH, Lockhart CH: Oral transmucosal fentanyl citrate for preanesthetic medication of pediatric day surgery patients with or without droperidol as a prophylactic anti-emetic. *Anesthesiology* 76:46, 1992.
71. Clark RF, et al: Delayed onset lorazepam poisoning successfully reversed by flumazenil in a child: Case report and review of the literature. *Pediatr Emerg Care* 1:32, 1995.
72. Sugarman JM, Paul RI: Flumazenil: A review. *Pediatr Emerg Care* 10:37, 1994.
73. Massanari M, Novitsky J, Reinstein LJ: Paradoxical reactions in children associated with midazolam during endoscopy. *Clin Pediatr* 36:681, 1997.
74. Proudfoot J: Analgesia, anesthesia and conscious sedation. *Emerg Med Clin North Am* 13:357, 1995
75. Terndrup TE, et al: A prospective analysis of intramuscular meperidine, promethazine, and chlorpromazine in pediatric emergency department patients. *Ann Emerg Med* 20:31, 1991.

CHAPTER

189 The Combative Patient

Gregory P. Moore and Louise Kao

PERSPECTIVE

Background

Dealing with combative patients is one of the most difficult challenges an emergency physician encounters. Often brought in against their will, such patients may be agitated, confrontational, and nearly impossible to examine. If not controlled, they may harm themselves or others, including the emergency department staff, other patients, and visitors. Although it is important to manage the combative patient, it is preferable to recognize signs of impending violence early in order to prevent its occurrence. The emergency physician should control the patient and the situation, diagnose and treat reversible causes of violence, and protect the patient and staff from harm. Emergency physicians are often called on to provide medical clearance before psychiatric admissions. The physician must recognize a medical etiology of an apparent psychiatric disorder to perform appropriate triage at disposition and avoid inadequate care. Medicolegal considerations include informed consent, battery, false imprisonment, and duty to warn. This chapter discusses these aspects of the management of the combative patient in the emergency department.

Epidemiology

Violence has been called our nation's shameful epidemic. Injury is the leading cause of death in persons younger than 44 years, and homicide is the second leading cause of death in persons aged 15 to 24 years.[1] Homicide rates in the United States are the highest of any industrialized country,[2] and rates of death from firearms are eight times higher in the United States.[3] For each death there are an estimated 19 additional injuries requiring hospitalization.[4] The estimated lifetime medical cost for treating all gunshot injuries in the United States in 1994 was $2.3 billion; taxpayers covered an estimated $1.1 billion of this expense.[5]

Because of its nature, the emergency department lends itself easily to becoming a setting for violent behavior. The emergency department is an environment of high stress owing to illness, prolonged waiting times, confusion, and frequent lack of communication. The 24-hour open door policy, availability of potential hostages, and widespread accessibility of drugs and weapons compound the problem.[6] In 1999, the Bureau of Labor Statistics estimated that there were 2637 nonfatal assaults on hospital workers, with the highest frequency of violent attacks occurring in the emergency department, psychiatric ward, waiting rooms, and geriatric units.[7] Up to 50% of human service providers become victims of violence sometime during their careers.[8,9] In a survey of 461 emergency medicine residents in 1994, 62% were concerned about their personal safety while working in the emergency department and 50% thought that security measures in their hospitals were inadequate.[10] A 1999 survey of psychiatry residents revealed that 73% reported being threatened and 36% had been physically assaulted in residency. Two thirds of them had received either no or inadequate training in managing combative patients.[11] Unfortunately, despite the obvious risks, we as providers are typically not trained in the identification and management of combative patients.

A 1988 survey of emergency department directors in 170 U.S. teaching hospitals with volumes of at least 40,000 visits per year showed that, of 127 responding hospitals, 32% reported at least one verbal threat daily, 18% reported at least one threat with a weapon daily, and 25% reported restraining at least one patient daily.[12] Within the previous 5 years, 7% of institutions had experienced a violent death in the emergency department, and 80% had a staff member injured by violence. The violent patient suffered as well, with 13% of hospitals reporting injuring patients while restraining them, including one strangulation death. Litigation was pending in 16% of surveyed emergency departments because of restraint of patients. However, only 40% of hospitals surveyed provided formal nursing education on this topic and only 62% had 24-hour security personnel in the emergency department. A 1994 survey of 44 pediatric emergency department directors revealed that more than half received one or more verbal threats a week, 77% reported one or more physical attacks on staff per year, and 25% reported actual injury to staff.[13] The survey found that 24-hour security was in place at only 54% of emergency departments. In addition, studies have shown that an emergency department census of 50,000 per year or more and an average waiting time of 2 hours or more were significantly associated with increased incidence of violence.[12,13]

Patients who are armed with lethal weapons pose a serious threat to emergency department staff. Weapons carriage in the emergency department population has been estimated at approximately 4% to 8%,[14,15] with one large university-county hospital emergency department reporting confiscating an average of 5.4 weapons a day using a metal detector.[16] At this center, 26.7% of major trauma patients seen over a 14-year period were armed with lethal weapons (84% knives and 16% guns). A total of 115 incidents of violence involving weapons occurred over this period, resulting in four fatalities of patients and six minor injuries to the staff.[16] They also documented a disturbing trend of decreasing average age of major trauma patients carrying weapons from a mean of 24 in 1979 to a mean of 19 in 1992. This finding parallels national surveillance data on firearm-related fatalities from 1992 to 1995, which reveal that firearm deaths are on the rise among males aged 15 to 24 years.[17] Clearly, the prevalence of weapons carriage in the emergency department represents a potential for rapid escalation of violence. Unfortunately, predicting weapons carriage in any particular patient is not an easy task.[18] As a result, one should assume that all violent patients are armed until proved otherwise, especially those presenting with major trauma.

Identification of potentially violent patients is difficult, with male gender, prior history of violence, and drug or alcohol abuse being the only positive predictors.[17,19-22] Ethnicity, diagnosis, age, marital status, and education are not reliable identifiers. A study conducted in an outpatient psychiatric setting found that the incidence of violent behavior did not vary with the experience of the psychiatrist.[19] Actuarial prediction of patients' violence in a 6-month time period using criteria such as age, drug use, and prior history of violence was substantially more accurate than prediction by evaluating attending psychiatrists.[23] How are we, as emergency physicians, to predict, prevent, and control violent outbursts in the emergency department? Appreciation of the potential for violence, preparedness, and proper utilization of verbal techniques and physical or chemical restraints allow us to assist the patient while preventing injury.

PRINCIPLES OF DISEASE

Pathophysiology

The pathogenesis of violent behavior is not well understood, as evidenced by the multitude of theoretical explanations. Theories postulated have explored environmental, historical, interpersonal, biochemical, electrical, genetic, hormonal, neurotransmitter, and alcohol and substance abuse disorders as potential etiologies.[24,25] Known psychiatric illness is also a risk factor, with schizophrenia (paranoid and nonparanoid), personality disorders, mania, and psychotic depression being most often associated with violent behavior.[22,24,26-28] Schizophrenics with delusions often become violent because they believe that others are attempting to harm them. They may also have auditory hallucinations commanding harm to others. Patients with antisocial and borderline personality disorder typically do not feel remorse for their violent actions. The manic patient is particularly dangerous because of emotional lability; pleasantness can quickly turn to aggression. However, the magnitude of the risk of violence associated with psychiatric illness is debatable.[29-32] Alcohol and substance abuse disorders are consistently found to be associated with violent behavior in both psychiatric and nonpsychiatric populations.

Biologically, the serotonin system has been postulated to control aggression and inhibition, with diminished serotonergic function thought to disinhibit aggression against the self and others.[33-35] Low levels of cerebrospinal fluid 5-hydroxyindoleacetic acid, a metabolite of serotonin, have been correlated with violent suicides or crimes.[36] Whole-blood serotonin, when measured in a representative birth cohort of 781 individuals, was significantly related to violence in men but not in women.[37] Generalized brain dysfunction has also been hypothesized to predispose to violent behavior by disrupting the regulation of aggression. Research on animals and humans who have suffered brain insults has implicated specific areas of the brain, particularly the prefrontal cortex and the temporal cortex.[38-40] Positron emission tomography of murderers in one study showed reduced glucose metabolism in the prefrontal cortex, superior parietal gyrus, left angular gyrus, and the corpus callosum as well as abnormal asymmetry between left and right hemispheres of the brain, providing further evidence for the existence of abnormal brain function in violent individuals.[41] The discovery of a disproportionately higher census of XYY males in institutionalized populations has led to genetic studies showing that XYY males have increased impulsiveness that may lead to increased aggression. Increased testosterone in males and hormonal fluctuation in females have also been implicated.[33]

MANAGEMENT

Risk Assessment

Evaluation of the combative patient begins with risk assessment and attention to safety measures. Violence usually erupts after a period of mounting tension. The astute practitioner may identify verbal and nonverbal cues and subsequently have the opportunity to defuse the situation.[28] Verbal cues include speech that is insistent, becoming progressively louder and ultimately threatening. Nonverbal cues include tense posture and motor restlessness. In a typical scenario, the patient first becomes angry, then resists authority, and finally becomes confrontational and may perform violent deeds. However, violent behavior may erupt without warning (especially with organic etiologies), and clinicians should not feel overly confident in their ability to sense impending danger. As a whole, practitioners tend to be poor predictors of impending violence. Despite this, one should respond and take appropriate precautions in response to a "gut feeling" that a dangerous situation may be developing.[6]

An obviously angry patient should always be considered potentially violent. Provocative behavior, an angry demeanor, pacing, loud speech, tense posture, gripping arm rails intensely, frequently changing body position, pounding walls or throwing things, and clenched fists are all signs of impending violence.[6,12] The patient should be removed from contact with other belligerent accomplices, as well as from other provocative patients, to prevent escalation. A quiet area with a window or direct observation is optimal. Because increased waiting times correlate positively with violent behavior,[7,12,13] one should consider seeing the potentially violent patient expeditiously to prevent escalation of aggression. Often, the aura of preferential treatment defuses patients' anger.

All patients should be disarmed before the interview. Metal detectors can be used for this purpose to remove weapons from all patients before emergency department entry. The practice of undressing all patients and placing them in a gown is useful both as a nonconfrontational search for weapons and for easy identification in the event that the patient escapes from the emergency department. Although searching patients for weapons may appear to be a violation of privacy, routine disarming of all patients presenting to the emergency department results in an increased feeling of safety for both patients and staff.[15,42]

The setting of the patient's interview should be one of privacy but not isolation.[6,26] Some emergency departments have seclusion rooms specifically intended for the purpose of interviewing potentially dangerous patients. Security should be nearby and the door should be left open to allow both intervention and escape. The patient and interviewer may be seated roughly equidistant from the door, or the interviewer may sit between the patient and the door. Blocking the door, however, poses a risk of harm to the clinician if the patient feels the need to escape. A physician who is trapped in the room with a violent patient is at high risk for personal injury. Ideally, two exits should be available and doors should swing outward. This arrangement facilitates escape but could increase the chance of injury to those standing outside the door. The clinician should have unrestricted access to the door and therefore should never sit behind a desk. The room should not contain heavy objects that may be thrown, such as ashtrays, or other potential weapons such as electrical cords, scalpels, needles, or hot liquids. The clinician should have a mechanism for alerting others that he or she is in danger, such as a panic button or a code word or phrase that instructs others to call for security (e.g., "I need Dr. Armstrong in here"). For personal protection, glasses, earrings, and necklaces should be removed and neckties should be removed or tucked into shirts. Personal accessories that may be used against the emergency physician, such as a stethoscope, scissors, or pocket knives, should be removed. The physician should be aware of any objects within the room or on the patient's body, such as pens, watches, or belts, that may be used as weapons.[6,43]

Verbal Management Techniques

The patient should be made as comfortable as possible, and the interviewer should adopt an honest and straightforward manner.[44] In some cases, an agitated patient may be aware of his or her impulse control problem and may welcome limit-setting behavior by the clinician (e.g., "I can help you with your problem, but I cannot allow you to continue threatening me or the staff").[6] The interviewer should act as an advocate for the patient. Offering a soft chair or something to eat or drink (not a hot liquid, which may be used as a weapon) may help to establish trust. A significant percentage of patients decompress at this point because offering food or drink appeals to their most basic human needs and attention to these needs builds trust. The interviewer should adopt a nonconfrontational demeanor and be an attentive and receptive listener without conveying weakness or vulnerability. The interviewer should respond verbally in a calm and soothing tone of voice. It is also important to avoid direct eye contact, avoid approaching the patient from behind, stand at least an arm's length away, and avoid sudden movements.[6]

A key mistake when interviewing such a patient is failing to address violence directly.[19,44] The patient should be asked relevant questions such as "Do you consider yourself a fighter?" or "Do you carry a gun?" Stating the obvious (e.g., "You look angry") may help the patient to begin sharing emotions. If the patient becomes more agitated, it is important to speak in a conciliatory manner and offer supportive statements such as "You obviously have a lot of will power and are good at controlling yourself" to help defuse the situation. If this is not successful, a respectful offer of medication or restraints to the patient may prevent further escalation.

Clinicians should be aware of their own reactions to potentially violent patients and avoid countertransference of anger toward them. Arguing, exhibiting machismo or condescension, commanding the patient to calm down, or threatening to call security may be seen as a challenge to such patients to "prove themselves" and have disastrous consequences. It is important not to lie to the patient (e.g., "I am sure you will be out of here in no time" when this is not the case) because violent consequences may follow when the lie is discovered. The innocent nurse or unsuspecting colleague who follows the interviewer may become the victim. It is especially important not to deny or downplay threatening behavior, which places the interviewer at increased risk for assault and injury. A chilling illustration of this principle involves a psychiatrist who was killed after entering the waiting room with a patient he knew was potentially violent and armed. He erroneously believed that the strength of the physician-patient relationship ensured his personal safety.[19] All threats should be taken seriously to prevent assault and injury.

If verbal techniques are unsuccessful and escalation of violence occurs, the physician should excuse him- or herself from the room and summon help using a predetermined code word or phrase or panic button.

Physical Restraints

Physical restraints should be considered when, despite a professional and proper approach to the combative patient, verbal techniques have been unsuccessful. The use of restraints can be humane and effective while facilitating diagnosis and treatment of the patient and preventing injury to the patient or medical staff.[45] Overall, the liability one incurs for restraining a patient against the patient's will is negligible compared with the potential liability for allowing a patient to lose control and hurt him or herself or others.[6]

Indications for emergency seclusion and restraint are (1) to prevent imminent harm to others, (2) to prevent imminent harm to the patient, (3) to prevent serious disruption of the treatment program or significant damage to the environment, and (4) as part of an ongoing behavior treatment program. Seclusion may be used to decrease environmental stimulation and at the patient's request. The clinician may find it helpful to classify patients into three categories: those with an organic disorder in which restraints facilitate evaluation, those with functional psychosis in which verbal techniques are less effective and restraints facilitate administration of neuroleptics, and those with personality disorders in which verbal techniques are not useful.[6]

Seclusion or restraint may be contraindicated because of a patient's clinical or medical condition. Seclusion should not be used in an unstable patient who requires close monitoring. Seclusion should also be avoided when the patient is suicidal, self-abusive, self-mutilating, or has had an ingestion or overdose.[28,46] Restraints are not to be applied for convenience only or as a punitive response for disruptive behavior, as injury to the patient and litigious consequences may follow. Having a colleague document agreement with the application of restraints is useful, as is the documentation of specific rather than general indications (e.g., "I restrained Mr. Smith because he told me he was going to beat me up and then took a swing at me" is preferable to "I restrained Mr. Smith because he was violent").

The implementation of restraints should be systematic and performed in accordance with an institutional or departmental protocol. Typical protocols begin with the examiner leaving the room to summon a trained restraint team when verbal techniques have proved unsuccessful. It may be helpful to consider the application of restraints as a procedure analogous to running an advanced cardiac life support code. The restraint team consists of at least five people, including a team leader. The leader is the only person giving orders and should be the individual with the most experience in implementing restraints, whether a physician, nurse, or security officer. Before entering the room, the leader outlines the restraint protocol and warns of anticipated danger (e.g., the presence of objects that may be used as weapons). All team members should remove personal effects that the patient could use against them. If the patient to be restrained is female, at least one member of the restraint team should be female to diminish potential allegations of sexual assault.

The team enters the room in force and displays a professional, rather than threatening, attitude.[6] Many violent individuals decompress at this point, as a large show of force protects their ego (i.e., "I would have fought back but there were too many against me"). The leader speaks to the patient in a calm and organized manner, explaining why restraints are needed and what the course of events will be (i.e., "You will receive a medical and psychiatric examination as well as treatment"). The patient is instructed to cooperate and lie down to have restraints applied. Some patients are relieved at the protection to self and others afforded by restraints when they feel themselves losing control. However, even if the patient suddenly appears less dangerous, when the decision to restrain has been made, it must be carried out. One should not negotiate with the patient at this point.

If physical force becomes necessary, one team member restrains a preassigned extremity by controlling the major joint (knee or elbow). The team leader controls the head. If the patient is armed, two mattresses can be used to charge and immobilize or sandwich the patient. Restraints are applied securely to each extremity and tied to the solid frame of the bed (not side rails, as later repositioning of side rails also repositions the patient's extremity). Leather restraints are optimal because they are physically strong and thus more efficacious in preventing escape and less constricting than typical soft restraints. For this reason, gauze should not be used. Soft restraints are helpful in restricting extremity use in the semicooperative patient but are unwarranted in the truly violent patient who is continuing to struggle and attempt escape. If chest restraints are used, it is vital that adequate chest expansion for ventilation is ensured. Applying a soft Philadelphia collar to the patient's neck prevents head banging and biting. Whenever possible, the treating physician should not actively participate in applying restraints to preserve the physician-patient relationship and not be viewed as adversarial. Restraining patients on their side helps prevent aspiration, although supine with the head elevated is more comfortable for the patient and allows a more thorough medical examination while providing some protection against aspiration.[28,47] When the patient is immobilized, announcing that "the crisis is over" has a calming effect on the restraint team and the patient.

After restraints have been applied successfully, the patient should be monitored frequently and positions changed to prevent neurovascular sequelae such as circulatory obstruction, pressure sores, and paresthesias as well as to avoid rhabdomyolysis associated with continued combativeness. A standardized form is recommended for this monitoring and should be developed by every emergency department that physically restrains patients (Figure 189-1). Documentation should include the specific indication for restraints and, if possible, a colleague's agreement that restraints were necessary. The restraint team should review their performance and discuss ways to improve efficiency in the future. Education and rehearsal by staff are imperative to maintain skills.

Sudden, unexpected deaths have been reported in patients who have been restrained.[48-51] Restraints applied by prehospital personnel in the prone or hobble (arms and legs restrained behind the patient)

LEATHER/SOFT RESTRAINT RECORD

DATE: ______________ TIME: ______________

Behavior Requiring Restraint: ______________

TYPE OF RESTRAINT: ☐ Leather ☐ Chest Vest ☐ Soft Limb Holders ☐ Pelvic Holder ☐ Body Holder ☐ Other ______________

LIMBS RESTRAINED: ☐ RUE ☐ LUE ☐ RLE ☐ LLE ☐ See Documentation from Referring Facility

POSITION: ☐ Prone ☐ Supine ☐ Side (circle) R L

MENTAL STATUS:

Oriented to:	Yes	No	Refuses
Person	☐	☐	☐
Place	☐	☐	☐
Time	☐	☐	☐

Reason for Restraint Explained to Patient

☐ Yes ☐ No (explain) ______________

Safety Check Done ☐ Yes ☐ No (explain) ______________

Alcohol/Drug Use Suspected: ☐ No ☐ Yes (explain) ______________

RN Signature: ______________

LEGEND
✓ = Need Assessed
– = Refused
\+ = Ate/Drank/Eliminated
NN= See Nurse's Notes
CC = Condom Catheter
NI = Not Impaired
Intake/Output/Circulation:
every 15 minutes for leathers,
every two hours for soft

DATE	TIME	EXTREMITIES RESTRAINED (If different from above)	TYPE (if changed from above)	INTAKE Indicated ✓, +, –, or NPO: FOOD	FLUID	OUTAKE ✓, +, –, foley or cc.: URINE	STOOL	CIRCULATION CHECK (circle)	RANGE OF MOTION (Indicate limb) every 2 hours	STAFF SIGNATURE
		LUE RUE LLE RLE						NI NN	LUE RUE LLE NN RLE	
		LUE RUE LLE RLE						NI NN	LUE RUE LLE NN RLE	
		LUE RUE LLE RLE						NI NN	LUE RUE LLE NN RLE	
		LUE RUE LLE RLE						NI NN	LUE RUE LLE NN RLE	
		LUE RUE LLE RLE						NI NN	LUE RUE LLE NN RLE	
		LUE RUE LLE RLE						NI NN	LUE RUE LLE NN RLE	
		LUE RUE LLE RLE						NI NN	LUE RUE LLE NN RLE	
		LUE RUE LLE RLE						NI NN	LUE RUE LLE NN RLE	

 Figure 189-1. Leather/soft restraint record.

position have resulted in deaths presumed by some to be due to positional asphyxia.[50] Research has cast some doubt on this theory.[52] Patients who are cocaine or stimulant intoxicated and restrained appear to be uniquely at risk for adverse outcomes.[48,49] Increased sympathetic tone and altered pain sensation have been postulated to allow exertion beyond normal physiologic limits in these patients, whereas sympathetic induced vasoconstriction may impede clearance of metabolic waste products. Alteration of respiratory mechanics in an acidemic patient resulting from a restraint position could be a contributing factor by impairing respiratory compensation. It seems prudent to recommend avoiding the prone restraint position altogether and using aggressive chemical sedation in the patient continuing to struggle in physical restraints.

The Joint Commission on Accreditation of Health Care Organizations (JCAHO) (PC.11.10 through PC 12.190, effective January 1, 2004) has written guidelines governing the use of restraint and seclusion for behavioral health patients, which must be reviewed by each hospital using these procedures. The reader is urged to review this publication. Educational materials regarding seclusion and restraint are available for purchase through their website: http://www.jcaho.org/index.html. To paraphrase, several essential elements must be provided for in a restraint situation including the following:

1. The implementation of restraint or seclusion is limited to emergencies where imminent risk of harm exists to patient or others.
2. Staff is trained and competent to apply restraint safely.
3. Staff is trained to minimize the use of restraint.
4. Patients in restraints are regularly evaluated and monitored.
5. Orders for restraint use are provided by licensed practitioners and are time limited.
6. Medical records document that the use of restraint or seclusion is consistent with organizational policy.

Rapid Tranquilization

Rapid tranquilization may be necessary to control an agitated patient and may be used in conjunction with physical restraints. The ideal pharmacologic agent for this purpose should be effective with multiple routes of administration, nonaddictive, immune to tolerance, and have a low side effect profile. In the 1900s, amobarbital was used but frequently was associated with respiratory depression. In the 1950s, chlorpromazine was found to have good efficacy; however, orthostatic hypotension, sedation, and tolerance to effects limited its usefulness. Rapid tranquilization with newer medications has been shown to be safe and effective in the management of psychotic and potentially assaultive patients.[36,53,55] Antipsychotic medications, also called neuroleptics, are useful for rapid tranquilization because of their high therapeutic index, lack of tolerance to the desired effects, and lack of addictive potential.[45,53] Classic antipsychotics block dopaminergic receptors and also have variable effects on cholinergic, adrenergic, histaminic, and serotonergic receptors. Antipsychotics can be divided into low potency (chlorpromazine, mesoridazine, thioridazine), mid-range potency (loxapine, molindone), and high potency (haloperidol, fluphenazine, thiothixene, trifluoperazine). The incidence of sedation, hypotension, and seizures is highest in the low-potency group and the incidence of extrapyramidal symptoms (EPSs) is greatest in the high-potency group.

Haloperidol (Haldol) is generally recommended as the drug of choice to sedate a violent patient, and rapid tranquilization is achieved using dosages of 2.5 to 10 mg intramuscularly (IM) at 30- to 60-minute intervals, with half doses used in elderly patients.[53-55] After IM injection, effects are typically seen in 10 to 30 minutes, with most patients requiring less than three doses to achieve the desired effect.[53] Although no ceiling dose has been established, it has been recommended that patients not receive more than six doses in 24 hours. However, 300 mg intravenously (IV) has been used over 24 hours without adverse effects (although the question of medication efficacy is raised with such dosing).[6] Using the lowest effective dose minimizes the risk of side effects. Of note, haloperidol is not approved for IV administration by the U.S. Food and Drug Administration (FDA); however, it has been used safety and effectively by this route with such widespread acceptance that FDA approval is most likely to be deferred indefinitely. The company is not likely to spend money to gain approval for a route of administration already in widespread use.

Droperidol (Inapsine), an analogue of haloperidol, has had a long history of success at doses of 5 to 20 mg IM with typically only one or two doses needed to control an agitated patient.[53,56-58] Intravenous dosing of droperidol starts at 1.25 to 2.5 mg per dose. One study showed that droperidol IM resulted in more rapid control of an agitated patient than the same dose (5 mg) of haloperidol IM; however, both drugs were equivalent after IV administration.[56] Compared with haloperidol, droperidol has a shorter duration of effect, a lesser incidence of EPSs, and a greater incidence of sedation and orthostatic hypotension.[55]

The most common side effects of haloperidol and droperidol include sedation, orthostatic hypotension, and EPSs. EPSs are not dose related, can occur after one dose, and may occur up to several days after administration.[55] After acute administration, patients may develop akathisia (extreme restlessness) or acute dystonia, which may be manifest as involuntary turning or twisting movements in the neck (torticollis), back (opisthotonos), and eyes (oculogyric crisis). Rarely, the mouth and tongue can be affected, compromising the airway.[53] The treatment for each of these symptoms is benztropine (Cogentin), 1 to 2 mg, or diphenhydramine (Benadryl), 25 to 50 mg, either IM or IV. Relief generally occurs within minutes. Haloperidol and droperidol have negligible anticholinergic properties and are often coadministered with anticholinergic agents (benztropine or diphenhydramine) in order to attenuate dystonia.[59]

Neuroleptic malignant syndrome is an idiosyncratic reaction that leads to autonomic instability. Symptoms include hyperthermia, hypertension, and lead-pipe rigidity of extremities. This reaction occurs in approximately 1% of patients receiving antipsychotic medications.[53] Clinicians should be familiar with this syndrome when administering antipsychotic medications. If neuroleptic malignant syndrome develops, supportive care should be administered and further neuroleptic medications withheld.

Some neuroleptic medications (especially phenothiazines such as chlorpromazine) may lower the seizure threshold; therefore, the use of neuroleptics in sympathomimetic-intoxicated patients has been controversial. In clinical practice, seizure activity occurring after haloperidol or droperidol administration appears to be a rare event. One retrospective review of 2468 patients receiving droperidol in an emergency department setting showed 3 patients with seizure activity.[58] A retrospective review of patients receiving droperidol for combative behavior revealed that of 101 sympathomimetic-intoxicated patients (78 cocaine, 23 amphetamine) who received droperidol, none had an adverse outcome.[60] In addition, haloperidol has been found in an animal model to prevent seizures in cocaine and amphetamine intoxication.[61]

Conduction disturbances, specifically prolongation of the QT interval and in some cases torsades de pointes, have been reported in patients sedated with haloperidol[62-65] and droperidol.[66-69] In December 2001, droperidol was given a "black box" warning by the FDA for cases of QT prolongation and torsades de pointes.[70] These cases originated from worldwide postmarketing surveillance and typically involved very high doses of droperidol (up to 100 mg IM). However, some cases were reported with low doses (<5 mg).[71,72] The FDA recommendations in the black box warning include a screening electrocardiogram (ECG) as well as cardiac monitoring when droperidol is administered. Clearly, obtaining an ECG of a combative patient before chemical restraint may be difficult if not impossible. Clinicians familiar with the safe use of droperidol for over 30 years have questioned the restriction of this medication.[71,73] Nonetheless, its usage has greatly decreased, and it is no longer available in a number of hospital formularies.

Atypical antipsychotic agents (risperidone, olanzapine, quetiapine, ziprasidone, and others) have largely replaced typical antipsychotics in the first-line treatment of schizophrenia because of increased efficacy for both positive and negative symptoms and a significantly decreased incidence of movement disorders.[55,59] In the past, the use of atypical antipsychotic agents to manage the acutely agitated or psychotic patient in the emergency department setting was limited by slow titration regimens and the lack of an intramuscular route of administration. Intramuscular formulations for olanzapine and ziprasidone have been developed and appear to offer promising additions to our current pharmacologic armamentarium when treating the combative patient.[55,74]

Olanzapine (Zyprexa) at 2.5 and 5.0 mg IM was equivalent to lorazepam 1 mg IM in controlling acute agitation in elderly patients with Alzheimer's disease or vascular dementia.[75] Olanzapine 10 mg IM was superior to lorazepam 2 mg IM in controlling acute agitation in patients with bipolar mania.[76] Olanzapine doses of 5, 7.5, and 10 mg IM were more rapidly effective than haloperidol 7.5 mg IM in controlling acute agitation in schizophrenic patients.[77,78] All of these studies were randomized, double blind, and placebo controlled. The most common side effect noted was mild hypotension. QTc prolongation was no different from that with placebo, and olanzapine was significantly less likely than haloperidol to produce dystonia and movement disorders. However, olanzapine has significant anticholinergic properties and could potentially exacerbate an anticholinergic delirium. Olanzapine IM has been recommended for FDA approval in the rapid control of acute agitation but is not available as of this writing.[79]

Intramuscular ziprasidone (Geodon) at doses of 10 and 20 mg has been found to be effective in reducing acute agitation in patients with underlying psychotic disorders.[80,81] A randomized, open-label study comparing ziprasidone and haloperidol for the treatment of acute psychosis found that ziprasidone (10 mg IM followed by 5 to 20 mg every 4 to 6 hours) was superior to haloperidol (2.5 to 10 mg IM and every 4 to 6 hours) in reducing agitation and improving scores on psychiatric assessments measured every 24 hours for 3 days. Improvement continued as patients were changed to oral medication in both groups. The most common side effect noted was dose-related sedation. Ziprasidone may prolong QTc up to 20 milliseconds from baseline with therapeutic use; however, to date there is no reported excess in sudden deaths and there are no reported cases of torsades de pointes with this agent. Ziprasidone IM has been FDA approved for the control of acute agitation in patients with schizophrenia. Recommended dosing is 10 mg IM every 2 hours or 20 mg IM every 4 hours, not to exceed 40 mg/day. Ziprasidone is not recommended for patients with known QTc prolongation or who are at risk for QTc prolongation.[74,82]

Although these newer intramuscular atypical antipsychotic agents appear to be effective in the chemical restraint of specific populations of agitated patients, their use in the emergency department management of the combative patient has not been defined at this point.

Benzodiazepines can also be used for rapid tranquilization of an agitated patient, with lorazepam (Ativan) proving superior to other benzodiazepines because of rapidity of action, effectiveness, short half-life, lack of active metabolites, and IM or IV route of administration.[26,45,53,83] Benzodiazepines are especially useful in patients who are agitated secondary to drug or alcohol intoxication and withdrawal while still maintaining efficacy in acute psychosis.[22] Recommended doses of lorazepam start with 2- to 4-mg increments IV, IM, or orally and are titrated upward as needed, up to 120 mg in 24 hours.[53] The most common side effects are sedation, confusion, ataxia, and nausea. Respiratory depression is the most significant risk when benzodiazepines are used in a patient who is already under the influence of a potential respiratory depressant such as alcohol.

Antipsychotics and benzodiazepines can be used alone or in combination. The combination of lorazepam with haloperidol has been studied prospectively and has been shown to be superior to either drug alone.[83] Ninety-eight agitated patients were enrolled in a randomized, double-blind, multicenter trial and their agitation was treated with either lorazepam 2 mg, haloperidol 5 mg, or both in combination. Doses were repeated as needed at hourly intervals, up to six times. Patients were re-evaluated hourly for efficacy, vital signs, and presence of side effects for a total of 12 hours. Patients receiving combination therapy improved significantly more in the first 3 hours than those receiving either drug alone, and more patients experienced EPSs in the haloperidol-alone group than in the combination group, possibly because of a greater number of doses needed. On the basis of these findings, combination therapy has been recommended as the treatment of choice for rapid tranquilization of the acutely agitated patient for optimal effect and minimal side effects. The use of 5 mg of haloperidol IV or IM with 2 mg of lorazepam IV or IM, repeated every 30 minutes to effect, is often recommended in the combative patient without contraindications to these medications.[45,55,74,84] Half doses should be used in elderly patients. These medications are compatible within the same syringe for up to 16 hours.[85]

Rapid tranquilization allows the emergency physician to calm patients so that they can cooperate in their evaluation and treatment and avoid harming themselves or others. The clinician should become familiar with several agents. Some argue that obscuring mental status with medication confuses clinical diagnosis and therefore these medications should be withheld until a diagnosis is made. However, diagnostic considerations must be weighed against placing the patient and medical staff at increased risk by withholding effective and safe medications. In addition, physical restraint alone, especially in a struggling patient, may increase the risks for patients' morbidity and mortality.

Assault

Unfortunately, physical assault may occur despite appropriate precautions and interventions. If assaulted, immediately summon help, preferably by use of a panic button. Maintain a sideward posture, keeping the arms ready for self-protection. If faced with a punch or a kick, deflect with an arm or a leg. If choking is attempted, tuck the chin in to protect the airway and carotids. If bitten, do not pull away but rather push toward the mouth and hold the attacker's nares shut to entice opening of the mouth. If threatened with a weapon, try to appear calm and comply with demands.[6] Adopt a nonthreatening posture and avoid sudden movements. Do not attempt to reach for the weapon. Avoid argument, despair, or whining. Attempt to establish a human connection with the hostage taker, as a hostage taker is less likely to murder a hostage if a relationship has been established.[26,86] Offering to administer to ill or injured hostages allows a hostage to appear less expendable. Do not bargain or make promises, and do not lie, as the consequences could be disastrous. Reassure the hostage taker that someone authorized to hear his or her complaints or demands should arrive promptly.[86] If a weapon is put down, do not reach for it but rather attempt to resolve the crisis verbally while awaiting security arrival. Legal authorities can be called on to provide a professional hostage negotiator if one is needed.

Each hospital should have a plan of action to be utilized in the case of extreme violence. The plan should include prevention and safety measures, a means for rapid notification of security and police personnel, evacuation plans, medical treatment, and crisis intervention.[6,86,87] A novel approach uses a violence management team trained in the preceding techniques to provide a mechanism for dealing with aggressive patients and protecting the staff.[88]

CLINICAL FEATURES

History and Physical Examination

Once the combative patient is controlled, the emergency physician needs to evaluate the patient for a possible organic cause of the agitated behavior. Separating functional from organic disease is a challenging but essential task when evaluating the combative patient. Even the patient with a prior psychiatric history should not be assumed to have a purely psychiatric diagnosis until an organic etiology has been ruled out. Organic causes of violent behavior are often reversible; therefore, correction of the underlying disorder may alleviate symptoms and prevent iatrogenic injury resulting from unnecessary sedation or restraint. In addition, patients who exhibit violent behavior that is caused or exacerbated by an organic problem may deteriorate rapidly if the medical issues are not addressed in a timely fashion. A focused history and physical examination assist the physician in differentiating functional from organic illness and facilitate a cost-effective and timely diagnostic evaluation.

Several historical features help to distinguish functional from organic illness. Patients older than 40 years who have a new onset of psychiatric symptoms are more likely to have an organic etiology for their illness.[89-91] Elderly patients are at higher risk for organic delirium because of medical illness or adverse reactions to medications. Patients with a history of drug or alcohol abuse may exhibit violent behavior as a manifestation of an intoxication or withdrawal syndrome. Acute onset of agitated behavior also points toward an organic etiology. Most psychiatric patients are alert and oriented and have a past psychiatric history. Table 189-1 lists clues for distinguishing functional from organic etiology of violent behavior.

The history of present illness should include psychiatric, medical, family, and social information including suicidal ideation, medication use, and any recent changes in prescribed medications. Often family and friends can provide valuable information, as the agitated patient may not be a reliable source of infor-

Table 189-1. Distinguishing Organic versus Functional Etiology of Violent Behavior

	Organic		
Clinical Feature	*Delirium*	*Dementia*	Functional
Onset	Acute	Gradual	Gradual
Age of onset	Any	>50 years	<40 years
Alertness	Altered	Normal	Normal or hyperalert
Orientation	Impaired	Normal	Normal
Hallucinations	Common, can be visual/auditory/tactile	None	Auditory in schizophrenia, otherwise uncommon
Symptom picture	Fluctuating	Stable	Stable
Abnormal vital signs	Common	Uncommon	Uncommon
Psychiatric history	No	No	Yes

Table 189-2. Vital Signs and Toxic Syndromes

Toxin	BP	P	RR	T	Pupil Size	Skin	Example
Sympathomimetic	↑	↑	↑	↑	↑	Wet	Cocaine
Anticholinergic	↑/↓	↑	↑/↓	↑	↑	Dry	Diphenhydramine
Cholinergic	↑/↓	↑/↓	—	—	↓	Wet	Pesticides
Opiates	↓	↓	↓	↓	↓	—	Morphine
Sedatives	↓	↓	↓	↓	↑/↓	—	Lorazepam
Withdrawal (ethanol, sedative-hypnotics)	↑	↑	↑	↑	↑	Wet	Benzodiazepine withdrawal

BP, Blood pressure; P, pulse; RR, respiratory rate; T, temperature; —, no change.
From Goldfrank LR, Flomenbaum NE, Lewin NA: Vital signs and toxic syndromes. In Goldfrank LR (ed): *Toxicologic Emergencies*, 6th ed. Stamford, Conn, Appleton-Lange, 1998, p 279.

mation. When available, they should be interviewed independently from the patient. Medical records may detail medical and psychiatric history as well as prior history of violence. Drug and alcohol use is an important part of the history, as substance abuse is highly correlated with violent behavior.

A thorough physical examination should be performed to search for an organic cause of violent behavior and uncover any resulting injury. Patients with persistently abnormal vital signs, a clouding of consciousness, or focal neurologic findings are more likely to suffer from organic disease and require further diagnostic evaluation. A careful head-to-toe examination should focus on general appearance (hygiene, nourishment, tremors), evidence of trauma, neurologic and mental status examination, and signs and symptoms of specific toxidromes (Table 189-2).[92]

Diagnostic Strategies

Diagnostic studies should be guided by the information obtained from the history and physical examination. This is an area of controversy, and although some authors advocate a standardized panel of laboratory and radiographic studies for patients with psychiatric symptoms, most recommend tailoring diagnostic studies on the basis of clinical findings.[90,93-96]

A rapid blood glucose determination and pulse oximetry should be obtained for all combative patients. Patients younger than 40 years with a prior psychiatric history and normal physical examination including vital signs, who are oriented and regain a calm demeanor without medical management, are unlikely to require further diagnostic testing.[95] Additional studies that may be useful in selected patients include serum electrolytes, blood and urine toxicology screening, serum ethanol, thyroid function panel, computed tomography scan or magnetic resonance imaging of the brain, and electroencephalography.[6,24,27,90] A lumbar puncture should be performed if a central nervous system infection is suspected. Specific medication levels may be determined when toxic levels would affect therapy. An ECG may be useful in elderly patients and in the setting of a suspected intentional ingestion.

An additional consideration in the diagnostic workup must be the concerns of the psychiatrist who ultimately evaluates the patient. Although serum ethanol and toxicology screening may not significantly affect a patient's medical management, the psychiatrist may use them to assess the degree to which alcohol or drug use contributes to the patient's behavioral issues.[90,97] Ideally, an agreement on a diagnostic strategy should be reached between the psychiatrist and emergency physician before referral. Unnecessary diagnostic testing prolongs emergency department length of stay and delays definitive psychiatric care.

Differential Considerations

Violent behavior often occurs in association with head trauma, hypoxia, hypoglycemia, electrolyte imbalance, infections (particularly herpes encephalitis), drug intoxication or withdrawal, adverse drug reactions, and metabolic and endocrine derangements.[6,26] Uncommon organic etiologies include seizures (temporal lobe, limbic); tumors, particularly those in the limbic system; limbic encephalitis; multiple sclerosis; porphyria; Wilson's disease; Huntington's disease; sleep disorders; hyperparathyroidism; and vitamin deficiencies (folate, B_{12}, niacin, and B_6).[29] In the emergency department setting, drug and alcohol intoxication and withdrawal are the most common diagnoses in combative patients.[28,47] The mnemonic FIND ME (*f*unctional, *i*nfectious, *n*eurologic, *d*rugs, *m*etabolic, *e*ndocrine) may be helpful to organize a diagnostic search for the etiology of violence. Box 189-1 illustrates various functional and organic entities associated with violent behavior.

BOX 189-1. Problems Associated with Violence

Psychiatric
- Schizophrenia
- Paranoid ideation
- Catatonic excitement
- Mania
- Personality disorders
  - Borderline
  - Antisocial
  - Delusional depression
  - Posttraumatic stress disorder
  - Decompensating obsessive-compulsive disorders
- Homosexual panic

Situational Frustration
- Mutual hostility
- Miscommunication
- Fear of dependence or rejection
- Fear of illness
- Guilt over disease process

Antisocial Behavior
- Violence with no associated medical or psychiatric explanation (these patients may be managed by the police or security)

Organic

Diseases
- Delirium
- Dementia
- Trauma
- CNS infection
- Seizures
- Neoplasm
- Cerebrovascular accident
- Vascular malformation
- Hypoglycemia
- Hypoxia
- AIDS
- Electrolyte abnormality
- Hypothermia or hyperthermia
- Anemia
- Vitamin deficiency
- Endocrine disorder

Drugs
- Unanticipated reaction to prescribed medication (especially sedatives in brain-injured or elderly patients)
- Alcohol (intoxication and withdrawal)
- Amphetamines
- Cocaine
- Sedative-hypnotic (intoxication or withdrawal)
- PCP
- LSD
- Anticholinergics
- Aromatic hydrocarbons (glue, paint, gasoline)
- Steroids

AIDS, acquired immunodeficiency syndrome; CNS, central nervous system; LSD, lysergic acid diethylamide; PCP, phencyclidine.

Medical Clearance

The emergency physician is often asked to provide "medical clearance" for the psychiatric or combative patient. It must be recognized that medical clearance is a misnomer in that the limited medical evaluation performed in the emergency department cannot exclude the presence of all possible medical conditions.[93,98] The incidence of organic disease in patients presenting with psychiatric complaints has been cited in the literature as varying from 24% to as high as 80%.[90,99,100] As a result, some authors have recommended that the term medical clearance be replaced with "medical screening" or that the term be avoided altogether and replaced instead with a thorough discharge note because the emergency department evaluation is focused on detecting only the medical problems that might be causing or contributing to the patient's violent behavior.[99] When the medical screening evaluation has been completed, it is essential for the emergency physician to communicate the findings to the consulting psychiatrist. The medical record should reflect that the emergency department evaluation makes it unlikely that an acute medical condition caused or contributed to the patient's behavior.

PREPARING THE EMERGENCY DEPARTMENT TO PREVENT VIOLENCE

Violence is an increasing problem; however, we as practitioners are largely underprotected and underprepared. A national telephone survey of 250 hospitals with emergency departments nationwide revealed that overall, 22.6% of hospitals have a 24-hour security presence in the emergency department, 14.1% have security present part of the day, and 63.3% do not have security formally assigned to the emergency department at any time during the day.[101] Only 21.4% control access to the emergency department during high risk hours, 38.7% use a security code, 40% have alarm buttons, 13.7% have a seclusion room, 36% use closed-circuit surveillance, and 1.6% use metal detectors. Security measures increase as emergency department census increases, both in teaching hospitals and in urban areas. The challenge for the emergency physician is to minimize the risk of violence in a cost-effective manner without creating a hostile or negative environment. Prevention of violence is best accomplished by developing a system that includes ongoing staff education, adequate personnel, and a well-designed physical structure. The personnel and features used in an institution's violence prevention program must be selected on the basis of the assessment of risk in each facility.

Security Personnel

A well-trained and responsive security force is a key element of any security system. Such personnel are a significant expense and their expertise is often sacrificed quickly during budget curtailments, and decisions regarding the type and number of guards are often made on an economic basis. The use of guns by hospital security personnel is controversial. Guards may be allowed to carry guns after completing extensive weapons training. Other devices, such as the taser, stun gun, and Mace, have been suggested as a less lethal alternative to guns.

Patient Searches

Searching patients for weapons on entering the emergency department is legal as long as searches are performed in a nondiscriminatory manner.[86] A warning sign should be prominently displayed, perhaps reading: "For the safety of patients and staff, individuals entering the emergency department may be screened for weapons." Almost all patients and families cooperate with searches and may actually feel safer as a result.[42] Clear written policies regarding searches and disposal of contraband must be distributed to the staff and closely followed.

Alarm Systems

Alarm systems are commonly used in the emergency department. The goal of any alarm system is to have a rapid appropriate response with a minimum of false alarms. A tiered alarm system is usually best. Panic buttons in each room activate a central buzzer in the department. Several designated emergency department personnel respond initially and then judge the level of response needed. Every emergency department should have at least one telephone with a direct line to police or security in case additional personnel are deemed necessary. A verbal code (e.g., "Dr. Armstrong to Room 9") is also a useful adjunct.[6]

Limited Access to the Emergency Department

Controlling flow into the emergency department can be an effective method of preventing violent acts. High-risk departments should limit access to one or two entrances, especially during the evening hours. Bulletproof glass barriers and buzzer access systems have been used as well.

Use of a Designated Room

American College of Emergency Physicians guidelines recommend that most emergency departments contain at least one secure examination room with shatterproof ceiling lights, a solid ceiling, heavy indestructible chairs, a well-secured restraint bed, two doors that can be locked from the outside, and an emergency distress button that can be activated unobtrusively.[88] If desired, this room can be set up for video monitoring by security or staff.

One large urban county hospital with a high incidence of violent behavior in the emergency department established a large security force, metal detectors, bulletproof Plexiglas in triage areas, a keypad security entry, controlled entryway into the emergency department, and metal bars to prohibit cars from driving into the department.[16] The hospital reported no incident of weapons-related violence or injury in the emergency department since these measures have been implemented.

Prevention

Violence is an event in which an ounce of prevention can be worth a pound of cure. The concepts of primary, secondary, and tertiary prevention can be applied to the emergency department environment.[12] Primary prevention refers to trying to control the factors in the environment that encourage the development of frustration and aggression. Long waiting times have been associated with development of violent behavior. Attempts to shorten waiting times and make the waiting room environment as pleasant as possible may be helpful in diminishing previolent aggression. The presence of surveillance cameras and a visible security force also act as deterrents (although their implementation is a form of tertiary prevention).

Secondary prevention of violence involves response to previolent agitation and aggression. Successful intervention involves early recognition of high-risk patients and timely implementation of de-escalation techniques. Staff should be trained to recognize previolent individuals and to evaluate them in a timely manner. Often the aura of preferential treatment defuses the situation.[88] The education of health personnel can be invaluable in preventing violence but often has been inexcusably overlooked. Training of staff in techniques for managing violence has been shown to lead to increased staff confidence and comfort while decreasing the rate of aggressive incidents.[102,103]

Tertiary prevention refers to limitation of the actual act of violence itself once it has occurred. Physical and chemical restraints are used, and security and police intervention are often needed. Emergency department protocols for dealing with the violent patient are important to minimize risks to the patient and staff. Security measures such as those outlined previously may be indicated in an emergency department with substantial risk for violence.

Violence has increasingly become a major public health issue, with focus on improved surveillance and universal preventive measures to target large populations.[104-106] Proposed intervention strategies include firearm legislation, public education, drug and alcohol rehabilitation programs, health professional education, community recreation programs for at-risk youth, mentoring programs, and control over exposure to violence in the media.[104] Physicians are increasingly aware of their role in reducing violence. Firearm regulations, hospital security mandates, and legislation for education of practitioners in the prevention and treatment of violence represent current controversies in which physicians should have a voice. As emergency physicians, we are faced with violence and the victims of violence on a daily basis and are uniquely positioned to help break the cycle of violence. A proposed agenda for violence prevention for emergency medicine includes improvements in medical education, research, and clinical practice as well as involvement with public education and advocacy.[107]

MEDICOLEGAL ISSUES

The primary medicolegal dilemmas faced in caring for the violent patient are informed consent versus patients' competence, patients' autonomy versus the safety of others (staff and society), and patients' confidentiality versus duty to third parties.

Consent and Competence

The combative or violent patient presents one of the most difficult situations for the emergency physician; proper medical care must be rendered while weighing legal dictates. The primary legal considerations in caring for combative patients can be divided into three areas: (1) the rights of patients, (2) duties of the health care providers, and (3) concern for third parties.

First consideration must be given to the rights of the patient. Traditionally, patients have the right to determine whether and when they want medical care and what medical care they desire.[6,47,108] Patients enter into contractual obligations with physicians by granting permission for medical care and treatment. This is referred to as consent for treatment. An analysis of what constitutes consent and the related topic of competence is helpful in determining what care should be provided to the combative patient in the emergency department.[109]

Consent is defined as a voluntary agreement by a person in the possession and exercise of sufficient mental capacity to make an intelligent choice to do something proposed by another. Consent is generally considered as either implied or expressed. Implied consent is defined as the signs, actions, facts, or inaction that raises the presumption of voluntary agreement. Thus, a patient presenting to an emergency department for assistance would generally be considered as providing implied consent.[109]

Individuals are entitled to make decisions about their health care if they are deemed competent. Competence is defined as the capacity or ability to understand the nature and effects of one's acts or decisions. Adults are presumed competent to grant consent for proposed medical treatment. An incompetent adult patient who is incapacitated by physical or mental illness and unable to understand the nature and consequences of his or her actions cannot give valid consent to proposed treatment. In the case of an incapacitated adult, consent must be obtained from someone who is authorized to consent. This may be someone that the patient requested when competent through a durable power of attorney, or if a court has decided the patient is incompetent, the patient's court-appointed guardian must authorize treatment. If a physician has determined that a patient is incapable of comprehending the nature and consequences of his or her conduct but the patient has not been judged incompetent, most courts accept the consent of the patient's next of kin. It is wise to document that the family desired and approved the proposed treatment. This "substituted consent" is not ideal because each individual is considered the true authority on deciding his or her care.[6,47,109]

The law usually presumes the patient's consent in an emergency. Courts have supported emergency physician actions, without consent, when the purpose was to preserve the patient's life or health.[47,110] They assume that a reasonable, competent, adult would want to be healthy. Specifically in the case of a violent patient, the emergency physician can safely assume that the act of presenting to an emergency department is at least an implied consent for evaluation and treatment. The emergency physician should quickly decide whether the patient is competent. If competent, the patient must give express consent before proceeding, but otherwise the physician is at liberty to provide care. Documentation of factors that led to the decision on competence as well as agreement of coworkers present is advisable and, if time permits, an actual court order is ideal. The more life threatening the emergency, the greater should be the physician's comfort in treatment. If competence cannot be determined, it is best to err on the side of treatment. Battery and false imprisonment are much easier to defend than passive negligence. In these situations, it is imperative to document that (1) an emergency existed, (2) there was inability to obtain consent, and (3) the treatment was for the patient's benefit.[6]

The standard of care in treating patients in the emergency department is defined by professional literature and practice standards in the national community of emergency medicine. In the treatment of the combative patient, the standard of care consists of diagnosis and treatment of conditions with an organic etiology (such as hypoglycemia, shock, intoxication, hypoxia, intracranial pathology) and the use of physical and chemical restraints to permit appropriate evaluation and treatment while protecting the patient and others from injury. When a patient's condition or illness requires knowledge, skill, or training outside the physician's field of expertise, consultation should be sought. Such practice and proper documentation should protect the emergency physician from negligence claims when dealing with a combative patient. The practitioner must be aware that the violent patient presents a unique challenge because of the psychological stress placed on the physician, the difficulty of establishing a normal therapeutic relationship; complex medical, psychiatric, and social issues; and the duty to maintain a safe emergency department environment.

Legal Case Precedents

There are a handful of definitive legal cases that address unique issues in management of the violent patient but also apply to other scenarios in care of patients. The emergency physician should become familiar with them to avoid future liability. In legal literature, an older case that has withstood challenge is more respected; in contrast, in medical literature newer data are weighted more heavily.

Battery

In 1980, a 44-year-old woman agreed to undergo an exploratory laparotomy to identify the etiology of vaginal bleeding. It was not an emergency; she was competent and signed a standard consent form. During the process, however, she repeatedly expressed a desire for her general surgeon to be present along with the obstetric surgeon. She called office personnel to request this and told the obstetric surgeon in preoperative meetings as well. Just before anesthesia was instituted, she stated that she did not want to be "put to sleep" until her surgeon was there. Nevertheless, she was anesthetized and operated on and a bilateral oophorectomy performed. During the surgery, her ureter was damaged and she suffered a protracted postoperative course. The patient sued for both medical malpractice and battery. The court found the physicians were not liable for malpractice (ureteral injury is a recognized and known complication) but awarded the patient damages of $75,000 for battery.[111]

Battery is the intentional infliction of a harmful or offensive bodily contact. Victims of battery do not necessarily have to be physically injured and may merely suffer damage to their dignity.[92] Courts are very protective of the "sanctity of the person," "bodily integrity," and "personal autonomy" as a fundamental personal right.[93] "Intentional" simply implies that the actor wanted to do the action, regardless of whether he or she was trying to help the patient. A physician must never physically invade or touch a competent patient without his or her consent, or the physician may be liable for battery. Recoverable damages can be "general," such as compensation for the harm done, and "special," such as compensation for medical charges, lost wages, and other expenses. These may not be covered by standard medical malpractice insurance.

The duty is much different when a patient is in an emergency situation and incompetent or represents a danger. In 1982 the Supreme Court supported the use of restraints to protect patients and others if it was in the best interest according to reasonable medical judgment.[112] In this case, a young, mentally handicapped male with repeated episodes of violence was restrained and involuntarily committed. The court stated, "We have established that the patient retains liberty interests in safety and freedom from bodily restraint. Yet these interests are not absolute, there are occasions in which it is necessary for the state to restrain the movement of residents—for example, to protect them as well as others from violence." The Model Penal Code allows "an exception from the assault statute for physicians . . . who act in good faith in accordance with accepted medical therapy."[113]

The importance of liability and responsibility for monitoring a patient after the patient has been restrained was illustrated in the case *Estate of Doe v ABC Ambulance*.[114] A 32-year-old schizophrenic threatened to kill his psychologist and was taken to the emergency department. When informed that he was going to be involuntarily admitted, he became violent. The patient was physically restrained in four-point restraints, chemically sedated, attached to a gurney on a backboard, and turned upside down. A towel was then placed over his mouth to prevent spitting and a sheet was laid over him to decrease outside stimulus. His complaints of inability to breathe were ignored. When he was being transferred later to the psychiatric ward, it was noticed that one of his protruding hands was blue. The patient was uncovered and found to be in cardiopulmonary arrest, from which he did not recover. His estate was awarded $2 million.

False Imprisonment

In 1991, a woman was held in a psychiatric facility for 3 days without her consent. No papers for involuntary commitment were completed. After this period, an evaluation determined her to be in danger and involuntary commitment papers were completed. She successfully sued the physicians and hospital that cared for her during the initial 3-day period (for both false imprisonment and battery) but absolved the later treating physicians.[115]

False imprisonment is the intentional infliction of a confinement and represents confinement and deprivation of personal liberty, for any length of time, without consent.[116] Damages may be awarded, even in the absence of physical harm, for inconvenience, mental suffering, and humiliation. Again, these may not be covered by standard medical malpractice insurance. All states have laws defining the procedure for holding patients against their will, and the emergency physician should become familiar with the statutes of the state in which he or she practices. In the preceding cases, it is clear that when physicians comply with state law and procedural paperwork, they are given great latitude in holding someone for a period of time to evaluate further and assess the danger. The emergency physician must immediately document and fill out appropriate forms when restraining or involuntarily committing a violent patient.

Duty to Warn Third Parties

Previously, physicians had a duty to care for and protect only the patient they had an established relationship with. The obligations of physicians caring for violent patients were dramatically changed by the famous court case of *Tarasoff v Regents of California* in 1976.[117] In that case, a man confided his intent to kill a woman to his psychologist. The psychologist called the police, who briefly detained the man and then released him. Two months later, he killed the woman, and her parents successfully sued the psychologist for not warning her of the danger. From this case, a "duty to warn" arose. The court stated that if a provider is aware of a "foreseeable" harm, the provider must either control the conduct of the potential offender or warn the intended victim. The courts have held that this duty to warn supersedes physician-patient confidentiality.

If a violent patient communicates intent to harm a foreseeable victim, the emergency physician should notify both law enforcement officials and the intended victim. For example, if the patient states, "I'm going to kill Sally Jones," or "I'm going to kill someone in the psychiatry clinic," a duty to warn is established. On the other hand, if the patient states, "I'm going to kill someone in the army," this does not represent an identifiable or foreseeable victim; thus, there is not a duty to warn.

Not all state courts honor the Tarasoff decision, but it was validated in a Missouri court case involving a paranoid schizophrenic.[118] In an inpatient group session, he admitted to having thoughts of stabbing his mother with a kitchen knife (a statement made several times over the years) but nevertheless was released that afternoon to the care of his parents without warning them. Later that night, the patient stabbed his father, who died, and his mother, who sustained severe injuries but lived. His mother sued the hospital for failure to warn. The defense claimed that after 25 years of illness, the family was already aware of the risk. A jury awarded $2 million to the mother. This case also reemphasizes the caveat that *all* threats of violence are taken seriously.

In general, the emergency physician should be aware of the concepts discussed here; however, medicolegal concerns should not dictate how a medical professional manages patients. Honest and reasonable concern and medical care for the patient's best interest are the best defense in navigating the legal minefield highlighted here.

DISPOSITION

After the violent patient has been evaluated medically, a decision must be made to either admit the patient, which may require the initiation of commitment proceedings, or discharge the patient. Admission should be considered for violent patients who state specific intentions to hurt themselves or others, refuse to answer questions, are under the influence of drugs or alcohol, are psychotic, have an organic brain syndrome, or refuse to cooperate.[6,20] Discharge may be appropriate if the violent behavior was caused by a temporary organic syndrome (e.g., intoxication) and the patient is now deemed to be in control and no longer violent. A violent psychiatric patient should not be discharged without psychiatric consultation and documented agreement with discharge. All discharged patients should be given specific follow-up evaluation. If a violent patient escapes the emergency department, legal authorities should be notified. If the patient threatened violence to a specific individual before escape, that individual should be notified as well. If the patient has committed a violent act, it is often possible to discharge the patient in police custody. Jail is a safe disposition as long as authorities are warned of potential danger. If the patient needs to be transferred, the accepting physician should be warned of possible violence.

KEY CONCEPTS

- Emergency department staff should be trained to recognize the early signs of impending violent behavior and to implement appropriate de-escalating techniques.
- Every emergency department should have a formal plan of action to deal with violent patients that integrates emergency department staff, hospital administration, security, and local authorities.
- Violent patients should be evaluated for possible medical and psychiatric conditions that might be causing or contributing to their behavior. The extent of this evaluation should be tailored to the patient and situation.
- An ounce of prevention is worth a pound of cure. There are a number of primary, secondary, and tertiary violence prevention techniques that every emergency department should consider.

REFERENCES

1. National Center for Injury Prevention and Control. Activity Report: 2001 Unintentional Injury Prevention Program. Centers for Disease Control and Prevention, Atlanta, GA. Available at: http://www.cdc.gov/ncipc/pub-res/unintentional_activity/00_preface.htm. Accessed February 4, 2004.
2. Reiss AJ, Roth JA: *Understanding and Preventing Violence*. Washington, DC, National Academy Press; 1993.
3. Krug EG, Powell KE, Dahlberg LL: Firearm related deaths in the United States and 35 other high and upper middle income countries. *Int J Epidemiol* 27:214, 1998.
4. Adams PF, Benson V: Current estimates from the National Health Interview Survey. *Vital Health Stat* 10:184, 1991.
5. Cook PJ, Lawrence BA, Ludwig J, Miller TR: The medical costs of gunshot injuries in the United States. *JAMA* 282:447, 1999.
6. Rice MM, Moore GP: Management of the violent patient: Therapeutic and legal considerations. *Emerg Med Clin North Am* 9:13, 1991.
7. National Institute for Occupational Safety and Health: Violence: Occupational Hazards in Hospitals. Centers for Disease Control. Available at: http://www.cdc.gov/niosh/topics/healthcare/#violence. Accessed February 4, 2004.
8. Schulte JM, et al: Violence and threats of violence experienced by public health field workers. *JAMA* 280:439, 1998.
9. Al-Sahlawi KS, et al: Violence against doctors: 1. A study of violence against doctors in accident and emergency departments. *Eur J Emerg Med* 6:301, 1999.
10. Anglin D, Kyriacou DN, Hutson HR: Residents' perspectives on violence and personal safety in the emergency department. *Ann Emerg Med* 23:1082, 1994.
11. Schwartz TL, Park TL: Assaults by patients on psychiatric residents: A survey and training recommendations. *Psychiatr Serv* 50:381, 1999.

12. Lavoie FW, Carter GL, Danzl DF, Berg RL: Emergency department violence in United States teaching hospitals. *Ann Emerg Med* 17:1227, 1988.
13. McAneney CM, Shaw KN: Violence in the pediatric emergency department. *Ann Emerg Med* 23:1248, 1994.
14. McNeil DE, Binder RL: Patients who bring weapons to the psychiatric emergency room. *J Clin Psychiatry* 48:230, 1987.
15. McCulloch LE, McNiel DE, Binder RL, Hatcher C: Effects of a weapon screening procedure in a psychiatric emergency room. *Hosp Community Psychiatry* 37:837, 1986.
16. Ordog GJ, et al: Weapons carriage among major trauma victims in the emergency department. *Acad Emerg Med* 2:109, 1995.
17. Cherry D, et al: Trends in fatal and nonfatal firearm related injury rates in the United States, 1985-1995. *Ann Emerg Med* 32:51, 1998.
18. Anderson AA, Ghali AY, Bansil RK: Weapon carrying among patients in a psychiatric emergency room. *Hosp Community Psychiatry* 40:845, 1989.
19. Dubin WR, Wilson SJ, Mercer C: Assaults against psychiatrists in outpatient settings. *J Clin Psychiatry* 49:339, 1988.
20. Beech DJ, Mercadel R: Correlation of alcohol intoxication with life-threatening assaults. *J Natl Med Assoc* 90:761, 1998.
21. Scott KD, Sachafer J, Greenfield TK: The role of alcohol in physical assault perpetration and victimization. *J Stud Alcohol* 60:528, 1999.
22. Citrome L, Volavka J: Violent patients in the emergency setting. *Psychiatr Clin North Am* 22:789, 1999.
23. Gardner W, Lidz CW, Mulvey EP, Shaw EC: Clinical versus actuarial predictions of violence of patients with mental illnesses. *J Consult Clin Psychol* 64:602, 1996.
24. Tardiff K: Diagnosis and management of violent patients. In Michels R, et al (eds): *Psychiatry*, vol 3. Philadelphia, Lippincott-Raven, 1997, pp 1-17.
25. Volavka J: The neurobiology of violence: An update. *J Neuropsychiatry Clin Neurosci* 11:307, 1999.
26. Tardiff K: The current state of psychiatry in the treatment of violent patients. *Arch Gen Psychiatry* 49:293, 1992.
27. Tardiff K: Unusual diagnoses among violent patients. *Psychiatr Clin North Am* 21:567, 1998.
28. Dubin WR, Weiss KJ: Emergency psychiatry. In Michels R, et al (eds): *Psychiatry*, vol 2. Philadelphia, Lippincott-Raven, 1997, pp 1-15.
29. Link BG, Andrews H, Cullen F: The violent and illegal behavior of mental patients reconsidered. *Am Sociol Rev* 57:275, 1992.
30. Swanson J, Borum R, Swartz M, Monahan J: Psychotic symptoms and disorders and the risk of violent behaviour in the community. *Crim Behav Ment Health* 6:317, 1996.
31. Arboleda-Florez J: Mental illness and violence: An epidemiological appraisal of the evidence. *Can J Psychiatry* 43:989, 1998.
32. Steadman HJ, et al: Violence by people discharged from acute psychiatric inpatient facilities and by others in the same neighborhoods. *Arch Gen Psychiatry* 55:393, 1998.
33. Burrowes KL, Hales RE, Arrington E: Research on biologic aspects of violence. *Psychiatr Clin North Am* 11:499, 1988.
34. Spoont MR: Modulatory role of serotonin in neural information processing: Implications for human psychopathology. *Psychol Bull* 112:330, 1992.
35. Alvarez JC, et al: Low blood cholesterol and low platelet serotonin levels in violent suicide attempters. *Biol Psychiatry* 45:1066, 1999.
36. Virkkunen M, et al: CSF biochemistries, glucose metabolism, and diurnal activity rhythms in alcoholics, violent offenders, fire setters, and healthy volunteers. *Arch Gen Psychiatry* 51:20, 1994.
37. Moffitt TE, et al: Whole blood serotonin relates to violence in an epidemiological study. *Biol Psychiatry* 43:446, 1998.
38. Damasio AR, Tranel D, Damasio H: Individuals with sociopathic behavior caused by frontal damage fail to respond autonomically to social stimuli. *Behav Brain Res* 41:81, 1990.
39. Mirsky AF, Seigel A: The neurobiology of violence and aggression. In Reiss AJ, Miczek KA, Roth JA (eds): *Understanding and Preventing Violence: Biobehavioral Influences*, vol 2. Washington, DC, National Academy Press, 1994, pp 59-172.
40. Goyer PF, et al: Positron emission tomography and personality disorders. *Neuropsychopharmacology* 10:21, 1994.
41. Raine A, Buschsbaum M, LaCasse L: Brain abnormalities in murderers indicated by positron emission tomography. *Biol Psychiatry* 42:495, 1997.
42. Mattox EA, Wright SW, Bracikowski AC: Metal detectors in the pediatric emergency department: Patron attitudes and national prevalence. *Pediatr Emerg Care* 16:163, 2000.
43. Kuhn W: Violence in the emergency department: Managing aggressive patients in a high-stress environment. *Postgrad Med* 105:143, 1999.
44. Hill S, Petit J: The violent patient. *Emerg Med Clin North Am* 18:301, 2000.
45. Allen MH: Managing the agitated psychotic patient: A reappraisal of the evidence. *J Clin Psychiatry* 61(Suppl 14):11, 2000.
46. Wynn R: Medicate, restrain or seclude? Strategies for dealing with violent and threatening behaviour in a Norwegian university psychiatric hospital. *Scand J Caring Sci* 16:287, 2002.
47. Lavoie FW: Consent, involuntary treatment, and the use of force in an urban emergency department. *Ann Emerg Med* 21:25, 1992.
48. Stratton SJ, Rogers C, Brickett K, Gruzinski G: Factors associated with sudden death of individuals requiring restraint for excited delirium. *Am J Emerg Med* 19:187, 2001.
49. Hick JL, Smith SW, Lynch MT: Metabolic acidosis in restraint associated cardiac arrest: A case series. *Acad Emerg Med* 6:239, 1999.
50. Reay DT, Fligner CL, Stilwell AD, Arnold J: Positional asphyxia during law enforcement transport. *Am J Forensic Med Pathol* 13:90, 1992.
51. Pollanen MS, Chaisson DA, Cairns JT, Young GJ: Unexpected death related to restraint for excited delirium: A retrospective study of deaths in police custody and in the community. *CMAJ* 158:1603, 1998.
52. Chan TC, et al: Restraint position and positional asphyxia. *Ann Emerg Med* 30:578, 1997.
53. Dubin WR, Feld JA: Rapid tranquilization of the violent patient. *Am J Emerg Med* 7:313, 1989.
54. Richards JR, Derlet R, Dundan D: Chemical restraint for the agitated patient in the emergency department: Lorazepam versus droperidol. *J Emerg Med* 16:567, 1998.
55. Currier GW, Trenton A: Pharmacological treatment of psychotic agitation. *CNS Drugs* 16:219, 2002.
56. Thomas HJ, Schwartz E, Petrilli R: Droperidol versus haloperidol for chemical restraint of agitated and combative patients: A prospective study. *Ann Emerg Med* 21:407, 1992.
57. Rosen CL, et al: The efficacy of intravenous droperidol in the prehospital setting. *J Emerg Med* 15:13, 1996.
58. Chase PB, Biros MH: A retrospective review of the use and safety of droperidol in a large, high-risk, inner-city emergency department patient population. *Acad Emerg Med* 9:1402, 2002.
59. Currier GW: Atypical antipsychotic medications in the psychiatric emergency service. *J Clin Psychiatry* 61(Suppl 14):21, 2000.

60. Branney SW, Colwell CB, Aschbrenner JK, Pons PT: Safety of droperidol for sedating out-of-control ED patients. *Acad Emerg Med* 3:527, 1996.
61. Derlet RW, Albertson TE, Rice P: The effect of haloperidol in cocaine and amphetamine intoxication. *J Emerg Med* 7:633, 1989.
62. Lawrence KR, Nasraway SA: Conduction disturbances associated with administration of butyrophenone antipsychotics in the critically ill: A review of the literature. *Pharmacotherapy* 17:531, 1997.
63. Wilt JL, Minnema AM, Johnson RF, Rosenblum AM: Torsade de pointes associated with the use of intravenous haloperidol. *Ann Intern Med* 119:391, 1993.
64. Tisdale JE, et al: The effect of intravenous haloperidol on QT interval dispersion in critically ill patients: Comparison with QT interval prolongation for assessment of risk of torsades de pointes. *J Clin Pharmacol* 41:1310, 2001.
65. Sharma ND, Rosman HS, Padhi ID, Tisdale JE: Torsades de pointes associated with intravenous haloperidol in critically ill patients. *Am J Cardiol* 81:238, 1998.
66. Lischke V, et al: Droperidol causes a dose-dependent prolongation of the QT interval. *Anesth Analg* 79:983, 1994.
67. Reilly JG, et al: QTc-interval abnormalities and psychotropic drug therapy in psychiatric patients. *Lancet* 355:1048, 2000.
68. Guy JM, et al: Torsades de pointes and prolongation of the duration of QT interval after injection of droperidol. *Ann Cardiol Angeiol (Paris)* 40:541, 1991.
69. Michalets EL, Smith LK, Van Tassel ED: Torsade de pointes resulting from the addition of droperidol to an existing cytochrome P450 drug interaction. *Ann Pharmacother* 32:761, 1998.
70. 2001 Safety Information Summaries. Available at: http://www.fda.gov/medwatch/safety/2001/safety01.htm#inapsi. Accessed February 4, 2004.
71. Kao LW, Kirk MA, Evers SJ, Rosenfeld SH: Droperidol, QT prolongation, and sudden death: What is the evidence? *Ann Emerg Med* 41:546, 2003.
72. McCormick CG: FDA Alert: Current FDA report on droperidol status and basis for the "black box" warning. *Am Soc Anesthesiol Newslett* 66:19, 2002.
73. Shale JH, Shale CM, Mastin WD: A review of the safety and efficacy of droperidol for the rapid sedation of severely agitated and violent patients. *J Clin Psychiatry* 64:500, 2003.
74. Bellnier TJ: Continuum of care: Stabilizing the acutely agitated patient. *Am J Health Syst Pharm* 59(17 Suppl 5):S12, 2002.
75. Meehan KM, et al: Comparison of rapidly acting intramuscular olanzapine, lorazepam, and placebo: A double-blind, randomized study in acutely agitated patients with dementia. *Neuropsychopharmacology* 26:494, 2002.
76. Meehan K, et al: A double-blind, randomized comparison of the efficacy and safety of intramuscular injections of olanzapine, lorazepam, or placebo in treating acutely agitated patients diagnosed with bipolar mania. *J Clin Psychopharmacol* 21:389, 2001.
77. Breier A, et al: A double-blind, placebo-controlled dose-response comparison of intramuscular olanzapine and haloperidol in the treatment of acute agitation in schizophrenia. *Arch Gen Psychiatry* 59:441, 2002.
78. Wright P, et al: Double-blind, placebo-controlled comparison of intramuscular olanzapine and intramuscular haloperidol in the treatment of acute agitation in schizophrenia. *Am J Psychiatry* 158:1149, 2001.
79. FDA Psychopharmacological Drugs Advisory Committee: Briefing document for Zyprexa IntraMuscular. Available at: http://www.fda.gov/ohrms/dockets/ac/01/briefing/3685b1_01_lilly.pdf. Accessed February 4, 2004.
80. Daniel DG, et al: Intramuscular (IM) ziprasidone 20 mg is effective in reducing acute agitation associated with psychosis: A double-blind, randomized trial. *Psychopharmacology* 155:128, 2001.
81. Lesem MD, et al: Intramuscular ziprasidone, 2 mg versus 10 mg, in the short-term management of agitated psychotic patients. *J Clin Psychiatry* 62:12, 2001.
82. Goodnick PJ: Ziprasidone: Profile on safety. *Expert Opin Pharmacother* 2:1655, 2001.
83. Battaglia J, et al: Haloperidol, lorazepam, or both for psychotic agitation? A multicenter, prospective, double blind, emergency department study. *Am J Emerg Med* 15:335, 1997.
84. Binder RL, McNiel DE: Emergency psychiatry: Contemporary practices in managing acutely violent patients in 20 psychiatric emergency rooms. *Psychiatr Serv* 50:1553, 1999.
85. Trissel L: *Handbook on Injectable Drugs*, 10th ed. Bethesda, Md, American Society of Health System Pharmacists, 1998.
86. Anonymous: *Emergency Department Violence: Prevention and Management*. Dallas, American College of Emergency Physicians, 1997.
87. Walsh-Kelly CM, Straid R: Impact of violence and the emergency department response to victims and perpetrator. *Pediatr Clin North Am* 45:449, 1998.
88. Brayley J, et al: The violence management team: An approach to aggressive behavior in a general hospital. *Med J Aust* 161:254, 1994.
89. Gallagher EJ: Neurologic principles. In Goldfrank LR, et al (eds): *Goldfrank's Toxicologic Emergencies*. New York, McGraw-Hill, 2002, pp 282-302.
90. Williams ER, Shepherd SM: Medical clearance of psychiatric patients. *Emerg Med Clin North Am* 18:185, 2000.
91. Reeves RR, Pendarvis EJ, Kimble R: Unrecognized medical emergencies admitted to psychiatric units. *Am J Emerg Med* 18:390, 2000.
92. Goldfrank LR, et al: Vital signs and toxic syndromes. In Goldfrank LR, et al (eds): *Goldfrank's Toxicologic Emergencies*. New York, McGraw-Hill, 2002, pp 255-260.
93. Henneman PL, Mendoza R, Lewis RJ: Prospective evaluation of emergency department medical clearance. *Ann Emerg Med* 24:672, 1994.
94. Herbert M: Assessment for medical clearance. *Ann Emerg Med* 25:852, 1995.
95. Korn CS, Currier GW, Henderson SO: "Medical clearance" of psychiatric patients without medical complaints in the emergency department. *J Emerg Med* 18:173, 2000.
96. Olshaker JS, et al: Medical clearance and screening of psychiatric patients in the emergency department. *Acad Emerg Med* 4:124, 1997.
97. Allen MH, Currier GW: Medical assessment in the psychiatric emergency service. *New Dir Ment Health Serv* 82:21, 1999.
98. Dubin WR, Weiss KJ, Zeccardi JA: Organic brain syndrome: The psychiatric imposter. *JAMA* 249:60, 1993.
99. Tintinalli JE, Peacock FW, Wright MA: Emergency medical evaluation of psychiatric inpatients. *Ann Emerg Med* 23:850, 1994.
100. Hall RCW, et al: Physical illness manifesting as psychiatric disease: Analysis of a state hospital inpatient population. *Arch Gen Psychiatry* 37:989, 1980.
101. Ellis GL, et al: ED security: A national telephone survey. *Am J Emerg Med* 12:155, 1994.
102. Nijman HL, Merckelbach HL, Allertz WF, Campo JM: Prevention of aggressive incidents on a closed psychiatric ward. *Psychiatr Serv* 48:694, 1997.
103. Fernandes CM, et al: The effect of an education program on violence in the emergency department. *Ann Emerg Med* 39:47, 2002.

104. Rae-Grant N, McConville BJ, Fleck S: Violent behavior in children and youth: preventive intervention from a psychiatric perspective. *J Am Acad Child Adolesc Psychiatry* 38:235, 1999.
105. Winett LB: Constructing violence as a public health problem. *Public Health Rep* 113:498, 1998.
106. Brener ND, Simon TR, Krug EG, Lowry R: Recent trends in violence-related behaviors among high school students in the United States. *JAMA* 282:440, 1999.
107. Muelleman RL, et al: An emergency medicine approach to violence throughout the life cycle. *Acad Emerg Med* 3:708, 1996.
108. Siner DA: Advance directives in emergency medicine: Medical, legal, and ethical implications. *Ann Emerg Med* 18:1364, 1989.
109. Bitterman RA: Medicolegal and risk management. In Marx JA, et al (eds): *Rosen's Emergency Medicine: Concepts and Clinical Practice*, vol 3, 5th ed. St Louis, Mosby, 2002, pp 2747-2760.
110. Moskop JC: Informed consent in the emergency department. *Emerg Med Clin North Am* 17:327, 1999.
111. *Pugsley v Privette* 220 Va. 892; 263 S.E.2d 60; 1980.
112. *Youngberg v Romeo* 457 U.S. 307; 1982.
113. Wexler DB: Seclusion and restraint: Lessons from law, psychiatry, and psychology. *Int J Law Psychiatry* 5:285, 1982.
114. *Estate of Doe v ABC Ambulance* in Medical Malpractice: Verdicts, Settlements, and Experts, vol 15, issue 7, p 15, 1999.
115. *Heath v Peachtree* Parkwood Hospital, Inc; 1991.
116. Restatement of Torts, Second, Section 36.
117. *Tarasoff v Regents of University of California* 17 Cal. 3d 425, 551 P.2d 334, 131 Cal. Rptr. 14; 1976.
118. *Dorothy McGrath et al v Barnes Hospital et al* in Medical Malpractice: Verdicts, Settlements, and Experts, vol 16, issue 5, p 54, 2000.

CHAPTER 190

The Difficult Patient

David W. Harrison and Robert J. Vissers

PERSPECTIVE

Certain patients who are seen in the emergency department consistently arouse negative reactions in health care providers. These negative reactions may be initiated by a patient's appearance, apparent attitude, interactive style, or presenting complaint. Difficult patients can rapidly disrupt the department's harmony and efficiency. Such patients are often referred to with a number of pejorative terms, including *gomer, crock, troll, dirtball,* and other even less complimentary slang terms of disdain. They may receive suboptimal medical care, impede patient flow, and influence the quality of care given to themselves and other patients, thus posing a medicolegal risk. Moreover, recurrent exposure to such patients, in the absence of a well-thought-out approach to dealing with them, may lead to escalating frustration for staff, promote unprofessional behaviors, and contribute to eventual burnout.

Historically, the medical literature has largely ignored the possibility of physicians harboring negative feelings toward any type of patient. Anger, hatred, and frustration are traditionally considered feelings that physicians should disown in favor of humor, compassion, and integrity. Although the latter are admirable attributes, to deny the presence of negative reactions is unrealistic. Physicians are as human as the patients they serve. Not until Freud coined the term *countertransference* were the negative reactions that patients can arouse in physicians actually recognized for their potential impact on care and used as diagnostic tools.

Good interpersonal skills have long been recognized as essential to the maintenance of the patient-physician relationship.[1] Although some clinicians have more natural abilities in this area than others, the myth that these skills are intuitive and cannot be taught is erroneous.[2] Teaching communication and relationship-building skills is now a priority of most medical schools and many primary care specialties.[3] The need for guidelines regarding the teaching and evaluation of interpersonal skills within emergency medicine residency programs has only recently been addressed.[4,5] The Accreditation Council for Graduate Medical Education (ACGME) has identified professionalism and communication skills as two of the six core competencies required in the curriculum of all U.S. residency programs, including emergency medicine, prompting greater interest in research and education in these areas.[6-8]

DISTINGUISHING PRINCIPLES

Scattered references to difficult patients can be found throughout the medical literature, where they are referred to as "problem patients," "disruptive medical patients," "unwanted patients," and, less diplomatically, "hateful patients."[9] Difficult patients are a very heterogeneous group. Individuals with personality disorders are commonly included in this category because of their rigid, maladaptive personality traits. However, difficult patients do not necessarily have personality disorders and may fall into one of several other familiar patient categories (e.g., drug seekers, hostile patients, malingerers, and emergency department repeaters).

There is no universally agreed upon definition of the difficult patient. We define the difficult patient as *one who interferes with the physician's ability to establish a normal patient physician relationship.* This impaired patient-physician relationship is often, but not necessarily, associated with negative feelings toward the patient.

PATHOLOGY OF THE PATIENT-PHYSICIAN RELATIONSHIP

An understanding of the difficult patient-physician relationship is hampered by a tendency to view it as a consequence of some inherent problem with the patient. Physician characteristics and the emergency department environment also play a role.[5,10,11]

Physician Factors

Impaired communication is a common problem in all forms of interpersonal relations and is often exaggerated in the medical setting. Patient satisfaction is highly correlated with patients' beliefs that clinicians listened to them and understood their request. Despite this, physicians continue to focus on their own medical agendas, which may be different from patients' concerns. When confronted with patients who have difficult social situations, physicians only exacerbate the problem when they refuse to deviate from their own rigid medical model.

It has been demonstrated that physicians often have preconceived stereotypes of how patients should behave when they are ill and rapidly categorize them as either the acceptable "truly sick" patient type or the "burdensome, difficult" patient type. People with "real disease" are excused for their symptoms. Patients falling outside the biomedical model are not. Patients may also be judged as difficult when cultural differences or language barriers interfere with mutual understanding between patient and physician.[12]

Giving insufficient information to patients about their diagnosis, treatment, and follow-up evaluation is another area of common communication breakdown. Studies show that in 20 minutes of patient-physician interaction, only 1 minute is reserved for educating patients about the illness.[13] Personal biases and prejudices also affect patient management.[10,14] The rapid formulation of an opinion based solely on appearances is a skill that physicians rely on to quickly form a "gestalt" about a patient. This is an essential skill for an emergency physician. However, to assume that such preconceived notions are influential only in a positive way is unrealistic.

Emergency Department Factors

The emergency department is an environment plagued with distractions and frequent interruptions, rarely approaching the comforting atmosphere that many patients need. A sense of urgency and strict time constraints are often present. Patient assessments are sometimes conducted in suboptimal environments, such as hallways. Patients may feel a lack of choice regarding their physicians or facilities. Opinion of the nursing staff may contribute to physicians' emotional bias. Physicians may similarly feel stressed by the prospect of losing control of the department while trying to deal with these particularly challenging patients.[12]

The Cycle of Impaired Patient-Physician Relationships

Difficult patients are deemed to make unreasonable demands on physicians (Figure 190-1). Physicians react with negative feelings and may direct negative actions toward the patient. Patients are sensitive to these negative reactions, feel threatened with abandonment, and attempt to sustain the relationship by escalating symptoms. Physicians experience greater frustration at the maladaptive behavior of the patients, and so the cycle is perpetuated.

The consequences of this impaired relationship for the patient include failure to have the real problems identified, missed medical diagnoses, "another poor experience" with the medical establishment, and premature or inappropriate discharge.[1] The negative impact on the staff is manifested by frustration, a sense of failure and defeat, burnout, litigation, and the development of unconstructive stereotypes and unrecognized prejudices.

STRATEGIES FOR MANAGING THE DIFFICULT PATIENT

This section discusses the management of difficult patients from three approaches: general strategies, dealing with negative reactions, and crisis intervention.

General Strategies

Box 190-1 lists several general strategies that are helpful in dealing with difficult patients.

Be Supportive

Being supportive is not always the natural response to difficult patients because of the negative feelings they arouse in the physician. Nevertheless, initiating the

BOX 190-1 General Strategies for Dealing with Difficult Patients

1. Be supportive.
2. Structure the interview.
3. Set limits.
4. Point out impasses.
5. Share your reactions.
6. Redirect the interview.
7. Take time out.
8. Use teamwork.
9. Understand the patient's agenda.

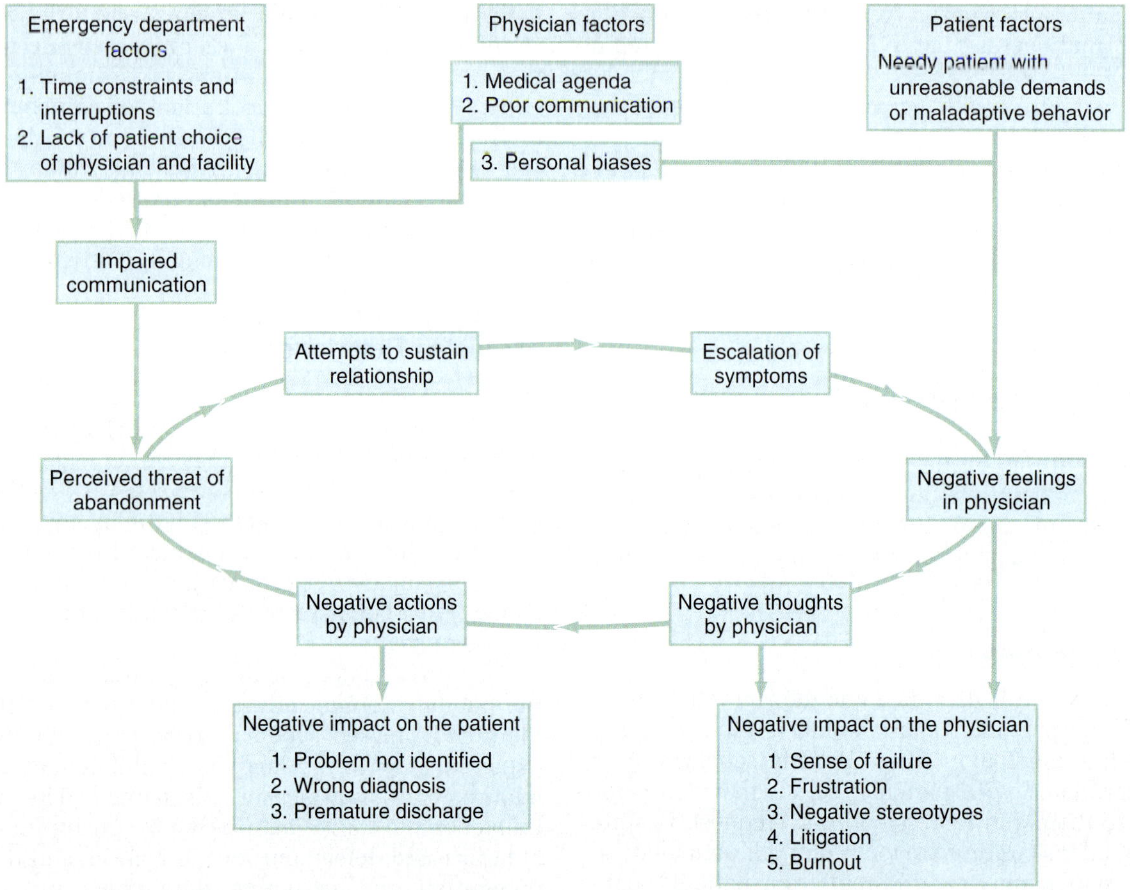

Figure 190-1. Cycle of the impaired patient-physician relationship.

interaction with a clear and explicit demonstration of concern and empathy may be the single most powerful tool at our disposal. Some physicians are concerned that being seemingly "soft" with a demanding or entitled patient may exacerbate the situation. To the contrary, expressing a respectful and empathetic concern for their problem effectively disarms many patients who were winding up for a long and arduous battle to be taken seriously. The possible news that there is no immediate solution available is more willingly received by patients who are convinced that they have been heard and the desire to help is sincere.

Connecting emotionally with the patient can take time. Initially addressing a smaller concern in a caring and respectful manner can build trust and create greater rapport and compliance. For example, a patient who seeks treatment for self-inflicted lacerations but who will not cooperate with a history aimed at assessing suicidal risk will often be more candid after the physician has rendered appropriate wound care in a nonjudgmental way.

Structure the Interview

Setting self-imposed time limits for contact with difficult patients helps control the anxiety associated with falling behind in a busy emergency department.[1] Flexibility in the structure of the assessment may be necessary. It is fair and appropriate to tell the patient of the need to excuse oneself to care for other patients. The fulfilled promise of returning to complete the next element of the assessment will help build trust and rapport.

Set Limits

It is helpful to share the ground rules of reasonable behavior with patients. For example, profane patients should be reminded that they are entitled to treatment, but that their language may offend other patients. The physician may suggest they censor their remarks or be escorted from the area.

Point Out Impasses

At times, patient expectations and physician limit setting produces an impasse. When this occurs, it may be necessary to agree to disagree. Some issues can be resolved by pointing out impasses and giving the patient a chance to help solve the problem. Impasses sometimes can be resolved if difficult issues are set aside and returned to later in the interview. This fundamental approach to negotiations is generally underutilized in the emergency department.

Share Your Reactions

Pointing out impasses may not be effective if a patient senses annoyance or frustration in the physician. It may be helpful at such times to share one's feelings explicitly with the patient while continuing treatment.

Redirect the Interview

Some patients love to talk about issues unrelated to the problem at hand. Pursuing trivial or chronic complaints should be avoided. Patients often require redirection to focus on issues that have some potential for resolution. Asking them to take a chronologic approach in discussing a specific concern may help keep them on track.

Take Time Out

Physicians occasionally feel unable to contain their frustration. One should feel comfortable retreating from the room and returning when both parties have regained their composure.

Use Teamwork

Individuals who intimidate or split the staff are much more easily managed from the outset with teamwork. This is especially important with violent patients requiring restraint where a show of strength in numbers may defuse potentially dangerous situations. A more subtle, but equally important, application of teamwork is in the management and discharge planning of patients with complex problems who require an especially well-organized, multidisciplinary approach involving medical and support services in the community. Occasionally, if available, the benefit of a "second opinion" from an emergency medicine colleague can help identify the difficult patient and allow the treating physician to regain clinical perspective.

Understand the Patient's Agenda

Sometimes physicians ask themselves "Why is this patient here?"[1] It is often productive to ask the patient the same question in a nonjudgmental fashion. The patient may have an easily satisfied, although unanticipated, agenda. This may be as simple as needing a bus ticket to get home or reassurance that there is no immediate danger of dying from some minor disorder. When the patient's needs are not as easily met, a clear understanding of the purpose of the visit may allow the opportunity to set more realistic goals.[15]

Dealing with Negative Reactions

Although negative reactions make dealing with difficult patients an unpleasant experience, they can also provide valuable diagnostic information. Physicians should accept these reactions as understandable responses to a patient's unpleasant behavior and use them to their advantage.[1]

Physicians typically have similar reactions to certain patient behaviors. The variations in these reactions depend on the individual physician's personality style, previous experiences, and unrecognized prejudices. Physicians must know their own reactions to specific behavioral patterns to use them as diagnostic aids.

Early recognition of these reactions may, in addition to their diagnostic value, allow the physician to analyze them as the first step in preventing the failed therapeutic relationship before it occurs.[10,12]

Negative Thoughts about the Patient

Negative thoughts about patients have the greatest potential to adversely affect patient care. Patients are often placed into a stereotyped category such as "drug addict," "malingerer," or "crock." The label may describe a particular patient more or less accurately, but in caring for difficult patients the potential exists for physicians to make inaccurate and potentially dangerous assumptions based on their biases linked to this label.

The process of assigning patients to epidemiologic categories is a normal part of clinical judgment. Certain categories are used to help define the likelihood of encountering diseases in particular patient populations, thereby influencing decisions regarding investigation, treatment, and disposition. The danger in dealing with difficult patients is that this process can result in inaccurate assumptions about patients and lead to compromised patient care.

Inaccurate assumptions about patients based on prejudicial, stereotyped labels have been called *cognitive distortions*. The following case example exemplifies the impact cognitive distortions can have on clinical decision making.

An injection drug user requests analgesia for severe neck pain after minor trauma. The physician labels the patient a drug seeker and assumes the complaints to be fictitious. After becoming aware of the physician's assumption, the patient becomes belligerent and aggressive. He is escorted from the emergency department by security. A few days later, he returns with quadriplegia resulting from a cervical epidural abscess.

The physician assumed the patient was malingering because of past experience with injection drug users without considering other legitimate explanations for the patient's behavior. This phenomenon, known as "all-or-none" thinking, leads to the real disease being overlooked.

Negative Self-Perceptions

Self-directed negative thoughts by physicians often reflect a sense of inadequacy or despair. Some patients contribute to the problem by criticizing their care in ways that reinforce the physician's feelings of inadequacy. Unreasonable expectations of patients coupled with their secret conviction that no one can really help and the all too prevalent rescue fantasies of physicians are a potent recipe for physician frustration, which in the long term can contribute to eventual burnout.

Negative Behaviors

Physician behaviors can be the most obvious manifestations of negative feelings and thoughts. Examples include rudeness, sarcasm, and indifference toward patients. A patient may receive an incomplete clinical evaluation, and unnecessary ancillary tests may be performed, as an attempt to compensate. Physical or chemical restraints, naloxone, or gastric lavage may be used inappropriately or punitively. Analgesics may be withheld or used sparingly. Faulty communication may result in misunderstood discharge instructions and poor compliance.

Although patients can suffer at the hands of physicians, the potential exists for the reverse to occur. Dissatisfied patients with incorrect diagnoses and poor follow-up instructions are prone to initiate successful malpractice suits against physicians.[1] Negative physician behaviors can also have an effect on the rest of the emergency department staff. Actions viewed by colleagues as inappropriate can compromise team morale and functioning. Physicians who are feeling angry, demoralized, and stressed may vent their frustrations on team members or consulting services, resulting in a further deterioration of the immediate situation, and potential damage to long-term working relationships.

Strategies for Managing Negative Reactions

Six strategies are helpful in managing physicians' negative reactions toward patients.

Maintain Appropriate Emotional Distance

Physicians should avoid reciprocating hostile reactions offered by patients. This may be difficult to resist and is best accomplished by maintaining sufficient emotional distance so as to avoid taking the patient's behavior personally. This "detached concern" must be balanced with sufficient emotional investment to convey a sense of caring and empathy toward the patient.[10]

Generate Alternatives to Negative Reactions

Instead of applying negative labels, physicians should attempt to view the patient as a victim of circumstance. Patients do not choose the social and genetic pool into which they are born. They do not choose to be abused children. They are entitled to high-quality care, delivered with courtesy and empathy, despite their behavior.

Attempt to Understand the Patient's Behavior as a Symptom

The second step in managing negative reactions is to recognize that patients relate to the world in a particular way because of their condition, culture, and circumstances. The condition may include a variety of medical and psychiatric problems, intoxication, cognitive impairment, or personality disorders or traits. The behaviors that one finds so disturbing should be recognized as the symptoms resulting from these conditions. Cultural differences and social circumstances can result in behaviors that seem irrational or difficult if the underlying issues are not understood. When attempting to maintain a compassionate approach to a particularly troubled and troubling patient, it is sometimes helpful to imagine how difficult one would find it to *be* that patient.

Look for the Cognitive Distortion

Cognitive distortions are best identified by looking for evidence that patients or situations are being stereotyped. Physicians should be aware of the effect that arbitrary inferences and all-or-none thinking have on interactions with patients and on clinical judgment.

Find a Rational Response to Cognitive Distortions

The initial reaction to the elderly schizophrenic patient presenting with chest pain might be to discount the symptoms as delusional. However, psychosis has not been demonstrated to be protective against ischemic heart disease, and the principle of considering the most potentially life-threatening diagnosis first serves both the patient and physician well in the emergency department.

Place Negative Reactions in Perspective by Viewing Them in Context

The emergency department is a stressful work environment. An expectation exists that emergency physicians will deal with problems quickly and effectively. Patients who thwart physicians' attempts to perform accordingly may be identified as undesirable. Such patients are difficult to view objectively when one is feeling overwhelmed. The frustration resulting from dealing with such difficult situations may produce an exaggerated response to a patient's behavior. Recognizing this may help reduce the loss of objectivity that leads to problems with patient care.

Although dealing with negative reactions is not the panacea for dealing with difficult patients, it provides the foundation for restructuring one's interactions with them in a way that will ultimately benefit the patient clinically and the physician emotionally.

Crisis Intervention

Some presenting complaints such as "can't sleep," "nervous stomach," "anxiety," and "can't cope" are especially likely to produce a sense of frustration and dread among caregivers. Attempts to deal with such complaints directly often prove unfruitful, partly because the patient's seemingly exaggerated affect interferes with effective communication. However, these are all signs of a patient presenting in crisis.[16]

Anatomy of a Crisis

A crisis occurs when a hazardous event is encountered and customary problem-solving strategies prove ineffective.[16] People experience crises of various intensities many times in their lives; common examples include the death of a loved one, the loss of a job, serious illness, and domestic violence. The usual response of an individual to such stress is to experience an inner tension that mobilizes coping skills. Different problem-solving behaviors are then tried based on previous experience.

If an effective means of resolving the crisis is chosen, the person returns to a more organized state. If a resolution to the crisis is not easily found, a period of disorganization follows. During this time, the person experiences intense emotions such as confusion, anxiety, fear, anger, and despair. It is during the state of emotionally charged disorganization that a person may seek help at the emergency department.

Patients in crisis will, by the nature of their complaints and behavior, fall into the category of "the difficult patient" whether or not they actually are a "difficult person." It is important to be able to apply certain techniques of crisis intervention when dealing with such patients.

Dealing with the Crisis

Recognizing the Crisis

The presenting complaint of a patient in crisis may be a description of an event, situation, emotion, or physical symptom that can be vague or specific (domestic violence, inability to cope, anxiety, unwell, headache). Patients who present with crisis-related symptoms are a heterogeneous group. At one end of the spectrum are patients who have chief complaints that describe some type of emotional suffering and who do not require a traditional "medical" workup. At the other extreme are patients who have very limited insight into the cause of their symptoms. They may need to be reassured in absolute terms about the absence of serious disease before their anxiety will be alleviated. Between these two extremes are patients who partially understand how their circumstances might be contributing to their suffering. They will accept the idea that "the effect of stress will often produce these kinds of physical symptoms." However, many patients justifiably are unwilling to accept this explanation until they believe their medical complaint has been adequately assessed. This usually requires no more than a careful history and physical examination. Some patients who are in severe crisis need to be taken through the steps of formal crisis intervention. Only then will they view their physical symptoms objectively enough to be reassured regarding the benign nature of their illness. Because of the complex nature and considerable time required for crisis intervention, it is often beyond the scope of practice of a busy emergency physician. Nevertheless, for the sake of completeness, a brief summary of the process is provided here (Box 190-2).

BOX 190-2. Five Basic Steps in Crisis Intervention

1. Recognizing the crisis
2. Gathering basic information
3. Understanding the development of the crisis
4. Reproducing the peak tension of the crisis
5. Finding the solution

Basic Information Gathering

The first step in crisis intervention, after recognition of the crisis, involves gathering general information about the patient's home environment, work situation, personal relationships, and social involvements. The purpose of basic information gathering is to place the patient and the crisis into context before exploring the crisis itself. This step is time consuming and cannot be rushed.

Understanding the Development of the Crisis

The physician next uses a structured interview to obtain information about the sequence of events leading up to the crisis and the nature of the crisis itself. The objective is to understand the situation while keeping the interview organized so that the patient can describe events without being overwhelmed by the emotion attached to them. This part of the interview should be conducted in a very directed fashion, with the emphasis placed on the factual content of the crisis. The physician should try to avoid exploring the situation's emotional impact on the patient until the next step in the process.

Reproducing the Peak Tension of the Crisis

Once the crux of the crisis has been identified, the physician should proceed to help the patient express the intense emotions associated with the situation. This provides catharsis for the patient. Through empathetic, active listening, whereby the physician reflects back to the patient the intense emotional upheaval of the circumstances, the person in crisis is allowed to experience the previously overwhelming emotions in a safe context. This places the physician in a position of trust and sets the stage for problem solving.

Finding the Solution

In the final phase of crisis intervention, the physician acts as a facilitator to help the patient and other involved parties find a solution to the problem. After gaining an understanding of the development of the crisis and its emotional and social implications, the physician reframes the circumstances in objective, realistic, and understandable terms for all those concerned. This may include emphasizing information previously overlooked by the patient and others and stressing the strengths of the patient.[16] Possible solutions to the crisis are then suggested, with participation from the involved parties, and the best plan for resolution is implemented. It is important that this be a joint effort and that the patient have some ownership of the solution. The physician should avoid the trap of "giving advice" to the patient. The purpose of crisis intervention is not to provide long-term emotional healing, but rather to offer a short-term solution that will allow the patient to better cope with the immediate problem.[17]

SPECIFIC APPROACHES FOR DEALING WITH DIFFICULT PATIENTS: PUTTING IT ALL TOGETHER

The various management strategies described here can be consolidated to formulate a practical approach to dealing with difficult patients. The first step is the recognition of specific behavior types, rather than traditional diagnoses. These behavior types describe the most difficult patients seen in the emergency department. Patients displaying some, but not all, characteristics of a certain behavioral type may still be amenable to the management strategies for that type.

Behavioral Classification

Individuals with personality disorders frequently present as difficult patients. Although reliably establishing the diagnosis of a personality disorder during the typical brief emergency department encounter is difficult, an awareness of those personality disorders having a high prevalence in the emergency department will ease communication with colleagues when the diagnosis has been previously established (Box 190-3).

An alternative to the traditional diagnostic categories for classifying difficult patients has been described.[18] It is based on four specific behavioral presentations and the negative reactions they produce. We have adapted this classification system, using more neutral terms. The behavioral categories are *dependent patients*, *entitled patients*, *intractable patients*, and *self-destructive patients*. Through recognition of the difficult patient's maladaptive behavior and identification of the physician's subsequent negative reactions, patients can be placed into one of these behavioral categories. The behavioral categories in turn suggest effective treatment strategies for each patient type (Table 190-1).

Dependent Patients

Dependent patients see physicians as inexhaustible sources of compassion and understanding. Their initially reasonable requests rapidly escalate into repeated demands for reassurance, affection, analgesia, or other forms of attention. They are excessive in their gratitude; however, the more care they receive, the more their needs multiply. Initially, the physician may feel powerful and unique. Dependent patients give the message, "You're the only doctor who cares" and the physician often believes it. As the demands escalate, the physician's patience diminishes and initial feelings of inflated self-esteem are replaced with feelings of frustration, exhaustion, and failure. This leads to a natural desire to discharge or refer these patients, along with their demands, to another unfortunate physician. The patient leaves feeling rejected and then begins the same vicious cycle with the next physician. Patients with certain personality disorders (dependent, borderline,

Table 190-1. Management Strategies: Putting It all Together

Behavioral Classifications	Traditional Diagnostic Categories Associated	Suggested Management Strategies
1. Dependent Patients Excessive needs for attention, reassurance, analgesia. Uses helplessness and seduction. Physician initially feels special, then drained and frustrated. Patient increases needs when ultimately rejected.	Personality disorders; dependent, histrionic, borderline Malingerers, chronic psychiatric patients	Try to view the patient's neediness as a symptom. Be supportive while setting limits on patient expectations. Follow-up with appropriate, consistent physician. May need crisis intervention.
2. Entitled Patients Fear of loss of power causes entitled behavior. Uses intimidation, name dropping, hostility, and threats. Physician feels intimidated, angry, sometimes inadequate. Potential for litigation.	Personality disorders: paranoid, narcissistic Substance abusers VIPs	Be supportive of entitlement to good care while setting limits on unreasonable demands. Allow patients to choose between reasonable treatment options. Avoid power struggles.
3. Intractable Patients Excessive needs for attention met by having insolvable problems with multiple visits, doctor shopping, poor compliance, and no hope for successful treatment. Physician feels frustrated, angry, but fears missing significant illness. Cycle of "help me, but nothing helps."	Personality disorders: antisocial, borderline Malingerers	Distinguish from other complicated patients and manage appropriately. Beware of cognitive distortions that may obscure significant illness. Be supportive while "sharing" pessimism and setting reasonable expectations.
4. Self-destructive Patients Disregard for own health and repeated visits for serious illness. Often overtly self-destructive, denying of illness. Physicians feel frustrated, helpless, angry, and guilty for wishing the patient success.	Borderline personality disorder Substance abusers Chronically suicidal patients	Provide appropriate medical care. Learn to deal with own negative and nihilistic reactions to patients. Look for signs of depression and consider psychiatric referral as needed.

VIPs, very important persons.

BOX 190-3. Commonly Encountered Personality Disorders

Borderline personality disorder is a pattern of instability of interpersonal relationships, self-image and affect, and marked impulsiveness beginning by early adulthood and present in a variety of contexts and may be indicated by five or more of the following:

1. Frantic efforts to avoid real or imagined abandonment
2. A pattern of unstable and intense interpersonal relationships characterized by alternating extremes of idealization and devaluation
3. Identity disturbance: markedly and persistently unstable self-image or sense of self
4. Impulsiveness in at least two areas that are potentially self-damaging (e.g., spending, sex, substance abuse, reckless driving, binge eating)
5. Recurrent suicidal behavior, gestures, threats, or self-mutilating behavior
6. Affective instability caused by a marked reactivity of mood (e.g., intense episodic dysphoria, irritability, or anxiety usually lasting a few hours and only rarely more than a few days)
7. Chronic feelings of emptiness
8. Inappropriate, intense anger or difficulty controlling anger (e.g., frequent displays of temper, constant anger, recurrent physical fights)
9. Transient, stress-related paranoid ideation or severe dissociative symptoms

Antisocial personality disorder is a pattern of disregard for and violation of the rights of others since the age of 15 years as indicated by three or more of the following:

1. Failure to conform to social norms with respect to lawful behaviors as indicated by repeatedly performing acts that are grounds for arrest
2. Deceitfulness, as indicated by repeated lying, use of aliases, or conning others for personal profit or pleasure
3. Impulsiveness or failure to plan ahead
4. Irritability and aggressiveness, as indicated by repeated physical fights or assaults
5. Reckless disregard for safety of self or others
6. Consistent irresponsibility, as indicated by repeated failure to sustain consistent work behavior or honor financial obligations
7. Lack of remorse, as indicated by being indifferent to or rationalizing having hurt, mistreated, or stolen from another

Dependent personality disorder is a pattern of pervasive and excessive need to be taken care of that leads to submissive and clinging behavior and fears of separation beginning by early adulthood and may be indicated by five or more of the following:

1. Has difficulty making everyday decisions without an excessive amount of advice and reassurance from others
2. Needs others to assume responsibility for most major areas of his or her life
3. Has difficulty expressing disagreement with others because of fear of loss of support or approval
4. Has difficulty self-starting projects or doing things (because of a lack of self-confidence in judgment or abilities rather than a lack of motivation or energy)
5. Goes to excessive lengths to obtain nurturing and support from others, to the point of volunteering to do things that are unpleasant
6. Feels uncomfortable or helpless when alone because of exaggerated fears of being unable to care for self
7. Urgently seeks another relationship as a source of care and support when a close relationship ends
8. Is unrealistically preoccupied with fears of being left to take care of self

Paranoid personality disorder is a pattern of distrust and suspiciousness of others such that their motives are interpreted as malevolent, beginning in early adulthood as indicated by four or more of the following:

1. Suspects, without sufficient basis, that others are being exploitive, harmful, or deceitful
2. Is preoccupied with unjustified doubts about the loyalty or trustworthiness of friends or associates
3. Is reluctant to confide in others because of unwarranted fear that the information will be used maliciously against him or her
4. Reads hidden demeaning or threatening meanings into benign remarks or events
5. Persistently bears grudges (i.e., is unforgiving of insults, injuries, or slights)
6. Perceives attacks on character or reputation that are not apparent to others and is quick to react angrily or to counterattack
7. Has recurrent suspicions, without justification, regarding the fidelity of spouse or sexual partner

Histrionic personality disorder is a pattern of excessive emotionality and attention seeking beginning by early adulthood as indicated by five or more of the following:

1. Is uncomfortable in situations in which the center of attention is someone else
2. Interaction with others is often characterized by inappropriate sexually seductive or provocative behavior
3. Displays rapidly shifting and shallow expression of emotions
4. Consistently uses physical appearance to draw attention to self
5. Has style of speech that is excessively impressionistic and lacking in detail
6. Shows self-dramatization, theatricality, and exaggerated expression of emotion
7. Is suggestible (i.e., easily influenced by others or circumstances)
8. Considers relationships to be more intimate than they actually are

Narcissistic personality disorder is a pattern of grandiosity, need for admiration, and lack of empathy beginning by early adulthood as indicated by five or more of the following:

1. Has a grandiose sense of self-importance (e.g., exaggerates achievements and talents, expects to be recognized as superior without commensurate achievements)
2. Is preoccupied with fantasies of unlimited success, power, brilliance, beauty, or ideal love
3. Believes self to be "special" and unique and can only be understood by, or should associate with, other special or high-status people (or institutions)
4. Requires excessive admiration
5. Has a sense of entitlement (i.e., unreasonable expectations of especially favorable treatment or automatic compliance with their expressed expectations)
6. Is interpersonally exploitive (i.e., takes advantage of others to achieve personal ends)
7. Lacks empathy, is unwilling to recognize or identify with the feelings and needs of others
8. Is often envious of others or believes that others are envious of them
9. Shows arrogant, haughty behaviors or attitudes

Adapted from American Psychiatric Association: *Diagnostic and Statistical Manual of Mental Disorders*, 4th ed. Washington, DC, American Psychiatric Association, 1994.

and histrionic), somatoform disorders, malingering, and chronic psychiatric disorders often are in this behavior category.[1,18]

Dependent patients are best managed early in the relationship before the help-rejection cycle is fully established. Some of their earliest identifying features are the negative reactions they produce in physicians. The replacement of physicians' strong feelings of self-esteem by frustration and failure is a diagnostic clue to this type of patient. Although it is important to be supportive with such patients, it is imperative to set limits as tactfully and firmly as possible. Physicians should point out their own limited time and resources. Reasonable expectations for the patient must be established while giving assurances that one will try to help. After appropriate management, disposition should be arranged, and written discharge instructions with defined criteria for return visits to the emergency department should be provided. The need for follow-up visits with the appropriate primary care provider should be emphasized.

Dependent patients are especially likely to seek solutions to their problems at the emergency department in times of crisis. Looking for the underlying issues and structuring the interview along the lines of crisis intervention can assist in finding a satisfactory resolution to the patient's problem.

Entitled Patients

Very important persons (VIPs) are often well-informed, independent professionals who may be knowledgeable in medical matters. They spend their professional lives in a position of authority and control. However, the traits that make them successful in the workplace can cause them to be demanding, fault-finding, and self-entitled patients.

Entitled patients also seem to have endless needs, but instead of helplessness or seduction, they use intimidation, hostility, and threats to attain their often unreasonable demands. Entitled patients fear being helpless and dependent on physicians. They use a shield of entitlement to protect themselves. An example is the lawyer who, in his refusal to accept his illness, roams from physician to physician demanding repeated tests and opinions, while threatening to sue the previous physician who had tried to help him. Physicians experience the natural responses of disgust, anger, and antagonism when faced with such patients. There may be an urge to enter into a power struggle with the patient. The other common temptation is to accept the patient's terms at the price of compromising his or her care. Occasionally, the physician may even experience shame at being unable to meet the patient's unrealistic demands. The maladaptive behaviors of entitled patients are commonly seen in people with paranoid and narcissistic personality disorders, as well as in addicted patients and VIPs.[19]

Because the behavior of the entitled patient stems from insecurity, it is important to be supportive. While reassuring patients that they are entitled to good medical care, physicians must set limits that unreasonable demands will not be met. Prolonged debates with the patient about diagnostic and therapeutic options should be avoided. Recommendations about management options should be offered and patients left to exercise their autonomy in choosing their preferred course. At the same time, physicians must communicate their acceptance of the patients' rights to exercise this control and that their decision will not jeopardize subsequent access to appropriate care.

Intractable Patients

Intractable patients, like dependent and entitled patients, have insatiable needs for emotional support. However, they are neither seductive nor dependent in their behaviors. They present the antithesis of entitlement; they believe nothing will help. Intractable patients desperately seek help despite the failure of all previous medical assistance. Their history is punctuated by multiple emergency visits and behaviors that are self-defeating, covert, and manipulative. These negative behaviors undermine treatment and antagonize physicians, creating feelings of anger, self-doubt, and frustration. Patients with borderline and antisocial personality disorders and malingerers often fall into this behavioral category.[19]

Malingerers are among the most difficult patients presenting to the emergency department. Malingering is the intentional production of false or grossly exaggerated physical or psychiatric symptoms, motivated by external incentives that are unrelated to illness.[20] These patients may be seeking narcotics, shelter, or compensation; may be attempting to avoid work or criminal prosecution; or may simply be lonely.

Malingering represents deceptive, manipulative behavior and is coded in the *Diagnostic and Statistical Manual of Mental Disorders*, 4th edition (DSM-IV) as a "problem" rather than a mental disorder.[19] This contrived behavior must be distinguished from the psychiatric illness of somatoform disorders. Somatization is the involuntary production of symptoms without the patient's awareness. Unlike malingerers, somatizers are not motivated by any conscious desire for secondary gain.

Repeaters are patients who inappropriately frequent the emergency department excessively to the point that most staff know them by name. Although chronic schizophrenics often fall into this category, this behavior can occur in any patient with poor coping skills and maladaptive responses to psychosocial stressors. The easy accessibility of the emergency department often makes it the only support system immediately available to chronically decompensated patients. Caring for these difficult patients often feels like an exercise in futility and can be a drain on limited resources.

Geriatric patients with multiple medical problems and those abandoned in the emergency department by caretakers who are no longer willing or able to meet their needs are also patient types that deserve special attention. Although these patients have problems that are often difficult to solve, the patients themselves are not necessarily difficult people.[21]

Intractable patients elicit strong negative reactions from physicians. Their multiple, vague complaints that defy diagnosis and successful treatment often cause them to be labeled as "crocks," along with dependent patients.

Intractable patients are sometimes identified by the feelings of futility that they produce in their caregivers. Physicians must avoid the temptation to overreact with cognitive distortions and dismiss the possibility of genuine illness in the patient. The physician must therefore distinguish intractable patients from other complicated patients, rule out conditions that require immediate intervention, and provide appropriate management and disposition. Alternatively, there may be a tendency to launch into extensive investigations inappropriately if the behavior type is not recognized. Collateral information from previous medical records and other caregivers is valuable in providing guidance as to how aggressive investigations should be.

Because this type of behavior stems from a need for a relationship and fear of rejection, it is important for physicians to be supportive. The belief that showing empathy will only encourage maladaptive behavior is generally untrue. To the contrary, an escalation of symptoms usually follows when these patients interpret a physician's lack of concern as rejection.

Nevertheless, limits should be set regarding patients' expectations. Physicians should use this strategy while acknowledging the difficulty of the patients' problems and sharing their deep concern, and perhaps even pessimism, regarding the outcome of the investigations and treatment. It is helpful to make statements such as, "You know, Mr. Jones, you obviously have a very difficult problem here. You've seen lots of doctors and had lots of tests and treatments that don't seem to be helping much. There is no way, given the limited resources available in the emergency department at 11 o'clock on a Friday night, that we are going to be able to get to the bottom of this. However, what I can do is examine you and do some tests to make sure that there is no new, serious problem going on tonight. Then you will be able to follow up with your regular doctor on Monday." In this way the physician can communicate both an interest in the patient and empathy for their condition while setting limits on expectations. Both the physician and patient then understand the "contract" and have a way of terminating the encounter satisfactorily.[15]

Self-Destructive Patients

Self-destructive patients are particularly difficult to treat. Unlike intractable patients, they do not seek help. Rather, they are repeatedly brought to the emergency department because of their neglectful and self-destructive behaviors. Their ability to deny their problems is profound and sets up the maladaptive cycle of "nothing is wrong and nothing will help." Yet their behaviors often require repeated heroic efforts to save their lives. Although their chronic self-destructive behaviors may temporarily meet their immediate needs of shelter and food and perhaps, paradoxically, some of the attention they outwardly reject, this lethal cycle usually leads to a premature death. The *substance abuser*, the *violent patient*, and the *suicidal patient* are included in this category of difficult patient.[9]

It is not surprising that emergency department staff respond to such patients negatively, feel frustrated and helpless, and may even secretly wish them success in their self-destructive efforts. These are among the most difficult patients to treat. In reality, physicians can do little apart from providing appropriate care for the multiple presentations characteristic of this type of patient. The greatest obstacle for physicians may be to come to terms with their own complacency about the survival or demise of such patients. The lack of real concern about whether they live or die or worse, actually wishing that they would die, is repugnant and produces feelings of self-recrimination. Our inability to relate to the self-destructive decisions made by these individuals contributes to our complacency about their plight. Remembering our own human weaknesses or risk-taking behaviors and viewing their seemingly incomprehensible behavior as a difference in degree rather than in kind may help us to have more empathy for them.[10] Being supportive is important. Signs of depression in the patient may indicate the need for psychiatric referral, which will usually be refused. Uncooperative patients who are overtly suicidal should be detained for psychiatric assessment.

SUMMARY

Dealing with difficult patients is a common problem in the emergency department. The impaired patient-physician relationships associated with them have multiple negative implications for both patients and physicians. Their management may be optimized by using the general principles for managing difficult patients, by dealing realistically with one's own negative reactions, and by using techniques of crisis intervention where appropriate. These strategies are best applied within the context of a behavioral classification that avoids pejorative terms and stereotypes, labels that differentiate them from "worthier" patients.[10] Although this approach is not a panacea for dealing with difficult patients, the framework may help physicians render appropriate care while minimizing personal frustration, medicolegal exposure, and eventual physician burnout.

One of the great challenges of medical practice is to maintain humanity when caring for these difficult and highly vulnerable individuals. By focusing on their humanity, we have the best chance of preserving our own.[10] It is easy to care for patients who generate sympathy and noble to care for those who do not.[12]

In the end, the ability to accept distressing behavior as a symptom and to treat even the most irritating individuals with compassion and kindness may be the key to surviving them. When asked how he had avoided burnout after decades in emergency medicine, one well-known patriarch of the specialty simply responded, "You've got to love the patients."[22] This is a tall order, and not meant in the literal sense. But the degree to which we can show caring and empathy, even to the unlovable, may be the key to maintaining the quality of our care, our satisfaction with the specialty, and our long-term survival in practice.

KEY CONCEPTS

- Difficult patients may elicit negative reactions in caregivers, resulting in undesirable implications for both themselves and their caregivers.
- Managing the difficult patient can be optimized by understanding the multiple factors contributing to the impaired physician-patient relationship.
- Behavioral classifications should be used instead of pejorative stereotypes when characterizing difficult behaviors.
- General and specific strategies, including understanding our own reactions, are helpful in dealing with the impaired physician-patient relationship.
- The ability to accept difficult behaviors as symptoms and treat even the most difficult patient with kindness is central to providing good care while avoiding personal frustration, medicolegal repercussions, and physician burnout.

REFERENCES

1. Andrew LB, Pollack ML (eds): *Wellness for Emergency Physicians.* Dallas, American College of Emergency Physicians, 1995.
2. Rosenweig S: The other half of the curriculum. *Ann Emerg Med* 20:591, 1991.
3. Yedidia MJ, Gillespie CC, Kachur E, et al: Effect of communications training on medical student performance. *JAMA* 290:1157, 2003.
4. Rosenweig S: Teaching the art of emergency medicine. *Ann Emerg Med* 20:71, 1991.
5. Marco CA, Smith CA: Conflict resolution in emergency medicine. *Ann Emerg Med* 40:347, 2002.
6. Hobgood CD, Riviello RJ, Jourilles N, Hamilton G: Assessment of communication and interpersonal skills competencies. *Acad Emerg Med* 9:1257, 2002.
7. Larkin GL, Binder L, Houry D, Adams J: Defining and evaluating professionalism: A core competency for graduate emergency medical education. *Acad Emerg Med* 9:1249, 2002.
8. Marco CA: Teaching professionalism to problem residents. *Acad Emerg Med* 9:1001, 2002.
9. Disruptive medical patients. In Hyman SE, Tesar G (eds): *Manual of Psychiatric Emergencies.* Boston, Little, Brown, 1994.
10. Simon JR, Dwyer J, Goldfrank LR: Ethical issues in emergency medicine. *Emerg Med Clin North Am* 17:353, 1999.
11. Iserson KV: Understanding the incomplete text: Interpreting the emergency department patient. *Am J Emerg Med* 10:361, 1992.
12. Adams J, Murray R: The difficult diagnosis. *Emerg Med Clin North Am* 16:689, 1998.
13. Waitzkin H: Doctor-patient communication: Clinical implications of social scientific research. *JAMA* 252:1441, 1984.
14. Birdwell BD, Herbers JE, Kroenke K: Evaluating chest pain: The patient's presentation style alters the physician's diagnostic approach. *Arch Intern Med* 153:1991, 1993.
15. Drossman DA: Psychological sound bites: Exercises in the patient-doctor relationship. *Am J Gastroenterol* 92:1418, 1997.
16. Gordon C: Crisis intervention: A general approach. In Hyman SE, Tesar G (eds): *Manual of Psychiatric Emergencies.* Boston, Little, Brown, 1994.
17. Kercher EE: Crisis intervention in the emergency department. *Emerg Med Clin North Am* 9:219, 1991.
18. Groves JE: Taking care of the hateful patient. *N Engl J Med* 296:883, 1978.
19. American Psychiatric Association: *Diagnostic and Statistical Manual of Mental Disorders,* 4th ed. Washington, DC, American Psychiatric Association, 1994.
20. Purcell DB: The somatic patient. *Emerg Med Clin North Am* 9:137, 1991.
21. Greenstein RA, Ness DE: Psychiatric emergencies in the elderly. *Emerg Med Clin North Am* 8:429, 1990.
22. Harrison DW: Emergency medicine as a martial art. *Ann Emerg Med* 17:115, 1999.

PART SIX

Emergency Medical Services

CHAPTER 191

Emergency Medical Service: Overview and Ground Transport

Thomas H. Blackwell

PERSPECTIVE

History of Emergency Medical Service

Napoleon's surgeon-in-chief, Barron Jean Larrey (1766-1842), may be credited with developing the first organized Emergency Medical Service (EMS) system. When the Prussians and Austrians declared war against the French, Larrey, assigned to the Army of the Rhine, noted that wounded soldiers were left unattended until fighting had ceased. Only then would surgeons enter the battlefield to attempt resuscitation. Convinced that mortality would decrease if the wounded were rapidly evacuated to field hospitals shortly after injury, Larrey positioned medical transport teams closer to the battleground to expeditiously remove those afflicted.[1] Using a similar strategy, Jonathan Letterman (1824-1872) improved military ambulance services and medical care during the American Civil War by organizing horse-drawn ambulance trains designed to rapidly transport wounded soldiers from the battlefield to proximate field hospitals.[2] Figure 191-1 depicts the early Larrey ambulance used during the Napoleonic Wars, the Rucker wagon used during the American Civil War, and a modern ambulance used today.

Before the advent of civilian ambulance services, the sick and injured were transported by any means available, including passerby motorists, wagons, farm machinery, delivery carts, buses, hearses, and taxicabs. In 1865, the Commercial Hospital in Cincinnati established the first hospital-based ambulance service. Four years later, the first city service began at New York's Bellevue Hospital.[3]

In 1957, as part of the annual survey on traffic safety, a select committee of the National Safety Council's Traffic Conference analyzed how injuries resulting from highway accidents were managed and made recommendations for improved services.[4] At the same time, physician advocates drafted papers on what they perceived constituted good emergency medical treatment.[5,6]

In 1965, the President's Commission on Highway Safety recommended a National Accident Response Program to decrease death and injury from highway accidents.[7] Results from a second national survey by the National Academy of Sciences–National Research Council were used to draft a White Paper titled *Accidental Death and Disability: The Neglected Disease of Modern Society.*[8] Published in 1966, this document described the hazardous conditions of provision of emergency care at all levels and outlined the necessary building blocks for future EMS maturation. These national efforts were the impetus for congressional legislation that directed the U.S. Department of Transportation (DOT)–National Highway Traffic Safety Administration (NHTSA) to develop a program for improving emergency medical care.

During the mid-1960s, prehospital cardiac care included field defibrillation programs in Belfast and cardiac arrest research in several U.S. cities.[9,10] In 1969, the first national conference on EMS convened and resulted in the development of a curriculum, certification process, and national registry for the emergency medical technician—ambulance (EMT-A). By 1972, the Department of Labor recognized the EMT as an occupational specialty.[11] Interested physicians and nurses later provided advanced educational courses and practical experience for EMTs, hence the beginning of paramedic providers.[12,13]

Additional programs prompted congressional passage of the EMS Systems Act of 1973 (PL 93-154), which authorized funding that dramatically improved the development of comprehensive regional EMS delivery systems. Efforts to improve pediatric emergency care took place in 1984 when Congress adopted the Emergency Medical Services for Children (EMS-C) initiative through the Health Services, Preventive Health Services, and Home Community Based Services Act of 1984 (PL 98-555).[14] An Institute of Medicine study released in 1994 promoted integration of the concept of EMS-C not just into existing EMS systems but also into comprehensive systems of care provision, including injury prevention, primary and definitive care, and rehabilitation services.[15]

Emergency Medical Service Systems

Multiple EMS system designs exist, all predicated on the type of community served. Though a local decision, all states incorporate an administrative office that governs or oversees the provision of EMS activities. Typically, the role is not to direct any individual service but to assist in planning, licensing services, and establishing or enforcing the scope and standards for practice. Other functions may include training, examining, certifying/recertifying providers, record keeping, collecting data, and auditing or investigating programs. A description of systems for the 200 most populous cities in the United States is periodically published in the *Journal of Emergency Medical Services.*[16] For simplicity, the following categorization of systems will be used: private and public agencies; basic life support

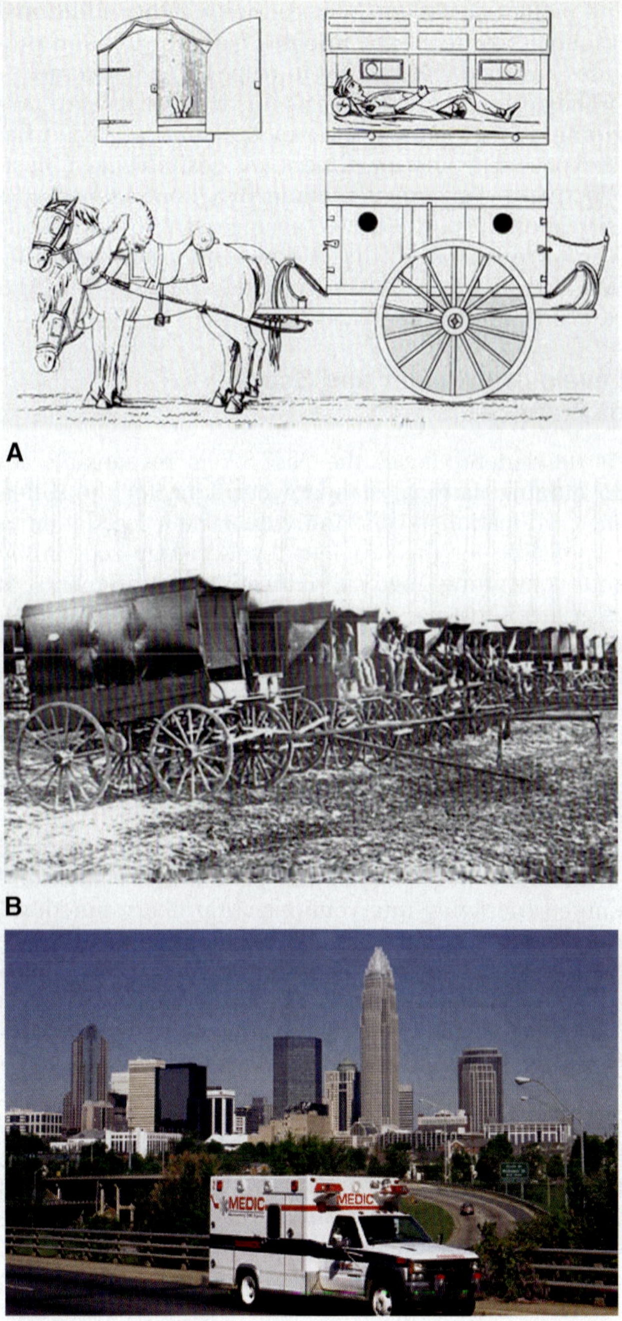

Figure 191-1. Larrey's flying ambulance **(A)**, Letterman's Rucker wagon **(B)**, and the modern ambulance **(C)** used today. (From the National Library of Medicine History of Medicine Division. Courtesy of Library of Congress, Prints & Photographs Division, LC-B8171-2585 DLC.)

(BLS) and advanced life support (ALS) services; and single-tiered, multitiered, and first responder (FR) systems.

Private and Public Agencies

When local government has not assumed primary responsibility for EMS services, communities may depend on private providers. Financial responsibility varies, but it is usually dependent on user fees. A local government subsidy may or may not supplement the operation. If multiple providers are serving one jurisdiction, calls may be allocated by rotation or specified zone coverage. Dispatching varies depending on the system, but it may be performed by the provider or by a central agency. Medical direction is often provided by a contracted physician or physician oversight board.

Hospital-based EMS systems are few in number and may be managed by a single hospital or hospital corporation. Not all hospital-based EMS programs are considered private in that the hospital may be a division under local or state government or operating under public authority. Like private models, financial responsibility is usually in the form of user fees, with or without additional subsidy. Dispatching may be provided by a local public safety agency, which may also be responsible for police and fire communications. An emergency physician from a sponsor or base hospital typically provides medical direction for these systems.

A public utility model is a hybrid between private and public design that allows local government to contract with a private or public provider. The successful bidder for service becomes a contracted entity that agrees to provide the specified services (ALS, BLS, or both) to the catchment area and, depending on the arrangement, may bill the patient directly or receive uniform reimbursement. Depending on local structure and interagency agreement, dispatching may be performed by an existing public safety organization or by the parent company. Medical direction is usually provided by a specified individual subject to contractual terms.

When government officials were faced with planning and establishing EMS systems during the early maturation period, many decided that the fire department was the logical choice to incorporate EMS. Fire stations were strategically located throughout the community, and personnel were already used to providing emergency responses. Firefighters could be cross-trained as a firefighter-paramedic or be dedicated to either fire or EMS function with the opportunity for transfer. Public EMS systems that were not incorporated into fire departments evolved into their own separate entity, referred to as a municipal third-service system. Such agencies are operated by local municipalities and are endorsed and supported by local government. Many cities have been successful in combining police, fire, and EMS under a global public safety agency, with all department heads or chiefs reporting to one manager or administrator. Financially, public EMS systems may be supported by a tax base, which may or may not be supplemented by user fees. Regardless of design, medical oversight for a municipal EMS system may be provided by a physician appointed and contracted by a local hospital, advisory council, or medical oversight board.

Basic Life Support and Advanced Life Support Services

BLS refers to the provision of emergency care without the use of advanced therapeutic interventions. Skills include airway management (oral and nasal airways, bag/mask ventilation), cardiopulmonary resuscitation (CPR), control of hemorrhage, fracture and spine immobilization, and assistance with childbirth. Defibrillation with an automated external defibrillator is often included in many BLS systems. Services are provided by emergency medical technicians, usually certified at the basic level (EMT-B).

BLS systems may be associated with poor survival rates from out-of-hospital cardiac arrest, especially those not incorporating automated external defibrillator technology.[17,18] Alternatively, there is debate on the effectiveness of ALS for medical and trauma emergencies.[19,20] Despite this evidence, few urban communities across the United States operate solely at the BLS level. Many rural and some suburban EMS services rely on volunteers who may not wish to become advanced-level providers. Because these services may have low call volumes, it becomes more difficult for personnel to maintain advanced skills and a proficient knowledge base.[21] In addition, such communities may not have access to medical supervision or hospital sponsorship for ALS care.

Systems categorized as ALS offer a more comprehensive level of service by highly educated providers, usually certified at the intermediate or paramedic level (EMT-I or EMT-P, respectively) or equivalent levels depending on individual state certifications. Provider skills include advanced airway interventions, placement of intravenous lines, administration of medications, cardiac monitoring and manual defibrillation, and certain invasive procedures. Most EMS systems in urban cities operate at the ALS level of care.

Single-Tiered, Multitiered, and First Responder Systems

In a single-tier system, every response, regardless of the call type, receives the same level of personnel expertise and equipment allocation (all BLS or ALS). Multitiered systems use a combination of ALS and BLS levels, depending on the nature of the call. Differences in cost and effectiveness between a mixed ALS-BLS service and an all ALS service have been debated. Currently, there has been a steady decrease in systems that provide mixed ALS-BLS care.[22,23] A single-tiered ALS response may prove to be cost-effective in specific locales, ensures the capability of providing a consistent advanced level of care to all patients regardless of illness or injury severity, and obviates the potential for undertriage or overtriage by 9-1-1 telecommunicators. Alternatively, a multitiered system may meet the needs of individual communities or agency infrastructure. This design often meets with employee satisfaction and has the potential to preserve ALS resources for higher-priority calls in that BLS transport of nonurgent patients allows for ALS ambulances to be available for potential critical responses.

Regardless of single-tiered or multitiered design, EMS systems usually include FR services as part of the response. The FR, usually a police officer or firefighter, is the nontransport BLS or ALS provider who quickly responds to the scene of an emergency to provide initial care before definitive medical care and transportation assets arrive. The FR quickly assesses the situation and patient or patients, determines whether additional resources are required, initiates patient care, and provides advance information to responding personnel.

The design of an EMS system is targeted toward providing quality patient care in the shortest time after unexpected injury or illness. A desirable and cost-effective design might include BLS nontransport FRs with short response times (average of 2 to 4 minutes) who have the capability of providing early defibrillation and airway support, coupled with ensuing ALS care and transport services.[24]

Levels of Provider and Scope of Practice

At the federal level, the NHTSA is responsible for developing national standard curricula for the different certification levels. Individual state legislation is responsible for the provider levels recognized, initial and continuing medical education requirements at each level, testing, and time intervals for course completion and recertification. The following outlines the DOT recommendations for the four common levels of provider along with suggested hours of training and incorporated skills (Table 191-1).

First Responder

The FR is typically the first to arrive at the scene of an incident. Initial scene and patient assessment and limited lifesaving interventions are primary functions. Along with CPR and basic airway management skills, the FR should be able to control hemorrhage and initiate spinal immobilization.

The four elements referred to as the "chain of survival" by the American Heart Association that decrease mortality from out-of-hospital cardiac arrest are early access to care, CPR, defibrillation, and advanced airway management and medications.[25] Because early defibrillation may improve survival from out-of-hospital cardiac arrest, the use of an automated external defibrillator should be a mandatory procedure for the FR.[26,27]

DOT recommends 40 hours of didactic instruction for the standard FR course and 16 to 36 hours for refresher training. Clinical rotation is not part of the curriculum.[28]

Emergency Medical Technician—Basic

The EMT-B is the minimum level required to staff a BLS ambulance and is commonly used for nonemergency and convalescent transport services. In addition to skills of the FR, the EMT-B is also involved in triage, more detailed patient assessment, and transportation. Like FRs, EMT-Bs should have the capability of providing early defibrillation.[29]

In 1995, NHTSA released the revised EMT-B curriculum. The initial course requires approximately 110 hours of instruction and includes 46 lessons, each with cognitive, effective, and psychomotor objectives.[30] Many states have expanded the course to include more skills such as use of an automated external defibrillator, epinephrine autoinjections, albuterol adminis-

Table 191-1. EMS Provider Level Training and Skills

EMS Provider Level	DOT Recommended Hours of Training	Skill Set
First responder	Initial: 40 hours Refresher: 16–36 hours	Initial scene and patient assessment Basic airway skills CPR Control of hemorrhage Spinal immobilization
EMT—basic	Initial: 110 hours Refresher: 24-hour refresher course, 48 hours of continuing education, and a BLS course every 2 years	First responder skills plus Triage and detailed patient assessment Automated external defibrillation May assist in some systems: use of epinephrine for anaphylaxis; albuterol for wheezing
EMT—intermediate	Initial: 300-400 hours and includes didactic and clinical experience	EMT-basic skills plus Endotracheal intubation Manual defibrillation IV line placement Limited pharmacologic treatments May in some systems: laryngeal mask airway
EMT—paramedic	Initial: 1000-1200 hours Refresher: 48-hour refresher course, 24 hours of yearly continuing education, and BLS and ALS courses at the pediatric and adult levels	EMT-intermediate skills plus Cardiac rhythm recognition Expanded pharmacologic treatment Needle decompression of a tension pneumothorax Needle or surgical cricothyrotomy Transthoracic cardiac pacing

ALS, advanced life support; BLS, basic life support; CPR, cardiopulmonary resuscitation; DOT, Department of Transportation; EMS, Emergency Medical Service; EMT, emergency medical technician; IV, intravenous.

tration by hand-held nebulizer or metered-dose inhaler, and intravenous fluid therapy. For recertification, DOT recommends a 24-hour refresher course, 48 hours of continuing education, and a BLS course every 2 years.

Emergency Medical Technician—Intermediate

The EMT-I was established to allow a more comprehensive approach to care when paramedic services were unavailable or unobtainable. Many states recognize the EMT-I certification, whereas others designate alternative, but comparable levels depending on specific skills and procedures. The intermediate level is useful for rural systems because it supplies an advanced level of service for less cost and educational time expended. The scope of practice for the EMT-I varies across the United States. Most systems allow the EMT-I to establish an intravenous line and to manually defibrillate. Limited medications and adjunctive airway devices (e.g., blind-insertion airway device or laryngeal mask airway) may be integrated skills.

DOT recommends 300 to 400 hours of initial education that includes didactic classroom lectures combined with hospital and field experience.[31]

Emergency Medical Technician—Paramedic

The EMT-P is the most advanced prehospital provider. Paramedics have the capability of addressing most prehospital emergencies. Their scope of practice includes a wide variety of therapeutics and procedures, including recognition of cardiac rhythms, expanded pharmacologic treatment, and advanced airway interventions. Other important invasive procedures include needle decompression of a tension pneumothorax, needle or surgical cricothyrotomy, and transthoracic cardiac pacing.

A recent revision of the national standard curriculum for the EMT-P calls for approximately 1000 to 1200 instructional hours, including didactic, clinical, and field education. All course content focuses on technical and professional competency. Additional modules are included that allow programs to incorporate an expanded scope of practice.[32] With the expansion of EMS technology and management career options, many paramedic educational programs have advanced from 1-year certificate curriculums to 2-year associate or 4-year baccalaureate degrees. Recertification requirements include a 48-hour refresher course, 24 hours of yearly continuing education, and BLS and ALS courses at the pediatric and adult levels.

Material Resources

Before the mid-1960s, few if any regulations governed system design, operations, and equipment. As EMS development progressed, guidelines for emergency vehicle specifications were adopted by DOT and equipment lists were proposed. Today, the American College of Surgeons, American College of Emergency Physicians (ACEP), and the EMS-C program continue to publish documents that recommend design, equipment, and medications for ambulances.[33,34]

Medications

During the 1980s, many believed that prehospital drug administration was unjustified and simply delayed hospital transport.[35,36] Moreover, there is still a lack of scientific evidence to support many of the practices that are currently used.[37] Despite this paucity of research, the American Heart Association continues to support the use of certain advanced cardiac life support (ACLS) medications, which are carried by most ALS services.[38] The wide variety of alternative medications is less uniform, including respiratory and anaphylaxis medications, preparations for altered mental status, analgesics, and antiemetics. Although fibrinolytics and agents for rapid sequence intubation (RSI) have not been universally accepted as standard for ground units, their use is increasing despite a lack of compelling evidence of improved outcome.

Equipment

Basic ambulance equipment should include items necessary for emergency procedures (e.g., airway support, hemorrhage control, fracture and spine immobilization, childbirth), personal protection, patient movement, and basic rescue procedures. Additional patient care equipment will be predicated on the level of provision outlined by the system design.

Ambulances

Three basic ambulance vehicle designs are recognized by DOT: type I, type II, and type III. Both type I and type III ambulances incorporate a modular patient compartment mounted on a conventional truck or van chassis, respectively. The type II vehicle is a standard van. The larger medium-duty vehicle, mounted on a business-class chassis, has become popular in recent years. This configuration requires less periodic maintenance and offers extended service time. Each ambulance manufacturer promotes various interior cabinetry, and all include sufficient lighting, outlets for 110-V equipment, suction, oxygen systems, and external audible and visual warning devices. The six-pointed blue star surrounding the Staff of Aesculapius, or the "Star of Life," is recognized worldwide as the standard symbol for EMS (Figure 191-2).[39]

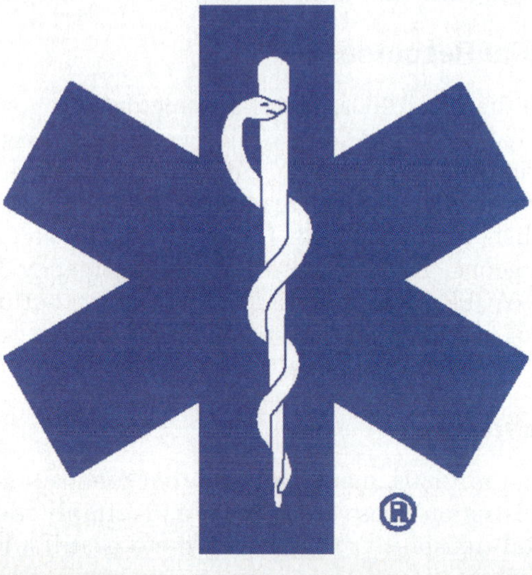

Figure 191-2. Star of Life symbol. (Courtesy of EMS Division, National Highway Traffic Safety Administration.)

Communications

Integral to prehospital care systems, EMS communications involve multiple components, all interlinked to facilitate expedient patient care. Effective communication systems include public information and education programs regarding general access to care, technology to ensure simplified access, means of call prioritization and management of available resources, protocols for providing emergency patient care instructions before EMS arrival, ability to communicate with allied agency and hospital personnel, educational opportunities for telecommunicators, and quality improvement processes.

Access

Since 1973, the 9-1-1 universal emergency access telephone number has been adopted by many communities throughout the United States. Basic 9-1-1 service simply connects a caller to a central communications center or public safety answering point. Enhanced 9-1-1 provides additional information by immediately displaying the caller's telephone number and address.

Emergency Medical Dispatch

Dispatching encompasses multiple elements that assist patients in receiving expeditious medical care.[40] It is estimated that 30% of EMS calls are for nonemergency conditions, with only 15% to 20% being considered calls for critical or life-threatening situations.[41]

The emergency medical dispatcher (EMD) is responsible for ascertaining the primary medical condition and severity. Communication centers that model their dispatch response protocols on priority use a finite list of common chief complaints, each having associated predetermined questions. Answers to these questions ultimately dictate a predefined response mode. Depending on the response assigned and system configuration, an ambulance (BLS or ALS) and possibly an FR resource are dispatched to respond in an emergency or nonemergency mode. When critical conditions are identified, the EMD may proceed in giving specific prearrival instructions to assist the caller in providing critical interventions before EMS arrival, including procedures such as opening and clearing an airway, performing CPR, controlling hemorrhage, and assisting with childbirth. Such assistance dramatically narrows the response time interval for receiving emergency medical care.

Systems Status Management

Depending on system size, the population served, and resources available, the use of systems status management has proved beneficial for many services. Based on historical data, high-performance or peak demand periods of the day coupled to service areas or call location can be identified so that coverage plans or posting assignments may be instituted. Such mechanisms place ambulances at predetermined locations where potential calls are likely to occur. Response vehicles may be equipped with an automatic vehicle locator that functions as a telemetry unit or with a global positioning satellite system that provides a site interface with the computer-aided dispatch system. This site information is helpful when staging or redeployment of vehicles is required during periods of high call volume or when limited resources are available.

Field Communications

While at the scene or during transport, EMTs usually have the capability of communicating with hospital staff. A consultative patient report may be given to receive medication or intervention orders or simply for notification of arrival. EMS providers should also have the capability of communicating with all allied public safety agencies for mutual aid purposes, mass casualty situations, or disaster responses. If air medical services are available, EMS and fire personnel must have the capability of communicating with the helicopter pilot and crew members. Scene personnel must relay landing zone information and potential hazards to the pilot and should provide a preliminary patient report to the medical crew.

MEDICAL DIRECTION

An EMS medical director is a physician with specialized interest and knowledge of patient care activities unique to the prehospital environment. Medical oversight must extend from the communications center through all components of field care. Typically, a contractual arrangement for services provides the physician with the administrative authority to implement patient care protocols, interact with all aspects of the system, and remove a provider from practice if medical care or behavior is substandard. Published guidelines describing the activities and performance of an EMS medical director have been prepared by the ACEP, National Association of EMS Physicians, NHTSA, and Health Resources and Services Administration.[42-44]

Medical direction consists of off-line (indirect) and on-line (direct) control. Off-line medical control includes protocol development, education of personnel, prospective and retrospective review of patient care, and other quality improvement processes. Direct medical control involves real-time interaction between a physician or designee and the field provider.

Indirect Medical Control

Medical accountability for patient care activities is the basis for indirect medical control and functions either before a patient is encountered (prospective) or after hospital transport has occurred (retrospective). Patient care guidelines and protocol development for EMTs and EMDs, continuing medical education, medicolegal policies, and quality/performance improvement processes are important elements.

Protocols

Perhaps the most important duty of the medical director is to develop patient care protocols. Protocols serve as pre-established practice guidelines that define the standard of care for most illnesses or injuries encountered in the prehospital setting. Operational issues such as hospital designation and destination policies, termination of resuscitation, and patient transport refusal may be included. Depending on state regulations, protocols may include standing orders for particular clinical situations such that EMTs may perform certain procedures or administer medications for predefined patient conditions before communication with hospital personnel. Protocol development should be driven by system resources and patient needs and should include guidelines for triage and care of specific patient populations, including trauma patients, newborns, and children.

Regardless of local communication protocols, prehospital providers should always be able to discuss a case with a physician for clarification or guidance when clinical questions or controversial situations arise. Furthermore, hospital notification is always important when critical patients are being transported.

Education

Medical directors should be familiar with and actively involved in local or regional educational programs for initial and continuing education courses for all levels of EMT certification. Course curriculum development and administration, evaluation, and revision processes should be understood. Systems that incorporate their own educational programs allow for modifications that reflect intrinsic needs of the system and the providers.

Field personnel and telecommunicators must be given regularly scheduled courses that improve competency in knowledge and skills. Instructional formats and resources to accomplish educational objectives may include didactic classroom lectures, skill laboratories, direct field observation, or distance learning models for self-paced opportunities. Standardized core content is important to maintain consistency and quality of care.

Quality/Performance Improvement

Once patient care protocols are developed and implemented, there must be mechanisms, such as retrospective review of patient care reports or direct field observation, to evaluate individual and system performance and patient outcome. Deviations from specific protocols may reflect problems with individual EMTs, medical control personnel, or the protocol itself, each requiring education and re-evaluation. Deficiencies, both operational and clinical, must be identified for appropriate remediation to occur, which may be in the form of counseling, educational instruction, or revisions of system design or patient care protocols.[45] Competency, knowledge retention, and skill performance are measurable parameters. Time standards (e.g., out-of-chute time [time from ambulance notification to deployment], response time, and scene time) are equally important measures.[46]

Direct Medical Control

Direct medical control is the concurrent direction of EMTs providing patient care. This may be in the form of radio or telephone communications or direct scene observation and may be considered centralized or decentralized. In a centralized system, a selected hospital is designated as the lead facility (base station hospital, resource hospital, or sponsor hospital) and is responsible for providing all direct medical control orders and notification regardless of the receiving facility. In a decentralized system, each hospital functions as a base station and provides direction to EMTs transporting patients to their facility.

Personnel responsible for direct medical control must be knowledgeable about the entire EMS system, receiving facilities, protocols, medication formulary and equipment, administrative and operational issues, and medicolegal implications for certain situations. Systems whose protocols include standing orders may require only direct communication for specific reasons. Thus, although these medical and administrative protocols may guide EMTs through most circumstances, medical control consultation may assist with medicolegal issues, situational problems at the scene, patient nontransport, or a multitude of potential ethical dilemmas that may be encountered. Regardless, direct medical control is usually invaluable for notifying a receiving facility for preparation of a treatment room and staff when critical or potentially critical patients are being transported.

PREHOSPITAL MEDICAL CARE AND CONTROVERSIES IN MANAGEMENT

Airway Support and Respiratory Emergencies

Interventions

Respiratory complaints account for a significant number of EMS responses. Basic measures to control and support a patient's airway include manual maneuvers (e.g., chin lift or jaw thrust), oral and nasopharyngeal devices, and use of bag/mask ventilation. At the advanced level, interventions may include endotracheal intubation, the use of alternative adjuncts (e.g., blind-insertion airway device or laryngeal mask airway), or surgical cricothyrotomy. RSI regimens, including neuromuscular blocking agents, have historically been used by air medical services but are now being implemented by ground EMS programs. Many studies have begun to challenge the effectiveness of prehospital intubation, particularly in view of an alarming incidence of esophageal intubation in some systems and poor outcomes with the use of RSI for head-injured patients.[47,48] One prospective, randomized study of pediatric prehospital airway management concluded that in the urban setting, bag/mask ventilation may be superior to intubation in certain patient groups.[49] Recent evidence has demonstrated the potential use of continuous or bilevel positive airway pressure for pulmonary edema and adult respiratory distress syndrome.[50]

Medications

Most advanced programs have adopted the use of clinically proven medications for bronchospasm, chronic obstructive pulmonary disease, and anaphylaxis, but no studies have demonstrated a benefit with the administration of these medications in the prehospital environment. Although some studies might be considered unethical (e.g., a prehospital study of epinephrine for anaphylaxis), others (e.g., prehospital use of β_2-agonists or steroids for asthma or loop diuretics for pulmonary edema) could easily be performed, with the results far from certain. Pending further studies, most systems have adopted the position that these medications do not harm patients in the prehospital setting, may be helpful, and do seem to provide comfort and clinical improvement for most patients experiencing varying degrees of respiratory distress.

Cardiovascular Emergencies

Interventions

Previous research has demonstrated the effectiveness of early defibrillation for terminating ventricular fibrillation and improving survival from sudden cardiac death.[51] Advances in technology have improved such that defibrillators, traditionally used by paramedics, are now used by a variety of public safety responders and bystanders. Design features, including a user-friendly system that automatically analyzes the cardiac rhythm, determines whether a shock is indicated, and charges and delivers the shock (or informs the operator when to do so), allow for widespread use of automated external defibrillators by emergency responders and laypersons with little or no knowledge of cardiac arrest. Public access defibrillation programs are being implemented throughout the country, with devices being placed in high-volume, populous, and secluded areas such as airports and airplanes, casinos, and office buildings.[52] Various models of automated external defibrillators incorporating different energy levels and shock waveforms are now being marketed; however, the effectiveness of each is still being scrutinized. Similarly, the effectiveness of public access defibrillation is currently being investigated.[53] Acquisition plus transmission of prehospital 12-lead electrocardiograms is becoming more prevalent as well. Though expensive to implement, several studies have revealed minimal delays in scene time while obtaining the electrocardiogram and a shorter time to intervention (administration of thrombolytic agents or admission to the catheterization laboratory) with the use of this technology.[54,55]

Medications

Traditional cardiac medications recommended by ACLS are used by most ALS systems. Recent investigations involving amiodarone as a prehospital agent to terminate refractory ventricular fibrillation have resulted in higher survival rates to hospital arrival; however, improvement in survival to discharge is still not significant.[56] Whether amiodarone should replace lidocaine for prehospital ventricular fibrillation requires further investigation, although many systems have already made this expensive change. The use of prehospital fibrinolytic agents for acute ST-elevation myocardial infarction has not gained wide acceptance and may be a useful intervention only for systems with prolonged transport times or when hospitals may not have catheterization or intervention facilities available. Future recommendations for prehospital use of these agents remains speculative.

Trauma Emergencies

Interventions

Interventions for specific medical emergencies, such as cardiac arrest (i.e. defibrillation, intubation, administration of intravenous medications), may be effectively performed while on the scene or before hospital transport. Alternatively, it is widely accepted that most interventions for traumatic injuries should be performed while en route to the hospital and that all effort should be expended to reduce on-scene time.

The issue of intravenous fluid administration has gained controversy over the past several years. High-volume intravenous fluid for hemodynamic instability resulting from traumatic injury has traditionally been the accepted standard in most prehospital care systems. Recent data, however, support a paradigm shift to restrictive or hypotensive resuscitation for penetrating truncal injuries. Restoration of hemodynamic stability with aggressive fluid resuscitation before definitive surgical hemostasis may lead to increased morbidity. Increasing mean arterial pressure to near-normal levels may result in hemodilution with an associated decrease in oxygen saturation and increased intravascular hydrostatic pressure resulting in disruption of an already fragile clot at the site of the insult and further hemorrhage.[57] Likewise, use of pneumatic antishock garments has been shown to increase mortality in penetrating torso injuries and is no longer recommended in urban EMS systems with short transport times. The benefit in rural systems with delayed prehospital times is ill defined, and the practice should probably be abandoned.

Similar to medical patients, definitive airway support by endotracheal intubation may be beneficial for severely injured patients, although the benefits of intubation in improving patient outcome have not been clearly delineated. To be successful, paramedics must exhibit the technical skills to rapidly place the endotracheal tube correctly, assess the placement, and move the intubated patient appropriately. In addition, providing the correct minute and tidal volumes is equally important. Overzealous personnel subconsciously delivering hyperventilatory rates may impair cardiac output and cause further tissue damage. Patients sustaining blunt head injury pose special problems that must be expeditiously addressed and resolved. Intubation provides a solid means of providing ventilatory assistance and airway protection, but the procedure and postintubation care may negate these potential benefits. Attempting to intubate head-injured patients may result in dental or soft tissue damage in patients with clenched teeth, and intracranial pressure may be exacerbated from an intact gag reflex or from subsequent regurgitation. Recent studies on the use of RSI in head-injured patients have revealed that patients experience significant hypoxia and bradycardia during the procedure and that outcome is actually worse.[48] Thus, the role of RSI in prehospital airway management in trauma patients is in question, just as it is for medical patients.

INTERFACILITY AND SPECIALIZED TRANSPORT

Transportation between health care facilities may take place for several reasons, including patient preference, unavailable diagnostic or therapeutic resources at the transferring facility, or a requirement of managed care organizations that patients be cared for in predesignated hospitals after stabilization. Hospital corporations engaged in networks or alliances that share resources and services will depend on interhospital transport systems to convey patients to allied institutions for specialized tests or procedures. Likewise, critical patients admitted to less specialized facilities may need to be transferred to tertiary care or designated trauma centers. Whereas long-distance transport may be best accomplished by air medical services, regional or local transport should use ground systems. These systems may be provided by either local EMS resources or those owned and operated by the hospital.

Interfacility transfer of patients for medically indicated reasons must fall under a set of requirements referred to as the Emergency Medical Treatment and Active Labor Act.[58] Although the EMS system providing the transport plays a key role, these guidelines primarily involve particular information and obligations that must be satisfied by the transferring and receiving facilities before transfer. An unstable patient should not be transferred to another facility at the request of a managed care organization unless the transferring hospital is incapable of providing standard care and the receiving hospital does have the capability of managing the condition and foreseeable complications. Box 191-1 lists various requirements that must be completed before transferring a patient to another facility.

BOX 191-1. EMTALA Requirements for Patient Transfers

Complete certification (risks and benefits) of transfer
Informed consent obtained from patient or family
Appropriate transportation (equipment and personnel) arranged
Treatment and stabilization performed
Acceptance from receiving facility ensured
Appropriate patient care data sent (fax or with patient)

EMTALA, Emergency Medical Treatment and Active Labor Act.

BOX 191-2. EMS Resource and Contact Information

American Ambulance Association	www.the-aaa.org
American College of Emergency Physicians	www.acep.org
Centers for Disease Control and Prevention	www.cdc.gov
Commission on Accreditation of Ambulance Services	www.caas.org
EMS Division, NHTSA	www.nhtsa.dot.gov/people/injury/ems
Maternal and Child Health Bureau, EMS-C	www.ems-c.org
National Association of EMS Educators	www.naemse.org
National Association of EMS Physicians	www.naemsp.org
National Association of EMTs	www.naemt.org
National Association of State EMS Directors	www.nasemsd.org
National Registry of EMTs	www.nremt.org

EMS, emergency medical service; EMT, emergency medical technician; NHTSA, National Highway Traffic Safety Administration.

Depending on patient condition, specialized transport services may function at the BLS or ALS level for providing emergency or nonemergency transportation. Patient transfers considered ALS may include interhospital (either emergency department or intensive care unit) neonatal or high-risk infant, critical cardiac, or trauma transport. The personnel configuration depends on the system design and level of care provided. Many programs use a nurse-paramedic combination. Patients requiring specialized care may need the services of specifically trained individuals, such as respiratory therapists, neonatal nurses, or other specialized critical care personnel. The presence of a physician is not mandatory but may be useful in select cases.

As with any EMS activity, all interfacility transport should be reviewed for appropriateness of transfer and medical care provided. In 1993, the Practice Management Committee of the ACEP updated the 1990 policy statement on interfacility transfer.[59]

THE FUTURE

The practice of prehospital medicine is expanding each and every day worldwide. The advancing scope of practice, alignment with public health initiatives, preparedness for domestic disasters, and specialty services are but a few of the ever-changing environments. Obstacles to expanding the domains of EMS will always include fiscal and organizational entities; however, providing quality, efficient, and responsible health care to the right patient, in the right setting, at the right time will always be laudable objectives for any system. As the world changes and call volumes increase, it is imperative that systems expand or reconfigure their performance to meet the increased societal demands for service. A variety of governmental and organizational institutions are available to the interested reader as a resource for understanding many of the issues facing EMS systems today and in the future. Box 191-2 lists contact information for many of these entities.

ACKNOWLEDGMENT

The author again wishes to thank Alex. Joey, and Marty for their understanding, tolerating, and accepting academia.

REFERENCES

1. Barkley KT: *The Ambulance.* Kiamesha Lake, NY, Load N Go Press, 1978.
2. Boyd DR: The conceptual development of EMS systems in the United States, part I. *Emerg Med Serv* Jan/Feb 1982.
3. Haller JS: The beginnings of urban ambulance service in the United States and England. *J Emerg Med* 8:743, 1990.
4. Hampton OP: Transportation of the injured: A report. *Bull Am Coll Surg* 45:55, 1960.
5. Committee on Trauma, American College of Surgeons: Minimal equipment for ambulances. *Bull Am Coll Surg* 46:136, 1961.
6. Hampton OP: Present status of ambulance services in the United States. *Bull Am Coll Surg* 50:177, 1965.
7. President's Commission on Highway Safety: *Health, Medical Care, and Transportation of the Injured.* Washington, DC, U.S. Government Printing Office, 1965.
8. Division of Medical Sciences, National Academy of Sciences–National Research Council: *Accidental Death and Disability: The Neglected Disease of Modern Society.* Washington, DC, National Academy of Sciences, 1966.
9. Pantridge JF, Geddes JS: A mobile intensive care unit in the management of myocardial infarction. *Lancet* 2:271, 1967.
10. Cobb LA, Alvarez H, Kopass MK: A rapid response system for out-of-hospital cardiac emergencies. *Med Clin North Am* 60:283, 1976.
11. U.S. Department of Transportation–National Highway Traffic Safety Administration: *Basic Training Program for Emergency Medical Technician—Ambulance.* Washington, DC, U.S. Department of Transportation, 1971.
12. Lewis RP, et al: Effectiveness of advanced paramedics in a mobile coronary care system. *JAMA* 241:1902, 1979.
13. Nagel EL, et al: Telemetry-medical command in coronary and other mobile emergency care systems. *JAMA* 214:332, 1970.
14. Law of the 98th Congress: *Health Services, Preventive Health Services, and Home Community Based Services Act of 1984, Public Law 98-555.* Washington, DC, 1984.
15. Institute of Medicine, National Academy of Sciences: *Emergency Medical Services for Children.* Washington, DC, National Academy of Sciences, 1993.
16. Monosky KA: 200-City survey. JEMS' annual report on EMS operational and clinical trends in the country's 200 most populous cities for 2002. *J Emerg Med Serv* 28:36, 2003.
17. Nichol G, et al: Effectiveness of emergency medical services for victims of out-of-hospital cardiac arrest: A metaanalysis. *Ann Emerg Med* 27:700, 1996.
18. Auble TE, Menegazzi JJ, Paris P: Effect of out-of-hospital defibrillation by basic life support providers on cardiac arrest mortality: A metaanalysis. *Ann Emerg Med* 25:642, 1995.
19. Pepe PE, et al: Cardiac arrest presenting with rhythms other than ventricular fibrillation. Contribution of resuscitative

effects toward total survivorship. *Crit Care Med* 21:1838, 1993.
20. Bickell WH, et al: Immediate versus delayed fluid resuscitation for hypotensive patients with penetrating torso injuries. *N Engl J Med* 331:1105, 1994.
21. McSwain NE: Controversies in prehospital care. *Emerg Med Clin North Am* 8:152, 1990.
22. Ornato JP, et al: The need for ALS in urban and suburban EMS systems [editorial]. *Ann Emerg Med* 19:1469, 1990.
23. Braun O, et al: Characteristics of midsized urban EMS systems. *Ann Emerg Med* 19:536, 1990.
24. Nichol G, et al: Cost-effectiveness analysis of potential improvements to emergency medical services for victims of out-of-hospital cardiac arrest. *Ann Emerg Med* 27:711, 1996.
25. Cummins RO, et al: Improving survival from sudden cardiac arrest: The "chain of survival." *Circulation* 83:1832, 1991.
26. American College of Emergency Physicians: Guidelines for implementation of early defibrillation/automated external defibrillator programs. *Ann Emerg Med* 22:740, 1993.
27. Haynes BE, et al: A statewide early defibrillation initiative including laypersons and outcome reporting. *JAMA* 266:545, 1991.
28. U.S. Department of Transportation–National Highway Traffic Safety Administration: *First Responder: National Standard Curriculum.* Washington, DC, U.S. Department of Transportation, 1996.
29. Weaver WD, et al: Use of automatic external defibrillator in the management of out-of-hospital cardiac arrest. *N Engl J Med* 319:661, 1988.
30. U.S. Department of Transportation–National Highway Traffic Safety Administration: *Emergency Medical Technician—Basic: National Standard Curriculum.* Washington, DC, U.S. Department of Transportation, 1994.
31. U.S. Department of Transportation—National Highway Traffic Safety Administration: *Emergency Medical Technician—Intermediate: National Standard Curriculum.* Washington, DC, U.S. Department of Transportation, 1999.
32. U.S. Department of Transportation–National Highway Traffic Safety Administration: *Emergency Medical Technician—Paramedic: National Standard Curriculum.* Washington, DC, U.S. Department of Transportation, 1998.
33. Committee on Trauma, American College of Surgeons: Essential equipment for ambulances—revised 1983. *Bull Am Coll Surg* 68:36, 1983.
34. American College of Emergency Physicians Position Paper: Optimal prehospital advanced life support skills, medications, and equipment. *Ann Emerg Med* 17:1109, 1988.
35. Smith JP, Bodai BI: The urban paramedic's scope of practice. *JAMA* 253:544, 1989.
36. Shuster M, Chong J: Pharmacologic intervention in prehospital care: A critical appraisal. *Ann Emerg Med* 18:192, 1989.
37. Callaham M: Quantifying the scanty science of prehospital emergency care. *Ann Emerg Med* 30:785, 1997.
38. American Heart Association: Guidelines for cardiopulmonary resuscitation and emergency cardiac care: Recommendations of the 1992 conference. *JAMA* 268:2171, 1992.
39. Department of Transportation–National Highway Traffic Safety Administration: *"Star of Life" Emergency Medical Care Symbol* (Publication No. HS-803-721). Washington, DC, U.S. Department of Transportation, 1979.
40. National Association of Emergency Medical Services Physicians Position Paper: Emergency medical dispatching. *Prehospital Disaster Med* 4:163, 1989.
41. Curka PA, et al: Emergency medical services priority dispatch. *Ann Emerg Med* 22:1688, 1993.
42. Alonso-Serra H, Blanton D, O'Connor RE: Position Paper, National Association of EMS Physicians: Physician medical direction in EMS. *Prehosp Med Care* 2:153, 1998.
43. American College of Emergency Physicians: Guidelines for medical direction of prehospital EMS. *Ann Emerg Med* 22:742, 1993.
44. U.S. Department of Transportation–National Highway Traffic Safety Administration, National Association of EMS Physicians, American College of Emergency Physicians, Health Resources and Services Administration–Maternal and Child Health Bureau: *Guide for Preparing Medical Directors.* 2001.
45. O'Connor RE, Megargel RE: The effect of a quality improvement feedback loop on paramedic skills, charting, and behavior. *Prehospital Disaster Med* 9:35, discussion 38, 1994.
46. Eckstein M, Alo K: The effect of a quality improvement program on paramedic on-scene times for patients with penetrating trauma. *Acad Emerg Med* 6:191, 1999.
47. Katz SH, Falk JL: Misplaced endotracheal tubes by paramedics in an urban emergency medical services system. *Ann Emerg Med* 37:62, 2001.
48. Davis DP, et al: The effect of paramedic rapid sequence intubation on outcome in patients with severe traumatic brain injury. *J Trauma* 54:444, 2003.
49. Gausche M, et al: Effect of out-of-hospital pediatric endotracheal intubation on survival and neurological outcome: A controlled clinical trial. *JAMA* 283:783, 2000.
50. Craven RA, et al: Use of bilevel positive airway pressure (BiPAP) in prehospital patients [abstract]. *Acad Emerg Med* 7:511, 2000.
51. Eisenberg MS, et al: Cardiac arrest and resuscitation: A tale of 29 cities. *Ann Emerg Med* 19:179, 1990.
52. Gratton M, Lindholm DJ, Campbell JP: Public-access defibrillation: Where do we place the AEDs? *Prehosp Emerg Care* 3:303, 1999.
53. Culley LL, et al: Public access defibrillation in out-of-hospital cardiac arrest: A community-based study. *Circulation* 109:1859, 2004.
54. Patel RJ, Vilke GM, Chan TC: The prehospital electrocardiogram. *J Emerg Med* 21:35, 2001.
55. Ferguson JD, et al: The prehospital 12-lead electrocardiogram: Impact on management of the out-of-hospital acute coronary syndrome patient. *Am J Emerg Med* 21:136, 2003.
56. Kudenchuk PJ, et al: Amiodarone for resuscitation after out-of-hospital cardiac arrest due to ventricular fibrillation. *N Engl J Med* 341:871, 1999.
57. Kowalenko T, et al: Improved outcome with hypotensive resuscitation of uncontrolled hemorrhagic shock in a swine model. *J Trauma* 33:349, 1992.
58. Bitterman RA: EMTALA. In Henry GL, Sullivan DJ (eds): *Emergency Medicine Risk Management: A Comprehensive Review,* 2nd ed. Dallas, American College of Emergency Physicians, 1997.
59. American College of Emergency Physicians: Appropriate interhospital patient transfer. *Ann Emerg Med* 22:766, 1993.

CHAPTER 191 Emergency Medical Service: Overview and Ground Transport

CHAPTER
192 Air Medical Transport

Howard Rodenberg and Ira J. Blumen

PERSPECTIVE

The history of air medical transport (AMT) began with the evacuation of wounded soldiers by balloon from Paris during the Franco-Prussian War. The French first used a fixed-wing aircraft (airplane) as an ambulance during World War I. In World War II, more than 1.1 million sick and wounded soldiers were airlifted to the United States during the last 3 years of the war. The Korean War introduced the rotor-wing aircraft (helicopter) to AMT. More than 20,000 wounded servicemen were strapped to litters outside the aircraft and transported from battalion aid stations to waiting hospital units. During the Vietnam War, Operation Dustoff transported more than 800,000 patients to hospitals.

The impact of AMT of the wounded soldier can be shown by comparing time to definitive care and mortality. During World War II, the average time from injury to definitive care was 6 to 12 hours, with a mortality rate of 6%. In Korea, the time was 2 to 4 hours, with 2% mortality. In Vietnam, the time was 65 minutes, and mortality was less than 1%.[1] Encouraged by the military experience, civilian AMT in the United States was propelled by the 1969 start of the first hospital-sponsored, fixed-wing air medical program. The first civilian helicopter emergency medical services (EMS) program in the United States was established in 1972.

AVIATION PHYSIOLOGY

A working knowledge of aviation physiology is vital to understanding the effects of AMT on pilots, flight crew, and patients.

Boyle's Law

The cornerstone of aviation physiology is *Boyle's law,* which states that the volume of a unit of gas (a specified number of molecules) is inversely proportional to the pressure on it. In concrete terms, Boyle's law means that as altitude increases (and atmospheric pressure decreases), the molecules of gas grow apart, and the volume of the gas expands. With descent (increasing atmospheric pressure), the molecules are condensed, and gas volume contracts.

Physiologic difficulties from expansion and contraction of gases within the closed spaces of the body may occur with any change in altitude. Squeeze injuries occur on descent and are common causes of barotitis and barosinusitis. Air trapped within the sinus or middle ear cavities cannot be equalized with ambient pressure, and the air within the space contracts, pulling mucosal and neurovascular elements with it. Reverse squeeze injuries occur on ascent. The decrease in barometric pressure leads to an increased volume of the air trapped within the space, exerting pressure on adjacent bony, neurovascular, or parenchymal structures. Ascent injuries also can include barotitis media, barosinusitis, conversion of a simple pneumothorax into a tension pneumothorax, and rupture of a hollow viscus by expansion of intestinal gas. The operation of medical equipment containing closed air space also can be affected. Intravenous flow rates, the pressure in air splints and in pneumatic antishock garment suits, and endotracheal tube cuff volumes may be altered with altitude.

Charles' Law

Charles' law follows from the volume effects of Boyle's law. *Charles' law* notes that as the temperature on a volume of gas rises, the volume of the gas also increases. The molecular dispersion seen with increases in gas volume at altitude (Boyle's law) means that at altitude, there is less chance of molecular collision with resulting generation of heat. Charles' law explains why the ambient temperature decreases with increased altitude.

Dalton's Law

Dalton's law states that the total barometric pressure at any given altitude equals the sum of the partial pressures of gases in the mixture ($P_t = P_1 + P_2 + P_3 \ldots P_n$). As pressure is reduced, expansion of gases creates increasing distances between molecules, and the quantity of oxygen available for respiration decreases. Although oxygen still constitutes 21% of the atmospheric pressure, each breath brings fewer oxygen molecules to the lungs, and hypoxia results (Table 192-1). The clinical effect of Dalton's law is manifested as a decrease in partial arterial oxygen tension with increasing altitude.

The most threatening feature of hypoxia is its insidious onset. Physiologic responses include an increased rate and depth of respirations and an increase in heart rate. With prolonged exposure, oxygen supply to the brain is insufficient to support cerebral metabolism. Signs and symptoms of cerebral hypoxia include headache, nausea, drowsiness, fatigue, and finally unconsciousness and death. Although the onset and severity of symptoms may vary with individuals, no

Table 192-1. Effects of Altitude on Oxygenation

Altitude (ft)	Barometric Pressure (mm Hg)	PAO_2 (mm Hg)	PaO_2 (mm Hg)	$PaCO_2$ (mm Hg)	Oxygen Saturation (%)
Sea level	760	159.2	103.0	40	98
8,000	565	118.4	68.9	36	93
10,000	523	109.6	61.2	35	87
15,000	429	89.9	45.0	32	84
18,000	380	79.6	37.8	30.4	72
20,000	349	73.1	34.3	29.4	66
22,000	321	67.2	32.8	28.4	60

PAO_2, partial pressure of alveolar oxygen; PaO_2, partial pressure of arterial oxygen; $PaCO_2$, partial pressure of arterial carbon dioxide.

one is exempt from the effects of hypoxia, including patients and air medical flight crew.

Henry's Law

Henry's law states that the mass of gas absorbed by a liquid is directly proportional to the partial pressure of the gas above the liquid. Henry's law has its most familiar applications in diving medicine, in which the increased pressure exerted on gases in the body at depth forces the gases into solution in the bloodstream. Rapid ascent from depth causes the gas to come out of solution within the bloodstream, resulting in decompression sickness or dysbarism. Henry's law does not carry the same weight in aviation medicine because the degree of change in atmospheric pressure per unit of distance is considerably less than the degree of change in water. Sudden decompression at high altitude similarly may result in dysbarism, however.

Additional Stresses of Flight

Other stresses of flight that can affect the patient or crew include temperature fluctuations, dehydration, noise, and vibration. Temperature changes may produce increases in metabolic rate and oxygen consumption. Prolonged exposure can result in motion sickness, disorientation, fatigue, and impaired performance.

As altitude increases and the air cools, the amount of moisture in the air decreases significantly. To prevent dehydration during AMT, fluid intake (oral or intravenous) must be monitored carefully, and all patients should receive humidified medical oxygen. Noise and vibration may represent the most ubiquitous stresses encountered in AMT; both may interfere with patient assessment or the function of medical equipment. Long-term exposure may result in fatigue, nausea, visual or vestibular disturbances, ear damage, and deterioration in task performance. Hearing protection should be worn during aircraft operations by the patient and crew.

PRINCIPLES OF AIR MEDICAL TRANSPORT SYSTEMS

Administrative Structure

Air medical services may take several forms. The most common type is hospital based, transporting from outlying referral centers or accident scenes to tertiary care centers. A single hospital or a consortium of institutions may sponsor flight programs. Private services usually involve fixed-wing aircraft (less often helicopters) and are based most often at an airport or other regional hub. These services often are funded on a fee-for-service or subscription basis. Additional subsidies from public and private organizations and from the sponsoring institutions are common. Public service agencies also may sponsor air medical services. Vehicles used by these programs are often multifunctional aircraft that serve in medical, search and rescue, fire suppression, and law enforcement roles. The Military Assistance to Safety and Traffic (MAST) program operated by the U.S. Armed Forces may transport ill or injured patients when no civilian service is available, and when MAST aircraft, equipment, and personnel are not being used for the unit's primary military mission. Funded by tax dollars, these programs often are operated at no cost to the patient.

Types of Missions

Air medical missions may involve primary or secondary response. Primary responses ("scene flights") are responses in which the aircraft serves as the sole means of patient transport to a receiving facility. Aircraft involved in secondary responses transport patients from outlying hospitals to facilities offering higher levels of care.

Air Medical Aircraft

Although the ground ambulance remains the primary means of prehospital and interfacility patient transport, the use of the air ambulance has grown significantly since the 1970s. No one aircraft is ideal for the needs of all air medical programs or for all patients. The vehicle selected should meet the mission requirements of the program for the types of patients to be transported and the anticipated service area.

Helicopters (Rotor-Wing Aircraft)

The helicopter offers several advantages over other transport vehicles. Traveling "as the crow flies" at speeds of 120 to 180 mph, helicopter transport time often cuts travel times by 75% compared with an equivalent distance by ground transport. The service area of helicopter programs is generally 150 to 200 miles from its base of operations. The rotor-wing aircraft has the ability to avoid common traffic delays and ground obstacles and can fly into locations that may be inaccessible to other modes of travel. Helicopter landing zone requirements are a disadvantage compared with ground ambulances but offer an advantage over the airport requirements of airplanes.

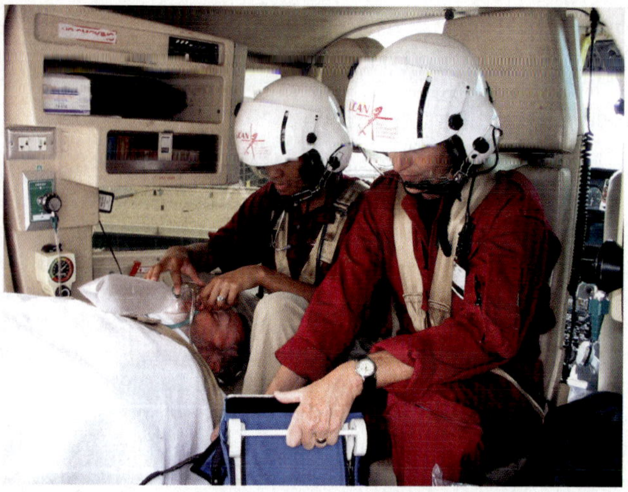

Figure 192-1. Confined spaces within helicopters may make performing procedures more challenging. (Photo courtesy of Ira Blumen, MD.)

Disadvantages to rotor-wing flight include the presence of noise and turbulence, which may interfere with patient evaluation, monitoring, and management. Weather considerations may limit significantly the availability of helicopter transport. In small and medium-sized helicopters, cramped patient compartments and weight limitations may compromise optimal patient care (Figure 192-1).

Many helicopter programs permit flight only under visual flight rules. When the weather conditions (ceiling and visibility) fall below established program minimums, a program may decline to undertake a transport for safety reasons. An increasing number of programs are equipping their helicopters and training their pilots for instrument flight rules, however, to allow safe travel in less favorable weather conditions. Instrument flight rule flight does not facilitate travel to the scene of an accident.

Airplanes (Fixed-Wing Aircraft)

Although rotor-wing missions attract more media attention, fixed-wing flights constitute a significant portion of AMT operations. Fixed-wing aircraft provide increased range; greater speed; and more patient, crew, and equipment capacity than rotor-wing vehicles. Decreased cabin noise and turbulence create fewer patient management problems, and pressurization can combat the impact of physiologic gas laws. Fixed-wing operations are limited, however, to areas that have airports, runways of appropriate length or condition, and refueling facilities. During fixed-wing transports, patient transfers require multiple vehicles (i.e., hospital to ambulance to airplane).

Various fixed-wing aircraft are available for medical transport. These range from unpressurized light planes with single- or twin-piston engines to pressurized turboprops and jets. The selection of the ideal aircraft depends on the nature of the air medical mission.

Air Medical Flight Crew

Air medical crew members represent the broad spectrum of health care providers. Most AMT programs in the United States provide critical care transport teams composed of one registered nurse (RN) and an additional crew member. Annual surveys show that the RN/paramedic team is most often used (>60%) in helicopter and airplane transports. Other combinations—RN/RN, RN/emergency medical technician (EMT), RN/physician, RN/respiratory therapist, and EMT-paramedic/EMT-paramedic—account for less than 10% each.[2]

Flight nurses generally have extensive experience in intensive care units or emergency departments. They may be specialized within the transport team to care for adult, pediatric, or neonatal patients. Paramedics often make their greatest contribution in the transport of critical patients from the scene of illness or injury. Respiratory therapists bring expertise in airway and ventilator management and oxygen delivery systems. Flight physicians may be residents, attending physicians, or medical directors of flight programs. Much research has focused on the specific benefit of the onboard physician.[3-6] Although the answer to this question remains controversial, what is clear is that the crew used by an AMT program must be explicitly tailored to the needs of the community and the patients it serves.

A poorly considered aspect of air medical staffing is the effect of the AMT environment on the ability of crew members to provide patient care. Human factors work has shown that most medical care procedures are rated more difficult to perform in an AMT vehicle than in other ground-based settings.[7] Auscultation of the lungs, palpation of pulses, performance of cardiopulmonary resuscitation, endotracheal intubation, and recognition of visual alarms all are impaired while aloft.[8-11] In addition, fatigue, motion sickness, an erratic pattern of work activity, and the high risk involved in AMT operations may affect task performance significantly.[12]

Medical Direction

All air medical services require the active involvement of a physician as air medical director, who is responsible for supervising, evaluating, and ensuring the quality of medical care provided by the AMT team. The air medical director must have the final authority over all clinical aspects of the air medical service. The medical director should ensure that the medical personnel have adequate training and qualifications to deliver appropriate medical care, that appropriate medical equipment and supplies are available, and that the correct vehicle is selected for transport. Medical care policies and procedures should be established, including specific provisions for on-line and off-line medical control. The Air Medical Physician Association and the National Association of EMS Physicians have established guidelines for the medical direction of an air medical service.[13]

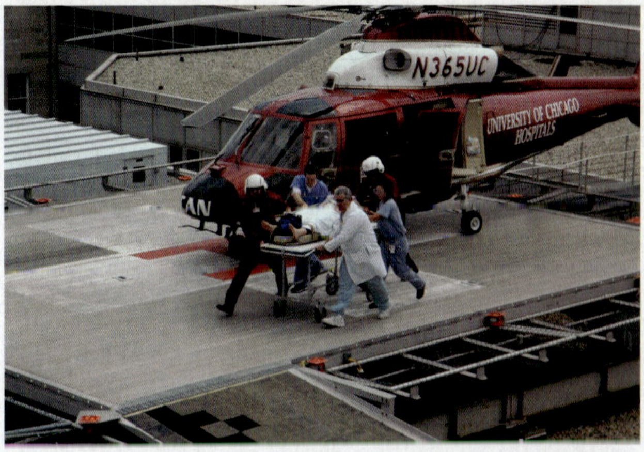

Figure 192-2. Landing zone safety is paramount to delivery of patients to hospitals. (Photo courtesy of Dan Lemkin, MD.)

Safety

Safety is the predominant concern of air medical operations, and ensuring safe conduct is a fundamental part of every flight program. Continual training of aircraft pilots and mechanics is essential, and both participate in ensuring the airworthiness of the vehicle. Medical personnel must be proficient in the emergency operations of the aircraft and the routine procedures in and around their helicopter or airplane. Crew fatigue and other self-imposed stresses that could affect safety, such as the use of prescription or over-the-counter medications, tobacco, and alcohol, must be scrupulously avoided.

Weather requirements or "minimums" must be strictly enforced. On receipt of a flight request, the pilot must verify the weather conditions and the condition of the aircraft. To ensure impartiality, the pilot should not be told of the patient's condition or acuity. The pilot always has the right to decline a mission because of aircraft or weather considerations. These decisions must not be influenced or reversed by administrators, flight crew, or other parties.

Landing Zones

Helicopter landing zones are inherently dangerous places. The most obvious risk of injury is from impact with rotor blades. This danger is heightened during ground operations, as the blades dip lowest to the ground at the slower rotor speeds associated with engine startup and shutdown. Injuries also may occur as a result of debris being propelled through the air by "rotor wash," increased noise levels and an inability to hear warnings, and slippery surfaces found on exposed landing sites.

Many hospitals have designated landing areas that are appropriately lit and secured (Figure 192-2), with fixed coordinates and predesignated liftoff and approach patterns. Most primary responses occur at unmarked sites, however. Ground personnel must be trained to designate and secure a safe landing zone for helicopter operations (Box 192-1). AMT programs have an obligation to help train ground staff on proper landing zone setup and conduct (Box 192-2).

BOX 192-1. Helicopter Safety and Air Medical Transport

- Vehicles and personnel should be kept at least 100 ft from the landing zone.
- Spectators should be kept at least 200 ft from the landing zone.
- No smoking or running is permitted within 50 ft of the helicopter.
- All items (e.g., IV lines, poles) should be kept below shoulder height.
- The flight crew opens and closes aircraft doors.
- The flight crew directs and supervises the loading and unloading of the patient and equipment.
- Ground personnel should use eye and ear protection.
- Approach the helicopter *only* when signaled to do so by the pilot or an on-board crew member.
- Approach and depart the helicopter *only* forward of the rear cabin door and in a crouched position with your head down.
- *Never approach or depart from the rear of the helicopter.*
- Stay clear of the tail rotor; it is virtually invisible and extremely dangerous.
- If the aircraft is parked on a slope, approach and depart on the downhill side (greatest clearance under the blades).
- Keep the landing zone clear of (or hold on to) all loose articles (e.g., hats, scarves, sheets, pillows).
- Protect patient from the dust and debris.
- Follow the flight crew's instructions at all times.
- In *disaster situations* and *mass casualty incidents,* victims, witnesses, and spectators may become hysterical or exhibit signs of an acute situational reaction. These individuals must be kept clear of the landing zone and helicopter *at all times.* Injured victims who exhibit this behavior should *not* be triaged for helicopter transport, or they should be transported *only* with adequate physical or chemical restraints in use.
- *If you do not know, ask.*

Courtesy of University of Chicago Hospitals Aeromedical Network (UCAN) and Illinois Association of Air and Critical Care Transport (IAACCT), 2005.

Emergency Medical Service

AMT should be an integral resource within a comprehensive Emergency Medical Service (EMS) system. Integration begins with the establishment of geographic service areas. Service areas may be determined based on program mission description, aircraft range and speed, the placement of specialty centers and receiving facilities, and the location and mission of air medical programs in adjacent regions. Population densities also are key factors. Helicopters are generally less useful in urban settings because of the proximity of health care facilities and a lack of open and safe landing zones. Paramedics, EMTs, and other public safety personnel should be provided with guidelines specifying when AMT should be considered. These protocols are best developed by EMS Medical Directors in close collaboration with their air medical colleagues.

BOX 192-2. Landing Zone (LZ) Requirements for Air Medical Transport

Landing Area

- LZ should be as close as possible to the scene or hospital entrance, but not so close that it may interfere with ground operations or patient care.
- LZ should be at least 100 × 100 ft.
- LZ should be as flat and level as possible.
- LZ *must* be clear of debris.

Hazards and Obstructions

- Identify all potential hazards that may be on the ground or near the approach/departure path of LZ.
- LZ should be clear of wires, poles, trees, buildings, vehicles, and spectators.
- Road cones, ropes, tape, and barricades are *not* recommended for use near LZ.
- Perimeter of LZ should be at least 50 ft away from potential obstructions and hazards.
- LZ should be located *upwind* from any hazardous material incident.

Approach and Departure Path

- Path should point into the wind and be free of obstruction to an altitude of 500 ft above the surface.
- Path should *not* pass over command posts, treatment areas, or operationally congested areas on the ground.

Day Operations

- Use radio communications and hand signals.
- Stand with your back to the wind.

Night Operations

- Use radio communications and lighting to designate LZ.
- Spotlights should be directed at the top of possible hazards, *not* toward the approaching or departing aircraft.
- Position a portable light, vehicle headlights, emergency vehicle flashing lights, flare, or chemical stick at each corner, with a fifth light upwind.
- Nonessential lights should be turned off.

Light Sources

- Lights *must* be clear of LZ.
- If portable, lights *must* be well secured.
- *Never* point lights toward an approaching or departing helicopter.

Wind Indicator

- Indicator may be a wind sock, flag, flare, or smoke.
- Indicator *must* be clear of LZ.
- If portable, indicator *must* be well secured.

Courtesy of University of Chicago Hospitals Aeromedical Network (UCAN) and Illinois Association of Air and Critical Care Transport (IAACCT), 2005.

CLINICAL CONCEPTS AND PATIENT CARE

Although virtually all types of patients have been transported by air medical services, definitive data indicating which patients benefit from flight are lacking. Many questions regarding the triage of patients to air or ground transport, the efficacy of air medical care, and the effects of AMT on morbidity and mortality in medical and surgical conditions remain unanswered.

BOX 192-3. Criteria for Air Medical Transport

1. Distance to the closest appropriate facility is too great for safe and timely transport by ground ambulance.
2. Patient's clinical condition requires that the time spent in transport be as short as possible.
3. Patient's condition is time critical, requiring specific or timely treatment not available at the referring hospital.
4. Potential for transport delay associated with ground transport is likely to worsen the patient's clinical condition.
5. Patient requires critical care life support during transport that was not available from the local ground ambulance service.
6. Patient is located in an area inaccessible to regular ground traffic, impeding ambulance egress or access.
7. Local ground units are not available for long-distance transport.
8. Use of local ground transport services would leave the local area without adequate EMS coverage.

Courtesy of University of Chicago Hospitals Aeromedical Network (UCAN), 2001.

In an effort to ensure that AMT resources are used wisely, the Air Medical Physician Association has established a detailed medical condition list for the appropriate use of AMT.[14] A more general approach to the need for AMT is illustrated in Box 192-3.

Trauma

The effect of helicopter EMS on trauma patient outcomes has been a topic of much study. Many studies show that overall mortality in patients transported by air medical services is significantly reduced, but others show no mortality reduction. More refined efforts note that the major advantage in mortality lies in transport of moderately to severely injured patients. Mortality can be reduced 35% if air transport is used in the appropriate subset of patients. Patients with minor injuries or very severe injuries do not gain additional survival benefit by use of air transport. Generally, patients with prolonged ground transport time from the trauma center obtain the most benefit from air medical services.[15-22]

Cardiac Disorders

Hypoxia at altitude causes a compensatory increase in pulse and respiratory rate, and the increased myocardial oxygen demand may result in cardiac decompensation. Studies of patients with acute myocardial infarction and unstable angina revealed that complications (e.g., hypotension, dysrhythmias, exacerbation of chest pain) could be managed effectively aloft. No problems have been seen during transport in series of patients with pacemakers or immediately after thrombolysis for myocardial infarction or stroke.[23-27] Major in-flight events among cardiac patients occur 12% to 41% of the time and physicans play an important role in safe transport.[3,25] It also has been documented that patients transported by air after resuscitation from cardiac arrest have improved outcomes over patients transported by ground crews.[28,29]

Pregnancy

AMT of a gravid woman is generally safe for the mother and fetus. Maternal inspired oxygen concentration is usually adequate to meet the metabolic demands of the fetus, but it may be prudent to provide maternal supplemental oxygen during flight. Transporting a woman in active labor is another major concern because delivery of the infant within the confines of the aircraft cabin may prove difficult.[30]

Neonates and Children

Pediatric and neonatal specialty centers often depend on air medical services for prompt transport of critically ill or injured patients to tertiary care centers with specialized pediatric services. These flight crews must have the experience, training, and competency to care for critical pediatric or neonatal patients and the appropriate equipment and medications. The Task Force on Interhospital Transport of the American Academy of Pediatrics has established guidelines for air and ground transport of pediatric and neonatal patients.[31]

EFFICACY AND COST-EFFICIENCY

Traditional research in air medical care has identified what can be done in the AMT setting. Work has shifted the focus from simple observational studies to measurement of the value of the interventions. The most basic consideration is if AMT makes a difference to patient care. Older, subjective studies show a benefit to AMT in only 10% to 20% of patients flown. Where AMT appears beneficial, the advantage seems related to the provision of on-site advanced life support care rather than to a unique advantage of the helicopter.[32] AMT has long been assumed to save additional lives in trauma; however, it is now recognized that improvements in outcomes are more likely related to the provision of on-site ALS care within a comprehensive trauma system rather than to the aircraft itself. Studies have challenged the benefit of AMT in interfacility transports in urban areas.[33,34] Although the speed of the aircraft is undoubtedly greater than that of any ground vehicles, small gains in transport time may be offset by higher costs without significant changes in patient outcome.[35-37]

Finally, there is increasing recognition that studies "proving" the efficacy of an AMT system must be taken within their own local contexts and that extrapolations and comparisons are often invalid. AMT systems must satisfactorily address operational needs for effective lines of referral and communication, smooth transfer processes, active clinical coordination, the availability of dedicated vehicles and equipment, and the integration of AMT services into a regional network of prehospital care.

FUTURE OF AIR MEDICAL TRANSPORT

AMT services work best when they are integral to and enhance an overall system of prehospital care. In most cases, the efficacy of AMT remains to be proven. Research into these issues is a key facet of the future of AMT. Efforts must be made to standardize research definitions and terms; explore novel uses of objective measures to evaluate components of AMT systems; and determine appropriate short-term, long-term, and comparative outcome measures for AMT.[38-40]

It also seems that advances in ground-based EMS are offsetting many of the assumed benefits of AMT, and, increasingly, the value of many prehospital interventions is being reassessed. Geographic issues, the regionalization of specialty services, the development of new highly time-sensitive therapies, and the need to transport patients quickly over long distances require systems to continue to assess the potential value of initiating or continuing AMT.

REFERENCES

1. Jacobs LM, Jacobs BB, Schwartz R: A medical helicopter transportation system for Connecticut. *Conn Med* 49:489, 1985.
2. Rau W: Medical crew survey. *AirMed* 5, 1999.
3. Kaplan L, Walsh D, Burney RM: Emergency aeromedical transport of patients with acute myocardial infarction. *Ann Emerg Med* 16:55, 1987.
4. Schwartz RJ, Jacobs LM, Lee M: The role of the physician in a helicopter emergency medical service. *Ann Emerg Med* 17:426, 1988.
5. McCloskey KA, King WD: Pediatric critical care transports: Is a physician always needed on the team? *Ann Emerg Med* 17:427, 1988.
6. Baxt WG, Moody P: The impact of a physician as part of the aeromedical prehospital team in patients with blunt trauma. *JAMA* 257:3246, 1987.
7. Myers KJ, Rodenberg H, Woodard D: Influence of the helicopter environment on patient care capabilities: Flight crew perceptions. *Air Med J* 14:21, 1995.
8. Hunt RC, et al: Adverse effects of helicopter flight on the ability to palpate carotid pulses. *Ann Emerg Med* 24:190, 1994.
9. Hunt RC, et al: Inability to assess breath sounds during air medical transport by helicopter. *JAMA* 265:1982, 1991.
10. Thomas SH, Stone CK, Bryan-Berge D: The ability to perform closed chest compressions in helicopters. *Am J Emerg Med* 12:296, 1994.
11. Fromm RE, Campbell E, Schlieter P: Inadequacy of visual alarms in helicopter air medical transport. *Aviat Space Environ Med* 66:784, 1995.
12. Wright MS, Bose CL, Stiles AD: The incidence and effects of motion sickness among medical attendants during transport. *J Emerg Med* 13:15, 1995.
13. Thomas SH, Williams KA, Claypool D: Medical director for air medical transport programs. Position paper of the National Association of EMS Physicians. *Prehosp Emerg Care* 6:155, 2002.
14. Air Medical Physician Association: Medical condition list and appropriate use of air medical transport: Position statement of the Air Medical Physician Association. *Prehosp Emerg Care* 6:464, 2002.

15. Baxt WG, et al: Hospital-based rotorcraft aeromedical emergency care services and trauma mortality: A multicenter study. *Ann Emerg Med* 14:859, 1985.
16. Eckstein M, et al: Helicopter transport of pediatric trauma patients in an urban emergency medical services system: A critical analysis. *J Trauma* 53:340, 2002.
17. Chappell VL, et al: Impact of discontinuing a hospital-based air ambulance service on trauma patient outcomes. *J Trauma* 52:486, 2002.
18. Cocanour CS, Fischer RP, Ursic CM: Are scene flights for penetrating trauma justified? *J Trauma* 43:83, 1997.
19. Cunningham P, et al: A comparison of the association of helicopter and ground ambulance transport with the outcome of injury in trauma patients transported from the scene. *J Trauma* 43:940, 1997.
20. Thomas SH, et al: Trauma helicopter emergency medical services transport: Annotated review of selected outcomes-related literature. *Prehosp Emerg Care* 6:359, 2002.
21. Jacobs LM, et al: Helicopter air medical transport: Ten-year outcomes for trauma patients in a New England program. *Conn Med* 63:677, 1999.
22. Phillips RT, Conaway C, Mullarkey D, Owen JL: One year's trauma mortality experience at Brooke Army Medical Center: Is aeromedical transportation of trauma patients necessary? *Milit Med* 164:361, 1999.
23. Bellinger RL, et al: Helicopter transport of patients during acute myocardial infarction. *Am J Cardiol* 61:719, 1988.
24. Fromm RE, et al: Bleeding complications following initiation of thrombolytic therapy for acute myocardial infarction: A comparison of helicopter-transported and non-transported patients. *Ann Emerg Med* 20:892, 1991.
25. Schneider S, et al: Critical cardiac transports: Air versus ground? *Am J Emerg Med* 6:449, 1988.
26. Fromm RE, et al: The incidence of pacemaker dysfunction during helicopter air medical transport. *Am J Emerg Med* 10:333, 1992.
27. Chalela JA, et al: Safety of air medical transportation after tissue plasminogen activator administration in acute ischemic stroke. *Stroke* 30:2366, 1999.
28. Werman HA, et al: Helicopter transport of patients to tertiary care centers after cardiac arrest. *Am J Emerg Med* 17:130, 1999.
29. Stone CK, et al: Interhospital transfer of cardiac patients: Does air transport make a difference? *Air Med J* 13:159, 1994.
30. Van Hook JW, et al: Aeromedical transfer of preterm labor patients. *Tex Med* 94:88, 1998.
31. American Academy of Pediatrics Task Force on Interhospital Transport: *Guidelines for Air and Ground Transportation of Neonatal and Pediatric Patients,* 2nd ed. Elk Grove Village, Ill, American Academy of Pediatrics, 1999.
32. Kurola J, et al: Paramedic helicopter emergency service in rural Finland—do benefits justify the cost? *Acta Anaesthesiol Scand* 46:779, 2002.
33. Arfken CL, et al: Effectiveness of helicopter versus ground ambulance services for interfacility transport. *J Trauma* 45:785, 1998.
34. Brampton WJ: Using helicopters for secondary transfer—does the patient benefit? *Anaesthesiol Reanimat* 26:102, 2001.
35. Nicholl JP, Beeby NR, Brazier JE: A comparison of the costs and performance of an emergency helicopter and land ambulances in a rural area. *Injury* 25:145, 1994.
36. Fetter WPF, et al: Neonatal transport by helicopter in the Netherlands: A 7-year overview. *Eur J Emerg Med* 2:88, 1995.
37. Safford SD, et al: A cost and outcomes comparison of a novel integrated pediatric air and ground transportation system. *J Am Coll Surg* 195:790, 2002.
38. Thompson CB, Schaffer J: Minimum data set development: Air transport time-related terms. *Int J Med Informatics* 65:121, 2002.
39. Rodenberg H: Effect of aeromedical aircraft on care of trauma patients: Evaluation using the revised trauma score. *South Med J* 85:1065, 1992.
40. Rodenberg H: The Revised Trauma Score: A means to evaluate aeromedical staffing patterns. *Aviat Space Environ Med* 63:308, 1992.

CHAPTER 193 Tactical Emergency Medical Support and Urban Search and Rescue

Richard Schwartz, John G. McManus, and Jeffrey Orledge

TACTICAL EMERGENCY MEDICAL SUPPORT

Perspective

Law enforcement agencies in the 21st century face an increase in terroristic threats and new challenges, including organized opposing forces, military-type weapons, direct fire, hostage and barricade situations, and potential toxic hazards. As these threats have increased, so has the recognition of the need for integrated medical support of tactical operations.[1-3] Tactical emergency medical support (TEMS) is the specialty of emergency medical services established to maintain safety, health, and welfare of Special Operations law enforcement units, such as special weapons and tactics (SWAT) teams, hostage rescue teams, and special emergency rescue teams.[4-6] These specially trained teams consist of highly trained and specially equipped law enforcement personnel who are tasked with mitigating and responding to many different high-risk criminal situations. Several emergency medical societies and programs have endorsed the practice of TEMS and have created training and education programs for emergency physicians, residents, and prehospital providers, enhancing their ability to provide preventive, urgent, and emergency care of patients in a functionally austere environment.[7-10]

Tactical Medical History

The principles of TEMS have largely been developed through lessons learned from military conflicts. Civilian TEMS structure most closely emulates the medical support structure of military special operations units such as Army Special Forces, Navy Seals, Army Rangers, and Air Force Pararescuemen.[7] These small, unique tactical units operate frequently outside the normal realm of military operations, remote from dedicated medical resources, often for long periods of time. Although modern TEMS units generally operate in the urban environment, where prompt evacuation to highly capable medical facilities is the rule, training must account for circumstances in which prolonged care must be provided on-site, when conflict circumstances preclude evacuation.

In the civilian setting, snipers, mass demonstrations, riots, and fire bombings gained notoriety as new forms of urban conflict in America during the late 1960s and early 1970s. Many of these incidents occurred in Los Angeles during and after the Watts Riot, leading to the formation of the first SWAT unit. As of 1996, there are more than 5000 SWAT teams in the United States supporting local, state, and federal agencies.[11] With the evolution of these specialized law enforcement tactical teams, the need for military-style emergency medical services (EMS) support began to emerge.[1] Although the Los Angeles Sheriff's Department had utilized SWAT-trained medics since 1971, it was not recognized as a standard practice until the early 1980s.[4]

Because of the dangerous environment, SWAT team members are at high risk for injury, with a casualty rate of 33 injuries per 1000 officer missions.[1] Suspects are injured at the rate of 18.9 injuries per 1000 officer missions, and bystanders are injured at the rate of 3.2 per 1000 officer missions. It was recognized that traditional EMS providers were not properly trained or equipped to enter these unique and sometimes remote austere environments to care for casualties.[1,3,4,12,13] In fact, basic EMS training still emphasizes that personnel should wait until the "scene is safe" before rendering medical care to patients. Past incidents such as those occurring at the Columbine High School in Littleton, Colorado, Ruby Ridge in Idaho, University of Texas in Austin, and the Mormon Library in Salt Lake City proved that sequestering medical personnel far from the area of operations leads to delays in definitive trauma care, with potentially higher rates of morbidity and mortality.[4,6,12,14,15] The tactical environment necessitates that the medical provider possess a unique training and skill subset to utilize a different set of field assessment and treatment priorities and strategies for monitoring and sustaining health maintenance. Provision of tactical medical care has now become an integral part of preplanning for federal, state, and local tactical teams in response to lessons learned.[3,7]

Goals of Tactical Emergency Medical Support

In the early years, the TEMS role was for care and evacuation of wounded. This role has now evolved with more emphasis on mission planning, primary care, preventive medicine, and emergency care of illness and injury. Although the primary goal of TEMS is to enhance the law enforcement mission, the tactical medical role involves a continuum of care to include maintenance of the team health, reconnaissance of environmental and situational aspects of the mission, coordination of local emergency medical support, creation of evacuation plan and routes, and assessment of future medical needs of the team, perpetrators, bystanders, and possible hostages.[2,7,16,17] Implementation of an effective tactical medical support program is now directed at achieving several important goals (Box 193-1). Today's tactical medical support is also expected to be tactically knowledgeable, mobile, and able to survive and provide and sustain appropriate care in a variety of hostile and adverse environments.

Tactical Team Structure, Training, and Integrated Medical Support

The structure and size of the SWAT team varies across the country according to location and purpose. Some teams have specific full-time roles for each individual, whereas other teams may have complete voluntary tactical teams with individuals serving several roles that rotate according to mission and availability of team members. The typical team is composed of assault teams, which make initial contact with suspects, and arrest teams, which support the assault team. There are also rescue teams, backup teams, and hostage and negotiation teams. A unit commander supervises the operation from a command post.[6,7]

The TEMS component of a tactical unit, like team structure, varies widely across the United States. Some SWAT teams use "standby" EMS personnel, and others have physician-only TEMS providers. Much like the military Special Forces, many civilian tactical law enforcement agencies are now integrating medical support into the tactical team to enhance mission success.[1,2,4]

Although not ideal, the minimal medical coverage at a tactical location should be the use of standby civilian

BOX 193-1. Goals of Tactical Emergency Medical Services

- Enhance mission accomplishment
- Prepare medical threat assessment
- Monitor the medical effects of environmental conditions
- Reduce death, injury and illness, and related effects, among team members, innocents, and perpetrators
- Reduce line of duty injury and disability
- Reduce lost work time
- Maintain good team morale
- Maintain health of team and provide preventive medicine
- Coordinate with surrounding agencies and hospitals
- Decrease liability
- Possess basic forensic knowledge and crime scene preservation

EMS personnel in a predetermined location. The "standby" EMS personnel treat casualties that are brought to them but are unable to assist in medical preplanning or inner perimeter rescue. This minimal medical support for tactical missions may be inadequate for some missions, given the high degree of potential injury and delay in definitive care.[3]

Law enforcement agencies using integrated medical support have varying medical qualifications. The use of EMT-Bs for medical coverage has the advantage of availability and modest cost. However, basic providers require medical control and have limited advanced lifesaving skill capabilities. Medical directors may be able to train basic providers with an enhanced skill set to provide appropriate medical care for tactical support. Paramedic providers also require medical control and have an even higher educational requirement for initial certification maintenance above the basic provider. However, the increased skill set possessed by advanced prehospital providers makes them favorable in a TEMS environment.[3] In a small number of jurisdictions, emergency physicians and residents provide medical oversight for TEMS units and are also deployed as medical operators in the tactical environment.[7,9] Although physician providers offer a broader scope of practice and do not require direct medical control, they usually have limited prehospital experience and also require tactical training.

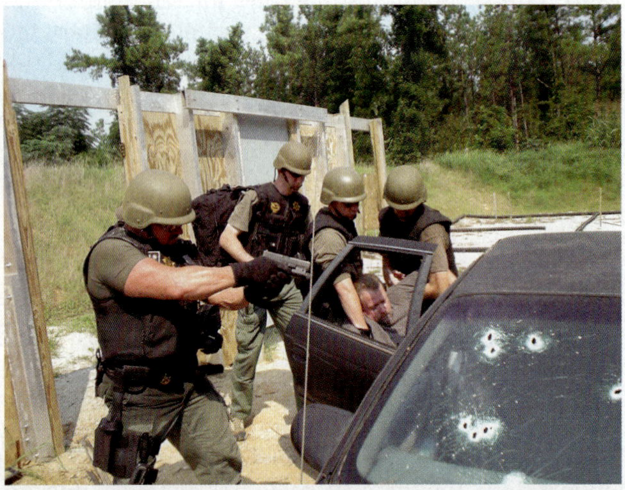

A

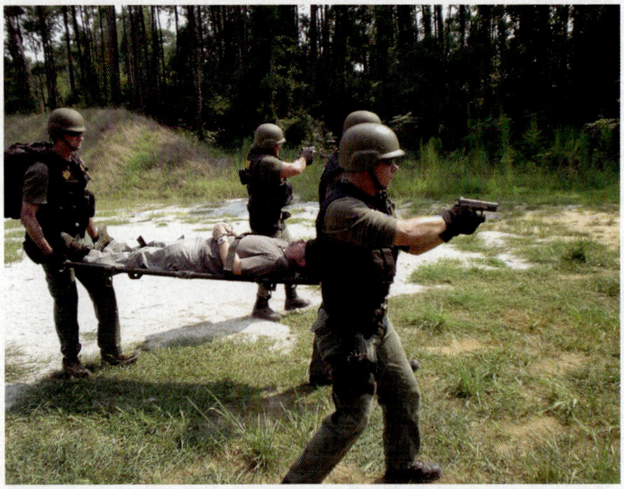

B

Figure 193-1. A, Special Response Team training for the extraction of an injured suspect. **B,** Note the suspect is secured with handcuffs to ensure the safety of the team and bystanders. (Courtesy of Richard Schwartz.)

Training Issues

The tactical environment is different than the traditional EMS environment. Traditional EMS doctrine teaches personnel to ensure the scene is "safe" before attempting to render care.[18] This principle is not possible in some tactical situations. Tactical training needs to take into account team tactics and movement, cover and concealment, equipment issues, nuclear/biological/chemical (NBC) training, rappelling, weapons familiarity, noise, and light discipline training.[7,19] Also, routine training needs to be done in basic rescue tactics, tactical room entries, open area rescues and tactics, movement under fire, cover and concealment, officer down drills, and, in some systems, firearm training (Figure 193-1).

Although Advanced Trauma Life Support (ATLS) may be applicable to the emergency department management of trauma patients in both civilian and military hospitals, it was not created for combat or tactical medicine.[13,20-23] ATLS was developed for physicians, not for out-of-hospital care. It assumes that hospital diagnostic and therapeutic equipment is available and, most importantly, does not recognize the existence of the tactical combat environment. The three goals of tactical combat care are (1) treat the casualty; (2) prevent additional casualties; and (3) complete the mission.[14,19] Tactical combat casualty care is divided into three distinct phases to provide the correct medical interventions at the correct time in the continuum of field care (Box 193-2).[31]

Care Under Fire

In terms of medical delivery in the civilian tactical environment, the area is usually divided into three zones: cold, warm, and hot.[3,19] These zones are based on tactical environment, threat level, and treatment options, which are based on a risk-benefit ratio relative to the medical provider and patient. The cold zone is a safe environment with no threat of injury. This zone is outside the inner perimeter, and regular EMS treatment principles usually apply. In the warm zone, threat is not considered immediate but still exists. Finally, the hot zone is characterized by possible direct exposure to hostile fire.

Care under fire refers to care being rendered in the "hot zone." In this zone, the medic and casualty are

BOX 193-2. Phases of Tactical Combat Care

1. Care under fire
2. Tactical field care
3. Casualty evacuation care (CASEVAC)

under direct effective hostile fire. Care in this phase is very limited, but not nonexistent. When care can be rendered, airway management, the first medical priority in routine prehospital medicine, is best deferred until the tactical field care phase due to difficulty maintaining the airway during evacuation under direct fire. Also, cardiopulmonary resuscitation and cervical spine immobilization have little to no role with treatment of penetrating injuries in this phase and are not a priority in the combat environment.[13,19,24-27] Recommended care is limited to achieving adequate hemostasis and evacuation of the casualty if possible.

Tactical Field Care

The second phase of care, tactical field care, is medical treatment rendered in the "warm zone." In this zone, the medic and casualty are still under threat of injury but not under direct fire. Care in this phase focuses on several areas that have been shown to increase morbidity and mortality in tactical environments if not addressed.[12,19] Airway establishment and maintenance is first addressed in this phase of treatment. Airway management depends on provider training, available equipment, time to evacuation, and type of environment. Next, breathing issues such as tension pneumothorax and open pneumothorax (sucking chest wound) need to be addressed in this phase of care. Circulatory issues such as tourniquet replacement with pressure dressings and correct fluid therapy are then addressed. Intravenous access needs to be established. The tactical environment often makes intravenous access difficult and alternate techniques and routes may be needed to establish access.[28-30] There has also been much controversy in both the civilian and military literature involving optimal type and amount of fluid resuscitation in caring for the trauma patient with controlled or uncontrolled hemorrhagic shock.[31-37] Advanced homostatic dressings can also be used for external hemorrhage not controlled with conventional therapy.[38] Adequate analgesia, prophylactic antibiotics, and appropriate use of cardiopulmonary resuscitation are also addressed in this phase.[13]

Combat Casualty Evacuation Care

Combat casualty evacuation care (CASEVAC) is the third phase of care that is being rendered to casualties in the "cold zone" and while they are evacuated to definitive medical care. Care now begins to closely approximate ATLS guidelines.[13,25] In the civilian setting, CASEVAC is provided en route via aeromedical transport or advanced life support ambulance and continued into the hospital setting, to which the casualties are transported as soon as they are evacuated from the hot or warm zone. Advanced life support care continues en route to the receiving facility, usually a level one trauma center (Figure 193-2).

Civilian Training Programs

Multiple commercial, local, state, and federal training programs exist.[3,6,7,39,40] One of the first and best known training programs for civilian tactical medical support is the Counter Narcotics and Terrorism Operational Medical Support Program. This program consists of a 58-hour course providing continuing education for prehospital providers having training at the emergency medical technician basic level or higher.[3,41] There are multiple other TEMS training courses available of varying length, and some emergency medical graduate medical education programs are incorporating TEMS into their curriculum.

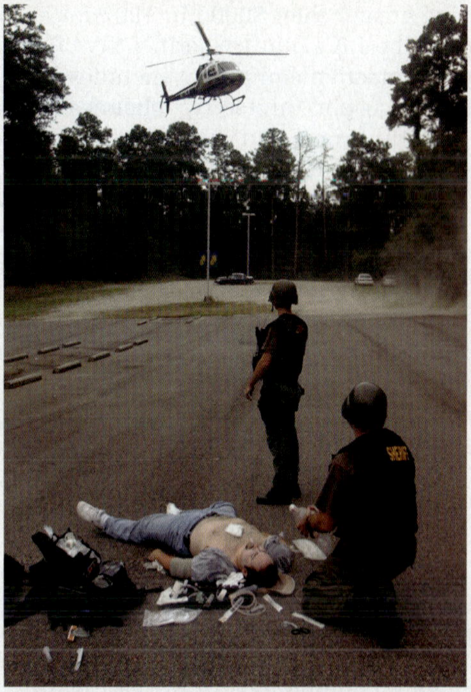

Figure 193-2. CASEVAC is usually provided via aeromedical transport or advanced life support ambulance in the civilian setting. (Courtesy of the *Augusta Chronicle,* Andrew Davis/Tucker.)

Tactical Emergency Medical Support Environment

Training

Practicing effective medical care in the tactical environment requires TEMS personnel to be well educated, trained, and equipped. Tactical EMS involves knowledge and skills that are not included in standard medical education. Integrated "team" training allows the medical support to understand their roles and learn all aspects of tactical law enforcement operations and fundamentals on how to approach the tactical medical arena. Unique medical scenario driven protocols should be developed and rehearsed with the tactical team. These specialized protocols may require advanced practice and require medical control approval that should also satisfy state or federal regulations.[3,41]

Equipment

The TEMS personnel must be familiar with and use tactical, protective, medical, and evacuation equipment. Equipping a TEMS provider can be costly, with the price being greater than $6000 in 1997 for each medic assigned to the LA County Sheriff's SWAT team.[7] The personnel protective equipment includes body armor, helmets, eye armor, protective chemical mask, and clothing. Body armor and protective suits raise heat stress and water consumption requirements. Protective gear also limits vision, communication, sensory input, and the ability to perform medical assessment and treatment.[19,41]

The medical equipment selected and carried by TEMS providers varies and is based on usage, size, weight, budget, training, experience, and mission type. Conventional EMS medications and equipment with bright markings and color coding is often discouraged in the tactical environment to maintain concealment. To optimize amount of equipment available, many TEMS providers separate the medical equipment by use or zones of care. First, they carry a small medical kit or "entry" bag that contains basic supplies utilized in the "hot" or "warm" zone. This small entry bag usually contains equipment such as gloves, tourniquets, simple airway devices, large-bore intravenous needles, and compressive dressings. Next, a larger "aid" bag is used to store equipment used to augment the entry bag and provide a higher level of medical care. This bag is often located in the warm zone or at the command post, if not carried. The aid bag usually contains mission-specific medical equipment, which is determined by the threat assessment, as well as advanced trauma equipment and supplies. Finally, type and location of evacuation equipment for the potential casualties must also be considered. There are several devices and litters that teams can utilize to effectively and safely transport casualties out of the tactical environment.

Remote Patient Assessment

Cases of hostages, barricaded suspects, and pinned down casualties, in which "hands-on" assessment is impossible, often prove to be challenging. Although assessment and management of casualties in these situations is difficult, it is not impossible. Remote patient assessment is another function of TEMS and is done when a person is injured and medical personnel must assess a patient from a distance. Several devices can aid in this remote assessment, including binoculars, gun scopes, night vision goggles, cameras, and microwave radar motion detectors. TEMS providers need to be trained to use visual assessment techniques.[41] If the scene presents a great risk to rescuers, then medical care may be limited to distant guidance and encouragement. Because military data have shown an inherent 20% mortality rate for medics who put themselves at risk, direct medical management should only be considered once the tactical situation permits.[19]

An extension of remote patient assessment has been termed "medicine across the barricade" and involves indirect patient care through skilled communication with a non-health care provider on site.[41]

Hazardous Materials

Incidents involving clandestine drug laboratories and weapons of mass destruction are also considerations in a TEMS environment. Decontamination becomes an issue if team members are exposed to a potential toxic substance. Rapid decontamination must be taught and practiced by tactical teams, because adequate decontamination is usually not available in the inner perimeter.[42,43]

Forensic Science

Basic knowledge of forensic science is important to recognize and preserve evidentiary items. Documentation of wound and blood patterns should be done. All evidence should be collected appropriately and the chain of custody honored.[44]

Medical Threat Assessment

Medical threat assessment is the accounting for all variables that may affect the health and welfare of the tactical team, the perpetrators, nearby civilians, and possible hostages. The medical threat assessment is an essential component of the preplanning phase and should be integrated into the tactical operation.[3,7,45] Medical information is gathered prospectively and continues "real time" during the entire operation. TEMS personnel help to advise the command on factors affecting medical conditions, such as current medical conditions of all personnel involved, environmental and terrain hazards (e.g., weather, obstacles), possible hostage scenarios, medical transport and communications, and potential toxic hazards (e.g., chemicals, plants, animals). The medical threat assessment also includes primary and secondary evacuation planning. Communication with local EMS elements about medical resources, casualty extrication and evacuation, routes of egress, and lines of communication should all be part of the medical assessment.[3,41,45] Once the medical threat assessment is complete, a plan is then developed based on the medical intelligence, addressing each possible situation while recognizing that the plan may change as the mission evolves.

Preventive Medicine

The maintenance of the tactical team's health is an important aspect of a TEMS program. Poor health has been shown to directly correlate with poor job performance and decreased mission accomplishment.[3,46-48] Ensuring that team members are medically and physically fit to participate in missions is essential to improve chances of success.[49] Key preventive medicine issues include monitoring of disease states and stress levels, field hygiene, sleep-wake cycle management during missions, maintenance of immunizations, injury prevention, monitoring of environmental risks, and making physical training recommendations.

Liability

Because special operations lends itself to high litigation and possible disability, TEMS providers need to ensure they have proper malpractice and disability coverage.[7] TEMS has become viewed as an essential component to provide "standard of care" tactical medicine. Both law enforcement and medical personnel have the responsibility of decreasing risk of injury.[2] Court cases have shown that officers who bring prisoners to health care institutions also have a duty to protect third parties from harm.[2,50]

KEY CONCEPTS

- The hostile environment that is intrinsic to urban SWAT team operations requires specialized training and planning for medical personnel.
- Integration of medical planning into both overall team preparation and specific mission planning is essential to an effective medical response in a threatening and dangerous environment.
- Determining medical capability for the hot, warm, and cold zones of a conflict area requires evaluation of local characteristics, the nature of the threat, team safety, and community resources.
- Appropriate use of tactical emergency medical support will aid in diminishing medical threats and improve overall chances of a successful mission.

URBAN SEARCH AND RESCUE

Perspective

"It was hard to breathe. The air was thick and choking. It looked as though black snow had fallen, covering everything." "It was as dark as a tunnel and the air was as thick as soup. Despite repeatedly scooping chunks of dust and debris from my mouth and nostrils, I inhaled and swallowed large quantities." "It took an hour to wash off the layers of dust which by now had become like a layer of concrete."

Drs. Kelly and Prezant, New York City Fire Department, during the 9/11 attacks against the World Trade Center

Urban Search and Rescue (US&R) is a relatively new concept. US&R is the science of responding to, locating, reaching, medically treating, and safely extricating victims entrapped by collapsed structures.[51] US&R is a "multi-hazard" discipline, because it can be needed in a variety of emergencies and disasters, including natural disasters (e.g., earthquakes, hurricanes) and human-made disasters (e.g., terrorist attacks, building and structure collapse, hazardous materials spills).[52] Prior to the 1980s, little information was available on the subject and the Federal Emergency Management Agency (FEMA) US&R teams had not yet been developed. However, since that time national awareness of disasters has increased and there is a demonstrated need for teams with specialized rescue and medical skills for the urban environment.[53]

Reviews of worldwide disasters have helped us understand the injury patterns that can be expected in events such as earthquakes and collapsed structures.[54-56] Immediately after a large earthquake or collapsed structure, there is usually a period of chaos. The local resources are overwhelmed, and most of the victims rescued at this time are rescued by uninjured bystanders. Patients requiring resuscitation during the "golden hour" unfortunately will likely not be reached in time.[1,53,56,57] However, there may still be a large number of injured people trapped in the rubble who will require rescue. Their survival depends on extrication and medical treatment within a short 24- to 48-hour time period, termed "the golden day."[54] After 48 hours, survival rates drop dramatically.[54] For responding resources to be effective, personnel must be highly trained, quickly deployable, mobile, and self-sufficient. The lessons learned have led to the development of the current US&R system in the United States.

History of Urban Search and Rescue in the United States

The current FEMA US&R system started with the Office of US Foreign Disaster Assistance (OFDA). The OFDA sent responders to earthquakes in Mexico City (1985), El Salvador (1986), and Armenia (1988), and the experiences of these responses led to the development of a specialized team for earthquake response. The first equipped, fully integrated team deployment happened in July 1990, when the OFDA sent a Disaster Assistance Response Team to Luzon Province, in the Philippines. The experiences of this team led to the development of the framework for the current US&R task force.[51]

Prior to 1990, FEMA was a disaster recovery agency. Hurricane Hugo and the Loma Prieta Earthquake focused national attention on the deficiency in disaster response. Since initial development, there have been a number of deployments of teams within the United States to various disasters, including hurricanes, earthquakes, and terrorist attacks.[51]

Components and Structure of an Urban Search and Rescue Team

The responding team must mobilize quickly to accomplish its objectives and must not place additional demands on the already stressed infrastructure.[1,52] An effective US&R team needs both properly trained personnel and appropriate equipment.

The equipment cache should allow the task force to be totally self-sufficient for the first 72 hours and to be capable of 24-hour operation for 10 days.[52,59] The FEMA equipment cache is divided into five groups: rescue equipment, medical equipment, technical equipment, communications equipment, and logistics equipment. The medical equipment cache was designed to treat the unique medical needs of trapped victims as well as the medical needs of the team itself. The medical cache contains enough supplies to be able to handle 10 critical cases, 15 moderate cases, and 25 minor cases. The cost of the entire cache is close to $2 million.[52,59]

Coordination and cooperation with local resources and other teams are critical.[51,60] The US&R team is integrated into the Incident Command System at the disaster. The leader is responsible for managing and supervising all team operations and for coordinating the team's efforts with the incident commander.[52,60]

The search team is responsible for developing and implementing a plan to search the area for victims. The search team can be subdivided into two teams, a *canine search team* and a *technical search team*. The canine team uses specially trained dogs to locate trapped victims. The technical team uses specialized microphones, listening devices, cameras, and fiber optic devices to locate victims in confined spaces. The search team is responsible for locating victims and identifying probable areas where victims may be found.[60]

The rescue team is composed of rescue specialists. Once a victim or potential victim is located, the rescue team is responsible for breaching the area and creating a safe entrance to, and exit from, the victim's position. Team members utilize specialized equipment for extricating the victim and have training in collapsed building rescue and hazardous materials.[60]

The technical team is composed of various specialists, including structural specialists, hazardous materials specialists, heavy rigging and equipment specialists, technical information specialists, and communications specialists.[60] These specialists work collaboratively to ensure a safe and efficient operation.

The logistics team is responsible for all the equipment needs, including inventory, issuing, and record keeping.[60]

Finally, there is the medical component, which is composed of medical personnel who are responsible for the medical needs of both the task force personnel and the victims. Typically, the medical personnel are emergency physicians and paramedics.[60,61]

Medical Team Operations in Urban Search and Rescue

A number of unique considerations must be addressed for US&R. As with TEMS, team physicians must realize that they will be operating outside of their usual environment and that they are not in charge overall. Typically, the physician on the team works with the team leader and the managers of the other components. To do this efficiently, the physician should be familiar with the capabilities and training of all the members on the team and the Incident Command System. Cross-training of team members is ideal.[51,53,60,61]

Medical Team Tasks

Predeployment. The job of the medical team in the predeployment phase is to ensure that the entire team is fit and functional for deployment and that the medical equipment cache is organized and up to date.[61] The perceived medical threats in the deployed area must also be addressed (e.g., endemic disease, water contamination, insect threats, existing medical support). A family and communication support system should also be set up before the deployment.

BOX 193-3. Medical Intelligence Gathering Prior to Deployment

- Type of disaster and predicted numbers and types of potential victims
- Capabilities of the team to deal with the medical aspects of the situation, including dealing with injured team members
- Local emergency departments level of functioning. Trauma center status and location
- Local EMS resources
- Location of planned triage staging area
- Communications with local resources (EMS, police, emergency departments, fire and rescue etc.)
- Weather, environment, or hazardous materials issues
- Availability of other resources (e.g., military, NDMS, DMAT)

DMAT, Disaster Medical Assistance Team; EMS, emergency medical service; NDMS, National Disaster Medical System.

Deployment. The medical team is responsible for much more than just treating the victims. Medical intelligence information needs to be collected and addressed (Box 193-3). A plan is required for transfer and transport of victims and for fatality management.

The medical action plan is critical for ensuring smooth operations and must be updated as conditions or knowledge change.[51,60,61] The medical component of a US&R team needs to be able to provide care for its own team members, whose needs may exceed those of the victims. The medical team also needs to assess adequacy of team members' rest and sleep and the psychological effects of the situation.[60,61] Public health issues, including integrity of food and water supply and waste management, are managed by the medical team. If there is a canine search component, the medical team should receive some sort of basic veterinary training before deployment.[60,61]

Confined Space Issues

A confined space is defined as any space with limited access and ventilation. The physician and medical team must be prepared to work in this setting during a deployment and must be aware of issues related to team and victim safety, air purification, and structural dynamics related to collapse or impending collapse.[51,58,60-62]

Specific Disorders in Urban Search and Rescue

Perspective

The US&R teams will typically be responding to the aftermath of earthquakes, collapsed structures, terrorist bombings, hurricanes, and other natural and human-made disasters.[51,52,61] Reviews of the literature have identified the types of medical problems and conditions that might be encountered.[51,52,61,63] Most of the medical conditions are those encountered in the emergency department and are handled similarly. There are a few clinical problems that occur with much greater frequency in the US&R environment: crush syndrome, compartment syndrome, particulate inhalation, hazardous materials exposures, and blast injuries.[51,61] Since the terrorist attacks of 9/11, there has also been an emphasis on preparing the US&R teams for the medical response to weapons of mass destruction.

Crush Injury and Crush Syndrome

Perspective

Compartment syndrome is defined as crush injury caused by swelling of tissue inside the confining fibrous sheath of a muscle compartment, which can cause further destruction of the intracompartment muscle and nerves (see Chapter 46). Fasciotomies in this setting are controversial; the potential benefit—to restore function and lessen rhabdomyolysis—has to be weighed against the much higher risks of infection and bleeding.[64,65] Crush syndrome is defined as the systemic manifestations caused by crushed muscle tissue. This typically occurs when blood flow is restored to the crushed tissue and the toxins are released systemically. It is estimated that between 3% to 20% of earthquake victims and up to 40% of survivors of multistory building collapses will develop crush syndrome.[64] Early hydration of the victim in the rubble before, during, and after extrication can lessen the renal effects of crush syndrome. Crush injury and crush syndrome can result from objects that have fallen on the patient or from the patient's own body weight. The length of time needed to develop crush syndrome depends on both the amount of pressure and patient factors. It can occur within 1 hour if the pressure is severe but usually takes 4 to 6 hours to develop. Typically, crush syndrome occurs in the lower extremities, the buttocks, or an entire upper extremity and the associated pectoral area.[61]

Pathophysiology of Crush Syndrome

The cause of muscular injury in crush injury is not fully understood and is controversial. It is thought that in crush injury, cellular blood flow at the local level is interrupted. These cells begin to function anaerobically, creating lactic acid and other toxins. The intracellular organelles' functions become disrupted and there is a shift of calcium into the cells.[66,67] This shift can lead to systemic hypocalcemia. The influx of calcium into the cell is thought to activate phospholipase A2 and other enzymes that eventually lead to the cell's death. The intracellular contents of the cell include lactic acid, potassium, myoglobin, uric acid, enzymes, leukotrienes, thromboxane, phosphate, and others. Once the cell's membrane is disrupted, the intracellular contents leak out locally. There is also increased capillary permeability. This can lead to edema and third spacing of fluid.[66,67] These effects occur locally until the tissue is released and reperfused. This is why victims can be trapped for days with severe crush injury and appear stable when reached by rescuers, only to deteriorate shortly after being rescued. There are reports of patients going into cardiac arrest shortly after rescue.[66-68] When the crushed area is released, there is the release of all the intracellular contents that have been building up locally into the systemic circulation, causing systemic symptoms. Lactic acid can cause a severe metabolic acidosis. Since 75% of the body's potassium is intracellular, the potassium released may be cardiotoxic. Hyperphosphatemia can aggravate hypocalcemia and cause metastatic calcifications. Uric acid, myoglobin, purines, and others can cause renal failure. Leukotrienes and other cellular toxins can lead to acute respiratory distress syndrome.[66-68] The major causes of early death due to crush syndrome are hypovolemia due to third spacing of fluid and dysrhythmias due to severe metabolic acidosis and hyperkalemia. Delayed causes of death include renal failure, acute respiratory distress syndrome, sepsis, ischemic organ injury, disseminated intravascular coagulation, and electrolyte disturbances.[64-67]

Management of Crush Syndrome

Early aggressive therapy is essential for prevention of crush syndrome and should begin before extrication.[66] All victims who have an obvious crush injury or are immobilized for 4 hours or longer should be considered to have crush injury. The severity of the crush syndrome may be related to the number of extremities with crush injury. In a Japanese study of earthquake victims, the incidence of acute renal failure due to crush syndrome was 50.5% with one extremity, 74.7% for two involved extremities, and 100% for three or more involved extremities.[64] Once a victim is located, the medical component needs to be actively involved with the rescue process and begin treatment before extrication. Cardiovascular instability is commonly seen in patients with crush syndrome.[67] As extrication is being done, continuous cardiac monitoring is recommended. Adequate hydration is recommended along with the usual management of hyperkalemia (insulin/glucose, ion exchange resins, β-agonists, and dialysis). The routine use of intravenous calcium in this setting is controversial. This is because not only is the potassium level elevated but there is also significant hyperphosphatemia. When additional calcium is given, there is the risk of forming metastatic calcifications of calcium phosphate. The current guidelines taught in the FEMA medical specialists course recommend intravenous calcium only for arrhythmias that do not respond to other measures or there is a documented severe hypocalcemia.[61]

The mainstay of treatment for crush syndrome and prevention of renal complications is forced diuresis. The fluid of choice is normal saline. There is considerable debate over the amount of fluid to be given. Large amounts of fluids may be needed because of significant third spacing. One to 1.5 L/hr has been suggested as a starting rate to use during the extrication process, with the rate being titrated to the patient's clinical status. It has been suggested that an average-sized adult may require up to 12 L/day of fluids to sustain a forced diuresis of 8 L/day to prevent renal complications. Continued monitoring of the patient's vital signs, hydration status, and urine output should be done to guide fluid administration until more invasive monitoring is available.[63] Alkalinization of the urine to prevent renal

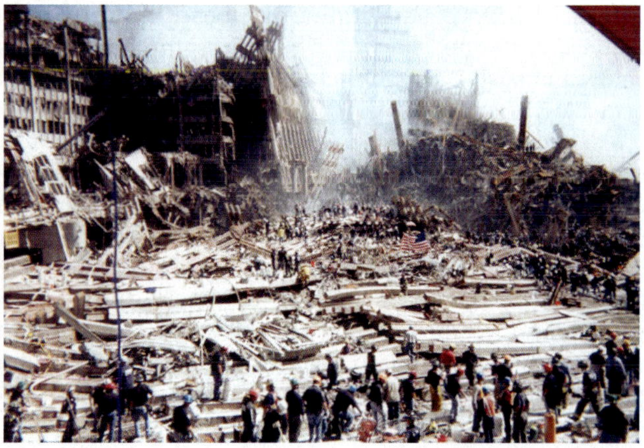

Figure 193-3. Massive amounts of dust and contaminants can exacerbate existing medical conditions, such as asthma and chronic obstructive pulmonary disease, during US&R operations. (Photo by Jeff Orledge.)

failure has been recommended in crush syndrome but has not been subjected to proper study, and the effects of the alkalinization, if any, are impossible to separate from those of the volume fluid used. Rhabdomyolysis and its relationship to renal failure are discussed in Chapter 125.

Other Medical Problems in Urban Search and Rescue

Another unique medical problem in US&R is dust and airway contamination. In every earthquake and collapsed building, a tremendous amount of dust is released in the air. During the first 48 hours of rescue efforts at the World Trade Center, 90% of the 10,116 New York City Fire Department rescue workers evaluated at the site reported an acute cough, often accompanied by nasal congestion, chest tightness, or chest burning, but only three required hospitalization for respiratory symptoms (Figure 193-3). During the 6 months after the attacks, 322 firefighters and one EMS worker had site-related cough severe enough to require more than 4 weeks of leave.[69]

The victim of a collapsed structure should be assumed to have some sort of dust contamination. This contamination can exacerbate existing respiratory disease such as asthma. The physician should evaluate the airway for any evidence of burns or hazardous materials exposure. During the extrication process, the patient's airway should be monitored and deterioration expected. If intubation is being considered, it is better to do it early before edema obstructs the airway, which makes the procedure more difficult. Medical management of the victim reached after prolonged entrapment is very different from the typical trauma setting. The "scoop and run" approach of the trauma patient is not always appropriate or possible.

Hypothermia can also be an issue for patients subjected to environmental conditions. Stabilization, extrication, and ongoing treatment should be directed at the prevention or reversal of hypothermia.

KEY CONCEPTS

- Urban Search and Rescue Teams (US&R) have many integrated components. Typically, the medical component is the smallest part of the team but has some of the greatest responsibilities.
- To be an effective part of the medical team, one needs to understand the incident command system, how the medical component interacts with the team, and the value of a good medical action plan.
- In many deployments, medical care of team members may constitute a much greater component of the medical activity than medical care of victims of the incident.
- Medical problems will be encountered in US&R, including:
  Crush syndrome
  Compartment syndrome
  Exacerbation of respiratory illness
  Hypothermia

REFERENCES

1. Heiskell LE, Carmona RH: Tactical emergency medical services: An emerging subspecialty of emergency medicine. *Ann Emerg Med* 23:778, 1994.
2. Vayer JS: Tactical emergency medicine. In Hogan DE, Bernstein JL (eds): *Disaster Medicine*. Philadelphia, Lippincott Williams & Wilkins, 2002.
3. Casualty Care Research Center: *Counter Narcotics and Terrorism Operational Medical Support Medical Director's Course Handbook*, 3rd ed. Bethesda, MD, Casualty Care Research Center, 2004.
4. Murphy M: FBI, SWAT Paramedics. *Tactical Edge J* 7:22, 1989.
5. Yeskey KS, Llewellyn CH, Vayer JS: Operational medicine in disasters. *Emerg Med Clin North Am* 14:429, 1996.
6. Rinnert KJ, Hall WL: Tactical emergency medical support. *Emerg Med Clin North Am* 20:929, 2002.
7. Vayer JA, Schwartz RB: Developing a tactical emergency medical support program. *Topics Emerg Med* 25:282, 2003.
8. Heck JJ, Pierluisi G: Law enforcement special operations medical support. *Prehosp Emerg Care* 5:403, 2001.
9. Bozeman WP: Tactical EMS: An emerging opportunity in graduate medical education. *Prehosp Emerg Care* 6:322, 2002.
10. Heck JJ, Pierluisi G: Law enforcement special operations medical support NAEMSP position paper. *Prehosp Emerg Care* 5:403, 2001.
11. Booth W: Exploding number of SWAT teams sets off alarms. *Washington Post* June 17, 1997 p A01.
12. Bellamy RF: The causes of death in conventional land warfare: Implications for combat casualty care research. *Mil Med* 149:55, 1984.
13. Butler FK, Hagmann J, Butler EJ: Tactical combat casualty care in special operations. *Mil Med* 161(Suppl):3, 1996.
14. Mabry RL, et al: United States Army Rangers in Somalia: An analysis of combat casualties on an urban battlefield. *J Trauma* 49:515, 2000.
15. Feero S, et al: Does out-of-hospital EMS time affect trauma survival? *Am J Emerg Med* 13:133, 1995.
16. Rasumoff D, Carmona R: Inside the perimeter: Evolving roles of the TEMS provider. *Tactical Edge J* 15:57, 1997
17. Rasumoff D, Carmona R: Inside the perimeter: Trends in TEMS. *Tactical Edge J* 14:52, 1996.
18. McSwain NE, et al: *The Basic EMT: Comprehensive Prehospital Care*. St. Louis, Mosby, 1990.

19. DeLorenzo RA, Porter RS: *Tactical Emergency Care.* Upper Saddle River, NJ, Prentice-Hall, 1999.
20. Llewellyn CH: The antecedents of tactical emergency medical support. *Topics Emerg Med* 25:274, 2003.
21. Smith JP, Bodai BI: The urban paramedic's scope of practice. *JAMA* 253:544, 1985.
22. Honigman B, et al: Prehospital advanced trauma life support for penetrating cardiac wounds. *Ann Emerg Med* 19:145, 1990.
23. Krausz MM, et al: "Scoop and run" or stabilize hemorrhagic shock with normal saline or small-volume hypertonic saline? *J Trauma* 33:6, 1992.
24. Butler FK, et al: Tactical management of urban warfare casualties in special operations. *Mil Med* 65(Suppl):1, 2000.
25. McSwain N (ed): *Military Medicine: Prehospital Trauma Life Support*, 5th ed. St Louis, Mosby, 2003, pp 316-331.
26. Arishita GI, Vayer JS, Bellamy RF: Cervical spine immobilization of penetrating neck wounds in a hostile environment. *J Trauma* 29:332, 1989.
27. Macmillian DS, Cone DC: Officer down. *Prehosp Emerg Care* 7:402, 2003.
28. Calkins MD, Fitzgerald G, Bentley TB, Burris D: Intraosseous infusion devices: A comparison for potential use in Special Operations. *J Trauma* 48:1068, 2000.
29. Dubrick MA, Holcomb JB: A review of intraosseous vascular access: Current status and military application. *Mil Med* 165:552, 2000.
30. Schwartz RB, Charity BM: Use of night vision goggles and low-level light source in obtaining intravenous access in tactical conditions of darkness. *Mil Med* 166:982, 2001.
31. Pepe PE, Mosesso VN, Falk JL: Prehospital fluid resuscitation of the patient with major trauma. *Prehosp Emerg Care* 6:81, 2002.
32. McSwain N (ed): *Military Medicine: Prehospital Trauma Life Support*, 5th ed. St Louis, Mosby, 2003, pp 316-331.
33. Bickell WH, et al: Immediate versus delayed fluid resuscitation for hypotensive patients with penetrating torso injuries. *N Engl J Med* 331:1105, 1994.
34. Wade CE, Dubick MA, Grady JJ: Optimal dose of hypertonic saline/dextran in hemorrhaged swine. *J Trauma* 55:413, 2003.
35. Dubick MA, Atkins JL: Small-volume fluid resuscitation for the far-forward combat environment: Current concepts. *J Trauma* 55:413, 2003.
36. Holcomb JB: Fluid resuscitation in modern combat casualty care: Lessons learned from Somalia. *J Trauma* 55:413, 2003.
37. Rhee P, Koustova E, Alam HB: Searching for the optimal resuscitation method: Recommendations for the initial fluid resuscitation of combat casualties. *J Trauma* 54(5 Suppl):S52, 2003.
38. Pusateri AE, et al: Advanced hemostatic dressing development program: Animal model selection criteria and results of a study of nine hemostatic dressings in a model of severe large venous hemorrhage and hepatic injury in swine. *J Trauma* 55:518, 2003.
39. Rasumoff D, Carmona R: An evaluation period for TEMS personnel: Do we need one? *Tactical Edge J* 13:03, 1995.
40. Law Enforcement Life Saver, Medical College of Georgia, 2003.
41. *Emergency Medical Technician Tactical Course Manual* 14th ed. Bethesda, MD: Uniformed Services University and Health Sciences, 1995.
42. Helskell LF, Tang DH: Medical aspects of clandestine drug labs. *Tactical Edge J* 12:51, 1994.
43. Heck JJ, Byers D: Chemical and biological agents: Implications for TEMS. *Tactical Edge J* 19:52, 2000.
44. Carmona RH, Rasumoff D: Forensic aspects of tactical emergency medical support. *Tactical Edge J* 10:54, 1992.
45. Dressler FL: Operational planning for the law enforcement medic. *Topics Emerg Med* 25:333, 2003.
46. Rasumoff D, Carmona R: Inside the perimeter: Understanding the risks and benefits in selection of mission-specific personnel protective equipment. *Tactical Edge J* 11:68, 1993.
47. Rasumoff D, Carmona R: Inside the perimeter: Diet and performance in the tactical environment. *Tactical Edge J* 12:82, 1994.
48. Sanders N: Should physical fitness qualifications be required for SWAT? *Tactical Edge J* 10:30, 1992.
49. Carmona R, Rasumoff D: Suggested Guidelines for TEMS Policy and SOP. *Tactical Edge J* 17:95, 1999.
50. Lessenger JE: Prisoners in the emergency department. *Ann Emerg Med* 14:179, 1985.
51. Barbera J, Cadoux C: Search, rescue, and evacuation. *Crit Care Clin* 7:321, 1991.
52. FEMA website. Available at www.fema.gov/usr/about.shtm
53. Barbera J, Lozano M: Urban Search and Rescue Medical Teams: FEMA Task Force System. *Prehosp Disast Med* 8:349, 1993.
54. Kunkle RF: Medical care of entrapped patients in confined spaces. In Proceedings of the International Workshop on Earthquake Injury Epidemiology for Mitigation and Response July 10-12. 1989. Baltimore, MD, The Johns Hopkins University Press, 1989, pp 338-344.
55. Noji EK: Natural disasters. *Disast Manag Crit Care Clin* 7:271, 1991.
56. Barbera A, Macintyre A: Urban search and rescue. *Emerg Med Clin North Am* 14:399, 1996.
57. FEMA website: US&R past deployments. Available at www.fema.gov/usr/about.shtm
58. Cone D: Rescue from the rubble: Urban search and rescue. *Prehosp Emerg Care* 4:352, 2000.
59. FEMA National US&R Response System Task Force Equipment Cache List Approved Jan. 28, 2000. FEMA website. Available at www.fema.gov/usr/about.shtm
60. National Urban Search and Rescue Response System Field operations guide; US Department of Homeland Security. FEMA Sept 2003. FEMA website. Available at www.fema.gov/usr/about.shtm
61. FEMA US&R Response system Task Force Medical Team Training Manual April 1997. FEMA website. Available at www.fema.gov/usr/about.shtm
62. Hew P, et al: Urban search and rescue. *Topics Emerg Med* 24:26, 2002.
63. Gans L, Kennedy T: Management of unique clinical entities in disaster medicine. *Emerg Med Clin North Am* 14:301, 1996.
64. Oda J, et al: Analysis of 372 patients with crush syndrome caused by the Hansshin-Awaji earthquake. *J Trauma Injury Infect Crit Care* 42:470, 1997.
65. Kazancioglu R, et al: The characteristics of infections in crush syndrome. *Clin Microbiol Infect* 8:1078, 2002.
66. Vandholder R, et al: Acute renal failure related to crush syndrome: Towards an era of seismo-nephrology. *Nephrol Dial Transplant* 15:1517, 2000.
67. Michaelson M: Crush injury and crush syndrome. *World J Surg* 16:899, 1992.
68. Kikta M, et al: Crush syndrome due to limb compression. *Arch Surg* 122:1078, 1987.
69. Centers for Disease Control and Prevention: Injuries and illnesses among New York City fire department rescue workers after responding to the World Trade Center attacks. *MMWR* (Special issue):51, 2002.

CHAPTER

194 Disaster Preparedness*

Carl H. Schultz, Kristi L. Koenig, and Eric K. Noji

PERSPECTIVE

Disasters affect all parts of the globe and cause harm to people, property, infrastructures, economies, and the environment. Harm to people includes death, injury, disease, malnutrition, and psychological stress. Recent natural catastrophes have included earthquakes in Iran (2003) and Armenia (1988) (Figure 194-1); a series of devastating hurricanes in the Caribbean (1998), including Hurricanes Mitch and Georges; severe flooding in Mozambique (2000), France (2003), and California (1998); tornadoes in Oklahoma and Texas (1999); and global adverse weather conditions related to the El Niño phenomenon (1997 and 1998). The future appears to be even more frightening. Increasing population density in floodplains and in earthquake- and hurricane-prone areas points to the probability of future catastrophic natural disasters with millions of casualties.

Factors that indicate an increasing probability of mass casualty incidents include (1) terrorist activity; (2) increasing population density in floodplains, seismic zones, and areas susceptible to hurricanes; (3) production and transportation of thousands of toxic and hazardous materials; (4) risks associated with fixed-site nuclear and chemical facilities; and (5) the possibility of catastrophic fires and explosions. For example, the U.S. Geological Survey has identified about 35 volcanoes in the western United States and Alaska that are likely to erupt in the future. Mt. Hood, Mt. Shasta, and the volcano underlying Mammoth Lakes in California are near population centers. Because of the rising population density in these areas, hazards from volcanic activity are increasing.

Given this probability and the increasing role of emergency medicine in disaster preparation, mitigation, response, and recovery, this chapter discusses disaster planning and operations with emphasis on the role of the emergency physician. The emergency physician has extensive responsibilities for community disaster preparedness and disaster medical services, particularly regarding terrorism.[1] In its June 2001 position paper, the American College of Emergency Physicians outlined the scope of emergency medicine's involvement in preparedness and response to terrorism and stated its belief that "hospital emergency departments will be the first and most critical line of defense for detection, notification, rapid diagnosis, and treatment" and furthermore that "emergency department personnel will become the *first responders* to a covert biological attack."

A committed emergency department alone is insufficient to provide hospitals with a successful disaster preparedness program. Institutional commitment by every hospital department and the administration is necessary to coordinate effectively with system-wide resources for disaster management.

NATURE OF DISASTERS

Definitions

One of the challenges facing those responsible for disaster preparation is that no standard definition of *disaster* exists. Some events that have been routinely classified as disasters clearly are not. For example, many would consider a plane crash a disaster, yet it may not even approach overwhelming the resources of the local responders. Because disaster medicine is multidisciplinary and depends on the integration of multiple levels of responders, the use of a common, precise terminology is essential.

In general terms, an event can be considered a disaster when it overwhelms response capabilities. These response capabilities can change in diverse environments or even in the same location at different times of the day or days of the week. For example, a multiple-vehicle accident with 6 critically injured patients and 12 patients with minor injuries could overwhelm both the emergency medical services system and the hospital in a small rural community. In an urban area with multiple hospitals that participate in a trauma system, however, this same event could be handled with routine resources. Thus, it is the functional impact on the specific area that is the key concept in determining whether a disaster exists.

Classic Terminology

Many terms have been used in an attempt to describe disasters. The words *internal* and *external* refer to a hospital setting to help distinguish whether an event has occurred within the hospital grounds (internal) or in the community (external). This concept distinguishes between preparing for casualties to arrive at the hospital versus dealing with casualties or resource problems within the hospital. This geographic distinction between internal and external may be useful, but it has severe limitations. Many events can be both

*The views expressed in this chapter do not necessarily represent the views of the Department of Veterans Affairs or of the United States Government.

internal and external to the facility at the same time (e.g., major earthquake or hurricane). Further, simply identifying the location of the event does not answer the critical question: How are response capabilities affected?

An etiologic descriptor for an event is another customary classification. It does not matter whether a disruption in the ability of the hospital to respond is caused by nature or by humankind. The key consideration is what needs to be done to mitigate and then to rectify the situation.

Some definitions have been based on the number of casualties. As previously described, the absolute number of patients is much less important than whether their needs exceed the resources to care for them. Another scheme divides disasters into three levels. Level I denotes a situation in which local resources are adequate to care for casualties. The 1999 attack on a Jewish community center by a lone gunman in California, for example, was handled effectively by local responders. Level II means that regional mutual aid is required to respond to the event. This was the case at the Hyatt Regency Hotel in Kansas City in 1981 when two skywalks collapsed, killing 114 people and injuring hundreds. Level III incidents require state and federal aid. The attack on the World Trade Center in 2001 (Figure 194-2) and Hurricane Andrew in 1992 were such events, causing such massive destruction that federal disaster medical assistance teams were deployed to New York and Florida, respectively, to provide medical personnel and supplies.

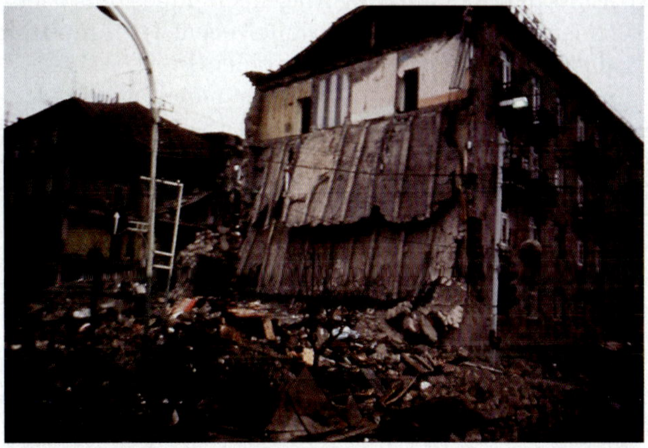

Figure 194-1. Natural catastrophes, such as this earthquake in Armenia (1988), have the potential to cause much injury and psychological stress.

One model being proposed eliminates the word *disaster* and replaces it with the acronym for potential injury-creating event, *PICE.* [2-3] The PICE nomenclature is an attempt to resolve the issue surrounding diverse meanings for *disaster.* Although not yet routinely accepted, this model is discussed here to help clarify important concepts in describing an event.

Potential Injury-Creating Event (PICE) Nomenclature

The acronym PICE and its modifiers concisely describe the critical features of most types or degrees of disaster.[2-4] The same occurrence can have different effects at different points in time; thus, as an event evolves over time, its description may change.

Modifiers are chosen from a standardized group of prefixes along with a stage to indicate the need for outside medical assistance (Table 194-1). The first prefix (column A) describes the potential for additional casualties. The second prefix (column B) describes whether local resources are overwhelmed and, if so, whether they must simply be augmented (disruptive)

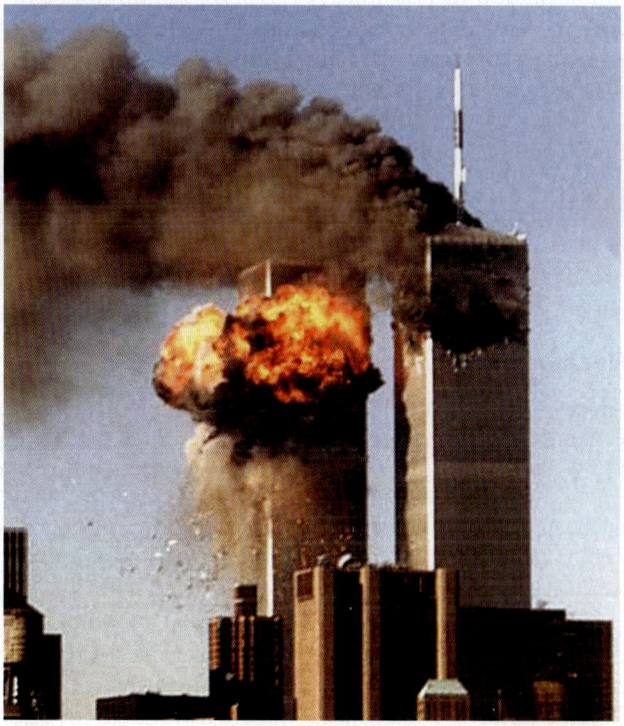

Figure 194-2. The World Trade Center attack of 2001 overwhelmed local resources and necessitated state and federal help.

Table 194-1. Potential Injury-Creating Event (PICE) Nomenclature

Prefix					
A	B	C	PICE Stage	Projected Need for Outside Aid	Status of Outside Aid
Static	Controlled	Local	0	None	Inactive
Dynamic	Disruptive	Regional	I	Small	Alert
	Paralytic	National	II	Moderate	Standby
		International	III	Large	Dispatch

or whether they must first be totally reconstituted (paralytic). The third prefix (column C) shows the extent of geographic involvement.[2-4]

The stage rating scale defines the likelihood that outside medical assistance will be needed either to augment or to completely reconstitute resources.[2-4] Stage 0 means that there is little or no chance. Stage I means that there is a small chance and requires placing outside medical help on alert. Stage II means that there is a moderate chance and outside help should be placed on standby. Stage III means local resources are clearly overwhelmed and requires the dispatch of outside resources and commitment of personnel. For example, a multivehicle accident with a dozen injuries and several deaths in a large city would be a stage 0, whereas in a small rural town it might be stage III (Table 194-2).

A PICE can be either static or dynamic. *Dynamic* implies an evolving situation in which it is too soon after the incident to determine the number of casualties and the impact on the hospital. Alternatively, a *static* situation results if 10 people are injured in an accident and little potential for further harm exists.[2-4]

In some situations, enhancing routine operations is not sufficient or possible. A PICE can completely overwhelm the capability to mount a normal response, so that a substitute plan for recovery must be used. Situations that require significant reconstitution of critical resources are termed *paralytic*.[2-4] Within the hospital, there are six critical elements necessary to provide a response (Box 194-1).[5,6] If one or more of these resources are compromised, they must be reconstituted or a substitute must be implemented. Such paralytic events can be either destructive or nondestructive (Box 194-2).[3]

Hazards Analysis

An important consideration in disaster planning is an awareness of the types of events for which the hospital or community is vulnerable. The classic example is the monumental risk from earthquakes in the central United States resulting from the combination of the New Madrid fault and the limited seismic safety requirements for buildings in that area. The planner must learn what types of support are available from outside agencies (e.g., hazardous materials decontamination from the fire departments, information from poison control centers). Although awareness of such resources is critical, contingency plans must be available when such assistance is not accessible.

Table 194-2. PICE Nomenclature Examples

World Trade Center Attack, 9/11/01	Dynamic, paralytic, local PICE, stage III
Los Angeles civil disturbance	Dynamic, paralytic, regional PICE, stage I
Northridge earthquake	Dynamic, disruptive, regional PICE, stage II
Oklahoma City bombing	Dynamic, disruptive, local PICE, stage I

After performing a hazard vulnerability analysis, emergency planners should consider the most probable events and prepare for them. There must also be planning for events that are rare but catastrophic.[7] The major peacetime threat to life and limb in the United States is probably a large earthquake in a densely populated area or a terrorist attack. The disaster planner must proactively identify all such hazards and prepare contingency plans for each.

TRIAGE

Triage comes from the French verb, *trier,* meaning "to sort." The concept of triage was used as far back as Napoleon's time to assign priorities to treatment of the injured when resources were limited. Priority is given to the most salvageable patients with the most urgent conditions. The emergency department uses triage in the hospital setting on a daily basis, but the focus of such triage must be changed under disaster conditions.[8] Standard emergency department triage is intended to identify the most seriously ill patients first and ensure that they receive rapid care. The goal of disaster triage is slightly different, that is, "to do the most good for the most people." It can be very difficult for physicians to realize that, to achieve the goal of maximizing benefit to an entire population of patients, they may need to let some patients die with only comfort care. Under true disaster conditions, cardiopulmonary resuscitation should not be performed.[9]

Routine Multiple-Casualty Triage

To assist in understanding triage techniques, it is useful to consider a routine prehospital event with multiple casualties (e.g., multivehicle accident).

In such situations, rescue personnel often use a simple triage and rapid treatment (START) technique that depends on a quick assessment of respiration, perfusion, and mental status.[10] Initially, all victims who

BOX 194-1. Six Critical Substrates for Hospital Operations

- Physical plant
- Personnel
- Supplies and equipment
- Communication
- Transportation
- Supervisory managerial support

BOX 194-2. Examples of Paralytic PICE

Destructive	Nondestructive
Bomb explosion	Snowstorm
Earthquake	Employee strike
Fire	Power failure
Civil unrest	Water supply cutoff

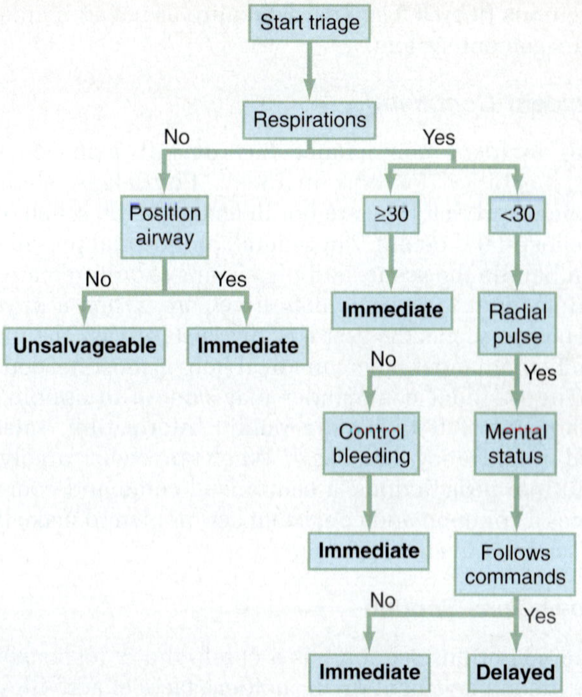

Figure 194-3. Simple triage and rapid treatment (START). Victims who can walk are identified first and triaged into the "minor" category. Those remaining are triaged using the algorithm. (Modified from Triage-START and SAVE. In *Medical Disaster Response Training Course Syllabus*. Dana Point, Calif, Medical Disaster Response, 1993.)

are able to walk are asked to move away from the immediate incident area. These patients are classified as green, or "walking wounded," and are reassessed after the more immediately critical patients are triaged.

As illustrated in Figure 194-3, a rescuer can move through each patient in seconds, quickly checking respiratory rate, pulse, and ability to follow commands (mental status), and divide them into the remaining three categories: (1) red (immediate), (2) yellow (delayed), and (3) black (deceased). The only patient care interventions provided during this process are the opening of an obstructed airway and direct pressure on obvious external hemorrhage. At this point, patients are generally transported to a hospital for definitive care. Most often, patients arrive with a color-coded triage tag and are reassessed and retriaged by the hospital staff.

Catastrophic Casualty Management

Triage during a widespread, catastrophic disaster differs from triage performed in routine prehospital and hospital settings. The number of victims is vastly increased, and medical resources are severely limited or even initially absent. Patients may remain on scene for an extended period and must be frequently reassessed. In addition, the triage process is decentralized, occurring at multiple sites, or compartments, simultaneously throughout the disaster zone. Rather than a single scene or localized disaster, this can be thought of as a compartmentalized disaster.[7] Lastly, patients tend to seek care at the closest hospital, a phenomenon known as *convergence*. Hospitals close to the disaster scene are overwhelmed, whereas hospitals located only a few miles away may receive few, if any, patients.

To address these considerations, the secondary assessment of victim endpoint (SAVE) system of triage was proposed.[11] The SAVE triage system is designed to identify patients who are most likely to benefit from care available under austere field conditions. When combined with the START protocol, SAVE triage is useful for any scenario in which multiple patients experience a prolonged delay in accessing definitive care.

The SAVE methodology is designed for use by health care providers within the disaster zone who begin caring for patients immediately but may not be able to transport patients to a definitive care facility for days. It is immediate and dynamic rather than delayed and static. Although there are many elements in common with other triage systems, rapid transport to a functional medical center within the ideal "golden hour" is impossible.

The SAVE triage methodology divides patients into three categories: (1) those who will die regardless of how much care they receive; (2) those who will survive whether or not they receive care; and (3) those who will benefit significantly from "austere" field interventions. Only those patients expected to improve receive more than basic care and comfort measures. Using SAVE, patients are separated into these three categories so resources can be focused appropriately. The decision to place patients in a particular group is based on field outcome expectations derived from existing survival and morbidity statistics.[11] An example is a situation in which three victims require chest tubes (two victims require one tube each and one victim requires two tubes), but only two chest tubes are available. The SAVE principles guide providers to place their last two chest tubes into the two victims that need it rather than into the single victim requiring two tubes.

During the triage process, individuals who would most benefit from early transport should be marked as "first out," in case an evacuation opportunity occurs. These would be victims with medical problems readily treatable at a hospital but untreatable and fatal in the field. A patient requiring surgery for intra-abdominal hemorrhage is a common example.

Since the issue of nuclear, biologic, and chemical terrorism has developed, new triage systems are under development. Responders must be protected from secondary contamination or exposure, and therefore, part of the triage algorithm must include a risk assessment and determination of whether, and what type of, personal protective equipment must be donned prior to accessing patients. A quick determination is critical to prevent patient deaths from traumatic injuries while awaiting medical care from responders concerned about their own health and safety. This is particularly true in a "combined event" scenario such as a radiologic dispersion device. Also associated with terrorism incidents are large numbers of *psychogenic casualties*, or those who believe they were exposed but actually were not. The emergency plan must include a mechanism to assess and sort these individuals so as not to overwhelm the emergency department. While performing triage, the emergency physician must also consider the effects of extremes of age, underlying disease, and multiple injuries when assessing the potential prognosis for a given patient.[12] The treatment of many nontraumatic emergencies fortunately can be accomplished with field interventions that do not consume extensive resources. Therefore, patients with such illnesses should usually be triaged to the treatment area.

Special Triage Categories

To maximize personnel resources, disaster victims who would normally be triaged to the observation area can be triaged to the treatment area if they possess special skills valuable to the medical team (e.g., medical expertise, translation skills). By increasing the number of functional team members, the effectiveness of the overall response will improve. The guiding principle supports the disaster triage goal of maximizing benefit to the most people.

PREHOSPITAL RESPONSE

Emergency Medical Services System Protocols

To prepare adequately, hospitals must be familiar with and involved in the development of county or regional plans. For example, some EMS systems use automatic systems such that each hospital may be expected to accept a predetermined number of critically ill or injured and minor patients without previous notification.

Physicians working at hospitals should be familiar with community disaster management operations, including the function of the emergency operations center.[6] Mutual aid agreements with other hospitals or regions should be considered for situations in which the hospital becomes overwhelmed or needs to be evacuated.

Incident Command System

The incident command system is a standard emergency management system used throughout the United States to provide a flexible command and control structure on which to organize a response.[13] By standardizing an organizational structure and using common terminology, the incident command system provides a management system that is adaptable to incidents involving a multiagency or multijurisdictional response. At the most basic level, there are five functional elements in the organizational structure: (1) incident command, (2) operations, (3) planning, (4) logistics, and (5) finance. The principles of the incident command system can also be applied to the hospital setting through the Hospital Emergency Incident Command System. With this type of organizational infrastructure and the flexibility to expand and collapse as needed, an orderly and efficient response to any incident can be accomplished. Since hospitals cannot anticipate every contingency, a system such as Hospital Emergency Incident Command System assists with planned improvisation. The Joint Commission on the Accreditation of Healthcare Organizations (JCAHO) standards require use of an incident management system.

Incident Command

The incident commander has overall management responsibility for the incident. Physicians should understand that they are not in charge at the scene of a prehospital incident.[14] In general, prehospital providers can handle the scene, and physicians should remain at the hospital to provide definitive care. When a physician is on scene, the best way to assist is to ask the incident commander where medical help is most needed.

The incident commander may choose to appoint a command staff to handle public information, safety, and interagency liaisons.[13] When an event involves multiple jurisdictions, a centralized command coordinates a common and consistent action plan to make the best use of available resources.

Operations Section

The operations section has a chief who is responsible for the management of all incident tactical activities.[13] This section can be expanded and subdivided into branches (e.g., law, fire, medical) and divisions. Operations also manages the resources assigned to staging areas. Ambulances, personnel, and supplies must be staged outside the perimeter of the scene and directed in as needed rather than converging on the disaster site, potentially disrupting activities, and blocking the exodus of patients. It is under the Operations Section that all medical triage and care is provided.

Planning Section

The planning section collects, evaluates, and disseminates information regarding incident operations and the status of resources. This section also develops action plans and conducts planning meetings.[13]

Logistics Section

The logistics section's chief is responsible for providing facilities, services, and material in support of the incident. This includes procuring equipment and supplies, providing food and medical support, and meeting transportation needs.[13]

Finance Section

The finance section is responsible for maintaining records on personnel and equipment time, providing payments to vendors for supplies and use of equipment, and determining the cost of various alternatives for strategic planning.

Organization of Prehospital Disaster Scene

The disaster site is organized into several distinct areas. The command post is the nerve center of the operation and contains the incident commander and section chiefs. A staging area for incoming personnel and equipment should be established on the outer perimeter. If air evacuation is needed, a safe landing zone must be identified. A casualty collection point and morgue should be designated. In conjunction with an incident command system, this structure brings order to the response.

PLANNING AND HOSPITAL RESPONSE

Comprehensive Emergency Management

The comprehensive emergency management all-hazard approach to disaster preparedness is now required by JCAHO. Comprehensive emergency management consists of four phases: (1) mitigation, (2) preparedness, (3) response, and (4) recovery.[14,15] *Mitigation* involves taking actions to reduce the impact of identified hazards. Training, drills, and cataloging resources are examples of *preparedness* activities. *Response* includes assessment of the situation and coordinating resources. Finally, *recovery* consists of a return to normal operations and debriefing to critique the response and provide psychological support to the rescuers.

As required by JCAHO, a hospital's disaster or "emergency management" plan must address events occurring both inside (internal) and outside (external) the institution.[15] Because some incidents trigger both internal and external plans, they should integrate seamlessly with each other.

Internal Disaster Plan

An *internal disaster* is any event that disrupts daily, routine hospital functions. This can represent an infrastructure failure (e.g., loss of electric power and water) or a threat to the safety of patients and hospital personnel (e.g., labor dispute). Because the internal disaster response varies from postponing elective surgery to facility evacuation, every hospital department must participate in the planning process. At a minimum, the internal plan should (1) clearly delineate the circumstances under which the plan is activated; (2) identify the command structure with defined lines of authority and responsibility; (3) describe a response strategy for each anticipated incident; (4) estimate an incident's impact on safety and hospital function, providing for evacuation if necessary; and (5) list essential information, such as critical telephone numbers (elevators, key personnel, pay telephones), community agencies (emergency medical services, police, public health), and sources of vital supplies (water, oxygen, drugs).[14]

After plan activation, the primary role of the emergency department is to assess and treat individuals with illness or injury. In the absence of casualties, other hospital departments primarily manage internal disasters. Nevertheless, the medical director of the emergency department should continuously monitor the response process.

In the unlikely event that evacuation of the emergency department is necessary, evacuation routes and relocation destinations that have been planned in advance maximize safety and efficiency. When resources are plentiful, emergency department patients in critical condition are assigned the highest priority for evacuation and transport. Less ill patients receive a lower priority.[16] When resources are limited (e.g., large-magnitude earthquake), the reverse strategy applies. The least critically ill patients receive the highest priority for evacuation.

External Disaster Plan

An external disaster is an event occurring in the community that results in a sudden influx of patients requiring emergency care at hospitals. This definition generally assumes that the incident has had no direct impact on hospital capacity or function. Participation in the planning and execution of the hospital disaster response is an important administrative responsibility.[9] Available data guiding development of disaster strategies are incomplete, but an effective disaster response can be created by reviewing the essential components of disaster plans and the previous experience of hospitals.[4,9,17] A member of the emergency department must have a leadership role in the planning and implementation of the external disaster plan.

Basic Components of Hospital Comprehensive Disaster Response Plan

Interdepartmental Planning Group

The interdepartmental planning group has the responsibility for hazard identification and disaster preparedness activities. Frequently referred to as the *disaster* or *emergency preparedness committee*, it is composed of representatives from all departments vital to the hospital's response, including administration, medical staff, nursing, safety, security, the emergency department, and engineering. Additional input may occasionally be necessary from outside agencies (e.g., fire department, hospital suppliers of goods and services, emergency medical services agency).

The committee must be structured to ensure that the plan is properly constructed, tested, and executed. Hospital resources must be provided to support the planning process and testing of the plan, and there must be a detailed educational program for all affected hospital staff.[15,18-20]

Resource Management

A full inventory of the hospital's resources must be available. In addition to equipment, space, and personnel within the institution, potential support from outside the hospital must be sought. It is also necessary to develop contingency plans to compensate for lost resources (e.g., failure of hospital computers during a power outage).

Strong relationships with community agencies (e.g., fire department, regional emergency medical services system) are important to ensure a coordinated disaster response. Hospitals located near companies using large amounts of hazardous materials are required by Title III of the Superfund Amendments and Reauthorization Act to participate in local emergency planning committees.[21]

Command Structure

An organized system establishing lines of authority and decision responsibility must be in place. This system should designate a command center where the disaster response can be coordinated and create a clear chain of command. This prevents confusion if certain individuals are missing, a common situation on nights and weekends. The command center should contain sufficient equipment to support command and control functions, even if the center must be moved as a result of hospital damage.

Media

The media can be an important source of information but can also significantly disrupt the hospital's disaster response. Therefore, arrangements should be made in advance for a designated individual to coordinate all media interactions and for these briefings to occur in a predetermined location. Media coordinators should inform reporters of the time they will receive their next update so they do not intrude on response operations while trying to obtain information. A strong media liaison can facilitate dissemination of important information to the public, as, for example, that no blood shortage exists so that individuals refrain from coming to the hospital to donate blood. Security should be involved in managing the media response to the hospital and in preventing media from interfering with triage and treatment of patients.

Communication

Communication systems are probably the most important, but also most vulnerable, component of a disaster plan.[9,22] Redundant systems are a must. Those responsible for mobilizing the emergency response require access to at least one other communication system besides the telephone (which is frequently one of the first systems compromised during a disaster). Two-way radios are often used, as are pay telephones, independent fax lines, and cellular phones. Another option is the evolving technology utilizing satellite phones and wireless hand-held devices to transmit e-mail messages. Runners are useful for intrahospital communication if all else fails.

Personnel

The disaster plan must include a roster of all critical positions and personnel and establish a reliable method for their mobilization. Several individuals should be assigned to each position in case some personnel cannot be reached. A protocol for managing volunteers is also crucial. A large group of uncontrolled volunteers descending on a hospital can be as disruptive as the disaster.[23] Some hospitals are credentialing volunteer health care providers in advance of a disaster so they will have emergency privileges should the need for their services arise.

Patient Management

A systematic approach to patient management is necessary to maximize resources. This includes protocols for decontamination, triage, patient prioritization, evacuation, and control of patients' families. Alternative use of hospital facilities must be anticipated, such as the conversion of a parking lot into a clinic area for suturing lacerations or a decontamination zone. Provisions for patient identification and treatment documentation are also important to facilitate federal and third-party reimbursement at the conclusion of the disaster.

Training Exercises

Disaster exercises are one of the more effective ways of familiarizing hospital staff with their responsibilities. All hospital departments should participate, and community agencies should be involved. The JCAHO requires two drills a year; these should mimic incidents that are likely to occur.

REVIEW OF HOSPITAL AND COMMUNITY DISASTER RESPONSE EXPERIENCE

Disaster plan implementation is complex and difficult. Much can be learned from reviewing previous disaster response experiences, resulting in improved implementation strategies. The following discussion highlights potential problem areas.

Focal Disasters

Most disasters experienced by hospitals are focal in nature. Hospital function is typically unimpaired. The majority of problems encountered are related to a sudden increase in patient volume and acuity or arrival of patients with illnesses not usually treated at that facility (e.g., burns, radiation exposure, sudden acute respiratory syndrome).

Hospitals frequently experience difficulty in effectively using and interfacing with community resources. Field triage must allocate patients rationally, and transfer agreements must be in place to facilitate interhospital movement of patients.

Media access must be controlled. During the Loma Prieta earthquake in 1989, a news helicopter occupied a nearby community hospital's only landing zone, preventing the possibility of landing a medical helicopter.

Redundant communication systems must be in place. Typical backup systems to the telephone are radios and cellular phones, but the frequencies can be overloaded in both systems. Two-way radios are reliable and should be part of the communications network.

Catastrophic Disasters

In a large-scale disaster, paramedics may be unavailable to assist in patient transfers or hospital evacuations. Disaster medical assistance teams and urban search and rescue teams will deploy, but their time to arrival on scene may be variable. Each individual hospital may have to fend for itself for 48 to 72 hours. Generator problems are frequent; they either fail altogether (as they did in Loma Prieta) or supply insufficient power to meet emergency needs (as in Northridge).[22,24] Evacuation plans must not require elevators for this reason. Telephone service will cease as lines are disrupted or deliberately restricted by the phone company. Cellular phones may function within a local area, but failure is likely if more distant sites within the city are dialed. Hospital radios designated for disaster use must have the hardware secured to prevent earthquake damage.

Under catastrophic conditions, mobilizing personnel is more difficult. Because telephone communication is unreliable, at least one additional system for contacting personnel at home must be in place. An alternative is to institute an automatic response system.

After earthquakes or explosions, immediate access to structural engineers is important. In the Northridge earthquake, eight hospitals in the Los Angeles area sustained enough damage to force evacuation of at least one patient. Four institutions completely evacuated their facilities in the first 24 hours, including two hospitals that met the most current structural earthquake standards. Further structural damage was subsequently identified and forced two additional hospitals to evacuate completely in the next 2 weeks. Ultimately, four of these hospitals were permanently closed and scheduled for demolition.[16]

Catastrophic earthquakes can cause extensive casualties, including large numbers of patients with crush syndrome and lacerations. Up to 90% of the victims with serious but survivable injuries are rescued by local responders and volunteer citizens in the first 24 to 48 hours.[25-26] Therefore, special medical teams such as disaster medical assistance teams and urban search and rescue teams may not significantly affect survival if they arrive after more than 48 to 72 hours. If hospitals are not functional and no backup plan exists, immediate advanced medical care will not be available, and many people will die. Therefore, planners must include a backup system to provide medical care at nonhospital sites.

Need for Local Response

Currently, it is not possible for outside assistance to arrive in force during the crucial first 48 hours. Therefore, an alternative source of immediate, sophisticated medical care is necessary. It appears this is best provided by local responders who arrive shortly after the event.[7,27] The Medical Disaster Response Project is the most advanced model of a local medical response to such a disaster. Developed by emergency physicians in southern California, the Medical Disaster Response Project has two components: (1) training of health care providers in the management of disaster victims under austere conditions, and (2) placement of sophisticated medical supplies at predesignated sites within the community.[7,28] Under this plan, victims could receive rapid, advanced medical care from surviving volunteer health care providers even if hospitals were destroyed.

Toxic Disasters (Hazardous Material)

Hospitals in the vicinity of major chemical industries, transportation corridors, or probable terrorist targets (e.g., Disneyland) should be aware of potential hazards from incidents involving chemical and radioactive substances and be prepared to decontaminate large numbers of individuals exposed to these hazardous substances. Effective decontamination of victims and the need for effective safety measures on the part of rescue personnel to prevent secondary contamination are critical.[29] Decontamination equipment must be stored near the emergency department and the staff must be trained in its use. This location must be known to personnel.[30] When such an emergency occurs, there is little time to search the hospital for the necessary supplies.

Ideally, patients contaminated with hazardous chemicals should first be brought to a predesignated decontamination area containing a warm water shower with a container to hold drainage water. Rescuers and victims should remove all clothing. These are bagged, tagged, and stored. Contaminated patients must never be brought into regular patient care areas because of the danger of contaminating other patients, hospital staff, and equipment. In 1994, paramedics unsuspectingly transported a patient contaminated with a degradation product of dimethyl sulfoxide to an emergency department in Riverside, California. Before detecting the presence of the hazardous material, six health care workers were exposed, including an emergency physician. This emergency physician experienced a near-fatal exposure and required intubation and an extensive stay in the hospital's intensive care unit. Uncontrolled spread of the toxin resulted in evacuation and temporary closure of the emergency department.[31]

The emergency department must close off the air intake vents in rooms containing contaminated patients so toxic products do not enter the ventilation system and circulate to other parts of the hospital. Rescue personnel and hospital staff should be protected by gowns, gloves, and masks, and, if necessary, supplied air respirators. The goals are to reduce the initial level of external contamination, contain the contamination that remains, and prevent further spread of these potentially dangerous substances to other patients and staff members.

NUCLEAR, BIOLOGIC, AND CHEMICAL TERRORISM

In addition to the familiar threat from hazardous materials, there is a new challenge: a potential attack by terrorists using nuclear, biologic, or chemical weapons (see Chapter 195). Although somewhat similar to hazardous materials situations, management of patients exposed to weapons of mass destruction (WMD) requires new knowledge and skills.

The most likely radiation source used by terrorists will probably not come from the detonation of a nuclear weapon. Instead, simple radiologic devices, such as those used by hospitals for radiation therapy, are believed to be the source of choice. They do not explode and give no warning of their presence. Terrorists can also dismantle such devices and incorporate the radioactive source into an explosive radiologic dispersion device ("dirty bomb"). Therefore, providers must recognize the presentation of patients suffering from radiation exposure to make the diagnosis. Patients who are irradiated but not externally or internally contaminated pose no threat to emergency department personnel.

One of the greatest challenges with respect to WMD is the detection of biologic weapons. Patients exposed to many of the biologic agents initially present with vague symptoms associated with flulike illnesses. Decontamination is not a priority unless the exposure is immediate; standard precautions are generally sufficient.

Unlike radiologic or biologic weapons, chemical agents produce symptoms quickly. The challenge is decontamination and treatment. Approximately 80% of mass casualty decontaminations are performed at hospitals. Therefore, hospitals must be prepared to decontaminate patients outside the emergency department. Personal protective equipment is also an issue for responders because of the risk of exposure during the decontamination process.[32]

DISASTER STRESS MANAGEMENT

Emergency health care providers experience high levels of stress responding to the needs of disaster victims. If this excessive stress exceeds the capacity of normal coping mechanisms, it can potentially interfere with job performance and produce disturbing symptoms. These symptoms include depression, sleep disturbances, increased use of alcohol and drugs, irritability, and anxiety.[33] Posttraumatic stress disorder can result.[34] In an attempt to reduce the psychological impact of these events on medical responders, a technique known as *critical incident stress debriefing* was introduced in 1983.[33] Subsequently, other models have been introduced.

In general, the longer the delay is between exposure to the critical incident and subsequent psychological intervention, the smaller the chance is for a successful outcome. Therefore, the critical incident stress debriefing process is designed for rapid implementation. During the incident, stress management staff or even a colleague can provide on-scene intervention. The goal is to assist the health care worker in regaining emotional control by facilitating communication of feelings and reactions through listening and support.

If a critical incident has profoundly affected multiple participants, and if symptoms are still present many hours later, a debriefing is held, which is a more extensive and formal version of a defusing. Debriefings are coordinated by mental health and peer support staff and focus on education and venting of emotions.[35] Data from previous experiences suggest that such intervention can assist providers in maintaining job performance and satisfaction, resulting in improved patient care.[36]

DISASTER RESPONSE ORGANIZATIONS

Department of Homeland Security

The Department of Homeland Security (DHS), a cabinet-level department formed after the terrorist attacks of September 11, 2001, is the federal government's lead organization for emergency management activities in the United States (the Federal Emergency Management Agency [FEMA] has been incorporated intact into DHS and retains its name). DHS has a coordinating responsibility for the entire spectrum of natural, technologic, and terrorist disasters. DHS assists state and local organizations to mitigate, prepare for, respond to, and recover from emergencies and is a major source of funding for these endeavors. Starting in 1992, the Federal Response Plan was used to coordinate federal assistance into 12 categories known as emergency support functions. Examples of emergency support functions include food, health and medical services, transportation, and communications. In 2003, the President of the United States directed that the DHS develop a National Incident Management System and a National Response Plan. Existing federal plans, including the Federal Response Plan, are being incorporated into the National Response Plan.

National Disaster Medical System

The National Disaster Medical System (NDMS) is a federally coordinated initiative designed to augment the emergency medical response capability of the United States in the event of a catastrophic disaster. This system is a cooperative program of four agencies in the federal government: (1) Department of Defense, (2) Department of Health and Human Services (HHS), (3) DHS, and (4) Department of Veterans Affairs (VA). DHS has the lead for the NDMS via FEMA. The NDMS provides an interstate medical mutual aid system linking the federal government, state and local agencies, and private sector institutions to address the medical needs of victims from catastrophic disasters. Its medical response element includes dozens of volunteer civilian disaster medical assistance teams that supplement the local medical infrastructure.

In a disaster, the NDMS is activated when state resources are overwhelmed and the governor makes a request for federal assistance. The disaster medical assistance teams must meet specific NDMS standards. Throughout the NDMS, emergency physicians are taking key roles in defining training standards, the deployment of clinical services, and the administration of field operations and in developing the concept of a civilian-federal disaster response capacity during national emergencies.[37]

Department of Veterans Affairs

The VA has not traditionally been regarded as a disaster response entity. However, one of VA's four mandated missions is emergency management. A unique feature of VA is that its facilities and personnel are situated nationwide, and these are used to support federal health and medical assistance to state and local governments during disasters. VA has highly trained specialty personnel that can support disaster medical activities. In addition to the vast pool of human resources, VA provides vast amounts of the pharmaceuticals and expendable supplies for on-site disaster support. Support is coordinated through DHS and HHS, as the lead federal agency for health and medical response.

Urban Search and Rescue

When a building collapses because of an earthquake, terrorist bombing, structural failure, or other reason, various challenges confront rescue and medical personnel.[38,39] Some victims require field amputations to facilitate extrication,[39] and use of urban search and rescue teams and effective emergency medical care is essential for successful lifesaving efforts.[40] This national system of multidisciplinary task forces is designed for rapid deployment to the sites of collapsed structures.[41,42] The medical team's responsibilities include caring for task force members, victims recovered by search and rescue activities, and the search team's dogs. There are now WMD-urban search and rescue teams trained by FEMA to respond to nuclear, biological, and chemical (NBC) terrorist attacks.

Centers for Disease Control and Prevention

The Centers for Disease Control and Prevention, based in Atlanta, is a U.S. federal agency under HHS. Its major responsibilities include preparing for and responding to public health emergencies (e.g., disasters) and conducting investigations into the health effects and medical consequences of these events. The major aims of the Centers for Disease Control and Prevention researchers are to assess the risks of death and injury and to develop strategies for preventing or mitigating the impact of future disasters. Other responsibilities of Centers for Disease Control and Prevention staff in the area of emergency preparedness and response include: (1) rapid assessment of the health and medical needs of disaster victims in the immediate post-disaster period; (2) development and maintenance of national systems for acute environmental hazard surveillance; and (3) provision of epidemiologic, sanitary, laboratory, and other relevant scientific support services to agencies involved in disaster planning and response.[43,44]

Metropolitan Medical Response Systems

Metropolitan Medical Strike Teams (MMSTs) are highly trained, readily deployable, and fully equipped groups of medical, fire, and rescue professionals. As a component of the larger Metropolitan Medical Response System, they support other local personnel in treating the victims of a chemical, biologic, or nuclear attack. At least 25 such teams are currently planned throughout the United States. Although composed of local personnel, MMSTs are under the direction of HHS. Their goal is to enhance local planning and response capability. However, hospital and community planners must still create an independent response because MMSTs require 90 minutes or longer to deploy.[45] MMSTs are equipped with chemical agent monitoring devices, protective equipment, and pharmaceutical supplies.

The Military

On April 17, 2002, Secretary of Defense Donald Rumsfeld announced the formation of the Northern Command, or NorthCom, to assume responsibility over all military forces that operate within the United States in response to external threats and in support of civil authorities. Furthermore, Secretary Rumsfeld stated that NorthCom will "help the department better deal with natural disasters, attacks on U.S. soil, or other civil difficulties. It will provide for a more coordinated military support to civil authorities such as FBI, FEMA and state and local governments."

FUTURE DIRECTIONS

The field of disaster medicine has become a major subspecialty within emergency medicine, and a section for disaster medicine has been organized within the American College of Emergency Physicians. There are also several national and international forums for the presentation of disaster medical research results. Since the American College of Emergency Physicians first defined a disaster medicine curriculum suitable for residencies and fellowships, a number of disaster medicine fellowships have been established in the United States. In the 21st century, disaster medicine will continue to develop as a professional activity in the United States.

KEY CONCEPTS

- The increasing likelihood of mass casualty incidents and high public expectations for an appropriate and timely response mandate careful and complete interagency planning.
- Mass casualty planning must account for the fact that traditional transport and communications systems will break down.
- Field personnel must be specifically trained in mass casualty triage and stabilization because austere field conditions change management strategies.
- All plans must protect caregivers and rescue personnel.
- Critical incident stress management may be highly desirable after an event and must be planned for in advance.
- Planners should establish and exercise a hospital-based incident management system.
- A plan must be in place to manage convergence of volunteers, address credentialing issues, and work with the media.

ACKNOWLEDGMENTS

The authors thank Connie J. Boatright, MSN, RN, Director, Education and Research, VA Emergency Management Strategic Healthcare Group (EMSHG); Peter W. Brewster, Emergency Preparedness Planning Specialist, EMSHG; and David S. Teeter, PharmD, Clinical Training Manager, EMSHG, for their assistance in writing and reviewing this manuscript.

REFERENCES

1. Waeckerle JF, et al: Executive summary: Developing objectives, content, and competencies for the training of emergency medical technicians, emergency physicians, and emergency nurses to care for casualties resulting from nuclear, biological, or chemical (NBC) incidents. *Ann Emerg Med* 37:587, 2001.
2. Bosner L, et al: Catastrophic events. In Kuehl AE (ed): *Prehospital Systems and Medical Oversight.* St. Louis, Mosby, 1994.
3. Koenig KL, Dinerman N, Kuehl AE: Disaster nomenclature: A functional impact approach: The PICE system. *Acad Emerg Med* 3:723, 1996. Available at http://www.homelandsecurity.org/journal/articles/displayArticle.asp?article=74.
4. Chaff L: Emergency preparedness. In *Safety Guide for Health Care Institutions,* 5th ed. Chicago, American Hospital Publishing, 1994.
5. Callum JR, Dinerman NM: Disaster preparedness. In Sheehy S (ed): *Emergency Nursing: Principles and Practice,* 3rd ed. St Louis, Mosby, 1992.
6. Aufderheide E: Resource management. In *Disaster Response: Principles of Preparation and Coordination.* St Louis, Mosby, 1989.
7. Koenig KL, Schultz CH: Disaster medicine: Advances in local catastrophic disaster-response. *Acad Emerg Med* 1:133, 1994.
8. Koenig KL: Triage: Do we need new concepts? [abstract] *Trauma Care* 13:44, 2003.
9. Waeckerle JF: Disaster planning and response. *N Engl J Med* 324:815, 1991.
10. Super G, et al: *START: Simple Triage and Rapid Treatment Plan.* Newport Beach, Calif, Hoag Memorial Hospital Presbyterian, 1994.
11. Benson M, Koenig KL, Schultz CH: Disaster triage: START then SAVE—a new method of dynamic triage for victims of a catastrophic earthquake. *Prehosp Disaster Med* 11:117, 1996.
12. Milzman DP, et al: Pre-existing disease in trauma patients: A predictor of fate independent of age and injury severity score. *J Trauma* 32:236, 1992.
13. Irwin RL: The incident command system (ICS). In Aufderheide E (ed): *Disaster Response: Principles of Preparation and Coordination.* St Louis, Mosby, 1989.
14. Schultz CH, Mothershead JL, Field M: Bioterrorism preparedness I: The emergency department and hospital. *Emerg Med Clin North Am* 20:437, 2002.
15. Joint Commission on the Accreditation of Healthcare Organizations: *Accreditation Manual for Hospitals.* Oak Brook Terrace, Ill, Joint Commission, 2001.
16. Schultz CH, Koenig KL, Lewis RJ: Implications of hospital evacuation after the Northridge, California, Earthquake. *N Engl J Med* 348:1349, 2003.
17. Kai T, Pretto E: Hospital preparedness in Osaka, Japan. *Prehosp Disaster Med* 8:S91, 1993.
18. Aufderheide E: *Community Medical and Hospital Disaster Planning Guidelines: An Interrogatory Format.* Dallas, American College of Emergency Physicians, 1995.
19. Drabek TE: *Emergency Management: The Human Factor.* Emmitsburg, Md, Federal Emergency Management Agency National Emergency Training Center, 1985.
20. The San Mateo County Health Services Agency: *Emergency Medical Services: Hospital Emergency Incident Command System,* 3rd ed. San Mateo, Calif, The San Mateo County Health Services Agency, 1998.
21. O'Neil K: Emergency department planning for hazardous materials victims: Getting started. *J Emerg Nurs* 20:41, 1994.
22. Estess PA, Angell LS: Watsonville Community Hospital responds to the 1989 Loma Prieta earthquake. *Plant Technol Safety Management Series* 2:21, 1990.
23. Cone DC, Weir SD, Bogucki S: Convergent volunteerism. *Ann Emerg Med* 41:457, 2003.
24. Earthquake Engineering Research Institute: *Northridge Earthquake: Preliminary Reconnaissance Report—January 17, 1994.* El Cerrito, Calif, The Institute, 1994.
25. Noji EK, Jones NP: Hospital preparedness for earthquakes. *Plant Technol Safety Manage Series* 2:13, 1990.
26. Pretto EA, et al: Disaster reanimatology potentials: A structured interview study in Armenia. III. Results, conclusions, and recommendations. *Prehosp Disaster Med* 7:327, 1992.
27. Noji EK: Evaluation of the efficacy of disaster response: Research at the Johns Hopkins University. *UNDRO News* July-August:11, 1987.
28. Schultz CH, Koenig KL, Noji EK: A medical disaster response to reduce immediate mortality following an earthquake. *N Engl J Med* 334:438, 1996.
29. Borak J, Callan M, Abbott W: *Hazardous Materials Exposure.* Englewood Cliffs, NJ, Brady, 1991.
30. Agency for Toxic Substances and Disease Registry: *Managing Hazardous Materials Incidents: Hospital Emergency Departments—A Planning Guide for the Management of Contaminated Patients, Atlanta, 1992.* Agency for Toxic Substances and Disease Registry.
31. Boodman SG: Health. *Washington Post,* Sept 13, 1994.
32. Koenig KL: Strip and shower: The duck and cover for the 21st century. *Ann Emerg Med* 42:391, 2003.
33. Mitchell J: When disaster strikes... the critical incident stress debriefing process. *J Emerg Med Serv* 8:36, 1983.
34. Burkle FM: Acute-phase mental health consequences of disasters: Implications for triage and emergency medical services. *Ann Emerg Med* 28:119, 1996.
35. Oster NS, Doyle CJ: Critical Incident Stress. In Hogan DE, Burstein JL (eds): *Disaster Medicine.* Philadelphia, Lippincott Williams & Wilkins, 2002.
36. Mitchell JT: Stress: The history, status and future of critical incident stress debriefings. *JEMS* 13:46, 1988.
37. Roth PB: Status of a national disaster medical response. *JAMA* 266:1266, 1991.
38. Kunkle RF: Medical care of entrapped patients in confined spaces. In *Proceedings of the International Workshop on Earthquake Injury Epidemiology: Implications for Mitigation and Response.* Baltimore, Johns Hopkins University, 1989.
39. Koenig KL, Schultz CH: The crush injury cadaver lab: A new method of training physicians to perform fasciotomies and amputations on survivors of a catastrophic earthquake [abstract]. *Ann Emerg Med* 21:613, 1992.
40. Noji EK: Medical consequences of earthquakes: Coordinating medical and rescue response. *Disaster Management* 4:32, 1991.
41. Better OS, Stein JH: Early management of shock and prophylaxis of acute renal failure in traumatic rhabdomyolysis. *N Engl J Med* 322:825, 1990.

42. Barbera JA, Lozano M: Urban search and rescue medical teams: FEMA task force system. *Prehosp Disaster Med* 8:349, 1993.
43. Patrick P, et al: The American Red Cross-Centers for Disease Control Natural Disaster Morbidity and Mortality Surveillance System [letter]. *Am J Public Health* 82:1690, 1992.
44. Noji EK: Role of the Centers for Disease Control in disaster preparedness and response [letter]. *Ann Emerg Med* 20:1397, 1991.
45. Institute of Medicine-National Research Council: *Chemical and Biological Terrorism: Research and Development to Improve Civilian Medical Response.* Washington, DC, National Academy Press, 1999.

CHAPTER

195 Weapons of Mass Destruction*

Carl H. Schultz and Kristi L. Koenig

PERSPECTIVE

The practice of emergency medicine now has another challenge: the possibility of an attack by terrorists using nuclear, biologic, chemical, or high-explosive weapons. Although conventional explosives remain the most common weapon used by terrorists, the risk from nuclear, biologic, and chemical agents will increase over time. The nomenclature for these weapons remains controversial. Some authors have proposed the use of *weapons of mass effect* or *weapons of mass disruption*. The military uses the acronym CBRNE, pronounced "see-burn-ee" and referring to *c*hemical, *b*iologic, *r*adiologic, *n*uclear, and *e*xplosive. This chapter uses *weapons of mass destruction* (WMD) because of its wide acceptance.

The results of an attack with WMD, although admittedly of low probability, are potentially catastrophic. According to a World Health Organization estimate, 50 kg of anthrax spores aerosolized above a city of 5 million people would result in 100,000 deaths, with an additional 150,000 people seriously infected. The cost of managing 100,000 cases of anthrax exposure is estimated at $26 billion by the Centers for Disease Control and Prevention (CDC).[1] Given these considerations, most authorities believe that preparedness for such threats must be improved.

Children are particularly vulnerable to these weapons. They breathe at a faster rate than adults, increasing their relative exposure to aerosolized agents. Some chemicals, such as sarin, are heavier than air, so tend to accumulate at the level where children are more likely to inhale them. Children have a greater surface area-to-volume ratio and their skin is thinner. This makes them more susceptible to agents that act on or through the skin. They have smaller fluid reserves and higher metabolic rates. Therefore, they are more vulnerable to dehydration from vomiting and diarrhea and suffer increased toxicity from a given exposure, such as to I^{131}.

The use of biologic and chemical agents dates back to biblical times, although the threat from radiation and nuclear detonation is relatively new. Assyrians poisoned the wells of their enemies using rye ergot in the 6th century BC. The Mongols catapulted bodies infected with bubonic plague over the walls of Caffa in the 14th century. A British officer proposed giving American Indians blankets taken from individuals infected with smallpox during Pontiac's Rebellion in 1763. During World War I, the Germans effectively used chlorine and mustard agent against the advancing Allied armies. The Japanese killed hundreds to thousands of Chinese citizens with bubonic plague during World War II by spraying towns with fleas infected with *Yersinia pestis.* Saddam Hussein employed mustard agent against the Iranians during the 1980s' Iran-Iraq War.

The use of WMD has been predominantly by the military during times of conflict. Recently, however, the use of these agents has taken an ominous turn. Nonaffiliated groups have begun using WMD directed at civilians to achieve political ends. The Bhagwan cult sprayed salad bars in Oregon with *Salmonella* in an attempt to influence an election in 1984.[2] The Aum Shinrikyo used the nerve agent sarin in an unsuccessful 1994 assassination attempt on three judges in Matsumoto, Japan. This same group used sarin again in the 1995 Tokyo subway attack that killed 11 people.[3] The United States experienced multiple anthrax hoaxes during 1997 and 1998, motivated by personal or political agendas. An actual anthrax attack using the U.S. mail occurred in the fall of 2001 and resulted in 11 deaths. The perpetrator's identity and motivation remain unknown. No one has yet used radiologic or nuclear devices in a successful terrorist attack, but at least one attempt has occurred. In addition, several highly radioactive sources have been stolen from U.S. medical facilities.

Many agents are potential candidates for weaponization, and some represent a substantial risk (Box 195-1).

*The views expressed in this chapter do not necessarily represent the views of the Department of Veterans Affairs or of the United States Government.

Management strategies for patients exposed to WMD are frequently similar to strategies for hazardous materials exposure. However, several features associated with WMD make these events unique (Box 195-2). Additional knowledge and skills are required in the evaluation and treatment of WMD victims. These plans represent only one small part of an overall comprehensive emergency management strategy for all hazards (see Chapter 194). A list of departments, bureaus, and agencies that can assist with planning and response to WMD events are listed in Table 195-1.

NUCLEAR AND RADIOLOGIC DEVICES

Terrorists selecting radiation as a means to inflict casualties are unlikely to employ nuclear weapons. These devices are heavily guarded, difficult to move due to their size and weight, and easy to detect. Although Russia acknowledges that 50 to 100 of its 1-kiloton "suitcase" nuclear weapons are missing, the problems of purchasing, moving, and detonating these devices are formidable. Sabotage at nuclear power stations is possible, but given tight security, multiple safety systems, and thick concrete housings surrounding the reactors, the threat is probably low.

Instead, simple radiologic devices, such as those used by hospitals for radiation therapy, are thought to be the source of choice. These sources are plentiful. They do not detonate on their own and give no warning of their presence, unless dispersed by a conventional explosive (radiologic dispersal device). Thefts of radiotherapy sources have occurred in the United States. Accidental dispersion from a stolen hospital therapy source in Brazil resulted in the screening of 112,000 people for contamination and found 249 exposed persons. Four ultimately died.[7] Placement of such a device at an information kiosk in a crowded mall during a busy holiday shopping season would silently expose countless persons to significant radiation.

Ionizing radiation, regardless of its type, causes injury at the cellular level, usually by damaging DNA. Rapidly dividing cells are the most sensitive. Patients develop symptoms within hours to days, depending on the dose. Common syndromes associated with radiation exposure include dermal burns, bone marrow failure, and gastrointestinal dysfunction (e.g., vomiting, gastrointestinal bleeding) (see Chapter 144). A U.S. Department of Homeland Security task force developed an expert consensus document on medical treatment of radiologic casualties.[4]

A basic emergency department radiation protocol must address decontamination, triage, staff safety, personal protective equipment (PPE), and diagnostic procedures that emphasize radiation monitoring. Victims presenting to the emergency department will suffer from three types of exposure: irradiation, internal contamination, and external contamination. Irradiated victims have been exposed to a beam of radiation, similar to someone undergoing a chest x-ray. They are not radioactive and pose no threat to emergency department personnel.

Contaminated patients are more problematic, and early involvement of the radiation safety officer is critical. This individual evaluates the degree of the victim's contamination and monitors radioactivity levels throughout the decontamination process. Inter-

BOX 195-1. Agents Currently Considered Likely Candidates for Use in Weapons of Mass Destruction

Chemical
Nerve agents
- Sarin
- Soman
- Tabun
- VX

Mustard agent

Biologic
Anthrax
Plague
Smallpox

Radiologic
Simple device
Dispersal device

BOX 195-2. Features of Weapons of Mass Destruction Threat

Fear
Lack of training for hospital personnel
Lack of equipment, including personal protection and diagnostic aids
Potential for mass casualties
Psychologic casualties
Crime scene requiring evidence collection and interaction with FBI
Potential for ongoing morbidity and mortality (dynamic situation)

Table 195-1. Resources and Contacts for Planning and Response to Events Involving Weapons of Mass Destruction

Organization	Website	Telephone
The Radiation Emergency Assistance Center/Training Site (REAC/TS)	www.orau.gov/reacts	865-576-3131
State and local health departments	www.statepublichealth.org/index.php www.cdc.gov/other.htm#states	
Centers for Disease Control and Prevention (CDC)	www.bt.cdc.gov	770-488-7100
Federal Bureau of Investigation (FBI)	www.fbi.gov	
Federal Emergency Management Agency (FEMA)	www.fema.gov	202-646-4600
U.S. Army Medical Research Institute of Chemical Defense	www.chemdef.apgea.army.mil/	

nally contaminated patients present a therapeutic challenge because they have radioactive material inside their bodies (lungs, gastrointestinal tract) or incorporated into their cells. They should be placed in an isolation room, where all secretions and bodily fluids can be collected. Various medications are available for administration to internally contaminated patients and can limit uptake or facilitate removal of certain radioactive elements. These medications include Radiogardase (Prussian blue) for cesium and thallium ingestions and diethylenetriamine pentaacetic acid (DTPA) for plutonium exposure. Health care providers can receive assistance by calling the Radiation Emergency Assistance Center/Training Site (REAC/TS) at 865-576-3131.

Externally contaminated victims have radioactive material on their skin or clothing and are decontaminated by removal of clothing and washing with soap and water. Washing by protected personnel must continue until monitoring by the radiation safety officer demonstrates absence of radioactivity. If present, wounds are decontaminated first. After the wounds are covered with a sterile, waterproof dressing, the remaining skin is washed. Hospitals must be prepared to decontaminate patients, because historical data suggest that up to 80% of patients do not receive this intervention before arrival.[2] Decontamination before hospital entry is crucial, because these individuals can expose caregivers to radiation and contaminate the entire hospital through the ventilation system. In such cases, decontamination takes precedence over emergency care. Removal of clothing and covering the head with a surgical cap can reduce contamination by 80% to permit stabilization in the decontamination unit, but complete decontamination should occur before exposure of unprotected staff to the patient.

Initial triage of radiation casualties is based on their overall pathologic condition, not on exposure. Even patients who have received a lethal dose of radiation do not die immediately. Therefore, a patient in acute distress from a myocardial infarction or urosepsis would be triaged ahead of a radiation victim with stable vital signs, regardless of the dose received. If a radiation casualty also suffers a severe injury or illness, immediate intervention is required. For example, most morbidity and mortality related to a radiologic dispersion device would be related to traumatic injuries from the explosion and not to radiation exposure.

In addition to patient contamination, the radiation safety officer is responsible for monitoring the exposure of hospital staff. All personnel involved in the care of contaminated patients should wear dosimeters, which measure the amount of radiation received by the wearer. The safety officer tracks the amount of radiation received by each staff member and can remove a health care worker from the area if the exposure is too high. Radiation monitoring is complex, and the radiation safety officer should be involved as early as possible. Hospitals should consider conducting disaster drills that include casualties suffering radiation injuries.

Although many radioactive elements are candidates for use in a terrorist attack, radioactive iodine (^{131}I) and related isotopes deserve additional discussion because of heightened interest. ^{131}I is found only after a nuclear detonation or in reactor fuel rods. While not impossible, the probability that terrorists could tap either of these sources is very small. The use of ^{131}I in a radiologic dispersal device is very unlikely, owing to its short half-life (8 days). Even if such a device could be made, it is extremely unlikely that the radiologic dispersal device could disperse sufficient radioactive material to pose an immediate health hazard.[5] Given these facts, the probability that any significant exposure of the population (especially children) to ^{131}I will occur is equally small. The large number of childhood thyroid cancers that occurred after the accident at the Chernobyl nuclear power plant was due mostly to situations that will not occur in the United States. These include delayed reporting of a breach in the reactor containment vessel preventing timely evacuation, failure to quarantine contaminated milk and vegetables, and significant iodine deficiency in the exposed children.[6] Nonetheless, concern regarding treatment to prevent thyroid cancer after potential exposure to ^{131}I remains. Current recommendations for treatment with potassium iodide, which blocks uptake of ^{131}I by the thyroid, are listed in Table 195-2. Caveats for using this table include increasing the amount of potassium iodide for adolescents approaching 70 kg to the adult dose (130 mg), and monitoring thyroid-stimulating hormone and free T_4 levels in neonates when possible. Nonpregnant adults older than 40 years are unlikely to benefit from this intervention.

BIOLOGIC WEAPONS

By convention, biologic weapons are divided into three groups: bacteria, viruses, and toxins. A characteristic shared by these agents is their ability to be dispersed

Table 195-2. Treatment with Potassium Iodide (KI) for Radioactive Iodine Exposure

Subpopulation	Predicted Exposure (rad)	KI Dose (mg)	Number of 130 mg Tablets
Adults >40 years	≥500	130	1
Adults 18–40 years	≥10	130	1
Pregnant/lactating women	≥5	130	1
Children 3–18 years	≥5	65	½
Children 1 month–3 years	≥5	32	¼
Neonates, birth–1 month	≥5	16	⅛

as an aerosol. Since this is the most effective means to expose a large population, aerosol dispersal is the most likely route that terrorists will use to deploy such weapons. Therefore, victims will have respiratory signs and symptoms. Dermal contact and ingestion are also potential pathways for exposure, and some agents are effective by these routes. People infected in the 2001 U.S. anthrax attack were inoculated via aerosol and dermal exposures. However, it is logistically more difficult to produce large casualty numbers using nonrespiratory portals of entry, so agents spread primarily by injection or through the gastrointestinal tract are less likely candidates for wide deployment. If the goal is to disrupt the economy or spread fear among the population, then almost any type of release will suffice, whether or not people actually die.

Patients exposed to biologic agents usually present with vague symptoms associated with flulike illnesses. Unless a biologic attack is announced or suspected, the emergency department staff may not realize they are treating victims. Indeed, it is not always possible to distinguish naturally occurring from engineered outbreaks of diseases. Therefore, personnel must be vigilant and at least consider the possibility of a bioweapon exposure when warning signs are present (Box 195-3). For example, large numbers of patients suddenly presenting with the "flu" not during flu season should cause concern. For these reasons, health surveillance will be paramount in identifying agents and potential sources. The emergency department must have a working relationship with local and state health departments as well as local law enforcement and stay appraised of CDC guidelines.

Several infectious agents with potential for use as biologic weapons can spread in a hospital environment. Examples include Ebola and smallpox.[2,7] Hospitals need protocols for PPE and patient isolation to ensure a safe environment. Fortunately, such protocols are similar to those applied to other infectious diseases (Box 195-4). Implementation of such precautions is credited with halting the in-hospital spread of the Ebola virus in the 1995 Zaire outbreak. Decontamination is not a priority unless the exposure is immediate. Standard (universal) precautions are generally sufficient, and special suits (e.g., levels A, B, and C) are unnecessary.[8]

Current assessment suggests that three biologic agents—anthrax, plague, and smallpox—represent the greatest threat.

Anthrax

Bacillus anthracis, a gram-positive spore-forming bacterium, is the causative agent of anthrax ("woolsorters' disease"). The spores are extremely hardy and can survive for years in the environment. The disease is caused by exposure to the spores, not the bacilli in their vegetative state. It is normally a disease of sheep, cattle, and horses and is rarely seen in developed countries because of animal and human vaccination programs. Disease in humans can occur when spores are inhaled, ingested, or inoculated into the skin. The spores germinate into bacilli inside macrophages. The bacteria then produce disease by releasing toxins (protective antigen, edema factor, and lethal factor) that cause edema and cell death.

Russia and the United States have successfully developed anthrax into a biologic weapon. The effectiveness of this agent was clearly demonstrated by two events: an accidental release of spores from a biologic weapons facility in the former Soviet Union town of Sverdlovsk in 1979 and the intentional distribution of anthrax spores through the mail along the eastern seaboard of the United States in 2001. After the Sverdlovsk release, at least 66 people died downwind from the compound during the next several weeks, and animal cases of anthrax were reported 30 miles away.[9,10] The ability of non-state-sponsored terrorist groups to develop anthrax as a weapon is uncertain. The Japanese organization Aum Shinrikyo made several attempts to disperse anthrax throughout Tokyo without success.[1] The perpetrator of the U.S. anthrax attack remains unidentified. However, many experts speculate that this individual was not a foreign national, given that the strain of anthrax used in the attack (Ames strain) was developed by the U.S. government.

Inhalational anthrax is the most lethal form of the disease and is caused by inhaling spores into the lungs. The mortality rate was thought to exceed 90%. However, the data from the 2001 anthrax exposure calls this figure into question (5 deaths in 11 cases). Although the actual mortality rate is unknown, it is probably in the 50% range.[11,12] The minimum number

BOX 195-3. Signs Suggesting Biologic Weapon Deployment

Syndromes
Pulmonary symptoms
Rashes
Sepsis syndrome
Influenza symptoms

Epidemiology
Multiple, simultaneous events
Dead animals
Large patient numbers with high toxicity and death rate

BOX 195-4. Recommendations for Prevention of In-Hospital Transmission of Contagious Agents

1. Isolate patient in single room with adjoining anteroom.
2. Have handwashing facilities and personal protective equipment (PPE) available in anteroom.
3. Use negative air pressure if possible.
4. Use strict barrier precautions: PPE, gowns, gloves, HEPA filter masks, shoe covers, protective eyewear.
5. Alert hospital departments that generate aerosols: laboratory (centrifuges), pathology (autopsies).

of spores required to produce disease is currently unknown. The original number quoted in the literature, 10^4 spores, appears high given recent experience.[13] After phagocytosis by macrophages, the spores germinate and are transported to the tracheobronchial lymph nodes, where the bacteria multiply. Over 2 to 10 days, patients develop a flulike illness, with malaise, fever, and nonproductive cough. This initial phase can be delayed for more than a month in some patients. Within 24 to 48 hours, abrupt deterioration occurs, with overwhelming sepsis, shock, hemorrhagic mediastinitis, dyspnea, and stridor. A chest radiograph obtained at this time may show a widened mediastinum and hilar adenopathy, but typical radiographic findings are not dramatic and could be missed (Figure 195-1). Computed tomography scanning of the chest is more sensitive and should be performed if the disease is suspected. Bloody pleural effusions can also occur, and examination of the lung fields frequently reveals consolidation. This can easily be confused with pneumonia (Figure 195-2). Death usually results within 3 days, and 50% of patients develop hemorrhagic meningitis. Human-to-human transmission has not been reported with inhalational anthrax.

Initial diagnosis is generally made clinically, based on a flulike or septic illness, a suspicious chest radiograph or computed tomography scan demonstrating hilar adenopathy, infiltrates, or pleural effusions, and a reason to consider anthrax in the first place (e.g., current outbreak, warning from authorities). Several clinical algorithms exist that attempt to separate patients with influenza from those with anthrax.[14,15] Unfortunately, they are based on a handful of anthrax cases, and their usefulness remains in doubt.[12] Sputum culture, Gram stain, and blood cultures are not helpful until late in the course of the disease. Tests to confirm the diagnosis of inhalational anthrax include the polymerase chain reaction for identification of anthrax markers in pleural fluid, serologic detection of immunoglobulin to protective antigen, and immunohistochemical testing of biopsy specimens.

In addition to inhalational anthrax, dermatologic anthrax can occur in any area where large numbers of spores are released, as was the case in the United States in 2001. This form of the disease occurs when spores are introduced into the skin, usually through open wounds or abrasions. The mortality rate is approximately 20% without treatment and 1% with treatment. Antibiotics do not affect the course of local disease but are used to prevent dissemination and death. After an incubation period of 1 to 5 days, a papule develops, progressing to form a large vesicle over the next several days. Severe edema occurs around the lesion and is associated with regional lymphadenitis. The lesions are not tender, and the patient may or may not be febrile (Figure 195-3). After about 1 week, the lesion ruptures, forming a black eschar (thus the name *anthrax,* Greek for "coal"). In the next 2 to 3 weeks, either the eschar sloughs off and the illness is over, or the organism disseminates and the patient dies. As with inhalational anthrax, the diagnosis is predominantly clinical. Confirmation is established by culturing of the lesion, punch biopsy, or serologic testing. A total of 11 cutaneous anthrax cases occurred in the United States after the 2001 attack.[16]

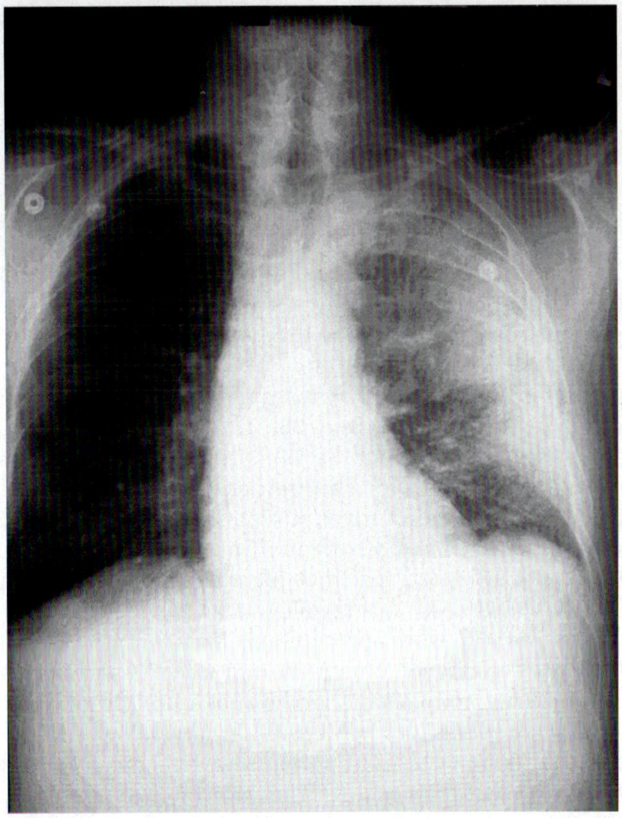

Figure 195-1. Chest radiograph of anthrax patient showing diffuse left lung consolidation consistent with pneumonia. There is no mediastinal widening. (Courtesy of the U.S. Centers for Disease Control and Prevention.)

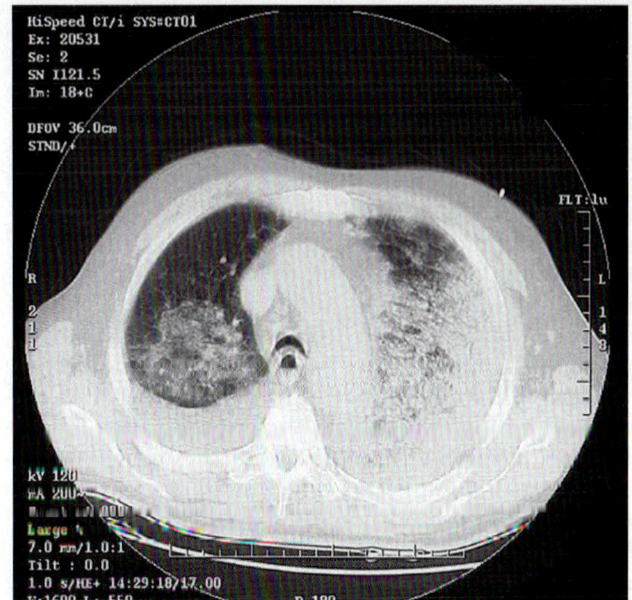

Figure 195-2. Chest computed tomography scan of an anthrax patient showing pulmonary consolidation and effusions. (Courtesy of the U.S. Centers for Disease Control and Prevention.)

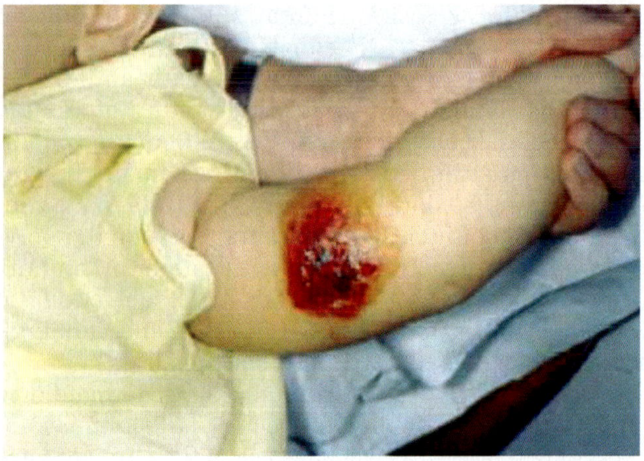

Figure 195-3. Child with cutaneous anthrax. (From Roche KJ, Chang MW, Lazarus H: Images in clinical medicine: Cutaneous anthrax infection. *N Engl J Med* 345:1611, 2001.)

A few cases of gastrointestinal anthrax and oropharyngeal anthrax are also likely after a terrorist attack. These rare manifestations usually occur with the ingestion of insufficiently cooked, contaminated meat. The mortality rate is approximately 50%. After ingestion, the spores are transported to regional lymphatic tissue, where symptoms develop after a 2- to 5-day incubation period. Patients with oropharyngeal anthrax present with sore throat and neck swelling from cervical and submandibular lymphadenitis. The tonsils also are frequently involved, and symptoms are associated with fever and toxicity. Dysphagia and respiratory distress often follow. Gastrointestinal anthrax begins with nausea, vomiting, and fever associated with mesenteric lymphadenitis. Patients then experience severe abdominal pain, hematemesis, ascites, and bloody diarrhea and may present with an acute abdomen.

BOX 195-5. Treatment for Anthrax

Cutaneous Anthrax *without* Toxicity

Adults	Ciprofloxacin, 500 mg PO bid
	or
	Doxycycline, 100 mg PO bid
	or
	Amoxicillin, 500 mg PO tid
Children	Ciprofloxacin, 20–30 mg/kg/day PO divided bid (max 1 g)
	or
	Doxycycline, 4.4 mg/kg/day PO divided bid (max 200 mg)
	or
	Amoxicillin, 20-40 mg/kg/day PO divided tid (max 1500 mg)

All doses given for 7-10 days.

Inhalational, Cutaneous, or Gastrointestinal Anthrax *with* Toxicity

Adults	Ciprofloxacin, 400 mg IV q12h
	or
	Doxycycline, 100 mg IV q12h
	or
	Penicillin G, 4 million units IV q4h
Children	Ciprofloxacin, 20–30 mg/kg/day IV divided q12h (max 1 g)
	or
	Doxycycline, 4.4 mg/kg/day IV divided q12h (max 200 mg)
	or
	Penicillin G, 100,000-400,000 U/kg/day IV divided q4h (max 24×10^6)

All doses given until toxicity resolves. Then switch to oral form. Treat for 60 days or until patient receives three doses of vaccine.

Postexposure Prophylaxis

Same drugs and dosage as for cutaneous anthrax *without* toxicity. Treat for 60 days or until patient receives three doses of vaccine.

Treatment

Traditional treatment for anthrax infection has been penicillin. However, weapons-grade anthrax is probably resistant to penicillin (although this was not the case with the U.S. attack). Current treatment recommendations reflect this fact (Box 195-5).[1,2] These consensus recommendations include fluoroquinolones and tetracycline for all children, regardless of age. Balancing the potential risks of such drugs against the consequences of infection by drug-resistant anthrax strains, the benefits justify the recommendations. Nontoxic victims with cutaneous anthrax can be treated as outpatients with oral ciprofloxacin or doxycycline for 7 to 10 days. Victims with inhalational, cutaneous, or gastrointestinal disease and toxicity require intravenous therapy with ciprofloxacin or doxycycline plus at least two other antibiotics (such as rifampin, clindamycin, imipenem, or an aminoglycoside). Patients can be switched to oral antibiotics when toxicity resolves. Other modalities that may be helpful include chest tube drainage of pleural effusions and possibly tracheal intubation and mechanical ventilation.[16] Surprisingly, the latter intervention did not improve mortality. All patients intubated after the U.S. anthrax attack died.[11,13]

Treatment must continue for 60 days or until the patient has received three doses of the anthrax vaccine, given on days 0, 14, and 28. The complete vaccine course requires 18 months. This treatment regimen is also recommended for children and pregnant women. If the anthrax strain proves susceptible, patients can be switched to intravenous penicillin or oral amoxicillin. In vitro studies suggest that ofloxacin or levofloxacin can be substituted for ciprofloxacin.[1]

For postexposure prophylaxis, oral ciprofloxacin (500 mg) or doxycycline (100 mg) twice a day is recommended. Amoxicillin can be substituted if sensitive strains are identified. Antibiotic prophylaxis must continue for 60 days or until patients have received at least three doses of the vaccine. The vaccine is approved by the U.S. Food and Drug Administration for adults but not for children. A recent review by the Institute of Medicine found the vaccine both safe and effective for prophylaxis against inhalational anthrax.[17]

Plague

Plague has been a human pathogen since antiquity. Many regions of the world, including Asia and India, are currently witnessing the third pandemic of plague, and this affliction is endemic in the western half of the United States. Plague is caused by *Yersinia pestis*, a gram-negative bacillus. It is normally a disease of rodents that is transmitted to humans through the bite of an infected flea or by inhalation. Three forms of the disease exist: pneumonic, bubonic, and septicemic plague. The bacteria do not form spores and die rapidly in the environment. However, they are viable for days in dry sputum, flea feces, and human remains. Dogs are relatively resistant to infection, but cats are highly susceptible and could form a reservoir for maintaining the disease in a human population. Recovery is followed by temporary immunity.

Primary pneumonic plague results when bacilli are inhaled into the lungs. It has a mortality rate approaching 100% if not treated early. Pneumonic plague will be the most frequently encountered form of the disease, since terrorists are likely to use aerosolization as the method of dispersal. After an incubation period of 2 to 3 days, victims develop sudden onset of fever, chills, and a flulike illness. This is followed within 24 hours by a fulminant pneumonia associated with hemoptysis, systemic toxicity, respiratory failure, circulatory collapse, and death. The pneumonia is classically lobar, but any x-ray pattern is possible, including acute respiratory distress syndrome. Six to 10% of victims develop plague meningitis. Coagulation abnormalities and hepatocellular injury occur. The coagulopathy is characterized by ecchymoses, disseminated intravascular coagulation, and acral gangrene ("black death"). The gangrene is caused by bacterial production of the coagulase enzyme in areas of the body where the temperature drops below 37° C. This causes blood to clot in fingers, toes, and the nose, with resultant infarction and gangrene. If the victims survive, long-term rehabilitation is required. Pneumonic plague is transmissible human to human.

Bubonic plague occurs when organisms are inoculated into the skin, usually from a flea bite. During the 2- to 3-day incubation period, the bacilli migrate to regional lymph nodes, where they multiply and cause inflammation and necrosis of lymphatic tissue, resulting in large, tender nodes, or buboes. Typically, buboes develop in the groin, axilla, or cervical region and are so painful that the patient will refrain from moving the affected area (Figure 195-4). Individuals experience fever, chills, and weakness. In approximately 25% of patients, vesicles or ulcerations occur at the site of the flea bite. The buboes are usually nonfluctuant but rarely can suppurate. Organisms can be aspirated from the nodes for diagnosis, but incision and drainage is not recommended because the lymphadenitis resolves with antibiotic treatment, and practitioners could become infected if exposed during the procedure.

Over the next week or more, the bacteria disseminate in approximately 50% of patients with bubonic plague. These victims develop septicemic plague or secondary

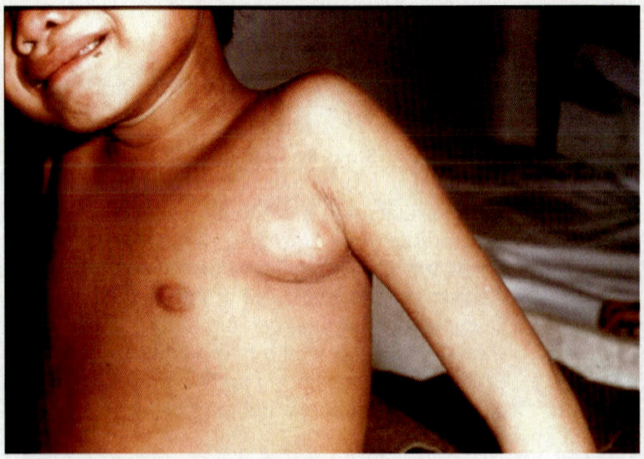

Figure 195-4. Child with bubonic plague demonstrating axillary bubo. (Courtesy of Frederick M. Burkle, Jr., MD, MPH.)

pneumonic plague and die if untreated. Those with septicemic plague experience endotoxemia, shock, disseminated intravascular coagulation, and coma. If bacteremia does not occur, most victims recover. A small percentage of those infected by fleas develop septicemic plague without detectable buboes. Direct human-to-human transmission does not occur with bubonic or septicemic plague. However, both these conditions can lead to secondary pneumonic plague, which is communicable. Therefore, initial isolation is recommended for all patients with plague.

Differential Diagnosis

The preliminary diagnosis of plague is clinical. Few diseases other than plague cause fulminant gram-negative pneumonia associated with hemoptysis in previously healthy individuals. The same can be said for diseases that cause lymphadenopathy. Cat-scratch disease, tularemia, and staphylococcal or streptococcal infections are all in the differential diagnosis. However, the extremely tender nature of the lymphadenopathy and the toxicity of the patient strongly suggest plague. Once the disease is suspected, Gram stain and culture of sputum, blood, cerebrospinal fluid, or lymph node aspirate are helpful. State health departments or the CDC can test specimens for the presence of the capsular antigen using direct fluorescent antibody staining. Polymerase chain reaction also holds promise. Unfortunately, all laboratory tests require several days to complete, so initial management decisions must be based on clinical findings.

Treatment

Antibiotic treatment is essentially the same for all three types of plague (Box 195-6).[18] The same caveats for the use of fluoroquinolones and tetracycline in children with anthrax also apply to plague. In the case of pneumonic and septicemic plague, treatment must be started within 24 hours of symptoms to improve outcome. Antibiotics are given for a minimum of 10 days. As patients improve, oral antibiotics are substi-

BOX 195-6. Treatment for Plague

Parenteral Therapy

Adults	Streptomycin, 1 g IM bid
	Gentamicin, 5 mg/kg once daily IM or IV
	Doxycycline, 100 mg IV bid
	Ciprofloxacin, 400 mg IV bid
	Chloramphenicol, 25 mg/kg IV qid
Children	Streptomycin, 15 mg/kg IM bid (max 2 g/day)
	Gentamicin, 2.5 mg/kg IM or IV tid
	Doxycycline, 2.2 mg/kg IV bid (max 200 mg/day)
	Ciprofloxacin, 15 mg/kg IV bid (max 1 g/day)
	Chloramphenicol, 25 mg/kg IV qid

Pregnant women: same as above but exclude streptomycin and chloramphenicol.

Oral Therapy

Adults	Doxycycline, 100 mg bid
	Ciprofloxacin, 500 mg bid
	Chloramphenicol, 25 mg/kg qid
Children	Doxycycline, 2.2 mg/kg bid (max 200 mg/day)
	Ciprofloxacin, 15 mg/kg bid (max 1 g/day)
	Chloramphenicol, 25 mg/kg qid

Pregnant women: same as above but exclude chloramphenicol.

tuted for intravenous therapy to complete the course. Respiratory isolation of patients with pneumonic plague is necessary for 4 days after beginning antibiotics to guarantee sterilization of sputum. Patients with septicemic and bubonic plague require isolation for 48 hours. If they do not develop pneumonia or draining lesions during this time, isolation can be discontinued. Nonseptic patients with mild bubonic plague can be treated at home with oral doxycycline or tetracycline for 10 days.

The mainstay of prophylaxis against plague remains oral antibiotics. A vaccine exists but has no value in an acute outbreak. It is effective only against bubonic disease and requires several months to impart immunity. The drugs for prophylaxis are tetracycline, doxycycline, ciprofloxacin, chloramphenicol, and possibly trimethoprim-sulfamethoxazole for children. The doses are the same as those listed in Box 195-5, except the duration of treatment is 7 days, not up to 10 days. Levofloxacin and ofloxacin can be substituted for ciprofloxacin.

Smallpox

Smallpox was eradicated in 1980 as a naturally occurring disease. The only known repositories of the variola virus, the etiologic agent of smallpox, are in the United States and Russia. However, the Russians were successful in weaponizing the virus, which may have been sold or smuggled out of the country.[7] The effectiveness of their weaponized strain was demonstrated in 1971, when an individual became infected while traveling on a ship 15 km downwind from a Soviet bioweapons test site (Vozrozhdeniye Island in the Aral Sea).[19] In addition, most of the world's population is no longer immune to infection because vaccination against small-

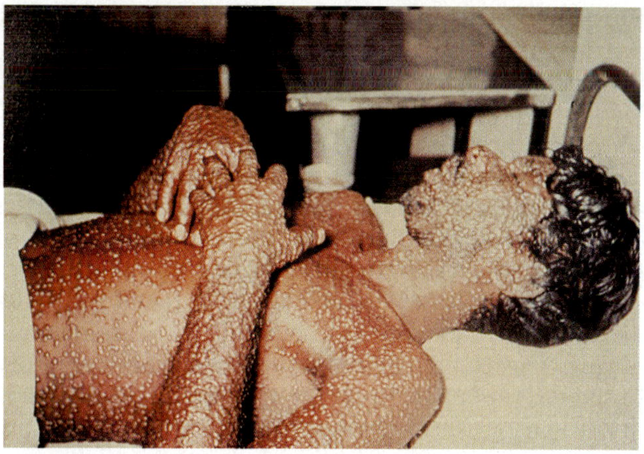

Figure 195-5. Man with smallpox. (From the U.S. Centers for Disease Control and Prevention Public Health Image Library. http://phil.cdc.gov/phil/detail.asp?id=131.)

pox ceased 20 years ago. Given its high infectivity and lethality, this makes smallpox an excellent biologic weapon.

The variola virus is spread as an aerosol. It can survive for 24 hours, possibly 48 hours, in the environment. The occurrence of smallpox in hospital employees whose only exposure was handling laundry from infected persons is testimony to its viability. Approximately 30% of exposed persons become ill. One infected person has the potential to infect up to 20 other individuals. Persons are infectious from the time the rash first appears until the scabs fall off (1-2 weeks). Anyone exposed to smallpox must be observed for 17 days to rule out infection.

The disease manifests clinically in several forms. Variola major and variola minor represent 90% of the cases. Variola major is the classic form, a more severe illness with a mortality rate of 30%. Variola minor is a milder form, with less toxicity, fewer pox, and a mortality rate of 1%. Two other forms of the disease, hemorrhagic and malignant (or flat) smallpox, are seen in 10% of cases; the mortality rate is greater than 90%. Patients with hemorrhagic smallpox develop symptoms earlier and become toxic quickly. Instead of pox, their rash is characterized by petechiae and hemorrhage. Death occurs in 5 to 6 days. Those with malignant smallpox have a similar course, but their rash is characterized by soft, flattened lesions that never progress to pustules. If they survive, the lesions resolve without forming scabs.

The infection begins when the virus is inhaled. After migrating to regional lymph nodes, the virus replicates for 3 to 4 days, then asymptomatically spreads to the spleen, bone marrow, other lymphoid tissue, and liver. A second viremia occurs 8 to 12 days later and is associated with fever, prostration, and headache. Mental status changes can occur. During this phase, lasting 2 to 3 days, the virus localizes to the skin and pharyngeal mucosa. A maculopapular rash soon appears, which becomes vesicular and finally pustular. The rash first appears on the face and forearms, later spreading to the legs and trunk. All the lesions in any one area of the body are the same age (Figure 195-5). Over the next

8 to 14 days, the pustules crust over and separate from the skin, leaving pitted scars.

A clinical algorithm developed by the CDC can assist in assessing the probability that an individual has smallpox. It relies on three major and five minor criteria. The major criteria are a febrile prodrome, classic smallpox lesions, and lesions in the same stage of development. The minor criteria are centrifugal distribution of pustules; first lesions on the oral mucosa, face, or forearms; toxic appearance; slow evolution of lesions; and pustules on the palms and soles. A patient with all three major criteria is at high risk and should be isolated and reported immediately. Patients with the febrile prodrome and either four minor criteria or one other major criteria are at moderate risk. Consultation with infectious disease and dermatology specialists should be sought and tests ordered to confirm varicella. If smallpox cannot be ruled out after these interventions, the patient should be treated as high risk. If a patient does not have the febrile prodrome or has the prodrome but no other major criteria and has fewer than four minor criteria, the individual is at low risk for smallpox. These patients can be managed as clinically indicated.[20]

Differential Diagnosis

As with anthrax and plague, the initial diagnosis of smallpox is clinical. The other illnesses resembling smallpox include chickenpox, herpes simplex, and monkeypox (now in the differential diagnosis because of a recent outbreak in the Midwest). Unlike variola, the rash associated with chickenpox (varicella) is seen first on the trunk, then spreads to the extremities and face. In addition, the pustules are in different stages of evolution in any one area of the body. If the first case seen is hemorrhagic or malignant smallpox, the diagnosis will probably be missed until more typical cases present. To confirm the diagnosis, vesicular fluid or scabs were traditionally sent for electron microscopic examination. Now, polymerase chain reaction techniques appear promising for rapid viral identification, with sensitivities and specificities in the 96% to 99% range.[21]

Treatment

No effective therapy currently exists for victims infected with smallpox who become symptomatic. However, potential antiviral agents, such as cidofovir, show promise. In mice exposed to a lethal cowpox challenge, administration of an oral lipid prodrug of cidofovir in modest doses once a day for 5 days produced 100% survival.[22] Vaccinia immunoglobulin (VIG) has no role in the treatment of active disease. Some practitioners suggest that most smallpox patients should be isolated at home or other nonhospital facilities, since the virus spreads easily in a hospital environment and the disease is currently untreatable.[7]

The best strategy for containing the disease is vaccination of the susceptible population. Vaccinating an immunocompetent individual within 3 days of exposure will prevent or significantly ameliorate illness. Vaccination up to 7 days may prevent death. Complications from vaccination with vaccinia virus occur and can be fatal. Groups at risk for these adverse consequences include pregnant women and those with eczema, human immunodeficiency virus infection, and immunosuppressive conditions (e.g., malignancy, steroid administration, hereditary immunodeficiencies). Given the seriousness of the disease, the current recommendation is to vaccinate these individuals and simultaneously administer 0.3 mg/kg of VIG intramuscularly. For persons developing complications from the vaccine (e.g., progressive vaccinia, ocular autoinoculation, eczema vaccinatum), the dose of VIG is 0.6 mg/kg IM and is divided over 24 to 36 hours. Ribavirin can be administered but is considered experimental. VIG is not indicated for vaccinia-associated encephalitis.

The smallpox vaccine supply situation has improved dramatically in the United States. The CDC now has 100 million doses of the traditional smallpox vaccine (Dryvax). These vials can be diluted 5:1 to produce a total of 500 million doses without any decrement in the vaccine's efficacy.[23] In early 2004, a British company delivered an additional 209 million doses of a second-generation vaccine derived from the same vaccinia virus used in Dryvax but grown in cell cultures. In addition, work is commencing on production of an improved modified vaccinia ankara vaccine. The virus used in the modified vaccinia ankara vaccine is so attenuated, it does not replicate in a human host. Officials hope this will make it safe for administration to immunocompromised individuals.

CHEMICAL WEAPONS

Unlike victims of biologic weapons, casualties exposed to chemical agents manifest symptoms quickly, from immediately to a few hours after contamination. Therefore, surveillance and recognition are less problematic. The challenge is decontamination and treatment.

Terrorism with chemical weapons produces casualties similar to those seen in hazardous materials incidents, and medical management is comparable. However, the unique features of such events, including the volume of patients and the risk of hospital contamination, necessitate additional preparation. For example, the Tokyo subway attack using sarin in 1995 resulted in 11 deaths and more than 5000 patients converging on local emergency departments. Although the majority of these patients had subclinical exposure or psychological symptoms alone, the health care system was severely taxed. Secondary contamination by direct contact or vaporization occurred in ambulances and at the hospitals.[3]

Health care facilities must have protocols in place to deal with the eventuality of chemically contaminated patients (Box 195-7).[24,25] Current recommendations for levels of PPE and types of decontamination facilities necessary in a hospital setting are inconclusive.[26]

The four basic classes of chemical agents are (1) nerve, (2) vesicant (blistering), (3) blood, and (4) pul-

BOX 195-7. Emergency Department Preparedness for Chemical Weapons of Mass Destruction

Community-based hospital planning
Personnel trained in recognition, mass casualty triage, and treatment
Decontamination facility with protocols (runoff water, warm water, etc.)
Personal protective equipment readily accessible and compliant with regulations
Rapid access to antidotes, cyanide kits, and anticonvulsants
Hospital incident management system in place
Knowledge of how to access experts quickly

BOX 195-8. Type and Degree of Nerve Agent Exposure

Vapor Exposure (Sarin)

Mild:	Rhinorrhea and miosis
Moderate:	Mild symptoms plus increased secretions, wheezing/dyspnea, muscle weakness/fasciculations, or gastrointestinal effects
Severe:	Apnea, seizures, loss of consciousness, flaccid paralysis, or major involvement of two organ systems

Liquid Exposure (VX)

Mild:	Localized sweating and fasciculations where a drop touches the skin; no miosis; may be delayed for 18 hours
Moderate:	Gastrointestinal effects; miosis uncommon; may be delayed for 18 hours
Severe:	Apnea, seizures, loss of consciousness, flaccid paralysis, or major involvement of two organ systems; occurs in less than 30 minutes at or above LD_{50}

monary (choking). Although all have potential for use as weapons, the nerve agents and vesicants are thought to represent the greatest threat.

Nerve Agents (Sarin, Tabun, Soman, VX)

Nerve agents are organophosphates. They inhibit the enzyme acetylcholinesterase, blocking the degradation of acetylcholine at the postsynaptic membrane. Acetylcholine accumulates, resulting in overstimulation of muscarinic and nicotinic receptors. Symptoms are receptor dependent. Stimulation of muscarinic receptors produces miosis, salivation, rhinorrhea, lacrimation, bronchorrhea, bronchospasm, vomiting, and defecation. The major life threat associated with this syndrome is ventilatory compromise from profound bronchorrhea and bronchoconstriction. Stimulation of nicotinic receptors produces muscle fasciculations, flaccid paralysis, tachycardia, and hypertension. Unlike typical organophosphates, exposure to nerve agents has not been associated with urination. In addition, bradycardia is rare, and miosis does not respond to systemic therapy.[9]

Nerve agents also cause direct central nervous system toxicity that manifests as seizures, coma, and apnea. In survivors, residual central nervous system effects manifest as psychological changes that can last for 4 to 6 weeks. These manifestations are caused by chemical effects, not stress.

A preliminary diagnosis of nerve agent exposure is based on clinical findings. Important features include muscle fasciculations and miosis, which are sufficient to justify treatment pending further evaluation. Diagnosis is confirmed by measuring red blood cell cholinesterase levels. This test is not readily available, however, so treatment must begin before test results are known.

The nerve agents most likely to be employed by terrorists are sarin (designated GB) and VX. Sarin exists as a liquid at room temperature but represents primarily a vapor threat because of its high volatility. Symptoms occur within seconds after inhaling vapor and peak at 5 minutes. There are no delayed effects; patients remaining asymptomatic 1 hour after possible exposure have not been contaminated. They can be sent home. VX is a thick liquid with low volatility. It represents a liquid threat only. Victims generally develop symptoms after skin exposure. The median lethal dose (LD_{50}) for VX is 10 mg, a droplet slightly larger than a pinhead. Death from doses of this size occurs in less than 30 minutes. Delayed symptoms occur, so individuals must be observed for 18 hours before potential contamination can be ruled out.

Decontamination of victims exposed to sarin vapor requires only removal of clothing. Persons contaminated with VX or liquid sarin must have their clothing removed and then must be decontaminated using showers. When the level of exposure or the involved agent is uncertain, full decontamination is prudent. Responders caring for patients in the presence of liquid sarin exposure may require level A or B protective suits.

Treatment

The treatment of nerve agent victims depends on the form, liquid or vapor, and level of exposure: mild, moderate, or severe (Box 195-8). Three drugs are the mainstay of treatment: atropine for the muscarinic effects (improves ventilation), pralidoxime chloride (2-PAM) for the nicotinic effects (reverses paralysis), and diazepam for the prevention and treatment of seizures (Box 195-9). If diazepam is unavailable, other benzodiazepines can be used. 2-PAM is most effective if administered within 4 to 6 hours of sarin exposure. After this period, the drug's impact wanes due to "aging," defined as the permanent attachment of sarin to the acetylcholinesterase enzyme. Hypertension can occur during 2-PAM administration and is controlled by intravenous phentolamine, 5 mg for adults and 1 mg in repeat doses for children.

An autoinjector kit (Mark I) approved by the Food and Drug Administration consists of two cartridges, one containing atropine (2 mg) and the other 2-PAM

BOX 195-9. Treatment for Nerve Agent Exposure*

Vapor

Mild:	Observe for 1 hour, then release; no treatment
Moderate:	One or two Mark I kits IM *or* Atropine, 2-4 mg IV, may repeat every 5-10 minutes as needed, *and* 2-PAM, 1 g IV over 30 minutes, may repeat every hour as needed
Severe:	Three Mark I kits IM and one diazepam autoinjector IM *or* Atropine, 6 mg IV, may repeat 2 mg boluses IV every 5-10 minutes, *and* 2-PAM, 1 g IV over 30 minutes, repeat every hour for total of 3 g, *and* diazepam, 5 mg IV, may repeat as needed

Liquid

Mild:	One Mark I kit IM *or* Atropine, 2 mg IV, *and* 2-PAM, 1 g IV over 30 minutes
Moderate:	Same as for vapor
Severe:	Same as for vapor

Pediatric Doses

Atropine, 0.02 mg/kg IV
2-PAM, 15 mg/kg IV over 20-30 minutes
Diazepam, 0.2-0.3 mg/kg IV

*Give atropine before attempting intubation. Otherwise, airway resistance will inhibit ventilation. Continue atropine until secretions are dry (usually ≤20 mg). In hypoxic patients, IV atropine has been reported to cause ventricular fibrillation, so consider using IM atropine.

(600 mg). Mark I kits are available as part of civilian pharmaceutical caches strategically located throughout the United States. An autoinjector containing 10 mg of diazepam also is available. Doses should be adjusted for pediatric and elderly patients. Using the Mark I kits to treat these populations can be problematic because of difficulty in adjusting the dose. An alternate solution is to inject the medication into a sterile vial. The drug can then be reaspirated in an appropriate amount for the patient's weight or age and administered.[27]

Vesicants (Mustard)

Vesicants (blistering agents) are chemical warfare agents that induce blister formation when contacting skin. Terrorists could use several of these compounds, but mustard is considered the chemical of choice. Mustard is a liquid at room temperature but has both liquid and vapor toxicity. Injury from mustard exposure occurs in 1 to 2 minutes, but symptoms do not develop for 4 to 8 hours. The exact mechanism is unknown, but the agent damages DNA, causing eventual cell death. Mustard has both local and systemic toxicity. Local effects occur from direct exposure to the skin, eyes, and airway. Systemic effects result from the impact of absorbed mustard on the bone marrow. Treatment is supportive and includes decontamination (to prevent secondary contamination) and airway maintenance. Although no specific antidote for mustard is currently available, a topical iodine preparation shows promise. When applied within 1 hour after mustard exposure to the skin of guinea pigs, an iodine-tetraglycol solution reduced vesicle formation and signs of inflammation.[28] Application more than 1 hour after exposure was not effective.

Eye damage from mustard exposure varies from conjunctivitis to corneal ulcer and perforation; however, only 1% of patients have permanent eye damage. Severe pain is frequently associated with mustard injury and causes significant blepharospasm. Irrigation is beneficial if performed within minutes of exposure but ineffective once symptoms occur. Standard treatment includes mydriatics, topical antibiotics, oral analgesics, and petroleum jelly applied to the lids to prevent adhesions. Topical steroids are indicated only within the first 24 hours.

The hallmark of mustard injury is skin blisters resembling second-degree burns. Within 4 to 8 hours of exposure, erythema and burning occur, followed by vesicle and bulla formation. Most vapor injuries do not involve the entire dermis, so wounds will not require skin grafting. If liquid exposure occurs to skin, full-thickness burns may result. The patient should be decontaminated by removing clothing and washing with water or a dilute bleach (1:10 hypochlorite) solution. Decontamination immediately after exposure prevents further injury to the patient, but delayed decontamination is indicated to protect staff. Treatment is supportive and includes standard burn wound management, analgesia, and tetanus prophylaxis. An important exception is fluid resuscitation. Fluid losses from mustard injury are much less than those associated with thermal burns. Therefore, standard burn formulas for fluid administration do not apply, and caution must be used to avoid overhydration.

The degree of airway injury after mustard exposure is dose dependent. Mild exposure causes irritation of the nose, sinuses, and pharynx and can be treated with cool, humidified mist. Moderate exposure extends to the larynx and upper trachea and may require treatment with oxygen, continuous positive airway pressure, or even intubation. Severe exposure involves the lungs, producing hemorrhagic necrosis of the bronchioles. Pulmonary edema is rare. Intubation is usually required, and patients may benefit from positive end-expiratory pressure and in-line bronchodilators. Steroids are of questionable benefit, and antibiotics should only be given for established infection.

Systemic toxicity from mustard is caused by bone marrow suppression. Absorbed mustard kills stem cells, causing the white blood cell count to fall after 3 to 5 days. Survival is rare if the white blood cell count falls below 200, which generally occurs when greater than 50% of the total body surface area is involved from exposure to liquid agent. Death after mustard exposure usually results from secondary infection.

Blood Agents (Cyanide)

Blood agents such as cyanide bind to cytochromes within mitochondria and inhibit cellular oxygen use. Low-dose exposures result in tachypnea, headache, dizziness, vomiting, and anxiety. Symptoms subside when the patient is removed from the source. At higher doses, the symptoms progress to seizures, respiratory arrest, and asystole within minutes of exposure.

Victims should be removed from the area, should have their clothing discarded, and should receive oxygen. If no improvement occurs, the cyanide antidote is given (amyl nitrate, sodium nitrite, sodium thiosulfate).

Pulmonary Agents (Phosgene, Chlorine)

Pulmonary or choking agents cause an inflammatory reaction when they come into direct contact with the eyes and upper airway. They can be life threatening if inhaled. No specific antidote exists. Treatment is mainly supportive and consists of removing the patient from the source, decontamination, airway maintenance, bronchodilators, and eye irrigation.

KEY CONCEPTS

- Emergency department preparedness for a radiation incident must address decontamination (an external, freestanding decontamination unit is best), triage, staff safety, PPE, and diagnostic procedures that emphasize radiation monitoring. The emergency personnel should make sure they know their radiation safety officer.
- Management of acute, life-threatening conditions takes priority over radiation-associated issues.
- Aerosol dispersal is a likely route that terrorists will use to deploy biologic weapons, so victims will present primarily with respiratory complaints.
- In addition to "flulike" symptoms, anthrax typically causes mediastinal widening, pulmonary consolidation, and pleural effusions best seen on chest computed tomography scans.
- Smallpox can spread in a hospital environment; thus, patients suspected of having smallpox should be admitted to locations separated from the rest of the hospital.
- Decontamination is a key activity in the management of patients exposed to chemical agents, and hospitals must provide this intervention.
- Nerve agents are organophosphates, and patients exposed to these agents are treated with large doses of atropine, repeated frequently, and pralidoxime.

REFERENCES

1. Inglesby TV, et al: Anthrax as a biological weapon: Medical and public health management. *JAMA* 281:1735, 1999.
2. Domestic Preparedness Training Program: *Hospital Provider Manual.* Edgewood Arsenal, Md, Chemical and Biological Defense Command, 1999.
3. Okumura T, et al: Report on 640 victims of the Tokyo subway sarin attack. *Ann Emerg Med* 28:129, 1996.
4. Koenig KL, Hatchett R (eds): Department of Homeland Security Working Group on Radiological Dispersal Device (RDD) Preparedness, Medical Preparedness and Response Sub-Group: Medical Response to Radiologic Casualties, May 2003. Available at http://www.va.gov/emshg.
5. Guidance for Protective Actions following a Radiological Terrorist Event. Position Statement of the Health Physics Society, McLean, Virginia, January 2004. Available at http://hps.org/hpspublications/papers.html#position. Accessed February 24, 2004.
6. Balk S, Miller RW: FDA Issues KI Recommendations. *AAP News* 20(3):00, 2002.
7. Henderson DA, et al: Smallpox as a biological weapon: Medical and public health management. *JAMA* 281:2127, 1999.
8. Schultz CH, Mothershead JL, Field M: Bioterrorism preparedness I: The emergency department and hospital. *Emerg Med Clin North Am* 20:437, 2002.
9. Friedlander AM: Anthrax. In Zajtchuk R, Bellamy RF (eds): *Textbook of Military Medicine.* Washington, DC, Office of the Surgeon General, US Army, 1997, pp 467-478.
10. Dixon TC, et al: Anthrax. *N Engl J Med* 341:815, 1999.
11. Jernigan JA, et al: Bioterrorism-related inhalational anthrax: The first 10 cases reported in the United States. *Emerg Infect Dis* 7:933, 2001.
12. Schultz CH: Chinese curses, anthrax, and the risk of bioterrorism. *Ann Emerg Med* 43:329, 2004.
13. Centers for Disease Control and Prevention: Update: Investigation of Bioterrorism-Related Inhalational Anthrax—Connecticut, 2001. *MMWR Morb Mortal Wkly Rep* 50:1029, 2001.
14. Hupert N, Bearman GML, Mushlin AI, Callahan MA: Accuracy of screening for inhalational anthrax after a bioterrorist attack. *Ann Intern Med* 139:337, 2003.
15. Kuehnert MJ, et al: Clinical features that discriminate inhalational anthrax from other acute respiratory illnesses. *Clin Infect Dis* 36:328, 2003.
16. Conference Summary: Clinical issues in the prophylaxis, diagnosis, and treatment of anthrax. *Emerg Infect Dis* 8:222, 2002.
17. Joellenbeck LM, et al: The anthrax vaccine—Is it safe? Does it work? Committee to Assess the Safety and Efficacy of the Anthrax Vaccine, Institute of Medicine, National Academy Press, Washington, DC, 2002, p 288. Available at http://www.nap.edu/catalog/10310.html. Accessed February 26, 2004.
18. Inglesby TV, et al: Plague as a biological weapon: Medical and public health management. *JAMA* 283:2281, 2000.
19. Tucker JB, Zilinskas RA: The 1971 Smallpox Epidemic in Aralsk, Kazakhstan, and the Soviet Biological Warfare Program. Occasional Paper No. 9. Chemical and Biological Weapons Nonproliferation Project, Center for Nonproliferation Studies, Monterey Institute of International Studies, Monterey, California, July 2002.
20. Evaluating patients for smallpox: Acute, generalized vesicular or pustular rash illness protocol. Available at http://www.bt.cdc.gov/agent/smallpox/diagnosis/pdf/spox-poster-full.pdf. Accessed February 27, 2004.
21. Sofi IM, et al: Real-time PCR assay to detect smallpox virus. *J Clin Microbiol* 41:3835, 2003.
22. De Clercq E: Cidofovir in the therapy and short-term prophylaxis of poxvirus infections. *Trends Pharmacol Sci* 23:456, 2002.
23. Frey SE, et al: Clinical responses to undiluted and diluted smallpox vaccine. *N Engl J Med* 346:1265, 2002.
24. Macintyre AG, et al: Weapons of mass destruction events with contaminated casualties: Effective planning for health care facilities. *JAMA* 283:242, 2000.
25. Burgess JL, et al: Emergency department hazardous material protocol for contaminated patients. *Ann Emerg Med* 34:205, 1999.
26. Koenig KL: Strip and shower: The duck and cover for the 21st century. *Ann Emerg Med* 42:391, 2003.
27. Henretig FM, Mechem C, Jew R: Potential use of autoinjector-packaged antidotes for treatment of pediatric nerve agent toxicity. *Ann Emerg Med* 40:405, 2002.
28. Wormser U, et al: Topical iodine preparation as therapy against sulfur mustard-induced skin lesions. *Toxicol Appl Pharmacol* 169:33, 2000.

PART SEVEN

The Practice of Emergency Medicine

CHAPTER 196

Guidelines in Emergency Medicine

J. Stephen Bohan

The essential daily work of the emergency physician consists of only three areas: acquiring data, making decisions, and performing procedures. Numerous other tasks are associated with each patient visit but none requires professional medical expertise.

Because of the many reasons for emergency department visits, the level of thought or decision making required varies accordingly. A few presentations (e.g., cardiac arrest, apnea) require almost reflexive action, after which further thought is required. Most visits require only a modest amount of information and rule-based action. As the population ages and is sustained by medical advances, the practice of emergency medicine is evolving from caring for relatively simple conditions (e.g., injuries, asthma, minor gastrointestinal complaints) to dealing with much more complex problems (e.g., altered cognition, medication interactions, multisystem failure). Decision making in this setting changes as well, moving from rule-based to integrative, employing substantive probabilistic reasoning.

The patient history dictates the course of the visit and directs all subsequent evaluation. The form of the patient's delivery of the history (e.g., coherent, interrupted by need to breathe, "raced") is as important as the content. Hypotheses are constantly formed and rejected by the interviewer during this process as the elements of the history are fed into and integrated with the database in the clinician's mind. This is an imperfect process for a variety of reasons. The story may be incomplete (in fact, an essential part of the assessment is to judge the level of completeness) and expressed in unfamiliar terms, tempered by gender or ethnicity, or affected by emotional or physical pain.

The physician's knowledge base may also be inadequate. The data on even the most common diseases and interventions are often ambiguous and may be derived from a patient base outside the emergency department. Even the best evidence gleaned from careful studies is often outdated at the time of publication or made irrelevant by the interim development of new medicines or tests. Finally, questions answered by research projects are not often the clinical question, for example, "Does this patient have coronary heart disease?" versus "Is it safe to send this patient home?"

Physicians acquire experience over time, which becomes the filter for information received and sent in the integrative process. More experience reduces the amount of information received and the number of hypotheses generated. Hypothesis selection is equally hampered by the lack of complete follow-up data. Emergency physicians may not be aware of the outcome of admitted patients and often do not know the outcome of discharged patients.

These impediments are largely structural, inherent in the nature of the clinical practice in an area of expanding knowledge. Adding to the increasing complexity of emergency medicine is the format of the patient-doctor interaction. In this multiple simultaneous patient model, the number of data sets to be managed grows proportionally but the capacity of the human mind to deal with them does not.

To deal with many data sets, physicians seek guidance from external sources, traditionally drawing from texts and teachers. Statements of authorities remained the only decision-making aids for millennia. Aggregation of expert opinions into consensus statements has a relatively short tradition in this country, dating from 1938 when the American Academy of Pediatrics published recommendations for management of infectious diseases.[1] Advances in science and technology since 1938 have created the demand for better decision-making aids. Some of these tools are cumbersome to use (e.g., differential diagnosis programs) and thus not of practical use to the emergency physician, whereas others (e.g., electrocardiographic interpretation programs in electrocardiographic machines) are simple and useful.

GUIDELINES

Published statements that make recommendations for action go by various names: *clinical policy, pathway, guideline*. These are often used interchangeably. Generically, they are "systematically developed statements to assist practitioners and patient decisions about appropriate health care for specific clinical circumstances."[2] Clinical decision rules are related recommendations that can be included in guidelines.

In general, the word *policy* carries the connotation of an inflexible rule, *pathway* suggests some time element, and *guideline* implies a recommendation. Guidelines can be applied to diagnostic or therapeutic interventions and often contain reminders about elements necessary before making a decision (e.g., contraindications).

At best, these documents are distillations of evidence and expert opinion supporting practices that have been shown to improve patient outcomes. At their worst, they are amalgamations of opinion often dubious in origin and execution, colored by political interests and of unproven benefit.

Guidelines have remarkable potential to benefit the patient-physician encounter.[3] They can promote interventions of proven benefit and discourage ineffective measures. They have the potential to reduce morbidity and mortality and to benefit health outcomes. They can reduce variation in practice, allowing optimal outcomes irrespective of which practitioner is consulted or where the consultation takes place. Guidelines can provide explicit recommendations when uncertainty exists about which test or treatment is best. This assistance can substantially reduce emergency physicians' intellectual and emotional burden.

Guidelines provide the basis for consensus building on the quality of the activity or endeavor. Quality improvement activities can then focus on adherence to or deviation from best practices. Adherence strongly affirms commitment to quality.

Guidelines may be inadequately or improperly developed, promoting untested or unproven interventions and encouraging ineffective or harmful care. Contradictory recommendations can be the source of conflict between patient and physician or among treating physicians. Guidelines may be overly influenced by opinion and may have goals other than patient benefit. Inflexible guidelines may serve the needs of populations but not the needs of the individual patient. A lack of flexibility can also disrupt the physician-patient relationship. Patients may interpret a guideline as an absolute and feel deprived of a test or treatment that is actually not suitable for their individual circumstance. Even if the content is coherent and reliable, guidelines may be poorly expressed or cumbersome to use and distracting to the user. Their presence may prevent the physician from considering alternative causes for symptoms or the patient's preferences. Guidelines may increase resource consumption or, when used for political advocacy, result in an inappropriate reallocation of resources. Lingering behind every guideline, despite disclaimers, is the threat of its use for legal purposes.

Despite these concerns, guidelines are proliferating at a rapid rate and becoming embedded in clinical practice. The decision to use a guideline is usually multifactorial. Commonly cited reasons are reduced variation, improved efficiency, improved heath outcomes, reduced costs, or some combination of these. Successful use of guidelines requires clear recognition and acknowledgment of the reason to use them.

Development

The first step is to choose whether to develop a new guideline or adopt an already existing one. As guidelines become more sophisticated, their development becomes more difficult and is often beyond the scope of competence of a single individual. The skills of the group assembled must be multifaceted and include the following: (1) literature search and retrieval, (2) epidemiology, (3) biostatistics, (4) health services research, (5) clinical practice, (6) group process, and (7) writing and editing.[4]

This group must be able to assess the nature of the evidence, the applicability of the evidence to the population of interest, and the fiscal implications of recommendations, including cost benefit and cost-effectiveness. Health policy expertise is required to assess the effect of the guideline on the health system. The group of experts needs both technical and administrative support to be effective. A checklist of the essential characteristics of valid guidelines has been assembled by an expert group.[5]

The question to be answered (e.g., "What should the practitioner do in this situation?") needs to be explicitly stated and highly refined, as do the questions that relate to the intermediate steps. Evidence that will form the answer to the questions must be gathered, assessed, graded, and translated into recommendations with each step guided by explicit criteria.

There are several schemes for grading evidence and assessing the strength of recommendations, none proven better than another. The one most commonly used in the emergency medicine literature is that employed by the American College of Emergency Physicians. The literature on which recommendations are based is rated as class 1, 2, or 3 depending on the quality of the study and its applicability to the question at hand. The best evidence (class I) is that drawn from randomized trials and meta-analyses of such trials. The Cochrane Library (www.cochrane.org) is a repository of such trials and analyses. The recommendation is then made and given a "strength" rating of level A (a high degree of certainty based principally on class 1 evidence), level B (a moderate degree of certainty as the result of mostly class 2 evidence), or level C (based on absent, inconclusive, or conflicting evidence).[6]

The American College of Cardiology (www.ACC.org), working with the American Heart Association and the European Society of Cardiology, has developed a variety of guidelines for care of conditions, some of which are particularly relevant to emergency medicine practice. Their development process is rigorous and includes members of other specialties and community practitioners.[7,8] While the levels of evidence approximate those of the American College of Emergency Physicians, the classes of recommendations differ significantly, being distributed over four levels, the last being "not useful/effective and may be harmful" (Figure 196-1). A summary (Figure 196-2) shows how these levels of evidence ("precision of estimate of treatment effect") relate to the classes of recommendations ("size of treatment effect") and demonstrates how the two elements come together to form a recommendation for best practice.

After the evidence is gathered and collected, there will be gaps in the knowledge base required to make recommendations. The method for incorporating opinion to fill these gaps needs to be made explicit, lest the process be suspect for bias. Finally, the guideline needs to have external review for content validity, clarity, and applicability.

Clinical Decision Rules

"A Clinical Decision Rule (CDR) is a clinical tool that quantifies the individual contributions that various

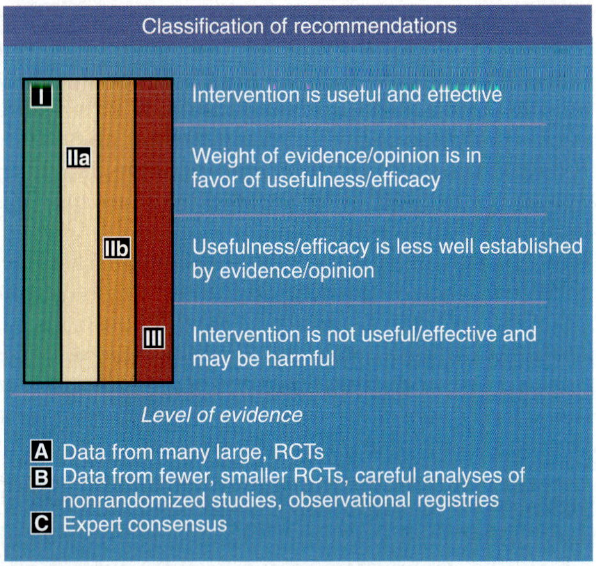

Figure 196-1. Classes of recommendations and level of evidence used in American College of Cardiology/American Heart Association clinical practice guidelines. RCT, randomized controlled trial. (From Gibbons RJ, Smith S, Antman E: American College of Cardiology/American Heart Association Clinical Practice Guidelines: Part 1: Where do they come from? *Circulation* 107:2979, 2003.)

components of the history, physical examination, and basic laboratory results make toward the diagnosis, prognosis, or likely response to treatment in a patient."[9] CDRs are an attempt to guide clinicians by simplifying and improving diagnostic accuracy and efficiency. Central to their development and use is their ability to establish pretest probability if certain conditions are met. This allows an estimate of risk for performing or not performing an action. Prior to use, CDRs need to be validated in multiple settings and their impact needs to be assessed, including their ease of use, rate of use, and effect on patient satisfaction.[10] CDRs are ranked as level 1, 2, or 3 depending on their compliance with these standards.[9] The Ottawa Ankle Rules is the only CDR to meet level 1 criteria. Other rules applicable to emergency medicine that have the potential of reaching level 1 and having a significant impact on practice habit are the San Francisco Syncope Rule,[11] the Canadian Head CT Rules,[12] the Canadian C Spine Rules,[13] and the NEXUS C Spine rule,[14] the latter two of which have been tested against each other.[15]

Sources and Adoption

The process of developing a guideline is dependent on the physical and fiscal capability (up to $1.2 million)

APPLYING CLASSIFICATION OF RECOMMENDATIONS AND LEVEL OF EVIDENCE
"Size of TREATMENT EFFECT"

"Estimate of certainty (precision) of treatment effect"

	Class I *Benefit >>> Risk* *No additional study needed* Procedure/treatment SHOULD be performed/administered	Class IIa *Benefit >> Risk* *Additional studies with focused objectives needed* IT IS REASONABLE to perform procedure/administer treatment	Class IIb *Benefit ≥ Risk* *Additional studies with broad objectives needed; additional registry data would be helpful* IT IS NOT UNREASONABLE to perform procedure/administer treatment	Class III *Risk ≥ Benefit* *No additional studies needed* Procedure/treatment should NOT be performed/administered SINCE IT IS NOT HELPFUL AND MAY BE HARMFUL
Level A *Multiple (3–5) population risk strata evaluated* *General consistency of direction and magnitude of effect*	• Recommendation that procedure or treatment is useful/effective • Sufficient evidence from multiple randomized trials or meta-analyses	• Recommendation in favor of treatment or procedure being useful/effective • Some conflicting evidence from multiple randomized trials or meta-analyses	• Recommendation's usefulness/efficiency less well established • Greater conflicting evidence from multiple randomized trials or meta-analyses	• Recommendation that procedure or treatment not useful/effective and may be harmful • Sufficient evidence from multiple randomized trials or meta-analysis
Level B *Limited (2–3) population risk strata evaluated*	• Recommendation that procedure or treatment is useful/effective • Limited evidence from single randomized trial or non-randomized studies	• Recommendation in favor of treatment or procedure being useful/effective • Some conflicting evidence from single randomized trials or non-randomized studies	• Recommendation's usefulness/efficacy less well established • Greater conflicting evidence from single randomized trial or non-randomized studies	• Recommendation that procedure or treatment not useful/effective and may be harmful • Limited evidence from single randomized trial or non-randomized studies
Level C *Very limited (1–2) population risk strata evaluated*	• Recommendation that procedure or treatment is useful/effective • Only expert opinion, case studies, or standard-of-care	• Recommendation in favor of treatment or procedure being useful/effective • Only diverging expert opinion, case studies, or standard-of-care	• Recommendation's usefulness/efficacy less well established • Only diverging expert opinion, case studies, or standard-of-care	• Recommendation that procedure or treatment not useful/effective and may be harmful • Only expert opinion, case studies, or standard-of-care

Figure 196-2. A summary shows how levels of evidence (precision of estimate of treatment effect) relate to the classes of recommendations (size of treatment effect) and demonstrates how the two elements come together to form a recommendation for best practice. (From Gibbons RJ, Smith S, Antman E: American College of Cardiology/American Heart Association Clinical Practice Guidelines: Part 1: Where do they come from? *Circulation* 107:2979, 2003.)

of large organizations.[5] As a result, most smaller organizations (individual hospitals and professional groups) adopt guidelines already developed by other organizations. This process, while simpler and quicker, must be no less careful. There are multiple sources and repositories of guidelines developed by government agencies, professional organizations, and individual institutions.

Table 196-1. Finding Guidlines

Databases	
Medline	"guideline" (publication type)
Healthstar	"Consensus Development Conference" (publication type)
EMBASE	"practice guidelines" (subject heading)
Websites	
www.ahrq.gov	Agency for Healthcare Research and Quality (formerly AHCPR)
www.guideline.gov	National Guideline Clearing House
www.acep.org	American College of Emergency Physicians
www.acc.org	American College of Cardiology
www.mssm.ecu	Mount Sinai School of Medicine
www.east.org	Eastern Association for the Surgery of Trauma

Searches for guidelines should start with published databases and websites of the repositories (Table 196-1). The American Medical Association publishes a compendium, which now contains more than 1800 policies contributed by more than 75 different organizations.[16] This compendium also delineates attributes that can guide the development and evaluation of practiced guidelines.

The National Guideline Clearing House (Table 196-2) is a repository and also offers comparisons of various guidelines on the same subject. The comparison of guidelines on pharyngitis is particularly illustrative, highlighting the various classifications of evidence used and noting the similarities and differences in recommendations and their implications.

The Eastern Association for the Surgery of Trauma produces exceptionally detailed and rigorously supported guidelines for management of trauma patients.[17]

Table 196-2. Classificaton Schemes for Standards of Evidence in Emergency Medicine

Recommendation	Level of Evidence
Schema I	
Class I	
Always acceptable, safe Definitely useful Proven in both efficacy and effectiveness Must be used in the intended manner for proper clinical indications	One or more large prospective studies are present (with rare exceptions) Study results consistently positive and compelling
Class IIa	
Safe, acceptable Clinically useful Considered treatment of choice	Generally higher levels of evidence Results are consistently positive
Class IIb	
Safe, acceptable Clinically useful Considered optional or alternative treatments	Generally lower or intermediate levels of evidence Generally, but not consistently, positive results
Class III	
Unacceptable Not useful clinically May be harmful	No positive high-level data Some studies suggest or confirm harm
Intermediate	
Continuing area of research No recommendations until further research	Evidence not available Higher studies in progress Results inconsistent, contradictory Results not compelling
Schema II	
Evidence-Based Standards	
Generally accepted principles for patient management that reflect a high degree of clinical certainty (i.e., based on "strength of evidence A" or overwhelming evidence from "strength of evidence B" studies that directly address all the issues).	Strength of Evidence A—Interventional studies including clinical trials, observational studies including prospective cohort studies, aggregate studies including meta-analyses of randomized clinical trials only.
Guidelines	
Recommendations for patient management that may identify a particular strategy or range of management strategies that reflect moderate clinical certainty (i.e., based on "strength of evidence B" that directly addresses the issue, decision analysis that directly addresses the issue, or strong consensus of "strength of evidence C").	Strength of Evidence B—Observational studies including retrospective cohort studies, case-controlled studies, aggregate studies including meta-analyses.
Options	
Other strategies for patient management based on preliminary, inconclusive, or conflicting evidence, or, in the absence of any published literature, based on panel consensus.	Strength of Evidence C—Descriptive cross-sectional studies, observational reports including case series, case reports, consensual studies including publishing panel consensus by acknowledged groups of experts.

Data in Schema I modified from American Heart Association by Pinnacle Publishing; data in Schema II from the American College of Emergency Physicians in its clinical policies.

Once obtained, the guideline should be assessed for validity. The methods for such assessments are published.[18] If the criteria for validity are comprehensive and rigorous and include not only the content but also explicitness about the development process, most published guidelines will not meet this standard. Fifty percent of a selection of guidelines developed in 1997 did not meet standards set by experts in guideline development. Only 40% specified outcomes of interest, and none met all 25 criteria for adequacy.[19]

Adoption should incorporate modifications to meet local needs, acknowledging any changes in strong recommendations. Attention should be paid to the reference population and how closely it mirrors the population (both of care givers and care receivers) to whom it will be applied.[20] The American College of Emergency Physicians is explicit as to the "Scope of Application," "Inclusion," and "Exclusion Criteria" for its clinical policies.[6] Guidelines should be reassessed for validity every 3 years.[21]

CONCEPT TO PRACTICE: CLINICAL PATHWAYS

Clinical pathways, also known as critical paths, critical pathways, care paths, or care maps, are the translation of guidelines into locally developed, functional tools that guide the process of care. They are the link between the establishment of a guideline and its use, usually employing printed management plans that display goals for patients and provide the sequence and timing of actions necessary to achieve these goals with optimal efficiency.[22,23] They have their origin in industrial management, where they are employed to increase efficiency in manufacturing by reducing variance. The focus is on the rate-limiting step in the manufacturing process.

Pathways differ from protocols in that the single purpose of protocols is to monitor and increase adherence to guidelines. Protocols often are often aimed at improving the quality of the care while pathways are predominately directed at promoting efficiency and reducing cost. Pathways are further distinguished by an element of constant monitoring and data evaluation intended to study not only compliance with the recommended action but also the process that links one action to another.[24] Since the process of care involves a variety of professional and nonprofessional staff, the development of pathways is characteristically multidisciplinary. The course of development for a pathway is similar to that of guidelines with the convening of a group, isolation of the issue to be addressed, gathering the evidence, reaching consensus, publication, and pilot implementation. A comprehensive description of one emergency department's experience, including examples of documentation tools, is available.[25]

In their most sophisticated expression, clinical pathways describe the tasks to be performed, timing and sequence of these tasks, and the people responsible for completing the task. This document is part of the patient's record. The goals here are simplicity, efficiency, increase in communication among members of the team, reduction of variation, and ease of audit. Often the record demands explanation of variance.

Clinical pathways have been an instrument in guiding and measuring emergency departments' response to the emergence of time-dependent therapies, particularly vascular emergencies. When goals such as "door to open artery time" become a standard, the response to such patients needs to be reworked and measured. Clinical pathways are important tools in achieving and maintaining a timely response, particularly when the description of the steps, the statement of important time intervals, and the necessary documentation are in a single document (Figure 196-3).

Clinical pathways are subject to the same criticism as guidelines in general: the tension between structure and flexibility, the surreptitious setting of "standards of care," and the demand for explanations of variance. Pathways carry the cost of development and implementation, are even less frequently validated than guidelines, and appear better suited to simple straightforward problems (e.g., procedures) than to complicated medical cases.

IMPLEMENTATION AND OUTCOMES

Before any beneficial outcome can be achieved, the guideline, pathway, or clinical decision rule must be used, and while the development or adoption of a guideline does not require a change in behavior, behavioral change is necessary for individuals to use and adhere to the guideline.[26,27] The literature is replete with failed efforts to achieve such change, which has brought attention to implementation. Simple dissemination is ineffective in modifying behavior in any meaningful way.[28-30] Even more elaborate strategies often fail.[8]

For example, the Joint National Committee on Hypertension first published its recommendations in 1977 and is currently on the seventh iteration of its guideline for management of blood pressure. Its recommendations are supported by the strongest of evidence. When primary care physicians were surveyed about their knowledge of the guidelines, about 40% of respondents were unaware of the guidelines. Of those who were aware, 75% stated that they would behave differently than the recommended guideline.[31]

Emergency physicians failed to adhere to evidence-based guidelines for the treatment of "isolated benign headache" 75% of the time.[32] One could assume that this was due to lack of awareness of the existence or content of the guideline, but the above-referenced study would belie that assumption.

This problem is not isolated to large national efforts. Dealing with only one intensive care unit, one group spent 4 months educating the staff on a version of guidelines for use of sedative and paralytic drugs based on the evidence-based guidelines of the Society of Critical Care Medicine. On review, only 23 of 100 consecutive patients were treated in a manner consistent with

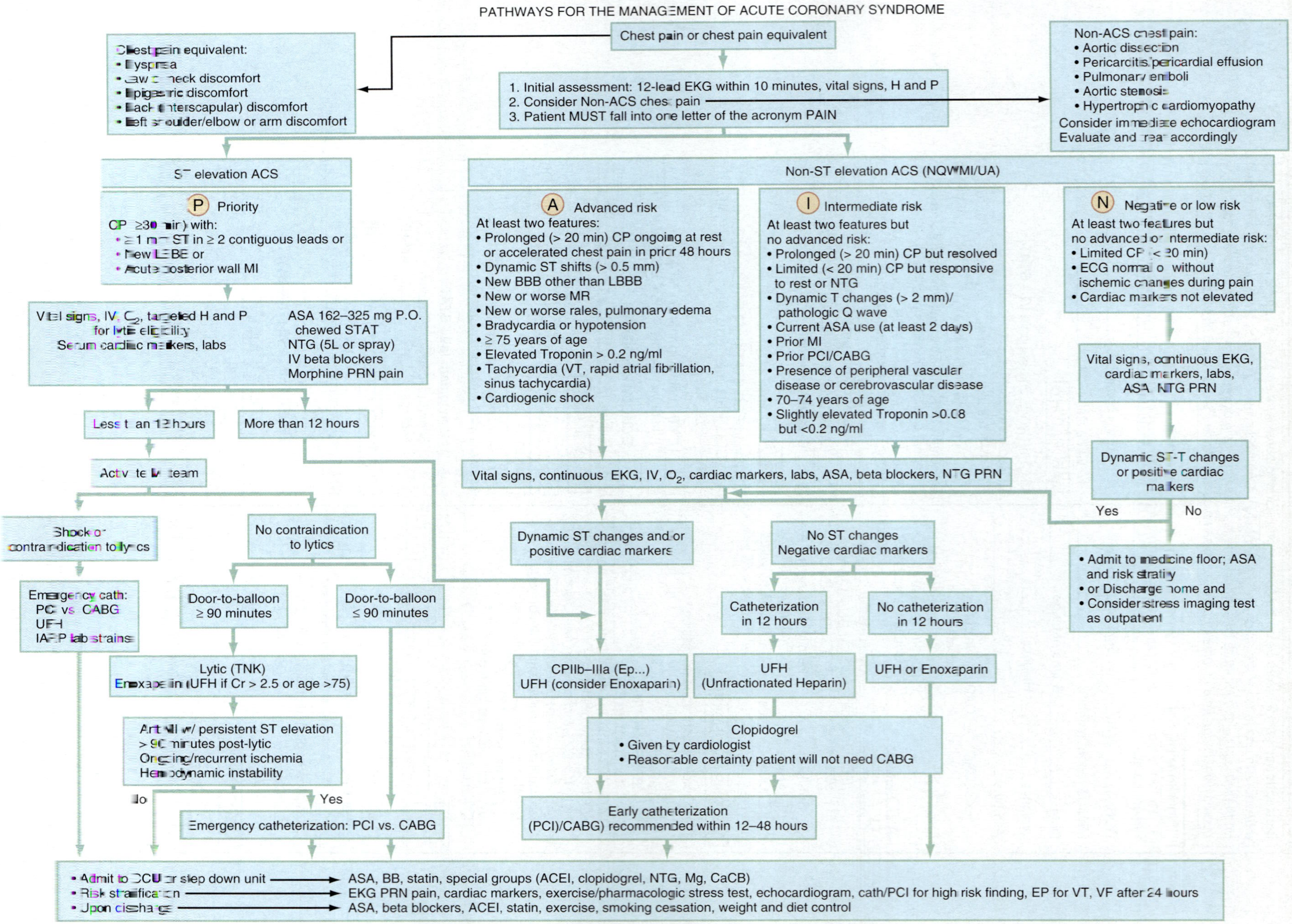

A

Figure 196-3. (See legend on next page.)

Instructions: *Check boxes below as appropriate. Strong consideration to be given for orders when it is indexed with any letter of the acronym* P A I N. *Checked boxes (☑) apply at all times. Twin boxes on the left* [Nurse][Time] *are for MD's initials and time of initialling. Twin boxes* [MD][Time] *on the right are for nurses' initials and time of initialling. These twin boxes should be filled up at all times by MDs and nurses.*

DEMOGRAPHICS:

Patient name: ____________

DOB:______ Age:_____ Sex: M☐ F☐

Medical record number: ____________

Date: ____________ & time of triage: ______

Weight: ________ Height: ________

Allergies: ____________

☐ Hx of CAD ☐ CAD equivalent
- ☐ Diabetes
- ☐ Carotid or peripheral arterial disease
- ☐ Abdominal aneurysm

Risk factors:

☐ Hypertension *(BP > 140/ 90 mm Hg)*

Smoking
- ☐ Active
- ☐ Quit < 2 years

☐ Diabetes

Dyslipidemia
- ☐ LDL > 130 mg/dL
- ☐ HDL < 40 mg/dL

Family Hx of early CAD *First degree relative:*
- ☐ *Male < 55 years*
- ☐ *Female < 65 years*

ROUTINE RN ORDERS:

☑ Obtain weight upon admission and daily weight
☑ Vital signs
  BP, HR, RR TID or ____________
  Temperature BID or ____________
☑ O_2 at 2 L/min via cannula for first 3 hours
☑ Check pulse oximeter
  If > 90% & chest pain free, discontinue O_2
  Notify MD if pulse oximeter < 90%
☑ Discontinue glucophage (Metformin)
☑ RN to provide teaching materials to patients with AMI
☑ Obtain old medical records
☑ Activity

[ ][ ] ____________ [ ][ ]
[ ][ ] Bedrest for first 24 hours then adv. as tolerated (if AMI) [ ][ ]

☑ Diet

[ ][ ] NPO, except medications [ ][ ]
[ ][ ] Low cholesterol, low saturated fat [ ][ ]
[ ][ ] Low sodium diet; 2 gm/day [ ][ ]
[ ][ ] Diabetic ________ calorie ADA [ ][ ]
[ ][ ] ____________ [ ][ ]

DISPOSITION:

[ ][ ] Observe in ED [ ][ ]
[ ][ ] Admit to: ___ CCU Service ___ Floor [ ][ ]

Attending: ____________

Intern/resident: ____________

Cardiology consult: ____________

☑ Code status: ____________

LABORATORY:

☑ CPK/CKMB and troponin I/T - **STAT**
☑ Repeat troponin at
  6–8 hrs. post adm at _/_/_ at _ AM/PM
  12–24 hrs. post adm at _/_/_ at _ AM/PM
☑ Repeat CPK-MB if troponin is positive and repeat CPK if CPK-MB is positive
☑ Na, K, Cl, creatinine, BUN, glucose, Mg, CBC, PT, PTT, LFT, lipid profile

[ ][ ] **CBC and lipid profile** in AM [ ][ ]
[ ][ ] **Urine toxicology screen** *(if indicated)* [ ][ ]
[ ][ ] **C-reactive protein** (12–24 hours) [ ][ ]

TESTS:

☑ **12 lead ECG STAT** (≤ 10 min) on arrival to ER or CCU, PRN chest discomfort & daily in AM for 3 days

[ ][ ] **CXR** - upright portable - **STAT** (unstable patients) - PA + L (if stable) [ ][ ]
[ ][ ] **ECHOCARDIOGRAM** [ ][ ]
[ ][ ] Other: ____________ [ ][ ]

IV SOLUTIONS:

[ ][ ] ____ at ____ ml/hr for ________ [ ][ ]

ANGIO +/– PCI: P A I

(PCI + stent preferred over lytic for ST elevation MI if timing is favorable)

[ ][ ] Send to **cath lab** - **STAT** [ ][ ]
[ ][ ] Schedule **cath** *(if high risk finding)* _/_/_ at ____ AM/PM [ ][ ]

THROMBOLYTICS: *(Target door to lytics ≤ 30 minutes)* P

STAT *(Start concurrently with IV Heparin or Enoxaparin)*

[ ][ ] **TENECTEPLASE (TNK-tPA)** [ ][ ]

< 60 kg	30 mg
60-69 kg	35 mg
70-79 kg	40 mg
80-89 kg	45 mg
≥ 90 kg	50 mg

B

Figure 196-3, cont'd Pathway (**A**) and standardized order set (**B, C**) for management of acute coronary syndromes with interventions supported by evidence annotated as "strong consideration." (From Herzog E, et al: The PAIN pathway as a tool to bridge the gap between evidence and management of acate coronary syndrome. *Critical Pathways in Cardiology* 3:20, 2004.)

HEPARINS: *(Select one)* P A I

☐ **UFH** (Unfractionated Heparin) [*when used concommitantly with GPIIb IIIa or lytic consider lowest dose*]
Bolus:____ units [60–70 units/kg (Maximum of 5,000 units)] IVP
Then: Infusion:____ units/hr [7–12 units/kg/hr *(Maximum of 1,000 units/hr)*]

☐ **Enoxaparin** 1 mg/kg SQ q 12h x 2 days ______ mg SQ every 12 h
☑ Hold Enoxaparin AM dose if scheduled for cath lab or invasive procedures.

ANTIPLATELET P A I N / P A I N

☑ Aspirin 162–325 mg PO/PR
For acute MI, first dose 325 mg, chew and swallow (nonenteric coated) ***STAT*** *[Give if not given in ED] Then 75–325 mg (enteric-coated) PO once daily*

☐ 162 mg
☐ 325 mg
☐ *Cannot take aspirin because*______

Clopidogrel *(avoid if CABG likely to follow)* P A
☐ 300 mg PO STAT then 75 mg PO once daily

GP IIb IIIa *(Select one)* P A
>> UFH should be used in conjunction with GPIIb IIIa

☐ **Integrilin**
Bolus 180 mcg/kg IVP______ mcg then Infusion 2 mcg/kg/min______ml/hr for 48–96 hrs or______
[If creatinine clearance < 50 ml/min or creatinine > 2 mg/dL give continuous infusion of 1 mcg/kg/min]

☐ **Abciximab** (*Give only prior to PCI*) *(0.25 mg/kg IV)*______ *mg IVP 10–20 min prior to PCI then [(0.125 mcg/kg/min) max 10 mcg/min]*______ *mog/min × 12 hours*

BETA BLOCKERS P A I

☐ **Metoprolol** 5 mg IVP; repeat q 5 min x 2 doses - **STAT**
☐ **Metoprolol** (25–100 mg) ________ mg PO q 12 h
☐ **Carvedilol** (3.125–25mg) mg ______ PO twice daily (favored if LV dysfunction)
☐ **Other**______
☑ Hold if SBP < 90 mm Hg or HR < 50 and notify MD
☐ *Cannot take beta blockers because* ______________

☐ *Severe bradycardia*
☐ *Hypotension*
☐ *Advanced heart block*
☐ *Decompensated heart failure*
☐ *Bronchospastic disease*

ACE INHIBITORS P A

For acute MI: definite for LV dysfunction, optional for preserved LV
If not on ACEI, start at low-dose. Titrate upward over 24–48 hrs. For acute MI, start as soon as patient is stabilized (after beta blockers, lytic or PCI) no sooner than 6 hours.

☐ **Captopril** 6.25 mg PO x 1 then 12.5 mg PO TID
☐ **Other**______
☑ Hold ACEI if SBP < 90 mm Hg and notify MD
☐ *Cannot take ACE inhibitors because*

NITROGLYCERIN P A
(Avoid if patient took Viagra in < 24 hrs or RV infarct)

☐ **Nitroglycerin IV**______ mcg/min × 24 hrs - **STAT** *(Titrate to chest pain only. Continue × 24–48 hrs for large MI, CHF, increased blood pressure, recurrent ischemia)*
☐ **Nitroglycerin** 0.4 mg SL q 5 minutes PRN for chest pain *(Repeat q 5 minutes × 2 doses. Notify MD if chest pain persists.)*
☑ Hold if SBP < 90 mm Hg. Notify MD.

STATINS ***(Prescribe to all ACS patients with LDL > 100 mg/dL)*** P A

☐ **Simvastatin**______
☐ **Atorvastatin**______
☐ **Other**______
☐ *Cannot take statins because*______

CALCIUM CHANNEL BLOCKERS

For ischemic pain if LV function is preserved and beta blockers are contraindicated, chest pain after cocaine use or Prinzmetal angina.

☐ ______________

PRN MEDS & OTHER MEDS

☐ **Morphine sulfate**______
☐ **Lorazepam**______
☐ **Docusate** 100 mg PO q 12 h______
☐ **Furosemide**___ mg every___ hours PO or IVP
☐ **Amniodarone** 150 mg IVP over 10 min, then, 1 mg/min x 6 hrs, then 0.5 mg/min
☐ **Lidocaine** ______________
☐ **Atropine** ______________
☐ **Magnesium** 1–2 gm IV over 5 min *(if low Mg, K or Torsade de Pointes)*
☐ **Pacemaker** (Transcutaneous)
☐ **Pacemaker** (Transvenous)
☐ **IADP** (for persistent shock, acute MR/VSD, post MI, refractory angina awaiting revascularization, refractory unstable VT/VP)
☐ **Electrical cardioversion**______

C

Figure 196-3, cont'd

the guidelines. Expanding the definition of *compliance* to include even partial compliance yielded only 58% treated in a compliant manner. The majority of practitioners actually thought they were following the guidelines.[33]

In managing cystitis, a managed care organization was successful in reducing resource use (urine analysis and high cost antibiotics) by shifting the central point of care away from the physician to a nurse, holding small group discussions, providing opinion leaders as educators and educating the (closed panel) patient population. They also pilot-tested the guideline to establish its acceptability and practicality. Despite these efforts, the guideline was not used in 47% of patient cases.[34]

The Ottawa Ankle Rules present a sobering example: "Clinicians expert in the use of the Ottawa Ankle Rules trained 16 other individuals to teach the use of the rules. These individuals returned to their Emergency Departments armed with slides, overheads, a 13 minute instructional video, and a mandate to train their colleagues locally and regionally in the use of the rules. Unfortunately, this program led to no change in the use of radiography."[9]

Despite one expert's apparently justified pessimism ("Modification of physician behavior has proven to be so daunting that no durable resolution of this problem seems likely in the near term."), successful implementations do occur.[35,36] Strategies that have been shown to achieve at least limited success in changing physician behavior require intensive and broad-reaching use of resources (The Cochrane Library contains the collection of literature on this subject in The Cochrane Effective Practice and Organization of Care Group). Multiple dimensions, both internal (knowledge, attitude, and behavior) and external (barriers), need to be addressed.[37,38] All concerned parties need to be involved, barriers need to be identified and removed, reminders need to be regular and appropriately timed, and social influence used. "Academic detailing" is of demonstrated utility, as are public statements by opinion leaders.[39] Marketing of guidelines can be directed to the patient as well as the physician, a strategy with successful precedent in the direct-to-patient advertisements of pharmaceutical companies. In some form and in some circumstances, the following have been effective in changing behavior: remuneration; restriction of resources (e.g., no expensive antibiotic without ID consult); and practice aids, including chart (paper or computer) reminders or different charting forms and chart audit.[39] Postimplementation interviews can be particularly revealing. Using computer-based order entry systems has been particularly effective.

Compliance with a guideline for unstable angina was associated with dramatically improved outcomes.[40] However, this association was not directly linked to dissemination of the guideline as distinct from changes in practice made for other reasons.

A group of physicians practicing in urgent care clinics of a large health system radically altered the number of hospital admissions in patients with community-acquired pneumonia when provided with an 8 × 11 inch form that required only summing "risk factors" to arrive at recommendations.[41] A home nurse visit was also made available and the logic was pilot tested before implementation. The form was used in 90% of cases and admissions were halved without any increase in mortality. The simplicity of the decision aid was noted in an analysis of the high compliance rate. However, the relative effect of the use of the guideline as opposed to the availability of the home nurse was not assessed.

This beneficial effect of the provision of simple tools has been confirmed in a controlled multihospital myocardial infarction care effort. Care measures were improved overall compared to nonintervention hospitals, but all of the benefit came from those who used the "tool kit" provided.[42] In an emergency department where symptom-based (as opposed to diagnosis-based) order sets and pathways resulted in fewer tests, fewer admissions, and shorter emergency department stays for subject patients compared to both historical controls with the same symptom presentation and contemporaneously when compared to symptoms not being studied.[43]

None of these successes have been tested for persistence of effect, nor were cost-benefit analyses done.

Norway, with a national hospital system, was successful in implementing a management guideline for mild head injuries and attributed the success of the project in part to targeting medical students and trainee physicians, as opposed to established practitioners, supporting the contention of the "old horse/new tricks" cliché.[44]

The conclusion is that interventions need at the very least to be focused, multimodal, easy for the user, and possibly accompanied by restrictions. They should be pilot-tested as well as accompanied by some reward, even if that is only feedback. Success may depend on the subject matter and the characteristics of the subject group, including demographics, qualifications, and even learning styles.[45] "...Even carefully designed educational interventions may not achieve the magnitude of change in behavior that was expected.... Practice behavior seems to be influenced by a wide range of factors other than research evidence."[46]

COMPUTER-BASED PROTOCOLS

The 4th century Greek philosopher Plato, in discussing the nature of political leadership, distinguished between task-based jobs and jobs centered on expertise, emphasizing flexibility and improvisation.[47] Using physicians as an example, he assessed the effect of codifying consensus and making it a rule. He concluded that it would be less than satisfactory because the rule would presuppose an average patient, not the individual sitting before the physician. This same reservation has resurfaced 17 centuries later.[48]

Additionally, the mode of the rule would reflect the thinking of the developer, not the thought processes of the clinician. This tension between constraint and freedom, between best practice and clinical judgment, remains today as one of the major impediments to successful implementation of guidelines. The challenge lies in reducing the opportunity for variability while simultaneously making allowances for patient individuality. Computers can go a long way in achieving this concept of "flexibility within boundaries."

Such a system has been demonstrated in the treatment of critical care unit patients, both in their need for hemodynamic support and in treatment of respiratory failure.[49] Decision support protocols are built into the computer order entry system at the patient's bedside. This system receives real-time physiologic data from monitoring equipment. The protocol is driven by the patient's physiologic parameters, and inappropriate options are not offered. No alternative method of entering orders exists, although overrides are possible, necessitating, however, an explanation of the reason for the override. Subjectivity in assessment of the patient's condition with respect to the question at hand (e.g., PEEP vs. no PEEP) is absent, in contradistinction to guidelines that simply provide recommendations and depend on the practitioner changing to the recommended behavior. In this model, the recommended action is the default one and the practitioner must take action to behave differently. Most paper-based guidelines require initiative to move to the recommended action while computer-based order entry systems that structure the care require initiative to deviate from the recommendation. Physician compliance with the recommended path of treatment was in the 95% range and reproducible over a wide number of hospitals.

Given the nature of clinical practice, computerized protocols must be explicit and unambiguous and include all possible outcomes under the rules. The site of operation must be the point of care, as the clinical decisions depend on accurate, precise, and timely data. Such data must be delivered to the practitioner in a convenient fashion that requires little or no effort while continuous collection of performance data allows for feedback to the user and iterative refinement to the developer. Simplicity and convenience are the hallmarks of such a system.

Computer-based systems have the potential to overcome many if not most of the deficiencies and objections of the traditional paper-based method. Variability of the patient's history is difficult to overcome; controlling the site of entry to diagnostic tests and therapies holds substantive promise for reducing variation and improving outcomes. Useful tests and preferred drugs can be displayed on the top screen while those of doubtful utility or those that are less cost-effective can only be accessed deeper in the system (Figure 196-4). Computer order entry has been shown, for instance, to dramatically reduce medication errors in hospitals.[50] When five emergency departments were asked to comply with a set of standards for six common chief complaints, the one department that embedded the

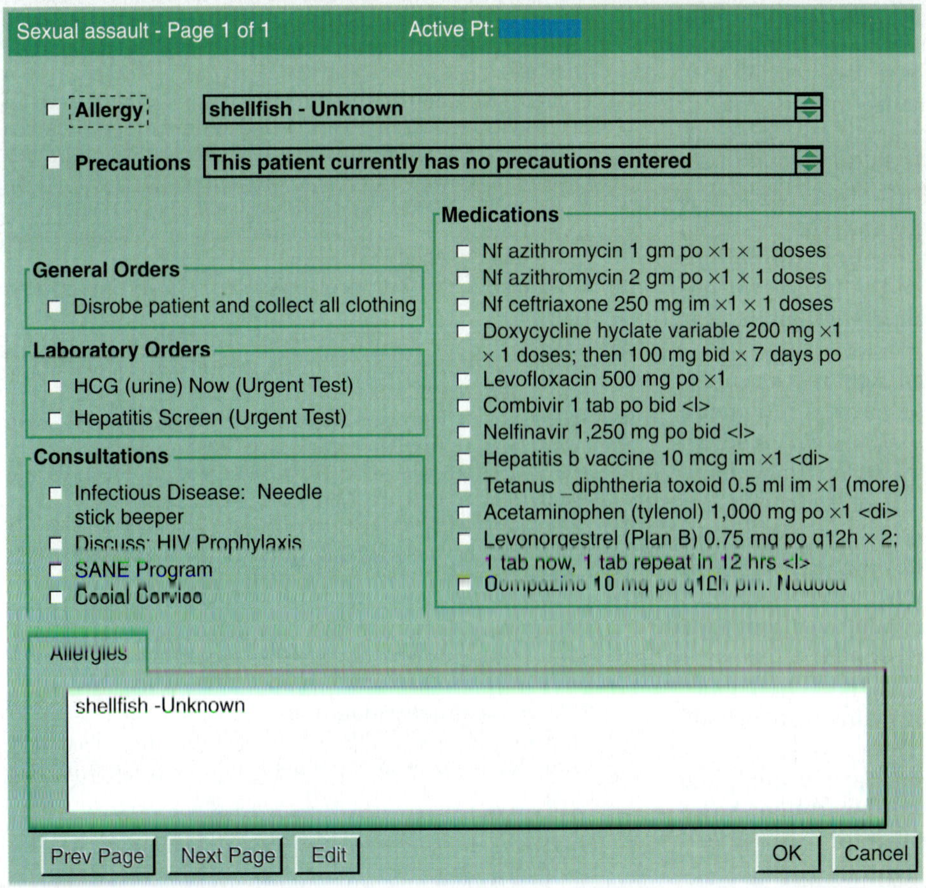

Figure 196-4. Order entry template for sexual assault.

standards in its electronic record performed the best by a considerable margin.[51] In this arrangement, the order sets become the pathways.

LEGAL AND ETHICAL CONSIDERATIONS

Guidelines have traditionally provided recommendations, not prescriptions, with most containing disclaimers that they are not standards. Large health care organizations support this approach. In Britain, the National Health Service states explicitly that "guidelines...cannot be used to mandate, authorize or outlaw treatment options. Regardless of the strength of the evidence, it will remain the responsibility of the practicing clinicians to interpret their application."[52] The World Health Organization similarly notes that "guidelines should provide extensive, critical and well balanced information on benefits and limitations of the various diagnostic and therapeutic interventions so that the physician may exert the most careful judgment in individual cases."[53] Statements such as these give comfort to the physician who feels constrained to do more or less than the guideline recommends. This latitude is usually intended specifically for the physician but in fact may be even more important for the patient.

Recently, this latitude appears to be waning. This may be the result of gradual accumulation of grade A evidence of sufficient magnitude to establish a clear and unequivocal standard. The most recent Advanced Cardiovascular Life Support Guidelines, now strictly evidence based, are more explicit:

"Our guidelines are no longer just *descriptive*—'This is how we do it here'—but can now be *prescriptive*—'This is how we should be doing it in the future.'"[54]

The implications of such a change in the role of guidelines on the practice of emergency medicine are substantial. Whether following guidelines provides a degree of immunity from accusations of malpractice is unknown, as is the converse, whether deviations from guidelines expose one to increased liability. Guidelines played a "relevant or pivotal role in the proof of negligence" in less than 7% of malpractice actions in this country.[55]

The latitude granted in all but the most recent guidelines was always directed at physician judgment, allowing discretion to suit the individual medical needs of the patient. The growth of patient autonomy brings new perspective to this latitude and to guidelines in general. What should happen if, in the face of guidelines on who may or may not receive renal dialysis, a patient demands the treatment? What duty does the patient's personal physician and the health system have to meet his demand? Likewise, should the answer be different if the patient's care for the potential treatment is to be paid for by the government, a private insurer, or the patient himself?

An example more relevant to emergency medicine might be the situation in which the department has a guideline on using computed tomography in a head injury case and a patient who does not meet eligibility criteria demands the test. Should the answer differ depending on the payer, time of day (scanner not busy versus scanner backed up), or strength of the demand? When, in fact, do expert recommendations become covert rationing and could such accusations be tempered by the inclusion on the development panel of lay persons as public representatives?[56] In the future, the incorporation of all stakeholders in the development and use of guidelines might produce a process that is inclusive of available evidence and considerate of the opinion of those most affected by the document, the patients.

REFERENCES

1. Drake L, et al: American Academy of Dermatology Guidelines of Care: Development and Process. *Arch Dermatol* 33:1369, 1997.
2. Field MJ, Lohr KN: *Clinical Practice Guidelines: Direction of a New Program.* Washington, D.C., National Academy Press, 1999.
3. Woolf S, et al: Clinical Guidelines: Potential benefit, limitations, and harms of clinical guidelines. *BMJ* 318:527, 1999.
4. Shekelle P, et al: Clinical guideline: Developing guidelines. *BMJ* 318:593, 1999.
5. Shiffman RN, et al: Standardized Reporting of Clinical Practice Guidelines: A Proposal from the Conference on Guideline Standardization. *Ann Intern Med* 139:493, 2003.
6. ACEP Clinical Policy Committee: Clinical Policy: Critical issues in the evaluation of adult patients presenting to the emergency department with acute blunt abdominal trauma. *Ann Emerg Med* 43:278, 2004.
7. Gibbons RJ, Smith S, Antman E: American College of Cardiology/American Heart Association Clinical Practice Guidelines: Part 1: Where do they come from? *Circulation* 107:2979, 2003.
8. Gibbons RJ, Smith S, Antman E: American College of Cardiology/American Heart Association Clinical Practice Guidelines: Part II: Evolutionary Changes in a Continuous Quality Improvement Project. *Circulation* 107:3101, 2003.
9. McGinn TG, et al: User's guides to the medical literature XXII: How to use articles about clinical decision rules. *JAMA* 284:79, 2000.
10. Gallagher EJ: Shooting an elephant. *Ann Emerg Med* 43:233, 2004.
11. Quinn JV, et al: Derivation of the San Francisco Syncope Rule to predict patients with short term serious outcomes. *Ann Emerg Med* 43:224, 2003.
12. Stiel IG, et al: The Canadian CT Head Rule for patient with minor head injury. *Lancet* 357:391, 2001.
13. Stiell IG, et al: Canadian C-spine rule study for alert and stable trauma patients. *JAMA* 286:1841, 2001.
14. Hoffman JR, et al: Validity of a set of clinical criteria to rule out injury to the cervical spine in patients with blunt trauma. *N Engl J Med* 343:94, 2001.
15. Stiell IG, Clement CM, McKnight RD: The Canadian C spine rule versus the Nexus low-risk criteria in patients with trauma. *N Engl J Med* 349:2510, 2003.
16. American Medical Association: *Policy Compendium.* Chicago, The Association, 1997.
17. Dunham DM, et al: Guidelines for emergency tracheal intubation immediately after traumatic injury. *J Trauma* 55:162, 2003.
18. Hayward RS, et al: Users' guides to the Medical Literature. VIII. How to use clinical practice guidelines: A. Are the recommendations valid? *JAMA* 274:574, 1995.

19. Shaney F, et al: Are guidelines following guidelines? The methodological quality of clinical practice guidelines in the peer reviewed medical literature. *JAMA* 281:1900, 1999.
20. Alrich R, et al: Using socioeconomic evidence in clinical practice guidelines. *BMJ* 327:1283, 2003.
21. Shakelle PG, Ortiz E, Rhodes D: Validity of the agency for Health Care Research and Quality Clinical Practice Guidelines: How quickly do guidelines become outdated. *JAMA* 286:1461, 2001.
22. Campbell H, Hotchkiss R, Bradshaw N: Integrated care pathways. *BMJ* 316:133, 1998.
23. Pearson S, Goulart-Fisher D, Lee T: Critical pathways as a strategy for improving care: Problems and potential. *Ann Intern Med* 123:941, 1995.
24. Every N, Hochman J, Becker R: Critical pathways: A review. *Circulation* 101:461, 2000.
25. Bridgeman T, Flores M, Rosenblath J: One emergency department's experience: Clinical algorithms and documentation. *J Emerg Nursing* 23:316, 1997.
26. Eccles M, et al: Effect of computerized evidence based guidelines on management of asthma and angina in adults in primary care: Cluster randomized controlled trial. *BMJ* 325:941, 2002.
27. Mendis D, et al: Management of spontaneous pneumothorax: Are British Thoracic Society guidelines being followed? *Post Grad Med J* 78:80, 2002.
28. Lewis L, Lasater L, Ruoff B: Failure of a chest pain policy to modify physician evaluation and management. *Ann Emerg Med* 259, 1995.
29. McGinn T, Guyatt G, Wyer P: Users' Guides to the Medical Literature: XXII. How to use articles about clinical decision rules. *JAMA* 284:79, 2000.
30. Oxman A, et al: No magic bullets: A systemic review of 102 trials of interventions to improve professional practice. *Can Med Assoc J* 153:1432, 1997.
31. Hyman D, Paulik V: Self-reported hypertension treatment practices among primary physicians. *Arch Intern Med* 160:2281, 2000.
32. Vinson DR: Treatment patterns of isolated benign headache in US emergency Departments. *Ann Emerg Med* 39:215, 2003.
33. Bair N, et al: Introduction of sedative, analgesic and neuromuscular blocking agent guidelines in a medical intensive care unit: Physician and nurse adherence. *Crit Care Med* 28:707, 2000.
34. Saint S, et al: The effectiveness of a clinical protocol guideline for the management of presumed uncomplicated urinary tract infection in women. *Am J Med* 106:636, 1999.
35. Gallagher EJ. How well do clinical practice guidelines guide clinical practice. *Ann Emerg Med* 40:394, 2002.
36. Grimshaw J, Russell I: Effect of clinical guidelines on medical practice: A systemic review of rigorous evaluations. *Lancet* 342:1317, 1993.
37. Cabana MD, et al: Why don't physicians follow clinical practice guidelines? A framework for improvement. *JAMA* 282:1458, 1999.
38. Grol R: Beliefs and evidence in changing clinical practice. *BMJ* 315:418, 1997.
39. Tamblyn R, Battista R: Changing clinical practice: Which interventions work? *J Contin Educ Health Prof* 13:273, 1993.
40. Giugliano R, et al: Association of unstable guidelines and with improved survival. *Arch Intern Med* 160:1775, 2000.
41. Dean N, et al: Implementation of admission decision support for community-acquired pneumonia: A pilot study. *Chest* 117:1368, 2000.
42. Mehta R, et al: Improving quality of care for acute myocardial infarction: The guidelines applied in practice (GAP) initiative. *JAMA* 287:1269, 2002.
43. Armon K, et al: The impact of presenting problem based guidelines for children with medical problems in an accident and emergency department. *Arch Dis Child* 89:159, 2004.
44. Muller K, et al: Minor head injuries: Impact of a national strategy for implementation of management guidelines. *J Trauma* 55:1029, 2003.
45. Stross J: Guidelines have their limits. *Ann Intern Med* 131:304, 1999.
46. Gunderson L: The effect of clinical practice guidelines on variations in care. *Ann Intern Med* 133:317, 2000.
47. Annas J, Waterfield R (eds): Plato: Statesman. Cambridge, Cambridge University Press, 1995.
48. Wears RL: Headaches from practice guidelines. *Ann Emerg Med* 39:334, 2002.
49. Morris A: Developing and implementing computerized protocols for standardization of clinical decisions. *Ann Intern Med* 132:373, 2000.
50. Bates DW, Leape L, Culen DJ: Effect of computerized physician order entry and a team intervention on prevention of serious medication errors. *JAMA* 280:1360, 1998.
51. Burnstin H, et al: Benchmarking and quality improvement: The Harvard Emergency Department Quality Study. *Am J Med* 107:437, 1999.
52. *NHS Executive Clinical Guidelines.* Leeds, NHSE, 1986.
53. Subcommittee of WHO/ISH, Mild Hypertension Liaison Committee: Summary of 1993 WHO/ISH guidelines for the management of mild hypertension. *BMJ* 707:1541, 1993.
54. American Heart Association: Part 6: Advanced cardiovascular life support, Section 1. Introduction to ACLS 2000: Overview of recommended changes in ACLS from Guidelines 2000 Conference. *Circulation* 102:1, 2000.
55. Hyams A, et al: Practice guidelines and malpractice litigation: A two way street. *Ann Intern Med* 122:450, 1995.
56. Norheim O: Health care rationing: Are additional criteria needed for assessing evidence based clinical practice guidelines? *BMJ* 319:1426, 1999.

CHAPTER 197

Medical Literature and Evidence-Based Medicine

Kelly D. Young and Roger J. Lewis

PERSPECTIVE

Medicine is an empiric science based on the experiences and insights of past and contemporary practitioners. Because the clinical experience of an individual physician is a small fraction of the experience of the medical profession as a whole, the advancement of medical science depends on physicians' abilities to assemble, organize, and disseminate information in order to learn from the experience of others.

The Medical Literature

During the last several decades, medical literature has exploded.[1,2] Thirty years ago, physicians could understand most medical publications. Currently, reports frequently use sophisticated statistical analyses that are unfamiliar to most clinicians.[3,4] Emergency physicians and other practitioners are increasingly aware that the quality of the research reported must be evaluated before the results can be considered valid and clinical practice altered. Also, the results of quality research may not be applicable if the population studied differs greatly from the patient population in the emergency physician's clinical practice. Even a clinician who possesses the analytical skills necessary to understand the modern medical literature will find it difficult to remain current, given the rate at which medical studies relevant to emergency medicine are published. Thus, the emergency physician must have a plan to identify, select, and read high-quality, relevant articles. Furthermore, the emergency physician must understand a number of principles to be able to analyze published studies critically.

The first step toward achieving these goals is to identify a small number of journals on which to focus.[5] Most high-quality studies relevant to emergency medicine are published in fewer than a dozen journals. Once a list of 6 to 12 journals is compiled, back issues can be skimmed to determine the average number of relevant articles in each issue. Those journals that publish the highest number of articles directly relevant to an emergency physician's clinical practice should then be selected.[5] An emergency physician in full-time clinical practice should probably focus on two to six journals per month. Regular pamphlet or audiotape updates reviewing recent literature relevant to emergency medicine can be purchased and used as a supplement to journal review. Articles should be pulled and read in full, however, before results are accepted and clinical practice altered.

Possible articles should then be screened to evaluate the relevance of the study question and population and to determine whether the methodology is of sufficient quality to warrant reading the article in more detail. Quality and clinical relevance vary greatly in the peer-reviewed literature.[5] Only articles that meet high standards for methodologic quality should be read in detail.[1,2] The emergency physician must learn to differentiate high-quality studies from poor-quality studies with unreliable results. Practitioners who understand the concepts presented in this chapter will have the basic foundation to differentiate good from poor studies and to focus their reading on those studies most likely to yield results that warrant a change in clinical practice.[6] Additional guidance can be obtained from the *Journal of the American Medical Association*'s Users' Guides to the Medical Literature series (http://medicine.ucsf.edu/resources/guidelines/users.html).[6]

A steadily increasing amount of attention is being paid to the importance of rigorous methodology in the design and execution of clinical trials.[3,7-9] A poorly designed statistical analysis can yield misleading results, but a trial is more likely to be weakened by a poorly chosen question, an inappropriate study population, or other methodologic errors that bias the results.[10-17] Thus, although some degree of statistical literacy is important, the practitioner must also understand nonstatistical issues in the design and analysis of clinical studies.[6,10-17]

TYPES OF CLINICAL STUDIES

Studies can be divided into two categories, cross-sectional and longitudinal (cohort), based on when the measurements are made on the study population.[12] In a cross-sectional study, data are obtained from a population of patients at a single point in time, whereas in a longitudinal study, data are obtained from a population of patients over a period of time.

Cross-Sectional Studies

Many epidemiologic studies are cross-sectional. Although a cross-sectional study cannot prove a causal relationship between a risk factor or treatment and an outcome, strong associations between identified variables in cross-sectional studies are suggestive of such effects.[18]

Many important observations can only be made using cross-sectional studies because, for practical and ethical reasons, some variables cannot be artificially manipulated to determine their effect on patient outcome.[18] Furthermore, the effect may be so delayed that a longitudinal study is impractical. An example is a study examining the association between cigarette use and lung cancer. It would be unethical to expose a nonsmoking population to the effects of cigarettes, and, even if one were to identify a population that voluntarily would use cigarettes, it would be impractical to observe subjects long enough for malignancies from cigarette smoking to appear. However, a cross-sectional study of self-reported cigarette use and the diagnosis of lung cancer that examines a population of subjects at a single point in time can easily demonstrate an association.

Longitudinal Studies

In a longitudinal, or cohort, study, a population of patients is enrolled in the study and measurements are made over a period of time.[11,12] Longitudinal studies can be observational, if no intervention is made, or they can be interventional.

Longitudinal Observational Studies

In a longitudinal observational study, data are collected from a group, or *cohort,* of patients over time, but no intervention is made. A longitudinal observational study can be either prospective or retrospective. In a *prospective* observational study, patients who meet specific eligibility criteria are identified, and data are prospectively gathered over time.[12] Prospective observational studies are valuable for defining the course of a particular disease treated with standard therapies and for identifying subgroups of patients with differing prognoses. If an association is noted between treatment and outcome in a prospective observational study, the association should be verified in a prospective interventional randomized clinical trial.

Although an observational study cannot prove a causal relationship, associations between initial patient characteristics or specific treatments and subsequent outcome can be detected. Such associations can be measured more accurately in a prospective longitudinal study than in a cross-sectional study, because both the original patient characteristics and the subsequent outcome are determined prospectively. When both the original patient characteristics and the outcome are determined prospectively, any associations observed are more likely to be true and not a result of bias.

In a *retrospective* observational study, medical records of patients with certain initial characteristics who are treated over time are reviewed and data abstracted. As with all retrospective studies, retrospective observational studies are subject to recording bias, problems with missing information, and other methodologic limitations. Because retrospective studies have these additional sources of bias and limitations, prospective studies provide higher quality evidence than retrospective studies. Prospective studies, however, are usually more difficult and time-consuming to perform.

Longitudinal Interventional Studies (Clinical Trials)

Interventional studies, which must be prospective, involve the artificial manipulation of a patient's therapy to determine the effect of an investigational treatment.[11,18] An interventional study can be controlled or uncontrolled, and, if controlled, it should be randomized.

In an *uncontrolled* interventional study, all patients who meet defined eligibility requirements are given the investigational therapy, and their outcomes are determined. Although such studies are useful for defining the rate of successful therapy in a well-defined population of subjects, the lack of a control group makes it difficult to estimate the relative effectiveness of the new therapy compared with another therapy. Previous experience with the standard treatment, in the form of a historical control group, can be used for comparison to the group receiving the new therapy. The use of such historical control groups is unreliable and often leads to an overestimate of the relative effectiveness of the new investigational therapy.[16] Medical care generally is becoming more effective, and thus the results of modern studies tend to yield better patient outcomes, even if the investigational treatment has no inherent advantage over the therapy received by the historical control patients.[16]

In a *controlled* clinical trial, some patients are given the new investigational treatment, and some patients (*control group*) are given a standard treatment.[11,12] The purpose of the control group is to define the effectiveness of the standard therapy in a group of patients as similar as possible to the group receiving the investigational therapy. To obtain two groups of patients who are nearly identical with respect to all characteristics that might influence the outcome of their disease, it is important that no external or subjective factors influence the assignment of treatment.[11,17] Each patient must have the same chance of receiving each therapy. For this reason, assignment to control or therapy groups should be randomized.

It is extremely important that control patients be given a therapy that is at least as effective as the best currently available treatment. It is unethical for a control group to receive an inferior treatment simply to demonstrate that a new treatment has some effectiveness.[19-22]

In general, longitudinal interventional studies provide the highest quality evidence, although this is controversial.[23-25]

RANDOMIZED LONGITUDINAL INTERVENTIONAL STUDY (CLINICAL TRIAL)

The steps in a randomized clinical trial assume that a worthwhile research question has been defined (Figure 197-1). No matter how well designed the study, if the research question is not well defined and not clinically useful, the intended audience will not find the study's results valuable.[26] The research question must also be

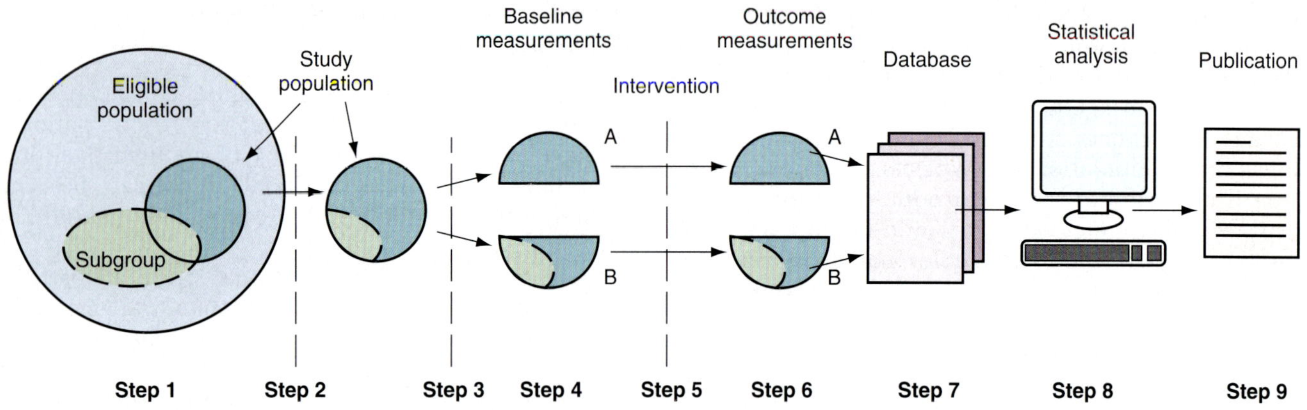

Step 1: Definition of the patient population	**Step 2:** Recruitment and enrollment of patients	**Step 3:** Randomization	**Step 4:** Measurement of baseline characteristics	**Step 5:** Treatment or intervention	**Step 6:** Collection of data on outcome	**Step 7** Data management	**Step 8:** Statistical analysis	**Step 9:** Presentation and publication of results
Problem 1: Heterogeneous population (confounding variables), poorly chosen inclusion criteria	**Problem 2:** Bias in recruitment, self-selection by potential subjects	**Problem 3:** Imbalance of important confounding characteristics, inadequate blinding	**Problem 4:** Imbalance of confounding characteristics is not detected	**Problem 5:** Unequal compliance or attrition	**Problem 6:** Subjects lost to follow-up, poorly defined outcomes	**Problem 7:** Data entry errors, data reduction errors or bias	**Problem 8:** Type I and type II errors, ill-advised comparisons or subgroup analysis, covariate imbalance	**Problem 9:** Overextra-polation of results, failure to recognize limitations of or biases in results
Solution 1: Population defined in terms of emergency department presentation, confounding characteristics considered in definition of population	**Solution 2:** Consecutive enrollment, records of nonenrolled but eligible patients	**Solution 3:** Effective randomization and blinding, stratified randomization	**Solution 4:** Planned prospective measurement of important confounding characteristics	**Solution 5:** Intention-to-treat analysis of final data, measurement of compliance, procedures to encourage compliance	**Solution 6:** Multistep plans to obtain follow -up data, unambiguous definitions of treatment outcome	**Solution 7:** Data verification, double data entry, value limited data entry, appropriate forms design	**Solution 8:** Small number of comparisons, planning of analysis, adequate sample size, multivariate modeling	**Solution 9:** Peer review, replication of results by other investigators, educated readership

Figure 197-1. Implementation and analysis of a prospective, randomized, controlled clinical trial.

prospectively defined; it is not appropriate to gather data and then devise a research question to fit the data. A good research question clearly defines four elements: (1) patient population and problem to be studied, (2) intervention to be applied to the treatment group, (3) comparison (control) intervention, and (4) outcome of interest.

Even if these four elements are well defined, the research question must still have relevance for the emergency physician. For example, a study that compares oral and parenteral antibiotics (treatment and comparison interventions) for the prevention of meningitis (outcome) in well-appearing febrile children with occult bacteremia confirmed by positive blood culture (patient population) is less useful to the emergency physician than a similar study including all well-appearing febrile children, since results of blood cultures are not typically available in the emergency department.

Step 1: Definition of Patient Population

Assuming an appropriate research question has been selected, the first step is to define the patient population to be studied.[27,28] The original patient population defined in the research question may be modified slightly by practical factors in study design. For example, although an investigator may want to study all asthmatic patients presenting to the emergency department, it may only be practical to study those presenting when investigators are available (*convenience sample*). Explicit inclusion and exclusion criteria must be defined before enrolling any patients, and these criteria must be uniformly applied in determining which patients are eligible to participate in the study. For the study to be most applicable to emergency medicine, the population should be defined in terms of clinical characteristics that are observable in the emergency department. On the other hand, groups of patients defined by their clinical characteristics in the emergency department are highly heterogeneous.[13] Some patients in the population may have more severe disease than other patients or may have a completely different cause for their symptoms.

When reading a study, one should look to see that the patient population is well defined and reasonably comparable to one's own patient population.[6] If important segments of the population are excluded (e.g., those with severe disease), the study results are not applicable to this subgroup. Researchers should not generalize their conclusions to patients not included in their study population.

Step 2: Recruitment and Enrollment of Patients

Once a patient population is defined, the next step is to recruit patients for enrollment in the study. To the extent possible, all patients meeting the predefined eligibility requirements for the study should be enrolled. The method of recruitment and enrollment should ensure that there is no systematic tendency to exclude a subgroup of patients from the study who meet the inclusion criteria. If such a *selection bias* exists, it will make the results of the study inapplicable to the types of patients that were excluded.[11,29] For example, if a study of head trauma patients specifies that informed consent must be obtained from the patient within the first half hour of presentation to the emergency department, there will be a systematic tendency to exclude patients with head trauma severe enough to result in an altered level of consciousness.

Even in a study that is appropriately designed, patients may self-select, resulting in selection bias. For example, patients of low socioeconomic status may be less likely than patients of high socioeconomic status to give consent for participation in clinical studies. Thus, although the disease itself may affect people in all socioeconomic strata, the study results may apply only to patients of high socioeconomic status similar to those who participated in the study.

To minimize selection bias, studies should aim to achieve consecutive enrollment of all patients who meet inclusion criteria. Furthermore, patients who meet eligibility criteria but are not subsequently enrolled should be counted to allow an estimation of the possible extent of any selection bias that might exist.[10] When reading a study, one should look for information on eligible patients who were not enrolled. A significant number of such patients may indicate selection bias. Researchers should explain why these patients were missed and should justify the validity of their results despite missed patients by showing, for example, that demographics and disease characteristics of missed patients were similar to those of enrolled patients.

Step 3: Randomization

The third step in conducting a clinical trial is to randomize enrolled patients to the different treatments being compared. The purpose of this randomized allocation is to create two groups of patients who, other than receiving different treatments, are as nearly identical as possible.[11]

Stratified randomization can be used to ensure that important confounding factors are equally distributed in the control and test groups.[11] In a stratified randomization, patients with the stratifying characteristic are randomized independently of those without the characteristic. For example, in a study of therapy for closed head injury, patients with severe closed head injury as defined by a low Glasgow Coma Scale score could be randomized independently of those patients with a higher Glasgow Coma Scale score. This would help ensure that the control and test groups have equal fractions of patients with severe and mild closed head injury.

Whenever possible, both the patient and the treating physician should be "blinded" (*double blinding*) to the therapy given.[11] Such blinding is important to ensure that both the patient and the investigating physician can make unbiased estimates of endpoints, including the occurrence of undesirable side effects. Recently, increasing importance has been placed on subjective outcomes, such as quality-of-life assessments made by the patient. Blinding is especially important to ensure that the patients' expectations regarding the effect of the new therapy do not influence their assessment of this type of outcome.

The quality of the randomization in a controlled clinical trial is important because studies that are inadequately randomized are more likely to "find" a positive treatment effect.[30] Similarly, studies in which blinding is inadequate, so that the patient or the treating physician might be able to determine the treatment the patient actually receives, are more likely to yield false-positive results.[15] When reviewing a clinical trial, one should look for truly random treatment assignment and adequate blinding procedures. For example, in a trial in which patients are enrolled if determined to be sufficiently "stable" by the physician and assignment to therapy or control is alternated, a physician with the bias that the therapy is not efficacious may avoid enrolling a patient by deeming the patient unstable if the physician knows that the next patient will be assigned to the treatment group. A better method of randomization would be assignment by a computerized randomization program, such that no pattern of assignment can be discerned by the enrolling personnel.

Step 4: Measurement of Baseline Characteristics

The fourth step is to measure the characteristics of patients enrolled in the study before therapy. The purpose of these baseline measurements is to detect imbalance between the control and test groups in characteristics that might influence each patient's chance for a successful outcome. Factors that might influence patient outcome and that are not controlled by the investigators are termed *confounding variables.* For example, the initial cardiac rhythm is a confounding variable in a study that compares different treatments for out-of-hospital cardiac arrest. If one group includes more patients in ventricular fibrillation while the other group has more patients in asystole, the intervention given to the first group will appear to be more efficacious. The influence of confounding characteristics must be anticipated, and those characteristics should be prospectively measured for all patients enrolled in the study. Subgroups of the overall patient population often have specific confounding characteristics (see Figure 197-1). If a clinically significant difference in outcome is ultimately detected between the two treatment groups, the baseline characteristics of the treatment groups should be compared to ensure that the observed difference in outcome did not occur because the two patient groups were not initially equivalent.[11] When reading a study, one should look to see that important confounders were measured and that they did not differ significantly between the groups studied.

Step 5: Treatment or Intervention

The next step is to administer the experimental treatment to the test group and the control treatment to the control group. Although the control and test patients should be nearly identical in their underlying characteristics, the two groups often have unequal compliance with therapy. For example, in a placebo-controlled study of an oral medication, those patients taking the active drug may find that it causes gastrointestinal discomfort, whereas those taking the placebo treatment might not experience such an effect. Therefore, patients taking the active agent may be less compliant with therapy. Unequal compliance complicates the interpretation of the outcome data.

Step 6: Collection of Data on Outcome

The sixth step is to determine the outcome of each patient. Definitions of treatment success and treatment failure must be explicitly defined before any data are collected. Sometimes a trial is initially designed to investigate the effects of therapy on one outcome, but during data analysis investigators notice an apparently significant effect on a different outcome. Such a serendipitous finding may be true but can also result from chance, because there are generally many such possible findings, and the study was not originally designed to investigate each of these possible outcomes. Such findings can be reported as interesting and warranting further investigation but should not be reported as reliable conclusions.

A difficulty with the collection of outcome data arises if too many subjects are lost to follow-up. This is more likely to occur in studies that evaluate the long-term effects of therapy. Patients who are lost to follow-up may have different characteristics than those patients who keep their follow-up appointments. For this reason, lack of complete follow-up in the study population can bias the results of the study.

Ensuring high rates of follow-up in studies of outpatient therapy is notoriously difficult. One approach is to create a multistep plan to obtain follow-up, with specific procedures to be followed if patients miss their first, second, or even third follow-up appointment. When reading a study, one should look at the percentage of patients lost to follow-up and look for a systematic effort to maintain good follow-up.

Step 7: Data Management

Once patients have been enrolled and have had their baseline characteristics measured, treatments administered, and outcomes determined, all this information must be organized and stored in a format that allows analysis of the data. Data should be collected on a form that limits and organizes the information. In general, information to be recorded on the data form should be highly structured, with categorical variables limited to a small number of possibilities and with very little (or no) unformatted "fill-in-the-blank" information requested. Such structure is required if the resulting data are to be analyzed statistically.

Errors may be introduced when data are entered into the database from data sheets. Bias can be introduced if certain types of data (e.g., written phrases in a patient questionnaire) must be reduced to a smaller number of categoric responses during the data entry procedure. Databases should be designed to ensure that the data listed are reasonable. For example, the electronic database should not allow entry of patient temperatures that are incompatible with life or negative blood pressures. When reviewing a study, one should look for data categorizations that are clear and clinically useful. For example, a study of post-resuscitation neurologic outcomes would be most useful to the emergency physician if patients were categorized as "normal," "mildly impaired," "severely impaired," or "dead," versus the more vague terms "good" or "poor" or by the results of a detailed neuropsychological battery of tests.

Step 8: Statistical Analysis

The next step is to analyze the data. Careful planning of the statistical analysis to be performed is required to minimize the chance of erroneous conclusions. Only a small number of comparisons should be made, and the study should be designed to have an adequate sample size to reliably detect a clinically important treatment effect.[31-35] The comparisons to be conducted must be defined prospectively, as well as any specific subgroups of patients that will be considered separately. Any imbalance in confounding baseline characteristics should be accounted for in the statistical analysis. Specific statistical tests are discussed later.

Step 9: Presentation and Publication of Results

Once the clinical trial data have been statistically analyzed, conclusions can be drawn from the results of the study. During the preparation of a manuscript describing the study and its conclusions, the investigators must be careful not to overextrapolate the results. Care must be taken to explain limitations in the study design and to enumerate factors that might bias the results of the study, or at least limit its applicability to different patient populations. One purpose of the peer review process is to ensure that appropriate care is taken in interpreting the clinical trial results.

The enthusiasm of most investigators and clinicians for the results of a clinical trial are partly determined by the direction of the results.[36] For example, a trial that shows a highly effective new therapy for a serious disease is interesting and exciting. On the contrary, a trial that shows that a previously unstudied therapy has no advantage over the currently accepted treatment may be less interesting. Because positive results are inherently more interesting, it is commonly believed that clinical trials yielding positive results are more likely to be published than those with negative results. This effect is termed *publication bias.*[37-39]

Recent studies, however, have shown that trials with negative results may be less likely to be submitted for publication but, once submitted, are as likely to be published as trials with positive results.[37,39] Thus publication bias may be the result of a *file drawer problem,* meaning that the results of studies with negative results sometimes end up in the file drawer, instead of in manuscripts submitted for publication.[40]

Publication bias and the file drawer problem are serious threats to the validity of the medical literature taken as a whole. If negative trials are selectively excluded from the medical literature, an ineffective treatment may appear to be at least partially effective because those (possibly poorly designed) studies that show some positive treatment effect are selectively submitted for publication. Meta-analyses or systematic reviews often utilize only published research. It may be unethical to subject patients to the risks and discomforts of participation in a clinical study and not publish the results, especially if participation did not result in any direct benefit to the patient.

Publication bias and other sources of bias can be especially problematic in pharmaceutical or commercially sponsored clinical research. Commercial studies are less likely to report unfavorable conclusions.[41] Data from industry-sponsored research may go unpublished or may be difficult to obtain for subsequent review.[42] When reading a clinical trial, one should look to see what agency or company funded the research and consider what biases, if any, might have been introduced.

DATA ANALYSIS

Classical Hypothesis Testing

Data from clinical trials are usually analyzed using *P* values and classical hypothesis testing.[3,7,8] In classical hypothesis testing, two hypotheses that might be supported by the data are considered. The first, called the *null hypothesis,* states that no difference exists between the groups being compared with respect to the measured outcome of interest.[7] For example, in a study examining the use of a new sympathomimetic agent for blood pressure support in patients with sepsis, the null hypothesis might be that there is no difference between the average systolic blood pressure achieved with the test agent and that achieved with the control agent. The *alternative hypothesis* states that the groups being compared are different.[7] In this example study, the alternative hypothesis might be that the test agent results in a 10 mm Hg greater average systolic blood pressure than the control agent. The magnitude of the difference between the two groups defined by the alternative hypothesis is called the *treatment effect* (Tables 197-1 and 197-2).

The treatment effect defined by the alternative hypothesis must be set before data are collected. The treatment effect should be large enough to be clinically important but small enough such that showing no difference between the groups rules out any clinically important treatment effect. In an interventional study, the difference defined is ideally the minimum treat-

Table 197-1. Steps in Classical Hypothesis Testing

Step	Description
Define the null hypothesis	There is no difference between the groups being compared. For example, in a clinical trial the null hypothesis might be that the response rate in the treatment group is equal to that in the control group.
Define the alternative hypothesis	The alternative hypothesis might be that the response hypothesis rate in the treatment group is greater than that in the control group by a given amount.
Calculate a *P* value	This calculation assumes that the null hypothesis is true. One determines the probability of obtaining the results found in the data, or other results even more inconsistent with the null hypothesis. This probability is the *P* value.
Accept or reject the null hypothesis	If the probability of observing the actual data, or more extreme results, under the null hypothesis is small ($P < \alpha$), then we should doubt that hypothesis. The idea is that if the probability under the null hypothesis of observing the actual results is very small, then there is a conflict between the null hypothesis and the observed data, and we should conclude that the null hypothesis is not true.
Accept the alternative hypothesis	If we reject the null hypothesis, we accept the alternative hypothesis by default.

Table 197-2. Terms Used in Design of Clinical Trials

Term	Definition
α	Maximum *P* value to be considered statistically significant; the risk of committing a type I error
α error	Type I error
Alternative hypothesis	Hypothesis considered an alternative to the null hypothesis; usually the alternate hypothesis is that there is an effect of the studied treatment on the measured variable of interest; also called *test hypothesis*
β	Risk of committing a type II error
β error	Type II error
Null hypothesis	Hypothesis that there is no effect of the studied treatment on the measured variable of interest
Power	Probability of detecting a treatment effect the size of the treatment effect sought (i.e., obtaining a *P* value $<\alpha$), given α, and the sample size of the clinical trial; power = $1 - \beta$
P value	Probability of obtaining results similar to those actually obtained, if the null hypothesis were true
Type I error	Obtaining a statistically significant *P* value when, in fact, there is no effect of the studied treatment on the measured variable of interest; also called *false positive*
Type II error	Not obtaining a statistically significant *P* value when, in fact, there is an effect of the treatment on the measured variable of interest that is as large or larger than the effect the trial was designed to detect; also called *false negative*

Modified from Lewis RJ: An introduction to the use of interim data analyses in clinical trials. *Ann Emerg Med* 22:1463, 1993.

ment effect thought to be clinically significant (i.e., that which would lead to a change in clinical practice). Sometimes a larger treatment effect is defined because designing a study to reliably detect the smallest clinically significant treatment effect would require too large a sample size.[32-35] When evaluating the results of a clinical trial, one should look for the size of the treatment effect that the trial was designed to detect.

Once the null and alternative hypotheses are defined, the null hypothesis is "tested" to determine which hypothesis (null or alternative) will be accepted as true. The process of testing the null hypothesis consists of calculating the probability of obtaining the observed results, or results that are even more inconsistent with the null hypothesis, assuming the null hypothesis is true. This probability is the *P* value.[7]

If the *P* value is less than some predefined value, denoted α (usually 5% or 0.05), the null hypothesis is rejected as false, and the alternative hypothesis is accepted as true. In other words, if the null hypothesis were true, the probability of obtaining data like that obtained or even more extreme results by chance alone is less than α.

Type I Errors

A type I error occurs when the investigator concludes that a difference has been demonstrated between two groups when no such difference exists.[7,8,43] It is a type of *false positive.* When data are analyzed using *P* values, a type I error occurs when a statistically significant *P* value is obtained but there is actually no underlying difference between the groups being compared. Because the *P* value is the probability of obtaining results equal to or more extreme than those actually observed, assuming there is actually no difference between the groups being compared, the risk of a type I error is equal to α, the maximum *P* value considered statistically significant, when the groups are fundamentally the same.[7,43]

Type II Errors, Power, and Sample Size

A type II error occurs when a difference exists between the two groups and that difference is as great as that defined by the alternative hypothesis, but when a nonsignificant *P* value is obtained.[7,32-35] In other words, there really is a difference between the two groups, but the trial failed to demonstrate this difference. A type II error is a type of *false negative* and is commonly denoted beta (β).

The *power* of a trial is the probability of detecting a treatment effect of a given size, if one truly exists.[32-35] Studies are usually designed to have a power of 0.80 or greater. Because the power of the trial is the chance of finding a true treatment effect, the quantity (1 – power) is the chance of missing a true treatment effect (i.e., risk of committing a type II error).[32,34] The value of (1 – β), or the power, and the magnitude of the treatment effect the clinical trial is designed to detect (defined by the alternative hypothesis) determine the sample size required for the study.[35]

The smaller the size of the treatment effect the study is designed to detect, the larger the required *sample size* will be for a given value of α (the maximum significant *P* value) and for a given power. For any given treatment effect, a smaller maximum significant *P* value or a larger power will also require a larger sample size. Surprisingly, clinical studies are often published with negative results even though the study did not have a sample size sufficient to detect reliably a clinically significant treatment effect.[32-35]

When reading a study, one should look for a statement about the power of the study. Generally, a power of 0.80 or greater is desirable. The treatment difference tested should not be too large, such that smaller clinically important treatment differences may still exist even after a "negative" result. Power and sample size should be estimated before beginning the study; a "post hoc power analysis" after the data have been collected is not recommended.

Statistical Tests

Depending on the characteristics of the data being analyzed, different statistical tests are used to determine the *P* value (Table 197-3). Student's *t* test and Wilcoxon rank sum test are used to compare continuous variables (e.g., serum glucose level, respiratory rate) between two groups of patients. If there are three or more groups of patients, one-way analysis of variance (one-way

Table 197-3. Common Statistical Tests

Statistical Test	Description
Student's *t* test	Used to test whether the means of measurements from two groups are equal, assuming that the data are normally distributed and that the data from both groups have equal variance.
Wilcoxon rank sum test (Mann-Whitney test)	Used to test whether two sets of observations have the same distribution; similar in use to the *t* test, but does not assume the data are normally distributed.
Chi-square test	Used with categoric-variables (two or more discrete treatments with two or more discrete outcomes) to test the null hypothesis that there is no effect of treatment on outcome; assumes at least five expected observations of each combination of treatment and outcome under the null hypothesis.
Fisher's exact test	Used similar to chi-squared test; may be used even when fewer than five observations are expected in one or more categories of treatment and outcome.
One-way analysis of variance (ANOVA)	Used to test the null hypothesis that three or more sets of continuous data have equal means, assuming the data are normally distributed and that the data from all groups have identical variances; may be regarded as a *t* test for three or more groups.
Kruskal-Wallis test	Nonparametric test analogous to one-way ANOVA; no assumption is made regarding normality of the data; may be regarded as a Wilcoxon rank sum test for three or more groups.

ANOVA) and the Kruskal-Wallis test are used to compare continuous variables between the groups. The chi-squared test and Fisher's exact test are used to detect associations between treatment and outcome when both the treatment and the outcome are categoric variables (e.g., placebo vs. active drug, lived vs. died, admitted vs. discharged).

Student's *t* test and one-way ANOVA are examples of parametric statistical tests. Parametric tests make assumptions about the underlying distribution of continuous variables. Both the Student's *t* test and ANOVA assume that the data are normally distributed (i.e., distributed in a bell-shaped curve around the central mean) and that the different groups yield data that have equal variance.

When the data to be analyzed are not normally distributed, the *P* value should be obtained using a nonparametric test.[7,8,44] Nonparametric tests are distribution free in that they do not rely on the data to have any particular underlying distribution. The nonparametric alternative to a *t* test for unpaired samples is the Mann-Whitney test, or Wilcoxon rank sum test. For a statistical comparison of paired measurements, the Wilcoxon signed rank test can be used. The nonparametric alternative to one-way ANOVA is the Kruskal-Wallis test. The *t* test may be used inappropriately when the data are unlikely to be normally distributed. If it is unclear whether the data are normally distributed, it is preferable to use the nonparametric test.

Confidence Intervals

Often the primary goal of a clinical trial is not simply to obtain a "yes-no" answer to the question of whether or not a treatment has any efficacy at all, but rather to estimate the magnitude of the treatment effect. This goal of measuring the effect of the treatment arises if another treatment is known to be effective. On the other hand, if no effective treatment is available, a new therapy may be adopted even if the study shows only the possibility of effectiveness.

When the primary goal of a study is to measure or estimate a treatment effect, the results should be reported using confidence intervals.[45-50] In general, a confidence interval is a range of treatment effects within which the true treatment effect falls with a given degree of certainty. For example, a 95% confidence interval will contain, within its limits, the true size of the treatment effect 95% of the time.[49-50]

Situations may arise in which a *P* value and confidence interval can lead to different qualitative interpretations of the same clinical trial results. Suppose one is studying a treatment for a disease that has no known effective therapy. If the 95% confidence interval for the treatment effect ranges from −2% to 30%, where the treatment effect is measured as the change in the absolute percentage of patients with a good outcome, many clinicians would interpret this as showing that, although the therapy may have little benefit, it has the possibility of having significant benefit (improving the outcome for up to 30% of patients). Thus, many clinicians would adopt the therapy as appropriate, given the lack of an effective alternative. If classical hypothesis testing had been used to analyze the same data, a nonsignificant *P* value would have been obtained. Many clinicians would then interpret the study as failing to show efficacy and conclude that the therapy was not appropriate for clinical use.[45-49]

When reading a study, one should look beyond the *P* values to the size of the treatment effect found and the width of the confidence intervals. If *P* is reported as significant (usually <0.05), one should make sure that the difference is clinically significant. For example, a difference in reduction of temperatures by 0.5° C between two antipyretics may not be clinically significant but would be statistically significant in a sufficiently large study. Issues such as cost, palatability, and adverse effects are likely to be more important in choosing between the two antipyretics. If *P* is reported as not significant (usually >0.05), the practitioner should ensure that the confidence interval is not so wide that a clinically important treatment effect is still possible, as in the previous example.

Multiple Comparisons

Whenever two groups of patients are compared statistically, even if they are fundamentally identical, a statistically significant *P* value can be obtained by chance.[7,43] If the maximum significant *P* value (α) is 0.05, there is a 5% chance that a statistically significant *P* value will be obtained when no true difference exists between the two patient populations. This risk of a false-positive *P* value occurs each time a statistical test is performed. When *multiple* comparisons are performed, whether they are "pairwise comparisons" of more than two groups of patients or the comparison of many different characteristics between two groups of patients, the risk of at least one false-positive *P* value is increased because the risk associated with each test is incurred multiple times (Table 197-4).[31,51,52] For a small number of tests, the overall risk of at least one type I error is roughly equal to the maximum significant *P* value used for each individual test multiplied by the total number of tests performed. This rough equality is the basis for the Bonferonni correction.[7,11,31]

The *Bonferonni correction* is a method for reducing the overall type I error risk for the whole study by

Table 197-4. Probability of at Least One Type I Error (False Positive) when Performing Multiple Comparisons*

Number of Comparisons	Probability of at Least One Type I Error
1	0.05
2	0.10
3	0.14
4	0.19
5	0.23
10	0.40
20	0.64
30	0.79

*Between identical groups with $\alpha = 0.05$.

reducing the maximum P value used for each of the individual statistical tests ("testwise risk"). The desired overall risk of a type I error (usually 0.05) is divided by the number of statistical tests to be performed, and this value is used as the maximum significant P value for each individual test. For example, if five comparisons are to be made, a maximum significant P value of 0.01 should be used for each of the five statistical tests.

The Bonferonni correction controls the overall risk ("studywise risk") of a type I error at the expense of an increased risk of a type II error. Because each statistical test is conducted using a more stringent criteria for a statistically significant P value, there is an increased risk that each test might miss a clinically important difference and yield a P value that is nonsignificant using the new criterion of $P < 0.01$.

Specific statistical tests have been developed to compare three or more groups of patients, such as the one-way ANOVA, Kruskal-Wallis test, chi-square test, and Fisher's exact test (see Table 197-3). These tests, which do not use the Bonferonni correction, can be useful for detecting differences among three or more groups with relatively high power while controlling the overall risk of a type I error. Their disadvantage is that, although they can detect a difference among three or more groups of patients, they do not define *which* pairwise differences are statistically significant. When reviewing positive studies with multiple study groups or multiple comparisons, one should consider the increase in type I error and check for the use of statistical methods accounting for multiple comparisons or appropriate for more than two study groups.

Interim Analyses of Accumulating Data

During a clinical trial, data accumulate sequentially and contain more and more information on the effectiveness of the treatments being compared. Often, however, these data are not analyzed until the trial has been completed and all patients have been enrolled. This type of fixed-sample-size design has the disadvantage of possibly enrolling more patients than are necessary to obtain a reliable result. It is often advantageous to plan one or more interim analyses of the data to be conducted before the full sample size has been reached, to see whether a reliable conclusion can be drawn from the data and the trial can be terminated early. Because this is a type of multiple comparison, such interim analyses must be planned in advance to avoid increasing the type I error rate.[11,52-54] When reading a study reporting results of an interim analysis, one should look to see that the interim analysis was planned, not performed because a casual observation of the data showed interesting or promising results.

Subgroups

Any group of patients is heterogeneous; this is especially true for groups of patients defined by presenting signs and symptoms in an emergency department setting. Some of the patients within such a group may have a more severe form of the disease in question, and some patients may have a coexisting disease that modifies the original disease process. Almost any group of patients can be considered to have multiple subgroups, each of which is more homogeneous than the overall group.

Because of this heterogeneity, a treatment effect that is detected within the entire group may or may not exist for a particular subgroup of the original population, or vice versa.[55-57] Therefore, the data from subgroups of patients are often analyzed separately. In some circumstances, this is important in determining which therapies are most effective in clinically important subgroups of patients.[55,56]

When subgroups of patients are to be analyzed, they should be defined prospectively. Unfortunately, studies with an overall negative result may emphasize a positive treatment effect found only in a subgroup defined after data collection. Although such findings may warrant brief discussion and further investigation, they are unreliable, because analyzing data from all possible after-the-fact subgroups requires the use of multiple statistical comparisons, which increases the chance that the finding represents a type I error.

Even if the subgroups were defined before the acquisition of any of the clinical trial data, testing for a treatment effect in each subgroup potentially increases the risk of a type I error. Also, because each subgroup of patients is smaller than the entire study population, the analysis of these subgroups may have low statistical power, which increases the chance of a type II error.

Additional problems can occur if the subgroups of patients are not defined properly.[55,56] A "proper" subgroup of patients is defined by signs, symptoms, or laboratory results that are available at the initial presentation and that are not modified by the treatments being compared. An "improper" subgroup of patients is defined by signs, symptoms, or laboratory findings that can, in principle, be modified by the treatments being administered. For example, in a study that compares different volumes of fluid resuscitation for patients with septic shock, an improper subgroup of patients might be defined by a low systolic blood pressure after fluid administration (the so-called refractory shock group). Conversely, a proper subgroup would be defined by a low systolic blood pressure before any fluid administration.

Because of the possible association between the subgroup assignment and the treatment being administered in an improperly defined subgroup, improper subgroups cannot be used to assess the effectiveness of therapies. It is a common error in many retrospective studies to compare such improper subgroups of patients. When reading a study reporting results in subgroups of patients, one should look to see that the subgroups were prospectively and properly defined and consider whether the characteristics defining the subgroup are available in the emergency department.

Multivariate Models

Multivariate modeling is a statistical tool used to determine the association between two or more independent (predictor) variables and a single dependent (outcome) variable. For example, a multivariate model might be used to determine the simultaneous effects of the patient's age and initial systolic blood pressure on the patient's chance of survival after penetrating abdominal trauma.

The two most common types of multivariate models in medical literature are multivariate linear regression models and multivariate logistic regression models. *Linear regression models* are used to determine the effects of two or more variables on a continuous outcome variable, such as blood pressure. *Logistic regression models* are generally used when the outcome is binary, such as survival (lived vs. died) or admission to the hospital (admitted vs. discharged).

Multivariate models offer several advantages over univariate analyses.[58-60] In a *univariate analysis*, the effect of a single predictor on the outcome is studied in isolation, often using the statistical tests discussed earlier in this chapter. Multivariate models are more akin to "real-life" clinical decision making, whereby a clinician considers several factors such as demographics (e.g., age, gender), history elements, and physical examination findings in deciding a patient's likely diagnosis or clinical course. They can determine which subsets of variables have significant effects on the outcome.

Multivariate models allow one to control for *confounders*, variables associated with the predictor one wishes to study that may also affect the outcome. For example, in studying the effect of alcohol intake on the outcome lung cancer diagnosis, tobacco smoking may confound the findings, since patients with high alcohol intake are more likely to also smoke, and smoking increases lung cancer. A multivariate model that includes both predictors, alcohol intake and smoking, allows one to look at the isolated effect of alcohol intake while holding the effects of other predictors (smoking) constant.[58]

An example of this phenomenon was illustrated in a recent study of the predictors of mortality in patients with ruptured abdominal aortic aneurysm.[61] Univariate analysis did not reveal the emergency department to operating room time interval to be a significant predictor of mortality, whereas in the multivariate model, prolonged emergency department to operating room time was clearly a significant predictor. Patients with longer emergency department to operating room times likely presented with other findings that made their diagnosis less clear, or the need for intervention appear less urgent, and were also associated with improved survival, such as higher initial systolic blood pressure and higher hematocrit. In the multivariate model, the effect of emergency department to operating room time could be assessed while holding such confounders as initial blood pressure and hematocrit constant.

The disadvantage of multivariate modeling is that it is more complex than univariate analysis. Certain statistical assumptions must be met, such as normal distribution of the outcome and independence of the predictor variables. Sometimes a single data point with an extreme value for a predictor or outcome variable, termed an *outlier*, exerts undue effects in the model. Regression diagnostics should be performed to assess that the statistical assumptions have been met and that no outliers are exerting undue effect.[58]

If two or more predictor variables interact (e.g., alcohol intake exerts an effect only in men, and not women, such that there is an interaction between the two predictors alcohol intake and gender), an *interaction term* must be included in the model. If two or more predictor variables give redundant information (e.g., the predictors age and arrest etiology may give redundant information for the outcome survival from pediatric cardiopulmonary arrest, since the vast majority of infants have an arrest etiology of sudden infant death syndrome), the model is said to have *multicollinearity*, and this may require revision of the model.[58]

Authors should report statistics that measure the "goodness of fit," or how well the model explains the observed data. However, the model may display good fit using these statistics and still be missing an important predictor variable or contain more predictor variables than necessary. Ultimately, investigators and readers need to have a basic understanding of the disease under study, to determine that all the likely significant predictors have been accounted for in the model.[58]

When reading studies using multivariate models, one should look for the use of independent predictor variables that make clinical sense. One should check the reporting of statistics measuring "goodness of fit" as well as discussion of regression diagnostics performed.

Importance of Prior Probabilities

Occasionally, statistical tests yield surprising results. Unexpected results are especially difficult to interpret using classical hypothesis testing. Consider a clinical trial that uses a randomized, double-blind controlled design to compare two antibiotics for prophylaxis of infectious complications of tube thoracostomy, with the development of local wound infections or empyema as the primary endpoint. Suppose no statistically significant difference is found in the rate of infectious complications, but a statistically significant difference in mortality is noted between the two treatment groups ($P = 0.03$). It seems inherently unlikely that the choice of prophylactic antibiotic would affect survival without affecting the infection rate. This is an example in which the apparent conclusion of the trial has a very low *a priori probability* of being true. In other words, the *a priori* probability that the choice of prophylactic antibiotic could influence survival after traumatic injuries without affecting infection rates is exceedingly small.

Two possible explanations exist for such results. First, the antibiotic may have a true effect on survival by a previously unknown mechanism. The results of the trial would then be a true positive. Second, the results of the study might be a type I error, with the statistically significant P value occurring by chance, even though the antibiotic has no effect on survival. The second explanation seems more likely than the first because the chance that the antibiotic exerted its effect through a previously unsuspected mechanism is so small. So, despite the fact that a statistically significant *P* value was obtained, it is unlikely that a true treatment effect exists. Classical hypothesis testing is most likely to be misleading when the alternative hypothesis being tested has a very low *a priori* probability of being true.[62]

The chance of any particular interpretation of data being correct depends both on the *a priori* probability of that conclusion being true and on the data supporting that conclusion.[62] An entire branch of statistical reasoning, bayesian statistics, has been developed to incorporate *a priori* information quantitatively into the interpretation of data. Bayesian analysis is analogous to usual clinical reasoning in which laboratory test results are interpreted in light of the patient's underlying risk of disease.[62,63] For example, the proper interpretation of nonspecific T-wave abnormalities in an electrocardiogram (ECG) depends on the patient from whom the ECG is obtained. If the ECG is obtained from a patient with multiple cardiac risk factors and typical ischemic chest pain, the T-wave abnormalities should be considered suggestive of myocardial ischemia. If, on the other hand, the ECG is obtained from a young, healthy adolescent with a very low chance of having cardiac disease, the T-wave abnormalities should be considered a normal variant. This use of *a priori* risk of disease in interpreting data is common in clinical practice. Similar logic should be used in the interpretation of data from clinical studies, especially when the conclusion would have been considered very unlikely before the study.[62-64]

When reviewing studies, one should consider the results in the context of one's knowledge base. Is there scientific basis for the results? Are the results in congruence with other research in this area? Have the results been corroborated in subsequent studies?

Data Dredging or Torturing

It is surprisingly common for large databases containing many hundreds or even thousands of patient records to be created without clear prior definition of what questions are to be asked of the data. A typical example of this type of database is a trauma registry. When such databases are analyzed, the number of different questions that could be asked (or hypotheses tested) is enormous. In the case of a trauma registry, many tens of variables potentially associated with an adverse outcome are collected. It is tempting to test statistically for an association of each of these variables with survival in an attempt to find combinations of variables that predict outcome. When such exploratory data analyses are performed without clearly defined hypotheses, the analyses may entail a very large number of statistical tests. Each one of these statistical tests carries the risk of a type I error. If enough hypotheses are tested, one is virtually assured of obtaining some statistically significant *P* values, even if none of the variables is associated with outcome.

Multiple comparisons are also made, although only implicitly, when large collections of data are visually inspected by an investigator searching for trends or associations. The investigator may make dozens of mental comparisons, most of which show little obvious difference among the groups being compared. Often, however, some "interesting" differences are noted and brought to the attention of the statistician for statistical testing. The statistician may then find a statistically significant difference but is unaware that many comparisons were made by the investigator in searching for one or a few promising comparisons.

This process of making a large number of implicit or explicit comparisons in searching for possibly important differences is called *data dredging* or, more pejoratively, *data torturing*.[65] Such undirected analysis of large databases virtually always yields statistically significant *P* values that are meaningless. Thus, even when working with large collections of data, it is essential that the comparisons to be made be defined before the inspection or collection of the data and that the total number of comparisons be kept to a minimum. The risk of false-positive results from data dredging are especially high when the hypotheses tested were unlikely to have been chosen before the data collection. In other words, hypotheses that are motivated by the same data used to test them are much less likely to be true than hypotheses that are defined before the data collection, based on independently known associations or concepts.

Not all studies performed on large preexisting databases are examples of data dredging. When reviewing such studies, one should look to see that the hypothesis was defined prior to any manipulation of the database. The hypothesis should be based on independent observations and corroborated by previous research (basic science, animal, or clinical).

Intention-to-Treat Analysis

The effectiveness of any therapy is determined both by the therapy's inherent efficacy and by the emergency physician's ability to administer the therapy to the patient. For example, in the case of an oral medication, the effectiveness will be decreased if patients find the medication's side effects to be intolerable and are noncompliant. Similarly, an invasive procedure will be less effective, on average, if it can only be performed successfully in a minority of patients. To estimate accurately the effectiveness a therapy will have in clinical practice, the emergency physician must properly account for those patients for whom a treatment is initiated but cannot be completed. This is the purpose of an intention-to-treat analysis.[66]

In an intention-to-treat analysis, patients are considered to be members of the treatment group to which they were originally assigned, regardless of whether they take the prescribed medication or the appropriate therapy is successfully administered to them.[66] For example, in a trial that examines the use of an oral agent, patients would be considered to be part of the test group if they were originally prescribed the test

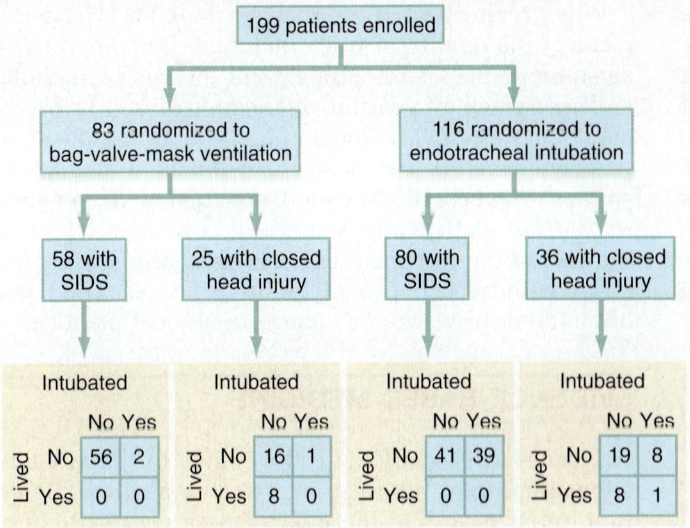

Figure 197-2. Results from a clinical trial comparing the use of bag/valve/mask ventilation to the use of endotracheal intubation in patients requiring advanced airway management in a prehospital setting. SIDS, sudden infant death syndrome.

medication, even if they freely admit to never having taken any of the tablets.

In a study of prehospital intubation, children were randomized to receive bag/valve/mask (BVM) ventilation alone or BVM ventilation followed by endotracheal intubation (Figure 197-2).[67] The populations of children were inherently heterogeneous; some children had sudden infant death syndrome, and others had closed head injury. The initial population was well randomized to the two interventions. Children with sudden infant death syndrome were substantially easier to intubate (because of their flaccid state) in the prehospital setting than children with closed head injury, but their overall survival rate was much lower.

The goal of the analysis of the data was to determine the effect of prehospital endotracheal intubation on survival. The correct way to group the data is to consider all patients initially assigned to the endotracheal intubation group as belonging to that group, whether or not they were successfully intubated. Thus, of 199 patients, 116 patients were assigned to the endotracheal intubation group, and 83 patients were assigned to the BVM ventilation group. Considering all patients in the endotracheal intubation group, whether or not they were successfully intubated, the overall survival rate is 7.7% (9/116). Similarly, considering all patients in the BVM ventilation group, the overall survival rate is 9.6% (8/83). Thus, the results of the study show a small trend toward improved survival with BVM ventilation.

Alternatively (but incorrectly), one might group the data according to the treatment actually received.[66] In this case, children initially assigned to the endotracheal intubation group, but not successfully intubated, might be considered to be members of the BVM ventilation group because that was the treatment they actually received. If one counts all children who received only BVM ventilation, the overall survival rate in that group is 10.8% (16/148). Similarly, if one considers only children who were *successfully* intubated as the members of the endotracheal intubation group, the overall survival rate in that group is only 2.0% (1/51). This type of analysis then suggests that endotracheal intubation is extremely harmful. Whenever there is an association between compliance or the ability to administer an intended treatment and the patient's baseline chance of a successful outcome, analysis by treatment received does not accurately estimate the effect of the therapy in an actual patient population.

Even when an intention-to-treat analysis is used to analyze study results, extrapolation of the results to the general population may be unreliable if the compliance in the general population is lower than that in the study population.[68] This is a common problem, because study populations tend to be highly compliant compared with the general population. When reviewing a study, one should look for an intention-to-treat analysis, rather than analysis by treatment received. Additionally, one should assess whether one's patient population is likely to be as compliant as the study population, or, in the case of a procedure, whether one is likely to be able to perform the procedure with the same rate of success.

Meta-analysis

Meta-analysis, or systematic review, is a statistical method for quantitatively combining the results of multiple clinical trials that investigate identical or similar therapies for a specific disease, to obtain more accurate estimates of the effectiveness of the treatment.[69] Unlike the traditional review article, a meta-analysis emphasizes the quantitative estimation of the treatment effect observed in all the available studies taken as a whole and usually provides an estimate of the reliability or quality of the results of each study. Meta-analyses can be powerful tools in practicing evidence-based medicine, since they collate the results of many or all available studies.[70]

Studies with poor design have been shown to be more likely to find an apparent positive treatment effect. A meta-analysis that includes many poorly designed studies tends to bias the results toward showing a positive treatment effect, even if no such effect exists. Methods for controlling and measuring the effect of poorly designed studies on the results of the meta-analysis have been developed and are often termed *sensitivity analyses*.[71] One method is to first perform the meta-analysis using only studies of the highest quality and then to sequentially include studies of lower and lower quality, to determine whether this causes a directional shift in the results. This approach requires a relatively objective measurement of study quality. Numerous scales and methods for defining study quality have been developed.[72,73]

Publication bias, whereby smaller studies with negative results (i.e., no treatment effect shown) are not submitted for publication, may affect the validity of the conclusions drawn by a meta-analysis.[70] Authors of meta-analyses must strive to include all available trials, often requiring search strategies beyond a simple MEDLINE search. Other methods may include hand searching of relevant review articles and identified studies' reference lists, contacting commercial sponsors and investigators to seek unpublished data, and searching nontraditional bibliographic databases.[74] Problems can arise when pharmaceutical companies withhold data from commercially sponsored trials.[42]

Funnel plots are used to assess for publication bias.[71] Authors plot trial size or quality score against treatment effect. One would expect a funnel-shaped plot, whereby smaller and lower quality trials have a wide base centered around the mean treatment effect, whereas larger and higher quality studies, because they provide more accurate estimates of the treatment effect, make up the narrower top of the funnel. If a portion of the funnel is missing, for instance the smaller studies with no treatment effect, this is indicative of publication bias.

Sometimes discrepancies arise between meta-analytic results and subsequent results from a large, randomized, clinical trial, leaving the reader wondering which results are correct.[75] Discrepancies may be due to bias introduced in the meta-analysis due to heterogeneity of studies included, poor quality of studies included, or publication bias.[75,76] Discrepancies may also be due to differences in inclusion or exclusion criteria, or in definitions of outcomes. For example, a meta-analysis of studies that included patients at high risk for preeclampsia found calcium supplementation to be effective prophylactic therapy, whereas a single large trial that included only low-risk patients found calcium supplementation to have no effect.[77] Because of the inclusion of multiple trials, a meta-analysis may incorporate results from thousands of patients, and small treatment effects may reach statistical significance. Such small treatment effects may be false positives arising from inadvertent bias in poorly designed studies, or from an artifact of the meta-analysis itself. Alternatively, the results may be true but clinically unimportant, or they may be true, clinically important, and warrant a change in clinical practice. The discerning reader must consider the size of the treatment effect and possible bias introduced by the meta-analysis methodology and studies included to determine which of the above is most likely.

When reviewing a meta-analysis, look for (1) assessment of the quality of trials included, (2) comprehensiveness of the search strategy for studies to include and assessment of possible publication bias, (3) narrow confidence intervals indicating a large number of patients, and (4) the majority of the highest quality studies to agree with the overall conclusion. Even when results are statistically significant, consider whether the size of the treatment effect is clinically significant and, combined with consideration of the costs and risks of the therapy, warrant a change in clinical practice.

EVIDENCE-BASED MEDICINE

Evidence-based medicine (EBM) refers to the systematic gathering of information from the medical literature, often regarding the effectiveness of a particular treatment or the diagnostic accuracy of a particular test, with the intent to apply that evidence in diagnostic or management decisions related to an individual patient.[78,79] Although a specialized vocabulary has evolved, including both old and new terms (Table 197-5), the practice of EBM essentially involves the systematic application of long-established principles of medical literature analysis that, until recently, were often unknown by or impractical for the medical practitioner.

The fundamental steps in EBM are (1) to define precisely the clinical question being asked in terms that can be addressed by clinical studies; (2) to gather the available medical literature related to the question defined; (3) to assess the relevance, validity, and quality of the evidence contained in each study; and (4) to summarize the available evidence so that diagnostic and management decisions can be made for the individual patient based on the recovered information.[78]

Step 1: Definition of Clinical Question

The first step in the practice of EBM is to define the clinical question clearly. The process of developing a well-formulated clinical question consists of several parts. First, the practitioner must define the population of patients similar to the individual patient motivating the search. The goal is to define a group of patients broad enough that they are likely to have been studied in clinical trials but specific enough that they are similar to the patient. Second, the practitioner must define the treatments or diagnostic approaches being considered. This involves defining the alternate approaches that might be used by reasonable practitioners in similar situations. Third, the practitioner must define the outcome of interest. The outcome of interest should be important to the patient and definable in terms of measurable quantities.

The steps required to define the clinical question in EBM practice are similar to the steps required to define a good hypothesis for a clinical trial: (1) the population for a clinical trial should be clearly defined, (2) the interventions to be used should be reasonable and well defined, and (3) a single clinically relevant and measurable outcome must be defined.

Table 197-5. Terms Used In Evidence-Based Medicine (EBM)

EBM Term	Definition
Bias	Tendency to yield a result that lies to one side or the other of the true value; an error that is not centered around zero.
Critically appraised topic (CAT)	Summary of the results of an analysis of the evidence relevant to a particular clinical question.
Likelihood ratio, negative (LR–)	Probability that a negative test result would occur in a patient with the disease in question, divided by the probability that a negative test result would occur in a patient without the disease in question (generally <1).
Likelihood ratio, positive (LR+)	Probability that a positive test result would occur in a patient with the disease in question, divided by the probability that a positive test result would occur in a patient without the disease in question (generally >1).
Negative predictive value	Fraction of patients with a negative test result who, in fact, do *not* have the disease in question.
Number needed to treat (NNT)	Number of patients who must be treated with the better of two treatments, so that one additional "good" outcome is obtained.
Odds	Probability of an outcome, divided by the probability of the outcome not occurring.
Odds ratio	Odds of the outcome of interest occurring in one group of patients, divided by the odds of the outcome of interest occurring in another group.
Positive predictive value	Fraction of patients with a positive test result who, in fact, *do* have the disease in question.
Post-test odds	Odds of the outcome of interest (e.g., particular disease being present), once a particular test result (positive or negative) is known to have occurred; equal to the pretest odds, times the likelihood ratio for the test result obtained.
Post-test probability	Probability of the outcome of interest, once a particular test result is known to have occurred.
Pretest odds	Odds of the outcome of interest, before the test result is known.
Pretest probability	Probability of the outcome of interest, before the test result is known.
Relative risk	Probability of an outcome in one group, divided by the probability of the same outcome in another group.
Reliability	Degree with which a clinical trial or diagnostic test is likely to yield consistent results when repeated.
Sensitivity	Fraction of patients with the disease in question who have a positive test result.
Specificity	Fraction of patients without the disease in question who have a negative test result.
Validity, external	Degree to which the results from a study accurately reflect what would happen to similar patients who were not enrolled, including patients at other locations.
Validity, internal	Degree to which a study accurately measures the outcomes for the enrolled study population.

Step 2: Collection of Evidence

The second step in the practice of EBM is to gather the available evidence.[78,80-83] Although a variety of resources might be used to accomplish this, the practitioner generally begins by searching one of the available electronic databases of published medical literature (e.g., MEDLINE). In addition, the physician may want to search one of the databases of known clinical trials (e.g., Cochrane collaborative) because these databases often include the results from studies that have not been published or are not available on MEDLINE. Initially, the goal is to cast a very wide net to gather as many of the available studies as possible.[78]

Step 3: Analysis of Studies for Validation, Reliability, and Relevance

The third step in the practice of EBM is to analyze each of the gathered studies to determine its validity, reliability, and relevance. The *validity* of a study is the degree with which the results are likely to represent "truth." When the clinical question involves the effect of a therapeutic intervention, a double-blind randomized clinical trial is generally believed to be the most valid type of study. The external validity of a study may be reduced if the patient population in the study is too dissimilar to the patient motivating the current activity, or if the clinical setting is substantially different from the physician's practice setting. Threats to internal validity include inadequate blinding, inadequate or no randomization, and use of historical controls, or worse, absence of controls.

The *reliability* of a study refers to the degree with which the results of the study are likely to be the same if the study were repeated in the same clinical setting using another group of similar patients. A study may have reduced reliability if the sample size is too small or if some of the study procedures were poorly defined and therefore difficult to repeat consistently (e.g., if some interventions were decided by individual treating physicians).

The *relevance* of a study is the degree with which the results, specifically the outcome or outcomes measured, directly address the clinical question being posed. Thus, a study is less relevant if the outcome used in the study is different than the outcome deemed most clinically important. For example, long-term survival may be the most clinically important endpoint for a particular condition, whereas the available clinical trials may use survival at 24 hours as their endpoint. This leaves open to question whether differences observed in survival at 24 hours would lead to differences in long-term survival.

Step 4: Summary of Most Useful Evidence

Based on these considerations, the practitioner of EBM proceeds to the fourth step, summarizing the available evidence from the studies that are the most valid, reliable, and relevant. For each of these studies, the size of the treatment effect or the accuracy of the diagnostic strategies should be noted. In the case of a binary outcome (e.g., lived vs. died, admitted vs. discharged), the *number needed to treat* is a useful measure of the size of the treatment effect.[79] The utility of diagnostic tests is best measured by positive and negative likelihood ratios. Other useful measures of diagnostic accuracy include sensitivity, specificity, positive predictive value, and negative predictive value.[84-86]

Step 5: Application to Patient and Critical Appraisal

Once the available evidence from high-quality studies is summarized, the practitioner is ready to apply the information to the care of the individual patient. To save the information, however, it is useful to create a summary of the entire EBM process, briefly describing each step and the results from each step. Such summaries are sometimes called *critically appraised topics*, which can be saved for future reference.[87] Such "short-cut reviews" performed by others are available in journals or on-line (www.ebem.org), but results must be interpreted in light of the specific study question, comprehensiveness of the search for evidence, and the appraisal process used.[88]

SUMMARY

For the educated reader, the medical literature provides an ever-expanding view of knowledge regarding the effectiveness of medical therapy. A qualitative understanding of the concepts described in this chapter allows the emergency physician to distinguish high-quality studies with results that warrant a change in clinical practice from poor-quality studies that, at best, only suggest important questions to be studied.

REFERENCES

1. Department of Clinical Epidemiology and Biostatistics, McMaster University Health Sciences Centre: How to read clinical journals. I. Why to read them and how to start reading them critically. *Can Med Assoc J* 124:555, 1981.
2. Haynes RB, et al: How to keep up with the medical literature. I. Why try to keep up and how to get started. *Ann Intern Med* 105:149, 1986.
3. Menegazzi JJ, Yealy DM, Harris JS: Methods of data analysis in the emergency medicine literature. *Am J Emerg Med* 9:225, 1991.
4. Wulff HR, et al: What do doctors know about statistics? *Stat Med* 6:3, 1987.
5. Haynes RB, et al: How to keep up with the medical literature. II. Deciding which journals to read regularly. *Ann Intern Med* 105:309, 1986.
6. Guyatt G, Rennie D (eds): *Users' Guides to the Medical Literature: A Manual for Evidence-Based Clinical Practice.* Chicago, American Medical Association, 2002.
7. Lewis RJ, Bessen HA: Statistical concepts and methods for the reader of clinical studies in emergency medicine. *J Emerg Med* 9:221, 1991.
8. Piantadosi S: *Clinical Trials: A Methodologic Perspective.* New York, John Wiley & Sons, 1997.
9. Altman DG, Goodman SN: Transfer of technology from statistical journals to the biomedical literature: Past trends and future predictions. *JAMA* 272:129, 1994.
10. Moher D, Schulz KF, Altman D, for the CONSORT Group (Consolidated Standards of Reporting Trials): The CONSORT statement: Revised recommendations for improving the quality of reports of parallel-group randomized trials. *JAMA* 285:1987, 2001.
11. Meinert CL: *Clinical Trials: Design, Conduct, and Analysis.* New York, Oxford University Press, 1986.
12. Hulley SB (ed): *Designing Clinical Research: An Epidemiologic Approach,* 2nd ed. Philadelphia, Lippincott Williams & Wilkins, 2001.
13. Bailey KR: Generalizing the results of randomized clinical trials. *Cont Clin Trials* 15:15, 1994.
14. Rosenbaum PR: Discussing hidden bias in observational studies. *Ann Intern Med* 115:901, 1991.
15. Schulz KF, et al: Empirical evidence of bias: Dimensions of methodological quality associated with estimates of treatment effects in controlled trials. *JAMA* 273:408, 1995.
16. Sacks H, Chalmers TC, Smith H: Randomized versus historical controls for clinical trials. *Am J Med* 72:233, 1982.
17. Chalmers TC, et al: Bias in treatment assignment in controlled clinical trials. *N Engl J Med* 309:1358, 1983.
18. Angell M: The interpretation of epidemiologic studies. *N Engl J Med* 323:823, 1990.
19. Hellman S, Hellman DS: Of mice but not men: Problems of the randomized clinical trial. *N Engl J Med* 324:1585, 1991.
20. Passamani E: Clinical trials: Are they ethical? *N Engl J Med* 324:1589, 1991.
21. Rothman KJ, Michels KB: The continuing unethical use of placebo controls. *N Engl J Med* 331:394, 1994.
22. Taubes G: Use of placebo controls in clinical trials disputed. *Science* 267:25, 1995.
23. Benson K, Hartz AJ: A comparison of observational studies and randomized, controlled trials. *N Engl J Med* 342:1878, 2000.
24. Concato J, Shah N, Horwitz RI: Randomized, controlled trials, observational studies, and the hierarchy of research designs. *N Engl J Med* 342:1887, 2000.
25. Pocock SJ, Elbourne DR: Randomized trials or observational tribulations? *N Engl J Med* 342:1907, 2000.
26. Kwiatkowski T, Silverman R: Research fundamentals. II. Choosing and defining a research question. *Acad Emerg Med* 5:1114, 1998.
27. Kramer MS: Medical research: A prescriptive view. *Pediatrics* 95:82, 1995.
28. Kahn CR: Picking a research problem: The critical decision. *N Engl J Med* 330:1530, 1994.
29. Kahn HA, Sempos CT: *Statistical Methods in Epidemiology.* New York, Oxford University Press, 1989.
30. Chalmers TC, et al: Evidence favoring the use of anticoagulants in the hospital phase of acute myocardial infarction. *N Engl J Med* 297:1091, 1977.
31. Smith DG, et al: Impact of multiple comparisons in randomized clinical trials. *Am J Med* 83:545, 1987.
32. Brown CG, et al: The beta error and sample size determination in clinical trials in emergency medicine. *Ann Emerg Med* 16:183, 1987.
33. Detsky AS, Sackett DL: When was a "negative" clinical trial big enough? How many patients you needed depends on what you found. *Arch Intern Med* 145:709, 1985.
34. Freiman JA, et al: The importance of beta, the type II error and sample size in the design and interpretation of the randomized control trial: Survey of 71 "negative" trials. *N Engl J Med* 299:690, 1978.
35. Moher D, Dulberg CS, Wells GA: Statistical power, sample size, and their reporting in randomized controlled trials. *JAMA* 272:122, 1994.
36. Koren G, Klein N: Bias against negative studies in newspaper reports of medical research. *JAMA* 266:1824, 1991.

37. Dickersin K, Min Y, Meinert CL: Factors influencing publication of research results: Follow-up of applications submitted to two institutional review boards. *JAMA* 267:374, 1992.
38. Begg CB, Berlin JA: Publication bias: A problem in interpreting medical data. *J R Statist Soc A* 151:491, 1988.
39. Dickersin K, et al: Publication bias and clinical trials. *Cont Clin Trials* 8:343, 1987.
40. Rosenthal R: The "file drawer problem" and tolerance for null results. *Psychol Bull* 86:638, 1979.
41. Friedberg M, et al: Evaluation of conflict of interest in economic analyses of new drugs used in oncology. *JAMA* 282:1453, 1999.
42. Johansen HK, Gotzsche PC: Problems in the design and reporting of trials of antifungal agents encountered during meta-analysis. *JAMA* 282:1752, 1999.
43. Brown GW: Errors, types I and II. *Am J Dis Child* 137:586, 1983.
44. Lewis RJ: Parametric statistical tests: Unnecessary assumptions, computers, and the search for the trustworthy p-value [editorial]. *Acad Emerg Med* 5:1048, 1998.
45. Simon R: Confidence intervals for reporting results of clinical trials. *Ann Intern Med* 105:429, 1986.
46. Simon R: Why confidence intervals are useful tools in clinical therapeutics. *J Biopharm Stat* 3:243, 1993.
47. Borenstein M: The case for confidence intervals in controlled clinical trials. *Cont Clin Trials* 15:411, 1994.
48. Goodman SN, Berlin JA: The use of predicted confidence intervals when planning experiments and the misuse of power when interpreting results. *Ann Intern Med* 121:200, 1994.
49. Young KD, Lewis RJ: What is confidence? Part I. The use and interpretation of confidence intervals. *Ann Emerg Med* 30:307, 1997.
50. Young KD, Lewis RJ: What is confidence? Part II. Detailed definition and determination of confidence intervals. *Ann Emerg Med* 30:311, 1997.
51. Klockars AJ, Sax G: *Multiple Comparisons.* Thousand Oaks, California, Sage Publications, 1986.
52. O'Brien PC, Shampo MA: Statistical considerations for performing multiple tests in a single experiment. Part 6. Testing accumulating data repeatedly over time. *Mayo Clin Proc* 63:1245, 1988.
53. Lewis RJ: An introduction to the use of interim data analyses in clinical trials. *Ann Emerg Med* 22:1463, 1993.
54. Lewis RJ, Bessen HA: Sequential clinical trials in emergency medicine. *Ann Emerg Med* 19:1047, 1990.
55. Yusuf S, et al: Analysis and interpretation of treatment effects in subgroups of patients in randomized clinical trials. *JAMA* 266:93, 1991.
56. Oxman AD, Guyatt GH: A consumer's guide to subgroup analyses. *Ann Intern Med* 116:78, 1992.
57. Lee KL, et al: Clinical judgment and statistics: Lessons from a simulated randomized trial in coronary artery disease. *Circulation* 61:508, 1980.
58. Glantz SA, Slinker BK: *Primer of Applied Regression & Analysis of Variance,* 2nd ed. New York, Appleton & Lange, 2000.
59. Hosmer DW, Lemeshow S: *Applied Logistic Regression.* New York, Wiley & Sons, 1989.
60. Concato J, Feinstein AR, Holford TR: The risk of determining risk with multivariable models. *Ann Intern Med* 118:201, 1993.
61. Hans SS, Huang RR: Results of 101 ruptured abdominal aortic aneurysm repairs from a single surgical practice. *Arch Surg* 138:898, 2003.
62. Lewis RJ, Wears RL: An introduction to the Bayesian analysis of clinical trials. *Ann Emerg Med* 22:1328, 1993.
63. Browner WS, Newman TB: Are all significant *P* values created equal? The analogy between diagnostic tests and clinical research. *JAMA* 257:2459, 1987.
64. Brophy JM, Joseph L: Placing trials in context using Bayesian analysis: GUSTO revisited by Reverend Bayes. *JAMA* 273:871, 1995.
65. Mills JL: Data torturing. *N Engl J Med* 329:1196, 1993.
66. Lee YJ, et al: Analysis of clinical trials by treatment actually received: Is it really an option? *Stat Med* 10:1595, 1991.
67. Gausche M, et al: Effect of out-of-hospital pediatric endotracheal intubation on survival and neurologic outcome: A controlled clinical trial. *JAMA* 283:783, 2000.
68. Andrade SE, et al: Discontinuation of antihyperlipidemic drugs: Do rates reported in clinical trials reflect rates in primary care settings? *N Engl J Med* 332:1125, 1995.
69. Olson CM: Understanding and evaluating a meta-analysis. *Acad Emerg Med* 1:392, 1994.
70. Klassen TP, Jadad AR, Moher DP: Guidelines for reading and interpreting systematic reviews. Part I. *Arch Pediatr Adolesc Med* 152:700, 1998.
71. Klassen TP, Jadad AR, Moher DP: Guidelines for reading and interpreting systematic reviews. Part III. *Arch Pediatr Adolesc Med* 152:915, 1998.
72. Chalmers TC, et al: A method for assessing the quality of a randomized control trial. *Cont Clin Trials* 2:31, 1981.
73. Moher D, et al: Assessing the quality of randomized controlled trials: An annotated bibliography of scales and checklists. *Cont Clin Trials* 16:62, 1995.
74. Klassen TP, Jadad AR, Moher DP: Guidelines for reading and interpreting systematic reviews. Part II. *Arch Pediatr Adolesc Med* 152:812, 1998.
75. Cappelleri JC, et al: Large trials vs. meta-analysis of smaller trials: How do their results compare? *JAMA* 276:1332, 1996.
76. Ioannidis JP, Cappelleri JC, Lau J: Issues in comparisons between meta-analyses and large trials. *JAMA* 279:1089, 1998.
77. DerSimonian R, Levine RJ: Resolving discrepancies between a meta-analysis and a subsequent large controlled trial. *JAMA* 282:664, 1999.
78. Sackett DL, et al: *Evidence-Based Medicine: How to Practice and Teach EBM*, 2nd ed. New York, Churchill Livingstone, 2000.
79. Cordell WH: Number needed to treat (NNT). *Ann Emerg Med* 33:433, 1999.
80. Corrall CJ, Wyer PC, Zick LS, Bockrath CR: Evidence-based emergency medicine. How to find evidence when you need it, part 1: Databases, search programs, and strategies. *Ann Emerg Med* 39:302, 2002.
81. Gallagher PE, Allen TY, Wyer PC: How to find evidence when you need it, part 2: A clinician's guide to MEDLINE—the basics. *Ann Emerg Med* 39:436, 2002.
82. Gallagher PE, Allen TY, Wyer PC: How to find evidence when you need it, part 3: A clinician's guide to MEDLINE—tricks and special skills. *Ann Emerg Med* 39:547, 2002.
83. Wyer PC, Allen TY, Corrall CJ: How to find evidence when you need it, part 4: Matching clinical questions to appropriate databases. *Ann Emerg Med* 42:136, 2003.
84. Fontanarosa PB: An evidence based approach to diagnostic testing in emergency medicine. *Emerg Med Clin North Am* 17:1, 1999.
85. Gallagher EJ: Clinical utility of likelihood ratios. *Ann Emerg Med* 31:391, 1998.
86. Gallagher EJ: Application of likelihood ratios to clinical decision rules: Defining the limits of clinical expertise. *Ann Emerg Med* 34:664, 1999.
87. Wyer PC: The critically appraised topic: Closing the evidence-transfer gap. *Ann Emerg Med* 30:639, 1997.
88. Wyer PC, Rowe BH, Guyatt GH, Cordell WH: The clinician and the medical literature: When can we take a shortcut? *Ann Emerg Med* 36:149, 2000.

CHAPTER 198

Observation Medicine and Clinical Decision Units

Malcolm Mahadevan and Louis Graff

PRINCIPLES OF OBSERVATION MEDICINE

Observation services are an extension of emergency department services specifically designed to address unmet patient needs. Observation services improve patient care by continuing the evaluation and management of selected emergency department patients who would otherwise require hospitalization for acute care services. With observation, 80% of these patients can be sent home without the need for hospitalization. The cost to evaluate and treat these patients is half that incurred by admission.[1,2] In addition, the physician threshold for extended evaluation (traditionally provided with hospitalization) is lowered. Patients with atypical signs and symptoms are more fully evaluated to rule out serious conditions such as acute myocardial infarction or acute appendicitis. Thus, in addition to lower costs, there is also a simultaneous decrease in the inadvertent release home of patients with serious disease.[1]

An emergency department observation unit is a designated area to provide these short-term services for up to 24 hours. Names given to observation units vary and include *chest pain unit*, *clinical decision unit*, and *rapid diagnostic treatment unit*. An emergency department–based observation unit is not a holding unit. A holding unit stems from hospital overcrowding and is an area where patients admitted to the hospital are held passively until they can be transferred to an inpatient hospital bed.

Two categories of patients benefit from extension of the 2- to 3-hour emergency department visit to up to 24 hours. One group is selected emergency department patients with a critical diagnostic syndrome (Box 198-1). These are patients whose diagnosis is unclear after the initial emergency department evaluation and who will benefit from further evaluation during observation. They are either admitted if found to have a serious disease or released home. The second group is emergency department patients with selected emergency conditions (see Box 198-1). Those patients not successfully treated during the traditional emergency department treatment period benefit from further treatment in an observation unit.

THE OBSERVATION APPROACH

The traditional emergency department encounter lasts between 2 and 3 hours. The physician performs a history and physical examination and orders laboratory and radiologic tests. When the test results return, the physician either admits the patient to the hospital or discharges the patient home.

The observation approach adds a third option at the completion of the emergency department evaluation. The patient is treated and further tested for up to 24 hours. After the observation period, patients are then admitted to the hospital or discharged home.

Observation begins with the physician writing the observation orders. The patient is transferred to the observation unit from the main emergency department. An observation unit chart is started with treatment and investigations are begun. The observation orders include the clinical impression, the reason for observation, the therapeutic evaluation plan, expected outcome, criteria and time frame for disposition, and the physician responsible for the patient's disposition. The responsible physician may be the emergency physician or the patient's private physician or a consultant.

Adequate staffing of the observation unit is crucial for the success of the program. The patient receives services for an average 12 to 24 hours beyond the emergency department visit. The amount of nursing staff required will be proportional to the type and intensity of treatment offered, the number of beds, whether the beds are monitored or nonmonitored, and the patient acuity. The average staff is one registered nurse per four to six patients in monitored beds and one registered nurse per six to nine patients in nonmonitored beds. The number of full-time equivalents of nursing staff is calculated to meet these staffing needs.

Staff nursing skills should be broad based and include the ability to care for patients of all ages with a wide spectrum of conditions. They should have the ability to provide critical care when needed and frequent assessments of patients under their care. Nurses should be able to provide prolonged patient and family interactions, including hygiene care, meals, and emotional support. These are all skills present in emergency nurses. When nonemergency nurses are recruited for the observation unit, they should be cross-trained, serving some shifts each month in the emergency department.

Additional physician staffing is also required for the observation unit. Managing emergency department patients in the observation unit for an additional 12 to 14 hours requires approximately a doubling of the physician service for that patient.[3] Calculations of the physician staffing for the amount of additional services

BOX 198-1. Conditions Appropriate for Observation

Evaluation: Critical Diagnostic Syndromes	Treatment: Emergency Conditions
Abdominal pain	Asthma
Chest pain	Atrial fibrillation
DVT	Congestive heart failure
Gastrointestinal bleed	Dehydration
Syncope	Infections
Trauma	Pneumonia
Blunt abdominal	Pyelonephritis
Blunt chest	
Penetrating abdominal	
Penetrating chest	
Head injury	

DVT, deep vein thrombosis.

will be approximately one full-time equivalent for every 2000 patients observed per year. As with the nurses, physicians in the observation unit must have broad-based knowledge and experience in the management of a wide variety of disease processes. Emergency physicians possess the skill sets necessary for observation medicine. The emergency physician is ultimately responsible for the care of the patient and needs to provide clear leadership at all times.

Patients and staff involved in the observation process should be well informed about the goals and benefits provided by the extended service. Well-written, condition-specific observation protocols ensure a continuum of care, with the transfer of patient care at shift change. The services provided in an emergency department observation unit are equivalent to inpatient services, albeit at an accelerated pace.

Consultants must be available to the observation unit as they would to any inpatient service. They provide therapeutic and management advice and assist in the serial examinations of patients as requested. The observation unit must identify needs, notify the consultant, assemble all the needed information, and carry out the consultant's recommendations within the shortest time frame possible.

Residents and medical students are included in the functioning of the observation unit, as exposure to the observation approach is an integral part of their training program. Emergency residents specifically need training in this area of emergency medicine through clinical practice, lectures, and review of published literature. Residents from other specialties benefit from the exposure by having a better understanding of its role and applicability in a select group of emergency department patients.

The amount and type of ancillary personnel needed in the observation unit depend on the size and type of services offered in the unit. An observation unit that offers chest pain evaluation may require different ancillary personnel than one that does not. Personnel may be from outside the department or function full time in the observation unit (e.g., respiratory therapists). They may also be personnel who have not traditionally been available to the emergency department, such as psychiatric nurses. Adequate secretarial and clerical staff are also crucial for proper functioning of the unit.

The structure of the observation unit will determine its clinical effectiveness and financial viability. Models for the structure of the observation unit are reviewed in the American College of Emergency Physicians textbook *ED Design*.[4] An observation unit that is properly designed and located adjacent to the emergency department will result in a 50% lowered cost compared with traditional hospital admission, while providing equivalent or improved quality of patient care.

Designating and empowering an emergency physician to manage the observation unit are critical for success. The complexity of patient care is multiplied when an emergency department adds observation services. The manager develops and implements clinical protocols for efficient quality patient care. The manager schedules and supervises the observation unit staff and leads the continuous quality improvement team monitoring the observation unit's functioning.

CLINICAL CONDITIONS

Evaluation of Critical Diagnostic Syndromes

Abdominal Pain

Traditional Approach

Abdominal pain is one of the most frequent complaints seen in the emergency department and accounts for 4% to 8% of all emergency department visits.[5] The typical emergency department evaluation of the abdominal pain patient includes a thorough history, physical examination, and the appropriate diagnostic tests. Within the short time frame of 2 to 3 hours, patients are given a provisional diagnosis and given a disposition home or to the hospital.

Problem with Traditional Approach

The emergency department evaluation is inadequate for many patients, and in 40% of emergency department patients, the origin of abdominal pain is never determined. Acute appendicitis is the most common abdominal surgical emergency and illustrates the inadequacies of the emergency department evaluation. The diagnosis of acute appendicitis is missed in 20% to 30% of cases (false-negative decisions). In addition, 20% to 30% of patients taken to surgery for acute appendicitis are found to have no abnormality (false-positive decisions).[5]

Observational Approach

With observation, the emergency department evaluation is extended from 2 to 3 hours to up to 23 hours (Box 198-2). After the initial history and physical examination of the patient, the physician makes an estimate of the probability that the patient actually has appendicitis. Those patients deemed to have an intermediate probability of disease are ideal candidates for the observational approach.[6] Patients who are immunocompro-

BOX 198-2. Observation Criteria for Abdominal Pain

Vital signs stable
Intermediate probability of appendicitis
or
Low probability of appendicitis with risk factor
Risk Factors
- Pregnant
- Elderly (>65 years old)
- Young (<3 years old)

mised or pregnant and those at the extremes of age can benefit from observation. Elderly people in particular can benefit from observation because surgical problems are often missed, owing to diminished diagnostic precision with increasing age.[7]

During the period of observation, the patient is usually kept fasted and hydrated intravenously. Serial abdominal examinations are repeated at 4-hour intervals and laboratory tests repeated as appropriate. Imaging and consultations are also arranged during this time frame. Patients without appendicitis will experience improvement of their pain and have had completion of diagnostic workup and exclusion of surgical disease.[8] Patients should be hospitalized if they have no improvement, have clinical deterioration, or have surgical pathology diagnosed by testing. In patients who do have appendicitis, signs and symptoms will continue or worsen.[8]

Physician decision making improves with observation. With observation, physicians' false-positive surgeries can nearly be eliminated. Intensive observation with serial physical examinations at least every 8 hours rather than once per day decreases the false-positive rate from 20% to 30% to 5%.[9,10] The use of a period of observation can also help identify many patients whose diagnosis may be missed during the initial emergency department evaluation. The appendicitis patient whose diagnosis is missed in the emergency department has few clinical signs or symptoms of appendicitis, making diagnosis difficult.[11] Physicians delaying disposition decisions on questionable cases can avoid these false-negative decisions. Because appendicitis patients develop more signs and symptoms during short-term observation and nonappendicitis patients clear their signs and symptoms, fewer patients have an unclear clinical picture after observation. More importantly, with observation physicians' false-negative decisions (missed appendicitis diagnosis) can be significantly reduced.[11] Missing the diagnosis on the initial physician evaluation leads to 72 hours of delay until surgery.[11] Complications (perforation, abscess formation) occur with delays in making the diagnosis of appendicitis and are proportional to the missed diagnosis rate.[11] Physicians who observe rather than discharge abdominal pain patients with low probability of appendicitis lower their missed diagnosis rate, avoiding potential perforations and abscess formation.

Chest Pain

Traditional Approach

The main focus of emergency department evaluation in chest pain patients is twofold: (1) assessment of the probability that the patient has acute myocardial infarction (AMI) or acute coronary ischemia (ACI) and (2) assessment of the risk of the patient having a life-threatening event. These two assessments help determine the appropriate setting for further testing and monitoring. The probability of AMI is traditionally assessed in the emergency department with a directed history, physical examination, electrocardiogram (ECG), and an initial measurement of creatine kinase-MB (CK-MB) and troponin I.[12]

Patients with clear evidence of AMI on ECG are potential candidates for immediate reperfusion therapy with either thrombolytics or emergency angioplasty. This subset is at high risk for life-threatening events and best managed in the coronary care setting with close monitoring. This approach has been shown to improve survival in patients with AMI.

Depending on the evaluating physician's threshold, chest pain patients without definite evidence of AMI at initial evaluation in the emergency department are generally admitted to the hospital to confirm or exclude ("rule in" or "rule out") ACI or AMI. Patients who are judged to have low probability of ACI after the initial evaluation are released home for outpatient follow-up monitoring.

Problem with Traditional Approach

The poor performance of initial diagnostic tests makes the evaluation of chest pain highly dependent on clinical judgment. It is well known that the initial ECG is diagnostic in only 50% of AMI patients,[13] and the initial CK-MB measurement has a sensitivity of only 35%.[14] The reliance on physician judgment has resulted in as many as 5% of AMI patients being discharged home.[1,15] AMI patients not identified at the initial evaluation and released from the emergency department have up to 25% serious risk of poor outcome.[1] This has led to emergency department physicians erring on the side of admitting patients to the hospital in an attempt not to miss the diagnosis in this group. The increased sensitivity of a more liberal admission policy results in two thirds of patients admitted for chest pain having a noncardiac cause for their symptoms.[1] The cost of this inefficiency has been estimated to run into billions of dollars.[4] In spite of this liberal admission policy, missed AMI is the leading cause for malpractice suits against emergency physicians.[16]

Observational Approach

The emergency physician can use the observation unit to extend the evaluation of patients with chest pain (Box 198-3). When used principally for such a purpose, the observation unit has been termed a *chest pain unit.* The chest pain unit has been successful in increasing the sensitivity and specificity of the evaluation process.[17] Patients with low to intermediate risk of AMI

BOX 198-3. Observation Criteria for Chest Pain

Nontraumatic chest pain
Low probability of disease or risk of adverse event
Stable vital signs
Normal cardiac markers
Nondiagnostic electrocardiogram
Cocaine-induced chest pain

are transferred to the observation unit. Patients unsuitable for observation unit evaluation include those who have a high probability of acute myocardial ischemia as evidenced by unstable vital signs, ECG findings of acute myocardial infarction, or persistent or recurring chest pain consistent with unstable angina.

The physician identifies patients with low probability for ACI by using one or more risk-stratification tools. Risk stratification based on classic risk factors alone has been shown to be a poor predictor[18] of short-term outcome. Risk stratification based on ECG findings is more reliable. The Brush ECG criteria[19] classify low risk as the absence of ST segment elevation or depression, T wave inversion or strain, new (or presumed new) Q waves, left bundle branch block, or paced rhythm. Another useful risk stratification tool is the Goldman protocol, which uses history, physical examination, and ECG findings[20] to classify patients into high (>70%), moderate, or low (<7%) risk. The Agency for Health Care Policy and Research criteria use the Goldman protocol to determine the risk of ischemia (low, moderate, or high) and the likelihood of complications.[21] Another tool is the acute cardiac ischemia time insensitive predictive instrument. This uses the ECG findings, patient age, patient gender, and the presence or absence of chest pain to assign a probability of acute ischemia.[22]

Patients admitted to the observation unit are first evaluated to rule out a myocardial infarction. They are serially tested with cardiac markers and ECGs. CK-MB estimation at 0, 3, 6, and 9 hours after presentation has 100% sensitivity, 98% specificity, and 100% negative predictive value in the detection of AMI.[17] Other useful serum cardiac markers are the troponins (I and T) and myoglobin. Patients who present more than 24 hours after symptom onset have negative CK-MB and myoglobin testing findings, but troponin T or I remains positive for up to 6 days. Patients are monitored with continuous ECG monitors equipped with dysrhythmia alarms and memory storage capabilities. Continuous ECG ST segment monitoring can detect dynamic ST segment changes indicative of ischemia, which, when present, indicates an increased likelihood for an adverse cardiac event.[23]

After evaluation to exclude AMI, the patient is evaluated for possible ACI. This may be performed before release of the patient from the emergency department or at follow-up evaluation within 72 hours of release from the emergency department. The most common testing modality used is exercise stress testing. Patients who obtain their target heart rate without ECG evidence of ischemia can be released home. They have an annual mortality rate of less than 1%.[24] The performance of exercise testing depends on the ability of the patient to exercise adequately, gender (women have higher false-positive rates), interpretability of the resting ECG, and the availability of the test. Other testing modalities include stress echocardiography and technetium (^{99m}Tc) sestamibi scanning.

Approximately one third of emergency department chest pain patients are candidates for observation, with 80% to 85% released home after observation.[1] This reduces the emergency department hospitalization rate from 60% to 70% to 40% to 50% of emergency department chest pain patients.[1] The cost of evaluation with observation is half that of traditional evaluation with hospitalization.[1] The safety and cost-effectiveness of the observation approach have been confirmed in four randomized clinical trials.[1,25-27] The use of observation units for chest pain evaluation is becoming the standard in American hospitals.

Deep Vein Thrombosis

Traditional Approach

The primary objectives for the treatment of deep vein thrombosis (DVT) are to prevent pulmonary embolism, reduce morbidity, and prevent or minimize the risk of developing postphlebitic syndrome. Patients with suspected DVT are usually hospitalized when diagnostic testing is unavailable in the emergency department or the diagnosis has been confirmed and further management is required. Traditionally, anticoagulation with unfractionated heparin has been administered by continuous intravenous infusion for 5 to 7 days while oral anticoagulation is instituted.[28] The anticoagulant response to this treatment varies markedly among patients, and therefore the dosage must be monitored by coagulation profiles.[29]

Problem with Traditional Approach

New modalities for investigation and treatment have made it possible to manage DVT on an outpatient basis rather than with hospitalization. There are new, less invasive investigative tests and newer therapeutic agents that do not require monitoring of coagulation profiles.

Observational Approach

The role of the observation unit in the management of patients suspected of having DVT is for diagnostic testing as well as initiation of therapy using low-molecular-weight heparin (LMWH) and patient education. Often the patient with suspected DVT presents during the night or a weekend when definitive tests for DVT (such as Doppler ultrasonography) are not available. The patient may have a positive D-dimer test finding, which requires a confirmatory definitive test because of its poor specificity.[30] In these circumstances, the patient can be anticoagulated for the short term with one dose of LMWH (enoxaparin 1 mg/kg bid) until the diagnosis can be clarified. If the diagnosis is confirmed, then the patient is admitted to the hospital or an outpatient approach considered. Patients considered for outpatient management are instructed on how to administer the medication. They are educated about DVT as well as its complications and possible side effects of the LMWH. Appropriate follow-up evaluation is also arranged before discharge. This approach has been shown to result in patients spending 67% less time in the hospital and having greater physical activity and social functioning than their standard heparin cohorts.[31] Outpatient management is not recommended if the patient has proven or suspected concomitant pulmonary embolism, significant comorbidities, extensive ileofemoral DVT, active bleeding, renal failure, or poor follow-up compliance. LMWH is administered by subcutaneous injection in doses adjusted for the patient's weight, without laboratory monitoring.

Outpatient testing with venous compression ultrasonography has become readily available.[32] It is both sensitive and specific for the diagnosis of proximal (femoropopliteal) DVT.[33] When repeated compression ultrasonography was compared with impedance plethysmography, compression ultrasonography was superior in detecting DVT.[32] It has been proven to be a safe method of deciding when to administer anticoagulation.[30] The value of D-dimer assay has also been shown to be a useful adjunct to compression ultrasonography in outpatient testing.

Upper Gastrointestinal Bleeding

Traditional Approach

Most patients with upper gastrointestinal bleeding are admitted to hospital after initial emergency department assessment and stabilization.

Problem with Traditional Approach

Upper gastrointestinal bleeding is a common and potentially life-threatening condition with an overall mortality rate of 6% to 10%.[34] However, most cases of upper gastrointestinal bleeding are self-limiting, and 80% of patients have only one bleeding episode.[35]

Observational Approach

Not all patients with upper gastrointestinal bleeding do poorly, suggesting that outpatient management is possible if patients at high risk for further bleeding can be identified. Prognostic indicators include the patient's age, heart rate, systolic blood pressure, orthostatic changes in blood pressure or pulse, color of stool or emesis, anticoagulant use, and comorbid conditions.[36] In an attempt to refine diagnostic accuracy, risk assessment, and disposition, several scoring systems have been developed. Some practitioners use hemodynamic stability, intensity of bleeding, and underlying health status as predictors of rebleeding, need for surgery, and mortality.[37] Some use a period of observation with early endoscopy to identify the patient who can be discharged early. Patients found to have clean-based ulcers at endoscopy have a rebleeding rate in the range of 0% to 2% and virtually never require urgent intervention for recurrent bleeding and can be released. Utilization of this approach has been proven to be both safe and cost-effective, including a prospective clinical trial that demonstrates that 24% of patients can avoid hospitalization with cost savings of $990 per patient.[38]

Syncope

Traditional Approach

Syncope, a common problem seen in the emergency department, is caused by a spectrum of disease entities. Emergency department evaluation includes a thorough history, physical examination, and 12-lead ECG. Patients with evidence of possible myocardial ischemia or a cardiac cause of their syncope are usually admitted to the hospital because cardiac syncope has a high risk of death (up to one third will have a poor outcome).[39] Those with concomitant heart failure have a 25% mortality rate at 30 days.[40] On the other hand, patients with noncardiac syncope have a low risk of adverse events (1%) and can be managed as outpatients.[39]

Problem with Traditional Approach

Attempts to exclude a possible cardiac cause for syncope usually result in 25% to 40% of patients being admitted to the hospital for further evaluation and management.[40] The emergency department evaluation with history, physical examination, and ECG identifies only 50% of patients with a serious cause of their syncope,[41] and this has often resulted in a liberal admission policy; however, one study found that only 12% of patients had a serious cause for syncope that justified hospitalization.[42]

Observational Approach

Extending the emergency department evaluation with a period of observation is a strategy to reduce unnecessary hospitalizations (Box 198-4). Patients with a cardiac syncope have a poor prognosis and need to be identified. These patients often do not have chest pain as a symptom, but may have ischemic changes on ECG, arm or shoulder pain, or prior history of exercise-induced angina. A "rule out myocardial infarction" evaluation with serial ECG and enzyme measurement may be the only way to identify these patients. Prolonged ECG monitoring can point to a specific cause in up to one fifth of patients, with half of all abnormalities detected in the first 24 hours.[43] The 1-year risk of

BOX 198-4. Observation Criteria for Syncope

Low to intermediate risk of adverse event
Stable vital signs
Loss of consciousness <10 minutes
No focal acute neurologic signs
Normal electrolytes and blood count
No objective evidence of inchemia or injury by electrocardiographic or cardiac markers

dysrhythmia or death in syncope patients correlates with four factors: an abnormal ECG, history of ventricular dysrhythmia, history of heart failure, and age greater than 45 years.[44] Patients with none of these risk factors have only a 4.4% rate of adverse events at 1 year and may be appropriate for outpatient evaluation. In contrast, patients with three or four risk factors have a 58% adverse outcome rate and should be admitted to the hospital. Patients with one or two risk factors have intermediate risk and may be appropriate for outpatient evaluation with observation. Patients unsuitable for observation include those who have abnormal neurologic findings, abnormal ECG or cardiac enzymes, history of trauma before syncope, or loss of consciousness for longer than 15 minutes.

During the observation period, serial examination of patients is carried out, including vital signs, with the majority of patients safely discharged home without hospitalization.[45] Continuous ECG monitoring, consultation, serial cardiac enzymes, and further tests such as two-dimensional echography of the heart, psychiatric assessment (associated with up to 25% of cases of syncope), and tilt table testing should be arranged when appropriate. Tilt table testing is a useful investigation in patients with recurrent syncope when heart disease is not suspected. Up to 60% of patients who have vagally mediated syncope can be detected by this modality.[46] The period of observation can also identify patients with cardiac dysrhythmias or sinus pauses who are candidates for more extensive diagnostic evaluation in the hospital.

Trauma

In a 1997 survey by the National Center of Health Statistics, it was estimated that there are 35 million trauma-related emergency department visits annually.[47] Patients with serious injuries require hospitalization for definitive therapy, whereas those with minor injuries can be discharged after treatment in the emergency department.

The problem with the traditional emergency department approach to trauma is that many patients have injury patterns or actual injuries that fall somewhere between the two scenarios just described. If these patients are released home, there is a risk that some will have poor outcomes as a result of a missed injuries. On the other hand, since the majority of these patients do not have serious injuries, admitting this group to the hospital will result in a waste of scarce health care resources.

For the last three decades, it has been evident that observation units are an efficient and useful strategy in the evaluation and management of trauma victims.[47] With observation, selected patients can be evaluated further to determine the need for admission. One study of 20,000 patients treated in an emergency department observation unit over a 12-month period found that 3% of emergency department trauma patients were admitted to the observation unit, with 86% safely discharged home without the need for admission.[48]

Blunt Abdominal Injury

Traditional Approach

Current emergency department practice in the management of these patients includes history taking, physical examination, blood analysis, plain radiography, ultrasonography, and computed tomography (CT). After initial stabilization and exclusion of other major injuries in the emergency department, most patients suffering blunt abdominal trauma are admitted to the hospital for further evaluation and monitoring.

Problem with Traditional Approach

Initial evaluation in the emergency department is inadequate for accurate disposition. One third of patients who do not have any symptoms suggestive of intra-abdominal injury may actually have significant injury.[49] Also, because none of the present modalities for investigating the presence of injury are 100% sensitive, many patients with initial negative investigation findings are hospitalized.

Observational Approach

Patients appropriate for observation are those who after initial emergency department evaluation have no clear evidence of serious injury on physical examination but remain at risk for serious injury because of mechanism of the injury or the individual's personal health (e.g., on anticoagulants). Evaluations during observation for up to 23 hours include repeat physical examinations, laboratory testing, imaging, and specialty consultations. Patients are admitted to the hospital if their condition deteriorates during the observation period or if, after testing, they are found to have serious internal injury. Patients with negative findings on evaluation and the ability to tolerate feeding can be safely released home. Patients who have sustained significant blunt abdominal trauma by mechanism of injury or have equivocal findings on abdominal examination should undergo further testing, such as CT scan, to detect occult injury.[50] Ultrasonography is being increasingly used in the initial evaluation of the patient with blunt abdominal trauma but has insufficient negative predictive value to be used to rule out serious intra-abdominal injury.[51] CT alone is not adequate to rule out serious injury, with sensitivity only 80% to 95%.[52] Observation alone in patients with blunt abdominal trauma is not sufficient, as up to 20% of patients with significant injury will not have abdominal tenderness or develop it even after a short period of observation.[52] Thus, the prudent approach to patients with significant blunt abdominal trauma without clear evidence of intra-abdominal injury is the utilization of a diagnostic test, such as CT, together with a period of observation.

Penetrating Abdominal Injury

Traditional Approach

Most patients with penetrating injury to the abdomen are hospitalized for further evaluation, which may include wound exploration in the operating room and additional diagnostic testing.

Problem with Traditional Approach

Many of these hospitalizations are unnecessary, as one third of patients with an abdominal stab wound do not have a breach of the peritoneum, and two thirds of these do not sustain visceral injury.[53]

Observational Approach

Observation in an observation unit can identify those patients who do not require surgical intervention. Patients undergo serial examinations by the physician, further diagnostic testing, and specialty consultation. Those without evidence of peritoneal perforation or visceral injury after evaluation are sent home after proper wound care.

The conservative approach to penetrating abdominal wounds was developed in the 1970s. Those without peritoneal breach can be safely sent home after wound care and a period of observation without the need for hospitalization. Those with stab wounds to the abdomen with peritoneal breach, but a negative finding on diagnostic peritoneal lavage can be safely managed in an observation unit.[53] Alternatives to the use of diagnostic peritoneal lavage for evaluating intra-abdominal injury include CT scan, laparoscopy, and ultrasonography.[54-56] Patients with significant intra-abdominal injuries identified during observation are admitted; the 70% to 90% without such injuries are released home.[53,57] Gunshot wounds are often more difficult to evaluate than stab wounds. However, patients who appear to have tangential gunshot wounds can avoid surgery with observation if they are hemodynamically stable and have initial negative test findings. Penetrating wounds manifest differently in children than in adults.[58] Initial diagnostic testing with CT and diagnostic peritoneal lavage in children detects only 50% of injuries, with only 30% of patients having localized tenderness. Observation can help avoid unnecessary surgery in patients without injury and avoid missing the diagnosis in those without clear evidence of injury.

Blunt Chest Trauma

Traditional Management

Many patients who have a history of blunt chest trauma in high-velocity accidents are admitted to the hospital to rule out myocardial or pulmonary contusion.

Problem with Traditional Approach

Very few patients admitted to the hospital with blunt chest trauma from high-velocity accidents without evidence of injury during emergency department evaluation are found to have serious injury during hospital evaluation.[59]

Observational Approach

Patients with isolated blunt chest injury who are otherwise stable with normal ECG are suitable for a period of observation to exclude myocardial injury. During the period of observation, patients are monitored with continuous ECG, specifically assessing for dysrhythmias. Serial enzyme determinations, such as troponin level, are also carried out to detect evidence of myocardial injury. Those patients with sternal fracture or other evidence of higher risk of intrathoracic injury should be considered for transesophageal echocardiogram.[60] Those with negative evaluations during the period of observation are released home for outpatient follow-up monitoring.

Much of the period of observation in patients with blunt chest trauma focuses on identifying the presence and prognosis of myocardial contusions. The overall incidence of cardiac-related complications in these patients is low (0.1%).[61] Patients with blunt cardiac trauma who have complications usually have an abnormal ECG or abnormal CK-MB or troponin level at presentation. Conversely, a normal ECG and CK-MB and troponin levels correlate with the lack of clinically significant complications.[62,63] Patients are unlikely to have complications who have isolated chest wall contusions and no abnormality of serial CK-MB, troponin, or ECG abnormalities or dysrhythmia over 6 to 12 hours of ECG monitoring.

Penetrating Chest Injury

Traditional Approach

Patients with chest trauma present with a spectrum of severity to the emergency department ranging from severe life-threatening injury requiring urgent operative intervention to hemodynamically stable patients with a negative initial evaluation. Most patients presenting with penetrating chest injuries are admitted to the hospital. Often, even those with a negative initial evaluation are admitted to exclude serious injury to the heart, lungs, and the major blood vessels.

Problem with Traditional Approach

The accuracy of this approach is limited, as many patients with evidence of injury are admitted but have no further deterioration or need for medical therapy. On the other hand, there are those without obvious evidence of serious injury who will have a negative outcome if released after the initial evaluation.

Observational Approach

A period of observation combined with diagnostic imaging can improve clinical decision making. Patients with evidence of a small pneumothorax or hemothorax can be monitored for deterioration. Those without evidence of serious injury but of concern to the physician can likewise be observed for complications. During the period of observation, patients are monitored for respiratory or hemodynamic compromise. Repeat chest radiographs can detect the development of hemothorax or pneumothorax. Patients who deteriorate during the period of observation require hospitalization.

The safety and efficacy of managing asymptomatic stab wound victims in the short-term observation unit have been clearly established in multiple studies.[64-66] A total of 5% to 15% will require hospitalization because of development of delayed pneumothorax, subcutaneous emphysema, hematemesis, or pneumopericardium.[64] In addition, the majority of stab wound victims with small pneumothoraces or hemothoraces will be treated solely with a chest tube without further surgical intervention. Major trauma centers can manage many of these patients as outpatients without hospitalization with use of a period of observation.

Patients with penetrating wounds to the cardiac area of the chest (between the nipples), region of the great vessels, or the thoracoabdominal area usually require more intensive testing to exclude not only injury to the heart, major vessels, and lungs but also to the diaphragm and the abdominal organs. Echocardiography may detect pericardial fluid or tamponade in patients with penetrating injury in close proximity to the heart.[67-69] Patients with small effusions may be observed in a monitored setting with serial examinations, whereas patients with large effusions should be treated surgically.[69] Patients with a negative echocardiography can be observed in the observation unit. Even patients with small effusions may have sustained a serious injury, so the intensity of monitoring needs to be high.

Head Injury

Traditional Approach

More than a half million head injuries occur annually in the United States; 75% are minor.[70] Traditional assessment of the head-injured patient includes initial risk assessment from the history and physical examination. Patients who have no loss of consciousness, no abnormal neurologic findings, and no risk factors for adverse events are discharged home after evaluation in the emergency department. Those patients with more severe head injury are usually evaluated with CT and hospitalized for either surgical intervention or monitoring.

Problem with Traditional Management

There is great variability in the evaluation of head-injured patients. The rate of CT scan usage for head-injured patients ranges from 15% to 70%. Of those patients scanned, 80% have no findings on CT scan.[71] The incidence of an abnormality being detected on CT scan for any patient with a Glasgow Coma Scale score of 15 and loss of consciousness in the emergency department ranges from 2.5% to 9.8%.[72] However, there has been no large study that addresses whether a low-risk patient with a Glasgow Coma Scale score of 15 and normal neurologic examination can be safely sent home without a CT scan. The evaluation and treatment of head-injured patients are already a great burden on health care finances, and the use of CT on all low-risk patients would only increase that burden.

Observational Approach

The low to moderate risk group can benefit from observation. These are patients with a significant mechanism of injury and no clear evidence of intracranial injury.[73] Patients with nonserious intoxications (e.g., alcohol) can also benefit from a period of observation. Most will not have a serious injury, and the intoxicated patient will clear the intoxication in less than 24 hours. During the observation period, serial neurologic examinations are performed. Patients with normal findings on serial examinations, without deterioration, can be sent home.

Patients with clear evidence of intracranial injury are not candidates for observation. This group includes patients with focal neurologic deficits, depressed or penetrating skull injuries, cervical spine injury, or abnormal CT scan. They are referred to neurosurgery and admitted to the hospital.

Treatment of Emergency Conditions

Asthma

Traditional Approach

More than 20 million people in the United States are afflicted with asthma. Acute exacerbation of asthma is a common presentation to the emergency department, with estimated annual admissions exceeding 450,000.[2] Traditionally, therapy is provided in the emergency department for 2 to 4 hours, consistent with national guidelines.[74] After an initial assessment (history, physical examination, peak expiratory flow rate [PEFR] or forced expiratory volume in 1 minute, oxygen saturation), treatment consists of β-agonists and steroids, where appropriate. Patients not successfully treated after 3 or 4 hours are hospitalized for further management.

Problems with Traditional Approach

With this approach, one third of patients presenting to the emergency department with asthmatic exacerbation are hospitalized.[75] This translates into an estimated medical cost of $1.2 billion annually.[76] Another pitfall in the traditional emergency department treatment of asthma is that short encounter times do not allow for identification and aggressive treatment of patients with a higher tendency for relapse. This leads to repeated emergency department visits, added medical costs, and diminished quality of life.

Observational Approach

An alternative to hospitalization for patients failing emergency department treatment is use of an extended, short-term intensive protocol of 8 to 12 hours in the observation unit.[2] With extended treatment, 80% of such patients can be discharged home.[2] Inclusion criteria for observation unit management are failure of standard initial emergency department management and continued respiratory distress and good response to emergency department management but high risk for relapse (Box 198-5). Increased risk of relapse is indicated by a history of numerous asthma-related emergency department or clinic visits within the past year, using more outpatient medications (including home nebulizers), and longer duration of symptoms.[75] Exclusion criteria include unstable vital signs, evidence of impending respiratory failure ($PaCO_2$ >45 mm Hg, PaO_2 <55 mm Hg), or severe airway restriction (PEFR <80 L/min after first inhaled β-agonist treatment).

BOX 198-5. Observation Criteria for Asthma

Failed standard emergency department management
Stable vital signs
Peak flow after third β-agonist >32% predicted
No concomitant illness (pneumonia, heart failure)
Successful emergency department management but high risk for relapse
Risk of relapse
- Second visit to emergency department within 10 days
- Previous intubation or intensive care unit admission
- Hospitalization in last year
- Three or more emergency department visits in 6 months
- Oral steroids for more than 6 months

Exclusion criteria also include factors that correlate with unsuccessful treatment during observation. These include a previous visit to the emergency department in the last 10 days, previous intensive care unit admission or intubation, hospitalization in the previous year, three or more emergency department visits in the last 6 months, use of oral steroids for more than half of the previous year, and peak flow after the third β-agonist treatment that is less than 32% of predicted.[2]

Therapy in the observation unit is a continuation of the emergency department treatment with handheld nebulized β-agonists every 2 to 4 hours and repeated steroids at 6 hours after initial therapy. Patients are managed up to 23 hours but generally are admitted to the hospital if they do not respond within 12 hours. Patients are released from the observation unit when they are not in respiratory distress, have minimal residual symptoms, and are at PEFR of 70% or greater of predicted or personal best. Before discharge, there should also be patient educational activities and assessment of inhaler techniques. Training can be provided as well. Patients should be initiated into daily diary keeping as well as a log of PEFR before and after treatment. Appropriate follow-up monitoring should also be arranged.

In recent years, there is increasing evidence in support of the observation unit in the management of acute asthma. This includes a prospective randomized clinical trial of observation versus traditional hospitalization of emergency department asthma patients who do not "break" in the first 3 to 4 hours.[2] Although there are no differences in relapse rate at 8 weeks, there are significant differences in the length of stay (9 hours vs 59 hours), patient satisfaction, quality of life, and cost savings of $1000 per patient. Patients treated in an observation unit have higher patient satisfaction according to four parameters: received service wanted, recommendation of service to others, satisfaction with service, and overall satisfaction compared with inpatient care.[2] Observation unit patients also report fewer problems with care received, communication, emotional support, physical comfort, and special needs.[2] Observation also has been shown to have utility in the management of pediatric patients with asthma. Of those who would otherwise require hospitalization, 30% to 70% can be successfully managed as outpatients with the observation unit.[77]

BOX 198-6. Observation Criteria for New-Onset Atrial Fibrillation

Normal electrolytes and blood count
Stable vital signs
No physical finding of heart failure
Jugular venous distention, ankle, edema, S3 gallop
No history of heart failure
No symptoms of myocardial ischemia
No objective evidence of ischemia by electrocardiographic or cardiac markers

Atrial Fibrillation

Traditional Approach

Atrial fibrillation is a relatively common condition that occurs in 2% to 3% of adults and is the most common sustained cardiac dysrhythmia in patients presenting to the emergency department.[78,79] The goals in management of acute atrial fibrillation are hemodynamic stabilization, symptom relief, prevention of thromboembolism, resolution of the dysrhythmia, and exclusion of serious pathologic causes of the dysrhythmia. The majority of patients who present to the emergency department with new-onset atrial fibrillation or acute atrial fibrillation are hospitalized.[80]

Problems with Traditional Approach

Recently, the necessity of admitting the majority of patients with acute atrial fibrillation has been questioned. It is recognized that new-onset atrial fibrillation for most patients is a transient dysrhythmia with no serious precipitants and a benign prognosis. One retrospective analysis of 216 patients admitted for atrial fibrillation found that a third of patients did not actually require admission to the hospital.[80]

Observational Approach

The observational approach to new and acute atrial fibrillation has been validated in a number of clinical trials.[81] The period of observation is usually 8 to 12 hours. During observation, patients are treated to rectify their dysrhythmia and evaluated for serious precipitants of their condition. After observation, 80% to 90% of patients can be discharged home without hospitalization.

Observation extends the emergency department evaluation of the patient for underlying medical conditions that may have precipitated the arrhythmia (Box 198-6). These include AMI, congestive heart failure, electrolyte abnormalities, and hyperthyroidism. AMI is excluded as a precipitant with serial cardiac enzyme testing over 6 to 9 hours. The period of observation is also used to detect structural heart disease with the use of echocardiography where appropriate. Patients are excluded from observation who have evidence after the emergency department evaluation of hemodynamic instability, comorbid conditions, heart failure, chest pain, or significant coronary artery disease.

Observation is also used to extend the emergency department treatment period of the patient. The spontaneous conversion rate for patients with acute atrial fibrillation is 50% to 70% within the first 24 hours.[82] Patients who spontaneously convert have a low rate of structural heart disease.[82] Those who do not spontaneously convert in the first 8 hours can be converted chemically or electrically.[83] After cardioversion, the patient needs to be observed. This is especially true for patients converted with the newer class III antidysrhythmic agents (e.g., ibutilide), which have the potential for serious side effects such as torsades de pointes (5% of patients), sinus bradycardia, and sinus arrest.[83,84] The risk of thromboembolism in patients with atrial fibrillation of less than 48 hours' duration is less than 1%, so patients who convert can be released home without need for anticoagulation.[85]

Congestive Heart Failure

Traditional Approach

Congestive heart failure (CHF) is highly lethal, with 37% of men and 33% of women dying within 2 years of diagnosis. The 6-year mortality rate is 82% for men and 67% for women, which corresponds to a death rate fourfold to eightfold greater than that of the general population of the same age.[86] Patients who present with CHF to the emergency department undergo history taking and physical examination and investigations including chest radiography. Treatment is begun with oxygenation, diuretics, inotropic agents, and vasodilators where appropriate. Most CHF patients treated in the emergency department are eventually hospitalized.

Problem with Traditional Approach

Congestive heart failure is highly prevalent, affecting about 1% of persons in their 50s and rising progressively with age to afflict 10% of persons in their 80s.[86] It is a growing problem; more than 2 million Americans have the disease and 400,000 new cases are diagnosed each year.[86] One third of the patients with CHF require hospitalization each year, one third get readmitted each year, and one third die within 2 years.[86] The annual cost to the health care system of managing patients with heart failure admitted to the hospital has been estimated at $28 billion.[87] Between 80% and 87% of patients diagnosed with CHF are hospitalized.[88]

Observational Approach

Observation is a strategy to avoid hospital admission with great cost savings (Box 198-7). Selected emergency department patients with CHF can be safely managed in an observation unit.[88,89] Patients appropriate for the observation unit are those with high probability of successful treatment with short-term extension of the emergency department visit. Patients should also have low severity of illness. They should not be hypoxic, should not have pulmonary edema or hypotension, and should not have objective evidence of AMI, hemodynamic instability, or serious comorbid conditions.[88,89] Recently, B type natriuretic peptide has been used to streamline decision making. Patients with B type natriuretic peptide levels between 100 and 500 pg/mL are suitable candidates for observation unit care because a good proportion of these patients would be able to be discharged home. The test has a negative predictive value of greater than 95%, and a positive predictive value of 70% to 95%. It correlates with pulmonary capillary wedge pressure, and since its half-life is less than ½ hour, serial measurements during observation can evaluate the effects of therapeutic interventions.[90,91]

BOX 198-7. Observation Criteria for Heart Failure

High probability of successful treatment
Physician clinical judgment that observation is safe and nil or one risk factor: hypoxia, hypotension or syncope, anasarca, pulmonary edema, or respiratory distress
No objective evidence of ischemia or injury: electrocardiographic or cardiac markers

Therapy and evaluation are a continuation of the initial 2- to 3-hour emergency department visit for up to 23 hours. Continuous ECG monitoring for dysrhythmias is done, as up to 30% of CHF patients have dysrhythmias.[92] Inotropic agents can be infused and the patient educated about preventable causes of the exacerbation. Therapy may include continuous infusion of loop diuretic (0.05-0.1 mg/kg/hr) titrated hourly to a net fluid balance of −1 mL/kg/hr. Most patients with acute exacerbation of chronic CHF have a preventable cause of their exacerbation, such as failure to take their medications or dietary indiscretion. The opportunity to provide patient education, medication review, and consultations with dietary and social service where necessary is fully utilized, as this has been shown to improve compliance with therapy.[93] Patients are discharged home when their symptoms are adequately controlled, all reversible causes of morbidity are treated or stabilized, and adequate outpatient support and follow-up care are arranged. With observation, the emergency department's focus can shift from providing only episodic care for CHF patients to providing more comprehensive and preventive care.[93]

Dehydration

Traditional Approach

Dehydration can be a presenting symptom of an underlying disease state and can affect the very young to the very old. Patients are often admitted for intravenous hydration to correct fluid and electrolyte imbalances or for further diagnostic evaluation.

Problem with Traditional Approach

Patients with dehydration are often hospitalized because short emergency department visits do not allow for full correction of fluid and electrolyte disorders or extensive evaluation for underlying causes. A common cause for return visits to the emergency

BOX 198-8. Observation Criteria for Dehydration

Stable vital signs
Limiting or treatable cause of illness
Mild to moderate electrolyte abnormalities
No cardiovascular compromise
Hyperemesis gravidarum

BOX 198-9. Observation Criteria for Pneumonia

Low risk of death (1% to 5%): clinical judgment or severity index
No risk factors for poor outcome: immunocompromised, neuromuscular disorder, pulmonary tuberculosis, cystic fibrosis
No objective evidence ischemia or injury: electrocardiographic or cardiac markers

department is dehydration due to inadequate emergency department therapy and evaluation.[94]

Observational Approach

The goals of observation unit therapy are adequate treatment of fluid and electrolyte abnormalities and identification of the underlying cause of symptoms. Appropriate patients for observation include those with acceptable vital signs and mild to moderate dehydration (Box 198-8). They should have self-limited or treatable causes not requiring hospitalization, with mild to moderate electrolyte abnormalities. Another group of patients that is appropriate for observation are those with hyperemesis gravidarum. Patients unsuitable for observation are those with unstable vital signs, cardiovascular compromise, underlying chronic medical illness, severe dehydration or electrolyte abnormalities, or associated conditions not amenable to short-term therapy (e.g., bowel obstruction, diabetic ketoacidosis, sepsis). Interventions include intravenous rehydration, serial examination and vital signs, and antiemetics. The time frame for observation is limited to 24 hours. The patient is released home when there are acceptable vital signs, resolution of symptoms, tolerance to oral fluids, and normal electrolytes. If the patient does not fulfill the discharge criteria or serious underlying pathology is found, the patient is admitted to the hospital.

Infections

Pneumonia

Traditional Approach

Each year, approximately 600,000 patients are admitted to the hospital with pneumonia, at a cost of about $4 billion.[95] Many of these patients are admitted after the initial emergency department evaluation. Physicians often rely on subjective criteria such as clinical appearance when selecting patients for hospital admission.[96]

Problem with Traditional Approach

There is great variation in the admission rates for pneumonia.[97] Emergency department physicians tend to overestimate the risk of death in patients with pneumonia, which has resulted in many low-risk patients being hospitalized unnecessarily.[96]

Observational Approach

Observation is appropriate for those patients the physician is concerned may not do well as outpatients (Box 198-9). This concern can be based on physician clinical judgment or by using a severity of illness index. Fine and associates[96] developed a prediction rule to estimate which pneumonia patients would be at higher risk for mortality. They reviewed medical records of more than 14,000 patients hospitalized with pneumonia and identified 14 key clinical variables (age, sex, coexisting illness, vital signs, and mental status) and seven key laboratory variables (blood urea nitrogen, glucose, hematocrit, arterial oxygen, and pleural effusion on chest radiograph). They then weighed each of these variables into a cumulative point total (PSI index) and assigned each patient to one of five mortality risk groups ranging from class I, which had a low risk (60-day mortality risk less than 0.5%) and can be treated as outpatients, to class V, which had a high risk (60-day mortality risk greater than 30%) and should be treated as inpatients. Patients in class III are at intermediate risk and traditionally one half are admitted and one half treated as outpatients. By use of the PSI to risk-stratify patients, physicians can avoid hospitalization of many low-risk patients.[98] Intermediate-risk patients (class III) are good candidates for a period of observation to clarify their need for hospitalization. Irrespective of the patient's risk as judged by PSI, some patients are not appropriate for observation but should be admitted: those with immunocompromise, pulmonary tuberculosis, high suspicion of pulmonary embolism, or hypoxia (Table 198-1).

During observation, patients are treated with intravenous antibiotics, oxygen therapy, and pulse oximetry monitoring. Hydration is given either orally or intravenously. After 10 to 12 hours of treatment in the observation unit, the patient is re-evaluated and a decision about disposition is made. Patients who deteriorate during the observation period or have a saturation of less than 90% on room air after observation should be admitted to the hospital.

Pyelonephritis

Traditional Approach

Pyelonephritis is a serious infection that frequently results in hospitalization for intravenous hydration and antibiotic administration.

Problem with Traditional Approach

Many patients who are admitted with pyelonephritis are judged retrospectively not to have had the condition. In addition, many patients who, on review, clearly have pyelonephritis are at very low risk for developing complications.

Table 198-1. Use of Pneumonia Severity Index (PSI) for Admission Decisions

Step 1: Assess Arterial Oxygenation for All Patients
Is pulse oximetry <90% or P_{O_2} <60 mm Hg?
YES: Inpatient therapy recommended **NO:** Go to Step 2

Step 2: Are Any of the Following Present?
- Patient 51 years of age or older,
- Coexisting medical conditions listed in Step 3, or
- Physical examination findings listed in Step 3

YES: Go to Step 3 **NO:** Risk-class I, go to Step 4

Step 3: Compute Risk Score (Sum of Applicable Points)

Risk Factor	*Points*
Demographic factors:	
Age in years (age −10 for women)	☐
Nursing home resident	10
Coexisting medical conditions:	
Neoplastic disease	30
Liver disease	20
Congestive heart failure	10
Cerebrovascular disease	10
Renal disease	10
Physical examination findings:	
Altered mental status	20
Respiratory rate ≥30/minute	20
Systolic blood pressure <90 mm Hg	20
Temperature <35° C or ≥40° C	15
Pulse ≥125/min	10
Laboratory and radiographic findings:	
Arterial pH <7.35	30
BUN ≥30 mg/dL	20
Sodium <130 mEq/L	20
Glucose ≥250 mg/dL	10
Hematocrit <30%	10
P_{O_2} <60 mm Hg or O_2 sat <90%	10
Pleural effusion by chest x-ray	10
Total Score (sum of all points):	☐

Step 4: Recommended Initial Site of Treatment

Risk Score	*Risk Class*	*Treatment Site*
Not Applicable	I	Outpatient
<71	II	Outpatient
71–90	III	Observation
91–130	IV	Inpatient
>130	V	Inpatient

BUN, blood urea nitrogen.

Observational Approach

Because of these two factors, the use of an outpatient approach for selected patients rather than hospital admission has been developed. Observation is appropriate for adult, nonpregnant women who appear to have uncomplicated pyelonephritis. Patients receive an initial dose of intravenous antibiotic, intravenous fluids, antiemetic, and antipyretic. Laboratory tests include complete blood cell count, urinalysis, and urine and blood cultures. Those patients who after 12 hours are clinically stable and able to tolerate oral fluids are released home.

Outpatient management of selected pyelonephritis patients with observation has been shown to be safe and effective. Only 5% to 25% of patients require hospitalization after the period of observation.[99,100] At 3-week follow-up examination, 2% to 6% have developed complications and require hospitalization.[99,100] With a period of observation and careful follow-up evaluation, selected patients with pyelonephritis can be successfully managed without hospital admission.[100]

REFERENCES

1. Graff LG, et al: Impact on the care of the emergency department chest pain patient from the Chest Pain Evaluation Registry (CHEPER) study. *Am J Cardiol* 80:563, 1997.
2. McDermott MF, et al: Comparison between emergency diagnostic and treatment unit and inpatient care in the management of acute asthma. *Arch Intern Med* 157:2055, 1997.
3. Graff L, et al: Emergency physician workload: A time study. *Ann Emerg Med* 22:1156, 1993.
4. Riggs L (ed): *Emergency Department Design.* Dallas, American College of Emergency Physicians, 1993.
5. Powers RD, Guertler AT: Abdominal pain in the ED: Stability and change over 20 years. *Am J Emerg Med* 13:301, 1995.
6. Pauker SG, Kassirer JP: The threshold approach to medical decision-making. *N Engl J Med* 302:1109, 1980.
7. Bender JS: Approach to the acute abdomen. *Med Clin North Am* 73:1413, 1989.
8. Graff LG, Radford MJ, Werne C: Probability of appendicitis before and after observation. *Ann Emerg Med* 20:503, 1991.
9. Thomson HJ, Jones PF: Active observation in acute abdominal pain. *Am J Surg* 152:522, 1986.
10. Banaszak P: Clinical quality improvement in a multihospital system: The Voluntary Hospitals of America/Pennsylvania experience. *Am J Med Qual* 8:56, 1993.
11. Graff L, et al: False-negative and false-positive errors in abdominal pain evaluation: Failure to diagnose acute appendicitis and unnecessary surgery. *Acad Emerg Med* 7:1244, 2000.
12. Hoekstra JW, et al: Emergency department CK-MB: A predictor of ischaemic complications—National Co-operative CK-MB project group. *Acad Emerg Med* 1:17, 1994.
13. McQueen MB, Holder K, El-Maraghi NRH: Assessment of the accuracy of serial electrocardiograms in the diagnosis of myocardial infarction. *Am Heart J* 105:258, 1983.
14. Lee TH, et al: Evaluation of creatine kinase and creatine kinase MB for diagnosing myocardial infarction: Clinical impact in the emergency room. *Arch Intern Med* 147:115, 1987.
15. Wears RL, et al: How many myocardial infarctions should we rule out? *Ann Emerg Med* 18:953, 1989.
16. Karcz A, et al: Massachusetts emergency medicine closed malpractice claims: 1988-1990. *Ann Emerg Med* 22:553, 1993.
17. Gibler WB, et al: A rapid diagnostic and treatment centre for patients with chest pain in the emergency department. *Ann Emerg Med* 25:1, 1995.
18. Jayes RL Jr, et al: Do patients' coronary risk factor reports predict acute cardiac ischaemia in the emergency department? A multicenter study. *J Clin Epidemiol* 45:621, 1992.
19. Brush JE Jr, et al: Use of the initial electrocardiogram to predict in-hospital complications of acute myocardial infarction. *N Engl J Med* 312:1137, 1985.
20. Goldman L, et al: A computer derived protocol to predict myocardial infarction in emergency department patients with acute chest pain. *N Engl J Med* 318:797, 1988.
21. Agency for Health Care Policy and Research: *Unstable Angina: Diagnosis and Management.* Publication No. 94-0002. Rockville, Md, US Department of Health and Human Services, 1994.
22. Selker HP, et al: Use of the acute cardiac ischemia time-insensitive predictive instrument (ACI-TIPI) to assist with

triage of patients with chest pain or other symptoms suggestive of acute cardiac ischemia: A multicenter, controlled trial. *Ann Intern Med* 129:845, 1998.
23. Decker WW, et al: Continuous 12-lead electrocardiographic monitoring in an emergency department chest pain unit: An assessment of potential clinical effect. *Ann Emerg Med* 41:342, 2003.
24. Mark DB, et al: Prognostic value of a treadmill exercise score in outpatients with suspected coronary artery disease. *N Engl J Med* 325:849, 1991.
25. Gomez MA, et al: An emergency department based protocol for rapidly ruling out myocardial ischemia reduces hospital time and expense: Results of a randomized study (ROMIO). *J Am Coll Cardiol* 28:25, 1996.
26. Farkouh ME, et al: A clinical trial of a chest-pain observation unit for patients with unstable angina. *N Engl J Med* 339:1882, 1998.
27. Goodacre S, et al: Randomised controlled trial and economic evaluation of a chest pain observation unit compared with routine care. BMJ 328:254, 2004, doi:10.1136/bmj.37956.664236.EE (published 14 January 2004)
28. Hirsh J: Heparin. *N Engl J Med* 324:1565, 1991.
29. Gotway MB, et al: Imaging evaluation of suspected pulmonary embolism. *Curr Prob Diagn Radiol* 28:129, 1999.
30. American College of Emergency Physicians: Clinical Policy: Critical issues in the evaluation and management of adult patients presenting with suspected lower-extremity deep venous thrombosis. *Ann Emerg Med* 42:124, 2003.
31. Koopman MM, et al: Treatment of venous thrombosis with intravenous unfractionated heparin administered in the hospital as compared with subcutaneous low-molecular-weight heparin administered at home. The Tasman Study Group. *N Engl J Med* 334:682, 1996.
32. Cogo A, et al: Compression ultrasonography for diagnostic management of patients with clinically suspected deep vein thrombosis: Prospective cohort study. *BMJ* 316:17, 1998.
33. Heijboer H, et al: A comparison of real-time compression ultrasonography with impedance plethysmography for the diagnosis of deep-vein thrombosis in symptomatic outpatients. *N Engl J Med* 329:1365, 1993.
34. Yavorski RT, et al: Analysis of 3,294 cases of upper gastrointestinal bleeding in military medical facilities. *Am J Gastroenterol* 92:231, 1995.
35. Fleisher D: Etiology and prevalence of severe persistent upper gastrointestinal bleeding. *Gastroenterology* 84:538, 1983.
36. Rockall TA, et al: Risk assessment after acute upper gastrointestinal haemorrhage. *Gut* 38:316, 1996.
37. Bordley DR, et al: Early clinical signs identify low risk patients with acute upper gastrointestinal hemorrhage. *JAMA* 253:3282, 1985.
38. Longstreth GF, Feitelberg SP: Successful outpatient management of acute upper gastrointestinal hemorrhage: Use of practice guidelines in a large patient series. *Gastrointest Endosc* 47:219, 1998.
39. Day SC, et al: Evaluation and outcome of emergency room patients with transient loss of consciousness. *Am J Med* 73:15, 1982.
40. Graff LG, et al: Correlation of the agency for health care policy and research congestive heart failure admission guideline with mortality: Peer review organization voluntary hospital association initiative to decrease events (PROVIDE) for congestive heart failure. *Ann Emerg Med* 34:429, 1999.
41. Linzer M, et al: Diagnosing syncope. Part 1. Value of history, physical examination, and electrocardiography. Clinical efficacy assessment project of the American College of Physicians. *Ann Intern Med* 126:989, 1997.
42. Junaid A, Dubinsky IL: Establishing an approach to syncope in the emergency department. *J Emerg Med* 15:593, 1997.
43. Bass E, et al: The duration of Holter monitoring in patients with syncope: Is 24 hours enough? *Arch Intern Med* 150:1073, 1990.
44. Martin TP, Hanusa BH, Kapoor WN: Risk stratification of patients with syncope. *Ann Emerg Med* 29:459, 1997.
45. Cunningham R, Mikhail MG: Management of patients with syncope and cardiac arrhythmias in an emergency department observation unit. *Emerg Med Clin North Am* 19:1051, 2001.
46. Silverstein MD, et al: Patients with syncope admitted to medical intensive care units. *JAMA* 248:1185, 1982.
47. McCaig LF, Burt CW: National Hospital Medical Care Survey: 2001 Emergency Department Summary. *Adv Data* 335:1, 2003.
48. Conrad L, et al: The role of an emergency department observation unit in the management of trauma patients, *J Emerg Med* 2:325, 1985.
49. Davis JJ, Cohn I Jr, Nance FC: Diagnosis and management of blunt abdominal trauma. *Ann Surg* 183:672, 1976.
50. Janzen DL, et al: Diagnostic accuracy of helical CT for detection of blunt bowel and mesenteric injuries. *Clin Radiol* 53:193, 1998.
51. Richards JR, et al: Sonographic assessment of blunt abdominal trauma: A 4-year prospective study. *J Clin Ultrasound* 30:59, 2002.
52. Livingston DH, et al: Admission or observation is not necessary after a negative abdominal computed tomographic scan in patients with suspected blunt abdominal trauma: Results of a prospective, multiinstitutional trial. *J Trauma* 44:273, 1998.
53. Henneman PL, et al: Diagnostic peritoneal lavage: Accuracy in predicting necessary laparotomy following blunt and penetrating trauma. *J Trauma* 39:1345, 1990.
54. Chiu WC, Shanmuganathan K, Mirvis SE, Scalea TM: Determining the need for laparotomy in penetrating torso trauma: A prospective study using triple-contrast enhanced abdominopelvic computed tomography. *J Trauma* 51:860, 2001.
55. Zantut LF, et al: Diagnostic and therapeutic laparoscopy for penetrating abdominal trauma: A multicenter experience. *J Trauma* 42:825, 1997.
56. Udobi KF, Rodriguez A, Chiu WC, Scalea TM: Role of ultrasonography in penetrating abdominal trauma: A prospective clinical study. *J Trauma* 50:475, 2001.
57. Rosemurgy AS, et al: Abdominal stab wound protocol: Prospective study documents applicability for widespread use. *Am Surg* 61:112, 1995.
58. Moss RL, Musemeche CA: Clinical judgment is superior to diagnostic tests in the management of pediatric small bowel injury. *J Pediatr Surg* 31:1178, 1996.
59. van Wijngaarden MH, Karmy-Jones R, Talwar MK, Simonetti V: Blunt cardiac injury: A 10 year institutional review. *Injury* 28:51, 1997.
60. Wiener Y, Achildiev B, Karni T, Halevi A: Echocardiogram in sternal fracture. *Am J Emerg Med* 19:403, 2001.
61. Foil MB, et al: The asymptomatic patient with suspected myocardial contusion. *Am J Surg* 160:638, 1990.
62. Maenza RL, Seaberg D, D'Amico F: A meta-analysis of blunt cardiac trauma: Ending myocardial confusion. *Am J Emerg Med* 14:237, 1996.
63. Collins JN, et al: The usefulness of serum troponin levels in evaluating cardiac injury. *Am Surg* 67:821, 2001.
64. Ammons MA, Moore EE, Rosen P: Role of the observation unit in the management of thoracic trauma. *J Emerg Med* 4:279, 1986.
65. Kerr TM, et al: Prospective trial of the six hour rule in stab wounds of the chest. *Surg Gynecol Obstet* 169:223, 1989.

66. Ordog GJ, Wasserberger J, Balasubramanium S, Shoemaker W: Asymptomatic stab wounds of the chest. *J Trauma* 36:680, 1994.
67. Aaland MO, Bryan FC 3rd, Sherman R: Two-dimensional echocardiogram in hemodynamically stable victims of penetrating precordial trauma. *Am Surg* 60:412, 1994.
68. Mandal AK, Sanusi M: Penetrating chest wounds: 24 years experience. *World J Surg* 25:1145, 2001.
69. Plummer D, et al: Emergency department echocardiography improves outcome in penetrating cardiac injury. *Ann Emerg Med* 21:709, 1992.
70. Kraus JF, Nourjah P: The epidemiology of mild uncomplicated head injury. *J Trauma* 28:1637, 1988.
71. Stiell I, et al: Variation in ED use of computed tomography for patients with minor head injury. *Ann Emerg Med* 30:14, 1997.
72. Jeret JS, et al: Clinical predictors of abnormality disclosed by CT after mild head trauma. *Neurosurgery* 32:9, 1993.
73. Masters SJ, et al: Skull x-ray examinations after head trauma: Recommendations by a multidisciplinary panel and validation study. *N Engl J Med* 316:84, 1987.
74. National Heart Lung and Blood Institute, National Asthma Education Programme: *Expert Panel Report 2: Guidelines for the Diagnosis and Management of Asthma.* National Institutes of Health publication no 97-4051. Bethesda, Md, NIH, 1997.
75. Emerman CL, et al: Prospective multicenter study of relapse following treatment for acute asthma among adults presenting to the emergency department. MARC investigators. Multicenter Asthma Research Collaboration. *Chest* 115:919, 1999.
76. Weiss KB, Gergen PJ, Hodgson TA: An economic evaluation of asthma in the United States. *N Engl J Med* 326:862, 1992.
77. McConnochie KM, et al: How commonly are children hospitalised for asthma eligible for care in alternative settings? *Arch Pediatr Adolesc Med* 153:49, 1999.
78. Kannel WB, et al: Epidemiological features of chronic atrial fibrillation. *N Engl J Med* 306:1018, 1982.
79. Feinberg WM, et al: Prevalence, age distribution, and gender of patients with atrial fibrillation: Analysis and implications. *Arch Intern Med* 155:469, 1995.
80. Mulcahy B, et al: New onset atrial fibrillation: When is admission medically justified? *Acad Emerg Med* 3:114, 1996.
81. Koenig BO, Ross MA, Jackson RE: An emergency department observation unit protocol for acute-onset atrial fibrillation is feasible. *Ann Emerg Med* 39:374, 2002.
82. Danias PG, et al: Likelihood of spontaneous conversion of atrial fibrillation to sinus rhythm. *J Am Coll Cardiol* 31:588, 1998.
83. Howard PA: Ibutilide: An antiarrhythmic agent for the treatment of atrial fibrillation or flutter. *Ann Pharmacother* 33:38, 1999.
84. Amin NB, et al: Sinus bradycardia and multiple episodes of sinus arrest following administration of ibutilide. *Heart* 79:628, 1998.
85. Weigner MJ, et al: Risk for clinical thromboembolism associated with conversion to sinus rhythm in patients with atrial fibrillation lasting less than 48 hours. *Ann Intern Med* 126:615, 1997.
86. Kannel WB, Ho K, Thom J: Changing epidemiological features of cardiac failure. *Br Heart J* 72:S3, 1994.
87. American Heart Association: *Heart Disease and Stroke Statistics—2005.* Dallas, American Heart Association National Center, 2005.
88. Graff L, et al: Correlation of the Agency for Health Care Policy and Research congestive heart failure admission guideline with mortality: Peer Review Organization Voluntary Hospital Association Initiative to Decrease Events (PROVIDE) for congestive heart failure. *Ann Emerg Med* 34:429, 1999.
89. Peacock WF: Acute emergency department management of heart failure. *Heart Fail Rev* 8:335, 2003.
90. Maisel AS, et al: Rapid measurement of B-type natriuretic peptide in the emergency diagnosis of heart failure. *N Engl J Med* 347:161, 2002.
91. Peacock WF: The B-type natriuretic peptide assay: A rapid test for heart failure. *Cleveland Clin J Med* 69:243, 2002.
92. Vinson JM, et al: Early readmission of elderly patients with congestive heart failure. *J Am Geriatr Soc* 38:1290, 1990.
93. West JA, et al: A comprehensive management system for heart failure improves clinical outcomes and reduces medical resource utilization. *Am J Cardiol* 79:58, 1997.
94. Gordon JA, et al: Initial emergency department diagnosis and return visits: Risk versus perception. *Ann Emerg Med* 32:569, 1998.
95. Garibaldi RA: Epidemiology of community-acquired respiratory tract infections in adults: Incidence, etiology, and impact. *Am J Med* 78:32, 1985.
96. Fine MJ, Auble TE, Yealy DM: A prediction rule to identify low-risk patients with community-acquired pneumonia. N Engl J Med 336:243, 1997.
97. McMahon LF Jr, Wolfe RA, Tedeschi PJ: Variation in hospital admissions among small areas: A comparison of Maine and Michigan. *Med Care* 27:623, 1989.
98. Marie TJ, et al: A controlled trial of a critical pathway for treatment of community-acquired pneumonia. CAPITAL Study Investigators. Community-Acquired Pneumonia Intervention Trial Assessing Levofloxacin. *JAMA* 283:749, 2000.
99. Roberts R: Management of patients with infectious diseases in an emergency department observation unit. *Emerg Med Clin North Am* 19:187, 2001.
100. Elkharrat D, et al: Relevance in the emergency department of a decisional algorithm for outpatient care of women with acute pyelonephritis. *Eur J Emerg Med* 6:15, 1999.

CHAPTER 199 Occupational Medicine and Occupational Health in the Emergency Department

Andrew R. Barnosky, Daniel K. Chapman, and Victor S. Roth

This chapter is intended (1) to highlight the administrative and philosophical aspects of occupational medicine practice that are relevant to the clinical practice of emergency medicine, (2) to provide an overview of surveillance methodologies and treatment strategies for health conditions relevant to the medical care of health care workers (occupational health), and (3) to provide background information on the aspects of the workers' compensation system that are relevant to the practice needs of the emergency physician and the appropriate care of workers.

OCCUPATIONAL MEDICINE

Overview of Occupational Medicine

The treatment of occupational injuries is an important aspect of both occupational medicine and emergency medicine. Each year in the United States, workers sustain an estimated 1 million eye injuries, 400,000 fractures, 21,000 amputations, and more than 2 million lacerations. Emergency departments throughout the country treat at least 3 million occupational injuries annually. Injuries that occur within the workplace occur at a rate more than twice the occurrence rate of those sustained within the home environment, and more than 200 million workdays are lost annually at a national cost that exceeds $25 billion.[1]

Occupational injuries most often result from an acute work-related event, and occupational illnesses are conditions that develop (acutely or chronically) in relation to an occupational exposure. Surveillance methodologies and comprehensive epidemiologic data for occupational illness lag behind those for injuries, yet it has been estimated that at least 400,000 new cases of disabling occupational illnesses and as many as 100,000 deaths from occupational diseases occur each year.[1]

Occupational medicine has been defined as "that branch of medicine dealing with the study, prevention, and treatment of workplace injuries and occupational diseases, and with the promotion of optimal health and safety in the workplace."[2] Given this definition, it is clear that there are tremendous areas of overlap and interface between the specialties of occupational medicine and emergency medicine, particularly in the acute phase of injury or illness management. Both occupational medicine physicians and emergency physicians are confronted on a daily basis with the triage, evaluation, diagnosis, and treatment of workers with work-related illnesses and injuries and a variety of issues regarding work restrictions, return-to-work decisions, judgments regarding emergency department discharge and hospital admission, and toxic exposure management and reporting requirements. Thus, it is appropriate for emergency physicians to have a working understanding of the aspects of occupational medicine that can enhance the care of patients with work-related injury or illness. Although it is not the purpose of this chapter to duplicate a review of specific injuries and illnesses covered elsewhere in this text, the principles of occupational medicine and the administrative practices of the specialty that have a bearing on emergency physicians are worthy of review.

Emergency physicians intuitively recognize that the vast majority of work-related conditions that are cared for on a daily basis in the emergency department represent *injuries*. Certainly, for most work-related injuries, there is often a cause-effect relationship that becomes apparent in the taking of the history, regardless of whether it is a new injury, exacerbation of a prior work-related injury, or the cumulative effect of a repetitive effort engaged in over time that has just begun to manifest pain to the extent that the patient perceives the need for medical intervention. Work-related *illnesses* are less well defined but no less important. Although the care of patients in the aftermath of a toxic or harmful exposure is the most frequent and obvious presentation for emergency physicians in this regard, illnesses caused by occupational exposure may arise in a variety of ways. The short text entitled *Occupational Medicine*[2] by Lomax and Johanning aptly describes five well-accepted principles of occupational medicine that physicians treating workers should keep in mind in their daily practice:

- Illnesses caused by occupational exposure usually arise in nonspecific ways that are often indistinguishable from those of illnesses that are unrelated to occupation. In taking the history of a patient presenting to the emergency department for care, incorporating routine questions regarding the individual's occupation is a good way to detect a potential relationship between the presenting symptoms and an occupational exposure.
- The clinical presentation of an occupational condition is often influenced by coexisting health problems. Although it is less relevant for patients presenting to an emergency department for initial care, it is nonetheless worthwhile to bear this in mind. If an occupational exposure is of long standing (e.g., lead exposure that worsens underlying hypertension), separating exposure-related factors

from those that are not exposure related may be practically impossible, yet understanding the possibility of a multifactorial etiology of disease may be advantageous in the overall initial evaluation and disposition of a patient.

- The dose relationship between a toxic exposure and the likelihood of developing a particular disease takes into account both the duration of a worker's exposure (usually measured in years) and the average concentration of the toxic agent to which the worker is exposed.
- People who have the same degree of exposure to a toxic agent differ significantly in the expression of symptoms and disease. In this regard, it is worthwhile to remember that significant differences in the genetic constitution and body chemistry of individuals may cause significant differences in the metabolism of a toxic agent and its effects on the individual.
- Some occupational diseases occur after a considerable latent period. Pleural asbestosis generally develops 15 to 20 years following chronic exposure to asbestos. After exposure to secondhand smoke, it may take a considerable time for the development of pulmonary carcinomas in susceptible individuals.

It is worthwhile to note that the goals of the physician providing care to a patient having a work-related injury should be analogous to those of all physicians caring for all patients, regardless of circumstance; that is, the primacy of the patient's welfare and the vision of optimal clinical outcomes should be considered paramount. Although the employer is undoubtedly a factor that needs to be integrated in the contextual features of the doctor-patient relationship when caring for workers, as with all other third-party payers in medicine, the patient is still the primary recipient of the fiduciary obligations of the physician. It needs to be recognized, however, that when a physician undertakes the care of a worker-patient, in addition to the traditional doctor-patient relationship that is formed at the outset, the physician may retain a parallel obligation of promoting the future health status of the patient's fellow workers. In this sense, the practice of occupational medicine not only entails the formation of a professional relationship between the physician and the patient but also recognizes the possibility of undertaking responsibilities for disclosing health risks that may affect the population of workers of which the patient is a member. Writing in *Ethical Dilemmas Facing Clinicians Who Provide Health Care to Workers*, Tabershaw has answered the question "Whose agent is the occupational physician?" in this way—"The physician works for no other purpose than the benefit of his patients. In occupational medicine, this is the worker. As with other third-party payers, the patient is still primary. The physician is not an 'agent' of industry."[3]

The American College of Occupational and Environmental Medicine's code of ethics stresses that (1) the highest priority is to be given to the health and safety of the individual (patient), (2) the physician must practice on a scientific basis with objectivity and integrity, and (3) the physician must give an honest opinion and avoid having his or her medical judgment influenced by any collective interest.[4]

Workers' Compensation

Emergency physicians are often the first members of the health care team to evaluate individuals with workplace-related injuries or illness. Recognizing that workers' compensation is the vehicle through which the costs of medical care and compensation for lost wages are managed for injured or ill workers, it is helpful to have a basic understanding of this integral compensation system.

Every country in the industrialized world has developed a system to compensate workers or their survivors for medical care costs and lost wages related to injuries or illnesses sustained in the workplace. In the great majority of industrialized nations, this compensation system evolved as an integral portion of each country's national social security system. In the United States, the health care evolution within our market-based economy fostered a workers' compensation model that developed along the lines of the indemnity insurance model, similar to the manner in which American health care in general had been financed. The workers' compensation insurance system began its evolution in the early 1900s in the United States as pressure began to mount to shift the impact of occupational injury and illness from the worker to the employer and society in general. This pressure came from increased numbers of successful lawsuits that had been brought by workers against employers for injuries sustained on the job, in addition to increased public awareness that an unfair burden was being placed on workers as the country began a new period of industrialization.[5] Prior to the early 1900s, American workers who were injured on the job were required to sue their employers for negligence, as in the absence of a successful lawsuit the families of workers generally bore the entire cost of the injury independently and were forced to live on charity.[6] The concept of having the employer assume the financial responsibility for the injury or death of an employee originated not in the United States but rather in Germany in 1884. The famed German manufacturer Bertha von Krupp successfully persuaded Chancellor Otto von Bismarck that taking care of workers was in the best interest of business and thus the economic stability of the country. This led to a series of historic events throughout the industrialized world that stimulated the development of similar "no-fault systems," in which employer negligence was not required for worker compensation and the employee gave up the right to sue the employer for negligence in exchange for the employer's agreement to pay the cost of medical care and to compensate the worker for lost time from work.[1(ppii,23)]

In light of this historical backdrop, workers' compensation in the United States today has become a state-mandated program that requires employers to have some form of insurance vehicle for covering employees for work-related injuries. The program guarantees that if an employee sustains an injury or illness arising out of the course of employment, the worker will receive medical care, wage compensation, and disability benefits. The benefit to the employee under this system is the absence of having to establish any negligence on the part of the employer; it is necessary to establish simply that the injury or disease is work related. The benefit to the employer under this system is the avoidance of litigation over accidental injuries that occur in the workplace; in addition, the cost of work-related injuries is spread across a larger risk pool, with the employer assuming only an appropriate actuarially adjusted proportion of the aggregate cost. Although the system attempts to mitigate the costs to a single employer of a catastrophic financial loss by spreading the risk through an insurance pool, experience rating of various groups allows employers to bear some burden of the disabling conditions of the workplace in the hope of improving job safety and health conditions for employees. In addition to workers' compensation systems providing injured employees with an income following the occurrence of an injury and in the period of recovery, the system attempts to ensure workers a competitive place within the employment market and strives to avoid time- and resource-intensive legal action.[1(ppii,23)] Finally, in the event of the death of the employee, survivors receive compensation for the present and future loss of the income provider (the configuration of such compensation varies according to the individual state statutes).

For an employee to receive workers' compensation benefits, the worker must have an injury or illness that arises "out of and in the course of employment." This term denotes a requirement when injury or illness is considered for compensability and simply means that the injury or illness must have occurred while the employee was involved in some activity related to his or her job or that the injury or illness may be considered as causally related to the performance of the individual's work. Recurrence of an earlier compensable injury is compensable as well, as may be a work injury that activates or exacerbates a preexisting condition.

Disability following a work-related injury may be partial or total and may likewise be temporary or permanent. *Temporary total disability* represents the situation in which the worker is expected to recover with treatment yet remains unable to work for a discrete period of time. The employee receives benefits during the time of recovery. *Permanent partial disability* represents the situation in which a worker is disabled to the extent that there is permanent loss of a discrete ability that limits the employee's ability to compete equally in the labor market. *Temporary partial disability* is the major category in which injured workers fall; it occurs when a worker is injured to the extent that the employee cannot perform his or her usual and customary duties but is capable of engaging in some form of modified duty during convalescence. *Permanent total disability* is the form of disability that renders an employee unable to work, is considered permanently and totally disabling, and is expected to extend into perpetuity. In some states, certain injuries (such as loss of both eyes or two limbs) are considered permanently and totally disabling.

Finally, a discussion of these issues would not be complete without mention of the difference between disability and impairment. *Impairment* is a measure of anatomic or functional loss as measured by a physician, and the judgment or opinion of the physician is then passed to disability raters, workers' compensation judges, commissioners, or hearing officers, who use this information to make a determination of "disability."[1(ppii,30)] *Disability*, contrasted with impairment, depends on the job that one is expected to do and hence that individual's ability to compete in the open job market. Impairment may or may not imply disability. For example, the loss of the distal phalanx of the left fifth finger is the same impairment on either a cellist or a cello maker, but the degree of disability would be far more substantial in the musician than the cello maker.

Return-to-Work Issues

When an employer requires occupational health (OH) care for an employee, the employer frequently utilizes the services of an emergency department or urgent care (UC) facility. Although many employers have relationships with OH providers, they augment service with an emergency department or UC facility after normal clinic business hours and on weekends. Sometimes, dedicated OH facilities are not geographically convenient and the emergency department or UC facilities may provide all work-related services including injury and illness care, preplacement and medical surveillance examinations, and drug and alcohol testing.

Employers have common expectations when sending an employee for OH care. Because maintaining productivity is a critical part of the business environment, employers desire that their employees be evaluated, treated, and returned to the workplace in a prompt and efficient manner. It is also an expectation that a thorough history of the injury or illness is obtained and that causation of the diagnosis is addressed when possible. Clear, concise, return-to-work (RTW) instructions should be provided to the employee and communicated to the employer in a timely fashion. Follow-up instructions should also be given to both employee and employer, whether involving return to the treating facility, an employer-designated OH provider, or, in some cases, another medical specialist. Finally, in regard to medical treatment practices and RTW issues, the emergency physician should be cognizant of the unique relationship in OH between the employee, employer, and provider.

As a matter of course, any patient presenting to an emergency facility has a thorough medical history taken. In the case of a patient presenting with an alleged occupational injury or illness, additional components of the medical history are required, not only to discern the nature of the injury or illness and the required treatment but also to allow a determination of the compensability of the presenting problem under the workers' compensation system applicable in the treatment facility's locale. Commonly, OH specialists are asked by the employer or workers' compensation representative to render an opinion about the work relatedness of a particular diagnosis. On occasion, emergency physicians may also be asked their opinion on these matters. A review of the presenting complaint and attendant history is an essential component of this decision-making process. It is important not only to ask the patient about the location and character of the complaints, inciting and relieving factors, onset of symptoms (insidious versus sudden), and mechanism of injury but also to inquire about specific job and work site issues such as type of work performed, duration with the current employer, recent task or process changes including recent increases in working hours, and previous injuries or illnesses associated with the employment. On the basis of this information, an opinion can be formed about the plausibility that the reported problem is related to the workplace tasks or that the history given by the employee is consistent with the nature of the presenting problem. In most systems, the provider merely presents this opinion, and the final determination about compensability is made by the insurer, which can in some cases also be the employer.

Treatment of work-related injuries and illnesses on an acute basis rarely varies from the treatment rendered for the same diagnosis in a non–work-related circumstance. A patient with an ankle sprain that occurs as a result of a workplace fall would be expected to be treated in a similar manner to a patient who falls at home and sustains an ankle sprain.

The critical difference between these two patients is that the emergency physician needs to formulate a plan for the injured employee that incorporates appropriate RTW instructions as well as a follow-up regimen based on the desires of the employer and in accordance with local laws. These plans need to be clearly communicated to both employee and employer on a timely basis. The provider should make every effort to return the injured or ill employee back to work after evaluation and treatment. When possible, the employee should be returned to his or her regular work. If, in the provider's opinion, the injury or illness precludes this, the employee can be returned to work with "restrictions." *Restrictions* are defined as instructions to both the employee and employer that limit certain activities yet allow the employer to place the employee at a task or tasks that enable the employee to work safely while also allowing the ability to recover from the specific injury or illness. A common example is a laborer with an acute onset of nonspecific musculoskeletal low back pain who presents to the emergency department. The laborer may not be able to perform the essential functions of his or her assigned tasks but could be returned to work with instructions limiting lifting to no more than 10 pounds, limiting bending and twisting activities, and alternating sitting and standing positions. The employer then has the option to utilize the employee in a productive and safe fashion while allowing the employee to recover. Restrictions should be as specific as possible so as to be easily interpretable by both employee and employer. Providers should avoid using terms such as "may perform light duty" or "no heavy lifting," which are too vague to be useful in making a placement decision.

Rarely, an occupational injury or illness may be severe enough to preclude the employee from any work-related activities. In this situation, the employee should be instructed not to return to work until seen in follow-up. The employer should be notified promptly of this decision so that appropriate follow-up arrangements can be made. Depending on the local workers' compensation statutes, employers may have designated OH providers that evaluate the employee the next business day to continue treatment and coordinate the patient's eventual return to work. In the United States, some state workers' compensation statutes permit employees to determine the physicians who provide their care, whereas other states allow employer-directed health care for occupational illness and injury. In situations in which employees may self-direct their care from the first day of injury or illness, instructions should still be given for prompt follow-up to ensure ongoing care and reduction of disability. Except in situations immediately threatening to life or limb, specialty and testing referrals should be deferred to the provider giving follow-up care. This allows better coordination of care and simplifies the emergency physician's main role, which is the acute evaluation and treatment of the presenting complaint.

Finally, in caring for patients with work-related injuries and illnesses, one should recognize the somewhat unique role the medical provider plays when dealing with OH issues. In most patient-provider relationships, the provider is considered to be an advocate of the patient with his or her sole obligation to the patient's needs. In an OH setting or when providing OH services, the provider not only has a duty to provide care for the individual patient but also has an obligation to communicate effectively with the employer representative and to make medical decisions that are in the best interest of the employee but also do not place the employer or other employees at the work site at risk. An example that illustrates this decision-making process may be useful. An individual presents to the emergency department or UC facility for a preplacement (new hire) examination. In the history taking, it is determined that the individual, who is being considered for a job involving primarily desk work but who is required to climb a 10-foot ladder twice per shift to obtain supplies, has insulin-dependent diabetes mellitus with fair control and infrequent hypoglycemic episodes. The remainder of the history is unremarkable and the physical examination is normal. It is clear that the individual can perform all aspects of the job, but the provider must take into consideration the risk to the individual as well as to coworkers should a hypoglycemic event resulting in loss of consciousness occur while the individual is climbing the ladder or is on top of the platform. The provider needs to protect the personal information of the individual while still communicating to the employer the need to have the individual avoid climbing and working at heights. The employer would, in this example, most likely determine the ladder-climbing function to be nonessential and have another qualified employee perform this limited task. In this example, the provider has determined restrictions that allow the employee to work safely, allow the employer and coworkers to be protected, and maintain the confidentiality of a personal medical condition. The emergency physician functioning in the role of OH provider needs to be cognizant of the different perspectives in the workplace, particularly when safety-sensitive positions are involved.

Drug and Alcohol Testing

In the United States, it has become increasingly common for employers to require drug or alcohol testing for their employees or prospective employees. Although many employers utilize an occupational medicine clinic for these testing services, some turn to the local emergency department or UC facility, especially if OH services are offered on site. Facilities that agree to collect specimens for drug and alcohol testing need to understand the reasons for testing, the different types of testing, and the collection methods available.

Drug and alcohol testing can be divided into two main categories, mandated and nonmandated. Mandated drug testing has its roots in Executive Order 12564,[7] which in 1986 directed each federal agency to establish a program to test its employees in safety-sensitive positions for illicit drugs. In April 1988, the Department of Health and Human Services published guidelines to ensure that drug testing was uniform, accurate, and confidential.[8] These became known as the National Institute on Drug Abuse (NIDA) guidelines.

In 1989, the Department of Transportation (DOT) adopted the NIDA guidelines for its drug testing procedures.[9] The adoption resulted in mandated testing for over 4 million employees covered by six different agencies. Each of these agencies also oversees private sector employees. The commonalties present in the DOT guidelines for drug testing ensure that (1) DOT procedures are followed for collection and analysis of the specimen as well as result reporting; (2) the five drugs tested for are marijuana, cocaine, amphetamines, opiates, and phencyclidine (PCP); (3) the types of testing include postaccident, preplacement, reasonable cause, random, and periodic; and (4) NIDA-certified laboratories are used for specimen analysis.

Although it is beyond the scope of this chapter to detail sample collection procedures for mandated drug and alcohol testing, it is crucial to understand these procedures if an emergency services program or facility is to undertake the responsibility for this testing. Although it is lengthy, the *Federal Register*[10] details all the necessary forms, collection procedures, and specimen handling including chain of custody and required staff competences for mandated drug and alcohol testing. Briefly, the collection site first needs to identify the employee by picture identification or a supervisor verifying the employee's identification. The proper chain of custody form needs to be completed by the collector and signed by the employee. Next, the sample is collected, which in the case of drug testing is a urine sample and in alcohol testing can be a breath or saliva sample. With urine specimens, the sample is sealed in front of the employee with a tamper-proof seal and then initialed. The sample is then sealed in a specimen bag and sent to a NIDA laboratory for processing, all the while maintaining established chain of custody procedures. All mandated urine collection must be done as split specimens, splitting the single provided sample into two separate containers. The second specimen is retained by the testing laboratory because the employee has the option of having the split specimen sent to a second NIDA laboratory for testing in the case of a positive test.

In the alcohol testing process, breath is sampled using a breath alcohol testing device, or evidential breath testing device, that has been properly maintained and calibrated. The testing must be done by a trained breath alcohol technician.[11] The results are immediately available and, if positive, which is defined by the DOT as 0.02% or greater, are confirmed with a second test after a 15-minute waiting period to clear any possible mouth alcohol. Alternatively, a sample of saliva can be collected by a breath alcohol technician or a screening test technician using a designated alcohol swab kit. Positive results must be confirmed using a breath alcohol testing device. The DOT guidelines do not address the use of blood specimens for alcohol testing. In the case of a positive alcohol test, the employer is immediately notified and the employee is removed, at least temporarily, from performing safety-sensitive functions. The employer then proceeds according to the applicable DOT guidelines.

Positive drug testing results stemming from mandated testing must be reviewed by a medical review officer (MRO). An MRO is a licensed physician who has received training and passed a certification examination covering the various areas of drug testing. The MRO notifies the employee before releasing the results to the employer. The MRO ensures that the testing was valid, ensures that the chain of custody was intact, and attempts to define an explanation for the test results. The employee may have a valid prescription that reasonably explains the positive drug test, in which case, once the prescription was verified by the MRO, the results would be reported as negative to the employer. When results are reported as positive to the employer, the employer is required to refer the individual to a designated substance abuse professional. This professional evaluates the employee and makes recommendations regarding education, treatment, follow-up testing, and aftercare.

The vast majority of drug and alcohol tests performed by employers are nonmandated tests that are addressed by specific company policies. It is highly advisable that companies develop a drug and alcohol testing policy if they choose to test their employees for drug or alcohol use, or both, so that testing and results are handled in a uniform manner. Typically, collection sites follow the DOT guidelines for collecting specimens because they are considered to be the "gold standard." Usually, split urine samples are not collected in nonmandated testing. The use of NIDA laboratories, MRO services, and substance abuse professional services is also not required in nonmandated testing, but most facilities and companies follow the thorough standards outlined in the comprehensive DOT drug testing guidelines. It is the responsibility of any medical facility that provides drug or alcohol testing to be familiar with the regulations and procedures involved before becoming involved in performing the various drug and alcohol tests.

OCCUPATIONAL HEALTH ISSUES IN THE EMERGENCY DEPARTMENT

The Material Safety Data Sheet

Emergency physicians are frequently the first physicians called upon to evaluate and treat patients for the acute adverse effects of a work-related chemical exposure. In such cases, a readily available source of information regarding chemical hazards is important in the evaluation, diagnosis, and treatment of patients involved in such exposures.[12]

In November 1983, the Occupational Safety and Health Administration (OSHA) promulgated the Federal Hazard Communication Standard (HazCom), a regulation covering a broad range of chemical hazards. The purpose of this standard was to "ensure that the hazards of all chemicals produced or imported by chemical manufacturers or importers are evaluated, and that information concerning their hazards is transmitted to affected employers and employees with the manufacturing sector."[13] In addition to containing provisions regarding labeling of chemical containers and appropriate training of the employees working with hazardous chemicals, HazCom, also known as the "worker's right to know law," requires that a chemical information sheet, the Material Safety Data Sheet (MSDS), be produced for all hazardous chemicals. An extensive number of MSDSs identify products considered hazardous by OSHA, with that number increasing daily. The MSDS lists a chemical's physical properties and health hazards, recommended measures to control exposure, and personal protective equipment required during use of the product.[14] An MSDS also contains vital emergency information, such as first aid measures and spill mitigation procedures. An MSDS provides emergency personnel with the proper procedures for treating a patient with a potential exposure to that product.

MSDSs are available from (1) the workplace in which the chemical is being used, (2) the manufacturer of the chemical, (3) the importer of the chemical, or (4) various Internet sites.

In most cases, when a worker is sent to the emergency department for medical evaluation following a chemical exposure, an appropriate MSDS is sent with the worker.

The primary way a company complies with HazCom is by maintaining an MSDS for each hazardous substance used or stored at its facilities. Unfortunately, companies that manufacture chemicals are not required to follow any specific format for the MSDS they provide to their customers, and MSDS formats can, and do, vary widely. Most MSDSs include eight main sections, as outlined in Box 199-1.

The quality of MSDSs is also a concern. Evidence from studies of MSDSs[15,16] indicates that the accuracy of information presented on MSDSs and their comprehensibility present major concerns when the sheets are used as sources of information when treating individuals for exposures.

Clinical Documentation Related to Material Safety Data Sheet Information

After reviewing the product MSDS and noting the potential clinical effects of exposure to a specific product, the physician should carefully document the history of the event and then conduct and document a pertinent clinical examination. In most cases, one would expect to see objective clinical manifestations of effects from exposure to be most evident soon after the exposure.

For example, if the MSDS indicates that the product used by the patient is an irritant, the treating physician should be meticulous in noting and documenting the presence or absence of irritant-type symptoms (such as burning sensations of the eyes, nose, or throat or shortness of breath) or signs (scleral injection, watery eyes, erythema of the nasal or pharyngeal mucous membranes, wheezing on lung auscultation). Such objective documentation of symptoms and positive or negative clinical findings can be used to support, or not support, future disability claims or litigation.

Blood-Borne Pathogens

The evaluation and treatment of hospital employees after accidental exposure to blood-borne pathogens often takes place in the emergency department.

A wide variety of blood-borne infections have the potential for transmission to health care workers. The infections of most concern are hepatitis B, hepatitis C, and human immunodeficiency virus (HIV). The most common routes of exposure are puncture wounds from needles and blood or body fluid splashes on mucous membranes or areas of abraded skin.

It is also important that emergency physicians and other emergency department personnel practice self-policing for occupational blood exposure. In a study of risk for occupational blood exposure in 24,000 hospital health care workers,[17] emergency department staff had the highest relative rate of occupational blood exposure, with nurses and laboratory staff found to be more exposed than physicians.

Despite widespread knowledge of universal precautions to prevent transmission of blood-borne pathogens, noncompliance with these precautions appears to be common. One study[18] concluded that "many health care workers seem not to take full advantage of barrier precautions in the emergency department." The study results determined that in trauma resuscitation, glove use compliance was high (98%)

BOX 199-1. Main Sections of a Typical Material Safety Data Sheet (MSDS)

Although there is no universal standard format for MSDSs and formats vary widely, most MSDSs contain eight main sections as outlined below:

Section I: Chemical Identity and Manufacturer

- This section contains the manufacturer's name, address, telephone number, and an emergency telephone number. The emergency physician may feel it necessary to contact the chemical manufacturer by telephone if immediate or additional information about the product is needed to treat the exposed employee appropriately.

Section II: Hazardous Ingredients

- This section contains generic names for each of the various chemicals contained in the product and the recommended maximum safe human exposure levels for each of these various chemical components.
- Even though a product may be considered hazardous, many of the individual chemical ingredients of the product listed on an MSDS may not be hazardous. However, the MSDS listing of the product components by the common (generic) names is still quite helpful, as it allows the emergency physician more readily to identify the individual hazardous components in the product and thus more quickly and appropriately treat the patient for the effects arising from exposure to the hazardous components of the product.
- The specific chemical identity of certain hazardous substances contained in a product may be withheld from the MSDS if that component is a proprietary ingredient. In that case, the MSDS must indicate the components that are being withheld from the MSDS as a trade secret. In addition, the MSDS must contain information concerning the properties and clinical effects of those components.
- In cases where the treating physician determines that a medical emergency warrants obtaining additional information about a specific product's proprietary chemical ingredient, the manufacturer, employer, or importer must immediately disclose that information.

Section III: Physical and Chemical Characteristics

- This section contains the physical and chemical characteristics of the product, including the odor, color, vapor pressure, vapor density, evaporation rate, freezing point, boiling point, water solubility, and specific gravity. In many cases, workplaces use several different chemical products. In such cases, if a chemical product to which a patient was exposed is unknown, using the company's MSDSs to identify the product's odor and color properties may enable the physician to recognize the product. Once the product is known, the chemical's other properties, such as vapor pressure, vapor density, and evaporation rate, help to determine the potential for human exposure and the likely route of that exposure. A product with a vapor density less than 1.0 will rise in air and is more likely to have a respiratory exposure route, while products with a vapor density greater than 1.0 will accumulate near the floor. Similar, a product with an evaporation rate greater than 1.0 is volatile and thus a more likely inhalation hazard than a product with an evaporation rate less than 1.0.[21]

Section IV: Fire and Explosion Hazard Data

- This section contains information on a product's flash point, flammability, and appropriate firefighting equipment.

Section V: Reactivity Data

- Hazardous decomposition products of the chemical are noted in this section. Such information aids the treating physician in cases where the chemical has broken down, which may take place under conditions of extreme heat (fire) or when mixed with water.

Section VI: Health Hazard Data

- After first reviewing Section II (Hazardous Ingredients), this is the section to which the emergency physician should turn when faced with a case of potential product exposure. This section incorporates information considered vital to the appropriate and timely treatment of the patient, including potential routes of exposure (dermal, respiratory, oral), appropriate first aid measures following exposure, acute health hazards based on the properties of the chemical, and chronic health hazards based on the properties of the chemical.

Section VII: Precautions for Safe Handling and Use

Section VIII: Control Measures

- These two sections of an MSDS are more relevant to people working with the product than to physicians treating an exposure to the product. However, because Sections VII and VIII outline safe handling techniques for the product and personal protective equipment (such as gloves, respirator, eye shields) that one should use when working with the product, it may be useful for the emergency physician to inquire whether those safety measures were in place and whether the recommended personal protective equipment was being used at the time the exposure event occurred.

but compliance with other barriers was much lower, including the use of eye protection (51%), gowns (41%), and masks (10%). Compared with emergency department nurses (31%), physicians made much more use of eye shield protection (61%).

On the other hand, a study of more than 6000 health care workers from large urban teaching hospitals[19] found that, compared with past years, the number of health care workers with immunity to hepatitis B has increased and the number of those who comply with surveillance after an exposure (initial baseline HIV test and follow-up testing) has improved. The authors claimed that these findings are encouraging and probably the result of the evolution of postexposure testing and treatment recommendations as well as a greater understanding of the diseases and their transmission.

The OSHA Bloodborne Pathogens Standard has probably played a significant role in increasing knowledge of disease transmission and highlighting the importance of following proper procedures to minimize the risk of accidental exposures. In 1991, OSHA issued the Bloodborne Pathogens Standard to protect workers from this risk. In response to the Needlestick Safety and Prevention Act passed by Congress in November 2000, OSHA revised the standard, effective April 2001. The revised standard clarified the need for employers to select safer needle devices and involved employees in identifying and choosing these devices. The revision also required employers to maintain a log of injuries associated with contaminated sharps.

The "U.S. Public Health Service guidelines for the management of occupational exposures to HBV, HCV, and HIV and recommendations for postexposure prophylaxis"[20] were updated in June 2001 and consolidated all previous U.S. Public Health Service recommendations for the management of health care personnel with an occupational exposure to blood and other body fluids that might contain hepatitis B virus (HBV), hepatitis C virus (HCV), or HIV.

The following recommendations are standard and relevant to treatment in the emergency department setting and were excerpted from the updated U.S. Public Health Service guidelines for the management of occupational exposures to HBV, HCV, and HIV and recommendations for postexposure prophylaxis.[19]

- Recommendations for HBV postexposure management include initiation of the hepatitis B vaccine series to any susceptible, unvaccinated person who sustains an occupational blood or body fluid exposure. Postexposure prophylaxis with hepatitis B immune globulin (HBIG) or hepatitis B vaccine series should be considered for occupational exposures after evaluation of the hepatitis B surface antigen (HBsAg) status of the source and the vaccination and vaccine response status of the exposed person. Guidance is provided to clinicians and exposed health care providers for selecting the appropriate HBV postexposure prophylaxis.
- Immune globulin and antiviral agents (e.g., interferon with or without ribavirin) are not recommended for postexposure prophylaxis of hepatitis C. For HCV postexposure management, the HCV status of the source and the exposed person should be determined, and for health care providers exposed to an HCV-positive source, follow-up HCV testing should be performed to determine whether infection develops.
- Recommendations for HIV postexposure prophylaxis include a basic 4-week regimen of two drugs (zidovudine [ZDV] and lamivudine [3TC], 3TC and stavudine [d4T], or didanosine [ddI] and d4T) for most HIV exposures and an expanded regimen that includes the addition of a third drug for HIV exposures that pose an increased risk for transmission. When the source person's virus is known or suspected to be resistant to one or more of the drugs considered for the postexposure prophylaxis regimen, selection of drugs to which the source person's virus is unlikely to be resistant is recommended.
- Occupational exposures should be considered urgent medical concerns to ensure timely postexposure management and administration of HBIG, hepatitis B vaccine, or HIV postexposure prophylaxis.

The guidelines also describe special circumstances (e.g., delayed exposure report, unknown source person, pregnancy in the exposed person, resistance of the source virus to antiretroviral agents, or toxicity of the postexposure prophylaxis regimen) in which consultation with local experts or the National Clinicians' Post-Exposure Prophylaxis Hotline, or both, is advised. The National Clinicians' Post-Exposure Prophylaxis Hotline (PEPline) at 1-888-HIV-4911 offers treating clinicians up-to-the-minute advice on managing occupational exposures (e.g., needlesticks, splashes) to HIV, hepatitis, and other blood-borne pathogens.

Exposure prevention (the use of gloves, masks, eye shields, gowns, and needle safety devices and proper disposal of sharps) remains the primary strategy for reducing occupational infections with blood-borne pathogens. Even with physicians' knowledge of these precautions, occupational exposures continue to occur. In addition to being the providers who most commonly treat such work-related exposures in health care workers, emergency physicians, as a group, have an elevated risk for occupational exposure to blood-borne infections. When an exposure takes place, the physician should report it immediately because HBIG, hepatitis B vaccine, and HIV postexposure prophylaxis are most likely to be effective if administered as soon as possible after the exposure.

The following recommendations for percutaneous or mucosal exposure to hepatitis B, hepatitis C, and HIV go into more detail about each individual exposure and are considered standard practice. The information is adapted directly from the U.S. Public Health Service guidelines updated report.

Management of Exposures to Hepatitis B

For percutaneous or mucosal exposures to blood, several factors must be considered when making a decision to provide prophylaxis, including the HBsAg status of the source and the hepatitis B vaccination and vaccine response status of the exposed person. Such exposures usually involve persons for whom hepatitis B vaccination is recommended. Any blood or body fluid exposure to an unvaccinated person should lead to initiation of the hepatitis B vaccine series.

The hepatitis B vaccination status and the vaccine response status (if known) of the exposed person should be reviewed. A summary of prophylaxis recommendations for percutaneous or mucosal exposure to blood according to the HBsAg status of the exposure source and the vaccination and vaccine response status of the exposed person appears in Table 199-1.

When HBIG is indicated, it should be administered as soon as possible after exposure (preferably within 24 hours). The effectiveness of HBIG when administered more than 7 days after exposure is unknown. When hepatitis B vaccine is indicated, it should also be administered as soon as possible (preferably within 24 hours and always administered in the deltoid muscle) and can be administered simultaneously with HBIG (at a different site).

For exposed persons who are in the process of being vaccinated but have not completed the vaccination series, vaccination should be completed as scheduled, and HBIG should be added as indicated (see Table 199-1). Persons exposed to HBsAg-positive blood or body fluids who are known not to have responded to a primary vaccine series should receive a single dose of HBIG and reinitiate the hepatitis B vaccine series with the first dose of the hepatitis B vaccine as soon as possible after exposure. Alternatively, they should receive two doses of HBIG, one dose as soon as possible after exposure and the second dose 1 month later. The option of administering one dose of HBIG and reiniti-

Table 199-1. Recommended Postexposure Prophylaxis for Exposure to Hepatitis B Virus

Vaccination and Antibody Response Status of Exposed Workers*	Treatment		
	Source HBsAg† Positive	*Source HBsAg† Negative*	*Source Unknown or Not Available for Testing*
Unvaccinated	HBIG‡ × 1 and initiate HB vaccine series§	Initiate HB vaccine series	Initiate HB vaccine series
Previously vaccinated			
Known responder‖	No treatment	No treatment	No treatment
Known nonresponder¶	HBIG × 1 and initiate revaccination or HBIG × 2**	No treatment	If known high risk source, treat as if source were HBsAg positive
Antibody response unknown	Test exposed person for anti-HBs†† 1. If adequate,‖ no treatment is necessary 2. If inadequate,¶ administer HBIG × 1 and vaccine booster	No treatment	Test exposed person for anti-HBs 1. If adequate,§ no treatment is necessary 2. If inadequate,§ administer vaccine booster and recheck titer in 1–2 months

*Persons who have previously been infected with HBV are immune to reinfection and do not require postexposure prophylaxis.
†Hepatitis B surface antigen.
‡Hepatitis B immune globulin; dose is 0.06 mL/kg intramuscularly.
§Hepatitis B vaccine.
‖A responder is a person with adequate levels of serum antibody to HBsAg (i.e., anti-HBs ≥ 10 mIU/mL).
¶A nonresponder is a person with inadequate response to vaccination (i.e., serum anti-HBs < 10 mIU/mL).
**The option of giving one dose of HBIG and reinitiating the vaccine series is preferred for nonresponders who have not completed a second three-dose vaccine series. For persons who previously completed a second vaccine series but failed to respond, two doses of HBIG are preferred.
††Antibody to HBsAg.
HB, hepatitis B; HBIG, HB immuneglobulin; HBsAg, HB surface antigen.

ating the vaccine series is preferred for nonresponders who did not complete a second three-dose vaccine series. For persons who previously completed a second vaccine series but failed to respond, two doses of HBIG are preferred.

Management of Exposures to Hepatitis C Virus

It is recommended that individual institutions establish policies and procedures for testing health care providers for HCV after percutaneous or mucosal exposures to blood. The following are recommendations for follow-up of occupational HCV exposures:

- For the source: perform testing for anti-HCV.
- For the person exposed to an HCV-positive source:
- Perform baseline testing for anti-HCV and ALT activity
- Perform follow-up testing (e.g., at 4 to 6 months) for anti-HCV and ALT activity (if earlier diagnosis of HCV infection is desired, testing for HCV RNA may be performed at 4 to 6 weeks)
- Confirm all anti-HCV results reported positive by enzyme immunoassay using supplemental anti-HCV testing (e.g., recombinant immunoblot assay).

For persons exposed to HCV in the occupational setting, appropriate counseling, testing, and medical follow-up should be made available.

Immunoglobulin and antiviral agents are not recommended for postexposure prophylaxis after exposure to HCV-positive blood. There is no guideline for the administration of therapy during the acute phase of HCV infection. Only limited data indicate that antiviral therapy may be beneficial if started early in the course of HCV infection.

Management of Exposures to Human Immunodeficiency Virus

Clinical Evaluation and Baseline Testing of Exposed Health Care Provider

Health care providers exposed to HIV should be evaluated within hours of exposure and should be tested for HIV at baseline to establish infection status at the time of exposure. If the source person is seronegative for HIV, baseline testing or further follow-up of the exposed person is normally not necessary. Serologic testing should be made available to all health care providers who are concerned that they might have been occupationally infected with HIV. If considering HIV postexposure prophylaxis, one should obtain information about medications the exposed person might be taking and any current or underlying medical conditions or circumstances (i.e., pregnancy, breast-feeding, or renal or hepatic disease) that might influence drug selection.

Postexposure Prophylaxis for HIV

The recommendations in Tables 199-2 and 199-3 apply to situations in which a person has been exposed to a source person with HIV infection or when information suggests the likelihood that the source person is HIV infected. These recommendations are based on the risk for HIV infection after different types of exposure and on limited data regarding the efficacy and toxicity of postexposure prophylaxis. Because most occupational HIV exposures do not result in transmission of HIV,

Table 199-2. Recommended HIV Postexposure Prophylaxis for Percutaneous Injuries

	Infection Status of Source				
Exposure Type	***HIV-Positive Class 1****	***HIV-Positive Class 2****	***Source of Unknown HIV Status†***	***Unknown Source‡***	***HIV-Negative***
Less severe§	Recommend basic two-drug PEP	Recommend expanded three-drug PEP	Generally, no PEP warranted; however, consider basic two-drug PEP‖ for source with HIV risk factors¶	Generally, no PEP warranted; however, consider basic two-drug PEP‖ in settings where exposure to HIV-infected persons is likely	No PEP warranted
More severe**	Recommend expanded three-drug PEP	Recommend expanded three-drug PEP	Generally, no PEP warranted; however, consider basic two-drug PEP‖ for source with HIV risk factors¶	Generally, no PEP warranted; however, consider basic two-drug PEP‖ in settings where exposure to HIV-infected persons is likely	No PEP warranted

*HIV-positive, class 1—asymptomatic HIV infection or known low viral load (e.g., <1500 RNA copies/mL). HIV-positive, class 2—symptomatic HIV infection, AIDS, acute seroconversion, or known high viral load. If drug resistance is a concern, obtain expert consultation. Initiation of postexposure prophylaxis (PEP) should not be delayed pending expert consultation, and, because expert consultation alone cannot substitute for face-to-face counseling, resources should be available to provide immediate evaluation and follow-up care for all exposures.
†Source of unknown HIV status (e.g., deceased source person with no samples available for HIV testing).
‡Unknown source (e.g., a needle from a sharps disposal container).
§Less severe (e.g., solid needle and superficial injury).
‖The designation "consider PEP" indicates that PEP is optional and should be based on an individualized decision between the exposed person and the treating clinician.
¶If PEP is offered and taken and the source is later determined to be HIV negative, PEP should be discontinued.
**More severe (e.g., large-bore hollow needle, deep puncture, visible blood on device, or needle used in patient's artery or vein).
AIDS, acquired immunodeficiency syndrome; HIV, human immunodeficiency virus.

Table 199-3. Recommended HIV Postexposure Prophylaxis for Mucous Membrane Exposures and Nonintact Skin Exposures

	Infection Status of Source				
Exposure Type*	***HIV-Positive Class 1†***	***HIV-Positive Class 2†***	***Source of Unknown HIV status‡***	***Unknown Source§***	***HIV-Negative***
Small volume‖	Consider basic two-drug PEP¶	Recommend basic two-drug PEP	Generally, no PEP warranted; however consider basic two-drug PEP¶ for source with HIV risk factors**	Generally, no PEP warranted; however, consider basic two-drug PEP¶ in settings where exposure to HIV-infected persons is likely	No PEP warranted
Large volume††	Recommend basic two-drug PEP	Recommend expanded three-drug PEP	Generally, no PEP warranted; however, consider basic two-drug PEP¶ for source with HIV risk factors**	Generally, no PEP warranted; however, consider basic two-drug PEP¶ in settings where exposure to HIV-infected persons is likely	No PEP warranted

*For skin exposures, follow-up is indicated only if there is evidence of compromised skin integrity (e.g., dermatitis, abrasion, or open wound).
†HIV positive, class 1—asymptomatic HIV infection or known low viral load (e.g., <1500 RNA copies/mL). HIV positive, class 2—symptomatic HIV infection, AIDS, acute seroconversion, or known high viral load. If drug resistance is a concern, obtain expert consultation. Initiation of postexposure prophylaxis (PEP) should not be delayed pending expert consultation, and, because expert consultation alone cannot substitute for face-to-face counseling, resources should be available to provide immediate evaluation and follow-up care for all exposures.
‡Source of unknown HIV status (e.g., deceased source person with no samples available for HIV testing).
§Unknown source (e.g., splash from inappropriately disposed blood).
‖Small volume (i.e., a few drops).
¶The designation, "consider PEP," indicates that PEP is optional and should be based on an individualized decision between the exposed person and the treating clinician.
**If PEP is offered and taken and the source is later determined to be HIV negative, PEP should be discontinued.
††Large volume (i.e., major blood splash).
AIDS, acquired immunodeficiency syndrome; HIV, human immunodeficiency virus.

BOX 199-2. Situations for Which Expert Consultation for HIV Postexposure Prophylaxis Is Advised

Delayed (i.e., later than 24–36 hours) exposure report
- The interval after which there is no benefit from postexposure prophylaxis (PEP) is undefined

Unknown source (e.g., needle in sharps disposal container or laundry)
- Decide use of PEP on a case-by-case basis
- Consider the severity of the exposure and the epidemiologic likelihood of HIV exposure
- Do not test needles or other sharp instruments for HIV

Known or suspected pregnancy in the exposed person
- Does not preclude the use of optimal PEP regimens
- Do not deny PEP solely on the basis of pregnancy

Resistance of the source virus to antiretroviral agents
- Influence of drug resistance on transmission risk is unknown
- Selection of drugs to which the source person's virus is unlikely to be resistant is recommended, if the source person's virus is known or suspected to be resistant to ≥1 of the drugs considered for the PEP regimen
- Resistance testing of the source person's virus at the time of the exposure is not recommended

Toxicity of the initial PEP regimen
- Adverse symptoms such as nausea and diarrhea are common with PEP
- Symptoms can often be managed without changing the PEP regimen by prescribing antimotility or antiemetic agents, or both
- Modification of dose intervals (i.e., administering a lower dose of drug more frequently throughout the day, as recommended by the manufacturer), in other situations, might help alleviate symptoms

HIV, human immunodeficiency virus.

potential toxicity must be carefully considered when prescribing postexposure prophylaxis. When possible, these recommendations should be implemented in consultation with persons who have expertise in antiretroviral therapy and HIV transmission (Box 199-2).

Timing and Duration of Postexposure Prophylaxis

Postexposure prophylaxis for HIV should be initiated as soon as possible. The interval within which postexposure prophylaxis should be initiated for optimal efficacy is not known. Starting the basic regimen immediately is probably better than delaying postexposure prophylaxis. Although animal studies suggest that postexposure prophylaxis is probably substantially less effective when started more than 24 to 36 hours after exposure, the interval after which no benefit is gained from postexposure prophylaxis for humans is not known. Therefore, if appropriate for the exposure, postexposure prophylaxis should be started even when the interval from exposure exceeds 36 hours. Initiating therapy after a longer interval (e.g., more than 1 week) might be considered for exposures that represent an increased risk for transmission. Because 4 weeks of ZDV appeared protective in occupational and animal studies, postexposure prophylaxis should probably be administered for 4 weeks, if tolerated.

Use of Postexposure Prophylaxis When HIV Status of Source Is Unknown

If the source person's HIV infection status is unknown at the time of exposure, use of postexposure prophylaxis should be decided on a case-by-case basis after considering the type of exposure and the likelihood of HIV infection in the source (see Tables 199-2 and 199-3). If these considerations suggest a possibility for HIV transmission and HIV testing of the source person is pending, initiating a two-drug postexposure prophylaxis regimen until laboratory results have been obtained and later modifying or discontinuing the regimen is reasonable. The following are recommendations regarding HIV postexposure prophylaxis:

- If indicated, start postexposure prophylaxis as soon as possible after an exposure.
- Reevaluate the exposed person within 72 hours after exposure, as additional information about the exposure or source person becomes available.
- Administer postexposure prophylaxis for 4 weeks, if tolerated.
- If the source person is determined to be HIV negative, discontinue postexposure prophylaxis.

Recommendations for HIV Postexposure Prophylaxis Drugs

Health care providers must strive to balance the risk for infection against the potential toxicity of the medications used when selecting a drug regimen for HIV postexposure prophylaxis. Because postexposure prophylaxis is potentially toxic, its use is not justified for exposures that pose a negligible risk for transmission (see Tables 199-2 and 199-3). Also, insufficient evidence exists to support recommending a three-drug regimen for all HIV exposures. Thus, two regimens for postexposure prophylaxis are provided:

- The "basic" two-drug regimen that is appropriate for most HIV exposures
- The "expanded" three-drug regimen that should be used for exposures with an increased risk for transmission (see Tables 199-2 and 199-3)

Most HIV exposures warrant a two-drug regimen using two nucleoside analogues (e.g., ZDV and 3TC, or 3TC and d4T, or d4T and ddI). Adding a third drug should be considered for exposures that pose an increased risk for transmission. Selection of the postexposure prophylaxis regimen should consider the comparative risk represented by the exposure and information about the exposure source, including history of and response to antiretroviral therapy based on clinical response, CD4+ T-cell counts, viral load measurements, and current disease stage. When the source person's virus is known or suspected to be resistant to one or more of the drugs considered for the postexposure prophylaxis regimen, selection of drugs to which the source person's virus is unlikely to be resistant is recommended. If this information is not immediately available, initiation of postexposure prophylaxis, if indicated, should not be delayed.

Changes in the postexposure prophylaxis regimen can be made after postexposure prophylaxis has been started. Reevaluation of the exposed person should be considered at 72 hours after exposure, as additional information about the exposure or source person becomes available.

Follow-up of Health Care Providers Exposed to HIV

Postexposure Testing. Health care providers with occupational exposure to HIV should receive follow-up counseling, postexposure testing, and medical evaluation, regardless of whether they receive postexposure prophylaxis. HIV antibody testing should be performed for at least 6 months after exposure (at 6 weeks, 12 weeks, and 6 months). Extended HIV follow-up (e.g., for 12 months) is recommended for health care providers who become infected with HCV after exposure to a source coinfected with HIV and HCV.

Although rare instances of delayed HIV seroconversion have been reported, the infrequency of this occurrence does not warrant adding to the anxiety level of the exposed persons by routinely extending the duration of postexposure follow-up past 6 months. However, this recommendation in an individual situation should be based on the clinical judgment of the exposed person's health care provider. HIV testing should be performed in any exposed person who has an illness that is compatible with an acute retroviral syndrome, regardless of the interval since exposure.

HIV antibody testing with enzyme immunoassay should be used to monitor for seroconversion. The routine use of direct virus assays to detect infection in exposed health care providers is not recommended. The high rate of false-positive results of these tests in this setting could lead to unnecessary anxiety or treatment. Despite the ability of direct virus assays to detect HIV infection a few days earlier than enzyme immunoassays, the infrequency of occupational seroconversion and increased costs of these tests do not warrant their routine use in this setting.

KEY CONCEPTS

- Material Safety Data Sheet (MSDS) provides emergency personnel with the proper procedures for treating patients with exposure to a product.
- Whether one provides prophylaxis for a potential hepatitis B exposure is determined by the HbsAg status of the source and the hepatitis B vaccination and vaccine response status of the exposed person.
- Those exposed to HIV should be evaluated within hours after exposure and should be tested for HIV at baseline to establish infection status at the time of exposure.
- A thorough history of an occupational injury is essential.
- A return-to-work (RTW) plan is required with all occupational injuries.
- Restrictions should be as specific as possible.
- Workers' compensation in the United States has become a state-mandated program that requires employers to have some form of insurance vehicle for covering employees for work-related injuries.

REFERENCES

1. LaDou J: *Occupational and Environmental Medicine*, 2nd ed. Stamford, Conn, Appleton & Lange, 1997.
2. Lomax JD, Johanning E: *Occupational Medicine*. Philadelphia, Lippincott Williams & Wilkins, 2001.
3. Taborshaw IR: Whose 'agent' is the occupational physician? *Arch Environ Health* 30:412, 1975.
4. American College of Occupational and Environmental Medicine Code of Ethical Conduct, October 25, 1993. Available at AMA Web page (http://www.ama-assn.org/ama/pub/article/7605-4825.html).
5. Rom WN: *Environmental and Occupational Medicine*. Boston, Little, Brown, 1992, p 1351.
6. Mueller KL: Occupational health in the emergency department. In Marx JA, et al (eds): *Rosen's Emergency Medicine: Concepts and Clinical Practice*, 5th ed. St. Louis, Mosby, 2002, p 2693.
7. Reagan R: Executive Order 12564: Drug-free federal workplace. *Federal Register* 51(September 27):32:889, 1986.
8. Department of Health and Human Services: Mandatory guidelines for federal workplace drug testing programs. *Federal Register* 53(April 11):11:970, 1988.
9. U.S. Department of Transportation: Procedures for transportation workplace drug testing programs. *Federal Register* 54(December 1):49:854, 1989.
10. *Federal Register* 65 (December 19):79:462, 579, 2000.
11. *Federal Register* 65 (December 19):79:503, 2000.
12. Greenberg MI, Cone DC, Roberts JR: Material safety data sheet: A useful resource for the emergency physician. *Ann Emerg Med* 27:347, 1996.
13. Hathaway BK: Understanding the material safety data sheet. *AAOHN J* 42:290, 1994.
14. Wysong M: Taking control of chemical management. *Occup Health Saf* 70:164, 2001.
15. Kolp P, Sattler B, Blayney M, Sherwood T: Comprehensibility of material safety data sheets. *Am J Ind Med* 23:135, 1993.
16. Hathaway BK: Understanding the material safety data sheet. *AAOHN J* 42:290, 1994.
17. Denis MA, et al: Risk of occupational blood exposure in a cohort of 24,000 hospital healthcare workers: Position and environment analysis over three years. *J Occup Environ Med* 43:370, 2001.
18. Madan AK, Rentz DE, Wahle MJ, Flint LM: Noncompliance of health care workers with universal precautions during trauma resuscitations. *South Med J* 94:277, 2001.
19. Behrman AJ, Shofer FS, Green-McKenzie J: Trends in bloodborne pathogen exposure and followup at an urban teaching hospital: 1987 to 1997. *J Occup Environ Med* 43:370, 2001.
20. Updated U.S. Public Health Service guidelines for the management of occupational exposures to HBV, HCV, and HIV and recommendations for postexposure prophylaxis. *MMWR Recomm Rep* 50(RR-11):1, 2001.

CHAPTER

200 Hyperbaric Medicine

Enoch T. Huang and Stephen R. Thom

PERSPECTIVE

Hyperbaric medicine deals with prevention of injury and illness due to exposure to elevated ambient pressures and with the therapeutic use of hyperbaric oxygen (HBO). HBO treatment involves intermittently breathing pure oxygen at greater than ambient pressure. In the 1980s and 1990s, HBO has been refined, with clarification of its mechanisms of action and clinical applications. Along with an expansion of the knowledge base, formalized education now exists so that physicians may obtain subspecialty board certification through the American Board of Medical Specialties. This chapter summarizes existing literature on uses for HBO therapy and some special issues related to care of patients in the emergency department.

ROLE OF HYPERBARIC MEDICINE IN EMERGENCY MEDICINE

HBO therapy is either a primary or an adjunctive intervention for a variety of disorders typically seen by emergency physicians (Box 200-1).[1,2] HBO is considered first-line, primary therapy for decompression sickness, cerebral air embolism, and carbon monoxide (CO) poisoning. Emergency physicians are adept in identifying these conditions and often initiate arrangements for patients to receive HBO therapy. In other cases, HBO is an adjunct to surgical intervention and antibiotics. Patients with necrotizing soft tissue infections, crush injuries, or compartment syndromes are admitted to an inpatient service, and hyperbaric physicians may not become involved until the latter stages of treatment. Early recognition of potential uses of HBO can occur in the emergency department, however, and may be limb saving or lifesaving. An increased awareness by emergency physicians of which patients might benefit from HBO could assist with earlier intervention.

HISTORY OF HYPERBARIC MEDICINE

Even before the discovery of oxygen in 1775, physicians recognized that the enriched air found in a hyperbaric chamber had beneficial effects (the oxygen tension found in air at twice the normal atmospheric pressure is equivalent to 42% oxygen). The manipulation of ambient pressure in the treatment of disease was used in 1662, although under the specious rationale that acute diseases would respond to higher pressures and chronic diseases would respond to lower pressures. During the next century, hyperbaric chambers grew in popularity. Surgeons observed that patients often required less sedation and had less tissue cyanosis after surgery performed in a hyperbaric environment. Growth culminated with creation of a six-story, "steel ball hospital" in Cleveland, Ohio, in 1926. This facility was capable of treating patients in 72 rooms over 12 floors at pressures of 3 atm absolute. The faddish nature of the treatments was rapidly emulated in Europe, and hyperbaric chambers became as popular as the mineral spas of the day. A precipitous drop in popularity later occurred as a result of overaggressive use and a paucity of knowledge on fundamental mechanisms.[1,2]

The recognition of decompression sickness dates to 1854, when coal miners leaving pressurized mine shafts complained of cramps and muscle pains. Physicians of the time noted that symptoms occurred only when miners left the mines and were relieved on returning to the mines. Despite early recognition of this pattern, however, use of recompression as treatment for the disease did not become established until 1889. Moir, an engineer supervising the creation of railroad tunnels underneath the Hudson River, began recompressing tunnel workers if they became symptomatic. Moir reduced the mortality rate of decompression sickness from 25% per year to only 1.6%.

Since the 1950s, hyperbaric medicine has grown at a steady pace as a result of an increased understanding of mechanisms of action and controlled clinical trials. The Undersea Medical Society is an organization founded in 1967 to serve the diving and undersea community. In 1976, it established a committee to undertake a systematic review of the research and uses of HBO. The organization changed its name to the Undersea and Hyperbaric Medical Society in 1986 to reflect the expanding medical uses of HBO. The committee report is updated periodically with review of the most recent literature regarding acceptable uses of HBO.[2]

BASIC MECHANISMS OF HYPERBARIC MEDICINE

Boyle's law states that under conditions of constant temperature and quantity of gas, there is an inverse relationship between volume and pressure. Increasing ambient pressure to 2 atm reduces the volume of an enclosed gas by half; this has a primary therapeutic effect when dealing with bubble-forming diseases, such

BOX 200-1. Accepted Indications for Hyperbaric Oxygen Therapy

- Air or gas embolism
- Carbon monoxide poisoning
- Clostridial myositis and myonecrosis
- Crush injury, compartment syndrome, acute traumatic ischemias
- Decompression sickness
- Enhancement of healing in selected wounds
- Exceptional blood loss anemia
- Necrotizing fasciitis
- Chronic refractory osteomyelitis
- Radiation necrosis
- Skin flap or graft compromise
- Thermal burns

Committee report. In Feldmeier JJ (ed): *Hyperbaric Oxygen Therapy.* Kensington, Md, Undersea and Hyperbaric Medical Society, 2003.

BOX 200-2. Mechanisms of Action of Hyperbaric Oxygen

Related to Hyperoxygenation of Tissues

- Angiogenesis in ischemic tissues[3-5] (mechanisms likely include oxygen behaving as intracellular signal transducer leading to augmentation of one or more growth factors)[6-8]
- Bacteriostatic/bactericidal actions[9,10]
- Carboxyhemoglobin dissociation hastened[11]
- *Clostridium perfringens* α toxin synthesis inhibited[12,13]
- Phagocytic bacterial killing improved[14]
- Temporary inhibition of neutrophil β_2 integrin adhesion[15-17]
- Vasoconstriction[18,19]

Related to Pressurization

- Reduction of gas bubble volume (Boyle's law)

as decompression sickness or arterial gas embolism. Outside of this limited application, Boyle's law gives way to *Henry's law,* which states that at a given temperature, the amount of gas dissolved in a solute is directly proportional to the partial pressure of the gas. By increasing ambient pressure, more oxygen can be dissolved in plasma. Oxygen should be viewed as a drug and the hyperbaric chamber as a dosing device. Elevating tissue oxygen tension is a primary effect. Although this effect may alleviate physiologic stress to hypoxic tissues, lasting benefits of HBO are related to abatement of underlying pathophysiologic processes by several mechanisms (Box 200-2).

HBO treatment is carried out in either a monoplace (single person) or multiplace (typically 2 to 14 patients) chamber. Pressures applied inside the chamber are usually 2 to 3 atm absolute (ATA), the sum of the atmospheric pressure plus additional hydrostatic pressure equivalent to 1 or 2 atm. Treatments typically are from 2 to 8 hours, depending on the indication, and may be performed one to three times daily. Monoplace chambers usually are compressed with pure oxygen. Multiplace chambers are pressurized with air, and patients breathe pure oxygen through a tight-fitting face mask, a hood, or endotracheal tube.

COMPLICATIONS AND CONTRAINDICATIONS

HBO therapy should not be considered unless proper supportive medial care can be delivered. Most chamber facilities today have equipment and treatment protocols analogous to an intensive care unit. The inherent toxicity of oxygen and potential for injury secondary to elevations of ambient pressure must be addressed whenever HBO is used therapeutically.

Barotrauma

Middle ear barotrauma is the most common adverse effect of HBO treatment.[20] As the ambient pressure within the hyperbaric chamber is increased, a patient must be able to equalize the pressure within the middle ear by autoinsufflation. If a pressure gradient develops across the tympanic membrane, pain followed by hemorrhage or serous effusion develops. Standard protocols for prevention include instructing patients on autoinsufflation techniques and sometimes using oral or topical decongestants. When autoinsufflation fails, tympanostomy tubes must be placed. The incidence of tube placement was reported to be roughly 4% in one series.[21] Other authors reported an overall incidence of aural barotrauma between 1.2% and 7%.[22,23]

Pulmonary barotrauma during HBO treatment is extremely rare, but should be suspected when any pulmonary or hemodynamic changes occur during or shortly after decompression. If pneumothorax is suspected, placement of a chest tube is appropriate. A preexisting pneumothorax should be treated with chest tube drainage before initiating therapy.

Oxygen Toxicity

Biochemical toxicity due to oxygen can be manifested by injuries to lungs, central nervous system, and eyes. Pulmonary insults can impair mechanics (elasticity), vital capacity, and gas exchange.[1,2] These changes occur rarely and are observed when treatment duration and pressures exceed typical therapeutic protocols. There is one report of reversible small airway changes in 4 of 21 patients treated daily for 90 minutes at 2.4 ATA for 21 days.[24] Most studies have failed to identify adverse pulmonary effects from standard protocols.[1,2,25]

Central nervous system oxygen toxicity is manifested as a grand mal seizure; this occurs with an incidence of approximately 1 to 4 in 10,000 patient treatments.[21,22] The risk is higher in hypercapnic patients and possibly patients who are acidotic or septic. An incidence of 7% (15 of 211 patients) was reported in a series of gas gangrene patients.[2,26] Seizures are relatively easy to manage in most cases; the inspired oxygen tension is reduced while leaving the patient at constant ambient pressure (to avoid pulmonary overexpansion injury when the patient is in the tonic convulsion phase). Pathologic changes in association with isolated oxygen-mediated seizures have not been found in studies with guinea pigs, rabbits, and humans.[2]

Progressive myopia has been reported in patients undergoing repetitive daily therapy, but this typically reverses within 6 weeks after termination of treatments.[27] Excessive treatments (>150 to 200 hours) have been associated with development of nuclear cataracts.[28] Although there is a theoretical risk for retrolental fibroplasia in neonates, there are no reports of this having occurred. Experimental and clinical evidence have not indicated that typical HBO therapy protocols have detrimental effects on neonates or the unborn fetus[29]; this is likely due to the relatively short duration of hyperoxia.

Other Risks

Confinement anxiety may occur and is typically managed with sedating agents. Any environment with an elevated concentration of oxygen presents a risk for fire. Scrupulous attention to avoiding an ignition source is standard in HBO therapy programs. Since the 1980s, no fires resulting in injury have been reported in the United States, but worldwide, 52 deaths have been reported.[30] Virtually all these were preventable. In 10 incidents, fire resulted when banned substances, such as cigarettes and lighters, were taken into the chamber.

CLINICAL APPLICATIONS

Arterial Gas Embolism and Decompression Sickness

Arterial gas embolism can occur whenever the vascular wall is disrupted, as in major trauma. Iatrogenic arterial gas embolism has been reported with cardiovascular, obstetric/gynecologic, neurosurgical, and orthopedic procedures; obtaining vascular access during hemodialysis; and opening of central venous catheters. Nonsurgical processes include pulmonary overexpansion during mechanical ventilation. In scuba divers, arterial gas embolism is due to pulmonary overexpansion on decompression. Decompression sickness (caisson disease, or the bends) is attributed to formation of nitrogen bubbles in the body on decompression. It occurs in miners and scuba divers on their return from high-pressure environments and in high-altitude aviators and astronauts when they leave their ambient environment and are exposed to reduced atmospheric pressure.[1,2]

Emergency treatment of gas bubble disorders includes standard support of airway, breathing, and circulation plus application of HBO. Referral as soon as possible is recommended. Even when treatments may be delayed, however, a trial of therapy is often recommended. Gas bubbles can persist in tissues for several days, and many reports note success when HBO is begun even after long delays.[2] Controlled animal trials support efficacy of HBO, but randomized clinical trials have not been done.[1,2,31]

Mechanisms of action of HBO in arterial gas embolism and decompression sickness treatment include the well-recognized reduction of gas volume based on Boyle's law, which can reduce vascular compromise acutely. Hyperoxygenation hastens inert gas diffusion, and there is a theoretical effect associated with leukocyte adherence to vascular endothelium damaged by bubbles. This latter mechanism has been suggested by several animal studies.[32,33]

Carbon Monoxide Poisoning

CO is the leading cause of injury and death by poisoning in the world.[1,2] The affinity of CO for hemoglobin to form carboxyhemoglobin is more than 200-fold greater than that of oxygen. CO-mediated hypoxic stress is a primary insult, but carboxyhemoglobin values correlate poorly with clinical outcome.[1,2,34] Alternative mechanisms to explain the toxicity of CO have been sought. Survivors of acute CO poisoning are at risk for developing delayed neurologic sequelae, including cognitive deficits, memory loss, dementia, parkinsonism, paralysis, chorea, cortical blindness, psychosis, personality changes, and peripheral neuropathy. Delayed neurologic sequelae typically occur 2 to 40 days after poisoning; the incidence is 25% to 50% after severe poisoning.[1,2,34]

Administration of supplemental oxygen is the cornerstone of treatment for CO poisoning. HBO causes carboxyhemoglobin dissociation to occur at a rate greater than that achievable by breathing pure oxygen at sea level pressure. Additional therapeutic mechanisms for HBO shown in animal models include an improvement in mitochondrial oxidative processes, inhibition of lipid peroxidation, and impairment of leukocyte adhesion to injured microvasculature. Five prospective, randomized trials have assessed clinical efficacy of HBO for acute CO poisoning.[34] Several trials failed to find benefit, but their clinical impact is limited due to methodologic weaknesses discussed in several publications. The current consensus is that HBO treatment significantly reduces the incidence of delayed neurologic sequelae and in retrospective comparisons seems also to diminish acute mortality.[1,2,34] Recommendations are for prompt referral and administration of three HBO treatments over the 24 hours after poisoning.[34]

Clostridial Myonecrosis (Gas Gangrene)

Successful treatment of gas gangrene depends on prompt recognition and aggressive intervention. Overall mortality rates of 11% to 52% have been reported. The impact of HBO has been assessed in 4 retrospective comparisons and 13 case series that have been discussed in previous reviews.[1,2,26] Because of difficulties with comparison among patient groups, evaluation of efficacy based on mortality or "tissue salvage" rates is difficult. Most authors comment on the clinical benefit of HBO treatment and share the opinion that temporal improvements of vital signs can be dramatic.

Progressive Necrotizing Infections

The use of HBO for treatment of necrotizing fasciitis and Fournier's gangrene has been reported in seven nonrandomized comparisons and three case series.[1,2,35–37] Variations in time of diagnosis and clinical status of patients on admission compromise the assessment of treatment benefits. Riseman and colleagues[38] reported that addition of HBO to surgical and antibiotic treatment reduced mortality versus surgery and antibiotics alone. Brown and coworkers[33] reported on a multicenter experience that documented a trend toward increased survival when treatment included HBO. Mechanisms of action may include suppressed growth of anaerobic microorganisms and improved bactericidal action of leukocytes, which function poorly in hypoxic conditions.[9,10,12–14] Animal trials to assess the mechanisms and efficacy of HBO have been problematic because synergistic bacterial processes are difficult to establish. HBO may potentiate antibiotic efficacy, and several animal models of polymicrobial bacteremia and sepsis have reported increased survival with HBO.[1,2]

Blood Loss Anemia

Intermittent HBO exposures have been applied to relieve temporarily physiologic stress from severe, acute anemia. This is a rare practice, but it is sometimes considered when transfusion is not possible due to crossmatching incompatibilities or religious beliefs. Anecdotal reports describe using 2.5 to 3 ATA of oxygen to increase arterial oxygen tension in plasma to meet metabolic needs.[2] Treatments are administered for only brief times when physiologic decompensation occurs because oxygen toxicity can be a problem. Short-term treatments, applied many times over several days, have been used to support life until red blood cells become available or until adequate red blood cell mass is generated endogenously.

Crush Injury and Limb Reperfusion

HBO has been used to a limited degree for acute traumatic peripheral ischemia and suturing of severed limbs. A single randomized, controlled trial (involving 36 patients) found HBO to reduce infection and wound dehiscence and to improve healing.[2,39] Changes in transcutaneous tissue oxygen measurements while exposed to HBO may be useful in predicting outcome.[40] The rationale for considering HBO is to improve temporarily oxygenation to hypoperfused tissues and because arterial hyperoxia would cause vasoconstriction that can diminish edema formation.[18,19] The use of HBO to reduce tissue edema and prevent myonecrosis has been shown most convincingly in the context of experimental compartment syndrome. Early use of HBO may reduce compartment pressures enough to avoid fasciotomy.[41]

Thermal Burns

Some burn centers employ adjunctive HBO to severe burns. Benefits with HBO, documented in animal models, include reducing partial-thickness to full-thickness skin loss, hastened epithelialization, and lower mortality.[1,2] Randomized clinical trials, albeit with small patient numbers, have reported improved rates of healing with shorter hospital stays and reduced costs. Uncontrolled series have reported efficacy, but some studies have failed to find benefit.[2] The rationale for treatment is to reduce tissue edema and increase capillary angiogenesis. The latter mechanism has not been shown directly with thermal injuries but is a well-documented effect in long-term applications of HBO for radiation injuries and microvascular deficiency wounds, which occur in many diabetics.[1,2]

EMERGING CONCEPTS

Critics of hyperbaric medicine have stated that it is a treatment in search of a disease. In the past, many uses of HBO have had little or no scientific merit, but more recent research and elucidation of mechanisms of action not only have justified current uses of HBO, but they have also stimulated interest in broader application of a simple treatment. There is increasing consideration of HBO for reperfusion injuries secondary to common pathophysiologic mechanisms in many organs, including leukocyte adhesion to injured vasculature.[15-17] Reactive oxygen species are involved with many aspects of wound healing.[6-8] The role of HBO as an adjunct when healing fails is a burgeoning field of research. Use of HBO in a variety of neurologic disorders, such as vegetative coma, multiple sclerosis, and cerebral palsy, continues to be discussed in the popular press, but fundamental mechanisms have been found wanting.

REFERENCES

1. Thom SR: Hyperbaric oxygen therapy. *J Int Care Med* 4:58, 1989.
2. Committee report. In Feldmeier JJ (ed): *Hyperbaric Oxygen Therapy*. Kensington, Md, Undersea and Hyperbaric Medical Society, 2003.
3. Marx RE, Johnson RP, Kline SN: Prevention of osteoradionecrosis: A randomized prospective clinical trial of hyperbaric oxygen versus penicillin. *J Am Dent Assoc* 111:49, 1985.
4. Kulonen E, Niinikoski J: Effect of hyperbaric oxygenation on wound healing and experimental granuloma. *Acta Physiol Scand* 73:383, 1968.
5. Uhl E, et al: Hyperbaric oxygen improves wound healing in normal and ischemic skin tissue. *Plast Reconstr Surg* 93:835, 1994.
6. Zhao L, et al: Effect of hyperbaric oxygen and growth factors on rabbit ear ischemic ulcers. *Arch Surg* 129:1043, 1994.
7. Bonomo S, et al: Hyperbaric oxygen as a signal transducer: Upregulation of platelet derived growth factor-beta receptor in the presence of HBO_2 and PDGF. *Undersea Hyperb Med* 25:211, 1998.
8. Feng JJ, Gibson JJ, Constant JS: Hyperoxia stimulates macrophage vascular endothelial growth factor (VEGF) production. *Wound Rep Reg* 6:122, 1998.
9. Brown OR: Reversible inhibition of respiration of *Escherichia coli* by hyperoxia. *Microbios* 5:7, 1972.
10. Hill GB, Osterhout S: Experimental effects of hyperbaric oxygen on selected clostridial species. *J Infect Dis* 125:17, 1972.
11. Pace N, Strajman E, Walker EL: Acceleration of carbon monoxide elimination in man by high pressure oxygen. *Science* 111:652, 1950.

12. Kaye D: Effect of hyperbaric oxygen on clostridia in vitro and in vivo. *Proc Soc Exp Biol Med* 124:360, 1967.
13. Van Unnik AJM: Inhibition of toxin production in *Clostridium perfringens* in vitro by hyperbaric oxygen. *Antonie Van Leeuwenhoek* 31:181, 1965.
14. Mader JT, et al: A mechanism for the amelioration by hyperbaric oxygen of experimental staphylococcal osteomyelitis in rabbits. *J Infect Dis* 142:915, 1980.
15. Chen Q, Banick PD, Thom SR: Functional inhibition of rat polymorphonuclear leukocyte β_2 integrins by hyperbaric oxygen is associated with impaired cGMP synthesis. *J Pharmacol Exp Ther* 276:929, 1996.
16. Thom SR: Functional inhibition of neutrophil β_2 integrins by hyperbaric oxygen in carbon monoxide mediated brain injury. *Toxicol Appl Pharmacol* 123:248, 1993.
17. Thom SR, et al: Inhibition of human neutrophil β_2 integrin-dependent adherence by hyperbaric oxygen. *Am J Physiol* 272:C770, 1997.
18. Bergofsky EH, Bertun P: Response of regional circulations to hyperoxia. *J Appl Physiol* 21:567, 1966.
19. Bird AD, Tefler AMB: Effect of hyperbaric oxygen on limb circulation. *Lancet* 1:355, 1965.
20. Carlson S, et al: Prevention of hyperbaric-associated middle ear barotrauma. *Ann Emerg Med* 21:1468, 1992.
21. Clements KS, Vrabec JT, Mader, JT: Complications of tympanostomy tubes inserted for facilitation of hyperbaric oxygen therapy. *Arch Otolaryngol Head Neck Surg* 124:278, 1998.
22. Plafki C, et al: Complications and side effects of hyperbaric oxygen therapy. *Aviat Space Environ Med* 71:119, 2000.
23. Trytko BE, Bennett M: Hyperbaric oxygen therapy: Complication rates are much lower than authors suggest. *BMJ* 318:1077, 1999.
24. Thorsen E, Aanderud L, Aasen TB: Effects of a standard hyperbaric oxygen treatment protocol on pulmonary function. *Eur Respir J* 12:1442, 1998.
25. Rusca F, et al: HBO therapy and pulmonary function tests. *Undersea Biomed Res* 18:112, 1991.
26. Hart GB, Lamb RC, Strauss MB: Gas gangrene: I. A collective review. *J Trauma* 23:991, 1983.
27. Lyne AJ: Ocular effects of hyperbaric oxygen. *Trans Ophthalmol Soc UK* 98:66, 1978.
28. Palmquist BM, Philipson B, Barr PO: Nuclear cataract and myopia during hyperbaric oxygen therapy. *Br J Ophthalmol* 68:113, 1984.
29. VanHoesen KB, et al: Should hyperbaric oxygen be used to treat the pregnant patient for acute carbon monoxide poisoning? A case report and literature review. *JAMA* 261:1039, 1989.
30. Sheffield PJ, Desautels DA: Hyperbaric and hypobaric chamber fires: A 73-year analysis. *Undersea Hyperb Med* 24:153, 1997.
31. McDermott JJ, et al: Effects of an increased PO_2 during recompression therapy for the treatment of experimental cerebral arterial gas embolism. *Undersea Biomed Res* 19: 403, 1992.
32. Helps SC, Gorman DF: Air embolism of the brain in rabbits pretreated with mechlorethamine. *Stroke* 22:351, 1991.
33. Martin JD, Thom SR: Vascular leukocyte sequestration in decompression sickness and prophylactic hyperbaric oxygen therapy in rats. *Aviat Space Environ Med* 73:565, 2002.
34. Hampson NB, et al: Carbon monoxide poisoning: Interpretation of randomized clinical trials and unresolved treatment issues. *Undersea Hyperb Med* 28:157, 2001.
35. Brown DR, Davis NL, Lepawsky M: A multi-center review of the treatment of major truncal necrotizing infections with and without hyperbaric oxygen therapy. *Am J Surg* 167:485, 1994.
36. Hollabaugh RS Jr, et al: Fournier's gangrene: Therapeutic impact of hyperbaric oxygen. *Plast Reconstr Surg* 101:94, 1998.
37. Shupak A, et al: Necrotizing fasciitis: An indication for hyperbaric oxygenation therapy? *Surgery* 118:873, 1995.
38. Riseman JA, et al: Hyperbaric oxygen therapy for necrotizing fasciitis reduces mortality and the need for debridements. *Surgery* 108:847, 1990.
39. Bouachour G, et al: Hyperbaric oxygen therapy in the management of crush injuries: A randomized double-blind placebo-controlled clinical trial. *J Trauma* 41:333, 1996.
40. Mathieu D, et al: Post-traumatic limb ischemia: Prediction of final outcome by transcutaneous oxygen measurements in hyperbaric oxygen. *J Trauma* 30:307, 1990.
41. Strauss MB, et al: Reduction of skeletal muscle necrosis using intermittent hyperbaric oxygen in a model compartment syndrome. *J Bone Joint Surg Am* 65:656, 1983.

CHAPTER 201 The Social Role of Emergency Medicine

James A. Gordon

> *Because of this exceptionally important social role of the physician, it [is] imperative that he be . . . a social worker.*[1]

For Andrija Stampar (1892-1958), a noted European physician and public health advocate, a person's social environment was as important to health as medical treatment. For many of today's physicians, however, the social and environmental components of health are considered distinct from traditional medicine. Why has this shift occurred? Part of the reason lies in the historical division between medicine and public health, a "schism"[1] of sorts. Although many attempts have been made in recent years to heal the schism, some of the most promising initiatives can be found in the nation's emergency departments, places that serve as a unique bridge between medicine and the public. Here, perhaps, the formal integration of public health and social services can provide an efficient model for promoting total community health.

MEDICINE AND PUBLIC HEALTH

Historical Division between Medicine and Public Health

Modern schools of public health take their origin from European departments of hygiene, which began to emerge in 1794. These departments were based within schools of medicine and became integrated into the medical curriculum. As medical science progressed, a distinct body of population-based knowledge began to emerge. The budding science of microbiology in the early 1900s led to the "germ theory" of disease, which led directly to advances in public sanitation and clean water supply. As more of a body of "public health" expertise developed during this time, forces conspired to separate traditional medicine from population- and environment-based concepts.

Beginning around 1910, leading advocates of the new field of public health began discussions about creating schools of public health separate from the medical schools. In 1913, the Rockefeller Foundation, instrumental in this process, began awarding grants of up to $25 million to create independent schools of public health at leading universities. Their funding created the first school of public health at Johns Hopkins University in 1918. Subsequently, Harvard acquired a school in 1918, the University of Toronto in 1924, and the University of Michigan in 1940, all with Rockefeller Foundation funding. As a precondition to receiving the funds, however, institutions were required to maintain building space and administrative structures completely separate from the medical schools.[1] Thus the "schism" was born.

Efforts to Reconcile Medicine and Public Health

Many leading figures of the day opposed the rather abrupt division between medicine and public health. They believed there should be a link between prevention and cure, and that social, occupational, and physical environments, along with education, were as important to health as clinical treatment. Leadership on both sides, it was believed, needed to emphasize an integrated approach to health as a continuum of care. Much time and energy has subsequently been spent trying to "heal the schism" created by the original funding stipulations. Over the past few decades, millions of dollars have been spent to promote an integrated view of health. Prominent philanthropic foundations, including the Rockefeller Foundation, have taken leadership roles in trying to ensure dissemination of basic epidemiologic and public health concepts within medical institutions, and to encourage greater cooperation between schools of medicine and public health.

Emergency Medicine as a Bridge between Medicine and Public Health

Emergency medicine offers unique advantages as a potential "bridge" between medicine and public health. Widely used, always open, and easily accessible, the emergency department is available to anyone who wishes to be seen, whether young or old, male or female, rich or poor. The number of emergency department visits in the United States has grown to more than 100 million per year as emergency care has become the only health care practice mandated by federal law to provide universal care (Emergency Medicine Treatment and Labor Act, or EMTALA). By virtue of the number, variety, and circumstances of the emergency patient population, emergency physicians share a unique relationship with their communities and remain among the only modern practitioners proficient in the broadest range of medical competencies. Often viewed as society's "safety net for the safety net,"[2] the emergency department is well positioned to help integrate medicine with a broad-based view of public health.

Despite managed care and other efforts to keep so-called nonurgent care out of the emergency department,[3] the number of emergency department visits continues to rise.[4] Although Medicaid recipients and the uninsured already account for a disproportionately high number of emergency department visits, even more of the country's uninsured are being forced to seek emergency department care as community clinics face an increasingly competitive health care marketplace. Moreover, worried emergency department patients continue to experience barriers to traditional primary care.[5] Under welfare reform, for example, Medicaid benefits are denied to new legal immigrants for at least 5 years, regardless of circumstance. Just as the legislation denies or reduces food assistance, welfare payments, disability income, and health insurance, however, it makes one notable exception: "No state may deny coverage of emergency medical services to either illegal or legal aliens."[6] As in prior federal legislation, the emergency department is singled out as the only component of the medical system, and, in this case, the only component of the entire social welfare system, that is absolutely protected for everyone.

EMERGENCY MEDICINE AND PUBLIC HEALTH

Public Health Issues and Approaches in the Emergency Department

The Society for Academic Emergency Medicine's Public Health and Education Task Force reported on the "public health approach to emergency medicine" in 1994.[7] They concluded that emergency departments are uniquely situated to help promote traditional public health and preventive medicine activities in a more proactive fashion. Because common public health issues frequently arise in the emergency department, organized emergency medicine has become active in helping to shape the federal "Healthy People" public health agenda.[8] Injury surveillance and prevention initiatives, for example, are well-suited to emergency departments as the primary site for treatment of trauma, including work-related and environmental injuries. Medical sequelae from alcohol and drug abuse, common in emergency patients, include not only traumatic injuries but also seizures, sudden death, and psychiatric illness. Smoking contributes to the respiratory failure, heart attacks, and asthma so often seen in emergency departments. Infectious diseases such as sexually transmitted diseases, hepatitis, tuberculosis, and human immunodeficiency virus are often seen and treated in emergency departments. Other important public health topics, including domestic violence and care for vulnerable populations, are also frequently the domain of the emergency department.

Various public health approaches have been described for use in the emergency department, including screening programs to identify individual and community needs, teaching and educational interventions, and active prevention, treatment, and referral programs.[7,9] Of all the cases of substance abuse seen in the emergency department, for example, only a fraction are detected and referred for appropriate follow-up.[10] Screening questions such as those developed for alcohol abuse, effective in identifying individuals at risk, might be applied more consistently and formally in the emergency department.[11] In the area of domestic violence, a significant number of battered women go unidentified without formal questioning.[12] The "teachable moment" can also be particularly germane to emergency practice. Brief advice to quit smoking, for example, has been shown to be effective during a limited medical encounter. The smoker who comes to the emergency department with an acute asthma exacerbation might listen to advice to quit smoking more in this setting than any other.[13] Other public health roles for the emergency department include active prevention (such as immunizations)[14] and treatment (e.g., for sexually transmitted diseases and other communicable diseases).

Public Health Research and Practice in the Emergency Department

Emergency departments represent a unique research consortium. Functioning at the interface of multiple systems, providers, and patients, the emergency department is a rich laboratory for public health research. Emergency departments provide not only a window on the health care needs of a diverse population but also a window on the overall performance of the health care system. As a primary component of the health care "safety net," data on the overall performance of the system can be clarified by looking at activity in the nation's emergency departments.[2] To assist in this endeavor, a template for the uniform data collection in emergency departments has been developed by a national working group in collaboration with the Centers for Disease Control and Prevention.[15] Called DEEDS (Data Elements for Emergency Department Systems), its public health applications include the surveillance of injury and disease patterns, analysis of social trends, and monitoring of health care and welfare reform.[16] Studying the nature and frequency of ambulance diversion from local emergency departments, for example, can serve to both define and monitor the impact of hospital crowding on patient safety.[2,17] Used proactively, information from ambulance transports could also help identify high-risk disease populations, coordinate local health care systems management, and design high-impact health education and intervention strategies.[18]

The Society for Academic Emergency Medicine's Public Health and Education Task Force also convened a Preventive Services Working Group in 1998 to study the feasibility of adopting U.S. Preventive Services Task Force recommendations in an emergency department setting.[19] Based on the availability of necessary resources, evidence supports several preventive interventions in the emergency department, including screening and referral for problem alcohol consumption, human immunodeficiency virus status (in high-prevalence, high-risk populations), and occult hypertension; brief counseling for smoking cessation; selective administration of the pneumococcal vaccine; and proactive primary care referral for children.[13,14,19-21] Project ASSERT (*a*lcohol, *s*ubstance abuse, *s*ervices, *e*ducation, *r*eferral, *t*reatment) is a successful emergency department–based initiative designed to implement many such interventions,[22] including efforts to detect and reduce domestic violence.[23] Investigators have found that emergency department waiting rooms are particularly effective sites for computerized health risk assessment and referral.[24] On a systems level, emergency departments have successfully partnered with state and local agencies to provide population-based firearms injury prevention data.[25,26] Nationally, an emergency department–based emerging infections sentinel network (EMERGEncy ID NET) was established to organize selected emergency departments into a cross-country screening network for infectious disease.[27] Other emergency departments have partnered with the Centers for Disease Control and Prevention to form injury control centers, designed to reduce injury-related morbidity and mortality. Such programs provide public and provider training on injury control and acute care, generate applied research to guide the direction of community-based injury control activities, and offer a variety of local and national information resources.[25]

EMERGENCY MEDICINE AND THE PUBLIC WELFARE

Social Service Issues and Approaches in the Emergency Department

The public sees no distinction between the rather academic notion of "public health and preventive medicine" and those social and human concerns integral to the maintenance of good health. A robust association between socioeconomic status and health has been demonstrated in multiple studies.[28] Not only can poor health lead to social problems, but social problems can lead to poor health. If the emergency department is uniquely positioned to help facilitate sociomedical integration, the challenge is to design a system to provide expanded social and human services in conjunction with clinical care, all without overburdening the existing care structure of the hospital and its community. A system of "social triage"[29] in the emergency department can offer some possibilities. Patients who seek treatment in the emergency department are already categorized and treated according to medical needs, but their pressing social concerns such as poverty, hunger, housing, and transportation are often ignored. What if those patients with pressing social needs could be referred to a "social triage center" of sorts for more comprehensive evaluation and care? The social triage center could be located in or near the emergency department, staffed by a social worker or service coordinator, and could be as small as a desk or as large as an office center. It would build on the current model of medical social work and case management, formalizing and expanding the emergency department as an integrated community resource.

Most communities lack this type of coordinating system, and those who do have it often exclude the hospital from the process. Although the emergency department serves as a de facto social service agency after hours and on weekends, relatively few social service resources are directed here. Some emergency departments do have full-time social workers, but many do not. Scattered efforts at social screening and intervention have been successfully implemented in various emergency departments,[22,24,30-35] but key services remain unavailable at critical times.[36-37]

Social Service Research and Practice in the Emergency Department

Some practitioners have suggested that intensive social intervention in the emergency department can decrease hospital utilization rates and costs.[38,39] A very low cost system of social triage would incorporate a short set of social screening questions into the existing emergency department registration and triage process and set aside a desk or cubicle for trained students or volunteers to provide community service referrals before discharge. A more comprehensive system would invite the local social service agency to "outstation" its workers in the emergency department. A hospital or emergency department can also choose to hire or assign its own social workers or service coordinators for such a project, in some cases combining and streamlining existing responsibilities, but in other cases delegating funds for new positions.[35] Even in the latter case, the potential impact of an effective social worker, including fewer "social" hospital admissions, fewer emergency department return visits, and more efficient use of nurse and physician time, can substantially offset staffing expenses.[38] Moreover, emergency department outreach workers who enroll uninsured children in state-sponsored health insurance programs can help the hospital recoup significant reimbursement dollars for previously uncompensated services.[40,41] Additional funding might also be provided through public-private partnerships in which government, health care systems, and local charities all participate together, each leveraging the unique contributions of the other.

Establishing such a community coordination and referral center is certainly not a novel concept. However, support for traditional safety net providers in this country has been reduced, whereas the role of the emergency department has only expanded. Some hospitals have identified the emergency department as a valuable site for multidisciplinary service coordination and discharge planning,[42,43] planning and studies of targeted social intervention in the emergency department have been promising.[22,24,30-35,40] Of course, no system can accommodate everyone, but relatively simple assistance during an emergency department visit can be crucial.[31,37,41,44] Crucial a multicenter study of uninsured children presenting to the emergency department, for example, demonstrated that simple outreach (handing out insurance applications in the emergency department) can nearly quadruple the odds of subsequent enrollment in government-sponsored children's health insurance.[31] Commenting on the promise of such an integrated approach, a former U.S. Surgeon General observed, "Families that are often hard to reach may be effectively contacted during an emergency visit. Given the potential for low-cost, high-impact outreach in this setting, EDs across the country ought to think of creative ways to leverage local resources in the national effort to provide health insurance for all children."[45] At the very least, all emergency departments should hand out insurance applications for uninsured children presenting for care.

As a specialty, emergency medicine has matured at a time when there is a critical need to integrate medical, public health, and social services to produce effective and cost-efficient health care. The emergency department can play an important role in this process and is uniquely situated to help bridge the historical gap between medicine and public health. Because of the emergency department's unique relationship with the public, it can play an important role in traditional aspects of public health and can become a leader in validating a sociomedical model of health care integration.

REFERENCES

1. White KL: Healing the schism: Epidemiology, medicine, and the public's health. In Lipkin M Jr (ed): *Frontiers of Primary Care Series.* New York, Springer-Verlag, 1991.
2. Gordon JA, Billings J, Asplin BR, Rhodes KV: Safety net research in emergency medicine: Proceedings of the Academic Emergency Medicine consensus conference on "the unraveling safety net." *Acad Emerg Med* 8:1024, 2001.
3. Derlet R: Prospective identification and triage of nonemergency patients out of an emergency department: A five year study. *Ann Emerg Med* 25:215, 1995.
4. McCaig LF, Burt CW: National Hospital Ambulatory Medical Care Survey: 2002 Emergency Department Summary. Advance data from vital and health statistics; no. 340, Hyattesville, Maryland, National Center for Health Statistics, 2004.
5. Young GP, et al: Ambulatory visits to hospital emergency departments: Patterns and reasons for use. *JAMA* 276:460, 1996.
6. American Public Welfare Association, National Governors Association, National Conference of State Legislators: An

analysis of the Personal Responsibility and Work Opportunity Reconciliation Act of 1996, Washington, DC, American Public Human Services Association, August 22, 1996, p 12.
7. Bernstein E, et al: A public health approach to emergency medicine: Preparing for the twenty-first century. *Acad Emerg Med* 1:277, 1994.
8. Society for Academic Emergency Medicine (SAEM) Public Health Task Force: Healthy People 2010 Emergency Medicine Module [informational lecture/slide presentation]. Available at http://www.saem.org/inform/hp2010.htm. Accessed February 5, 2004.
9. Rhodes KV, et al, for the SAEM Public Health and Education Task Force Preventive Services Working Group: Preventive care in the emergency department, part I: Clinical preventive services—are they relevant to emergency medicine? *Acad Emerg Med* 7:1036, 2000.
10. Lowenstein SR, et al: Behavioral risk factors in emergency department patients: A multisite survey. *Acad Emerg Med* 5:781, 1998.
11. D'Onofrio G, et al, for the SAEM Substance Abuse Task Force: Patients with alcohol problems in the emergency department, part 1: Improving detection. *Acad Emerg Med* 5:1200, 1998.
12. Rhodes KV, Levinson W: Interventions for intimate partner violence against women: Clinical applications. *JAMA* 289:601, 2003.
13. Bernstein SL, Becker BM: Preventive care in the emergency department: Diagnosis and management of smoking and smoking-related illness in the emergency department: A systematic review. *Acad Emerg Med* 9:720, 2002.
14. Stack SJ, et al: An emergency department-based pneumococcal vaccination program could save money and lives. *Ann Emerg Med* 33:299, 1999.
15. National Center for Injury Prevention and Control: Data elements for emergency department systems, Release 1.0, Atlanta, 1997, Centers for Disease Control and Prevention. Available at http://www.cdc.gov/ncipc/pub-res/deedspage.htm. Accessed February 5, 2004.
16. Garrison HG, et al: Emergency department surveillance: An examination of issues and a proposal for a national strategy. *Ann Emerg Med* 24:849, 1994.
17. Asplin BR, et al: A conceptual model of emergency department crowding. *Ann Emerg Med* 42:173, 2003.
18. Hsiao AK, Hedges JR: Role of the emergency medical services system in regionwide health monitoring and referral. *Ann Emerg Med* 22:1696, 1993.
19. Irvin CB, et al, for the SAEM Public Health and Education Task Force Preventive Services Work Group: Preventive care in the emergency department, part II: Clinical preventive services—an emergency medicine evidence-based review. *Acad Emerg Med* 7:1042, 2000.
20. D'Onofrio G, Degutis LC: Preventive care in the emergency department: Screening and brief intervention for alcohol problems in the emergency department—a systematic review. *Acad Emerg Med* 9:627, 2002.
21. Rothman RE, et al: Preventive care in the emergency department: Should emergency departments conduct routine HIV screening? A systematic review. *Acad Emerg Med* 10:278, 2003.
22. Bernstein E, et al: Project ASSERT: An ED based intervention to increase access to primary care, preventative services, and the substance abuse treatment system. *Ann Emerg Med* 30:181, 1997.
23. Anglin D, Sachs C: Preventive care in the emergency department: Screening for domestic violence in the emergency department. *Acad Emerg Med* 10:1118, 2003.
24. Rhodes KV, et al: Better health while you wait: A controlled trial of a computer-based intervention for screening and health promotion in the emergency department. *Ann Emerg Med* 37:284, 2001.
25. Gordon JA, et al: Emergency department initiatives to improve the public health. *Acad Emerg Med* 5:935, 1998.
26. Kellermann AL, Bartolomeos KK: Firearm injury surveillance at the local level: From data to action. *Am J Prev Med* 15:109, 1998.
27. Talan DA, et al: EMERGEncy ID NET: An emergency department-based emerging infections sentinel network. The EMERGEncy ID NET Study Group. *Ann Emerg Med* 32:703, 1998.
28. Bunker JP, et al (eds): *Pathways to Health: The Role of Social Factors.* Menlo Park, Calif, Henry J. Kaiser Family Foundation, 1989.
29. Gordon JA: The hospital emergency department as a social welfare institution. *Ann Emerg Med* 33:321, 1999.
30. Gordon JA, Dupuie TA: Child health insurance outreach through the emergency department: A pilot study. *Acad Emerg Med* 8:1088, 2001.
31. Gordon JA, Emond JA, Camargo CA: The State Children's Health Insurance Program: A multicenter trial of outreach through the emergency department. *Am J Pub Health* 95:250, 2005.
32. Ling LJ, et al: New models for emergency and ambulatory care at academic health centers—Part I: New York City. *Acad Emerg Med* 2:836, 1995.
33. Grossman LK, et al: Decreasing nonurgent emergency department utilization by Medicaid children. *Pediatrics* 102:20, 1998.
34. Gerson LW, et al: Multicenter study of case finding in elderly emergency department patients. *Acad Emerg Med* 2:729, 1995.
35. Goldberg RM, et al: Health promotion and disease prevention in the emergency department. In Bernstein E, Bernstein J (eds): *Case Studies in Emergency Medicine and the Health of the Public.* Sudbury, Mass, Jones and Bartlett Publishers, 1996, pp 316-328.
36. Birnbaum A, et al: Domestic violence: Diurnal mismatch between need and availability of services. *Acad Emerg Med* 3:246, 1996.
37. Gordon JA, et al: Where health and welfare meet: Social deprivation among patients in the emergency department. *J Urban Health Bull N Y Acad Med* 78:104, 2001.
38. Gordon JA: Cost-benefit analysis of social work services in the emergency department: A conceptual model. *Acad Emerg Med* 8:54, 2001.
39. Wrenn K, Rice N: Social-work services in an emergency department: An integral part of the health care safety net [including "Further thoughts from the reviewers"]. *Acad Emerg Med* 1:247, 1994.
40. Mahajan P, Stanley R, Ross KW, et al: Evaluation of an emergency department-based enrollment program for uninsured children. *Ann Emerg Med* 45:245, 2005.
41. Gordon JA: The science of common sense: Integrating health and human services in the hospital emergency department. *Ann Emerg Med* 45:251, 2005.
42. Hart RG, et al: Discharge information for emergency department patients [letter to the editor]. *Ann Emerg Med* 27:392, 1996.
43. Jerome GV, et al: A structured approach to developing a community organization database [letter to the editor]. *Acad Emerg Med* 3:984, 1996.
44. Kersey MA, et al: The prevalence and effects of hunger in an emergency department patient population. *Acad Emerg Med* 6:1109, 1999.
45. Richmond JB: Comment on "Should the ED Promote Child Health Insurance?" *Pediatric Emerg Crit Care* 14:47, 2001.

CHAPTER 202 Information Technology in Emergency Medicine

Jonathan M. Teich and William H. Cordell

PERSPECTIVE

During the Industrial Age, we used machines to improve our lives by extending the capacity of our muscles. During the Information Age, we are improving our lives by extending the capabilities of our minds.[1] Health care today is one of the most information-intensive professions and service industries. Emergency clinicians, who are fundamentally knowledge workers, should have a basic knowledge of the current principles and tools of information management.[2] This chapter emphasizes key concepts regarding information management in emergency medicine and discusses emerging information technologies.

TERMINOLOGY

Data are numbers, text, graphics, images, and voice stored in a form that can be processed by a computer.[3] *Information* is the meaningful interpretation of data. It is important to distinguish between information technologies and information management. Through the early 1980s, the term *computer* covered just about the whole field of information processing. Today, information technologies encompass a rapidly expanding range of equipment, applications, services, and basic technologies falling into three primary categories: computers, telecommunications, and multimedia data.[3] The term *information management* refers to the capture, storage, sharing, analysis, display, and standardization of information. The term *medical informatics* refers to the scientific discipline that has arisen at the interface of computer science, data analysis, and health care. This field of study encompasses a broad range of issues in the management and use of biomedical information, including medical computing as well as the study of the nature of medical information.[4]

USES OF INFORMATION IN HEALTH CARE

The goal of information management in emergency medicine is to quickly and conveniently present current, valid, and relevant data of all types in an appropriate format, when and where they are needed, for those persons authorized to use them.[5] A growing body of research has shown that adverse outcomes do occur from lack of information and, conversely, that information systems can improve care and efficiency and reduce cost and adverse events.[6-12] Compared with other businesses and services, health care organizations are late in applying information technologies to their core function of patient care. The original clinical systems were passive bookkeeping systems designed to report data when requested. More advanced systems have gone past simple reporting functions to provide education, clinical guidance and decision support, and advanced communication functions.[13-15] Computerized medical records designed for documentation of ambulatory care have been developed,[16,17] some with clinical decision support capabilities.[18] Conceptually, clinical information management tasks can be categorized by broad functional areas discussed in the following sections.

Retrieving and Viewing Data

Much of the emergency physician's time is spent tracking down results of laboratory tests and other diagnostic studies and waiting for the chart to review prior visit documentation. Often, more time is spent searching for and recording information than synthesizing and analyzing the information.[19] Information systems can very effectively improve access to data by automating the rote tasks of collecting and organizing information, ensuring that a physician is rapidly and completely informed about a patient's history and about the status of the current encounter. The physician's time is then saved for abstraction and reasoning, tasks that humans perform much better than computers. This improved access must be balanced by meticulous attention to confidentiality concerns. With appropriate safeguards and permissions, however, information that is vital for clinical care can be made readily available. In most cases, this information is *passive* (i.e., viewed upon request with a results-viewer program). In some cases, a computer system can provide *active* delivery of new information, by alerting the clinician that new data are available (as in a tracking system), or even delivering the information directly to a mobile computer or pager carried by the clinician.

Some communities have established connected systems that make data from any of several local hospitals available to emergency departments in any one of the hospitals.[20] This trend is likely to grow, as better technology and public health concerns have made increased access both possible and necessary. The government-sponsored National Health Information Infrastructure project is concerned with methods of increasing access to necessary information across traditional barriers.

Communicating

Communication functions convey information from one person to another, or automatically from a machine (such as a laboratory system) to a person. The information can come as text messages, images, videos, or many other forms. Communication tasks include entry notifications, follow-up referrals, prescription ordering, financial eligibility verification, and automatic alerts (e.g., when a laboratory test result is markedly abnormal).

Electronic mail (e-mail) is probably the best-known form of computer-facilitated communication. Although some clinicians use e-mail for communicating patient information to other clinicians, security vulnerabilities may make this inadvisable. E-mail messages go through several intermediate stations between sender and recipient and can be intercepted if left unencrypted. Viruses, worms, and other destructive programs can be carried through e-mail, causing potential hazards for the security of the entire computer network. Secure messaging systems designed specifically for health care are generally considered to be a preferred alternative for communicating sensitive information.

Communication can also occur between information systems, through standard protocols. Emergency care could be enhanced by automatic communication of information from emergency medical services computers (where they are used), hospital inpatient records, and ambulatory-care records; in turn, emergency department data can be instantly communicated out to public health surveillance centers, greatly facilitating detection of epidemics. A variety of efforts are underway at the national and international levels to develop standards so that disparate computer systems can exchange this information easily and securely.

Communications between machines can be delivered over private lines, but secure transmission over the Internet has become more popular because of substantially lower cost and near-universal access. *Extensible markup language (XML)* is a popular way of representing data for Internet transmission. Telemedicine is a newer form of practice interaction that is highly dependent on sophisticated communication systems.

Documenting

In a typical encounter, documentation includes the recording of physician encounter notes, procedure notes, nursing observations and assessments, orders, treatments and results, tests and studies, and discharge summaries. Documentation is often time-consuming and inconvenient, especially because federal requirements have tied reimbursement to highly detailed and structured recording of all evaluation and management. Documentation is also frequently redundant, as each clinician enters data that may have been recorded previously.

Computers may help standardize data entry and make it a more satisfactory process. The use of preformatted, problem-specific, structured emergency department records has been shown to improve documentation.[11,21,22] Documentation of some items of long persistence, such as past medical history and family history, can be partially transferred from previously recorded information, resulting in faster and more complete documentation; this must be undertaken prudently, to ensure that the data being transferred are still relevant and accurate. Some documentation can be entered by patients themselves or by parents of pediatric patients.[12] Patients may even be more forthcoming in giving information to a computer than to a physician interviewer.[23]

Electronic medical information systems hold several other advantages over paper-based systems, including ease of data retrieval, legibility, and access by more than one person at a time.[24] Clinical encounters, especially in emergency medicine, often involves data entry by several persons concurrently. Because computers can be linked together in a network, each item of documentation can be recorded at the location of the actual event and viewed by all other clinicians at their own locations.

Making Decisions

Considerable experience to date has shown that computers can improve medical decision making by presenting pertinent data, information, and knowledge when it is needed, where it is needed, and in an appropriate format.[25] This "just-in-time" presentation of relevant information[26] is responsible for the potent effect of what are called *clinical decision support (CDS) systems*. CDS is a valuable component of a modern clinical information system. CDS systems analyze incoming clinical data such as test results and new orders, use logic to detect potentially hazardous conditions (such as an allergy to a drug being ordered), notify the physician, and suggest actions to remedy the situation.[15]

Although early work focused on programs that could facilitate diagnosis, the focus in CDS has shifted to more practical goals. Common CDS interventions include alerts that notify the physician about important or worrisome new data and reminders that show information about an action that is due but has not yet taken place. Computerized physician order entry systems can facilitate the use of CDS, a practice shown to have significant impact on quality and cost of care.[8,27]

Reactive CDS interventions provide immediate feedback and critiques at the time clinicians are making decisions. *Proactive* CDS systems have also been used to promote the use of guidelines and plans of care that have been preestablished for a given clinical situation or chief complaint (e.g., the diagnostic evaluation of suspected pulmonary embolism). Such broader interventions can be used to promote the use of evidence-based medicine by ensuring that the clinician caring for an individual patient is immediately made aware of current, pertinent, patient-focused evidence at the moment a critical decision is being made.

Education

Patient education is often neglected, given the rushed pace of modern medicine. However, proper attention to follow-up education is an important way to help patients care for themselves at home, potentially reducing adverse events and preventing unnecessary visits. Delivery of patient education materials is one of the most effective and widely adopted forms of information management in medicine. These materials traditionally have come in the form of printed brochures and handouts. Maintaining a computerized version of this information ensures that the desired material is always easy to find and up to date. Audio and video educational programs can also be delivered via computer. In addition, the materials can be automatically referenced. For example, when a particular diagnosis code is documented, the computer may bring up a list of relevant educational materials.

With the advent of widespread Internet access by patients, many sites now offer general educational materials to the public, although the quality and reliability of this information can be quite variable.[28] Online or computer-based education can also be made available to the clinician.

Online Reference Databases. Many major reference works, journals, and reference databases (including pharmacopeia and poisoning treatment information) are now available on health care networks as well as for bedside use on handheld or tablet computers. Using the *application service provider* model, the reference information does not need to be stored on the local network at all. The publisher can constantly update the content on its own website and subscribers can access the information through an Internet browser. Other publishing models include publishing reference information in a paper-based format supplemented with continual on-line updating (as is the case with the textbook you are reading).

Simulator Technology. *Simulation* is the employment of high-fidelity mannequins, partial task trainers, and interactive computer software to address the cognitive, psychomotor, and affective domains of medical education. Real-life patient scenarios are developed, allowing participants to suspend disbelief while managing simulated patients in a patient-safe environment. Simulator technology has advanced significantly in recent years, with a variety of realistic monitoring outputs, simulations that respond appropriately to subtle variations in treatment, and comprehensive recording. Debriefing of performance allows participants to analyze their experience in high-acuity situations in a controlled educational setting (Figure 202-1). In the future, standardized scenarios may have a role in competency-based residency and certification examinations.

Computer-Based Emergency Medicine Review and Testing. The American Board of Emergency Medicine moved to a computer-based review and testing system in 2004 to support its new continuous certification program for emergency physicians. Compared to in-person testing, with all of the issues and expenses of siting, proctoring, paper-handling, and certification recording, the computerized testing process is much more capable of supporting the increased testing volume.

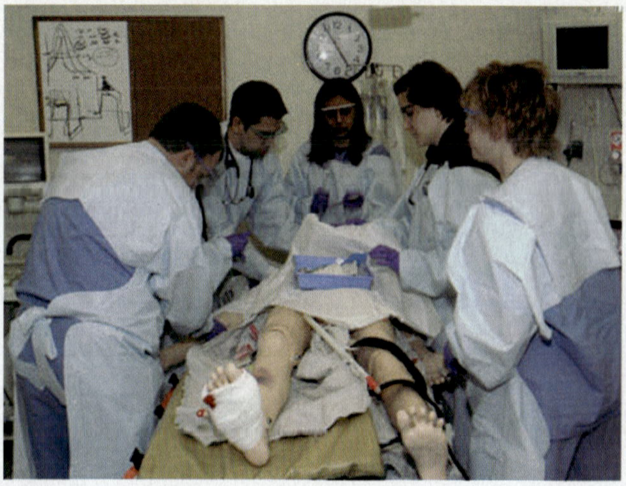

Figure 202-1. A team of physicians performs acute management on a patient simulator. (Courtesy of Charles Pozner, MD.)

Analysis of Practice

Physicians today are being held accountable for the costs of diagnostic and therapeutic management, the quality of results, and the satisfaction of customers.[19] To achieve this, clinicians and managers must be able to measure, track, and analyze the costs, processes, and outcomes of care. Aggregate analysis is essential in determining clinical patterns, areas of needed care improvement, hidden system problems, and the pursuit of research. Tools that perform regular assessment of practice patterns, spot significant trends, and allow ad hoc queries are increasingly vital to the effectiveness of the department.

INFORMATION MANAGEMENT IN THE EMERGENCY DEPARTMENT

Emergency medicine presents unique challenges in information handling. Emergency clinicians care for multiple patients in an unscheduled, high-acuity environment with a rapid stream of observations, tests, and treatments. In the course of every patient visit, emergency physicians use information resources to communicate with those who have prior information, view patient data, document findings and plans, guide clinical decision making, educate patients and themselves, and communicate with the next caregiver.[2] Each step of an emergency department encounter can contain several elements of basic and advanced information management and be a source of aggregate data for research and management (Table 202-1). In this section, we review some of the most common clinical information technology tools available in emergency departments.

Access to Prior Information

At the basic level, the patient or family (in person), ambulatory physicians (by telephone), emergency medical services, and the paper hospital chart supply most prior information. If electronic health records are

Table 202-1. Elements of Basic and Advanced Information Management that May Be Contained in Each Step of an Emergency Department Encounter

Step of Encounter	Element of Information Management
Prehospital	**Basic**
	Emergency medical services observations and treatments
	Advanced
	Home care protocols and home monitoring
	Personal health records and management tools
	Telephone triage protocols
	Emergency medical services-to-base station communication
	Analysis of Aggregate Data
	Referral patterns
Patient arrival and triage	**Basic**
	Prearrival information from primary physician
	Registration, demographic, financial information
	Advanced
	Information from electronic medical record
	Information from regional health information network
	Smart cards
	Documentation templates for triage data entry
	Coded vocabulary for syndrome classification
	Analysis of Aggregate Data
	Case mix and volume
	Patient registries
Evaluation	**Basic**
	Test and study results, documentation
	Hospital paper chart
	Advanced
	Complaint-specific protocols and guidelines
	Alerts for new events and/or abnormal results
	Patient tracking systems
	Access to relevant reference information
	Structured documentation
	PACS (picture archiving and communication system)
	Telemedicine
	Analysis of Aggregata Data
	Predictive value of tests
Treatment	**Basic**
	Documentation
	Order writing by hand
	Advanced
	Computerized order entry and communication
	Order sets
	Alerts for potential errors and adverse drug events
	Analysis of Aggregate Data
	Time to treat
	Outcomes analysis vs. ordering patterns
Disposition/discharge	**Basic**
	Communication to primary care physician and admitting unit
	Patient instructions
	Advanced
	Discharge orders
	Prescription entry and communication
	Automated patient instructions
	CPT (Current Procedural Terminology) coding from documentation
	Referral eligibility
	Automatic messages to referring and follow-up providers
	Analysis of Aggregate Data
	Outcomes
	Disposition patterns
Follow-up	**Basic**
	manual checking of late results
	Advanced
	Automated laboratory follow-up
	Public health reporting tools
	Compliance checking
	Analysis of Aggregata Data
	Return visits to the emergency department
	Syndromic surveillance

in place, a wide variety and great depth of prior patient data are available. The emergency physician can see a summary of the patient's problems, medications, allergies, test results, recent visit notes, discharge summaries, and more, in moments.

Even if the electronic health records are not part of the same computer system as that used in the emergency department, it is possible to gather this information through communications protocols. To do this, both the sending and receiving systems must be aware of the protocols, which must also guard that the access is appropriate from a security and privacy standpoint. This sort of data communication is uncommon at present, but an increasing number of communities have expressed interest. Another way to get entry notifications is through a secure messaging system. Typically, the referring clinician can access a secure website page from home or office and enter or transfer the relevant information on that page. The information is then available to appropriate persons in the emergency department.

Information During the Emergency Department Visit

Tracking Systems. An emergency department tracking system provides a continuous real-time view of key information for all the patients in the department. Typically, this is viewed as either a list of patients, or a pictorial representation of the department, with each patient depicted as one line or one block, respectively. For each patient, the tracking system may show whether any tests are pending, the patient's current admission status, the patient's location, referral or pre-entry information, and the status of orders, diagnostic studies, and other factors. In more advanced systems, color coding can reveal at a glance which patients are in need of priority attention; this is a boon to the emergency physician who needs to know which patient should get attention next. For example, a green border may mean the patient has been admitted; a yellow border may indicate a patient who has not yet been seen by a physician; and a brown border may denote a patient who has pending orders for the nurse. Inside the card, red letters may show that the patient has a highly abnormal ("panic") laboratory value.[15] A staff physician can look at the tracking system and immediately see which patients fit any these criteria. By clicking on a patient, the clinician can assign patients, enter orders, view the patient's test results and other medical records, and perform other critical and common functions.

Computerized Physician Order Entry (CPOE). CPOE systems are computer programs in which orders are entered directly on the computer by a physician. Nurses, pharmacists, and other key personnel use the computer to view and process orders. In the inpatient setting, CPOE systems have been shown to enhance efficiency, reduce costs, and prevent serious medical errors and adverse events.[6,8,9] CPOE in the emergency department setting is relatively uncommon but holds promise to achieve the same or even greater gains. Because a tracking or monitoring system clearly shows which patients have pending orders, communication between doctor and nurse often proceeds more smoothly, and fewer orders are accidentally missed. In addition, clinical decision support logic can provide immediate feedback regarding allergies, drug interactions, duplicate orders, and other hazardous situations.

A CPOE system designed optimally for the emergency department will look different from those designed for inpatient care. For example, compared with inpatient care, emergency department practice typically involves a smaller range of orders and sets of orders that are often ordered together for a given presenting complaint. Therefore, it is possible to produce *order sets* or *order templates* associated with each chief complaint, in which the most likely orders appear together on a single screen (Figure 202-2). This greatly increases speed and convenience.

Picture Archiving and Communications Systems (PACS) and Imaging Systems. In a PACS, images from radiography, computed tomography, magnetic resonance imaging, and other imaging modalities are stored digitally, instead of on film. Typically, a radiologist can view the images with an expensive workstation featuring a high-resolution display that allows extremely high-quality images to be studied carefully for maximum diagnostic accuracy. Meanwhile, less expensive but still high-quality displays can be scattered throughout the department, elsewhere in the hospital, or even off site, wherever it is most convenient. PACS viewer controls permit variation of contrast, brightness, and other visual parameters to further facilitate interpretation; three-dimensional reconstructions systems are even available in some sites.

The PACS systems can be quite expensive, and, unlike most computer applications, in which disk storage is essentially unlimited and inexpensive, the storage of high-resolution images still has limits. However, the savings in time, workflow, and film costs and the improved speed and accuracy possible in many situations make PACS systems increasingly popular in modern emergency departments. In some more remote settings, a regional PACS system captures data from multiple emergency departments, allowing a single central radiology department to provide image interpretation services for all.

Documentation Systems. In a typical emergency department, documentation, including required information for billing, is done either by direct handwriting or by dictation. Handwriting can be very time-consuming, and thus handwritten notes are often very terse, sometimes lacking the necessary documentation elements needed for appropriate billing. Additionally, handwritten notes are often difficult to read. Dictation and transcription solve these problems but can be very expensive.

Information technology permits a number of alternatives. Among these are structured documentation, in which notes are created by following structured outlines and checking boxes for positive and negative findings; voice recognition systems, in which entire notes are dictated and transcribed by computer, with high but imperfect accuracy; and facilitated transcription

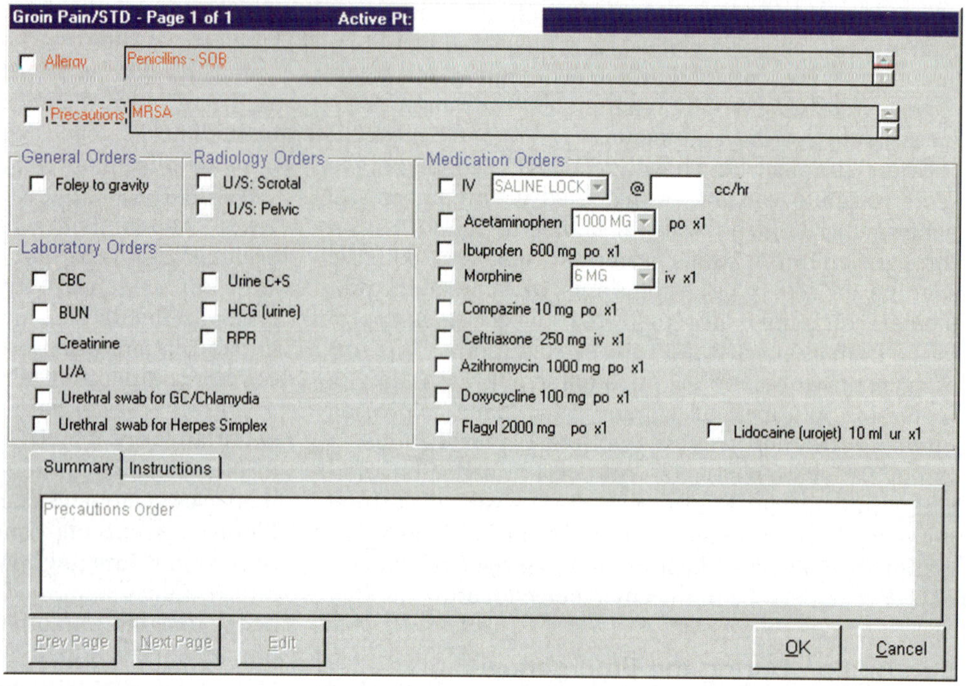

Figure 202-2. An ordering template from a computerized provider order entry (CPOE) system that has been designed for emergency department workflow. One of several dozen templates will appear automatically, based on the chief complaint at triage. Because of the relatively limited range of orders in an emergency department, most common orders can be selected from this one screen. (Courtesy of Brigham and Women's Hospital.)

systems, in which the voice recognition step is followed by processing by a human transcriptionist, who can make corrections at a much lower cost than it would take to do complete manual transcription. Experimental systems also permit the patient or the patient's family member to produce some of the documentation by completing forms and questionnaires in the waiting room or the examination room. The primary attraction of structured documentation systems currently is that they make it easier to generate appropriate justification for higher level billing codes.

Information at the End of the Emergency Department Visit

Discharge Instructions. Preprinted discharge instructions are usually more complete and easier to read than handwritten instructions. Although some hospitals keep preprinted paper instruction sheets available in racks, maintaining the stocks of these instructions is difficult, and the instructions are difficult to change and customize. A number of commercial and noncommercial producers provide large collections of discharge instructions for different problems, procedures, and medications online. The sheets never run out of stock and can be updated more easily. The physician or nurse can select one or more instruction sheets, input additional information (such as special instructions, or the doctor's name) easily, and print out the sheets for the patient. Instructions can also be sent to the patient via e-mail (or, more appropriately, through secure messaging) so that the patient cannot lose the information. Additional valuable features in some systems include the ability to select relevant instructions directly from an order set, and automatic documentation in the record that the instructions were given, which is useful for documentation and also for liability protection.

Notification to the Referring Physician. Using secure messaging, a note can be automatically sent to the primary or referring physician immediately upon completion of the emergency department visit. This note can include information that has already been captured during the registration, clinical care, or discharge processes, such as complaint, diagnosis, attending physician's name, test results, and disposition.

Commercial and Proprietary Emergency Department Systems

At the time of this writing, about two dozen vendors specialize in emergency department systems, including tracking, CPOE, documentation, billing, and other functions. A few others include some of these functions as part of an integrated hospital information system, although the emergency department functions are less customized. Actual usage of these commercial systems is still quite small, perhaps only in 3% to 6% of all hospitals. Still, government, private sector, regulatory agency, and overall patient safety and quality concerns continue to drive increased adoption of these systems. In some states, malpractice insurance premium discounts are offered to emergency physicians who use computers for documentation and other functions.

SECURITY AND CONFIDENTIALITY OF PATIENT INFORMATION

The ability to safeguard a patient's privacy is paramount in any information system, whether paper-based or electronic.[29] As applied to information systems, security protections refer to methods to prevent physical intrusion, theft of data, or attack on the system's integrity. Confidentiality protections limit whether a given user of the system can get access to a given patient's data. Effective information management is a balancing act between confidentiality and ease of access.

Computerized medical records present new opportunities and challenges for privacy protection. Computerized records, when improperly protected, could accelerate the chances of a widespread privacy violation, particularly in a large health care network,[30] because all information is theoretically available at each workstation on the network. On the other hand, in the paper chart world, security is greatly compromised because anyone in physical proximity to the chart can open it and view it without leaving any record that they did so. Technological solutions, such as encoding and digital certificates, make it possible to provide strong protection for information in a computerized medical record, if they are used conscientiously.

Confidentiality is enforced by authentication, authorization, and auditing. *Authentication* refers to the methods the system uses to ensure that a user is actually who he or she claims to be. *Authorization* refers to the privileges and restrictions for each user once authenticated. The most familiar form of authentication is the combination of a user name and password. Because the password is presumably a secret known only to the individual associated with the user name, it is very difficult for another person to try to forge that individual's identity and gain that user's authorizations. This method can be defeated if the password is deliberately or inadvertently shared, is written down in a location where it can be seen by others, or is so simple that it can be found through an unauthorized search.

Highly confidential systems use a second form of authentication such as a physical token (e.g., magnetically coded identification card or identification card with a second, rapidly changing password) or a biometric input device (e.g., fingerprint scanner or retinal pattern reader). Auditing systems ensure that a record is kept of all entries and accesses to critical information. They also provide a means of retrospectively tracing the flow of information in the event of a confidentiality violation. Such systems may also include trend analyses that detect unusual patterns of activity (such as a sudden increase in information accesses when a very important person [VIP] is treated).

Health care information computer networks can be accessed from outside the hospital via telephone or Internet connections, so the data on and functional integrity of these networks must be protected from accidental and deliberate threats. Many clinicians and patients are unaware of these potential security threats. For example, e-mail is increasingly being used to communicate patient information. E-mail messages, however, go through many different computers around the world on their way from sender to recipient. In most cases, it is relatively easy for a person at one of these intermediate stations to gain access to the contents of the message. *Encryption* (scrambling of information during transmission to prevent interception of messages), use of secure Internet message storage, and increased public awareness are necessary to ensure the safe communication of confidential information.[31]

Security is as much a management discipline as a technical issue.[3] Management procedures are particularly important and include confidentiality and security policy establishment and enforcement, staff education, monitoring, and sanctions. In an observational study of health care workers' conversations on hospital elevators, inappropriate comments and violations of patient confidentiality occurred with disturbing frequency.[32] An observational study conducted in an emergency department similarly found that breaches of privacy and confidentiality occurred by all members of the health care team.[33]

HIPAA (Healthcare Insurance Portability and Accountability Act)

HIPAA is an acronym for the Healthcare Insurance Portability and Accountability Act (also known as the Kennedy-Kassebaum Act, Public Law 104-191) that was enacted in 1996. HIPAA includes provisions that require hospitals, physicians, and managed care companies to adopt medical information security, privacy, and data standards or face penalties. HIPAA directed the Department of Health and Human Services to publish new rules to ensure the standardization of electronic health data and develop security standards to protect the confidentiality and integrity of individually identifiable health information.

In essence, the Act stipulates that patient-specific information should be available only to health workers who have a need to know it—those who are involved in the direct care, administrative services, or billing for that patient. The privacy provisions of the HIPAA are still open to some interpretation and confusion as of this writing, causing both under- and overprotectiveness in various transactions. Emergency access to data for immediate health- and life-protecting needs is specifically protected in the Act. Other typical emergency department transactions, such as learning about patient visits to other medical centers, should normally be referred to hospital counsel.

STANDARDS

Different clinical information systems may use a variety of dictionaries, nomenclatures, and indexes to describe common clinical elements such as medications, conditions, laboratory tests, and admission data. Standard definitions are necessary for exchange of data among these systems for clinical use,[34] for appropriate grouping of data in multisite research studies,[35] and for building reusable guidelines and protocols that interact directly with the information systems to promote optimal care and prevent errors. Variations in the way that data are entered in different emergency department record systems and even within individual systems impede the use of emergency department records for patient care and deter their reuse for secondary applications, including public health surveillance, research, and quality improvement.[36]

Historically, standards have been slow to arise in medical information systems. A small number of standards have become widely adopted, including Health Level 7 (HL-7), a standard for exchanging data among medical information systems, and the International Classification of Diseases (ICD-9 and ICD-10) for recording diagnoses. In many other areas, however, widely used standards have not appeared. This is in part due to the lack of a central dominant entity to create de facto standards. Recently, a number of development efforts have been undertaken to promote standards in key areas such as laboratory test data,[37] clinical decision support rules, and specifically for emergency medicine (the Data Elements for Emergency Department Systems, or DEEDS).[35] Commercial manufacturers of clinical information systems are increasingly supporting these standards.

NETWORKS

Emergency medicine is a specialty that relies on communication across wide areas. Emergency physicians have for decades directed midlevel providers (emergency medical technicians and paramedics) using telecommunication technologies (radios, phones, and telemetry devices). Poison control centers, typically tightly linked with emergency medicine, use information-intensive resources and telecommunications to provide directed care from a central location for poisoned patients over large geographic areas. In information management, communication is facilitated when all of the parties to a transaction have access to a common network.

Computers inside a hospital are generally arranged in a local area network (LAN), which provides access to common data from a variety of locations, such as sharing the same master patient list and letting all department coordinators use it. A LAN connects devices in close physical proximity, such as those in an office, clinic, or emergency department. A regional health information network (RHIN) links health records among a potentially vast array of clinics, hospitals, pharmacies, laboratories, managed care organizations, and other entities over a wide geographic area.[29] Whereas LANs generally operate within one institution, RHINs may connect many institutions in the same community. RHINs also allow for the collection, storage, retrieval, and analysis of large amounts of health care data for outcomes research and quality assurance.

The biggest hurdles in networking communities may be political rather than technological. Institutions and individuals, often in financially competing systems, must gain trust and confidence in one another to allow the sharing of information. These hurdles are being overcome as more and more organizations realize the mutual benefits of sharing clinical information. A RHIN that links information from all emergency departments in a large metropolitan area over a secure network has been implemented,[38] and others are in development.

THE INTERNET IN HEALTH CARE

The Internet, a global "network of networks," has transformed global information management and communication.[39] The rise of the Internet in the late 1990s was a spectacular phenomenon affecting almost all areas of business, communication, and education. For health care, the Internet offers great potential to coordinate health resources and improve patient care. But it must be used judiciously, because its open format allows both useful and harmful information to be presented with equal ease and visual sophistication.

Fundamentally, the Internet, particularly the World Wide Web, is important because of three practical factors: It provides a standard method for presenting data that can be seen by anyone with a single simple program; it provides standardized access to data and information regardless of the geographic location of the data; and the availability of standard search engines makes it easy to find this information.

Typical clinical information systems now include a significant component of web-based information. In some cases, the entire information system is actually stored off-site in a well-maintained, high-performance data center, while the users of the system enter and view their information through secure websites. In other cases, the primary information systems are sited within the hospital or medical center, and the Internet is used for communication, reference material, knowledge resources, and patient information.

Patients anxious to participate in decisions about their own treatment have turned to the Internet to confirm diagnoses, validate physician-recommended treatments, and seek alternative therapies. Although increased information for patients has been linked to improved outcomes, there are inherent dangers associated with the kind of unauthenticated information available on the Web. This provides an opportunity for the academic health sciences community to take the lead in ensuring that patients have access to reliable health information and that "patient informatics" be integrated into the teaching of clinical skills.[40]

OTHER INFORMATION TECHNOLOGIES

The preceding section illustrates how information technologies can contribute to the core components of an emergency department encounter. Several other technologies facilitate department management, coordination of prehospital services, public health, education, and remote care. Some of the most common or most promising examples are described here.

Coverage and Scheduling

Some specialized systems facilitate creation of work schedules for doctors, nurses, and other staff, taking into consideration the complex needs of staffing one or more emergency departments around the clock. Typically, these systems take online schedule-request forms as input, apply simple and complex scheduling rules (e.g., favoring forward rotation of shifts to minimize circadian rhythm disturbance), and generate a complete, balanced schedule. Schedule changes and shift exchanges can be made on the computer, so that the correct schedule is immediately available at all workstations on the network.

Diversion Management

As emergency department diversion becomes a more frequent reality of modern practice, it is critical for emergency medical services coordinators to have an accurate picture of which hospitals are and are not open to new patients, to know where a patient in a given location should be directed. A small number of specialized diversion management systems help provide reports, views, and other controls to help manage hospital availability on a local or regional basis.[41]

Prehospital Information Systems

Although most of the current discussion has to do with information technology used in the emergency department itself, another new development is the availability of information systems for emergency medical services personnel. Using small portable wireless devices such as laptop and tablet computers, these systems allow emergency medical technicians and paramedics to document and monitor patients more efficiently, to capture information directly from electronic monitoring equipment, and potentially to upload their findings to the hospital's own system upon arrival. As mentioned previously, such systems are still uncommon and to some extent experimental. However, the technology has great potential to provide benefits in efficiency, communication, accuracy, and safety, and as technology costs continue to drop, it is reasonable to expect that such systems will be more common in the future.

Integration with Electron Medical Record

With increasing concerns about patient safety, medical errors, and improving patient quality, more hospitals and more practices are purchasing electronic medical record systems, which maintain a lifetime record of a patient's health status, treatments, test results, and other information. Most forecasts call for the number of electronic medical record systems implemented to increase significantly over the next decade. Some of these systems have been adapted for use in the emergency department. Although such systems are, in general, not customized to emergency department workflow, they can be useful for results viewing, some types of documentation, and access to information from other ambulatory encounters.

Syndromic Surveillance and Public Health Reporting

In the United States, public health tracking of new epidemics has always been a concern, but the terrorist attacks and anthrax episodes of 2001 have stimulated enormous interest in enhancing *syndromic surveillance,* the ability to detect unusual regional illness patterns rapidly. A large number of regional projects are underway to develop such systems, and information technology is at the center of most such efforts. Typically, a surveillance system requires (1) a coding scheme that allows related illnesses or presentations to be classified together, (2) documentation and communication of all such patient presentations from one or several emergency departments to a central processing center, (3) detection logic that can spot significant variations from the expected incidences of these presentations, and (4) an alerting system to let authorities know when such a variation has occurred.[42-48] Current work is focused on developing optimal coding schemes and detection logic for maximum sensitivity and specificity. Although the high interest and funding of these projects is based on terrorist events, very similar information technology can be used to detect influenza patterns, new respiratory syndromes, and other significant public health incidents.

The Role of Informatics in Disasters, War, and Terrorism

The United States and countries around the world are currently facing several new, concurrent large-scale health crises as a result of terrorist activity.[48] Three major health issues have risen sharply in urgency: bioterrorism, the threat of widespread delivery of agents of illness; mass disasters, local events that produce large numbers of casualties and overwhelm the usual capacity of health care delivery systems; and the delivery of optimal health care to remote military field sites. In addition to biosurveillance and bioagent detection, information technologies can improve the emergency medicine-disaster response by coordinating information from field to hospital, rapid acquisition of multipatient information from the disaster site, and telemedicine and telepresence (remote guidance) for procedures.

Telemedicine

The future of emergency medicine lies beyond the confines of the emergency department.[49] Medical care from a distance is one of the most promising applications of advanced communication technology.[50] Telemedicine, broadly defined, is the use of telecommunications technologies to provide medical information and services across long distances or natural barriers. Telemedicine systems use high-speed communications lines, video conferencing, and custom peripheral devices (e.g., high-resolution cameras, stethoscopes, and otoscopes) to deliver specialty health care to areas where it is not otherwise available.

Most telemedicine applications for patient care are consultations with the patient at one site and the consulting specialist at another. The interaction may involve the exchange of voice communications, transmission and review of medical records and diagnostic testing results, transmission of still images or video clips in a "store-and-forward" mode (in which data are acquired and transmitted for review at a later time), and real-time interactive video. Despite widespread interest in distance medicine, relatively few patients have been treated with the use of these technologies.[51] Emergency teleconsultations[49,52] and Internet consultations[53] have been described, and telemedicine applications in prehospital and disaster medicine[54] as well as "home delivery" of care and monitoring are being explored.

SUMMARY

The implications of information technologies are enormous for emergency patients, emergency clinicians, and the specialty of emergency medicine. In 1968, Weed wrote, "It has been said that preoccupation with the medical record and the computer leads to neglect of the 'humanitarian' side and the 'art' of medical practice. The most humanitarian thing a physician can do is to precisely know what he is doing, and make the patient as comfortable as he can in the face of problems that he cannot solve." More than three decades later, we continue to strive to take advantage of these marvelous technological changes, hoping that the greatest "byproduct" of improved information management in emergency medicine may simply be more time to spend with the patient.[19]

Emergency clinicians need to understand the information workflow of emergency medical practice and research and be aware of the role information technologies can play in improving care delivery. Just as we do not need to understand how a telephone works to make good use of it, clinicians do not need technical medical computing or programming skills to become effective computer users.[4] However, the clinician does need to know how to frame requirements and understand the basic services that information technologies can provide.

At a systems level, emergency departments could be transformed into "knowledge hubs,"[5] where clinical practice, care delivery, and information resources are integrated. Emergency departments could also play a leadership role in developing and testing enterprise-wide clinical information systems.[55] As computers become fast, cheap, and ubiquitous, it perhaps seems obvious that they could help improve patient care and practice efficiency. The truth is that optimal use of information technology is far from automatic. Creative and rigorous efforts will be required to make information a benefit and not a burden.[2]

REFERENCES

1. McDonald M: Health in the age of telecognition. In Bezold C, et al (eds): *2020 Visions: Health Care Information Standards and Technologies*. Rockville, Md, United States Pharmacopeia Convention, 1993.
2. Teich JM, Waeckerle JF: Emergency medical informatics. *Ann Emerg Med* 30:667, 1997.
3. Keen PGW: *Every Manager's Guide to Information Technology: A Glossary of Key Terms and Concepts for Today's Business Leader*, 2nd ed. Boston, Harvard Business School Press, 1995.
4. Shortliffe EH, et al: *Medical Informatics: Computer Applications in Health Care*. Reading, Mass, Addison-Wesley, 1990.
5. Cordell WH, et al: Strategies for improving information management in emergency medicine to meet clinical, research, and administrative needs. *Acad Emerg Med* 5:162, 1998.
6. Bates DW, et al: Potential identifiability and preventability of adverse events using information systems. *J Am Med Inform Assoc* 1:404, 1994.
7. Petersen LA, et al: Using a computerized sign-out program to improve continuity of inpatient care and prevent adverse events. *Jt Comm J Qual Improv* 24:77, 1998.
8. Bates DW, et al: Effect of computerized physician order entry and a team intervention on prevention of serious medication errors. *JAMA* 280:1311, 1998.
9. Teich JM, et al: The Brigham integrated computing system (BICS): Advanced clinical systems in an academic hospital environment. *Intl J Med Inf* 54:197, 1999.
10. Bates DW, Gawande AA: Improving safety with information technology. *N Engl J Med* 348:2526, 2003.
11. Buller-Close K, Schriger DL, Baraff LJ: Heterogeneous effect of an Emergency Department Expert Charting System. *Ann Emerg Med* 41:644, 2003.
12. Porter SC, et al: Parents as direct contributors to the medical record: Validation of their electronic input. *Ann Emerg Med* 35:346, 2000.
13. Tierney WM, et al: Physician inpatient order writing on microcomputer workstations: Effects on resource utilization. *JAMA* 269:379, 1993.
14. Johnston ME, et al: Effects of computer-based clinical decision support systems on clinician performance and patient outcome: A critical appraisal of research. *Ann Intern Med* 120:135, 1994.
15. Kuperman G, et al: Detecting alerts, notifying the physician, and offering action items: A comprehensive alerting system. In *Proceedings of the AMIA Annual Fall Symposium*. 1996, p 704.
16. Rind DM, Safran C: Real and imagined barriers to an electronic medical record. *Proceedings of the Annual Symposium on Computer Applications in Medical Care*. 1993, p 74-78.
17. Borst F, et al: Fifteen years of medical encoding in the Diogene HIS. *Medinfo* 8:43, 1995.
18. Safran C, et al: Development of a knowledge-based electronic patient record. *MD Comput* 13:46, 1996.
19. Smith MS, Feied CF: The next-generation emergency department. *Ann Emerg Med* 32:65, 1998.
20. Overhage JM, et al. A randomized, controlled trial of clinical information shared from another institution. *Ann Emerg Med* 39:14, 2002.
21. Humphreys T, et al: Preformatted charts improve documentation in the emergency department. *Ann Emerg Med* 21:534, 1992.
22. Wrenn K, et al: The use of structured, complaint-specific patient encounter forms in the emergency department. *Ann Emerg Med* 22:805, 1993.
23. Wald JS, et al: Patient entries in the electronic medical record: An interactive interview used in primary care. In *Proceedings of the Annual Symposium on Computer Applications in Medical Care*. 1995, p 147.
24. Cordell WH: Information technologies for emergency medicine. *Acad Emerg Med* 1:194, 1994.

25. Wong ET, Abendroth TW: Reaping the benefits of medical information systems. *Acad Med* 71:353, 1996.
26. Chueh H, Barnett GO: "Just-in-time" clinical information. *Acad Med* 72:512, 1997.
27. Teich JM, et al: Effects of computerized physician order entry on prescribing practices. *Arch Intern Med* 160:2741, 2000.
28. Jadad AR, Gagliardi A: Rating health information on the Internet: Navigating to knowledge or to Babel? *JAMA* 279:611, 1998.
29. Goodman K: The ethics of CHINs. *Physicians and Computers* October:16-24, 1997.
30. Woodward B: The computer-based patient record and confidentiality. *New Engl J Med* 333:1419, 1995.
31. Sands DZ, et al: Use of electronic mail in a teaching hospital. In *Proceedings of the Annual Symposium on Computer Applications in Medical Care.* 1993, p 306.
32. Ubel PA, et al: Elevator talk: Observational study of inappropriate comments in a public space. *Am J Med* 99:190, 1995.
33. Mlinek EJ, Pierce J: Confidentiality and privacy breaches in a university hospital emergency department. *Acad Emerg Med* 4:1142, 1997.
34. Halamka JD, et al: CareWeb, a web-based medical record for an integrated health care delivery system. *Int J Med Inf* 54:1, 1999.
35. Pollock DA, et al: Data elements for emergency department systems, release 1.0 (DEEDS): A summary report. DEEDS Writing Committee. *J Emerg Nurs* 24:35, 1998.
36. National Center for Injury Prevention and Control: Data elements for emergency department systems, release 1.0. Atlanta, Centers for Disease Control and Prevention, 1997.
37. McDonald CJ, et al: What is done, what is needed and what is realistic to expect from medical informatics standards. *Int J Med Inf* 48:5, 1998.
38. Overhage JM, et al: Design and implementation of the Indianapolis Network for Patient Care and Research. *Bull Med Libr Assoc* 83:48, 1995.
39. Frisse M: Medical informatics' promised land: Are we there yet? *Acad Med* 74:1301, 1999.
40. Bader SA, Braude RM: "Patient informatics": Creating new partnerships in medical decision making. *Acad Med* 73: 408, 1998.
41. Barthell EN, et al: Assuring community emergency care capacity with collaborative Internet tools: The Milwaukee experience. *J Public Health Manag Pract* 9:35, 2003.
42. Travers DA, et al: Emergency department data for bioterrorism surveillance: Electronic data availability, timeliness, sources and standards. In *Proceedings of the AMIA Symposium.* 2003, p 664.
43. Mandl KD, et al: Implementing syndromic surveillance: A practical guide informed by the early experience. *J Am Med Inform Assoc* 11:141, 2004.
44. Lober WB, et al: J Syndromic surveillance using automated collection of computerized discharge diagnoses. *Urban Health* 80:97, 2003.
45. Lober WB, et al: Roundtable on bioterrorism detection: Information system-based surveillance. *J Am Med Inform Assoc* 9:105, 2002.
46. Gesteland PH, et al: Rapid deployment of an electronic disease surveillance system in the state of Utah for the 2002 Olympic Winter Games. In *Proceedings of the AMIA Symposium.* 2002, 285.
47. Barthell EN, et al:. The Frontlines of Medicine Project: A proposal for the standardized communication of emergency department data for public health uses including syndromic surveillance for biological and chemical terrorism. *Ann Emerg Med* 39:422, 2002.
48. Teich JM, et al: The informatics response in disaster, terrorism, and war. *J Am Med Inform Assoc* 9:97, 2002.
49. Lambrecht CJ: Emergency physicians' roles in a clinical telemedicine network. *Ann Emerg Med* 30:670, 1997.
50. Balas EA, et al: Electronic communication with patients: Evaluation of distance medicine technology. *JAMA* 278: 152, 1997.
51. Schafermeyer, RW: Telemedicine and emergency medical care: Improved care delivery, or just another video game? [editorial]. *Ann Emerg Med* 30:682, 1997.
52. Shafqat S, et al: Role for telemedicine in acute stroke: Feasibility and reliability of remote administration of the NIH stroke scale. *Stroke* 30:2141, 1999.
53. Garshnek V, Burkle FM Jr: Telecommunications systems in support of disaster medicine: Applications of basic information pathways. *Ann Emerg Med* 34:213, 1999.
54. Kedar I, et al: Internet based consultations to transfer knowledge for patients requiring specialised care: Retrospective case review. *BMJ* 326:696, 2003.
55. Feied CF, et al: Emergency medicine can play a leadership role in enterprise-wide clinical information systems. *Ann Emerg Med* 35:162, 2000.

CHAPTER 203 Multiculturalism and Care Delivery

Edward Bernstein, Judith Bernstein, and Thea James

Every day, in emergency departments across the nation, physicians encounter challenging cases that require an appreciation of cultural differences. Lack of understanding of the role of cultural factors can have an adverse effect on physician-patient communication and trust. Health outcomes can also be negatively affected, as demonstrated by a large body of literature on racial and ethnic disparities in types of interventions and outcomes for heart and lung disease. Race, culture, ethnicity, class, gender, economic conditions, spirituality, and sexual orientation define health, illness, and health care access and outcomes for our

Table 203-1. Changing Demographics in the United States

Racial Groups (in millions)	1990	2003	2010	2020	2030	2060
Total population	249	283	300	323	325	432
Hispanic	9.0	12.7	14.6	16.3	19.4	26.6
Non-Hispanic black	11.8	12.3	12.5	12.9	13.0	13.2
American Indian and Alaskan Native	0.7	0.7	0.8	0.8	0.8	0.8
Asians and Pacific Islander	2.8	4.2	4.8	5.7	6.7	9.8
Non-Hispanic white	75.7	70.1	67.3	64.3	60.1	49.6

From U.S. Census Bureau, 2000. Available at http://www.census.gov/population/www/projections/natsum-T5.html. Accessed January 26, 2004.

patients. Missing these cues is as serious as leaving a major diagnosis out of a differential.[1,2]

In the arena of medical diagnosis and treatment, emergency physicians are trained to expect and welcome a wide range of diagnoses and perform advanced technical procedures. The challenges brought by cultural barriers are more difficult to overcome than technical challenges, however, because emergency-physician training has not included comparable knowledge, exposure, skills, and problem-solving experience related to cultural competence. Yet the American College of Emergency Physicians (ACEP) Code of Ethics, 1998-99, commits us to "protect the rights and best interests of the most vulnerable, . . . [and] secure access to emergency and other basic health care for all."[3] This code also recognizes that "denial of emergency care or delay in providing emergency services on the basis of race, religion, ethnic background, social status, type of illness or injury, or ability to pay is unethical." Lewis Goldfrank, past president of the Society of Academic Emergency Medicine (SAEM) and a member of the Institute of Medicine, and Robert Knopp, Associate Editor of *Annals of Emergency Medicine,* comment in an editorial about ethnic disparities in emergency department analgesia prescription that, "With the legacy of racism and the growing body of medical evidence indicating differential care in the emergency department and other medical specialties, we believe that the burden of responsibility has now shifted so that the medical profession must now demonstrate that physicians are providing appropriate and timely care for all. . . . Our integrity as a profession and as a nation hangs in the balance."[4] The purpose of this chapter is to provide the knowledge base in cultural competence that is essential to meet patient needs, improve health outcomes, reduce racial and ethnic disparities, and achieve professional goals.

RATIONALE FOR CULTURAL COMPETENCE

Changing Demographics: New Challenges for Emergency Physicians

We live in a global community, and both the U.S. population and the types of health problems seen by emergency physicians are constantly changing. In 2000, the U.S. Census Bureau estimated that 31 million, or 11% of the 285 million people in the United States, were foreign born (from 138 countries) and 18% of the population speaks a language other than English at home.[5] Hispanics currently represent 13% of the population, non-Hispanic blacks 12.3%, American Indians and Alaskan Natives 0.8%, Asians and Pacific Islanders 4.2%, and non-Hispanic whites 69.7%. It is projected that by 2030 the population will grow to 351 million, with 19.4% Hispanics, 13% non-Hispanic blacks, 0.8% American Indians and Alaskan Natives, 6.7% Asians and Pacific Islanders, and 60.1% non-Hispanic whites. Racial and ethnic minority representation in the United States will exceed 30% within a decade and 40% by 2030, and Hispanic and Asian groups will grow at a much greater rate. There will be no minority group by mid-century (Table 203-1).[6]

These figures do not speak to the diversity within these groups. The category *Hispanic*, for example, is an ethnic grouping counted in the race category of the census, but it fails to capture the significant range of diversity represented by Spanish speakers. Hispanics may share some cultural practices and speak similar versions of the Spanish language but have major differences in their history, socioeconomic status, cultural identity, what they call themselves (Hispanic or Latino), vocabulary, levels of acculturation, health beliefs, habits, access to care, and health outcomes.

What do these changes in demographics mean to practicing emergency physicians? As the populations we care for become more diverse, our patients' health problems will diversify as well. The ACEP Code of Ethics challenges us, in these circumstances, to advocate for equity, recognize the current ethnic and racial health disparities targeted by *Healthy People 2010* (the public health agenda for the nation), and work with other health organizations and providers to contribute to eliminating these disparities.[7]

Racial and Ethnic Disparities in Health Care Access and Outcomes

In the last decade, both financial and nonfinancial barriers to access for racial and ethnic minority populations have been documented. These include high rates of uninsurance, lack of prenatal care, hospitalizations for ambulatory-sensitive diagnoses (an indicator of reduced access to primary care), and concentration of minorities in areas of physician shortage.[8] In 2003, the Institute of Medicine (IOM) produced a report commissioned by the U.S. Congress in which more than 100

Table 203-2. Racial and Ethnic Differences in Age Adjusted Mortality Rates, 2001 (per 100,000)

	Hispanic	Black, Non-Hispanic	American Indian and Alaskan Native	Asian and Pacific Islander	White, Non-Hispanic
All mortality	659.0	1101.0	686.7	492.0	843.0
Infant mortality/1000 births	5.4	13.5	9.7	4.7	5.7
Heart disease	192.0	316.9	159.6	137.6	246.0
Cerebrovascular disease	44.9	78.8	41.3	51.2	56.0
Liver disease	15.8	9.3	40.4	3.5	9.0
Unintentional injury	30.7	15.4	51.3	17.4	36.2
Suicide	5.7	5.5	10.5	5.4	12.5
Homicide	8.3	21.2	6.8	4.2	4.0
Diabetes	36.7	22.8	40.4	16.9	22.1
Acquired immunodeficiency syndrome	6.2	22.8	2.7	0.7	2.1
Malignant neoplasms	132.2	243.1	131	119.5	197.4

From CDC/NCHS National Vital Statistics System. Available at http://www.cdc.gov/nchs

studies assessing the quality of care for racial and ethnic minorities living in this country were analyzed.[9] According to this IOM report, minorities received fewer needed services and procedures than whites, after controlling for insurance status, income, and other access factors. These findings applied to a wide range of health conditions such as cancer, cardiovascular disease, human immunodeficiency virus and acquired immunodeficiency syndrome, diabetes, and mental illness. Racial differences in refusal rates were small and did not adequately explain the disparities. The findings identified cultural and linguistic barriers, fragmentation of the health care system, and differences in sites of care delivery and insurance coverage as explanatory factors. The authors suggest that unconscious bias, prejudice, stereotyping, and physician uncertainty of severity may influence clinical decision making and allocation of services and procedures. The report concludes that "racial and ethnic disparities in healthcare exist, and because they are associated with worse outcomes in many cases, are unacceptable."

The IOM report also discussed important nonfinancial barriers to access, such as the unequal distribution of physicians in areas where minority populations live. In particular, the number of racial and ethnic minorities living in medically underserved areas is three times the proportion of minorities in the population overall. Poor urban communities with high African American and Hispanic representation averaged 24 physicians per 100,000 people, compared with 69 physicians per 100,000 in communities with low representation. African American physicians are five times more likely to treat African American patients than other physicians, Hispanic physicians are 2.5 times more likely to treat Hispanics, and minority physicians are more likely to serve patients with Medicaid or no insurance.[10] However, enrollment of minorities in health profession schools has been declining for African Americans, Hispanics, American Indians, and Alaskan Natives. In fact, the American Association of Medical Colleges reported that in four states with restrictions against affirmative action, in the year following enactment, there was a 17% decline in applications and a 26% decline in matriculation to medical schools from under-represented minority groups.[11] Dr. Jordan Cohen, President of the American Association of Medical Colleges, argues that "to achieve diversity in the health profession is not someone else's problem; it is a problem for the profession, for all of us who are concerned about the future of access to health care and the quality of health care that we are going to be able to provide our society."[12]

The National Institutes of Health National Center for Minority Health and Health Disparities, created by Congressional Public Law 106-525 to oversee research in health care disparities, reports that improvements in health have not been universal over the last two decades. "Striking disparities in the burden of illness and death" exist for African Americans, Hispanics, Native Americans, Alaskan Natives, Asians, and Pacific Islanders. Members of these groups have shorter life expectancy and higher rates of cardiovascular disease, cancer, infant mortality, birth defects, asthma, diabetes, stroke, sexually transmitted disease, and mental illness (Table 203-2).[10,11]

Factors Contributing to Disparities in Health Outcomes

In the last decade, reports have appeared regularly in major peer-reviewed journals about disparities in the use of diagnostic tests and procedures and in access to appropriate treatment modalities.

Test and Treatment Options: Physician-Patient Communication Failure?

Recent studies document clearly that both Hispanics and African Americans receive fewer analgesics for extremity fractures than white patients in the emergency department setting, despite evidence of no difference across race and ethnicity in ability to discriminate painful sensation.[15-19]

Evidence from other specialties corroborates that differences in provision of medically appropriate procedures and therapies are often related to race and ethnicity. In the case of preventive measures, for example, elderly black and Hispanic people are less likely to receive influenza and pneumococcal vaccine, and Hispanics are less likely to have a blood pressure check or a cholesterol level assessment within the last 2 years.[20] In the domain of surgery, the operative rate for certain lung cancers was 76.7% for whites and 64% for blacks, and the 5-year survival was 34.1% and 26.4%, respectively.[21] The authors concluded that if black patients had undergone surgery, the 5-year survival rate would have been similar. An accompanying editorial suggests that the medical establishment take some responsibility for the racial discrimination that results in inadequate emphasis on prevention or insufficiently aggressive care for black patients.[22]

These issues also apply to disparities between black and white populations with respect to cardiovascular disease. After adjusting for severity and coexisting conditions, African Americans are less likely to undergo bypass surgery or angioplasty than whites, and differences were more significant for those predicted to benefit most from revascularization.[23] A recent multicenter emergency department study found racial disparities in access to cardiac catheterization for African Americans and other non-whites with acute myocardial infarction and unstable angina. Surprisingly, the researchers also found that African American patients were less likely to receive a timely electrocardiogram or an assay for cardiac markers, and doctors were less likely to prescribe anti-ischemic medications.[24]

Discrimination and Health Outcomes

Deleterious health consequences that result from racial discrimination have been well documented.[25] In a recent study of the nation by state, in those states where more respondents to the *General Social Survey* indicated that blacks lacked innate ability, there was a closely associated increase in age-adjusted black mortality that was considerably stronger than the correlation for mortality and socioeconomic status.[26] Mechanisms used to cope with the stress of racism have been shown to backfire by adding to health risks, as in the case of smoking, substance abuse, and overeating.[27,28] Racism-induced stress has been shown to be negatively associated with many disease entities such as diabetes, hypertension, depression, and preterm birth.[29-33] Similar experiences have been described for homosexuals vis-à-vis homophobia.[34]

Race-Based Medical Decision Making

Racism, sexism, and homophobia can interfere with the establishment of trust and the delivery of effective medical care if providers create or establish barriers based on their own internal biases, prejudices, and negative reactions to racial or cultural characteristics, such as skin color or clothing styles. Patients read these reactions clearly during an encounter with a provider. A barrier is created, and the opportunity for a good medical outcome may be lost. Provider biases against persons with certain stigmatized diseases, such as human immunodeficiency virus and substance abuse, can also create barriers to effective health care. When primary-care physicians viewed scripted video interviews with hypothetical patients with chest pain who had similar symptoms, risk factors, vital signs, and thallium stress test and electrocardiographic findings, they were less likely to refer African American women for cardiac catheterization than men and whites, even though the scripts varied only by race and gender.[35]

Failure of Trust

Patients from minority communities have reason to be skeptical about the validity of medical research and the appropriateness of medical recommendations. Participants in the Tuskegee study, for example, were not notified when effective treatment for syphilis became available, because researchers wished to investigate the natural course of the disease.[36] Middle-class African American patients often rate their interactions with non-black physicians as less participatory than when the doctor is of the same race as the patient.[37,38] Yet this option for physician-patient congruence is rarely available to minority patients because only 4% of physicians are black, whereas 12% of the population is black.[9]

In the *Agency for Health Quality Research National Healthcare Disparities Report*, blacks and Hispanics were found to be more critical of the patient-provider relationship than whites. A higher percentage of adult blacks and Hispanics rated their health care at less than 6 on a scale of 1 to 10 in the past year and believed that they would have gotten better care if they were of a different race or ethnicity. The report provided evidence confirming perceptions of a lower quality of medical care. For example, when black and Hispanic adults older than 65 years of age were hospitalized for pneumonia, they were less likely than comparable whites to have blood culture samples drawn and antibiotics administered in accordance with current recommendations. Hispanics with myocardial infarction were less likely to have been administered aspirin or a β-blocker on admission and discharge. In comparison to white dialysis patients, fewer blacks and Hispanics in need of a kidney were registered on waiting lists for transplant or had received a transplant within 3 years.[39]

Language and Effective Medical Care

According to the 2000 U.S. census, 47 million Americans (18%) speak a language other than English at home, 21.3 million speak English less than very well, and 10.7 million speak English not at all or not well.[5] Patients with limited English proficiency are more likely to defer needed services, leave against medical advice, miss appointments, fail to adhere to treatment regimens, lack a regular provider, and report poorer health status.

Transcribed audiotapes of medical encounters in a pediatric emergency department setting were studied to ascertain differences in communication error rates for patients who were aided by professional hospital interpreters as compared to those who had an ad hoc interpreter (family, friend, or nonprofessional hospital worker) and those who had no interpreter available. They found that communication errors occurred equally among the ad hoc and the no interpreter groups. These errors included left out words (52%), incorrect words (16%), substituted words (13%), interjected personal views (10%), and added words (8%). The errors of ad hoc interpreters were more likely to result in clinically significant medical errors, such as omitting drug allergies and giving inaccurate instructions on dosing and route of administration.[40] The use of untrained nonprofessional employees as interpreters results in serious translation errors, including omissions, additions, and substitutions for what the patient is trying to say, and the use of relatives, particularly children, may violate privacy and disrupt family norms of authority.[41,42]

A cross-sectional survey at a public hospital emergency department suggested that there is a patient-perceived need for interpreter services, and the highest patient satisfaction ratings are obtained when patients can communicate directly with their physicians.[43] Satisfaction ratings for patients using ad hoc interpreters are lower, and rates are lowest when an interpreter should have been used but was unavailable. In one retrospective study of Spanish, Haitian Creole, and Portuguese Creole speaking patients presenting to the emergency department with chest pain, headache, and abdominal pain, the investigators found that the use of trained interpreters was associated with increased intensity of emergency department services, reduced emergency department return rate, increased clinic utilization, and lower charges over the next 30 days, without any simultaneous increase in length of stay or cost of visit.[44]

A state-wide emergency department patient satisfaction survey in Massachusetts indicated that non-English speakers were less satisfied with their emergency department care, were less willing to return for care, and reported more problems with emergency care.[45] The authors state that interpreter service is likely to improve the satisfaction of this group.

CULTURAL COMPETENCE: A TOOL FOR ENHANCING EMERGENCY DEPARTMENT CARE

Defining Culture, Ethnicity, and Race

Culture has always been an ambiguous term, hard to define because of confusion about the distinctive characteristics of culture, ethnicity, and race. Culture is most simply the "sum total of socially inherited characteristics of a human group that comprises anything one generation can tell, convey or hand down to the next; in other words the non-physical inherited traits we possess."[46] *Ethnicity*, sometimes understood as country of origin, is defined as "a collectivity within a larger society having real or putative common ancestry, memories of a shared historical past, and a cultural focus on one or more symbolic elements defined as the epitome of their peoplehood."[47]

Race is itself a social construction, a socially assigned arbitrary identity given to people on the basis of visual appearance. Racism structures society and hence the experience of delivering and receiving medical care. The social concept of blacks as an inferior race was propagated by 19th century biologists determined to justify profits from slavery.[48] Although their pseudoscientific methods have been thoroughly refuted, race is still a major determinant of history, culture, economics, and health outcomes in the United States, and racial categorization persists into modern times. Manning Marable, Professor of History and Director of the Institute of African-American Studies at Columbia University, describes race (blackness) as "the projection of white folk upon us, rather than what black people are really about."[49]

Culture is a specific subset of behaviors, patterns, beliefs, thoughts, values, customs, traditions, attitudes, and communication styles shared by members of a group or community that define their reality. Race describes only socially assigned categories of physical appearance. Ethnicity describes country of origin. Therefore, interchangeable use of the terms *culture, race,* and *ethnicity* is inappropriate and can create barriers to effective medical care, especially in the brief, focused time period and chaotic setting of the emergency department.

The Cultural Competence Continuum: A Measure of Proficiency

Culturally competent health care is defined as both the individual provider's and the health care organization's abilities to deliver effective medical care to people of different cultures, and is based on demonstration of sensitivity, valuing of cultural differences, and self-awareness of cultural background and biases. Cultural competence increases the chance of understanding the perspectives of our patients so we can provide services that are consistent with their needs. Possible benefits include improved health outcomes, maximal use of limited resources, and increased customer retention and access to care.[50]

Cross and Barzon[51] provide a model for improving individual and organizational cultural competence that uses a self-assessment continuum, which ranges from cultural destructiveness to cultural incapacity, to cultural blindness, through precompetence, to basic and advanced competence. On the lower end of the continuum is *cultural destructiveness*, which promotes institutional racism and specifically excludes certain groups from access to medical education and to medical care. Individuals at this end of the continuum actively collaborate with the immigration authorities to deport patients or deny emergency care to undocumented immigrants seeking medical care. In 1995, ACEP went on record to oppose "federal and state initiatives which require physicians and health care facilities to refuse care to undocumented persons or to report suspected undocumented persons to immigration authorities."[3]

The history of medicine in the United States contains many unfortunate examples of destructive practices. For example, the Sims procedure for fistula repair was developed by performing 30 medically unnecessary surgeries on slaves over a 2-year period.[52] The legacy of such destructive acts and the double standard it reflects cannot be easily overcome. Even today, African American physicians in training are often assumed to be technicians, transporters, or other nonprofessional medical workers, not doctors—despite white coat, name tag, and stethoscope.[53]

The second category in Cross and Barzon's schema, *cultural incapacity,* is characterized by micro- rather than macro-aggression. It includes calling African American women by their first names or "dear" or "doll," assuming a paternalistic stance, projecting certain negative characteristics or stereotypes or lower expectations onto minority individuals, or resenting the need for interpreters for non-English speakers. Persons operating at this level may not be conscious of racist attitudes but will make patients feel unwelcome.

The middle category, *cultural blindness,* promotes the delusion that staff and institution are completely free of biases about color, race, culture, and ethnic differences. The construct at this level is that "everyone should be treated the same." Although moving toward a more respectful position, this level of competency fails to recognize the positive contributions of diversity or the pervasiveness of bias within medical institutions. Administrators operating in an institution at this level may see no reason to hire, train, or retain a diverse staff, or to be open to minority health belief models that may value spiritual and herbal practices. There is an implicit sense that the dominant culture has little to learn or incorporate from others, a form of ethnocentric superiority and a denial of the potential for problems related to discrimination or ignorance.

Cultural precompetence, the starting point for competence, requires that an organization begin asking questions, engage in self-assessment, and start a process of improvement to go beyond needs assessment into concrete action and reallocation of resources. *Basic cultural competence,* which encompasses a long-term commitment to improve, requires that organizations establish a mission statement, policies for care of diverse groups, and programs for staff training, recruitment, and retention and provide concrete manifestations that patients from diverse backgrounds are welcome. This type of organization has signs in many languages, provides multilingual telephone services and interpreters, includes ethnic and racial variables in its database, has culturally sensitive visiting policies, and evaluates quality of care given to the diverse groups on an ongoing basis. Practitioners of *advanced cultural competence* are innovators who conduct research and evaluate and disseminate new models of care.

Evolution of New Standards for Health Care

In response to the identification of unacceptable differences in both health care provision and health care outcomes, state Medicaid regulations and Health Plan Employer Data and Information Set criteria now reflect the need to establish quality performance measures to ensure access to appropriate services for culturally diverse populations.[54] A new standard of care has been established that requires institutions and practitioners to provide for medical needs in the patient's primary language and in a manner compatible with patients' health beliefs and practices. Health care institutions and providers are asked to collect data stratified by race, ethnicity, and language and to institute quality improvement efforts when cross-cultural differences in outcomes of care, process indicators, or patient satisfaction are detected. They are asked to develop culturally competent systems of care based on an assessment of the organization's mission, goals, policies, practices and services, staff training needs, and the current diversity of the staff.

After the assessment process, health care organizations must identify opportunities to improve the cultural competence of the organization and its delivery of health care services to a diverse population. At the top of the list is the improvement of interpreter services. Hospitals are asked to establish minimum performance standards for interpreters that include training in culturally specific medical language and code of ethics. These requirements have now been codified as a set of standards for culturally and linguistically appropriate services by the Office of Minority Health and the Agency for Health Care Research and Quality and published in the Federal Register (December 15, 2000).[55] In Spring 2000, the Massachusetts legislature took a positive step in the direction of compliance with these standards by passing a law requiring all emergency departments to provide interpreter service, and authorizing the state to provide Medicaid reimbursement for interpreter services.

Culturally Competent Approach to Language Barriers

In 1996, the SAEM Task Force on Physician-Patient Communication identified lack of a common language as the single most common barrier to communication in the emergency department. Professional medical interpreters were recommended for the following reasons: (1) confidentiality, (2) medical knowledge and a common vocabulary with the provider, and (3) fluency. Two emergency department case reports illustrate this point[56]:

A 50-year-old Mexican-American man who spoke only Spanish was seen in the emergency department because of "chest pain." Because no translator was available, an electrocardiogram and chest radiograph were ordered. The electrocardiogram was normal; the chest radiograph showed a widened mediastinum suggestive of a dissecting aortic aneurysm. An aortogram was subsequently performed, which demonstrated a normal aorta. At some point, a Spanish-speaking physician was able to elicit a 1-year history of difficulty swallowing and regurgitation of food. A barium swallow was performed, which revealed achalasia.

A 22-year-old Vietnamese man arrived in the emergency department unresponsive and comatose with small, reactive pupils. Naloxone hydrochloride and 50% dextrose in water were administered without response. The medical history, obtained from a family member who spoke some English, consisted of brief answers to specific questions, and was not helpful diagnostically. A lumbar puncture and examination of the cerebrospinal fluid ruled out meningitis. A clerk later recalled that a child with the same last name was admitted the previous day for headache, nausea, and vomiting caused by carbon monoxide poisoning. In retrospect, it was clear that the history obtained from a family member who was under stress and giving vague answers to pointed questions was inadequate. The authors conclude that "a trained bicultural translator can effectively elicit the history as conceptualized by the patient or family and translate it both linguistically and in the format of Western Medicine."

This last example also illustrates that bilingualism is necessary but not sufficient. There are nuances and sociocultural assumptions in both languages as well as nonverbal cues that must be communicated along with words for effective diagnosis, treatment, and disposition. The medical interview is the heart of the medical encounter between physician and patient, yet in an interpreted interaction, neither patient nor physician is in a position to judge the accuracy or completeness of a lay interpreter's translation. Clearly, omissions, additions, opinions, guesses, and distortions can lead to serious mistakes and unnecessary diagnostic procedures.

Standards and certification for medical interpreters are needed to ensure consistency and quality. The Massachusetts Medical Interpreter Association recommends that standards cover interpretation, the cultural interface, and ethical behavior. Because the meaning inherent in the message is rooted in culturally specific beliefs, values, assumptions, customs, and norms, and language is itself an expression of culture, it may be necessary for a medical interpreter to go beyond a literal interpretation to explain unstated assumptions and to find new ways of communicating untranslatable words or concepts. In addition to maintaining confidentiality, the medical interpreter has an ethical burden to uphold the trust of both parties and assure them that the considerable power associated with the interpreter's role will not be abused, and that information will be faithfully conveyed without interjecting the subjective opinions and thoughts of the interpreter. Even with such qualified interpreters, the emergency physician still needs to monitor the flow of the interview, and from time to time to clarify meaning and ensure understanding. This can be done by the interpreter's repeating what he or she thought the patient meant, and asking the patient to repeat what the interpreter said. It is important to observe the interaction for phrase length as an indication of material not translated or added by the translator.

Using Cultural Competence to Cross the Barrier of Different Beliefs, Values, and Life Experiences

The SAEM task force report also recognized that different cultures have different ways of viewing the world, but cautioned that it is dangerous to hold strong preexisting assumptions about any cultural group, because variations within cultures often exceed variations between them. A patient who is thoroughly acculturated into American society may be offended by a health care provider's attribution of traditional beliefs. Even in the context of a busy emergency department encounter, it is necessary and feasible to get to know the individual patient sufficiently to make a rough assessment about level of acculturation, or at least to ask rather than to assume.

With this caveat in mind, it is important to be aware of differences between cultures in preferences for interpersonal space, direct gaze, deference to elders in decision making, family involvement, and traditional healing practices. Some cultures require a greater interpersonal distance than others. Some change the interpersonal space when things are not going well by, for example, by sitting down. In some communities such as the Navajo, it is rude to look at someone directly, and in others it is rude not to do so. It is important to know who will make the decisions regarding patient care, because it may be elders, community leaders, spouses, or parents, and not the patient, as is usual in the Western medical model. Similarly, alternative definitions of the family should be respected. If the patient wants to have extended or non-genetically related family present, then emergency physicians should support that wish in order to reduce stress and facilitate effective medical decision making, which may mean negotiating with emergency department staff to bend visiting regulations or change culturally insensitive rules.

In some cultures, the diagnosis of specific diseases can be particularly problematic. For example, in African American and Puerto Rican communities, cancer is often perceived as a fatal disease. Patients may therefore avoid initial evaluation or choose no treatment when diagnosed, even when the cancer is identified at an early stage and the prognosis is good. A health care provider who understands these health beliefs and concerns can work collaboratively with patients and provide health information in a format that the patient can accept.

Alternative healing systems have strong cultural roots. In 1997, the U.S. population made an estimated 629 million visits to providers of alternative health care, over 243 million more than to conventional health care providers and an increase of 47% since 1990. An estimated 44% used at least one complementary alternative therapy in 1997.[57]

Folk medicine is too diverse for providers to know all possible practices, but emergency physicians need to know some of the more common therapies and ask their patients about them. Ignorance is not bliss. More than a few emergency physicians have called social workers to investigate children with apparent bruises caused by coining, which involves vigorous rubbing of the skin with coins and warm oil (tiger balm) to release the "bad wind" (reduce fever). These parents, who have attempted to help their children by using health care practices that are widely accepted in their communities of origin, feel accused, and the trust between the physician and the family may be irrevocably lost. Similarly, herbal remedies can be effective or at least harmless, but on occasion they can be toxic, as in the case of clay ingestion by pregnant women, the use of marijuana tea to treat asthma, and powders containing high concentrations of lead oxide to treat *empacho,* a condition in which it is believed that a substance (usually food or saliva) gets "stuck" to the walls of the stomach or intestines, causing an obstruction.

Specific uses of folk medicine need to be elicited respectfully in a careful history and evaluated. Then, recommendations can be presented nonjudgmentally, and alternative folk remedies that are benign can be prescribed along with needed allopathic medications.

The practitioner and the patient will inevitably bring different beliefs and values to the medical encounter; the key to cultural competence is respectful negotiation of these differences without imposing the power of physician expertise, thus protecting patient autonomy. If patients are satisfied, they will carry out follow-up recommendations and return to the emergency department in the future when they need emergency care.

In a review of Hispanic cultural practices, Flores and colleagues suggest a five-step approach for the pediatric emergency department that is applicable to all of emergency medicine: the physician should (1) explain that he or she is aware that a given folk illness exists; (2) ask whether the parent or patient has ever heard of it; (3) ask whether the patient has the folk illness now; (4) ask what treatment the patient is receiving for the condition; and (5) suggest alternatives to harmful folk remedies, accommodate wherever possible (nonjudgmentally) to folk illness beliefs and practices, and integrate the use of harmless folk remedies into the treatment plan.[58]

Interpreting the Culture of Medicine to Patients from Diverse Backgrounds

There are inherent conflicts between the culture of medical care, particularly emergency department culture, and the cultures of many of our patients. Physicians are expert in diagnosing and treating *diseases,* which represent abnormal structures or functions of the human body (the pathophysiology of disease states). On the other hand, patients experience *illness,* a subjective, feeling state that is interpreted through the lens of culture and has a personal and social meaning. The patient is an expert in his or her own illness and its effects on daily living, whereas a physician is expert in the effects of diseases on organ systems. Both ways of looking at the world have validity, but they are radically different.[59] Unfortunately, the culture of medicine tends to recognize only its own interpretation and perspective. A culturally competent approach recognizes both and works to integrate the best of both worlds.

A patient may have very high blood pressure, or human immunodeficiency virus infection, or early cervical cancer and not experience symptoms. If patients do not feel sick and experience no alteration in functioning, they may not accept a physician's diagnosis. There may be conflict between the patient's perception of causality and the physician's, as in the case of the differences between the medical diagnosis of hypertension and the commonly accepted view of hypertension as "high blood" in the African American community.[60]

On the other hand, a patient may feel sick—be ill, weak and dizzy, with extreme fatigue or abdominal pain—yet the physician is unable to diagnose a disease despite a thorough history, physical examination, testing, and appropriate consultation. For example, "susto," an illness recognized by Mexican-Americans, causes listlessness, insomnia, depression, and anorexia and is believed to be caused by exposure to a frightening experience. Treatment requires the patient to speak openly about the events that led to the "susto," followed by bed rest and a ritual that includes prayers, incantations, and "barridas" (sweeping of the body with an egg, a candle, or herbal teas).[61]

To be most effective, physicians need to investigate how patients view the causality of their illnesses and how they experience them in order to negotiate a therapeutic intervention. Exploration might take the form of comments and questions such as, "Help me to see through your eyes how you understand this problem. Have you or someone you know experienced it before?" Some cultures, for example, experience different types of imbalance as the source of illness: yin and yang in Chinese medicine; wind, water, and fire in Ayurvedic (East Indian) medicine; hot and cold in many traditional medicine models; or spiritual disharmony, as in the case of those who view illness as a punishment from God for sins. In each of these cases, harmony is the goal of medical care. Medications that have side effects of anxiety or elevated pulse (e.g., sympathomimetics for treatment of asthma) might not be understood or acceptable because they are perceived as creating even more disharmony.

If the reaction of the emergency physician implies disbelief and disrespect for the patient's perceptions, the result may be loss of faith in Western medicine and subsequent failure to seek treatment for life-threatening illnesses. The alternative is for the physician to accept the patient's experience at face value as uniquely his or hers, or, when possible, reframe it in terms of medical knowledge. This process permits the physician to validate the patient's experience, and in this case to provide a referral for psychotherapy if traditional measures do not alleviate the problem. Then both physician and patient will be satisfied with the outcome of the encounter.

Role Expectations in Western Medicine: Opportunity for Misunderstanding

The culture of medicine, especially in emergency medicine, has its own set of patient expectations, rules and regulations, language, and dress distinctions that reflect a hierarchy of authority, a characterization of patients as good or bad, and different sets of behaviors toward patients depending on the category to which they have been assigned. The "good emergency patient" is acutely ill but waits patiently until called without complaining, requesting pain medications, getting angry, or being loud or disruptive. The "good patient" understands the triage system and provides a clear, concise, pertinent history with enough information for accurate diagnosis. The "good patient" does not take up physician time with minor complaints, feelings, or tangentially related information. The "good patient" accepts invasive examinations and procedures without protest, agrees to admission or to a discharge plan, does not require long explanations of rationale for treatment, and has a support system in place for a safe discharge. A "good patient" who does not speak English brings someone to interpret, someone who can bridge the cultural divide and help with transportation upon discharge. A "good patient" does not moan, scream for a nurse or doctor, or act violently. A "good patient" does not have family members who are emotionally upset, stir up trouble, or challenge providers. A "good patient" uses seat belts, maintains personal hygiene and normal weight, takes prescribed medications, avoids drugs and cigarettes, and exercises. "Good patients" share a trust, understanding, and belief in scientific, modern, technological medicine and its value. Because they comprehend the physician's explanation of causality—for instance, bacterial infection as a cause of pneumonia—they agree to a discharge plan and adhere to a treatment regimen. They understand medical jargon and require very little explanation and ask a minimum of questions. "Good patients" help maintain the flow through the emergency department, whereas their opposites obstruct the flow. "Good patients" get better; the "bad patient" keeps coming back, has chronic recurrent conditions, and has confusing or hard-to-resolve problems.

So it is not surprising and no fault of their own that people coming from different cultures may find it impossible not to violate one of the many rules and regulations of the emergency department. Every medical encounter is potentially a cross-cultural experience, and negotiating the divide is a challenge for both patients and providers. But it is not enough just to make allowances for many patients' ignorance of the rules of American medical culture. Cultural competence involves a reframing of many of these unstated rules because they prevent us from looking beneath the surface and addressing real problems. When a patient comes in with vague complaints, there may be a social stressor that has tipped the balance of mental health. There may be circumstances that the patient does not feel comfortable sharing with the provider because of cultural, racial, or language barriers, or there may have been an overload of negative stimuli related to racial and ethnic discrimination—a crisis for the person and the body this person inhabits.[62,63] People from minority cultures experience stressful events daily that the white provider, secure in his or her socioeconomic status and membership in the dominant majority, can only imagine: being passed by the 15th taxi in a row because "it's not safe to pick up blacks"; being followed in a department store because you and your friend were speaking Spanish; to have to "dress up" to go to the store to avoid a possible humiliating moment; or standing in line to register at a hotel, dressed in professional clothing, and being asked by a white person in line, "Hey, can you take my baggage to my room?" In each of these cases, assumptions were made about the person on the basis of a stereotype related to physical appearance or presumed country of origin. There is mounting evidence that these types of negative encounters engender clinical depression and anxiety and contribute to hypertension and other medical sequelae. If a patient self-defines as having an emergency by showing up at the emergency department, the problems that cause that person to come deserve our respect.

A study of racial and ethnic patterns of hospital emergency departments found that four times as many African Americans and Hispanics as whites report the emergency department as a source of care.[64] Patients who "overuse or abuse" the emergency department are seen as "bad patients," but the reasons given in this study are entirely rational (Box 203-1). These reasons may explain, at least in part, why the emergency departments of our nation had an estimated 107 million visits in 2001.

BOX 203-1. Rational Explanations for Minority Populations' Use of the Emergency Department as a Preferred Source of Care

1. Individuals need not request an appointment to receive care.
2. Emergency departments provide sophisticated medical technology.
3. Emergency departments operate 24 hours a day.
4. Emergency department services are often covered by health insurance and other options are not.
5. Emergency departments have a tradition of free care.
6. Economically disadvantaged people may try to avoid seeking medical care, hoping to get better without it, until the problem becomes an emergency.
7. Many communities lack culturally competent private practitioners.
8. Emergency departments are often close to inner-city neighborhoods, whereas many primary care providers have abandoned the city center environs for the suburbs.

Adapted from Thornton MC, White Means SI: Racial and ethnic patterns of hospital emergency department use. In Lillie Blanton M, Leigh W (eds): *Achieving Equitable Access: Studies of Health Care Issues Affecting Hispanics and African Americans.* Washington, DC, University Press of America, 1994.

To practice good medicine in this health care and social environment, emergency physicians must critically question and reframe the moralistic good patient/bad patient paradigm. We, like our patients, are at the whim of forces beyond our control, and both patients and practitioners will experience higher levels of satisfaction if these issues are addressed directly. Patients must take responsibility for their own behaviors whenever possible, but physicians can and should work with health care institutions to adopt policies that improve access to culturally competent health care. These actions can help create a safe environment for both practitioners and patients.

RECOMMENDATIONS

Diversity among the emergency department patient population poses a challenge to emergency physicians. Recognition of cultural differences, knowledge about diverse cultures, awareness of the health impact of cultural beliefs and practices, and sensitivity to patients' needs can reduce access barriers and improve clinical outcomes and hospital-community relationships, while reducing the number of repeat visits and the cost of health care. Diversity education also creates a rich environment for conceptualizing and researching health problems.

There are many opportunities for emergency departments and their institutions to improve care for patients in multicultural communities. These include plans to address problems related to (1) lack of protocols for patient care; (2) lack of resources for translation and cross-cultural interpretation; (3) pressure to maintain flow and efficiency with cultural competence, which can be seen as an added burden; (4) lack of cross-cultural teaching guidelines and standards in medical education; (5) inadequate recruitment and retention of minority residents, faculty, and practitioners; and (6) lack of pathways for communication and collaborative work with communities.

Concrete recommendations, based on the culturally and linguistically appropriate services standards, have been proposed for pediatric emergency settings and can be applied universally: (1) institutions should employ trained medical interpreters and a diverse workforce; (2) pharmacies should label prescriptions and provide medical instructions in the patient's primary language; (3) administrators should post multilingual signs and ensure that handouts and forms are translated; (4) quality improvement programs should collect and analyze data and provide information to monitor outcomes based on race/ethnicity; and (5) a diverse group of patients should be enrolled in research studies to improve outcomes.[65]

Recommendations from the IOM report for a series of additional legal, regulatory, and policy measures were highlighted in a recent *Academic Emergency Medicine* editorial entitled, "Training of medical professionals and the delivery of health care as related to cultural identity groups." These recommendations include the following: (1) patients in public managed care organizations should have the same patient bill of rights as patients in the private HMOs; (2) the number of health care providers who are themselves members of racial and ethnic minority groups should be increased; (3) resources must be adequate to enforce penalties for civil rights violations; (4) incentives to promote disparities should be stringently limited; (5) health care professionals should have opportunities for cross-cultural education; (6) patient participation in decision making should be enhanced through education; (7) community health care workers/advocates should assist patients to negotiate the health care system successfully; (8) the diversity of faculty and residents must be improved; (9) a cross-cultural curriculum should be developed for residency training and continuing education; and (10) physicians must educate themselves and the general public about the need to eliminate racial and ethnic disparities in health care.[66]

SUMMARY

Changing demographics manifest themselves in a diverse emergency department patient population, and emergency department practitioners must learn to be culturally competent and promote systemic change to provide quality care. Essential cultural competence tools for providers include recognition of cultural differences, respect for individual opinions and perspectives about health and illness, and, most important, ability and willingness to negotiate differences in order to offer the best opportunity for good health care outcomes. Culturally appropriate health care systems must be incorporated into emergency departments, which serve as the gateway to our health care institutions.

BOX 203-2. Basic Skills in an Intercultural Curriculum

Communicate an interest in and respect for the patient's culture.

Tactfully and respectfully ask for general cultural information (such as herbal remedies, acupuncture, coining, moxibustion, or other cures attempted).

Elicit the patient's understanding of and beliefs about illness or health problems.

Request information regarding folk medicine beliefs, for instance, mal ojo (the evil eye or evil spirit) among Mexican-Americans, voodoo among Haitians, yin and yang among Chinese patients, rootwork among African-Americans, and spiritism (the ability of spirits to make people sick or cure them) among Puerto Ricans.

Interpret verbal and nonverbal behaviors in a culturally relevant manner.

Negotiate a culturally appropriate health care plan with the patient and his or her family as partners.

Demonstrate an ability to work as a team with a medical interpreter in the bilingual medical encounter.

From Goldstein E, et al: Intercultural medicine. In Jensen N, Van Kirk J (eds): *A Curriculum for Internal Medicine Residency*. Philadelphia, American College of Physicians, 1995.

BOX 203-3. Policies for Institutional Improvement

Educate emergency department personnel about the circumstances of patients' lives and the interesting cultures that have evolved to deal with these circumstances using a variety of formats:

1. A series of hospital inservices to provide information about each specific patient group that uses the institution
2. Small focus groups with patients to improve our understanding of our patients needs, and begin the process of freeing providers from racial and ethnic stereotypes that create barriers to good medical care
3. Training utilizing videotapes and role-playing exercises to enhance movement along the cultural competence continuum

Meet with community organizations to build trust and create partnerships for preventive education.

Hire employees who reflect the cultures, ethnicity, and socioeconomic background of emergency department patients to improve the quality of services.

Provide interpreter services, visual aids, and other educational materials in a variety of languages, and multilingual health education classes.

Participate as an institution in community health fairs.

Basic skills proposed in an intercultural curriculum developed by Goldstein and associates[67] for internal medicine residents can apply equally to emergency physicians (Box 203-2). Policies that will promote cultural competence, increase patient satisfaction, and improve health outcomes include those listed in Box 203-3.

REFERENCES

1. Fadiman A: *The Spirit Catches You and You Fall Down: A Hmong Child, Her American Doctors, and the Collision of Two Cultures.* New York, Farrar, Straus & Giroux, 1997.
2. Davis K: *The Quality of American Health Care: Can We Do Better?* New York, Commonwealth Fund, 2001.
3. The American College of Emergency Physicians, 1998-99 Ethics Committee: *Code of Ethics for Emergency Physicians.* Dallas, The American College of Emergency Physicians, 1999.
4. Goldfrank LR, Knopp RK: Racially and ethnically selective analgesia: Is this racism? *Ann Emerg Med* 35:79, 2000.
5. US Census Bureau, Profile of Selected Social Characteristics: 2000. Available at: http://factfinder.census.gov/servlet/QTTable?_bm=y&-geo_id=D&-qr_name=DEC_2000_SF4_U_DP2&-ds_name=D&-_lang=en&-redoLog=false. Accessed January 26, 2004.
6. US Census Bureau (NP-T5) Projections of the Resident Population by Race, Hispanic Origin, and Nativity: Middle Series, 1999 to 2100. Washington D.C., U.S. Department of Commerce Available at http://www.census.gov/population/www/projections/natsum-T5.html. Accessed January 26, 2004.
7. U.S. Department of Health and Human Services: *Healthy People 2010: National Health Promotion, and Disease Prevention Objectives.* Washington, DC, Public Health Service, 2000.
8. National Center for Health Statistics: Health, United States, 1998 chartbook on socioeconomic status health. Hyattsville, MD, U.S. Government Printing Office, 1998. Available at http://raceandhealth.hhs.gov.
9. Smedley BD, Stith AY, Nelson AR (eds): *Unequal Treatment: Confronting Racial and Ethnic Disparities in Health Care.* Washington, DC: National Academy Press, 2003. Available at http://books.nap.edu/books/030908265X/html/index.html. Accessed January 27, 2004.
10. Komaromy M, et al: The role of black and Hispanic physicians in providing health care for underserved populations. *N Engl J Med* 334:1305, 1996.
11. Cohen J: Statistics don't lie: Anti-affirmative action is bad for our health. *Acad Med* 72:1084, 1997.
12. Cohen JJ: Disparities in Health Care: An Overview. *Acad Emerg Med* 10:1155, 2003.
13. National Center for Minority Health and Health Disparities: Annual Report on Health Disparities Research-Fiscal Year 2001. Available at http://ncmhd.nih.gov/our_programs/strategic/pubs/AnnReportFY01Binder1.pdf. Accessed January 26, 2004.
14. Arisas E, et al: Deaths: Final data for 2001. National vital statistics reports; vol 52 no3. Hyattsville, MD, National Center for Health Statistics, 2003. Available at http://www.cdc.gov/nchs/data/nvsr/nvsr52/nvsr52_03.pdf. Accessed January 26, 2004.
15. Todd KH, Samaroo N, Hoffman JR: Ethnicity as a risk factor for inadequate ED analgesia. *JAMA* 269:1537, 1993.
16. Todd KH, Samaroo N, Hoffman JR: The effect of ethnicity on physician estimates of pain severity in patients with isolated extremity trauma. *JAMA* 271:925, 1994.
17. Todd KH, Deaton C, D'Adamo AP, Goe L: Ethnicity and analgesic practice. *Ann Emerg Med* 35:11, 2000.
18. Zatzick DF, Dimsdale JE: Cultural variations in response to painful stimuli. *Psychosom Med* 52:544, 1990.
19. Chan A, Woodruff RK: Comparison of palliative care needs of English and non-English-speaking patients. *J Palliat Care* 15:26, 1999.
20. CDC: Racial/ethnic disparities in influenza and pneumococcal vaccination levels among persons aged >65 years: United States, 1989-2001. *MMWR* 52:958, 2003.
21. Bach PB, Cramer LD, Warren JL, Begg CB: Racial differences in the treatment of early-stage lung cancer. *N Engl J Med* 341:1198, 2000.
22. King TE, Brunetta P: Racial disparity in rates of surgery for lung cancer [editorial; comment]. *N Engl J Med* 341:1231, 1999.
23. Peterson ED, et al: Racial variation in the use of coronary-revascularization procedures: Are the differences real? Do they matter? *N Engl J Med* 336:480, 1997.
24. Venkat A, et al: The impact of race on acute management of chest pain. *Acad Emerg Med* 10:1199, 2003.
25. Taukli-Williams J, Carrillo J: The impact of psychosocial stressors on African American and Latino preschoolers. *J Natl Med Assoc* 87:473, 1995.
26. Kennedy BP, et al: (Dis)respect and black mortality. In Kawachi I, Kennedy B, Wilkinson R (eds): *The Society and Population Health Reader.* New York, The New Press, 1999.
27. Romano PS, Bloom J, Syme LS: Smoking, social support and hassles in an urban African American community. *AJPH* 81:1415, 1991.
28. Walcott-McQuigg JA: The relationship between stress and weight-control behavior in African American women. *J Natl Med Assoc* 87:427, 1995.
29. Jackson JS, et al: Racism and the physical and mental health status of African Americans: A thirteen year national panel study. *Ethn Dis* 6:13247, 1996.
30. Murrell NL: Stress, self-esteem, and racism: Relationships with low birth weight and preterm delivery in African American Women. *J Natl Black Nurses Assoc* 8:45, 1996.
31. Auslander WF, Thompson SJ, Dreitzer D, Santiago JV: Mothers' satisfaction with medical care: Perceptions of

racism, family stress, and medical outcomes in children with diabetes. *Health Soc Work* 22:190, 1997.
32. Dressler WW: Social identity and arterial blood pressure in the African American community. *Ethn Dis* 6:176, 1996.
33. Thompson VL: Perceived experiences of racism as stressful life events. *Commun Ment Health J* 32:223, 1996.
34. Kreiger N, Sidney S: Prevalence and health implications of anti-gay discrimination: A study of black and white women and men in the CARDIA cohort. Coronary artery risk development in young adults. *Int J Health Serv* 27:157, 1997.
35. Schulman KA, et al: The effect of race and sex on physicians' recommendations for cardiac catheterization. *N Engl J Med* 340:618, 1999.
36. Corbie-Smith G: The continuing legacy of the Tuskegee Syphilis Study: Considerations for clinical investigation. *Am J Med Sci* 317:5, 1999.
37. Cooper-Patrick L, et al: Race, gender, and partnership in the patient-physician relationship. *JAMA* 282:583, 1999.
38. vanRyn M, Burke J: The effects of race and socioeconomic status on physicians' perceptions of patients. *Soc Sci Med* 50:813, 2000.
39. Agency for Health Care Quality: *National Healthcare Disparities Report.* Washington, DC, Department of Health and Human Services, 2003.
40. Flores G, et al: Errors in medical interpretation and their potential clinical consequences in pediatric encounters. *Pediatrics* 11:6, 2003.
41. Baker D, et al: Use and effectiveness of interpreters in an emergency department. *JAMA* 275:783, 1996.
42. Tang SY: Interpreter services in healthcare: Policy recommendations for healthcare agencies. *J Nurs Adm* 29:23, 1999.
43. Baker DW, Hayes R, Fortier JP: Interpreter use and satisfaction with interpersonal aspects of care for Spanish-speaking patients. *Med Care* 36:1461, 1998.
44. Bernstein J, et al: Trained medical interpreters in the emergency department: Effects on services, subsequent charges and follow-up. *J Immigrant Health* 4:171, 2002.
45. Carrasquillo O, Orav J, Brennan TA, Burstin HR: Impact of language barriers on patients' satisfaction in an emergency department. *J Gen Int Med* 14:282, 1999.
46. Fejos P: Man, magic and media. In Goldston I (ed): *Medicine and Anthropology.* New York, International University Press, 1959.
47. Schermerhorn R: Comparative ethnic relations: A framework for theory and research. Chicago, University of Chicago Press, 1978.
48. Fullilove MT: Comment: Abandoning "race" as a variable in public health research—An idea whose time has come. *Am J Public Health* 88:1297, 1998.
49. Stuart J: The African-American century: A roundtable. *Am Legacy* Winter:18, 2000.
50. National Alliance for Hispanic Health: A Primer for Cultural Proficiency: Toward Quality Health Services for Hispanics. Washington, DC, Estrella Press, 2001. Available http://bhpr.hrsa.gov/diversity/cultcomp.htm.
51. Cross TL, Barzon B, Jacobs CG, Doller B: *Towards a Culturally Competent System of Care: A Monograph on Effective Services for Minority Children Who are Severely Emotionally Disturbed.* Washington, DC, Child and Adolescent Service System Program (CASSP) Technical Assistance Center, Georgetown University Child Development Center, 1989.
52. Barker-Benfield J: *The Horrors of the Half Lived Life: Male Attitudes toward Women and Sexuality in the 19th Century.* New York, Harper and Row, 1976.
53. Shervington DO, Bland IJ, Myers A: Ethnicity, gender identity, stress, and coping among female African American medical students. *J Am Med Wom Assoc* 51:153, 1996.
54. Massachusetts Division of Medical Assistance: *Appendix G: Cultural Competence QIP Reporting.* Boston, DMA, 1997.
55. Office of Minority Health: *National Standards for Culturally and Linguistically Appropriate Services in Health Care.* Final Report. Rockville, MD, US DHHS, 2001. Available at http://www.omhrc.gov/omh/programs/2pgprograms/finalreport.pdf.
56. Weaver C, Sklar D: Diagnostic dilemmas and cultural diversity in the ER. *West J Med* 133:356, 1980.
57. Wolsko PM, et al: Insurance coverage, medical conditions, and visits to alternative medicine providers: Results of a national survey. *Arch Intern Med* 162:281, 2002.
58. Flores G: Culture and the patient-physician relationship: Achieving cultural competency in health care. *J Pediatr* 136:14, 2000.
59. Downs K, Bernstein J, Marchese T: Providing culturally competent primary care for immigrant and refugee women: A Cambodian case study. *J Nurse-Midwifery* 42:499, 1997.
60. Snow L: Walkin' Over Medicine. San Francisco, Westview Press, 1992.
61. Flores C: Hispanic immigrants: Health care access and outcomes. In Bernstein E, Bernstein J (eds): *Case Studies in Emergency Medicine and the Health of the Public.* Boston, Jones & Bartlett, 1996.
62. West CM, Kantor GK, Jasinski JL: Sociodemographic predictors and cultural barriers to help-seeking behavior by Latina and Anglo American battered women. *Violence Vict* 13:361, 1998.
63. Jones DR, et al: Affective and physiological responses to racism: The roles of afrocentrism and mode of presentation. *Ethn Dis* 61:109, 1996.
64. Thornton MC, White-Means SI: Racial and ethnic patterns of hospital emergency department use. In Lillie-Blanton M, Leigh W (eds): *Achieving Equitable Access: Studies of Health Care Issues Affecting Hispanics and African Americans.* Washington, DC, University Press of America, 1996.
65. Flores G: Providing culturally competent pediatric care: Integrating pediatricians, institutions, families, and communities into the process. *J Pediatr* 143:1, 2003.
66. Scott CJ, Martin M, Hamilton G: Training of medical professionals and the delivery of health care as related to cultural identity groups. *Acad Emerg Med* 10:1149, 2003.
67. Goldstein E, et al: Intercultural medicine. In Jensen N, Van Kirk J (eds): A Curriculum for Internal Medicine Residency. Philadelphia, American College of Physicians, 1995.

CHAPTER 204

Process Improvement and Patient Safety in the Emergency Department

Pat Croskerry, Marc J. Shapiro, Shawna J. Perry, and Robert L. Wears

PERSPECTIVE

The overall process of patient care in the emergency department begins with the initial decision by the patient (or caregiver or family) to seek emergency assistance and ends with the patient's disposition and follow-up. The care process is highly complex, with many separate components, people, and interfaces with other processes in the health care organization (Figure 204-1). This complexity, among other things, provides many opportunities for process failures, "errors," and adverse outcomes. Although process failures in health care have been studied for decades,[1] most of that effort originated from outside of the field of health care,[1] and consequently health care professionals were largely unaware of it.

This began to change in the early 1990s, when the Harvard Medical Practice Study[2] reported that almost 4% of hospitalized patients suffered significant adverse events during their care, and that almost 30% of these were due to human "error." The study noted that failures in emergency department care accounted for only about 3% of all adverse events, but went on to estimate that more than 90% of adverse emergency department events were judged to be preventable (the highest proportion for any site of care). The study was replicated several years later, with roughly similar results.[3] These studies and others ultimately led the Institute of Medicine to issue a report in 1999 entitled *To Err Is Human: Building a Safer Health System*.[4] This report, unlike the previous studies, provoked the interest of the media and the general public and thrust the issue of safety in health care onto the national agenda. Although the report was controversial, its one great accomplishment was that it introduced some of the fundamental concepts regarding safety in complex systems into the world of health care for the first time. The most transforming concept was the idea that failures (or "errors") in care were not the result of bad decisions or bad individuals but were instead intrinsic properties of the processes of care in which health care professionals work. Thus, efforts to reduce these failures should be focused on changing the processes of care rather than identifying, retraining, or punishing the workers.

In the field of health care, the response to the Institute of Medicine report was mixed. Most health care professionals focused on the projected number of deaths due to "error," arguing that they were either too high[5,6] or too low[7], and a third, smaller group argued that the concept of "error" was essentially contestable, and thus an approach aimed at counting "errors" was fundamentally flawed.[8] Although the transforming concept of system failure was introduced, it has not been fully understood nor completely accepted, for several reasons. First, it is vague and complicated and goes against the natural human tendency to believe that individuals cause outcomes. Second, it smacks of irresponsibility and offends our sense of free agency, in that we would prefer not to view ourselves as trapped in a system moving inexorably toward a bad outcome. Nevertheless, emergency physicians have begun the long and difficult process of looking at our own practices, processes, and environments, using new tools from the "science of safety"[9] to improve our performance.

In emergency medicine, professional organizations have developed task forces, interest groups, or special sections on safety and quality to provide a focus for these activities. A basic curriculum for teaching about safety has been developed[10]; safety case reports have been instituted as a regular feature in an emergency medicine journal[11]; and some interesting lines of research on the processes of emergency care have begun. Chisholm[12] reported that emergency physicians are interrupted, on average, about once every 6 minutes, and that two thirds of those interruptions cause a change in task; this is important because both interruptions and task switching frequently lead to process failures. Coiera and colleagues[13] studied emergency physicians in Australia and reported high communication loads and similar levels of interruptions. Morey[14] reported that specific training of emergency physicians and nurses to work together in teams led to reductions in failures and improved performance. Wears[15] has noted ergonomic shortcomings in the workplace and pointed out their potential for contributing to failures in care. Fordyce[16] reported that self-detected errors occurred in almost 20% of all emergency department cases, but that only 2% were associated with adverse events. Fordyce's work emphasizes that errors are ubiquitous but only rarely combine with other factors to produce adverse events, and it supports the notion that focusing on eliminating errors is not likely to be a productive strategy for improvement.

SOURCES OF FAILURE IN EMERGENCY CARE

There are many characteristics of emergency medical practice that make it vulnerable to failures[14,17-24] (Table 204-1). This section focuses on some of the principal

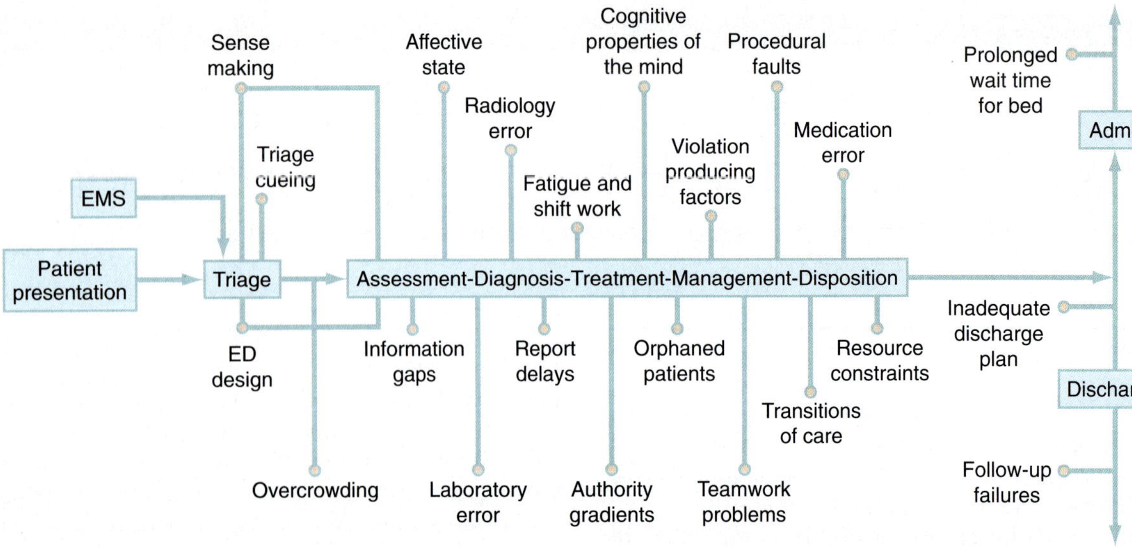

Figure 204-1. Process mapping showing sources of failures. The overall process is highly simplified and presented as a linear model of a patient's trajectory. (The actual process is much more complex, involving multiple simultaneous patients at different stages, and loops within a given patient's trajectory). Sources of failure may occur in parallel or at multiple stages in the sequence and are often additive in their overall effect on patient safety.

factors that contribute to adverse outcomes and how they might be better managed to improve safety.

Emergency Department Design/Human Factors and Ergonomics

Two frequently overlooked contributors to lowered safety in any work environment are the design of the workspace and the engineering of the tools and procedures used to do the work.[25] This is especially true for emergency departments, as the majority were not designed for the care actually being delivered there. Emergency department caregivers then adapt to the space by creating "work-arounds" to cope with the limitations and impediments.

The same process occurs with the tools, equipment, procedures, and protocols. There is rarely consistency in equipment across or between areas; for instance, the blood pressure monitor in the emergency department is often not the same type of model as that used in radiology. Additionally, the equipment is likely not to have a "user-centered design," and in-service training often lags behind the introduction of technology into the treatment area.

The contribution of poor design factors to the difficulty in maintaining safety in a health care environment is generally overlooked by staff; coping with these difficulties is generally accepted as "part of the job."[15] However, despite their best efforts, the coping ability of workers is finite and can be frittered away by a multitude of tiny failures, each of which diverts valuable time and attentional energy from that available to be spent on clinical issues. This increases the risk of a failure that may not seem directly linked to the workplace, the procedures, or the equipment.

Table 204-1. Characteristics of the Emergency Department that Affect Performance

Instrinic*	Extrinsic†
Human cognitive properties	High communication load
High levels of uncertainty	Poor teamwork
High decision density	Overcrowding
High cognitive load	Production pressures
Narrow windows of opportunity	High ambient noise levels
Multiple interruptions/distractions	Information gaps
Low signal-to-noise ratio‡	Report delays
Surge phenomena§	Inadequate staffing
Novel or infrequently occurring conditions	Poor feedback
Patient factors (e.g., language, delirium)	Inexperience
	Inadequate supervision
	Sleep deprivation/sleep debt
	Fatigue
	Multiple transitions of care
	Poorly designed procedures

**Instrinsic* factors are intimately part of the nature of emergency care, and as such are not amenable to change but instead must be compensated for.
†*Extrinsic* factors are in principle manageable and typically relate to resource constraints.
‡*Low signal to noise ratio* refers to the low likelihood of a critical diagnosis compared with a benign diagnosis for similarly presenting symptoms and findings (e.g., subarachnoid hemorrhage *vs* tension headache).
§*Surge phenomena* refers to the rapid changes in volume and acuity, routinely experienced in many EDs.

Overcrowding

Emergency department overcrowding has long been recognized as a major source of time-delay failures and a threat to patient safety.[26] It is important to understand that such delays are not simply an inconvenience to the patient but may give rise to significant adverse events.

For example, patients with atypical presentations for severe illnesses who have been mistriaged to low levels of acuity may experience inordinate and occasionally fatal delays. In other cases, such as community-acquired pneumonia, cellulitis, lacerations, and others, more expedient care may significantly improve the course of the illness. A significant proportion of patients who leave without being seen may have serious illness and incur delays in diagnosis and treatment. At the other end of the process, when the patient is ready for admission to the hospital from the emergency department, further time delay errors may occur (see Figure 204-1). Not only do such delays create throughput problems for the emergency department and contribute to front-end loading or "entry-block," they also give rise to discontinuities in care and may lead to adverse events. Recently, the problem of overcrowding has been recognized by the Joint Commission on Accreditation of Healthcare Organizations, and a new leadership standard has been issued, effective January 2005.[27] Specifically, the standard will require hospital leadership to measure crowding and patient flow problems regularly and to develop measures to address them, but provides little specific guidance.

Information Gaps

Missing information is common in emergency care and can significantly affect quality of care.[28] Hospital records, especially discharge summaries, details of past medical history, and other important information is often difficult to access in an expedient fashion. Even referral notes sent in by family doctors with the patient may not reach the emergency physician. Emergency physicians must then sometimes act on the basis of incomplete or erroneous information and become used to doing so, so that information is sometimes not even sought when it might have been retrieved.

Performance Shaping Factors

Blaming individuals for "errors" in the emergency department contributes little to an understanding of risk, vulnerability, and failure. A wide variety of ambient, systemic conditions in the emergency department contribute to the majority of adverse events and near-misses that occur (see Table 204-1). Some performance shaping factors can be considered to be "intrinsic," part and parcel of the milieu of emergency medicine and thus not amenable to direct control. These factors must be managed by strategies of buffering or mitigating their effects. In contrast, other "extrinsic" performance shaping factors typically reflect limitations of resources. When resources are limited, a trade-off can occur in the ability of the emergency department to provide safety and quality in patient care. This condition is referred to as RACQITO (Resource Availability Continuous Quality Improvement Trade-Off),[29] a concept derived from speed–accuracy trade-offs described in industrial settings.

BOX 204-1. Violation-Producing Factors

Gender
Mood
Ill-health
Risk seeking/risk aversion
Normalization of deviance
Maladaptive group pressures (group-think)
Maladaptive copying behavior
Underconfidence/overconfidence
Perceived authorization to deviate
Authority gradient effects (obeying authority figure or absence of disapproving authority figure)
Likelihood of detection

Based on an original schema by Williams,[64] adapted for emergency medicine by Croskerry and Wears.[20] A summary can also be found in Reason.[30]

Violation Producing Factors

While at first one might think that violations of organizational policies, rules, and procedures would always be culpable causes of failures and adverse events, the modern approach to safety has pointed out that some violations are actually necessary for the safe functioning of the system, and others fall somewhere in between.[30] Aside from recklessness, drug use on the job, moral failings, and other egregious acts, research in other domains has identified factors that are associated with rule and safety violations (Box 204-1). Fluctuations in mood can occur for a variety of reasons and will result in inconsistent clinical performance; males are more likely to break safety rules and engage in more risk-taking behavior than females.[30] Risk-seeking and risk-averse attitudes have been associated aspects of decision making in the emergency department.[31] The "normalization of deviance"[32] is an accumulated tolerance of small variances from safe operating conditions that develops over time and ultimately compromises safety. The effects of perceived authority can lead to violations, either through the absence of a disapproving authority, a directive supporting violation from an authority figure, or from an individual's self-perception that he or she is authorized to disregard or deviate from prescribed procedures.

Teamwork

Good teamwork is essential to the safe practice of emergency medicine, but emergency caregivers are not trained or evaluated as teams. Teamwork training in other fields, such as aviation, has been successful in reducing failures related to poor communication, authority gradients (both within and between professions), and cross-monitoring.[33] Work on transferring teamwork training principles into emergency medicine has suggested that teamwork failures were involved in roughly 40% of malpractice cases.[34] The lack of cross-monitoring team members and the failure of advocacy or assertion of corrective actions were two of the most frequent factors identified. A multidisciplinary teamwork training course showed a significant improvement in quality of team behaviors and a sixfold decrease in observed clinical errors.[14] Teamwork is not a specific fix for any one type of error but should be viewed as an adaptable human factors program with a set of teachable skills and behaviors capable of increasing system resilience, a hallmark of high-reliability organizations.

Teamwork training requires a change of culture, which can be difficult for emergency department staff. Institutional and emergency department leadership must be fully committed to process before implementing teamwork training for all staff. Resistance on the part of senior clinicians to behavioral change is likely to be encountered, and it will be necessary to demonstrate the clinical relevance of this training. High-fidelity medical simulation supported by audiovisual feedback offers the educational methodology to help clinicians see the necessity of behavioral change. Audiovisual debriefing of simulation scenarios is a powerful educational methodology to motivate behavioral change and improve teamwork.[35] A major unanswered question is how to embed teamwork behaviors into medical training and how to sustain the behaviors over time.

Authority Gradients

Almost all human groups have some form of authority gradient among their members. This can be based on profession (doctors have greater authority than nurses), organizational rank (attending physicians have more authority than residents) or a variety of less relevant factors. Ideally, information between team members should flow freely, but this may not occur if low-authority members are inhibited by differences in seniority, stature, expertise, profession, or social status. There are clear examples of cases in which authority gradients have been responsible for adverse events.[36] A cultural change is required to create an atmosphere in which all team members feel comfortable expressing their viewpoint, especially if it is a dissenting one, and one in which authority figures have the ability to recognize the value of perspectives other than their own, to the extent that they elicit, rather than merely accept, alternative views. Senior clinicians are in a powerful position to bridge gradients through the use of clinical narratives from their own experience that illustrate errors and judgment failures.[37]

Cognitive Properties of the Mind

The human mind has characteristic dispositions to respond to particular stimuli and contexts in specific ways. A great deal of effort has gone into identifying and describing these; more than 30 *cognitive dispositions to respond* have been described.[17] A number of strategies have been proposed to reduce the adverse outcomes associated with cognitive dispositions to respond.[38]

The overall process of patient care in the emergency department is driven by a process of making clinical sense out of multiple sets of fragmented, tangential, and interrupted stimuli. This is aimed at making an accurate diagnosis if possible, or if not (more commonly), a useful framing of the problem, which in turn determines management and disposition. Although many diagnoses, such as lacerations, dislocations, fractures, and foreign bodies, are self-evident, others (chest pain, fever, headache, abdominal pain) are often associated with high levels of diagnostic uncertainty and are more likely to lead to problems. Cognitive biases can frequently be identified in retrospect following diagnostic failures,[39] but the problem of hindsight bias makes this identification problematic.[40]

In addition to cognitive mental properties, the emotional state of the physician can affect his or her decision making; this has been referred to as *visceral bias*.[17] To date, relatively little attention has been directed at the important role of affective bias in decision making. Although processes such as countertransference, fundamental attribution error,[29] and, in particular, the economy of perception that underlies stereotyping are well understood in psychology, health care workers are typically less aware of them in their own work. It is important, too, to recognize that health care workers are as vulnerable to psychiatric illness as anyone else. Emotional dysregulation and other affective or psychiatric disorders should be promptly detected by supervisors and appropriate support and follow-up arranged.

Fatigue and Shift Work

Both fatigue and shift work contribute to performance failures,[41] but relatively little research has been directed at their respective impacts on clinical performance in the unique milieu of the emergency department. Although the two are often considered together, they are different entities and exert both qualitatively and quantitatively different effects on performance.[42] Fatigue has a number of determinants separate from those associated with shift work (Figure 204-2).

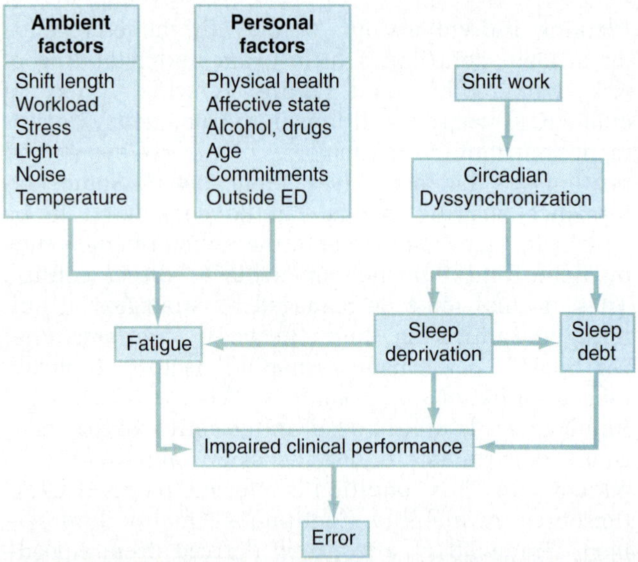

Figure 204-2. Relationships between shift work, fatigue, and performance.

Performance declines as work hours increase,[43] but the optimal shift length in the emergency department is unknown and difficult to delineate for several reasons. The relationship with workload or acuity is not well appreciated, and some workers exhibit perverse incentives, for example preferring to work longer shifts in order to get more days off. More recovery time between shifts might be expected to enhance job performance, but these issues remain relatively unexplored. A survey of emergency physicians found a preference for 8-hour over 12-hour shifts,[44] but it is not known whether job satisfaction in the emergency department translates into improved clinical performance and fewer adverse events. Other ambient conditions within the emergency department, competing commitments outside the emergency department, age, ill-health, and other factors all contribute to fatigue.

Shift work has extensive, well-documented, detrimental effects on health[45] that, in turn, have an impact on well-being and job performance. Importantly, it leads to disruption of circadian rhythms that inevitably result in sleep deprivation. Circadian dyssynchronicity largely occurs through missing sleep in the *anchor period*, approximately midway through the sleep phase when core temperature and arousal level are at their lowest. It has been stated that the performance degradation of someone who has been up all night is roughly equal to that of person with a blood alcohol level of 0.1%[46] (Box 204-2).

The acute effects of sleep deprivation are well known, but the chronic effects are less appreciated. Invariably, working a night shift results in less sleep the following day, and subsequent sleep is often disrupted and fragmented in the struggle to restore the circadian rhythm before the night-shift cycle repeats itself. This results in the accumulation of a *sleep debt* that has a significant impact on performance. A study of anesthesia residents on a normal work schedule, with no on-call duty in the preceding 48 hours, showed daytime sleepiness scores comparable to those of patients with narcolepsy or sleep apnea.[47] The on-call schedule of these subjects (five periods per month) entailed considerably less sleep deprivation and fragmentation than an average emergency physician's schedule. Increasing age is associated with decreased tolerance for sleep deprivation.[48]

The appropriate management of shift work and fatigue to improve patient safety is not well understood, and further research is needed in this area. The specialty as a whole has yet to address it collectively. In most high-hazard industries, the assumption is that fatigue and long, aberrant work hours lead to poor performance, and the burden of proof is in the hands of those who believe that such work practices are safe. In the health care industry, concerns over discontinuity of care and difficulties in changing medical culture have pushed the burden of proof into the hands of those who wish to change the status quo. Given that medical personnel, like all human beings, function suboptimally when fatigued, efforts to reduce fatigue and sleepiness should be undertaken, and the burden of proof should be in the hands of the advocates of the current system to demonstrate that it is safe.[49] In the meantime, shift scheduling should be optimized to reduce the impact of circadian disruption, and emergency department personnel should practice good sleep hygiene. Some basic approaches have been reviewed (Box 204-3).[43,45]

BOX 204-2. Effects of Sleep Deprivation[46]

- Longer reaction time
- Lapses in attention or concentration
- Lost information
- Errors of omission
- Poor short-term memory
- Poor mood (increased confusion, stress, and irritability)
- Reduced motivation
- Distractibility
- Sleepiness
- Poor psychomotor performance:
  - at circadian low points
  - when sedentary
  - on long, difficult, or externally paced tasks
  - with no feedback
  - in unchanging surroundings, particularly with reduced light or sound, or with low motivation, interest, or novelty

BOX 204-3. Rational Approaches to Shift Work[43,45]

- Optimize circadian-friendly schedules
  - Forward rotating (clockwise with circadian rhythms)
  - Rapid changes
  - Minimize consecutive nights (1 or 2)
  - 24 to 48 hours off after nights
  - Allow social time, including some weekends
  - 8-hour shifts (absolute maximum 12 h)
  - Institute regular, predictable template
- Employ proper sleep hygiene
  - Use a sleep-friendly room: room-darkening blinds, white noise or earplugs, no phones, family aware
  - Maintain a regular sleep routine
  - Try anchor sleep
  - Avoid caffeine, alcohol, and drugs
  - Prophylactic naps
- Modulate circadian rhythms
  - Exercise
  - Consider bright light
- Eat healthy
  - Eat a balanced diet
  - Avoid junk food
  - Keep regular mealtimes
- Promote a healthy life and work style
  - Promote a personal healthy lifestyle
  - Educate friends and family about shift work issues
  - Educate colleagues about shift work issues
  - Advocate for department improvements in working conditions
  - Advocate for shift worker friendly community services
- Avoid pharmaceuticals
  - Use caffeine in moderation, prn
  - Do not use sedatives or stimulants
  - Avoid alcohol before sleep

PROBLEM AREAS IN EMERGENCY CARE

Certain processes in emergency care are generally held to be common sources of failure. These problem areas include triage, technical procedures, transitions in patient care, orphaned patients, laboratory and radiographic tests, and medications.

Triage

The point of entry of all patients into the emergency department is through triage. Triage is, by definition, an abbreviated decision making process and can never be completely safe. Illness and injury have a variety of presentations that will occasionally be atypical or otherwise misleading. An additional problem is that there is a low "signal to noise" ratio for a number of serious conditions (i.e., when the incidence of a serious condition is far exceeded by that for a benign condition, but their clinical presentations are similar). Inevitably, the triage process involves trade-offs between sensitivity and specificity. Under-triage for a particular patient would have a greater potential for an adverse event than over-triage, whereas over-triage affects resource utilization and may have an impact on the care of other patients.

The predominant triage system in the United States involves three levels, categorizing patients into emergency, urgent, or nonurgent. This system tends to have a higher rate of under-triage when compared to a five-level system.[35] Australia, Canada, and the United Kingdom have adopted national five-level systems with improved intra- and inter-rater reliability. A five-level triage system, the Emergency Severity Index has since been developed in the United States, with excellent inter-rater reliability.[50] None of the five-level triage systems have shown consistency with children.

Triage assessments are important contributors to process failures and adverse events. Beyond treatment delays, which can occur with under-triage or be produced by over-triage, an incorrect assessment may be the triggering event that initiates a chain of failures. Geography can become destiny, and an inappropriate triage to a specific treatment area may create a bias in the treating clinician's mind.

Technical Procedures

Patients who require a procedure in the emergency department tend to be at greater risk of adverse events.[16] Since some critical procedures are rarely required (e.g., cricothyrotomy), the acquisition and especially the maintenance of a requisite level of skill is an important problem in emergency medicine. Simulation techniques have considerable potential here[51] but require both capital and human investment to be effective.

Transitions in Patient Care

The need for 24-hour access to care and the fragmented nature of health care delivery requires the occurrence of transitions of care between providers, either within the emergency department (at shift changes) or between the emergency department and other care areas (when patients are admitted, transferred, or discharged).

The emergency department shift "sign-over" or "handoff" is generally thought of as a communication activity performed for the transfer of clinical information, but it also embodies the transfer of responsibility and authority from one emergency department provider to another. The sign-over also conveys general situational awareness (e.g., the state of the department, hospital, city) and provides a forum for reviewing decision making and treatment plans. At present, there has been little study of these transitions of care, despite their ubiquity and importance to the specialty.[52] Sign-overs are highly variable in their content, the number of individuals involved, the physical configuration (e.g., walking, stationary, at bedside), the tools utilized to facilitate the transition (e.g., white boards, medical records, written notes), and length of the transition process. Although widely regarded as providing a major contribution to adverse events, sign-overs also provide an opportunity for review of decision making by clinicians and have been documented as opportunities for recovery by bringing "fresh eyes" to a patient's case.[18,52]

Studies of sign-overs in the emergency department are currently in their infancy. Some potential threats to high-quality transitions have been identified, but a clear understanding of how to minimize these threats has not yet been established, although some common sense approaches seem obvious. Problem areas include the following:

- Interruptions during the turnover (e.g., phone calls, sidebar conversations) can cause a loss of focus and lead to the omission of important information.
- Lack of consistent structure to the turn-over. While the traditional case presentation narrative is generally followed (chief complaint, history, physical examination, initial laboratory results, impression, plan), the case presentation format does not automatically remind participants of pending or as yet uncompleted tasks.
- Patients are commonly "marked" in ways that can sometimes be helpful but sometimes is harmful, especially for at-risk groups such as the homeless, psychiatric patients, alcoholics, or drug abusers.

Orphaned Patients

Orphaned patients are those who have suffered temporary loss or diminished supervision or accountability for their care. This may occur at several stages in the process. Patients who are seen and assessed at triage and then wait in the waiting area are temporarily orphaned. Those who are brought in by paramedics sometimes remain on stretchers for hours before being admitted to the emergency department. The well-being of these patients critically depends on the efficacy of initial assessment and on judicious interval reassessment by the triage nurse. With prolonged wait times, occult conditions can mature to serious and potentially catastrophic levels. Patients who leave without being seen or before treatment is completed have "orphaned" themselves. Patients may be temporarily orphaned out of the emergency department for radiographic studies or other special tests. Occasionally, patients get "lost in the shuffle" and are overlooked at shift change, or they may get "lost" after one or more consultations with other services. A significant cause of orphaning in some emergency department is when no beds are available for admitted patients. In such cases, patients may be put in holding areas in or adjacent to the emergency department and have been known to languish for days, receiving sporadic care from a succession of caregivers who know increasingly less about their condition.

Laboratory

The interface between the emergency department and its ancillary services is critically important. Failures can occur at three phases of laboratory's process. Preanalytic errors mostly occur through inappropriate collection of specimens: technique, timing, and identification of both patient and specimen. Analytic errors refer to those that arise directly from the testing process within the laboratory. Postanalytic errors occur after the test result has been obtained and take the form of keyboard entry errors; excessive turn-around time; data that have been overlooked, have been lost, or fail to reach the physician; and clinical misinterpretation of the data. A blood bank study found that the majority of failures occurred in the pre- and postanalytic stages, with less than 5% in the analytic stage.[53] Overall, the laboratory defect rate is less than 1%, but the number of exposures is very large. Of the failures that do occur, up to 50% may have a moderate, and up to 8%, a severe, impact on patient care.[54]

Radiology

Radiographic imaging is a critical aspect of diagnosis and management in the emergency department. Although patient identification and wrong-side problems are important, the majority of failures lie in interpretation. Assuming the radiologist's interpretation to be the criterion standard, the rate of errors in interpretation by emergency department physicians and residents may be as high as 16% for plain radiographs and more than double that for computed tomography scans.[55] Clearly, not all misinterpretations are consequential, and emergency physicians typically seek the advice of the radiologist when they recognize difficult interpretations, but the majority of hospitals do not have continuous on-site coverage by radiologists. Prompt review of all films by a radiologist will detect significant errors, but effective procedures are required to ensure timely and appropriate follow-up. Programs of focused feedback and review have been effective in substantially reducing the rate of clinically important misinterpretations.[56]

Medications

Medication errors constitute the largest proportion of failures in most general studies, with failures occurring in all six steps of the process (prescription, transcription, dispensing, administration, monitoring, discharge).[57] In many situations, emergency departments take on the dispensing role, obviating input from the pharmacy, where many errors are corrected. In addition, team communication errors can contribute to many failures: missed medications, wrong medications, and duplicate dosing. Pediatric patients are at higher risk; drug errors are no more common than in adults, but they are typically more serious.[58,59]

The presence of a pharmacist on the clinical team has been shown to reduce medication errors in several settings.[60] There is great interest in the potential for computer technologies, such as bar-coding or computerized physician order entry, to enhance medication safety, but despite some successful demonstrations, widespread implementation has not occurred, and some practitioners fear that such systems will introduce new problems to replace old ones.[61] In addition, the Institute for Safe Medication Practices has recommended certain problematic practices be avoided in writing orders or prescriptions,[62] and the Joint Commission on Accreditation of Healthcare Organizations has incorporated those recommendations into its standards (Table 204-2). Success in this area will require more

Table 204-2. Abbreviations and Notations to Avoid[62]

Abbreviation or Notation	Correction	Reason
AU	each ear	mistaken for OU
DC or D/C	discharge or discontinue	confusion between two definitions
HCTZ	hydrochlorthiazide	mistaken for hydrocortisone 250
$MgSO_4$	magnesium sulfate	mistaken for morphine sulfate
MSO_4	morphine sulfate	mistaken for magnesium sulfate
µg	microgram	mistaken for "mg" when written
qd, qid, qod	daily, 4 times/day, or every other day	mutually confused
qhs	nightly or at bedtime	mistaken for "qh"
OD	once daily	mistaken for OD (oculus dexter)
U	units	mistaken for a zero (4U seen as 40)
IU	units	mistaken for "IV"
cc	mL	mistaken for "U" (units)
no leading zero (.5 mg)	use leading zeros for decimal doses (0.5 mg)	decimal point missed (read as "5 mg")
trailing zero (5.0 mg)	avoid trailing zero for whole number doses (5 mg)	decimal point missed (read as "50 mg")
name letters and dose numbers too close (inderal 40 mg)	leave large space between name and dose	misread as "inderal 140 mg"

than just individual attentiveness; nurses, unit secretaries, and pharmacists will have to feel comfortable challenging improper usage by physicians.

CONCLUSION

Safely managing patients in the emergency department depends on a multiplicity of processes. All appear vulnerable to failure, yet all have the potential for improvement through judicious process management. Efforts by front-line workers will not be sufficient, and so considerable effort will be required at the "blunt end" of the system.[63] The number and complexity of emergency department processes requires a conscious awareness and understanding of process management, and emergency departments may benefit from personnel specifically trained in this regard.

Safety in complex, dynamic environments such as emergency departments is itself dynamic. It is a "non-event," since it is the absence of things that should not occur anyway. It cannot be banked for future use but is dynamically created by emergency department workers in a well-designed and supportive organizational environment. Achieving safe performance in such settings is analogous to fighting a guerilla war: there are no dramatic victories, but there are occasional horrific defeats, and there is no end in sight. Success will require constancy of purpose, a willingness to adopt new ideas and tools from outside of health care, and continued effort and investment.

REFERENCES

1. Bosk C: *Forgive and Remember: Managing Medical Failure.* Chicago, University of Chicago Press, 1979.
2. Brennan TA, et al: Incidence of adverse events and negligence in hospitalized patients. Results of the Harvard Medical Practice Study I. *N Engl J Med* 324:370, 1991.
3. Studdert DM, et al: Negligent care and malpractice claiming behavior in Utah and Colorado. *Med Care* 38:250, 2000.
4. Kohn LT, Corrigan JM, Donaldson MS (eds): *To Err is Human: Building a Safer Health System.* Washington, DC, National Academy Press, 1999.
5. McDonald CJ, Weiner M, Hui SL: Deaths due to medical errors are exaggerated in institute of medicine report. *JAMA* 284:93, 2000.
6. Dunn JD, Wears RL: The November Special Issue on Errors [letter]. *Acad Emerg Med* 8:686, 2001.
7. Leape LL: Institute of medicine medical error figures are not exaggerated. *JAMA* 284:95, 2000.
8. Wears RL: Beyond error. *Acad Emerg Med* 7:1175, 2000.
9. Wears RL: The science of safety. In Zipperer L (ed): *Lessons in Patient Safety.* Chicago, National Patient Safety Foundation, 2001.
10. Cosby KS, Croskerry P: Patient safety: A curriculum for teaching patient safety in emergency medicine. *Acad Emerg Med* 10:69, 2003.
11. Croskerry P, Shapiro MJ: "Profiles in patient safety": A new feature. *Acad Emerg Med* 9:324, 2002.
12. Chisholm CD, Collison EK, Nelson DR, Cordell WH: Emergency department work place interruptions: Are emergency physicians multi-tasking or interrupt driven? *Acad Emerg Med* 7:1239, 2000.
13. Coiera EW, et al: Communication loads on clinical staff in the emergency department. *Med J Aust* 176:415, 2002.
14. Morey JC, et al: Error reduction and performance improvement in the emergency department through teamwork training: Evaluation results of the MedTeams project. *Health Serv Res* 37:1553, 2002.
15. Wears RL, Perry SJ: Human factors and ergonomics in the emergency department. *Ann Emerg Med* 40:206, 2002.
16. Fordyce J, et al: Errors in a busy emergency department. *Ann Emerg Med* 42:324, 2003.
17. Croskerry P: Achieving quality in clinical decision making: Cognitive strategies and detection of bias. *Acad Emerg Med* 9:1184, 2002.
18. Beach C, Croskerry P, Shapiro M: Profiles in patient safety: Emergency care transitions. *Acad Emerg Med* 10:364, 2003.
19. Chisholm CD, Pencek AM, Cordell WH, Nelson DR: Interruptions and task performance in emergency departments compared with primary care offices. *Acad Emerg Med* 5:470, 1998.
20. Croskerry PG, Wears RL: Safety in Emergency Medicine. In Markovchick V, Pons P (eds): *Emergency Medicine Secrets,* 3rd ed. Philadelphia, Hanley and Belfus, 2003.
21. Gaba DM, Howard SK: Patient safety: Fatigue among clinicians and the safety of patients. *N Engl J Med* 347:1249, 2002.
22. Derlet R, Richards J, Kravitz R: Frequent overcrowding in U.S. emergency departments. *Acad Emerg Med* 8:151, 2001.
23. Stiell A, Forster AJ, Stiell IG, van Walraven C: Prevalence of information gaps in the emergency department and the effect on patient outcomes. *CMAJ* 169:1023, 2003.
24. Croskerry P: The feedback sanction. *Acad Emerg Med* 7:1232, 2000.
25. Gosbee J: Human factors engineering and patient safety. *Qual Saf Health Care* 11:352, 2002.
26. Richardson LD, Asplin BR, Lowe RA: Emergency department crowding as a health policy issue: past development, future directions. *Ann Emerg Med* 40:388, 2002.
27. New Leadership Standard on Managing Patient Flow for Hospitals. Available at http://www.ed-qual.com/News/JCAHO_Patient_Flow_Standard.htm. Accessed April 7, 2004.
28. Stiell IG, et al: The Canadian CT Head Rule for patients with minor head injury. *Lancet* 357:1391, 2001.
29. Croskerry P: The cognitive imperative: Thinking about how we think. *Acad Emerg Med* 7:1223, 2000.
30. Reason J: *Managing the Risks of Organizational Accidents.* Aldershot, UK, Ashgate Publishing Co, 1997.
31. Pearson SD, et al: Triage decisions for emergency department patients with chest pain: Do physicians' risk attitudes make the difference? *J Gen Intern Med* 10:557, 1995.
32. Vaughan D: *The Challenger Launch Decision: Risky Technology, Culture and Deviance at NASA.* Chicago, University of Chicago Press, 1996.
33. Helmreich RL, Merritt AC: *Culture at Work in Aviation and Medicine.* Aldershot, UK, Ashgate, 1998.
34. Risser DT, et al: The potential for improved teamwork to reduce medical errors in the emergency department. The MedTeams Research Consortium. *Ann Emerg Med* 34:373, 1999.
35. Small SD, et al: Demonstration of high-fidelity simulation team training for emergency medicine. *Acad Emerg Med* 6:312, 1999.
36. Vincent C: Hemivulvectomy: The wrong side removed. Available at http://www.webmm.ahrq.gov/spotlightcases.aspx?ic=33 (Accessed October 23, 2003).
37. Chisholm CD, Croskerry P: A case study in medical error: The use of the portfolio entry. *Acad Emerg Med* 11:388, 2004.
38. Croskerry P: Cognitive forcing strategies in clinical decision making. *Ann Emerg Med* 41:110, 2003.
39. Graber M, Gordon R, Franklin N: Reducing diagnostic errors in medicine: What's the goal? *Acad Med* 77:981, 2002.

40. Henriksen K, Kaplan H: Hindsight bias, outcome knowledge and adaptive learning. *Qual Saf Health Care* 12:46ii, 2003.
41. Miller DP, Swain AD: Human error and human reliability. In Salvendy G (ed): *Handbook of Human Factors.* New York, Wiley, 1986, p 219.
42. Dodge R: Circadian rhythms and fatigue: A discrimination of their effects on performance. *Aviat Space Environ Med* 53:1131, 1982.
43. Jha AK, Duncan BW, Bates DW: Fatigue, sleepiness, and medical errors. In *Making Health Care Safer: A Critical Analysis of Patient Safety Practices.* Evidence Report/Technology Assessment No. 43; AHRQ Publication 01-E058. Rockville, MD, Agency for Healthcare Research and Quality, 2001. Available at http://www.ahcpr.gov/clinic/ptsafety/chap46a.htm.
44. Thomas H Jr, Schwartz E, Whitehead DC: Eight- versus 12-hour shifts: Implications for emergency physicians. *Ann Emerg Med* 23:1096, 1994.
45. Frank JR: Shiftwork and emergency medicine practice. *Can J Emerg Med* 4:421, 2002.
46. Bonnet MH: Sleep deprivation. In Kryger M, Roth T, Dement WC (eds): *Principles and Practice of Sleep Medicine.* Philadelphia, WB Saunders, 2000.
47. Howard SK: Sleep deprivation and fatigue: Are we sleepy people keeping people asleep? *CSA Bulletin* 49(1), 2000.
48. Reid K, Dawson D: Comparing performance on a simulated 12 hour shift rotation in young and older subjects. *Occup Environ Med* 58:58, 2001.
49. Gaba DM: Physician work hours: The "sore thumb" of organizational safety in tertiary health care. In *Proceedings of the Second Annenberg Conference on Enhancing Patient Safety and Reducing Errors in Health Care.* Rancho Mirago, CA, National Patient Safety Foundation; 1998, p 142.
50. Tanabe P, Gimbel R, Yarnold PR, Adams JG: The Emergency Severity Index (version 3) 5-level triage system scores predict ED resource consumption. *J Emerg Nurs* 30:22, 2004.
51. Jha AK, Duncan BW, Bates DW: Simulator-based training and patient safety. In *Making Health Care Safer: A Critical Analysis of Patient Safety Practices.* Evidence Report/Technology Assessment No. 43; AHRQ Publication 01-E058. Rockville, MD, Agency for Healthcare Research and Quality, 2001. Available at http://www.ahcpr.gov/clinic/ptsafety/chap45.htm (Accessed April 1, 2004).
52. Wears RL, et al: Shift changes among emergency physicians: Best of times, worst of times. In *Proceedings of the Human Factors and Ergonomics Society 47th Annual Meeting.* Denver, CO, Human Factors and Ergonomics Society, 2003, p 1420.
53. Boone DJ, et al: Transfusion medicine monitoring practices: A study of the College of American Pathologists/Centers for Disease Control and Prevention Outcomes Working Group. *Arch Pathol Lab Med* 119:999, 1995.
54. Bonini P, Plebani M, Ceriotti F, Rubboli F: Errors in laboratory medicine. *Clin Chem* 48:691, 2002.
55. Kripalani S, Williams MV, Rask K: Reducing errors in the interpretation of plain radiographs and computed tomography scans. In Making Health Care Safer: A Critical Analysis of Patient Safety Practices. Evidence Report/Technology Assessment No. 43; AHRQ Publication 01-E058. Rockville, MD, Agency for Healthcare Research and Quality, 2001. Available at http://www.ahcpr.gov/clinic/ptsafety/chap35.htm.
56. Espinosa JA, Nolan TW: Reducing errors made by emergency physicians in interpreting radiographs: Longitudinal study. *BMJ* 320:737, 2000.
57. Croskerry P, et al: Profiles in patient safety: Medication errors in the emergency department. *Acad Emerg Med* 11:289, 2004.
58. Selbst SM, Fein JA, Osterhoudt K, Ho W: Medication errors in a pediatric emergency department. *Pediatr Emerg Care* 15:1, 1999.
59. Kaushal R, et al: Medication errors and adverse drug events in pediatric inpatients. *JAMA* 285:2114, 2001.
60. American Society of Health-systems Pharmacists: Top-priority actions for preventing adverse drug events in hospitals. Recommendations of an expert panel. *Am J Health Syst Pharm* 53:747, 1996.
61. Ash JS, Berg M, Coiera E: Some unintended consequences of information technology in health care: The nature of patient care information system-related errors. *J Am Med Inform Assoc* 11:104, 2004.
62. Abbreviations to Avoid. *ISMP Medication Safety Alert* 6:1, 2001.
63. Turnbull JE: Process management and systems thinking for patient safety. *J Innovative Management* 7:5, 2001.
64. Williams JC: Assessing and reducing the likelihood of violation behaviour—preliminary investigation. In *Proceedings of an International Conference on the Commercial and Operations Benefits of Probabilistic Safety Assessments.* Edinburgh, Institute of Nuclear Engineers, 1997.

Section II **PHILOSOPHICAL ISSUES OF PRACTICE**

CHAPTER 205 Bioethics

Kenneth V. Iserson

WHAT IS BIOETHICS?

Ethics is the application of values and moral rules to human activities. *Bioethics* is a subsection of ethics that uses ethical principles and decision making to solve actual or anticipated dilemmas in medicine and biology. Bioethics seeks to find reasoned and defensible solutions to the moral problems clinicians face.

Bioethics and professional etiquette are two distinct bodies of values and standards. Bioethics deals with relationships between practitioners and patients, practitioners and society, and society and patients. Professional etiquette specifically relates to standards governing the relationships and interactions between practitioners. Although the two areas occasionally overlap, they rely on different standards, values, and methods of solving problems.

Some of the problem areas specifically within the realm of professional etiquette include billing, referrals, advertising, competition, conflicts of interest, professional courtesy, employment and supervision of auxiliary personnel, use of secret remedies and exclusive methods, and the location and appearance of an office, emergency department, or urgent care center. These are quite different from the basic moral values and patient-centered issues that are the concerns of bioethics.

LAW VERSUS ETHICS

It is said that good ethics makes good law, but good law does not necessarily make good ethics. Since societal values are incorporated both within the law and within ethical principles and decisions, how does bioethics differ from law? Laws are rules of conduct established by legislatures, administrative agencies, courts, or other governing bodies. They often vary from locale to locale and are enforceable in the jurisdiction where they prevail. Ethics incorporates the broad values and beliefs of correct conduct. Although bioethical principles do not change because of geography (at least not within one culture), interpretation of the principles may evolve as societies change. The same evolution occurs within the law. One example is the issue of elective abortion, which, although once illegal in most U.S. jurisdictions, is now legal in most circumstances and jurisdictions. All of the underlying ethical principles do not have universal support, just as the values implicit in many of these legal changes have divided U.S. society.

Significant overlap exists between legal and ethical decision making. Frequently there is concurrence on basic issues. On occasion, clarity within the law can lead to clearer thinking in bioethics (and vice versa). Both law and bioethics, for example, use the term *rights,* as in "patients' rights" and "the right to die." This term, often used to advance an ethical argument about medical care, is frequently misunderstood or applied erroneously. A legal right is a demand that a person can make on another person (*in personam* rights) or a claim against the state for recognition and enforcement of this demand (*in rem* rights). Most rights involved in bioethical discussion are *in rem* rights. These generally are negative rights because they entail someone else's duty to refrain from doing something. Occasionally, as in the case of the right of an accident victim to be helped by bystanders, there is a positive right—a right to another person's positive actions. A common source of ethical conflict is between active rights, rights to act or not act as one chooses, and passive rights, rights to not be acted upon by others in certain ways. This often produces dilemmas because of conflicts between the rights of liberty and safety.[1] One conflict in both law and ethics is the question of the presence of absolute rights, which would be complete, without exception, and unconditional, such as those espoused by Locke or present in the Constitution's Bill of Rights. The issue has been hotly debated over the years in the U.S. Supreme Court and in the ethical literature.[2]

Without a Duty to Act, There Can Be No Rights

Both a moral and a logical correlation exist between the rights and the duties of individuals; one cannot exist in the absence of the other. In general, a duty is an action required by the rights of others, by law, by higher authority, or by conscience.[2] This obligation to act can be based on an individual's personal values, professional position, or other commitment.[3] For the physician, this duty to act is a role responsibility, at least when holding oneself out as a physician, and possibly at all times. The role-duty link occurs "whenever a person occupies a distinctive place or office in a social organization, to which specific duties are attached to provide for the welfare of others or to advance in some specific way the aims or purposes of the organization."[4] In this circumstance, performance is not predicated on a guarantee of compensation but on a concern for another person's welfare.[5] The emergency physician has just such a duty.

Modern bioethics developed during the last four decades because the law has often remained silent, inconsistent, or morally wrong on matters vital to the biomedical community. The rapid increase in biotechnology, the failure of both the legal system and the legislatures to deal with new and pressing issues, and the increasing liability crisis drove the medical community to seek answers to some of the difficult questions practitioners were having to work through on a daily basis. In some instances, practitioners thought that laws governing their practice were wrong because they failed to acknowledge relevant moral principles. These concerns came at a time when the Western world, especially the United States, began turning away from a uniform reliance on religious values and turning toward more generic secular values for answers. The medical community was no exception. Several generally accepted values emerged that have guided ethical thinking and been instrumental in forming health care policies in the United States and other Western countries during the past three decades.

VALUES

Values are the standards by which human behavior is judged and are acquired from indoctrination into our birth culture. These values are learned, usually at an early age, from observing behavior and through secular (including professional) and religious education. Although many of these learned values overlap, each source often claims moral superiority over the others, whether the values are generic and cultural, legal norms, religious and philosophical traditions, or professional principles.[6] Societal institutions incorporate and promulgate values, often attempting to solidify old values even in a changing society. In a pluralistic society, clinicians who treat individuals having multiple and differing value systems must be sensitive to others' beliefs and traditions.

Although each individual is entitled and perhaps even required to have a personal system of values, certain values have become generally accepted by the medical community, courts, legislatures, and society at large. Autonomy and individual dignity are two such values that have been considered fundamental and are often given overriding importance. Although some groups disagree about each of the generally accepted values, this dissension has not affected their application to medical care.

Societal and Professional Values

The basic tenet taught to all medical students is nonmaleficence: "First, do no harm." This credo, often stated in the Latin form, *primum non nocere,* derives from knowing that patient encounters with physicians can harm as well as help. With the physician's fallibility recognized, patient autonomy is and has been for the past three decades the overriding professional and societal bioethical value. Patient autonomy means recognizing an adult individual's right to accept or reject recommendations for medical care (even to the extent of refusing all care) if capable of appropriate decision making. It is the counterweight to the medical profession's long-practiced paternalism (or parentalism) wherein the practitioner determined what was "good" for the patient, regardless of whether the patient agreed. Coupled with paternalism is coercion, the threat or use of violence to influence behavior or choice. The joining of the august figure in white with implied or explicit threats has been and still is a potent force for counteracting any potential patient autonomy. The thrust of modern bioethics is to respect patients by honoring their autonomy (Box 205-1).

BOX 205-1. Commonly Accepted Societal and Bioethical Values

Autonomy: Self-determination: a person's ability to make personal decisions, including those affecting personal medical care. Autonomy is the opposite of paternalism.

Beneficence: Doing good. A duty to confer benefits. Production of benefit.

Confidentiality: The presumption that what the patient tells the physician will not be revealed to any other person or institution without the patient's permission.

Distributive justice: Fairness in the allocation of resources and obligations. This value is the basis of and is incorporated into society-wide health care policies.

Nonmaleficence: Not doing harm, prevention of harm, and removal of harmful conditions.

Personal integrity: Adhering to one's own reasoned and defensible set of values and moral standards.

At the patient's bedside, beneficence (doing good) and confidentiality (holding information in confidence) have been long-held and nearly universal tenets of the medical profession. Similarly, personal integrity (the adherence to one's own moral and professional standards) is basic to thinking and acting ethically.

The concept of comparative or distributive justice suggests that a society's comparable individuals and groups should share similarly in the society's benefits and burdens. Many society-wide decisions affecting thoughts and actions about the allocation of limited health care resources are based on this principle. Yet for individual clinicians to arbitrarily limit or terminate care on a case-by-case basis at patients' bedsides is an erroneous extrapolation of the idea that there may be a need to limit health care resource expenditures.[7] Distributive justice is a policy concept rather than a clinical model.

A controversial value within the medical community is truth-telling. Many people who believe that the patient, no matter what the circumstances, has the right to know the truth have championed absolute honesty. Yet honesty must be tempered with compassion; honesty does not equate to brutality. There are multiple tales of champions of absolute fidelity who were appalled by their own physicians' lack of sensitivity when relating unfavorable medical news to them.[8] Those who champion truth-telling as an important value justifiably complain that it is often not done well. Requiring that the truth be told with a modicum of sensitivity does not denigrate the requirement that the truth be told. Physicians sometimes do not universally accept truth-telling within the medical profession because of poor role models, lack of training in interpersonal interactions, and bad experiences, rather than a discounting of the value itself.[9]

Physicians accept a lack of truth-telling, depending on the circumstances. When failure to disclose the truth may physically harm patients, such as in the infamous Tuskegee experiments on black men with syphilis, it is not only immoral but also probably illegal to withhold the information. Likewise, if failure to disclose information is strictly for the physician's benefit, such as not telling a patient about a dismal prognosis or a medical error, the clinician's behavior suggests serious ethical and legal deficits. The issues become somewhat murkier when truth-telling involves a third party, such as a sex partner who is being exposed to an infectious disease.[9]

Emergency physicians' professional values have been incorporated into organization codes, such as the American College of Emergency Physicians' *Code of Ethics,* and as a more personal oath developed by the Society for Academic Emergency Medicine.[10,11] Ethical codes from other medical organizations differ widely, in both their content and their specificity.[12]

Religious Values

Organized religions are recognized as keepers of society's values. Even though various religions appear dissimilar, most hold the Golden Rule, "Do unto others

BOX 205-2. Commonly Accepted Moral Rules

Moral rules govern actions based on ethics and codes of conduct. These can justifiably be enforced and their violation punished. Although none of these rules is absolute, they all require one not to cause evil. Somewhat paradoxically, however, they may neither require preventing evil nor doing good.

1. Do not kill.
2. Do not cause pain.
3. Do not disable.
4. Do not deprive of freedom.
5. Do not deprive of pleasure.
6. Do not deceive.
7. Keep your promise.
8. Do not cheat.
9. Obey the law.
10. Do your duty.

Modified from Gert B: *Morality: A New Justification of the Moral Rules.* Oxford, Oxford University Press, 1988.

as you would have them do unto you," as a basic tenet. Other moral rules common to most religions are listed in Box 205-2. Problems surface in trying to apply religion-based rules to specific bioethical situations. For example, although "Do not kill" is generally accepted, the activities that constitute killing, active or passive euthanasia, or merely reasonable medical care vary with the interpretation of the world's religions, as they do with the interpretations of various philosophers.[13]

Some practitioners have a conflict with specific professionally or societally accepted values on a religious, philosophic, or practical basis. When such a conflict exists in a practitioner's mind, it is deemed morally and legally acceptable, within certain constraints, for the individual to follow a course of action based on a personal value system. When conflicts over values exist, however, it is essential for the practitioner to recognize the patient's identity, dignity, and autonomy, to avoid the error of blindly imposing one's own values on others. Even when the physician initially plans to follow a course consistent with societally accepted values, it is desirable to review the case's specific circumstances and the hierarchical importance of the values involved. In each specific case, the ethical analysis must recognize all practicable courses of action and the benefits and detriments of each, while at the same time respecting the patient's values.

One classic dilemma is the exsanguinating adult patient, awake and still with medical decision-making capacity, who explicitly refuses to accept any blood or blood product based on religious beliefs. The physician, with a professional duty and moral commitment to preserve life, does not agree with the patient's decision. Yet society (through the benchmark of court decisions) has repeatedly sided with the patient. In this case, the patient's autonomy and right to practice religion are recognized as the overriding values. This case becomes somewhat less clear when the patient does not have decision-making capacity, is a minor, or appears to be under external pressures to make a life-threatening decision.

The stark dichotomy of ethical thought and values is often most vividly demonstrated in discussions of good and evil. The following is a current set of definitions that might help the physician find solutions to ethical problems. *Good* can be defined as what no rational person will avoid without a reason. Examples include freedom, pleasure, health, wealth, and knowledge. *Evil* can be defined as what all rational persons desire to avoid for themselves and for others they care about. Examples include untimely death, pain, disability, and loss of freedom or pleasure.[14] In the example above, rational individuals, on a deeply held religious basis, sometimes do choose a likelihood of death in refusing a blood transfusion over the permanent pain and anguish they feel would ensue if they should violate their religious injunction.

BIOETHICAL DILEMMAS

A problem for many physicians is deciding what constitutes an ethical problem. The most straightforward example of an ethical quandary is the dilemma. A *dilemma* is a choice of two or more courses of action, each representing a conflicting value to which one adheres. A dilemma is often explained as being "damned if you do and damned if you don't." In the following example the attending physician can be said to be on the horns (two prickly but seemingly equal choices) of a dilemma:

A 60-year-old man stabbed himself in the abdomen because he had intractable pain from terminal pancreatic cancer, unrelieved by any medical therapy. A well-meaning friend, who happened to be in the house when the event occurred, called the paramedics, who brought the man to the emergency department. Although the man will obviously bleed to death if not given aggressive care, neither the patient, who is still alert and oriented, nor his wife, who is present, wants any treatment other than pain control. A review of his chart confirms that his physicians are at a loss as to how to alleviate his pain and that he is expected to die within the next several weeks.[15] The physician believes in respecting a patient's autonomy, yet usually questions patients' decision-making capacity when they attempt suicide. Such patients' actions seem to raise the question of whether, in fact, they have a right or an ability to be autonomous. This physician also believes strongly in beneficence: helping those in need, relieving pain, and saving lives when possible. Beneficence suggests alternative courses of action: palliative care or aggressive therapeutic intervention. Merely using analgesics and other comfort measures will abet a suicide; initiating aggressive medical and surgical interventions will prolong a dying process that the physician's colleagues have found to be unresponsive to even palliative treatment. Which value takes precedence: patient autonomy or beneficence? And if beneficence, in what direction is it to be aimed, toward relieving suffering, prolonging life, or a third option that could include

Table 205-1. Relative Differences Between Emergency Practice and Primary Care Practice

Emergency Department	Primary Care
Patient is often brought in by ambulance, police, or family.	Patient chooses to enter medical care system.
Patient does not choose physician.	Patient chooses physician.
Emergency department personnel must gain patient's trust.	Physician and nurses already enjoy patient's confidence and trust.
Emergency department personnel do not know patient, family, values.	Physician and nurses often know patient, family, values.
Patient experiences an acute change in health.	Patient has chronic medical problems.
Anxiety, pain, alcohol, and altered mental status are common.	Anxiety, pain, alcohol, and altered mental status are less common.
Decisions are made quickly.	There is usually time for reflection and deliberation.
Physician makes decisions independently.	Physician has a greater opportunity to consult with patient, family, other physicians, ethics committees, lawyers, courts, ethicists.
Physician represents institution and medical staff.	Physician represents self or medical group.
Work environment is open and less controlled.	Work environment is private and controlled.
Emergency department personnel frequently have a stressful work schedule.	Work schedule is often set or canceled by physician.

Modified from Sanders AB: Unique aspects of ethics in emergency medicine. In Iserson KV et al, eds: *Ethics in Emergency Medicine*, 2nd ed, Tucson, Ariz, Galen Press, 1995.

both? Bioethics deals with problems that are neither black nor white, only gray.

Other examples of ethical problems and conflicts in emergency medical care include questions regarding resuscitation efforts, especially when patients and families may not want resuscitation; teaching, particularly in critical situations or using the newly dead; emergency medical services control, when administrative rules and good patient care conflict; helping others, when one's own life may be placed at risk; involvement in physician-assisted suicide[16,17]; and patient access, limited financial and personnel resources in the face of obvious patient need. Even if these problems do not fit into the classic form of a dilemma, they can be recognized as bioethical problems because they require the clinician to make a choice between two (or more) accepted values.

BIOETHICS IN EMERGENCY MEDICINE

The emergency physician has a markedly different relationship with patients than do other practitioners, especially others providing primary care (Table 205-1).[18-20]

Emergency physicians often care for patients who are unfamiliar to them and to the institution. Although practitioners who either know their patients or who care for them in less acute settings often have other mechanisms for making ethical decisions, emergency physicians often have limited options. Although there may be arguments over which is the optimal course of action with a specific set of values, there is often general agreement over what may constitute ethically wrong actions. The method of ethical case analysis described in Box 205-3[21] provides the emergency physician in need of a fast answer to an ethical dilemma a method of avoiding an ethically incorrect course of action.

Stopping at the first step, using a known precedent, is the most productive way to use this method.

BOX 205-3. A Rapid Approach to Emergency Ethical Problems

Is this a type of ethical problem for which you have already worked out a rule, or is it at least similar enough so that the rule could reasonably be extended to cover it?

- YES — Follow the rule.
- NO — Is there an option that will buy you time for deliberation without excessive risk to the patient?
  - YES — Take that option.
  - NO —
    1. Apply Impartiality Test.
    2. Apply Universalizability Test.
    3. Apply Interpersonal Justifiability Test.

Modified from Iserson KV: An approach to ethical problems in emergency medicine. In Iserson KV, et al (eds): *Ethics in Emergency Medicine*, 2nd ed. Tucson, Ariz, Galen Press, 1995.

However, this takes planning, reading, and thinking about ethical problems. Many physicians are unprepared to do this. Just as with the indications for any emergency procedure, emergency physicians should be prepared with a course of action for at least the most common ethical dilemmas they may face in the emergency department. But even the prepared clinician can encounter cases without relevant known precedents.

With no precedent to rely on and no way to "buy time," the practitioner must select a possible course of action and test it for ethical validity. The three tests involved in the method are the Impartiality Test, the Universalizability Test, and the Interpersonal Justifiability Test. The Impartiality Test asks whether the practitioner would accept this action if in the patient's place. In essence this is a form of the Golden Rule. The Universalizability Test asks whether the practitioner would feel comfortable having all practitioners perform this action in all relevantly similar circumstances. This generalizes the action to all colleagues, asking whether a rule for the contemplated behavior is reasonable. The Interpersonal Justifiability Test asks whether the practitioner can supply good reasons to others for the action. Will peers, superiors, or the public be satisfied with the answers? If all three tests can be answered in the affirmative, then the practitioner has a reasonable probability that the proposed action falls within the scope of ethically acceptable actions.

BIOETHICAL DILEMMAS IN EMERGENCY MEDICAL PRACTICE

Withholding and Withdrawing Treatment

In emergency medicine, a significant difference rightfully persists between withholding and withdrawing life-sustaining medical treatment. The justification for this stems, in part, from the nature of emergency medical practice and the unique manner in which clinicians apply many ethical principles. Because emergency physicians often lack vital information about their patients' identities, medical conditions, and wishes, withholding emergency medical treatment is much more problematic than later withdrawing unwanted or useless interventions. Once an emergency physician obtains enough information to confirm a patient's wishes or medical condition, medical treatment can be appropriately withdrawn, if indicated. Without this information, the presumption must be for intervention. Society has specific expectations from emergency medical practitioners. Due to the nature of emergency medicine, both in the prehospital and the emergency department settings, there are higher standards for withholding than for withdrawing medical treatment.[22]

Prehospital Resuscitation

A number of unique bioethical problems arise because of the emergency physician's interactions with the emergency medical services system.

Emergency medical services systems were developed in the early 1970s because many Americans died due to a lack of adequate and systematic prehospital care and transportation to medical facilities. The systems that have been developed, including their progressive upgrading in training, skill levels, and equipment, have made great strides in remedying these problems. Yet another, more insidious dilemma arose: how to treat patients entering the emergency medical services system who neither want nor benefit from medical care. The worst-case scenario is the terminally ill patient, for whom comfort care is all that can be provided, whose panicked relative calls 911 in the last dying moments. The response is predictable and painful to all involved.[23,24] The dilemma is between nonmaleficence toward this patient and beneficence for all potential patients needing resuscitation. If arbitrary (by nonphysician and other than patient-surrogate) determinations can be made about who will and will not be resuscitated in the prehospital setting, then there is a possibility of failing to care for patients who might have benefited because of other people's agendas. One potential solution is the better and more widespread use of advance directives.

Advance Directives

Several types of legal and quasilegal documents come under the term *advance directives.* These are indicators of what is to be done for a patient in extremis who is no longer able to give or withhold permission for treatment. Advance directives are usually written to avoid prolonging an inevitable, often painful or nonsentient dying process. Physicians are most familiar with the do-not-resuscitate (DNR) order, normally initiated in hospitals, nursing homes, and hospices. (The DNR order is not strictly an advance directive but does serve to transmit conditional orders to other health care personnel.)

DNR Order

A physician-written DNR order in the hospital chart informs other medical personnel that they should not institute CPR in the event of cardiopulmonary arrest. Ideally, this order is put on charts only after consultation with the patient (possessing decisional capacity), family or other surrogate decision makers, and usually involves chronically ill patients with a poor prognosis for long-term survival. The newer acronyms, DNIR (do not initiate resuscitation) or DNAR (do not attempt resuscitation), more honestly suggest that resuscitation attempts do not always succeed. These orders usually work well within a specific institution, but if patients are transferred, often from a nursing facility or hospice to the emergency department, the act of transfer or activation of the emergency medical services system negates the order. This can be directly contrary to a patient's wishes for terminal care. However, if a patient arriving in the emergency department still has the capacity to make a decision concerning resuscitation, part of an emergency physician's duty is to document such a decision in the patient's chart, including the specific actions to be limited, the circumstances of the discussion, and the individuals present during the discussion.[23-25] Many institutions have now recognized that simple DNAR forms are inadequate descriptions for other health care personnel to interpret and have changed to limitation-of-treatment forms specifying exactly what is not to be done for a patient.[26]

Prehospital Directives

During the past several years, 43 states have enacted methods whereby patients outside of health care facilities can avoid unwanted resuscitation attempts.

(Those not having such policies are Delaware, the District of Columbia, Iowa, Mississippi, Nebraska, North Dakota, Pennsylvania, and Vermont.[27]) These usually take the form either of a prehospital DNAR order or, in a few cases, a prehospital advance directive. Often confused, the two forms differ greatly in their philosophies. The prehospital DNAR order is a physician-originated document. A patient or legal surrogate generates the prehospital advance directive with little or no involvement from health care personnel. Both instruct emergency medical services personnel who have been erroneously called at the time of death not to attempt to resuscitate the patient (or to stop resuscitation efforts if they have already begun when such a form is found). Both types of form have proved effective.[24,28-31] The most common reason for having physician-initiated forms is the specter of murders and suicides being aided by patient-initiated documents. In practice, this has not occurred.[32]

Living Will

The living will is a relatively standardized form adopted in most states and the District of Columbia. (Massachusetts, Michigan, and New York do not have statutes.[27]) This document requests that health care workers not perform (or in some cases, *do perform* despite apparent medical futility[33]) future resuscitative measures. It goes into effect only if the individual lacks decision-making capacity; until that point, the patient must consent to medical treatment, regardless of anything said in a living will. Living wills normally require both that a physician certify an individual as terminally ill and that the designee has the mental capacity to understand its provisions. (Arizona, in a break with tradition, does not use the "terminally ill" criteria, since the law's drafters found that all extant definitions were unclear. No ill effects have resulted.[30]) States allow varying levels of specificity in the document, including, in some cases, the refusal of artificial nutrition and hydration.

Although most emergency physicians have encountered relatives waving living wills at them during a resuscitation, a consistent part of these documents specifies that the patient's physician must have seen and accepted the document's provisions in advance. This requirement establishes a physician contact who will act on the patient's behalf. For physicians, it protects those whose value systems will not allow them to abide by the documents' provisions. It also encourages families and physicians to discuss the circumstances surrounding the time of death and the actions they can take.

The emergency physician will rarely, if ever, be in the position of having accepted a living will's provisions in advance. In the setting of an emergency department resuscitation, the best that a living will can do, assuming that the patient is correctly identified, is to suggest what the patient's wishes were. However, the document in no way restricts the emergency physician's actions.[32]

Durable Power of Attorney

A more commonly used advance directive is the durable power of attorney with medical provisions. Forty-nine states and the District of Columbia have statutes authorizing such directives. (Alaska does not have such a statute.[27]) The durable power of attorney has existed for some time and was initially designed to allow business affairs to be continued when individuals were out of contact with civilization for long periods. The document in its usual form takes effect immediately. However, when it is used as a medical advance directive, specific provisions take effect when the individual no longer has the capacity to make medical decisions. The document specifies a surrogate decision maker. It allows more flexibility than living wills, because the surrogate can make any health care decisions that the patient would ordinarily make.

Nonstandard Advance Directives

Emergency physicians occasionally encounter medallions, tattoos, or other indicators that seem to be advance directives.[34,35] These may cause consternation, since they fall outside society's bounds for indicating life-determining decisions. What should clinicians do if these indicators come to light during resuscitations? To be useful, advance directives must be available to the treating clinicians when they are needed, must be a product of the patient's (or sometimes the surrogate's) deliberations, must be understandable, and must cover the patient's current medical situation. Nonstandard directives, usually abbreviated or abstract (such as a tattooed symbol for "do not defibrillate"), fail to meet these requirements. Of special concern is that the nature of such indicators may make it unclear whether the patient or surrogate either understood how their "directive" might be interpreted or whether it was still what they desired. In general, emergency physicians should not rely on these indicators to make critical patient decisions.

Decision-Making Capacity and Consent

Decision-Making Capacity

Many ethical dilemmas in emergency medical care dissolve upon ascertaining a patient's decision-making capacity, often linked with consent to (or more often refusal of) a medical procedure. A basic canon of both ethics and law, as stated by Justice Cardozo, is that "every human being of adult years and sound mind has a right to determine what shall be done with his own body . . ."[36] These situations can often be clarified by understanding what is meant by decision-making capacity and how it relates to consent.

In clinical practice, the word *competence* is often used to mean *capacity*. *Competence* is a legal term and can only be determined by the court. *Capacity* refers to a patient's ability to make decisions about accepting health care recommendations. Capacity is always decision-relative rather than global. For example,

BOX 205-4. Components of Decision-Making Capacity

1. Knowledge of the options.
2. Awareness of consequences of each option.
3. Appreciation of personal costs and benefits of options in relation to relatively stable values and preferences. (When ascertaining this, emergency physicians should ask patients why they made a specific choice.)

Modified from Buchanan AE: The question of competence. In Iserson KV, et al (eds): *Ethics in Emergency Medicine,* 2nd ed. Tucson, Ariz, Galen Press, 1995.

although an inebriated person can have the capacity to decline to have a small laceration sutured, especially if there is evidence that there has been prior refusal without remorse, the same individual may not have the capacity to accept an elective operation or refuse to have an emergency lifesaving procedure or operation. To have adequate decision-making capacity in any one circumstance, an individual must understand the options, the consequences of acting on the various options, and the costs and benefits of these consequences by relating them to a relatively stable framework of personal values and priorities (Box 205-4).[37,38]

Disagreeing with the physician's recommendation is not in itself grounds for determining that the patient is incapable of making a decision. In fact, even refusing lifesaving medical care may not prove the person incapable of making valid decisions if it is done on the basis of firmly held religious beliefs, such as in the case of the Jehovah's Witness patient refusing a blood transfusion described previously.

Consent

There are two general types of consent: implied and informed. Both are operative in the emergency setting. Implied consent (more properly, presumed consent) covers necessary lifesaving procedures that it is presumed any reasonable person would wish to have. This can easily be related to the value concepts of good and evil discussed previously. Implied consent can be operative in a patient who retains decision-making capacity, as when an arm is held out to give blood, or in a patient without this capacity, such as the individual with a gunshot wound to the abdomen who arrives in an unconscious state.

Informed consent (or informed refusal) assumes that a patient who has decision-making capacity is given all the pertinent facts regarding the risks and benefits of a particular procedure, understands them, and voluntarily agrees (or declines) to undergo the procedure. It is in this matter that confusion often reigns. Does the patient have the capacity to understand? Is this capacity to be questioned only if there is refusal of "good" medical care? Furthermore, what procedures require informed, as opposed to implied, consent? Does suturing always require informed consent, or only when it is complex? Does a lumbar puncture require it? The requirement for informed consent varies in practice and law from area to area and even among practitioners and institutions in the same areas.

Surrogate Decision Makers

When patients do not have the capacity to make medical decisions for themselves and they lack advance directives naming a surrogate or giving specific instructions, someone must make the decision for them. Four major classes of decision-makers have been proposed and actually used in these cases: family, bioethics committees, physicians, and courts.

Family

Traditionally, and usually in practice, the family—especially the spouse—acts as a surrogate decision maker when a patient does not have the capacity to make medical decisions. It should be understood, however, that even when there is a strong family tie, emotional or fiscal factors may sway the surrogate decision maker from certain courses of action the patient would wish taken.

Surrogates make decisions based on two distinct patterns: substituted judgment and best interests. Substituted judgment is used when there is an assumption that the surrogate knows enough about the patient's values to make a decision similar to that which the patient would make. It is not clear that anyone knows that much about another person.[39] Surrogates use the best interest standard when they do not know what the patient would want done in a particular situation but, as in the case of Karen Ann Quinlan, the patient once had the capacity to make such decisions.[40] They use the patient's prior statements and behavior to document the patient's values as well as possible, and then make a decision as close as possible to what the patient would have wanted. Some states may require explicit written directives for surrogates to follow.[41,42] The best-interest standard also applies, as in the Saikewicz case, when the patient has never had adequate decision-making capacity.[43] Unless there is already a court-appointed guardian, these situations often end up in court.

Children represent a special situation. Individuals younger than the age of majority (or unemancipated) are usually deemed incapable of making independent medical decisions. Nevertheless, in most cases the same rules that apply to adult capacity apply to children. The more serious the consequences, the more capacity and understanding of the options, consequences, and values involved are required of them to make, or assent to, a decision. Even if a parent is present, it is not always clear that the adult is acting in the best interest of the child. In such cases, child protective services may become involved. Disagreements between parents are possible. In some cases, this results in the involvement of bioethics committees or the courts.

Surrogate Lists

If a patient lacks decision-making capacity and has no advance directive, many states provide that specific individuals automatically become the person's surrogate. In practice, this almost always means that the patient's spouse acts in that capacity. Some states now have a statutory surrogate list to simplify the process. The most extensive of such lists specifies, in order: spouse (not divorced or legally separated), a majority of adult children who can be reasonably contacted, parents (of an adult), domestic partner, sibling, close friend, and attending physician in consultation with a bioethics committee.[44]

Bioethics Committees and Consultants

Multidisciplinary committees have developed in most large hospitals to help solve bioethical dilemmas, often involving surrogate decision making. In this process, they also act to reconfirm prognoses and to mediate between dissenting parties. Some smaller hospitals have bioethics consultants rather than committees to perform many of the same functions.

Physicians

In the past, physicians made unilateral decisions for their patients, regardless of whether the patients had the capacity to decide for themselves. This still occurs, of course, especially in the unexpected and stressful setting of the acute illnesses and injuries seen in emergency departments. There is a tendency for physicians to determine that a patient does not have the capacity to make medical decisions simply because the patient disagrees with the clinician. If the patient's decision-making capacity is questioned in the emergency department, the clinician, often without assistance, is forced to make a decision. In emergency cases, this cannot be avoided. But when it is possible to "buy time," clinicians should take the time (see Box 205-3).

When making unilateral decisions, physicians should recognize that they are not omniscient. They should acknowledge that prognoses are often incorrect, medical knowledge is finite, and, whenever possible, they need to respect patient autonomy, a basic societal value.

Courts

The courts often act as the final adjudicators of disagreements over medical care. They appoint legal guardians and, in select cases, set precedent that is followed as health law. The courts, however, are usually neither expeditious nor necessarily cognizant of bioethical principles. They are solely instructed to follow the societal values codified in the law. Many courts have suggested that, whenever possible, health care decisions should remain at the bedside, rather than in legal chambers.[40-42]

Teaching

The emergency department is a major teaching environment for young physicians and paramedical personnel. Because the sickest and most diverse patients enter through the emergency department, the balance between training and treatment raises some thorny bioethical issues.

Resuscitation

The most time-dependent of all activities, and arguably the best training periods in the emergency department, occur during resuscitations. The patients who require this care have implicitly been guaranteed that all appropriate medical knowledge and skill will be brought to bear to attempt to save their lives. This implied promise leads to a moral dilemma. If the most proficient individuals always lead resuscitations and perform procedures, the patient would receive the beneficence, as well as nonmaleficence, they presumed they would get. Yet this practice would deprive future patients of trained clinicians who could bestow the same quality care.

This controversy has raged for many years. The appropriate balance seems to be that training in emergency departments can ethically proceed, as it does in other areas of medicine, if there are safeguards in the form of on-site, supervising, experienced clinicians available to ascertain that the patients get the best possible appropriate care. It has also been suggested that medical students and residents might be certified for cognitive and procedural skills in a manner similar to other hospital physicians. This certification would enable faculty to know when individuals are capable of performing resuscitations, as well as other medical procedures, on their own.[45] Some training centers have adopted this process.

Rarely discussed, but a common practice in some teaching hospitals, has been the custom of allowing trainees with little skill or knowledge to learn and practice procedures on those undergoing resuscitation only when a patient is deemed "unsalvageable."[46] This practice does a disservice to the patient, since prolonging resuscitative attempts solely for this purpose may lead to a clinical state that prolongs the death. It also harms the family and society by making them pay for unnecessary procedures.

Notifying Survivors

Emergency physicians, who deal with sudden death on a daily basis, must pass their knowledge of how to care for survivors, the newest patients, on to the next generation. Professionals whose job includes delivering news about sudden unexpected deaths need to learn how to perform this task before doing it. Unfortunately, most medical "short courses" dealing with resuscitation, such as Advanced Cardiac Life Support (ACLS), Advanced Trauma Life Support (ATLS), and Pediatric Advanced Life Support (PALS), have not incorporated death notification into their training programs or manuals.

Occasionally, physicians give the job of death notification to residents, medical students, or nurses. Although all three groups should be present to learn the techniques involved, to have an opportunity to hear what is said and how it is said, and to observe an attending physician showing some sensitivity, they should not be left to do death notifications on their own. That is a form of professional abandonment and, in a teaching hospital, the worst form of student abuse.[47,48]

Postmortem Teaching

A less commonly discussed part of emergency medical teaching is the use of recently deceased patients to teach or practice emergency techniques, such as intubations and central line placement. Although there is controversy about whether this practice is ethical, it seems that if medical treatment could not save the patient, then the emergency physician's responsibility is to hone skills for the next patient in need of expertise in resuscitative techniques. This is not to condone the desecration of a body. Rather, it suggests that because clinicians learned the techniques used during the dead patient's attempted resuscitation on other dead or living patients, this (now dead) patient owes the next patient the same courtesy. No one would advocate practicing unneeded procedures on living patients, and there are many who argue against using experimental animals. The religious or ethical beliefs of some emergency department personnel may make practicing or teaching these procedures in such circumstances problematic.[49-51]

Bowing to fear of adverse publicity, national medical groups have asserted that postmortem teaching should not be performed in any case without the explicit survivor consent.[52] This has essentially halted such teaching in most emergency departments.

Disasters and Triage

In situations with limited medical resources, be they personnel, equipment, or time (and it always boils down to a lack of time), clinicians use "triage" to determine which patients receive treatment. Clinicians have long recognized that they must have rules to equitably distribute medical resources in situations of scarcity. Triage procedures, following the concept of equity, are designed to provide equivalent treatment for those with equivalent needs, that is, to treat similar patients similarly. Triage represents a more explicit and often more drastic allocation of medical resources than normally occurs. What type of treatment a patient receives during disasters depends on the triage "lottery" rules in place.

Four potential triage models are possible, based, in part, on the circumstances that govern our lives. They each have an ethical basis.

1. Treating the most serious, or potentially serious, illnesses and injuries first is the most common medical triage model, since time, rather than actual physical resources, is what is being allocated.
2. First-come, first-served, also called the statistical lottery, is a part of normal, non-crisis medical triage. This model is unworkable in catastrophic situations, since it ignores the "life expectancy, urgency of need, and likelihood of survival."[53] A bias-free selection method, it would lead to gross inequities in resource distribution in these extreme scenarios.
3. Social worth as a basis for triage consideration depends on an individual's luck in the natural and social lotteries. Natural lotteries are the wide range of talents, abilities, disabilities, deformities, and illnesses among individuals. Social lotteries are the disparity in how individuals are chosen to be the recipients of attention, jobs, love, care, or other benefits. Medical triage protocols generally ignore the criteria of social worth, although individuals considered "VIPs" often seem to get faster, if not better, treatment.
4. Patients' best prognosis is only applied to instances of severe resource limitation, such as battlefield and post-catastrophe triage, sometimes called "lifeboat" or "nightmare" situations. During this type of triage, clinicians decide whom to save when not all can be saved. They justify this on utilitarian principles—using available resources to maximally benefit the most people.

Triage models differ depending on whether they are being used in routine civilian medical practice, battlefield situations, disaster settings, or after biochemical, chemical, or radiologic terrorist attacks on civilian populations. The ethical basis for prioritizing the allocation of scarce resources, especially after biologic attacks, also differs, with designated responders (fire, police, emergency medical services, and, in some instances, emergency department personnel) getting priority due to their lifesaving "multiplier effect."

Although these rules for sorting patients and distributing resources are standardized for most situations, the key for implementing nonroutine triage is to develop, with bioethics consultation, the criteria to use before the crisis occurs.[54,55]

Resuscitation Research

Physicians in a new and advancing specialty have an obligation to advance the knowledge base from which they practice. This can be done only through research, a significant component of which must necessarily be clinically based. Federally mandated institutional review boards (IRBs) must approve any research involving human subjects, including research in emergency departments and, possibly, in prehospital care.[56] The IRBs try to guarantee that patients asked to participate in research see an adequate informed-consent document and prospectively sign it. It has been suggested that, even if the patient is conscious, in the midst of a medical emergency it is unclear whether truly free and informed consent can be given.[57,58] In both trauma and cardiac resuscitation research this is, of course, impossible. It is usually difficult or impossible to obtain retrospective patient or, if appropriate, prospective surrogate consent. So as not to deny critically ill and injured patients the opportunity to participate in possibly beneficial research trials, the U.S. Food and Drug Administration and Department of Health and Human Services issued new regulations, effective in 1996, that allow "emergency research" without informed consent. These regulations contain extensive patient safeguards, including community consultation, public disclosure, and intensive oversight.[59] The public, however, does not seem to be enthralled with the idea of waiving consent for these studies.[60]

The ethical basis for these regulations is that if it is not harmful to them, and especially if it is potentially helpful, most "reasonable" patients would acquiesce to the research, given the basic values of good and evil (see Box 205-2).[61-63] This appropriately paternalistic attitude among physician researchers is analogous to the same attitude in other acute care situations. In these instances, individuals suffering unexpected events with a high probability of rapid mortality or serious morbidity without medical intervention generally demand that the physician delivering acute care act in the patient's best interest, immediately and without discourse. This is one instance in which society demands that the clinician act paternalistically. If there is a chance that the patient could benefit from a therapeutic course of action in such circumstances, most people would demand that it be done. They would feel similarly for acute care research, especially when accepted or standard therapy is futile, and possibly when the investigators believe that equipoise (therapeutic equality) exists between the two tested forms of therapy. Protection for the patient in these cases is derived from the IRB, which among other things must guard against the possibility of organ-specific success but failure to benefit the entire person, such as producing a patient in a persistent vegetative state after "successful" CPR.

Questions exist, however, about the ethics of randomized trials in clinical research. Alternative methods have been proposed but as yet are not fully accepted by either clinicians or statisticians.[64-66] Not all such methods are applicable to research in acute care. Beyond IRB authorization for research is a moral responsibility for the individual researcher to ensure that the research protocol and execution are ethical. This responsibility extends to the journals in which the research is published.[67]

Restricted Access to Emergency Medical Care

According to the President's Commission for the Study of Ethical Problems in Medicine and Biomedical Research, society has a moral obligation to ensure that everyone has access to adequate health care without being subject to excessive burdens.[68] The need for health care is unequally distributed in the population and highly unpredictable. Few could afford this care if left to their own devices; therefore, mechanisms are in place to share the risk.[69]

The ethical dilemma for emergency physicians comes in basically two forms, one precipitated by the institution in which the emergency department is housed and one by outside third-party payers. It is prudent and ethical to err on the side of providing for the patient's needs.

Institutions may pressure emergency physicians to limit treatment, ancillary tests, or admissions for patients without the ability to pay. Although this may seem patently immoral, another question must be asked: if the institution were to become bankrupt and close its doors, would care be available for anyone? Hospitals have closed their doors because of financial losses; many hospitals, especially in inner-city areas, are on the verge of bankruptcy. There is a moral obligation to the community to keep a health care facility viable, but the balance is a tricky one. Some institutions have suggested refusing care to patients coming to the emergency department, sending some patients away for clinic appointments at a later time.[70]

Some prepaid health maintenance organizations (HMOs) use "gatekeepers" to keep patients in need of emergency medical care away from immediate assistance at institutions other than the HMO parent hospital. Moreover the HMO's income may depend on *not* hospitalizing patients, *not* using ancillary tests, and *not* permitting emergency department visits; the patient's medical needs must receive highest priorities.

ROLE OF BIOETHICS COMMITTEE

A good resource to aid in ethical decision making is the bioethics committee.[71] Bioethics committees, or institutional ethics committees, have a relatively short history. Yet there is already a modicum of uniformity in the types of activities that these committees perform. Beginning with the 1971 *Medico-Moral Guide* of the Canadian bishops, the 1973 Massachusetts General Hospital Critical Care Committee, and the 1977 Montefiore Medical Center (New York) bioethics committee, the movement to have a base for hospital ethical decision making has arisen.

After the Quinlan decision, the prevalence of institutional ethics committees increased.[40] Recently there have been some attempts to legislate the functions of hospital ethics committees. A Maryland statute requires the ethics committee to be involved in cases with life-threatening conditions. Other states specify a role for the committees, and in 1995 the Joint Commission on Accreditation of Healthcare Organizations began requiring that hospitals ensure that ethics committees' functions are accomplished.[72]

Currently, ethics committees are primarily located in hospitals and serve either the entire hospital or a special unit, such as a neonatal intensive care nursery. They usually have four main functions. First, they coordinate education on bioethical issues (for the committee members, hospital physicians and staff, patients, families, and local hospital community) about the ethical dimensions of clinical care. Second, they help institute mandatory or suggested policies or guidelines concerning bioethical issues (policies and guidelines for health care professionals regarding decision-making processes in problematic cases and resource allocation). Third, they consult prospectively and retrospectively on clinical cases and offer advice and conclusions to those directly involved, most often concerning the treatment or nontreatment of patients who lack decision-making capacities. Ethics committees usually do not act as the primary decision makers. Rather, they serve in a consulting, informational, and advisory capacity, supporting the primary decision-making role of the patient-family-physician triad, especially for urgent decisions about withholding, withdrawing, or continuing life-sustaining medical care. Experienced bioethics committees find that some of their cases, both concurrent (and usually stat) and retrospective, come from the emergency department and emergency medical services. Finally, they counsel hospital staff, patients, and families on ethical issues. This counseling is often done through educational forums and meetings to air and resolve disagreements among staff, patients, and families about clinical care decisions. In essence, the function of the ethics committee is to consider and help resolve unusual, complicated ethical problems.[71]

The experience of many suggests that ethics per se does not have the sole role in committee discussions of concrete cases. Because conflict is the essential element in issues brought before ethics committees, it is thought that a large part of their work comprises clarifying the facts and fostering communication.

Bioethics, at least as a method of formal thinking about clinical activities, is a new province within emergency medicine. The concepts and decision-making processes are designed to clarify and direct patient-physician interactions, to decide on right versus wrong decisions, and to discover morally acceptable paths to follow. Yet the mere act of pondering the issues involved will inevitably lead to more questions. These are the same questions—about aspects of the practice, administration, and biotechnology of emergency care—that will be asked by the entire society in the decades to come. Thinking about some of these questions now will allow the specialty to find answers and to proactively put its house in order.[57]

REFERENCES

1. Iserson KV: Ethics of wilderness medicine. In Auerbach P (ed): *Wilderness Medicine: Management of Wilderness and Environmental Emergencies,* 4th ed. St. Louis, Mosby, 2001, p 1820.
2. Feinberg J: *Social Philosophy.* Englewood Cliffs, NJ, Prentice-Hall, 1973.
3. Black HC: *Blacks Law Dictionary,* 7th ed. St Paul, Minn, West Publishing, 1999.
4. Hart HLA: *Punishment and Responsibility.* Oxford, Oxford University Press, 1976.
5. Ladd J: Legalism and medical ethics. *J Med* 4:70, 1979.
6. Graber GC: Basic theories in medical ethics. In Monagle JF, Thomasma DC (eds): *Medical Ethics.* Rockville, Md, Aspen, 1995.
7. Landesman BM: Physician attitudes toward patients. In Iserson KV et al (eds): *Ethics in Emergency Medicine,* 2nd ed. Tucson, Ariz, Galen Press, 1995.
8. Kübler-Ross E: *On Death and Dying.* New York, Macmillan, 1969.
9. Novack DH, et al: Physicians' attitudes toward using deception to resolve difficult ethical problems. *JAMA* 261:2980, 1989.
10. American College of Emergency Physicians Ethics Committee: *Code of Ethics for Emergency Physicians.* Dallas, ACEP, 2003.
11. Larkin GL, SAEM Ethics Committee: A code of conduct for academic emergency medicine. *Acad Emerg Med* 6:45, 1999.
12. Iserson KV: Principles of biomedical ethics. *Emerg Clin North Am* 17:283, 1999.
13. McCormick RA: Theology and bioethics. *Hastings Cent Rep* 19:5, 1989.
14. Gert B: *Morality: A New Justification of the Moral Rules,* Oxford, Oxford University Press, 1988.
15. Gorovitz S: Suicide. In Iserson KV, et al (eds): *Ethics in Emergency Medicine,* 2nd ed. Tucson, Ariz, Galen Press, 1995.
16. Moskop J, Iserson KV: Emergency physicians and physician-assisted suicide, part I: A review of the physician-assisted suicide debate. *Ann Emerg Med* 38:570, 2001.
17. Moskop J, Iserson KV: Emergency physicians and physician-assisted suicide, part II: Emergency care for patients who have attempted physician-assisted suicide. *Ann Emerg Med* 38:576, 2001.
18. Iserson KV: The problem patient. In Hamilton G, et al (eds): *Emergency Medicine: An Approach to Clinical Problem Solving.* Philadelphia, WB Saunders, 1991.
19. Sanders AB: Unique aspects of ethics in emergency medicine. In Iserson KV, et al (eds): *Ethics in Emergency Medicine,* 2nd ed. Tucson, Ariz, Galen Press, 1995.
20. Simon JR, et al: The difficult patient. *Emerg Med Clin North Am* 17:353, 1999.
21. Iserson KV: An approach to ethical problems in emergency medicine. In Iserson KV, et al (eds): *Ethics in Emergency Medicine,* 2nd ed. Tucson, Ariz, Galen Press, 1995.
22. Iserson KV: Withholding and withdrawing medical treatment: An emergency medicine perspective. *Ann Emerg Med* 28:51, 1996.
23. Iserson KV: Getting advance directives to the public: A role for emergency medicine. *Ann Emerg Med* 20:692, 1991.
24. Iserson KV: Prehospital advance directives: A better way. *J Emerg Med* 23:419, 2002.
25. Iserson KV: Federal advance directives legislation: Potential effects on emergency medicine. *J Emerg Med* 9:67, 1991.
26. University Medical Center, Tucson, AZ: Limitation of Medical Care Form. In Monagle JF, Thomasma DC: *Medical Ethics: Policies, Protocols, Guidelines & Programs.* Gaithersburg, Md, Aspen, 2003, p 5:98.
27. Partnership for Caring: Legal developments. Available at http://www.partnershipforcaring.org/resources/ Accessed October 2003.
28. Crimmins TJ: Prehospital do-not-resuscitate orders. In Iserson KV, et al (eds): *Ethics in Emergency Medicine,* 2nd ed. Tucson, Ariz, Galen Press, 1995.
29. Iserson KV: Foregoing prehospital care: Should ambulance staff always resuscitate? *J Med Ethics* 17:19, 1991.
30. Iserson KV: A simplified prehospital advance directive law: Arizona's approach. *Ann Emerg Med* 22:1703, 1993.
31. Iserson KV: If we don't learn from history . . . ethical failings in a new prehospital directive. *Am J Emerg Med* 13:241, 1995.
32. Iserson KV, et al (eds): *Ethics in Emergency Medicine,* 2nd ed. Tucson, Ariz, Galen Press, 1995.
33. Marco CA, Larkin GL, Moskop JC, Derse AR: Determination of "futility" in emergency medicine. *Ann Emerg Med* 35:604, 2000.
34. Iserson KV: Nonstandard advance directives: A pseudoethical dilemma. *J Trauma* 44:139, 1998.
35. Iserson KV: The "no code" tattoo: An ethical dilemma. *West J Med* 156:309, 1992.
36. *Schloendorff v Society of New York Hospital,* 105 NE 92, 93, 1914.
37. Moskop JC: Informed consent in the emergency department. *Emerg Med Clin North Am* 17:327, 1999.
38. Buchanan AE: The question of competence. In Iserson KV, et al (eds): *Ethics in Emergency Medicine,* 2nd ed. Tucson, Ariz, Galen Press, 1995.

39. Sonnenblick M, et al: Dissociation between the wishes of terminally ill patients and decisions by their offspring. *J Am Geriatr Soc* 41:599, 1993.
40. *In re Quinlan*, 70 NJ 10, 355 A2d 647, 1976; *cert denied*, 429 US 922, 1976.
41. *Cruzan v Director, Missouri Department of Health*, US 58 LW 4916, 1990.
42. *Rasmussen v Fleming*, 154 Ariz 207, 741 P2d 674, 1987.
43. *Superintendent of Belchertown v Saikewicz*, 373 Mass 728, 370 NE 2d 417, 1977.
44. Arizona Living Wills and Health Care Directives Act, *Ariz Rev Stat Ann* ss36-3201 to 36-3287, 2000.
45. Iserson KV: The supervision of physicians in training: An educational and ethical dilemma. *Med Teacher* 10:195, 1988.
46. Kaldjian LC, et al: Insertion of femoral-vein catheters for practice by medical house officers during cardiopulmonary resuscitation. *N Engl J Med* 341:2088, 1999.
47. Iserson KV: *Grave Words: Notifying Survivors about Sudden, Unexpected Deaths.* Tucson, Ariz, Galen Press, 1999.
48. Iserson KV: *Pocket Protocols: Notifying Survivors About Sudden Unexpected Deaths.* Tucson, Ariz, Galen Press, 1999.
49. Iserson KV: *Death to Dust: What Happens to Dead Bodies?* 2nd ed. Tucson, Ariz, Galen Press, 2000.
50. Iserson KV: Postmortem procedures in the emergency department: Using the recently dead to practice and teach. *J Med Ethics* 19:92, 1993.
51. Iserson KV: Law versus life: The ethical imperative to practice and teach using the newly dead emergency department patient. *Ann Emerg Med* 25:91, 1995.
52. American Medical Association Council on Ethical and Judicial Affairs: Policy E-8.181 *Performing Procedures on the Newly Deceased for Training Purposes.* Chicago, AMA, 2001.
53. Rhodes R, Miller C, Schwartz M: Transplant recipient selection: Peacetime vs. wartime triage. *Cambridge Q* 4:327, 1992.
54. Iserson KV, Pesik N: Ethical resource distribution after biological, chemical or radiological terrorism. *Cambridge Q Healthcare Ethics* 12:55, 2003.
55. Pesik N, Keim ME, Iserson KV: Terrorism and the ethics of emergency medical care. *Ann Emerg Med* 37:642, 2001.
56. Department of Health and Human Services: *Regulations of the DHHS on the Protection of Human Subjects.* Code 45, CFR 46.
57. Fish SS: Research ethics in emergency medicine. *Emerg Clin North Am* 17:461, 1999.
58. Williams BF, French JK, White HD: Informed consent during the clinical emergency of acute myocardial infarction (HERO 2 consent substudy): A prospective observational study. *Lancet* 15:918, 2003.
59. Investigator responsibilities: 21 CFR 50.24 and 45 CFR 46.10(I).
60. DeIorio NM, et al: Attitudes and knowledge of ED patients and visitors regarding waiver of consent resuscitation research. *Acad Emerg Med* 9:383, 2002.
61. Iserson KV: Human subjects in trauma research. In Iserson KV, et al (eds): *Ethics in Emergency Medicine*, 2nd ed. Tucson, Ariz, Galen Press, 1995.
62. Fost NC: Human subjects in cardiopulmonary resuscitation research. In Iserson KV, et al (eds): *Ethics in Emergency Medicine*, 2nd ed. Tucson, Ariz, Galen Press, 1995.
63. Spivey WH, et al (eds): Informed consent for biomedical research in acute care medicine. *Ann Emerg Med* 20:1251, 1991.
64. Weinstein MC: Allocation of subjects in medical experiments. *N Engl J Med* 291:1278, 1974.
65. Hellman S: Randomized clinical trials and the doctor-patient relationship. *Cancer Clin Trials* 2:189, 1979.
66. Spivey WH: Informed consent for clinical research in the emergency department. *Ann Emerg Med* 18:766, 1989.
67. Iserson KV: Physician ethics in human research: The role of medical publications. *Ann Emerg Med* 19:828, 1990.
68. President's Commission for the Study of Ethical Problems in Medicine and Biomedical Research: *Securing Access to Health Care, vol 1: The Ethical Implications of Differences in the Availability of Health Services.* Washington, DC, US Government Printing Office, 1983.
69. Iserson KV, Kastre T: Are emergency departments a "safety net" for the medically indigent? *Am J Emerg Med* 14:1, 1996.
70. Derlet RW, Nishio DA: Refusing care to patients who present to an emergency department. *Ann Emerg Med* 19:262, 1990.
71. Iserson KV, et al: The future functions of HECs. *Hosp Ethics Committee Forum* 1:63, 1989.
72. Joint Commission for the Accreditation of Healthcare Organizations: *1995 Accreditation Manual for Hospitals.* Chicago, JCAHO, 1994.

CHAPTER 206 End of Life

Jean T. Abbott and Susan Stone

PERSPECTIVE

The emergency department is frequently the site of critical turns in people's health. It is the place where sudden, unexpected deaths occur and bad news must be delivered to survivors. It is also increasingly a source of care for patients struggling with chronic diseases, individuals in the late stages of terminal illness, and people actively involved in the dying process. The emergency physician often does not know whether an emergency presentation is an unexpected event or an expected one and, as a result, must possess the skills necessary to handle both circumstances.

Death in the emergency department is different from death in other areas of the hospital, for the following reasons: (1) deaths are likely to be unexpected; (2) the patient, family, and their values are often unknown to the emergency department staff; (3) trust needs to be established rapidly; and (4) the emergency physician often has to act on limited medical information.[1] These factors add to an already stressful medical interaction for the emergency care team. In an emergency, the emergency physician's initial response must be to treat aggressively and resuscitate patients in extremis in the absence of countermanding advance directives. Much of the core of emergency medicine is devoted to preventing untimely death in people with severe trauma, a "heart too young to die," or another sudden unexpected life threat. When resuscitative and rescue efforts fail, or when the natural end to life comes, the emergency specialist must be prepared to work with the staff and with the patient's loved ones to assist in giving this profound human event the meaning and respect it deserves.

Other skills are important in end-of-life care. The emergency physician needs to manage unexpected medical downturns in patients with chronic or terminal diseases and help people who have arrived at the end of their lives. Establishing goals of care and implementing or supporting palliative treatments may be important. This requires the skills of discerning the burdens of illness for an individual, determining the kind of relief being sought in the emergency department, understanding how to best care for each patient, and perhaps even how a "good death" would look to a patient with terminal disease. These skills are vital to achieving the wide range of goals for medical care of patients.

PRINCIPLES OF DISEASE

Epidemiology of Death and Dying

One hundred years ago, the predominant pattern of dying was a rapid, precipitous death from infectious diseases and accidents. With modern medical advances, chronic diseases have become part of the last years of most people's lives. Three diseases—heart disease, cancers, and stroke—accounted for 60% of deaths in the United States in 2000, whereas unintentional injury accounted for only 4% of deaths.[2] Most people live with some limitation in their ability for self care for 2 to 4 years before they die. Four common trajectories of dying have been described (Figure 206-1). Sudden death (due to cardiac arrest, trauma, or other sudden event) occurs in only 10% of people. The other trajectories are more common and occur with roughly equal frequency. The predictable decline in patients with "terminal illness" over 6 months or less provided the basis for the hospice concept for dealing with deaths from cancer and AIDS. In cases of organ failure (chronic obstructive pulmonary disease [COPD], heart failure, renal failure, and other progressive serious medical diseases), gradual decline is punctuated by intermittent exacerbations (entry-reentry decline). The time of death for people with these progressive and ultimately fatal diseases is not very predictable, and it often happens rather unexpectedly during an acute deterioration. These patients are frequently treated for acute deterioration in emergency departments. This population should and can execute advance directives indicating whom they would like to make medical

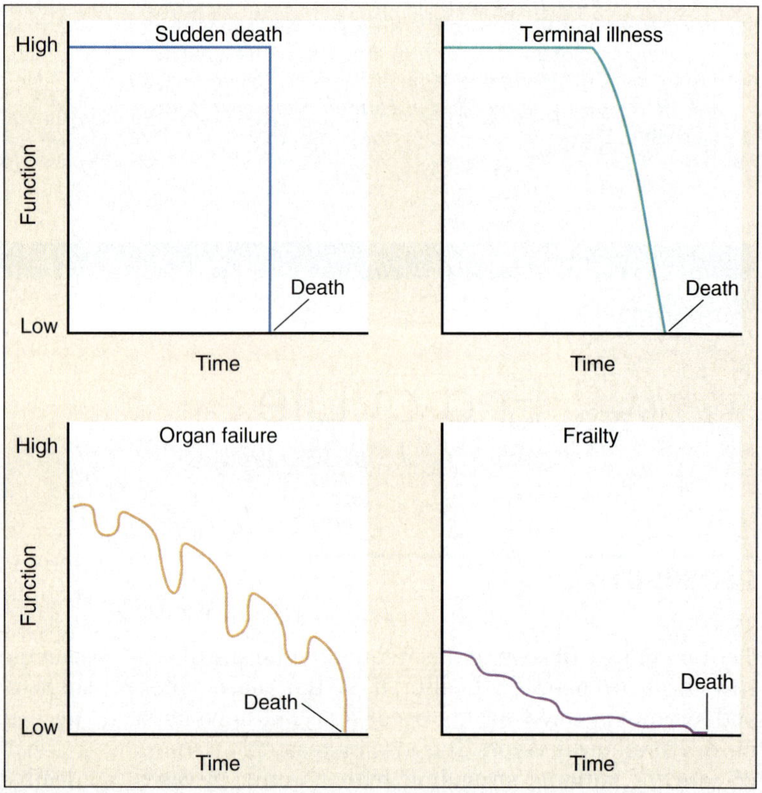

Figure 206-1. Theoretical trajectories of dying. (From Lunney JR, Lynn J, Hogan C: Profiles of older Medicare decedents. *J Am Geriatr Soc* 50:1108, 2002.)

decisions if they are incapacitated and what treatments they would like with subsequent acute episodes. The fourth trajectory of gradual decline or "frailty" is associated with some form of dementia in one half of people and has a lingering course that can extend over many years, stressing and wearing out caregivers and other support systems as decline in functional abilities progresses.[3]

In Western culture, death has become medicalized over the last 50 years.[4] Modern technology has often allowed human control over the timing, site, and pace of dying. Death occurs in an institution for more than 80% of people.[5] Frequently, the dying process is accompanied by invasive diagnostics and medical interventions, even when death is expected, and these interventions may increase suffering at the end of life. Patients, families, and physicians all feel value in fighting death; death is often seen in our society as the failure of scientific know-how to keep people alive, rather than the natural end to a life. Medicine places high value on the tasks of helping people through acute exacerbations of their chronic illnesses, modifying diseases that cannot be cured, and treating people to maximize what they can do in the time that remains to them. We need to become less fearful of death, so that we can not only help our patients make the best of the last years of their lives but also recognize and help them, and their families, deal with death as the natural ending of life.

Definitions of Death

Biologic definitions of death are currently the subject of considerable debate. Twenty years ago, cardiorespiratory failure defined death, as this was rapidly followed by brain death (which could not be directly measured) caused by failure of oxygenation and perfusion. Death was a biologic, distinct event, because all vital systems stopped when one failed.

Currently, cardiopulmonary "death" is not necessarily inevitable or irreversible. Ventilation can be maintained externally, and even circulatory support through pharmacologic means or pump assist can sometimes buttress an inadequate heart. Because of this, the alternative concept of "brain death" has been developed. The brain-based determination of death is derived from the irreversible failure of clinical function of the whole brain, including apnea, profound coma with unresponsiveness, and absence of brain stem reflexes.[6] The most common causes of brain death in adults are traumatic brain injury and subarachnoid hemorrhage. In children, they are accidental or nonaccidental trauma and asphyxia.[7] These are events that are seen with some frequency in the emergency department, although the criteria and irreversibility standards for brain death are seldom met in the first hours after the resuscitative effort. One important impetus for the development of a concept of brain death was the need to define a biologic and ethical boundary to life for procuring organs for transplantation. Declaration of brain death allows harvesting of organs with patient or family consent while continuing cardiopulmonary support and organ perfusion.

Difficulties with the definition of brain death have increased as we have learned more sophisticated measures of neurologic function. It is rare, particularly in non-trauma patients, for complete brain death to occur, even though people may have irreversible and severe brain damage and permanent unconsciousness.[8] Newer protocols to increase the pool of organ donors have bypassed brain "death" by defining a "non-heart beating" organ donor. In patients in whom the prognosis for meaningful survival is dismal, but complete brain death will not occur before cardiopulmonary arrest, life-sustaining support of pulmonary and cardiac function is withdrawn by permission or request of the patient or surrogates. Death is declared after an interval of 2 to 10 minutes (depending on the protocol). This assures the family and clinicians that death of the patient is inevitable but minimizes warm-ischemic time for organs, allowing multiorgan harvesting to be achieved.[6] Some ethicists have suggested that it is time to go back to a simple cardiopulmonary definition of death, allowing patients and families to donate organs when the patient is in a terminal state or irreversibly brain damaged, but prior to formal "death" pronouncement. This presumes there is a medical and ethical judgment that the patient is terminal and will not be harmed, and donation is the informed wish of the patient or family.[8]

The public often confuses our medical language around death, perhaps because we are not clear about the concepts either. We "allow the person to die" when we remove the ventilator and cardiac support, but we may do that because the patient is dead by brain criteria already. When a patient has no "higher" brain function or cognition, the public may consider him or her to be "dead" even though whole brain death requires failure of the brainstem in addition to cortical function. The confusion over medical definitions of death is made greater by cultural and religious variations in conceptions of death. In addition, the different criteria may lead to suspicion among the public that these definitions are "malleable" and serve physician agendas, rather than respecting the patient.[9] In the emergency department, cardiopulmonary death is the only definition that we recognize. The use of the term *brain dead* is to be avoided.[9] Brain death requires time to diagnose and confirm. In the patient who is breathing and who has a pulse (which often is the successful result of our resuscitative efforts), it is more important to introduce the family to concepts of prognosis, brain injury, and the further steps that will occur over the succeeding hours that will give physicians and family a clearer picture of whether an injury or insult is fatal or not.

Futility

Physicians are not required to offer treatments that have no benefit.[10,11] Unfortunately, we often do not have enough data in the prehospital setting or in the emergency department to make this judgment. In the case of cardiopulmonary resuscitation (CPR), the emergency physician must proceed with full resuscitative measures without knowing the benefit or burden of this course, unless there is a clear understanding that this is contrary to the patient's wishes. The term "futility" is best avoided in medical discussions of critical patients. *Futility* is sometimes defined as treatment for which no survivors have been reported in similar circumstances in well-designed studies. Other authorities have attempted to quantify futility as a less than 1% chance of resulting in meaningful survival.[10] These criteria are vague and not useful to the emergency physician in deciding whether to resuscitate an elderly or cachectic-appearing patient. Rarely does the emergency physician have information about the patient's overall condition that would allow such a determination, even if the physician were to accept the quantitative definition, which continues to be debated.

The term *futility* can also be used qualitatively, implying that "meaningful" life will not result from the proposed intervention. This use of this term is problematic also because it is a unilateral judgment about values that a patient and family may or may not hold about what constitutes important and significant life. As shorthand for a very low likelihood of success, the emergency physician should only use the term nontechnically (if at all) in a discussion about the purposes or likelihood of success of a given proposed procedure or treatment plan with the patient or family.[11]

Quality of Life and a "Good" Death

As technology gives us the ability to stabilize serious and noncurable diseases and manipulate the timing of death, and as people are increasingly exercising their autonomy in deciding how to control their dying, more is being written and discussed about what constitutes a "good death." There is evidence that the quality of life for persons who live into their 80s is better than it was 20 years ago.[12] For that, medicine can be proud. But there are also serious deficiencies in end-of-life care. A majority of people wish to die at home, although nearly 80% die in an institution. Progressive debility prior to death is common and feared: three fourths of patients are nonambulatory, one third are incontinent, and 40% are cognitively impaired when they die.[13] In the famous SUPPORT study of more than 9000 patients with life-threatening diseases and a 6-month mortality rate of about 50%, only half the physicians knew when patients did not want CPR, and families reported that half the conscious patients were experiencing significant pain at the time of death.[14]

In the emergency department, emergency resuscitation is performed unless patients' wishes to the contrary are clearly known. Information that CPR, intubation, or other invasive treatments are not desired can be conveyed in the form of written advance directives, a state-authorized "No-CPR" or DNAR (do not attempt resuscitation) directive, clear indications from the patient's medical durable power of attorney for medical affairs, or communication with the patient's physician. Unfortunately, less than one quarter of people have written advance directives of any type. Prior conversations and verbal indications of wishes between patients and family or physicians are also uncommon and are rarely available in a truly emergency situation. The lack of knowledge of patients' wishes is particularly worrisome because most people (patients and surrogates) do not understand what "do everything" means. In one study, authors discovered that many people did not realize that successful resuscitation often led to the patient's being placed on life support equipment.[15] In another study of public awareness of CPR, only one third realized that intubation was part of resuscitation, and less than half understood that it included defibrillation.[16]

Family and other surrogates are poor at predicting care that their loved one would want or not want. In one study comparing patient and surrogate choices about life support, surrogates guessed patient wishes only 59% of the time, little better than chance. The best predictor of accurate knowledge of patient wishes in that study and others was a specific discussion between the patient and surrogate about values and wishes.[17]

Physicians and other health care providers likewise have a difficult time judging quality of life and patient wishes at the end of life. In an elegant and classic study, Gerhart and colleagues[18] surveyed emergency care providers' hypothetical attitudes toward quality of life after spinal cord injuries and compared their responses to those of high-level spinal cord injury survivors. Only 18% of providers (emergency medical technicians, nurses, and physicians) imagined they would be glad to be alive after a severe spinal cord injury, whereas 92% of survivors were glad to be alive. Eighty-six percent of the quadriplegics felt that their quality of life was average or better, whereas only 17% of emergency care providers predicted they would have as affirmative a view of their quality of life in the same condition. It is important to remember that people's assessment of what is a "good life" changes with time, age, and the realities of illness.

What priorities most commonly occupy patients at the end of life? When the end of life is near, patients have both medical and nonmedical concerns about their dying. Singer[19] suggests that five topics predominate in people who are dying: having pain and other symptoms adequately relieved, avoiding inappropriate prolongation of dying, achieving control, relieving others of the burden of their dying, and strengthening personal relationships. The only way to know what is important and what brings joy to patients' lives, particularly in the face of chronic or disabling disease, is by asking the patients and those close to them.[20]

The Goals of Medicine

Medical authorities and philosophers have long debated the proper goals of medicine. Physicians are most familiar with the goal of curing. Certainly in emergency medicine, the prevention of premature death and the diagnosis and treatment of diseases are primary. The wealth of technologies, medicines, and other interventions that have developed in the past 20 years have provided us with an impressive armamentarium for attacking disease. They have also left us with a sizeable population of persons who live with chronic diseases. Ellen Fox reminds us of the complexity of our task in medicine: "Although cure is unquestionably an appropriate goal of medicine, other goals are important as well: promoting health, preventing illness and injury, restoring functional capacity, avoiding premature death, relieving suffering, and caring for those who cannot be cured."[21] In Western society, the curative model predominates and physicians are rewarded for being analytic and rational. The disease, not the person, becomes the object of analysis. Symptoms are clues to diagnosis rather than objects to be treated in and of themselves.[21] Fox points out that the palliative care emphasis on "relief of suffering, control of symptoms, and restoration of functional capacity" is really just the other end of a spectrum of care that a physician provides. Most patients have reversible elements to their disease process, and even the patient with streptococcal pharyngitis wants symptom relief. So the goal of medicine may be to discern where to place the emphasis for the patient: the curative and palliative models need to be titrated in varying proportions to maximize care for the individual.[21]

If the physician recognizes the goal of relieving suffering, he or she needs to understand the difference between *pain* and *suffering*. Eric Cassell first introduced the idea that a primary goal of medicine was the relief of suffering in a landmark article in the *New England Journal of Medicine* in 1982.[22] Cassell's main point is that pain happens to bodies, but suffering happens to persons. Suffering derives from the meaning behind the pain or other symptom. It is unique to each person and can only be understood from the patient's perspective. Suffering is "the state of severe distress associated with events that threaten the intactness of the person." There are patients who are in severe distress without any physical pain, and persons who "handle" their pain with very little assistance. Patients suffer, as Cassell points out, "when they feel out of control, when the pain is overwhelming, when the source of the pain is unknown, when the meaning of the pain is dire, or when the pain is chronic."[22] Understanding how to relieve suffering requires the physician to question the patient, to listen empathetically, and to honor the nonbiologic needs of such patients.

Palliative and Hospice Medicine

As the population continues to age and the number of persons living with chronic illnesses rises, quality at the end of life has become increasingly important. Several movements have attempted to rebalance the curative versus palliative models of medical care by emphasizing patient-centered care that maximizes quality of life, particularly as the burden of chronic or irreversible disease becomes great. The hospice movement, which started in England in the 1960s, sought to provide a haven of medical care for persons dying of cancer. Home and inpatient hospice programs now exist throughout this country and are funded through most insurance plans. Patients are usually only eligible for hospice, however, if a physician certifies that the patient's life expectancy is less than 6 months and if the patient agrees to forego any nonhospice interventions. Only about 20% of patients die while receiving hospice services, including less than half of patients with cancer. In addition, referrals occur a median of 20 days before death, leaving insufficient time for many of the interventions that hospice can offer.[23]

A far larger number of people are not ever hospice eligible, since they die during a less predictable acute complication of a chronic noncancer illness (see Figure 206-1).[3] Their prognosis at any point in time is uncertain, even when their diseases are not curable and the appropriate goals of care may switch primarily to enhancing the quality of their remaining life, keeping them as active as possible, and controlling symptoms. This broader movement in end-of-life care is referred to as *palliative care*. The World Health Organization defines palliative care as "active total care of patients whose disease is not responsive to curative treatment. Control of pain, of other symptoms, and of psychological, social and spiritual problems is paramount. The goal of this care is to offer the best possible quality of life for patients and their families."[24] The Palliative Care movement, with programs in many hospitals and linkages to hospice organizations, has developed recently to fill the gap in end-of-life care for patients not qualifying for hospice and for patients with incurable debilitating illness (e.g., COPD, congestive heart failure) that require symptom control.

Emergency Medicine and End-of-Life Care

Emergency physicians encounter death more frequently than physicians in many other specialties. Emergency medicine developed as a specialty, in large part, because of recognition of the critical time element involved, and the diagnostic and intervention skills needed, to rescue people from premature death and disability. As society has evolved, so has the specialty. Resuscitation and restoration to functional living will always be a primary goal of our practice and our research. But seriously ill patients are frequently treated in the emergency department with urgent complaints for which time does not allow deliberation about choices of care through conversations with patients or family. With an increasing population of persons with severe chronic disease, cure may not be possible; however, often interventions are available that can improve the quality of remaining life. Also, at the end of the course of chronic disease, death is not always unwelcome. Achieving our emergency medicine goals requires a complex set of skills. The rest of this chapter is devoted to aspects of end-of-life care that should be part of every emergency physician's skill set: delivering bad news, death notification, establishing and honoring patient goals of care and advance directives, symptom control, and palliation.

SPECIFIC DISORDERS AND CONCERNS

Prehospital Considerations

Historically, prehospital systems were designed to provide immediate resuscitation, stabilization, and transport of seriously ill or injured persons to emergency departments. Aggressive and early resuscitation, through CPR, airway management, defibrillation, fluid resuscitation, and trauma stabilization, has resulted in significant benefits and reduced mortality in the patient with critical illness for whom survival is time-dependent and potentially reversible causes of illness or injury threaten life. Emergency medical service systems are also called to assist when elderly patients whose death is not unexpected die or are in extremis. To fully respect the right of patients to determine what treatments they receive, prehospital providers should always ask if patients have a DNAR (do not attempt resuscitation) directive and honor those written requests that can be identified at the scene and are recognized in the provider's protocols. In the absence of clear directives, full prehospital resuscitation should be initiated, and the patient should be transported to the emergency department for further treatment and clarification of any limitations in desired interventions.

Emergency medical service is also activated for patients with acute decompensation of chronic medical conditions such as heart failure or COPD, as well as for symptoms that occur in the context of terminal conditions when caregivers at the scene cannot cope. Patients at the end of life may desire aggressive interventions for acute exacerbations of chronic illnesses, or they may desire supportive care or transportation only to achieve a nonviolent end to their life. In emergency situations, it may not be possible to determine the patient's underlying medical conditions, in what stage of their life cycle they currently live, or if they desire professional aid in their dying process without invasive interventions. In some situations, however, a titrated response is possible and noninvasive supportive care (such as positioning, suctioning, oxygen, or mask ventilation) during transport can buy time until the emergency department can clarify the patient's goals of care.

Field Death Pronouncement

Several medical circumstances have been identified in which prehospital providers should not initiate or continue CPR because of uniformly poor outcomes and no benefit from intervention. Previous American Heart Association (AHA) guidelines stated that CPR could be justifiably withheld or discontinued in patients with nontraumatic cardiac arrest in circumstances when no survivors after CPR have been reported in well-designed studies. Since there are always exceptional cases, the most recent AHA committee recommendations emphasize that all patients deserve the right of a trial of CPR unless an appropriate DNAR order is in place or clear signs of irreversible death, such as decapitation, lividity, or rigor mortis, are present.[25] The National Association of Emergency Medical Services physicians supports this approach. Termination of resuscitation efforts in nontraumatic cases should be made in agreement with online medical direction and predicated on access to witnesses or family, provider comfort with death notification and grief counseling, as well as safety and logistic considerations.[26] If questions about resuscitation exist, CPR and advanced cardiac life support should be initiated and the patient transported. It can often be easier to withdraw care in the emergency department than to withhold care at the scene.[27]

Honoring Advance Directive Wishes to Withhold Resuscitation

Emergency medical service providers must operate under policies that allow instances for withholding resuscitation at the end of life. The 1991 Patient Self-Determination Act recognizes the need for health care providers to honor informed decisions by patients who wish not to be resuscitated. Identifying valid directives to withhold CPR or intubation is problematic for prehospital providers, because information about patient wishes and underlying diseases is frequently confusing, DNAR requests cannot be validated easily, and rapid intervention is frequently required. Many state-based programs have been developed to try to identify patients requesting no CPR through bracelets or official registered forms on their persons, allowing supportive care without resuscitative efforts if the patient arrests.[28] Several concerns persist: patient wishes can change over time, nonstandard forms of DNAR requests (such as medic alert bracelets, notes on prescription pads, or tattoos) cannot be recognized, and relative-bystanders may not be accurately relaying the wishes of the patient.[29]

Attempts to honor patients' requests at the end of life should be a goal for both prehospital providers and emergency physicians. Most providers have experienced situations in which attempted resuscitation is later determined to have been against the patient's wishes. In a Seattle review of prehospital cardiac arrests in which all patients received full resuscitative efforts, 7% of patients were ultimately determined to have had "unwanted" resuscitation, and 25% of patients experienced resuscitation in the context of severe chronic disease.[30] In one survey of emergency medical technicians, more than 20% had experienced ethical conflicts over the execution, honoring, or validity of DNAR wishes or orders at the scene.[31] Interestingly, another survey among prehospital providers in the Northeast found that the providers understood and agreed on withholding resuscitative efforts in terminally ill patients with advance directives. The majority of respondents in this survey believed that a statute would minimize confusion and provide legal authorization for what they found to be important but were powerless to initiate.[32]

The American College of Emergency Physicians (ACEP) has recognized the difficulties with respecting patients' desires to forgo resuscitative efforts and issued guidelines for developing out-of-hospital DNAR policies.[33] In some states, statutory authority for emergency medical services personnel to honor DNAR orders has been developed, but provisions vary widely. Written statements or identification bracelets must be consistent, easily recognizable, legally acceptable in that state, and clear about what resuscitative measures the patient would and would not wish to receive.[34] A family member or friend who is present at the scene and has valid medical durable power of attorney for health care documentation may make decisions to initiate or refuse treatment measures on behalf of the patient. Otherwise, verbal requests to limit resuscitation cannot be accepted, since it is impossible to confirm that these represent the patient's current wishes.[34] The "default" response to a 911 summons is a full attempt at resuscitation, in the absence of clear directives to the contrary. The prehospital provider needs to be aware of the standards for honoring DNAR requests in their state.[35,36]

Special Issues in the Prehospital Setting

In the prehospital arena, care of the dead and dying involves treating not only the patient but also the family and friends with respect. This respect is most often shown by skillful attempts at resuscitation, but, when death is expected, the prehospital provider may provide the medical expertise in helping to make this important passage occur with grace. The underlying theme to these scenarios is that triage extends beyond the patient or deceased. The patient's family and friends also require appropriate care and attention. This may be in the form of referral for counseling, chaplain services, simple consolation, or transport to a hospital site where more resources are available.

Palliative Care and Home Hospice. Provision of comfort care becomes more important in patients with critical illness near the end of life. Although protocols exist as part of hospice care that avoid activating the emergency medical services system, scenarios routinely occur in which the patient is in the dying process and family panic or cannot handle some terminal situation. There may be anxiety in the last hours of life, a feeling of helplessness, or concern for the patient's perceived or real suffering. There may also be disagreement between family members about the best way to help the dying person. It is important to review DNAR documents and, if necessary, transport the patient to the hospital when it is not clear what would be best for the patient. An "all-or-none" response by emergency medical services should be expanded to incorporate patients' wishes in a non-arrest situation near the expected end of their lives. Often the prehospital provider has less invasive treatment, such as oxygen, suctioning, and noninvasive ventilatory support, to offer the patient and family in distress. The family may request death pronouncement at home, but prehospital providers should involve medical control to affirm this. Transport and comfort care should always be offered if the family wishes or if the setting appears uncomfortable for those involved in the dying process.

Cultural Considerations. Cultural sensitivity is important at critical times like the death or dying of a family member. People from different backgrounds can have different rituals or customs around death. While the prehospital provider cannot be expected to know what these are, it is important to ask the family if they have special needs, procedures, or rites that need to be observed during the last moments of a loved-one's life and to try to respect these.

Suicide. Although respect for patient wishes is a core value in our society, suicidal patients are frequently impaired. We believe that suicidal depression is usually treatable and can be reversed.[37] Patients near death from suicide should receive full resuscitative efforts unless there is a specific exception, such as physician-assisted suicide in Oregon, with formal documentation and an alternative protocol for prehospital providers to follow. If the patient is dead and meets criteria for not starting resuscitation (dependent lividity, or pulselessness after decapitation from a gunshot wound), the medical examiner can be notified. The scene needs to be protected to allow an investigation, if needed, since the history is rarely clear or complete during the emergency call. Decisions should be made after consultation with the medical control physician.

Multiple Victim Incidents. When equipment and personnel are overextended, field triage is required. The field team must make judgments about who will benefit most from care. Dealing with multiple casualties may mean choosing not to attempt resuscitation of someone who probably would not survive and utilizing the limited facilities and personnel to help those who probably could survive with intervention. Most health care workers are unfamiliar and uncomfortable with these decisions. At these times, cardiopulmonary criteria of pulselessness, absent respirations, and unresponsiveness are recommended to pronounce death. A physician should be involved, and the entire team will benefit from debriefing and review after disasters in which pronouncement at the scene is required.

Pregnancy. In the case of a pregnant trauma patient, fetal survival is best ensured by aggressive care of the mother. Some unborn babies will die despite major or minor maternal injuries, but field rescue of the baby with pronouncement of the mother is rarely appropriate and not advised without physician control. A pulseless woman in the third trimester of pregnancy should be transported to the nearest emergency department capable of performing a perimortem cesarean section for attempted resuscitation of both mother and baby.

Pediatric Deaths—Sudden Infant Death Syndrome. Death of a child is among the most difficult experiences that we confront in our lives. Pediatric deaths, regardless of the cause, should have the benefit of complete resuscitative efforts, including transport. Child abuse should always be considered as a possibility. Transport may be done more for the psychological benefit to the family than in the hope of survival. As sudden infant death syndrome has become more widely recognized and understood by the public, some families resent the "extraordinary measures" attempted in the resuscitation of their infant once the diagnosis is recognized and the consequences are inevitable. Many desire to be with their infant in his or her last moments. Prehospital personnel should respond to these requests with understanding and compassion; however, the site of pronouncement of death should be in the hospital for almost all pediatric deaths.

Death in the Emergency Department

Delivering Bad News

Every emergency physician will be required to communicate bad news to patients, family members, and caregivers. The manner in which this is done helps shape the course of subsequent grief and coping, strengthens trust, and fosters collaboration in planning between the medical team and the patient and family. However, many providers feel inadequately prepared to deliver bad news, particularly when a life-threatening illness or family death is encountered. These skills take time and experience to learn. The best ways to learn are through explicit instructional sessions, role playing, use of standardized patients, and the example of colleagues who are comfortable with "caring" for their patients.[1,38-40]

Empirical studies and theoretical constructs for how to understand best practice in delivering bad news are remarkably lacking. One theoretical construct has been suggested by Ptacek and Eberhardt.[41] The goal of skillfully breaking bad news is to reduce the severity and the duration of stress and encourage engagement of coping mechanisms. This holds for both the physician and patient or their caregivers. In the emergency department, the staff and physicians' stress often peaks just before transmission of the bad news. Skilled resuscitation, diagnosis, and treatment of patients are key to keeping the external sources of stress manageable. Experience, practice, and self-examination constitute the best way of reducing the negative feelings associated with the anticipatory stress of delivering bad news.[41] For the patient and family, the emergency department is typically the place where bad news is sudden and unexpected. This can certainly make the strain even more severe and overwhelming. Trust between emergency department caregivers and critically ill patients or their survivors, who were unlinked strangers just a few minutes before, does not come easily. Surveys of patients and families indicate that desirable features of receiving bad news include privacy when receiving news, the ability to express emotions safely, information that is free of unclear language or medical jargon, empathetic and caring attitude, allowance for hope, and ability to ask and receive good medical information.[41] The steps listed in Box 206-1 and explained in detail in the following paragraphs are designed to shape the interaction to facilitate the patient's or survivors' work through this stress and movement towards coping. This six-step template was adapted from Buckman's work and adopted also by the Education for Physicians on End-of-Life Care teaching project.[23,42] It mirrors the consensus recommendations of experts, although clearly more critical evaluation and studies are needed to understand what does and does not work in this setting.[41] Key to moving through the process of delivering bad news is the ability to listen, pause, and let oneself be guided by the patient and family in regard to the pace, amount of information, and style that will work best to let these particular persons feel and hear what they need.

BOX 206-1. Delivering Bad News

The steps listed below can help you think critically about how best to communicate at a time when stress is high. See the text for details about each step.

Step 1. Physician preparation
Step 2. What does the patient know?
Step 3. How much does the patient want to know?
Step 4. Sharing the information
Step 5. Responding to feelings
Step 6. Planning and follow-up

Adapted from Buckman R: *How to Break Bad News: A Guide for Health Care Professions.* Baltimore, Johns Hopkins University Press, 1992.

Step 1. Physician Preparation

Before the physician interacts with the family or patient, preparatory steps are important. These include confirming all medical facts of the case, clarifying the name of the patient, being aware if there is uncertainty about the patient's identity, and knowing the relationships between the patient and those with whom one will be talking. The physical site for the conversation is important; the environment should be quiet and allow for private exchange of information and should be located where the patient and family can safely express emotions. Sometimes this is very difficult in the chaos of the emergency department, but there is usually a family room or other quiet area to use. If the patient can be included, moving the patient to a private area may be possible, or key members of the patient's support group can be gathered around the bedside.

Physicians should identify themselves and their position, address the patient (when present) or the key persons receiving the news directly, and refer to the patient by name. One should sit down close to the patient, make direct eye contact with the patient (or close relatives), and be physically and mentally open to their concerns and needs.

Step 2. What Does the Patient Know?

It is useful to know what the patient or family understands prior to the delivery of news. An introductory question can be used, such as "What do you understand about your illness?" or "What have you been told happened to your spouse/sibling (use name)?" This information helps the physician to see the event as the patient and family are seeing it thus far and adjust the way he or she delivers the news to their understandings. In the emergency department, when patients and families may expect "the worst," this tactic can be perceived as delaying. In a less critical situation, however, asking about prior testing, conversations with physicians, and understanding of the patient's illness can help the subsequent information fit into the patient's perspective and expectations.

Step 3. How Much Does the Patient Want to Know?

Every patient has the right to accept or refuse medical treatments based on informed consent. This is also true for information. Most of our patients appreciate the direct, simple truth about their condition and prognosis. There will, however, be some patients who do not want to accept the information that the provider is about to deliver. These patients may wish to designate a friend or family member to represent them. This should be respected if possible. It is important to remember that individuals process information and make decisions in many different ways, based on their own cultural and religious views, and previous experiences. The Western principles of truth telling and individual decision-making are cultural values and may be foreign to some families and communities.

Sometimes the family learns of a diagnosis and prognosis before the patient and requests that the patient not be told of the diagnosis. The physician's alliance with both patient and family is important, although responsibility to the patient is primary. Physicians should explore why families do not want the patient told bad news: is it a cultural tradition, are they afraid of what harm it will cause the patient, or have they had prior bad experiences? The physician is still required to ask the patient how much he or she would like to know. Sometimes it is helpful for physicians to invite family to join with them as they ask this of the patient. This important information should be learned using an independent interpreter (rather than family member) if the patient does not speak the same language as the physician.

Step 4. Sharing the Information

In general, patients and families want to know bad news in a timely fashion.[41] This is sometimes uncomfortable, particularly when important information may not yet be known—a common occurrence in the emergency department. At the very least, it is recommended that patients and family be given a preparatory warning after introductions, such as, "I am afraid I have some bad news." When delivering the information, one should use simple nonmedical language and make sure that the patient comprehends the information. Space should be allowed for patients and family to absorb the news, to react, and to begin to ask questions. The patient and family stress response will lag behind that of the physician, because the physician has had at least a few minutes to adjust to the current situation, but the family has not.[41]

While using the phrase "I'm sorry" can be a reflection of empathy, it can be misinterpreted. Some physicians have suggested using expressions such as "I wish things were different" instead, as a sign of solidarity.[43] Providing survival data when the discussion is about a severe or terminal diagnosis may be better reserved for a later time, but one should know how to access this information, and the physician's message should include some realistic hope and also reassurance that the patient will not be abandoned by the medical care team, even when cure or survival is unlikely.

Step 5. Responding to Feelings

The reaction to bad news is often unpredictable and can range from sadness to rage. One should be aware of the wide varieties of responses that will be seen. The patient and family should be allowed to express their feelings, even if it is uncomfortable. Acute grief is painful but important. The emergency physician must be prepared both for persons who turn inward and those who rage outwardly. Practicing and reflecting on these situations allows the physician to deliver bad news and support the survivors. In the emergency department, it is often helpful to invite members of the team into this meeting (e.g., social worker, nurse, or chaplain) who will not be pulled away to other care needs, can provide emotional support, and can help the family navigate through the early stages of grief, as well as the technical details necessary.

Step 6. Planning and Follow-up

The emergency department is an entry point to the hospital if the patient survives. Family should be encouraged to stay with the patient, particularly if it is possible that the end of life is near. Prognosticating may be difficult, given the limited information we accumulate in the initial assessment. When emergency department management has stabilized a patient with an acute, critical turn, it may be appropriate to look ahead to decompensation that could occur later in the hospitalization. Some authors have suggested a "hope for the best, and prepare for the worst" kind of conversation.[44] The physician can share the success, however transient, of the emergency department interventions and the positive news and hope that this provides. At the same time, he or she can prepare the patient or family for the possibility of later setback or even arrest, and have them consider what actions may or may not be appropriate if "the worst" happens. If the patient does not have written advance directives, the emergency department can facilitate the conversation, initiate written wishes, or at least prewarn the patient that the admitting physician will need to have an early conversation about future plans and goals for the patient. The physician should assure the patient and family of what the next steps will be, including admission or discharge from the hospital, consultation with specialists, support group referral, or chaplain services. It is important to make sure the patient and family do not feel abandoned. Even when dying is near, providing active care and comfort is a major task for the medical team.

Death Notification

One of the most difficult forms of "bad news" to deliver is death notification. Emergency physicians need to practice this skill specifically (Box 206-2).

Death notification usually occurs after an unsuccessful resuscitation attempt. Physicians should be

BOX 206-2. Elements of an Empathic Death Disclosure

Introduce self/role.
Sit down.
Assume comfortable communication distance.
Use acceptable tone/rate of speech.
Make eye contact.
Maintain open posture.
Give advanced warning of bad news.
Deliver news of death clearly (use "dead"/"died").
Tolerate survivor's reaction.
Explain medical attempts to "save" patient.
Use no medical jargon; use language that is clear and easily understood.
Offer viewing of deceased.
Offer to be available to survivor.
Conclude appropriately.

From Quest TE, et al: The use of standardized patients within a procedural competency model to teach death disclosure. *Academic Emerg Med* 9:1326, 2002.

sure they are presentable and wear a name badge. If possible, one should identify who has arrived, their relation to the patient, and what they know. Other members of the medical team may have met them already and can be a source of background information. Arrangements should be made so that 5 to 10 undisturbed minutes with the family are available by having a colleague cover the emergency department or by the physician's excusing himself or herself briefly from other patients. If an interruption cannot be prevented, the family should be assured that the physician will return, and the physician should do so as expeditiously as possible.

Sometimes the family initiated the 911 call and knew that their loved one had died at that time. On the other hand, a family summoned to the emergency department may have absolutely no idea that they are about to be informed that their loved one has been critically injured or has died. For this reason, it is useful to have an emergency department nurse or colleague advise the family briefly about the general nature of the event and the status of resuscitation as soon as possible. When giving the news, physicians should use clear "dead" or "died" language to be sure that there are no misunderstandings about the outcome being conveyed. The emergency physician needs to assure the survivors, if at all possible, that their responses to the emergency were appropriate, that the medical care team did all that was possible, and that the victim did not experience unnecessary discomfort. Appreciation of their presence in the emergency department, or even in the resuscitation room, is also important to emphasize.

The physician can try to mobilize continuing support for survivors, being sure that key people close to the survivors are being called, and that there is room for all the family and friends to be present. A family spokesperson may need to be identified, particularly for later questions and details. Hospital chaplains are very helpful in this situation and are trained to address concerns of patients and families of varying faiths or no structured faith. Clergy may also be important to the family, and clinicians should ask (if a chaplain is not present to facilitate this) if a specific religious resource person would be appropriate to call.

Phone Notification. If the first contact with survivors of an emergency department death is by telephone, it is recommended that the survivor be told to come to the emergency department if at all possible.[1] Although family members may ask or even demand to know if death has occurred, allowing some time for assimilation of news by delaying information about the final outcome has been found to be better in the grieving process.[45] Nonphysician staff are particularly useful to summon survivors and can inform the relative that the patient has been involved in an accident or is seriously ill and that things are not going well.

When the notification is to somebody who is more than an hour away or otherwise unable to physically come to the emergency department to receive the bad news, it must be given by phone. The physician should (1) make sure that the relative has someone present in the room if possible, (2) ask the relative to be seated, and (3) name the person involved. One should start with brief information about the circumstances and warn the person that one has bad news before breaking it to them. Even a few seconds of preparation in these circumstances can serve to partially attenuate the acute psychic pain. Based on the response, there may be a need to ask, "Are you able to talk for a few minutes?" Some individuals may be unwilling or unable to continue after they hear the initial news, and they should be given an "out," but a definite time to reconnect must be established (e.g., 10 to 15 minutes).[1,45] Long-distance loved ones cannot view the body to facilitate confirmation and acceptance and inevitably have questions not addressed in the initial conversation. The relative should be given a telephone contact of someone who actually cared for the patient. Otherwise, if a relative calls back, a lack of information about what transpired on another shift may cause frustration, or even feed the person's denial or false hope that this tragedy has not happened.

Viewing the Body. At some time immediately after death, an opportunity to view the body should be offered to the family. This may be the first exposure to the body for the survivors and can make concrete what has up to now been only abstract and unreal. Although a majority of survivors find viewing the body helpful, no attempt should be made to force this procedure on survivors, and they should not be made to feel that it is wrong not to view the body. If viewing is presented as an alternative and an aid in the mourning process, it is usually considered helpful.

If possible, the body should be moved to a small room, preferably away from the main treatment area. This not only ensures privacy but also makes the family feel more at ease. Family members should be warned of what to expect, such as color and temperature changes, injuries or invasive premortem procedures, and the presence of endotracheal and intravenous tubing. With sufficient preparation, most people are not shocked by the appearance.

A staff member should remain in the room or within close range of the viewing at all times. This contact allows the staff to help make the viewing an important and supportive aspect of the grieving process. At times, it may be necessary to touch the body to assure the family that this is appropriate. Survivors should be allowed to remain with the body for as long as seems appropriate. When gross disfigurement has occurred, the viewers should be warned about this, and the body should be discretely covered where necessary. Survivors may even find that helping to clean and prepare the body (particularly with a pediatric death), holding a loved one, or preparing for transport may allow a final expression of caring.

Family Observing the Resuscitation. It is increasingly common to invite a close family member to attend resuscitation attempts. This has been endorsed in the 2000 AHA Emergency Cardiac Care guidelines.[25] Whereas some family members find this very helpful in understanding that "everything has been done" for their loved one, others may be uncomfortable. A staff person who is dedicated to supporting that person should always accompany family members. In difficult resuscitation attempts, when major trauma has occurred or the diagnosis and circumstances are unclear, the physician and caregivers should feel comfortable requesting that family wait with staff outside the resuscitation room to avoid the distraction of nonmedical people during critical decision making.

Sedation for Survivors. Requests for tranquilizers, sedatives, sleeping medications, or just "something for the nerves" are common. The grieving process is important and difficult work. Prescriptions for a light sedative for a few days may be appropriate but usually require evaluation of the survivor by the physician directly. The survivor needs to know that the psychic pain is to be expected and where to turn for help and support during this difficult time.[1]

Autopsy and Closure. The "event" of death notification should be concluded with a physician expression of condolences and concern for the survivors—all of us can honestly express the wish that we did not need to be the bearer of such life-changing news.[43] In many hospitals, chaplains or social workers or nurses are trained in informing the family about arrangements for the body, including notification of a mortician and interface with a coroner, which is not uncommon in emergency department deaths. If the staff desires an autopsy, this is an appropriate time to request permission. Autopsies not only are valuable in contributing to the advancement of knowledge, education, quality assurance, and public education but also can be indispensable in minimizing guilt and blame associated with the death of a loved one. Additionally, findings of unknown pathology may be important for family members if there is a genetic factor.

Consent for Procedures on the Newly Dead. The use of the newly dead to teach procedural skills is currently being debated in the medical community. It is important to educate residents in procedural skills, and emergency physicians often need to review procedures that they perform very rarely. Newly dead have been a silent source of learning in the past. While there is some evidence that the public generally supports the practice, serious questions about respect for bodies and the need for informed consent have also been raised.[46] The AMA recently published a policy that affirms that consent should be obtained from survivors.[47] In emergency medicine, it has been argued that obtaining consent is not feasible: finding authorizing survivors is difficult, voluntary consent is questionable in a stressful situation of sudden death, and time pressures require early resumption of other emergency department activities. Some have tried to distinguish between invasive or major procedures (thoracotomy, peritoneal lavage, venous cutdown) and minor or less invasive ones, such as intubation. The current ACEP position is that informed consent must be obtained from relatives before any procedures are performed on the newly dead. The performance of involuntary, nontherapeutic invasive procedures, including those performed during CPR, should be regarded as an ethically unacceptable departure from a standard of care that emphasizes the centrality of respect for the patient, the patient's well-being, and the requirement for informed consent.[47-49]

The Grief Response

Grief is defined as emotional pain induced by sorrow and loss. It is associated with a constellation of symptoms and behaviors that are influenced by cultural and personal issues, other current life stressors, and the relationship of the survivor to the deceased. Survivors are often the "patients" toward whom the emergency physician needs to direct his or her best expertise in the case of an emergency department death. Giving bad news and sharing in the beginnings of the grief response are among the most difficult situations physicians need to handle. The emergency physician must recognize that patients and loved ones also experience grief responses when a sudden downturn of health that brings a patient to the emergency department is seen as a threat to life and wellness, not just when patients die.

Much has been written about the grief responses of both dying persons and their survivors. Experienced health care workers who have been involved in delivering bad news know that the acute grief response is unpredictable. It is important to understand the range of what can be expected and be able to identify those groups at risk for complicated grief. Recognition of higher risk survivors may help stimulate referral and decrease the risk of development of major depression and other stress disorders.

The initial response to any death, whether expected or unexpected, is acute psychic pain that is associated with shock, disbelief, numbness, and inability to process further information.[1] Some persons display anger, loud screaming, crying, and occasionally acute anxiety or syncope. Alternatively, the physician may observe a false calm or no reaction. In addition to the initial emotional shock, other more cognitive reactions, including denial, guilt, sadness, fear, shame, and anger, may be exhibited. Reactions may be based on the cultural and personal backgrounds of the survivors. This wide range of expressions is normal and expected; there is no "right" way to grieve. In the emergency department, outward reactions will many times be perceived as problematic and disruptive. The goal of the emergency physician is to help as much as survivors allow and to avoid taking personally the survivors' anger, resentment, and other outward emotional expressions, even if directed at the emergency department staff.[1] Likewise, it is important to accept that there will be survivors who leave the department still in denial and not emoting; they may need and want to postpone their grieving for what they feel is a more appropriate gathering.

Guilt often plays a role in acute grief. To not be in control and to have a loved one die is uncomfortable, particularly in our society, where death is often seen as a failure. Self-blame is common and all the more difficult when a survivor was involved in interactions that directly preceded or were responsible for the victim's death. Guilt is especially profound in pediatric deaths, after which parents may withdraw from each other in their pain. Emotional expressions of grief also include denial, intellectualization, numbness, relief, anxiety, and confusion.[1,23,50]

A variety of delayed emotional and physical symptoms can occur as the individual assimilates the reality that death has occurred. Physical symptoms include fatigue, anorexia, palpitations, hyperventilation, restlessness, headache, irritability, and insomnia. Emotional symptoms, in addition to guilt, anger, depression, and denial, include difficulty in concentrating, lack of organization, fear, and preoccupation with the deceased. These grief responses are to be expected. Special memories can trigger the grief response after the initial grieving period, and the memory and emotional pain of the loss may last a lifetime. Symptoms of grief, including psychic pain, numbness, intrusive thoughts, and disorganization continue to recur during the recovery of most survivors, gradually becoming attenuated but recurring over months or years without clear "stages."[51]

For most survivors, the emotional reaction to a loss lasts 6 to 12 months. Four tasks necessary to achieve resolution of grief after a major loss have been described.[50] (1) The bereaved needs to accept that the death has actually occurred. The emergency physician can facilitate this with clear communication and the option of viewing the body and helping the survivor construct the story of this major life event. (2) The survivor needs a chance to feel the pain of the loss, which is why sedation should be given for only a few days at most. (3) The survivor must acknowledge the impact of the loss and the changes that it brings to his or her life; this work takes months. (4) Finally, the survivor must return to activities and relationships and recommit his or her energy to living life. While the emergency physician only sees the very beginning of this process, understanding "normal" grieving gives the emergency physician a framework for understanding his or her role in the process.

BOX 206-3. Risk Factors for Complicated Grief Reactions

Spousal death:
- Long-term marriage
- Children involved
- Strong dependence in relationship
- Significant economic consequences for loss

Conflict (especially recent) or ambivalent relationship with deceased
Pediatric death
Long geographic distance between deceased and survivor
Social isolation or prior mental illness in survivor
Presence of elderly or dependent care receivers in the family unit

Adapted from Iserson KV: *Grave Words: Notifying Survivors About Sudden, Unexpected Deaths.* Tucson, Ariz, Galen Press, 1999.

Complicated Grief. Complicated grief is the existence of dysfunctional symptoms that interfere with a return to re-engagement in the community over a prolonged period of time, usually years. It is associated with adverse health, increased morbidity, and inability to find joy or even to function in the community. It is different than depression and is not treated effectively within that construct.[51] Risk factors for difficulty navigating the work of grieving can sometimes be recognized, even in the emergency department (Box 206-3). The emergency physician should enlist social workers, chaplains, and others in establishing a plan for continued support. The physician may be able to alert the survivors' primary physician, or even the at-risk survivor directly, that ongoing work will be required to see this grief to resolution.

Grief Reactions in Staff. The impact of death in emergency medicine is significant for the staff, including physicians. Stressors that exacerbate grief and the emotional impact of emergency department work include exposure to premature deaths of young people, victims of random and senseless violence, care to those who may have caused an accident or injury, and care that must be delivered rapidly on the basis of scant knowledge, but which other professionals can later second-guess. Each of us also carries a personal history that may include circumstances that make particular emergencies hit a raw nerve of which our colleagues may not be aware, as, for instance, an alcoholic father, a sibling who has committed suicide, or a friend killed by a drunk driver.

Because of the sometimes overwhelming contact with death and dying in the emergency department, it is important to have intradepartmental mechanisms for helping address staff grief responses. At morbidity and mortality conferences, some discussion should be allotted to ethical, sociologic, and emotional sequelae of the cases being presented. The morbidity and mortality process itself helps "make sense" of difficult situations and is part of our grieving process. Case conferences, including a full range of medical personnel, chaplains, and social workers, are useful to articulate and share sadness, anger towards patients, and other emotional and cognitive work required for healing. This is particularly important to offer staff after major community disasters. Although for some people denial is a positive coping mechanism, for others the opportunity to share and express emotions is needed to begin to move forward and resume the work of caring for patients.

Transplantation

The number of organ donations in the United States lags behind the ever-increasing numbers of persons awaiting transplantation. The number of *potential* organ donors in the United States is estimated at 8000 to 15,000 annually. In 1999, there were 72,000 patients on the organ network waiting list, 6000 of whom died waiting for organs. Half were awaiting a kidney, 30% a liver, 12% a heart, and 10% a lung. Estimates are that only one third of the potential is being realized by the current organ donation system. Two major problems account for the lack of donation. First, approximately 25% of the families of eligible donors are not given the option of donation. Educational interventions have successfully increased the rates of donation. Second, more than half of the families approached decline donation. Nondonor families have a poor understanding of brain death and may feel they have insufficient time and privacy to make their decision. Frequently, they are later dissatisfied with their decision against donation. Success is greater when death announcements are "decoupled" from request for organ donation and when trained professionals can ask in a private setting.[52]

In 1998, the U.S. Centers for Medicare and Medicaid Services, in response to the shortage of organ donors, changed federal regulations to require that hospitals notify their local organ procurement organization in a timely manner about patients whose death is "imminent," so that all families can be presented with the option of organ and tissue donation. The regulation requires trained "designated requestors" to make the request for organ donation and requires that any persons who discuss organ donation with families be trained to do so. The change is partly in recognition of the fact that many hospital staff who care for potential donors and their families are unfamiliar, uncomfortable, or lack sufficient training in the knowledge and skills necessary to present the options of organ and tissue donation to families.[54]

Ischemia-resistant tissues, such as corneas, eyes, skin, bone, veins, and heart valves, can be retrieved 10 to 24 hours after death if the body has been refrigerated within 4 hours after death. Age limits for organ and tissue donation range up to 80 years, although patients older than 55 years are judged on an individual basis. Organs and tissues not routinely used for transplantation are those from patients with cancer (except eye lenses, which are avascular) or those with human immunodeficiency virus. Marginal candidates include patients with hepatitis, diabetes, and severe hypertension. The organs that are routinely transplanted include the kidneys, liver, heart, lungs, pancreas, and less often the small bowel.[1]

Emergency physicians are in a unique position to begin the process of preparing survivors for the mandated request by an organ procurement organization.[51] Since the emergency physician is the person informing survivors of the death of a patient, their conversation should be primarily focused on the events surrounding that death. Emergency physicians should, however, be prepared to answer questions if families ask about organ donation and let them know that an organ procurement organization will be discussing those issues with them. Families often feel gratified and comforted by the thought that that a loved one can, in death, perhaps help another person. If the deceased has signed a donor card, and particularly if the wish to donate was discussed prior to death, agreement of the survivors is more likely. At present, in most states, consent for organ donation is requested even in cases in which the individual has signed an organ donor card. It is hoped that in the near future the expressed wishes of the deceased will not be allowed to be overridden by survivors. State statutes governing the details of the consent process for donation vary.[1]

PALLIATIVE CARE IN THE EMERGENCY DEPARTMENT

Providing quality palliative end-of-life care is important in the emergency department. The evidence that we do not know what others want at the time of critical illness is discussed in the first part of this chapter. In the case of a cardiopulmonary arrest or major trauma resuscitation, attempts at curative intervention should always be performed unless the emergency physician has clear instructions from the patient or surrogate to the contrary. In less critical situations, however, guidance about the goals and direction of emergency department care is needed, and management strategies should be "patient-centered."[23] Although some would argue that it is time-consuming and unnecessary to develop a nuanced approach to emergency department patient care, it is no longer appropriate to treat patients maximally and "let the admitting doctor sort these issues out." Comfort and quality of life become a higher priority for many patients with severe chronic diseases, such as cancer, COPD, heart failure, renal insufficiency, or dementia. Some of the procedures that are normal interventions of emergency department care may not be appropriate in this subset of patients.

Establishing Goals of Care

The primary skill that emergency physicians must have in managing patients near the end of life is the ability to communicate. In a true emergency, such conversations must take a back seat to resuscitation interventions. In many patients, however, it is not imperative to treat before discussion or diagnosis. The emergency physician has several methods for establishing what treatments patients want near the end of life.

Reviewing and Honoring Advance Directives. Asking patients about advance directives is now federally mandated, as is having somebody available to assist patients with documenting end-of-life wishes in all patients who are admitted to the hospital. The Patient Self Determination Act of 1991 was enacted to assure patients that they could control the kind of care they get at the end of life (see Chapter 205). Living wills are rarely directly applicable to emergency department care, since they are usually predicated on certification of a number of days in a clearly terminal state. They, as well as more detailed advance directives of other varieties, do not usually foresee the particular medical emergency that precipitates an emergency department visit. Their existence, however, indicates that a patient has considered how medical care should or should not look. Advance directives may indicate that aggressive life-saving interventions are in order, or that a patient is in the dying process and wants to be kept comfortable. While the details or procedures listed in advance directives are rarely pertinent to the needs of the moment, they provide a good entry point for discussions with the patient or family about what the goals of care should be at this particular time. People's wishes change over time, and written advance directive requests should be reconfirmed at the time of an acute crisis, although with an honest readiness on the part of the emergency physician to accept the limitations that a patient may have requested previously. The emergency physician should be well versed in the technicalities of the various forms of written, legal advance directives that exist.

Processing Verbal Requests. Verbal requests to titrate or limit procedures can be made by the patient or the patient's surrogate. The emergency department must determine whether the patient has decision-making capacity, and, if not, who should be the spokesperson for the patient. Invasive tests and procedures may not be performed on patients without their consent. In emergency situations, we rely on the emergency exception to informed consent and act to preserve life, or at least to buy time to consider options. Many situations in the emergency department, however, do not require immediate intervention, or they allow for a less invasive alternative (such as mask ventilation for respiratory failure) while goals for the emergency department visit are discussed.

Initiating a Conversation on Goals of Care. Emergency physicians see many sick patients who do not have written advance directives but are temporarily stable enough to having meaningful conversations about what their needs and goals are, where they perceive they are in the course of their disease, whether they wish to cure an intercurrent problem, which symptoms require management, and how much effort they wish to have undertaken should resuscitation be needed to preserve their life. Patients with seemingly lethal conditions may be aggressively pursuing curative or at least disease-modifying options, whereas the heavy burden of suffering other patients are experiencing is not obvious until you ask about their illness. The only way to determine the patient's needs is to ask.

Questions that can be useful for initiating this conversation are listed in Table 206-1. The emergency physician has the disadvantage of needing to learn the answers to some of these questions in a fast-paced

Table 206-1. Representative Questions for Initiating the Discussion About End-of-Life Issues

Domain	Representative Questions*
Goals	Given the severity of your illness, what is most important for you to achieve? How do you think about balancing quality of life with length of life in terms of your treatment? What are your most important hopes? What are your biggest fears?
Values	What makes life most worth living for you? Would there be any circumstances under which you would find life not worth living? What do you consider your quality of life to be like now? Have you seen or been with someone who had a particularly good death or particularly difficult death?
Advance directives	If with future progression of your illness you are not able to speak for yourself, who would be best able to represent your views and values? (health care proxy) Have you given any thought to what kinds of treatment you would want (and not want) if you become unable to speak for yourself in the future? (living will)
Do-not-resuscitate order	If you were to die suddenly, that is, you stopped breathing or your heart stopped, we could try to revive you by using cardiopulmonary resuscitation (CPR). Are you familiar with CPR? Have you given thought as to whether you would want it? Given the severity of your illness, CPR would in all likelihood be ineffective. I would recommend that you choose not to have it, but that we continue all potentially effective treatments. What do you think?
Palliative care (pain and other symptoms)	Have you ever heard of hospice (palliative care)? What has been your experience with it? Tell me about your pain. Can you rate it on a scale of 1 to 10? What is your breathing like when you feel at your best? How about when you are having trouble?
Palliative care ("unfinished business")	If you were to die sooner rather than later, what would be left undone? How is your family handling your illness? What are their reactions? Has religion been an important part of your life? Are there any spiritual issues you are concerned about at this point?

*Physicians should give the patient an opportunity to respond to each question. Base follow-up questions and responses on careful listening to the patient, using the patient's own words whenever possible.

From Quill JE: Initiating end of life discussions with seriously ill patients: Addressing the "elephant in the room." *JAMA* 284:2502, 2000.

setting, during an acute downturn in the patient's health, and with no prior relationship with this patient. On the other hand, it may be easier to "take stock" and have this conversation in just such a setting. Pulling up a chair, sitting with the patient and family, and spending a few minutes clarifying the patient's values and view of the present and the future may make a big difference in designing the patient's care and disposition.

It is useful to start the "goals of care" conversation with a global understanding of this person's illness, values, fears, and expectations. This makes the "procedures" part of the conversation flow naturally. The physician can guide the patient and family about what treatments will be useful in the context of overall goals and values. Antibiotics may be appropriate for an acute pneumonia, but they may not be indicated in a patient with advanced dementia who has been bedridden and unable to communicate for several years. Intubation will be acceptable for some COPD patients, whereas others have struggled on the ventilator before and do not wish to experience that discomfort again. Intravenous hydration is useful for dehydration but may just increase secretions in the patient who is actively dying. All these interventions need to be seen in the context of caring for the patient and enabling them to achieve their goals.

Initiating Advance Directives and DNAR Orders. Several authors have suggested that emergency departments may be an important link in initiating advance directives because they are the portal of access for patients to the hospital.[55] Wrenn and Brody described a small series of patients for whom the emergency physician wrote DNAR orders on admission.[56] Balentine and colleagues described another series, with few negative responses from the families who were approached.[57] Both papers point out that fragmentation in health care may mean that prior wishes are not translated into hospitalized settings, and the emergency department may be the best place to establish or renew documentation of the patient's wish to forgo resuscitation at the outset of the hospitalization.

Treating Symptoms Requiring Palliation

When a patient is suffering from a disease that is not curable, he or she may still want a variety of medical interventions as part of care: antibiotics for intercurrent infections, drainage of effusions that cause shortness of breath, wound care for decubiti, decompression of bowel obstructions, and aggressive pain management. On the other hand, the best way of maximizing patient function and quality of remaining life may require de-emphasizing diagnosis and primarily addressing symptoms. The most common reason that patients with end stage illness seek care in the emergency department is for control of intolerable symptoms such as nausea, vomiting, dyspnea, severe constipation or diarrhea, and pain (Box 206-4).

BOX 206-4. Palliative Medical Treatment Options to Enhance Quality of Life

- Pain control
- Control of fluid and electrolyte imbalance
- Nausea/vomiting/constipation management
- Radiation therapy for bone pain, cord compression, hemorrhage from tumors
- Drainage tubes for malignant effusions/obstructions
- Treatment of intercurrent infections
- Management of incontinence
- Supplemental oxygen
- Anxiolytics, anti-depressives, appetite stimulants when appropriate

The emergency physician experiences several concerns when attempting to treat symptoms in frail persons near the end of life. One of the more "foreign" concepts to most emergency physicians is the treatment of symptoms without diagnosing the underlying cause, even though this is often the appropriate option. Additionally, the concern over "drugging" patients or overtreating them is common. Worry about unintended consequences may lead to underdosing medications, leaving patients without their desired relief. This problem frequently arises with the use of opioids to control pain. Concerns about respiratory depression arise, leading to inadequate pain control, even though the risk of respiratory depression is minimal when the dose is titrated to the patient's desired endpoint. The EPEC curriculum is an excellent resource for learning about strategies that are unique to palliative caring for patients.[23] The following "pearls" from that program may be useful.

Pain. For patients presenting with acute pain or chronic pain of moderate intensity (rated 5/10 or above) opioid use is appropriate (see Chapter 187). A thorough medication history must be obtained to determine tolerance and dose adjustments that may be needed. Multiple agents used together are often more effective, combining long-acting agents (e.g., methadone) and "as needed" boluses for acute exacerbations. The use of nonsteroidal anti-inflammatory drugs may be helpful in potentiating the effects of opiates in cancer patients. Differentiating neuropathic pain is also important, because medications such as gabapentin or tricyclics may be added. Rising serum levels of opioids stimulate the chemotactic trigger zone, causing nausea. Minimizing fluctuations by using long-acting agents whenever possible can limit this form of nausea. It is important to clearly explain to the patient and caretakers about the regimen, as well as monitoring parameters and expected side effects, and also to coordinate changes in treatment regimens with the primary physician.[23]

Nausea and Vomiting. Nausea and vomiting arise from the gastrointestinal tract, cerebral cortex, vestibular apparatus, or the chemoreceptor trigger zone in the fourth ventricle. The neurotransmitters involved include serotonin, dopamine, acetylcholine, and histamine. Successful treatment of nausea and vomiting revolves around selecting the drugs that will target the right receptors. In addition to usual antiemetics, dexamethasone, octreotide (which reduces secretions and may be useful in cases of intestinal obstruction), and tetrahydrocannabinol may be important adjuncts to control nausea.[23,58]

Constipation. Constipation is multifactorial near the end of life; causes include decreased mobility, medications, mechanical obstruction, and dehydration. Stimulant laxatives, then osmotic laxatives should be tried in escalating doses, and combinations may be needed. Opioids can be a major problem; tolerance does not develop to this side effect of chronic and high-dose use. Every attempt should be made to prevent rather than treat constipation by anticipating the need for stimulant softener combinations when using opioids chronically. In cases of mechanical small bowel obstruction, medical management with clear liquids, loperamide, and octreotide results in resolution in a majority of patients.[23]

Anorexia and Cachexia. Anorexia and cachexia develop in patients with advanced diseases and may be more stressful for the family than the patient. Parenteral nutrition does not necessarily reverse this, nor does it affect life expectancy, although infections of the esophagus should be considered and appetite stimulants are sometimes useful.[23]

Shortness of Breath. Shortness of breath can also be part of the last stages of airway disease or cancer involving the lungs. There are many causes, and several treatment choices should be tried. Alternatives include symptomatic treatment with oxygen (which may not work if central triggers are operating), anxiolytics, and opioids, which may decrease the sensation of breathlessness. In the actively dying patient, morphine and atropine can be used to dry secretions and slow breathing rates and calm the work of breathing.[23]

Special Situations and Diseases

Advanced Dementia

Alzheimer's dementia is a prolonged and relentless chronic disease that can last up to 20 years. With severe dementia, patients may be combative, incontinent, and unable to ambulate. In the terminal phases of the disease, they are bedridden, mute, and dysphagic and suffer from intercurrent infections.[59] In the demented patient, invasive procedures often require restraints and sedation, and the emotional burden to the patient is high. Even hospitalization, administration of intravenous fluids or antibiotics, and other common interventions are frightening to patients with dementia. Percutaneous gastrostomy tubes do not prolong life in these patients, and their qualitative benefits are questionable. Feeding tubes do not prevent aspiration, provide palliation, or improve function in a progressive severe disease like dementia.[60,61] For the emergency physician, this means that even the simplest procedures, such as administration of antibiotics, should be thoughtfully chosen and discussed beforehand with surrogates when there is time to do so. Addressing concerns of caregivers is also particularly important in dealing with families of dementia patients. Depression is common in caregivers, the burden of caring for patients is very heavy, and grieving may occur before death, as the person that they knew disappears in front of them.

Renal Failure

Dialysis has been a technical success in prolonging life for patients without kidney function. Because it is now so common, physicians do not realize that the annual mortality rate is 23%, reflecting the incidence of severe chronic diseases in these patients. The emergency physician rarely has a chance to discuss this treatment modality with patients, since the usual emergency department visit is for emergency complications of electrolyte or fluid imbalance. Understanding that dialysis is a choice and not a mandatory intervention, however, may be a useful attitude to affirm in discussing long-term choices with patients and families in the emergency department. In the patient with dementia or cancer, electing to not treat renal failure is an option many patients and families may not understand.[62]

Heart Failure and Chronic Obstructive Pulmonary Disease

Although the physiologic parameters of terminal heart failure and COPD are well described, death from these diseases is commonly unexpected and may occur as part of a sudden acute deterioration that is not remediable. When death occurs, it is important to remind the survivors that the underlying disease is the real cause of mortality.

On the other hand, if the acute decompensation becomes stabilized in the emergency department, the emergency physician may be the best person to have a conversation concerning advance directive with the patient and family to establish, at a minimum, what kind of resuscitation measures should be performed if the patient suffers a cardiac or respiratory event in the hospital and who should make decisions on behalf of the patient if he or she should become incapacitated at some time during the admission. In patients with chronic diseases of the entry/re-entry type (see Figure 206-1), the time after an emergency has resolved (at least temporarily) is often the best time to establish what interventions would be appropriate if decompensation occurs again. In terminal stages, these patients may receive an undue focus on diagnostics when compared with cancer patients, particularly if the mortality rate associated with these conditions is not acknowledged. Palliative care or hospice referral is often useful in assisting the patient with understanding and acknowledging prognosis and establishing intentional and realistic projects and goals for their remaining life.

ACKNOWLEDGMENTS

We thank Drs. Ben Honigman, John Armstrong II, and Peter Rosen for their hard work in prior editions of this chapter.

KEY CONCEPTS

- In an emergency, the emergency physician must act rapidly, presuming curative goals, and it is often impossible to withhold initial interventions.
- The emergency physician should honor advance directives and patient wishes whenever possible, including withdrawal of invasive support if the patient's desire to not receive such treatments is determined after initial emergency department intervention.
- Suffering is not the same as physical pain: persons suffer, particularly when symptoms threaten their future.
- Patients have individual perceptions of burdens and benefits when they live with their illnesses. One cannot predict a person's quality of life and whether treatment is "right" for a patient without asking.
- At the time of admission, the minimum information needed from patients and families when they have a disease that may be fatal can be gained by asking the following questions: What kind of resuscitation do you wish to receive if an emergency occurs after admission? Whom do you want to make decisions for you if you cannot?
- A discussion of goals of care is more effective if it starts by clarifying the patient's broad values and goals. From the broad discussion, the provider can suggest what procedures may or may not be useful in attaining the patient's goals.
- The purposes of hospitalization for persons with severe terminal diseases should be clear and in line with the patient's values.

REFERENCES

1. Iserson KV: *Grave Words: Notifying Survivors about Sudden, Unexpected Deaths.* Tucson: Galen Press, 1999.
2. Mokdad AH, et al: Actual causes of death in the United States, 2000. *JAMA* 291:1239, 2004.
3. Lunney JR, et al: Patterns of functional decline at the end of life. *JAMA* 289:2387, 2003.
4. Clark D: Between hope and acceptance: The medicalisation of dying. *BMJ* 324:905, 2002.
5. McCue JD: The naturalness of dying. *JAMA* 273:1039, 1995.
6. Bernat JL: The defense of the whole-brain concept of death. *Hasting Cent Rep* 28:14, 1998.
7. Wijdicks EFM: The diagnosis of brain death. *N Engl J Med* 233:1215, 2001.
8. Truog RD: Is it time to abandon brain death? *Hastings Center Report* 27:29, 1997.
9. Capron AM: Brain death: Well settled yet still unresolved. *N Engl J Med* 344:1244, 2001.
10. Council on Ethical and Judicial Affairs, AMA. Medical futility in end-of-life care. *JAMA* 281:937, 1999.
11. Helft PR, Siegler M, Lantos J: The rise and fall of the futility movement. *N Engl J Med* 343:293, 2000.
12. Liao Y, et al: Quality of the last year of life of older adults: 1986 vs 1993. *JAMA* 283:512, 2000.
13. Lentzer HR, et al: The quality of life the year before death. *Am J Public Health* 82:1093, 1992.
14. SUPPORT Investigators: A controlled trial to improve care for seriously ill hospitalized patients. *JAMA* 274:1591, 1995.
15. Schneiderman L, et al: Relationship of general advance directive instructions to specific life-sustaining treatment preferences in patients with serious illness. *Arch Intern Med* 152:2114, 1992.
16. Thurber DF: Public awareness of the nature of CPR: A case for values-centered advance directives. *J Clin Ethics* 7:55, 1996.
17. Suhl J, et al: Myth of substituted judgment: Surrogate decision making regarding life support is unreliable. *Arch Intern Med* 154:90, 1994.
18. Gerhart KA, et al: Quality of life following spinal cord injury: Knowledge and attitudes of emergency care providers. *Ann Emerg Med* 23:807, 1994.
19. Singer PA, Martin DK, Kelner M: Quality end-of-life care: patients' perspectives. *JAMA* 281:163, 1999.
20. Quill TE: Initiating end-of-life discussions with seriously ill patients: Addressing the "elephant in the room." *JAMA* 284:2502, 2000.
21. Fox E: Predominance of the curative model of medical care: a residual problem. *JAMA* 278:761, 1997.
22. Cassell EJ: The nature of suffering and the goals of medicine. *N Engl J Med* 306:639, 1982.
23. Emmanuel LL, von Gunten DF, Ferris FD (eds): The Education for Physicians on End-of-Life Care (EPEC) Curriculum. Robert Wood Johnson Foundation, The EPEC Project, 1999.
24. World Health Organization website, 1990. Available at http://www.who.int/dsa/justpub/cpl.htm
25. American Heart Association: ACLS Provider Manual (70–2502). American Heart Association, 2001.
26. Bailey ED, Wydro GC, Cone DC: Termination of resuscitation in the prehospital setting for adult patients suffering nontraumatic cardiac arrest: position paper, NAEMSP. *Prehospital Emerg Care* 4:190, 2000.
27. Iserson KV: Withholding and withdrawing medical treatment: An emergency medicine perspective. *Ann Emerg Med* 28:51, 1996.
28. Leon MD, Wilson EM: Development of a statewide protocol for the prehospital identification of DNR patients in Connecticut including new DNR regulations. *Ann Emerg Med* 34:263, 1999.
29. Iserson KV, Sanders AB, Mathieu D: *Ethics in Emergency Medicine*, 2nd ed. Tucson, Galen Press, 1995.
30. Dull SM, et al: Expected death and unwanted resuscitation in the prehospital setting. Ann Emerg Med 23:997, 1994.
31. Heilicser B, Stocking C, Siegler M: Ethical dilemmas in emergency medical services: The perspective of the emergency medical technician. *Ann Emerg Med* 27:239, 1996.
32. Partridge RA, et al: Field experience with prehospital advance directives. *Ann Emerg Med* 32:589, 1998.
33. ACEP: "Do not attempt resuscitation" orders in the out-of-hospital setting. ACEP Policy Resource and Education Paper, 2003. Available at http://acep.org/3,437,0.html
34. NAEMSP: National guidelines for statewide implementation of EMS "Do not resuscitate" (DNR) programs. NAEMSP 1993. Available at http://naemsp.org/Position%20Papers/DNRPrograms.html
35. Adams JG: Prehospital do-not-resuscitate orders: A survey of state policies in the United States. *Prehospital Disaster Med* 8:317, 1993.
36. Sabatino CP: Survey of state EMS-DNR laws and protocols. *J Law Med Ethics* 27:297, 1999.
37. Sullivan MD, Youngner SJ: Depression, competence, and the right to refuse lifesaving medical treatment. *Am J Psychiatry* 151:971, 1994.
38. Groopman J: Dying words: How should doctors deliver bad news? *New Yorker* 62:Oct 28, 2002.
39. Iserson KV: The gravest words: Sudden-death notifications and emergency care. *Ann Emerg Med* 36:75, 2000.
40. Quest TE, et al: The use of standardized patients within a procedural competency model to teach death disclosure. *Acad Emerg Med* 9:1326, 2002.
41. Ptacek JT, Eberhardt TL: Breaking bad news: A review of the literature. *JAMA* 276:496, 1996.
42. Buckman R: *How to Break Bad News: A Guide for Health Care Professions.* Baltimore, Johns Hopkins University Press, 1992.

43. Quill TE, Arnold RM, Platt F: "I wish things were different." *Ann Intern Med* 135:551, 2001.
44. Back AL, Arnold RM, Quill TE: Hope for the best, and prepare for the worst. *Ann Intern Med* 138:439, 2003.
45. Leach RM: Death notification: Practical guidelines for health care professionals. *Crit Care Nurs Q* 19:21, 1995.
46. Oman KS, Armstrong JD 2nd, Stoner M: Perspectives on practicing procedures on the newly dead. *Acad Emerg Med* 9:786, 2002.
47. AMA: E-8.181 Performing procedures on the newly deceased for training purposes. June 2001. Available at http://www.ama-assn.org/apps/pf_online/pf_online?f_n=browse&doc=policyfiles/CEJA/E-8.181.HTM&&s_t=&st_p=&nth=1&prev_pol=policyfiles/CEJA/E-7.05.HTM&nxt_pol=policyfiles/CEJA/E-8.01.HTM&. Accessed March 23, 2004.
48. Berger JT, Rosner F, Cassell EJ: Ethics of practicing medical procedures on newly dead and nearly dead patients. *J Gen Intern Med* 17:774, 2002.
49. ACEP Information Paper: Teaching procedures on the newly dead. 2003. Available at http://www.acep.org/1,32652,0.html. Accessed March 24, 2004.
50. von Gunten CF, Ferris FD, Emanuel LL: Ensuring competency in end-of-life care: Communication and relational skills. *JAMA* 284:3051, 2000.
51. Prigerson HG, Jacobs SC: Caring for bereaved patients: "All the doctors just suddenly go." *JAMA* 286:1369, 2001.
52. Gortmaker SL, et al: Organ donor potential and performance. *Crit Care Med* 24:432, 1996.
53. Williams MA, et al: The physician's role in discussing organ donation with families. *Crit Care Medicine* 31:1568, 2003.
54. Henderson SO, et al: Organ procurement in an urban level 1 emergency department. *Ann Emerg Med* 34:466, 1998.
55. Adams J, Wolfson AB: Ethical issues in geriatric emergency medicine. *Emerg Med Clin North Am* 8:183, 1990.
56. Wrenn K, Brody SL: Do-not-resuscitate orders in the emergency department. *Am J Med* 92:129, 1992.
57. Balentine J, et al: Emergency department do-not-attempt-resuscitation orders: Next-of-kin response to the emergency physician. *Acad Emerg Med* 3:54, 1996.
58. Baines MJ: ABC of palliative care: Nausea, vomiting and intestinal obstruction. *BMJ* 315:1148, 1997.
59. Hurley AC, Volicer L: Alzheimer disease: "It's okay, mama, if you want to go, it's okay." *JAMA* 288:2324, 2002.
60. Post SG: Tube feeding and advanced progressive dementia. *Hasting Cent Rep* 31:36, 2001.
61. Finucane TE, Christmas C, Travis K: Tube feeding in patients with advanced dementia: A review of the evidence. *JAMA* 282:1365, 1999.
62. Cohen LM, Germain MJ, Poppel DM: Practical considerations in dialysis withdrawal: "To have that option is a blessing." *JAMA* 289:2113, 2003.

CHAPTER 207

Medicolegal and Risk Management

Robert A. Bitterman

PERSPECTIVE

Emergency Medical Treatment and Active Labor Act

Federal and state laws govern much of the practice of emergency medicine. The federal Emergency Medical Treatment and Active Labor Act (EMTALA, also known as COBRA or the "antidumping" law) dictates how emergency physicians must triage, register, examine, provide workup, treat or stabilize, discharge or transfer, utilize hospital resources, and involve medical staff expertise when caring for patients presenting to the emergency department.[1-3] State laws further control the practice of emergency medicine through such issues as consent, reporting requirements, confidentiality requirements, forensic and police matters, civil commitments, and emergency medical services (EMS) statutes.

Practicing good medicine may have been enough to avoid legal entanglements historically, but not today. Knowledge of the law is now essential owing to the magnitude and complexity of controlling legal authority and the significant penalties levied for noncompliance, such as criminal sanctions, civil monetary penalties, and exclusion from participation in government programs such as Medicare and Medicaid.

EMTALA regulates every aspect of how hospitals and emergency physicians must triage, register, and examine individuals who present to the emergency department seeking medical attention. The law was originally passed in 1985 to prevent private hospitals from transferring ("dumping") medically unstable, indigent patients to public hospitals. Subsequent amendments to the law, government regulations, and court decisions greatly expanded the reach of EMTALA, which now sets a national standard of care for emergency services.[2-4] It is extremely important for the emergency physician to understand how EMTALA defines and how regulatory agencies and the courts interpret the concepts of emergency medical condition, medical screening examination, stabilization, and patient disposition.

Emergency Medical Condition

Any individual who comes to an emergency department requesting examination or treatment must be provided an appropriate *medical screening examination* (MSE).[5] The purpose of the MSE is to determine whether the patient has an emergency medical condition (EMC). EMTALA defines an EMC as "acute symptoms of sufficient severity (including severe pain) such that the absence of immediate medical attention could reasonably be expected to result in any of the following:

1. Placing the health of the individual (or, with respect to a pregnant woman, the health of the woman or her unborn child) in serious jeopardy, or
2. Serious impairment to bodily functions, or
3. Serious dysfunction of any bodily organ or part."[6]

Or, in the case of a pregnant woman who is having contractions, the following:

4. There is inadequate time to effect a safe transfer to another hospital before delivery, or the transfer may pose a threat to the health or safety of the woman or the unborn child.[7]

This is vague, broad language. Competent physicians can reasonably disagree whether certain symptoms are acute, immediate, or serious enough to be EMCs. The courts hold that the relevant factor is whether the hospital *perceived* the patient to have an EMC, not whether the patient actually had an EMC, and not whether the emergency physician or hospital should have known that the EMC existed. The focus is whether the hospital in fact *actually determines* the patient has an EMC. The standard is subjective.[8] If the physician and hospital perform an appropriate MSE and in good faith determine that no EMC exists, the courts will not retrospectively review that decision; rather, it will be a simple state malpractice issue of whether the examination and diagnosis met the applicable standard of care.

SCREENING REQUIREMENTS

If the MSE does not reveal an EMC, further care of that patient is not dictated by EMTALA, so the law's provisions governing stabilizing treatment, transfer of the patient, involvement of on-call physicians, and the control of managed care patients no longer apply. This interpretation emphasizes the critical importance of emergency physicians in documenting the presence or absence of an EMC during a patient's initial emergency department evaluation.

Everyone who presents to the emergency department must be screened. Whether the patient is indigent, a member of a managed care plan, or covered by Medicare, Medicaid, or private insurance is irrelevant; the hospital must provide everyone who presents for care with an MSE.[5] This includes all patient populations, such as illegal aliens, minors, and private patients of the hospital's medical staff but excludes persons who are already patients of the hospital, such as inpatients or outpatients undergoing a scheduled procedure at the hospital who are brought to the emergency department for emergency care.[2] The screening of minors is discussed later in the section on consent.

Private Patients and Triage

In many hospitals, members of the hospital's medical staff often meet their private patients in the emergency department. These patients are examined and treated by their private physicians, not the emergency physician on duty. Such practice is entirely appropriate to maintain physician-patient relationships and allowable under EMTALA. However, the hospital should have prearranged procedures for handling private patients that do not unduly delay the patient's MSE or the hospital could be liable under EMTALA for failure to provide an "appropriate" MSE. Delay of treatment in such instances also frequently results in hospital liability through state malpractice actions.

All private patients should be triaged according to the hospital's established protocols. If the triage nurse determines that the patient requires immediate care, the emergency physician on duty should provide the necessary treatment until the patient's private physician arrives in the emergency department to assume the patient's care.

If triage determines that the patient does not require immediate care, the emergency physician should see the patient in the order consistent with the usual practice of the emergency department, generally in the order of acuity or time of arrival. If the private physician comes to the emergency department and sees the patient before the emergency physician, the examination by the private physician constitutes the required MSE by the hospital. Furthermore, there has been no undue delay of the MSE for any nonmedical reason. However, if the patient's private physician has not arrived by the time the emergency physician would normally examine the patient, the emergency physician should perform a MSE. If no EMC is evident, the patient can wait for his or her physician to arrive. If an EMC exists, the emergency physician should undertake appropriate stabilizing treatment until the patient's physician arrives.[9]

In *Clark v. Baton Rouge General Medical Center* a patient came to the emergency department to meet a neurologist. While waiting, the patient began vomiting, and the patient's daughter repeatedly requested help. The emergency department staff and the emergency physician refused to examine or treat the patient because she already had a physician coming in to see her, and the hospital did not have a contract with her insurance carrier. The court held that the daughter's pleas for help constituted a valid request for the MSE under EMTALA, condemned the conduct of the hospital and physician, and awarded her damages for the hospital's failure to provide a MSE as required by law.[10]

Hospital Property

The Centers for Medicare and Medicaid (CMS), previously known as the Health Care Financing Administration, deems anyone on hospital property to have come to the emergency department.[11,12] CMS defines hospital property to be the entire main hospital campus, including parking lots, sidewalks, and driveways, and any ambulance owned and operated by the hospital, even if the ambulance is not on hospital grounds.[11] CMS exempts a number of on-campus areas from compliance with EMTALA, generally those areas that typically do not provide emergency care, such as physicians' offices, skilled nursing facilities, other entities that participate separately under Medicare, and other nonmedical facilities on campus.[2] CMS also exempts application of the law to off-campus facilities and other "departments of a provider" that were never intended or structured to manage emergency medical conditions, such as dialysis centers, rehabilitation units, laboratories and radiology centers, or primary care clinics. These facilities should have written policy and procedures for appraisal of emergencies and arranging transfers when appropriate.

It is unclear whether hospital owned and operated off-campus urgent care centers must comply with EMTALA. CMS intended to require urgent care centers to comply with the law, but the actual language of the new regulations effective November 2003 suggests otherwise. Hospitals should examine how their relationship with the urgent care centers is legally structured in conjunction with the new regulations to determine whether the law applies in their individual case.[2,13]

The legal determinations of when someone on hospital property is covered by EMTALA are complex, but clearly physical presence on the hospital grounds coupled with a request for examination requires the hospital to provide an MSE. The physical presence of an individual on hospital property by itself is insufficient to require the hospital to provide an MSE. There must also be a request for examination or treatment, which can be made by *anyone* on behalf of the patient; the request does not have to come from the patient, a family member, or a legal guardian.[5]

Also, if an individual is unable to verbally request care, the individual's behavior may constitute a request if the hospital's personnel are aware of the behavior and a prudent layperson would believe that the individual's behavior indicated a need for examination or treatment.[2]

The CMS divides hospital property into dedicated emergency departments and all other property that is not a dedicated emergency department.

A dedicated emergency department is defined as any department or facility of the hospital, regardless of whether it is on or off campus, that is licensed by the state as an emergency department; is held out to the public as a place that provides care for emergency medical conditions on an unscheduled basis; or actually does provide care for emergency medical conditions a certain percentage of the time.[2]

Units qualifying as dedicated emergency departments include a hospital's typical emergency department, labor and delivery unit, psychiatric intake center, and potentially urgent care centers. CMS intended EMTALA to apply to urgent care centers; however, urgent care centers do not hold themselves out as able to provide care for true emergency medical conditions, as that term is defined by the statue. Thus, in the author's opinion, the typical urgent care center will not likely meet the new regulatory definition of a dedicated emergency department and therefore will not have to comply with EMTALA. CMS may readdress this issue further.

Presentations to the hospital's dedicated emergency department only require a request for examination or treatment of a medical condition; it is not required that the presentation be for an emergency medical condition to trigger EMTALA's screening duty. Presentations to hospital property other than the dedicated emergency department do, however, require the request to be for an emergency medical condition before EMTALA applies.[2]

Other Emergency Department Functions

Hospital emergency departments serve many functions other than the evaluation and treatment of patients with true medical emergencies. Physicians on the hospital staff may use the emergency department in the off-hour periods to provide injections or obtain laboratory tests or radiographs on their patients. Police use the emergency department to obtain blood alcohol samples on allegedly intoxicated automobile drivers. Some hospitals may use the emergency department to provide urine drug screens on injured workers, prescription refills, allergy shots, rabies vaccinations, blood transfusions, or other community services, such as blood pressure screening or flu shots.

TESTING REQUESTS AND REQUIREMENTS

The test category includes urine or serum drug screening, routine laboratory tests, and x-ray films. In each case, no immediate medical decision making is required. The patient's physician determines the indication for the studies and is responsible for the patient's care, including following up on the test or x-ray results. The patient is not requesting "examination or treatment for a medical condition" by the hospital's emergency department, so the hospital does not need to provide an MSE.

Such patients should not be sent through triage and should not have their vital signs taken, and the hospital should not create the usual emergency department chart for them. They should not be asked to sign the usual emergency department "consent for treatment" forms, which could imply they were requesting examination and treatment. Separate paperwork should be used to document the visit, the particular test performed, the patient's informed consent for the testing, and a specific statement that the patient is not requesting an MSE, any communication with the private physician, and the patient's signature.

Some individuals come to the emergency department on their own, not at the request of their physician, and request a test (e.g., for pregnancy, human immunodeficiency virus). These persons should all be given an MSE before any test is conducted. If the person declines the MSE, he or she should be referred elsewhere to obtain the requested test: outpatient clinic, personal physician, public health clinic, or local drugstore for a pregnancy test. Documentation that the individual declined the offered MSE is essential.

Minor Treatments

The minor treatment category includes allergy shots, tetanus shots, rabies vaccines, blood letting or blood transfusions, chemotherapy infusion for cancer or possible organ transplant rejection, reinsertion of a feeding tube or Foley catheter, prescription refills, suture removals, antibiotic injections, and narcotic injections for chronic pain syndromes. Patients presenting to the emergency department requesting treatment should be given an MSE. In each instance, the common denominator is the element of medical decision making.

Antibiotic and narcotic injections require special comment. Physicians, particularly in rural hospitals, send their patients to the emergency department and then call in phone orders for parenteral medications. The patients are not examined by the emergency physician on duty. This practice should be avoided, and it may violate EMTALA because the hospital does not provide the patient the same MSE as for any patient with the same complaint. It is irrelevant if the patient's private physician examined the patient in the office immediately before sending the patient to the emergency department. This requirement of EMTALA may not be cost-efficient medicine, but both CMS and the courts agree that the hospital must provide an MSE to any individual who comes to the emergency department and requests examination or treatment for a medical condition.[1,14]

All patients presenting for minor treatments should be triaged, registered, and managed as other emergency department patients are. The emergency physician should evaluate the patient to determine whether the patient's condition meets the definition of an EMC before the hospital administers any medications. CMS and the courts will assume these patients requested examination or treatment, and the hospital must demonstrate that either (1) these patients did not request that an MSE be performed or (2) the emergency physician's evaluation did not reveal an EMC.

The CMS recently attempted to eliminate application of EMTALA to persons coming to the emergency department for reasons other than seeking emergency care. However, the language of the new regulations really did not change anything. The hospital still must perform an MSE of the extent necessary to determine whether an EMC exists, regardless of whether the patient's presenting complaint appears to be for a non emergency condition.[2,13]

Direct Emergency Department Admissions

Direct patient admissions in the emergency department are always problematic. In the three most common scenarios, the patient (1) is sent in after being examined by the physician in the office, (2) is sent in after phone contact with their physician, or (3) is accepted by phone-in transfer from a different hospital emergency department or inpatient setting. In all cases, the patient's physician intends to see the patient later, after the admission, and not in the emergency department. Medically, each scenario is different and may require a different level of acute medical intervention. Legally, however, each is now the same under EMTALA because of CMS's new regulations.[2,3,13] EMTALA no longer applies to the treatment or stabilization of inpatients, regardless of whether they are directly admitted to the floor, directly admitted via the emergency department, or boarded in the emergency department awaiting bed placement. Even if the inpatient is brought down to the emergency department, the law does not apply.[2,15]

An inpatient is defined as "an individual who is admitted to a hospital for bed occupancy for purposes of receiving inpatient hospital services . . . with the expectation that he or she will remain at least overnight."[2] It does not matter if the situation changes later and the patient can be discharged or transferred to another hospital and does not actually use the bed overnight. The key element is that the patient must be formally admitted with a documented admission order. A physician's intent to admit or the patient's acuity indicating "obviously will be admitted" is not enough to satisfy the definition. Documentation is critical.[2,15]

The CMS does not consider patients admitted to "observation status" to meet the regulatory definition of "admitted" patients (not admitted for purposes of receiving inpatient services), and thus EMTALA still applies to the care of observation patients, such as patients managed in emergency department chest pain units.[2,15]

Therefore, under the new regulations, direct admits sent through or held in the emergency department from a physician's office, a nursing home, or in transfer from another emergency department or another hospital inpatient setting are no longer covered by EMTALA, even though they have come to the hospital's emergency department.

Preventive Services

Blood pressure screening and vaccination services do not require an MSE. The patient is not requesting examination or treatment for a medical condition. The patient is attempting to prevent illness prophylactically, not seek treatment of an illness. These vaccinations are distinct from tetanus boosters because boosters are typically administered in response to injury and are a component of medical decision making and treatment.

Sexual Assault Cases

Hospital emergency departments frequently assist the police in the collection of evidence related to alleged sexual assault cases. If the individual is at the emergency department solely to provide evidence for the criminal investigation and is not requesting examination or treatment for a medical condition, no MSE is required. However, if the individual complains of pain or injury or wants pregnancy or sexually transmitted disease prophylaxis, the person is requesting examination or treatment for a medical condition and must be provided an MSE.[16]

Prescriptions

In small communities, local pharmacies are frequently not open continuously. Hospital pharmacies, sometimes through the hospital emergency department, often fill prescriptions for patients in the off hours. Patients presenting to the emergency department for these prescriptions do not need an MSE. If the prescription is filled through the emergency department, the hospital should have the patients sign a form indicating they are not requesting an MSE, for the same reasons and in the same manner as when tests are done in the emergency department at the request of physicians.

This situation is different than patients presenting to the emergency department requesting prescription refills. Patients requesting refills are not seeking pharmacy services but rather medical decision making services from a physician by asking for a prescription renewal to treat an underlying medical condition.[2,9]

Blood Alcohol Tests

For both medical and legal reasons, the emergency physician should offer an MSE to all individuals presenting to the emergency department for police-requested blood alcohol samples. This scenario is different from that of patients presenting to the emergency department to have blood tests done as ordered by their physicians. Persons in police custody have not been examined by a physician, and the results of the test will not be returned to a physician to care for the patient. The police officer brought the patient because of aberrant behavior, suspected to be caused by alcohol intoxication. Many diseases mimic alcohol intoxication, including hypoglycemia, cerebral hypoxia, head injury, metabolic abnormalities, and other toxins besides alcohol. Medically, alcohol intoxication should not automatically be presumed as the cause of the patient's condition just because it is so common. The emergency physician should examine the individual to determine if an EMC exists.[9]

The patient may refuse the MSE and request that only the blood be drawn. If the patient appears competent, this can be done. The refusal of the MSE must be documented, as noted for other testing done in the emergency department, with additional documentation of the risks and benefits of the offered MSE and careful notation of the patient's competence. If the patient is too intoxicated to make medical decisions, the physician must retain the patient until the patient is competent enough to make rational decisions. Only physicians should assess and document an individual's competence; other hospital personnel should not be allowed to make these decisions.[9]

Again, under EMTALA, the "request for examination or treatment" can be made by anyone on behalf of the patient. The police officer's request for blood alcohol sampling may be sufficient to constitute the request for an MSE.

MEDICAL SCREENING EXAMINATION

Implementation

EMTALA does not specify whether a physician, nurse, or other health care provider must perform the MSE. CMS regulations require that the screening examination be done by "qualified medical personnel"[17] and that the hospital's governing body formally designate, in writing, who is a qualified person to perform medical screening on behalf of the hospital.[17,18] CMS's *State Operations Manual* (SOM) specifies that the hospital cannot allow the medical director of its emergency department to designate who is qualified to perform screenings on behalf of the hospital.[19]

Triage by a nurse is not considered an MSE. Neither CMS nor the courts accept triage as adequate to determine whether an EMC exists.[2,9]

It is strongly recommended that hospitals require physicians be responsible for all MSEs performed in the emergency department. Either the physician personally performs the screening or is directly responsible for examinations performed by physician assistants, nurse practitioners, or housestaff. It is appropriate to use physician assistants and nurse practitioners to screen patients who are determined by nurse triage to have less acute or severe conditions. However, the physician on duty should be ultimately responsible for all patients.

Ancillary Services

The law requires hospitals to provide the screening examination "within the capabilities of the hospital's emergency department, including ancillary services routinely available to the emergency department."[5] According to CMS, this means that the scope of a MSE may "range from a simple process involving only a brief history and physical examination to a complex process that also involves performing ancillary studies and procedures such as (but not limited to) lumbar punctures, clinical laboratory tests, computed tomography scans, diagnostic tests and procedures."[20]

Since the stated purpose of the MSE is to determine whether an EMC exists, CMS and the federal courts hold that the hospital must conduct whatever examination is necessary to make that determination.[21] It may take only a visual glance to rule out any EMC in a patient with a rash. However, if it takes a complete neurologic examination, computed tomography scan, and lumbar puncture to decide whether that patient has a serious underlying infection, then those procedures are considered part of the MSE.

Thus, if the emergency department usually has ultrasonography, computed tomography, ventilation/perfusion scans, and similar tests available, it must use those resources if necessary to determine whether the patient has an EMC. However, the hospital is obliged only to utilize the resources ordinarily available to its emergency department.[5] Neither the statute nor the regulations mandate that hospitals expand resources or offer additional services to emergency department patients. An exception may be the use of interpreters for patients not fluent in the English language, which is now required by the Medicare conditions of participation.[22,23]

The CMS views the ancillary services available to the emergency department to include the services of on-call physicians if their expertise is required to decide if the patient has an EMC.[2,9,13,20,22,24] If the emergency physician cannot determine whether a patient has an EMC, the physician must use the on-call physicians to help make that determination. For example, if it takes an on-call surgeon to decide whether a patient has an "acute abdomen," the surgical evaluation becomes an integral part of the hospital's MSE.

Standard Procedures

The federal courts hold that there are two components to an appropriate MSE: (1) the examination must be "reasonably calculated to identify critical medical conditions," and (2) the "exact same level of screening must be uniformly provided to all patients who present with substantially similar complaints."[21] In other words, a hospital satisfies the requirements of EMTALA if it conducts standard screening procedures, uniformly, to all patients with similar complaints and circumstances.

Liability and Motive

Each hospital determines its own standard screening procedures. By necessity, each hospital's standard will be individualized, because each hospital emergency department has varying capabilities and different ancillary services available. Once a hospital defines its standard screening process, however, it must apply that process uniformly to all patients presenting with similar complaints, and material departure from its standard screening procedure constitutes inappropriate screening under EMTALA. Since motive is not a relevant issue in the federal courts (except the 6th Circuit) or during CMS investigations, liability results from any material deviation of the hospital's screening process, regardless of the hospital's motive and regardless of the reason for the deviation. For example, a Florida hospital's screening policy stated triage would be conducted within 3 minutes after a patient's arrival at the emergency department. When one patient was not triaged until 45 minutes after arrival, it constituted a violation of the law because the hospital did not follow its own policy.[9]

Once hospitals define their own standard screening process, they will be held to that standard, by both plaintiffs and the government enforcers. Investigators and plaintiff attorneys will subpoena and closely examine the hospital's policies and procedures, medical staff bylaws, emergency department departmental rules and regulations, practice guidelines, and other written information on the screening process. They will compare the written process to what actually transpired.

Guidelines

Practice guidelines or protocols, including managed care manuals, adopted by emergency departments or hospitals may be treated essentially the same as the hospital's own policies and procedures. They are also routinely used to demonstrate that the hospital "failed to follow its own rules" when hospitals and physicians do not adhere to their adopted parameters. In fact, practice guidelines are used against physicians and hospitals much more frequently than they are used to their benefit in malpractice litigation.[25]

Registration and Authorization

All managed care patients presenting to the emergency department must be screened, regardless of whether they are members of a commercial managed care organization (MCO), a Medicare MCO, or a state-sponsored Medicaid managed care plan. MCOs may acknowledge that screening is required, but they frequently expect hospitals to provide different levels of screening for their enrollees. Managed care plans may request that the hospital merely "eyeball the patient" or perform a clinical examination sufficient to determine whether or not the patient can safely be triaged to a managed care facility. Neither CMS nor the courts condone this practice, emphasizing that the scope of the MSE not only must be *reasonably calculated* to determine whether an EMC exists but also must be *uniform* for all those who present with substantially similar complaints.[26,27]

Furthermore, hospitals should never delay a patient's MSE in order to obtain prior authorization from an MCO. Managed care authorization is authorization for payment only; it is not authorization for treatment. CMS's regulations are clear: "Managed healthcare plans cannot deny a hospital permission to examine or treat their enrollees. They may only state what they will and will not pay for, and regardless of whether a hospital is to be reimbursed for the treatment, it is obligated to provide the services specified in EMTALA."[19] Hospitals are legally obliged to provide the MSE, and they will be held to that standard regardless of the financial pressures placed on them by MCOs.

In its new regulations, CMS explicitly banned prior authorization for managed care plans before completion of the MSE and commencement of stabilizing treatment.[2] Hospitals may only obtain authorization for payment from insurance entities "concurrently" with stabilization of the patient.[2]

Patients often ask questions about their obligation to pay for emergency services, particularly whether their insurance will cover the visit or how much it will cost to receive care at the emergency department. Regardless of EMTALA, all patient questions should be answered forthrightly, honestly, and completely by the hospital staff. *Patients* control the interaction between themselves and health care providers, not hospitals or physicians, not the MCO, and not the government. After the hospital answers the patient's questions, the patient is responsible for making informed decisions about further aspects of care.

If a patient chooses to withdraw a request for examination or treatment and leave the emergency department, hospitals must carefully handle the interaction related to the "voluntary withdrawal" (see consent section). Generally, routine financial questions can be answered by registration personnel or triage nurses trained to give "stock answers," not discourage or coerce the patient in any way, and to encourage the patient to stay and defer economic discussions until after an MSE is performed. Whenever the patient intends to leave, the staff should involve the physician on duty.

Regardless of managed care status, "VIP" status, private patient status, or any other classification, all patients should be processed in the same manner. CMS still allows hospitals to conduct reasonable registration procedures in the emergency department, including collecting insurance data. A reasonable registration process may include obtaining demographic data, name of the patient's physician, and whether the patient is insured and what type of insurance. During the registration process, the patient can sign the hospital's usual "informed consent to be examined" form and a routine form that holds the patient financially accountable for any charges not covered by the patient's insurance carrier.[2]

The key is to create parallel tracks for medical and financial issues and to ensure that the financial track never interferes with the medical care in any way. Bedside registration is probably necessary under the existing regulatory scheme to avoid "no-delay" violations, as CMS would consider any delay in access to the MSE due to diversion to the registration area to be against the law. Waiting for examination and treatment because the emergency department is overwhelmed is not a violation, but waiting for examination because the registration clerks are collecting insurance information could be.[2]

The CMS continues to warn hospitals not to coerce patients into leaving before they receive their federally guaranteed right to an MSE, stating "reasonable registration processes may not unduly discourage individuals from remaining for further evaluation."[2]

Collection of co-pays, down payments, advanced beneficiary notifications (ABNs), or signatures on managed care financial forms may constitute such "economic coercion" if not done very carefully. Hospitals must also ensure that staff behavior does not create a hostile environment or constructive denial of the MSE.

The triage team, physician and nursing staff, and all clinical personnel should not know the patient's insurance status throughout the initial screening and stabilizing treatment. This removes insurance status as an issue should the government later claim that the staff was motivated in some way or treated the patient disparately on the basis of financial condition. It is easier to prove that actions were not predicated on the patient's financial status when one lacks knowledge of that status than to prove that one's actions were medically appropriate despite knowing the patient had no insurance.

After the MSE and initiation of stabilizing treatment, economic considerations can be considered in determining the patient's future care, such as the admission, transfer, or discharge and follow-up.

In its new regulations, CMS also added a new rule, a "no delay in examination or treatment" rule, which states that it is acceptable for an emergency physician to contact the patient's private physician for medical advice "as long as this consultation does not inappropriately delay" screening or stabilizing services.[2] This new rule will increase hospital regulatory liability, potential civil monetary penalties, and potential civil lawsuits for conduct totally outside the scope of the statute. The language of the law unambiguously states that delay of patient care must be on account of the patient's insurance status to be a violation of EMTALA.[13]

Documentation

EMTALA is a technical law, and compliance with the technicalities requires proper documentation. Furthermore, clinical outcomes are irrelevant under government enforcement, and compliance is not presumed; the hospitals must prove compliance through documentation.

Central Log

Hospitals must maintain a central log of all patients presenting to the emergency department requesting examination or treatment. The log must contain the name and disposition of the patient, including whether the patient refused treatment, whether the hospital refused to provide an MSE or treatment, and whether the patient was admitted, treated and stabilized, transferred, or discharged.[28] The purpose of the log is to permit CMS and the state surveyors to select and review individual records to investigate whether the hospital is in compliance with the law.[19]

The log must include all individuals presenting to the hospital's dedicated emergency departments, whether on campus or off campus.[2,28,29] These areas now include the typical emergency department, freestanding emergency centers, labor and delivery suites, ambulatory care or fast tract areas contained in the emergency department, and psychiatric intake centers.[2] The logs are not required to be collated into a single document but must be retrievable at CMS's request.

Medical Record

All areas of the hospital used to conduct the MSE must create a medical record for the patient and keep a log of those presenting for examination and treatment.[30] If members of the hospital medical staff see their patients in the emergency department, either on a scheduled or an unscheduled basis, the hospital must create a medical record and require the physician to document the care provided in that record. The physician's private office records documenting care provided at the hospital are insufficient.

Most important, the emergency physician should document whether an EMC was determined to exist on *every* patient seen in the emergency department, even if the initial chief complaint is seemingly trivial. Again, the purpose of the required MSE is to determine legally if an EMC is present. To facilitate documentation, emergency department charts should have two boxes imprinted right on the chart; one for "EMTALA EMC present" and one for "EMTALA EMC absent." The person performing the MSE should check the appropriate box for each patient, and completion of this documentation should be a prime part of the emergency department's quality improvement monitoring program.

STABILIZATION REQUIREMENTS

Once the hospital determines that an individual has an EMC, EMTALA requires the hospital to either stabilize the EMC, or, if it lacks the capability to stabilize the patient, to transfer the patient to another medical facility that can provide the necessary treatment.[31]

When and if the patient is "stabilized" have enormous ramifications for hospitals and physicians, because once patients are stabilized, EMTALA no longer applies.[32] After stabilization, hospitals are free to refuse further treatment or to transfer stabilized patients for purely economic reasons. On-call physicians can refuse to treat or admit stable patients or insist that stable patients be transferred due to their lack of or type of insurance. An MCO can refuse further payment to the hospital and request that the stabilized patient be transferred to one of its contracting facilities.[33,34]

Health care providers must remember that other federal, state, or local standards may govern further treatment or transfer of emergency patients. State laws may prohibit hospitals from transferring patients for any reason except that they are incapable of handling the patient's medical problem.

Two elements must be present to trigger EMTALA's stabilization requirement: (1) the patient must have an EMC, as defined by law, and (2) the hospital must determine that an EMC exists. However, the mere existence of an EMC is not sufficient to invoke the duty to stabilize; the hospital must also have actual knowledge that the EMC is present. *Actual knowledge* is a legal term that means the examining physician subjectively believed an EMC existed. It is not the commonly understood objective standard used in malpractice cases, where liability is predicated on whether the physician knew or reasonably should have known the patient had an emergency condition. Whether the physician's judgment was negligent, or even grossly negligent, is irrelevant under EMTALA. The *subjective perception* of the examining physician controls whether EMTALA's stabilization requirement is triggered.

The appellate courts have uniformly held that if an EMC is not detected, the hospital has no stabilization duty and cannot be charged with failure to stabilize the patient's condition.[9,35,36] Furthermore, consideration or suspicion that an EMC may exist does not rise to the level of actual knowledge. If the hospital fails to detect an EMC through its standard screening procedures, the patient has only a state malpractice claim of "failure to diagnose" and not a federal cause of action for "failure to stabilize" the emergency condition. Once the physician or hospital does diagnose an EMC, however, the courts will allow a failure-to-stabilize claim to be brought in federal court under EMTALA.

The elements of EMTALA are distinctly different from ordinary malpractice, and hospitals and physicians should understand the differences. Documentation in the medical record of "no EMC present" eliminates all further liability under EMTALA. Understanding and implementing the documentation paradigm of EMTALA is the new risk management agenda for hospitals and their physicians.

The screening section of EMTALA only mandates the hospital to provide those services within the capability of the *emergency department,* including ancillary services routinely available to the emergency department.[5] In the stabilization section, however, the level of services required is within the capabilities of staff and facilities available at the hospital.[37]

The capabilities of the hospital staff include whatever level of care the personnel of the hospital can provide within the training and scope of their professional licenses and hospital privileges.[20] To ensure that hospitals have physician staff available to stabilize patients, the U.S. Congress mandated that Medicare-participating hospitals must have on-call physicians available to provide treatment necessary to stabilize the individual with an EMC.[38]

Thus, whenever the emergency department determines that a patient has an EMC, the hospital must, within the full capabilities of its staff, facilities, and medical staff, including on-call physicians, stabilize the patient.[37] If the hospital is unable to stabilize the patient, a physician must certify that a transfer is medically indicated and arrange an "appropriate" transfer to a higher-level facility.

The treating physician should always decide whether a patient's EMC is stable or unstable. If two physicians disagree over whether the patient is stable but only one of the physicians is at the bedside caring for the patient, the on-site physician should make the decision.[2,9] It is *not* appropriate for an on-call physician, a "managed care gatekeeper" physician, a physician at a receiving facility, or even the patient's regular attending physician to disagree with the decision of the on-site physician over the phone. If one of these outside physicians wants to overrule the determination of the on-site physician, he or she must come to the hospital and personally examine the patient.

EMTALA defines the term *stabilized* as follows: "no material deterioration in the condition is likely, within reasonable medical probability, to result from or occur during the transfer of the individual from a facility."[39] For a pregnant woman having contractions who is determined to have an EMC, stabilized means that the woman has delivered (including the placenta).

This is a *legal* definition of stabilization, not a medical definition. The standard of care for any patient diagnosed with an EMC will be judged by this legal definition, not by the usual medical malpractice standards. This is a national standard under federal law, not a local standard under state malpractice law.[9,40]

The "stabilized" question typically arises only when the patient deteriorates during or after the transfer and experiences an adverse medical result. It is likely to appear, particularly in hindsight, that the patient was not completely stabilized before transfer. Health care providers should remember that their compliance will usually be judged by an unsympathetic jury, aided by hindsight, in the context of a patient who has suffered an adverse medical outcome. Unfortunately, the court system, not the health care system, will ultimately determine when a patient is legally "stabilized."[9,40]

In *Roberts v. Galen* the U.S. Supreme Court ruled that a plaintiff need not show improper motive for a transfer in order to prevail on a failure-to-stabilize claim under EMTALA. The plaintiff merely must prove that the patient was not properly stabilized before the transfer.[9,40] It should be noted that all discharges from the emergency department are legally transfers under EMTALA.[41]

EMTALA's requirement to provide on-call physicians no longer extends to inpatients diagnosed with an EMC.[2] Other Medicare conditions of participation govern inpatient care, and hospitals certainly should implement policies and procedures for providing emergency specialty services to patients who develop EMCs after admission to the inpatient setting.[2]

DISPOSITION REQUIREMENTS

Admission

Once the emergency physician determines that the patient needs to be admitted, the patient's physician should be contacted. It is appropriate to arrange admission through the physicians who have contracted with the patient's MCO plan and through the patient's chosen private physician rather than the hospital's listed on-call physician. If the on-call physician for the patient or the emergency department disagrees with the emergency physician's judgment, it is incumbent on the on-call physician to come to the emergency department to personally examine the patient. This fact should be mutually understood by all physicians on the medical staff and the administration, and written into staff or hospital policies.

The CMS believes that when an on-call physician is at an office, it is *not* acceptable to refer emergency patients to the offices for examination and treatment. "The physician must come to the hospital to examine the patient."[20] Since the law applies to the hospital, CMS demands that all screening examinations and stabilization occur at the hospital, unless the hospital is incapable of performing those tasks. It has enforced its interpretation by finding numerous hospitals in violation of the law for sending emergency department patients to physicians' offices.[42]

Medical Specialty Exceptions

Exceptions to the referral ruling include ophthalmologists, who usually have better equipment in their offices than the emergency department for examining patients with eye complaints to determine whether an EMC is present. In essence, movement to the office in these cases becomes a medically indicated transfer to receive a higher level of services than the hospital can provide. CMS accepts such movement, as long as the emergency department arranges a formal transfer in compliance with EMTALA.

The CMS's interpretation is extremely unsatisfactory to most specialists, particularly orthopedic surgeons. It is standard practice in most hospitals for the emergency physician to splint many displaced fractures and send the patient to the on-call orthopedic surgeon's office for reduction of the fracture and further necessary treatment. CMS believes that the orthopedic surgeon must perform the reduction and treatment at the hospital in each case because their offices have no resources that the hospital lacks.

The CMS's rule applies only to patients with an EMC that is unstable.[9] If the emergency department "stabilizes" the fracture, EMTALA no longer applies. Thus, it is reasonable to send patients to the office for further treatment, as long as they meet the legal definition of "stable at the time of discharge" from the emergency department. Whether the patient is stable to go to the orthopedist's office depends solely on the judgment of the examining emergency physician. If the patient has accompanying injuries or is too uncomfortable to be moved, or if the emergency physician believes the injury is such that the patient should not travel, the orthopedic surgeon should care for the patient in the emergency department.[9]

Follow-Up

Obtaining follow-up care for emergency department patients, particularly indigent persons and Medicaid recipients, is a significant problem for almost every hospital. However, EMTALA does not encompass the on-call physician's office in this scenario. If the patient does not have an EMC or is stable at discharge, EMTALA does not apply from that point forward. Again, all discharges from the hospital are legally defined as transfers. In this scenario, the patient is being transferred home in stable condition, so EMTALA does not apply.

Common follow-up cases include the patient with pneumonia; the child with a febrile illness without a source; the weekend athlete with a torn medial collateral knee ligament, undisplaced radial head fracture, or shoulder dislocation successfully reduced by the emergency physician; and the patient with undifferentiated abdominal pain. The common denominator in each case is that the emergency physician believes the patient does *not* have an existing EMC that needs immediate care by the on-call physician, at the hospital, at that time.

The key issue in follow-up cases is whether the patient is stable at the time of discharge from the emergency department. If so, EMTALA does not apply further, and the on-call physician has no legal duty under EMTALA to see the patient in the office. The real issue is the level of commitment the hospital and medical staff want to make to their community. If the administration, the board, and the medical staff are comfortable with their decision, and if they have acted in the best interests of the patients they serve, they should have no trouble defending their actions to CMS or anyone.

Whatever decision the hospital and physicians make regarding emergency department follow-up, they should explicitly define those responsibilities in the medical staff bylaws or hospital rules and regulations, so that everyone understands what it means to be "on call" for the emergency department at that hospital.

Emergency department discharge instruction sheets should also include a *fail-safe clause* advising patients to return to the emergency department if the patient's condition deteriorates before seeing the referral specialist or if the arrangements for follow-up fail for any reason. Such a statement could help the hospital avoid liability when the on-call specialist fails to implement the prescribed follow-up plan.[43]

Transfer

Under EMTALA, any patient movement away from the hospital is legally defined as a "transfer."[44] Thus, all patients discharged from an emergency department are considered, from a legal perspective, to have been transferred, and all the transfer requirements of the law apply. Sending a patient home who is determined retrospectively to be unstable is considered a transfer of an unstable patient, and as such, a violation of law. To avoid such retrospective analyses, emergency physicians should document that no EMC was found and/or that the patient was stable on discharge. If the patient leaves without permission, the hospital has not legally transferred the patient.

Stable patients can be transferred to contract hospitals for further medical care, but unstable patients cannot. CMS's new interpretive guidelines should help hospitals deal with managed care entities, particularly when the parties disagree as to whether a patient is stable for transfer. Accordingly, "If there is disagreement between the treating physician and an off-site physician (e.g., a physician at the receiving facility or the patient's primary care physician if not physically present at the first facility) about whether the patient is stable for transfer, the medical judgment of the treating physician usually takes precedence over that of the off-site physician."[20]

Managed care physicians would have to appear in the emergency department to examine the patient and assume responsibility for the patient's care if they wanted to countermand the judgment of the initial examining physician. This means the managed care physicians must have appropriate credentials to handle emergency cases and be privileged to practice at that hospital.

Before transferring any patient out of the emergency department, the emergency physician must first determine whether the patient is stable, as defined by law. EMTALA regulates the transfer of unstable patients only; it does not apply to the transfer of stable patients.[2,9] If no EMC is found, the patient is considered stable. The determination of whether a patient is stable must be made at the time of transfer to be valid under the law.[35] Unstable patients can be transferred for only one of two reasons: the transfer is medically indicated, or the patient requests the transfer.[9] There is no "managed care transfer of an unstable patient" or even of a stable patient.

Patients are usually transferred out of the emergency department because the transferring facility lacks the capability or the resources necessary to treat the patient's EMC. Examples include head-injured patients in a hospital without a neurosurgeon on staff, pregnant women who need the services of a high-risk obstetric center, or the multiple-trauma patient treated initially in a rural emergency department who requires treatment at a level-one trauma center.

EMTALA defines such transfers as "medically indicated transfers" because the purpose of each transfer is to obtain a higher level of medical care necessary to treat the patient's condition that is not available at the transferring facility. EMTALA governs almost every aspect of medically indicated transfers, including requiring hospitals to adopt and enforce policies to ensure compliance with federal transfer laws and mandating specific actions by the transferring and receiving hospitals (Box 207-1).[1-3,9,46,47]

Some states have enacted their own transfer laws.[48] Most state laws parallel EMTALA, but some are more burdensome, so physicians who are responsible for patient transfers should be aware of controlling laws and regulations in their own state as well as federal law.

BOX 207-1. Recommended Patient Transfer Procedures

Duties of Transferring Facility

1. Stabilize the patient, if possible.
2. Complete a physician certificate of transfer.
3. Obtain the patient's informed consent to the transfer.
4. Arrange for another hospital to accept the patient in transfer.
5. Send appropriate data to the accepting facility (medical records, test results, transfer forms).
6. Effect the transfer through qualified personnel and transportation equipment.
7. Maintain records of all transfers.

Duties of Facility Accepting Transfer

1. Accept all appropriate requests for transfer.
2. Maintain records of all transfers.
3. Report all EMTALA transfer violations.

CONSENT FOR MEDICAL CARE

Informed Consent

The doctrine of "informed consent" is a fundamental principle of the American legal system. "Every human of adult years with a sound mind has a right to determine what should be done with his own body."[49] Physicians may not examine or treat any person without consent, and that consent must be informed. This means that the patient must be given all pertinent ("material") information concerning the nature, risk, and alternatives of the treatment before the patient can be deemed to have effectively consented to the medical intervention.

Physicians should always endeavor to obtain informed consent but must remain cognizant of the significant limitations and number of exceptions to the doctrine, especially in the emergency setting. Delaying treatment in an emergency to obtain informed consent is a much more serious and common medicolegal problem than failure to obtain proper informed consent.

The law of informed consent contains a great deal of uncertainty, with many gray areas. Different states have different views, either in their statutory laws (legislation) or in their common law (judge-made law or precedent), on the meaning of "informed consent" in the care of the emergency patient. Most cases are unique and depend on the specific circumstances.

Emergency physicians rarely have time to seek legal consultations, let alone wait for a court to render a decision concerning the legal nuances of consent issues. In these situations, it is helpful for emergency physicians to use a *when-in-doubt rule* to guide their immediate actions. The rule simply states that when emergency physicians are in doubt regarding the legality of a situation, "they should do what they believe to be in the patient's best interest and worry about the legal consequences later." Although emergency physicians risk criminal and civil charges of false imprisonment, battery, and even negligence suits for failure to obtain appropriate informed consent, the courts almost universally rule in favor of physicians who act in good faith on behalf of their patients in emergency situations. Successful civil litigation regarding an issue of consent theory against an emergency physician acting reasonably, and consistent with the appropriate standard of care, is extremely rare. An emergency physician is much more likely to be sued for failure to treat while waiting for consent than for providing reasonable treatment without consent.

Federal Versus State Laws

Both federal laws (e.g., EMTALA) and state laws govern consent.[5,31] EMTALA comes into play primarily in the evaluation of minors and when patients refuse an examination, stabilizing treatment, or transfer. State consent laws vary widely and may be set by statutes, case law, or both. The concepts discussed next are generally applicable to emergency care, but physicians should be cognizant of the consent laws particular to their own state.

The law presumes that an adult is mentally competent to make medical decisions and that the competent adult is entitled to sufficient information to make an informed decision concerning the physician's proposed course of examination and treatment.[50] Under the doctrine of *informed consent,* physicians have the duty to disclose the following information to patients[50-52]:

1. The patient's condition and/or diagnosis;
2. The nature and purpose of the proposed treatment, including the likelihood of success in the physician's practice;
3. Reasonable alternative measures related to the diagnosis and treatment, including the probable outcome of those alternatives;
4. The particular known inherent risks that are material to make an informed decision about whether to accept or reject the proposed treatment, including the consequences of refusing that treatment.

"Reasonable Person" versus "Professional Disclosure" Standard

The states are split on the standard used to determine what should be disclosed for patients to make informed decisions, but the modern trend is toward the "reasonable person standard" of disclosure. Under this standard, a physician must disclose all the information that a reasonable person would require to make a decision under the facts and circumstances of the case. Under the second standard, still in use in some states, termed "the professional disclosure standard," a physician must provide the same information that other physicians in the community would provide to patients in the same or similar circumstances. This is generally less stringent than the reasonable person standard.[52,53]

Physicians do not need to disclose every remote risk associated with a procedure or risks that are common knowledge or obvious to the patient, such as the risk of infection after wound repair.[54] The law only requires disclosure of risks that are material, judged by their seriousness or chance of occurrence. Courts define material information as information that "the physician knows or should know would be regarded as significant by a reasonable person in the patient's position when deciding to accept or reject the recommended medical procedure."[55]

Some states legally require physicians to disclose specific risks, such as death.[56] Some states statutorily require a physician to meet both the reasonable person standard and the professional disclosure standard.[57,58]

Physician's Role in Process

The physician who proposes to undertake the procedure must be the one to obtain the patient's informed consent. The duty to obtain consent cannot be delegated, so physicians cannot ask nurses or other health care providers to obtain patients' consent on their behalf. The physician who will care for the patient is best qualified to discuss the treatment and its risks and benefits with the patient. Nurses, as well as physicians not skilled in performing the procedure, cannot obtain valid informed consent.

The physician should write or dictate into the patient's medical record a summary of the discussion held with the patient and the family concerning the elements of informed consent. Particular attention should be made to documenting those material risks discussed with the patient before obtaining the patient's consent.

Consent is a *process,* not a signature. A written, signed, separate consent form is not legally required under the doctrine of informed consent; however, hospitals may require emergency physicians to complete standardized consent forms and obtain the patient's signature. The signed form is not a substitute for the consent process. It cannot replace the exchange of information that occurs between the physician and the patient and the family, the answering of questions, and the ultimate agreement of the patient to undergo the medical or surgical intervention.[50]

A signed, written consent form, however, does constitute some evidence of a valid consent. In some states, a written signed consent form is presumed to be valid consent unless that presumption is rebutted by proof that the consent was obtained by fraud, deceit, or misrepresentation of a material fact.[59]

Implied Consent in Emergency Situations

If an unconscious or incapacitated patient cannot express consent, the law will assume the patient consented to treatment for the emergency situation. Implied legal consent is premised on two principles: (1) duty to obtain informed consent is excused if death or irreparable harm may result if the physician delays providing treatment, and (2) the law assumes that a reasonable, competent, lucid adult would consent to lifesaving treatment.[60,61]

The emergency treatment allowed is limited to the circumstances of the emergency, however, and only treatment required to resolve the emergency should be undertaken without consent. Similarly, the emergency condition must require immediate medical attention, with insufficient time to inform the patient or seek consent from another person.[62]

The courts disagree on the definition of a "true emergency," and whether the emergency exception applies in a given case depends on the definition accepted by the court and the application of that definition to the particular set of facts. Fortunately, the courts will generally stretch the doctrine to protect physicians who act in good faith in caring for a patient with a perceived emergency condition.[63,64] This is one situation where use of the "when-in-doubt rule" and documentation of the physician's concerns will weigh greatly in the court's determination of whether the physician acted appropriately without obtaining informed consent. Physicians can further protect themselves by obtaining a second opinion that a true emergency exists.

Minors

Minors Accompanied by a Parent or Legal Guardian

Parents and legal guardians have the right to consent on behalf of their minor children. However, they must act reasonably and in the best interests of their children. If they do not, their right to consent may be abrogated by the state or the courts. Parents are not allowed to refuse treatment for life-threatening injuries to a child. The management of injured children whose parents refuse to give their consent to treatment is discussed later.

Either natural parent of the minor child may provide legally binding consent. If one parent agrees with a proposed treatment and the other does not, consent may be accepted from the agreeing parent. Even if separated or divorced, either parent may give consent unless one parent has been judicially granted sole legal custody of the child, in which case only the custodial parent may consent. The child's biologic father, even if never married to the mother, may also consent for his child.

Unaccompanied Minors

EMTALA mandates that all persons presenting to an emergency department requesting care be examined to determine whether an emergency condition is present.[5] This federal law takes precedence over all state consent laws regarding the initial evaluation of a minor child. In essence, the child's mere presence at an emergency department requesting an examination or treatment constitutes legal consent to examine the child to determine whether an EMC is present. Furthermore, the hospital should never delay this initial screening evaluation in order to wait for consent.

If an EMC is discovered through the initial screening examination,[5,31] the physician may treat the emergency under either state or federal legal theories. First, under state laws the standard emergency exception doctrine applies. State laws allow physicians to proceed with treatment whenever an emergency exists. Although no uniform legal definition of emergency exists among the states, state laws tend to define an emergency very liberally, such as "any threat to the minor's life or health." The courts almost always affirm a physician's judgment regarding an emergency condition and rarely question the treatment given to a minor without parental consent.[63,65] Preserving life, preventing permanent disability, alleviating pain and suffering, and avoiding eventual harm have been used as guidelines for emergency treatment without consent.[63] Any minor presenting to the emergency department should be triaged and provided an MSE to determine whether an emergency exists.

Under EMTALA, if an EMC is present, the hospital and physicians must provide "stabilizing treatment."[31] Federal law also gives the physician broad discretion to decide what treatment should be performed and in what time frame it should be accomplished. The stabilization requirement includes transfer to an institution capable of handling the minor's injuries if necessary. Thus, under federal law, a minor could be examined, stabilized, or transferred to another institution without consent ever being obtained from the family; in this instance, the care would be not only in the patient's best interest, but also legally correct.[5,31]

Generally, if the MSE does not reveal an emergency condition, physicians need to obtain proper consent from the minor's parents or legal guardian. However, state laws and the courts have applied a number of exceptions to allow minors to seek treatment on their own without parental consent. These exceptions vary widely from state to state, and most are applied through a facts and circumstances analysis on a case-by-case basis by the courts. Under the *mature minor* exception, minors who possess an understanding and appreciation of the nature and consequences of the treatment and appear competent to make their own decisions are allowed to consent, despite not having reached the defined age for maturity (usually 18 years).[66] A mature minor is usually 15 to 17 years old.

The *emancipated minor* provides another exception to the need for parental consent. If the minor is living independently, is self-supporting, or is in the U.S. Armed Forces, the courts may recognize the minor as emancipated and able to consent on his or her own behalf. Again, this is determined by the courts on a case-by-case basis.[67] Additionally, most states have statutory reasons, such as sexually transmitted diseases, pregnancy, or domestic violence injuries, which allow minors to seek care without the consent of their parents.[68-70]

Incompetent or Incapacitated Adults

If an individual has been declared legally incompetent by a court, consent must be obtained from the person's court-appointed legal guardian. In addition, individuals may appoint legal surrogates to make legal decisions for them should they become incompetent. State-sanctioned living wills, advance directives, and durable medical powers of attorney all transfer consent powers from an individual who becomes incompetent to a legally appointed surrogate.[71]

If an incompetent adult has neither a legal guardian nor an appointed surrogate, physicians typically look to the patient's family for consent to treatment. However, consent to treatment by the family, even the patient's spouse, is generally not acceptable under American law, unless the spouse or family member has been appointed legal guardian by a court of proper jurisdiction.[72] Marriage does not confer one spouse the legal capacity to consent to medical treatment for the other spouse, even when the ill or injured spouse is incompetent.

Some states recognized this problem and enacted "family consent statutes," which outline a hierarchy of family members who can provide consent when the family member becomes incapacitated.[73] However, even when families have no legal standing to consent for the incompetent relative, it is always wise to involve family in the medical decision-making process. Communication and concern for the family avoid misunderstandings, surprise, and anger, which are the primary reasons for litigation. Fortunately, if an emergency exists, no authorization from family is necessary to provide such reasonable care as is necessary to correct the life-threatening situation. Once the emergency is resolved, consent should be obtained from someone authorized to act on behalf of the incompetent patient. If there is no appointed legal guardian or surrogate and no state statute on family consent, the physician will need to seek consent authorization from the courts. The courts may appoint a guardian at that time, generally a family member, or after judicial review of the issues the court itself may grant consent on behalf of the incapacitated person.[74]

Prisoners

Competent prisoners generally do not surrender the right to consent by virtue of being incarcerated. However, a state or court may compel treatment based on interests perceived as paramount to the prisoner's interests.[75] The elements usually necessary to treat self-inflicted injuries over the objection of the competent prisoner include the following[76]:

1. The injury to the prisoner was willful and intentionally self-inflicted.
2. The proposed treatment is necessary is preserve or restore the health of the prisoner.
3. The prisoner is competent to act on his or her own behalf.
4. The prisoner refuses to give consent.
5. The physician reduces the medical indications for treatment to writing in the prisoner's medical record.

Alcohol-Intoxicated Patients

Alcohol intoxication itself may not render a patient incompetent to give informed consent.[77] The emergency physician must evaluate each situation individually to determine whether the patient is incapacitated by alcohol to the extent that he or she is no longer able to understand the proposed treatment, risks and benefits, and rational alternatives. In essence, one cannot disregard the general rules for determining whether the individual is competent to make informed decisions just because the patient is intoxicated with alcohol. However, the when-in-doubt rule is particularly applicable in these cases because alcohol intoxication is often associated with occult serious illness or injury.

Alcohol intoxication, particularly if documented by a measured blood alcohol concentration (BAC), is strongly suggestive to courts and juries of impaired mental status, even though health care workers recognize that many alcoholics are entirely rational and competent at fairly high BACs.[78] Conversely, low BACs do not guarantee competence because other processes (e.g., hypoglycemia, blood loss, other illicit substances) may cause the patient to be incompetent.[79] Thus, the patient's clinical capacity is more important than the specific level of alcohol in determining competence.

One advantage of obtaining a BAC is that the level may be used in a criminal charge against the individual who may have been driving and caused a motor vehicle crash. Approximately 14 states allow physicians' discretion to report an intoxicated driver to authorities on the basis of a BAC.[80] States may also allow blood samples to be drawn only for medical purposes, later to be subpoenaed by the prosecutor for use against the driver in a driving-while-intoxicated prosecution or other criminal charges.[81]

It is important to recognize that the state "legal limit" of intoxication is not a measure of a patient's competence. The legal level for driving has little, if anything, to do with the capacity to make informed decisions. However, this is sometimes difficult for judges and juries to understand, and the emergency physician can actually use the level to support a judgment that the patient was not competent to make informed decisions in a particular instance. At other times, it is better not to have a "number" so that the only relevant criterion for determining the patient's competence is the physician's judgment.

Patients Given Pain Medications

Obtaining informed consent from patients treated with pain medications before a procedure is a common issue. Similar to alcohol intoxication, the mere fact that a patient has been given narcotic analgesia does not render the patient incapable of consenting to surgical procedures. Plaintiff attorneys can always argue "the patient was too snowed with drugs to give consent"; on the other hand, they can equally argue that the patient was "in too much pain to consent and would have agreed to anything to stop the pain." In such cases, the patient's ability to understand the ramifications pertaining to the procedure should be assessed and acted on, involving the family in the process if possible. The physician should document that the patient's premedicated state was considered when judging the patient's competence to make an informed decision.

REFUSAL OF MEDICAL CARE

Informed Refusal

The corollary to a patient's right to give informed consent is the patient's right to refuse medical care, even if such refusal results in death. In *Cruzan v. Director, Missouri Department of Health,* the U.S. Supreme Court determined that a competent adult has a constitutionally protected right to refuse medical care.[82] However, that right is not absolute. Under particular circumstances, courts will consider countervailing compelling state interests, such as preventing suicide, preserving life, and protecting innocent third parties.

Physicians who honor a competent patient's decision to refuse treatment will not be subject to liability for any resulting bad outcome.[83,84] Today, the physician is more likely to be successfully sued for treating patients over their objections or without their consent, even when the treatment is lifesaving.[85] Before allowing a competent patient to refuse care, however, the emergency physician should evaluate and if possible address the patient's reasons for refusal.

When a competent adult refuses indicated medical intervention, it often is the result of fear, anger, misunderstanding, or some other failure in communications in the physician-patient relationship. Before allowing a patient to refuse care, the physician should try to determine and resolve the underlying reasons behind the patient's refusal. The attending physician must always be involved when a patient refuses medical care or expresses the intent to leave against medical advice.[86]

As with consent, refusal of medical care is a process, not a signature. It must be an informed refusal; merely having the patient sign an "informed consent to refuse examination, treatment, or transfer" form or an "against medical advice" form is not sufficient. The four essential components of the process are discussed next.

Determining Competence

The physician must determine that the patient is competent to make decisions. A normal mental status examination without evidence of diminished mental capacity from closed head injury, severe pain, hypoxia, hypotension, alcohol intoxication, mental retardation, or mind-altering substances is good evidence of competency. Noting the patient's rationale for refusing care, even if it is not reasonable, provides additional evidence of competency.

Ensuring an Informed Decision

To be legally binding, a decision to refuse a test or treatment or to sign out against medical advice must be an informed decision. The physician must explain the severity of the patient's condition, the potential complications, and the alternative treatments available. The physician should use terms that the patient can understand and provide the patient an opportunity to ask questions. The patient must understand that the risks of refusing care include the possibility of permanent disability and death. Ideally, a witness should be present when the physician informs the patient and any family members.

Involving Others

The patient's family, friends, and personal physician should be involved whenever possible. These persons should hear the same message as the patient, because they may be able to persuade the patient to accept the recommended therapy. If the patient expressly forbids the emergency physician to speak with others, as is the patient's legal right, this should be explained to them and documented in the medical record.

Documenting Appropriately

Appropriate documentation of the refusal process is necessary to protect the physician and hospital from inappropriate litigation. The patient should be asked to sign the refusal form.[2,9]

If the patient refuses to sign the form, that fact should be documented, and the form signed by a hospital representative who witnessed the patient's refusal. The medical record should reflect the patient's mental status examination and competency to make informed decisions, the risks and benefits of recommended treatments, the available alternatives, and the participating family or friends. Documenting the patient's rationale for refusing treatment, that the patient was treated to the extent allowed by the patient, and that the patient was invited to return for care at any time offers added protection.

Federal Rules

EMTALA requires hospitals to take and document specific actions when patients refuse medical screening, treatment and stabilization, or transfer. The government and the federal courts presume that the patient requested emergency care and place the burden of proof on the hospital to demonstrate that the patient voluntarily refused care.[2,9,87]

There are essentially two scenarios in which patients leave the hospital after refusing examination or treatment. First, some patients simply pick up and leave, unknown to anyone affiliated with the hospital. If witnessed, the patient does not respond to requests to return for the examination or to discuss the issues with the hospital staff. Hospitals generally refer to these as patients who "left without being seen" (LWBS) or "left before examination." In the second scenario, the hospital is aware that the patient is about to leave and has an opportunity to interact before the patient leaves. Hospitals generally refer to this as "leaving against medical advice." The Office of the Inspector General (OIG) and CMS refer to both these scenarios as "voluntary withdrawal" of the patient's request for evaluation and treatment.[2,9,88]

Leaving Without Being Seen

If a patient walks out before the MSE and later has an adverse medical result, the burden will be on the hospital to prove that the individual left voluntarily and was not denied examination or treatment by the hospital. The OIG and CMS admonish hospitals regarding LWBS patients, stating that "hospitals should be very concerned about patients leaving without being screened. Since every patient that presents seeking emergency services is entitled to a screening examination, a hospital could violate the patient anti-dumping statute if it routinely keeps patients waiting so long that they leave without being seen, particularly if the hospital does not attempt to determine and document why individual patients are leaving, and reiterate to them that the hospital is prepared to provide a medical screening if they stay."[9,17]

Hospitals need to have a policy and practice for LWBS patients that adequately documents pertinent findings and protects the hospital from liability. In most hospitals, the staff calls the patient and checks the waiting area at least three times before declaring that the patient has left the department. These serial checks should be documented and timed on the patient's record, and once it is evident that the patient is no longer present, the record should be reviewed on a timely basis by the physician on duty. If the reviewing physician discovers something of concern regarding the patient's chief complaint or triage data, the individual can be contacted and encouraged to return to the emergency department. The registration papers, triage records, nursing documentation at triage, and the physician's review and documentation of that review should all be kept in the patient's permanent record. These records should be retained for a minimum of 5 years to protect the institution should the interaction ever be the subject of a retrospective EMTALA investigation or litigation on behalf of the individual.[2,9]

Leaving Against Medical Advice

If the hospital is aware that an individual intends to leave before completion of the MSE or stabilizing treatment for whatever reason (e.g., tired of waiting, changes mind, concerned over cost of care), the hospital must handle and document the interaction carefully to avoid EMTALA or medicolegal liability.[2,9,89,90] In each case the following steps should be taken:

1. *Inform the patient of the hospital's obligation under the law.* The emergency department staff should inform individuals of their rights under the EMTALA to receive medical screening and any necessary stabilizing treatment from the hospital regardless of their ability to pay for that service.
2. *Determine the patient's competence.* Only legally competent individuals can refuse necessary medical care. For example, an alcohol-intoxicated individual who presents to the hospital with a medical complaint cannot be allowed to leave the hospital without examination and treatment until it is determined that he is legally competent to make such a decision.
3. *Explain the risks and the benefits to the patient.* For individuals to make an informed consent to voluntarily withdraw their request for services, they must understand the benefits and the risks of withdrawal before refusing examination and treatment. These risks and benefits should be specific to the individual's chief complaint.
4. *Secure the patient's written informed consent to refuse care.* The hospital should take all reasonable steps to secure the individual's written and informed consent (i.e., obtain signature) to refuse medical care. A standard form should be used that contains space for documenting the patient's competence, the risks and benefits discussed, and whether the patient's family was available to be involved in the discussions. If the patient refuses to sign the form and simply walks out after the interaction with the hospital, the person who discussed the issues with the patient and witnessed the patient's refusal should sign the form and document the interaction.
5. *Offer the patient alternative care.* The emergency department staff should suggest that patients see their

private physician soon. Also, patients should return to the emergency department for care if their symptoms worsen or if they simply change their mind.

6. *Document the interaction in the patient's hospital record.* The medical record, preferably a dictated and transcribed medical record, should accurately relate the interaction between the hospital and the individual refusing the MSE. The record reflects the hospital's conformity to the law and the patient's leaving of his or her own accord, specifically, the risks of refusing the examination and the reasons for the patient's refusal. Documenting the reasons for refusal provides evidence that the hospital did not economically coerce or in any way financially deter the patient from remaining for the MSE. The chart must clearly indicate that the patient did not leave the department based on a "suggestion" by the hospital concerning any financial issues.

Parent or Guardian Who Refuses Care or Blood Transfusions for a Minor

Generally, state laws support parental control of health issues affecting their children. However, the state will not allow parents to deny children needed emergency medical care under the doctrine of *parens patriae,* the state's paternalistic interest in children.[91] All states empower emergency physicians to intercede under their child abuse and child neglect laws.[92] When a child's injuries are potentially life threatening, the emergency physician can take custody of the child under the child abuse laws and provide indicated treatment, including blood transfusions. When deciding whether to act, the when-in-doubt rule definitely applies, and all jurisdictions statutorily protect physicians from criminal and civil liability for acting in good faith to protect children.[92]

The courts have specifically addressed the issue of Jehovah's Witness parents attempting to refuse emergency blood transfusions for their minor children. All jurisdictions hold that a parent's right to freedom of religion does not include the right to deny life-sustaining medical intervention for their children.[93,94] One judge best summarized the feelings of the courts: "Not even a parent has unbridled discretion to exercise his or her religious beliefs when the state's interest in preserving the health of the children within its borders weighs in the balance."[95]

Some states specifically address the issue of overriding parental refusal of indicated medical intervention by statute. In North Carolina, for example, if the parents refuse to consent to treatment, and the delay to obtain a court order would seriously worsen the child's physical condition or endanger the child's life, and if a second physician agrees that the procedure is necessary to prevent immediate harm, a physician can render treatment without parental consent. If a second physician cannot be contacted before initiating treatment, the physician may still perform the indicated procedure without parental consent.[96]

Conversely, courts refuse to rule against the parents' wishes when the child's medical condition is not serious or life threatening.[97] If there is no life threat or potential for serious impairment, the parents' refusal should be respected. Parental refusal of indicated nonemergency medical treatment is usually statutorily defined as "child neglect," which is not legally sufficient to take custody of the child. Child neglect should still be reported to the appropriate authorities; treatment for the child can then be obtained under a court order.[92]

Jehovah's Witnesses

Adult Blood Transfusions

The approximately 1 million Jehovah's Witnesses in the United States believe that blood transfusion destroys their relationship with God and forfeits their chance for eternal life; accepting transfusion is not a minor infraction of their faith.[98] They do not accept whole blood, packed cells, platelets, white cells, plasma, or autotransfusion of stored blood. Most will allow the use of crystalloids, albumin, hemophiliac preparations, immunoglobulins, dialysis, and heart-lung machines.[98,99]

Jehovah's Witnesses and the issue of blood transfusion present very difficult medicolegal issues in the emergency department.[100] State courts may have widely divergent views on the issue, and no clear-cut answers exist. However, the current trend is granting patients greater autonomy to refuse blood, even when the state asserts compelling interests to override a person's refusal.

General principles of consent and the when-in-doubt rule apply, but hospitals and medical staff should also (1) develop policies and procedures in advance to resolve potential conflicts with the Jehovah's Witness patients in the community; (2) coordinate the management of each case with hospital legal counsel, in contact with a judge who can issue court orders when appropriate, if time allows; (3) have other physician consultants write notes of agreement regarding the need to give blood; and (4) communicate effectively with patients and family, in advance when possible.

Competent Adult

The courts have found that "the competent adult has the right to refuse a transfusion regardless of whether his refusal to do so arises from fear of adverse reaction, religious belief, recalcitrance, or cost."[101] This applies "even though we may consider a patient's beliefs unwise, foolish, or ridiculous."[102] However, even this right is not absolute. If the individual's refusal conflicts with compelling state interests such as the preservation of life, the prevention of suicide, or the protection of innocent third parties, the courts may order transfusions despite the individual's objections.[100,103,104]

Previously, typical scenarios in which the courts overrode a competent person's refusal included cases of pregnant women to protect the life of the fetus, mothers of young children to promote the general welfare of the children, and a sole supporting father or mother to avoid offspring from becoming wards of the state.[104-106] Several court decisions, however, have significantly restricted the hospital's or state's ability to assert compelling interests challenging a competent individual's right of self-determination.[107-110]

Unconscious or Medically Incompetent Adult

In an emergency, if the Jehovah's Witness's beliefs are unknown, physicians may transfuse the patient because consent will be implied under the emergency doctrine.[111,112] It is irrelevant if the spouse, mother, or other family members adamantly refuse to allow the transfusion for religious reasons. The state's compelling interest in preserving life outweighs the family's expression of the patient's religious preferences.[111]

In the past, when a Jehovah's Witness's beliefs and transfusion preferences were known in advance, but the patient was incompetent at the time of the emergency, the courts tended to support transfusion until the patient became competent and could refuse transfusion contemporaneously.[93,113] However, the law in this area is in a state of flux, particularly because of the enigmatic question: If a card carried by the patient identifies him as a member of the Jehovah's Witnesses and sets out his religious objection to blood transfusion, should this be considered adequate evidence for physicians to rely upon to withhold blood transfusions in an emergency?

The trend today is toward accepting the card as a form of advanced directive that is binding on hospitals and physicians. In at least six states, if the card is dated and signed before two witnesses, it is statutorily valid.[114,115] Even if the blood refusal card does not conform to a state's advance directive statute, it should be considered strong evidence, but not necessarily determinative, of the Jehovah's Witness's wishes. Advance directives are merely a means to express an individual's rights and are not the exclusive means to express those rights legally.[60,103] Jehovah's Witnesses are learning to use state statutorily defined advance directive methods to legally express their intentions.[116]

Interestingly, no Jehovah's Witness has successfully sued a health care provider to recover damages in cases in which blood was withheld on the basis of an apparently valid blood refusal card.[117] Also, "criminal, civil, or professional misconduct liability has never been imposed on health care providers for forgoing treatment the patient did not want."[118]

REPORTING REQUIREMENTS

All states require the hospital emergency department to report certain events or illnesses to local public health authorities. The state's primary intent is to prevent the spread of communicable diseases, protect its citizens from disease and violence, and prosecute criminal acts. In each instance, the state statute overrides the patients' rights to confidentiality of their medical records. The statutes typically also provide physicians immunity from civil liability or criminal prosecution if the reporting is done in good faith.[119]

All emergency departments should maintain up to date lists of diseases and incidents that must be reported to the state. Also, the process to ensure appropriate reporting and identification of who is responsible for reporting should be detailed in departmental policy.

Communicable Diseases

Typical communicable diseases that must be reported include those of epidemiologic concern, such as sexually transmitted disease (e.g., gonorrhea, syphilis, chlamydial infection, nongonococcal urethritis, human immunodeficiency virus infection, acquire immunodeficiency syndrome), and highly communicable illnesses (e.g., tuberculosis, hepatitis, pertussis). Emergency physicians also have a duty to warn patients with communicable diseases against activities that may spread the disease and must instruct them to inform contacts to seek evaluation and treatment. Physicians should adequately document such instructions in the medical record to prevent liability to third parties for failure to warn appropriately.

Violent Acts

Wounds, injuries, and illness resulting from criminal acts of violence must be reported to state agencies.[120] Bullet wounds, powder burns, stab wounds, intentional poisonings, child abuse or neglect, sexual assaults, spousal abuse, domestic violence, and any suspicious injuries generally must be reported.

Deaths

All deaths must be reported to state or local authorities. Additionally, death under certain circumstances must be reported to the county medical examiner. These circumstances include (1) deaths from violence, poisoning, accident, suicide, or homicide; (2) any sudden death in someone in apparently good health or when unattended by a physician; (3) any death occurring in a jail, prison, correctional institution, or in police custody; and (4) any death occurring under suspicious, unusual, or unnatural circumstances.[121] Fetal deaths may also have to be reported, usually if over 20 weeks' gestation or the typical gestational period of possible viability.[122]

When a death requires a report to the medical examiner, the integrity of the scene and the body should be preserved. Emergency department staff should disturb the body as little as possible, secure the patient's belongings and any potential evidentiary materials, and leave in place medical interventions such as endotracheal tubes, nasogastric tubes, and central or peripheral intravenous lines. The medical examiner will determine whether the state will assert authority over the body, order an autopsy, or release the body to the family.[121]

Animal Bites

Most states require the reporting of animal bites, particularly dog and cat bites, to the local public health department. The states also generally require the reporting of bites by any animals known to be potential carriers of rabies, such as bats, raccoons, skunks, foxes, and cattle. The obvious intent of such statutes is to prevent cases of human rabies and to control the spread of rabies within the animal community.[123]

Substance Abuse and Chronic Diseases

Some states require the reporting of substance abuse or certain chronic diseases, such as cancer.[124]

REFERENCES

1. 42 USC 1395dd.
2. EMTALA Final regulations. 68 Federal Register 53221-53264. 2003. Available at *http://www.access.gpo.gov/su_docs/fedreg/a030909c.html.*
3. HHS CMS/Survey and Certification Group. S&C-04-34, Revised Final EMTALA Guidelines, May 13, 2004. Available at *http://www.cms.hhs.gov/medicaid/survey-cert/sc0434.pdf.*
4. The Medicare Prescription Drug Improvement and Modernization Act. Public Law 108-173, December 8, 2003.
5. 42 USC 1395dd(a).
6. 42 USC 1395dd(e)(1)(A).
7. 42 USC 1395dd (e)(1)(B).
8. *Harris v Health and Hospital Corp,* 852 F.Supp 701 (SD Ind 1994)
9. Bitterman RA: *Providing Emergency Care Under Federal Law: EMTALA.* Dallas, American College of Emergency Physicians, 2001.
10. 65 *Fed Reg* 18548 (2000).
11. *Clark v Baton Rouge General Medical Center,* 657 So2d 741 (La App 1995).
12. 42 CFR 489.24(b).
13. Bitterman RA. *Providing Emergency Care Under Federal Law: EMTALA, 2004 Supplement.* Dallas, American College of Emergency Physicians, 2004.
14. *Vickers v Nash General Hospital,* 78 F3d 139 (4th Cir 1996).
15. 68 Federal Register 53221, 53263; 42 CFR 489.24(d)(2) and 489.24(b).
16. *CM v Tomball Regional Hospital,* 961 SW2d (Tex App 1997).
17. 42 CFR 489.24(a).
18. 42 CFR 482.55.
19. 59 *Fed Reg* 32099, 32113, 32116. 1994.
20. CMS Interpretive Guidelines, V15-24. 1998.
21. *Correa v Hospital of San Francisco,* 63 F3d 1184 (1st Cir 1995).
22. 64 *Fed Reg* 36070, 61353, 61359. 1999.
23. 42 CFR 482.13(a)(1).
24. CMS State Operations/Survey and Certification Group S&C-02-34, On-call requirements-EMTALA (June 13, 2002); S&C-02-35, Simultaneously on call (June 13, 2002).
25. Hyams AL, et al: Practice guidelines and malpractice litigation: a two way street. *Ann Intern Med* 122:450, 1995.
26. *Brooker v Desert Hospital Corp,* 947 F2d 412 (9th Cir 1991).
27. *Gatewood v Washington Healthcare Corporation,* 933 F2d 1037 (DC Cir 1991).
28. 42 CFR 482.20(3).
29. 42 CFR 413.65(g)(1)
30. 42 CFR 482.24(b).
31. 42 USC 1395dd(b).
32. *Cherukuri v Shalala,* 1999 Fed App 0160P (6th Cir).
33. Wanerman R: The EMTALA paradox. *Ann Emerg Med* 40:464, 2002.
34. Bitterman RA: Explaining the EMTALA paradox [editorial]. *Ann Emerg Med* 40:470, 2002.
35. *Cleland v Bronson Healthcare Group, Inc,* 917 F2d, 271-272 (6th Cir 1990).
36. *Bryant v Adventist Health System,* 289 F3d 1162 (9th Cir 2002); and *Harry v Marchant,* 291 F3d 767 (11th Cir 2002).
37. *Lopez-Soto v Hawayek,* No 98-1594, 1999 WL 188283 (1st Cir 1999).
38. 42 USC 1395cc(a)(1)(I)(iii).
39. 42 USC 1395dd(e)(3)(B).
40. *Smith v. Botsford General Hospital,* Case No: 00-71459, US District Court, Eastern District, Southern Division of Michigan (April 2003).
41. *Roberts v Galen of Virginia, Inc,* 119 S Ct 685 (1999), 525 US 249, 142 L ED2d 648.
42. Frew SA: On-call physicians: The no. 2 cause of COBRA problems. *Emergency Physicians Monthly* May 1997, p 7.
43. Morgan D: Emergency room follow-up care and malpractice liability. *J Legal Med* 16:373, 1995.
44. 42 USC 1395dd(e)(4).
45. 42 USC 1395dd(c)(1)(A)(ii).
46. 42 USC 1395cc(a)(1)(I)(i).
47. HHS/CMS Program Memorandum S&C-02-06, Hospital capacity-EMTALA (November 29, 2001).
48. California Health and Safety Code 1317.5 (West 1990).
49. *Schloendoff v The Society of New York Hospital,* 211 NY 125 (NY 1914).
50. Katz J: *The Silent World of Doctor and Patient.* New York, Free Press, 1984.
51. *Cobbs v Grant,* 502 P2d 1 (Calif 1972)
52. Furrow B, et al: The liability of health care professionals. In *Health Law.* St Paul, Minn, West, 1995.
53. *Wells v Van Nort,* 125 NE 910 (Ohio 1919).
54. *Percle v St Paul Fire and Marine Insurance Co,* 349 So2d 1289 (1977).
55. *Truman v Thomas,* 611 P2d 902 (1980).
56. Iowa Code Ann 147.137 (West 1989).
57. Ala Code 6-5-484 (1990).
58. NC Gen Stat 90-21.13.
59. NC Gen Stat 90-21.13(b).
60. *Canterberry v Spence,* 464 F2d 772 (DC Cir), *cert denied* 409 US 1064 (1972).
61. *Dunham v Wright,* 423 F2d 940 (3rd Cir 1970).
62. *Wheeler v Barker,* 208 P2d 6068 (1949).
63. *Sullivan v Montgomery,* 279 NYS 575 (1935).
64. *Thomson v Sun City Community Hospital,* 668 P2d 605 (1984).
65. Tsai AK, et al: Evaluation and treatment of minors: Reference on consent. *Ann Emerg Med* 22:1211, 1993.
66. *Cardwell v Bechtol,* 1724 SW2d 739 (TN 1987).
67. Cal Civ Code 62 (West 1979); Wyo Stat 14-1-101 (1981).
68. Colo Rev Stat 13-22-103 (1979).
69. Mass Gen Laws Ann 112, 12F (West 1975).
70. NC Gen Stat 130A-135, 90-21.5(a).
71. Collin F, et al: *Durable Powers of Attorney and Health Care Directives,* 3rd ed. American College of Legal Medicine, 1997.
72. *In re Quinlan,* 335 A2d 647 (1976).
73. Ark Stat Ann 41-41-2 (1994); Idaho Code 39 4305 (1975); *Wells v Van Nort,* 125 NE 910 (Ohio 1919).
74. Cal Probate Code 3200-3211(West 1991); Va Code 37.1-134.2 (1982).
75. *Commissioner of Corrections v Myers,* 399 NE2d 452 (1979).
76. NC Gen Stat 148-46.2.
77. *Miller v. Rhode Island Hospital,* 625 A2d 778 (RI 1993).
78. Siegel DM: Consent and refusal of treatment. *Emerg Med Clin North Am* 11:833, 1993.

79. Ethering JM: Emergency management of acute alcohol problems. *Can Fam Physician* 42:2423, 1996.
80. Reporting Patients' Blood Alcohol Levels. *Emerg Med News* 18:1, 1996.
81. Mich Comp Laws Ann 257.625a(9).
82. *Cruzan v Director, Missouri Department of Health,* 497 US 261, 279 (1990).
83. *Rodriguez v Pinol,* 634 So2d 681 (Fla Ct App1994).
84. *Wons v Public Health Trust,* 500 So2d 679, 686 (Fla Dist Ct App 1987).
85. *Rogers v Sells,* 178 Okla 103 (1936).
86. Dubow D, et al: Emergency department discharges against medical advice. *J Emerg Med* 10:513, 1992.
87. *Stevison v Enid Healthcare System, Inc,* 920 F2d 710 (10th Cir 1999).
88. 64 Federal Register 61353 (1999). This is the Department of Health and Human Services OIG/CMS Special Advisory Bulletin on the Patient Anti-Dumping Statute, November 10, 1999.
89. 42 CFR 489.24(c)(2).
90. 42 USC 1395dd(b)(2)(3).
91. Goldstein J: Medical care for the child at risk: State supervision of parental autonomy. *Yale Law J* 86:645, 1977.
92. llivan DJ: Patient discharge against medical advice. *Emerg Dept Legal Lett* 7:91, 1996.
93. *In re Estate of Dorone,* 534 A2d 1271 (Pa 1985).
94. *Jehovah's Witness of Washington v Kings County Hospital,* 278 F Supp 488 (DC 1967), *affirmed per curiam* 390 US 598 (1968).
95. *Nowak v Cobb County-Kennestone Hosp Authority,* 74 F2d 1173 (1996).
96. NC Gen Stat 90-21.1-3.
97. *In re Green,* 292 A2D 387 (Pa 1972).
98. Cox M, Lumly J: No blood or blood products. *Anesthesia* 50:583, 1995.
99. Migden DR, Braen GR: The Jehovah's Witness blood refusal card: Ethical and medicolegal considerations for emergency physicians. *Acad Emerg Med* 5:815, 1998.
100. Spence RK: The Jehovah's Witness patient and medicolegal aspects of transfusion medicine. *Semin Vasc Surg* 7:121, 1994.
101. *St. Mary's Hospital v Ramsey,* 465 So2d 666 (1985).
102. *In re Brooks Estate,* 205 NE2d 435 (1965).
103. Hartman KM: Exceptions to informed consent in emergency medicine. *Hosp Physician* March:53, 1999.
104. *In re Osborne,* 294 A2d 372 (DC Ct App 1972).
105. *Hamilton v McAuliffe,* 352 A2d 634 (MD 1976).
106. *In re Winthrop Univ Hosp,* 490 NYS2d 996 (Sup Ct 1985); and *In re Melideo,* 390 NY S2d 523 (1976).
107. *Fosimire v Nicholeau,* 551 NE2d 77 (NY 1990).
108. *In re Dubreuil,* 629 So2d 819 (Fla 1993).
109. *In re Fetus Brown,* 1-96-2316 (Ill App Ct 1997).
110. *Stamford Hosp v Vega,* 236 Conn 646 (1996).
111. *John F Kennedy Mem Hosp v Heston,* 279 A2d 670 (NJ 1971).
112. *University of Cincinnati Hospital v Edmond,* 506 NE2d 299 (1986).
113. *Werth v Taylor,* 475 NW2d 426 Mich App (1991).
114. Colo Rev Stat Ann 15-14-504(b),(b)(3),505(2),506(1); Fla Stat Ann 765.101(1); Ky Rev Stat Ann 311.621(2),637(6); Me Rev Stat Ann Tit 18A, 5-801(a),801(I),802(a),804; Md Code Ann, Health-Gen 5-601(b),602(c),603,611(e)(2); 79 Op Att'y Gen 94-028 n13 (Md 1994); NM Stat Ann 24-7A-1(A),2,4,16(A).
115. Md Ann Code 43 135C (1980).
116. Ridley DT: Honoring Jehovah's Witnesses' advanced directives in emergencies. *Acad Emerg Med* 5:824, 1998.
117. Zeitz E: Legal reasoning and medical decision making [editorial]. *Acad Emerg Med* 5:755, 1998.
118. Refusing and foregoing treatment. In *Treatise on Health Care Law.* 18.07[2] (1997).
119. NC Gen Stat 7A-550, 130A-142.
120. NC Gen Stat 90-21.20.
121. NC Gen Stat 130A-383.
122. NC Gen Stat 130A-114.
123. NC Gen Stat 130A-196.
124. NC Gen Stat 130A-209, 211.

CHAPTER 208 Wellness, Stress, and the Impaired Physician

Richard Goldberg

PERSPECTIVE

Wellness can be defined as the optimal state of health and well-being achieved through the active prevention of illness.[1] Emergency medicine as a specialty was still in its formative years when concerns were first expressed regarding the stressful and unhealthful aspects of emergency practice and the impact such stressors could have on wellness and career longevity.[2,3] While experience has shown that large numbers of emergency physicians enjoy long and fulfilling careers, questions remain about how best to cope with the excessive demands of emergency practice.[4]

This chapter presents a survey of wellness issues facing the emergency physician, dividing them into three main sections: Major stressors, physician burnout and impairment, and strategies for promoting wellness in emergency practice.

CAUSATIVE FACTORS: MAJOR STRESSORS IN EMERGENCY MEDICINE

What features of the practice of emergency medicine are potentially unhealthful? A large number of stressors have been cited in the literature, applying both to practicing emergency physicians and physicians in training.[5,6] Ultimately, they relate to four aspects of emergency practice: (1) difficult patient and professional relationships, (2) diversity of practice elements, (3) diminished resources, and (4) difficult decisions.

Difficult Patient and Professional Relationships

Although the ability to provide care for a variety of critically ill patients is a major source of gratification for most emergency physicians, there may be no other medical specialty in which the physician-patient relationship is so potentially problematic. Many patients presenting to the emergency department are highly stressed, often suffering the effects of both pain and apprehension. They may have language barriers, organic brain syndromes, or other altered states that render them more difficult to evaluate. They may be "frequent fliers," presenting with conditions requiring inordinate amounts of time and resources. They may also be dangerous, manifesting any of a variety of emotional disorders, including hypochondriasis, chemical dependency, sociopathic behaviors, and psychoses.[7]

Issues of personal safety have become major concerns among emergency department personnel for a variety of reasons, including acts of violence, verbal threats, heightened exposure to a variety of infectious diseases, and, more recently, agents of bioterrorism.[8,9] Dealing with such difficult patients can arouse in the emergency physician a variety of negative emotions, including feelings of helplessness, inadequacy, fear, vindictiveness, anger, or even hatred. Such feelings, however understandable, may become considerable sources of stress.[10,11]

Professional relationships may also be stressful. Emergency physicians practice "fishbowl medicine," conducting the entire range of their practice habits in full view of the medical staff. Disputes can arise regarding management and disposition decisions, spheres of practice ("turf"), and referral practices. In addition, although perhaps less prevalent an attitude than in the early days of the specialty, some physician colleagues regard emergency physicians as "journeyman housestaff" with commensurate clinical skills. The issue of professional status also surfaces in dealings with hospital administrators, who are sometimes unwilling to prioritize appropriately the needs of the emergency department.[6]

Relations with other emergency department personnel are also subject to strain. Because of the contractual nature of the typical emergency practice, the emergency physician does not have the same sense of workplace "ownership" as physicians in office practice. Nurses and ancillary personnel are usually not hired by the emergency physician, and disputes can arise over issues of responsibility and control.[6,12]

Diversity of Practice Elements

Diversity may be the overriding characteristic of emergency practice, particularly in terms of hours, patients, pace, and acuity. Work schedules typically include a mixture of irregularly assigned days, nights, weekends, and holidays. The practice environment is often chaotic. Emergency department workers are subjected to a barrage of intrusive noises, including alarms, monitors, and telephones, as patients of all ages and presentations arrive for evaluation at unpredictable intervals. This diversity is often cited by medical students and residents embarking on careers in emergency medicine as a challenging, even beguiling feature of the specialty. The older practitioner, after years of struggling to maintain some semblance of order within the department, is much more likely to view diversity as a major stressor.[5,6,12]

Diminished Resources

In recent years, most hospitals and emergency departments have had to implement cost-cutting measures as a means of coping with the impact of managed care contracts, dwindling government reimbursements, and the need to provide substantial amounts of uncompensated care. These measures have resulted in a number of important resource limitations with which the emergency physician must contend. These include (1) diminished staffing of nurses, ancillary personnel, and social services; (2) burdensome cost-containment policies and documentation requirements regarding access to diagnostic and treatment modalities, specialty consultations, and hospital admissions; (3) inadequate policies providing for the care and disposition of medically indigent patients; and (4) diminished reimbursement for services rendered.[5,6,12]

Difficult Decisions

Emergency physicians are continually making critical decisions based on incomplete or ambiguous information. Difficulties in the decision-making process, concerns regarding patient safety, and fears regarding medical mistakes as well as litigation are additional stressors of major importance.[5,6,12]

CONSEQUENCES: THE BURNED-OUT OR IMPAIRED PHYSICIAN

Burnout

The term *burnout* was introduced by Freudenberger in 1975 to refer to feelings of job dissatisfaction caused by work-related stress.[13] Burnout is of special relevance to physicians because it undermines the personal relationship between caregiver and recipient that is essential to effective service. People in advanced phases of burnout are likely to experience decreased productivity, less satisfaction with work, higher turnover, lower self-esteem, more physical symptoms, more troubled family relationships, and a variety of affective changes, such as hostility, anxiety, and depression. Symptoms of burnout are thought to be potential precursors of more severe manifestations of impairment, including alcoholism, drug abuse, and suicide.[14]

Several studies have documented moderate to high levels of burnout among certain populations of emergency physicians,[4,15] and few emergency physicians would dispute the particular significance of burnout as an occupational hazard. However, burnout is not an inevitable consequence of emergency practice. A randomized survey of 958 emergency physicians conducted by the American Board of Emergency Medicine in 1999 found the respondents to be primarily in middle age and quite satisfied with their careers; work stressors were graded as only moderate in intensity.[16]

Additional information regarding the burnout process in emergency medicine is available either by accessing the website of the American College of Emergency Physicians or by directly contacting the College's Practice Management Department (800/798-1822).

Physician Impairment

Physician impairment exists when a physician's professional performance is adversely affected because of illness, including mental or physical illness, aging, alcoholism, or chemical dependence.[17] It is estimated that 17,000 practicing physicians are afflicted with substance abuse problems and that 100 deaths annually among physicians are directly attributable to chemical dependency.[18] Several studies suggest that alcohol and substance abuse may be higher in emergency medicine residents and practicing emergency physicians than in other practitioners or specialties.[19,20]

Impairment in a physician colleague is often difficult to detect. A pattern of events rather than a single precipitating incident may be the key to making the diagnosis. Problems in the workplace are often preceded by a history of family difficulties, including frequent arguments, periods of separation, extramarital affairs, and divorce. Associated frequent job changes and intervals between employment may also be present. Finally, hospital duties are affected as patient care responsibilities become neglected and poor medical judgment is exhibited. The problem may develop over a long period because strong elements of denial exist among family and associates, as well as the impaired physician.[18]

As an ethical principle, emergency physicians are obliged to deal fairly and honestly with colleagues and take appropriate actions to protect patients from health care providers who are impaired or incompetent or who engage in fraud or deception.[21] Programs to detect and treat physician impairment have now been established in every state. A few states have recovery programs that are legislatively mandated, being administered by state medical boards, state medical societies, or independent organizations. A carefully structured program of reentry into the work environment is critical to the recovery process. The prognosis for recovery appears to be excellent when long-term monitoring occurs.[18,22]

COPING TECHNIQUES: WELLNESS STRATEGIES FOR THE EMERGENCY PHYSICIAN

The very qualities that characterize medically successful physicians (perfectionism, drive to succeed, willingness to work long and irregular hours, and ideals of individual service and sacrifice) dispose them to neglect their own physical and emotional needs.[23] The formulation of any comprehensive wellness strategy is based on the concept of lifestyle balance and involves the integration of professional goals and responsibilities with needs for self-care and development.[23-25] Cultivation of lifestyle balance involves four basic elements (Box 208-1).

BOX 208-1. Lifestyle Balance: Wellness Strategies for the Emergency Physician

1. Promote wellness in the professional environment.
   a. General measures
   b. Strategies for shift work
   c. Strategies for managing difficult and violent patients
   d. Professional support groups
2. Cultivate close family and social relationships.
3. Develop and maintain physical fitness.
4. Cultivate methods of relaxation and renewal.

Promoting Wellness in the Work Place

A strong predictor of job satisfaction among professionals with highly demanding jobs is the degree to which they have control over their workplace.[14] Emergency physicians can introduce more control over elements of their practice by (1) ensuring adequate physician and support staffing to accommodate patient load, (2) ensuring adequate input in the development of departmental policies and procedures, (3) cultivating relationships among physicians and staff, and (4) mitigating noise, light, space, and structural discomforts.[15,26]

A major workplace issue for emergency physicians is the irregularity of scheduled hours. Shift changes are often cited as a major cause of dissatisfaction within the specialty.[12,15] Shift work is associated with a variety of adverse effects on physical and emotional health. These include an increased incidence of ulcer disease, depression, mood swings, drug and alcohol abuse, altered immune response, chronic hypertension, cardiovascular mortality, infertility in women, divorce, and work-related accidents and errors.[27] A variety of shift work strategies have been proposed as a means of mitigating these effects (Box 208-2).[28]

Professional support groups also can help emergency physicians with issues of control over stressful aspects of their practice. The American College of Emergency Physicians has a Wellness Section devoted to consideration of such issues and has sponsored policies and programs to address them. The College also has a speaker's bureau, consisting of members who are available to address a variety of wellness-related issues.

A particularly important form of support group relates to *critical incident stress debriefing*. Critical incidents are traumatic events that have sufficient emotional power to overcome the usual coping abilities of people exposed to them. Emergency physicians are constantly being exposed to critical incidents,

BOX 208-2. Shift Work Strategies

1. Work the same shift as much of the time as possible and keep the same sleep patterns. Compensation should be increased for those willing to work night shifts for extended periods.
2. Work isolated night shifts, with minimal circadian disruptions.
3. Consider the *Thomas schedule* for groups.[64] One physician works an extended night schedule 1 month or longer, with isolated nights off being covered by the other group members.
4. Schedule shift rotations in a clockwise direction, with 1-month minimum time per rotation.
5. Eight-hour shifts are preferable to 12-hour shifts.
6. Sleep in a darkened room; minimize disruptions.
7. For those unable to maintain consistent sleep patterns, use compromise strategies such as anchor sleep, split sleep periods, or napping to mitigate circadian disruptions.
8. Start the awake period with a high-protein meal, switching to complex carbohydrates toward bedtime. Avoid caffeine and high-calorie, high-fat snack food before sleep. Eat meals regularly.
9. Use bright light (>10,000 lux) for 2 hours after arising as an adjunct in adjusting to new shifts.
10. Exercise regularly.
11. Plan regular quality time with family and friends.
12. Do not try to live a day shift lifestyle while working night shifts.

including serious multiple-casualty incidents, pediatric injuries or deaths, line-of-duty deaths, injuries to emergency personnel, events with excessive media interest, and events involving victims known to emergency personnel. Rescue personnel exposed to such incidents can be subject to the cognitive, emotional, and physical sequelae comprising the posttraumatic stress syndrome. Components of this syndrome include a continual reexperiencing of the event in thoughts, dreams, or daily life; an avoidance of any stimuli associated with the event; a sense of numbness of one's emotions; and a wide variety of other symptoms, including sleep disturbance, irritability, and loss of emotional control.[29]

The concept of debriefing has evolved over the past 20 years based on the combined experiences of a variety of emergency services and military personnel. The two main goals of debriefings are to lessen the emotional impact of distressing critical incidents and to accelerate recovery from such events before stress reactions occur. As originally described, debriefings are structured group meetings that emphasize venting of emotion and discussion of other reactions to a critical event.[30] Formal critical incident stress debriefing teams are available in many communities through local emergency medical services agencies. Debriefings can also occur on an informal basis in the emergency department. Such sessions can take the form of impromptu meetings of emergency and rescue personnel involved in specific incidents in which the details of a particular event and its associated emotional content are expressed.[29]

BOX 208-3. American Heart Association Dietary Guidelines

1. Restrict total fat to ≤30% of total calories.
2. Restrict saturated fat to <10% of total calories.
3. Limit the total intake of cholesterol-raising fatty acids (saturated and trans fats) to ≤10% of calories.
4. Limit cholesterol intake to <300 mg/day.
5. Replace cholesterol-raising fatty acids with whole grains and unsaturated fatty acids from fish, vegetables, legumes, and nuts.
6. Limit sodium intake to ≤2400 mg/day (≤6.0 g/day of salt).
7. If alcohol is consumed, limit intake to two drinks/day for men, one drink/day for women.
8. Eat at least two servings of fish per week.
9. Eat five or more servings of vegetables and fruits per day.
10. Eat six or more servings of grain products per day.
11. Emphasize daily intake of low-fat or nonfat dairy products.

Family and Social Relationships

Many physicians are overly dedicated to their work and prone to delay sources of gratification. These qualities can interfere with the development of family and social relationships, a problem that may be compounded for emergency physicians by their irregular hours.[31-33] The ability to develop and sustain intimate relationships may be the most critical element in any wellness formula. The simplest and most profound way to maintain one's mental health while actively absorbed in a demanding career is to establish and cultivate a viable relationship with a caring, emotionally expressive spouse or significant other. The promotion of a close family relationship involves, at the very least, a willingness to assign and prioritize protected time with spouse and other family members. For many physicians, it also involves a conscious effort to develop communication skills, particularly with respect to active listening and the open expression of feelings.[33]

Physical Fitness

Physical fitness is an important concern for emergency physicians, given the rigors of a typical emergency practice. Unfortunately, the obstacles to developing a comprehensive fitness program may be considerable. Factors such as irregular hours, hectic work pace, and the variable quality of hospital menus complicate the task of establishing and maintaining exercise regimens and healthy dietary habits. The impact of proper diet and exercise on a variety of wellness parameters is clearly established. Documented benefits of an appropriate diet include lower cholesterol levels, weight control, augmented blood pressure control, and a lower incidence of certain cancers. The American Heart Association periodically provides dietary guidelines (Box 208-3).[34]

The benefits of a regular and vigorous exercise program include enhanced exercise tolerance, cardiovascular fitness, lower blood pressure, increased high-density lipoproteins, decreased triglyceride levels, augmented weight reduction efforts, lessened anxiety and depression, and improved glucose tolerance. According to current American Heart Association guidelines, cardiovascular fitness is best maintained by a program of aerobic exercise (the repetitive use of large muscle groups) three to six times per week for at least 30 minutes per session. Strength-developing activities (resistance training) should be performed at least twice per week, using 8 to 10 exercises that use the major muscle groups of the legs, trunk, arms, and shoulders. Eight to 12 repetitions of each exercise, using one or two sets, is recommended. The exercises should be vigorous, sufficient to raise heart rate to at least 50% of maximum (average maximum heart rate for an individual is 220 minus age).[35]

Relaxation and Renewal

In dealing with the innumerable stresses of emergency practice, emergency physicians must be equipped with considerable emotional resources, derived in part from strong peer and personal support systems. Methods of relaxation and renewal are important additional elements.[6,15,24]

Emergency physicians must continually cultivate the ability to remain functional and emotionally equilibrated in facing the turbulence of the typical emergency department. Physiologic correlates of stress, such as increased heart and respiratory rates, oxygen consumption, and serum lactate level, can be normalized by a variety of relaxation techniques. These include prayer, Zen, yoga, transcendental meditation, autogenic training, and progressive relaxation. Studies indicate that the regular use of such techniques can allow individuals to gain considerable control over the relaxation process.[36-38]

A final element in the promotion of wellness and lifestyle balance is the concept of *renewal*. Physicians typically develop a work ethic that makes it difficult to disengage from medical responsibilities. A single-minded devotion to career ultimately is impoverishing, and by neglecting restorative activities, physicians tend to lose their emotional resilience.[24,39] The concept of renewal involves the ability to prioritize and establish time for rest and revitalization, as well as spiritual, emotional, and intellectual growth. Out of the maelstrom that comprises a typical day in the emergency department, emergency physicians should look to sources of renewal as key elements in their formula for lifestyle balance.

SUMMARY

Many aspects of the practice of emergency medicine are potentially unhealthful. Emergency physicians can hope for less stressful, more fulfilling careers by adopting strategies to enhance personal and professional well-being.

REFERENCES

1. Margen S, et al (eds): *The Wellness Encyclopedia*. Boston, Houghton Mifflin, 1991.
2. Wasserberger J, et al: Violence in the emergency department. *Top Emerg Med* 14:71, 1992.
3. Crippen DW: Emergency medicine redux: The rise and fall of a community medical specialty. *Ann Emerg Med* 13:539, 1984.
4. Goldberg R, et al: Burnout and its correlates in emergency physicians: Four years experience with a wellness booth. *Acad Emerg Med* 3:1156, 1996.
5. Chapman DM: Burnout in emergency medicine: What are we doing to ourselves? *Acad Emerg Med* 4:245, 1997.
6. Zun L, Cobernick M, Howes DS: Emergency physician stress and morbidity (clinical conference). *Am J Emerg Med* 6:370, 1988.
7. Groves JE: Taking care of the hateful patient. *N Engl J Med* 298:883, 1978.
8. Dorevitch S, Forst L: The occupational hazards of emergency physicians. *Am J Emerg Med* 18:300, 2000.
9. Blanchard JC, Curtis KM: Violence in the emergency department. *Emerg Med Clin North Am* 17:717, 1999.
10. Gorlin R, Zucker HD: Physicians' reactions to patients: A key to teaching humanistic medicine. *N Engl J Med* 308:1059, 1983.
11. Simon JR, Dwyer J, Goldfrank LR: The difficult patient. *Emerg Med Clin North Am* 17:353, 1999.
12. Keller KL, Koenig WJ: Sources of stress and satisfaction in emergency practice. *J Emerg Med* 7:293, 1989.
13. Freudenburger HJ: The staff burn-out syndrome in alternative institutions. *Psychother Theory Res Pract* 12:73, 1975.
14. Maslach C, Jackson SE: Patterns of burnout among a national sample of public contact workers. *J Health Hum Res Admin* 7:289, 1984.
15. Lloyd S, Streiner D, Shannon S: Burnout, depression, life and job satisfaction among Canadian emergency physicians. *J Emerg Med* 12:559, 1994.
16. Reinhart MA, Munger BS, Rund DA: American Board of Emergency Medicine Longitudinal Study of Emergency Physicians. *Ann Emerg Med* 33:22, 1999.
17. American College of Emergency Physicians Policy Statement: *Physician impairment*. Approved by Board of Directors, September, 1990. Available at http://www.acep.org
18. Centrella M: Physician addiction and impairment: Current thinking. A review. *J Addictive Dis* 13:91, 1994.
19. Hughes PH, Baldwin DC Jr, Sheehan V: Resident-physician substance abuse, by specialty. *Am J Psychiatry* 149:1348, 1992.
20. McNamara RM, Sanders AB, Ling L, et al: Substance use and alcohol abuse in emergency medicine training programs, by resident report. *Acad Emerg Med* 1:47, 1994.
21. Sanders A, et al: American College of Emergency Physicians ethics manual. *Ann Emerg Med* 20:1153, 1991.
22. Boisauvin EV, Levine RE: Identifying and assisting the impaired physician. *Ann J Med Sci* 322:31, 2001.
23. Quill TE, Williamson PR: Healthy approaches to physician stress. *Arch Intern Med* 150:1857, 1990.
24. Covey S: *The Seven Habits of Highly Effective People: Restoring the Character Ethic*. New York, Simon & Shuster, 1989.
25. Margulies JL, Pollack ML: Developing a healthy lifestyle. In Andrew LB, Pollack ML (eds): *Wellness for Emergency Physicians*. Dallas, American College of Emergency Physicians, 1995.
26. Margulies JL: Control issues. In Andrew LB, Pollack ML (eds): *Wellness for Emergency Physicians*. Dallas, American College of Emergency Physicians, 1995.
27. LaDou J: Health effects of shiftwork. *West J Med* 137:525, 1982.

28. Whitehead DC, Thomas H Jr, Slapper DR: A rational approach to shift work in emergency medicine. *Ann Emerg Med* 21:1250, 1991.
29. Oster NS, Doyle CJ: Critical incident stress and challenges for the emergency workplace. *Emerg Med Clin North Am* 18:339, 2000.
30. Mitchell JT: The history, status and future of critical incident stress debriefing. *JEMS* 13:47, 1988.
31. Gabbard GO, Menninger RW: *Medical Marriages.* Washington, DC, American Psychiatric Press, 1988.
32. Gabbard GO, Menninger RW: The psychology of postponement in the medical marriage. *JAMA* 261:2378, 1989.
33. Coombs RH: Marital status and personal well-being, a literature review. *Fam Relations* 40:97, 1990.
34. Krauss RM, et al: AHA dietary guidelines revision 2000: A statement for healthcare professionals from the nutrition committee of the American Heart Association. *Circulation* 102:2284, 2000.
35. Fletcher GF, Balady G, Blair S, et al: Statement on exercise: Benefits and recommendations for physical activity programs for all Americans. A statement for healthcare professionals from the committee on exercise and cardiac rehabilitation of the council on clinical cardiology, American Heart Association. *Circulation* 94:857, 1996.
36. Benson H, Rosner EA, Marzetta BR, Klemchuk HM: Decreased blood pressure in pharmacologically treated hypertensive patients who regularly elicited a relaxation response. *Lancet* 1:289, 1974.
37. Benson H, Klipper MZ: *The Relaxation Response.* Avenel, NH, Wings Books, 1992.
38. Levitt MA, Derrick GR: An evaluation of psychological parameters of stress in the emergency department. *Am J Emerg Med* 9:217, 1991.
39. Coombs RH, Fawzy FI: The impaired physician syndrome: A developmental perspective. In Scott C, Hawk J (eds): *Heal Thyself: The Health of Health Professionals.* New York, Brunner/Mazel, 1986.

Index

Note: Page numbers followed by b, f, and t refer to boxes, figures, and tables, respectively.

A priori probability, 3055-3056
"A" wave, jugular venous, in tricuspid stenosis and regurgitation, 1307
Abandonment of elderly, 1010
Abciximab, in myocardial infarction, 1186
Abdomen
  acute, in spinal cord injury, 2907
  anterior, 490
  contusions of, 494
  infection in, antibiotics for, 217
Abdominal aortic aneurysm, 1330-1340
  back pain in, 265t
  clinical features of, 1332-1333
  diagnostic strategies in, 1334-1336, 1334f-1336f, 1337-1338
  differential diagnosis in, 1336, 1336b
  disposition in, 1340
  epidemiology of, 1330, 1331t
  false, 1330, 1340
  management of, 1336-1339
  pathophysiology and natural history of, 1330-1331
  repair of
    endovascular, 1338-1339, 1339f
    late complications of, 1339-1340
    survival rate for, 1339
    traditional, 1338, 1339f
  ruptured, 1331
    abdominal pain in, 214t
    clinical features of, 1332-1333
    management of, 1336-1338
  types of, 1330, 1331f
Abdominal cramps
  in *Aeromonas hydrophila* gastroenteritis, 1467
  in *Bacillus cereus* food poisoning, 1471
  in *Clostridium difficile* enterocolitis, 1475
  in *Clostridium perfringens* food poisoning, 1471
  in coccidian gastroenteritis, 1478
  in *Escherichia coli* food poisoning, 1474
  in hemorrhagic *Escherichia coli* serotype O157:H7 gastroenteritis, 1466
  in intestinal amebiasis, 1480
  in Meckel's diverticulum, 2613
  in *Plesiomonas shigelloides* gastroenteritis, 1468
  in scombroid fish poisoning, 1472
  in staphylococcal food poisoning, 1470
  in *Vibrio* fish poisoning, 1472
  in *Vibrio parahaemolyticus* gastroenteritis, 1466
  in viral gastroenteritis, 1476
Abdominal distention
  in acute mesenteric ischemia, 1447
  in colonic volvulus, 1498
  in gastric volvulus, 1394
  in *Giardia* gastroenteritis, 1479
  in large bowel obstruction, 1496
  in malrotation with midgut volvulus, 2606
Abdominal examination
  in abdominal pain, 213, 215
  in abdominal trauma, 493-494
  in chest pain, 187t
  in constipation, 239
  in diarrhea, 233
  in fever, 135
  in multiple trauma, 309-310, 310f
  in nausea and vomiting, 202t
  in pelvic pain, 240, 250t
  in vaginal bleeding, 256t
Abdominal mass
  in abdominal aortic aneurysm rupture, 1333
  in abdominal trauma, 494
  in children, 2646
Abdominal migraine, 2679
Abdominal pain, 209-218. *See also* Pelvic pain.
  ancillary studies in, 215-216, 216t
  differential considerations in, 212-214, 212f, 214t-215t, 216-217, 216t
  disposition in, 217-218
  empiric management of, 217, 218f-219f
  epidemiology of, 209
  extraabdominopelvic causes of, 211b
  history in, 213, 213b
  in abdominal trauma, 493
  in acute mesenteric ischemia, 1447
  in acute pancreatitis, 1429
  in adrenal insufficiency, 1997
  in appendicitis, 1452
  in *Bacillus anthracis* gastroenteritis, 1469
  in *Campylobacter* gastroenteritis, 1460
  in cholangitis, 1421
  in cholecystitis, 1420
  in cholelithiasis, 1418
  in chronic pancreatitis, 1435
  in ciguatera fish poisoning, 1473
  in coccidian gastroenteritis, 1477, 1478
  in colonic ischemia, 1504
  in colonic volvulus, 1498
  in diabetic ketoacidosis, 1963
  in diverticular disease, 1493
  in ectopic pregnancy, 2743
  in elderly person, 2828-2829, 2828t
  in esophageal perforation, 1385
  in gastric volvulus, 1394
  in gastritis, 1391
  in *Giardia* gastroenteritis, 1479
  in hemorrhagic *Escherichia coli* serotype O157:H7 gastroenteritis, 1466
  in inflammatory bowel disease, 1501
  in intussusception, 1442
  in irritable bowel syndrome, 1491
  in large bowel intussusception, 1500
  in large bowel obstruction, 1496
  in pancreatic carcinoma, 1437
  in parasitic infection, 2113
  in pelvic inflammatory disease, 1570
  in peptic ulcer disease, 1392
  in peritoneal dialysis patient, 1553
  in pregnancy, 2733, 2752-2756, 2753t
  in radiation proctocolitis, 1505
  in salmonellosis, 1463
  in shigellosis, 1464
  in small bowel obstruction, 1442
  in spontaneous bacterial peritonitis, 1412
  in staphylococcal food poisoning, 1470
  in systemic lupus erythematosus, 1811
  in uterine inversion, 2820
  in women, 1453, 1453t
  in *Yersinia enterocolitica* gastroenteritis, 1465
  locations of, 212f
  nonspecific, 211t
  observation in, 3063-3064, 3064b
  opioids for, 2925-2926
  pathophysiology of, 209-212, 210t-211t, 211b
  pediatric
    differential considerations in, 2611, 2612t
    in appendicitis, 2619
    in hemolytic uremic syndrome, 2654
    in Henoch-Schönlein purpura, 2615, 2653
    in inflammatory bowel disease, 2616
    in intussusception, 2610
    in osteogenesis imperfecta, 2700
    in renal stones, 2646
  physical examination in, 213, 215
  rapid assessment and stabilization in, 213
  white blood cell count in, 1889
Abdominal radiography. *See* Radiography, abdominal.
Abdominal surgery, small bowel obstruction after, 1441
Abdominal tenderness
  in abdominal trauma, 494
  in genitourinary trauma, 515
Abdominal trauma, 489-512
  anatomy and physiology in, 490
  cardiac tamponade in, 473
  clinical features in, 492-495
  diagnostic peritoneal lavage in, 499-501, 500t
  differential considerations in, 501-502
  epidemiology of, 489-490
  history in, 492-493
  iatrogenic, 492
  in elderly person, 346
  laboratory tests in, 495
  laparoscopy in, 501, 508
  local wound exploration in, 501
  management of, 502-510
  observation in, 3067-3068
  pancreatitis following, 1428
  pathophysiology of, 490-492
  pediatric, 340-342
    blunt, 492, 510
    epidemiology of, 489-490
    history in, 493
  physical examination in, 493-495
  prehospital care in, 502
  radiologic imaging in, 495-499, 496f-499f
Abdominal viscera, in pregnancy, 317
Abducens nerve, 1665t
Abductor digiti minimi, 580-581, 581f
Abductor digiti quinti nerve, compression of, heel pain in, 836-837
Abductor pollicis brevis, 580, 581f
Abductor pollicis longus, 581, 582f, 583f
Abrasion
  corneal, 289, 289f, 292, 294t, 933, 1047, 1047f
  facial, 390
  pattern
    in motor vehicle crashes, 964
    in physical assault, 962, 962f
  scalp, 372
Abrasion collar, in long-range handgun wounds, 957, 957f
Abruptio placentae, 319-320, 2747-2748, 2809-2810
Abrus precatorius, 2471-2472, 2472f
Abscess, 2202-2207
  amebic, 1415-1416, 2106-2107
  anorectal, 1513-1515, 1513t, 1514f
  Bartholin, 1560, 2205, 2205f
  Bezold, 1072
  brain
    after head trauma, 370-371
    ancillary studies in, 1720
    cerebrospinal fluid analysis in, 1716-1719, 1717t, 1718t, 1719f
    complications of, 1716
    diagnosis of, 1716-1720
    differential considerations in, 1720, 1721b
    disposition in, 1723
    epidemiology of, 1711
    etiology of, 1712
    headache in, 174t, 1641, 2678
    in cancer patient, 1920
    in otitis media, 1068
    lumbar puncture in, 1716, 1716b
    management of, 1722, 1723
    neuroimaging studies in, 1719-1720
    pathophysiology of, 1713, 1713f

Abscess *(Continued)*
    risk factors for, 171b
    signs and symptoms of, 1714-1715
  Brodie's, 2184
  collar-button, 617, 617f
  cutaneous, 2202-2204, 2203t
  epidural
    in vertebral osteomyelitis, 2184-2185
    spinal, 1684
  epiglottitic, 1115
  extradural, in otitis media, 1068
  hepatic, 1414-1417, 1415f, 1416f, 2113
  horseshoe, 1515
  in carbuncle, 2204
  in diverticular disease, 1494-1495
  in furuncle, 2204
  in hidradenitis suppurativa, 2204-2205
  intersphincteric, 1513t, 1514, 2206
  intra-abdominal, in appendicitis, 1453, 1458
  ischiorectal, 1513t, 1514, 2206
  necrotizing, 1515
  parapharyngeal, 1121-1123, 1122f
  paraspinal cold, in tuberculosis, 2159
  pelvirectal, 2206
  perianal, 2206
  periapical, 1028, 1030f, 1031, 1032
  periodontal, 1031, 1033
  perirectal, 1513t, 1514, 2205-2206, 2206f
  peritonsillar, 1117-1118, 1118f
  pilonidal, 2206-2207
  postanal, 1513t, 1514-1515
  pulmonary, 1033, 1134, 1134f
  pyogenic, 1414-1415, 1415f
  retrobulbar, 288, 295t
  retropharyngeal, 1120-1121, 1120f, 1121f, 2522-2523, 2523f
  spinal, 1684, 1712, 1715, 1716
  subperiosteal
    in mastoiditis, 1072
    in osteomyelitis, 2175
  supralevator, 1513t, 1514
  tubo-ovarian, 248, 251t
Absence seizure, 1621
Absinthe, 2412
Abuse
  child, 968-976
    abdominal trauma in, 490
    bruises consistent with, 969-971, 969f, 970f, 970t, 2502b
    diagnostic strategies in, 973-974
    differential considerations in, 974-975, 975f, 2699-2701
    disposition in, 976
    epidemiology of, 968-969, 969t
    facial trauma in, 383
    head trauma in, 349, 367
    historical indicators of, 2501b
    history of, in sexual assault cases, 979
    immersion scalds in, 916
    in Munchausen's syndrome by proxy, 1761, 1763, 1763t, 1765
    management of, 975-976
    physical abuse in, 969-971, 969f, 970f, 970t, 972, 973, 974-975
    radiography in, 2699
    reporting of, 976
    sexual abuse in, 969, 971, 972-973, 974, 975
    sexually transmitted disease and, 973-974, 974t
    signs and symptoms of, 971-973
    skeletal aspects of, 2698-2701
  elder, 1008-1015
    caregiver interview in, 1013
    clinical features of, 1011-1013, 1011b, 1012b
    definitions and types of, 1009-1010
    diagnostic strategies in, 1013
    documentation of, 1013
    epidemiology of, 1009
    etiology and risk factors for, 1010-1011, 1010b
    future directions in, 1015
    institutional, 1009, 1015
    interventions and referrals in, 1013-1014
    reporting requirements in, 1014-1015
    screening for, 1011, 1011b
  intimate partner, 994-1006
    barriers to diagnosis of, 998
    clinical features of, 996-998
    definitions of, 995, 995t
Abuse *(Continued)*
    disposition in, 1004-1005, 1005b
    documentation of, 1000-1001, 1003-1004
    during pregnancy, 997, 2734-2735, 2734t
    epidemiology of, 995-996
    improving emergency department response to victims of, 1005-1006
    legal considerations in, 1004-1005
    referral in, 1004
    risk assessment in, 1000, 1002b, 1003b
    risk factors for injury related to, 996
    screening for, 998-999, 999b, 1000f, 1001f, 1002b
    use of emergency department in, 996
    validation of patient's experience in, 999-1000
  of persons with disabilities, 1015
  sexual. *See* Sexual abuse; Sexual assault.
Acalculous cholecystitis, 1421, 2620, 2621
Acanthamoeba infection
  neurologic disorders in, 2107
  visual disturbances in, 2110
Acanthosis nigricans
  in diabetes mellitus, 1972
  internal malignancy associated with, 1862-1863
Acarbose, during pregnancy and lactation, 2790
Acceleration-deceleration injury, 352
Accessory muscles of respiration
  in asthma, 1084, 2534, 2535t
  in chronic obstructive pulmonary disease, 1100
Accessory ossicles of foot, 821-822, 822f
Accessory pathway, 1203
  atrial flutter with, 1229
  in Lown-Ganong-Levine syndrome, 1237
  in Wolff-Parkinson-White syndrome, 1235-1237, 1236f, 1237f
Accident prevention. *See* Injury prevention and control.
Accidental hypothermia, 2236-2252
  advanced life support in, 2245-2246
  cardiovascular agents for, 2246
  clinical features of, 2241-2242, 2242b
  diagnostic strategies in, 2242-2244
  disposition in, 2251
  dysrhythmia in, 2237-2238, 2246
  laboratory evaluation of, 2242-2244, 2243f
  management of, 2244-2251
  outcome of, 2251
  pathophysiology of, 2237-2239, 2238f, 2239t
  predisposing factors in, 2239-2241, 2240b
  rewarming techniques in, 2247-2251, 2247b, 2250b
  septicemia following, 2247
  volume resuscitation in, 2245
Acclimatization
  to heat stress, 2255-2256
  to high altitude, 2297-2298, 2297b, 2298f
Acebutolol, 1209, 1321t
  overdose of, 2373t, 2374
Acetabular fracture, 728-729, 728b, 731, 731f, 732f, 757
Acetaminophen, 2927
  alcohol interactions with, 2875-2876
  during pregnancy and lactation, 2781
  for migraine, 1633, 1633t, 2680
  for osteoarthritis, 1787
  for pediatric fever, 2511, 2514, 2515
  hepatotoxicity of, 1413
  in children, 2935
  in elderly person, 2826
  metabolism of, 2331-2332, 2332f
  overdose of, 2331-2337, 2332f
    antidotes to, 2329t
    chronic exposure in, 2334b, 2335
    clinical features of, 2332-2333
    diagnosis of, 2333-2335, 2333b, 2334b
    disposition in, 2337
    in children, 2335
    management of, 2333b, 2334b, 2335-2337
    risk assessment using treatment nomogram in, 2333-2335, 2334f
Acetazolamide
  for acute mountain sickness, 2301-2302
  for central retinal artery occlusion, 1057
  for closed-angle glaucoma, 1056
  for hyperuricemia, 1914
  for increased intraocular pressure, 292
Acetic acid, for neutralization of alkali burn, 932
Acetone
  isopropyl alcohol metabolism to, 2402, 2403f
  on breath, in diabetic ketoacidosis, 1964
Acetylcholine
  in delirium, 1646-1647
  in dementia, 1657
Acetylcholinesterase inhibitors, 2457-2462, 2458b
  for myasthenia gravis, 1706
N-Acetylcysteine
  for acetaminophen overdose, 2331-2332, 2332f, 2333b, 2334b, 2336-2337
  for contrast agent-induced renal failure, 1537
  in pregnancy, 2336-2337
  intravenous, 2336
Achalasia, 1397, 1398
Achilles tendon
  injury to, 1799-1800
  rupture of, 818, 1800
Acid, weak, for neutralization of alkali burn, 932
Acid burn, 931-933
  esophageal perforation from, 483
  ocular, 1046
  oral, 2381, 2383
  pathophysiology of, 930
Acid-base disorders, 1922-1932. *See also* Acidosis; Alkalosis; Ketoacidosis.
  diagnosis of, 1924
  in hypothermia, 2242-2243, 2243f
  in salicylate overdose, 2340
  mixed, 1931, 1931b
  physiologic buffers and, 1923
  pulmonary compensation in, 1923
  renal compensation in, 1923-1924
Acid-fast bacillus smear, in tuberculosis, 2147, 2154, 2154f
Acidosis. *See also* Ketoacidosis.
  anion gap, 1927-1929, 1927b
    delirium in, 1651
    in cyanide poisoning, 2437
    in ethylene glycol poisoning, 2399, 2400-2401
    in methanol poisoning, 2396, 2397
    seizure in, 1622
  double-gap
    differential diagnosis in, 2397
    in ethylene glycol poisoning, 2400
    in methanol poisoning, 2397
  hypokalemia in, 1938
  lactic, 1928-1929
    in crush injury, 3007
    in sepsis, 2216
    in shock, 42-43, 43f
  metabolic, 1926-1930, 1927f, 1931b
    dialysis for, 1549
    etiology of, 1927-1929, 1927b
    in abdominal trauma, 495
    in acute renal failure, 1539, 2650
    in cyanide poisoning, 2437
    in diarrhea, 2624
    in salicylate overdose, 2340
    management of, 1929-1930
    physiologic compensation in, 1929
    renal compensation in, 1923-1924
    with high anion gap, 1927-1929, 1927b
    with normal anion gap, 1927b, 1929
  paradoxical central nervous system, from sodium bicarbonate, 1930
  respiratory, 1924-1926, 1925b, 1925f, 1931b
    causes of, 1925b
    clinical features of, 1924-1925
    in chronic obstructive pulmonary disease, 1100
    management of, 1925-1926
    physiologic compensation in, 1925
Acoustic neuroma, 147t, 1668-1669
Acquired immunodeficiency syndrome. *See* HIV/AIDS.
Acrocyanosis, 1347, 1357
Acrodermatitis chronica atrophicans, in Lyme disease, 2124-2125
Acromial process fracture, 679, 680
Acromioclavicular joint
  anatomy of, 670-671, 671f
  dislocation at, 685-687, 686f, 687f
  osteoarthritis in, 687
Acromioclavicular ligaments, 670, 671f
ACTH (adrenocorticotropic hormone)
  for gouty arthritis, 1786
  for infantile spasms, 2666

Action potential of myocardial cells, 1200, 1201f, 1202f
Activated charcoal
in acetaminophen overdose, 2336
in amphetamine abuse, 2896
in anticholinergic poisoning, 2349-2350
in barbiturate overdose, 2483
in beta blocker overdose, 2374
in bipyridyl compound poisoning, 2466
in NSAID overdose, 2340
in opioid overdose, 2455
in overdosed/poisoned patient, 2330
in PCP intoxication, 2893
in salicylate overdose, 2341
Activated protein C
for sepsis, 2221-2222
for septic shock, 53
Active compression-decompression–cardiopulmonary resuscitation, 89, 98
Active external rewarming, 2248
Acute abdomen, in spinal cord injury, 2907
Acute chest syndrome, in sickle cell disease, 1880
Acute confusional state, 2679. *See also* Confusion.
Acute coronary syndromes, 1154-1195. *See also* Angina; Myocardial infarction.
atypical presentations in, 1158-1159, 1159t
chest pain centers and, 1181-1182
chest pain in, 183, 186, 186b, 188, 189f, 190t-191t
chest radiography in, 1174, 1175f
clinical features of, 1157-1161, 1158t, 1159t
cocaine-related, 2391
creatine kinase MB isoenzyme in, 1175f, 1176t, 1177-1178
diagnostic strategies in, 1161-1181
echocardiography in, 1179
electrocardiography in, 1161-1174
abnormalities in, 1161-1163, 1162f-1164f, 1162t
additional lead, 1171-1173, 1172f, 1173f
adjuncts in, 1171-1174
anatomic location of infarct on, 1164-1166, 1164t, 1165f-1167f
body surface mapping and, 1174
limitations of, 1174
noninfarct ST segment elevation and, 1166-1170, 1167f-1172f
NSTEMI and, 1170-1171
QT dispersion and, 1174
serial, 1173-1174, 1173f
epidemiology of, 1155
graded exercise testing in, 1180-1181
historical perspective of, 1154-1155
in pregnancy, 2763t, 2766-2767
management algorithm for, 189f
management of, 1182-1195
angiotensin-converting enzyme inhibitors in, 1185
antiplatelet therapy in, 1185-1187
antithrombotic therapy in, 1187-1188
aspirin in, 1185
beta blockers in, 1184-1185
calcium channel blockers in, 1185
clinical pathways for, 3039f-3041f
direct thrombin inhibitors in, 1188
glycoprotein IIb/IIIa receptor inhibitors in, 1186, 1194
heparins in, 1187-1188
morphine in, 1184
nitroglycerin in, 1184
pharmacologic, 1184-1188, 1195
reperfusion in, 1189-1195
thienopyridines in, 1186-1187
time to treatment and, 1182-1184, 1183f, 1184f
missed diagnosis of, 1160
pathophysiology of, 1156-1157
physical examination in, 1159, 1159t
prehospital care in, 1157
radionucleotide scanning in, 1179-1180
risk factors for, 186b
serum markers in, 1174-1179, 1175f, 1176t
spectrum of disease in, 1155-1156
transfer of patient with, 1195
troponins in, 1175-1177, 1175t, 1176t
Acute lung injury. *See* Pulmonary edema, noncardiogenic.
Acute mountain sickness (AMS), 2300-2303, 2301b. *See also* Altitude; High altitude illness.
Acute mountain sickness (AMS) *(Continued)*
clinical presentation in, 2301
epidemiology of, 2296
management of, 2301-2302
pathophysiology of, 2299-2300, 2299f
prevention of, 2302-2303
Acute necrotic ulcerative gingivitis (ANUG), 1033, 1033f
Acute radiation syndrome, 2317t, 2321-2322, 2321f
Acute renal failure. *See* Renal failure, acute.
Acute respiratory distress syndrome (ARDS), 1141, 1141b
in ethylene glycol poisoning, 2399
in pancreatitis, 1429
in sepsis, 2214, 2214b
mechanical ventilation in, 32
pulmonary contusion vs., 461
Acute seroconversion syndrome, in HIV infection, 2075
Acute stress disorder, 1746b
Acute tubular necrosis, 1534b, 1535-1537, 1536b
in rhabdomyolysis, 1977, 1977f
urinary findings in, 1527t
Acyclovir
during pregnancy and lactation, 2785
for bacterial meningitis, 2665
for Bell's palsy, 1667
for febrile, neutropenic cancer patient, 2838t
for genital herpes, 1557t, 1559, 1858
for herpes simplex esophagitis, 1387
for herpes simplex meningoencephalitis, 1722
for herpes simplex virus infection, 2042
for herpes zoster, 2043
for varicella, 1859, 2043
in HIV/AIDS, side effects of, 2079t
indications for, 2038
prophylactic, in monkey bites, 888, 889t
Adaptive immune response, 2832-2834
Addison's disease, 1994, 1996, 1997
Adductor pollicis, 580, 581f
Adenocarcinoma, pancreatic, 1437-1438
Adenopathy. *See* Lymphadenopathy.
Adenosine
during pregnancy and lactation, 2788
for dysrhythmia, 1212-1213, 2586b
for junctional tachycardia, 1234
for pediatric resuscitation, 101t, 104
for supraventricular tachycardia, 2588, 2589f
for wide-complex tachycardia, 1240
side effects of, 1212
Adenosine deaminase test, in tuberculosis, 2155
Adenosine triphosphate depletion
in cerebral ischemia, 65
in rhabdomyolysis, 1977
Adenovirus infection, 1289, 2034t, 2045
Adhesive capsulitis, 682, 698-699, 699t, 1797
Adhesive strips for ankle immobilization, 571, 572f
Adhesive-tipped swab for foreign body removal from ear, 863
Adie's tonic pupil, 1061
Adipocytes, glucose metabolism in, 1956
Adjustment disorder
depression vs., 1740
with anxiety, 1749
Admission. *See* Hospitalization.
Adnexal mass
in ectopic pregnancy, 2743
pelvic pain in, 250t
Adolescent
abdominal pain in, 2611, 2612t
alcohol consumption in, 2877
antituberculous agents for, 2166, 2167b
consent to treatment on behalf of, 3167-3168
depression in, 1737
developmental milestones in, 2496t, 2497
gastrointestinal bleeding in, 2613-2614, 2614t
refusal of medical care for, 3171
substance abuse in, 2883, 2884
suicide by, 1769
violence and, 1017-1022
vomiting in, 203, 208t, 2606t
Adrenal hemorrhage, 1995, 1995b
Adrenal insufficiency, 1994-1998
acute, 1994-1996, 1995b
autoimmune, 1996
chronic, 1996
clinical features of, 1995-1997, 1996t
Adrenal insufficiency *(Continued)*
diagnosis of, 1997-1998
in sepsis, 2214
management of, 1998
Adrenergic medications
for asthma, 1086-1088, 1087t, 2539, 2539t, 2540-2541
for chronic obstructive pulmonary disease, 1105
Adrenocorticotropic hormone
for gouty arthritis, 1786
for infantile spasms, 2666
Adrenocorticotropic hormone stimulation test, in adrenal insufficiency, 1997-1998
Adult infectious botulism, 2013, 2015
Adult Protective Services, 1014
Adult resuscitation. *See* Resuscitation.
Advance directives, 3132, 3133, 3142
honoring, 3144-3145, 3152
initiating, 3153
nonstandard, 3133
Advanced life support
in hypothermia, 2245-2246
in ICD patient, 1256-1257
in pacemaker patient, 1255
in pediatric resuscitation, 99, 99f
prehospital, 78
Advanced life support (ALS) systems, 2986
Adynamic ileus, 1440, 1441b, 1443
Aeroesophageal foreign body, 2529-2530
Aeromonas hydrophila
dysenteric colitis in, 229t
gastroenteritis in, 1461t, 1462t, 1467-1468
Aerophobia, in rabies, 2065
Aerosol exposure, ocular trauma from, 1046
Affect, flattened, in schizophrenia, 1728
Affective disorders. *See* Mood disorders.
Affective processes, in clinical decision making, 130, 131t
Afterdepolarization
dysrhythmias from, 1205
early vs. delayed, 1201, 1202f
Afterload, in heart failure, 1260-1261, 1260f, 1261f
Age. *See also* Adolescent; Child; Elderly person; Infant; Neonate.
fertility rate and, 2722
fibrinolytic therapy eligibility and, 1190
gestational. *See* Gestational age.
high-altitude illness and, 2296
risk for injury and death by, 942t, 949t
Agent Orange, 2463, 2463b
Aggression, 1768. *See also* Abuse; Combative patient; Violence.
Aging. *See* Elderly person.
Agitation
in amphetamine abuse, 2896
in anticholinergic poisoning, 2349
in delirium, 1653-1654
in depression, 1737
in PCP intoxication, 2891, 2892
in substance abuse, 2886
in thought disorders, 1730
violent behavior and. *See* Combative patient.
Agonal respiration, 97
Agoraphobia, 1746b, 1749
Agranulocytosis, antipsychotic-induced, 2448
AIDS. *See* HIV/AIDS.
Air
compressed, esophageal perforation from, 483
contaminated, in scuba diving–related disorders, 2283
Air bags, 946-947
in pregnancy, 2735-2736
injury from, 964, 965f
Air casts, for ankle immobilization, 571, 573f, 817
Air contrast enema, in intussusception, 2611
Air hunger, in chronic obstructive pulmonary disease, 1100
Air leak, persistent, 466
Air medical transport, 2994-2999
administrative structure in, 2995
aviation physiology and, 2994-2995, 2995t
clinical concepts and patient care in, 2998-2999
criteria for, 2998b
efficacy and cost effectiveness of, 2999
flight crew in, 2996
future of, 2999

Air medical transport *(Continued)*
medical direction in, 2996
safety issues in, 2997, 2997b, 2997f, 2998b
types of missions in, 2995
Air pollution, in COPD exacerbation, 1099
Air trapping, in airway foreign body aspiration, 866
Aircraft for medical transport, 2995-2996, 2996f
Airway. *See also* Airway management; Intubation; Mechanical ventilation; Ventilatory Support.
adult vs. child, 2519, 2520f
angioedema of, 1835
cellulitis of, in epiglottitis, 1115
contamination of, in urban search and rescue, 3008
decision to intubate, 2-3
difficult
approach to, 8-9, 9f
cricothyrotomy for, 22-23, 23f
esophagotracheal combitube for, 20, 20f
fiberoptic intubation of, 20-21, 22f
identification of, 3-4, 3b, 4b, 5f
in children, 2502, 2502b
intubating laryngeal mask airway for, 19, 19f
lighted stylet for, 19-20, 20f
retrograde intubation of, 20
special airway devices for, 18-23, 19f-23f
failed, 8, 9, 10f
special airway devices for, 18-23, 19f-23f
failure to maintain or protect, as indication for intubation, 2
foreign body in, 864-870, 867f-869f, 2529-2530, 2550-2551, 2551f
inflammation of
in asthma, 1080-1081, 1080f, 1083, 2532-2533
in chronic obstructive pulmonary disease, 1097-1098
reflex closure of, in physically disabled patient, 2907-2908
remodeling of, in asthma, 1081, 1083
rewarming of, 2248-2249, 2249t
surgical, 22
in multiple trauma, 306
in neck trauma, 445
Airway management. *See also* Airway; Intubation; Mechanical ventilation; Ventilatory support.
crash airway algorithm for, 7, 8f
in anaphylaxis, 1830
in cardiac arrest, 87
in central nervous system infection, 1721
in comatose patient, 158
in dental infection, 1032
in elderly trauma patient, 348
in facial trauma, 389
in foreign body aspiration, 868-870
in heatstroke, 2264
in hemoptysis, 280
in laryngotracheal trauma, 447-448
in multiple trauma, 306
in myasthenia gravis, 1706
in neck trauma, 444-445
in neonatal resuscitation, 122
in organophosphate poisoning, 2460
in pregnant trauma patient, 322
in seizure, 166, 1626
in sepsis, 2218-2219
in severe head trauma, 358-359
in smoke inhalation, 921-922
in spinal injuries, 436
in subarachnoid hemorrhage, 1637
in thermal burns, 921-923
pediatric
in anaphylaxis, 2549
in cardiac arrest, 97-98, 105-109, 106f, 107b, 107t
in epiglottitis, 2523-2524
in neck trauma, 445
in status epilepticus, 2672
in trauma, 329, 332t
in upper airway obstruction, 2521, 2521f
prehospital, 2990, 2991
Airway muscles, weakness of, 138-139
Airway obstruction
difficult airway and, 4
in adult epiglottitis, 1115
in asthma, 1081
in chronic obstructive pulmonary disease, 1097, 1098
Airway obstruction *(Continued)*
in foreign body impaction, 864-870, 867f-869f, 2529-2530, 2550-2551, 2551f.
in pharyngitis, 276-277
measurement of, 1084-1085
pediatric, 2502, 2502b, 2519-2530, 2532-2552
evaluation of, 2498, 2498f, 2521, 2521f
in aeroesophageal foreign body, 2529-2530
in anaphylaxis, 2546-2550
in asthma, 2532-2544
in bronchiolitis, 2544-2546
in congenital lesions, 2522, 2524-2525, 2524f, 2527-2528, 2528f
in croup, 2525-2527, 2526f, 2527b
in epiglottitis, 2523-2524, 2524f
in foreign body aspiration, 2550-2551, 2551f
in laryngeal disease, 2524-2525, 2524f
in retropharyngeal abscess, 2522-2523, 2523f
in subglottic tracheal disease, 2525-2527
in supraglottic disease, 2522-2524
in tracheal disease, 2527-2529, 2529t
pathophysiology of, 2519, 2520f
stridor in, 2519-2520, 2521t
Airway pressure release ventilation, 33
Airway tuberculosis, 2151
Akathisia, antipsychotic-induced, 1732, 2446-2447
Akinesia, antipsychotic-induced, 1732
Alanine aminotransferase
in acute pancreatitis, 1431, 1431t
in alcoholic hepatitis, 1409
in amebic abscess, 1416
in viral hepatitis, 1404
Alarm systems, in emergency department, 2966
Albendazole, for *Enterobius vermicularis* gastroenteritis, 1482
Albumin
administration of, after burn injury, 923
as cardiac marker, 1178
glycosylated, in diabetes mellitus, 1959
Albuterol
for acute renal failure, 2650
for asthma, 1086-1087, 1087t, 1088, 2538, 2539t, 2543t
for chronic obstructive pulmonary disease, 1105
for hyperkalemia
in acute renal failure, 1539
in chronic renal failure, 1545, 1545t
Alcohol. *See also* Ethanol.
drug interactions with, 2875-2877, 2876t
for wound cleansing, 848t
metabolism of, 2859
occupational testing for, 3080-3081
Alcohol consumption
cardiovascular effects of, 2866
deaths related to, 300
during pregnancy, 2791-2792, 2791b, 2877-2878
endocrine effects of, 2871
gastrointestinal and hepatic effects of, 2867-2869
hematologic effects of, 2873-2874, 2873t
hypothermia and, 2240, 2874-2875
in adolescents, 2877
in ciguatera fish poisoning, 1473
in elderly person, 2877
metabolic effects of, 2871-2872, 2872t
neurologic effects of, 2869-2870
oncologic effects of, 2874
physiologic effects of, blood alcohol levels and, 2859, 2859t
psychiatric effects of, 2875
pulmonary effects of, 2866-2867
rhabdomyolysis from, 1979
risks and benefits of, 2867b
submersion injuries and, 2312, 2314
trauma and, 2878
Alcohol intoxication, 2327t, 2328
as diagnosis of exclusion, 2859-2860
as injury risk factor, 948-949
consent and, 3168-3169
disposition in, 2879
management of, 2860
opioid/sedative/ethanol syndrome and, 2327t, 2328
violence and, 1018
Alcohol withdrawal syndrome, 2860-2863
clinical features of, 2860-2861
differential considerations in, 2860
disposition in, 2879
hypertension in, 1314
management of, 2861-2863
pathophysiology of, 2860
seizure in, 1623, 2863
Alcoholic cardiomyopathy, 2866
Alcoholic cirrhosis, 2868
Alcoholic fatty liver, 2868
Alcoholic hepatitis, 2868
Alcoholic ketoacidosis, 1927-1928, 1964-1965, 2872-2873
Alcoholic liver disorders, 1407, 1409, 2867-2868
cirrhosis in, 1410
hepatitis in, 1405, 1409
Alcoholic pancreatitis, 2868
acute, 1426, 1427-1428
chronic, 1434-1435
Alcohol-in-combination, emergency department visits related to, 2884f
Alcoholism, 2858-2880, 2859-2860
definition and natural history of, 2858
dementia in, 1658
differential considerations in, 2859-2860
hypertension in, 1314
hypomagnesemia in, 1947
hypophosphatemia in, 1951
immune defects in, 2841-2842
infection in, 2842, 2870-2871
neuropathy in, 1692, 2869
psychiatric and social problems in, 2879-2880
screening test for, 2858
sideroblastic anemia in, 1873
suicide and, 1769
Alcohol-related seizure, 1623, 2863-2866, 2863b, 2879
Aldosterone, 527
in heart failure, 1262
in hypertension, 1311, 1312f
in sodium homeostasis, 1933
Aldosterone receptor blockers, 1321t
Alexia, in ischemic stroke, 1609
Alexithymia, in somatoform disorders, 1753
Alfentanil, 2922t, 2923
Alice in Wonderland syndrome, 2679
Aliphatic petroleum distillates, toxicity of, 2428, 2429t
Alkalemia, in pregnancy, 1926
Alkali burn, 931-933
esophageal perforation from, 483
ocular, 1046, 1046f, 2384
oral, 2381, 2381f, 2382-2383, 2382f
pathophysiology of, 930
Alkaline batteries
impaction of, 1384
ingestion of, 2384-2385
Alkaline phosphatase
in acute pancreatitis, 1431, 1431t
in amebic abscess, 1416
in hepatitis, 1404
in peritoneal lavage, 501
in pregnancy, 2726
in pyogenic abscess, 1415
Alkalinization, urinary. *See* Sodium bicarbonate.
Alkalosis
metabolic, 1930-1931, 1931b
causes of, 1930, 1930b
from vomiting, 201
renal compensation in, 1924
saline-resistant, 1931
saline-responsive, 1930-1931
respiratory, 1926, 1931b
causes of, 1926, 1926b
during acclimatization to high altitude, 2297-2298
hypophosphatemia in, 1951
in chronic obstructive pulmonary disease, 1100
in salicylate overdose, 2340
Allen's test, 586, 588f, 1346
Allergens, sensitization to, 1819
Allergic airway inflammation, in asthma, 1080-1081, 1080f, 1083
Allergic conjunctivitis, 296t
Allergic contact dermatitis, 1851-1852, 1851f, 1852f
Allergic granulomatosis and angiitis, 1816

Allergic rhinitis, exercise-induced asthma and, 1082
Allergic sinusitis, 1123
Allergy. *See also* Anaphylaxis; Hypersensitivity reactions.
  classification of reactions in, [illegible]
  immune system and, 1820-1822, 1820f
  immunopathology of, 1819
  incidence of, 1819
  pathophysiology of, 1822-1824, 1822f
  to antibiotics, 1826
  to aspirin/NSAIDs, 1828
  to bupivacaine, 846-847
  to contrast media, 1828
  to foods, 1826, 1848, 2547, 2548
  to herbal medicines, 2477, 2477t
  to hymenoptera stings, 1827, 2547
  to insulin, 1972
  to latex, 1826-1827, 2543
  to local anesthesia, 846-847, 1827, 2931
  to miscellaneous medications, 1827
  to opioid analgesics, 1828
  to pyrethrins and pyrethroids, 2467
  to sulfites, 1827
  to whole blood and immunoglobulins, 1827
Allis technique for hip reduction, 758-759, 759f
Alloantibodies, extrinsic, in hemolytic anemia, 1882
Allopurinol
  for gouty arthritis, 1786
  for hyperuricemia, 1914
All-terrain vehicle accidents, facial trauma from, 382
Almitrine, for chronic obstructive pulmonary disease, 1106
Aloe vera, for frostbite, 2232
Alogia, in schizophrenia, 1728
Alpha (α) error, 3051t, 3052
Alpha particles, 2319, 2320f
Alpha-adrenergic agonists
  central, 1321t
  for alcohol withdrawal syndrome, 2862
Alpha-adrenergic blocking agents, 1321t
  for hypertensive emergencies, 1319
Alphavirus, 2047-2048
Alprazolam, 2484, 2484t
ALTE (apparent life-threatening event), 2714, 2718-2720, 2718b, 2719b.
Alteplase. *See* Tissue plasminogen activator (t-PA).
Alternating current, electrical injury and, 2268
Alternative hypothesis, 3051, 3051t
Alternative medicine, cultural competent approach to, 3113-3114
Alternobaric vertigo, in scuba diving–related disorders, 2286, 2287t
Altitude. *See also* Acute mountain sickness (AMS); High-altitude illness.
  and underlying medical conditions, 2307-2309
  barometric pressure and, 2297
  definitions of, 2296
  dehydration and, 2995
  oxygenation and, 2307, 2307f, 2994, 2995t
  oxyhemoglobin dissociation curve and, 2296, 2297f, 2298
Aluminum antacids
  for hyperphosphatemia, 1953
  for upper gastrointestinal disorders, 1398
Alum-precipitated toxoid test, in vasa previa, 2810
Alveolar bone fracture, 1040
Alveolar gas equation, 2297, 2297b
Alveolar infiltration, in pulmonary contusion, 460, 460f
Alveolar osteitis, acute, 1034
Alzheimer's disease
  anxiety in, 1748
  clinical features of, [illegible]
  diagnosis of, 1661
  epidemiology of, 1655
  palliative care in, 3154
  pathophysiology of, 1655
  treatment of, 1661-1662
Amanita muscaria mushroom, 2412-2413, 2412f
Amanita phylloides, 2479
Amantadine
  for influenza, 1139, 2035, 2037
  for neuroleptic malignant syndrome, 2449
Amblyomma americanum tick, 2121f

Ambulances
  air, 2995-2996, 2996f
  ground, 2988, 2988f
Amebiasis
  abscess in, 1415, 2106-2107
  drug therapy for, [illegible]
  dysenteric colitis in, 229t
  dysentery in, 235, 1477t, 1480-1481
  hepatic abscess in, 1415-1416, 2112
  in HIV/AIDS, 1482-1483
  intestinal symptoms in, 1477t, 1480-1481
  pulmonary symptoms in, 2110
American College of Cardiology, clinical practice guidelines of, 3035, 3036f
American College of Emergency Physicians, clinical practice guidelines of, 3035
American Heart Association
  clinical practice guidelines of, 3035, 3036f
  dietary guidelines of, 3177, 3177b
American Medical Association
  clinical practice guidelines published by, 3037
  medical literature guidance of, 3046
American Sign Language, 2905
Amikacin
  for febrile, neutropenic cancer patient, 2838t
  for tuberculosis, 2163t
Amiloride hydrochloride, 1321t
Aminoglycosides
  acute tubular necrosis from, 1536
  during pregnancy and lactation, 2784
  for febrile, neutropenic cancer patient, 2838t
Aminophylline
  for anaphylaxis, 1831b, 1832-1833
  for asthma, 1090, 1090t
  for chronic obstructive pulmonary disease, 1105
Aminosalicylic acid
  for inflammatory bowel disease, 1502
  for tuberculosis, 2163t, 2164-2165
Aminosidine, for intestinal amebiasis, 1481
Amiodarone, 1209
  during pregnancy and lactation, 2788
  for atrial fibrillation, 1232b, 1233
  for cardiac arrest, 92
  for dysrhythmia, 2586b
  for hypertrophic cardiomyopathy, 1295-1296
  for pediatric resuscitation, 101t, 104-105
  for ventricular fibrillation and pulseless ventricular tachycardia, 112-113
  for ventricular tachycardia, 1242
  hepatotoxicity of, 1414
  hypothyroidism from, 1990
  prehospital use of, 2990-2991
  side effects of, 1209, 1210b
  thyrotoxicosis from, 1986
Amitriptyline
  for neuropathic pain, 1692
  metabolism of, 2352
  prophylactic, for migraine, 2680-2681
Amlodipine, 1321t
  for postpartum cardiomyopathy, 2821
  overdose of, 2377t
Ammonia, anhydrous, injury from, 934-935
Ammunition, handgun, 954, 954f
Amnesia
  alcohol-induced, 2869
  in delirium, 1649
  in dementia, 1658-1659
  in head trauma, 363
Amniorrhexis, 2807-2808, 2808t
Amniotic fluid, meconium in, 120, 120f
Amniotic fluid embolism, 2751-2752, 2821
Amniotic membrane, premature rupture of, 2807-2808, 2808t
Amniotic membrane patching, in acute ocular chemical injury, 933
Amoxapine
  metabolism of, 2352
  overdose of, 2354
Amoxicillin
  for Lyme disease, 1789, 2127t, 2128
  for otitis media, 1068, 1069, 1070t
  for pneumonia, 2557, 2558t, 2563
  for sinusitis, 1125
  prophylactic, for pediatric bacteremia, 2506
Amoxicillin-clavulanate
  for otitis media, 1068, 1069, 1070t
  prophylactic, in cat bites, 888
Amperage, electrical injury and, 2269, 2269t

Amphetamines
  abuse of, 2893-2896, 2894t, 2895b
  designer, 2408-2409, 2410-2411
  during pregnancy, 2793
  overdose of, 2392
Amphotericin
  hepatotoxicity of, 1414
  in HIV/AIDS, side effects of, 2079t
Amphotericin B
  for cryptococcal meningitis, 2081
  for febrile, neutropenic cancer patient, 2838-2839, 2838t
  for fungal meningitis, 1722
Ampicillin
  during pregnancy and lactation, 2784
  for meningococcal disease, 2023
  for pediatric fever, 2513-2514
AMPLE history, 330b
Amplification, of bodily functions, 1756
Ampulla, Vater's, carcinoma of, 1423
Amputation
  fingertip, 610, 610f
  foot, 838
  in frostbite, 2234
  in hand trauma, 612-613, 613b
  in peripheral vascular injury, 543
  penile, 532-533
Amrinone
  for acute pulmonary edema in hypotensive patient, 1270t, 1274
  for cardiogenic shock, 54
  for heart failure, in infants and children, 2583t, 2584
Amsel criteria, in bacterial vaginosis, 1568
Amyl nitrite, for cyanide poisoning, 939, 2438
Amylase
  in abdominal trauma, 495
  in acute pancreatitis, 1430
  in peritoneal lavage, 501
Amyloid angiopathy, intracerebral hemorrhage from, 1609
Amyloidosis
  cardiac, 1297
  pericarditis in, 1287
Amyotrophic lateral sclerosis, 1704
  clinical characteristics of, 1680t
  motor neuron disease in, 1700
Anabolic steroids, hepatotoxicity of, 1414
Anaerobic cellulitis, 2199, 2208
Anaerobic organisms, lower respiratory infection due to, 1130
Anal fissures, 1508, 1512-1513, 1512f, 1513t
Anal pruritus, 1509, 1517-1518, 1517b
  causes of, 1517, 1517b
  in *Enterobius vermicularis* gastroenteritis, 1481
  in parasitic infection, 2113-2114
Anal reflexes, in head trauma, 357
Analgesia, 2913-2935
  acute vs. chronic pain and, 2913-2914, 2914b
  definition of terms related to, 2914b
  during pregnancy and lactation, 2781, 2784
  during rewarming of frostbite, 2232
  evaluation and documentation of pain and, 2916-2917, 2917b, 2917t
  for abdominal pain, 217
  for acute pancreatitis, 1433
  for appendicitis, 1456
  for back pain, 264, 267, 710
  for chest pain, 184
  for chronic pancreatitis, 1436
  for dental caries pain, 1031
  for epididymitis, 2639
  for femoral and hip fractures, 749
  for knee trauma, 776
  for migraine, [illegible]
  for pleural effusion, 1151
  for procedures, 2938-2954, 2940t-2941t. *See also* Procedural sedation and analgesia.
  for red and painful eye, 291
  for reduction of glenohumeral joint dislocation, 689
  for renal stones, 2646
  for rib fracture, 455-456
  for sickle cell disease, 1880
  for thermal burns, 924
  for urolithiasis, 1591-1592
  in child, 2935-2936, 2946-2947, 2952-2954
  in elderly person, 2826-2827, 2936
  in ventilated patient, 31

Analgesia *(Cotinued)*
intravenous regional anesthesia for, 2934
local anesthesia for, 2930-2933, 2931t, 2932b, 2932t
nitrous oxide–oxygen mixtures for, 2929-2930
nonopioid/NSAID, 2926-2928, 2927b, 2927f
nonpharmacologic interventions for, 2934
of face, Dejeune onion skin pattern of, 420
oligoanalgesia and, 2917-2918
opioid, 2918-2926
adjuvant agents with, 2921
agonist-antagonist group of, 2924-2925, 2924b
common therapeutic mistakes in, 2918-2921, 2919b
for abdominal pain, 2925-2926
intramuscular, disadvantages of, 2919-2920, 2919b
mechanism of action of, 2918, 2918t
oral, 2925
parenteral, 2921-2924
pathophysiology of pain and, 2914-2916, 2915f, 2915t, 2916f, 2916t
patient-controlled, 2920
prehospital, 2936
priorities of pain management and, 2918
sites and mechanisms of, 2916, 2916t
skeletal muscle relaxants for, 2928-2929
topical anesthesia for, 2933-2934
Analysis of variance, one-way, 3052-3053, 3052t
Anaphylactic shock
causes of, 47
treatment of, 52b, 54
Anaphylactoid purpura, 2615, 2615f
Anaphylactoid reaction, 1819
Anaphylaxis, 1818-1834. *See also* Allergy; Hypersensitivity reactions.
biphasic, 1828
classification of reactions in, 1821-1822
clinical features of, 1825t, 1828-1829, 2547-2548
complications of, 2548
diagnosis of, 1829, 2548
differential considerations in, 1829-1830, 2548-2549
disposition in, 1833-1834, 2549-2550
dyspnea in, 179t
epidemiology of, 2547
etiology of, 1819, 1824-1828, 1824b
idiopathic, 1828
immune complex–mediated agents in, 1827
immune system and, 1820-1822, 1820f, 1821f
immunoglobulin E–mediated
agents associated with, 1826-1827
signal transduction system in, 1822-1823, 1822f
immunopathology of, 1819
in children, 2546-2550
incidence of, 1819
management of, 1830-1833, 1831b, 2549
mediators of, 1823, 1823b
nonimmunologic activators of, 1828
pathophysiology of, 1822-1824, 1822f, 2547
physically induced, 1828
physiologic effects of, 1824, 1825t
prevention of, 1833-1834, 1834b
risk factors for, 1819-1820
to horse serum–derived antivenin, 901
to snake venom, 898
transfusion-related, 60
Anastomotic aneurysm, after abdominal aortic aneurysm repair, 1340
Anatomic abnormalities, neonatal resuscitation in, 121
Anatomic differences, in children vs. adults, 329, 329b, 329t, 335b
Anatomic snuffbox, 581, 583f, 625
Ancef, for catheter-related infections, 1363
Ancillary services, in medical screening examination, 3160-3161
Anembryonic gestation, 2740
Anemia, 1867-1884
after head trauma, 353
aplastic, 1875-1876, 1875t
decreased red blood cell production in, 1870-1876, 1870b, 1871t
definition of, 1867
differential diagnosis in, 1869-1884, 1870b, 1871t
emergent, 1868-1869, 1869b
Anemia *(Cotinued)*
heart failure in, 1268
hemolytic, 1868t, 1876-1884
abnormal sequestration in, 1884
ancillary evaluation of, 1877, 1877b
aplastic crisis in, 2046, 2046f
clinical features of, 1876-1877
differential diagnosis in, 1878-1884, 1879b
drug-induced, 1883, 1883b
environmental causes of, 1883-1884
extrinsic alloantibodies in, 1882
extrinsic autoantibodies in, 1882-1883, 1883b
extrinsic mechanical causes of, 1883
in alcoholism, 2874
intrinsic enzyme defects in, 1878-1879, 1879b
intrinsic hemoglobin abnormality in, 1879-1882. *See also* Sickle cell disease.
intrinsic membrane abnormality in, 1879
jaundice in, 246
laboratory studies in, 1877-1878, 1877b, 1877f, 1878f
microangiopathic, 1883
in acute renal failure, 1540
in alcoholism, 2873-2874
in chronic renal failure, 1543
in lead poisoning, 2421
in pregnancy, 2724, 2763t, 2767-2768
in systemic lupus erythematosus, 1808
in thalassemia, 1872-1873, 1872f
in trichuriasis, 2107
increased red blood cell destruction in, 1868t, 1876-1884
iron deficiency, 1871-1872, 1871f, 1872t
in alcoholism, 2873-2874
in pregnancy, 2763t, 2767-2768
macrocytic and megaloblastic, 1873-1875, 1874f, 1874t, 1875t, 2768, 2873
microcytic, 1871-1873
myelophthisic, 1876, 1876f
nonemergent, 1869, 1870b
normochromic and normocytic, 1875-1876, 1875t, 1876f
of chronic disease, 1873, 1876
pathophysiology of, 1867-1868, 1868b, 1868f
pernicious, optic neuropathy from, 1060
sickle cell, 1879-1882
altitude and, 2308
clinical features of, 1880-1881, 1881f, 1881t
in pregnancy, 2763t, 2768
management of, 1881-1882
pathophysiology of, 1879-1880
urinary tract infection in, 1578
sideroblastic, 1873, 2874
Anemone, 909
Anesthesia, 2914b
dissociative, in syringomyelia, 1683
general, for critically ill asthmatic patient, 1093
in Colles' fracture, 633, 634f
in frostbite, 2230
in red and painful eye, 291
in wound care, 845-847
intravenous regional, 2934
isoflurane, for status epilepticus, 1627-1628, 1627t
local, 2914b, 2930-2933, 2931t, 2932b, 2932t
allergy to, 846-847, 1827, 2931
buffering in, 846, 2932-2933, 2932b
in calcific tendinitis, 698
in wound care, 846
ophthalmic, 1063b, 1064
profiles of agents used for, 2930-2931, 2931t, 2932t
toxicity of, 2931-2932
topical, 2933-2934
Aneurysm
aortic. *See* Aortic aneurysm.
atherosclerotic, infection in, 1356, 1357t
carotid artery, parapharyngeal abscess and, 1123
cerebral, and subarachnoid hemorrhage, Hunt and Hess scale for, 1636, 1636t, 1637
coronary artery, in Kawasaki disease, 2025, 2026, 2594
false. *See* Pseudoaneurysm.
left ventricular, ST segment elevation in, 1167, 1168f
Aneurysm *(Continued)*
pathophysiology of, 1343
peripheral arterial
infected, 1356-1357, 1357t
lower extremity, 1354
traumatic, 1357
upper extremity, 1354-1355
visceral, 1355-1356
renal artery, urolithiasis vs., 1591
traumatic, 1357
Angiitis, allergic, 1816
Angina. *See also* Acute coronary syndromes; Chest pain.
atypical, 1158-1159, 1159t
classic, 1158, 1158t
clinical features of, 1157-1161, 1158t, 1159t
differential diagnosis in, 1159, 1159t
history in, 1157-1159
hypertension and, 1316
in aortic stenosis, 1306
in hemodialysis patient, 1551
increasing or progressive, 1156
Ludwig's, 1028, 1032, 1118-1119
new-onset, 1156
pathophysiology of, 1156-1157
prehospital care in, 1157
rest, 1156
septicemia after, 1123
stable, 1155-1156
unstable
definition of, 1156
in differential diagnosis of chest pain, 190t-191t
management of
antiplatelet therapy in, 1185-1187
beta blockers in, 1184-1185
heparins in, 1187-1188
morphine in, 1184
missed diagnosis of, 1160
ST segment depression in, 1163f
variant (Prinzmetal), 1156
Vincent's, 1033, 1111-1112, 1113
Anginal equivalent symptoms, 1158
Angioedema, 1834-1835
hereditary, 1835
in anaphylaxis, 1825t, 2547
Angiography
computed tomography
in anthrax exposure, 3025, 3025f
in cervical vascular injury, 449
in peripheral arteriovascular disease, 1348
in pulmonary embolism, 1375-1377, 1377b
coronary, in aortic rupture, 480-481
digital subtraction
in peripheral vascular injury, 543
intravenous, in aortic rupture, 480-481
in abdominal trauma, 499
in acute mesenteric ischemia, 1448, 1448f
in colonic ischemia, 1504
in frostbite, 2231
in gastrointestinal bleeding, 224
in ischemic stroke, 1613
in pelvic fracture, 732-734, 733f
in pregnant trauma patient, 321t
in proximity wounds, 543
in severe head trauma, 362, 362t
magnetic resonance
in ischemic stroke, 1613
in peripheral arteriovascular disease, 1348
Angioma, spider, in hepatitis, 1404
Angioplasty, coronary, percutaneous transluminal. *See* Percutaneous coronary intervention.
Angiostrongylus costaricensis, 2113
Angiotensin, 527
in heart failure, 1262
in hypertension, 1311, 1312f
in sodium homeostasis, 1933
Angiotensin II receptor blockade, 1322t
during pregnancy and lactation, 2788
for chronic heart failure, 1276
Angiotensin-converting enzyme inhibitors, 1322t
angioedema from, 1835
during pregnancy and lactation, 2788
for acute coronary syndromes, 1185
for chronic heart failure, 1270t, 1275-1276
for dilated cardiomyopathy, 1294
for hypertension, 1320
for postpartum cardiomyopathy, 2821
Anhedonia, in depression, 1736

Anhydrous ammonia, injury from, 934-935
Animal bite, 882-892
  antibiotic prophylaxis in, 887-889, 887t
  cats in, 883-884, 888
  disposition in, 889-890
  dogs in, [illegible]
  domestic herbivores in, 885
  epidemiology of, 882
  ferrets in, 884-885
  infected, treatment of, [illegible]
  infection risks in, 885-886, 885t
  management of, 886-889, 886b, 887t, 889b, 889t
  osteomyelitis after, 2176
  pigs in, 885
  primates in, 884, 888-889, 889b, 889t
  reporting requirements for, 3172-3173
  rodents in, 884
  systemic infection in, 885
  wild animals in, 885
Anion gap
  calculation of, 1931
  in mixed acid-base disorders, 1931
  in rhabdomyolysis, 1981
Anion gap acidosis, 1927-1929, 1927b
  delirium in, 1651
  in cyanide poisoning, 2437
  in ethylene glycol poisoning, 2399, 2400-2401
  in methanol poisoning, 2396, 2397
  seizure in, 1622
Anisakiasis, 2100t, 2113
Anisocoria, 1061-1062
Ankle
  edema of, heat-induced, 2258-2259
  immobilization of, 571, 572f, 573f
  tendinopathy of, 1799-1800
Ankle trauma, 808-820
  anatomy and physiology in, 808, 809f, 810f
  clinical features of, 808, 810
  diagnostic strategies in, 810-811, 810f, 811f
  dislocation without fracture in, 820
  fracture in, 811-815, 812b, 812f-815f
  ligament injuries in, 815-818, 817b, 817f
  pathophysiology of, 808, 810f
  physical examination, 810
  soft tissue injuries in, 815-820
  tendon injuries in, 818-820, 819f
Ankle-brachial index, 541-542
Ankylosing spondylitis, 1789
Annular ligament, 647, 648f
Annulus fibrosus, 702, 702f
Anogenital examination
  in genitourinary trauma, 515
  in sexual assault victim, 986-988, 987f, 987t, 988t
Anogenital warts, 1563-1564, 1564f
Anorectal disorders, 1507-1522. *See also* Anorectal pain.
  abscesses and fistulas in, 1513-1515, 1513t, 1514f
  anal fissures in, 1508, 1512-1513, 1512f, 1513t
  anatomy and physiology in, 1507-1508, 1508f
  clinical features of, 1508-1509, 1508b
  fecal incontinence in, 1516-1517, 1516b
  foreign bodies and, 875-877, 876f, 1521-1522, 1522f
  hemorrhoids in, 1509-1512, 1510t, 1511b, 1511t, 1512f
  hidradenitis suppurativa in, 1515-1516
  history in, 1508-1509, 1508b
  in HIV/AIDS, 1520, 1520b, 2084
  levator ani syndrome in, 1516
  management of, 1509-1522
  pain and itching in, 1509
  physical examination in, 1509
  pilonidal disease in, 1515
  procidentia in, 1521, 1521f
  proctalgia fugax in, 1509, 1516
  pruritus ani in, 1509, 1517-1518, 1517b
  rectal bleeding in, 1508
  sexually transmitted disease and, 1518-1520, 1518t
  swelling and masses in, 1508-1509
Anorectal pain, 1509.
  in anal fissures, 1512-1513
  in appendicitis, 1452
  in hemorrhoids, 1510
  in levator ani syndrome, 1516
Anorexia
  in appendicitis, 2619
  in chronic renal failure, 1542
  palliative care for, [illegible]
Anoscopy, 1509
  in gastrointestinal bleeding, 224
  in sexual assault victim, 988
ANOVA, 3052-3053, 3052t
Anserine bursitis, 795-796, 1803-1804
Antacids
  during pregnancy and lactation, 2790
  for gastroesophageal reflux, 1389
  for peptic ulcer disease, 1392
  for upper gastrointestinal disorders, [illegible]
Antalgic gait
  in femoral neck stress fracture, 755-756
  pediatric, 764-765
Anterior chamber, nonpenetrating trauma to, 1048-1049, 1048f, 1049f
Anterior chamber angle recession, 1049
Anterior cord syndrome, 419f, 420, 1678, 1678f
Anterior cruciate ligament injury, 790-791, 792
  intercondylar eminence fracture and, 779
  meniscal tears and, 792, 793
  Segond fracture and, 777, 777f
  stability testing in, 773, 774
  tibial femoral knee dislocation and, 788
  tibial plateau fracture and, 778
Anterior drawer test
  of ankle, 816-817
  of knee, 773
Anterior elbow dislocation, 664f, 665-666
Anterior fat pad in elbow, 651, 651f
Anterior humeral line, 651, 651f
Anterior interosseous nerve, 586 589, 589f
Anterior superior iliac spine, avulsion of, 750, 750f
Anterior talofibular ligament, injury to, 816-817
Anterior tibial artery, 797
  anatomy of, 771
  injury to, 547
Anterior uveitis, 287, 287f, 289, 295t
Anteroposterior radiographs, in spinal injuries, 424, 426, 426f, 427f
Anthrax
  as biological weapon, 3021, 3024-3026, 3025f, 3026b, 3026f
  cutaneous, 1860, 1861f, 3025, 3026f
  gastrointestinal, 1461t, 1462t, 1468-1469, 3026
  inhalational, 3024-3025, 3025f
  oropharyngeal, 1469, 3026
  vaccine for, 3026
Antiallergy agents, ophthalmic, 1063b
Antiasthmatic agents, during pregnancy and lactation, 2789-2790
Antibiotics
  after miscarriage, 2742
  allergy to, 1826
  anaphylaxis to, 2547
  Clostridium difficile enterocolitis from, 1470t, 1474-1475
  diarrhea from, 233
  during pregnancy and lactation, 2758, 2784
  for abdominal infections, 217
  for acute necrotic ulcerative gingivitis, 1033
  for acute pancreatitis, 1434
  for acute septic arthritis, 2706, 2706t
  for adult epiglottitis, 1115
  for *Aeromonas hydrophila* gastroenteritis, 1461t, 1468
  for AIDS-related diarrhea, 1484, 1485t
  for anorectal sexually transmitted disease, 1519
  for anthrax exposure, 3026, 3026b
  for appendicitis, 1457
  for *Bacillus anthracis* gastroenteritis, 1461t, 1469
  for bacterial endocarditis, 2591
  for bacterial meningitis, 1721-1722, 1721t, 2663-2664, 2664t
  for bursitis, 1803
  for catheter-related infections, 1363
  for cellulitis, 2107, 2107t
  for central nervous system abscess, 1722
  for central nervous system infections in cancer patient, 1920
  for cholangitis, 1422
  for chronic obstructive pulmonary disease, 1106
  for *Clostridium difficile* enterocolitis, 1475
  for cystic fibrosis, 2564-2565
  for diphtheria, 2004
  for diverticular disease, 1494-1495, 1494b, [illegible]
Antibiotics *(Continued)*
  for *Escherichia coli* food poisoning, 1474
  for esophageal perforation, 1386
  for febrile cancer patient, 1908b, 1909
  for fever, 137
  for impetigo, [illegible]
  for infected aneurysm, 1356
  for infectious diarrhea, 229t-230t, 235
  for infective endocarditis, 1302
  for inflammatory bowel disease, [illegible]
  for intussusception, 2612
  for isosporiasis, 1478
  for Ludwig's angina, 1032, 1119
  for Lyme disease, 1292, 1789, 2127-2128, 2127t
  for malrotation with midgut volvulus, 2608
  for mastoiditis, 1072
  for meningococcal disease, 2023
  for neck masses, 1076
  for necrotizing enterocolitis, 2609
  for necrotizing otitis externa, 1071
  for neutropenia, 2516
  for neutropenic cancer patient, 2837-2839, 2838t
  for open fracture, 558
  for orofacial infections, 1032
  for osteomyelitis, 2187, 2189t
  for otitis externa, 1071
  for otitis media, 1068-1069, 1069t, 1070t
  for pacemaker-induced infection, 1250
  for peritonitis in dialysis patient, 1552-1553, 1553t
  for peritonsillitis, 1118
  for pertussis, 2006
  for plague, 3027-3028
  for *Plesiomonas shigelloides* gastroenteritis, 1461t, 1468
  for pneumococcal disease, 2018-2019
  for pneumonia, 1136-1139, 1138t, 1139t, 2557, 2558t, 2562-2563
  for prostatitis, 1586
  for purulent pericarditis, 1286
  for retropharyngeal abscess, 1121
  for Rocky Mountain spotted fever, 2136, 2136t
  for salmonellosis, 1461t, 1463
  for sepsis, 2221, 2221t
  for septic arthritis, 1785, 2178t, 2192
  for septic shock, 53
  for shigellosis, 1461t, 1464
  for sinusitis, 1125
  for small bowel obstruction, 1444
  for spinal epidural abscess, 1684
  for spinal infection, 712
  for spontaneous bacterial peritonitis, 1413
  for streptococcal pharyngitis, 1112-1113
  for tar removal, 927
  for tetanus, 2011
  for toxic shock syndrome, 2030, 2201
  for traveler's diarrhea, 1486-1487
  for urinary tract infections, 2643-2644
  for *Vibrio* fish poisoning, 1472
  for *Yersinia enterocolitica* gastroenteritis, 1465
  in asthma, 1090
  in comatose patient, 163
  injections of, medicolegal issues in, 3159
  ophthalmic, 1063b, 1064
  preoperative, in arterial injury, 544
  prophylactic
    for anthrax exposure, 3026
    for bacteremia, 2506
    for infective endocarditis, 1302, 1303b, 1303t
    for meningococcal disease, 2024
    for red and painful eye, 292
    for rheumatic fever, 2597
    for traveler's diarrhea, 1486-1487
    in abdominal trauma, 502
    in animal bite, 887-889, 887t
    in frostbite, 2232
    in hand amputation and ring avulsion injuries, 613
    in HIV/AIDS, 2089
    in human bites, 891-892
    in hypothermia, 2247
    in open ankle fractures, 814
    in open tibial shaft fracture, 800-801
    in severe head trauma, 381
    in wound management, 854 855
  resistance to, plasmids and, 1575
  topical, for burn injury, [illegible]

Antibodies
B cell, 2832
diversity of, 1821
Lyme disease, 2125
meningococcal, 2021
Antibody-antigen specificity, 1821
Anticholinergic agents
for anaphylaxis, 1832
for asthma, 1089, 2539t, 2541
for chronic obstructive pulmonary disease, 1105
for dysphagia, 1398
for nausea and vomiting, 206
for vertigo, 146
overdose of, 2345-2350, 2346b, 2346t, 2347f
alcohol withdrawal syndrome vs., 2860
antidotes to, 2329t
clinical presentation in, 2347-2348, 2347t
diagnosis of, 2349
differential diagnosis in, 2348, 2348b
disposition in, 2350
management of, 2349-2350
types of, 2345, 2346b, 2346t
Anticholinergic toxidrome, 2327, 2327t, 2347-2348
Anticoagulation
during pregnancy and lactation, 2757, 2785-2786
for acute mesenteric ischemia, 1449
for cerebral venous thrombosis, 1671
for dilated cardiomyopathy, 1294
for ischemic stroke, 1615-1616
in deep venous thrombosis, 1370
in peripheral arteriovascular disease, 1349
in pulmonary embolism, 1377
postresuscitation, 86
Anticonvulsant therapy
for alcohol withdrawal syndrome, 2862
for neuropathic pain, 1692
for seizure, 166-167, 166t
during pregnancy and lactation, 2763t, 2769, 2786-2787
immediate, 1626-1628, 1627t
in children, prophylactic, 2674-2676, 2675t
in intracerebral hemorrhage, 1616
long-term, 1628-1629, 1629t
for status epilepticus, 1627-1628, 1627t, 2672-2673, 2672t
for trigeminal neuralgia, 1664, 1666
in developmentally disabled patient, 2898-2899
prophylactic, in head trauma, 361, 361b, 370
side effects of, 1628t, 2674-2675
withdrawal of, 2676
Antidepressants
discontinuation syndrome with, 2365-2366
FDA-approved, 2353t
for depression, 1741
for somatoform disorders, 1758
overdose of, 2352-2366, 2354t
bupropion in, 2361, 2361t
cyclic antidepressants in, 2352-2357, 2353b, 2353f, 2354b, 2355f, 2357t
mirtazapine in, 2362-2363
monoamine oxidase inhibitors in, 2363-2365, 2363b-2365b, 2364t
neurologic complications of, 2354t, 2356
selective serotonin reuptake inhibitors in, 2357-2360, 2358b, 2358t, 2359b, 2360t
trazdone in, 2361-2362
venlafaxine in, 2362, 2362t
suicide and, 1768
Antidiuretic hormone
for cardiac arrest, 92
for gastrointestinal bleeding, 225
for heart failure, 1262-1263
for pediatric resuscitation, 100, 103t
for sepsis, 2213, 2219t, 2220
in sodium homeostasis, 1933
Antidote, 2329t
antivenin as
Latrodectus, 906
scorpion, 908
snake, 900-902, 900t
cyanide, 2329t, 2437-2438, 2440
in benzodiazepine poisoning, 2326, 2329t, 2485-2486, 2485b
in opioid overdose, 2948-2949
Antidromic tachycardia, in Wolff-Parkinson-White syndrome, 1235, 1237
"Antidumping" law, 3156
Antidysrhythmic devices. *See* Implantable cardioverter-defibrillator; Pacemaker(s).
Antidysrhythmic drugs
adenosine as, 1212-1213
class IA, 1206
class IB, 1206-1207
class IC, 1207-1208
class II, 1208-1209, 1208t
class III, 1209-1210
class IV, 1210-1211
classification of, 1204-1213, 1205b
digitalis as, 1211-1212, 1211t
during pregnancy and lactation, 2787-2788
for adult resuscitation, 92-93
for chronic heart failure, 1277
for pediatric resuscitation, 109-113, 110f-113f, 110t
heart failure from, 1269
magnesium as, 1212
prodysrhythmic effects of, 1205-1206
Antiemetic agents
during pregnancy and lactation, 2790
for nausea and vomiting, 203, 206, 208b, 208t
Antiepileptic agents. *See* Anticonvulsant therapy.
Antifibrillatory agents, 1209-1210
Antifreeze
bittering agents in, 2402
ingestion of, 2398-2402, 2401t
Antifungals, during pregnancy and lactation, 2785
Antigen detection, in central nervous system infection, 1718-1719
Antigen detection kits, cerebrospinal fluid, in bacterial meningitis, 2662
Antihelmintics, 2098t
Antihemophilic factor antibodies, in hemophilia A, 1901
Antihistamines
during pregnancy and lactation, 2789-2790
for anaphylaxis, 1831b, 1832
for nausea and vomiting, 206
for scombroid fish poisoning, 1472
for upper airway angioedema, 1835
for urticaria, 1848
Antihypertensive drug therapy
agents used in, 1321t-1322t
ambulatory, 1320, 1320t
during pregnancy and lactation, 2762, 2763t, 2765t, 2788-2789
for aortic dissection, 1328-1329
for eclampsia, 2751
for hypertensive emergencies, 1317-1319, 1317t
for hypertensive urgency, 1320
for intracerebral hemorrhage, 1616
for ischemic stroke, 1614, 1614t
in children, 2652-2653, 2653t
Antiinflammatory drugs
after cerebral ischemia, 72
in frostbite, 2233
nonsteroidal. *See* Nonsteroidal antiinflammatory drugs.
Antilymphocyte monoclonal antibody preparations, for organ transplant patient, 2850-2851
Antimalarial drugs, 2098t
for systemic lupus erythematosus, 1809
Antimotility agents
for AIDS-related diarrhea, 1484
for diarrhea, 235, 236t
Antimuscarinic agents, overdose of, 2345-2349. *See also* Anticholinergic agents, overdose of.
Antimyosin scanning, in myocarditis, 1290
Antinuclear antibodies, in systemic lupus erythematosus, 1808
Antioxidant therapy, after cerebral ischemia, 71
Antiparasitic agents, 2098-2099, 2098t, 2100t-2103t
Antiparkinsonian drugs
anticholinergic toxicity of, 2345, 2346, 2346b, 2347t
for prevention of antipsychotic-induced extrapyramidal symptoms, 1731
Antiphospholipid antibody syndrome, 1809-1810t
Antiplatelet therapy
for acute coronary syndromes, 1185-1187
for acute mesenteric ischemia, 1449
for ischemic stroke, 1615
postresuscitation, 86
Antiprotozoals, 2098t
Antipsychotic agents, 2446t
agranulocytosis from, 2448
atypical
for agitation in delirious patient, 1654
for rapid tranquilization, 2962
complications of, 1732-1733
extrapyramidal symptoms from, 2445, 2446-2447, 2449
for agitation in delirious patient, 1654
for mood disorders, 1741
for rapid tranquilization, 2961-2962
for thought disorders, 1730-1731, 1731b
neuroleptic malignant syndrome from, 2445, 2447, 2447t, 2448, 2448t, 2449, 2961-2962
overdose of, 2446, 2448-2449
QT prolongation and torsades de pointes from, 2447, 2449
seizures from, 2448, 2962
side effects of, 2961-2962
tardive dyskinesia from, 2445, 2447
toxicity of, 2445-2450, 2446t
Antipyretics, 137
Antiretroviral therapy, 2039, 2087-2089, 2087t
during delivery, 2810
for HIV postexposure prophylaxis, 2091-2092, 3085t, 3086-3087
in pregnancy, 2088-2089, 2764t, 2774
rifamycins and, drug interactions between, 2166
Antiseptics, for wound cleansing, 847-848, 848t
Antisocial personality disorder, 2979b
in alcoholism, 2875
malingering and, 1763
Antistreptococcal antibody titers, in rheumatic fever, 1304
Antithrombotic therapy
in acute coronary syndromes, 1187-1188
in frostbite, 2232-2233
Antitoxin. *See also* Immunization; Vaccine.
botulism, 1707-1708, 2016
diphtheria, 1113, 2004
equine, allergy to, 1827
Antituberculous agents
during pregnancy and lactation, 2168, 2785
first-line, 2162, 2163t, 2164
fixed-dose combinations if, 2164
for drug-resistant tuberculosis, 2166-2167, 2167b, 2167t
for extrapulmonary tuberculosis, 2168
for initial therapy, 2165-2166, 2165t
for latent infection, 2168-2169, 2168t
in children and adolescents, 2166, 2167b
in HIV/AIDS, 2166
noncompliance with, risk factors for, 2162
second-line, 2163t-2164t, 2164-2165
susceptibility testing for, 2154-2155
Antivenin
Latrodectus, 906
scorpion, 908
snake, 900-902, 900t
Antiviral agents
during pregnancy and lactation, 2785
for myocarditis, 1290
for pneumonia, 1139
ophthalmic, 1063b, 1064
prophylactic, in monkey bites, 888-889, 889t
Antiviral chemotherapy, 2035-2039, 2036t-2037t
Anton's syndrome, 1060
Anxiety
endogenous, 1745
exogenous, 1745, 1746b
in cardiovascular disease, 1746-1747
in drug intoxication and withdrawal states, 1748
in endocrine disease, 1747
in neurologic disorders, 1747-1748
in primary psychiatric disorders, 1748-1749
in pulmonary disease, 1747
medical illness manifesting as, 1745-1746, 1746b
somatoform disorders vs., 1757
Anxiety disorders, 1744-1752
clinical features of, 1745, 1745b
definitions of, 1746b
differential considerations in, 1745-1749, 1746b
disposition in, 1751-1752
epidemiology of, 1744

Anxiety disorders *(Continued)*
  generalized, 1746b
  management of, 1749-1751
    pharmacological, 1750-1751, 1750t
    psychological, 1751
  not otherwise specified, 1746b
  pathophysiology of, 1744-1745
  substance-induced, 1746b
Anxiolytics, 1750-1751, 1751t
Aorta
  coarctation of, 1312, 2578-2579
  penetrating atherosclerotic ulcers of, 1325
Aortic aneurysm
  abdominal, 1330-1340
    back pain in, 265t
    clinical features of, 1332-1333
    diagnostic strategies in, 1334-1336, 1334f-1336f, 1337-1338
    differential diagnosis in, 1336, 1336b
    disposition in, 1340
    epidemiology of, 1330, 1331t
    false, 1330, 1340
    management of, 1336-1339
    pathophysiology and natural history of, 1330-1331
    repair of
      endovascular, 1338-1339, 1339f
      late complications of, 1339-1340
      survival rate for, 1339
      traditional, 1338, 1339f
    ruptured, 1331
      abdominal pain in, 214t
      clinical features of, 1332-1333
      management of, 1336-1338
    types of, 1330, 1331f
  thoracic
    chronic, 482
    superior vena cava syndrome in, 1909
Aortic arch
  congenital anomalies of, dysphagia in, 1383
  right-sided, 2574
Aortic clamping
  in abdominal aortic aneurysm rupture, 1337
  in abdominal trauma, 502
  in aortic rupture, 481
Aortic compression, for postpartum hemorrhage, 2819
Aortic dissection, 1324-1329
  abdominal aortic aneurysm vs., 1330
  anatomy and physiology in, 1324
  arterial embolism vs., 1352
  back pain in, 261, 265t
  chest pain in, 183, 186b, 190t-191t
  clinical features of, 1325-1326
  diagnostic strategies in, 1326-1328, 1326t, 1327f, 1327t
  differential diagnosis in, 1328
  disposition in, 1329
  epidemiology of, 1324
  hypertension in, 1317
  management of, 1328-1329
  pathophysiology of, 1324-1325
  risk factors for, 186b
  Stanford classification of, 1325, 1325f
Aortic media, degeneration of, in aortic dissection, 1324-1325
Aortic regurgitation, 1307
  heart failure in, 1265
  in aortic dissection, 1326
  in pregnancy, 2763t, 2767
Aortic rupture, 476-482, 477f-479f, 481b, 510, 511f
Aortic stenosis, 1306-1307
  heart failure in, 1265
  in pregnancy, 2763t, 2767
Aortic wall, intramural hemorrhage within, 1325
Aortoenteric fistula
  after abdominal aortic aneurysm repair, 1340
  in abdominal aortic aneurysm rupture, 1333
Aortography
  in aortic dissection, 1327
  in aortic rupture, 480-481
Aortoiliac occlusive disease, 1345, 1350
Aortovenous fistula, in abdominal aortic aneurysm rupture, 1333
APACHE-II system in acute pancreatitis, 1452
Apgar score, 122, 122t
Aphasia, in ischemic stroke, 1609
Aphthous stomatitis, 1036
Aphthous ulcers
  in Behçet's disease, 1814
  in HIV/AIDS, 2083
Aplastic anemia, 1875-1876, 1875t
Aplastic crisis
  in hemolytic anemia, 2046, 2046f
  in sickle cell disease, 1880
Apley's test, in meniscal tears, 774
Apnea
  definition of, 2714
  from etomidate, 2947
  in neonates, 119
  in pneumonia, 2562
  respiratory depression with, in GHB intoxication, 2489
  sleep, hypertension in, 1313
Apocrine glands, 915, 2255
  abscess of, in hidradenitis suppurativa, 2204-2205
Apolipoprotein E gene, in dementia, 1657
Apophyseal injuries/disorders, 2700-2711, 2711f
Apophysitis, 2709-2710
  of elbow, 2710-2711
  of hip, 2711
Apoptosis, after cerebral ischemia, 66
Apparent life-threatening event, 2714, 2718-2720, 2718b, 2719b
Appearance
  in chest pain, 187t
  in dyspnea, 178t
  in headache, 172t
  in nausea and vomiting, 202t
  in pediatric assessment triangle, 2497-2498, 2498t
  in vaginal bleeding, 256t
  toxic, as indication for lumbar puncture, 2659
Appendectomy, laparoscopic, 1457-1458
Appendicitis, 1451-1458
  abdominal pain in, 210t
  complications of, 1453-1454
  diagnosis of, 1454-1455
  differential diagnosis in, 1455, 1456t
  disposition in, 1458
  epidemiology of, 1451
  historical perspective in, 1451
  imaging studies in, 1454-1455, 1455f, 1456
  in children, 1452-1453, 2509b, 2618-2620, 2620f
  in elderly person, 1453
  in pregnancy, 1453, 2752-2754, 2754f
  in women, 1453, 1453t
  management of, 1456-1458, 1457f
  nausea and vomiting in, 205t
  observation in, 1455, 3063, 3064
  pathophysiology of, 1451-1452
  pelvic pain in, 251t
  perforation in, 1452, 1453, 1458
Appendicolith, 2619, 2620f
Appendix, perforation of, 1452, 1453, 1458
Appendix testis
  in children, 2641
  torsion of, 1597
Appetite disturbance, in depression, 1737
Apprehension sign
  in anterior subluxation of glenohumeral joint, 690, 691f
  in patellar dislocation, 786
Aqueous humor, 1055
Arachidonic acid, metabolism of, 1081f
Arbovirus
  group A, 2047-2048
  group B, 2049-2050
Arcanobacterium haemolyticum, in pharyngitis, 1111, 1113, 1114
Arenavirus, 2034t, 2055-2056
Argentine hemorrhagic fever, 2055-2056
Aripiprazole, 2446t
  for thought disorders, 1731
Arm. *See also* Forearm *entries.*
  decompression of, in burn injury, 935
  delivery of, in shoulder dystocia, 2815
Aromatic petroleum distillates, toxicity of, 2428, 2429t
Arousal
  disorders of, in sudden infant death syndrome, 2718
  physiology of, 156
Arrhythmia. *See* Dysrhythmia.
Arsenic poisoning, 2329t, 2423-2424, 2424b
Arterial anatomy, 1342
Arterial aneurysm, peripheral
  infected, 1356-1357, 1357t
  lower extremity, 1354
  traumatic, 1357
  upper extremity, 1354-1355
  visceral, 1355-1356
Arterial blood gases
  during cardiopulmonary resuscitation, 80-81
  in asthma, 1085, 2537
  in chronic obstructive pulmonary disease, 1100
  in comatose patient, 162
  in cyanosis, 271
  in electrical and lightning injuries, 2276
  in hypothermia, 2242, 2243f
  in infants and children, 2572-2573
  in pulmonary contusion, 461
  monitoring of, 36-39
    capnography/capnometry in, 37-39, 38f
    pulse oximetry in, 30-37
    transcutaneous and conjunctival, 36
Arterial disease, in hypertension, 1312-1313
Arterial embolism, 1352-1353
  differential diagnosis in, 1352
  management of, 1352-1353
  pathophysiology of, 1343-1344
  physical examination in, 1346, 1347t
  vs. thrombosis in situ, 1347t
Arterial gas embolism
  in scuba diving–related disorders, 2285-2286
  recompression therapy for, 2288-2292, 2288b, 2289f-2291f
  vs. pulmonary decompression sickness, 2288, 2288t
Arterial injury
  in hip trauma, 761
  peripheral, 536-547. *See also* Arteriovascular disease, peripheral.
    clinical features of, 539-541, 540f
    diagnostic strategies in, 541-543
    disposition in, 547
    epidemiology of, 536-537
    of lower extremity, 546-547
    of upper extremity, 544-546
    pathophysiology of, 537-539, 538f
    treatment of, 543-544
Arterial insufficiency, 539, 1345-1346, 1350-1352
Arterial occlusion, acute, 1345, 1345f, 1352-1354, 1353f
Arterial pressure index, in peripheral vascular injury, 541-542
Arterial spasm, reversible, posttraumatic, 538
Arterial supply
  to distal humerus and elbow, 648, 648f
  to femur and hip, 737, 737t, 738f
  to foot, 821
  to forearm, 640t
  to hand, 585-586, 587f, 588f
  to knee, 771
  to lower leg, 797
  to lower limb, 540f
  to nose, 1073, 1073f
  to pelvis, 717-718
  to upper limb, 540f
  to wrist, 622, 625f
Arterial thrombosis, 1344, 1347, 1347t, 1353-1354
Arteriography
  in cervical vascular injury, 449
  in knee trauma, 774
  in pelvic fracture, 732-734, 733f
  in peripheral arteriovascular disease, 1348
  in peripheral vascular injury, 542-543
  in popliteal artery injury, 546-547
  in subclavian artery injury, 545
  in thoracic outlet syndrome, 1360
  in tibial femoral knee dislocation, 788
Arteriosclerosis, hypertension in, 1312
Arteriovascular disease, peripheral, 1342-1366
  acute arterial occlusion in, 1345, 1345f, 1352-1354, 1353f
  arterial anatomy and, 1342
  arterial embolism in, 1343-1344, 1346, 1347t, 1352-1353
  arterial thrombosis in, 1344, 1347, 1347t, 1353-1354
  arteriosclerosis obliterans in, 1350-1351
  arteriovenous fistula in, 538-539, 541, 1344, 1347, 1360

Volume 1 pp 1–1024 • Volume 2 pp 1025–2226 • Volume 3 pp 2227–3180

Arteriovascular disease, peripheral *(Continued)*
- atheroembolism in, 1343-1344, 1353, 1353f
- Buerger's disease in, 1351-1352
- chronic arterial insufficiency in, 1345-1346, 1350-1352
- clinical features of, 1344-1347
- diagnosis of, 1348
- drug abuse–related, 1360-1361
- history in, 1344-1346, 1345f
- inflammatory, 1344, 1347
- management of, 1348-1350
- pathophysiology of, 1342-1344
- physical examination in, 1346-1347, 1347t
- thoracic outlet syndrome in, 1358-1360, 1358f, 1359f
- trauma in, 1344
- vasospastic disorders in, 1344

Arteriovenous anastomoses rewarming, 2248
Arteriovenous bridge fistula, prosthetic, 1365-1366
Arteriovenous fistula, 538-539, 541, 1344, 1347, 1360
Arteriovenous malformations
- hemorrhage in, 1609
- seizure in, 1624

Arteriovenous rewarming, continuous, 2250t, 2251
Arteritis
- giant cell (temporal)
  - headache in, 1638
  - ischemic stroke vs., 1611
  - pericarditis in, 1284
- pathophysiology of, 1344
- Takayasu's, 1813

Arthralgia, in Henoch-Schönlein purpura, 2615, 2653
Arthritis, 1776-1792. *See also* Osteoarthritis; Rheumatic disease.
- anatomy and physiology in, 1777, 1777f
- arthrocentesis in, 1780-1781
- clinical findings in, 1778-1779, 1779f, 1779t
- diagnosis of, 1779-1782, 1780t
- differential considerations in, 1782, 1782b
- disposition in, 1792
- electrocardiography in, 1782
- gonococcal, 1787-1788, 2190-2191
- gouty, 1785-1786
- historical perspective of, 1776-1777
- in chronic renal failure, 1543
- in hepatitis B, 1788
- in Lyme disease, 1788-1789, 2124, 2126
- in seronegative spondyloarthropathies, 1789-1790
- management of, 1782-1792, 1783f, 1784f
- monarticular, 1782-1787, 1783f
- pathophysiology of, 1777, 1777f
- polyarticular, 1303-1304, 1784f, 1787-1792, 1790b, 2596
- pseudogout and, 1786-1787
- radiological findings in, 1779-1780, 1780t
- reactive, 1789-1790, 1791, 2192
- rheumatoid, 1791-1792
  - in pregnancy, 2776
  - myocarditis in, 1297
  - pericarditis in, 1284
  - skin lesions in, 1862t
- rubella, 1788
- septic, 1782-1785, 2174
  - clinical features of, 1784-1785, 2188-2191
  - complications of, 2190
  - differential considerations in, 2191-2192
  - disposition in, 2193
  - etiology and microbiology of, 2177-2179, 2178t
  - gonococcal, 2190-2191
  - history and physical examination in, 2188
  - in atypical joints, 2191
  - in disseminated gonococcal infection, 1566
  - in hand, 618
  - in knee, 796
  - in tuberculosis, 2159
  - joint aspiration and joint fluid analysis in, 2188-2190, 2189f
  - management of, 1785, 2178t, 2192-2193
  - pathophysiology and epidemiology of, 1782-1784, 2177
  - pediatric, 2190, 2509b, 2704-2706, 2705t, 2706t

Arthritis *(Continued)*
  - pediatric limp from, 764
  - with existing joint disease, 2191
- synovial fluid analysis in, 1781-1782, 1781t
- viral, 1788

Arthritis-dermatitis syndrome, 1566, 1788, 1843-1844, 1843f
Arthrocentesis
- in arthritis, 1780-1781
- in knee trauma, 774

Arthrography, in knee trauma, 774-775
Arthrometer, in anterior cruciate ligament injury, 774
Arthropathy
- back pain in, 703, 705-706
- psoriatic, 1790

Arthroplasty, hip
- partial, 751, 752b
- total, 749-750, 750f

Arthropod envenomation, 903-908
Arthroscopy
- in ankle trauma, 811
- in intercondylar eminence fracture, 780
- in knee trauma, 774
- in meniscal tears, 793
- in septic arthritis, 2189

Arthrotomy, for infected hip, 2192
Articular cartilage destruction, in septic arthritis, 2177
Articular humeral fractures, 661-664, 661f-663f
Articular surface, fracture extension into, 553
Artificial tears, 1063b, 1064
Ascariasis, 2100t, 2113
Ascending aortic rupture, 476, 477
Ascending reticular activating system, 156
Ascending sensory tracts, 1676, 1676f, 2915, 2915f, 2916f
Ascites
- in chronic schistosomiasis, 2112, 2113f
- in cirrhosis, 1410, 1411
- in pancreatitis, 1427
- in spontaneous bacterial peritonitis, 1412

Ashman phenomenon, 1203, 1223, 1230, 1232f
Aspartate aminotransferase
- in acetaminophen overdose, 2335
- in acute pancreatitis, 1431, 1431t
- in alcoholic hepatitis, 1409
- in amebic abscess, 1416
- in viral hepatitis, 1404

Aspergilloma, in tuberculosis, 2151, 2151f
Aspergillus
- in febrile, neutropenic cancer patient, 2836
- in infective endocarditis, 1301
- in osteomyelitis, 2178-2179

Asphalt burns, petroleum-derived, 926-927, 937
Asphyxia, traumatic, in chest wall trauma, 459
Asphyxiants, simple, inhalation of, 2432-2433
Asphyxic asthma, sudden, 1084
Aspiration
- after vomiting, 202
- cavernosal, in priapism, 2636
- foreign body, 864-870, 867f-869f, 2529-2530, 2550-2551, 2551f
- in hydrocarbon poisoning, 2428, 2431
- in physically disabled patient, 2907-2908
- in submersion injuries, 2312-2313
- meconium, resuscitation in, 120, 120f, 122
- of tooth, 395, 866
- pneumonia and, 1136

Aspiration pneumonia, in children, 2560
Aspiration techniques
- for confirmation of endotracheal tube placement, 6
- in bursitis, 1802
- in gonococcal arthritis, 2191
- in knee trauma, 776
- in osteomyelitis, 2182
- in peritonsillar abscess, 1118
- in pneumothorax, 1147
- in radial head and neck fracture, 664
- in septic arthritis, 2188-2190, 2189f, 2192
- in septic olecranon bursitis, 667

Aspirin
- allergy to, 1828
- during pregnancy and lactation, 2776, 2781
- for acute coronary syndromes, 1185
- for chest pain, 184
- for ischemic stroke, 1615
- for Kawasaki disease, 2027, 2596

Aspirin *(Continued)*
- for migraine, 2680
- for polycythemia, 1885
- for systemic lupus erythematosus, 1808
- gastritis from, 1390
- metabolism of, 2339-2340, 2340f
- overdose of, 2339-2342, 2340f
  - chronic exposure in, 2340
  - clinical features of, 2341, 2341b
  - diagnosis of, 2341
  - disposition in, 2342
  - management of, 2341-2342, 2341b
- thrombocytopathy from, 1898-1899

Aspirin-exacerbated respiratory disease, 1082
Asplenia, immune defects in, 2842-2843
Assault
- by combative patient, 2963
- sexual. *See* Sexual assault.

Assisted-living facilities, institutional abuse in, 1009, 1015
Asterixis, in hepatic encephalopathy, 1411
Asthma, 1078-1094. *See also* Status asthmaticus.
- acute severe, near fatal, and fatal, 1091-1093
- adrenergic medications for, 1086-1088, 1087t, 2538, 2539t, 2540-2541
- altitude and, 2307
- anticholinergic agents for, 1089, 2539t, 2541
- anxiety in, 1747
- clinical features of, 1083-1084
- corticosteroid-resistant, 1089
- corticosteroids for, 1087t, 1088-1089, 2539t, 2541-2543, 2543t
- critically ill patient with
  - intubation and ventilator strategies for, 1092-1093
  - noninvasive strategies for, 1091-1092
  - refractoriness to treatment in, 1093
- definition of, 1078
- diagnosis of, 1083, 1084-1085, 1086t
- differential diagnosis in, 1086b
- disposition in, 1093-1094, 1094b
- dyspnea in, 179t
- epidemiology of, 1078-1079, 1079f
- exercise-induced, 1082
- genetic findings in, 1082-1083
- historic components in, 1084
- in aspirin-exacerbated respiratory disease, 1082
- in pregnancy, 1091, 2761-2762, 2763t, 2765t
- intubation in, 2542
- leukotriene modifiers for, 1090, 2542, 2543t
- magnesium sulfate for, 1087t, 1089-1090
- management of, 1086-1093, 1087t
  - guidelines for, 1083
  - home strategies for, 1086
  - inpatient vs. observation or clinical decision unit, 1093
  - planning discharge in, 1094, 1094b
  - severity of attack and, 1086, 1087t
- menstruation-associated, 1082
- methylxanthines for, 1090, 1090t
- monitoring strategies in, 1085
- mortality in, 1078
  - risk factors for, 1084b
- observation in, 3069-3070, 3070b
- oxygen therapy for, 1086, 1091-1092, 2538
- pathology of, 1083
- pathophysiology of, 1080-1083, 1080f, 1081f
- pediatric, 2532-2544
  - clinical features of, 2534-2536
  - complications of, 2535-2536, 2536b
  - diagnosis of, 2536-2537, 2536f, 2537f
  - differential diagnosis in, 2537, 2538b
  - disposition in, 2542-2544
  - epidemiology of, 2532
  - factors associated with, 2533-2534, 2534b
  - history in, 2534, 2534b
  - management of, 2537-2542, 2539t, 2540f, 2543t
  - pathophysiology of, 2532-2533
  - physical examination in, 2534-2535, 2535t
  - prehospital care in, 2537
  - severity assessment score for, 2503t
- physical examination in, 1084, 1086t
- prediction of relapse in, 1093
- psychological factors in, 1082
- pulmonary barotrauma and, 2285
- rapid sequence intubation in, 16
- reflux-induced, 1388-1389
- severity of, classification of, 2534t

Asthma *(Continued)*
sudden asphyxic, 1084
symptoms of, 1083-1084
Astrovirus, 2034t, 2057-2058
Asystole
in hypothermia, [illegible]
pediatric, 111-112, 112f, 2586t, 2590
treatment of, 84-85
Ataxia
cerebellar
in high-altitude cerebral edema, 2306
pediatric, 2681, 2682
in multiple sclerosis, 1673
pediatric, 2681-2682, 2681b
Ataxia telangiectasia, 2682
Atelectasis, in asthma, 2537, 2537f
Atenolol, 1321t
during pregnancy and lactation, 2788
for alcohol withdrawal syndrome, 2862
overdose of, 2373t
Atheroembolism, 1343-1344, 1353, 1353f
Atherosclerosis
coronary artery disease and, 1157
in diabetes mellitus, 1970
infected aneurysm in, 1356, 1357t
pathophysiology of, 1342-1343
Athetoid cerebral palsy, 2904
Athletes
injuries in. *See* Sports injuries.
young, sudden death in, 2597-2599, 2597b
Atlantoaxial dislocation
anterior, 399, 401, 402f
rotary, 405-406, 408f
Atlantoaxial instability, in Down syndrome, 2901
Atlantoaxial separation, in retropharyngeal abscess, 1121
Atlanto-occipital dislocation, 399, 401, 402f
Atlas
posterior neural arch fracture of, 410, 410f
radiography of, 424, 424f-425f
Atmospheres absolute, 2280
Atmospheric cooling power, 2255
Atopic dermatitis, 1841-1842
Atopy
in anaphylaxis, 1820, 2547
in asthma, 2533
Atovaquone, in HIV/AIDS, side effects of, 2079t
Atracurium, in intubation, 14
Atrial clot, 1232
Atrial dysrhythmias, 1216
in cocaine overdose, 2390
in myocardial contusion, 469
Atrial fibrillation, 1230-1233, 1231f, 1232b, 1232f
etiology of, 1230-1231, 1232b
in hyperthyroidism, 1987
in hypertrophic cardiomyopathy, 1296
in hypothermia, 2238
in infants and children, 2589
in mitral stenosis, 1306
ischemic stroke in, 1608
observation in, 3070-3071, 3070b
treatment of, 1231-1233, 1232b
Atrial fibrillation-flutter, 1231
Atrial flutter, 1229-1230, 1230f-1231f
in infants and children, 2589
with accessory pathway, 1229
Atrial parasystole, 1226
Atrial rupture, 470-472
Atrial septal defect, 2578
Atrial tachycardia, 1228-1229, 1228f, 1229f
multifocal, 1228, 1229f
nonparoxysmal, 1228
paroxysmal, 1228
Atrioventricular block, 1218-1221
antipsychotic-induced, 2447
first-degree, 1218, 1219f
in beta blocker overdose, 2374-2375
in Lyme disease, 2123-2124, 2128
second-degree
Mobitz type I (Wenckebach), 1218-1219, 1218t, 1219b, 1220f
Mobitz type II, 1218t, 1219-1220, 1220f
third-degree (complete), 1220-1221, 1221f
Atrioventricular dissociation, isorhythmic, 1221
Atrioventricular node
conduction and, 1202, 1202t, 1203, 1203f
digitalis effects on, 2368
Atrium, penetrating injury to, 472
Atrophic vaginitis, 1909
Atropine
for anaphylactic patient on beta blockers, 1831b, 1833
for asystole, 85
for beta blocker overdose, 2375
for bradycardia, [illegible]
for calcium channel blocker–induced hypotension, 2377-2378
for cardiac arrest, 93
for complete atrioventricular block, 1221
for digitalis toxicity, 2371
for dysrhythmia, 2586b
for nerve agent exposure, 3030-3031, 3031t
for organophosphate poisoning, 2460
for pediatric resuscitation, 99, 100, 101t-102t, 103-104
for pulseless electrical activity, 84
for sinoatrial block, 1218
for sinus node dysfunction, 1218
in rapid sequence intubation, 11b
mydriasis from, 1061
Attachment apparatus, 1027, 1027f
Attitudinal bias, 130
Attribution error, 130
Auditing systems for confidential medical records, 3103
Auditory symptoms, in vertigo, 144
Aura, migraine with, 2678, 2678b
Auscultation
cardiac, in infants and children, 2571-2572, 2572b
for confirmation of endotracheal tube placement, 7
of pregnant abdomen, 2728
Austin Flint murmur, in aortic regurgitation, 1307
Authentication, in confidential medical records, 3103
Authority gradients, as source of failures in emergency department, 3122
Authorization, in confidential medical records, 3103
Autoimmune adrenal insufficiency, 1996
Autoimmune hemolytic anemia, 1882-1883, 1883b
Autoimmune response, in systemic lupus erythematosus, 1806, 1808
Autoimmune thrombocytopenic purpura, 1897-1898
Automatic external defibrillators, in pediatric resuscitation, 113
Automaticity, altered, dysrhythmias from, 1204, 1204f
Automobile cooling system, and body's heat dissipation mechanisms, 2256-2258, 2256f
Automotive products, bittering agents in, 2402
Autonomic arousal, 1745
Autonomic dysreflexia, in spinal cord injury, 2906
Autonomic nervous system, 2459f
Autonomic neuropathy
diabetic, 1971
in alcohol withdrawal syndrome, 2861
in tetanus, 2009
Autonomy, 3129, 3129b
Auto-pedestrian collisions. *See* Pedestrian collisions.
Autotransfusion, 59
in hemothorax, 465
in multiple trauma, 307-308
Avascular necrosis
after fracture, 562
after talar fracture, 824
in knee trauma, 782
in scuba diving–related disorders, 2286
of femoral head, 739-741, 741b, 742f
after femoral neck fracture, 740, 742f, 750-751
pediatric, 767
of proximal femoral epiphysis, 2706-2707, 2707f
Aviation physiology, 2994-2995, 2995t
Aviator's fracture, 550t
Avolition, in schizophrenia, 1728
AVPU system, 330b
Avulsion, tooth, 380-390, 395, 1037-1040, 1038f, 1039f
Avulsion fracture, 553, 554f
femoral, 750, 750f
fibular, 818
Avulsion fracture *(Continued)*
of elbow, 2711, 2711f
of greater tuberosity, in glenohumeral joint dislocation, 688
of tibial tubercle, 798, 798f
pelvic, 780-781, 781f
sprains and, 566
Avulsion injuries
nail bed, 611
ring, in hand trauma, 612-613, 613b
scalp, 372
Awake oral intubation, 12
Axillary artery, 540, 540f
aneurysm of, 1354-1355
injury to, 545
Axillary nerve
anatomy of, 672
injury to, after anterior glenohumeral joint dislocation, 687, 690
Axillary vein injury, 545
Axis, radiography of, 424, 424f-425f
Axonal injury
in child abuse, 971
in head trauma, 374
Axonotmesis, 559
Azathioprine, 2844
for inflammatory bowel disease, 1502
for myasthenia gravis, 1706
for organ transplant patient, 2850
in pregnancy, 2776
toxicity of, 1417
Azidothymidine, in pregnancy, 2764t, 2774
Azithromycin
during pregnancy and lactation, 2784
for AIDS-related diarrhea, 1484
for *Campylobacter* gastroenteritis, 1461, 1461t
for chancroid, 1559t, 1563
for *Chlamydia trachomatis* infection, 1559t, 1565
for chronic obstructive pulmonary disease, 1106
for granuloma inguinale, 1559t, 1563
for Lyme disease, 1789, 2127t, 2128
for *Mycobacterium avium* infection in HIV/AIDS, 2076
for nongonococcal urethritis, 1565
for pertussis, 2006
for pharyngitis, 1113
for pneumonia, 2558t
for salmonellosis, 1463
in HIV/AIDS, side effects of, 2079t
Azotemia. *See also* Uremia.
evaluation of, 1533f, 1537
prerenal, 1527t, 1532-1533, 1533b, 1538
Aztreonam, for febrile, neutropenic cancer patient, 2837, 2838t

B cell antibodies, 2832
B cells
development of, 1820-1821, 1820f
in asthma, 1080, 1080f
Babesiosis, 2104-2105, 2113, 2138-2140, 2139f
Babinski's sign
in cerebral herniation, 355
in head trauma, 357
Baby oil, for tar removal, 927
Bacille Calmette-Guérin (BCG) vaccine, 2170-2171, 2170b
Bacillus anthracis, 3024
Bacillus anthracis gastroenteritis, 1461t, 1462t, 1468-1469
Bacillus cereus food poisoning, 1470t, 1471
Bacitracin ointment, for burn wounds, 926
Back, 490
examination of, in back pain, 263
gunshot wounds to, 506-507
stab wounds to, 505
Back blows, for airway foreign body, 2530
Back pain, 260-267
ancillary studies in, 264
chronic, 713
diagnostic approach to, 261-264, 261b, 262b, 263f
differential diagnosis in, 262t, 263f, 264, 265t-266t
disposition in, 267
empiric management of, 264, 266f, 267

Back pain *(Continued)*
epidemiology of, 260-261
functional, 703, 706
history in, 261b, 262
in diskitis, 1684
in elderly person, 707
in epidural abscess, 261, 265t, 703, 706, 712, 1684
in epidural hematoma, 1683
in epidural spinal cord compression, 1919
in pregnancy, 2733
in spinal cord tumor, 1685
in transverse myelitis, 1682
low, 701-715
anatomy and physiology in, 702, 702f
clinical features of, 703-707, 704t, 705f
differential considerations in, 709, 710b
disposition in, 713
epidemiology of, 701-702
laboratory tests in, 707
management of, 710-713, 711f
pathophysiology of, 702-703
pathophysiology of, 261
pediatric, 703, 707, 713
physical examination in, 261b, 262-264
radiologic imaging in, 707-709, 708b, 708f-709f
rapid assessment and stabilization in, 261-262, 263f
referred, 703, 706
skeletal muscle relaxants for, 2928-2929
uncomplicated, 703-704, 710-711
Baclofen
for gastroesophageal reflux, 1390
for spasticity in cerebral palsy, 2904
for spasticity in multiple sclerosis, 1673
Bacteremia. *See also* Sepsis.
definition of, 2212b
gonococcal, 1566
in AIDS-related diarrhea, 1483
in infective endocarditis, 1301
meningococcal, 2021, 2023
pediatric fever and, 2505-2506, 2512, 2515
pneumococcal, 2019
Bacterial infection
hyperpyrexia in, 2506
in bone or joint infections, 2177-2178, 2178t
in botulism, 2012-2016
in cancer patient with impaired cell-mediated immunity, 2839-2840
in conjunctivitis, 296t
in COPD exacerbation, 1099
in croup, 2528-2529, 2529t
in diarrhea, 228, 230b
in diphtheria, 2001-2004, 2003b
in endocarditis, prophylaxis for, 2590-2591, 2591b
in febrile cancer patient, 1908
in Kawasaki disease, 2024-2027, 2025b
in meningitis. *See* Meningitis, bacterial.
in meningococcal disease, 2020-2024
in organ transplant patient, 2848-2849, 2849f
in otitis media, 1066-1067
in peritonitis, 245-246, 1412-1413, 1441
in peritonsillitis, 1117
in pertussis, 2004-2007, 2005f, 2006b
in pharyngitis, 274-275, 275t, 1109
in pneumococcal disease, 2016-2020, 2020b
in pneumonia, 1129, 1130-1131
pediatric, 2555, 2556-2557, 2556f, 2557f, 2558t, 2563t
in prostatitis, 1586
in sinusitis, 1123, 1124, 1125
in tetanus, 2007-2012, 2008f, 2010b, 2012t, 2013t
in toxic shock syndrome, 2027-2031, 2028b, 2029b, 2029t
in tracheitis, 2528-2529, 2529t
in vaginosis, 1567t, 1568-1569, 2758
of hip and femur, pediatric limp from, 764
serious, in children, signs of, 2658, 2659t
Bacterial pathogens
in central nervous system infection, 1711t
in contaminated blood products, 60-61
in cutaneous abscess, 2203, 2203t
in dental plaque, 1028
Bacteriology, in urinary tract infection, 1574-1575
Bacteriuria, 1573, 2757-2758
Bacteroides fragilis, in Ludwig's angina, 1032
Bad news, delivering, 3146-3147, 3146b
Bag/mask ventilation. *See also* Mask ventilation.
difficult, evaluation of, 4, 4b
in adult resuscitation, 87
in neonatal resuscitation, 122
in pediatric resuscitation, 108
Baker's cyst, 796, 797f
BAL (British anti-Lewisite), for mercury poisoning, 2426
Balanoposthitis, 2637-2638, 2638f
Balantidiasis, 2100t
Ballistic injury, nonpenetrating, in chest wall trauma, 458-459
Ballistics, handgun wound, 954-955
Balloon-tipped catheter for foreign body removal, 862f, 863, 872-873
Ballottement, 2728
Bandage immobilization, 568-571
Bankart's fracture, in glenohumeral joint dislocation, 688
Barbiturates
after cerebral ischemia, 71-72
as induction agents, 15-16
for GHB withdrawal, 2490
for procedural sedation and analgesia, 2940t-2941t, 2945-2946
in children, 2953
for severe head trauma, 360-361
overdose of, 2481-2483, 2482b, 2482f
withdrawal from, 2482
Barium enema
in appendicitis, 1454
in colonic ischemia, 1504
in colonic volvulus, 1498f
in diverticular disease, 1493
in intussusception, 2611, 2611f
Barlow provocative test, in developmental hip dysplasia, 2701, 2702b
Barodontalgia, in scuba diving–related disorders, 2286
Barometric pressure, altitude and, 2297
Barosinusitis, in scuba diving–related disorders, 2282
Barotitis, 2281-2282, 2282f, 2286-2287, 2287t, 2292
Barotrauma, 2281
external ear, 2282, 2292
facial, 2282, 2293
gastrointestinal, 2286
inhalational, cocaine-induced, 2388
inner ear, 2282, 2287-2288, 2287t, 2292
middle ear, 2281-2282, 2282f, 2286-2287, 2287t, 2292
pulmonary, 2285-2286, 2293
Barrett's metaplasia, 1389
Bartholin abscess, 1560, 2205, 2205f
Bartholin cyst, 1559-1560
Barton bandage, for chronic temporomandibular joint dislocation, 1042
Bartonella, in infective endocarditis, 1301
Barton's fracture, 550t, 635-636, 636f
Bartter's syndrome, 1938
Basal ganglia lesions, in methanol poisoning, 2396
Base deficit
in abdominal trauma, 495
in shock, 46, 47
Basic life support systems, 2985-2986
Basic life support techniques, in pediatric resuscitation, 97-99
Basilar artery migraine, 1632, 2679
ataxia in, 2681
vertigo in, 2683
Basilar impression, in osteogenesis imperfecta, 2700-2701
Basilar skull fracture, 357, 358b, 373
meningitis after, 370
Basophil(s), 2834
activated, mediators of, 1823, 1823b
normal values for, 1886t
Battered child syndrome, 973
Batteries
impaction of, 1384
ingestion of, 871, 873, 2384-2385
Battering. *See* Abuse.
Battery, 2967
Baumann's angle, 651-652, 651f, 2694, 2695f
Bayesian statistics, 3056
Bazin's disease, 1816
Beanbag shotgun shells, ballistic injury associated with, 458-459
Beau's lines, in Kawasaki disease, 2026
Bed rest
for high-altitude pulmonary edema, 2304
for myocarditis, 1290
Bee pollen, adverse effects of, 2476t
Bee stings. *See* Hymenoptera stings.
Behavior
as symptom, 2976
grossly disorganized, in schizophrenia, 1728
of difficult patient, classification of, 2978-2981, 2978t. *See also* Difficult patient.
violent. *See* Combative patient; Violence.
Behavioral disorders. *See also* Psychiatric disorders.
in bacterial meningitis, 2658, 2659
in hyperthyroidism, 1987
in PCP intoxication, 2414, 2415-2416
seizures vs., 2668
Behavioral risk factors, in injury prevention and control, 947-948
Behçet's disease, 1814-1815
Belladona alkaloids, anticholinergic toxicity of, 2345, 2346, 2346b, 2347t
Bell's palsy, 1666-1667, 1668, 2123
Benazepril hydrochloride, 1322t
Bendroflumethiazide, during pregnancy and lactation, 2788
Bends, 2279, 2284
Beneficence, 3129, 3129b
Benign early repolarization, ST segment elevation in, 1166-1167, 1167f, 1168f
Benign paroxysmal positional vertigo, 147t, 2683
Benign rolandic epilepsy, 2666
Bennett's fracture, 550t, 599-600, 599f
Benzalkonium chloride, for rabies postexposure prophylaxis, 2068
Benzathine penicillin
for Lyme disease, 1789
for rheumatic fever, 1791
for scarlet fever, 1851
for streptococcal pharyngitis, 1304
for syphilis, 1856
Benznidazole, for Chagas' disease, 2112
Benzocaine, topical, 2933
Benzodiazepines
as induction agents, 16
during pregnancy and lactation, 2787
for agitation, 1654, 2349
for alcohol withdrawal syndrome, 2861-2862, 2863
for alcohol-related seizure, 2864, 2865
for anxiety disorders, 1750-1751, 1751t
for back pain, 267
for bupropion-induced seizure, 2361
for cocaine overdose, 2391
for GHB withdrawal, 2490
for PCP intoxication, 2416, 2892
for procedural sedation and analgesia, 2940t-2941t, 2944-2945
in children, 2953
for psychedelic-induced intoxication, 2408
for rapid tranquilization, 2962-2963
for seizure, 166, 166t, 1626, 1627t
for status epilepticus, 2672-2673, 2672t
for tetanus, 2010-2011
for thought disorders, 1731
in heatstroke, 2265
in ventilated patient, 30
overdose of, 2483-2486, 2484t
antidote to, 2326, 2329t, 2485-2486, 2485b
prophylactic, in severe head trauma, 361
reversal agents for, 2949
withdrawal from, 2486, 2486b
Benztropine
anticholinergic toxicity of, 2345
for acute extrapyramidal symptoms, 2449
for mood disorders, 1741
Bepridril, overdose of, 2376, 2377t
Bereavement, depression vs., 1740
Best interests, 3134
$Beta_2$ agonists
during pregnancy and lactation, 2762, 2765t, 2789
for anaphylactic shock, 54
for anaphylaxis, 1831b, 1832

Beta$_2$ agonists *(Continued)*
for asthma, 1086-1088, 1087t, 2538, 2539t, 2540-2541
for bronchiolitis, 2546
for chronic obstructive pulmonary disease, 1105
for hyperkalemia, 1941
for pneumonia, 2562
Beta blockers, 1208-1209, 1208t, 1321t
contraindications to, 1208
during pregnancy and lactation, 2788
for acute coronary syndromes, 1184-1185
for alcohol withdrawal syndrome, 2862
for anxiety disorders, 1751
for aortic dissection, 1328
for atrial fibrillation, 1232-1233
for atrial flutter, 1229
for atrial tachycardia, 1228
for chloral hydrate poisoning, 2487
for chronic heart failure, 1276-1277
for dilated cardiomyopathy, 1294
for glaucoma, 1063b
for hypertension, 1320
for hypertensive emergencies, 1318-1319
for hypertrophic cardiomyopathy, 1295
for junctional tachycardia, 1234
for migraine prophylaxis, 1634
for premature ventricular contractions, 1225
for tetanus, 2011
for thyroid storm, 1989
for torsades de pointes, 1241
for ventricular tachycardia, 1242-1243
for Wolff-Parkinson-White syndrome, 1237
heart failure from, 1269
overdose of, 2373-2376, 2373t, 2374b, 2375b
Beta (β) error, 3051t, 3052
Beta particles, 2319, 2320f
Betamethasone valerate, for phimosis, 2636
Beta-mimetics, for premature labor, 2806-2807, 2806b
Betaxolol, 1321t, 2373t
Betel nut
adverse effects of, 2476t
drug interactions with, 2478t
Bethanecol, for nausea and vomiting in children, 206
Beverages, MAOI toxicity and, 2364, 2364b
Bezoar
gastrointestinal, 873, 875
urinary tract, 877
Bezold abscess, in mastoiditis, 1072
Bias
attitudinal, 130
cognitive, 3122
confirmation, 132
definition of, 3059t
publication, 3050-3051, 3058
selection, 3049
visceral, 3122
Bicarbonate
in metabolic acidosis, 1929
in metabolic alkalosis, 1930
in respiratory acidosis, 1925
in respiratory alkalosis, 1926
inhalational, for irritant gas exposure, 2434-2435
sodium. *See* Sodium bicarbonate.
Bicarbonate–carbonic acid buffer system, 1923
Biceps muscle lesions, 697-698, 697f
Biceps tendon
long head of, 672, 673f, 697
rupture of, 668, 697-698
short head of, 697
subluxation and dislocation of, 698
Bicipital tendinopathy, 1797
Bicipital tenosynovitis, 697, 697f
Bier block, 2034
Bigeminy, 1222, 1222f
Bile acid administration, for cholelithiasis, 1419
Bile duct(s)
common, obstruction of, in cholangitis, 1421, 1422f
extrahepatic, carcinoma of, 1423
Bilevel positive airway pressure, 28, 28f
in critically ill asthmatic patient, 1092
Biliary cirrhosis, 1410
Biliary colic, in cholelithiasis, 1418
Biliary pancreatitis, 1426, 1427, 1428, 1433, 1434
Biliary tract carcinoma, 1422
Biliary tract disorders, 1418-1423
abdominal pain in, 210t
in children, 2620-2621
nausea and vomiting in, 204t
obstructive, jaundice in, 243, 244f
Bilious vomiting, in malrotation with midgut volvulus, 2606
Bilirubin
in acute pancreatitis, 1431, 1431t
in hemolytic anemia, 1878
in hepatitis, 1404
in infants and children, 2601-2603, 2602t, 2603b, 2603t, 2604f-2605f
in pyogenic abscess, 1415
metabolism of, 243
Bimalleolar fractures, 813
Bioethics, 3127-3138
dilemmas in, 3130-3131, 3132-3137
emergency medicine guidelines and, 3044
in decision-making capacity and consent, 3133-3135, 3134b
in disasters and triage, 3136
in emergency medicine, 3131-3137, 3131b, 3131t
in HIV/AIDS, 2089-2090
in medical teaching/training, 3135-3136
in occupational medicine, 3077
in prehospital resuscitation, 3132-3133
in resuscitation research, 3136-3137
in withholding and withdrawing treatment, 3132
legal issues vs., 3128
professional etiquette vs., 3128
values and, 3128-3130, 3129b, 3130b
Bioethics committees
as surrogate decision-makers, 3135
role of, 3137-3138
Bioethics consultants, as surrogate decision-makers, 3135
Biofeedback, for anxiety disorders, 1751
Biologic weapon(s), 3023-3029, 3024b
anthrax as, 3021, 3024-3026, 3025f, 3026b, 3026f
botulinum toxin as, 2013
disaster preparedness for, 3018
infectious agents as, 3024, 3024b
plague as, 3027-3028, 3027f, 3028b
smallpox as, 3028-3029, 3028f, 3029f
warning signs of, 3024, 3024b
Biological factors, in suicide, 1767-1768
Biomechanical properties of skin, 843
Biomechanical risk factors, in injury prevention and control, 946-947
Biomechanics of head trauma, 352
Biophysical profile of fetus, 2802, 2802t
Bioprosthetic valve, complications of, 1308
Biopsy
endomyocardial
in dilated cardiomyopathy, 1294
in myocarditis, 1290, 1290f
rectal, in AIDS-related diarrhea, 1484
skin, in Rocky Mountain spotted fever, 2135
small bowel, in AIDS-related diarrhea, 1484
Bipolar disorder
clinical features of, 1738-1739
differential considerations in, 1740-1741
epidemiology of, 1735
hypomanic episode in, 1738
manic episode in, 1738-1739, 1738b
mixed, 1739
pathophysiology of, 1735-1736
stabilization in, 1741
treatment of, 1742
Bipyridyl compound poisoning, 2465-2466, 2465b
Bird's beak sign, in colonic volvulus, 1498f
Birth, transitional circulation at, 118-119, 119t, 2568
Birth defects
alcohol-related, 2791-2792, 2791b
drug-induced, 2779-2780, 2780b
Birth trauma, postpartum hemorrhage from, 2818
Bismuth
for diarrhea, 236t
for traveler's diarrhea, 1400
for upper gastrointestinal disorders, 1399
Bisoprolol fumarate, 1321t, 2373t
Bispectral Index monitoring, during procedural sedation and analgesia, 2919
Bisphosphonates
for hypercalcemia, 1946
for hypercalcemic cancer patient, 1916
Bite
animal, 882-892
antibiotic prophylaxis in, 887-888, 887t
cats in, 883-884, 888
disposition in, 889-890
dogs in, 882-883, 887-888
domestic herbivores in, 885
epidemiology of, 882
ferrets in, 884-885
infected, treatment of, 889-890
infection risks in, 885-886, 885t
management of, 886-889, 886b, 887t, 889b, 889t
pigs in, 885
primates in, 884, 888-889, 889b, 889t
reporting requirements for, 3172-3173
rodents in, 884
systemic infection in, 885
wild animals in, 885
antibiotic prophylaxis for, 854-855
human, 890-892, 891t, 892b
antibiotic prophylaxis in, 891-892
antiviral prophylaxis in, 891
in child abuse, 969
in clenched-fist injuries, 611
in extensor tendon injuries at metacarpophalangeal joint, 608
in sexual assault, 986b
infected, treatment of, 892, 892b
tetanus prophylaxis in, 891, 891t
to penis, 534
rabies transmission from, 2065
venomous, 894-911
arthropods in, 903-908
marine animals in, 908-909, 910
scorpions in, 907-908
snakes and other reptiles in, 895-903, 897f, 897t, 900t
spiders in, 905-907
venom delivery in, 895
Bite marks, in physical assault, 962, 962f
Bitolterol, for asthma, 2538, 2539t
Bittering agents, in automotive products, 2402
Bivalirudin, in myocardial infarction, 1188
BK virus, 2045-2046
Black widow spider bite, 905-906, 2329t
Bladder
anatomy of, 519
decompression of, for urinary retention, 1599
distention of, in spinal cord injury, 2906
dysfunction of, in multiple sclerosis, 1672
neurogenic, in spinal cord injury, 2908
physical examination of, 1572-1573
stones in, 1593
trauma to, 519-526, 521f-526f, 719
Bladder neck obstruction, 1538
Blanch sign of Steele, in slipped capital femoral epiphysis, 2708
Blastic crisis, in chronic myeloid leukemia, 1888
Blastomyces dermatitidis, in pneumonia, 1130
Bleach, ingestion of, 2380-2381
Blebs, in frostbite, 2231
Bleeding. *See also* Hemorrhage.
after hemodialysis, 1549
from arteriovenous fistula or graft, 1366
gastrointestinal, 220-227. *See also* Gastrointestinal bleeding.
in facial trauma, 389, 390
in hemothorax, 465
in neck trauma, 444
in peripheral vascular injury, 539
in radiation proctocolitis, 1505
nasal, 394
rectal, 1508
in Meckel's diverticulum, 2618
with defecation, 1508
vaginal, 254-259. *See also* Vaginal bleeding.
Bleeding diathesis
in alcoholism, 2874
in disseminated intravascular coagulation, 1903
in hyperviscosity syndrome, 1913
in pregnancy, 2753t
Bleeding disorders, 1892-1904
ancillary studies in, 1894-1895, 1894b
clinical features of, 1894-1895, 1894b

Bleeding disorders *(Continued)*
differential diagnosis and management of, 1895-1904
disposition in, 1904
in alcoholism, 2874
in coagulopathies, 1899-1904
in platelet disorders, 1896-1899, 1896b
in vascular disorders, 1896, 1896b
pathophysiology of, 1892-1894, 1893b, 1893f
Bleeding time, in bleeding disorders, 1895
Blepharitis, 293t, 1055
Blinding in clinical trials, 3049
Blindness. *See also* Visual loss.
cortical, 1060
legal, 2905
postconcussive, 367
river, 2109, 2109f
Blister
burn, 925
fracture, 563
in frostbite, 2232, 2233f
in mustard exposure, 3031
Blocking agents, for internal radioactive contamination, 2324
Blood
leukodepleted, in hemorrhagic shock, 52
occult, tests for, in gastrointestinal bleeding, 222
vomiting of, 221
Blood agents, as chemical weapons, 939, 3031-3032
Blood alcohol concentration (BAC), 2859
Blood alcohol tests, police-requested, medicolegal issues in, 3160
Blood banking, 57
Blood component therapy, 56-61
clinical features in, 58
decision making in, 58-59
outcomes in, 59-61
pathophysiologic principles in, 57-58, 58t
therapeutic modalities in, 59
Blood culture
in acute septic arthritis, 2705
in AIDS-related diarrhea, 1483-1484
in bacterial meningitis, 2662
in central nervous system infection, 1720
in gastrointestinal anthrax, 1469
in infected aneurysm, 1356
in infective endocarditis, 1301-1302
in meningococcal disease, 2022
in pediatric fever, 2510
in pneumococcal disease, 2018
in pneumonia, 1135, 2561
in sepsis, 2216-2217
Blood dyscrasias, oral manifestations of, 1036
Blood flow. *See also* Circulation.
cerebral, 350-352, 351f
after brain resuscitation, 68
autoregulation of, 351
loss of, 354
during cardiopulmonary resuscitation, 67
during cerebral ischemia, 62, 63f-64f
in hypothermia, 2238
in stroke, 1606-1607
restoration of, after cardiac arrest, 62-64
during cardiopulmonary resuscitation, 76-77
renal, in hypothermia, 2239
to skin, in pediatric assessment triangle, 2498t, 2499, 2499f
Blood gases, arterial. *See* Arterial blood gases.
Blood loss, anemia from, 1868
Blood pressure. *See also* Hypertension; Hypotension.
in pregnancy, 316, 317t, 2725, 2727
management of
guidelines for, 3038
in aortic rupture, 481
in peripheral vascular injury, 543
measurement of, 1310-1311
monitoring of, 35-36
normalization of, in sepsis, 2218
pediatric, 2495, 2495t, 2571, 2571t, 2578, 2651t
Blood products, bacterial contamination of, 60-61
Blood protein buffers, 1923
Blood sample, in anemia, 1869
Blood smear
in anemia, 1869
in babesiosis, 2140
in bleeding disorders, 1894
Blood smear *(Continued)*
in hemolytic anemia, 1877, 1877f, 1878f
in sickle cell disease, 1881, 1881f
Blood supply
to face, 385, 385f
to femur and hip, 737, 737t, 738f
to foot, 821
to forearm, 640t
to hand, 585-586, 587f, 588f
to knee, 771
to lower leg, 797
to nose, 1073, 1073f
to pelvis, 717-718
to shoulder, 672
to wrist, 622, 625f
Blood tests
in chronic obstructive pulmonary disease, 1101
in gastrointestinal bleeding, 222
in septic arthritis, 2189
Blood transfusion, 56-61
adjuncts in, 58
clinical features in, 58
decision making in, 58-59
hepatitis C infection risk in, 1403
hypocalcemia after, 1943
in autoimmune hemolytic anemia, 1883
in gastrointestinal bleeding, 222
in hemolytic uremic syndrome, 2655
in kernicterus prophylaxis, 2603, 2604f
in multiple trauma, 307-308
in pelvic fracture, 723, 728, 731
in peripheral vascular injury, 543
in placenta previa or abruptio placentae, 2748
in sickle cell disease, 1880
in thalassemia, 1872-1873
massive, 57-58
outcomes in, 59-61
pathophysiologic principles in, 57-58, 58t
refusal of, 3171-3172
therapeutic modalities in, 59
thrombocytopenia after, 1897
viral infection transmission and, 57t, 61
Blood typing, 57, 58
Blood urea nitrogen (BUN), 1527
dialysis and, 1549
in acute renal failure, 2649
in hypothermia, 2243
in nausea and vomiting, 203
Blood volume, in pregnancy, 316-317, 317t, 2724, 2724f
Blood-borne pathogen exposure, 3081-3087, 3084t, 3085t, 3086b
Bloodborne Pathogen Standard, 3082
Blood-brain barrier, 350
Bloody show, in labor and delivery, 2798-2799
Bloody stool, 221
in hemolytic uremic syndrome, 2654
in hemorrhagic *Escherichia coli* serotype O157:H7 gastroenteritis, 1466
in inflammatory bowel disease, 2616
in intussusception, 2610
in *Plesiomonas shigelloides* gastroenteritis, 1468
Blowout fracture, orbital wall, 393
"Blue bloater," 1099
Blue cohosh, adverse effects of, 2476t
Blue leg, painful, 1370
Blue toe syndrome
in abdominal aortic aneurysm, 1332
in arteriosclerosis obliterans, 1350
in atheroembolism, 1343, 1353, 1353f
Blunt trauma
abdominal
diagnostic studies in, 507-508, 507t
epidemiology of, 489
history in, 493
management of, 508-510, 508f, 509t, 510f, 511f
observation in, 3067
pathophysiology of, 491-492
physical examination in, 494-495
chest
aortic injury in, 476-482, 477f-479f, 481b
cardiac injury in, 467-472
esophageal injury in, 483-484
flail chest and, 457
observation in, 3068
from lightning, 2271
in physical assault, 960-962, 961f-962f
Blunt trauma *(Continued)*
in pregnancy, 318, 2734
in sternal fracture, 456
ocular, 1044-1051
peripheral vascular injury in, 536-547
clinical features of, 539-541, 540f
diagnostic strategies in, 541-543
disposition in, 547
epidemiology of, 536-537
of lower extremity, 546-547
of upper extremity, 544-546
pathophysiology of, 537-539, 538f
treatment of, 543-544
renal, 527, 528-530, 530f
to ear, 392
to neck
pathophysiology of, 442
pharyngoesophageal injuries in, 446-447
vascular injuries in, 448-450
ureteral, 530
Bockhart, impetigo of, 2202
Body
cooling of
for comatose survivors of cardiac arrest, 69
for heatstroke, 2263-2264, 2264b, 2265f
rewarming of. *See* Rewarming.
skin tension lines of, 844f
viewing of, after death, 3148-3149
Body lice, 1853-1854, 1853f
Body packing/stuffing
cocaine, 2391-2392
management of, 874-875, 2886
opioid, 2454
Body surface area assessment, in burn injury, 919-920, 920f
Body surface mapping, in acute coronary syndromes, 1174
Body temperature
abnormalities of. *See* Fever; Heat illness; Hyperthermia; Hypothermia.
changes in, during air medical transport, 2995
determination of, in children, 2508
regulation of. *See* Thermoregulation.
Boehler's angle, 827, 827f
Boerhaave's syndrome, 201-202, 206t, 484
Bolivian hemorrhagic fever, 2056
Bone
anatomy of, 2174-2175, 2175f
as buffer, 1923
fracture of. *See* Fracture.
growing, 554, 556f, 2689
infection of. *See* Osteomyelitis.
needle aspiration of, in osteomyelitis, 2182
of distal humerus and elbow, 647, 647f
of foot, 820-821, 820f
of forearm, 639
of hand, 577-578, 579f-580f
of hip and femur, 736-737, 737f
of knee, 770, 771f
of lower leg, 797
of wrist, 622, 623f
periosteal formation of, 2699
plastic deformation of, 2690
Bone bruise, in knee, 781
Bone cancer, hypercalcemia in, 1914
Bone marrow transplantation
for aplastic anemia, 1875-1876
for sickle cell disease, 1881
Bone pain, in osteomyelitis, 2179
Bone scan
in ankle trauma, 811
in arthritis, 1780
in foot trauma, 822
in fracture, 558
in frostbite, 2231
in hip fracture, 746, 748f
in knee trauma, 774
in Legg-Calvé-Perthes disease, 2707
in lower leg stress fractures, 804
in osteomyelitis, 2180-2181, 2180f, 2181f
in scaphoid fracture, 628
in septic arthritis, 2189-2190
in stress fracture of foot, 838
Bone tumor, osteomyelitis vs., 2186
Bonferonni correction for reducing risk of type I error, 3053-3054
Bonfils Intubating Fiberscope, 21, 22f
Bony fish injuries, 910-911
Borborygmi, in *Giardia* gastroenteritis, 1479

Borderline personality disorder, 2979b
  depression vs., 1740
  suicide and, 1769
Bordetella pertussis/parapertussis, 2004-2007, 2005f, 2006b, 2559-2560
Borrelia burgdorferi, 3118. *See also* Lyme disease.
Borrelia spp., in relapsing fever, 2129
Bosworth fracture, 550t
Botanical poisoning. *See* Plant poisoning.
Botulinum toxin, 2013, 2014
  for anal fissures, 1513
Botulism, 1707-1708, 2012-2016
Bougienage, for foreign body removal, 873, 2617
Boutonniére deformity, 607, 607f
Bovine pustular stomatitis virus, 2040
Bowel. *See* Intestinal *entries;* Intestine(s); Large intestine; Small intestine.
Bowel sounds, in abdominal trauma, 494
Bowstring sign, in lumbar radiculopathy, 704
Boxer's fracture, 550t, 597, 597f
Boyle's law, 2280, 2281f, 2994
Brachial artery
  anatomy of, 540, 540f, 648, 648f
  injury to, 545, 665
Brachial plexus, 672, 1676
  compression of, thoracic outlet syndrome from, 1358
  injury to, 1692-1693, 1693b
    axillary artery injury and, 545
    scapula fracture and, 680
    subclavian artery injury and, 545
  testing of, 674, 674t
Bracing, functional, for ankle immobilization, 571
Bradycardia, 1215
  in beta blocker overdose, 2374-2375
  in hypothermia, 2237
  pediatric, 111, 111f, 2585, 2586t
  sinus, 1215-1216, 1216f
    from succinylcholine, 13
    in hypothyroidism, 1992
Bradycardia-tachycardia syndrome, 1231
Brain. *See also* Cerebral *entries.*
  anatomy and physiology of, 350-352, 351f
  cellular damage to, in head trauma, 352-353, 353f
  contusion of, 374
  diffuse axonal injury in, 374
  inflammation of. *See* Encephalitis.
  membranes of, inflammation of. *See* Meningitis.
  pediatric, vulnerability of, 366
  swelling of. *See* Cerebral edema.
  traumatic injury to. *See* Head trauma; Traumatic brain injury.
Brain abscess
  after head trauma, 370-371
  ancillary studies in, 1720
  cerebrospinal fluid analysis in, 1716-1719, 1717t, 1718t, 1719f
  complications of, 1716
  diagnosis of, 1716-1720
  differential considerations in, 1720, 1721b
  disposition in, 1723
  epidemiology of, 1711
  etiology of, 1712
  headache in, 174t, 1641, 2678
  in cancer patient, 1920
  in otitis media, 1068
  lumbar puncture in, 1716, 1716b
  management of, 1722, 1723
  neuroimaging studies in, 1719-1720
  pathophysiology of, 1713, 1713f
  risk factors for, 171b
  signs and symptoms of, 1714-1715
Brain damage
  seizure and, 2665
  violent behavior and, 2957
Brain death, 3141
Brain resuscitation, 62-73
  clinical outcomes in, 72-73
  experimental therapies in, 70-72
  pathophysiology of cerebral ischemia and, 62-67, 63f-64f
  standard strategies for, 67-70, 69t
Brain tumor
  ataxia in, 2681
  cerebral herniation in, 1918
Brain tumor *(Continued)*
  headache in, 1637-1638, 2678
  in pregnancy, 2732
Brainstem
  assessment of, in head trauma, 357
  in arousal, 156
Brainstem encephalitis, ataxia in, 2681
Brainstem reflex examination, in comatose patient, 159t, 160-161
Branham's sign, 1347
Brassaia, 2472
BRAT diet, for diarrhea, 235
Braxton-Hicks contractions, 2728, 2798
Breast
  cancer of
    hypercalcemia in, 1914
    superior vena cava syndrome in, 1909
  changes in, during pregnancy, 2724, 2728
Breast milk jaundice, 2601-2603, 2602t, 2603b, 2603t, 2604f-2605f
Breast feeding, in HIV/AIDS, 2774
Breath sounds
  in tension pneumothorax, 462
  in tuberculosis, 2150
Breath-holding spells
  definition of, 2714
  seizures vs., 2668
Breathing
  management of
    in cardiac arrest, 87
    in elderly trauma patient, 348
    in pediatric resuscitation, 98, 108-109
    in pediatric trauma, 329-330, 332t
  periodic, in acute mountain sickness, 2301, 2302
  work of, in pediatric assessment triangle, 2498-2499, 2498f, 2498t, 2499f
Breathlessness. *See* Dyspnea.
Breech presentations, in labor and delivery, 2811-2813, 2811b, 2812f, 2813b
Bretylium, 1209
"Bridegroom's palsy," 1695
Broca's aphasia, in ischemic stroke, 1609
Brodie's abscess, 2184
Bromocriptine, for neuroleptic malignant syndrome, 2449
Bronchial artery embolization, for hemoptysis, 282
Bronchial hyperresponsiveness, in asthma, 2533
Bronchiectasis
  hemoptysis in, 280
  in chronic obstructive pulmonary disease, 1102-1103
Bronchiolitis, in children, 2509b, 2544-2546
Bronchitis
  chronic, 1097, 1100
  high-altitude, 2304
  laryngotracheal, 2525-2527, 2526f, 2527b
Broncholithiasis, hemoptysis in, 280
Bronchopleural fistula, 466
Bronchopulmonary dysplasia, 2565, 2565f
Bronchorrhea, in organophosphate poisoning, 2459
Bronchoscopy
  in acute inhalation injury, 921
  in foreign body removal, 870, 2551
  in hemoptysis, 282
  in neck trauma, 445
  in tracheobronchial injury, 466
  in tuberculosis, 2154
Bronchospasm
  heroin-induced, 2452-2453
  in anaphylaxis, 1825t, 1829-1830
  in irritant gas exposure, 2434
Bronchostenosis, tuberculous, 2151
Bronchus, ruptured, subcutaneous emphysema and, 459
Broselow emergency tape, in pediatric resuscitation, 106, 114f 115f
Brow presentations, in labor and delivery, 2815-2816
Brown recluse spider bite, 906-907
Brown-Séquard syndrome, 418, 419f, 420, 1677-1678, 1678f
Brudzinski sign
  in bacterial meningitis, 2059
  in central nervous system infection, 1714
Brugada criteria, 1237, 1239f
Bruises, in child abuse, 969-971, 969f, 970f, 970t, 2502b
Bruit, in arteriovenous fistula, 539, 541
Bruit de moulin, in myocardial rupture, 471
Brush ECG criteria, for risk stratification in acute coronary ischemia, 3065
B-type natriuretic peptide
  as cardiac marker, 1178
  in asthma, 1085
  in chronic obstructive pulmonary disease, 1101, 1102
  in heart failure, 1269-1270
  in pulmonary embolism, predictive value of, 1377, 1378t
Bubo, in tularemia, 2131
Bubonic plague, 3027, 3027f
Buccal space infection, 1028-1029
Bucket-handle fracture, 727, 729f
Bucket-handle tears, meniscal, 792
Buckle fracture, 800, 2690, 2690f
Buddy-taping
  of metacarpal or phalangeal fractures, 595, 595f
  of phalangeal fractures, 834
Budesonide
  for asthma, 1089
  for viral croup, 2526-2527
Buerger's disease, 1351-1352
Buerger's sign, 1346
Buffer systems, physiologic, 1923
Buffer therapy. *See* Sodium bicarbonate.
Buffering, in local anesthesia, 846, 2932-2933, 2932b
Bufo toad, tryptamines obtained from, 2407
Bulk agents, for constipation, 241t, 242
Bullae, 1839t
  giant, pneumothorax vs., 1146
  in frostbite, 2231
  in pemphigus vulgaris, 1857, 1857f
  in varicella, 1858, 1859f
  subpleural, in pneumothorax, 1145
Bullet
  handgun, 954, 954f
  rubber, ballistic injury associated with, 458-459
Bullet resistant vests, ballistic injury associated with, 458-459
Bullosis diabeticorum, 1972
Bullous impetigo, 1842, 1843, 2202
Bullous myringitis, 1066-1067
Bullying behavior, 1017
Bumetanide, 1321t
  for acute renal failure, 2650
Bundle branch fascicles, 1202
Bunyavirus, 2034t, 2055
Bupivacaine, 2931t, 2932t, 2933
  allergy to, 846-847
  for femoral and hip fractures, 749
  for local anesthesia, 846
  in knee trauma, 776
  in radial head and neck fracture, 664
Buprenorphine, 2924-2925, 2924b
Bupropion, overdose of, 2361, 2361t
Burkholderia cepacia, in cystic fibrosis, 2564-2565
Burn
  chemical, 929-939
    acid and alkali burns in, 931-933
    anhydrous ammonia in, 934-935
    caustics in, 2380-2385, 2381f, 2381t, 2382f
    cement burns in, 935
    chemical terrorism and, 937-939, 938t
    community preparedness and HAZMAT response in, 930-931
    elemental metals in, 937
    esophageal perforation from, 483
    formic acid in, 934
    hydrocarbon-related, 936-937
    hydrofluoric acid in, 933-934
    nitrates in, 936
    pathophysiology of, 930
    phenol and derivatives in, 935-936
    tar burns in, 937
    white phosphorus in, 936
  classification of, 913
  epidemiology of, 913-914, 914f
  feathering, 2273, 2273f
  in acute radiation syndrome, 2322
  in elderly person, 347
  in electrical and lightning injuries, 2267-2277
    clinical features of, 2271 2274, 2272f
    complications of, 2274
    differential considerations in, 2275

Burn *(Continued)*
    disposition in, 2277
    management of, 2275-2277, 2276b
    mechanisms of, 2270-2271, 2270b
    perioral, 391
    physics of, 2267-2270, 2268t, 2269t
  in mustard exposure, 3031
  kissing, 2272, 2272f
  management of, 920-927
  pathophysiology of, 915-919
  powder, 953
  thermal, 913-928
    airway management and respiratory care in, 921-923
    anatomy of skin and, 914-915
    burn shock and, 918
    burn wound assessment in, 919-920, 920f
    burn wound care in, 924-927, 925f
    catheterization of patient in, 923
    depth of burn injury in, 918-919, 919f
    disposition in, 927, 927b
    epidemiology of, 913-914, 914f
    fluid resuscitation in, 921, 922-923
    gastrointestinal disorders in, 924
    in child abuse, 969-970, 970f, 970t
    in lightning injury, 2273
    in physical assault, 963, 964f
    metabolic response to therapy in, 919
    ocular, 1046
    pain management in, 924
    patient categorization in, 920
    pediatric considerations in, 923
    physiologic changes in, 917-918
    prehospital care in, 921
    thermodynamics of burn injury in, 915-917, 915t, 916f, 917t
    transportation of patient in, 923-924
    white phosphorus in, 936
    zones of tissue injury in, 917, 917f
Burn center, patient transfer to, 927, 927b
Burn shock, 918
Burnout, in emergency physician, 3175-3176
Burow's solution, for tinea corporis, 1839-1840
Bursa
  aspiration of, 1802
  elbow, 649
  radiohumeral, 649
  radioulnar, flexor tendons and, 585, 586f
  trochanteric, calcification of, 742, 744f
Bursitis, 568, 1801-1804
  anserine, 1803-1804
  calcific, of femur and hip, 742, 744f
  common sites for, 1796f
  iliopsoas, 1803
  ischiogluteal, 1803
  knee, 795-796
  olecranon and prepatellar, 1801-1803
  septic, 1801-1803
  subacromial, 693-696, 694t, 695f, 1803
  subcalcaneal, 836
  trochanteric, 1803
Burst fracture of vertical body, 411-412, 411f-413f, 426, 427f
Buspirone
  for anxiety disorders, 1751, 1751t
  for opioid withdrawal, 2456
  overdose of, 2486
Butanediol, overdose of, 2488b, 2489
Butorphanol, 2924, 2924b
Butter, for tar removal, 927
Button (disk) batteries, ingestion of, 871, 873, 875, 2384-2385
Buttonhole deformity, 607, 607f
Butyrophenones
  cardiotoxicity of, 2445
  for alcohol withdrawal syndrome, 2862
  for psychedelic-induced intoxication, 2408
  for psychostimulant intoxication, 2410
Bypass, cardiopulmonary. *See* Cardiopulmonary bypass.
Bypass graft
  coronary artery, previous, fibrinolytic therapy eligibility and, 1191
  for peripheral arteriovascular disease, 1350

Cachexia, palliative care for, 3154
Café coronary, 865, 1383
Caffeine
  for postdural puncture headache, 1641
  sudden infant death syndrome and, 2719-2720
CAGE questions, for alcoholism, 2858
Caisson's disease, 2279, 2284
Calcaneofibular ligament injury, 816, 817
Calcaneus
  fracture of, 826-827, 826f, 827f
  stress fracture of, 836, 837
Calcification
  in bursitis of femur and hip, 742, 744f
  in hip trauma, 741-742, 743f-755f
  in pancreatitis, 1435-1436, 1436f
  in peritendinitis of femur and hip, 742
  in tendinitis, 698
  in tendinopathy, 568, 1797-1798
  of gallstones, 1418, 1418f
Calcitonin
  for hypercalcemia, 1915, 1946
  in calcium homeostasis, 1941
Calcium
  for beta blocker overdose, 2375
  for hyperkalemia
    in acute renal failure, 1539
    in chronic renal failure, 1545, 1545t
  for hypermagnesemia, 1950
  for hypocalcemia, 1539, 1943-1944
  for pediatric resuscitation, 101t, 104
  imbalance of. *See* Hypercalcemia; Hypocalcemia.
  in cerebral ischemia, 65
  in phosphate homeostasis, 1950-1951
  in resting membrane potential, 1199-1200, 1200f
  in shock, 45
  normal physiology of, 1941-1942
  serum, measurement of, 1942
Calcium antacids, for upper gastrointestinal disorders, 1398
Calcium apatite crystals, in pseudogout, 1787
Calcium channel blockers, 1210-1211, 1321t
  after cerebral ischemia, 71
  antidotes to, 2329t
  during pregnancy and lactation, 2788
  for acute coronary syndromes, 1185
  for atrial fibrillation, 1232-1233
  for atrial flutter, 1229
  for atrial tachycardia, 1228
  for chronic heart failure, 1276
  for dysphagia, 1398
  for hypertrophic cardiomyopathy, 1295
  for junctional tachycardia, 1234
  for premature labor, 2807
  for premature ventricular contractions, 1225
  for ventricular tachycardia, 1243
  for Wolff-Parkinson-White syndrome, 1235, 1237
  heart failure from, 1269
  overdose of, 2376-2379, 2377b, 2377t, 2378b
Calcium chelation, hypocalcemia from, 1943
Calcium chloride
  for calcium channel blocker–induced hypotension, 2377-2378
  for cardiac arrest, 93
  for hyperkalemia, 1940-1941, 2650
  for verapamil-induced hypotension, 1210
Calcium disodium edetate, for radioactive lead poisoning, 2324
Calcium disodium ethylenediaminetetraacetic acid, for lead poisoning, 2422
Calcium gluconate
  for hydrofluoric acid burns, 933
  for hyperkalemia, 1940-1941
Calcium hydroxide dust particles, in scuba diving–related disorders, 2283
Calcium hydroxide paste, for dentin fractures, 1037
Calcium hydroxyapatite crystals, in calcific tendinopathy, 1797
Calcium oxalate crystals, in ethylene glycol poisoning, 2398, 2399-2400
Calcium oxalate kidney stones, 1587
Calcium pumps, 1976, 1977f
Calcium pyrophosphate crystals
  in pseudogout, 1786
  in synovial fluid, 1782
"Calcium sign," in aortic dissection, 1326
Calculus
  gallbladder, 1418-1419, 1418f, 1419f. *See also* Cholelithiasis.
  renal, 1586-1593, 1586b, 1589f-1592f, 1593b. *See also* Urolithiasis.
  vesical, 1593
Calf veins, 1368
  isolated thrombosis of, 1370
Calicivirus, 2034t, 2057-2058
California encephalitis, 2055
Callus formation, in fracture healing, 564
Calpains
  in cerebral necrosis, 66
  inhibitors of, after cerebral ischemia, 72
Calyces, 527, 527f
Calymmatobacterium granulomatis, in granuloma inguinale, 1563
Cam walker, for ankle immobilization, 571
Campylobacter infection
  in dysenteric colitis, 229t
  in gastroenteritis, 1460-1461, 1461t, 1462t, 2625
Canalicular system, lacerations involving, 1051, 1051f
Cancer. *See also site of cancer, e.g.,* Breast, cancer of.
  acute tumor lysis syndrome in, 1911-1912, 1911b, 1912b
  adrenal insufficiency in, 1996
  alcoholism and, 2874
  central nervous system infections in, 1920
  cerebral herniation in, 1918
  dyspnea in, 179t
  encephalopathy in, 1920-1921
  epidural spinal cord compression in, 1919-1920
  fever in, 1907-1909, 1908b
  HIV/AIDS and, 2079
  hypercalcemia in, 1914-1916, 1915b, 1944-1945
  hyperuricemia in, 1913-1914
  hyperviscosity syndrome in, 1912-1913
  hypophosphatemia in, 1951-1952
  immune defects in, 2834-2841, 2836t, 2838t
  neoplastic cardiac tamponade in, 1916-1918
  neutropenia in, 2834-2839, 2836t, 2838t
  oncologic emergencies in, 1907-1921
  pediatric fever in, 2516
  seizures in, 1919
  skin lesions associated with, 1862-1864
  superior vena cava syndrome in, 1909-1911, 1910f
Cancrum oris, 1033
Candesartan, 1322t
Candida albicans
  in catheter-related infections, 1363
  in diaper dermatitis, 1852
  vaginitis in, in pregnancy, 2758
Candida bezoar, 877
Candida infection
  in cancer patient with impaired cell-mediated immunity, 2840
  in esophagitis, 1386, 1387
  in febrile, neutropenic cancer patient, 2836
  in HIV/AIDS, 2083-2084
  in infective endocarditis, 1301
  in osteomyelitis, 2178
  in pericarditis, 1286
  in pharyngitis, 275, 1112, 1113
  skin lesions in, 1840-1841
Candidiasis
  cutaneous, 1841
  esophageal, 2083-2084
  oral, 2083
  vulvovaginal, 1567t, 1568
Canine search team, 3006
Canine space infection, 1028
Cannabis plants, 2411
"Can't intubate, can't oxygenate" situation, 8
Canthal tendon, lacerations involving, 1051
Capacity, decision-making, 3133-3134, 3134b
Capillary refill, delayed, in peripheral vascular injury, 539
Capitate
  anatomy of, 622, 623f, 625
  fracture of, 630
Capitellum
  anatomy of, 647, 647f
  fracture of, 661-662, 661f
    in little leaguer's elbow, 663, 663f

Capitolunate angle, 626, 627f
Capnocytophaga canimorsus infection, in dog bites, 883, 887-888
Capnography/capnometry, 37-39, 38f
  during cardiopulmonary resuscitation, 81-82, 81f
Capreomycin, for tuberculosis, 2163t
Capsaicin, toxicity of, 2472
Capsicum annum, 2472
Capsule
  hip, 736, 736f
  shoulder, 672, 673f
Capsulitis, adhesive, 682, 698-699, 699t, 1797
Captopril, 1322t
  during pregnancy and lactation, 2788
Caput medusae, in cirrhosis, 1410
Carbamate poisoning, 2329t, 2458b, 2461-2462
Carbamazepine
  during pregnancy and lactation, 2786
  for neuropathic pain, 1692
  for seizure, 2675, 2675t
  for tic douloureux, 1034
  for trigeminal neuralgia, 1664, 1666
  side effects of, 1628t
Carbon dioxide
  arterial pressure of
    end-tidal carbon dioxide and, 37-38
    in metabolic acidosis, 1929
    in metabolic alkalosis, 1930
    in pregnancy, 318
    in respiratory acidosis, 1925
    in respiratory alkalosis, 1926
    minute ventilation and, 1923
  end-tidal, 37-39, 38f
    during cardiopulmonary resuscitation, 81-82, 81f
    for confirmation of endotracheal tube placement, 6, 6f
    in children, 2504
    monitoring of, during procedural sedation and analgesia, 2942-2943
  partial pressure of
    altitude and, 2297, 2297b
    cerebral blood flow and, 351, 351f
    transcutaneous, 36
  retention of, in chronic obstructive pulmonary disease, 1100
Carbon monoxide poisoning, 2438-2441
  cyanosis in, 271-272
  headache in, 174t
  in scuba diving–related disorders, 2283
  metabolic acidosis in, 1927
  nausea and vomiting in, 206t
  rhabdomyolysis in, 1979
  risk factors for, 171b
  with cyanide poisoning, 2440-2441
Carbon tetrachloride, toxicity of, 2887
Carbonated beverages, for esophageal obstruction, 1384
Carbonic acid–bicarbonate buffer system, 1923
Carbonic anhydrase inhibitors
  for glaucoma, 1063b
  metabolic acidosis from, 1929
Carboxyhemoglobin toxicity
  cyanosis in, 271-272
  in burn injury, 922
Carbuncle, 1843, 2204
Carcinoma
  biliary tract, 1423
  hepatocellular, 1417
  pancreatic, 1437-1438
  scrotal, 2642
  testicular, 2642
Cardiac. *See also* Heart *entries*.
Cardiac agents. *See* Cardiovascular drugs.
Cardiac amyloidosis, 1297
Cardiac arrest, 75-94
  airway and breathing management in, 87
  algorithm for, 89f
  asystole and, 84-85
  cardiopulmonary resuscitation in, 88-90
  defibrillation in, 90-91
  epidemiology of, 76
  etiology of, 77-78, 78t
  factors preceding, 77
  history and physical examination in, 78-79, 79t
  in anaphylaxis, 1825t
  in critically ill asthmatic patient, 1093
  in electrical and lightning injuries, 2272, 2274
Cardiac arrest *(Continued)*
  in pulmonary embolism, 1379-1380
  monitoring in, 79-82, 80f-82f, 80t
  neurologic recovery after, 62-73
    clinical outcomes in, 72-73
    experimental therapies in, 70-72
    pathophysiology of cerebral ischemia and, 62-67, 63f-64f
    standard strategies for, 67-70, 69t
  outcomes in, 93
  pacing in, 91
  pathophysiology of, 76-77
  pediatric, 97-116
    adenosine for, 101t, 104
    advanced life support techniques in, 99, 99f
    airway management in, 97-98, 105-109, 106f, 107b, 107t
    amiodarone for, 101t, 104-105
    antidiuretic hormone for, 100, 103t
    atropine for, 99, 100, 101t-102t, 103-104
    basic life support techniques in, 97-99
    breathing management in, 98, 108-109
    calcium for, 101t, 104
    circulatory management in, 98-99, 109-113
    defibrillation and cardioversion in, 113
    epinephrine for, 111, 114
    etiology of, 109-113, 109t, 110f-112f, 110t
    family presence during, 114-116
    glucose for, 100, 101t, 103
    lidocaine for, 102t, 105
    magnesium for, 104
    pharmacologic therapy in, 100-105, 101t-103t, 109-113
    postresuscitation stabilization in, 113-114, 113f
    procainamide for, 103t, 105
    rapid sequence intubation in, 107-108, 107b, 107t
    sodium bicarbonate for, 100, 101t
    tape measurement system in, 114, 114f-115f
  pharmacologic therapy in, 91-93
  postresuscitation management of, 85-87, 86, 88f
  pulseless electrical activity and, 84
  therapeutic modalities in, 87-93
  ventricular fibrillation and pulseless ventricular tachycardia and, 84
Cardiac auscultation, in infants and children, 2571-2572, 2572b
Cardiac cellular electrophysiology, 1199-1201, 1200f-1202f
Cardiac compression model of chest compression, 77, 98
Cardiac conduction, 1201-1203, 1202t, 1203f
Cardiac dysrhythmia. *See* Dysrhythmia.
Cardiac enzymes, in myocardial contusion, 469
Cardiac examination
  in chest pain, 187t
  in chronic obstructive pulmonary disease, 1100
  in dyspnea, 178t
  in spinal cord injury, 310
Cardiac glycosides, in oleander, 2474
Cardiac index, 1259
Cardiac markers
  in acute coronary syndromes, 1174-1179, 1175f, 1176t
  in chest pain, 188
  in infants and children, 2575
  multiple use of, 1175-1179
Cardiac massage, open-chest, 89-90
Cardiac monitoring. *See also* Electrocardiography.
  during cardiopulmonary resuscitation, 79-82, 80f-82f, 80t
  in hypothermia, 2245
  in myocardial infarction, 1173-1174, 1173f
Cardiac output
  during acclimatization to high altitude, 2298
  in heart failure, 1261
  in myocardial contusion, 468
  in pregnancy, 2725
Cardiac pacing. *See* Pacemaker(s); Pacing.
Cardiac sarcoidosis, 1297
Cardiac surgery
  in pregnancy, 2788
  pericarditis after, 1283
Cardiac tamponade, 1285-1286, 1286f
  acute, 473-476, 474f, 475f, 476t
  heart failure in, 1265
Cardiac tamponade *(Continued)*
  in children, 340
  in hemodialysis patient, 1550-1551
  in myocardial rupture, 471
  in uremic pericardial effusion, 1282
  neoplastic, 1016-1018
Cardiac trauma, 467-482
  acute pericardial tamponade in, 473-476, 474f, 475f, 476t
  blunt, 467-472
  blunt aortic injury in, 476-482, 477f-479f, 481b
  chronic thoracic aneurysm and, 482
  in children, 340
  intracardiac injuries in, 472
  myocardial concussion in, 467
  myocardial contusion in, 467-470
  myocardial rupture in, 470-472
  penetrating, 472-476
  pericarditis after, 1283
Cardinal presentation(s)
  abdominal pain as
    diagnostic approach to, 212-216, 212f, 214t-216t
    differential considerations in, 212-214, 212f, 214t-215t, 216-217, 216t
    disposition in, 217-218
    empiric management of, 217, 218f-219f
    pathophysiology of, 209-212, 210t-211t, 211b
  back pain as, 260-267
    diagnostic approach to, 261-264, 261b, 262b, 263f
    differential diagnosis in, 262t, 263f, 264, 265t-266t
    disposition in, 267
    empiric management of, 264, 266f, 267
  chest pain as, 183-188
    ancillary studies in, 185-186, 188t
    diagnostic table in, 188, 190t-191t
    differential considerations in, 183-184, 184t
    disposition in, 188, 192f
    epidemiology of, 183
    history in, 185, 186b, 186t
    management of, 188, 192f
    pathophysiology of, 183
    physical examination in, 185, 187t
    rapid assessment and stabilization in, 184-185, 184f
  coma and depressed level of consciousness as, 156-164
    diagnostic approach to, 157-162, 158b, 159t, 160f, 162f, 163f
    disposition in, 163
    empiric management of, 162-163
  confusion as, 150-155
    diagnostic approach to, 150-153, 151b, 152f, 153f
    differential diagnosis in, 153, 154b, 154f
    disposition in, 154-155
    empiric management of, 154, 155f
  constipation as, 237-242
    diagnostic approach to, 238-239, 238b
    differential diagnosis in, 239, 240f
    disposition in, 242
    empiric management of, 239-242, 240f, 241t, 242b
    pathophysiology of, 237
  cyanosis as, 268-273
    diagnostic approach to, 268-271, 270b, 270f
    differential diagnosis in, 270b, 271-273, 272f
    disposition in, 273
    empiric management of, 273
    pathophysiology of, 268, 269b, 269f
  diarrhea as, 227-236
    diagnostic approach to, 228-233, 230b, 231b
    differential diagnosis in, 228, 230b-231b, 234
    disposition in, 235-236
    empiric management of, 234-235, 234f, 236t
    pathophysiology of, 228, 229t-230t
  dizziness and vertigo as, 142-149
    diagnostic approach to, 143-146, 143b, 143t, 145b, 145t, 148f
    differential diagnosis in, 143, 143b, 143t, 146, 147t-148t
    disposition in, 146, 149
    management of, 148, 148t
    pathophysiology of, 142-143
  dyspnea as, 175-181
    diagnostic approach to, 176-177, 176t, 178t-180t

- Cardinal presentation(s) *(Continued)*
    - differential considerations in, 177, 179t, 180
    - disposition in, 181
    - empiric management of, 180-181, 182f
  - fever as, 134-137
    - diagnostic approach to, 135-137, 135b, 135t
    - differential considerations in, 135, 135b, 135t, 137
    - disposition in, 137
    - empirical management of, 137
  - gastrointestinal bleeding as, 220-227
    - diagnostic approach to, 220-223, 221b
    - differential diagnosis in, 220, 221b, 223
    - disposition in, 225-227, 225b, 226t
    - management of, 223-225, 223f
  - headache as, 169-175, 173t
  - hemoptysis as, 279-283, 281b, 282f
  - jaundice as, 243-246
    - diagnostic approach to, 243-244, 244f, 245f
    - differential diagnosis in, 245, 246t
    - empiric management of, 245-246, 247f
  - nausea and vomiting as, 200-207
    - diagnostic approach to, 201-203, 202t
    - differential considerations in, 201-202, 201t, 203, 204t-206t, 207f
    - disposition in, 207, 209
    - management of, 203, 206, 207f, 208b, 208t
    - pathophysiology of, 200-201, 201f
    - pediatric considerations in, 203, 208t
    - physical examination in, 202t
    - rapid assessment and stabilization in, 201t
  - pelvic pain as, 248-253
    - diagnostic approach to, 248-250, 250t
    - differential diagnosis in, 249b, 250, 251t-252t
    - empiric management of, 250, 252-253, 252f, 253f
  - pharyngitis as, 274-279
    - diagnosis of, 275-278, 276t, 277f, 277t
    - differential diagnosis in, 278
    - management of, 278-279, 278f
    - pathophysiology of, 274-275, 275t
  - red and painful eye as, 283-297
    - diagnostic approach to, 283-288, 284b, 285b, 287f
    - differential diagnosis in, 288-290, 288f-291f
    - disposition in, 293t-297t, 297
    - empiric management of, 290-292, 293t-297t
  - seizure as, 164-168
    - diagnosis of, 165-168, 165t
    - differential considerations in, 165-166, 165t
    - disposition in, 168
    - empiric management of, 166-167, 166t, 168
  - syncope as, 193-198
    - diagnostic approach to, 193-196, 194b, 195b, 195t, 196t
    - differential diagnosis in, 194b, 196, 196t, 197t, 198f
    - disposition in, 198
    - empiric management of, 196, 198, 199f
  - vaginal bleeding as, 254-259
    - diagnostic approach to, 254-257, 255t, 256t
    - differential diagnosis in, 255t, 257, 257t-258t
    - disposition in, 259
    - empiric management of, 257, 259, 259f, 260f
  - weakness as, 138-141
    - diagnostic approach to, 138-139, 139f, 139t, 140b, 140t
    - differential diagnosis in, 138, 139t, 140, 140b
    - disposition in, 141
    - empiric management of, 140-141, 141b
- Cardioembolic ischemic stroke, 1608
- Cardiogenic pulmonary edema, 32, 1261-1262
- Cardiogenic shock
  - causes of, 47
  - definition of, 49, 49b
  - in myocardial infarction, 1160, 1194
  - reperfusion therapy in, 1194
  - treatment of, 52b, 54, 113-114, 113f, 1273
- Cardiomegaly, with pulmonary edema, 1174, 1175f
- Cardiomyopathy, 1293-1297
  - alcoholic, 2866
  - amyloidosis and, 1297
  - connective tissue disorders and, 1297-1298
  - dilated, 1293-1294
    - heart failure in, 1264
    - peripartum cardiomyopathy and, 1297
  - heart failure in, 1264
  - hypertrophic, 1294-1296
- Cardiomyopathy *(Continued)*
    - heart failure in, 1264
    - sudden death in, 1298, 2597-2598
  - inflammatory. *See* Myocarditis.
  - ischemic, 1264
  - peripartum, 1297
  - postpartum, 2821
  - restrictive, 1296-1297
    - constrictive pericarditis vs., 1288
    - heart failure in, 1264
  - sarcoidosis and, 1297
- Cardiopulmonary arrest, 79
- Cardiopulmonary bypass
  - during cardiac arrest, 90
  - for rewarming in accidental hypothermia, 2250-2251, 2250t
  - in aortic rupture, 481
  - in myocardial rupture, 471-472
- Cardiopulmonary decompensation, in pulmonary embolism, 1378, 1379f
- Cardiopulmonary resuscitation
  - active compression-decompression, 89, 98
  - before defibrillation, 90
  - blood flow during, 76-77
  - brain resuscitation and, 67-68
  - capnography in, 39
  - cough, 90
  - for cardiac arrest, 88-90
  - for submersion victim, 2313-2314
  - in hypothermia, 2245-2246
  - in pediatric resuscitation, 98-99
  - interposed abdominal compression, 89, 98
  - previous, fibrinolytic therapy eligibility and, 1191
  - vestibule or circumferential, 89
  - withdrawing or discontinuing, 3144, 3152
- Cardiothoracic injury, pediatric, 338-340
- Cardiothoracic ratio, in infants and children, 2573
- Cardiovascular collapse
  - from local anesthesia, 2932
  - in anaphylaxis, 1824, 1825t, 2548
  - in carbon monoxide poisoning, 2439
  - in cyclic antidepressant poisoning, 2352
  - in pneumococcal disease, 2018
- Cardiovascular depression, in septic shock, 46
- Cardiovascular disorders
  - after head trauma, 371
  - altitude and, 2308
  - anxiety in, 1746-1747
  - in chronic renal failure, 1542
  - in developmentally disabled patient, 2902
  - in diabetes mellitus, 1970
  - in HIV/AIDS, 2086
  - in hyperviscosity syndrome, 1913
  - in Kawasaki disease, 2025, 2026
  - in opioid overdose, 2453
  - in parasitic infection, 2111-2112
  - in pregnancy, 2766-2767
  - in Rocky Mountain spotted fever, 2134
  - in sepsis, 2213-2214
  - in serotonin toxicity, 2357t, 2360
  - in systemic lupus erythematosus, 1807
  - in thermal burns, 918
  - pediatric, 2567-2599
    - chest radiography in, 2573-2574, 2573f, 2574f
    - circulatory changes related to, 2568-2569
    - compensatory responses associated with, 2569, 2569b
    - history in, 2570-2571, 2570b
  - syncope in, 2685
- Cardiovascular drugs
  - during pregnancy and lactation, 2787-2789
  - for hypothermia, 2246
  - in elderly person, 2826
  - overdose of, 2368-2379
  - prehospital use of, 2990-2991
  - syncope from, 195b
- Cardiovascular emergencies
  - air medical transport in, 2998-2999
  - prehospital care in, 2990-2991
- Cardiovascular system
  - aging and, 345
  - in accidental hypothermia, 2237-2238, 2238f
  - in acclimatization and endurance training, 2256
  - in electrical and lightning injuries, 2272
  - in pregnancy, 316-317, 317t, 2725
  - in thyrotoxicosis, 1986-1987
  - sepsis and, 2219-2220
- Cardiovascular trauma, 467-482. *See also* Cardiac trauma.
- Cardioversion
  - for atrial fibrillation, 1231-1232
  - for pulseless electrical activity, 84
  - for supraventricular tachycardia, 2587-2588
  - for torsades de pointes, 1244
  - for ventricular tachycardia, 1242
  - for wide-complex tachycardia, 1239
  - for Wolff-Parkinson-White syndrome, 1235, 1237
  - in pediatric resuscitation, 113
- Carditis
  - in acute rheumatic fever, 2596
  - in Lyme disease, 2123-2124, 2128
- Care paths, 3038, 3039f-3041f
- Care under fire in tactical emergency medical support, 3002-3003
- Caregiver interview, in elder abuse, 1013
- Caries, 1028-1029, 1030-1032, 1030f, 1031f
- Carnitine, for diphtheria, 1291
- Carotid artery
  - aneurysm of, parapharyngeal abscess and, 1123
  - dissection of
    - after head trauma, 357-358
    - headache in, 1638-1639, 1639f
  - injury to, 448
  - stroke involving, 1607, 1609
- Carotid duplex scanning, in ischemic stroke, 1613
- Carotid pulse, during cardiopulmonary resuscitation, 79
- Carotid sinus massage
  - for dysrhythmias, 1214, 1215
  - in digitalis toxicity, 2371
- Carpal bones
  - anatomy of, 577-578, 579f, 622, 623f
  - radiography of, 625-626, 626f, 627f
- Carpal injuries, 627-632
  - capitate fracture in, 630
  - hamate fracture in, 629
  - lunate fracture in, 629
  - pisiform fracture in, 629
  - scaphoid fracture in, 627-629, 628f
  - trapezium fracture in, 630
  - trapezoid fracture in, 630
  - triquetral fracture in, 629
- Carpal instability, 630-632, 630f-633f
- Carpal tunnel, 578
- Carpal tunnel syndrome, 639, 639f, 1696-1697, 1697b, 1697f
  - in hypothyroidism, 1992
  - in pregnancy, 2733
  - thoracic outlet syndrome vs., 1360
- Carpal tunnel view of wrist, 627, 627t
- Carpometacarpal joint
  - dislocation of
    - finger, 603, 603f
    - thumb, 604
  - motions of, 578f
- Carrying angle of elbow, 649, 649f, 650f
  - loss of, after supracondylar fracture, 657-658
- Cartridge, handgun, 954, 954f
- Carvedilol, 1321t, 2373t
- Caspase inhibitors, after cerebral ischemia, 72
- CAST fracture, 975
- Cast immobilization
  - in Achilles tendon rupture, 818
  - in carpal bone fractures, 628, 628f, 629
  - in gastrocnemius strain, 804
  - in humeral shaft fracture, 654-655, 654f
  - in intercondylar eminence fracture, 780
  - in Lisfranc injuries, 830
  - in medial malleolar fracture, 813
  - in metatarsal head and neck fractures, 832
  - in metatarsal shaft fractures, 831
  - in metatarsophalangeal dislocation, 835
  - in patellar fracture, 785
  - in peroneal tendon dislocation or tear, 819
  - in posterior malleolar fracture, 813
  - in sesamoid fractures, 835
  - in Smith's fracture, 634-635
  - in tibial plateau fracture, 779
  - in tibial tubercle fracture, 799
- Castration anxiety, 1746b
- Casts
  - air, for ankle immobilization, 571, 573f, 817
  - fatty
    - in proteinuria, 1532
    - in urinary sediment, 1526, 1526f

Casts *(Continued)*
in glomerulonephritis, 1534
in urinary sediment, 1525-1527, 1526f
plaster, 571-573
Cat
bites by, [illegible]
rabies in, 2064, 2064f
Cataracts
in electrical injuries, 2272
in substituted phenol poisoning, 2464
Catastrophic casualty management, 3013-3014
Catatonia, in schizophrenia, 1728
Catecholamines
for acute pulmonary edema in hypotensive patient, 1273-1274
for beta blocker overdose, 2375
for calcium channel blocker overdose, 2378
for digitalis toxicity, 2368
in anxiety disorders, 1744
in torsades de pointes, 1244
Caterpillar bites, 908
Catfish envenomation, 910
Cathartics, for botulism, 2016
Catheter
balloon-tipped, in foreign body removal, 862f, 863, 872-873
Foley
in burn injury, 923
in foreign body removal, 2617
in genitourinary trauma, 515, 517, 518f
in peripheral vascular injury, 543
Groshong, 1363-1364, 1365f
Hickman-Broviac, problems related to, 1361-1363, 1362b, 1362f, 1365f
laceration of, 1363
occluded indwelling, differential diagnosis in, 1362b
Quinton-Mahurkar, 1362f, 1364-1365
Word, for Bartholin abscess, 1560
Catheterization
central venous
in adult resuscitation, 91-92
in pediatric resuscitation, 99
postresuscitation, 87
in thermal burn, 923
pulmonary artery, in shock, 50
urinary
in children, 2643
in genitourinary trauma, 515, 517, 518f
in hypothermia, 2244-2245
in urinary retention, 1599-1600
Catheter-related infection, 1363
in peritoneal dialysis patient, 1553
of urinary tract, 1578-1579
Cationic protein, in asthma, 1081
Cauda equina syndrome, 420, 1678f, 1679
back pain in, 261, 265t, 703, 706, 712
in pelvic fracture, 720
pseudoclaudication in, 1350
Causalgia, 562
Causes of death, 942t
Causes of injury deaths, 949t
Caustic keratoconjunctivitis, 288, 288f, 293t
Caustics
dermal exposure to, 2384
esophagitis from, 1386, 1387-1388
ocular exposure to, 2384
oral exposure to, 2380-2385, 2381f, 2381t, 2382f
Cavernosal aspiration, for priapism, 2636
Cavitation
in pneumonia, 1134, 1134f
nontuberculous, 2157
tuberculous, 2153, 2153f
CD4 (helper) cell, 2833
CD4 count, in case definition of AIDS, 2071, 2072b
CD8 (suppressor) cell, 2833
Cecal bascule, 1497
Cecal volvulus, [illegible]
Cefazolin, for peritonitis in dialysis patient, 1553, 1553t
Cefdinir, for otitis media, 1069
Cefepime, for febrile, neutropenic cancer patient, 2837, 2838t
Cefixime
for gonococcal arthritis, 1788
for gonorrhea, 1559t, 1566
Cefotaxime
for gonococcal dermatitis, 1843
for Lyme disease, 2127t, 2128
Cefotaxime *(Continued)*
for meningococcal disease, 2023
for pediatric fever, 2513-2514, 2515
for pneumococcal disease, 2019
for pneumonia, 2558t
Cefotetan, for pelvic inflammatory disease, 1571t
Ceftizoxime, for gonococcal dermatitis, 1843
Ceftriaxone
for anorectal sexually transmitted disease, 1519
for bacterial meningitis, 1721, 1722
for chancroid, 1559t, 1563
for epididymitis, 1597t, 2639
for fever, 2513, 2514, 2515
for gonococcal arthritis, 1788
for gonococcal dermatitis, 1843
for gonorrhea, 1559t, 1566
for Lyme disease, 1789, 2127t, 2128
for mastoiditis, 1072
for meningococcal disease, 2023
for meningococcal meningitis, 1723
for otitis media, 1069, 1070t
for pelvic inflammatory disease, 1571t
for pneumococcal disease, 2019
for pneumonia, 2558t
for prostatitis, 1586
prophylactic
for bacteremia, 2506
for meningococcal disease, 2024
Cefuroxime
for bacterial meningitis, 1721, 1722
for Lyme disease, 1789
for mastoiditis, 1072
for otitis media, 1068, 1070t
for pneumococcal disease, 2019
for pneumonia, 2558t
prophylactic, in cat bites, 888
Celecoxib, 2928
Celiac trunk, 1445
Cell membrane, myocardial, electrophysiology of, 1199-1201, 1200f-1202f
Cell stimulation therapy, for febrile, neutropenic cancer patient, 2839
Cell-mediated immunity, 2833
defects in, 2833
from corticosteroids, 2843
in cancer patient, 2839-2840
in renal failure, 2842
immunosenescence of, 2826
in tuberculosis, 2148
Cellophane tape test, in *Enterobius vermicularis* gastroenteritis, 1481
Cellular phone, pacemaker oversensing due to, 1254
Cellularity, cerebrospinal fluid, in bacterial meningitis, 2661-2662, 2661t
Cellulitis, 2196-2199, 2196t, 2197t
clostridial (anaerobic), 2208
gram-negative and anaerobic, 2199
in erysipelas, 2198
in head and neck spaces, 1027, 1028-1029, 1030f, 1117
influenzae, 2199
nonclostridial crepitant, 2208
orbital, 293t, 2197-2198
periorbital (preseptal), 1055, 2197-2198
peritonsillar, 1117-1118, 1118f
retropharyngeal, 1120-1121, 1120f, 1121f
staphylococcal, 2198-2199
streptococcal, 2198
submandibular, 1028, 1032, 1118-1119
synergistic necrotizing, 2209
upper airway, in epiglottitis, 1115
Cement burn, 935, 2381
Cementum, 1026, 1027f
Centerfire rifle wounds, forensic evaluation of, 959, 959f, 960f
Centers for Disease Control and Prevention, 2016, 3010
Centipede bites, 908
Centor criteria, in pharyngitis, 1112
Central cord syndrome, 417-418, 419f, 1077, 1078f
Central herniation
after head trauma, 356
in cancer patient, 1910
Central log of patients presenting to emergency department, 3162
Central nervous system. *See also* Brain; Spinal cord.
aging and, 345
Central nervous system *(Continued)*
cyclic antidepressant effects on, 2354b
degenerative diseases of, seizure in, 1624
in acute radiation syndrome, 2321-2322
in decompression sickness, 2284
in electrical and lightning injuries, 2273-2274
in fetal alcohol syndrome, 2791b, 2792
in heatstroke, 2262
in hypothermia, 2238
in lead poisoning, 2421
in submersion victim, 2313
in systemic lupus erythematosus, 1807
in thermoregulation, 2255
in tuberculosis, 2160-2161, 2161f
lymphoma of, in HIV/AIDS, 2082
oxygen toxicity in, in scuba diving–related disorders, 2283
tumor of, seizure in, 1624
vasculitis of, seizure in, 1624
Central nervous system abscess
ancillary studies in, 1720
cerebrospinal fluid analysis in, 1716-1719, 1717t, 1718t, 1719f
complications of, 1716
diagnosis of, 1716-1720
differential considerations in, 1720, 1721b
disposition in, 1723
epidemiology of, 1711
etiology of, 1712
locations of, 1710-1711
lumbar puncture in, 1716, 1716b
management of, 1722, 1723
neuroimaging studies in, 1719-1720
pathophysiology of, 1713, 1713f
signs and symptoms of, 1714-1715
Central nervous system acidosis, from sodium bicarbonate, 1930
Central nervous system depression
in barbiturate overdose, 2482
in benzodiazepine poisoning, 2484
in chloral hydrate poisoning, 2487
in flunitrazepam overdose, 2486
in hydrocarbon poisoning, 2429
in opioid overdose, 2452
Central nervous system infection, 1710-1723
acute and subacute
ancillary studies in, 1720
cerebrospinal fluid analysis in, 1716-1719, 1717t, 1718t, 1719f
complications of, 1715-1716
diagnosis of, 1716-1720
differential considerations in, 1720, 1721b
disposition in, 1723
epidemiology of, 1711
etiology of, 1711-1712, 1711b, 1712b
lumbar puncture in, 1716, 1716b
management of, 1721-1723, 1721t
neuroimaging studies in, 1719-1720
pathophysiology of, 1713, 1713b
signs and symptoms of, 1714-1715
after head trauma, 370-371
definitions in, 1710-1711
in cancer patient, 1920
in HIV/AIDS, 2079-2082, 2080f
slow virus, 2058
dementia in, 1657-1658, 1659
Central pontine myelinolysis, in hyponatremia, 1935
Central retinal artery occlusion, 283, 284f, 1057, 1057f
Central retinal vein occlusion, 1057, 1057f
Central venous catheterization
in adult resuscitation, 91-92
in pediatric resuscitation, 99
postresuscitation, 87
Central venous oxygen saturation, during cardiopulmonary resuscitation, 82, 82t
Central venous pressure
in cardiac tamponade, 473
in multiple trauma, 304, 307
in shock, 51
postresuscitation, 87
Central venous pressure lines, in sepsis, 2217
Cephalexin, for impetigo, 1843
Cephalosporins
allergy to, 1826
during pregnancy and lactation, 2784
for febrile, neutropenic cancer patient, 2838t
for orofacial infections, 1032

Cephalosporins (Continued)
for peritonitis in dialysis patient, 1552, 1553t
for pharyngitis, 1113
Cerebellar artery syndrome, posteroinferior, 420
Cerebellar ataxia
in high-altitude cerebral edema, 2306
pediatric, 2681, 2682
Cerebellar degeneration, alcoholic, 2870
Cerebellar disturbances
in hypothyroidism, 1992
in multiple sclerosis, 1672
in vertigo, 145
Cerebellar hemorrhage, 147t, 378
Cerebellotonsillar herniation, after head trauma, 356
Cerebral. *See also* Brain.
Cerebral anatomy, mood disorders and, 1735
Cerebral aneurysm, and subarachnoid hemorrhage, Hunt and Hess scale for, 1636, 1636t, 1637
Cerebral artery
embolism to, in scuba diving–related disorders, 2285
stroke involving, 1607, 1609
Cerebral atrophy, in dementia, 1656-1657
Cerebral blood flow, 350-352, 351f
after brain resuscitation, 68
autoregulation of, 351
loss of, 354
during cardiopulmonary resuscitation, 67
during cerebral ischemia, 62, 63f-64f
in hypothermia, 2238
in stroke, 1606-1607
restoration of, after cardiac arrest, 62-64
Cerebral demyelination, in hyponatremia, 1935
Cerebral edema
after head trauma, 354
during cerebral ischemia, 64-65
high-altitude, 2296, 2299-2300, 2299f, 2305-2306, 2305b
in diabetic ketoacidosis, 1967
in salicylate overdose, 2340
in spinal cord injury, 2906
Cerebral hemodynamics, 350-352, 351f
Cerebral hemorrhage. *See* Intracerebral hemorrhage.
Cerebral herniation
after head trauma, 354-356, 355f
in cancer patient, 1918
Cerebral hypoperfusion
after brain resuscitation, 68
syncope and, 193, 194b
Cerebral hypoxia, during air medical transport, 2994-2995
Cerebral ischemia
neurologic recovery after, 62-73
clinical outcomes in, 72-73
experimental therapies in, 70-72
standard strategies for, 67-70, 69t
pathophysiology of, 62-67, 63f-64f
Cerebral malaria, 2104f, 2105
Cerebral palsy, 2903-2904
failure to thrive in, 2900
musculoskeletal disorders in, 2901-2902
Cerebral perfusion pressure, 352
during cardiopulmonary resuscitation, 80, 80f
Cerebral resuscitation, 62-73
clinical outcomes in, 72-73
experimental therapies in, 70-72
in near-hanging and strangulation, 451
pathophysiology of cerebral ischemia and, 62-67, 63f-64f
standard strategies for, 67-70, 69t
Cerebral thrombovasculitis, in Rocky Mountain spotted fever, 2134
Cerebral vasospasm, in traumatic subarachnoid hemorrhage, 377
Cerebral venous catheterization, problems related to, 1361-1366, 1362b, 1362f, 1364f, 1365f
Cerebral venous thrombosis, 1670-1671
Cerebritis, lupus, 1807
Cerebrospinal fluid
analysis of
in bacterial meningitis, 2661-2662, 2661t
in central nervous system infection, 1716-1719, 1717t, 1718t, 1719f
in delirium, 1652
in Guillain-Barré syndrome, 1690-1691
in headache, 173t
Cerebrospinal fluid (Continued)
in HIV/AIDS, 2080
in multiple sclerosis, 1672-1673
in subarachnoid hemorrhage, 1636-1637
leakage of, in midface fracture, 394
physiology of, 350
Cerebrospinal fluid shunt, in developmentally disabled patient, 2899
Cervical disk herniation, thoracic outlet syndrome vs., 1360
Cervical lymphadenopathy
in African trypanosomiasis, 2106
in Kawasaki disease, 2026
in peritonsillitis, 1117
in pharyngitis, 1109, 1110f
Cervical motion tenderness
in pelvic inflammatory disease, 1570
pelvic pain in, 250t
Cervical os, 250t
Cervical rib syndrome, thoracic outlet syndrome in, 1358
Cervical spine
anatomy of, 400f
cartilage space assessment of, 424
neurologic examination of, 415-417
pediatric, anatomic differences in, 335b
pseudosubluxation of, 421
subluxation of, 401, 404, 404f-405f, 427, 428f
Cervical spine immobilization, 435, 436
in comatose survivors of cardiac arrest, 70
in multiple trauma, 308
in spinal injuries, 435-436
Cervical spine injury
airway management in, 436
computed tomography in, 427, 429-431, 429b, 429f-432f
extension, 410-411, 410f-411f
vertebral artery injury from, 420, 420f
facial trauma and, 386
flexion, 399, 401-404, 402f-405f
head trauma with, 358
in children, 336-338, 337f
in elderly person, 413, 415f
in intubation, 17-18
in multiple trauma, 308-309
in neck trauma, 445
magnetic resonance imaging in, 431-435, 433f-436f
radiographic evaluation of, 420-427, 422f-428f
anteroposterior view in, 424, 426, 426f, 427f
cross-table lateral view in, 421, 424, 425f, 426f
flexion-extension views in, 428
indications for, 420-421
oblique views in, 426-428, 426f, 427f, 428f
odontoid view in, 424, 424f-425f
standard trauma series in, 421, 422f-424f
rotational, 405-409, 408f-410f
shear, 405, 406f-407f
stabilization in, 435-436
vascular damage in, 413, 415f
vertical compression, 411-413, 411f-414f
Cervical vertebrae, 399, 400f
Cervicogenic headache, 1642
Cervix
examination of
during labor, 2799, 2799f
in sexual assault victim, 987
in pregnancy, 2723
Cesarean section
in abruptio placentae, 2809
in circumvallate placenta, 2810
in face, brow, and compound presentations, 2816
in HIV-infected patient, 2810
in multiple gestations, 2816
in placenta previa, 2809
in umbilical cord prolapse, 2817
in uterine rupture, 2820-2821
in vasa previa, 2810
perimortem, 325-326
vaginal birth after, 2820
Cesium ingestion, radiogardase for, 3023, 3023t
Cestode infection, 2099t
Cetirizine, during pregnancy and lactation, 2790
Chadwick's sign, 2723, 2728, 2798
Chagas' disease, 2103t
fever in, 2105
myocarditis in, 1291, 2111-2112
Chain of custody in sexual assault cases, 985b
Chalazion, 293t, 1054, 1055f
Chalcosis, 1052
Chamomile, adverse effects of, 2476t
Chance's fracture, 550t
Chancre, syphilitic, 1560-1561, 1560f, 1855, 1855f
Chancroid, 1518t, 1519, 1557t, 1559t, 1562-1563, 1562f
Changuinola virus, 2047
Chaparral, adverse effects of, 2476t
Charcoal, activated. *See* Activated charcoal.
Charcot's triad in cholangitis, 1421
Charles' law, 2280, 2994
Chauffeur's fracture, 550t
Cheek injury, 391
Chelating agents
for arsenic poisoning, 2424
for internal radioactive contamination, 2324
for iron overdose, 2420
for lead poisoning, 2422-2423
for mercury poisoning, 2426
for rhabdomyolysis, 1982
Chemical injuries, 929-939
acid and alkali burns in, 931-933
anhydrous ammonia in, 934-935
caustics in, 2380-2385, 2381f, 2381t, 2382f
cement burns in, 935
chemical terrorism and, 937-939, 938t. *See also* Chemical weapons.
community preparedness and HAZMAT response in, 930-931
elemental metals in, 937
formic acid in, 934
hydrocarbon-related, 936-937
hydrofluoric acid in, 933-934
in pesticide poisoning, 2452-2469
nitrates in, 936
ocular, 1046, 1046f
pathophysiology of, 930
phenol and derivatives in, 935-936
tar burns in, 937
white phosphorus in, 936
Chemical peels, 935
Chemical vaginitis, 1569
Chemical weapons, 937-939, 938t, 3029-3032, 3030b, 3031b
blood agents (cyanide) as, 939, 3031-3032
disaster preparedness for, 3018
nerve gases as, 939, 3030-3031, 3030b, 3031b
pulmonary agents (phosgene, chlorine) as, 939, 3032
vesicants (mustard) as, 938-939, 3031
Chemoreceptor trigger zone, in nausea and vomiting, 200
Chemotaxis, 2834
Chemotherapy, acute tumor lysis syndrome in, 1911
Chemtrec (Chemical Transportation Emergency Center), 931
Cherenkov radiation, 2317
Chernobyl nuclear reactor incident, 2317
Cherry-red spot, in central retinal artery occlusion, 283, 284f, 1057, 1057f
Chest
examination of, in dyspnea, 178t
flail, 457-458, 457f, 458b, 460
low, 490
gunshot wounds to, 506
stab wounds to, 505
Chest compressions
abdominal trauma after, 492
cardiac compression model of, 77, 98
closed, 89
for critically ill asthmatic patient, 1093
for submersion victim, 2314
in hypothermia, 2245
in neonatal resuscitation, 123
in pediatric resuscitation, 98-99, 109
in ventricular fibrillation and pulseless ventricular tachycardia, 84
open, 89-90
thoracic pump model of, 77, 98
Chest pain, 183-188. *See also* Angina.
ancillary studies in, 185-186, 188t
cocaine-related, 2390-2391, 2390b, 2392, 2392b
diagnostic table in, 188, 190t-191t
differential diagnosis in, 183-184, 184t, 1159, 1159t

Chest pain (Continued)
disposition in, 188, 192f
epidemiology of, 183
history in, 185, 186b, 186t
in aortic dissection, 1325
in aortic rupture, 478
in dilated cardiomyopathy, 1293
in esophageal motility disorders, 1396-1397
in esophageal perforation, 1395
in esophagitis, 1387
in gastroesophageal reflux, 1388
in hemodialysis patient, 1551
in hypertrophic cardiomyopathy, 1295
in mitral valve prolapse, 1305
in myocarditis, 1290
in neoplastic cardiac tamponade, 1917
in pericarditis, 1280-1281
in pneumothorax, 1145
in pregnancy, 2732-2733
in pulmonary embolism, 1372, 1380
in tuberculosis, 2149
management of, 188, 192f
nonmyocardial, guidelines for, 192f
observation in, 3064-3065, 3065b
pathophysiology of, 183
pediatric, 2570-2571, 2592
physical examination in, 185, 187t
rapid assessment and stabilization in, 184-185, 184f
Chest pain centers, 1181-1182, 3064-3065, 3065b
Chest Pain Evaluation in the Emergency Room (CHEER), 1181-1182
Chest radiography. *See* Radiography, chest.
Chest thrusts, for airway foreign body, 2530
Chest trauma. *See* Thoracic trauma.
Chest tube
abdominal trauma after, 492
in children, 339
in hemothorax, 465
in pleural effusion, 1151-1152
in pneumothorax, 463, 464, 464b, 1147-1148
Chest wall trauma, 454-459
costochondral separation in, 457
flail chest in, 457-458, 457f, 458b
nonpenetrating ballistic injury in, 458-459
observation in, 3068-3069
pneumothorax and, 461
rib fracture in, 454-456, 454b, 455f
sternal fracture in, 456-457
subcutaneous emphysema and, 459-460
traumatic asphyxia in, 459
Chickenpox. *See* Varicella.
Chilblains, 2228, 2230
Child, 2494-2720. *See also* Adolescent; Infant; Neonate.
abdominal pain in
differential considerations in, 2611, 2612t
in appendicitis, 2619
in hemolytic uremic syndrome, 2654
in Henoch-Schönlein purpura, 2615, 2653
in inflammatory bowel disease, 2616
in intussusception, 2610
in osteogenesis imperfecta, 2700
in renal stones, 2646
abuse of. *See* Child abuse.
acetaminophen poisoning in, 2335
acute bacterial meningitis in, 2657-2665
clinical features of, 2658-2659, 2658t
diagnosis of, 2659-2663, 2660b, 2661f, 2661t
differential considerations in, 2663, 2663b
management of, 2663-2665, 2664t
pathophysiology of, 2657-2658
acute mountain sickness in, 2301, 2302
acute renal failure in, 2649-2651, 2649b
acute rheumatic fever in, 2596-2597, 2596f
acute septic arthritis in, 2704-2706, 2706f, 2706t
air medical transport of, 2999
airway obstruction in, 2502, 2502b, 2519-2530, 2532-2552
altered consciousness in, 2502-2503
analgesia in, 2935-2936, 2946-2947, 2952-2954
anaphylaxis/anaphylactoid reactions in, 2546-[illegible]
anatomic and physiologic differences in, 329, 329b, 329t, 335b, 2494-2495
appendicitis in, 1452-1453, 2509b, 2618-2620, 2620f
Child (Continued)
assessment of
appearance in, 2497-2498, 2498t
circulation to skin in, 2498t, 2499, 2499f
clinical interview in, 2500-2501, 2501b
hands-on, 2499-2500
physical examination in, 2501
special health care needs and, 2503-2504
triage tools in, 2500, 2500t
work of breathing in, 2498-2499, 2498f, 2498t, 2499f
asthma in, 2532-2544
clinical features of, 2534-2536
complications of, 2535-2536, 2536b
diagnosis of, 2536-2537, 2536f, 2537f
differential diagnosis in, 2537, 2538b
disposition in, 2542-2544
epidemiology of, 2532
factors associated with, 2533-2534, 2534b
history in, 2534, 2534b
management of, 2537-2542, 2539t, 2540f, 2543t
pathophysiology of, 2532-2533
physical examination in, 2534-2535, 2535t
prehospital care in, 2537
severity assessment score for, 2503t
ataxia in, 2681-2682, 2681b
athletic, sudden death of, 2597-2599, 2597b
atrial septal defect in, 2578
automobile restraint seats for, 947, 948
back pain in, 703, 707, 713
bacterial endocarditis in, 2590-2591, 2591b
benzodiazepine poisoning in, 2484-2485
beta blocker overdose in, 2375
biliary tract disorders in, 2620-2621
blood pressure in, 2495, 2495t, 2571, 2571t, 2651t
bronchiolitis in, 2509b, 2544-2546
bronchopulmonary dysplasia in, 2565, 2565f
burns in
in child abuse, 969-970, 970f, 970t
unintentional, 975
calcium channel blocker overdose in, 2378-2379
cardiac arrest in, 97-116
adenosine for, 101t, 104
advanced life support techniques in, 99, 99f
airway management in, 97-98, 105-109, 106f, 107b, 107t
amiodarone for, 101t, 104-105
antidiuretic hormone for, 100, 103t
atropine for, 99, 100, 101t-102t, 103-104
basic life support techniques in, 97-99
breathing management in, 98, 108-109
calcium for, 101t, 104
circulatory management in, 98-99, 109-113
defibrillation and cardioversion in, 113
epinephrine for, 111, 114
etiology of, 109-113, 109t, 110f-112f, 110t
family presence during, 114-116
glucose for, 100, 101t, 103
lidocaine for, 102t, 105
magnesium for, 104
pharmacologic therapy in, 100-105, 101t-103t, 109-113
postresuscitation stabilization in, 113-114, 113f
procainamide for, 103t, 105
rapid sequence intubation in, 107-108, 107b, 107t
sodium bicarbonate for, 100, 101t
tape measurement system in, 114, 114f-115f
cardiovascular disorders in, 2567-2599
chest radiography in, 2573-2574, 2573f, 2574f
circulatory changes related to, 2568-2569
compensatory responses associated with, [illegible]
history in, 2570-2571, 2570b
physical examination in, 2571-2575, 2571t, 2572b
causes of death in, 942t, 949t
chest pain in, 2570-2571, 2592
cholecystitis in, 1421
cholelithiasis in, 1419
cigarette ingestion by, 2474
coarctation of the aorta in, 2578-2579
congenital heart disease in, 2575-2582
acyanotic, 2577-2579, 2577f
chest radiography in, 2573-2574, 2574f
Child (Continued)
clinical features of, 2575-2576, 2575t
cyanotic, 2579-2581, 2579f, 2581b
diagnosis of, 2576, 2576b
ductal-dependent, 2576-2577, 2576b, 2577b
incidence of, 2575, 2575t
management of, 2576-2577, 2576b, 2577b
postoperative complications of, 2581
respiratory syncytial virus infection and, 2581-2582, 2582b
consent to treatment on behalf of, 3167-3168
constipation in, 2612-2613
croup in, 2525-2527, 2526f, 2527b
cyanosis in
central, cardiac vs. pulmonary, 2569, 2569b, 2572
in tetralogy of Fallot, 2580
pathophysiology of, 269t, 2569
cystic fibrosis in, 2564-2565, 2565f
death of
in emergency department, 2717
prehospital issues related to, 3145-3146
depression in, 1737
developmental differences in, 2495-2497, 2496t
diarrhea in, 227, 2623-2634, 2628b, 2628t
difficult airway in, 2502, 2502b
digitalis poisoning in, 2372, 2372t
dysrhythmias in, 2584-2590, 2584b, 2586b, 2587f-2589f
Eisenmenger syndrome in, 2578
electrocardiography in, 2574-2575, 2574t
emergency department visits by
readiness for, 2504
reasons for, 2494, 2495t
epiglottitis in, 2523-2524, 2524f
factitious disorder in, 1762
fever in, 2505-2517
ancillary tests in, 2508-2510
bacteremia and, 2505-2506, 2512, 2515
chest radiography in, 2510
clinical features of, 2508-2510
disposition in, 2517
history in, 2508
hyperpyrexia and, 2506
in cancer patient, 2516
in congenital heart disease, 2517
in heat exhaustion and heatstroke, 2510
in HIV/AIDS, 2516
in Kawasaki disease, 2511, 2512b
in septic shock, 2511
in sickle cell anemia, 2516-2517
in toxic ingestion, 2510-2511
in toxic shock syndrome, 2511, 2511b
in ventriculoperitoneal shunts, 2517
lumbar puncture and, 2660
management of, 2511-2516, 2513b
of unknown origin, 2507, 2507b
pathophysiology of, 2505
petechiae and, 2507-2508
physical examination in, 2508, 2509b
prehospital care in, 2511
seizure and, 2507, 2666-2667, 2674, 2674b
temperature determination in, 2508
foreign bodies in
airway, 2529-2530, 2550-2551, 2551f
gastrointestinal, 2616-2617, 2617f
fracture in, 554-557
apophyseal, 2709-2711, 2711f
child abuse and, 970, 970t, 2698-2701
clavicle, 2692-2693, 2693f
condylar, 660
diaphyseal, 2699
distal radius, 637-639, 637f, 638f, 638t
elbow avulsion, 2711, 2711f
epicondylar, 662-663, 662f
femoral, 763-764, 763f
greenstick, 554, 556f
hand, 600
healing of, 781
metaphyseal, 2699
Monteggia, 2697
multiple, in osteogenesis imperfecta, 2700-2701, 2700f, 2700t
nose, 392
patterns of, 554-557, 557t, 2690-2692, 2690f, 2692f, 2691t
radius, 644, 644f
rib, 2699
skull, 334-335, 2699

Child (Continued)
supracondylar, 655-659, 656f-658f
supracondylar humeral, 2693-2697, 2694f-2696f, 2694t
toddler's, 2698, 2698f
torus, 554, 556f
trochanteric, 767
ulnar, 644, 644f
unintentional, 975
gastroesophageal reflux in, 2609-2610
gastrointestinal bleeding in, differential considerations in, 220, 221b, 2613-2614, 2614t
gastrointestinal disorders in, 2601-2621
general approach to, 2494-2504
genitourinary disorders in, 2635-2655
headache in, 2676-2681
acute, 2677
chronic-nonprogressive, 2679
chronic-progressive, 2677-2678
clinical features of, 2676-2677, 2677b
cluster, 2679
diagnosis of, 2679, 2680b
differential considerations in, 2677b
management of, 2680-2681
migraine, 2678-2679, 2678b
pathophysiology of, 2676
heart failure in, 2582-2584, 2583t
hematuria in, 2644-2645, 2645b
hemolytic uremic syndrome in, 2654-2655
Henoch-Schönlein purpura in, 2615, 2615f, 2653-2654
hip dysplasia in, 2701-2702, 2702b, 2702f
hip pain in, 764-765, 2702-2709, 2703b
Hirschsprung's disease in, 2612-2613
human bites in, 890
hypertension in, 2651-2653, 2651b, 2651t, 2652b, 2653t
hypertrophic pyloric stenosis in, 2603-2606, 2605f, 2606t
infectious diarrhea in, 2623-2634
clinical features of, 2626
complications of, 2626
dehydration in, 2629, 2629t
diagnosis of, 2626-2627
differential diagnosis in, 2627, 2627t
disposition in, 2628-2629, 2628b
epidemiology of, 2623-2624
etiology of, 2624-2626, 2628t
fluid and electrolyte management for, 2629-2634, 2630t, 2632b-2634b
management of, 2628, 2628t
pathophysiology of, 2624
inflammatory bowel disease in, 2615-2616
intubation of, 18, 99, 106-107, 108-109, 2519
intussusception in, 2509b, 2610-2612, 2611f, 2612t
iron overdose in, 2418-2419
jaundice in, 2601-2603, 2602t, 2603b, 2603t, 2604f-2605f
Kawasaki disease in, 2593-2596, 2594b, 2595f
lead poisoning in, 2421
Legg-Calvé-Perthes disease in, 2706-2707, 2707f
lower airway obstruction in, 2532-2552
in anaphylaxis, 2546-2550
in asthma, 2532-2544
in bronchiolitis, 2544-2546
in foreign body aspiration, 2550-2551, 2551f
marijuana intoxication in, 2411
Meckel's diverticulum in, 2613-2615, 2614t
musculoskeletal disorders in, 2689-2711
anatomy and physiology in, 2689
apophyseal, 2709-2711, 2711f
child abuse and, 970, 970t, 2698-2701
physeal, 2690, 2691f, 2691t, 2692, 2692f
myocarditis in, 2591-2592
nephrotic syndrome in, 2648-2649
neurologic disorders in, 2657-2686
noninvasive monitoring in, 2504
nursemaid's elbow in, 666, 666f, 2697-2698, 2697f
Osgood-Schlatter syndrome in, 2710
osteogenesis imperfecta in, 2700-2701, 2700f, 2700t
osteomyelitis in, 2183-2184, 2184f
pancreatitis in, 1428, 2618, 2618t
penile disorders in, 2635-2638, 2637f-2638f
peptic ulcer disease in, 1392

Child (Continued)
pericarditis in, 2592-2593, 2593f
periosteal new bone formation in, 2699
pertussis in, 2559-2560
pharmacokinetics of drugs in, 2935, 2952
plant poisoning in, 2471
pneumonia in, 2554-2564
aspiration, 2560
bacterial, 2555, 2556-2557, 2556f, 2557f, 2558t, 2563t
chlamydial, 2559, 2559f, 2563t
complications of, 2562
diagnosis of, 2560-2561, 2561f
differential diagnosis in, 2561, 2562b
epidemiology of, 2555
in immunocompromised host, 2560
management of, 2558t, 2562-2564
mycoplasmal, 2558-2559, 2563t
pathophysiology of, 2555
physical examination in, 2556
signs and symptoms of, 2555-2556
viral, 2555, 2557-2560, 2563t
poststreptococcal glomerulonephritis in, 2647-2648
procedural sedation and analgesia in, 2946-2947, 2952-2954
proteinuria in, 2646-2647
red and painful eye in, 292
refusal of medical care for, 3171
renal disorders in, 2635-2655
renal stones in, 2645-2646
renal tumor in, 2646
respiration in, physiology of, 338
resuscitation of, 97-116
adenosine for, 101t, 104
advanced life support techniques in, 99, 99f
airway management in, 97-98, 105-109, 106f, 107b, 107t
amiodarone for, 101t, 104-105
antidiuretic hormone for, 100, 103t
atropine for, 99, 100, 101t-102t, 103-104
basic life support techniques in, 97-99
breathing management in, 98, 108-109
calcium for, 101t, 104
cardiac rhythm and etiology of arrest in, 109-113, 109t, 110f-112f, 110t
circulatory management in, 98-99, 109-113
defibrillation and cardioversion in, 113
epinephrine for, 111, 114
family presence during, 114-116
glucose for, 100, 101t, 103
lidocaine for, 102t, 105
magnesium for, 104
pharmacologic therapy in, 100-105, 101t-103t, 109-113
postresuscitation stabilization in, 113-114, 113f
procainamide for, 103t, 105
rapid sequence intubation in, 107-108, 107b, 107t
sodium bicarbonate for, 100, 101t
tape measurement system in, 114, 114f-115f
termination of, 116
retropharyngeal abscess in, 2522-2523, 2523f
scrotal masses and swelling in, 2638-2642, 2639f-2640f
seizure in, 367, 2665-2676
after head trauma, 334
anticonvulsant therapy for, 2674-2676, 2675t
clinical features of, 2665-2667, 2666b
diagnosis of, 2670-2671
disposition in, 2674-2676, 2674b, 2675t
etiology of, 2667-2670, 2668b-2670b
febrile, 2507, 2666-2667, 2674, 2674b
management of, 2671-2673, 2671b, 2672t
pathophysiology of, 2665
precipitators of, identification and treatment of, 2673
secondary survey in, 2502
status epilepticus and, 2667, 2668b, 2672-2673, 2672t
septic arthritis in, 2190
Sever's disease in, 2710
shock in, 2499, 2503
slipped capital femoral epiphysis in, 2707-2709, 2708f
small bowel obstruction in, 1441
stroke volume in, decreased, causes of, 2569, 2569b

Child (Continued)
submersion injuries in, 2311, 2314-2315
surrogate decision-making for, 3134
syncope in, 2685-2686
tetralogy of Fallot in, 2579-2581, 2579f, 2580f, 2581b
thermal burns in, 923, 969-970, 970f, 970t
transient synovitis in, 2703-2704
trauma in, 328-342
abdominal, 340-342
blunt, 492, 510
epidemiology of, 489-490
history in, 493
cardiothoracic, 338-340
cervical spine, 336-338, 337f
clinical features of, 329-330
disposition in, 342
epidemiology of, 328
facial, 382, 383
general management principles in, 331-333, 332b, 332t, 333t
head, 333-336, 334b, 335b, 366-368, 369b
hip, 763-767, 763f, 765f-767f
primary survey in, 329-330, 329t, 331t-333t
renal, 528
secondary survey in, 330, 330b, 333, 333b, 2501, 2501b, 2502b
surgical indications in, 332b
upper airway obstruction in, 2519-2530
evaluation of, 2521, 2521f
in congenital lesions, 2522, 2524-2525, 2524f, 2527-2528, 2528f
in croup, 2525-2527, 2526f, 2527b
in epiglottitis, 2523-2524, 2524f
in foreign body aspiration, 2529-2530
in laryngeal disease, 2524-2525, 2524f
in retropharyngeal abscess, 2522-2523, 2523f
in subglottic tracheal disease, 2525-2527
in supraglottic disease, 2522-2524
in tracheal disease, 2527-2529, 2529t
pathophysiology of, 2519, 2520f
stridor in, 2519-2520, 2521t
urinary tract infection in, 1573, 1583-1585, 2510, 2642-2644, 2643b, 2643t
clinical features of, 1583, 1583t
diagnosis of, 1583-1584, 1584f
treatment of, 1584-1585
ventricular septal defect in, 2577
vertigo in, 2682-2685, 2683b, 2684b, 2684f
violence and, 1017-1022
vital signs in, 2495, 2495t
vomiting in, 203, 206, 208t, 2605, 2606t, 2627t, 2628b
vulnerability of, to weapons of mass destruction, 3021
Child abuse, 968-976
abdominal trauma in, 490
bruises consistent with, 969-971, 969f, 970f, 970t, 2502b
diagnostic strategies in, 973-974
differential considerations in, 974-975, 975f, 2699-2701
disposition in, 976
epidemiology of, 968-969, 969t
facial trauma in, 383
head trauma in, 349, 367
historical indicators of, 2501b
history of, in sexual assault cases, 979
immersion scalds in, 916
in Munchausen's syndrome by proxy, 1761, 1763, 1763t, 1765
management of, 975-976
physical abuse in, 969-971, 969f, 970f, 970t, 972, 973, 974-975
radiography in, 2699
reporting of, 976
sexual abuse in, 969, 971, 972-973, 974, 975
sexually transmitted disease and, 973-974, 974t
signs and symptoms of, 971-973
skeletal aspects of, 2698-2701
Child maltreatment, 968
Child neglect, refusal of medical care and, 3171
Child restraint seats, 947, 948
Childbirth. *See* Labor and delivery.
Chili pepper, drug interactions with, 2478t
Chinese liver fluke, 2100t
Chi-squared test, 3052t, 3053
Chlamydia conjunctivitis, 297t

Chlamydia pneumoniae, 1130, 1132, 2559
in myocarditis, 1292
in pharyngitis, 1109, 1111, 1113
Chlamydia psittaci, in pneumonia, 1131
Chlamydia trachomatis
dysuria in, 1579-1580, 1579t
in epididymitis, 1595, 1596
in pharyngitis, 1111, 1113
in pneumonia, 2559
in pregnancy, 2758
in sexually transmitted disease, 1518t, 1519, 1559t, 1562, 1564-1565
in urinary tract infection, 1579-1580, 1579t
Chloral hydrate
for procedural sedation and analgesia, in children, 2954
overdose of, 2487
Chloramphenicol
during pregnancy and lactation, 2784
for meningococcal disease, 2023
for pneumonia, 2558t
for Q fever, 2137
for Rocky Mountain spotted fever, 1850, 2136, 2136t
Chlorazepate, 2484, 2484t
Chlordiazepoxide, 2484, 2484t
for alcohol withdrawal syndrome, 2862-2863
Chlorhexidine
for prickly heat, 2259
for skin disinfection, 847
Chlorinated hydrocarbon poisoning, 2462-2463, 2462b
Chlorine, as chemical weapon, 3032
Chlorophenoxy compound poisoning, 2464-2465, 2465b
Chloroquine, for systemic lupus erythematosus, 1809
Chlorothiazide, 1321t
Chlorpheniramine, for anaphylaxis, 1831b, 1832
Chlorpromazine, 2446t
hepatotoxicity of, 1414
in heatstroke, 2265
seizures from, 2962
Chlorpropamide
overdose of, hypoglycemia from, 1961
rash from, 1972
Chlorprothixene, 2446t
Chlorthalidone, 1321t
during pregnancy and lactation, 2788
Choanal atresia, 121, 2522
Choking, in airway foreign body aspiration, 865, 866
Cholangiopancreaticoduodenography, endoscopic retrograde, in abdominal trauma, 499
Cholangiopancreatography, endoscopic retrograde
in acute pancreatitis, 1433
in chronic pancreatitis, 1436
in gallstone pancreatitis, 1434
in jaundice, 244
pancreatitis after, 1428
Cholangiopathy, AIDS, 1423
Cholangioscopy, endoscopic, in cholangitis, 1422
Cholangitis, 1421-1422, 1422f
Cholecystitis, 1419-1421, 1419f
acalculous, 1421, 2620, 2621
emphysematous, 1421
jaundice in, 246
Cholecystography, oral, in cholelithiasis, 1419
Choledocholithiasis, 246
Cholelithiasis, 1418-1419, 1418f, 1419f
in children, 2620-2621
in cholangitis, 1421, 1422f
in cholecystitis, 1419f, 1420
in pregnancy, 1419, 2754-2755
pancreatitis in, 1426, 1427, 1428, 1433, 1434
Cholestasis
in drug-induced liver disorders, 1414
in pregnancy, 1416, 1417, 2726
jaundice in, 243, 244f, 246
Cholesteatoma, in otitis media, 1067
Cholesterol gallstones, 1418
Choline acetyltransferase, in dementia, 1657
Cholinergic syndrome
in organophosphate poisoning, 2459, 2459b
in overdosed/poisoned patient, 2327t, 2328
mushrooms associated with, 2479
Cholinergic urticaria, 1848
Cholinesterase inhibitors, for myasthenia gravis, 1706
Chondrocalcinosis, in hypothyroidism, 1992
Chondrolysis, in slipped capital femoral epiphysis, 2709
Chondromalacia patellae, 786
Chopart's joint
anatomy of, 820, 820f
injuries to, 827
Chorea
in acute rheumatic fever, 2596
in rheumatic fever, 1304
Choreoathetoid movement, in cocaine overdose, 2388
Choreoathetosis, paroxysmal, 2668
Chorioamnionitis, 2759, 2808, 2808b
Chorionic membrane, premature rupture of, 2807-2808, 2808t
Choroid, 1045f
Chromic gut suture, 852t
Chromosomal abnormalities, miscarriage and, 2740
Chronic disease, reporting requirements for, 3173
Chronic obstructive pulmonary disease, 1097-1107
acute decompensation in, causes of, 1101-1103, 1103t
acute exacerbations of
causes of, 1099, 1103t
management of, 1103-1106, 1103t-1105t
altitude and, 2307, 2308
anxiety in, 1747
clinical features of, 1099-1100
definition of, 1097
diagnosis of, 1100-1101
differential diagnosis in, 1101-1103
disposition in, 1106, 1106t
dyspnea in, 179t
epidemiology of, 1097
mechanical ventilation in, 31-32
natural history of, 1099, 1099f
palliative care in, 3154
pathophysiology of, 1097-1098
pharmacologic therapy for, 1105-1106
physical examination in, 1099-1100
pneumonia in, 1132
pneumothorax in, 1102, 1143-1144, 1145
staging severity of, 1098-1099, 1098t
symptoms of, 1099
ventilation and oxygenation in, 1103-1105, 1103t-1105t
Chronic pain syndromes, 2913-2914, 2914b
Chronic recurrent multifocal osteomyelitis (CRMO), 2184
Churg-Strauss syndrome, 1816
Chvostek's sign, in hypocalcemia, 1943
Cicuta maculata, 2472, 2472f
Cicutoxin, 2472
Cidofovir, 2038
Cigarette burn, in child abuse, 969, 969f
Ciguatera fish poisoning, 1470t, 1473-1474
Cilastatin, for febrile, neutropenic cancer patient, 2838t
Ciliary flush, in traumatic iridocyclitis, 1049, 1049f
Ciliary muscle, 1045f
Cimetidine, 1390t
for anaphylactic shock, 54
for anaphylaxis, 2549
for hymenoptera stings, 904
for scombroid fish poisoning, 1472
Cimino-Brescia fistula, 1365-1366
Ciprofloxacin
for anthrax exposure, 3026, 3026b
for *Campylobacter* gastroenteritis, 1461
for *Escherichia coli* food poisoning, 1474
for gonococcal arthritis, 1788
for gonococcal dermatitis, 1843-1844
for granuloma inguinale, 1560t, 1563
for infectious diarrhea, 235
for meningococcal meningitis, 1723
for *Plesiomonas shigelloides* gastroenteritis, 1468
for prostatitis, 1586
for salmonellosis, 1463
for shigellosis, 1461t, 1464
for traveler's diarrhea, 1487
for urinary tract infection, 1582
for *Vibrio* fish poisoning, 1472
prophylactic, for meningococcal disease, 2024
Circadian rhythm disruption, from shift work, performance and, 3123, 3123b
Circuit, AC vs. DC, electrical injury and, 2268
Circulation. *See also* Blood flow.
fetal, 2568, 2568f
in beta blocker overdose, 2375
in cardiac arrest, 88-90
in elderly trauma patient, 348
in pediatric resuscitation, 98-99, 109-113
in pediatric trauma, 330, 332t
in pregnant trauma patient, 322-323
neonatal, 2568-2569
persistent fetal, 119
transitional, at birth, 118-119, 119t, 2568
Circumcision, complications of, 2638
Circumferential cardiopulmonary resuscitation, 89
Circumflex fibular artery, 771
Circumflex humeral arteries, 672
Circumvallate placenta, 2810
Cirrhosis, 1410-1411
alcoholic, 2868
hepatocellular carcinoma and, 1417
immune defects in, 2841-2842
infections in, 2842
pipe-stem, in chronic schistosomiasis, 2112, 2113f
prerenal azotemia in, 1532-1533
with ascites, 1410, 1411, 1412
Cisapride, for nausea and vomiting, 206
Citalopram, metabolism of, 2357
Citrate, hypocalcemia from, 1943
Civil protection order, in intimate partner violence and abuse, 1005
Clarithromycin
during pregnancy and lactation, 2784
for Lyme disease, 2127t, 2128
for *Mycobacterium avium* infection in HIV/AIDS, 2076
for pertussis, 2006
for pharyngitis, 1113
for pneumonia, 2558t
in HIV/AIDS, side effects of, 2079t
Clark v. Baton Rouge General Medical Center, 3157
Claudication
exercise-induced, in arteriosclerosis obliterans, 1350
intermittent, in chronic arterial insufficiency, 1345
Clavicle
anatomy of, 670, 671f
fracture of, 676-679, 676f-679f
in children, 2692-2693, 2693f
subclavian artery injury and, 545
Clavicular splint, 569, 677, 678f
Clawhand, 586, 588f
Clay shoveler's fracture, 401, 403f, 550t
Clearblue One Step pregnancy test, 2729
Clenched-fist injury, 611, 890
Clenched-fist view of wrist, 627, 627t
Clindamycin
for babesiosis, 2140
for bacterial vaginosis, 1567t, 1568
for orofacial infections, 1032
for otitis media, 1069
for pelvic inflammatory disease, 1571t
for pneumonia, 2558t
for toxic shock syndrome, 2030, 2201
in HIV/AIDS, side effects of, 2079t
Clinical decision making
diagnostic approach and, 125-130, 127f, 128b, 129f
errors in, 130-133, 131t, 133b
Clinical decision rules in emergency medicine, 3035-3036
Clinical decision support (CDS) systems, 3098
Clinical decision unit, 1093. *See also* Observation medicine.
Clinical documentation, in material safety data sheet, 3081, 3082b
Clinical interview, in pediatric assessment, 2500-2501, 2501b
Clinical pathways, 3038, 3039f-3041f
decision making errors in using, 131t, 132
Clinical practice guidelines. *See* Guidelines for emergency medicine.
Clinical protocols, 3038
Clinical question, in evidence-based medicine, 3036

Clinical reasoning, 126
Clinical studies, 3046-3047
Clinical trials, 3047-3051, 3048f
Clonazepam, 2484, 2484t
  during pregnancy and lactation, 2787
  for seizure, 2675t
  side effects of, 1628t
Clonidine, 1321t
  during pregnancy and lactation, 2789
  for alcohol withdrawal syndrome, 2862
  for opioid withdrawal, 2455-2456
  withdrawal of, hypertension from, 1313-1314
Clonorchis sinensis, 2100t
Clopidogrel
  for acute coronary syndromes, 1186-1187
  for chest pain, 184
  thrombocytopenia from, 1898
Closed-fist injury, 611, 890
Closed-loop obstruction of small bowel, 1440
Close-range handgun wounds, 956, 956f
Clostridial cellulitis, 2208
Clostridial myonecrosis, 2208-2209
Clostridium botulinum poisoning, 1707-1708, 2012-2016
Clostridium difficile infection
  in antibiotic-associated enterocolitis, 1470t, 1474-1475
  in dysenteric colitis, 230t
  in pseudomembranous colitis, 2625
Clostridium difficile toxin test, 233
Clostridium perfringens food poisoning, 1470-1471, 1470t, 2625-2626
Clostridium tetani, 2007, 2008-2009. *See also* Tetanus.
Clot solubility testing in bleeding disorders, 1895
Clotrimazole
  during pregnancy and lactation, 2785
  for candidal esophagitis, 1387
  in HIV/AIDS, side effects of, 2079t
Cloxacillin, for staphylococcal scalded skin syndrome, 1845
Clozapine
  for psychosis in demented patient, 1662
  for thought disorders, 1731
  toxicity of, 2446, 2446t, 2448
"Club drugs," 2883-2884
Clubbing, in cyanosis, 270-271, 270f
Cluster headache, 1634-1635, 2679
Coagulation
  disseminated intravascular, 1903-1904, 1904t
    after head trauma, 371
    in anaphylaxis, 1825t
    in meningococcal disease, 2022
    in pregnancy, placental abruption and, 319-320
    in rhabdomyolysis, 1981
    in sepsis, 2214
  for epistaxis, 1074
  hypothermic, 2243-2244
  in pregnancy, 2725
  in wound healing, 842
  regulation of, 1894
  zone of, in burn injury, 917, 917f
Coagulation factors, 1892, 1893b, 1893f, 1894
  assays of, in bleeding disorders, 1895
  replacement of, for disseminated intravascular coagulation, 1904
Coagulation pathway
  disorders of. *See* Coagulopathy.
  in hemostasis, 1892, 1893f, 1894
Coagulation studies, 1894-1895, 1894b
Coagulopathy, 1899-1904
  in disseminated intravascular coagulation, 1903-1904, 1904t
  in heatstroke, 2262, 2265
  in hemophilia A, 1899-1902, 1901t, 1902t
  in hemophilia B, 1903
  in pancreatitis, 1430
  in rhabdomyolysis, 1981, 1983
  in sepsis, 2214
  in submersion victim, 2313
  in von Willebrand's disease, 1902-1903
  oral hemorrhage and, 1042
Coal tar burns, 926-927, 937
Coarctation of the aorta, 1312, 2578-2579
Cobalt blue lamp test of corneal damage, 287-288
COBRA, 3156
Cocaethylene, 2876
Cocaine
  alcohol interactions with, 2876
  cardiac effects of, 1292-1293
  during pregnancy, 2792-2793
  formulations of, 2386, 2387t
  metabolism of, 2386
  mydriasis from, 1061
  overdose of, 2386-2392
    body packing/stuffing and, 2391-2392
    clinical features of, 2386-2388, 2387b
    diagnosis of, 2388-2389
    differential diagnosis in, 2389, 2389b
    disposition in, 2392, 2392t
    emergency department visits related to, 2884f
    management of, 2389-2391, 2389b, 2390b
  pathophysiology of, 2386, 2387f
  rhabdomyolysis from, 1979
  seizure from, 1623
  topical, 846, 2933
Cocaine test, in Horner's syndrome, 1061-1062
Coccidia, gastroenteritis from, 1476-1479, 1477t
Coccidioides immitis
  in cancer patient with impaired cell-mediated immunity, 2840
  in pneumonia, 1130
Coccyx, 400f
  fracture of, 725
Cochleovestibular apparatus damage, in middle ear barotrauma, 2282
Cochrane Library, clinical practice guidelines in, 3035, 3042
Codeine, 2920, 2921t, 2925
  during pregnancy and lactation, 2784
  for migraine, 2680
  respiratory effects of, 2453t
Coffee bean sign
  in colonic volvulus, 1499
  in small bowel obstruction, 1443
Cognitive dispositions as source of failures in emergency department, 3122
Cognitive distortions, difficult patient and, 2975, 2976
Cognitive impairment
  assessment of, 151, 152f, 153f
    in delirium, 1649-1650, 1650f
    in systemic lupus erythematosus, 1811
    in thought disorders, 1730
  in delirium, 1649
  in dementia, 1658-1659
  in depression, 1737
  in elderly person, 2827
  in multiple sclerosis, 1672
Cognitive processes, in clinical decision making, 130, 131t, 132
Cognitive-behavioral therapy, for anxiety disorders, 1751, 1751t
Coining, 3114
Coital headache, 1642
Colchicine
  for gouty arthritis, 1786
  for pseudogout, 1787
Cold agglutinins, in autoimmune hemolytic anemia, 1883
Cold diuresis, 2239
Cold intolerance, in hypothyroidism, 1991
"Cold sores," 2230
Cold stress. *See also* Frostbite; Hypothermia.
  injuries associated with
    central, 2236-2252
    peripheral, 2228-2235
  physiology of, 2228-2229, 2236-2237, 2237f
Cold urticaria, 1848
Cold water treatment, of burned skin, 921
Cold-water head dunking, for dysrhythmias, 1214-1215
Colic
  biliary, in cholelithiasis, 1418
  in lead poisoning, 2421
  nonsteroidal antiinflammatory drugs for, 2926
  renal, 1586-1593, 1586b, 1589f-1592f, 1593b. *See also* Urolithiasis.
Colitis
  antibiotic-associated, *Clostridium difficile,* 1470t, 1474-1475
  dysenteric, infectious causes of, 228, 229t-230t
  ulcerative, 1500-1503, 1502b, 1502f, 1503b
    in children, 2615-2616
    skin lesions in, 1862t
Collagen, in wound healing, 842-843
Collagen vascular disease, oral manifestations of, 1035, 1035f
Collar-button abscess, 617, 617f
Collateral geniculate artery injury, in tibial femoral knee dislocation, 788
Collateral ligament
  of ankle, 808, 809f
  of knee
    anatomy of, 770, 771f
    injury to, 791-792
    stress test of, 774
  radial, 647, 648f
    injury to, 604
  stress test of, 774
  ulnar, 647, 648f
    injury to, 604
Colles' fracture, 632-633, 634f, 635f
  reverse, 633-635, 635f
Colloid solutions
  for anaphylaxis, 1833
  for hemorrhagic shock, 52
  for septic shock, 53
Colon
  congenital aganglionosis of, 2612-2613
  distention of, in large bowel obstruction, 1496, 1496f
  diverticula of, 1492-1495, 1494b, 1495b
  ischemia of, 1503-1504
  pathologic dilation of, 1501, 1502f
  trauma to, 489, 490
  volvulus of, 1497-1499, 1498f, 1499b, 1499f
Colonic inertia, in elderly person, 237
Colonoscopy
  in colonic ischemia, 1504
  in large bowel obstruction, 1496-1497
Colorado tick fever, 2047, 2140-2141
Colorectal cancer, large bowel obstruction in, 1495
Colostrum, 2724, 2728
Colposcopy, in sexual assault examination, 987, 987b
Coma, 156-164
  alcohol-induced, 2869
  diagnostic approach to, 157-162, 158b, 159t, 160f, 162f, 163f
  disposition in, 163
  drug-induced, 1991
  empiric management of, 162-163
  epidemiology of, 156
  hypothyroid, 1991
  in anticholinergic poisoning, 2348
  in barbiturate overdose, 2482
  in carbon monoxide poisoning, 2439
  in cardiac arrest survivors
    acute coronary syndrome diagnosis and, 86
    resuscitative hypothermia for, 68-70, 69t, 85-86
  in cyclic antidepressant poisoning, 2354t, 2356
  in eclampsia, 2749
  in hepatic encephalopathy, 1411
  in high-altitude cerebral edema, 2306
  in hyperviscosity syndrome, 1913
  in intracerebral hemorrhage, 1610
  in rabies, 2066
  in Rocky Mountain spotted fever, 2134
  myxedema, 1990, 1990b, 1991, 1991b, 1993-1994
    hypothermia and, 2239
  pathophysiology of, 156
  scoring methods for, 157, 157t
Combat casualty evacuation care (CASEVAC), 3003, 3003f
Combative patient, 2956-2969
  assault by, 2963
  diagnostic studies in, 2964
  differential considerations in, 2964-2965, 2965b
  disposition of, 2969
  epidemiology of, 2956-2957
  functional vs. organic etiology of, 2963, 2964t
  history taking and physical examination of, 2963-2964, 2964t
  medical clearance of, 2965
  medicolegal issues of, 2967-2969
  pathophysiology of, 2957
  physical restraints for, 2958-2961, 2960f
  preparation of emergency department for, 2965-2967

Combative patient *(Continued)*
rapid tranquilization of, 2961-2963
risk assessment and, 2957-2958
verbal management techniques for, 2958
Combustible liquids, flash points of, 915, 915t
Comfrey, adverse effects of, 2476t
Commercial emergency department information technology systems, 3102
Comminuted fracture, 552, 552f, 2690, 2691f
Commitment, involuntary, in suicide, 1773
Common bile duct obstruction, in cholangitis, 1421, 1422f
Common cold
coronavirus infection in, 2051
pharyngitis in, 1110
Common femoral artery
anatomy of, 540, 540f
bifurcation of, arterial embolism at, 1343
Common peroneal mononeuropathy, 1698-1699, 1698f
Common peroneal nerve, 771
Commotio cordis
in children, 340
sudden death in, 2599
Commotio retinae, 1050
Communicable diseases, reporting requirements for, 3172
Communication
in disaster response, 3015
in emergency medical services, 2988-2989
information technology for, 3098
with hearing impaired patient, 2905
with visually impaired patient, 2905
Community, disaster response experience in, 3016-3017
Community preparedness, in chemical injuries, 930-931
Comparative justice, 3129, 3129b
Comparison radiographs, in fracture, 557-558
Compartment pressure, measurement of, 561-562, 561f
Compartment syndrome, 559-562, 560b, 561b, 561f
crush injury and, 3007-3008
in foot, 838-839
in hand, 614, 614f
in lower leg, 804
in peripheral vascular injury, 539
in rhabdomyolysis, 1977-1978, 1980, 1983, 1983f
in thigh, 749
in tibial femoral knee dislocation, 789
Compartments
of knee, 770, 771f
of lower leg, 797
of thigh, 737, 737t, 738f
Competence
capacity vs., 3133-3134, 3134b
determination of, in refusal of medical care, 3169
elder abuse and, 1014
impaired, consent in, 3168
of combative or violent patient, 2967
Complement
activation of, in cerebral ischemia, 66
deficiencies of, 2833
in anaphylaxis/anaphylactoid reactions, 2547
Complement pathway, 2832-2833
Complementary medicine, cultural competent approach to, 3113-3114
Complete blood count
in abdominal pain, 215, 216t
in arthritis, 1779
in bacterial meningitis, 2662
in bleeding disorders, 1894
in central nervous system infection, 1720
in delirium, 1651
in headache, 173t
in nausea and vomiting, 203
Complete fracture, 2690, 2691f
Complex regional pain syndrome, 562-563
Compound presentations, in labor and delivery, 2815-2816
Compressed air, esophageal perforation from, 483
Compression
for epistaxis, 1074
for snakebite management, 899
rhabdomyolysis from, 1978
Compressive optic neuropathy, 1000
Computed tomography
before lumbar puncture, 1716, 1716t
in abdominal aortic aneurysm, 1335, 1336f, 1338
in abdominal trauma, 496-498, 497f, 498f
in acute mesenteric ischemia, 1447-1448
in acute pancreatitis, 1432-1433
in airway foreign body aspiration, 866-867
in ankle trauma, 811
in aortic dissection, 1327, 1327f, 1327t
in aortic rupture, 479-480, 479f
in appendicitis, 1454-1455, 1455f, 1456, 2619-2620
in arthritis, 1780
in back pain, 708
in bacterial meningitis, 2662-2663
in brain abscess, 371
in brain contusion, 374
in central nervous system infection, 1719-1720
in cerebral venous thrombosis, 1670
in cervical vascular injury, 440
in chronic pancreatitis, 1436
in colonic ischemia, 1504
in comatose patient, 162
in delirium, 1651
in dementia, 1661
in depressed skull fracture, 373
in diverticular disease, 1493
in elderly trauma patient, 347
in electrical and lightning injuries, 2275-2276
in epidural hematoma, 375, 375f, 376f
in esophageal foreign body, 872
in esophageal obstruction, 1383
in esophageal perforation, 1385
in facial fracture, 388, 389, 394f
in flail chest, 457
in foot trauma, 822
in fracture, 558
in gastrointestinal foreign body, 874
in headache, 172, 173t, 2679
in head-injured child, 368
in hemoptysis, 281
in HIV/AIDS, 2079-2080
in intracerebral hemorrhage, 1613
in ischemic stroke, 1612, 1612f
in jaundice, 244
in knee trauma, 774
in large bowel obstruction, 1496
in laryngotracheal trauma, 447
in minor head trauma, 364
in moderate head trauma, 363
in multiple trauma, 312, 313
in ocular foreign body, 860, 860f
in osteomyelitis, 2181
in pediatric head trauma, 336
in pelvic fracture, 721-722, 723
in pelvic pain, 250
in peripheral vascular injury, 542
in pneumonia, 1133
in pneumothorax, 463
in pregnant trauma patient, 321, 321t
in pulmonary contusion, 460-461
in red and painful eye, 288
in renal disorders, 1528, 1528f
in renal trauma, 528, 529f
in rib fracture, 455
in seizure, 168, 1625, 2671
in septic arthritis, 2190
in severe head trauma, 362, 362t
in sinusitis, 1124, 1125f
in skull fracture, 372
in small bowel obstruction, 1443
in soft tissue foreign body, 879
in spinal injuries, 427, 429-431, 429b, 429f-432f, 430-431, 431f
in sternoclavicular joint dislocation, 684, 684f
in subarachnoid hemorrhage, 1636, 1637f
in subdural hematoma, [illegible]
in *Toxoplasma gondii* infection, 2081, 2082f
in ureteral trauma, 531
in urinary tract infection, 1578
in urolithiasis, 1589, 1589f
of parapharyngeal abscess, 1122, 1122f
of pyogenic abscess, 1415, 1415f
of retropharyngeal abscess, 1121, 1121f
Computed tomography angiography
in anthrax exposure, 3025, 3025f
in bacterial meningitis, 1716, 1716t
in cervical vascular injury, 440
Computed tomography angiography *(Continued)*
in peripheral arteriovascular disease, 1348
in pulmonary embolism, 1375-1377, 1377b
Computed tomography urogram, in renal stones, 2645-2646
Computed tomography venography, in pulmonary embolism, 1377
Computer-based protocols, for emergency medicine guidelines, 3042-3044, 3043f
Computerized physician order entry (CPOE) systems, 3043, 3043f, 3101, 3102f
Conception, estimated date of, 2727
Concussion
in children, 335
in head trauma, 365-366, 367
myocardial, 467
Conduction system, 1201-1203, 1202t, 1203f
Conductive hearing loss, 1072
Conductive heat transfer, 2255
Condylar fracture
distal, 770-777
in adults, 660-661, 661f
in children, 660
tibial, 777-779, 777f-778f
Condylomata lata, in syphilis, 1561, 1561f
Condylomata acuminata, 1518t, 1519-1520, 1559t, 1563-1564, 1564f, 2045
Cone shells, 910
Confidence intervals, 3053
Confidentiality
as value, 3129, 3129b
of patient information, 3102-3103
Confirmation bias, 132
Confounding variables, 3049, 3055
Confusion, 150-155, 156
acute, 2679
after moderate head trauma, 363
diagnostic approach to, 150-153, 151b, 152f, 153f
differential diagnosis in, 153, 154b, 154f
disposition in, 154-155
empiric management of, 154, 155f
epidemiology of, 150
guidelines for evaluation of, 1645-1646
in delirium, 1645-1655
in dementia, 1655-1662
in rabies, 2065-2066
pathophysiology of, 150
Confusional Assessment Method, in delirium, 1650, 1650f
Congenital heart disease, 2575-2582
acyanotic, 2577-2579, 2577f
chest radiography in, 2573-2574, 2574f
clinical features of, 2575-2576, 2575t
cyanotic, 2579-2581, 2579f, 2581b
diagnosis of, 2576, 2576b
ductal-dependent, 2576-2577, 2576b, 2577b
incidence of, 2575, 2575t
management of, 2576-2577, 2576b, 2577b
pediatric fever in, 2517
postoperative complications of, 2581
respiratory syncytial virus infection and, 2581-2582, 2582b
Congestive heart failure. *See* Heart failure.
Congo-Crimean hemorrhagic fever, 2055
Conium maculatum, 2472, 2473f
Conjunctiva, 1045f
foreign body in, 1048
laceration of, 1051
nonpenetrating trauma to, 1046-1048, 1047f, 1048f
Conjunctival blood gas monitoring, 36
Conjunctivitis
gonococcal, 1566
in anaphylaxis, 1825t
in Kawasaki disease, 2025-2026
red and painful eye in, 296t-297t
Connective tissue disorders
myocarditis in, 1297-1298
pericardial disease in, 1284
Conn's syndrome, hypokalemia in, 1938
Conoid ligament, 670-671, 671f
Conscience anxiety, 1746b
Conscious sedation, 2914b
Consciousness
altered, 156-164. *See also* Coma; Mental status, altered.
after head trauma, 354, 363-364
definitions of, 156-157

Consciousness *(Continued)*
diagnostic approach to, 157-162, 158b, 159t, 160f, 162f, 163f
disposition in, 163
empiric management of, 162-163
epidemiology of, 156
host defense impairment in, 1129
in beta blocker overdose, 2374
in central nervous system infection, 1714
in children, 2502-2503
in cyclic antidepressant poisoning, 2352
in high-altitude cerebral edema, 2306
in neoplastic cardiac tamponade, 1917
in scuba diving–related disorders, 2285
pathophysiology of, 156
clouding of, 156
Consent
federal vs. state laws governing, 3166
for procedural sedation and analgesia, 2940
implied, 3134, 3167
in alcohol intoxication, 3168-3169
in delirious patient, 1654-1655
in impaired competence, 3168
in patient given pain medications, 3169
in sexual assault cases, 978, 979b
informed, 3134, 3166
emergency research without, 3136-3137
for procedures on newly dead, 3149
physician's role in, 3166-3167
minors and, 3167-3168
of combative or violent patient, 2967
prisoners and, 3168
"reasonable person" vs. "professional disclosure" standard in, 3166
Constipation, 237-242
acute vs. chronic, 238b
complications of, 239
definition of, 237, 237t
diagnostic approach to, 238-239, 238b
differential diagnosis in, 239, 240f
disposition in, 242
empiric management of, 239-242, 240f, 241t, 242b
epidemiology of, 237
in children, 2612-2613
in colonic volvulus, 1497, 1498
in spinal cord injury, 2907
palliative care for, 3154
pathophysiology of, 237
Constrictive pericarditis, 1288
heart failure in, 1265
neoplastic, 1917
restrictive cardiomyopathy vs., 1296
Consultation
in HIV postexposure prophylaxis, 3086b
in observation unit, 3063
in poisoning, 2331
in spinal cord injury, 311
Consumption, galloping, 2151
Contact burn, 913-928. *See also* Thermal burn.
Contact dermatitis, skin lesions in, 1851-1852, 1851f, 1852f
Contact dermatoconjunctivitis, 296t
Contact handgun wounds, 955-956, 955f, 956f
Contact lens
corneal complications of, 1054
superficial punctate keratitis from, 1054
Contaminated air, in scuba diving–related disorders, 2283
Contamination. *See also* Decontamination.
of airway, in urban search and rescue, 3008
of blood products, 60-61
of herbal medicines, 2476-2477
radioactive
external, 2320
internal, 2320, 2324
management of, 2322-2324, 2323f
wound, 2321
Continence
loss of, 1516-1517, 1516b
physiology of, 1507
Contingency management
for factitious disorder, 1764-1765
in HAZMAT incidents, 931
Continuous positive airway pressure (CPAP), 27-28
in acute pulmonary edema, 1271, 1271f
in sleep apnea in chronic heart failure, 1277
Continuous positive airway pressure (CPAP) *(Continued)*
in submersion victim, 2314
mask, 28
Contraception, emergency, after sexual assault, 991, 991t
Contractility, in heart failure, 1260f, 1261
Contraction-relaxation cycle, 1259
Contrast agents
acute tubular necrosis from, 1536-1537
prevention of, 1539
allergy to, 1828
anaphylaxis to, 2547
Contrast studies
in abdominal trauma, 499, 499f
in bladder trauma, 521-525, 521f-526f
in esophageal foreign body, 871-872
in esophageal perforation, 485, 485f
in gastrointestinal foreign body, 873-874
in urethral trauma, 517-519, 518f-520f
Contrecoup contusion, 352, 374
Controlled mechanical ventilation (CMV), 27
Contusion
eyelid, 1044
foot, 838
in facial trauma, 390, 391
in head trauma, 335, 374
pattern
in pedestrian collisions, 966
in physical assault, 961-962, 961f, 962f
renal, 530, 530f
testicular, 534
Conus medullaris syndrome, 1678f, 1679
Convective heat transfer, 916, 917t, 2255
Convenience sample, 3048
Conversion disorder, 1755, 1755b
Convulsion, in shigellosis, 1464
Convulsive status epilepticus, 2667
Cooling system, automobile, and body's heat dissipation mechanisms, 2256-2258, 2256f
Cooling techniques
for comatose survivors of cardiac arrest, 69
for heatstroke, 2263-2264, 2264b, 2265f
Coombs and Gell classification of hypersensitivity reactions, 1821-1822
Coombs test, in hemolytic anemia, 1878
Co-oximetry, in carbon monoxide poisoning, 2439
COPD. *See* Chronic obstructive pulmonary disease.
Copper, corneal foreign body containing, 1052
Copper reduction tests, in diabetes mellitus, 1959, 1959b
Copper sulfate, for white phosphorus burn, 936
Copperheads, 896
Coprine in mushrooms, ethanol and, 2479
Cor pulmonale, in chronic obstructive pulmonary disease, 1100
Coracoacromial arch, 671f, 672
Coracoclavicular ligaments, 670-671, 671f
Coracoid process
anatomy of, 671f, 672
fracture of, 679, 680
Coral snakes, 896, 898
Core rewarming, active, 2248-2251
Core temperature, monitoring of
in heatstroke, 2263
in hypothermia, 2244
Core temperature afterdrop, in hypothermia, 2238
Corn syrup, infant botulism from, 2013
Cornea, 1045f
abrasions of, 289, 289f, 292, 294t, 933, 1047, 1047f
clouding of
in alkali burn, 1046, 1046f
in closed-angle glaucoma, 1056, 1056f
damage to, testing of, 287-288
diseases of, 1053-1054, 1054f
foreign body in, 289, 289f, 292, 294t, 297, 1047, 1047f, 1048f
herpes simplex virus infection of, 289, 290f, 295t
laceration of, 1051, 1051f
nonpenetrating trauma to, 1046-1048, 1046f, 1047f, 1048f
ulcers of, 289, 289f, 294t, 1052, 1052f, 1054
Corner stitch suture, 851
Coronary angiography, in aortic rupture, 480-481
Coronary angioplasty, percutaneous transluminal. *See* Percutaneous coronary intervention.
Coronary artery
aneurysm of, in Kawasaki disease, 2025, 2026, 2594
anomalous, sudden death in, 1298
congenital anomalies of, sudden death in, 2597
dilation of, in Kawasaki disease, 2594
embolism to, in scuba diving–related disorders, 2285
laceration of, 472
Coronary artery bypass graft, previous, fibrinolytic therapy eligibility and, 1191
Coronary artery disease
alcohol consumption and, 2866
altitude and, 2308
atherosclerotic plaques in, 1157
cardiac arrest in, 77
echocardiography in, 1179
epidemiology of, 1155
graded exercise testing in, 1180-1181
historical perspective of, 1155
in systemic lupus erythematosus, 1807
Coronary stents, in myocardial infarction, 1195
Coronary vasospasm, in acute coronary syndromes, 1157
Coronavirus, 2034t, 2050-2051
Coronoid fossa, 647, 647f
Corpus cavernosa
anatomy of, 532, 532f
rupture of, 533-534, 534f
Corpus luteum cyst rupture
ectopic pregnancy vs., 2745
pelvic pain in, 251t
Corpus spongiosum, 532, 532f
Corrigan's pulse, in aortic regurgitation, 1307
Cortical blindness, 1060
Cortical dysfunction, in confusion, 150
Corticospinal tract, lateral, 1676, 1676f
Corticosteroids. *See also specific agents, e.g.,* Prednisone.
adrenal insufficiency from, 1994-1995
allergy to, 1827
during pregnancy and lactation, 2762, 2765t, 2776, 2789
for adhesive capsulitis, 699, 699t
for anaphylactic shock, 54
for anaphylaxis, 1833, 2549
for asthma, 1087t, 1088-1089, 2539t, 2541-2543, 2543t
for atopic dermatitis, 1842
for bacterial meningitis, 1722, 2664-2665
for Behçet's disease, 1815
for Bell's palsy, 1667
for bronchiolitis, 2546
for bursitis, 1803
for calcific tendinitis, 698
for caustic ingestion, 2383
for chronic obstructive pulmonary disease, 1105-1106
for epicondylitis, 667
for granulomatous vasculitis, 1814
for Henoch-Schönlein purpura, 2615
for hypercalcemia, 1946
for hypercalcemic cancer patient, 1916
for hypothermia, 2246
for inflammatory bowel disease, 1502, 2616
for knee bursitis, 796
for meningococcal disease, 2023-2024
for microscopic polyangiitis, 1814
for migraine, 1633t, 1634
for multiple sclerosis, 1673
for myasthenia gravis, 1706
for myxedema coma, 1994
for nephrotic syndrome, 2648
for optic neuritis, 1059-1060
for organ transplant patient, 2850, 2851f
for pharyngitis, 1113
for polyarteritis nodosa, 1814
for PROM, 2808
for Rocky Mountain spotted fever, 2136-2137
for sciatica, 711
for sepsis, 2222
for septic shock, 54
for severe head trauma, 361
for spinal injuries, 438
for subacromial syndromes, 696

Corticosteroids *(Continued)*
  for superior vena cava syndrome, 1911
  for systemic lupus erythematosus, 1808-1809
  for thyroid storm, 1989
  for tuberculosis, 2168
  for viral croup, 2526-2527
  immunosuppressive effects of, 2843-2844
  medical indications for, 1995, 1996b
  ophthalmic, 1063b, 1064
  toxicity of, 1417
Corticotropin. *See* Adrenocorticotropic hormone.
Cortisol, in glucose regulation, 1957
Cortisone acetate, for adrenal insufficiency, 1998
Corynebacterium diphtheriae, 1110-1111, 2001, 2002. *See also* Diphtheria.
Costochondral separation, 457
Costoclavicular ligaments, 670, 671f
Costoclavicular syndrome, 1359
Cotton fever, in intravenous drug abuse, 2454
Cotton's fracture, 550t
Cough
  as host defense, 1128-1129
  in airway foreign body aspiration, 865, 866
  in asthma, 1083
  in bacterial tracheitis, 2528
  in bronchiolitis, 2545
  in chronic obstructive pulmonary disease, 1099, 1100
  in high-altitude pulmonary edema, 2303
  in pertussis, 2005
  in pneumonia, 2556
  in tuberculosis, 2149
  in viral croup, 2525
  whooping, 2559-2560
Cough cardiopulmonary resuscitation, 90
Cough headache, 1642
Counter Narcotics and Terrorism Operational Medical Support Program, 3003
Counterimmunoelectrophoresis, in central nervous system infection, 1718
Coup contusion, 374
Couplet, 1222
Coupling interval, 1222
Courts, as surrogate decision-makers, 3135
Cowpox virus, 2040
Coxiella burnetii, 1131, 2137
Coxsackie A virus infection, exanthems in, 1849
Coxsackie B virus infection
  in myocarditis, 1289
  in pancreatitis, 1428
Coxsackievirus, 2057
Coyote, rabies in, 2062-2063, 2064
Cozen's test, in lateral epicondylitis, 1798
Crack cocaine, 2386, 2387t
"Crack dancing," 2388
Cramps
  abdominal. *See* Abdominal cramps.
  heat, 2258, 2258b
Cranial decompression, in severe head trauma, 361
Cranial nerve examination, in head trauma, 357
Cranial neuropathy, 1664-1670, 1665t
  diabetic, 1669-1670
  eye movement disorders in, 1062-1063
  in ethylene glycol poisoning, 2399
  in Lyme disease, 2123
  in tetanus, 2009
Cranial osteomyelitis, after head trauma, 371
Craniofacial abnormalities, in fetal alcohol syndrome, 2791b, 2792
Cranium, anatomy and physiology of, 350
C-reactive protein
  as cardiac marker, 1178
  in appendicitis, 1454
  in immune response, 2831
  in osteomyelitis, 2179
Creatine, in nausea and vomiting, 203
Creatine kinase
  in electrical and lightning injuries, 2276
  in rhabdomyolysis, 1980-1981, 1981f, 1983, 1990f
Creatine kinase MB isoenzyme
  in acute coronary syndromes, 1176f, 1176t, 1177-1178
  in chest pain, 188
  in cocaine-related chest pain, 2388
Creatinine
  dialysis and, 1549
  in acute renal failure, 2649
  serum, 1527
Cremasteric reflex, 1594
  loss of, in testicular torsion, 1595
Crescent sign, in Legg-Calvé-Perthes disease, 2707, 2707f
Creutzfeldt-Jakob disease, 1657-1658, 1659, 2058
Cricoid cartilage fracture, 447
Cricothyrotomy
  difficult, evaluation of, 4
  for failed airway, 9, 10f
  in airway foreign body removal, 870, 2530
  in multiple trauma, 306
  in neck trauma, 445
  percutaneous, 22-23, 23f
  surgical, 22
  with transtracheal jet ventilation, 22, 22f
Crisis intervention, for difficult patient, 2976-2977, 2977b
Critical care unit, computer order entry system for, 3043, 3043f
Critical diagnostic syndromes, observation of, 3063-3069
Critical incident stress debriefing, 3018, 3176-3177
Critically appraised topic, 3059t, 3060
Crohn's disease, 1500-1503, 1502b, 1503b, 2615-2616
Cromolyn
  during pregnancy and lactation, 2789
  for chronic asthma, 2542, 2543t
Crossed straight leg raise test, in lumbar radiculopathy, 704
Cross-sectional studies, 3046-3047
Crotamiton, for scabies, 1855
Croup, 2051
  bacterial (membranous), 2528-2529, 2529t
  screening for, 2509b
  spasmodic, 2527
  viral, 2525-2527, 2526f, 2527b, 2529t
Cruciate ligament injury, 790-791, 792
  intercondylar eminence fracture and, 779
  meniscal tears and, 792, 793
  Segond fracture and, 777, 777f
  tibial femoral knee dislocation and, 788
  tibial plateau fracture and, 778
Crush injuries, 3007-3008
  antibiotic prophylaxis in, 854
  in foot trauma, 838
Crutches
  for ankle sprain, 817
  for proximal fibula fracture, 802
Cruzan v. Director, Missouri Department of Health, 3169
Cryoglobulinemia
  hyperviscosity syndrome in, 1912
  mixed, 1815
Cryotherapy
  for condylomata acuminata, 1564
  for orthopedic injuries, 573-574
  for tendinopathy, 1801
  for trigeminal neuralgia, 1666
Cryptococcal meningitis, 2081
Cryptococcus neoformans
  in cancer patient with impaired cell-mediated immunity, 2840
  in HIV/AIDS, 2081
Cryptogenic cirrhosis, 1410
Cryptosporidium gastroenteritis, 1476-1478, 1477t
  in HIV/AIDS, 1478, 1482, 1484, 2084
Crystallization, extracellular, in frostbite, 2229, 2229b
Crystalloids
  for anaphylactic hypotension, 2549
  for bacterial meningitis, 2663
  for cardiac tamponade, 475
  for gastrointestinal bleeding, 221
  for hemorrhagic shock, 52
  for pediatric infectious diarrhea, 2631
  for pulmonary contusion, 461
  for septic shock, 53
Crystalluria, in ethylene glycol poisoning, 2398, 2399-2400
Cubitus valgus, 659
Cubitus varus, 657-658
Cuboid
  dislocation of, 828
  fracture of, 828
Culdocentesis
  in ectopic pregnancy, 2745
  in vaginal bleeding, 256t, 257
Cultural blindness, 3112
Cultural competence, 3107-3117. *See also* Racial/ethnic differences.
  as tool for enhancing emergency department care, 3111-3116
  continuum of, 3111-3112
  institutional policies promoting, 3117, 3117b
  rationale for, 3108-3111, 3108t, 3109t
  recommendations for, 3116
  standards for, 3112-3113
  to cross barrier of different beliefs, values, and life experiences, 3113-3114
  to cross language barrier, 3112-3113
Cultural considerations, in prehospital end-of-life care, 3145
Cultural destructiveness, 3111-3112
Cultural incapacity, 3112
Cultural precompetence, 3112
Culture
  blood
    in acute septic arthritis, 2705
    in AIDS-related diarrhea, 1483-1484
    in bacterial meningitis, 2662
    in central nervous system infection, 1720
    in gastrointestinal anthrax, 1469
    in infected aneurysm, 1356
    in infective endocarditis, 1301-1302
    in meningococcal disease, 2022
    in pediatric fever, 2510
    in pneumococcal disease, 2018
    in pneumonia, 1135, 2561
    in sepsis, 2216-2217
  in central nervous system infection, 1719
  in diphtheria, 2003
  in febrile, neutropenic cancer patient, 2837
  in genital herpes, 1558-1559
  in gonorrhea, 1566
  in osteomyelitis, 2182
  in pertussis, 2006
  joint fluid, in septic arthritis, 2189
  sputum
    in chronic obstructive pulmonary disease, 1101
    in pneumonia, 1134-1135
    in tuberculosis, 2154-2155
  stool
    in *Aeromonas hydrophila* gastroenteritis, 1468
    in AIDS-related diarrhea, 1483
    in *Bacillus anthracis* gastroenteritis, 1469
    in *Campylobacter* gastroenteritis, 1460
    in *Clostridium difficile* enterocolitis, 1475
    in coccidial gastroenteritis, 1478
    in diarrhea, 233
    in *Giardia* gastroenteritis, 1479
    in hemorrhagic *Escherichia coli* serotype O157:H7 gastroenteritis, 1467
    in infectious diarrhea, 2626-2627
    in intestinal amebiasis, 1480
    in pediatric fever, 2510
    in *Plesiomonas shigelloides* gastroenteritis, 1468
    in salmonellosis, 1463
    in shigellosis, 1464
    in *Vibrio* fish poisoning, 1472
    in *Vibrio parahaemolyticus* gastroenteritis, 1466
    in *Yersinia enterocolitica* gastroenteritis, 1465
  throat, in pharyngitis, 1111, 1112
  urine
    in epididymitis, 2639
    in pediatric fever, 2509-2510
    in urinary tract infection, 1576-1577, 1577b
Culture (human), definition of, 3111
Cuneiform
  dislocation of, 828
  fracture of, 828
Curling's ulcers, in burn injured patient, 924
Current, direct vs. alternating, electrical injury and, 2268

Cushing's reflex/phenomenon, after head trauma, 354
Cutaneous abscess, 2202-2204, 2203t
Cutaneous anthrax, 1860, 1861f, 3025, 3026f
Cutaneous candidiasis, 1841
Cutaneous larva migrans, 2100t, 2109
Cutaneous mastocytosis, 1835
Cutaneous presentations. *See* Skin lesions; Skin rash.
Cutis marmorata, 2284, 2499, 2499f
Cyanide antidote kit, 2329t, 2437-2438, 2440
Cyanide poisoning, 2436-2438, 2437f
  antidotes to, 2329t, 2437-2438, 2440
  as chemical weapon, 939, 3031-3032
  carbon monoxide poisoning vs., 2439
  carbon monoxide poisoning with, 2440-2441
  cyanosis in, 271
Cyano-acrylate adhesive-tipped swab, for foreign body removal from ear, 863
Cyanosis, 268-273
  ancillary studies in, 271
  central, 269, 270b, 2889-2890
  diagnostic approach to, 268-271, 270b, 270f
  differential diagnosis in, 270b, 271-273, 272f
  disposition in, 273
  empiric management of, 273
  history in, 268-269
  in airway foreign body aspiration, 866
  in high-altitude pulmonary edema, 2303
  in nitrite abuse, 2889-2890
  pathophysiology of, 268, 269b, 269f
  pediatric
    cardiac vs. pulmonary, 2569, 2569b, 2572
    in tetralogy of Fallot, 2580
    pathophysiology of, 269t, 2569
  peripheral, 269, 270b
  physical examination in, 269-271, 270f
  pseudocyanosis and, 268
Cyanotic congenital heart disease, 2579-2581, 2579f, 2581b
Cyclic antidepressants
  central nervous system effects of, 2354b
  overdose of, 2352-2357, 2353f, 2354b, 2355f, 2357t
  peripheral nervous system effects of, 2353b
  pharmacodynamic effects of, 2353b
Cyclobenzaprine, for back pain, 2928-2929
Cyclooxygenase inhibitors, 1082, 2342
Cyclooxygenase-2 inhibitors, 2927-2928, 2927b, 2927f
  in aspirin-exacerbated respiratory disease, 1082
Cyclophosphamide
  for Goodpasture syndrome, 1816
  for granulomatous vasculitis, 1814
  for mixed cryoglobulinemia, 1815
Cycloplegics, 1063b, 1064
  for red and painful eye, 292, 297t
Cycloserine, for tuberculosis, 2163t, 2164-2165
Cyclospora cayetanensis gastroenteritis, 1477t, 1478-1479
Cyclosporine, 2844
  drug interactions with, 2850, 2850t
  during pregnancy and lactation, 2776
  for inflammatory bowel disease, 1503
  for myasthenia gravis, 1706
  for organ transplant patient, 2849-2850, 2850t
  nephrotoxicity of, 2850
  toxicity of, 1417
Cyclothymic disorder, 1739
CYP450 enzymes, in acetaminophen metabolism, 2332, 2332f
Cyproheptadine, for serotonin toxicity, 2360
Cyst, 1839t
  Baker's, 796, 797f
  Bartholin, 1559-1560
  corpus luteum, ruptured
    ectopic pregnancy vs., 2745
    pelvic pain in, 251t
  hydatid, 2102t, 2105-2106, 2106f, 2111, 2113
  leptomeningeal, in head-injured child, 368
  ovarian, 251t
  popliteal, 796, 797f
Cystic duct obstruction, cholecystitis in, 1420
Cystic fibrosis
  in children, 2564-2565, 2565f
  pneumonia in, 1132
Cystic myelopathy, in spinal cord injury, 2909
Cysticercosis, 2102t, 2105
Cystine kidney stones, 1587
Cystitis, 1573
  dysuria in, 1580-1581
  guidelines for management of, 3042
  in children, 2642, 2643, 2644
  in men, 1585
  in urinary tract infection, 1575
  treatment of, 1581-1582, 1581t
Cystography, retrograde
  computed tomography, in bladder trauma, 521, 525, 526f
  conventional, in bladder trauma, 521, 521f-526f
Cystostomy, for urinary retention, 1600, 1600f
Cytoid body, in malignant hypertension, 1315
Cytokines
  as anaphylaxis mediators, 1823, 1823b
  during resuscitation from hemorrhagic shock, 46
  in asthma, 1080, 1080f, 1081
  in bacterial meningitis, 2662
  in cerebral ischemia, 66-67
  in sepsis, 2213
  in shock, 43, 44f, 45
Cytomegalovirus infection, 2043-2044
  drugs for, 2036t
  in cancer patient with impaired cell-mediated immunity, 2840
  in esophagitis, 1387
  in gastroenteritis, 1482, 1484
  in HIV/AIDS, 1482, 1484, 2076, 2086
  in organ transplant patient, 2847-2848
  in pneumonia, 1130
  in retinitis, 2086
Cytotoxic cerebral edema
  after head trauma, 354
  in high-altitude cerebral edema, 2300
Cytotoxic diarrhea, 228
Cytotoxic hypersensitivity reactions, 1821

D-400, drug interactions with, 2478t
Dacroadenitis, 293t
Dacryocystitis, 293t, 1055, 1055f
Dalton's law, 2280, 2994-2995, 2995t
Dance's sign, in intussusception, 2611
Danger Assessment instrument, 1000, 1003b
Danger space, 1117
Danis-Weber classification of ankle fractures, 814f
Dantrolene
  for neuroleptic malignant syndrome, 1733, 2449
  for phenelzine overdose, 2365
Dapsone, in HIV/AIDS, side effects of, 2079t
Darkfield microscopy, in syphilis, 1561, 1856
Dashboard fracture, 550t
Data, definition of, 3097
Data access, information technology for, 3097
Data analysis in evidence-based medicine, 3051-3058, 3051t, 3057f
  confidence intervals in, 3053
  data dredging or torturing in, 3056
  hypothesis testing in, 3051-3058, 3051t, 3057f
  intention-to-treat analysis in, 3056-3057, 3057f
  interim analyses of accumulating data in, 3054
  meta-analysis in, 3057-3058
  multiple comparisons in, 3053-3054
  multivariate models in, 3054-3055
  prior probabilities and, 3055-3056
  statistical tests in, 3052-3053, 3052t
  subgroups in, 3054
Data collection, 3050
Data dredging or torturing, 3056
Data management, 3050
Databases, electronic, 3059, 3099
Datura stramonium poisoning, 2345, 2346, 2473, 2473f
D-dimer analysis
  in cerebral venous thrombosis, 1671
  in deep venous thrombosis, 1369-1370
  in pulmonary embolism, 1374-1375
DDT (dichlorodiphenyltrichloroethane), 2462-2463, 2462b
De Quervain's tenosynovitis, 1799
Death. *See also* End of life.
  autopsy after, 3149
  brain, 3141
  cardiopulmonary, 3141
Death *(Continued)*
  causes of, 942t
  definitions of, 3141
  epidemiology of, 3140-3141, 3140f
  field pronouncement of, 3144
  "good," 3142
  grief response after, 3149-3151, 3150b
  in emergency department, 3146-3151, 3146b, 3148b
  injury, causes of, 949t
  new, consent for procedures after, 3149
  of child
    in emergency department, 2717
    prehospital issues related to, 3145-3146
  reporting requirements for, 3172
  sedation for survivors after, 3149
  triage marker of, 2251
  viewing body after, 3148-3149
Death notification
  by phone, 3148
  empathy in, 3147-3149, 3148b
  training in, bioethical dilemmas in, 3135
Debacterol, for aphthous stomatitis, 1036
Debridement
  in open tibial shaft fracture, 801
  in wound management, 847
  surgical, in osteomyelitis, 2187
Decelerations, in fetal heart rate, 2801, 2803f
Decerebrate posturing
  in cerebral herniation, 355, 356
  in head trauma, 357
Decision analysis, 132
Decision making
  diagnostic approach and, 125-130, 127f, 128b, 129f
  errors in, 130-133, 131t, 133b
Decision-makers, surrogate, 3134-3135
Decision-making capacity, 3133-3134, 3134b
Decision-making process, as stressor for emergency physician, 3175
Decompression
  in burn injury, 925, 925f
  in cardiopulmonary resuscitation, 89, 98
  in pneumothorax, 1147
  in severe head trauma, 361
  in small bowel obstruction, 1444
  in thoracic outlet syndrome, 1360
  in urinary retention, 1599
  surgical, in spinal stenosis, 712
Decompression sickness, 2283-2285
  flying and, 2293-2294, 2293f
  recompression therapy for, 2288-2292, 2288b, 2289f-2291f
  type I, 2279, 2284
  type II, 2284-2285
Decongestants
  for sinusitis, 1125
  ophthalmic, 1063b
Decontamination
  gastrointestinal, 2330. *See also specific type, e.g.,* Activated charcoal.
    in anticholinergic poisoning, 2349
    in barbiturate overdose, 2483
    in bipyridyl compound poisoning, 2466
    in hydrocarbon poisoning, 2431
    in iron overdose, 2420
    in mercury poisoning, 2426
    in opioid overdose, 2455
  in bipyridyl compound poisoning, 2466
  in chlorinated hydrocarbon poisoning, 2463
  in HAZMAT incidents, 931
  in mustard exposure, 3031
  in nerve agent exposure, 3030
  in organophosphate poisoning, 2460
  in pyrethrin and pyrethroid exposure, 2467
  in radiation exposure, 2322-2323, 2323f, 3023
  in toxic disasters, 3017
Decorticate posturing, in head trauma, 357
Decubitus ulcer
  in developmentally disabled patient, 2903
  in physically disabled patient, 2907
  in spinal injuries, 438
Deep fascia
  anatomy of, 842
  cervical, 442-443, 1027
Deep fascial space infection in hand, 617-618, 617f
Deep partial-thickness burn, 918-919, 919f
Deep peroneal nerve, 797

Deep sedation, 2938, 2939b
Deep tendon reflexes
examination of, in spinal injuries, 417, 417t
in head trauma, 357
pseudomyotonic, in hypothyroidism, 1992
Deep vein thrombosis. *See* Venous thrombosis.
DEET
overdose of, 2468-2469
prophylactic, for tick-borne illness, 2147
Defasciculation, in rapid sequence intubation, 11b
Defecation
bleeding with, 1508
normal, 237
physiology of, 1507-1508
Defense Against Weapons of Mass Destruction Act, 938
Deferoxamine
for iron overdose, 2420
for thalassemia, 1872-1873
Defibrillation
in cardiac arrest, 90-91
in hypothermia, 2246
in infants and children, 2586b
in pacemaker patient, 1255
in pediatric resuscitation, 113
in ventricular fibrillation and pulseless ventricular tachycardia, 84, 112
prehospital, 2990
Degenerative joint disease. *See* Osteoarthritis.
Degloving injuries, penile, 532
Dehydration. *See also* Hypovolemia.
clinical assessment of, 2627t
during air medical transport, 2995
heat illness and, 2256
in AIDS-related diarrhea, 1483
in diabetic ketoacidosis, 1962, 1964, 1966
in hypercalcemia, 1945
in hyperglycemic hyperosmolar nonketotic coma, 1968, 1969
in pediatric infectious diarrhea, 2629, 2629t
in *Plesiomonas shigelloides* gastroenteritis, 1468
in pneumonia, 2562
observation in, 3071-3072, 3072b
types of, by serum sodium, 2629t
Delayed primary wound closure, 849
Delbet classification of pediatric femoral fractures, 763, 763f
Delirium, 156, 1645-1655
clinical findings in, 1648-1651, 1650f
confusion vs., 150
dementia vs., 1645, 1653, 1660
diagnosis and ancillary studies in, 1651-1652
diagnostic criteria for, 1645, 1645b
differential diagnosis in, 1652-1653, 1652t, 2348, 2348b
disposition in, 1655
etiology of, 1647-1648, 1647t
in anticholinergic poisoning, 2348
in HIV/AIDS, 2086
management of, 1653-1655
pathophysiology of, 1645-1647
Delirium tremens, 1653, 2861
Delivery. *See* Labor and delivery.
Delta gap
calculation of, 1924
in mixed acid-base disorders, 1931
Delta wave, in Wolff-Parkinson-White syndrome, 1235
Delusional disorder, 1729
Delusions
in amphetamine abuse, 2894
in depression, 1737
in schizophrenia, 1727
Dementia, 1655-1662
advanced, palliative care in, 3154
AIDS, 2081
Alzheimer's. *See* Alzheimer's disease.
clinical features of, 1658-1660, 1659t, 1660t
cortical vs. subcortical, 1659, 1659t
delirium vs., 1645, 1653, 1660
depression vs., 1740-1741
diagnosis of, 1660-1661, 1661b
diagnostic criteria for, 1654, 1654b
differential diagnosis in, 1660
etiology of, 1656, 1656b
pathophysiology of, 1656-1658
Dementia *(Continued)*
pseudodementia (depression) vs., 1656, 1659-1660, 1660t
treatment and disposition in, 1661-1662
Demyelinating polyneuropathy, 1690-1691, 1690b
Demyelination
in hyponatremia, 1935
in multiple sclerosis, 1681-1682
in transverse myelitis, 1682
Dengue, 2049-2050
Dental bacterial plaque, 1028
Dental caries, 1028-1029, 1030-1032, 1030f, 1031f
Dental disorders, in developmentally disabled patient, 2903
Dental emergencies. *See also* Oral medicine.
nontraumatic, 1027-1029, 1030f
traumatic, 1036-1042
Dental infection
airway management in, 1032
extension of, into head and neck, 1027, 1028-1029, 1030f, 1032
Ludwig's angina and, 1032, 1118-1119
Dental pain. *See* Oral pain.
Dentin fracture, 1037
Dentition. *See* Tooth (teeth).
Department of Homeland Security, 3018
Department of Transportation drug testing guidelines, 3080
Department of Veterans Affairs, 3018-3019
Dependent patient, 2978, 2978t, 2980
Dependent personality disorder, 2979b
Depolarization, 1200
Depolarizing agents, in intubation, 13-14
Depressed skull fracture, 373
Depression
asthma and, 1082
clinical features of, 1736-1738, 1736b, 1737b
criteria for, 1736, 1736b
differential considerations in, 1740-1741
dysthmic, 1738
epidemiology of, 1735
in alcoholism, 2875
in children and adolescents, 1737
in elderly person, 1737-1738, 2827
in HIV/AIDS, 2086-2087
in pseudodementia, 1656, 1659-1660, 1660t
in seasonal affective disorder, 1738
masked (hidden), 1737
panic attack in, 1748-1749
pathophysiology of, 1735-1736
postpartum, 1738, 2821-2822
psychosocial theories of, 1736
somatoform disorders vs., 1756-1757
stabilization in, 1741
substance-induced, 1739-1740, 1740b
suicide and, 1737, 1768, 1769
treatment of, 1741-1742
Dermacentor andersoni tick, 908
Dermacentor variabilis tick, 908, 2118f, 2121f
Dermatitis
atopic, 1841-1842
contact, 1851-1852, 1851f, 1852f
diaper, 1852
erythematous, 1863f
gonococcal, 1566, 1843-1844, 1843f, 2191
in arthritis-dermatitis syndrome, 1566, 1788, 1843-1844, 1843f
infectious eczematoid, in otitis media, 1067-1068
seborrheic, in HIV/AIDS, 2085
Dermatoconjunctivitis, 296t
Dermatographism, in urticaria, 1848, 1848f
Dermatologic presentations. *See* Skin lesions; Skin rash.
Dermatomes, sensory, 418f
Dermatomyositis, 1708
internal malignancy associated with, 1863
neuromuscular dysphagia in, 1396
skin lesions in, 1862t, 1863f
Dermatophyte infections, 1838-1840, 1839f, 1840f
Dermis, 842, 914
Dermopathy, diabetic, 1861f, 1862t, 1863f, 1971-1972
Descending aortic rupture, 476-477
Desferrioxamine, for rhabdomyolysis, 1982
Designer amphetamines, 2400-2409, 2410-2411
Desmopressin
for hemophilia A, 1902
for von Willebrand's disease, 1903
Detergents, ocular trauma from, 1046
Detorsion, in colonic volvulus, 1499
Developmental milestones, 2495-2497, 2496t
Developmentally disabled patient, 2898-2904, 2900t-2902t
abuse of, 1015
cardiovascular disorders in, 2902
cerebral palsy in, 2903-2904
cerebrospinal fluid shunts in, 2899
dental disorders in, 2903
failure to thrive in, 2900-2901
fractures in, 2901
gastrointestinal disorders in, 2903
musculoskeletal disorders in, 2901-2902
psychiatric disorders in, 2903
pulmonary disorders in, 2903
seizures in, 2898-2899
skin disorders in, 2903
Devil's claw, drug interactions with, 2478t
Dexamethasone
for acute mountain sickness, 2302
for adrenal insufficiency, 1998
for asthma, 2539t, 2541
for bacterial meningitis, 1722, 2664-2665
for cerebral herniation, 1918
for epidural spinal cord compression, 1919
for high-altitude cerebral edema, 2306
for meningococcal disease, 2024
for septic arthritis, 2193
for thyroid storm, 1989
for viral croup, 2526, 2527
Dexamethasone suppression test, in dementia, 1661
Dexon suture, 852t
Dextran, low-molecular-weight, in frostbite, 2233
Dextromethorphan
respiratory effects of, 2453t
toxicity of, 2413-2414, 2415, 2416
Dextrose
for acute renal failure, 2650
for alcohol intoxication, 2860
for alcohol withdrawal syndrome, 2861
for alcoholic ketoacidosis, 2873
for burn injured children, 923
for comatose patient, 157-158
for hypoglycemia, 1961
for neonatal resuscitation, 123t, 124
for pediatric infectious diarrhea, 2631
for Wernicke-Korsakoff syndrome, 2869
Dezocine, 2924, 2924b
Diabetes insipidus
causes of, 1936b
hypernatremia in, 1935, 1936
Diabetes mellitus, 1955-1974
anxiety in, 1747
carpal tunnel syndrome in, 1697
classification of, 1957, 1957b
clinical features of, 1958-1959
cranial mononeuropathy in, 1669-1670
delirium in, 1649
diagnosis of, 1959-1960, 1959b
epidemiology of, 1958
etiology and pathophysiology of, 1958
gestational, 1957, 2772
hyperglycemic hyperosmolar nonketotic coma in, 1968-1970, 1968b, 1969b
hypoglycemia in, 1960-1961, 1960b, 1961b
hypomagnesemia in, 1948
immune defects in, 2841
in alcoholism, 2871
in pancreatitis, 1435
in pregnancy, 1972, 2764t, 2771-2772
infectious complications in, 1971, 2841
ketoalkalosis in, 1963
late complications of, 1970-1972
mononeuropathy multiplex in, 1699
myocardial infarction in, atypical presentations associated with, 1159
nephropathy in, 1970
in pregnancy, 1972
neuropathy in, 1691-1692, 1970-1971
in pregnancy, 1972
lower extremity ulcers in, 1351, 1971
new trends in, 1973
oral manifestations of, 1035
retinopathy in, 1970
in pregnancy, 1972
skin lesions in, 1861f, 1862t, 1863f, 1971-1972
urinary tract infection in, 1578

Diabetic foot, 1971
osteomyelitis in, 2185-2186
Diabetic ketoacidosis, 1928, 1962-1967
complications of, 1967
diagnosis of, 1963-1964
differential considerations in, 1964-1965
disposition in, 1967
etiology of, 1963
hypophosphatemia in, 1951
in pregnancy, 1972, 2771-2772
laboratory tests in, 1964, 1964t
management of, 1965-1967, 1965b
nausea and vomiting in, 205t
pathophysiology of, 1962-1963, 1962t, 1963f
Diagnostic approach, clinical decision making and, 125-130, 127f, 128b, 129f
Diagnostic-therapeutic trial, in clinical decision making, 128
Dialysate, bloody, causes of, 1553
Dialysis
for acute renal failure, 2650
for acute tumor lysis syndrome, 1912, 1912b
for barbiturate overdose, 2483
for beta blocker overdose, 2375
for bipyridyl compound poisoning, 2466
for chronic heart failure, 1277
for chronic renal failure, 1547-1554
complications of, 1549-1554, 1550b, 1552b, 1553t
emergency, indications for, 1548-1549, 1548b
for hyperkalemia, 1941
for isopropyl alcohol poisoning, 2404
for lithium toxicity, 2444
for pulmonary edema in chronic renal failure, 1546, 1548
for rewarming in accidental hypothermia, 2249, 2250t, 2251
for salicylate overdose, 2342
for toxic alcohol poisoning, 2401-2402
for uremic pericarditis, 1282
vascular access for, problems related to, 1364-1366
Dialysis disequilibrium syndrome, 1622
Diaper dermatitis, 1852
Diaphoresis
in asthma, 1084
in ciguatera fish poisoning, 1473
Diaphragm
in pregnancy, 317
injury to, laparotomy and, 504
Diaphragmatic hernia
neonatal resuscitation in, 121
traumatic, in children, 340, 341
Diaphyseal fracture, 2699
Diaphysis, 2175, 2175f
Diarrhea, 227-236
acute vs. chronic, 228
ancillary studies in, 233
diagnostic approach to, 228-233, 230b, 231b
differential diagnosis in, 228, 230b-231b, 234
disposition in, 235-236
empiric management of, 234-235, 234f, 236t
epidemiology of, 227-228
from abnormal motility, 228
history in, 232
hypokalemia from, 1938
in *Aeromonas hydrophila* gastroenteritis, 1467
in *Bacillus anthracis* gastroenteritis, 1469
in *Bacillus cereus* food poisoning, 1471
in *Campylobacter* gastroenteritis, 1460
in ciguatera fish poisoning, 1473
in *Clostridium difficile* enterocolitis, 1475
in *Clostridium perfringens* food poisoning, 1471
in coccidial gastroenteritis, 1477, 1478
in *Escherichia coli* food poisoning, 1474
in *Giardia* gastroenteritis, 1479
in hemolytic uremic syndrome, 2654
in hemorrhagic *Escherichia coli* serotype O157:H7 gastroenteritis, 1466
in HIV/AIDS, 1482-1484, 1482t, 1483b, 1485t, 2084
in inflammatory bowel disease, 1501, 2616
in intestinal amebiasis, 1480
in intussusception, 2610
in parasitic infection, 2112, 2112f, 2113f
in *Plesiomonas shigelloides* gastroenteritis, 1468
in salmonellosis, 1463
Diarrhea *(Continued)*
in scombroid fish poisoning, 1472
in shigellosis, 1464
in staphylococcal food poisoning, 1470
in *Vibrio* fish poisoning, 1472
in *Vibrio parahaemolyticus* gastroenteritis, 1466
in viral gastroenteritis, 1476
in *Yersinia enterocolitica* gastroenteritis, 1465
infectious, 228, 230b
pediatric, 2623-2634
treatment of, 229t-230t, 235
inflammatory, 228, 229t-230t
metabolic acidosis in, 2624
noninfectious, 228, 231b
osmotic, 228, 2624
pathophysiology of, 228, 229t-230t
pediatric, 227, 2623-2634, 2628b, 2628t. *See also* Children, infectious diarrhea in.
physical examination in, 232-233
rapid assessment and stabilization in, 228, 232
secretory, 228, 2624
severe, with blood and mucus. *See* Dysentery.
traveler's, 1484-1487, 1486t, 1487b
Diastolic dysfunction
in heart failure, 1267
in restrictive cardiomyopathy, 1296
Diathermic rewarming, 2250
Diazepam, 2484, 2484t
for alcohol withdrawal syndrome, 2862, 2863
for alcohol-related seizure, 2864, 2865
for cocaine overdose, 2389
for febrile seizure, 2667
for nerve agent exposure, 3030
for psychostimulant intoxication, 2410
for seizure, 166, 166t, 1626, 1627t
in cancer patient, 1919
in children, 2675t
for status epilepticus, 2672-2673, 2672t
for tetanus, 2011
for vertigo, 146
in ventilated patient, 30
prophylactic, in severe head trauma, 361
Dichloroacetic acid, for condylomata acuminata, 1564
Dichlorophenoxyacetic acid, 2465b
Diclofenac, 2927
Dicloxacillin
during pregnancy and lactation, 2784
for folliculitis, 1843
for impetigo, 1843
for staphylococcal scalded skin syndrome, 1845
Didanosine, 2079t
Dieffenbachia, 2473, 2473f
Diet
BRAT, for diarrhea, 235
diabetic, 1973
during pregnancy, 2736
high-fiber, for diverticular disease, 1494
in acute pancreatitis, 1433-1434
in burn injury, 918
Dietary guidelines
for traveler's diarrhea prophylaxis, 1486
of American Heart Association, 3177, 3177b
Dietary supplements, 2475-2477, 2476t
Diethylcarbamazine, for loiasis, 2110
Diethylenetriamine pentaacetic acid, for plutonium exposure, 3023
Difficult airway
approach to, 8-9, 9f
cricothyrotomy for, 22-23, 23f
esophagotracheal combitube for, 20, 20f
fiberoptic intubation of, 20-21, 22f
identification of, 3-4, 3b, 4b, 5f
in children, 2502, 2502b
intubating laryngeal mask airway for, 19, 19f
lighted stylet for, 19-20, 20f
retrograde intubation of, 20
special airway devices for, 18-23, 19f-23f
Difficult patient, 2972-2982
as stressor for emergency physician, 3175
behavioral classification of, 2978-2981, 2978t
combative patient as, 2956-2969. *See also* Combative patient.
definition of, 2972-2973
emergency department factors in, 2973
impaired patient-physician relationship and, 2973, 2974f
Difficult patient *(Continued)*
management of, 2973-2981
crisis intervention in, 2976-2977, 2977b
dealing with negative reactions in, 2975-2976
general strategies in, 2973-2975, 2973b
personality disorder classification of, 2978, 2979b
physician factors in, 2973
Diffuse axonal injury
in child abuse, 971
in head trauma, 374
Digital radiography, in fracture, 557
Digital subtraction angiography
in peripheral vascular injury, 543
intravenous, in aortic rupture, 480-481
Digitalis lanata, 2476
Digoxin (digitalis)
as antidysrhythmic drug, 1211-1212, 1211t
during pregnancy and lactation, 2787
for acute pulmonary edema in hypotensive patient, 1270t, 1274
for atrial flutter, 1229
for chronic heart failure, 1276
for heart failure, 2583, 2583t
for junctional tachycardia, 1234
hyperkalemia from, 1940
misconceptions about, 1212
overdose of, 2368-2373
acute vs. chronic, 2369, 2370t
antidotes to, 2329t
clinical features of, 2369, 2370b
diagnosis of, 2369-2370
differential diagnosis in, 2370
disposition in, 2372-2373
dysrhythmias associated with, 2369b
in children, 2372, 2372t
management of, 2370-2371, 2372b
pathophysiology of, 2368-2369, 2369b
risk of, factors associated with, 2369b
side effects of, 1211-1212, 1212b
Dihydrocodeine, respiratory effects of, 2453t
Dihydroergotamine, for migraine, 1633t, 1634
Dihydropyridines, 1321t
Dilated cardiomyopathy, 1293-1294
heart failure in, 1264
inflammatory. *See* Myocarditis.
peripartum cardiomyopathy and, 1297
Dilation and curettage, after miscarriage, 2742
Dilation and evacuation, in ectopic pregnancy, 2745
Diloxanide, for intestinal amebiasis, 1481
Diltiazem, 1211, 1321t
during pregnancy and lactation, 2788
for atrial flutter, 1229
for dysphagia, 1398
overdose of, 2376, 2377t
Dilutional thrombocytopenia, 1898
Dimenhydrinate, for vertigo, 146
Dimercaprol
for arsenic poisoning, 2424
for lead poisoning, 2422
2,3-Dimercaptosuccinic acid
for arsenic poisoning, 2424
for lead poisoning, 2422
for mercury poisoning, 2426
Dinitrocresol, 2463, 2463b
Dinitrophenol, 2463, 2463b, 2464
Diphenhydramine
anticholinergic toxicity of, 2345
for acute extrapyramidal symptoms, 2449
for anaphylactic shock, 54
for anaphylaxis, 1831b, 1832, 2549
for drug eruptions, 1845
for hymenoptera stings, 904
for local anesthesia, 847, 2931
for OTC sleep aid overdose, 2487-2488, 2488t
for scombroid fish poisoning, 1472
for upper airway angioedema, 1835
for vertigo, 146
Diphenoxylate
for diarrhea, 236t
overdose of, 2456
respiratory effects of, 2453t
Diphtheria, 2001-2004, 2003b
myocarditis in, 1291
pharyngitis in, 1110-1111, 1113
vaccine for, 2002, 2004, 2012, 2012t
Diphyllobothrium latum, 2102t, 2107

Diplegia, spastic, in cerebral palsy, 2904
Dipstick tests, in diabetes mellitus, 1959, 1959b
Dipylidium caninum, 2102t
Dipyridamole, for Kawasaki disease, 2027
Diquat poisoning, 2465-2466, 2465b
Direct antiglobulin test, in hemolytic anemia, 1878
Direct current, electrical injury and, 2268
Direct patient admission, medicolegal issues in, 3159
Direct thrombin inhibitors, in acute coronary syndromes, 1188
"Dirty bomb," 2316
Disability. *See also* Developmentally disabled patient; Physically disabled patient.
  assessment of, in pediatric trauma, 330, 330b, 331t, 332t
  in elderly trauma patient, 348
  vs. impairment, 3078
  work-related, types of, 3078
Disaster
  bioethical dilemmas in, 3136
  internal vs. external, 3010-3011
  PICE nomenclature vs., 3011-3012, 3011t, 3012b, 3012t
  role of informatics in, 3105
  scene of, organization of, 3014-3015
Disaster preparedness, 3010-3019
  comprehensive emergency management in, 3015
  definitions in, 3010-3012
  disaster response organizations and, 3018-3019
  external disaster plan in, 3015
  for catastrophic disasters, 3016-3017
  for focal disasters, 3016
  for nuclear, biologic, and chemical terrorism, 3017-3018
  for radiation exposure, 2323
  for toxic disasters, 3017
  for weapons of mass destruction, 3017-3018
  future directions in, 3019
  hazards analysis in, 3012
  hospital response in, 3015-3016
  internal disaster plan in, 3015
  nature of disasters and, 3010-3012
  need for local response in, 3017
  planning in, 3015-3016
  prehospital response in, 3014-3015
  stress management and, 3018
  triage in, 3012-3014, 3013f
Disaster preparedness committee, 3015
Discharge instructions
  in procedural sedation and analgesia, 2943
  in wound management, 855-856, 856b
  preprinted, 3102
Discoid rash, in systemic lupus erythematosus, 1806
Discontinuation syndrome, with antidepressants, 2365-2366
Discrimination, and health outcomes, 3109-3110
Disease and injury prevention. *See* Injury prevention and control.
Disease transmission
  in HIV/AIDS, 990, 990b, 2073, 2810
  in tuberculosis, 2147, 2169-2171, 2170b
  via human bite, 891
Disequilibrium syndrome, in hemodialysis patient, 1551
Dishwashing detergents, ingestion of, 2380, 2381t
Disinfection, skin, in wound care, 847
Disk herniation
  lumbar, 702-703, 704-705, 711-712
  magnetic resonance imaging in, 432, 433f
  radicular pain in, 264
Diskectomy, surgical, 711
Diskitis, in children, vertebral osteomyelitis vs., 2185
Dislocation, 564-566, 565f. *See also* Fracture-dislocation; Instability.
  ankle, 820
  atlantoaxial or atlanto-occipital, 399, 401, 402f, 405-406, 408f
  biceps tendon, 698
  carpal, 630-631, 630f-632f
  distal radioulnar joint, 636-637, 640-641, 640f
  elbow, 664-666, 664f, 665f
  facet
    bilateral, 404, 405f
    unilateral, 406, 408f-409f, 409
Dislocation *(Continued)*
  foot
    cuneiform, cuboid, or navicular, 828
    interphalangeal, 835-836
    Lisfranc, 828-831, 829f, 830f
    metatarsophalangeal, 835
    subtalar, 825-826, 825f
    total talar, 826
  hand, 600-604, 601f-603f
  hip, 756-759, 757f-759f
    arterial injury in, 761
    avascular necrosis after, 740
    pediatric, 763
    prosthetic, 749, 750f, 760
  in electrical and lightning injuries, 2273
  in Monteggia's fracture, 642, 642f
  knee
    patellar, 785-786, 785b
    tibial femoral, 787-790, 789f
  lens, 1049
  peroneal tendon, 818-819, 819f
  proximal tibiofibular joint, 802-803
  shoulder, 683-693
    acromioclavicular, 685-687, 686f, 687f
    glenohumeral, 687-693, 688f-694f
    scapulothoracic, 693
    sternoclavicular, 683-685, 684f-685f
  temporomandibular joint, 396, 1041-1042, 1041f
  testicular, 534
  thumb
    carpometacarpal joint, 604
    interphalangeal joint, 564, 565f, 603
Disopyramide, 1206, 2787
Displacement
  in extension supracondylar fracture, 656-657
  in femoral neck fracture, 751, 752b
  in medial epicondylar fracture, 662-663
  in olecranon fracture, 663
  in proximal humerus fractures, 681, 681f, 682f
Disposition requirements, 3164-3165, 3165t
Disseminated intravascular coagulation, 1903-1904, 1904t
  after head trauma, 371
  in anaphylaxis, 1825t
  in meningococcal disease, 2022
  in pregnancy, placental abruption and, 319-320
  in rhabdomyolysis, 1981
  in sepsis, 2214
Dissociative agent intoxication, 2413-2426, 2414t, 2415t
Dissociative anesthesia, in syringomyelia, 1683
Dissociative sedation, 2914b, 2938, 2939b
Distal femur
  anatomy of, 770, 771f
  epiphyseal fracture of, 780-781
  fracture of, 776-777
Distal fibula, avulsion fracture of, 818
Distal humerus
  anatomy of, 647, 647f
  fracture of, 655-661
    condylar, 660-661, 661f
    intercondylar, 659-660, 659f
    lateral condyle, 660
    medial condyle, 660
    supracondylar, 655-659, 656f-658f
      in children, 2693-2697, 2694f-2696f, 2694t
    transcondylar, 659, 659f
Distal interphalangeal joint
  dislocation of, 564, 565f, 601, 601f
  extensor tendon injury at, 605-607, 606f, 607f
Distal phalanx
  extensor tendon injury at, 605-607, 606f, 607f
  fracture of, 593-594, 593f
Distal radioulnar joint, 622, 623f, 639-640
  dislocation of, 636-637
    in Galeazzi's fracture, 642-643, 643f
Distal radius
  injuries to, 632-639, 634f-638f
    Barton's fracture in, 635-636, 636f
    Colles' fracture in, 632-633, 634f, 635f
    Hutchinson's fracture in, 636, 636f
    pediatric, 637-639, 637f, 638f, 638t
    radioulnar joint disruption in, 636-637
    Smith's fracture in, 633-635, 635f
  ulnar slant of, 625, 626f
  volar tilt of, 626, 626f
Distal tibiofibular syndesmotic ligament injury, 816, 817
Distributive justice, 3129, 3129b
Disulfiram, alcohol interactions with, 2876-2877
Diuresis
  cold, 2239
  forced, in crush injury, 3007
Diuretics, 1921t
  during pregnancy and lactation, 2788
  for acute pulmonary edema, 1270t, 1272
  for chronic heart failure, 1276
  for hyperkalemia in chronic renal failure, 1546
  for hypernatremia, 1936
  for hyponatremia, 1935
  for intracerebral hemorrhage, 1616
  for superior vena cava syndrome, 1911
  hypercalcemia from, 1945
  hypokalemia from, 1937
  hypomagnesemia from, 1947
  hypophosphatemia from, 1951
  metabolic alkalosis from, 1930
Dive history, focused, 2286b
Divers Alert Network (DAN), 2288
Diversion management, computerized, 3105
Diversity education, 3116, 3116b. *See also* Cultural competence.
Diversity of practice elements, as stressor for emergency physician, 3175
Diverticular disease, 1492-1495, 1494b, 1495b, 2848
Diverticulitis, abdominal pain in, 210t
Diverticulum, Meckel's, in children, 2613-2615, 2614t
Diving reflex, 2312
Diving-related disorders. *See* Scuba diving–related disorders.
Dizziness, 142-149
  diagnostic approach to, 143-146, 143b, 143t, 145b, 145t, 148f
  differential diagnosis in, 143, 143b, 143t, 146, 147t-148t
  disposition in, 146, 149
  management of, 146, 149f
  pathophysiology of, 142-143
DMSA (2,3-Dimercaptosuccinic acid)
  for arsenic poisoning, 2424
  for lead poisoning, 2422
  for mercury poisoning, 2426
DNA synthesis, in megaloblastic anemia, 1873
DNA viruses, 2034t, 2039-2046
DNAR (do-not-attempt-resuscitate) order, 3132, 3133
  in advance directives, honoring, 3144-3145
  initiating, 3153
DNIR (do-not-initiate-resuscitate) order, 3132
DNR (do-not-resuscitate) order, 3132
Dobutamine
  for acute pulmonary edema in hypotensive patient, 1270t, 1273-1274
  for anaphylaxis, 1833
  for heart failure, 2583t, 2584
  for sepsis, 2219t, 2220
  in pediatric resuscitation, 114
Documentation
  in injury prevention and control, 945-946
  information technology for, 3098, 3101-3102
  of child abuse, 972-973
  of elder abuse, 1013
  of facial trauma, 388
  of gunshot wounds, 953
  of informed consent, 3167
  of intimate partner violence and abuse, 1000-1001, 1003-1004
  of medical screening examination, 3162-3163
  of physical restraint use, 2959, 2960f
  of refusal of medical care, 3169-3170
  of sexual assault, 985b, 989, 989b
  of suicide attempt, 1774
  of testing in emergency department, 3158
Dog
  bites by, 854, 882-883, 887-888
  rabies in, 2061, 2062-2063, 2063f, 2064
Dog-ear deformity repair, 851
Doll's eye reflex, 161, 357, 2503
Domestic elder abuse, 1009
Domestic herbivore bite, 885
Domestic violence. *See* Intimate partner violence and abuse.
Domperidone, for nausea and vomiting in children, 206
Donepezil, for dementia, 1661

Donovanosis, 1559t, 1563
Donq quai, drug interactions with, 2478t
Dopamine
  for acute pulmonary edema in hypotensive patient, 1270t, 1273
  for acute renal failure, 1538, 2650
  for anaphylaxis, 1833
  for burn injury, 923
  for calcium channel blocker overdose, 2378
  for cyclic antidepressant poisoning, 2356
  for heart failure, 2583-2584, 2583t
  for hypothermia, 2246
  for sepsis, 2219t, 2220
  for septic shock, 53
  in mood disorders, 1735
  in neonatal resuscitation, 123t, 124
  in pediatric resuscitation, 114
  suicide and, 1768
Dopamine antagonists, during pregnancy and lactation, 2790
Dopexamine, for sepsis, 2222
Doppler ultrasonography
  color flow, 542, 774
  in knee trauma, 774
  in peripheral arteriovascular disease, 1346, 1348
  in peripheral vascular injury, 541
  in testicular torsion, 1595, 2640
  in testicular trauma, 534, 535f
Dorsal Barton's fracture, 550t
Dorsal compartment of forearm, 640, 640t
Dorsal extrinsic ligaments of wrist, 622, 624f
Dorsal horn, in pain transmission, 2914-2915, 2915f
Dorsal intercalated segment instability (DISI), 631-632, 633f
Dorsal rhizotomy, for spasticity in cerebral palsy, 2904
Dorsal subaponeurotic space infection, 617, 618
Dorsal surface of hand, 576, 577f, 608
Dorsal vein of penis, 532, 532f, 534
Dorzolamide, for increased intraocular pressure, 292
Double blinding, 3049
Double decidual sac sign, 2730
Double vision, in botulism, 2014
Double-break pelvic fracture, 727
Double-bubble sign
  conditions associated with, 2607
  in hypertrophic pyloric stenosis, 2604, 2605f
  in malrotation with midgut volvulus, 2607
Double-gap acidosis
  differential diagnosis in, 2397
  in ethylene glycol poisoning, 2400
  in methanol poisoning, 2397
Douching, during pregnancy, 2736
Down syndrome, 2900t, 2901
Doxapram, for chronic obstructive pulmonary disease, 1106
Doxazosin, 1321t
Doxepin, for upper airway angioedema, 1835
Doxorubicin, cardiotoxicity of, 1292
Doxycycline
  during pregnancy and lactation, 2785
  for anorectal sexually transmitted disease, 1519
  for anthrax exposure, 3026, 3026b
  for *Campylobacter* gastroenteritis, 1461
  for *Chlamydia trachomatis* infection, 1559t, 1565
  for ehrlichiosis, 2138
  for epididymitis, 1597t, 2639
  for granuloma inguinale, 1559t, 1563
  for Lyme disease, 1789, 2127, 2127t, 2128
  for lymphogranuloma venereum, 1559t, 1562
  for malaria, 2104
  for nongonococcal urethritis, 1565
  for Q fever, 2137
  for Rocky Mountain spotted fever, 1850, 2136, 2136t
  for syphilis, 1856
  for *Vibrio* fish poisoning, 1472
  prophylactic, for tularemia, 2131
Doxylamine, in OTC sleep aids, overdose of, 2487-2488, 2488t
Dracunculus medinensis, skin disorders in, 2100t, 2108-2109
Drain cleaner, ingestion of, 2380, 2381t
Drainage
  in paronychia, 615, 615f
Drainage *(Continued)*
  in pericoronitis, 1035
  in septic arthritis, 2192, 2706
  of Bartholin cyst abscess, 2205, 2205f
  of cutaneous abscess, 2204
  of felon, 615, 616f
  of periodontal abscess, 1031, 1033
  of peritonsillar abscess, 1118
  of retropharyngeal abscess, 1121
Drains, in wound management, 855
Dressings
  for burn wounds, 925, 926
  in wound management, 855
  Jones compression, 570-571
Dressler syndrome, 1283
Drive-by shootings, 1020-1021
Drooling
  in developmentally disabled patient, 2903
  in epiglottitis, 2523
Drop arm test
  in rotator cuff tear, 696
  in rotator cuff tendinopathy, 1797
Droperidol, 2446t
  conduction disturbances from, 2962
  for delirium, 1654
  for PCP intoxication, 2416
  for rapid tranquilization, 2961-2962
  for thought disorders, 1730
  side effects of, 2961-2962
Drotrecogin alfa, for septic shock, 53
Drowning
  definition of, 2311
  submersion injuries and, 2311-2315
Drug(s). *See also* Medications.
  abuse of. *See* Substance abuse.
  anxiety from, 1746b, 1748
  aplastic anemia from, 1875, 1875t
  ataxia from, 2681
  birth defects from, 2779-2780, 2780b
  chronic renal failure from, 1544
  coma from, 1991
  cyanosis from, 269t
  delirium from, 1647-1648
  dementia from, 1656, 1658
  diarrhea from, 231b
  gingival hyperplasia from, 1036
  heart failure from, 1269
  hemolytic anemia from, 1883, 1883b
  hepatic injury from, 1413-1414, 1414t
  hypomagnesemia from, 1948
  immune thrombocytopenia from, 1897
  interactions of
    substance abuse and, 2884
    with alcohol, 2875-2877, 2876t
    with herbal medicines, 2477, 2478t
    with labor and delivery, 2811t
    with MAOIs, 2364, 2364b
  lupus erythematosus from, 1809, 1809t
  mood disorders from, 1739-1740, 1740b, 1740f
  myasthenia gravis exacerbation from, 1706, 1706b
  overdose of. *See* Poisoning/overdose.
  pancreatitis from, 1428, 1429b
  pharmacokinetics of
    in children, 2935, 2952
    in elderly person, 2826
  psychosis from, 1727b, 1728-1729
  reactions to
    in elderly person, 2826-2827
    in HIV/AIDS, 2079t, 2087
  rhabdomyolysis from, 1979
  safety of, during pregnancy and lactation, 2781-2790, 2782t-2783t
  seizures from, 1623, 2669-2670, 2670b
  syncope from, 195, 195b
  toxicity of
    cardiac arrest and, 77
    in chronic renal failure, 1544, 1544b
    in heart transplant patient, 2852
    in organ transplant patient, 2849-2851, 2850t, 2851f
  transfer of
    across placenta, 2780-2781
    during lactation, 2781
  urinary retention from, 1599, 1599b
  with anticholinergic effects, 2345, 2346t
  withdrawal from. *See* Withdrawal.
Drug Alert Warning Network (DAWN), 2883
Drug eruptions, skin lesions in, 1844-1845, 1844f, 1845f, 1846t-1847t
Drug testing, occupational, 3080-3081
Drusen, in macular degeneration, 1059, 1059f
Dry mouth, in botulism, 2014
Dry skin, in HIV/AIDS, 2084-2085
Dry socket, 1034
Duchenne dystrophy, 2900t
Duchenne's sign, 586, 588f
Ductus arteriosus, closure of, 2568
  cardiac lesions associated with, 2576-2577, 2576b, 2577b
Duke criteria for infective endocarditis, 1302
Duodenal atresia, malrotation with midgut volvulus vs., 2607
Duodenal C-loop, in malrotation with midgut volvulus, 2607, 2607f, 2608f
Duodenal perforation, 496, 497f
Duodenal rupture, 485, 485f
Duodenal ulcers, 1391-1394
Duplex ultrasonography, 449, 542
Dupuytren's fracture, 550t
Durable power of attorney, 3133
Dural leak, bacterial meningitis associated with, 1712
Dural penetration, as indication for lumbar puncture, 2660
Dural sinus, 350
Duroziez's murmur, in aortic regurgitation, 1307
Dust contamination, in urban search and rescue, 3008
Duty to act, legal rights and, 3128
Duty to warn third parties, 2967-2968
Dying. *See* Death; End of life.
Dynamic splinting, of metacarpal or phalangeal fractures, 595, 595f
Dysarthria, in ischemic stroke, 1609
Dysbarisms, 2280-2281, 2281f. *See also* Scuba diving–related disorders.
Dysentery, 2624
  amebic, 235, 1477t, 1480-1481
  in shigellosis, 1464
  infectious causes of, 228, 229t-230t
Dysesthesia, in ciguatera fish poisoning, 1473
Dysmetria, 145
Dyspepsia
  in peptic ulcer disease, 1391, 1392
  nonulcer, 1393
Dysphagia, 1395-1398
  clinical features of, 1396-1397
  diagnosis of, 1397-1398
  esophageal, 1397
  in esophageal obstruction, 1383
  in esophagitis, 1387
  in gastroesophageal reflux, 1388
  in neck masses, 1076
  management of, 1398
  oropharyngeal, 1396-1397
  pathophysiology of, 1395-1396, 1396b
Dyspnea, 175-181
  acute, differential diagnosis in, 1101-1103
  ancillary studies in, 177, 180t
  at rest, in high-altitude pulmonary edema, 2303
  chest pain associated with, 185, 186t
  diagnostic approach to, 176-177, 176t, 178t-180t
  differential considerations in, 176, 176t, 177, 179t, 180
  disposition in, 181
  empiric management of, 180-181, 182f
  epidemiology of, 176
  exertional, 176, 1269
  history in, 176-177
  in abdominal trauma, 493
  in aortic stenosis, 1306
  in asthma, 1083, 2534, 2535t
  in chronic obstructive pulmonary disease, 1099
  in dilated cardiomyopathy, 1293
  in heart failure, 1269
  in hemodialysis patient, 1551
  in neoplastic cardiac tamponade, 1917
  in pleural effusion, 1150
  in pneumothorax, 1145
  in pregnancy, 2725, 2753t
  in pulmonary embolism, 1372
  palliative care for, 3154
  pathophysiology of, 176
  physical examination in, 177, 178t, 179t

Dyspnea *(Continued)*
rapid assessment and stabilization in, 181f
symptoms associated with, 177
terminology related to, 175-176
Dysproteinemia, hyperviscosity syndrome in, 1912
Dysrhythmia, 1199-1244
after head trauma, 371
alcohol consumption and, 2866
anxiety in, 1746-1747
atrial, 1216
bradycardia, sinoatrial and atrioventricular block as, 1215-1221
cardiac cellular electrophysiology and, 1199-1201, 1200f-1202f
cardiac conduction and, 1201-1203, 1202t, 1203f
chaotic, causes of, 1227b
classification of, 1213
electrocardiography in, 1213-1214, 1214b, 1214f
extrasystoles and parasystole as, 1221-1226
from altered automaticity, 1204, 1204f
from phenol chemical peel, 935
from succinylcholine, 13
heart failure in, 1268
in amphetamine abuse, 2895
in anaphylaxis, 1825t
in asthma, 2536
in chloral hydrate poisoning, 2487
in cocaine overdose, 2388, 2390
in crush injury, 3007
in hydrofluoric acid poisoning, 934
in hypercalcemia, 1945
in hyperkalemia, 1940
in hyperthyroidism, 1987
in hypertrophic cardiomyopathy, 1295
in hypomagnesemia, 1948-1949
in hypothermia, 2237-2238, 2246
in hypothyroidism, 1992
in myocardial contusion, 468-469
in submersion victim, 2313
maneuvers for diagnosis and treatment of, 1214-1215
mechanisms for formation of, 1204-1205, 1204f
narrow-complex tachycardia as, 1226-1235
pediatric, 2584-2590, 2584b, 2586b, 2587f-2589f
in cardiac arrest, 109-113, 109t, 110f-113f, 110t
unstable, 110, 110t
pharmacologic treatment of, 1204-1213, 1205b. *See also* Antidysrhythmic drugs.
preexcitation and accessory pathway syndromes as, 1235-1237
pseudodysrhythmias and, 1215, 1215f
reentry mechanisms for, 1204-1205, 1204f
sinus, 1216, 1216f
stable, initial assessment of, 1213-1215, 1214b, 1214f
triggered, 1205
unstable, signs and symptoms of, 1213
wide-complex tachycardia as, 1237-1244
Dysthmic disorder, 1738
Dystonia, antipsychotic-induced, 1732, 2446
Dysuria
differential diagnosis in, 1579-1581, 1579t, 1580f
in children, 2643, 2643t

E code in injury prevention and control, 945-946
Ear
anatomy of, 384
blunt trauma to, 392
discharge from
in malignant otitis externa, 1071
in otitis externa, 1070
in otitis media, 1067
examination of, in facial trauma, 388
external
barotrauma to, 2282, 2292
infection in. *See* Otitis externa.
foreign body in, [illegible]
in decompression sickness, 2284
inner, barotrauma to, 2282, 2287-2288, 2287t, 2292
laceration of, [illegible]
Ear *(Continued)*
middle
barotrauma to, 2281-2282, 2282f, 2286-2287, 2287t, 2292
infection in. *See* Otitis media.
pain in. *See* Otalgia.
Ear squeeze, 2281-2282, 2282f, 2286-2287, 2287t, 2292
Early asthmatic response, 1091
Earthquakes, disaster preparedness for, 3016, 3017
Eastern Association for the Surgery of Trauma, clinical practice guidelines of, 3037
Ebb phase, in recovery from burn injury, 919
Ebola virus, 2054
Ecchymoses, in chronic renal failure, 1543
Eccrine glands, 915, 2255
Echinacea, adverse effects of, 2476t
Echinococcal infection, pulmonary disorders in, 2110-2111
Echinococcus granulosus, 2102t, 2105-2106, 2106f, 2111, 2113
Echinococcus multilocularis, 2102t
Echocardiography
during cardiopulmonary resuscitation, 82
in acute coronary syndromes, 1179
in aortic dissection, 1327, 1327t
in aortic rupture, 480, 480f
in cardiac tamponade, 474, 1285
in cyanosis, 271
in high-altitude pulmonary edema, 2304
in hypertrophic cardiomyopathy, 1295
in infective endocarditis, 1302
in ischemic stroke, 1613
in multiple trauma, 313
in myocardial contusion, 469
in neoplastic cardiac tamponade, 1917
in pericardial effusion, 1285, 1285f
in pericarditis, 1282
in pulmonary embolism, 1377, 1378t
in restrictive cardiomyopathy, 1296
Echovirus, 2057
Eclampsia, 1627, 2749-2751, 2750b
Economic violence, 1018
Ecstasy. *See* MDMA (methylenedioxymethamphetamine).
Ecthyma, impetigo vs., 2202
Ectopic pregnancy, 2742-2746
ancillary studies in, 2745
clinical features of, 2743
diagnosis of, 2743-2744
differential considerations in, 2745
hormonal assays in, 2744
management of, 2745-2746, 2746f
miscarriage vs., 2741
risk factors for, 2743, 2743b
ultrasonography of, 2730, 2744, 2744b
Eczematoid dermatitis, in otitis media, 1067-1068
Eczematous rash, drug-induced, 1844, 1847t
Edema
anorectal, 1508-1509
burn, 917
cerebral. *See* Cerebral edema.
heat, 2258-2259
in aortic rupture, 478
in *Bacillus anthracis* gastroenteritis, 1469
in diphtheria, 2003
in frostbite, 2229, 2231
in hypothyroidism, 1992
in nephrotic syndrome, 1531
in spinal cord injury, 2906, 2907
in superior vena cava syndrome, 1910
laryngeal, in anaphylaxis, 1825t, 2548
peripheral, in parasitic infection, 2107-2108
pulmonary. *See* Pulmonary edema.
renal causes of, 2648
scrotal, in children, 2638-2642, 2639f-2640f, 2641
Edrophonium test, in myasthenia gravis, 1705
Education
diversity, 3116, 3116b. *See also* Cultural competence.
patient
information technology for, 3098-3099
on back pain, 710-711
on wound management, [illegible]
Educational materials, on emergency seclusion and restraint, 2961
Educational programs, in emergency medical services, 3080
Efavirenz, for HIV/AIDS, 2088
Effective refractory period, 1200, 1202f
Effervescent agents, for esophageal obstruction, 1384
Effusion
otitis media with, 1066, 1069-1070
pericardial, 1284-1285, 1285f
in cardiac tamponade, 474, 474f
in chronic renal failure, 1540
in HIV/AIDS, 1287
in hypothyroidism, 1993
in myocardial contusion, 468
in pregnancy, 1287
malignant, 1283-1284
transudative vs. exudative, 1285
uremic, 1282
pleural, 1134, 1148-1153
clinical features of, 1150-1151, 1151f
exudative vs. transudative, 1149-1150, 1152, 1152b
in pneumonia, 2561, 2562
in superior vena cava syndrome, 1911
in systemic lupus erythematosus, 1808
in tuberculosis, 2152, 2152f, 2158-2159
loculated, 1148
malignant, 1149, 1153
management of, 1151-1153, 1152b
parapneumonic, 1148, 1149, 1152, 1153
pathophysiology of, 1148-1150, 1149b, 1149f
Egg embryo–grown vaccine, allergy to, 1827
Ehlers-Danlos syndrome, aortic dissection in, 1324-1325
Ehrlichiosis, 2137-2138
Eighty percent rule, in neck masses, 1075
Eikenella corrodens infection, in human bites, 890
Eisenmenger syndrome, 2578
Elastoplast, for ankle immobilization, 571
Elbow
apophysitis of, 2710-2711
avulsion fracture of, 2711, 2711f
examination of, 649-650, 649f, 650f
in arthritis, 1778
immobilization of, 569
little leaguer's, 663, 663f, 2710-2711
nursemaid's, 666, 666f, 2697-2698, 2697f
ossification centers in, 652, 652f, 653t, 2694, 2694f, 2694t
pain in, in apophysitis, 2710
tendinopathy of, 668, 1798-1799
tennis, 667, 1798-1799, 2710-2711
Elbow trauma, 647-668
anatomy in, 647-649, 647f, 648f
biceps tendon rupture in, 668
clinical features of, 649-650, 649f, 650f
dislocation in, 664-666, 664f, 665f
epicondylitis in, 667, 1798-1799, 2710-2711
humeral fractures in, 652-664
articular surface, 661-664, 661f-663f
distal, 655-661, 656f-661f
shaft, 652-655, 653f, 654f
management of, 652
olecranon bursitis in, 667, 1801-1803
radial head subluxation in, 666, 666f, 2697-2698, 2697f
radiography in, 641f, 650-652, 651f
Elderly person, 2824-2830
abdominal injuries in, 346
abdominal pain in, 2828-2829, 2828t
abuse of, 1008-1015
caregiver interview in, 1013
clinical features of, 1011-1013, 1011b, 1012b
definitions and types of, 1009-1010
diagnostic strategies in, 1013
documentation of, 1013
epidemiology of, 1009
etiology and risk factors for, 1010-1011, 1010b
future directions in, 1015
institutional, 1009, 1015
interventions and referrals in, 1013-1014
reporting requirements in, 1014-1015
screening for, 1011, 1011b
alcohol consumption in, 2877
anxiety in, [illegible]
appendicitis in, 1453
as intractable patient, 2980
auto-pedestrian collisions in, 345
back pain in, 707

Elderly person *(Continued)*
  burns in, 347
  causes of death in, 942t, 949t
  central retinal artery occlusion in, 1057, 1057f
  chronic salicylate toxicity in, 2340
  constipation in, 237
  delirium in, 1649
  depression in, 1737-1738
  diagnostic strategies in, 2828
  extremity injuries in, 346-347
  falls in, 344, 2829-2830
  fever in, 134
  head trauma in, 346
  heat illness in, 2256
  high-altitude illness in, 2296
  history taking in, 2827
  hypothermia in, 2239-2240, 2241
  immunizations in, 2829
  infections in, 2828
  macular degeneration in, 1059, 1059f
  motor vehicle crashes in, 344-345
  myocardial infarction in, 2828
  pancreatitis in, 1428
  pharmacologic considerations in, 2826-2827
  physical examination of, 2827-2828
  physiologic changes in, 345, 2825-2826, 2825t
  pneumonia in, 1131, 2828
  psychosocial considerations in, 2827
  rib fracture in, 456
  seizure in, 1624
  soft tissue injuries in, 347
  spinal cord injury in, 346
  spinal injuries in, 413, 415f
  substance abuse in, 2883
  suicide in, 1767, 1769-1770
  transcondylar fracture in, 659, 659f
  trauma in, 344-348, 2829
    background of, 344
    clinical features of, 347
    diagnostic strategies in, 347
    disposition in, 348
    epidemiology of, 344-345
    management of, 348
    pathophysiology of, 345
    specific disorders and injuries related to, 345-347
Electrical alternans
  in cardiac tamponade, 474, 474f, 1285, 1286f
  in neoplastic cardiac tamponade, 1917
Electrical arc, 2270-2271
Electrical field strength, 2270
Electrical injuries, 2267-2277
  cardiac arrest in, 78
  clinical features of, 2271-2274, 2272f
  complications of, 2274
  differential considerations in, 2275
  disposition in, 2277
  in pregnancy, 2277
  management of, 2275-2277, 2276b
  mechanisms of, 2270-2271, 2270b
  perioral, 391
  physics of, 2267-2270, 2268t, 2269t
  rhabdomyolysis from, 1978
Electrocardiography
  during cardiopulmonary resuscitation, 79
  during procedural sedation and analgesia, 2943
  electrophysiologic correlates of, 1202, 1203f
  in acute coronary syndromes, 1161-1174
    abnormalities in, 1161-1163, 1162f-1164f, 1162t
    additional lead, 1171-1173, 1172f, 1173f
    adjuncts in, 1171-1174
    anatomic location of infarct on, 1164-1166, 1164t, 1165f-1167f
    body surface mapping and, 1174
    limitations of, 1174
    noninfarct ST segment elevation and, 1166-1170, 1167f-1172f
    NSTEMI and, 1170-1171
    QT dispersion and, 1174
    serial, 1173-1174, 1173f
  in aortic dissection, 1326, 1326t
  in arthritis, 1782
  in asthma, 1085
  in atrial flutter, 1229, 1230f-1231f
  in cardiac tamponade, 474, 474f, 1285, 1286f
  in chest pain, 185-186, 188t
  in chronic obstructive pulmonary disease, 1101
  in cocaine overdose, 2388
Electrocardiography *(Continued)*
  in cyanosis, 271
  in cyclic antidepressant poisoning, 2354, 2355f
  in dilated cardiomyopathy, 1293
  in dysrhythmias, 1213-1214, 1214b, 1214f
  in electrical and lightning injuries, 2272, 2275, 2276b
  in gastrointestinal bleeding, 223
  in headache, 173t
  in heart transplant patient, 2853, 2853f
  in high-altitude pulmonary edema, 2304
  in hypertrophic cardiomyopathy, 1295
  in hypothermia, 2237, 2238f
  in lithium toxicity, 2442
  in mitral regurgitation, 1306
  in mitral stenosis, 1305
  in mitral valve prolapse, 1305
  in myocardial contusion, 468-469
  in myocarditis, 1289
  in nausea and vomiting, 203
  in neoplastic cardiac tamponade, 1917
  in pacemaker patient, 1248-1250, 1249f, 1250f, 1255
  in pericarditis, 1281-1282, 1281f, 2592-2593, 2593f
  in pregnancy, 318, 2725
  in pulmonary embolism, 1373, 1373f, 1378, 1379f
  in syncope, 195, 196t
  in ventricular tachycardia, 1238-1239, 1241f-1243f
  15-lead, 1171-1173, 1172f, 1173f
  pauses on
    compensatory, 1224f
    noncompensatory, 1222, 1223
  prehospital, 2990
Electroconvulsive therapy, for depression, 1742
Electroencephalogram
  in ataxia, 2682
  in seizure, 168, 2671
Electrolyte disturbances, 1933-1953. *See also specific electrolyte disturbances, e.g.,* Hyperkalemia.
  alcohol-induced, 2871-2872, 2872t
  in asthma, 1085
  in bacterial meningitis, 2662
  in chronic obstructive pulmonary disease, 1102
  in comatose patient, 161-162
  in delirium, 1648, 1649
  in diabetic ketoacidosis, 1962
  in hyperglycemic hyperosmolar nonketotic coma, 1968, 1969
  in hypothermia, 2243
  in infants and children, 2573
  in nausea and vomiting, 203
  in pediatric gastroenteritis, 2630-2634, 2630t, 2632b-2634b
  in rhabdomyolysis, 1979-1980, 1982
  in sepsis, 2216
Electromagnetic spectrum, 2318, 2318f
Electromechanical dissociation, 84, 112
Electromyography
  in botulism, 2015
  needle, 1689
Electronic databases, 3059
Electronic fetal monitoring, 2800
Electronic medical information systems, 3098
Electronic thermometer, 2508
Electrophysiological studies, 1689
Electroporation theory, 2267
Electrothermal burns, 2270
Electrothermal heating formulas, 2268b
Elemental metals, skin injuries from, 937
Elephantiasis, 2107-2108
Elevated arm stress test, in thoracic outlet syndrome, 1359
Ellis classification of tooth fracture, 1036, 1036f
Embolectomy
  for acute arterial embolism, 1352
  for pulmonary embolism, 1379
Embolism
  amniotic fluid, 2751-2752, 2821
  arterial, 1352-1353
    differential diagnosis in, 1352
    management of, 1352-1353
    pathophysiology of, 1343-1344
    physical examination in, 1346, 1347t
    vs. thrombosis in situ, 1347t
Embolism *(Continued)*
  arterial gas
    in scuba diving–related disorders, 2285-2286
    recompression therapy for, 2288-2292, 2288b, 2289f-2291f
    vs. pulmonary decompression sickness, 2288, 2288t
  atheroembolism and, 1343-1344, 1353, 1353f
  fat, 563
  pulmonary. *See* Pulmonary embolism.
  superior mesenteric artery, 1445-1446, 1446b
  thromboembolism and, 1308, 1343-1344
  venous air, in neck trauma, 444, 450
Embolization
  in acute coronary syndromes, 1157
  in pelvic fracture, 732-734, 733f
  of bronchial arteries, for hemoptysis, 282
Emergence phenomena, from ketamine, 2946-2947
Emergency department
  as factor in difficult patient-physician relationship, 2973
  death in, 2717, 3146-3151, 3146b, 3148b
  dedicated, regulatory definition of, 3158
  design of, 3120
  information management in, 3099-3102, 3100t, 3102f
  minority populations' use of, 3115-3116, 3115b
  nonemergency functions of, 3158-3160
  occupational health issues in
    blood-borne pathogen exposure protocol and, 3081-3087, 3084t, 3085t, 3086b
    material safety data sheet and, 3081, 3082b
  overcrowding in, 3120-3121
  pediatric-ready, 2504
  performance shaping factors in, 3120t, 3121-3123
  process improvement and patient safety in, 3119-3126
    problem areas and, 3124-3126, 3125t
    sources of failure and, 3119-3123, 3120f, 3120t
  promoting wellness in, 3176-3178, 3176b, 3177b
  violence in, 2956-2969. *See also* Combative patient.
    epidemiology of, 2956-2957
    gang, 1021-1022
    management of, 2957-2963
    medicolegal issues related to, 2967-2969
    prevention of, 2965-2967
Emergency medical condition, 3156-3157
Emergency medical dispatcher, 2988
Emergency medical services, 2984-3032, 2987-2988
  air medical transport in, 2994-2999. *See also* Air medical transport.
  bioethical dilemmas in, 3132-3133
  communications in, 2988-2989
  disaster preparedness in, 3010-3019. *See also* Disaster preparedness.
  educational programs in, 2989
  end of life issues in, 3144-3146
  future directions in, 2992
  history of, 2984
  interfacility and specialized transport in, 2991-2992, 2991b, 2992b
  material resources in, 2987-2988, 2988f
  medical direction of, 2989-2990
  prehospital care and management controversies in, 2990-2991
  provider levels and scope of practice in, 2986-2987, 2987t
  quality/performance improvement in, 2989
  resource and contact information for, 2992
  systems for
    air medical transport integration with, 2997
    design of, 2984-2986, 2985f
    protocols in, 3014
    status management of, 2988-2989
  tactical emergency medical support in, 3000-3005. *See also* Tactical emergency medical support.
  urban search and rescue in, 3005-3008, 3006b, 3008f
  weapons of mass destruction and, 3021-3032
Emergency medical services medical director, 2989-2990
Emergency medical technician–basic, 2986-2987, 2987t

Emergency medical technician–intermediate, 2987, 2987t
Emergency medical technician–paramedic, 2987, 2987t
Emergency Medical Treatment and Active Labor Act (EMTALA), 2991, 3156
Emergency medicine
  bioethics in, 3131-3137, 3131b, 3131t. *See also* Bioethics.
  certification in, information technology for, 3099
  clinical decision rules in, 3035-3036
  clinical pathways in, 3038, 3039f-3041f
  cultural competence and, 3107-3117
    as tool for enhancing emergency department care, 3111-3116
    continuum of, 3111-3112
    institutional policies promoting, 3117, 3117b
    rationale for, 3108-3111, 3108t, 3109t
    recommendations for, 3116
    standards for, 3112-3113
    to cross barrier of different beliefs, values, and life experiences, 3113-3114
    to cross language barrier, 3112-3113
  disaster preparedness in, 3010-3019. *See also* Disaster preparedness.
  end of life issues in, 3143-3154. *See also* Death; End of life.
  evidence-based, 3046-3060
    data analysis in, 3051-3058, 3051t, 3057f
    hypothesis testing in, 3051-3058, 3051t, 3057f
    medical literature and, 3046
    practice guidelines in, 3036f, 3037t
    randomized clinical trials in, 3047-3051, 3048f
    steps in, 3058-3060
    terms in, 3058, 3059t
    types of clinical studies in, 3046-3047
  failures in, 3119-3126
    problem areas for, 3124-3126, 3125t
    sources of, 3119-3123, 3120f, 3120t
  forensic, 952-966
  guidelines for, 3034-3044
    computer-based protocols for, 3042-3044, 3043f
    development of, 3035, 3036f
    implementation and outcomes of, 3038, 3042
    legal and ethical considerations in, 3044
    sources and adoption of, 3036-3038, 3037t
  information gaps in, 3121
  information technology in, 3097-3106
    Internet and, 3104
    networks and, 3104
    security and confidentiality of patient information and, 3102-3103
    standards and, 3103-3104
    telemedicine and, 3105-3106
    terminology in, 3097
    uses of, 3097-3099, 3104-3106
  injury control in, 940-950, 945b. *See also* Injury prevention and control.
  medicolegal issues in, 3156-3173. *See also* Medicolegal issues.
  observation in, 3062-3073
    approach in, 3062-3063
    in abdominal pain, 3063-3064, 3064b
    in asthma, 3069-3070, 3070b
    in atrial fibrillation, 3070-3071, 3070b
    in chest pain, 3064-3065, 3065b
    in congestive heart failure, 3071, 3071b
    in deep vein thrombosis, 3065-3066
    in dehydration, 3071-3072, 3072b
    in head trauma, 3069
    in infection, 3072-3073, 3072b, 3073t
    in syncope, 3066-3067, 3066b
    in trauma, 3067-3069
    in upper gastrointestinal bleeding, 3066
    of critical diagnostic syndromes, 3063-3066
    of emergency conditions, 3069-3073
    principles of, 3062, 3063b
    staffing requirements for, 3062-3063
  occupational medicine and, 3076-3081
    drug and alcohol testing in, 3080-3081
    overview of, 3076-3077
    return-to-work issues in, 3078-3080
    workers' compensation and, 3077-3078
  restricted access to, bioethical dilemnas in, 3137
Emergency medicine *(Continued)*
  stressors in, 3174-3175
  teamwork in, failure of, 3121-3122
Emergency physician
  and primary care physician, differences between, 3131, 3131t
  as advocate for injury prevention and control, 948, 950
  as factor in difficult patient-physician relationship, 2973
  as surrogate decision-maker, 3135
  burnout in, 3175-3176
  delivery of bad news by, 3146-3147, 3146b
  diagnostic and management decisions made by, 125, 126b. *See also* Clinical decision making.
  grief response in, 3150-3151
  impaired, 3176
  major stresses for, 3174-3175
  negative reactions of, 2975-2976
  role of, in informed consent, 3166-3167
  wellness strategies for, 3176-3178, 3176b, 3177b
Emergency preparedness committee, 3015
Emergency seclusion and restraint, 2958-2961, 2960f
Emesis. *See* Vomiting.
EMLA (eutectic mixture of local anesthetics), 846, 2933
Emotional abuse, of elder, 1010
Emotional lability, in delirium, 1649
Emotional upset, heart failure from, 1268
Empathy, in death notification, 3147-3149, 3148b
Emphysema
  in chronic obstructive pulmonary disease, 1100
  in esophageal perforation, 1385
  orbital, 1044, 1045f
  subcutaneous
    chest wall trauma and, 459-460
    in esophageal perforation, 484
    in scuba diving–related disorders, 2286
    tracheobronchial injury and, 466, 466f
Emphysematous cholecystitis, 1421
Empty can test, in rotator cuff tendinopathy, 1797
Empyema
  in pleural effusion, 1152, 1153
  in pneumonia, 2562
  in tuberculosis, 2150-2151
  subdural, in otitis media, 1068
Enalapril, 1322t
  during pregnancy and lactation, 2788
  for hypertensive emergencies, 1319
Enamel, 1026, 1027f
  fractures involving, 1036-1037
Encainide, 1208, 2788
Encephalitis, 1710
  alcohol withdrawal syndrome vs., 2860
  arboviral, 2047-2048
  brainstem, ataxia in, 2681
  California, 2055
  headache in, 174t, 1641
  in cancer patient, 1920
  in rabies, 2065
  otic, 1068
  risk factors for, 171b
  St. Louis, 2049-2050
  viral
    ancillary studies in, 1720
    cerebrospinal fluid analysis in, 1716-1719, 1717t, 1718t, 1719f
    complications of, 1715
    diagnosis of, 1716-1720
    differential considerations in, 1720, 1721b
    disposition in, 1723
    epidemiology of, 1711
    etiology of, 1712
    lumbar puncture in, 1716, 1716b
    management of, 1722, 1723
    neuroimaging studies in, 1719-1720
    pathophysiology of, 1713
    signs and symptoms of, 1714
Encephalomyelitis, postinfectious demyelinating, ataxia in, 2681
Encephalopathy
  hepatic, 1411-1412, 1411t
    clinical stages of, 245t
    grades of, 1411t
    in cirrhosis, 1411
    jaundice in, 240
Encephalopathy *(Continued)*
  HIV, 2081
  hypertensive, 1314-1315
    headache in, 1641
    pediatric, 2650, 2652
    seizure in, 1622
  in cancer patient, 1920-1921
  in Lyme disease, 2124
  in pertussis, 2000
  lead, 2421, 2422
  progressive multifocal, 2045-2046
    dementia in, 1658, 1659
    in HIV/AIDS, 2082
  spongiform
    dementia in, 1657-1658, 1659
    from inhaled heroin, 2452
  uremic, 1542
End of life, 3139-3154. *See also* Death.
  death notification and, 3147-3149, 3148b
  emergency medicine and, 3143-3154
  epidemiology of death and dying and, 3140-3141, 3140f
  futility and, 3141-3142
  goals of medicine and, 3142-3143
  grief response in, 3149-3151, 3150b
  hospice medicine at, 3143
  initiating discussion about issues in, 3152-3153, 3152t
  palliative care at, 3143, 3151-3154, 3152t
  prehospital considerations in, 3144-3146
  quality of life and, 3142
  transplantation requests at, 3151
Endobronchial tuberculosis, 2151
Endocarditis, 1300-1302
  clinical features of, 1301
  diagnostic strategies in, 1301-1302, 1302b
  in prosthetic valve patient, 1308
  in Q fever, 2137
  in systemic lupus erythematosus, 1807
  management of, 1302, 1302b
  pathophysiology of, 1301
  prophylaxis for, 1302, 1303b, 1303t
  risk factors for, 1302, 1303b
Endocrine disorders
  anxiety in, 1747
  dementia from, 1656
  diarrhea in, 231b
  in chronic pancreatitis, 1435
  in sepsis, 2214
Endocrine system
  alcohol consumption and, 2871
  in mood disorders, 1735-1736
Endoleak, after abdominal aortic aneurysm repair, 1340
Endometriosis
  pelvic pain in, 251t
  postpartum, 2821
  thoracic, 1144
Endomyocardial biopsy
  in dilated cardiomyopathy, 1294
  in myocarditis, 1290, 1290f
Endophthalmitis
  posttraumatic, 1052, 1052f
  red and painful eye in, 290, 296t
Endorphin, 2451
Endoscopic cholangioscopy, in cholangitis, 1422
Endoscopic retrograde cholangiopancreaticoduodenography, in abdominal trauma, 499
Endoscopic retrograde cholangiopancreatography
  in acute pancreatitis, 1433
  in chronic pancreatitis, 1436
  in gallstone pancreatitis, 1434
  in jaundice, 244
  pancreatitis after, 1428
Endoscopy
  esophageal perforation from, 482
  in AIDS-related diarrhea, 1404
  in diverticular disease, 1494
  in esophageal foreign body removal, 872
  in esophageal obstruction, 1383-1384
  in esophageal perforation, 485
  in esophagitis, 1387
  in gastrointestinal bleeding, 224
Endothelial cells
  in hemostasis, 1892, 1893f
  injury to, in frostbite, 2229
Endothelin-1, in heart failure, 1203

Endotracheal intubation. *See also* Airway management; Mechanical ventilation.
  approach to, 7-8, 7f-9f
  assessment of access for, 4, 5f
  capnography in, 38-39
  confirmation of tube placement in, 6-7, 6f
  elevated intracranial pressure and, 17, 18t
  hemodynamic consequences of, 16-17
  in acute pulmonary edema, 1271, 1271f
  in adult epiglottitis, 1115
  in adult resuscitation, 87, 91
  in airway foreign body removal, 870
  in anaphylaxis, 1830
  in asthma, 1092
  in botulism, 2016
  in chronic obstructive pulmonary disease, 1103-1113, 1105t
  in flail chest, 458, 458b
  in hypothermia, 2244
  in Ludwig's angina, 1119
  in neonatal resuscitation, 122
  in submersion victim, 2314
  in tracheobronchial injury, 466
  of difficult airway
    approach to, 8-9, 9f
    cricothyrotomy for, 22-23, 23f
    esophagotracheal combitube for, 20, 20f
    fiberoptic, 20-21, 22f
    identification in, 3-4, 3b, 4b, 5f
    intubating laryngeal mask airway for, 19, 19f
    lighted stylet for, 19-20, 20f
    retrograde, 20
    special airway devices for, 18-23, 19f-23f
  outcomes in, 23
  pediatric, 99, 106-107, 108-109, 330, 2519
  pharmacologic agents in, 13-16
  potential cervical spine injury in, 17-18
  prehospital, 2990, 2991
  rapid sequence, 9-12, 10b
    in asthma, 16
    in elevated intracranial pressure, 17, 18t
    in head trauma, 358-359
    in neck trauma, 444
    in shock, 51
    indications for, 7-8
    paralysis with induction phase in, 11
    pediatric, 18, 107-108, 107b, 107t
    post-intubation management in, 11-12
    prehospital, 2990, 2991
    preoxygenation in, 10, 10f
    preparations for, 9-10
    pretreatment agents for, 10, 11b
    tube placement in, 11
    vs. blind nasotracheal intubation, 12
    with competitive neuromuscular blocking agent and etomidate, 14-15, 15t
  status asthmaticus and, 16, 17t
Endotracheal suctioning
  in meconium aspiration, 120, 120f, 122
  in ventilated patient, 31
Endovascular cooling, for comatose survivors of cardiac arrest, 69
Endovascular surgery
  for abdominal aortic aneurysm, 1337, 1338-1339, 1339f
  for aortic rupture, 482
End-stage renal disease. *See* Renal failure.
Endurance training, cardiovascular system in, 2256
Enema
  for constipation, 241t, 242
  in appendicitis, 1454
  in colonic ischemia, 1504
  in colonic volvulus, 1498f
  in diverticular disease, 1493, 1494
  in intussusception, 2611, 2611f
  in large bowel obstruction, 1496-1497
Enophthalmos, in red and painful eye, 286
Enoxaparin
  for prostatis, 1586
  with tenecteplase, in myocardial infarction, 1194-1195
Enriched Air Nitrox (EAN), 2279-2280
Entactogen intoxication, 2408-2411, 2409f
Entamoeba histolytica infection
  amebic abscess in, 1415, 2106-2107
  amebic dysentery in, 235, 1477t, 1480-1481
  drug therapy for, 2100t
  dysenteric colitis in, 229t
Entamoeba histolytica infection *(Continued)*
  hepatic abscess in, 1415-1416, 2113
  in HIV/AIDS, 1482-1483
  intestinal symptoms in, 1477t, 1480-1481
  pulmonary symptoms in, 2110
Enteritis. *See also* Gastroenteritis.
  bacterial, 1469-1475, 1480t
    acute, 2625-2626
    invasive, 1460-1469, 1461t, 1462t
    toxin-induced, 1469-1475, 1480t
  in HIV/AIDS, 1482-1484, 1482t, 1483b, 1485t
  protozoal, 1476-1482, 1477t
  viral, acute, 1475-1476
Enteritis necroticans, 1471
Enterobius vermicularis infection, 1479-1482
  drug therapy for, 2100t
  gastroenteritis in, 1479-1482
  pruritus ani in, 2113-2114
Enterocolitis
  antibiotic-associated, *Clostridium difficile,* 1470t, 1474-1475
  in infants and children, 2613
  necrotizing, 2608-2609, 2609f
Enteromonas hominis gastroenteritis, 1477t
Enteropathy, HIV-induced, 1482
Enterovirus infection, 1289, 2057
Entitled patient, 2978t, 2980
Entrance wounds
  centerfire rifle, 959, 959f
  handgun, 955-958, 955f-957f
Envenomation grading, 900-901. *See also* Venomous animal injuries.
Environmental control for tuberculosis, 2169-2170
Environmental exposures
  accidental hypothermia in, 2236-2252
  electrical and lightning injuries in, 2267-2277
  frostbite in, 2228-2235
  heart failure from, 1268
  heat illness in, 2254-2265
  high altitude illness in, 2296-2309
  radiation injuries in, 2316-2325
  scuba diving and dysbarism in. *See* Scuba diving–related disorders.
  submersion injuries in, 2311-2315
Environmental factors
  in COPD exacerbation, 1099
  in hemolytic anemia, 1883-1884
Environmental somatization syndrome, 1753
Enzyme analysis, in electrical and lightning injuries, 2276
Enzyme defects, in hemolytic anemia, 1878-1879, 1879b
Enzyme-linked immunosorbent assay
  for HIV, 2073-2074
  in Lyme disease, 2125
  pregnancy test using, 2728-2730, 2729f
Eosinophil(s), 2834
  in asthma, 1081, 1083
  normal values for, 1886t
Eosinophilic peritonitis, 1552
Eosinophilic pneumonia, tropical, 2110
Ephedrine/ephedra
  abuse of, 2893
  overdose of, 2393
Epicondyles, 770, 771f
  anatomy of, 647, 647f
  fracture of, 662-663, 662f
Epicondylitis, 667
  lateral, 1798
  medial, 1798-1799, 2710-2711
Epidemiology, in injury prevention and control, 945-946
Epidermal appendages, depth of, burn injury and, 917
Epidermis, 842, 914
Epididymal appendage, torsion of, 1597
Epididymis
  anatomy of, 1594, 1594f
  physical examination of, 1573
Epididymitis, 1595-1597, 1597t, 2638-2639, 2639f
Epidural abscess
  back pain in, 261, 265t, 703, 706, 712, 1684
  in vertebral osteomyelitis, 2184-2185
  magnetic resonance imaging in, 708, 709f
  spinal, 1684
Epidural hematoma, 374-375, 375f, 376f
  back pain in, 265t
  in cancer patient, 1919-1920
Epidural hematoma *(Continued)*
  in children, 335
  spinal, 1683-1684
Epidural spinal cord compression, in cancer patient, 1919-1920
Epigastric pain
  differential diagnosis in, 1393
  in acute pancreatitis, 1429
  in chronic pancreatitis, 1435
  in pancreatitis, 2618
Epiglottic abscess, 1115
Epiglottis, adult vs. child, 2519, 2520f
Epiglottitis, 2529t
  adult, 1114-1116, 1115f, 1116f
  pediatric, 2523-2524, 2524f
  screening for, 2509b
Epilepsia partialis continua, 1621
Epilepsy. *See also* Seizure.
  benign rolandic, 2666
  brain damage and, 2665
  childhood and juvenile, 2666
  classification of, 2665-2667, 2666b
  electroencephalogram in, 2671
  febrile seizures and, 2666-2667
  gestational, 1624
  ictal events in, clinical features of, 1620-1622
  migraine and, 2679
  psychomotor, 1621
  risk of, after seizure, 2674
  temporal lobe, vertigo in, 148t
Epileptic syndromes, 2665-2667, 2666b
Epileptiform discharges, 2671
Epinephrine
  for anaphylactic shock, 54
  for anaphylaxis, 1830, 1831b, 1832, 2549
  for asthma, 1088, 2539t, 2541
  for asystole, 85
  for bradycardia, 2585
  for bronchiolitis, 2546
  for cardiac arrest, 92
  for digital trauma, 2932
  for dysrhythmia, 2586b
  for heart failure, 1263, 2583t, 2584
  for hymenoptera stings, 904
  for neonatal resuscitation, 123-124, 123t
  for pediatric resuscitation, 111, 114
  for sepsis, 2219t, 2220
  for viral croup, 2526
  in glucose regulation, 1957
  topical, 846
EpiPen, 1834, 2550
Epiphyseal injuries
  classification of, 555-556, 557t
  distal radius, 638-639, 638f
  proximal humerus, 682-683, 683f
  proximal tibial, 780-781
Epiphyseal-shaft angle of Southwick, in slipped capital femoral epiphysis, 2709
Epiphysis, 2175, 2175f
  of hand
    anatomy of, 578, 580f
    fracture of, 600
  proximal femoral, avascular necrosis of, 2706-2707, 2707f
  slipped capital femoral, 765-767, 765f, 766f, 2707-2709, 2708f
Epipremnum aureum, 2473
Episcleritis, red and painful eye in, 289-290, 290f, 295t
Episioproctotomy, in shoulder dystocia, 2815
Episiotomy, 2804
  in shoulder dystocia, 2815
  in vaginal breech delivery, 2813
Epistaxis, 863, 1072-1075, 1073f, 1074t
Epithelialization, in wound healing, 843
Eplerenone, 1321t
Eponychium, 589
Eprosartan, 1322t
Epstein-Barr virus, 2044
  in organ transplant patient, 2848
  in pharyngitis, 1111
Eptifibatide, in myocardial infarction, 1186
Epulis, in pregnancy, 2726
Equine antitoxins, allergy to, 1827
Ergonovine, after miscarriage, 2742
Errors in medical inquiry and clinical decision making, 130-133, 131t, 133b
Erysipelas, 2198

Erythema, 1839t, 1844
in Kawasaki disease, 2026
malar, in systemic lupus erythematosus, 1863f
palmar, in pregnancy, 2724
Erythema induratum, 1816
Erythema infectiosum, 1850, 2046, 2046f
Erythema marginatum, in rheumatic fever, 1304
Erythema migrans, in Lyme disease, 2122, 2122f
Erythema multiforme
drug-induced, 1846t
internal malignancy associated with, 1863
skin lesions in, 1852-1853, 1853f
Erythema nodosum, 1816-1817
drug-induced, 1847t
internal malignancy associated with, 1863-1864
skin lesions in, 1856-1857, 1856f
Erythematous dermatitis, in dermatomyositis, 1863f
Erythrocyte. *See* Red blood cell *entries.*
Erythrocyte sedimentation rate
in acute septic arthritis, 2705
in arthritis, 1779
in back pain, 707
in headache, 173t
in osteomyelitis, 2179
in pediatric fever, 2509
in pregnancy, 318
in red and painful eye, 288
in temporal arteritis, 1060
in transient synovitis, 2703
Erythrocytosis, 273, 1884-1885, 1884f, 1885b
Erythroderma, internal malignancy associated with, 1864
Erythromelalgia, 1357
Erythromycin
alcohol interactions with, 2875
during pregnancy and lactation, 2784
for *Campylobacter* gastroenteritis, 1461, 1461t
for diphtheria, 2004
for epididymitis, 2639
for folliculitis, 1843
for granuloma inguinale, 1559t, 1563
for impetigo, 1842-1843
for Lyme disease, 1292, 1789, 2127t, 2128
for lymphogranuloma venereum, 1559t, 1562
for orofacial infections, 1032
for pertussis, 2006
for pharyngitis, 1113
for pneumonia, 2558t
for relapsing fever, 2129-2130
for scarlet fever, 1851
for syphilis, 1856
for toxic shock syndrome, 2030
hepatotoxicity of, 1414
Erythropoietin, in anemia, 1868
Escape rhythms, idiojunctional, 1216, 1218
Escharotomy, in burn care, 921, 924-925, 925f
Escherichia coli
enterohemorrhagic, dysenteric colitis in, 229t
in food poisoning, 1470t, 1474
in gastroenteritis, 2626
in urinary tract infection, 1574
Escherichia coli serotype O157:H7 infection, in hemorrhagic gastroenteritis, 1461t, 1462t, 1466-1467
Escherichia coli serotype O157:H7 toxin test, 233
Escitalopram, 2357
Esmolol, 1209
for aortic dissection, 1328
for hypertensive emergencies, 1319, 2653
in aortic rupture, 481
overdose of, 2373t
Esomeprazole, 1390t
Esophageal dilation, perforation from, 482-483
Esophageal disorders
alcohol consumption and, 2867
gastroesophageal reflux in, 1388
in HIV/AIDS, 2083-2084
of motility, 1395-1396, 1397
Esophageal dysphagia, 1397
Esophageal intubation, detection of, 6-7, 6f
Esophageal obturator airway
abdominal trauma after, 492
esophageal perforation from, 483
Esophageal sphincter, lower, defective, in gastroesophageal reflux, 1388
Esophageal stricture, from caustic ingestion, 2383
Esophageal web, 1383
Esophagitis, 1386-1388
causes of, 1386
clinical features of, 1387
diagnosis of, 1387
in gastroesophageal reflux, 1388
in HIV/AIDS, 2083
management of, 1387-1388
Esophagotracheal combitube, for intubation of difficult airway, 70, 70f
Esophagus
anatomy and physiology of, 1382
cancer of, from caustic ingestion, 2383
compression of, 1383
diffuse spasm of, 1397
foreign body in, 868f, 869f, 870-873, 1382-1384, 2617, 2617f
nutcracker, 1397
obstruction of, 1382-1385
pain in, causes of, 1387
perforation/rupture of, 482-485, 482b, 484b, 485f, 1385-1386
anatomy and physiology in, 482
chest pain in, 183, 187, 190t-191t
conditions that mimic, 484b
diagnosis of, 484-485, 485f
epidemiology of, 482
etiology of, 482-484, 482b
management of, 485
spontaneous, from vomiting, 201-202, 206t, 484
trauma to, 446-447
from caustic ingestion, 483, 2381, 2382f, 2383
subcutaneous emphysema and, 459
Essex-Lopresti fracture, 550t
Estate of Doe v ABC Ambulance, 2967
Estrazolam, 2484t
Etanercept, 2844
Ethambutol
for *Mycobacterium avium* infection in HIV/AIDS, 2076
for tuberculosis, 2162-2163, 2163t, 2164t
Ethanol. *See also* Alcohol *entries.*
butanediol with, 2489
chloral hydrate with, 2487
coprine-containing mushrooms with, 2479
flunitrazepam with, 2486
for toxic alcohol poisoning, 2401, 2401t
Ethibond suture, 852t
Ethical case analysis in emergency medicine, 3131-3132, 3131b
Ethical codes, 3129
Ethical issues in medicine and biology. *See* Bioethics.
Ethionamide, for tuberculosis, 2163t, 2164-2165
Ethmoid sinus, 1123
Ethmoid sinusitis, 1124
Ethmoidal arteries, 1073, 1073f
Ethnic differences. *See* Racial/ethnic differences.
Ethnicity, definition of, 3111
Ethosuximide
during pregnancy and lactation, 2787
for pediatric seizure, 2675t
side effects of, 1628t
Ethyl chloride, 2933
Ethylene glycol poisoning, 2398-2402, 2401t
antidotes to, 2329t
metabolic acidosis in, 1928
pharmacology and metabolism in, 2398, 2399f
Ethylene oxide, allergy to, 1827
Etidocaine, 2931t
Etidronate, for hypercalcemia, 1946
Etomidate
as induction agent, 15
for procedural sedation and analgesia, 2940t-2941t, 2947-2948, 2951t, 2952
for rapid sequence intubation, 15, 15t, 359
Eucalyptus oil, 2475
Euphorbia pulcherrima, 2474
Eustachian tube dysfunction, in otitis media, 1066
Euvolemic hypernatremia, 1936
Euvolemic hyponatremia, 1934, 1935
Evaporation, heat transfer by, 2255
Evidence collection
in child abuse, 972-973
in gunshot wounds, 960
in intimate partner violence and abuse, 1000-1001, 1003-1004
Evidence collection *(Continued)*
in motor vehicle crashes, 965, 965f
in pedestrian collisions, 966b
in sexual assault cases, 984-989, 985b-987b, 987f, 987t, 988f, 988t
Evidence based medicine, 3046-3060
data analysis in, 3051-3058, 3051t, 3057f
hypothesis testing in, 3051-3058, 3051t, 3057f
medical literature and, 3046
practice guidelines in, 3036f, 3037t
randomized clinical trials in, 3047-3051, 3048f
steps in, 3058-3060
terms in, 3058, 3059t
types of clinical studies in, 3046-3047
Evisceration, in abdominal stab wound, laparotomy and, 504
Exanthem, 1848-1851
drug-induced, 1844, 1846t
in Rocky Mountain spotted fever, 2133-2134, 2133f, 2134f
Exanthem subitum, 1850, 2044
Exchange resins, for hyperkalemia, 1941
Exchange transfusion
for Goodpasture syndrome, 1816
for hyperviscosity syndrome, 1913
for kernicterus prophylaxis, 2603, 2604f
for myasthenia gravis, 1707
for thrombotic thrombocytopenic purpura, 1898
Exercise
anaphylaxis from, 1828
asthma from, 1082
during pregnancy, 2736
hematuria from, 1603-1604
rhabdomyolysis from, 1978
Exercises, shoulder
in clavicle fracture, 677, 679f
in proximal humerus fractures, 682
Exertional dyspnea, 176
Exertional headache, 164?
Exertional heatstroke, 2256, 2262
Exertional rhabdomyolysis, 1978
Exit blot, pacemaker failure to capture due to, 1253
Exit wounds
centerfire rifle, 959, 959f
handgun, 958-959, 958f
Exophthalmos, in red and painful eye, 286
Exotoxin(s)
in diphtheria, 2002
in toxic shock syndrome, 2029
Expiratory volume, 30
Exposure, in pediatric trauma, 330, 333t
Extension injuries, of cervical spine, 410-411, 410f-411f
Extension supracondylar fracture, 655-659, 656f-658f
Extension teardrop fracture, 410-411
Extensor carpi radialis brevis, 581, 582f, 583f
Extensor carpi radialis longus, 581, 582f, 583f
Extensor carpi ulnaris, 582, 582f, 583f
Extensor digiti minimi, 582, 582f, 583f
Extensor hallucis longus tendon, 838
Extensor indicis proprius, 581-582, 582f, 583f
Extensor pollicis brevis, 581, 582f, 583f
Extensor pollicis longus, 581, 582f, 583f
Extensor retinaculum
of ankle, 808, 809f
of knee, 770, 771f
Extensor tendons
of hand
anatomy of, 581-582, 582f, 583f
trauma to, 605-608, 605f-607f
of knee
anatomy of, 770, 771f
trauma to, 782-784, 783f, 784f
External disaster plan, 3015
External ear
barotrauma to, 2282, 2292
infection of. *See* Otitis externa.
External radiation exposure, 2320
External radioactive contamination, 2320
External rewarming, 2247, 2248
External rotation stress test, of ankle, 817
External rotation technique, for reduction of anterior glenohumeral joint dislocation, 689, 689f
Extra-articular fracture, of thumb metacarpal, 599

Extracorporeal blood rewarming, 2250-2251, 2250t
Extracorporeal membrane oxygenation
for sepsis, 2222
in pediatric resuscitation, 98-99
Extracorporeal shock wave lithotripsy
for cholelithiasis, 1419
for urolithiasis, 1593
Extradural abscess, in otitis media, 1068
Extrahepatic bile duct carcinoma, 1423
Extraocular movement disorders, 1062-1063
Extraocular muscle function, in red and painful eye, 286
Extraperitoneal bladder rupture, 526
Extrapyramidal symptoms
dementia with, 1657
from antipsychotic agents, 2445, 2446-2447, 2449
prevention of, 1731
Extrasystoles, 1221-1225
Extravascular hemolytic transfusion reaction, 60
Extreme altitude, 2296
Extremity(ies)
examination of
in chest pain, 187t
in cyanosis, 270-271, 270f
in dyspnea, 178t
in peripheral vascular injury, 541
lower
aneurysm of, 1354
escharotomy of, 924
immobilization of, 569-571, 570f, 572f, 573f
isolated mononeuropathy of, 1694b, 1697-1699
ulcers of, 1350-1351, 1972
vascular injury of, 546-547
venous anatomy of, 1368-1369
trauma to
in elderly person, 346-347
in electrical and lightning injuries, 2273, 2277
upper
aneurysm of, 1354-1355
deep venous thrombosis of, 1370
distal, neurologic examination of, 2694t
escharotomy of, 924-925, 925f
fracture of, in elderly person, 346
immobilization of, 569, 569f
isolated mononeuropathy of, 1693-1697, 1694b
vascular injury of, 544-546
vascular disease of. *See* Peripheral arteriovascular disease; Venous thrombosis.
Extrinsic ligaments of wrist, 622, 624f
Exudative pericardial effusion, 1285
Exudative pleural effusion, 1149-1150, 1152, 1152b
Exudative retinal detachment, 1058
Eye, 1044-1064
acute visual loss and, 1056-1061, 1057f-1059f
anatomy of, 283, 284f, 384, 1045f
anisocoria and, 1061-1062
conjunctivitis of
gonococcal, 1566
in anaphylaxis, 1825t
in Kawasaki disease, 2025-2026
red and painful eye in, 296t-297t
corneal disease and, 1053-1054, 1054f
epidemiology of, 1044
examination of
in altered consciousness, 2502-2503
in facial trauma, 387-388
in red and painful eye, 285-288, 285b
extraocular movement disorders and, 1062-1063
eyelid and ocular soft tissue disorders and, 1054-1055, 1055f
foreign body in, 859-861, 860f, 861f
glaucoma and, 1055-1056, 1056f
HIV/AIDS and, 2085-2086
hypertension and, 1055
laceration of, 392
Lyme disease and, 2124
nystagmus and, 1062
ophthalmic drugs for, 1063-1064, 1063b
opioid overdose and, 2453
optic disk abnormalities and, 1062
pressure of. *See* Intraocular pressure.
Eye *(Continued)*
red and painful
ancillary studies in, 288
diagnostic approach to, 283-288, 284b, 285b, 287f
differential diagnosis in, 288-290, 288f-291f
disposition in, 293t-297t, 297
empiric management of, 290-292, 293t-297t
epidemiology of, 283
history in, 285
in infants and children, 292
physical examination in, 285-288, 285b
traumatic, 283, 290, 292, 297
trauma to, 1044-1052. *See also* Ocular trauma.
vertigo and, 2685
Eye drops, 1063
Eye movements
disorders of, 1062-1063
examination of, in comatose patient, 159t, 160-161
Eyebrow laceration, 392
Eyelid
contusion of, 1044
disorders of, 1054-1055, 1055f
laceration of, 392, 1051, 1051f
super glue adhered to, 1046
thermal burns of, 1046
Fab antivenin, in snakebite, 901
Fab fragments
for digitalis toxicity, 2371, 2372b
for oleander poisoning, 2474
Face
analgesia of, Dejeune onion skin pattern of, 420
anatomy of, 383-386, 383f-386f
barotrauma to, in scuba diving–related disorders, 2282, 2293
blood supply to, 385, 385f
edema of, in superior vena cava syndrome, 1910
nerve supply to, 383-384
skin of, 384-385, 384f
skin tension lines of, 843f
trauma to, 382-396
anatomy and physiology in, 383-386, 383f-386f
clinical features of, 386-388
disposition in, 396
epidemiology of, 382-383
fractures and dislocations in, 392-396, 394f, 395f
history in, 386-387
imaging of, 388-389
management of, 389-391
pathophysiology of, 386, 387f
penetrating, 386, 387f
physical examination in, 387-388
prehospital care in, 389-390
soft tissue injuries in, 390-392
Face presentations in labor and delivery, 2815-2816
Facet dislocation
bilateral, 404, 405f
unilateral, 406, 408f-409f, 409
Facial auditory nerve oxalosis, in ethylene glycol poisoning, 2399
Facial expression, lines of, 384, 384f
Facial flushing, in scombroid fish poisoning, 1472
Facial nerve, 1665t
paralysis of, 1666-1668
clinical features of, 1667-1668
diagnosis of, 1668
disposition in, 1668
in otitis media, 1067
pathophysiology of, 1666-1667
tumor of, paralysis from, 1667
Facial pain
in multiple sclerosis, 1673
in trigeminal neuralgia, 1664
Facial rash
in dermatomyositis, 1708
in systemic lupus erythematosus, 1806
Facial skeleton, 383, 383f
Factitious disorder, 1761-1765
by proxy, 1761, 1763, 1765
clinical features of, 1761-1762
Factitious disorder *(Continued)*
diagnosis of, 1764
differential considerations in, 1764, 1764b
disposition in, 1765
management of, 1764-1765
somatoform disorders vs., 1757
Factor VII deficiency, 1899
Factor VIII deficiency
assay for, 1899-1900
in hemophilia A, 1900-1902
in von Willebrand's disease, 1902-1903
Factor VIII replacement
for hemophilia A, 1900-1902, 1901t, 1902t
for von Willebrand's disease, 1902-1903
Factor IX deficiency, 1902
Failure to thrive, in developmentally disabled patient, 2900-2901
Failures in emergency care, 3119-3126
problem areas for, 3124-3126, 3125t
sources of, 3119-3123, 3120f, 3120t
Fainting, 2685
Falls
in elderly person, 344, 2829-2830
in pregnancy, 318
injury control in, 943t
mechanism of injury of, 302, 303t
False imprisonment, 2967
False labor, 2798
False negative, 3052
False positive, 3052
Famciclovir
for genital herpes, 1557t, 1559, 1858
for herpes simplex esophagitis, 1387
indications for, 2038
Familial periodic paralysis, 1709
Family
as surrogate decision-maker, 3134
during pediatric resuscitation, 114-116, 3149
in pediatric trauma, 330
Family relationships, promotion of, as wellness strategy for emergency physicians, 3177
Famotidine, 1390t
for anaphylaxis, 2549
Fascial anatomy, 842
Fascial planes of head and neck, 1027, 1030f, 1116
Fasciculations, from succinylcholine, 13-14
Fasciitis, 2196t, 2207-2208
Fasciola hepatica, 2101t, 2113
Fascioliasis, fever in, 2105
Fasciolopsis buski, 2101t
Fasciotomy, for compartment syndrome, 562, 1983
Fasting, preprocedural, 2939-2940
Fasting hypoglycemia, 1961-1962
Fat embolism, 563
Fat pads
in elbow and humeral trauma, 651, 651f
in supracondylar fracture, 2694-2695, 2695f
Fatigue
in multiple sclerosis, 1673
in myasthenia gravis, 1705
performance and, 3122-3123, 3122f, 3123b
Fatty casts
in proteinuria, 1532
in urinary sediment, 1526, 1526f
Fatty liver
alcoholic, 2868
in pregnancy, 1417, 2755-2756
Feathering burn, 2273, 2273f
Febrile seizures, 2507, 2666-2667, 2674, 2674b
Febrile transfusion reaction, 60
Fecal impaction
in developmentally disabled patient, 2903
in spinal cord injury, 2907
management of, 1497
Fecal incontinence, 1516-1517, 1516b
Fecal leukocytes, in diarrhea, 233, 2627
Federal Hazard Communication Standard, 3081
Feeding intolerance, in necrotizing enterocolitis, 2608
Felbamate, 1628t
Felodipine, 1321t
overdose of, 2377t
Felon, 615-616, 616f
Female
HIV/AIDS in, 2072
myocardial infarction in, atypical presentations associated with, 1159
urine collection methods in, 1575

Feminism, in alcoholism, 2871
Femoral aneurysm, 1354
Femoral artery and vein
  anatomy of, 737, 738f
  injury to, 546
Femoral condyles, 770, 771f
Femoral fracture
  arterial injury in, 761
  arthroplasty for, 749-750, 750f
  avulsion, 750, 750f
  distal, 776-777
  distal epiphyseal, 780-781
  occult, 746, 748f
  open fracture care in, 748-749, 749t
  pain management in, 749
  pediatric, 763-764, 763f
  proximal, 750-752, 750f-751f, 752b
  stress, 755-756
  traction and immobilization in, 746, 748
  with minimal or no trauma, 755
Femoral head
  anatomy of, 736, 737f
  arterial supply to, 737, 738f
  avascular necrosis of, 739-741, 741b, 742f
    after femoral neck fracture, 740, 742f, 750-751
    pediatric, 767
  development of, 763, 763f
  dislocation of, 756-759, 757f-759f
  fracture-dislocation of, 759-760, 760f
Femoral neck
  anatomy of, 736, 737f
  development of, 763, 763f
  fracture of, 750-752, 750f-751f, 752b
    avascular necrosis after, 740, 742f, 750-751
    displaced, 751, 752b
    radiologic evaluation in, 746, 747f, 751f
    stress type, 755-756
Femoral nerve, 737
Femoral nerve block, for femoral and hip fractures, 749
Femoral neuropathy, in hip trauma, 762
Femoral pulse, during cardiopulmonary resuscitation, 79
Femoral shaft fracture, 755
  pediatric, 763-764
  subtrochanteric, 753-755, 754f
Femoral trauma, 735-768
  anatomy in, 736-738, 736f-738f, 737t
  clinical features of, 742-744
  diagnostic strategies in, 746, 747f, 748f
  epidemiology of, 735-736
  femoral and hip fractures in, 746-756
    arthroplasty for, 749-750, 750f
    avulsion type, 750, 750f
    compartment syndrome in, 749
    femoral shaft, 755
    greater or lesser trochanteric, 753, 753f
    history in, 742-743
    intertrochanteric, 752-753, 752f
    open fracture care in, 748-749, 749t
    pain management in, 749
    pathophysiology of, 739
    physical examination in, 743-744
    proximal femoral, 750-752, 750f-751f, 752b
    stress type, 755-756
    subtrochanteric, 753-755, 754f
    traction and immobilization in, 746, 748
    with minimal or no trauma, 755
  femoral head fracture-dislocation in, 759-760, 760f
  hip dislocation in, 756-759, 757f-759f
  hip prosthesis dislocation in, 749, 750f, 760
  management of, 746-750
  muscular injuries in, 761-762
  neurologic injuries in, 762-763
  pathophysiology of, 739-742, 739f-745f
  pediatric considerations in, 763-767, 763f, 765f-767f
  radiologic evaluation in, 746, 747f, 751f
  soft tissue injuries in, 761-763
  vascular injuries in, 762
Femur
  anatomy of, 736-738, 736f-738f, 737t
  underlying lesions of, 741-742, 743f-755f
  immobilization of, 569-570, 570f
  neoplastic disease in, 742, 745f
  osteoporosis of, 739, 739f-741f
Fenamate, overdose of, 2940
Fennel, adverse effects of, 2476t
Fenoldopam, for hypertensive emergencies, 1318
Fentanyl, 2922t, 2923
  for procedural sedation and analgesia, 2940t-2941t, 2944, 2952-2953
  in intubation of patient with elevated intracranial pressure, 17
  in rapid sequence intubation, 11b
  respiratory effects of, 2453t
  sympatholytic dose of, 17
  with midazolam, for procedural sedation and analgesia, 2950, 2951t
Ferret bite, 884-885
Ferritin, serum, in pregnancy, 2768
Ferrous sulfate, for iron deficiency anemia, 1871
Fertility rate, age-specific, 2722
Fertilization, hormonal role in, 2723
Fetal alcohol syndrome, 2791-2792, 2791b, 2877-2878, 2901t
Fetal anticonvulsant syndrome, 2769
Fetal heart rate monitoring, in pregnant trauma patient, 39, 319, 323-324, 324f
Fetal pole, ultrasonography of, 2730, 2731f
Fetal stations, in labor and delivery, 2799, 2799f
Fetomaternal hemorrhage, Kleihauer-Betke test for, 321
Fetopelvic disproportion, 2811
Fetor hepaticus, in hepatic encephalopathy, 1411
Fetus
  abruptio placentae and, 2747-2748
  antenatal assessment of, 2800-2802, 2803f
  ballottement or palpation of, 2728
  biophysical profile of, 2802, 2802t
  circulation in, 2568, 2568f
  death of
    first- or second-trimester, 2740
    sonographic criteria for, 2741, 2741b
  diabetes effects on, 2772
  evaluation of, in pregnant trauma patient, 323-324, 323f, 323t, 324f
  hyperthyroidism effects on, 2773
  maternal chronic medical illness effects on, 2761-2776, 2763t-2764t
  maternal drug therapy and, 2779-2780, 2780b
  maternal substance abuse and, 2791, 2791b
  radiographic identification of, 2730
  skull of, bony landmarks of, 2800f
  trauma to, 319
  ultrasonography of, 2741, 2741b, 2741t
  umbilical cord entanglement with, 2817-2818
Fever, 134-137
  altered mental status and, 136, 2509b
  diagnostic approach to, 135-137, 135b, 135t
  differential considerations in, 135, 135b, 135t, 137
  disposition in, 137
  empirical management of, 137
  epidemiology of, 134
  hyperthermia vs., 2258
  in *Aeromonas hydrophila* gastroenteritis, 1467
  in alcoholism, 2870-2871
  in amebic abscess, 1415
  in anticholinergic poisoning, 2348
  in arthritis, 1778
  in *Bacillus anthracis* gastroenteritis, 1469
  in *Campylobacter* gastroenteritis, 1460
  in central nervous system infection, 1714
  in cholangitis, 1421
  in *Clostridium difficile* enterocolitis, 1475
  in Colorado tick fever, 2141
  in diarrhea, 232
  in elderly person, 134, 2827-2828
  in hemorrhagic *Escherichia coli* serotype O157:H7 gastroenteritis, 1467
  in HIV/AIDS, 2076
  in hyperthyroidism, 1986
  in infective endocarditis, 1301
  in intestinal amebiasis, 1480
  in Kawasaki disease, 2025
  in meningococcal disease, 2021
  in neutropenic cancer patient, 2834-2839, 2836t, 2838t
  in osteomyelitis, 2179
  in otitis media, 1067
  in pancreatitis, 1429
  in pertussis, 2006
  in *Plesiomonas shigelloides* gastroenteritis, 1468
  in pneumococcal disease, 2010
Fever (*Continued*)
  in purulent pericarditis, 1286
  in pyogenic abscess, 1414
  in Q fever, 2137
  in rheumatic fever, 1304
  in Rocky Mountain spotted fever, 2133
  in salmonellosis, 1463
  in septic arthritis, 1785, 2188
  in shigellosis, 1464
  in sickle cell disease, 1880-1881
  in staphylococcal food poisoning, 1470
  in toxic shock syndrome, 2029
  in *Vibrio parahaemolyticus* gastroenteritis, 1466
  in viral gastroenteritis, 1476
  in *Yersinia enterocolitica* gastroenteritis, 1465
  pathophysiology of, 134-135
  pediatric, 2505-2517
    ancillary tests in, 2508-2510
    bacteremia and, 2505-2506, 2512, 2515
    chest radiography in, 2510
    clinical features of, 2508-2511
    disposition in, 2517
    history in, 2508
    hyperpyrexia and, 2506
    in appendicitis, 2619
    in bacterial meningitis, 2658, 2659
    in bacterial tracheitis, 2528
    in cancer patient, 2516
    in congenital heart disease, 2517
    in epiglottitis, 2523
    in heat exhaustion and heatstroke, 2511
    in hemolytic uremic syndrome, 2654
    in HIV/AIDS, 2516
    in Kawasaki disease, 2511-2512, 2512b
    in pneumonia, 2556
    in septic shock, 2511
    in sickle cell anemia, 2516-2517
    in toxic ingestion, 2511
    in toxic shock syndrome, 2511, 2511b
    in ventriculoperitoneal shunts, 2517
    lumbar puncture and, 2660
    management of, 2511-2516, 2513b, 2515f
    of unknown origin, 2507, 2507b
    pathophysiology of, 2505
    petechiae and, 2507-2508
    physical examination in, 2508, 2509b
    prehospital care in, 2511
    seizure and, 2507, 2666-2667, 2674, 2674b
    temperature determination in, 2508
  plus petechiae, as indication for lumbar puncture, 2660
  relapsing, 2129-2130
Feverfew, adverse effects of, 2476t
Fiber, dietary, for constipation, 241t, 242
Fiberoptic bronchoscopy, in acute inhalation injury, 921
Fiberoptic intubation, 20-21, 22f
Fibrin clot formation, 1892, 1893f, 1894
Fibrin deposition, in thrombosis, 1368
Fibrinogen
  in bleeding disorders, 1895, 1903
  in disseminated intravascular coagulation, 1903-1904
  in placenta previa, 2748
  in pregnancy, 318
Fibrinolysis, in anaphylaxis, 1825t
Fibrinolytic therapy
  for acute arterial occlusion, 1349
  for stroke, 1613t, 1615, 1615b
  in cocaine overdose, 2391
  in myocardial infarction, 1189-1192, 1192b
    contraindications to, 1192b
    eligibility criteria for, 1190-1192
    reduced-dose, in PCI candidates, 1195
    selection of agent for, 1189-1190
    with glycoprotein inhibitor, 1194
  in pulmonary embolism, 1377-1378, 1378t, 1379
  prehospital use of, 2991
Fibroproductive lesions, in tuberculosis, 2153
Fibula
  anatomy of, 797
  fracture of
    avulsion, 818
    distal, 818
    proximal, 801-802, 802f, 814f
    stress, 804
Fibular compression test, 818

Field care, tactical, 3003
Field communications in emergency medical services, 2988-2989
Field death pronouncement, 3144
Fifth disease, 1850, 2046, 2046f
Fifth metatarsal base fracture, 832, 833f, 834
Fight bite, 611, 890
Figure-of-eight splint
for clavicle fracture, 2693
in clavicle fracture, 677, 678f
in sternoclavicular joint dislocation, 684
Filariasis, 2100t, 2107-2108
File drawer problem, in clinical trials, 3051
Filovirus, 2034t, 2054
Financial exploitation, of elder, 1010
Finger
amputations and ring avulsion injuries of, 612-613, 613b
boutonniére deformity of, 607, 607f
carpometacarpal joint dislocation of, 603, 603f
decompression of, in burn injury, 925
distal interphalangeal joint dislocation of, 601, 601f
distal phalanx fracture of, 593-594, 593f
examination of, in arthritis, 1779
extensor tendon injuries in, 605-608, 605f-607f
felon of, 615-616, 616f
flexor tendon injuries in, 608-609
herpetic whitlow of, 616
metacarpal fractures of, 595-599, 597f-598f
metacarpophalangeal joint dislocation of, 602-603, 602f, 603f
motions of, 578f
proximal and middle phalangeal fractures of, 594-595, 594f-596f
proximal interphalangeal joint dislocation of, 601-602
radiography of, 592f
swan neck deformity of, 607, 607f
trigger, 585, 618
vascular injuries of, 613-614
Finger drop, in radial mononeuropathy, 1695
Finger sweeping, for airway foreign body removal, 869
Finger traps, in Colles' fracture, 633, 635f
Fingernail
paronychia and, 614-615, 615f
structural framework of, 589
Finger-snapping test, in lateral epicondylitis, 1798
Fingertip
anatomy of, 589, 589f
injuries to, 609-611, 610f
Finkelstein's test, in De Quervain's tenosynovitis, 1799
Fioricet, for migraine, 2680
Fiorinal, for migraine, 2680
Fire ant stings, 904, 905, 1827
Fire burn, 913-928. *See also* Thermal burn.
Fire corals, 909
Fire departments, EMS systems incorporated into, 2985
Fire victim, simultaneous carbon monoxide and cyanide poisoning in, 2440-2441
Firearm injuries. *See also* Gunshot wounds; Shotgun wounds.
death from, 300
epidemiology of, 489
nonpowder, 1019
street gangs and, 1021
suicide and, 1768
youth, 1018-1019
Firethorn, 2475
First responder, 2986, 2987t
First stage of labor, 2799-2800, 2799f-2802f
First-degree atrioventricular block, 1218, 1219f
First-degree burn, 918, 919f
First-trimester fetal death, 2740
First-trimester vaginal bleeding, 2740-2741, 2746f
Fish poisoning
ciguatera, 1470t, 1473-1474
scombroid, 1470t, 1472-1473
Vibrio, 1470t, 1471-1472
Fisher's exact test, 3052t, 3053
Fissure, anal, 1508, 1512-1513, 1512f, 1513t
Fistula
anorectal, 1513, 1515
aortoenteric
Fistula *(Continued)*
after abdominal aortic aneurysm repair, 1340
in abdominal aortic aneurysm rupture, 1333
aortovenous, in abdominal aortic aneurysm rupture, 1333
arteriovenous, 538-539, 541, 1344, 1347, 1360
arteriovenous bridge, prosthetic, 1365-1366
bronchopleural, 466
perilymphatic, vertigo in, 2685
Fitz-Hugh–Curtis syndrome, 1570
Fixation
in humeral shaft fracture, 655
in metacarpal or phalangeal fractures, 595
in open tibial shaft fracture, 801
in pelvic fracture, 731-732
Flail chest, 457-458, 457f, 458b, 460
Flammable liquids, 915
Flank, 490
gunshot wounds to, 506-507
stab wounds to, 505
Flank pain
in renal stones, 2646
in urolithiasis, 1588, 1590, 1593b
Flash burn, 2272
Flash points, of combustible liquids, 915, 915t
Flatulence, in intestinal amebiasis, 1480
Flavivirus, 2034t, 2049-2050
Flecainide, 1208, 2788
Flexion injuries of cervical spine, 399, 401-404, 402f-405f
Flexion supracondylar fracture, 657f, 658-659
Flexion teardrop fracture, of cervical spine, 401, 403f
Flexion-extension radiographs, in spinal injuries, 427
Flexor carpi radialis, 582, 584f
Flexor carpi ulnaris, 582, 584f
Flexor digiti minimi, 580-581, 581f
Flexor digitorum profundus, 582, 584-585, 584f, 585f, 609
Flexor digitorum superficialis, 582, 584, 584f, 585f, 609
Flexor hallucis longus tendinitis, 820
Flexor hallucis longus tendon, 838
Flexor pollicis brevis, 580, 581f
Flexor pollicis longus, 582, 584f
Flexor pulley system, 582, 584f
Flexor retinaculum, 808, 809f
Flexor tendons, of hand, 582, 584-585, 584f, 585, 585f, 586f
relationship to radial and ulnar bursae, 585, 586f
trauma to, 608-609
Flexor tenosynovitis, 616-617
Flight crew in air medical transport, 2996
Flip test, in lumbar radiculopathy, 704
Floaters, eye, 1040
Flori-Methane spray, 2933
Flow phase in recovery from burn injury, 919
Fluconazole
during pregnancy and lactation, 2785
for candidal esophagitis, 1387
for cryptococcal meningitis, 2081
for esophageal candidiasis, 2083-2084
for tinea capitis, 1839
for vulvovaginal candidiasis, 1567t, 1568
in HIV/AIDS, side effects of, 2079t
Fludrocortisone acetate, for adrenal insufficiency, 1998
Fluid
depletion of. *See* Dehydration; Hypovolemia.
excess of. *See* Hypervolemia.
Fluid and electrolyte disturbances
in delirium, 1648, 1649
in diabetic ketoacidosis, 1962
in hyperglycemic hyperosmolar nonketotic coma, 1968, 1969
in pediatric gastroenteritis, 2630-2634, 2630t, 2632b-2634b
Fluid challenge, for acute pulmonary edema in hypotensive patient, 1273
Fluid intake, heat illness and, 2256
Fluid restriction, for hyponatremia, 1935
Fluid resuscitation
for diabetic ketoacidosis, 1966
for diarrhea, 235
for hyperglycemic hyperosmolar nonketotic coma, 1969
for hypermagnesemia, 1950
Fluid resuscitation *(Continued)*
for hyperuricemia, 1914
for hypovolemic hypotension, 360
for rhabdomyolysis, 1982
for salicylate overdose, 2341-2342
for sickle cell disease, 1881
in abdominal aortic aneurysm rupture, 1337
in cardiac tamponade, 475
in crush injury, 3007-3008
in elderly trauma patient, 348
in gastrointestinal bleeding, 221
in heatstroke, 2264-2265
in hemorrhagic shock, 52
in hypothermia, 2245
in lithium toxicity, 2443
in multiple trauma, 307
in neonatal resuscitation, 123t, 124
in pulmonary contusion, 461
in sepsis, 2218, 2219, 2219t
in septic shock, 53
in severe head trauma, 360
in shock, 52
in thermal burns, 921, 922-923
in toxic shock syndrome, 2030
pediatric
in cardiac arrest, 109
in hypertrophic pyloric stenosis, 2605-2606
in infectious diarrhea, 2629-2634, 2630t, 2632b-2634b
in necrotizing enterocolitis, 2609
prehospital, 2991
Fluid retention, from high altitude exposure, 2298
Fluke infection, 2100t-2101t
Flu-like illness, in anthrax exposure, 3025
Flumazenil
for benzodiazepine reversal, 2949
in benzodiazepine overdose, 2326
in children, 2953
in comatose patient, 163
Flunitrazepam, overdose of, 2486
Fluoride poisoning. *See* Hydrofluoric acid.
Fluorine-18-deoxyglucose positron emission tomography, in osteomyelitis, 2181
Fluoroquinolones
during pregnancy and lactation, 2785
for *Escherichia coli* food poisoning, 1474
for pneumonia, 1136
for tuberculosis, 2164t, 2165
for urinary tract infection, 1581t, 1582, 1583
prophylactic, in cat bites, 888
Fluoroscopy, in esophageal foreign body removal, 872-873
Fluoxetine, 2357
Fluphenazine, 2446t
injectable, for psychotic relapse, 1732
Flurazepam, 2484, 2484t
Flush syndromes, anaphylaxis vs., 1829
Flutter waves, 1229, 1230f-1231f
Flying, decompression sickness and, 2293-2294, 2293f
Focused assessment with sonography for trauma (FAST), 312-313, 723
Fogarty catheter embolectomy, for acute arterial embolism, 1352
Fogarty catheter thrombectomy
for arterial thrombosis, 1354
for peripheral arteriovascular disease, 1349
Folate/folic acid
deficiency of
causes of, 1873b
megaloblastic anemia from, 1873-1875, 1874f, 1874t, 1875t
supplementation of, in pregnancy, 2768
Foley catheter
in burn injury, 923
in foreign body removal, 2617
in genitourinary trauma, 515, 517, 518f
in peripheral vascular injury, 543
Folinic acid
for toxic alcohol poisoning, 2402
for *Toxoplasma gondii* infection, 2082
Folk/alternative medicine, cultural competent approach to, 3113-3114
Folliculitis, skin lesions in, 1843
Follow-up
in clinical trials, 3050
in disposition requirements, 3164-3165
Fomepizole, for toxic alcohol poisoning, 2401

Food allergy, 1826, 1848, 2547, 2548
Food bolus impaction, management of, 872
Food poisoning
  Bacillus cereus, 1470t, 1471
  bacterial, 1469-1475, 1480t
  ciguatera, 1470t, 1473-1474
  Clostridium botulinum, 2012-2016
  Clostridium perfringens, 1470-1471, 1470t
  Escherichia coli, 1470t, 1471
  in salmonellosis, 1461-1463, 1461t, 1462t
  reporting requirements for, 1463b
  scombroid, 1470t, 1472-1473
  staphylococcal, 1469-1470, 1480t
  Vibrio, 1470t, 1471-1472
Foods
  MAOI toxicity and, 2364, 2364b
  tyramine-containing, 1313, 1314b
Foot
  diabetic, 1971
  edema of, heat-induced, 2258-2259
  in Kawasaki disease, 2026
  pain in, 836-837
  puncture wounds to
    antibiotic prophylaxis for, 855
    osteomyelitis after, 2185
  trench, 2228, 2230-2231
Foot drop, in common peroneal mononeuropathy, 1699
Foot trauma, 820-839
  anatomy and physiology in, 820-821, 820f
  calcaneal fracture in, 826-827, 826f, 827f
  clinical features of, 821
  compartment syndrome in, 838-839
  contusions and sprains in, 838
  crush injuries, amputations, and major vascular injuries in, 838
  cuboid fracture in, 828
  cuneiform fracture in, 828
  diagnostic strategies in, 821-822, 822f
  dislocation of cuneiform, cuboid, or navicular bones in, 828
  interphalangeal dislocations in, 835-836
  Lisfranc injuries in, 828-831, 829f, 830f
  metatarsal base fractures in, 832-834, 833f
  metatarsal head and neck fractures in, 832
  metatarsal shaft fractures in, 831-832
  metatarsophalangeal dislocations in, 835
  midtarsal joint injuries in, 827
  navicular fracture in, 827-828
  osteochondral fracture of talar dome in, 824-825, 825f
  pain in, 836-837
  phalangeal fractures in, 834
  sesamoid fractures in, 834-835
  stress fractures in, 837-838
  subtalar dislocation in, 825-826, 825f
  talar fracture in, 822-824, 823f, 824f
  tendon injuries in, 838
  total talar dislocation in, 826
Foramen magnum, 350
Foramen ovale, closure of, 2568
Forced air warming systems, 2248
Forced expiratory volume in 1 second (FEV_1)
  in asthma, 1084, 1086t, 2535t, 2536
  in chronic obstructive pulmonary disease, 1098, 1098t, 1101
Forced vital capacity
  in chronic obstructive pulmonary disease, 1098, 1098t
  weakness and, 139
Forearm arterial injury, 545-546
Forearm splint, 569
Forearm trauma, 639-644
  anatomy in, 639-640, 640t
  clinical features of, 640
  Galeazzi's fracture in, 642-643, 643f
  Monteggia's fracture-dislocation in, 642, 642f
  plastic deformation in, 644, 645f
  radiography in, 640-641, 640f
  shaft fractures of radius and ulna in, 641
  ulnar shaft fracture in, 641-642
Forefoot
  anatomy of, 820, 820f
  interphalangeal dislocations of, 835-836
  metatarsal base fractures of, 832-834, 833f
  metatarsal head and neck fractures of, 832
  metatarsal shaft fractures of, 831-832
  metatarsophalangeal dislocations of, 835
  pain in, 837
Forefoot *(Continued)*
  phalangeal fractures of, 834
  sesamoid fractures of, 834-835
Foreign body, 859-879
  anorectal, 875-877, 876f, 1521-1522, 1522f
  assessment for, 845, 850
  gastrointestinal, 870-877, 2616-2617, 2617f
  genitourinary, 877-878
  in airway, 864-870, 2529-2530, 2550-2551, 2551f
    clinical features of, 864-865
    history in, 865-866
    imaging of, 866-868, 867f-869f
    management of, 868-870
    physical examination in, 866
  in bowel, 873-875, 875f
  in children
    airway, 2529-2530, 2550-2551, 2551f
    esophageal, 2617, 2617f
    gastrointestinal, 2616-2617, 2617f
  in ear, 861-863, 862f
  in esophagus, 868f, 869f, 870-873, 1382-1384, 2617, 2617f
  in hand, 618-619
  in lower leg, 805
  in nose, 863-864
  in pharynx, 870-873
  in stomach, 873-875, 875f, 1384-1385
  lead, 2423
  management of, 859
  ocular, 859-861, 860f, 861f, 1051-1052
    conjunctival, 1048
    corneal, 292, 297, 1047, 1047f, 1048f
  oropharyngeal, 1384
  soft tissue, 878-879
Forensic emergency medicine, 952-966
  in auto-pedestrian collisions, 965-966, 966b, 966f
  in gunshot wounds, 953-960, 954f-960f
  in motor vehicle trauma, 963-966, 964b, 965f-966f, 966b
  in physical assault, 960-963, 961b, 961f-964f
  in sexual assault, 984-989, 985b-987b, 987f, 987t, 988f, 988t
Forensic science, tactical emergency medical support and, 3004
Formaldehyde
  ingestion of, 2384
  methanol metabolism to, 2395, 2396f
Formic acid
  methanol metabolism to, 2395, 2396f
  poisoning from, 934
Formication, in amphetamine abuse, 2894
Formoterol, for asthma, 1088
Forward elevation maneuver, for reduction of anterior glenohumeral joint dislocation, 689
Foscarnet
  for AIDS-related diarrhea, 1484
  for cytomegalovirus esophagitis, 1387
  for herpes zoster, 2043
  in HIV/AIDS, side effects of, 2079t
  indications for, 2038
Fosinopril, 1322t
Fosphenytoin
  for alcohol-related status epilepticus, 2865
  for seizure, 166, 166t, 1627, 1627t
  for status epilepticus, 2672t, 2673
  prophylactic, in severe head trauma, 361
  side effects of, 1628t
Fournier's syndrome, 2208
Four-pillar anterior ring injuries, pelvic, 725, 726f
Fourth stage of labor, 2805
Fourth-degree burn, 919, 919f
Fourth-nerve palsy, eye movement disorders in, 1062-1063
Fox, rabies in, 2062, 2062f, 2063f
Foxglove plant, 2368, 2369f
Fractional excretion of sodium (FENa), 1527-1528, 1527t, 1528b
Fracture, 552-564
  alignment of, 552-553
  alveolar bone, 1040
  angulation of, 553, 554f
  ankle, 811-815, 812b, 812f-815f
  avascular necrosis after, 562
  blisters associated with, 563
  clavicle, 676-679, 676f-679f
    in children, 2692-2693, 2693f
    subclavian artery injury and, 548
Fracture *(Continued)*
  closed, 552
  comminuted, 552, 552f, 2690, 2691f
  compartment syndrome in, 559-562, 560b, 561b, 561f
  complete vs. incomplete, 550
  complex regional pain syndrome after, 562-563
  complications of, 558-564, 563b
  cricoid cartilage, 447
  diagnostic modalities in, 557-558
  displacement of, 552-553, 553f
  eponyms for, 550t-551t, 554
  facial, 392-396, 394f, 395f
    dental and alveolar, 395
    forehead, 393
    imaging of, 388-389, 394f
    mandible, 394-395, 395f
    midface, 393-394, 394f
    orbit, 393
    temporomandibular joint, 395-396
    zygoma, 394
  fat embolism syndrome after, 563
  foot
    calcaneal, 826-827, 826f, 827f
    cuboid, 828
    cuneiform, 828
    Lisfranc, 828-831, 829f, 830f
    metatarsal base, 832-834, 833f
    metatarsal head and neck, 832
    metatarsal shaft, 831-832
    navicular, 827-828
    phalangeal, 834
    sesamoid, 834-835
    stress, 837-838
    talar, 822-824, 823f, 824f
    talar dome, osteochondral, 824-825, 825f
  forearm, 641-644
  hand
    distal phalanx, 593-594, 593f
    mechanism of injury in, 592-593, 592f
    metacarpal, 595-600, 597f-599f
    pediatric, 600
    proximal and middle phalangeal, 594-595, 594f-596f
    terminology in, 592-593, 592f
  healing of, 564, 781
  hemorrhage associated with, 559, 559t
  hip, 746-756
    arthroplasty for, 749-750, 750f
    avulsion type, 750, 750f
    compartment syndrome in, 749
    femoral shaft, 755
    greater or lesser trochanteric, 753, 753f
    history in, 742-743
    intertrochanteric, 752-753, 752f
    open fracture care in, 748-749, 749t
    pain management in, 749
    pathophysiology of, 739
    physical examination in, 743-744
    proximal femoral, 750-752, 750f-751f, 752b
    stress type, 755-756
    subtrochanteric, 753-755, 754f
    traction and immobilization in, 746, 748
    with minimal or no trauma, 755
  humeral, 652-664
    articular surface, 661-664, 661f-663f
    distal, 655-661, 656f-661f
    proximal, 680-682, 681f, 682f
    proximal epiphyseal, 682-683, 683f
    shaft, 652-655, 653f, 654f
    supracondylar, 2693-2697, 2694f-2696f, 2694t
  immobilization after
    casts for, 571-573, 573f
    complications of, 563, 564b
    splinting and bandaging for, 568-571, 569f, 570f
  in developmentally disabled patient, 2901
  in electrical and lightning injuries, 2273
  in spinal cord injury patient, 2909
  infection and, 558, 558b
  knee
    distal femur, 776-777
    patellar, 784-785, 785t
    proximal intra-articular tibial, 777-781
  laryngeal, in near-hanging and strangulation, 451
  lower leg
    proximal extra-articular tibial, 797-799

Fracture *(Continued)*
proximal fibula, 801-802, 802f
stress, 803-804
tibial shaft, 799-801, 801f
mandibular, 394-395, 395f
nasal, 391-392
nasoethmoid, 393-394
nerve injuries in, 559, 559t
nomenclature in, 550t-551t, 552-554, 552b, 553f-555f
oblique, 552, 552f
odontoid
type II, 405, 406f-407f
type III, 432f
with anterior dislocation, 399, 401, 402f
open, 552, 558, 558b
orbital, 393, 1044, 1045f
osteomyelitis after, 2185
pathologic, 553
pediatric, 554-557
apophyseal, 2709-2711, 2711f
child abuse and, 970, 970t, 2698-2701
clavicle, 2692-2693, 2693f
condylar, 660
diaphyseal, 2699
distal radius, 637-639, 637f, 638f, 638t
elbow avulsion, 2711, 2711f
epicondylar, 662-663, 662f
femoral, 763-764, 763f
greenstick, 554, 556f
hand, 600
healing of, 781
metaphyseal, 2699
Monteggia, 2697
multiple, in osteogenesis imperfecta, 2700-2701, 2700f, 2700t
nose, 392
patterns of, 554-557, 557t, 2689-2692, 2690f-2692f, 2691t
radius, 644, 644f
rib, 2699
skull, 334-335, 2699
supracondylar, 655-659, 656f-658f
supracondylar humeral, 2693-2697, 2694f-2696f, 2694t
toddler's, 2698, 2698f
torus, 554, 556f
trochanteric, 767
ulnar, 644, 644f
unintentional, 975
pelvic, 717-734
acetabular, 728-729, 728b, 731, 731f, 732f
anatomy in, 717-718, 718f
and blunt abdominal trauma, 509, 510f
classification of, 723, 723b
clinical features of, 718-720
diagnostic peritoneal lavage in, 722-723, 722f
epidemiology of, 717
general management of, 722f, 723
gynecologic injury in, 720
hemorrhage in, 718
evaluation of, 722-723, 722f
management of, 731-734, 731b, 733f
high-energy, 726-728, 727b, 733f
in bladder trauma, 520-521
in elderly person, 346
low-energy, 723-726, 724f
neurologic injury in, 719-720
open, 719
penetrating injuries in, 720
posterior urethral trauma and, 516, 516f
prehospital care in, 718
radiologic imaging in, 720-722, 721f
retrograde urethrogram and, 517-518
thoracic aortic injury in, 720
urologic injury in, 719
visceral and soft tissue injuries in, 719
penile, 533-534, 534f
peripheral vascular injury in, 544, 559
rib, 454-456, 454b, 455f
anatomy in, 455f
aortic rupture and, 479
flail chest and, 457
in children, 2699
in chronic obstructive pulmonary disease, 1102
pneumothorax and, 461-462
pulmonary contusion and, 460

Fracture *(Continued)*
shoulder, 676-683
clavicle, 676-679, 676f-679f
proximal humeral epiphysis, 682-683, 683f
proximal humerus, 680-682, 681f, 682f
scapula, 679-680, 680f
skull, 372-374
basilar, 373
clinical assessment and significance of, 372
depressed, 373
frontal, 393
in children, 334-335, 2699
linear, 372-373
open, 373-374
spinal
anatomy and physiology in, 399, 402f
back pain in, 706
computed tomography in, 429-430, 429f
disposition in, 439
extension, 410-411, 410f-411f
flexion, 399, 401-404, 402f-405f
minor, 439
rotational, 405-409, 408f-410f
vertical compression, 411-413, 411f-414f
with cord impingement, back pain in, 265t
spiral, 552, 552f
sternal, 456-457
stress, 553
thermal therapy for, 573-574
tibial
epiphyseal, 780-781
proximal
extra-articular, 797-799
intra-articular, 777-781
shaft, 799-801, 801f
stress, 803-804
subcondylar, 797-798
tibial plateau, 777-779, 777f-778f
tibial spine, 779-780, 780f
tibial tubercle, 798-799, 798f
tooth, 395, 1036-1037, 1036f
transverse, 552, 552f
wrist, 627-630, 632-636, 637-639
Fracture-dislocation, 564
Monteggia's, 551t, 642, 642f, 2697
of femoral head, 759-760, 760f
thoracic spine, 410f
Frailty, trajectory of dying in, 3140f, 3141
Francisella tularensis, 1131, 2130-2132
Free radical scavengers, after cerebral ischemia, 71
Free radicals, in necrosis after cerebral ischemia, 66
Free wall rupture, in myocardial infarction, 1160
Freeze-thaw phase of frostbite, 2229, 2229b
Freiberg's disease, 837
Frenzel maneuver for middle ear barotrauma, 2292
Freon gas abuse, frostbite from, 296f, 2887
Fresh frozen plasma, 59, 307
Friction rub
pericardial, 1281, 2592
pleural, 1150
Friedreich's ataxia, 2682
Frontal sinus, 1123
Frontal sinusitis, 1126
Frontal skull fracture, 393
Frontotemporal dementia, 1657
Frostbite, 2228-2235
clinical features of, 2230-2231
diagnostic strategies in, 2231
disposition in, 2233-2234
from freon gas abuse, 296f, 2887
management of, 2231-2233, 2232b
pathophysiology of, 2229, 2229b
predisposing factors in, 2229-2230, 2230b
sequelae of, 2234, 2234b
temperature regulation physiology and, 2228
Frostnip, 2230
Frozen shoulder, 682, 698-699, 699t, 1797
Full-thickness burn, 919, 919f
Fulminant hepatitis, 1404
Fundic soufflé, 2728
Funduscopic examination, in red and painful eye, 287

Fundus, normal, 1045f
Fungal infection
during pregnancy and lactation, 2785
in cancer patient with impaired cell-mediated immunity, 2840
in febrile cancer patient, 1908
in HIV/AIDS, 2079
in meningitis
complications of, 1715-1716
management of, 1722
pathophysiology of, 1713
signs and symptoms of, 1714
in organ transplant patient, 2848
in otitis externa, 1070-1071
in pharyngitis, 275, 1112, 1113
in pneumonia, 1130
in sinusitis, 1123, 1124, 1126
of bone or joint, 2178-2179
skin lesions in, 1838-1840, 1839f, 1840f
Fungal pathogens, in central nervous system infection, 1711t
Fungus ball, in tuberculosis, 2151, 2151f
Funic reduction in umbilical cord prolapse, 2817
Funnel plots for assessment of publication bias, 3058
Furazolidone, for *Giardia* gastroenteritis, 1479-1480
Furosemide, 1321t
for acute pulmonary edema, 1270t, 1272
for acute renal failure, 2650
for heart failure, 2583
for high-altitude pulmonary edema, 2304
for hypercalcemia, 1915, 1946
for hypermagnesemia, 1950
for hyponatremic hypovolemia, 2631-2632
for nephrotic syndrome, 2648
Furuncle, 1843, 2204
Furunculosis, in otitis externa, 1071
Fusospirochetes, in necrotizing ulcerative oral diseases, 1033
Futility, end of life and, 3141-3142

GABA (γ-Amino butyric acid) agonists, after cerebral ischemia, 71-72
GABA (γ-Amino butyric acid) receptor complex, 2481, 2482
Gabapentin
for neuropathic pain, 1692
for pediatric seizure, 2675t
side effects of, 1628t
Gadolinium-enhanced magnetic resonance imaging, in osteomyelitis, 2182, 2182f
Gait abnormalities
antalgic, 764-765, 765f
cerebellar, 145
in developmental hip dysplasia, 2702
in femoral neck stress fracture, 755-756
in slipped capital femoral epiphysis, 2708
Galeal laceration, 372, 850
Galeazzi's fracture, 550t, 642-643, 643f
Galeazzi's sign, in developmental hip dysplasia, 2701, 2702f
Gallbladder
carcinoma of, 1423
enlarged, in pancreatic carcinoma, 1437
hydrops of, in children, 2620
in pregnancy, 2726
inflammation of, 1419-1421, 1419f
porcelain, 1423
Gallium-labeled bone scan, in osteomyelitis, 2181, 2181f
Galloping consumption, 2151
Gallstone ileus, small bowel obstruction in, 1441
Gallstones, 1418-1419, 1418f, 1419f. *See also* Cholelithiasis.
Galveston formula, for fluid resuscitation of pediatric burn patient, 923
Gamekeeper's thumb, 604
Gamma globulin. *See* Immunoglobulin preparations.
Gamma rays, 2319, 2320f
Gamma/neutron exposure, 2319-2320
Ganciclovir
for AIDS-related diarrhea, 1484
for cytomegalovirus esophagitis, 1387

Ganciclovir *(Continued)*
in HIV/AIDS, side effects of, 2079t
indications for, 2038
Gang violence, 1017-1018, 1020-1022
Ganglion, hand, 618
Ganglionopathy, 1700, 1700b
Gangrene
gas, 2208-2209
in frostbite, 2229
local gas, 2208
Meleney's synergistic, 2208
Ganser's syndrome, 1729
Garlic, drug interactions with, 2478t
Gartland classification for extension-type supracondylar fracture, 2694t
Gas(es), pulmonary irritant, inhalation of, 2433t, 2434-2435, 2434f
Gas embolism
in scuba diving–related disorders, 2285-2286
recompression therapy for, 2288-2292, 2288b, 2289f-2291f
vs. pulmonary decompression sickness, 2288, 2288t
Gas gangrene, 2208-2209
Gas laws, 2280-2281, 2281f, 2994-2995, 2995t
Gas-forming agents, for food bolus impaction management, 872
Gasoline, dermal exposure to, 936-937
Gastric acid secretion, inhibitors of, 1390t, 1398-1399
Gastric emptying
in pregnancy, 2726
prolonged, gastroesophageal reflux in, 1388
Gastric fluid aspiration, pneumonia vs., 1136
Gastric infarction, 1394
Gastric injury, from alkali ingestion, 2381, 2381f, 2382f
Gastric lavage
in anticholinergic poisoning, 2349
in gastrointestinal bleeding, 224
in mercury poisoning, 2426
in overdosed/poisoned patient, 2330
Gastric mucosa damage, causes of, 1391, 1391b
Gastric outlet obstruction
in hypertrophic pyloric stenosis, 2603
in peptic ulcer disease, 1393
Gastric tonography, in shock, 50-51
Gastric tube, in gastrointestinal bleeding, 223-224
Gastric ulcers, 1391-1394
Gastric volvulus, 1394-1395
Gastritis, 1390-1391
nausea and vomiting in, 204t
peptic ulcer disease vs., 1393
Gastrocnemius strain, 804
Gastroenteritis
abdominal pain in, 211t
Aeromonas hydrophila, 1461t, 1462t, 1467-1468
Bacillus anthracis, 1461t, 1462t, 1468-1469
Bacillus cereus, 1470t, 1471
bacterial, 1469-1475, 1480t
acute, 2625-2626
invasive, 1460-1469, 1461t, 1462t
toxin-induced, 1469-1475, 1480t
Campylobacter, 1460-1461, 1461t, 1462t, 2625
ciguatera, 1470t, 1473-1474
Clostridium perfringens, 1470-1471, 1470t
Cryptosporidium, 1476-1478, 1477t
Cyclospora cayetanensis, 1477t, 1478-1479
diarrhea and, 234
Entamoebaa histolytica, 1477t, 1480-1481
Enterobius vermicularis, 1479-1482
Escherichia coli, 1470t, 1474, 2626
Giardia, 1477t, 1479-1480
hemorrhagic *Escherichia coli* serotype O157:H7, 1461t, 1462t, 1466-1467
hepatitis A, 2625
in HIV/AIDS, 1482-1484, 1482t, 1483b, 1485t, 2084
in salmonellosis, 1461-1463, 1461t, 1462t, 2625
in shigellosis, 1461t, 1462t, 1464-1465, 2625
Isospora belli, 1476-1478, 1477t
nausea and vomiting in, 204t
pediatric, 2623-2634
clinical features of, 2626
complications of, 2626
dehydration in, 2629, 2629t
diagnosis of, 2626-2627
differential diagnosis in, 2627, 2627t
Gastroenteritis *(Continued)*
disposition in, 2628-2629, 2628b
epidemiology of, 2623-2624
etiology of, 2624-2626, 2628t
fluid and electrolyte management in, 2629-2634, 2630t, 2632b-2634b
management of, 2628, 2628t
pathophysiology of, 2624
Plesiomonas shigelloides, 1461t, 1462t, 1466
protozoal, 1476-1482, 1477t
rotavirus, 1475-1476, 2624-2625
scombroid, 1470t, 1472-1473
staphylococcal, 1469-1470, 1480t, 2626
Vibrio, 1470t, 1471-1472, 2626
Vibrio parahaemolyticus, 1461t, 1462t, 1465-1466
viral, acute, 1475-1476, 2624-2625
Yersinia enterocolitica, 1461t, 1462t, 1465, 2625
Gastroesophageal reflux, 1388-1390
causes of, 1388, 1388b
clinical features of, 1388-1389
complications of, 1389
diagnosis of, 1389
hypertrophic pyloric stenosis vs., 2605
in apparent life-threatening event, 2718
in asthma, 1083-1084
in developmentally disabled patient, 2903
in infants and children, 2609-2610
in sudden infant death syndrome, 2715
management of, 1389-1390, 1390t
Gastrointestinal anthrax, 3026
Gastrointestinal barotrauma, in scuba diving–related disorders, 2286
Gastrointestinal bleeding, 220-227
alcohol consumption and, 2867
ancillary studies in, 222-223
diagnostic approach to, 220-223, 221b
differential diagnosis in, 220, 221b, 223
disposition in, 225-227, 225b, 226t
epidemiology of, 229
history in, 221
in abdominal stab wound, 504
in acute renal failure, 1540
in *Bacillus anthracis* gastroenteritis, 1469
in burn-injured patient, 924
in cirrhosis, 1411
in hemodialysis patient, 1550
in iron overdose, 2419
management of, 223-225, 223f
observation in, 3066
pediatric, differential considerations in, 220, 221b, 2613-2614, 2614t
physical examination in, 222
rapid assessment and stabilization in, 220-221
risk stratification in, 225-226, 225b, 226t
Gastrointestinal disorders, 1382-1423. *See also specific disorders, e.g.,* Appendicitis.
alcohol consumption and, 2867
diarrhea in, 231b
hypomagnesemia in, 1948
in acute mountain sickness, 2301
in arsenic poisoning, 2423
in chloral hydrate poisoning, 2487
in chronic renal failure, 1542
in developmentally disabled patient, 2903
in HIV/AIDS, 2082-2084
in hyperthyroidism, 1987
in multiple sclerosis, 1672
in opioid overdose, 2453
in parasitic infection, 2112-2114
in sepsis, 2214
in spinal injuries, 438
in systemic lupus erythematosus, 1808
in thermal burns, 918
in tuberculosis, 2161-2162
pelvic pain in, 249b
upper, pharmacological agents for, 1398-1399
Gastrointestinal foreign bodies, 870-877, 2616-2617, 2617f
Gastrointestinal system
in acute radiation syndrome, 2322
in pregnancy, 317, 2726
Gastrointestinal vasculitis, in systemic lupus erythematosus, 1808
Gastropathy, 1390-1391
Gastrostomy tube, in developmentally disabled patient, 2900-2901
Gatifloxacin
for tuberculosis, 2164t, 2165
for urinary tract infection, 1582
"Gay bowel syndrome," 1518
Gaze deviations, in comatose patient, 160-161
Gelatin sponge, for epistaxis, 1074
Gene activation, in cerebral ischemia, 66
General anesthesia, 1093, 2938, 2939b
Generalized anxiety disorders, asthma and, 1082
Genetic factors
in asthma, 1082-1083
in violent behavior, 2957
Genetic factors in mood disorders, 1736
Genital discharge, in sexually transmitted diseases, 1564-1571
Genital herpes, 1557-1559, 1557t, 1558f, 1559t, 1858
Genital ulcers, 1557-1564
in Bartholin cyst and abscess, 1559-1560
in chancroid, 1557t, 1559t, 1562-1563, 1562f
in condylomata acuminata, 1559t, 1563-1564, 1564
in granuloma inguinale, 1559t, 1563
in herpes simplex virus infection, 1557-1559, 1557t, 1558f, 1559t, 1858
in lymphogranuloma venereum, 1557t, 1559t, 1562
in syphilis, 1557t, 1559-1562, 1559t, 1560f, 1561f
Genital warts, 1518t, 1519-1520, 1563-1564, 1564f, 2045
Genitalia
examination of
in genitourinary trauma, 515
in sexual assault, 986-988, 987f, 987t, 988t
male, anatomy of, 516f
Genitourinary disorders, 1524-1604. *See also specific disorders, e.g.,* Renal failure.
foreign body and, 877-878
in infants and children, 2635-2655
in opioid overdose, 2453
in spinal injuries, 438
in tuberculosis, 2159
Genitourinary infection. *See also* Sexually transmitted disease.
in pregnancy, 2757-2759
Genitourinary trauma, 514-535
bladder injuries in, 519-526, 521f-526f
clinical features of, 515
Foley catheter placement in, 515, 517, 518f
in sexual assault, 986-988, 987f, 987t, 988t
penile injuries in, 532-534, 532f-534f
renal injuries in, 526-530, 527f, 529f-530f
staining techniques in, 988-989, 988f
testicular injuries in, 534-535, 535f
ureteral injuries in, 530-531, 531f-532f
urethral injuries in, 515-519, 516f-520f
Gentamicin
during pregnancy and lactation, 2784
for catheter-related infections, 1363
for febrile, neutropenic cancer patient, 2838t
for pediatric fever, 2513
for pneumonia, 2558t
for tularemia, 2131
Geriatric patient. *See* Elderly person.
German measles. *See* Rubella.
Germander, adverse effects of, 2476t
Gerstmann-Strassler syndrome, 2058
Gestation(s)
anembryonic, 2740
multiple
incidence of, 2722
labor and delivery in, 2816
Gestational age, 2722-2723
fetal viability and, 323, 323t
fundal height and, 2800, 2802f
uterine size and, 323, 323f
Gestational diabetes mellitus, 1957, 2772
Gestational epilepsy, 1624
Gestational hypertension, 2749-2751, 2750b
Gestational sac, ultrasonography of, 2730, 2730f, 2731f
GHB (γ-Hydroxybutyrate)
overdose of, 2488-2490, 2488b
withdrawal from, 2490
Ghon focus, in tuberculosis, 2152, 2152f
Giant cell arteritis
headache in, 1638
ischemic stroke vs., 1611
pericarditis in, 1284

Giardia antigen test, in diarrhea, 233
Giardia infection
drug therapy for, 2101t
in gastroenteritis, 1477t, 1479-1480
Gila monster, 896, 898-899, 902
Ginger, adverse effects of, 2476t
Gingiva, 1027, 1027f
hyperplasia of, drug-induced, 1036
laceration of, 1040
lesions of, in leukemic states, 1036
resorption of, 1032-1033
spontaneous hemorrhage of, 1042
Gingival sulcus, 1027, 1027f
Gingivitis, 1032-1033, 1033f
Ginkgo
adverse effects of, 2476t
drug interactions with, 2478t
Ginseng
adverse effects of, 2476t
drug interactions with, 2478t
Glandular injuries, in neck trauma, 450
Glandular tularemia, 2131
Glans penis, 532, 532f
Glasgow Coma Scale
for adults, 157, 157t
for pediatric patient, 331t, 334
in head trauma, 356-357, 357t
Glatiramer acetate, for multiple sclerosis, 1673
Glaucoma, 1055-1056
acute, headache in, 1640
acute angle closure
headache in, 174t
red and painful eye in, 288, 289f, 295t
risk factors for, 171b
closed-angle, 1056, 1056f
low-tension, 1055
open-angle, 1055-1056
pharmacologic management of, 1063b, 1064
Glenohumeral joint
anatomy of, 672, 673f
anterior subluxation of, 690, 691f
dislocation of, 687-693, 688f-694f
anterior, 687-690, 688f-690f
inferior, 692-693, 692f-694f
posterior, 691-692, 691f, 692f
Glenohumeral ligaments, 672, 673f
Glenoid fossa
anatomy of, 672, 673f
fracture of, 680
Glenoid labrum, 672, 673f
Glenoid rim fracture, in glenohumeral joint dislocation, 688
GlideScope, 21f
Glipizide
during pregnancy and lactation, 2790
for new-onset hyperglycemia, 1973
Global massage, for central retinal artery occlusion, 1057
Globe. *See* Sclera.
Globin production, decreased, in thalassemia, 1872
Globus symptom, in neck masses, 1076
Glomerular filtrate, composition of, 1524
Glomerular filtration rate, 1524, 2725-2726
Glomerular proteinuria, 1531
Glomerulonephritis
acute renal failure in, 1534, 1534b
hypertension in, 1312
in Goodpasture syndrome, 1816
poststreptococcal, 2647-2648
Glossopharyngeal nerve, 1665t
Glucagon
for anaphylactic patient on beta blockers, 1831b, 1833
for beta blocker overdose, 2375
for calcium channel blocker overdose, 2378
for diabetic ketoacidosis, 1963
for esophageal obstruction, 1384
for food bolus impaction management, 872
for hypoglycemia, 1961
in glucose regulation, 1956-1957
Glucocorticoids. *See also* Corticosteroids.
excess of, hypertension in, 1313
replacement of, for adrenal insufficiency, 1998
Gluconeogenesis, 1956
Glucose
administration of
for alcohol intoxication, 2860
for alcohol withdrawal syndrome, 2861
Glucose *(Continued)*
for alcoholic ketoacidosis, 2873
for hyperkalemia, 1941
for Wernicke-Korsakoff syndrome, 2869
in coma, 157-158
in neonatal resuscitation, 123t, 124
in pediatric resuscitation, 100, 101t, 103
cerebrospinal fluid
in bacterial meningitis, 2661
in central nervous system infection, 1718
dipstick blood, in diabetes mellitus, 1960
disturbances of. *See* Hyperglycemia; Hypoglycemia.
impaired fasting, 1957
impaired tolerance, 1957
in pregnancy, 2771
metabolism of, in pregnancy, 2724
normal physiology of, 1955-1957
regulation of, 1956-1957
serum
in bacterial meningitis, 2662
in comatose patient, 157, 161
in diabetes mellitus, 1959
in diabetic ketoacidosis, 1964, 1964t
urine, in diabetes mellitus, 1959, 1959b
Glucose oxidase tests, in diabetes mellitus, 1959, 1959b
Glucose transporter (GLUT) proteins, 1958
Glucose-6-phosphate dehydrogenase deficiency, in hemolytic anemia, 1878-1879, 1879b
α-Glucosidase inhibitors, 1973
Glue, ocular trauma from, 1046
Glue sniffer's rash, 2430
Glutamate, in cerebral ischemia, 65
Glutamate antagonists, after cerebral ischemia, 71
Glutamine, in hepatic encephalopathy, 1411
Gluteus muscle strain, 761
Glyburide
during pregnancy and lactation, 2790
for new-onset hyperglycemia, 1973
Glycemic control, 1973
Glycogenolysis, 1956
Glycoprotein IIb/IIIa receptor inhibitors
in acute coronary syndromes, 1186
in myocardial infarction
with fibrinolytic therapy, 1194
with percutaneous coronary intervention, 1186, 1194
thrombocytopenia from, 1897
Glycosuria, in pregnancy, 2725-2726
Glyphosate poisoning, 2467-2468
Goal-directed therapy
for postresuscitation care, 87, 88f
for shock, 50-52, 51f
Goiter, toxic
diffuse, 1985-1986, 1987
in pregnancy, 2764t, 2772-2773
multinodular, 1986
uninodular, 1986
Goldenseal, adverse effects of, 2476t
Goldman protocol, for risk stratification in acute coronary ischemia, 3065
Gonococcal arthritis, 1787-1788, 2190-2191
Gonococcal dermatitis, 1566, 1843-1844, 1843f, 2191
Gonococcal pharyngitis, 1111, 1112, 1113
Gonorrhea, 1518t, 1519, 1559t, 1565-1567, 1565f
diagnosis of, 1566
disseminated, 1566
epididymitis in, 1595
in pregnancy, 2758-2759
septic arthritis in, 1784
treatment of, 1559t, 1566-1567
"Goodness of fit" measurement, 3055
Goodpasture syndrome, 1816
Gouty arthritis, 1785-1786
Graded exercise testing, in acute coronary syndromes, 1180-1181
Graft infection, after abdominal aortic aneurysm repair, 1339-1340
Grafting, vascular, for peripheral arteriovascular disease, 1349-1350
Graft-versus-host-disease, transfusion-associated, 60
Gram stain
in bacterial meningitis, 1718, 1718t, 2662
in cutaneous abscess, 2203-2204
in gonorrhea, 1566
Gram stain *(Continued)*
in meningococcal disease, 2022
in pneumococcal disease, 2018
in sepsis, 2217
in septic arthritis, 2189
in urinary tract infection, 1576
Gram-negative bacteria
in cellulitis, 2199
in febrile, neutropenic cancer patient, 2835
in sepsis, 2212
Gram-positive bacteria
in febrile, neutropenic cancer patient, 2835-2836
in sepsis, 2212
Grandiosity, in mania, 1739
Granular casts, in urinary sediment, 1526, 1526f
Granules, in hemostasis, 1892, 1893f
Granulocyte, 1886, 2834
Granulocyte colony-stimulating factor, recombinant, for febrile, neutropenic cancer patient, 2839
Granulocyte count, radiation dose and, 2321
Granulocytopenia, in febrile cancer patient, 1907-1909, 1908b
Granuloma inguinale, 1559t, 1563
Granulomatosis, allergic, 1816
Granulomatous disease
hypercalcemia in, 1945
oral manifestations of, 1035
Granulomatous vasculitis, 1814
Graupel, lightning and, 2267
Graves disease, 1985-1986, 1987, 2764t, 2772-2773
Gravidity, 2722
Gray (Gy), 2321
Grease, in high-pressure injection injuries to hand, 612
Greater trochanter fracture
intertrochanteric, 752-753, 752f
isolated, 753, 753f
pediatric, 767
subtrochanteric, 753-755, 754f
Greater tuberosity fracture, in glenohumeral joint dislocation, 688
Green tobacco sickness, 2374
Greenstick fracture, 554, 556f, 2690
distal radius, 637
midclavicular, 677, 678f
tibial shaft, 800
Grief response, 3149-3151, 3150b
complicated, 3150, 3150b
depression vs., 1740
in staff, 3150-3151
Griseofulvin, for tinea capitis, 1839
Groin pull, in hip trauma, 761-762
Groshong catheter, 1363-1364, 1365f
Ground substance, 914
Group A beta-hemolytic streptococcus (GABHS) infection
in pharyngitis, 1109, 1110, 1111, 1112-1113, 1114
in pneumonia, 2557
Growing skull fracture, in head-injured child, 368
Growth disturbances, in proximal tibial epiphyseal injuries, 781
Growth factors, hematopoietic, for acute radiation syndrome, 2324
Growth hormone, in glucose regulation, 1957
Growth plates, in hip, 763, 763f
Grunting, in pediatric assessment, 2498
Guaiac test, 222
Guanabenz, 1321t
Guanfacine, 1321t
Guanidine hydrochloride, for botulism, 2016
Guar gum, drug interactions with, 2478t
Guidelines for emergency medicine, 3034-3044
clinical decision rules and, 3035-3036
clinical pathways and, 3038, 3039f-3041f
computer-based protocols for, 3042-3044, 3043f
decision making errors in using, 131t, 132
development of, 3035, 3036f
implementation and outcomes of, 3038, 3042
legal and ethical considerations in, 3044
medical screening examination and, 3161
on emergency seclusion and restraint, 2961
sources and adoption of, 3036-3038, 3037t

Guillain-Barré syndrome
neuropathy in, 1690-1691
sensory ataxia in, 2682
weakness in, 138, 140, 141
Guilt, in grief response, 3150
Guinea worm skin disorders, 2100t, 2108-2109
Gums, in pregnancy, 2726
Gunshot residue test, 960
Gunshot wounds. *See also* Firearm injuries.
abdominal
diagnostic studies in, 505
history in, 493
management of, 505-507, 506f
pathophysiology of, 490-491
physical examination in, 494
forensic aspects of, 953-960, 954f-960f
mechanism of injury of, 302, 303t
nonpenetrating ballistic injury from, 458-459
observation in, 3068
peripheral vascular, 537
to head, 368-370
to neck, 441
transcervical, 446
Gunstock deformity, after supracondylar fracture, 657-658
Gut suture, 852t
Gutter splint
in epiphyseal hand fracture, 600
in metacarpal or phalangeal fractures, 595, 596f
in metacarpal shaft fracture, 599
Guyon's canal, 586
Gynecologic injury
in intimate partner violence and abuse, 997
in pelvic fracture, 720
Gynecologic problems, in pregnancy, 2752, 2753t
Gyromitrin, in mushrooms, 2479

HACEK group, in infective endocarditis, 1301
Haddon's strategies, for injury prevention and control, 943, 943t, 944t
Haemophilus ducreyi, in chancroid, 1562, 1563
Haemophilus influenzae
in bacteremia, 2506
in bone or joint infections, 2177, 2178t
in epiglottitis, 1115, 1116
in meningitis, 1723
in pneumonia, 1129, 1132, 2557
vaccine for, 1723
Hair follicle, 915
Hair perm relaxers, caustic injuries from, 2381
Hair removal, in wound care, 847
Hairpin splint, in distal phalanx fracture, 593, 593f
Hairy leukoplakia, in HIV/AIDS, 2083
Halazepam, 2484t
Hallucination
from ketamine, 2946-2947
in delirium, 1649
in depression, 1737
in schizophrenia, 1727
Hallucinogen intoxication, 2406-2416. *See also specific drugs.*
dissociative agents in, 2413-2426, 2414t, 2415t
entactogens in, 2408-2411, 2409f
marijuana and miscellaneous plants and fungi in, 2411-2413, 2412f
mushrooms in, 2478-2479
serotonin-like agents in, 2406-2408, 2407f
Hallux
fracture of, 834
interphalangeal dislocation of, 836
pain in, 837
Halogenated hydrocarbons, 2428, 2429t
Haloperidol, 3116t
for agitation in delirious patient, 1654
for agitation in demented patient, 1662
for alcohol withdrawal syndrome, 2862, 2863
for mood disorders, 1711
for PCP intoxication, 2416, 2892
for rapid tranquilization, 2961-2962
for thought disorders, 1730
hepatotoxicity of, 1414
injectable, for psychotic relapse, 1732
side effects of, 2961-2962
with lorazepam, for rapid tranquilization, 2963
Halothane, hepatotoxicity of, 1414
Hamate
anatomy of, 622, 623f
fracture of, 629
Hamman crunch
in esophageal perforation, 484
in subcutaneous emphysema, 459
Hamman's sign
in esophageal perforation, 1385
in pneumopericardium, 1200
Hammer fracture, 814
Hamstring injury, 761
Hand, 576-619
bites of
antibiotic prophylaxis for, 854-855
human, 611, 890-892, 891t, 892b
infection risks in, 885
examination of, 590, 590b
foreign body in, 618-619
ganglion in, 618
motions of, 576, 577f-578
nontraumatic injury to, 618
stenosing tenosynovitis in, 618
structural framework of, 576-589
blood supply and, 585-586, 587f, 588f
fingertip and, 589, 589f
muscle and tendon function and, 578, 580-585, 581f-585f
nail and, 589
nerve supply and, 586, 587, 588f, 589f
skeleton and, 577-578, 579f-580f
skin cover and, 576-577
synovial spaces and, 585, 586f
surface anatomy of, 576, 577f
Hand symptoms
in Kawasaki disease, 2026
in pregnancy, 2733
Hand trauma, 592-618
amputations and ring avulsion injuries in, 612-613, 613b
clenched-fist injuries in, 611
clinical features of, 589-590, 590b
compartment syndrome in, 614, 614f
diagnostic strategies in, 590-591, 591f, 592f
dislocations and ligamentous injuries in, 600-604, 601f-603f
epidemiology of, 576
fingertip injuries in, 609-611, 610f
fracture in
distal phalanx, 593-594, 593f
mechanism of injury in, 592-593, 592f
metacarpal, 595-600, 597f-599f
pediatric, 600
proximal and middle phalangeal, 594-595, 594f-596f
terminology in, 592-593, 592f
high-pressure injection injuries in, 611-612
infection in, 614-618, 615f-617f
mutilating injuries in, 609
nerve injuries in, 614
radiologic evaluation of, 590-591, 591f, 592f
soft tissue injuries in, 600
tendon injuries in, 604-609, 605f-607f
vascular injuries in, 613-614
Handguns
forensic aspects of, 954-955, 954f
wounds inflicted by, forensic evaluation of, 955-960, 955f-960f
youth violence and, 1018-1019
Hand-held metal detector, in esophageal foreign body, 872
Hanging and near-hanging, 450-451
Hanging cast technique, in humeral shaft fracture, 654-655, 654f
Hanging weight method, for reduction of anterior glenohumeral joint dislocation, 689, 689f
Hangman's fracture, 410, 411f, 421, 550t
Hank's solution, 1038-1039, 1039f
Hantaviruses, 1131, 2055
Haptoglobin, in hemolytic anemia, 1877-1878
Hare traction splint, 569-570, 570f, 746, 748
Haversian canals, 2175, 2175f
Hawkin's sign, in rotator cuff tendinopathy, 1707
Hazard Communication Standard (HazCom), 3001
Hazardous materials
disaster preparedness and, 3012, 3017
tactical emergency medical support and, 3004
HAZMAT response, in chemical injuries, 930-931
Head and neck. *See also* Ophthalmologic conditions; Oral medicine; Otolaryngologic conditions.
cancer of
central nervous system infections in, 1920
hypercalcemia in, 1914
examination of
in fever, 135
in head trauma, 357-358, 358b
in sexual assault victim, 986
in vertigo, 144-145
fascial planes of, 1027, 1030f, 1116
in electrical and lightning injuries, 2272
lymph nodes in, 1075, 1075f
space infections of, 1027, 1028-1029, 1030f, 1032, 1116-1117, 1116f
parapharyngeal, 1121-1123, 1122f
peritonsillar, 1117-1118, 1118f
retropharyngeal, 1120-1121, 1120f, 1121f
submandibular, 1028, 1032, 1118-1119
Head bobbing, 2498
Head compression, 352
Head position, in comatose survivors of cardiac arrest, 70
Head tilt–chin lift maneuver, in pediatric resuscitation, 97
Head trauma, 349-379. *See also* Traumatic brain injury.
abdominal trauma and, 509-510, 511f
alcohol consumption and, 2878
anatomy and physiology in, 350-352
ataxia in, 2681
biomechanics of, 352
brain cellular damage and death in, 352-353, 353f
central nervous system infections after, 370-371
cerebral hemodynamics and, 350-352, 351f
complications after, 370-371
concussion in, 365-366
contusion in, 374
diffuse axonal injury in, 374
epidemiology of, 349
epidural hematoma and, 374-375, 375f, 376f
facial nerve paralysis from, 1667
facial trauma and, 386
headache following, 1640
hemophilia A and, 1902
history in, 356
in child abuse, 970-971
in elderly person, 346
inflicted, 349, 367
intracerebral hematoma and, 378, 378f
intracranial hematoma and, 371
management of, 358-366
medical complications in, 371
minor, 363-365, 364b
moderate, 362-363
neurologic complications in, 370-371
neurologic examination in, 356-357, 357t
observation in, 3069
pathophysiology of, 353-356, 355f
pediatric, 333-336, 334b, 335b, 366-368, 368b
penetrating, 368-370
physical examination in, 356-358, 358b
scalp wounds in, 371-372
seizure in, 370, 373, 1623, 2669
in children, 334, 367
prophylaxis against, 361, 361b
severe, 358-362, 359f
skull fractures in, 372-374
subdural hematoma and, 375-377, 376f
subdural hygroma and, 377
traumatic intracerebellar hematoma and, 378
traumatic subarachnoid hemorrhage and, 377
vertigo in, 144, 147t, 2684
Headache, 169-175, 1631-1643
acute, 2677
after moderate head trauma, 363
ancillary studies in, 172, 173t
cervicogenic, 1642
chronic-progressive, 2677-2678
classification of, 1631, 1632b
cluster, 1634-1635, 2679
coital, 1641
cough, 1642
differential considerations in, 170, 170t, 171b, 173-175, 174t
disposition in, 175

Headache (Continued)
epidemiology of, 169
exertional, 1642
history in, 170-172, 170t
hypertensive, 1641
in acute glaucoma, 1640
in acute mountain sickness, 2300, 2301
in bacterial meningitis, 2659
in brain tumor, 1637-1638, 2678
in carotid and vertebral artery dissection, 1638-1639, 1639f
in central nervous system infection, 1714
in cerebral venous thrombosis, 1670
in giant cell arteritis, 1638
in high-altitude illness, 1642
in idiopathic intracranial hypertension, 1639-1640
in intracerebral hemorrhage, 1610
in intracranial infection, 1641
in pneumonia, 2556
in polycythemia, 1884
in Q fever, 2137
in Rocky Mountain spotted fever, 2134
in scombroid fish poisoning, 1472
in spinal cord injury, 2906
in subarachnoid hemorrhage, 1635-1637, 1636t, 1637f, 2677
in trigeminal neuralgia, 1642
in *Vibrio parahaemolyticus* gastroenteritis, 1466
isolated benign, guidelines for management of, 3038
management of, 175
medication-induced, 1642
migraine. *See* Migraine.
orofacial pain in, 1034
pathophysiology of, 169
pediatric, 2676-2681
clinical features of, 2676-2677, 2677b
diagnosis of, 2679, 2680b
differential considerations in, 2677b
management of, 2680-2681
pathophysiology of, 2676
physical examination in, 172, 172t
postdural puncture, 1641
postpartum, 2732
posttraumatic, 1640
primary, 1631-1635
rapid assessment and stabilization in, 170
secondary, 1635-1642
tension, 1635, 2679
Healing
fracture, 564, 781
wound, 842-843
Health beliefs/values, racial/ethnic differences in, culturally competent approach to, 3113-3114
Health care
culturally competent, 3111-3116. *See also* Cultural competence.
information in, uses of, 3097-3099
Internet in, 3104
racial/ethnic differences in access to, 3108-3111, 3109t
Health care workers
hepatitis B exposure protocol for, 1406, 1408f, 3083-3084, 3084t
HIV exposure protocol for, 2091-2092, 3083, 3084-3087, 3085t, 3086b
Health insurance status, medical screening examination and, 3162
Health Level 7, 3104
Health promotion
for emergency physician, 3176-3178, 3176b, 3177b
in pregnancy, 2735-2737
Hearing impaired patient, 2904-2905
Hearing loss
acute, as indication for lumbar puncture, 2660
in otitis media, 1067
sensorineural, in acoustic neuroma, 1668
sudden, 1072, 1073b
vertigo and, 144, 2684b, 2684f
Heart. *See* Cardiac; Cardiovascular; Coronary.
Heart disease. *See* Cardiovascular disorders; Coronary artery disease; Valvular heart disease.
Heart failure, 1258-1278
acute, 1266
acute pulmonary edema in, 1261-1262, 1270-1274. *See also* Pulmonary edema, acute
Heart failure (Continued)
alcohol consumption and, 2866
cellular mechanisms of, 1259-1261, 1260f, 1261f
chronic, 1266, 1274-1277, 1275t
classification of, 1266-1267, 1267b
clinical evaluation of, 1267-1270, 1268b
compensatory mechanisms in, 1262-1263
constrictive pericarditis vs., 1288
definition of, 1258
diagnostic testing in, 1269-1270
drug-induced, 1269
epidemiology of, 1259
forward vs. backward, 1267
high-output vs. low-output, 1266
history in, 1269
in aortic regurgitation, 1307
in cardiomyopathy, 1264
in coronary artery disease, 1263-1264
in dilated cardiomyopathy, 1293
in Kawasaki disease, 2026
in myocarditis, 1264-1265, 1268
in pericardial disease, 1265
in pulmonary disease, 1265-1266
in valvular heart disease, 1265, 1268
myocardial hypertrophy in, 1262
myocardial pathophysiology in, 1263
neurohormonal alterations in, 1262-1263
observation in, 3071, 3071b
palliative care in, 3154
pediatric, 2582-2584, 2583t
physical examination, 1269
pleural effusion in, 1149
precipitating causes of, 1267-1269, 1268b
prerenal azotemia in, 1532-1533
rapid-onset, 1270
right-sided vs. left-sided, 1266-1267
stroke volume in, 1260, 1260f, 1262
systemic vascular resistance in, 1262
systolic vs. diastolic dysfunction in, 1267
thyrocardiac, 1987
transfusion-related, 60
treatment of, 1270-1277, 1270t
vs. chronic obstructive pulmonary disease, 1101, 1102
without pulmonary congestion, 1274
Heart murmur
in aortic regurgitation, 1307
in aortic rupture, 478
in aortic stenosis, 1306
in arteriovenous fistulas, 1347
in chronic obstructive pulmonary disease, 1100
in hypertrophic cardiomyopathy, 1295
in infective endocarditis, 1301
in mitral regurgitation, 1306
in mitral stenosis, 1305
in mitral valve prolapse, 1305
in myocardial rupture, 471
in tetralogy of Fallot, 2580
in tricuspid stenosis and regurgitation, 1307
innocent (functional), 2572
pediatric, 2571-2572, 2572b
Heart rate
fetal, antenatal assessment of, 2800-2802, 2803f
fever and, 135
in heart failure, 1261
in pregnancy, 2727
pediatric, 2495, 2495t, 2571, 2571t
Heart rhythm, disorders of. *See* Dysrhythmia.
Heart sounds
fetal, 2727-2728
in aortic regurgitation, 1307
in chronic obstructive pulmonary disease, 1100
in hypertrophic cardiomyopathy, 1295
in mitral stenosis, 1305
in pacemaker malfunction, 1254
in pneumopericardium, 1288
pediatric, 2571
Heart transplant, 2851-2854, 2852f, 2853f
Heartburn
in gastroesophageal reflux, 1388
in pregnancy, 2726
Heat capacity of material, burn injury and, 915
Heat cramps, 2258, 2258b
Heat edema, 2258-2259
Heat exhaustion, 2259-2260, 2259t
heatstroke vs., 2261
pediatric fever in, 2510
Heat illness. *See also* Hyperthermia.
fever vs., 2258
minor, 2258-2259
pathophysiology of, 2256-2258
predisposing factors in, 2256-2258, 2256f
rhabdomyolysis in, 1978-1979
Heat intolerance, in hyperthyroidism, 1986
Heat loss
increased, hypothermia and, 2240, 2240b
mechanisms of, 2236, 2255
minimization of, in burn care, 921
Heat production
decreased, hypothermia and, 2239-2240, 2240b
increased, heat illness and, 2257
physiology of, 2254-2255
Heat rash, 2259
Heat regulation, 2255-2256
Heat stress
acclimatization to, 2255-2256
physiology of, 2254-2256
Heat syncope, 2259
Heat transfer
burn injury and, 916
mechanisms of, 916, 917t, 2254-2255
Heat transfer coefficient, 916, 917t
Heated irrigation, for rewarming, 2250
Heatstroke, 2260-2265
classic, 2261-2262
clinical features of, 2261-2263, 2261b, 2261t
diagnostic strategies in, 2263, 2263b
exertional, 2256, 2262
Heatstroke, hyperthyroidism vs., 1988
management of, 2263-2265, 2264b, 2265f
pediatric fever in, 2510
physiology of, 2260-2261
Heavy metal poisoning, 2418-2426
arsenic in, 2423-2424, 2424b
iron in, 2418-2421, 2419t, 2420f, 2420t
lead in, 2421-2423, 2422t
mercury in, 2424-2426, 2425b, 2425t
Heel pain
in Sever's disease, 2710
subcalcaneal, 836-837
HEENT (head, eyes, ears, nose, and throat findings)
in headache, 172t
in nausea and vomiting, 202t
Hegar's sign, 2728, 2728f
Heimlich device, 1147
Heimlich maneuver, for foreign body removal, 2530
Helicobacter pylori infection
in gastritis, 1390, 1391
in peptic ulcer disease, 1392, 1394, 1394b
Helicopters for medical transport, 2995-2996, 2996f
in severe head trauma, 358
in trauma, 2998
landing zone safety issues of, 2997, 2997b, 2997f, 2998b
Heliox
for asthma, 2542
for chronic obstructive pulmonary disease, 1106
for critically ill asthmatic patient, 1091-1092
Heliox diving, 2280
Helium intoxication, solvent abuse vs., 2888
HELLP syndrome, in pregnancy, 245, 2749
Helmet use, in pregnancy, 2735-2736
HELPER mnemonic for shoulder dystocia, 2816b
Hemangioma, subglottic, 2525
Hemarthrosis
in anterior cruciate ligament injury, 790-791
in distal femur fracture, 777
in intercondylar eminence fracture, 779
in patellar dislocation, 786
in tibial plateau fracture, 777-778
Hematemesis, 221
Hematochezia, 221
Hematocrit
in abdominal trauma, 495
in acute pancreatitis, 1431
in gastrointestinal bleeding, 222
in hypothermia, 2243
normal values for, 1868t
pediatric, 2573
Hematologic disorders, 1878-1904. *See also specific disorders, e.g.,* Anemia.
alcohol-induced, 2873-2874, 2873t

Hematologic disorders *(Continued)*
in HIV/AIDS, 2087
in pregnancy, 2767-2768
in sepsis, 2214
in systemic lupus erythematosus, 1808
in thermal burns, 918
Hematologic studies
in abdominal trauma, 495
in hypothermia, 2248
in sepsis, 2216
Hematoma
epidural, 374-375, 375f, 376f
back pain in, 265t
in cancer patient, 1919-1920
in children, 335
spinal, 1683-1684
in fracture healing, 564
in peripheral vascular injury, 539
in tibial femoral knee dislocation, 788
intracerebral, 378, 378f
mediastinal, sternal fracture and, 456
orbital, 393
pelvic, 718
penile, 534
perirenal, 498f
retrobulbar, red and painful eye in, 288, 295t
retroperitoneal, pelvic fracture and, 500
subdural, 375-377, 376f
headache in, 2678
in children, 335
subungual
nail bed laceration and, 594
nail bed trauma and, 610-611
Hematoma block, in Colles' fracture, 633, 634f
Hematopoietic growth factors, for acute radiation syndrome, 2324
Hematopoietic response
in acute radiation syndrome, 2322
to high altitude, 2298
Hematopoietic system, development of, 1820f
Hematuria, 1528-1530, 1601-1604
causes of, 1529, 1529b, 1529t, 1601, 1601b, 1602b, 1603t
clinical features of, 1530, 1601-1602, 1602b
differential considerations in, 1603-1604
evaluation of, 1529-1530
exercise-induced, 1603-1604
imaging studies in, 1530, 1603
in bladder trauma, 520
in glomerulonephritis, 1534
in pelvic fracture, 719
in renal trauma, 528
in spinal cord injury, 310
in ureteral trauma, 530-531
in urologic trauma, 515
laboratory studies in, 1530, 1602-1603
pediatric, 2644-2645, 2645b
in Henoch-Schönlein purpura, 2615
in proteinuria, 2647
in renal stones, 2645
pseudohematuria and, 1604
Heme pigment, in urine, 1525
Hemiarthroplasty, for displaced femoral neck fracture, 751, 752b
Hemiparesis, in cerebral herniation, 355
Hemiplegic migraine, 1632, 2678-2679
Hemlock
poison, 2472, 2473f
water, 2472, 2472f
Hemodialysis
complications of, 1549-1552, 1550b, 1552b
for acute renal failure, 2650
for acute tumor lysis syndrome, 1912, 1912b
for barbiturate overdose, 2483
for beta blocker overdose, 2375
for bipyridyl compound poisoning, 2466
for chronic renal failure, 1547
for isopropyl alcohol poisoning, 2404
for rewarming in accidental hypothermia, 2250t, 2251
for salicylate overdose, 2342
for toxic alcohol poisoning, 2401-2403
vascular access for, problems related to, 1364-1366
Hemodynamics
cerebral, 350-352, 351f
during pregnancy, 316-317, 317t
of intubation, 16-17
Hemoglobin
as buffer, 1923
glycosylated, in diabetes mellitus, 1959
in carbon monoxide poisoning, 2438
in gastrointestinal bleeding, 222
in pregnancy, 2724, 2725f
intrinsic abnormality of, in sickle cell disease, 1879-1882
normal values for, 1866t
pediatric, 2573
Hemoglobinemia, march, 1883
Hemoglobinopathies, traumatic hyphema and, 1049
Hemoglobin-oxygen dissociation curve
altitude and, 2296, 2297f
in cyanosis, 268, 269f
shift of, during acclimatization to high altitude, 2298
Hemoglobin-oxygen transport, impaired, anemia from, 1866
Hemoglobinuria, paroxysmal nocturnal, 1879
Hemolysis
extravascular, 1877
in burn injury, 917
in hypophosphatemia, 1952
in prosthetic valve patient, 1308
intravascular, 1876-1877
Hemolytic anemia, 1868t, 1876-1884
abnormal sequestration in, 1884
ancillary evaluation of, 1877, 1877b
aplastic crisis in, 2046, 2046f
clinical features of, 1876-1877
differential diagnosis in, 1878-1884, 1879b
drug-induced, 1883, 1883b
environmental causes of, 1883-1884
extrinsic alloantibodies in, 1882
extrinsic autoantibodies in, 1882-1883, 1883b
extrinsic mechanical causes of, 1883
in alcoholism, 2874
intrinsic enzyme defects in, 1878-1879, 1879b
intrinsic hemoglobin abnormality in, 1879-1882. *See also* Sickle cell disease.
intrinsic membrane abnormality in, 1879
jaundice in, 246
laboratory studies in, 1877-1878, 1877b, 1877f, 1878f
microangiopathic, 1883
Hemolytic disorders
in alcoholism, 2874
jaundice in, 243, 244f
Hemolytic transfusion reaction
extravascular, 60
intravascular, 59-60
Hemolytic uremic syndrome
in hemorrhagic *Escherichia coli* serotype O157:H7 gastroenteritis, 1467
pediatric, 2654-2655
Hemoperfusion
in barbiturate overdose, 2483
in bipyridyl compound poisoning, 2466
Hemoperitoneum, 498, 498f, 499
diagnosis of, 507
iatrogenic, 492
Hemophilia A, 1900-1902, 1901t, 1902t
Hemophilia B, 1903
Hemopneumothorax, spontaneous, 1146
Hemoptysis, 279-283
diagnostic approach to, 280-281
differential diagnosis in, 281, 281t
disposition in, 282-283
epidemiology of, 279
in tuberculosis, 2149, 2151, 2162
management of, 282, 282f
massive, definition of, 279
pathophysiology of, 280
Hemorrhage. *See also* Bleeding.
adrenal, 1995, 1995b
cerebellar, vertigo in, 147t
fetomaternal, Kleihauer-Betke test for, 321
hypertensive, 1608-1609, 1608b
in abdominal trauma, 502
in aortic rupture, 479, 479f, 480, 480f
in arteriovenous malformations, 1609
in cardiac tamponade, 473
in fracture, 550, 550t
in hand trauma, 613-614
in hemodialysis patient, 1550
in multiple trauma, 308, 312, 313f
in myocardial rupture, 471
Hemorrhage *(Continued)*
in pediatric trauma, 330, 332t
in pelvic fracture, 718
evaluation of, 722-723, 722f
management of, 731-734, 731b, 733f
in penetrating cardiac trauma, 472
in peptic ulcer disease, 1393
in peripheral vascular injury, 539, 543
intracerebral
alcohol consumption and, 2869-2870
anatomy and physiology in, 1607
cerebral herniation in, 1918
clinical features of, 1610-1611, 1610t, 1611f
diagnosis of, 1613
differential diagnosis in, 1611-1612
disposition in, 1617
epidemiology of, 1608-1609, 1608b
in pertussis, 2006
management of, 1616
pathophysiology of, 1607
volume of, measurement of, 1611, 1611f
intracranial
dysrhythmia after, 371
hypertension in, 1316
oral, 1036, 1042
orbital, 1046
pelvic pain and, 250
postpartum, 258t, 2818-2820
pulmonary, in Goodpasture syndrome, 1816
retinal, 1050
high-altitude, 2306-2307, 2307f
in child abuse, 971
retrobulbar, 1046
spinal cord, magnetic resonance imaging in, 434, 434f
subarachnoid, 1635-1637, 1636t, 1637f
diagnosis of, 1636-1637, 1637f
dysrhythmia after, 371
headache in, 174t, 1637, 2677
Hunt and Hess scale for, 1636, 1636t
in pregnancy, 2732
risk factors for, 171b
spinal, 1682
traumatic, 377
treatment of, 1637
subconjunctival, 285, 296t, 1048, 1048f
vitreous, 1050, 1058-1059
Hemorrhagic fever viruses, 2055-2056
Hemorrhagic gastroenteritis, in *Escherichia coli* serotype O157:H7 infection, 1461t, 1462t, 1466-1467
Hemorrhagic shock
causes of, 44f, 45-46
definition of, 49, 49b
in subclavian artery injury, 545
treatment of, 52-53, 52b
Hemorrhoidal arteries, 1507
Hemorrhoids, 1509-1512, 1510t, 1511b, 1511t, 1512f, 2726
Hemosiderosis, transfusional, 61
Hemostasis
disorders of. *See* Bleeding disorders.
physiology of, 1892-1894, 1893b, 1893f
Hemothorax
in children, 339
traumatic, 464-465, 465b, 465f, 1152
Henderson-Hasselbalch equation, 1923
Hennebert fistula test, in middle ear barotrauma, 2282
Henoch-Schönlein purpura, 1815, 2615, 2615f, 2653-2654
Henry's law, 2280-2281
Heparin
during pregnancy and lactation, 2757, 2766, 2785, 2786
for arterial thrombosis, 1354
for cerebral venous thrombosis, 1671
for cervical vascular injury, 449
for deep venous thrombosis, 1370
for disseminated intravascular coagulation, 1904
for ischemic stroke, 1615-1616
for peripheral arteriovascular disease, 1349
for pulmonary embolism, 1377
in acute coronary syndromes, 1187
low-molecular-weight
advantages of, 1188
during pregnancy and lactation, 2757, 2786

Heparin *(Continued)*
for deep vein thrombosis, 3065-3066
in acute coronary syndromes, 1187-1188
thrombocytopenia from, 1897
Hepatic abscess, 1414-1417, 1415f, 1416f, 2113
amebic, 1415-1416
pyogenic, 1414-1415, 1415f
Hepatic artery aneurysm, 1355
Hepatic encephalopathy, 1411-1412
clinical stages of, 245t
grades of, 1411t
in cirrhosis, 1411
jaundice in, 246
Hepatitis
alcoholic, 1405, 1409, 2868
chronic, 1416
fulminant, 1404
halothane-induced, 1414
in developmentally disabled patient, 2903
in pregnancy, 2755, 2775
serologic markers in, 1405t
transmission of, in human bites, 891
viral, 1402-1406
clinical features of, 1404
diagnosis of, 1404-1405, 1405t
disposition in, 1405-1406
epidemiology of, 1402-1404, 1403f, 1403t
management of, 1405-1406
pathophysiology of, 1404
postexposure prophylaxis for, 1406, 1407t, 1408f
Hepatitis A, 1402, 1403f, 1405, 2035t, 2057, 2625
Hepatitis B, 1402-1403, 1403f, 1403t, 1405, 1406, 1407t
arthritis in, 1788
chronic, with hepatitis D infection, 1404
drugs for, 2036t
hepatocellular carcinoma and, 1417
in organ transplant patient, 2848
in pregnancy, 2775
occupational exposure protocol for, 1406, 1408f, 3083-3084, 3084t
prophylaxis against, after sexual assault, 990, 990b
vaccine for, 1406, 2035t
Hepatitis B immune globulin, for postexposure prophylaxis, 1406, 3083-3084, 3084t
Hepatitis B surface antigen, 1402-1403, 1403f, 1403t
Hepatitis B surface antigen status, postexposure prophylaxis and, 3083-3084, 3084t
Hepatitis C, 1403, 1405, 1406, 1408f, 2050
drugs for, 2036t
in kidney transplant patient, 2855
in organ transplant patient, 2848
in pregnancy, 2775
occupational exposure protocol for, 3083, 3084
Hepatitis D, 1404, 1405
Hepatitis E, 1403-1404, 2058
Hepatitis G, 1404
Hepatocellular carcinoma, 1417
Hepatomegaly, in hepatitis, 1404
Hepatorenal syndrome, in cirrhosis, 1411
Hepatosplenomegaly, in tricuspid stenosis and regurgitation, 1307
Herbal medicines, 2475-2477, 2476t
allergic reactions to, 2477, 2477t
contamination of, 2476-2477
drug interactions with, 2477, 2478t
misidentification of, 2475-2476
Hernia
diaphragmatic
neonatal resuscitation in, 121
traumatic, in children, 340, 341
hiatal, gastroesophageal reflux in, 1388
inguinal, 1598, 2641-2642
obturator, 1441
small bowel obstruction related to, 1441
Herniation
cerebral
after head trauma, 354-356, 355f
in cancer patient, 1918
disk
lumbar, 702-703, 704-705, 711-712
magnetic resonance imaging in, 432, 433f
radicular pain in, 264
impending, in multiple trauma, 308
Herniation syndromes, in children, 335 336
Heroin
during pregnancy, 2793-2794
emergency department visits related to, 2884f
pharmacology of, 2452
respiratory effects of, 2452-2453, 2453t
route of administration of, 2451-2452
toxicity of, 2452-2453
withdrawal from, 2452, 2455-2456
Herpes B virus, 2044-2045
Herpes simplex virus infection, 2040-2042
Bell's palsy and, 1667
corneal involvement in, 289, 290f, 295t, 1054, 1054f
drugs for, 2036t
genital, 1557-1559, 1557t, 1558f, 1559t, 1858
in cancer patient with impaired cell-mediated immunity, 2840
in encephalitis, 1712
in esophagitis, 1387
in HIV/AIDS, 2085
in organ transplant patient, 2848
in pharyngitis, 1110, 1112, 1114
in pregnancy, 2758
in sexually transmitted disease, 1518t, 1519
skin lesions in, 1857-1858, 1858f
Herpes zoster, 2042-2043
ophthalmic, 1054
skin lesions in, 1859-1860, 1860f
Herpes zoster oticus, 1071, 1667
Herpesvirus, 2034t, 2040-2045. *See also specific type, e.g.,* Herpes simplex virus infection.
Herpesvirus simiae, 884, 888-889, 889b, 889t, 2044-2045
Herpetic whitlow, 616
Heterotopic ossification
after tibial femoral knee dislocation, 790
of femur and hip, 741-742, 743f-754f
Heterotopic pregnancy, 2743
Hexachlorophene, for wound cleansing, 848t
Hiatal hernia, gastroesophageal reflux in, 1388
Hickman-Broviac catheter, problems related to, 1361-1363, 1362b, 1362f, 1365f
Hidradenitis suppurativa, 1515-1516, 1843, 2204-2205
High altitude
definition of, 2296
oxygenation at, 2307, 2307f
High-altitude cerebral edema (HACE), 2305-2306, 2305b
clinical presentation in, 2306, 2306f
epidemiology of, 2296
management of, 2306
pathophysiology of, 2299-2300, 2299f
High-altitude illness, 2296-2309. *See also* Acute mountain sickness (AMS).
acclimatization and, 2297-2298, 2297b, 2298f
and underlying medical conditions, 2307-2309
environmental considerations in, 2297
epidemiology of, 2296
headache in, 1642
pathophysiology of, 2298-2300, 2299f, 2300f
High-altitude pulmonary edema (HAPE), 2303-2305, 2303b
ancillary tests in, 2300f, 2303-2304
clinical presentation in, 2303
differential diagnosis in, 2304
disposition in, 2305
epidemiology of, 2296
management of, 2304-2305, 2305f
pathophysiology of, 2298-2299, 2299f, 2300f
prevention of, 2305
re-entry, 2303
High-altitude retinal hemorrhage, 2306-2307, 2307f
High-frequency flow interruption ventilation, in burn care, 922
High-frequency ventilation, 33
High-pressure injection injuries, to hand, 611-612
High-pressure irrigation, for wound cleansing, 848
High-velocity missiles
abdominal injuries from, 491
in youth violence, 1019
Hill-Sachs deformity, 688, 688f
reverse, 691, 692f
Hilum, 527, 527f
Hindfoot
anatomy of, 820, 820f
calcaneal fracture of, 826-827, 826f, 827f
Hindfoot *(Continued)*
pain in, 836-837
subtalar dislocation of, 825-826, 825f
talar dome of, osteochondral fracture of, 824-825, 825f
talar fracture of, 822-824, 823f, 824f
total talar dislocation of, 826
Hip
anatomy of, 736-738, 736f-738f, 737t
apophysitis of, 2711
calcifying lesions of, 741-742, 743f-755f
development of, 763, 763f
developmental dysplasia of, 2701-2702, 2702b, 2702f
examination of, in arthritis, 1779, 1779f
immobilization of, 569-570, 570f
neoplastic disease in, 742, 745f
normal radiograph of, 746, 747f
osteoarthritis of, 739, 739f-741f
Hip adductor strain, 761
Hip arthroplasty
partial, 751, 752b
total, 749-750, 750f
Hip dislocation, 756-759, 757f-759f
arterial injury in, 761
avascular necrosis after, 740
pediatric, 763
prosthetic, 749, 750f, 760
Hip pain
atraumatic, differential diagnosis of, 756b
pediatric, 2702-2709, 2703b
in acute septic arthritis, 2704-2706, 2705t, 2706t
in apophysitis of hip, 2711
in Legg-Calvé-Perthes disease, 2706-2707, 2707f
in slipped capital femoral epiphysis, 765-767, 765f, 766f, 2707-2709, 2708f
in transient synovitis, 2703-2704
limp from, 764-765
Hip prosthesis, dislocation of, 749, 750f, 760
Hip trauma, 735-768
anatomy in, 736-738, 736f-738f, 737t
clinical features of, 742-744
diagnostic strategies in, 746, 747f, 748f
epidemiology of, 735-736
femoral and hip fractures in, 746-756
arthroplasty for, 749-750, 750f
avulsion type, 750, 750f
compartment syndrome in, 749
femoral shaft, 755
greater or lesser trochanteric, 753, 753f
history in, 742-743
in elderly person, 347
intertrochanteric, 752-753, 752f
open fracture care in, 748-749, 749t
pain management in, 749
pathophysiology of, 739
physical examination in, 743-744
proximal femoral, 750-752, 750f-751f, 752b
stress type, 755-756
subtrochanteric, 753-755, 754f
traction and immobilization in, 746, 748
with minimal or no trauma, 755
femoral head fracture-dislocation in, 759-760, 760f
hip dislocation in, 756-759, 757f-759f
hip prosthesis dislocation in, 749, 750f, 760
management of, 740-750
muscular injuries in, 761-762
neurologic injuries in, 762-763
pathophysiology of, 739-742, 739f-745f
pediatric considerations in, 763-767, 763f, 765f-767f
radiologic evaluation in, 746, 747f, 751f
soft tissue injuries in, 761-763
vascular injuries in, 762
HIPAA (Healthcare Insurance Portability and Accountability Act), 3103
Hirschsprung's disease, 2612-2613
Hirudin, in myocardial infarction, 1188
His bundle, 1202
Histamine
in anaphylaxis/anaphylactoid reactions, 1823, 1823b, 2547, 2548
in asthma, 1080f, 1081
Histamine receptor antagonists, for anaphylactic shock, 54

Histamine$_1$-receptor blockers
anticholinergic toxicity of, 2346b
for anaphylaxis, 2549
overdose of, 2487-2488, 2488t
Histamine$_2$-receptor blockers
for acute pancreatitis, 1434
for anaphylaxis, 2549
for gastroesophageal reflux, 1389, 1390t
for upper gastrointestinal disorders, 1390t, 1398-1399
Histoplasma capsulatum
in cancer patient with impaired cell-mediated immunity, 2840
in pneumonia, 1130
Histoplasma infection, of pericardium, 1286
Histrionic personality disorder, 1755, 2979b
HIV virion, 2073
HIV/AIDS, 2056, 2071-2093
acalculous cholecystitis in, 1421
anorectal disorders in, 1520, 1520b, 2084
antibiotic prophylaxis in, 2089
antiretroviral therapy for, 2039, 2087-2089, 2087t
bone or joint infections in, 2179
cardiovascular disease in, 2086
case definition of, 2071, 2072b
central nervous system lymphoma in, 2082
cholangiopathy in, 1423
classification and staging of, 2075
complications of, 2076-2087, 2076t, 2078b, 2079t
Cryptococcus neoformans in, 2081
dementia in, 1658, 1659
diarrhea in, 1482-1484, 1482t, 1483b, 1485t, 2084
disposition in, 2089, 2090b
drug reactions in, 2079t, 2087
drugs for, 2036t-2037t, 2039
encephalopathy in, 2081
enteropathy in, 1482
epidemiology of, 2071-2073, 2072b, 2072f
esophageal disorders in, 2083-2084
ethical issues in, 2089-2090
gastrointestinal disorders in, 2082-2084
headache in, 1641
hematologic disorders in, 2087
historical background of, 2071
immunization in, 2089
in pregnancy, 2764t, 2774, 2810
initial evaluation in, 2075
intussusception in, 1441-1442
liver disorders in, 2084
Mycobacterium tuberculosis in, 1136, 1140-1141, 2078-2079
myelopathy in, 1683
myocarditis in, 1292
neurologic disorders in, 2079-2082, 2080f
neuropathy in, 1692, 2082
nonoccupational exposure protocol for, 2092
occupational exposure protocol for, 2091-2092, 3083, 3084-3087, 3085t, 3086b
ophthalmologic conditions in, 2085-2086
oropharyngeal disorders in, 2083
pancreatitis in, 1428
parasitic co-infections in, 2114
pediatric fever in, 2516
pericardial disease in, 1287
pneumonia in, 1135-1136, 1136f, 1138-1139, 1140-1141, 2077-2078
point-of-care testing for, 2074-2075, 2810
primary HIV infection in, 2075
progression of, predictors of, 2076
progressive multifocal leukoencephalopathy in, 2082
psychiatric considerations in, 2086-2087
pulmonary disease in, 2076-2079, 2076t
renal disorders in, 2086
rhabdomyolysis in, 1979
sexually transmitted disease in, 2087
skin disorders in, 2084-2085
skin lesions in, 1861f, 1862t
suicide in, 1770
systemic symptoms of, 2076, 2078b
tests for, 990, 2073-2075, 2810, 2087
Toxoplasma gondii infection in, 2081-2082, 2092t
transmission of, 2073
during labor and delivery, 2810
in human bites, 891
in sexual assault, 990, 990b
HIV/AIDS *(Continued)*
tuberculosis in, 1136, 1140-1141, 2078-2079, 2149, 2153-2154, 2166
tuberculosis meningitis in, 2082
with hepatitis C infection, 1403
HIV-associated nephropathy (HIVAN), 2086
Hives, 1834, 1834f, 1835
drug-induced, 1844-1845, 1844f, 1846t-1847t
skin lesions in, 1847-1848, 1848f
transfusion-related, 60
HMG CoA reductase inhibitors, rhabdomyolysis from, 1979
HMPAO scan, in osteomyelitis, 2181
Hoarseness
in airway foreign body aspiration, 866
in neck masses, 1076
in viral croup, 2525
Hodgkin's lymphoma, radiation-induced pericarditis in, 1284
Hohl's classification of tibial plateau fractures, 778f, 779
Holiday heart syndrome, 1230-1231
Holly plant, 2474
Homan's sign, in deep venous thrombosis, 1369
Home monitoring for apparent life-threatening event or SIDS, 2720
Homeland Security, 3018
Homicide
intimate partner, 995-996
youth, 1017, 1019
Honey, infant botulism from, 2013
Honeybee stings. *See* Hymenoptera stings.
Hookworm infection, 2101t, 2107
Hordeolum, 293t, 1054
Horizontal mattress suture, 850
half-buried, 851
Horner's syndrome, 416, 420, 1061-1062
Hornet stings. *See* Hymenoptera stings.
Horse serum–derived antivenin, 901
Horseshoe abscess, 1515
Hospice care, 3143, 3145
Hospital property, screening requirements related to, 3157-3158
Hospitalization
direct, medicolegal issues in, 3159
for alcohol-related problems, 2879-2880
for burn injury, 927, 927b
for chronic obstructive pulmonary disease, 1106t
for croup, 2527, 2527b
for hemophilia A, 1902
for nonemergent anemia, 1870b
for pelvic inflammatory disease, 1571
for pneumonia, 1138, 1140
for seizure, 2674
for suicide attempt, 1773
for systemic lupus erythematosus, 1811-1812
for tuberculosis, 2169
for urolithiasis, 1592-1593, 1593b
in disposition requirements, 3164
of febrile, neutropenic cancer patient, 2839
Hospitals
critical operational substrates for, 3012b
disaster response experience in, 3016-3017
disaster response plan for, 3015-3016
EMS programs based in, 2985
Host defenses, against pneumonia, 1128-1129
Hot tar burns, 926-927
Housemaid's knee, 795
Human bite, 890-892, 891t, 892b
antibiotic prophylaxis in, 891-892
antiviral prophylaxis in, 891
in child abuse, 969
in clenched-fist injuries, 611
in extensor tendon injuries, at metacarpophalangeal joint, 608
in sexual assault, 986b
infected, treatment of, 892, 892b
tetanus prophylaxis in, 891, 891t
to penis, 534
Human chorionic gonadotropin assays
in ectopic pregnancy, 2744, 2745
in pregnancy, 2738-2739, 2739f, 2741, 2741t
in vaginal bleeding, 256-257, 256t
Human granulocytic ehrlichiosis, 2137-2138
Human herpesvirus-3. *See* Herpes zoster; Varicella zoster virus.
Human herpesvirus-4. *See* Epstein-Barr virus.
Human herpesvirus-5. *See* Cytomegalovirus.
Human herpesvirus-6, 2044
Human herpesvirus-7, 2044
Human herpesvirus-8. *See* Kaposi's sarcoma.
Human immunodeficiency virus infection. *See* HIV/AIDS.
Human monocytic ehrlichiosis, 2137-2138
Human papillomavirus infection, 2034t, 2045
drugs for, 2037t
genital warts from, 1518t, 1519-1520
in condylomata acuminata, 1563-1564, 1564f
in HIV/AIDS, 2085
Human T-cell leukemia virus type 1, 2056
Hume fracture, 550t
Humeral head
anatomy of, 647
compression fracture of, 688, 688f
impaction fracture of, 691, 692f
manipulation of, in reduction of glenohumeral joint dislocation, 689, 689f
Humeral trauma, 647-668
anatomy in, 647-649, 647f, 648f, 672, 673f
biceps tendon rupture in, 668
clinical features of, 649-650, 649f, 650f
elbow dislocation in, 664-666, 664f, 665f
epicondylitis in, 667, 1798-1799, 2710-2711
fractures in, 652-664
articular surface, 661-664, 661f-663f
distal, 655-661, 656f-661f
proximal, 680-682, 681f, 682f
proximal epiphyseal, 682-683, 683f
shaft, 652-655, 653f, 654f
supracondylar, 2693-2697, 2694f-2696f, 2694t
management of, 652
olecranon bursitis in, 667, 1801-1803
radial head subluxation in, 666, 666f, 2697-2698, 2697f
radiography in, 641f, 650-652, 651f
soft tissue injuries in, 667-668
Humerus, immobilization of, 569
Humidity, evaporative heat loss and, 2255
Humoral immunity, 2832
defects in, in cancer patient, 2840-2841
Hunter serotonin toxicity criteria, 2359b
"Hunting response," 2228
Huntington's disease, 1747
Hutchinson's fracture, 636, 636f
Hutchinson's sign, in ophthalmic herpes zoster, 1054
Hyaline casts, in urinary sediment, 1526, 1526f
Hydatid cyst, 2102t, 2105-2106, 2106f, 2111, 2113
Hydatidiform mole, 2746-2747
Hydralazine, 1321t
during pregnancy and lactation, 2765t, 2788-2789
for hypertension of pregnancy, 1317
for hypertensive emergencies, 1318, 2653, 2765t
Hydrazine, overdose of, antidotes to, 2329t
Hydrocarbons
abuse of, 2886-2889, 2887t, 2888f, 2889b
chlorinated, poisoning from, 2462-2463, 2462b
dermal exposure to, 936-937, 2430, 2431
for tar removal, 927
poisoning from, 2428-2432, 2429t, 2430f, 2431f
Hydrocele
acute, 1598
in children, 2641
Hydrochlorothiazide, 1321t
during pregnancy and lactation, 2788
for hypertension, 1320
Hydrocodone, 2453t, 2920, 2921t, 2925
Hydrocortisone
for adrenal insufficiency, 1998
for anaphylactic shock, 54
for asthma, 1088
for diaper dermatitis, 1852
for hypercalcemia, 1940
for myxedema coma, 1994
for sepsis, 2222
for septic shock, 54
for thyroid storm, 1990
in hypothermia, 2246
Hydrofluoric acid
antidotes to, 2329t
dermal exposure to, 933-934, 2384
hypocalcemia from, 1943
ingestion of, 934, 2380, 2381t, 2383

Hydrogen peroxide
for acute necrotic ulcerative gingivitis, 1033
for wound cleansing, 848t
ingestion of, 2384
Hydrogen sulfide poisoning, antidotes to, 2329t
Hydroids, stinging, 909
Hydromorphone, 2453t, 2920, 2921t, 2923-2924
Hydronephrosis, in urolithiasis, 1589, 1589f, 1590f
Hydrophobia, in rabies, 2065
Hydrotherapy
in acid and alkali burns, 932, 933
whirlpool, for frostbite, 2234
Hydroxyamphetamine, in Horner's syndrome, 1062
Hydroxychloroquine, for systemic lupus erythematosus, 1809
Hydroxyurea, for sickle cell disease, 1881
Hydroxyzine, 2446t
adjuvant, with opioids, 2921
for urticaria, 1848
Hymenal trauma, in sexual assault, 987
Hymenolepsis nana, 2102t
Hymenoptera stings, 903-905
allergy to, 1827, 2547
rhabdomyolysis from, 1979
Hyoscyamine, anticholinergic toxicity of, 2345
Hyperabduction syndrome, thoracic outlet syndrome in, 1359
Hyperaldosteronism
hypokalemia in, 1938
in hypertension, 1311
metabolic alkalosis in, 1930
Hyperammonemia, in hepatic encephalopathy, 1411
Hyperamylasemia, in hypothermia, 2243
Hyperbaric oxygen therapy
for carbon monoxide poisoning, 2439-2440
for frostbite, 2233
for high-altitude cerebral edema, 2306
for high-altitude pulmonary edema, 2304, 2305f
for myonecrosis, 2209
for nitrite abuse, 2891
for peripheral arteriovascular disease, 1350
for scuba diving–related disorders, 2288-2292, 2288b, 2289f-2291f
for simultaneous carbon monoxide and cyanide poisoning, 2440-2441
Hyperbilirubinemia
in hepatitis, 1404
in pyogenic abscess, 1415
pediatric, 2601-2603, 2602t, 2603b, 2603t, 2604f-2605f
Hypercalcemia, 1944-1947
causes of, 1944-1945, 1944b
clinical features of, 1945-1946, 1945b
dialysis for, 1548
in adrenal insufficiency, 1997
in cancer patient, 1914-1916, 1915b
in hyperthyroidism, 1988
in hypothyroidism, 1993
in rhabdomyolysis, 1981
management of, 1946-1947, 1946b
nonneoplastic, 1914, 1914b, 1915, 1915f
Hypercapnia, permissive
for chronic obstructive pulmonary disease, 1104
for critically ill asthmatic patient, 1092
Hypercarbia, in scuba diving–related disorders, 2283
Hyperchloremia, in respiratory alkalosis, 1926
Hyperemesis gravidarum, 204t, 206, 2756
Hyperemia zone, in burn injury, 917, 917f
Hyperglycemia
after cerebral ischemia, 70
in alcoholism, 2871
in hyperthyroidism, 1988
in hypothermia, 2243
in pancreatitis, 1429-1430
in peritoneal dialysis patient, 1554
new-onset, 1973
seizure in, 1622
Hyperglycemic hyperosmolar nonketotic coma, in diabetes mellitus, 1968-1970, 1968b, 1969b
Hyperhidrosis, in frostbite, 2234
Hyperinfection syndrome, in organ transplant patient, 2849
Hyperkalemia, 1939-1941
cardiac arrest in, 77
causes of, 1939-1940, 1940b
dialysis for, 1548
from succinylcholine, 14, 14t
in acute renal failure, 1539, 2650
in acute tumor lysis syndrome, 1911
in adrenal insufficiency, 1997
in chronic renal failure, 1545-1546, 1545t
in crush injury, 3007
in digitalis toxicity, 2370
in familial periodic paralysis, 1709
in hemodialysis patient, 1551
in hemolytic uremic syndrome, 2655
in hypothermia, 2243
in rhabdomyolysis, 1981
management of, 1940-1941
Hyperlipidemia, in nephrotic syndrome, 1531, 2648
Hypermagnesemia, 1949-1950, 1949b
dialysis for, 1548-1549
in acute renal failure, 1539
Hypernatremia, 1935-1937
causes of, 1935-1936, 1936b
clinical features of, 1936
euvolemic, 1936
hypervolemic, 1936
hypovolemic, 1936, 2629t, 2632, 2634b
management of, 1936-1937
seizure in, 1622, 2669
Hyperoxia test of cardiac vs. pulmonary cyanosis, 2572
Hyperparathyroidism
hypercalcemia in, 1915, 1944
hypertension in, 1313
Hyperphosphatemia, 1952-1953, 1953b
hypocalcemia in, 1943
in acute renal failure, 1539
in acute tumor lysis syndrome, 1911
in hemolytic uremic syndrome, 2655
in rhabdomyolysis, 1981
Hyperpigmentation, mucocutaneous, in Addison's disease, 1997
Hyperpnea, 176
in tetralogy of Fallot, 2581
Hyperpyrexia, pediatric fever and, 2506
Hypersensitivity reactions. *See also* Anaphylaxis.
at insulin injection sites, 1971
cytotoxic, 1821
delayed, 1821-1822
immediate, 1821
immune complex, 1821
in tuberculosis, 2148
Hypersensitivity vasculitis, 1815-1817
Churg-Strauss syndrome as, 1816
erythema nodosum as, 1816-1817
Goodpasture syndrome as, 1816
Henoch-Schönlein purpura as, 1815, 2615, 2615f
mixed cryoglobulinemia as, 1815
panniculitis as, 1817
serum sickness as, 1815-1816
Hypersplenism, hemolytic anemia in, 1884
Hypertension, 1310-1322
altitude and, 2308
arterial disease in, 1312-1313
chronic, in pregnancy, 2762, 2763t, 2765t
definition of, 1310
determination of, 1310-1311
diastolic vs. systolic, 1310
essential, 1311
fibrinolytic therapy eligibility and, 1191
gestational, 2749-2751, 2750b
headache in, 1641
heart failure in, 1267-1268
in amphetamine abuse, 2895
in aortic dissection, 1317
in aortic rupture, 478
in chronic renal failure, 1316-1317
in glucocorticoid excess, 1313
in intracranial hemorrhage, 1316
in MAOI toxicity, 2365
in myocardial ischemia, 1316
in pheochromocytoma, 1313
in pregnancy, 1317, 2727, 2765t
in pulmonary edema, 1316
in sleep apnea, 1313
in spinal cord injury, 2906
in stroke syndromes, 1315-1316
Hypertension *(Continued)*
in systemic lupus erythematosus, 1807
in thyroid and parathyroid disease, 1313
intracranial
after head trauma, 353-354, 367
headache and, 174t, 2677-2678
idiopathic, 1639-1640, 1640b
in developmentally disabled patient, 2899
in high-altitude cerebral edema, 2306
in pediatric patient, 334, 334b
intubation and, 17, 18t
risk factors for, 171b
treatment of, 360, 367
lower extremity ulcers in, 1351
malignant, 1315
acute renal failure in, 1535
dialysis for, 1548
mild or transient, 1320, 1322
ocular, 1055
pathophysiology of, 1311-1314
pediatric, 2651-2653, 2651b, 2651t, 2652b, 2653t
pulmonary
altitude and, 2308
from high altitude exposure, 2298-2299
in pregnancy, 2762, 2766
renal disease in, 1311-1312
renin-angiotensin-aldosterone system in, 1311, 1312f
renovascular, 526-527, 1311
venous
from arteriovenous fistula or graft, 1366
in superior vena cava syndrome, 1910
Hypertensive emergencies
clinical presentation in, 1314-1317, 1314b
in cocaine overdose, 2388, 2390
in PCP intoxication, 2893
in pregnancy, 2762, 2763t, 2765t
management of, 1317-1319, 1317t
pediatric, 2652, 2653, 2653t
Hypertensive encephalopathy, 1314-1315
headache in, 1641
pediatric, 2650, 2652
seizure in, 1622
Hypertensive hemorrhage, 1608-1609, 1608b
Hypertensive urgency
clinical presentation and management of, 1319-1322, 1320t, 1321t-1322t
pediatric, 2651, 2652-2653
Hyperthermia. *See also* Heat illness.
after brain resuscitation, 68
delirium in, 1648
fever vs., 2258
in amphetamine abuse, 2894, 2896
in anticholinergic poisoning, 2348, 2349
in cocaine overdose, 2388, 2389-2390, 2390b
in cyclic antidepressant poisoning, 2354t, 2356
in PCP intoxication, 2414-2415, 2416, 2892
in psychostimulant overdose, 2408, 2410-2411
in substituted phenol poisoning, 2464
malignant, 14, 2257
succinylcholine-induced, 14
Hyperthyroidism, 1985-1989
anxiety in, 1747
apathetic, 1986, 1988, 1988t
clinical features of, 1986-1987, 1987b
diagnosis of, 1987-1988
differential considerations in, 1988, 1988t
etiology of, 1985-1986, 1986b
factitious, 1986
heart failure in, 1268
hypertension in, 1313
in pregnancy, 2764t, 2772-2773
in thyrotoxic periodic paralysis, 1709
management of, 1988, 1989, 1989t
skin lesions in, 1862t
Hypertonic saline
for elevated intracranial pressure, 360
for multiple trauma patient, 307
for seizure in acute renal failure, 2650
Hypertriglyceridemia
in alcoholism, 2871
in diabetic ketoacidosis, 1964
in pancreatitis, 1428
Hypertrophic cardiomyopathy, 1294-1296
heart failure in, 1264
sudden death in, 1298, 2597-2598
Hypertrophic pyloric stenosis, in infants and children, 2603-2606, 2605f, 2606t

Hyperuricemia
in acute renal failure, 1539-1540
in acute tumor lysis syndrome, 1911, 1912
in alcoholism, 2871
in cancer patient, 1913-1914
in rhabdomyolysis, 1981
Hyperventilation, 176
for cerebral herniation, 1918
for elevated intracranial pressure, 360, 367
for intracerebral hemorrhage, 1616
for scuba diving–related disorders, 2292
functional vs. organic, 1749
hypophosphatemia from, 1951
in chronic obstructive pulmonary disease, 1100
in cyclic antidepressant poisoning, 2356
Hyperventilation syndrome, 2668
Hyperventilation tetany, heat cramps vs., 2258
Hyperviscosity
cyanosis in, 273
in cancer patient, 1912-1913
in polycythemia, 1884
Hypervitaminosis A, fracture in, 2701
Hypervolemia
dyspnea in, 179t
hypernatremic, 1936
hyponatremic, 1934, 1935
in acute renal failure, 1540
in polycythemia, 1884
Hyphema
red and painful eye in, 290, 296t
traumatic, 1048-1049, 1048f
Hypnosis
for anxiety disorders, 1751
for pain management, 2934
Hypnotic, 2914b. *See also* Sedative hypnotics.
Hypoalbuminemia
in nephrotic syndrome, 2648
in rhabdomyolysis, 1981
pediatric, 2646
Hypobaria, in acute mountain sickness, 2300
Hypobaric hypoxia, 2297, 2298-2299, 2299f
Hypocalcemia, 1942-1944
alcohol-induced, 2871, 2872t
causes of, 1942-1943, 1942b
clinical features of, 1943, 1943b
in acute renal failure, 1539
in acute tumor lysis syndrome, 1911
in ethylene glycol poisoning, 2400
in hydrofluoric acid poisoning, 934
in pancreatitis, 1430
in rhabdomyolysis, 1976-1977, 1977f, 1981
management of, 1943-1944
seizure in, 1622, 2669
Hypocapnia, neurologic effects of, 351, 351f
Hypocarbia, ventilation-induced, 351, 351f
Hypochondriasis, 1755-1756
Hypogammaglobulinemia, in cancer patient, 2840-2841
Hypoglossal nerve, 1665t
Hypoglycemia
alcohol-induced, 2860, 2871
clinical features of, 1960-1961
confusion and, 150
diagnosis of, 1961
fasting, 1961-1962
hyperthyroidism vs., 1988
hypothermia and, 2239
in adrenal insufficiency, 1997, 1998
in alcoholic hepatitis, 1409
in chronic pancreatitis, 1435
in diabetes mellitus, 1960-1961, 1960b, 1961b
in hypothermia, 2243
in hypothyroidism, 1993, 1994
in neonates, 119
in nondiabetic patient, 1961-1962, 1962b
in opioid overdose, 2454
in overdosed/poisoned patient, 2326
in pregnancy, 1972
management of, 1961, 1961b
postprandial, 1961
seizure in, 166, 1622, 2669
unawareness of, 1960
vertigo in, 116t
Hypoglycemic agents, oral, 1972-1973
alcohol interactions with, 2877
overdose of, hypoglycemia from, 1961
rash from, 1972
Hypogonadism, male, in alcoholism, 2871
Hypokalemia, 1937-1939
alcohol-induced, 2871, 2872t
causes of, 1937-1938, 1938b
clinical features of, 1938-1939
hypomagnesemia in, 1947
in digitalis toxicity, 2370
in familial periodic paralysis, 1709
in hypercalcemic cancer patient, 1915-1916
in hypothermia, 2243
in respiratory alkalosis, 1926
management of, 1939
metabolic alkalosis in, 1930
rhabdomyolysis in, 1979
vomiting-induced, 201
Hypomagnesemia, 1947-1949
alcohol-induced, 2871, 2872t
causes of, 1947-1948, 1948b
clinical features of, 1948-1949
in digitalis toxicity, 2371
management of, 1949
seizure in, 1622, 2669
Hypomanic episode, 1738
Hyponatremia, 1933-1935
alcohol-induced, 2871, 2872t
causes of, 1933-1934, 1934b
clinical features of, 1934
diagnosis of, 1934
euvolemic, 1934, 1935
hypervolemic, 1934, 1935
hypovolemic, 1933-1934, 1935, 2629t, 2631-2632, 2633b
in adrenal insufficiency, 1997
in hypothyroidism, 1993, 1994
in nephrotic syndrome, 2648
management of, 1935
MDMA-induced, 2408
rhabdomyolysis in, 1979-1980
seizure in, 1622, 2669
Hyponychium, 589
Hypoparathyroidism
anxiety in, 1747
hypocalcemia in, 1942
seizure in, 1622
Hypophosphatemia, 1951-1952, 1951b, 1952b
alcohol-induced, 2871-2872, 2872t
rhabdomyolysis in, 1979
Hypotension
acute pulmonary edema with, 1273-1274
after brain resuscitation, 68
after head trauma, 353
fibrinolytic therapy eligibility and, 1191
from propofol, 2947
gastritis in, 1391
hypovolemic, 360, 367
in abdominal aortic aneurysm rupture, 1333
in adrenal insufficiency, 1997
in barbiturate overdose, 2482
in beta blocker overdose, 2374-2375
in cardiac tamponade, 473
in cyclic antidepressant poisoning, 2352, 2354-2356
in head trauma, 359-360, 370
in heatstroke, 2264, 2265f
in hemodialysis patient, 1550-1551, 1550b
in hip trauma, 743-744
in hypothyroidism, 1994
in isopropyl alcohol poisoning, 2403
in MAOI toxicity, 2365
in opioid overdose, 2453
in pregnancy, 316, 2725
in pulmonary embolism, 1372
in shock, 45
neurogenic, secondary to spinal shock, 437
orthostatic
from antipsychotic agents, 1732
in spinal cord injury, 2900
Hypotensive resuscitation, in peripheral vascular injury, 543
Hypotensive shock, in anaphylaxis, 2548
Hypothalamic-pituitary-adrenal axis
in mood disorders, 1735 1736
in sepsis, 2214
suppression of, adrenal insufficiency from, 1997-1998
Hypothalamus, in temperature regulation, 134
Hypothenar hammer syndrome, 1355
Hypothenar mass or eminence, 576, 577f
Hypothenar muscles, 580-581, 581f
Hypothermia
accidental, 2236-2252
advanced life support in, 2245-2246
cardiovascular agents for, 2246
clinical features of, 2241-2242, 2242b
diagnostic strategies in, 2242-2244
disposition in, 2251
dysrhythmia in, 2237-2238, 2246
laboratory evaluation of, 2242-2244, 2243f
management of, 2244-2251
outcome of, 2251
pathophysiology of, 2237-2239, 2238f, 2239t
predisposing factors in, 2239-2241, 2240b
rewarming techniques in, 2247-2251, 2247b, 2250b
septicemia following, 2247
volume resuscitation in, 2245
alcohol consumption and, 2874-2875
cardiac arrest from, 78
definition of, 2236
delirium in, 1648
in barbiturate overdose, 2482
in hypothyroidism, 1992, 1994
in neonates, 119
in opioid overdose, 2454
in submersion injuries, 2312, 2314
in urban search and rescue, 3008
oxygenation considerations during, 2249, 2249t
physiology of cold exposure and, 2236-2237, 2237f
resuscitative, 85-86
mild, 68-70, 69t
profound and selective, 70
rhabdomyolysis in, 1979
zones of, 2239t
Hypothermic coagulation, 2243-2244
Hypothesis testing, 3051-3058, 3051t, 3057f
Hypothetico-deductive process, clinical decision making by, 127, 127f, 131t, 132
Hypothyroidism, 1990-1994
causes of, 1990, 1990b
clinical features of, 1990-1992, 1991b, 1991t
congenital, 2773
diagnosis of, 1992-1993
differential considerations in, 1993
heart failure in, 1268
hypertension in, 1313
in lithium toxicity, 2443
in pregnancy, 2773
management of, 1993-1994
seizure in, 1622
skin lesions in, 1862t, 1863f
Hypotonic diuresis, in hyperglycemic hyperosmolar nonketotic coma, 1968
Hypoventilation
controlled
for chronic obstructive pulmonary disease, 1104
for critically ill asthmatic patient, 1092
in hypothyroidism, 1994
in pediatric cervical spine injury, 338
Hypovolemia. *See also* Dehydration.
differential diagnosis in, 2629, 2629t
from vomiting, 201
gastritis in, 1391
hypernatremic, 1936, 2629t, 2632, 2634b
hyponatremic, 1933-1934, 1935, 2629t, 2631-2632, 2633b
in acute renal failure, 1540, 2650
in adrenal insufficiency, 1997, 1998
in burn injury, 917
in chronic renal failure, 1543
in crush injury, 3007
in ectopic pregnancy, 2745
in gastrointestinal bleeding, 222-223
in hypercalcemia, 1945
in hyperglycemic hyperosmolar nonketotic coma, 1968
in septic shock, 46-47
isonatremic, 2629t, 2631, 2632b
Hypovolemic hypotension, in head trauma, 360, 367
Hypovolemic shock
in cardiac tamponade, 473
in diabetic ketoacidosis, 1966
mechanical ventilation in, 32
Hypoxemia
acute, differential diagnosis in, 1101-1103
confusion and, 150

Hypoxemia *(Continued)*
from high altitude exposure, 2298-2299, 2299f
in chronic obstructive pulmonary disease, 1100, 1104-1105
in pulmonary embolism, 1372
Hypoxia
after brain resuscitation, 68
after head trauma, 353
during air medical transport, 2994-2995
hypobaric, 2297, 2298-2299, 2299f
in cyanide poisoning, 2436
in neonates, 119
in simple asphyxiant inhalation, 2433
neurologic effects of, 351-352
rhabdomyolysis in, 1979
Hypoxic (tet) spells, in tetralogy of Fallot, 2580-2581, 2580f, 2581b
Hypoxic ventilatory response, during acclimatization to high altitude, 2297-2298
Hypsarrhythmia, infantile spasms with, 2665-2666
Hysterectomy, for postpartum hemorrhage, 2819
Hysterical conversion reactions, visual loss in, 1060-1061
Hysterical neurosis, conversion type, 1755, 1755b

Iatrogenic injury
abdominal trauma as, 492
esophageal perforation as, 482-483
peripheral vascular, 536-537
Ibotenic acid, 2479
Ibuprofen, 2927
for back pain, 710
for migraine, 2680
in frostbite, 2232
in HIV/AIDS, side effects of, 2079t
overdose of, 2343
Ibutilide, 1209-1210
for atrial fibrillation, 1232b, 1233
Ice packs
for dysrhythmias, 1214-1215
for heatstroke, 2264
for supraventricular tachycardia, 2588
Ice test, in myasthenia gravis, 1705-1706
Ice therapy. *See* Cryotherapy.
Ichthyosis, acquired, internal malignancy associated with, 1864
Icterus gravidarum, 2726
Idiojunctional escape rhythms, 1216, 1218
Ileocecitis, in *Yersinia enterocolitica* gastroenteritis, 1465
Ileocolic intussusception, 2611
Ileoileal intussusception, 2611
Ileus
adynamic, 1440, 1441b, 1443
gallstone, small bowel obstruction in, 1441
segmental, 1440
Ilex, 2474
Iliac artery and vein injury, 546
Iliac wing fracture, 724
Iliopsoas bursitis, 1803
Iliopsoas strain, 761
Iliotibial band syndrome, 793-794
Ilium, 717, 718f
Imidazole, for tinea versicolor, 1840
Imipenem, for febrile, neutropenic cancer patient, 2838t
Imipramine
for neuropathic pain, 1692
metabolism of, 2352
Imiquimod, for condylomata acuminata, 1564
Immersion burn, 916
in child abuse, 969-970, 970f, 970t
in physical assault, 963, 964f
Immersion foot, 2228, 2230-2231
Immersion syndrome, 2311-2312
Immersion therapy
for heatstroke, 2264
for rewarming, 2232, 2248
Immobilization
casts for, 571-573, 573f. *See also* Cast immobilization.
complications of, 563, 564b
in acromioclavicular joint dislocations, 686
in ankle sprain, 817
in anterior glenohumeral joint dislocation, 690
Immobilization *(Continued)*
in biceps tendon rupture, 697
in bicipital tenosynovitis, 697
in clavicle fracture, 677, 678f
in condylar fracture, 660-661
in epiphyseal hand fracture, 600
in extension supracondylar fracture, 655-656
in femoral and hip fractures, 746, 748
in flexion supracondylar fracture, 659
in humeral shaft fracture, 654-655, 654f
in knee extensor tendon injuries, 783
in knee ligament injuries, 792
in mallet finger, 606, 606f
in metacarpal or phalangeal fracture, 595, 595f, 596f
in metatarsal base fracture, 833
in olecranon fracture, 663
in Osgood-Schlatter disease, 799
in patellar dislocation, 786
in posterior elbow dislocation, 665
in proximal fibular fracture, 802
in proximal humeral epiphyseal fracture, 683
in proximal humeral fracture, 682
in proximal tibial epiphyseal injuries, 781
in proximal tibiofibular joint dislocation, 803
in rotator cuff tear, 696
in scapula fracture, 680
in snakebite management, 899
in sprain, 566
in sternoclavicular joint dislocation, 684
in tibial femoral knee dislocation, 789
in tibial shaft fracture, 800
in ulnar shaft fracture, 642
in wound management, 855
splinting and bandaging for, 568-571, 569f, 570f, 572f, 573f. *See also* Splint immobilization.
Immune complex hypersensitivity reactions, 1821
Immune complexes
in Henoch-Schönlein purpura, 1815
in vasculitis, 1812-1813
Immune complex–mediated agents, in anaphylaxis, 1827
Immune response
acute-phase, 2831-2832
adaptive, 2832-2834
in asthma, 1080-1081, 1080f
in bone or joint infection, 2176
in Kawasaki disease, 2025
in systemic lupus erythematosus, 1806, 1808
in tuberculosis, 2148
non–microbe-specific, 2831-2832
pneumonia and, 1129
reticuloendothelial system in, 2832
Immune system
characteristics of, 1821
development of, 1820-1821, 1820f
in elderly person, 2826
in pregnancy, 2724-2725
physical barriers in, 2831
disruption of, in cancer patient, 2841
suppression of. *See* Immunocompromised patient.
Immune thrombocytopenia, 1896-1897
Immune-mediated transfusion reactions, 59-60
Immunization. *See also* Vaccine.
during pregnancy, 2736
for viral infection, 2033-2034, 2035t
in bronchopulmonary dysplasia, 2565
in elderly person, 2829
in HIV/AIDS, 2089
Immunocompromised patient, 2831-2844, 2832t
adaptive immunity in, 2832-2834
alcoholism and, 2841-2842
antibiotic prophylaxis in, 854
cancer and, 2834-2841, 2836t, 2838t
delirium in, 1649
diabetes mellitus and, 2841
immunosuppressive therapy in, 2843-2844
infection in, 2834-2843, 2835t
non–microbe-specific immunity in, 2831-2832
organ transplantation and. *See* Organ transplant patient.
pneumonia in, 1132, 2560, 2841
renal failure and, 2842
respiratory tract infection in, 2841
reticuloendothelial system in, 2832
splenectomy and functional asplenia and, 2042-2043
Immunoglobulin(s)
anaphylactic-type reactions to, 1827
classes of, 1821, 2832
structure of, 1821, 1821f
Immunoglobulin A, 2832
Immunoglobulin E, 2832
in anaphylactic shock, 47
in anaphylaxis, 2547
in asthma, 1080, 1080f
Immunoglobulin E antibodies, 1819
Immunoglobulin E–mediated anaphylaxis
agents associated with, 1826-1827
signal transduction system in, 1822-1823, 1822f
Immunoglobulin G, 2832
Immunoglobulin M, 2832
Immunoglobulin preparations
for hepatitis B postexposure prophylaxis, 1406, 3083-3084, 3084t
for Kawasaki disease, 2027, 2596
for measles, 1849
for myasthenia gravis, 1707
for myocarditis, 1290
for rabies, 2068, 2068b
for tetanus, 856, 857t, 2011
for toxic shock syndrome, 2030-2031, 2201
for varicella, 1859
Rh (anti-D), in pregnancy, 2742, 2752
Immunomodulatory therapy, for myasthenia gravis, 1707
Immunopathology, 1819, 1821-1822
Immunoprophylaxis, for hepatitis, 1406, 1407t
Immunosenescence, 2826
Immunosuppressive therapy
agents used in, 2843-2844
for diabetes mellitus, 1973
for myasthenia gravis, 1706
for myocarditis, 1290
for organ transplant patient, 2849-2851, 2850t
for systemic lupus erythematosus, 1809
Impact seizure, 334
in children, 367
in head trauma, 2669
Impaction fracture, 553, 555f
Impairment, disability vs., 3078
Impalement, in facial trauma, 386, 387f
Impartiality Test, in ethical case analysis, 3131-3132
Impetigo, 1842-1843, 2201-2202
Impingement, nerve root, 702-703
Impingement syndrome of shoulder, 693-696, 694t, 695f, 1796-1797
Impingement test, 694, 695f
Implantable cardiac devices, 1246-1257. *See also* Pacemaker(s).
Implantable cardioverter-defibrillator, 1255-1257
advanced life support in patient with, 1256-1257
complications of, 1256
disposition in, 1257
for chronic heart failure, 1277
indications for, 1246-1247, 1247b
malfunction of, 1256, 1256b, 1257b
terminology and components in, 1255-1256
Implements in situ, in abdominal stab wound, 504, 505
Implied consent, of combative or violent patient, 2967, 3134
Impotence, pelvic fracture and, 719
Imprisonment, false, 2967
Impulses, grouped, causes of, 1219, 1219b
Inborn errors of metabolism, ataxia in, 2682
Incarceration, penile, 532, 533f
Incident command system, 3014
Incised wounds, in physical assault, 963
Incision and drainage
in paronychia, 615, 615f
in pericoronitis, 1035
of Bartholin cyst abscess, 2205, 2205f
of cutaneous abscess, 2204
of felon, 615, 616f
of periodontal abscess, 1031, 1033
of retropharyngeal abscess, 1121
Incontinence, fecal, 1516-1517, 1516b
Incorporation, radioactive, 2320
Indapamide, 1321t
India ink staining of cerebrospinal fluid, in central nervous system infection, 1718, 1719f

Indinavir, in HIV/AIDS, side effects of, 2079t
Indirect immunofluorescence assay (IFA)
  in babesiosis, 2140
  in ehrlichiosis, 2138
  in Rocky Mountain spotted fever, 2135
Indium-labeled bone scan, in osteomyelitis, 2181
Indomethacin, 2927
  during pregnancy and lactation, 2784
  for gouty arthritis, 1790
  for premature labor, 2807
  for reactive arthritis, 1790
Induction agents, 15-16, 2914b
Induration, 1839t
Infant. *See also* Neonate.
  abdominal pain in, differential considerations in, 2611, 2612t
  acute bacterial meningitis in, 2657-2665
    clinical features of, 2658-2659, 2658t
    diagnosis of, 2659-2663, 2660b, 2661f, 2661t
    differential considerations in, 2663, 2663b
    management of, 2663-2665, 2664t
    pathophysiology of, 2657-2658
  acute septic arthritis in, 2704-2706, 2705t, 2706t
  airway foreign body in, 869-870, 2530
  apnea in, 2714
  apparent life-threatening event in, 2718-2720, 2718b, 2719b
  atrial septal defect in, 2578
  automobile restraint seats for, 947, 948
  bacterial endocarditis in, 2590-2591, 2591b
  botulism in, 1707, 2013, 2015-2016
  burn injury in, 923
  cardiovascular disorders in, 2567-2599
    chest radiography in, 2573-2574, 2573f, 2574f
    circulatory changes related to, 2568-2569
    compensatory responses associated with, 2569, 2569b
    history in, 2570-2571, 2570b
    physical examination in, 2571-2575, 2571t, 2572b
  causes of death in, 942t, 949t
  chest pain in, 2570-2571
  choanal atresia in, 2522
  coarctation of the aorta in, 2578-2579
  congenital heart disease in, 2575-2582
    acyanotic, 2577-2579, 2577f
    chest radiography in, 2573-2574, 2574f
    clinical features of, 2575-2576, 2575t
    cyanotic, 2579-2581, 2579f, 2581b
    diagnosis of, 2576, 2576b
    ductal-dependent, 2576-2577, 2576b, 2577b
    incidence of, 2575, 2575t
    management of, 2576-2577, 2576b, 2577b
    postoperative complications of, 2581
    respiratory syncytial virus infection and, 2581-2582, 2582b
  cyanosis in
    central, cardiac vs. pulmonary, 2569, 2569b, 2572
    in tetralogy of Fallot, 2580
    pathophysiology of, 2569
  developmental milestones in, 2496-2497, 2496t
  diarrhea in, 2628b, 2628t
  dysrhythmias in, 2584-2590, 2584b, 2586b, 2587f-2589f
  Eisenmenger syndrome in, 2578
  electrocardiography in, 2574-2575, 2574t
  fever in
    management of, 2512-2514, 2513b
    pathophysiology of, 2505
  gastroesophageal reflux in, 2609-2610
  gastrointestinal bleeding in, differential considerations in, 220, 221b, 2613-2614, 2614t
  gastrointestinal disorders in, 2601-2621
  heart failure in, 2582-2584, 2583t
  hip dysplasia in, 2701-2702, 2702b, 2702f
  Hirschsprung's disease in, 2612-2613
  HIV/AIDS in, 2774
  hypertrophic pyloric stenosis in, 2603-2606, 2605f, 2606t
  hypomagnesemia in, 1948
  increased intracranial pressure in, 334, 334b
  infectious diarrhea in, 2623-2634
    clinical features of, 2626
    complications of, 2626
    dehydration in, 2629, 2629t

Infant *(Continued)*
    diagnosis of, 2626-2627
    differential diagnosis in, 2627, 2627t
    disposition in, 2628-2629, 2628b
    epidemiology of, 2623-2624
    etiology of, 2624-2626, 2628t
    fluid and electrolyte management in, 2629-2634, 2630t, 2632b-2634b
    management of, 2628, 2628t
    pathophysiology of, 2624
  intussusception in, 2509b, 2610-2612, 2611f, 2612t
  jaundice in, 2601-2603, 2602t, 2603b, 2603t, 2604f-2605f
  Kawasaki disease in, 2593-2596, 2594b, 2595f
  malrotation with midgut volvulus in, 2606-2608, 2607f, 2608f
  myocarditis in, 2591-2592
  necrotizing enterocolitis in, 2608-2609, 2609f
  neurologic disorders in, 2657-2686
  peptic ulcer disease in, 1392
  pericarditis in, 2592-2593, 2593f
  periodic breathing in, 2495
  pneumonia in, 1131
  red and painful eye in, 292
  renal and genitourinary disorders in, 2635-2655
  renal function in, 923
  stroke volume in, decreased, causes of, 2569, 2569b
  sudden death of. *See* Sudden infant death syndrome.
  temperature determination in, 2508
  tetralogy of Fallot in, 2579-2581, 2579f, 2580f, 2581b
  upper airway obstruction in, 2519-2530
    evaluation of, 2521, 2521f
    in congenital lesions, 2522, 2524-2525, 2524f, 2527-2528, 2528f
    in croup, 2525-2527, 2526f, 2527b
    in epiglottitis, 2523-2524, 2524f
    in foreign body aspiration, 2529-2530
    in laryngeal disease, 2524-2525, 2524f
    in retropharyngeal abscess, 2522-2523, 2523f
    in subglottic tracheal disease, 2525-2527
    in supraglottic disease, 2522-2524
    in tracheal disease, 2527-2529, 2529t
    pathophysiology of, 2519, 2520f
    stridor in, 2519-2520, 2521t
  urinary tract infection in, 1583, 1583t, 2510, 2642-2644, 2643b, 2643t
  ventricular septal defect in, 2577
  vomiting in, 203, 208t, 2605, 2606t, 2627t, 2628b
  wheezing in, 2532-2533
Infantile spasms, 2665-2666
Infarction
  gastric, 1394
  lung, pulmonary embolism with, 1373
  myocardial. *See* Myocardial infarction.
  renal, urolithiasis vs., 1591
  spinal cord, 1683
  splenic, in sickle cell disease, 2308
Infection. *See also* Bacterial infection; Fungal infection; Parasitic infection; Viral infection.
  catheter-related, 1363
    in peritoneal dialysis patient, 1553
    of urinary tract, 1578-1579
  cerebrospinal fluid shunt–related, in developmentally disabled patient, 2899
  facial nerve paralysis from, 1666-1667
  fever in, differential diagnosis in, 135, 135t
  fracture and, 558, 558b
  from pacemaker, 1250
  heart failure in, 1268
  hypothermia and, 2241
  in acute renal failure, 1540
  in alcoholism, 2870-2871
  in atherosclerotic aneurysm, 1356, 1357t
  in burn injury, 918
  in chronic renal failure, 1543, 1546-1547
  in diabetes mellitus, 1971
  in elderly person, 2838
  in febrile cancer patient, 1907-1909, 1908b
  in hand trauma, 614-618, 615f-617f
  in heart transplant patient, 2853-2854
  in kidney transplant patient, 2855
  in liver transplant patient, 2854-2855
  in lung transplant patient, 2856

Infection *(Continued)*
  in neutropenic cancer patient, 2834-2839, 2836t, 2838t
  in organ transplant patient, 2847-2849, 2847b
  observation in, 3072-3073, 3072b, 3073t
  of arteriovenous fistula or graft, 1366
  of vascular access for hemodialysis, 1549-1550
  rhabdomyolysis in, 1979
  seizure in, 1029
  susceptibility to, in sickle cell disease, 1880-1881
  thrombocytopenia in, 1897
  wound
    prophylaxis against, 854-855
    risk factors for, 844-845, 844b
Infectious agents
  as biologic weapons, 3024, 3024b
  in organ transplant patient, 2847b
Infectious diarrhea, 228, 230b
  pediatric, 2623-2634
    clinical features of, 2626
    complications of, 2626
    dehydration in, 2629, 2629t
    diagnosis of, 2626-2627
    differential diagnosis in, 2627, 2627t
    disposition in, 2628-2629, 2628b
    epidemiology of, 2623-2624
    etiology of, 2624-2626, 2628t
    fluid and electrolyte management in, 2629-2634, 2630t, 2632b-2634b
    management of, 2628, 2628t
    pathophysiology of, 2624
  treatment of, 229t-230t, 235
Infectious diseases, 2001-2225. *See also specific diseases, e.g.,* Tuberculosis.
Infectious eczematoid dermatitis, in otitis media, 1067-1068
Infectious esophagitis, 1386, 1387
Infectious mononucleosis, 1110, 1112, 1114
  cytomegalovirus in, 2043
  Epstein-Barr virus in, 2044
Infectious parotitis, 1428, 2052
Infective endocarditis, 1300-1302
  clinical features of, 1301
  diagnostic strategies in, 1301-1302, 1302b
  in prosthetic valve patient, 1308
  management of, 1302, 1302b
  pathophysiology of, 1301
  prophylaxis for, 1302, 1303b, 1303t
  risk factors for, 1302, 1303b
Inferior mesenteric artery, 1445
Infiltration therapy, for hydrofluoric acid burns, 933
Inflammation
  after cerebral ischemia, 66-67
  allergic, in asthma, 1080-1081, 1080f, 1083
  in septic shock, 47
  in shock, 43, 44f, 45
  macular disorders from, 1059
  of bursa. *See* Bursitis.
  of joint. *See* Arthritis.
  of tendon. *See* Tendinitis/tendinopathy.
  systemic, in burn injury, 917-918
Inflammatory bowel disease, 1500-1503, 1502b, 1502f, 1503b
  Aeromonas hydrophila gastroenteritis and, 1467
  arthritis in, 1790
  in children, 2615-2616
  pericarditis in, 1287
Inflammatory diarrhea, 228, 229t-230t
Inflammatory disorders. *See also specific disorders, e.g.,* Arthritis.
  allergy, anaphylaxis, and hypersensitivity in, 1818-1835
  arthritis as, 1776-1792
  bursitis as, 1801-1804
  myopathy in, 1708
  tendinopathy as, 1794-1801
  vasculitis as, 1812-1817
Inflammatory mediators
  in anaphylaxis, 1823, 1823b, 2547
  in asthma, 1081
  in sepsis, 2313
Inflammatory pancreatitis, 1435
Inflammatory pseudotumor, 203t
Infliximab, 2844
  for inflammatory bowel disease, 1503
Influenza, 2054-2055
  drugs for, 2057t

Volume 1 pp 1–1024 • Volume 2 pp 1025–2226 • Volume 3 pp 2227–3180

Influenza *(Continued)*
  in pneumonia, 1130, 1139
  pharyngitis in, 1110
  rhabdomyolysis in, 1979
  vaccine for, 2035t, 2055
Influenzae cellulitis, 2199
Information management
  definition of, 3097
  in emergency department, 3099-3102, 3100t, 3102f
  prehospital, 3099, 3101, 3105
Information technology in emergency medicine, 3097-3106
  Internet and, 3104
  networks and, 3104
  security and confidentiality of patient information and, 3102-3103
  standards and, 3103-3104
  telemedicine and, 3105-3106
  terminology in, 3097
  uses of, 3097-3099, 3104-3106
Informed consent, 3134, 3166
  emergency research without, 3136-3137
  for procedures on newly dead, 3149
  physician's role in, 3166-3167
Informed refusal of medical care, 3169-3170
Infrapatellar bursitis, 795-796
Infraspinatus muscle, 672, 673f
Inguinal hernia, 1598, 2641-2642
Inguinal lymphadenopathy, in lymphogranuloma venereum, 1562
Inhalation
  of anhydrous ammonia, 935
  of carbon monoxide, 2438-2441
  of cocaine, 2388
  of cyanide, 2436-2438, 2437f
  of heroin, 2451, 2452
  of hydrocarbons, 2428-2432, 2430f
  of hydrofluoric acid, 933
  of hydrogen sulfide, 2436-2438, 2437f
  of pulmonary irritants, 2433t, 2434-2435, 2434f
  of pyrethrins and pyrethroids, 2467
  of simple asphyxiants, 2432-2433
  of tobacco. *See* Smoking.
  smoke, 2435-2436
    carbon monoxide with cyanide poisoning in, 2440-2441
Inhalational anthrax, 3024-3025, 3025f
Injection pain, reducing, 2932-2933, 2932b
Injection therapy
  in adhesive capsulitis, 699, 699t
  in knee bursitis, 796
Injections, antibiotic and narcotic, medicolegal issues in, 3159
Injury prevention and control, 940-950
  acute trauma care and, 948
  advocacy of public policy for, 948, 950
  epidemiology and documentation in, 945-946
  in elderly person, 2829-2830
  in gang violence in emergency department, 1021-1022
  in pregnancy, 2735-2737
  in youth violence, 1020
  methods of prevention in, 944-945
  prehospital care in, 948
  principles of, 940, 941f, 943-945, 943t, 944t
  public health and, 943-944, 944t
  risk factor assessment in, 946-948
  scientific approach to, 940, 941b
Injury severity score (ISS), 300, 302b
Inner ear
  barotrauma to, 2282, 2287-2288, 2287t, 2292
  in decompression sickness, 2284
Innominate bone, 717, 718f
Inotropic agents, for sepsis, 2219t, 2220-2221
Inpatient, definition of, 3159
Insect repellent
  overdose of, 2468-2469
  prophylactic, for tick-borne illness, 2142
Insect sting kit, allergy to, 1827
Insect stings. *See* Hymenoptera stings.
Insecticide poisoning. *See* Pesticide poisoning.
Insomnia
  in acute mountain sickness, 2301, 2302
  in depression, 1737
  seizures vs., 2668
Inspiratory muscles, weakness of, 139
Inspiratory stridor, in pediatric assessment, 2498
Instability. *See also* Dislocation; Fracture-dislocation.
  atlantoaxial, 2901
  carpal, 630-632, 630f-633f
  shoulder, 674
Instinctual anxiety, 1746b
Institutional abuse, 1009, 1015
Institutional review boards, 3136, 3137
Instrument testing, for anterior cruciate ligament injury, 774
Insufficiency fracture, of femoral neck, 750-752, 750f-751f, 752b
Insufflation technique, for nasal foreign body, 864
Insulin
  allergy to, 1972
  deficiency of, diabetic ketoacidosis from, 1962
  in glucose regulation, 1956
  release of, 1956
Insulin preparations, allergy to, 1827
Insulin pumps, 1973
Insulin resistance
  in diabetes mellitus, 1966
  in pregnancy, 2724
Insulin therapy
  during pregnancy and lactation, 2790
  for calcium channel blocker overdose, 2378
  for diabetic ketoacidosis, 1965-1966
  for hyperkalemia, 1941
  skin problems associated with, 1971-1972
Integrity, personal, 3129, 3129b
Intention-to-treat analysis, 3056-3057, 3057f
Interaction term, 3055
Interclavicular ligaments, 670, 671f
Intercondylar eminence fracture, 779-780, 780f
Intercondylar fracture, 659-660, 659f
Intercostal retractions, in pediatric assessment, 2498, 2498f
Interdental papillae, edematous, in acute necrotic ulcerative gingivitis, 1033
Interferon-α, recombinant, indications for, 2038-2039
Interferon-β, for multiple sclerosis, 1673
Interferon-γ, in tuberculosis, 2155
Interleukin-4, in asthma, 1080, 1080f
Interleukin-13, in asthma, 1080, 1080f
Interleukin(s), in sepsis, 2213
Intermediate-range handgun wounds, 956-957, 956f
Intermittent claudication, in chronic arterial insufficiency, 1345
Intermittent mechanical ventilation (IMV), 27
Internal cervical os, miscarriage and, 2740
Internal disaster plan, 3015
Internal elastic lamina, 1342
Internal iliac arteries, 717-718
Internal radioactive contamination, 2320, 2324
International Classification of Diseases, 3104
International normalized ratio
  in bleeding disorders, 1895
  in hepatitis, 1404
Internet, in health care, 3104
Interossei muscles, 580, 581f
  decompression of, in burn injury, 925, 925f
Interosseous membrane, 797
Interpersonal Justifiability Test, in ethical case analysis, 3132
Interphalangeal joint, 578, 579f
  dislocation of
    distal, 601, 601f
    in foot, 835-836
    in thumb, 564, 565f, 603
    proximal, 601-602
  extensor tendon injury at
    distal, 605-607, 606f, 607f
    proximal, 607-608, 607f
  motions of, 578f
  stability testing of, 601
Interposed abdominal compression–cardiopulmonary resuscitation, 89, 98
Interpreter services
  and effective medical care, 3110-3111
  as standard of cultural competence, 3112-3113
  requirements for, 3161
  sign language, 2905
Interscapular pain, in aortic rupture, 478
Intersphincteric abscess, 1513t, 1514, 2206
Interstitial nephritis, acute, 1534-1535, 1534b
Intertriginous infections, in HIV/AIDS, 2085
Intertrochanteric fracture, 752-753, 752f
Intervertebral disk, 702, 702f
  herniation of
    lumbar, 702-703, 704-705, 711-712
    magnetic resonance imaging in, 432, 433f
    radicular pain in, 264
Intestinal amebiasis, 1477t, 1480-1481
Intestinal fluke, 2101t
Intestinal transit time, in pregnancy, 2726
Intestine(s). *See also* Gastrointestinal *entries;* Large intestine; Small intestine.
  decompression of, for small bowel obstruction, 1444
  distention of, in small bowel obstruction, 1440
  foreign body in, 873-875, 875f
  inflammation of. *See* Enteritis; Gastroenteritis.
  ischemia of. *See* Mesenteric ischemia.
  obstruction of
    abdominal pain in, 214t
    in Hirschsprung's disease, 2612
    in hypertrophic pyloric stenosis, 2603-2606, 2605f, 2606t
    in intussusception, 2610
    in malrotation with midgut volvulus, 2606-2608, 2607f, 2608f
    large bowel, 1495-1497, 1496f
    nausea and vomiting in, 205t
    small bowel, 1440-1444, 1441b, 1443f
  perforation of, in seat belt injuries, 491
  whole-bowel irrigation of
    in beta blocker overdose, 2374
    in cocaine body packing/stuffing, 2391
    in iron overdose, 2420
    in lithium toxicity, 2444
    in opioid overdose, 2455
    in overdosed/poisoned patient, 2330
Intimal flap
  in aortic rupture, 479, 479f, 480, 480f
  in peripheral vascular injury, 538
Intimate partner violence and abuse, 994-1006
  barriers to diagnosis of, 998
  clinical features of, 996-998
  definitions of, 995, 995t
  disposition in, 1004-1005, 1005b
  documentation of, 1000-1001, 1003-1004
  during pregnancy, 997
  epidemiology of, 995-996
  facial trauma from, 382-383
  improving emergency department response to victims of, 1005-1006
  in pregnancy, 2734-2735, 2734t
  legal considerations in, 1004-1005
  referral in, 1004
  risk assessment in, 1000, 1002b, 1003b
  risk factors for injury related to, 996
  screening for, 998-999, 999b, 1000f, 1001f, 1002b
  use of emergency department in, 996
  validation of patient's experience in, 999-1000
Intoxication. *See* Poisoning/overdose.
Intra-abdominal abscess, in appendicitis, 1453, 1458
Intra-aortic balloon pump counterpulsation, for cardiogenic shock, 54
Intra-arterial drug abusers, vascular abnormalities in, 1360-1361
Intra-arterial pressure monitoring, in heart failure, 1269, 1270t, 2773
Intra-articular fracture, of thumb metacarpal, 599-600, 599f
Intracardiac injection, in adult resuscitation, 92
Intracardiac injuries, traumatic, 472
Intracerebral hematoma, 378, 378f
Intracerebral hemorrhage
  alcohol consumption and, 2869-2870
  anatomy and physiology in, 1607
  cerebral herniation in, 1918
  clinical features of, 1610-1611, 1610t, 1611f
  diagnosis of, 1613
  differential diagnosis in, 1611-1612
  disposition in, 1617
  epidemiology of, 1608-1609, 1608b
  in pertussis, 2006
  management of, 1616
  pathophysiology of, 1607
  volume of, measurement of, 1611, 1611f
Intracranial abscess. *See* Brain abscess.
Intracranial hemorrhage
  dysrhythmia after, 371
  hypertension in, 1316

Intracranial hypertension
after head trauma, 353-354, 367
headache and, 174t, 2677-2678
idiopathic, 1639-1640, 1640b
in developmentally disabled patient, 2899
in high altitude cerebral edema, 2306
in pediatric patient, 334, 334b
intubation and, 17, 18t
risk factors for, 171b
treatment of, 360, 367
Intracranial infection, headache in, 1641
Intracranial lesion
delirium in, 1649
dementia in, 1660
in head-injured child, 367
Intracranial pressure
cerebral perfusion pressure and, 352
elevated. *See* Intracranial hypertension.
Intracranial trauma, repetitive, dementia from, 1656
Intractable patient, 2978t, 2980-2981
Intramuscular opioid analgesia, disadvantages of, 2919-2920, 2919b
Intraocular pressure
in red and painful eye, 286-287
increased
from succinylcholine, 14
in central retinal artery occlusion, 1057
in glaucoma, 1055, 1056
in retrobulbar hemorrhage, 1046
in traumatic hyphema, 1048
reversal of, 292
normal, 1055
Intraosseous access
in adult resuscitation, 92
in pediatric resuscitation, 99
Intraperitoneal air, 496, 496f, 504
Intraperitoneal bladder rupture, 526
Intraperitoneal hemorrhage, 493, 498, 498f
in multiple trauma, 312, 313f
peritoneal lavage in, 499-501, 500t
Intraperitoneal injury
penetrating renal trauma and, 528
single vs. multiple, 502
vs. necessary laparotomy, 502
Intrathoracic dislocation, 697, 698f
Intravascular hemolytic transfusion reaction, 59-60
Intravenous drug abuse
cotton fever in, 2454
infective endocarditis in, 1300-1301
skin lesions associated with, 1864, 1865f
vascular abnormalities in, 1360-1361
Intravenous fluid therapy, in pediatric infectious diarrhea, 2630-2634, 2632b-2634b
Intravenous immunoglobulin. *See* Immunoglobulin preparations.
Intravenous pyelography
in renal trauma, 528
in ureteral trauma, 531, 531f
Intravenous regional anesthesia, 2934
Intrinsic ligaments of wrist, 622, 624f
Intubation. *See also* Mechanical ventilation.
approach to, 7-8, 7f-9f
awake oral, 12
confirmation of tube placement in, 6-7, 6f
decision criteria for, 2-3
elevated intracranial pressure and, 17, 18t
esophageal, detection of, 6-7, 6f
fiberoptic, 20-21, 22f
hemodynamic consequences of, 16-17
in abdominal trauma, 494
in acute pulmonary edema, 1271, 1271f
in adult epiglottitis, 1115
in adult resuscitation, 87, 91
in airway foreign body removal, 870
in anaphylaxis, 1830
in asthma, 1082
in barbiturate overdose, 2483
in botulism, 2016
in caustic ingestion, 2383
in chronic obstructive pulmonary disease, 1103-1113, 1105t
in facial trauma, 389, 390
[illegible]
in hypothermia, 2244
in Ludwig's angina, 1119
in multiple trauma, 306
in neonatal resuscitation, 122

Intubation *(Continued)*
in orofacial infections, 1032
in sepsis, 2219
in submersion victim, 2314
in tracheobronchial injury, 466
in weakness and ventilatory insufficiency, 141, 141b
induction agents in, 15-16
measurement of potential difficulty in, 4-5
nasogastric
esophageal perforation from, 483
in abdominal trauma, 494
in acute pancreatitis, 1433-1434
in burn injury, 923
in gastric volvulus, 1394
in gastrointestinal bleeding, 223-224
in hypothermia, 2244
in neck trauma, 444
in small bowel obstruction, 1444
nasotracheal, 12
esophageal perforation from, 483
in multiple trauma, 306
in neck trauma, 444
neuromuscular blocking agents in, 13-15
of difficult airway
approach to, 8-9, 9f
cricothyrotomy for, 22-23, 23f
esophagotracheal combitube for, 20, 20f
fiberoptic, 20-21, 22f
identification in, 3-4, 3b, 4b, 5f
intubating laryngeal mask airway for, 19, 19f
lighted stylet for, 19-20, 20f
retrograde, 20
special airway devices for, 18-23, 19f-23f
oral access for, assessment of, 4, 5f
outcomes in, 23
pediatric, 18
in asthma, 2542
in bacterial tracheitis, 2529
in status epilepticus, 2672
pharmacologic agents in, 13-16
potential cervical spine injury in, 17-18
prehospital, 2990, 2991
rapid sequence, 9-12, 10b
in asthma, 16
in elevated intracranial pressure, 17, 18t
in head trauma, 358-359
in neck trauma, 444
in shock, 51
indications for, 7-8
paralysis with induction phase in, 11
pediatric, 18, 107-108, 107b, 107t
post-intubation management in, 11-12
prehospital, 2990, 2991
preoxygenation in, 10, 10f
preparations for, 9-10
pretreatment agents for, 10, 11b
tube placement in, 11
vs. blind nasotracheal intubation, 12
with competitive neuromuscular blocking agent and etomidate, 14-15, 15t
retrograde, 20
status asthmaticus and, 16, 17t
with sedation alone, 12
without pharmacologic agents, 12-13
Intussusception
in Henoch-Schönlein purpura, 2615
in infants and children, 2509b, 2610-2612, 2611f, 2612t
large bowel, 1499-1500
small bowel, 1441-1442
Inverse ratio ventilation (IRV), 33
Inversion stress test, 817
Involucrum, in osteomyelitis, 2175
Iodine exposure, as weapon of mass destruction, 3023, 3023t
Iodine therapy, for thyroid storm, 1909
Iodine tincture, ingestion of, 2381
Iodoquinol, for intestinal amebiasis, 1481
Ionizing radiation, 2318f, 2319
Iothalamate meglumine contrast medium, in retrograde cystography, 521, 525
Ipratropium
during pregnancy and lactation, 2762, 2765t, 2790
for anaphylaxis, 1832
for asthma, 1087t, 1089, 2539t, 2541
for chronic obstructive pulmonary disease, 1105

Irbesartan, 1322t
Iridocyclitis, traumatic, 1049, 1049f
Iridodialysis, traumatic, 1049
Iridodonesis, in lens dislocation, 1049
Iris, 1045f
flat or plateau, closed angle glaucoma from, 1056
nonpenetrating trauma to, 1048-1049, 1048f, 1049f
Iron
caustic effects of, 2419
corneal foreign body containing, 1047, 1048f, 1052
metabolic acidosis from, 1928
overdose of, 2418-2421, 2419t, 2420f, 2420t
antidotes to, 2329t
preparations of, 2419t
requirements for, in pregnancy, 2724
Iron deficiency anemia, 1871-1872, 1871f, 1872t
in alcoholism, 2873-2874
in pregnancy, 2763t, 2767-2768
Irradiation
definition of, 2319
microwave, 2319
for rewarming in accidental hypothermia, 2250
vs. contamination and incorporation, 2319-2320
whole body, acute radiation syndrome after, 2317t, 2321-2322, 2321f
Irrigation
for foreign body removal from ear, 863
heated, for rewarming, 2250
in acid and alkali burns, 933
in anhydrous ammonia exposure, 935
in cement burn, 935
in hydrofluoric acid exposure, 933, 934
in ocular burns, 1046
in red and painful eye, 290-291
of wound, 848
Irritability
in bacterial meningitis, 2658
in pediatric assessment, 2498
Irritable bowel syndrome, 1490-1492, 1491b, 1492b
Irritant laxatives, for constipation, 241t, 242
Irritants, ocular trauma from, 1046
Ischemia
cerebral
neurologic recovery after, 62-73
clinical outcomes in, 72-73
experimental therapies in, 70-72
standard strategies for, 67-70, 69t
pathophysiology of, 62-67, 63f-64f
colonic, 1503-1504
in frostbite, 2229, 2229b
limb-threatening
in acute arterial occlusion, 1345
management of, 1351
mesenteric. *See* Mesenteric ischemia.
myocardial. *See* Myocardial ischemia.
of tissue, in compartment syndrome, 560-561, 560b, 561b, 561f
transient. *See* Transient ischemic attack (TIA).
warm, in peripheral vascular injury, 537
Ischemic central retinal vein occlusion, 1057
Ischemic heart disease. *See* Acute coronary syndromes; Coronary artery disease; Myocardial infarction; Myocardial ischemia.
Ischemic optic neuropathy, 1060
Ischemic penumbra, 1607
Ischemic stroke
acute drug therapy for, 1615-1616, 1615t
anatomy and physiology in, 1607
antihypertensive drug therapy for, 1614, 1614t
cardioembolic, 1608
clinical features of, 1609-1610, 1610t
diagnosis of, 1612-1613, 1612f
differential diagnosis in, 1611
disposition in, 1616-1617
epidemiology of, 1607-1608, 1607t
fibrinolytic therapy for, 1615, 1615t
in central retinal artery occlusion, 1057
management of, 1613-1616, 1613t, 1614t, 1616b
pathophysiology of, 1606-1607
thrombotic, 1607-1608
time goals in, 1613t
Ischial tuberosity avulsion fracture, 724, 724f

Ischiogluteal bursitis, 1803
Ischiorectal abscess, 1513t, 1514, 2206
Ischium, 717, 718f
Isoenzyme analysis, in electrical and lightning injuries, 2276
Isoflurane anesthesia, for status epilepticus, 1627-1628, 1627t
Isolation
  in plague, 3027-3028
  in pneumonia, 1136, 1140-1141
  in tuberculosis, 2147, 2169-2170
Isonatremic hypovolemia, 2629t, 2631, 2632b
Isoniazid
  during pregnancy and lactation, 2785
  for tuberculosis, 2162, 2163t
  hepatotoxicity of, 1413
  in HIV/AIDS, side effects of, 2079t
  metabolic acidosis from, 1928
  overdose of, antidotes to, 2329t
Isopropyl alcohol poisoning, 2402-2404, 2403f
Isoproterenol
  for anaphylactic patient on beta blockers, 1831b, 1833
  for calcium channel blocker overdose, 2378
  for torsades de pointes, 1244
Isorhythmic atrioventricular dissociation, 1221
Isospora belli gastroenteritis, 1476-1478, 1477t, 2084
Isradipine, 1321t, 2377t
Itraconazole
  for candidal esophagitis, 1387
  for tinea capitis, 1839
  in HIV/AIDS, side effects of, 2079t
Ivermectin
  for *Onchocerca volvulus* infection, 2109
  for pediculosis, 1854
Ivory soap, for rabies postexposure prophylaxis, 2068
Ixodes tick, 2117, 2118, 2118f, 2121f, 2139

J wave, in hypothermia, 2237, 2238f
Jacksonian march, 1621
Japanese encephalitis virus, 1723
Jarisch-Herxheimer-type reaction
  in Lyme disease, 2128
  in relapsing fever, 2130
Jaundice, 243-246
  diagnostic approach to, 243-244, 244f, 245f
  differential diagnosis in, 245, 246t
  empiric management of, 245-246, 247f
  epidemiology of, 243
  in cholangitis, 1421
  in drug-induced liver disorders, 1414
  in hepatitis, 1404
  in hyperthyroidism, 1987
  in pancreatic carcinoma, 1437
  in pregnancy, 2726, 2753t
  in pyogenic abscess, 1414-1415
  neonatal, 2601-2603, 2602t, 2603b, 2603t, 2604f-2605f
Jaw-thrust maneuver, in pediatric resuscitation, 97
JC virus, 2045-2046
Jefferson fracture, 412-413, 414f, 421, 550t
Jehovah's Witnesses, refusal of medical care by, 3171-3172
Jellyfish, 909
Jequirty pea, 2471-2472, 2472f
Jerk test, in knee trauma, 774
Jimson weed poisoning, 2345, 2346, 2473, 2473f
Jobe's sign, in rotator cuff tendinopathy, 1797
Joint
  anatomy of, 2175
  arthrocentesis of, 1780-1781
  aspiration of
    in gonococcal arthritis, 2191
    in septic arthritis, 2188-2190, 2189f, 2192
  clinical anatomy of, 1777, 1777f
  contractures of, in cerebral palsy, 2901
  dislocation of. *See* Dislocation.
  examination of, 1778-1779, 1779f
  infection of. *See* Septic arthritis.
  inflammation of. *See* Arthritis.
  injury to, in electrical and lightning injuries, 2273
  subluxation of. *See* Subluxation.
Joint fluid analysis, in septic arthritis, 2188-2190, 2189f
Joint pain
  causes of, 1778, 1778t
  in gouty arthritis, 1785
  in hypothyroidism, 1992
  in osteoarthritis, 1787
  in septic arthritis, 1784-1785, 2188
Joint prosthesis, infection after, 2191
Jones compression dressing, 570-571
Jones criteria for rheumatic fever, 1303, 1304b, 1790b, 2596, 2596f
Jones fracture, 550t, 832
Judgment, substituted, 3134
Jugular vein injury, 448
Jugular venous "A" wave, in tricuspid stenosis and regurgitation, 1307
Jugular venous distention
  in constrictive pericarditis, 1288
  in tension pneumothorax, 462
Jumper's knee, 794
Junctional parasystole, 1226
Junctional tachycardia, 1233-1235, 1233f, 1234f
  nonparoxysmal, 1234
  paroxysmal, 1233-1234, 1233f, 1234f, 1235
  reentrant, 1233
Junin virus, 2055-2056
Juniper, adverse effects of, 2476t
Justice, distributive, 3129, 3129b
Juvenile epilepsy, 2666

Kanamycin, for tuberculosis, 2163t
Kaopectate, for diarrhea, 236t
Kaposi's sarcoma, 1861f, 2044, 2079, 2083, 2085
Karlea, drug interactions with, 2478t
Kawasaki disease, 2024-2027, 2025b
  diagnostic criteria for, 2512b
  myocarditis in, 1293
  pediatric, 2593-2596, 2594b, 2595f
  pediatric fever in, 2511, 2512b
Kayexalate, for hyperkalemia, 1545-1546, 1545t, 1941
Kelly clamp, for oropharyngeal foreign body removal, 1384
Kemerovo virus, 2047
Keratitis
  epithelial, corneal, 1054
  red and painful eye in, 289, 289f, 290f, 294t-295t
  superficial punctate, 294t, 1054
  ultraviolet, 1046-1047
Keratoconjunctivitis
  in herpes zoster, 1054
  red and painful eye in, 288, 288f, 293t, 295t
Keratotomy, radial, altitude and, 2309
Keraunoparalysis, in lightning injuries, 2274
Kerion, 1839
Kernicterus
  in hyperbilirubinemia, 2602
  prevention of, 2603, 2604f-2605f
Kernig sign
  in bacterial meningitis, 2659
  in central nervous system infection, 1714
Kernohan's notch syndrome, in cerebral herniation, 355
Ketamine
  abuse of, 2893
  as induction agent, 16
  for critically ill asthmatic patient, 1092
  for hypoxic (tet) spells, 2581
  for procedural sedation and analgesia, 2940t-2941t, 2946-2947, 2950, 2951t, 2953
  toxicity of, 2413, 2415
Ketoacidosis
  alcoholic, 1927-1928, 1964-1965, 2872-2873
  diabetic, 1928, 1962-1967
    complications of, 1967
    diagnosis of, 1963-1964
    differential considerations in, 1964-1965
    disposition in, 1967
    etiology of, 1963
    hypophosphatemia in, 1951
    in pregnancy, 1972, 2771-2772
    laboratory tests in, 1964, 1964t
    management of, 1965-1967, 1965b
    nausea and vomiting in, 205t
    pathophysiology of, 1962-1963, 1962t, 1963f
Ketoconazole
  during pregnancy and lactation, 2785
  for candidal esophagitis, 1387
  for esophageal candidiasis, 2083
  for tinea versicolor, 1840
  hepatotoxicity of, 1414
  in HIV/AIDS, side effects of, 2079t
Ketones, urine, in diabetes mellitus, 1959
Ketoprofen, for gouty arthritis, 1786
Ketorolac, 2927
  for abdominal pain, 217
  for migraine, 2680
  for urolithiasis, 1591-1592
Ketosis, in isopropyl alcohol poisoning, 2403
Khat, 2393, 2893
Kidney. *See also* Renal *entries.*
  anatomy of, 527, 527f
  blood supply to, 527, 527f
  gluconeogenesis in, 1956
  physical examination of, 1572, 1573f
  size of, in chronic renal failure, 1543, 1543b
  transplantation of, 2855
  ureter, and bladder films (KUB)
    in bladder trauma, 521, 522f, 523f, 524f
    in urethral trauma, 518
    in urolithiasis, 1590, 1592f
Kidney stones, 1586-1593, 1586b, 1589f-1592f, 1593b. *See also* Urolithiasis.
Kienbock's disease, 629
Kiesselbach's area, 1073f
Killer bees, 904
Kindling, 1623
Kingella kingae, in bone or joint infections, 2177, 2178t
Kinky-hair syndrome, fracture in, 2701
Kissing burn, 2272, 2272f
Klebsiella pneumoniae, 1130, 1132
Kleihauer-Betke test, for fetomaternal hemorrhage, 321
Klein's line, in slipped capital femoral epiphysis, 2708
Knee
  bursitis of, 795-796
  dislocation of, popliteal artery injury and, 546
  immobilization of, 570-571
  osteoarthritis in, 796
  septic arthritis in, 796
  tendinitis of, 794, 795
  tendinopathy of, 1799
Knee pain
  differential diagnosis in, 771-772
  in bursitis of knee, 795
  in iliotibial band syndrome, 794
  in lateral patellar compression syndrome, 794
  in patellofemoral pain syndrome, 786-787
  in peripatellar tendinitis, 794
  in plica syndrome, 794-795
  in popliteus tendinitis, 795
  in tibial tubercle fracture, 798
Knee trauma, 770-796
  anatomy and physiology in, 770-771, 771f
  arthrocentesis in, 774
  arthroscopy in, 774
  bone bruise in, 781
  clinical features of, 771-774
  collateral ligament injuries in, 791-792
  cruciate ligament injuries in, 790-791
  distal femur fracture in, 776-777
  extensor tendon injuries in, 782-784, 783f, 784f
  meniscal tears in, 792-793
  osteochondritis dissecans in, 781-782
  osteonecrosis in, 782
  overuse injuries in, 793-796
  patellar dislocation in, 785-786, 785b
  patellar fracture in, 784-785, 785f
  patellofemoral pain syndrome in, 786-787
  physical examination in, 772-773, 772b, 772f
  proximal intra-articular tibial fractures in, 777-781
    epiphyseal, 780-781
    tibial plateau, 777-779, 777f-778f
    tibial spine, 779-780, 780f
  radiologic evaluation in, 774-775
  soft tissue injuries in, 790-792
  stability testing in, 773-774
  tibial femoral knee dislocation in, 787-790, 789f
Koplik's spots, in measles, 1849, 2053, 2053f
Korsakoff's psychosis, 2869

Kruskal-Wallis test, 3052t, 3053
Kuru, 2058
Kussmaul's respiration
  in diabetic ketoacidosis, 1963
  in metabolic acidosis, 1929
Kussmaul's signs, in neoplastic cardiac tamponade, 1917
Kyphosis, in pregnancy, 2727
Labetalol, 1341t
  during pregnancy and lactation, 2765t, 2788
  for aortic dissection, 1328
  for hypertensive emergencies, 1318-1319, 2653, 2765t
  for intracranial hemorrhage–related hypertension, 1316
  for tetanus, 2011
  overdose of, 2373t, 2374
Labor and delivery, 2797-2822
  abruptio placentae and, 2809-2810
  amniotic fluid embolism and, 2821
  bloody show in, 2798-2799
  breech presentations in, 2811-2813, 2811b, 2812f, 2813b
  chorioamnionitis in, 2808, 2808b
  circumvallate placenta and, 2810
  complicated, 2810-2816
  delivery preparations and techniques in, 2802, 2804
  drug interactions in, 2811t
  emergency, epidemiology of, 2797
  episiotomy in, 2804, 2813, 2815
  face, brow, and compound presentations in, 2815-2816
  false vs. true labor in, 2798
  human immunodeficiency virus transmission during, 2810
  in multiple gestations, 2816
  in spinal cord injured patient, 2769
  limitations of emergency department for, 2797
  malpresentations in, 2811-2816, 2811b, 2811t, 2812f, 2813b, 2814f, 2815f, 2816b
  maternal complications of, 2818-2822
  normal, 2798-2805
  nursery care after, 2798, 2798b
  patient transfer considerations in, 2797-2798
  placenta previa and, 2808-2809
  postpartum cardiomyopathy and, 2821
  postpartum depression and, 2821-2822
  postpartum endometriosis and, 2821
  postpartum hemorrhage and, 258t, 2818-2820
  premature, 2805-2807, 2806b, 2807b
  PROM in, 2807-2808, 2808t
  routine adjuncts to, risk-benefit analysis of, 2805t
  shoulder dystocia in, 2811, 2813-2815, 2814f, 2815f, 2816b
  stages of, 2799-2805, 2809f
    first, 2799-2800, 2799f-2802f
    second, 2800-2804, 2802b, 2802t, 2803f
    third, 2804-2805
    fourth, 2805
  substance abuse and, 2791, 2791b
  third-trimester complications associated with, 2805-2810
  umbilical cord–related emergencies in, 2817-2818, 2817t
  uterine inversion and, 2820
  uterine rupture and, 2820
  vasa previa and, 2810
Laboratory studies
  as source of failures in emergency department, 3125
  during cardiopulmonary resuscitation, 82
  for pregnancy detection, 2728-2730, 2729f
  in abdominal trauma, 495
  in accidental hypothermia, 2242-2244, 2243f
  in acute pancreatitis, 1430-1432, 1431t, 1432b
  in anemia, 1869
  in arthritis, 1770
  in back pain, 204, 707
  in comatose patient, 161-162
  in confusion, 152-153
  in cyanosis, 271
  in delirium, 1051-1052
  [illegible]
  in diabetic ketoacidosis, 1904, 1904t
  in disseminated intravascular coagulation, 1903, 1904t
  in elderly trauma patient, 347
Laboratory studies (Continued)
  in electrical and lightning injuries, 2276
  in fever, 137
  in gastrointestinal bleeding, 222-223
  in hematuria, 1530, 1602-1603
  in hemolytic anemia, 1877-1878, 1877b, 1877f, 1878f
  in hemoptysis, 281
  in jaundice, 240-244, 244t
  in multiple trauma, 304
  in neuromuscular disorders, 1704-1705
  in osteomyelitis, 2179
  in pediatric fever, 2508-2510
  in pediatric pneumonia, 2560-2561
  in pediatric seizure, 2671
  in pediatric trauma, 332-333
  in pneumonia, 1134-1135
  in pregnancy, 318, 2728-2730, 2729f
  in pregnant trauma patient, 324
  in proteinuria, 1532
  in renal trauma, 528
  in seizure, 168
  in severe head trauma, 361
  in tuberculosis, 2151-2152
  in urinary tract infection, 1575-1577, 1577b
  in urolithiasis, 1588-1589
  in vertigo, 145
  in weakness, 139
  renal, 1524-1528, 1526f, 1527t, 1528b, 1528f
Labyrinthitis
  in otitis media, 1067
  vertigo in, 146, 147t, 2683
Laceration
  cheek, 391
  conjunctival, 1051
  corneal, 1051, 1051f
  coronary artery, 472
  ear, 392
  eye, 392
  eyelid, 1051, 1051f
  liver, 497f
  management of, 842-857. *See also* Wound management.
  mouth, 391
  of extensor mechanism over distal interphalangeal joint, 607, 607f
  pattern
    in motor vehicle crashes, 964, 965f
    in physical assault, 962, 962f
  penile, 532
  renal, 530, 530f
  scalp, 371-372, 850
  testicular, 534
Lachman's test, in anterior cruciate ligament injury, 773
Lacrimal glands, 385
Lacrimal sac, infection of, 1055, 1055f
Lactate
  in acute mesenteric ischemia, 1447
  in cyanide poisoning, 2437
  in shock, 47
  postresuscitation levels of, 87
Lactate clearance index, in shock, 50
Lactate dehydrogenase
  in acute tumor lysis syndrome, 1911
  in hemolytic anemia, 1878
  in hepatitis, 1404
Lactation
  asthma during, 1091
  drug therapy during, safety of, 2781-2790, 2782t-2783t
  drug transfer during, 2781
Lactic acid, cerebrospinal fluid, in central nervous system infection, 1718
Lactic acidosis, 1928-1929
  in crush injury, 3007
  in sepsis, 2216
  in shock, 42-43, 43f
Lactobezoar, 879
Lactulose, for hepatic encephalopathy, 1412
Lacunar stroke, 1600
Ladd's bands, 2606
Laënnec's cirrhosis, 1410
Lambert-Eaton myasthenic syndrome, 1705
[illegible]
Lamivudine, in HIV/AIDS, side effects of, 2079t
Lamotrigine
  during pregnancy and lactation, 2787
Lamotrigine (Continued)
  for pediatric seizure, 2675t
  side effects of, 1628t
Landing zone safety issues for helicopters, 2997, 2997b, 2997f, 2998b
Langer's lines, 384, 384f
Language, developmental milestones in, 2495-2497, 2496t
Language barriers
  and effective medical care, 3110-3111
  culturally competent approach to, 3112-3113
Lansoprazole, 1390t
Laparoscopy
  in abdominal trauma, 501, 508
  in appendicitis, 1455, 1457-1458
  in ectopic pregnancy, 2745
  in pelvic pain, 250
  in small bowel obstruction, 1444
Laparotomy
  in abdominal aortic aneurysm, 1338, 1339f
  in acute mesenteric ischemia, 1448
  in blunt abdominal trauma, 507-510, 507t, 508f, 509t
  in children, 510
  in penetrating abdominal trauma
    from gunshot wounds, 505-507, 506f
    from stab wounds, 503-505, 503f, 503t
Large intestine. *See also* Anorectal disorders; Colon; Rectum.
  disorders of, 1490-1506
  diverticular disease of, 1492-1495, 1494b, 1495b
  inflammatory bowel disease and, 1500-1503, 1502b, 1502f, 1503b
  intussusception of, 1499-1500
  irritable bowel syndrome and, 1490-1492, 1491b, 1492b
  obstruction of, 1495-1497, 1496f
    causes of, 1499b
    in volvulus, 1497-1499, 1498f, 1499b, 1499f
    pseudo-obstruction and, 1495-1496, 1497
  radiation proctocolitis and, 1505-1506
Larkspur, adverse effects of, 2476t
Laryngeal disease, pediatric upper airway obstruction in, 2524-2525, 2524f
Laryngeal dystonia, antipsychotic-induced, 2446
Laryngeal edema, in anaphylaxis, 1825t, 2548
Laryngeal foreign body, 870
Laryngeal fracture, in near-hanging and strangulation, 451
Laryngeal injury, in smoke inhalation, 2435
Laryngeal mask airway, 18-19, 19f
  in airway foreign body removal, 870
  in neonatal resuscitation, 123
  intubating, 19, 19f
Laryngeal papilloma, 2045, 2525
Laryngeal tuberculosis, 2151
Laryngeal web, 2525, 2525f
Laryngitis, 1114
Laryngomalacia, 2524, 2524f
Laryngoscopy
  direct
    awake, 8
    evaluation of suitability for, 4, 5f
  failed, 8
  fiberoptic, in neck trauma, 445
  grades in, intubation difficulty and, 5
  in adult epiglottitis, 1115, 1115f
  in confirmation of endotracheal tube placement, 6-7
  reflex sympathetic response to, 16-17
  video and rigid fiberoptic, 21, 22f
Laryngotracheal stenosis, 2525
Laryngotracheal trauma, 447-448
Laryngotracheobronchitis, viral, 2525-2527, 2526f, 2527b
Larynx, adult vs. child, 2519, 2520f
Lasègue's sign, in lumbar radiculopathy, 704
Lassa fever virus, 2037t, 2055
Late asthmatic response, 1081
Lateral collateral ligament
  anatomy of, 770, 771f, 808, 809f
  injury to, 791-792
  [illegible]
Lateral compression pelvic fracture, 727, 729f
Lateral condyle
  anatomy of, 647, 647f, 770, 771f
  fracture of, 660-661, 661f

Lateral corticospinal tract, 1676, 1676f
Lateral elbow dislocation, 665
Lateral epicondylitis, 1798
Lateral femoral cutaneous mononeuropathy, 1698
Lateral malleolus
anatomy of, 808, 809f
fracture of, 812-813, 813f
Lateral meniscus injury, 792-793
Lateral patellar compression syndrome, 794
Lateral pharyngeal space, 1027, 1117
Lateral radiographs of spinal injuries, 421, 424, 425f, 426f
Lateral retinacula, 770, 771f
Lateral spinothalamic tract, 1676, 1676f
Lateral talocalcaneal ligament injury, 816
Lateral tibiofemoral compartment, 770, 771f
Latex agglutination, in central nervous system infection, 1718-1719
Latex allergy, 1826-1827, 2547
Law enforcement, tactical emergency medical support in, 3000-3005
Laxatives
abuse of, 239
for constipation, 241t, 242
Löffler's syndrome, 2110
Le Fort fracture, 387, 393, 551t
Le Fort-Wagstaffe fracture, 551t
Lead
blood level of, as biomarker, 2422
encephalopathy caused by, 2421, 2422
foreign body containing, 2423
poisoning from, 2421-2423, 2422t
antidotes to, 2329t
sideroblastic anemia in, 1873
Lead snowstorm, from centerfire rifle wound, 959, 960f
Learned helplessness, 1736
Leaving against medical advice, 3170-3171
Leaving without being seen, 3170
Lebombo virus, 2047
Left bundle branch block
myocardial infarction in, predictors of, 1167, 1170f
ST segment elevation in, 1167, 1169, 1169f, 1170f
Left ventricular aneurysm, 1167, 1168f
Left ventricular free wall rupture, 1160
Left ventricular hypertrophy, 1169-1170, 1172f
Left ventriculoplasty, for chronic heart failure, 1277
Left-sided heart failure, 1266-1267
Leg. *See also* Lower leg.
blue, painful, 1370
decompression of, in burn injury, 925
position of, in hip trauma examination, 744
swelling of, in spinal cord injury, 2907
Leg pain
in disk herniation, 705
lower, differential diagnosis of, 803
Legal case precedents, for combative or violent patient, 2967-2968
Legal issues, 3156-3173
combative patient and, 2967-2969
consent to medical care and, 3166-3169
disposition requirements and, 3164-3165, 3165t
emergency medical condition and, 3156-3157
Emergency Medical Treatment and Active Labor Act and, 3156
in blood transfusion, 58
in intimate partner violence and abuse, 1004-1005
in patient transfer during labor and delivery, 2797
medical screening examination and, 3160-3163
of combative patient, 2967-2969
refusal of medical care and, 3169-3172
reporting requirements and, 3172-3173
screening requirements and, 3157-3158
stabilization requirements and, 3163-3164
testing requests and requirements and, 3158-3160
Legal rights, 3128
Legg-Calvé-Perthes disease, in children, 2706-2707, 2707f
Legionella infection
in cancer patient with impaired cell-mediated immunity, 2839-2840
in rhabdomyolysis, 1979
Legionella pneumoniae, 1130, 1132
Legionella pneumophila, myocarditis in, 1292
Leishmaniasis
cutaneous, 2108, 2108f
drug therapy for, 2101t
fever in, 2105
Lemierre's syndrome, parapharyngeal abscess and, 1123
LEMON approach for evaluation of difficult airway, 3-4, 3b, 4b, 5f
Lennox-Gastaut syndrome, 2666
Lens, 1045f
dislocation of, 1049
subluxation of, 1049
Leopold's maneuvers, 2800, 2801f, 2813
Leptomeningeal cyst, in head-injured child, 368
Leriche's syndrome, 1345
Lesser trochanter fracture
intertrochanteric, 752-753, 752f
isolated, 753, 753f
pediatric, 767, 767f
subtrochanteric, 753-755, 754f
LET (lidocaine, epinephrine, and tetracaine), 2933
Lethality Checklist in intimate partner violence and abuse, 1000, 1003b
Lethargy, in pediatric assessment, 2498
Leucovorin, for toxic alcohol poisoning, 2402
Leukemia
acute tumor lysis syndrome in, 1911
central nervous system infections in, 1920
chronic myeloid, 1887-1888, 1887f
fever and granulocytopenia in, 1908
gingival lesions in, 1036
hypercalcemia in, 1914
hyperuricemia in, 1913
hyperviscosity syndrome in, 1912
hypogammaglobulinemia in, 2840-2841
immune thrombocytopenia in, 1897
lymphocytosis in, 1888
Leukemoid reaction, 1888
Leukocyte. *See* White blood cell *entries.*
Leukocyte esterase, urinary, in urinary tract infection, 1575-1576
Leukocytosis
causes of, 1887b
in amebic abscess, 1416
in appendicitis, 1454
in asthma, 1085
in pertussis, 2006
in pyogenic abscess, 1415
lymphocytic, 1887b, 1888
neutrophil, 1887-1888, 1887b, 1887f
Leukoencephalopathy
progressive multifocal, 2045-2046
dementia in, 1658, 1659
in HIV/AIDS, 2082
spongiform, from inhaled heroin, 2452
Leukopenia, 52, 1888-1889, 1889t
Leukopheresis, for hyperviscosity syndrome, 1913
Leukoplakia, hairy, in HIV/AIDS, 2083
Leukotriene modifiers
during pregnancy and lactation, 2789
for aspirin-exacerbated respiratory disease, 1082
for asthma, 1090, 2542, 2543t
Leukotrienes
as anaphylaxis mediators, 1823, 1823b
in aspirin-exacerbated respiratory disease, 1082
in asthma, 1080f, 1081, 1081f
Levalbuterol, for asthma, 1087, 1087t, 2538
Levator ani syndrome, 1516
Levator scapulae muscle, 672, 673f
Levator tendon lacerations, 1051
Levitaractam, for seizure, 2675t
Levofloxacin
for tuberculosis, 2164t, 2165
for urinary tract infection, 1582
Levorphanol, respiratory effects of, 2453t
Levothyroxine
for hypothyroidism, 1993-1994
in hypothermia, 2246-2247
Lewy body dementia, 1656, 1657
Libman-Sachs vegetations, in systemic lupus erythematosus, 1807
Lice, 1853-1854, 1853f
Lichen sclerosis et atrophicus, 975
Lichen tropicus, 2259
Lichenification, 1839t, 1842
Licorice
adverse effects of, 2476t
drug interactions with, 2478t
Lidocaine, 1206-1207, 2931, 2931t, 2932, 2932t
allergy to, 846-847
buffered, 2932-2933
cardiac, 847
central nervous system toxicity of, 2932
during pregnancy and lactation, 2787-2788
epinephrine, and tetracaine combination, 2933
for anal fissures, 1513
for cardiac arrest, 92-93
for digitalis toxicity, 2371
for dysrhythmia, 2586b
for intubation of asthmatic patient, 16
for knee bursitis, 796
for local anesthesia, 846
for pediatric resuscitation, 102t, 105
for premature ventricular contractions, 1225
for rapid sequence intubation, 11b, 359
for reduction of glenohumeral joint dislocation, 689
for rotator cuff tear, 696
for ventricular fibrillation and pulseless ventricular tachycardia, 113
for ventricular tachycardia, 1242
for wide-complex tachycardia, 1239-1240
topical, 846, 2933
Life experiences, racial/ethnic differences in, culturally competent approach to, 3113-3114
Life or limb threats, in clinical decision making, 128
Lifestyle modification, for gastroesophageal reflux, 1389
Life-threatening event, apparent, 2714, 2718-2720, 2718b, 2719b
Ligamentous injuries
carpally, 630-632, 630f-633f
in ankle trauma, 815-818, 817b, 817f
in hand, 600-604, 601f-603f
spinal, 434, 435f, 439
Ligaments
of ankle, 808, 809f, 810f
of distal humerus and elbow, 647-648, 648f
of hip, 736, 736f
of knee, 770-771, 771f
of lumbosacral spine, 702, 702f
of pelvis, 717, 718f
of shoulder, 670-671, 671f, 672, 673f
of wrist, 622, 624f
Ligamentum flavum, 702
Ligase chain reaction test, in tuberculosis, 2155
Ligature strangulation, 450
Lighted stylet, for intubation of difficult airway, 19-20, 20f
Lightning injuries, 2267-2277
and distribution of lightning, 2268f
clinical features of, 2271-2274, 2273f
complications of, 2274
differential considerations in, 2275
disposition in, 2277
management of, 2275-2277, 2276b
mechanisms of, 2271, 2271b
physics of, 2269-2270
rhabdomyolysis from, 1978
Light's criteria, in pleural fluid analysis, 1152, 1152b
Likelihood ratio, 3059t
Limaprost, in frostbite, 2232
Limb ischemia, in tibial femoral knee dislocation, 788
Limb-threatening ischemia
in acute arterial occlusion, 1345
management of, 1351
Limp
child with, 764-765, 765f
in Legg-Calvé-Perthes disease, 2706
in slipped capital femoral epiphysis, 2708
Lindane, for *Phthirus pubis* infestation, 1569
Linear burns, 2273
Linear regression models, 3055
Linear skull fracture, 372-373
Lingual tonsillitis, 1114, 1114f
Linton tube, for gastrointestinal bleeding, 225
Lip
laceration of, 391, 1040
skin of, 384-385
Lip reading, 2905

Lipase
  in acute pancreatitis, 1430-1431
  serum
    in abdominal trauma, 495
    in nausea and vomiting, 203
Lipid-lowering therapy, rhabdomyolysis from, 1979
Lipoatrophy, insulin, 1971
Lipohyalinosis, 1608
Lipohypertrophy, insulin, 1971
Lipovnik virus, 2047
Lisfranc's joint
  anatomy of, 820, 820f
  fractures and dislocations of, 551t, 828-831, 829f, 830f
  sprains of, 838
Lisinopril, 1322t
Listeria infection, in cancer patient with impaired cell-mediated immunity, 2839-2840
Lister's tubercle, 581, 583f, 625
Lithium
  drug interactions with, 2442, 2443t
  for bipolar disorder, 1742
  hypercalcemia from, 1945
  toxicity of, 2442-2444, 2443t
Lithotripsy, extracorporeal shock wave
  for cholelithiasis, 1419
  for urolithiasis, 1593
Little leaguer's elbow, 663, 663f, 2710-2711
Livedo reticularis, 1347, 1357
Liver. *See also* Hepatic *entries.*
  alcohol metabolism in, 2859
  cancer of, 1417
  enlarged, in hepatitis, 1404
  fatty
    alcoholic, 2868
    in pregnancy, 1417, 2755-2756
  gluconeogenesis in, 1956
  in immune response, 2831
  injury to
    acetaminophen-induced, 2332-2333, 2334, 2335, 2336, 2337
    drug-induced, 1413-1414, 1414t
    in children, 342
    in heatstroke, 2262
  transplantation of, 1417-1418, 2337, 2854-2855, 2854f
  trauma to, 489, 490, 491, 497f
Liver disorders, 1402-1418
  alcoholic, 1407, 1409, 2867-2868
    cirrhosis in, 1410
    hepatitis in, 1405, 1409
  chronic, end stage, 1410-1411. *See also* Cirrhosis.
  drug-induced, 1413-1414, 1414t
  encephalopathy in, 1411-1412, 1411t
  in HIV/AIDS, 2084
  in pregnancy, 1416-1417, 2755-2756
  inflammatory. *See* Hepatitis.
  spontaneous bacterial peritonitis in, 1412-1413
Liver enzymes
  in acetaminophen overdose, 2335
  in acute pancreatitis, 1431, 1431t
  in alcoholic hepatitis, 1409
  in amebic abscess, 1416
  in viral hepatitis, 1404
Liver function tests
  in abdominal trauma, 495
  in nausea and vomiting, 203
Living will, 3133
Lizards, venomous, 896, 898-899, 902
LOAD mnemonic, in rapid sequence intubation, 10, 11b
Lobar atelectasis, in chronic obstructive pulmonary disease, 1102
Local anesthesia, 2914b, 2930-2933, 2931t, 2932b, 2932t
  allergy to, 846-847, 1827, 2931
  buffering in, 846, 2932-2933, 2932b
  in calcific tendinitis, 698
  in wound care, 846
  ophthalmic, 1063b, 1064
  profiles of agents used for, 2930-2931, 2931t, 2932t
  toxicity of, 2931-2932
Local area network (LAN), 3104
Local disaster preparedness, 3017
Local gas gangrene, 2208
Local wound exploration, in abdominal trauma, 501
Locus ceruleus
  in anxiety disorders, 1744
  in mood disorders, 1735
Logistic regression models, 3055
Loiasis
  drug therapy for, 2100t
  visual disturbances in, 2110
Loma Prieta earthquake, 2016, 2017
Longitudinal studies, types of, 3047
Long-range handgun wounds, 957, 957f
Loop diuretics, 1321t
  for acute pulmonary edema, 1270t, 1272
  for chronic heart failure, 1276
Loperamide
  for diarrhea, 236t
  for traveler's diarrhea, 1487
Loratadine, during pregnancy and lactation, 2790
Lorazepam, 2484, 2484t
  for agitation in delirious patient, 1654
  for alcohol withdrawal syndrome, 2862, 2863
  for alcohol-related seizure, 2864, 2865
  for anxiety disorders, 1750
  for neuroleptic malignant syndrome, 2449
  for psychedelic-induced intoxication, 2408
  for psychostimulant intoxication, 2410
  for rapid tranquilization, 2962-2963
  for seizure, 166, 166t, 1626, 1627t, 1919
  for status epilepticus, 2672-2673, 2672t
  for thought disorders, 1731
  prophylactic, in severe head trauma, 361
Lordosis, in pregnancy, 2727
Losartan, 1322t
Low-back pain. *See* Back pain.
Lower airway obstruction, pediatric, 2532-2552
  in anaphylaxis, 2546-2550
  in asthma, 2532-2544
  in bronchiolitis, 2544-2546
  in foreign body aspiration, 2550-2551, 2551f
Lower esophageal sphincter, defective, in gastroesophageal reflux, 1388
Lower extremity
  aneurysm of, 1354
  escharotomy of, 924
  immobilization of, 569-571, 570f, 572f, 573f
  isolated mononeuropathy of, 1694b, 1697-1699
  ulcers of, 1350-1351, 1971
  vascular injury of, 546-547
  venous anatomy of, 1368-1369
Lower gastrointestinal bleeding, 220-227
  diagnostic approach to, 220-223, 221b
  differential diagnosis in, 220, 221b, 223
  disposition in, 225-227, 225b, 226t
  management of, 223-225, 223f
Lower leg
  arteries of, 540f, 797
  trauma to, 796-805
    anatomy and physiology in, 797
    compartment syndrome and, 804
    foreign bodies and, 805
    Osgood-Schlatter disease in, 799
    proximal extra-articular tibial fracture in, 797-799
    proximal fibula fracture in, 801-802, 802f
    proximal tibiofibular joint dislocation in, 802-803
    soft tissue injuries in, 547, 804-805
    stress fracture in, 803-804
    tibial shaft fracture in, 799-801, 801f
Lower respiratory tract infection
  in bronchiolitis, 2544-2546
  in pertussis, 2004-2007, 2005f, 2006b, 2559-2560
  in pneumococcal disease, 2016-2020, 2020b
  in pneumonia, 1128-1141, 2554-2564. *See also* Pneumonia.
Lower sulcus examination, in red and painful eye, 286
Lower urinary tract trauma
  bladder injuries in, 519-526, 521f-526f
  urethral injuries in, 515-519, 516f-520f
Low-molecular-weight dextran, for frostbite, 2233
Low-molecular-weight heparin
  advantages of, 1188
  during pregnancy and lactation, 2757, 2786
Low-molecular-weight heparin *(Continued)*
  for acute coronary syndromes, 1187-1188
  for deep vein thrombosis, 3065-3066
Lown classification of premature ventricular contractions, 1225, 1225t
Lown-Ganong-Levine syndrome, 1237
Low-output states, arterial embolism vs., 1352
Loxapine, 2446t
LSD (lysergic acid diethylamide), 2406-2408, 2407f
Lubeluzole, after cerebral ischemia, 71
Lubricants, for constipation, 241t, 242
Ludington's test, in biceps tendon rupture, 697
Ludwig's angina, 1028, 1032, 1118-1119
Lugol's iodine solution, for thyroid storm, 1989
Lumbar disk herniation, 432, 433f, 702-703, 704-705, 711-712
Lumbar plexus, 718
Lumbar puncture
  headache after, 1641
  in alcohol-related seizure, 2864
  in central nervous system infection, 1716, 1716b
  in cerebral venous thrombosis, 1670-1671
  in delirium, 1652
  in headache, 172, 173t
  in subarachnoid hemorrhage, 1636
  pediatric
    contraindications to, 2660
    in bacterial meningitis, 2659-2662, 2660b, 2661f, 2661t
    in febrile seizure, 2507
    in headache, 2679
    in seizure, 2671
    procedure for, 2660-2661, 2661f
  traumatic, 1717-1718
Lumbar spine
  anatomy of, 400f, 702, 702f
  vertebral osteomyelitis in, 2184
Lumbar vertebrae, 399, 400f
Lumbosacral plexopathy, 1692-1693, 1693b
Lumbosacral plexus, 1676
Lumbosacral spine, 702, 702f
Lumbrical muscles, 580, 581f
Lunate
  anatomy of, 622, 623f, 625
  dislocation of, 630, 632f
  fracture of, 629
Lung. *See also* Cardiopulmonary; Pulmonary; Respiration; Respiratory.
  abscess in, 1033, 1134, 1134f
  cancer of
    hypercalcemia in, 1914
    superior vena cava syndrome in, 1909
  collapsed. *See* Pneumothorax.
  examination of
    in chest pain, 187t
    in dyspnea, 178t
    in fever, 135
  fetal, 119
  infarction of, pulmonary embolism with, 1373
  transplantation of, 2855-2856
  uremic, 1542
Lung disease. *See* Pulmonary disorders; *specific diseases, e.g.,* Pneumonia.
Lung infection. *See* Respiratory tract infection.
Lung injury. *See* Pulmonary trauma.
Lungfluke, 2101t, 2110-2111
Lunotriquetral ligament, 622, 624f
Lunula, 589
Lupus erythematosus
  drug-induced, 1809, 1809t
  systemic, 1805-1812
    clinical features of, 1806-1808, 1806b
    diagnosis of, 1808
    disposition in, 1811-1812
    epidemiology of, 1805
    immune thrombocytopenia in, 1896-1897
    in pregnancy, 1810, 2775-2776
    management of, 1808-1810
    myocarditis in, 1297
    oral manifestations of, 1035, 1035f
    panniculitis in, 1817
    pathophysiology of, 1806
    pericarditis in, 1284
    skin lesions in, 1862t, 1863f
Luxatio erecta, 692-693, 692f-694f
Lye, ingestion of, 2380, 2381, 2381t

Lying, pathologic, in Munchausen's syndrome, 1762
Lyme disease, 2118-2129
acute disseminated infection in, 2123-2124, 2128
arthritis in, 1788-1789, 2124, 2126
carditis in, 2123-2124, 2128
clinical features of, 2119, 2121f, 2122-2125
diagnosis of, 2125
differential considerations in, 2126
early, 2122-2123, 2122f, 2123t, 2127-2128
epidemiology of, 2119, 2120f
facial paralysis in, 1667, 1668
in pregnancy, 2128-2129
late, 2124-2125, 2128
management of, 2126-2128, 2127t
mononeuropathy multiplex in, 1699-1700
myocarditis in, 1291-1292
neurologic disorders in, 2123, 2128
ophthalmologic disorders in, 2124
vaccine for, 2126-2127
vertigo in, 2683
Lymph node(s)
in head and neck, 1075, 1075f
regional, in tularemia, 2131
Lymphadenitis, tuberculous, 2158
Lymphadenopathy
cervical
in African trypanosomiasis, 2106
in Kawasaki disease, 2026
in peritonsillitis, 1117
in pharyngitis, 1109, 1110f
in genital herpes, 1558
in plague, 3027
in rubella, 1850
in tuberculosis, 2152, 2152f
inguinal, in lymphogranuloma venereum, 1562
mediastinal, differential diagnosis in, 2157
Lymphangitis, traumatic, of penis, 534
Lymphatic system, of hand, 586
Lymphocyte(s), function of, 1886
Lymphocyte count
and hematopoietic involvement in radiation exposure, 2322
normal values for, 1886t
radiation dose and, 2317t, 2321
Lymphocytic choriomeningitis virus, 2055
Lymphocytic leukemia
acute, 1888
chronic, 1888
Lymphocytosis, 1887b, 1888
in leukemia, 1888
in pneumonia, 2561
Lymphogranuloma venereum, 1518t, 1519, 1557t, 1559t, 1562
Lymphohematogenous dissemination of tuberculosis, 2147-2148
Lymphoma
acute tumor lysis syndrome in, 1911
central nervous system, in HIV/AIDS, 2082
central nervous system infections in, 1920
Hodgkin's, radiation-induced pericarditis in, 1284
hyperuricemia in, 1913
immune thrombocytopenia in, 1897
superior vena cava syndrome in, 1909
Lymphomatoid granulomatosis, 1814
Lymphoproliferative disorders, in HIV/AIDS, 2079
Lysergic acid diethylamide, 2406-2408, 2407f
Lyssavirus, rabies from, 2065
"Lytic" cocktail, for procedural sedation and analgesia, in children, 2954

Mach effect, 558
Machupo virus, 2056
Macrocytic anemia, 1873-1875, 1874f, 1874t, 1875t
Macrocytosis, in alcoholism, 2873
Macroglobulinemia, Waldenstrom's, hyperviscosity syndrome in, 1912
Macroglossia, 2522
Macrolides
during pregnancy and lactation, 2784
for otitis media, 1069
Macrophage, 2834
Macula, 1045f
Macular disorders, 1059, 1059f, 1970
Macular purpura, 1839t
Macules, 1839t, 1844-1848
MADFOCS mnemonic, 1720t
Magnesium
as antidysrhythmic drug, 1212
for alcohol withdrawal syndrome, 2863
imbalance of. *See* Hypermagnesemia; Hypomagnesemia.
normal physiology of, 1947
Magnesium antacids, for upper gastrointestinal disorders, 1398
Magnesium sulfate
for asthma, 1087t, 1089-1090, 2542
for atrial flutter, 1229
for atrial tachycardia, 1228
for cardiac arrest, 93
for diabetic ketoacidosis, 1966
for digitalis toxicity, 2371
for dysrhythmia, 2586b
for eclamptic seizure, 1627-1628, 1627t
for hypomagnesemia, 1949
for junctional tachycardia, 1234
for pediatric resuscitation, 104
for premature ventricular contractions, 1225
for tetanus, 2011
for torsades de pointes, 113, 1244
for ventricular tachycardia, 1242
in pregnancy
for asthma, 2762
for eclamptic seizure prophylaxis, 2750, 2751
for myocardial infarction, 2766
for premature labor, 2806, 2806b
Magnesium wasting, in alcoholic hepatitis, 1409
Magnet, for pacemaker malfunction, 1251-1252, 1251b, 1252f-1254f
Magnetic resonance angiography
in ischemic stroke, 1613
in peripheral arteriovascular disease, 1348
Magnetic resonance cholangiopancreatography, in pancreatitis, 1433
Magnetic resonance imaging
in abdominal trauma, 499
in airway foreign body aspiration, 867
in ankle trauma, 811
in aortic dissection, 1327t, 1328
in appendicitis, 1455
in arthritis, 1780
in back pain, 708, 709f
in central nervous system infection, 1719-1720
in cerebral venous thrombosis, 1670
in deep venous thrombosis, 1370
in delirium, 1651
in epidural abscess, 708, 709f
in foot trauma, 822
in fracture, 558
in frostbite, 2231
in headache, 2679
in hip fracture, 746
in ischemic stroke, 1613
in knee extensor tendon injuries, 783
in knee ligament injuries, 791
in knee trauma, 774-775
in Legg-Calvé-Perthes disease, 2707
in meniscal tears, 793
in minor head trauma, 365
in multiple sclerosis, 1673, 2910
in osteomyelitis, 2181-2182, 2182f
in peripheral vascular injury, 542
in pregnancy, 2730
in pregnant trauma patient, 321
in scaphoid fracture, 628
in seizure, 2671
in septic arthritis, 2190
in severe head trauma, 362, 362t
in soft tissue foreign body, 879
in spinal carcinoma, 712-713
in spinal cord disorders, 1680
in spinal injuries, 431-435, 433f-436f
in tendinopathy, 1801
in vertebral osteomyelitis, 2182f, 2185
in vertigo, 146
Magnetic resonance spectroscopy, in multiple sclerosis, 2910
Magnetic resonance venography, in cerebral venous thrombosis, 1670
Magnolia officinalis, 2476
Ma-huang
abuse of, 2893
adverse effects of, 2476t
drug interactions with, 2478t
Maisonneuve fracture, 551t, 802, 802f, 814f
Major basic protein, in asthma, 1081
Major burn injury, 920
Major histocompatibility complex antigens, 2833
Malabsorption
alcohol consumption and, 2868-2869
in chronic pancreatitis, 1435
Malaise
in infective endocarditis, 1301
in pneumonia, 2556
Malar erythema, in systemic lupus erythematosus, 1863f
Malaria
anemia in, 2107, 2107f
cerebral, 2104f, 2105
drug therapy for, 2101t-2102t
fever in, 2099, 2103-2104, 2104f
visual disturbances in, 2110
Malathion, for *Phthirus pubis* infestation, 1569
Male
cystitis in, 1585
genitalia of, anatomy of, 516f
hypogonadism in, 2871
pyelonephritis in, 1585
sexual assault of, 992
urinary tract infection in, 1573, 1574, 1585-1586
urine collection methods in, 1575
Malgaigne fracture, 551t, 727
Malignant disease. *See* Cancer.
Malignant hypertension, 1315
acute renal failure in, 1535
dialysis for, 1548
Malignant hyperthermia, 14, 2257
Malignant otitis externa, 1071
Malingering, 1761-1765, 2980
clinical features of, 1763
diagnosis of, 1764, 1764b
differential considerations in, 1764
disposition in, 1765
management of, 1765
somatoform disorders vs., 1757
visual loss and, 1061
Mallampati score, 4, 5f
Malleolar fractures, 812-813, 813f
Mallet finger, 605-607, 606f, 607f
Mallory-Weiss tears, from vomiting, 201
Malnutrition
hypothermia and, 2239
in AIDS-related diarrhea, 1483
Malpighian layers, 914
Malpresentations, in labor and delivery, 2811-2816, 2811b, 2811t, 2812f, 2813b, 2814f, 2815f, 2816b
Malrotation
of metacarpal or phalangeal fracture, 594, 594f, 595f
of phalangeal fractures, 595
with midgut volvulus, 2606-2608, 2607f, 2608f
Malunion, 564
in Colles' fracture, 633
in phalangeal fracture, 595
Mammalian bite. *See* Animal bite; Human bite.
Managed care, medical screening examination and, 3161-3162
Management decision making, 127, 131t, 132
Mandible, 384
anatomy of, 1026, 1027f
dislocation of, 1041-1042, 1041f
fracture of, 394-395, 395f
Mandibular division of trigeminal nerve, 384
Maneuvers for diagnosis and treatment of dysrhythmias, 1214-1215
Mania, 1738-1739, 1738b
differential considerations in, 1741
stabilization in, 1741
substance-induced, 1740, 1740b
Mannitol
for acute renal failure, 1538, 2650
for cerebral herniation, 1918
for ciguatera fish poisoning, 1473-1474
for closed-angle glaucoma, 1056
for elevated intracranial pressure, 360, 367
for heatstroke, 2264
for hyperuricemia, 1914

Mannitol *(Continued)*
  for rhabdomyolysis, 1982
  neuroprotective effects of, 360
  preoperative, in arterial injury, 544
Mann-Whitney test, 3053
Mantoux test, 2150-2157, 2157b, 2150t
Manual strangulation, 450
Maoexipril, 1322t
Maprotiline, overdose of, 2352, 2354
Marburg virus, 2054
March fracture, 551t
March hemoglobinemia, 1883
Marfan syndrome, 2901t
  aortic dissection in, 1324-1325
  sudden death in, 2597
Marijuana use, 2411-2412
  during pregnancy, 2792
  emergency department visits related to, 2884f
Marine animal envenomations, 908-911
Mask, for tuberculosis exposure prophylaxis, 2170
Mask continuous positive airway pressure, 28
Mask ventilation. *See also* Bag/mask ventilation.
  heated, 2249
  laryngeal. *See* Laryngeal mask airway.
  mechanical, 29
Masked depression, 1737
Mass
  abdominal
    in abdominal aortic aneurysm rupture, 1333
    in abdominal trauma, 494
    in children, 2646
  adnexal
    in ectopic pregnancy, 2743
    pelvic pain in, 250t
  anorectal, 1508-1509
  hypothenar, 576, 577f
  neck, 1075-1076, 1075f, 1076b
  red blood cell, in thermal burns, 918
  scrotal, 1593-1598
    anatomy and physiology in, 1594, 1594f
    differential considerations in, 1594-1598
    in children, 2638-2642, 2639f-2640f
Masseter spasm
  from succinylcholine, 14
  in tetanus, 2009
Mast cells
  activated, mediators of, 1823, 1823b
  in asthma, 1080-1081, 1080f
Mastication, muscles of, 1026, 1027f
Mastocytosis, 1835
Mastoiditis, 1071-1072
Material exploitation of elder, 1010
Material resources, in emergency medical services, 2987-2988, 2988f
Material safety data sheet, 3081, 3082b
Mauriceau maneuver, 2813
Maxillary division of trigeminal nerve, 384
Maxillary sinus, 1123
  teardrop sign in, from orbital wall fracture, 1044, 1045f
Maxillary sinusitis, 1034, 1124, 1124f, 1125f
McBurney's point, 1451, 1452
McGill forceps, for oropharyngeal foreign body removal, 1384
McMurray's test, in meniscal tears, 774
McRoberts' maneuver, in shoulder dystocia, 2815, 2815f
MDMA (methylenedioxymethamphetamine), 2408-2409, 2410-2411
  abuse of, 2894, 2895
  overdose of, 2392-2393
  rhabdomyolysis from, 1979
Mean corpuscular hemoglobin (MCH), 1871t
Mean corpuscular hemoglobin concentration (MCHC), 1871t
Mean corpuscular volume (MCV), 1871t
Measles, 2052-2053, 2053f
  Kawasaki disease vs., 2601
  screening for, 2509b
  skin lesions in, 1019
  vaccine for, 2035t, 2053
Mebendazole, for *Enterobius vermicularis* gastroenteritis, 1482
Mechanical obstruction of small bowel, 1440
Mechanical ventilation
  abdominal trauma after, 492
  basic approaches to, 26-27
  evolving therapies in, 33
Mechanical ventilation *(Continued)*
  in asthma, 1092-1093
  in burn care, 922
  in chronic obstructive pulmonary disease, 1103-1113, 1105t
  in flail chest, 450, 450b
  in sepsis, 2219
  in submersion victim, 2314
  in tetanus, 2011
  initial settings and ongoing monitoring in, 29-30, 29t
  intubation for. *See* Intubation.
  mask, 29
  outcomes in, 33
  patient management in, 30-31
  special clinical circumstances in, 31-32
  techniques in, 27-28
Meckel's diverticulum, 2613-2615, 2614t
Meckel's scan, 2613
Meclizine, for vertigo, 146
Meconium aspiration, resuscitation in, 120, 120f, 122
Media
  in disaster response, 3015
  violence and, 1018
Medial collateral ligament
  anatomy of, 770, 771f, 808, 809f
  injury to, 778, 791-792
  stress test of, 771
Medial condyle
  anatomy of, 647, 647f, 770, 771f
  fracture of, 660-661, 661f
Medial elbow dislocation, 665
Medial epicondyle
  avulsion of, in little leaguer's elbow, 663, 663f
  fracture of, 662-663, 662f
Medial epicondylitis, 1798-1799, 2710-2711
Medial malleolus
  anatomy of, 808, 809f
  fracture of, 813, 814f
Medial meniscus, injury to, 792-793
Medial orbital wall fracture, 393
Medial patellar retinaculum injury, patellar dislocation and, 785
Medial retinacula, 770, 771f
Medial tibiofemoral compartment, 770, 771f
Median nerve, 586-587, 588f, 589f, 622, 625f, 648, 648f
  compression of, in pregnancy, 2733
  injury to
    in Colles' fracture, 633
    in posterior elbow dislocation, 665
    palmaris longus laceration and, 609
    neuropathy of, 639, 639f, 1696-1697, 1697b, 1697f
    palsy of, 587, 588f
Mediastinal crunch, in pneumopericardium, 1288
Mediastinal hematoma, sternal fracture and, 456
Mediastinal irrigation, for rewarming in accidental hypothermia, 2250
Mediastinal widening
  abdominal trauma and, 510, 511f
  in aortic rupture, 478-479, 478f
Medical clearance, of combative patient, 2965
Medical decision making
  information technology for, 3098
  racism in, 3110
Medical director, EMS, 2989-2990
Medical disorders
  abdominal trauma vs., 501-502
  anxiety associated with, 1745-1746, 1746b
  depression associated with, 1739, 1739b
  in intimate partner violence and abuse, 997
  psychosis associated with, 1728-1729, 1728b, 1729t
  somatoform disorders vs., 1757, 1757b
Medical information, 3097
Medical information systems, electronic, 3098
Medical inquiry, in clinical decision making, 125-126, 127f, 130, 131t, 132
Medical liability
  in tactical emergency medical support, 3004-3005
  motive and, 3161
Medical literature
  electronic databases of, 3059
  evaluation of, 3046. *See also* Evidence-based medicine.
  publication bias in, 3050-3051, 3058
Medical procedures
  abdominal trauma from, 492
  esophageal perforation as, 482-483
Medical records
  electronic
    confidentiality and, 3103
    integration with, 3105
  of patient presenting to emergency department, 3162-3163
Medical review officer (MRO), [illegible]
Medical screening examination, 3160-3163
  documentation of, 3162-3163
  implementation of, 3160-3161
  patient withdrawal of request for, 3162
  registration and authorization in, 3161-3162
  requirements for, 3157-3158
  use of ancillary services in, 3160-3161
Medical specialty exceptions in disposition requirements, 3164
Medical students, in observation unit, 3063
Medical teaching/training, bioethical dilemnas in, 3135-3136
Medical threat assessment in tactical emergency medical support, 3004
Medication errors, 3125-3126, 3125t
Medications. *See also* Drug(s).
  abbreviations and notations to avoid for, 3125, 3125t
  [illegible] injuries from, 3001
  in prehospital care, 2987-2988, 2990-2991
Medicine, goals of, 3142-3143
Medicolegal issues, 3156-3173
  combative patient and, 2967-2969
  consent to medical care and, 3166-3169
  disposition requirements and, 3164-3165, 3165t
  emergency medical condition and, 3156-3157
  Emergency Medical Treatment and Active Labor Act and, 3156
  in blood transfusion, 58
  in intimate partner violence and abuse, 1004-1005
  in patient transfer during labor and delivery, 2797
  medical screening examination and, 3160-3163
  of combative patient, 2967-2969
  refusal of medical care and, 3169-3172
  reporting requirements and, 3172-3173
  screening requirements and, 3157-3158
  stabilization requirements and, 3163-3164
  testing requests and requirements and, 3158-3160
Meditation, for anxiety disorders, 1751
Medulla, vomiting center in, 200, 201f
Mefenamic acid, overdose of, 2343
Megacolon, toxic, 1501, 1502f, 2613, 2616
Megaloblastic anemia, 1873-1875, 1874f, 1874t, 1875t
  in alcoholism, 2873
  in pregnancy, 2768
Melasma gravidarum, 2728
Melena, 221
Meleney's synergistic gangrene, 2208
Membrane potential, 1199-1200, 1200f
Memory loss
  alcohol-induced, 2869
  in delirium, 1649
  in dementia, 1658-1659
  in head trauma, 363
Menarche, median age of, 2722, 2723f
Ménière's disease
  acoustic neuroma vs., 1669
  vertigo in, 146, 147t, 2683
Meningioma, acoustic neuroma vs., 1669
Meningismus
  in HIV/AIDS, 2079
  in Rocky Mountain spotted fever, 2134
Meningitis, 1710
  after basilar fracture, 370
  ancillary studies in, 1720
  bacterial
    ancillary studies in, 1720
    cerebrospinal fluid analysis in, 1716-1719, 1717t, 1718t, 1719f
    complications of, 1715
    diagnosis of, 1716-1720
    differential considerations in, 1720, 1721b
    disposition in, 1723
    epidemiology of, 1711

Meningitis *(Continued)*
etiology of, 1711-1712, 1711b, 1712b
lumbar puncture in, 1716, 1716b, 2659-2662, 2660b, 2661f, 2661t
management of, 1721-1723, 1721t
neuroimaging studies in, 1719-1720
pathophysiology of, 1713
pediatric, 2657-2665
clinical features of, 2658-2659, 2658t
diagnosis of, 2659-2663, 2660b, 2661f, 2661t
differential considerations in, 2663, 2663b
management of, 2663-2665, 2664t
pathophysiology of, 2657-2658
rash in, 2658, 2659
signs and symptoms of, 1714
cerebrospinal fluid analysis in, 1716-1719, 1717t, 1718t, 1719f
complications of, 1715-1716
cryptococcal, 2081
diagnosis of, 1716-1720
differential considerations in, 1720, 1721b
disposition in, 1723
epidemiology of, 1711
etiology of, 1711-1712, 1711b, 1712b
fungal
complications of, 1715-1716
management of, 1722
pathophysiology of, 1713
signs and symptoms of, 1714
headache in, 174t, 1641
host factors predisposing to, 1714t
in cancer patient, 1920
in Lyme disease, 2123
in meningococcal disease, 1711-1712, 1714, 1715, 1720, 1721t, 1722-1723, 2021-2022
in otitis media, 1068
in pneumococcal disease, 1711, 1714, 1715, 1720, 1721t, 1723, 2019
in tuberculosis, 2160-2161
complications of, 1715
in HIV/AIDS, 2082
management of, 2161
signs and symptoms of, 1714
spinal, 2161
lumbar puncture in, 1716, 1716b
management of, 1721-1723, 1721t
neuroimaging studies in, 1719-1720
noninfectious causes of, 1712b
pathophysiology of, 1713
risk factors for, 171b
seizure in, 1623, 2669
signs and symptoms of, 1714
viral, 2663, 2664
ancillary studies in, 1720
cerebrospinal fluid analysis in, 1716-1719, 1717t, 1718t, 1719f
complications of, 1715
diagnosis of, 1716-1720
differential considerations in, 1720, 1721b
disposition in, 1723
epidemiology of, 1711
etiology of, 1712, 1712b
lumbar puncture in, 1716, 1716b
management of, 1722, 1723
neuroimaging studies in, 1719-1720
pathophysiology of, 1713
signs and symptoms of, 1714
Meningococcal disease, 2020-2024
Henoch-Schönlein purpura vs., 2615
in children, 2506, 2507, 2509b
meningitis in, 1711-1712, 1714, 1715, 1720, 1721t, 1722-1723, 2021-2022
pediatric bacteremia in, 2506
Meningococcal vaccine, 1723, 2024
Meningoencephalitis
arboviral, 2049
in Lyme disease, 2123
seizure in, 1623
Meningomyelocele, neonatal resuscitation in, 121
Meniscal tears, 792-793
anterior cruciate ligament injury and, 790
stability testing in, 774
Menkes' kinky-hair syndrome, fracture in, 2701
Menstruation
asthma associated with, 1082
catamenial pneumothorax and, 1144
current, fibrinolytic therapy eligibility and, 1192
toxic shock syndrome and, 2028
Mental illness. *See* Psychiatric disorders.
Mental retardation, abuse of persons with, 1015
Mental space infection, 1029
Mental status, altered. *See also* Consciousness, altered.
alcohol-induced, 2869
categories of, 153, 154f
confusion as, 150
definitions of, 156-157
differential diagnosis in, 2397
fever and, 136, 2509b
headache and, 170
in adrenal insufficiency, 1997
in hemodialysis patient, 1551-1552, 1552b
in hyperglycemic hyperosmolar nonketotic coma, 1968
in ischemic stroke, 1609
in isopropyl alcohol poisoning, 2403
in methanol poisoning, 2396
in nonconvulsive status epilepticus, 2667
in PCP intoxication, 2891, 2892
in toxic shock syndrome, 2029
treatable causes of, mnemonic for, 157, 157t
Mental status examination, 151, 152f, 153f
in delirium, 1649-1650, 1650f
in systemic lupus erythematosus, 1811
in thought disorders, 1730
Meperidine, 2922t, 2923
during pregnancy and lactation, 2784
for acute pancreatitis, 1433
for migraine, 1633t, 1634
oral, 2920, 2925
pharmacology of, 2452
toxicity of, 2452, 2453t
vs. morphine, 2920-2921, 2920t
Mepivacaine, 2931t, 2932t
Meralgia paresthetica, 1698, 2733
6-Mercaptopurine, for inflammatory bowel disease, 1502
Mercury
antidotes to, 2329t
poisoning from, 2424-2426, 2425b, 2425t
sources of, 2425b
Meropenem, for febrile, neutropenic cancer patient, 2838t
Mersilene suture, 852t
Mesalamine, for inflammatory bowel disease, 1502
Mescaline, 2409, 2409f
Mesenteric adenitis, appendicitis vs., 2620
Mesenteric artery, superior, 1445
embolism of, 1445-1446, 1446b
thrombosis of, 1446
Mesenteric ischemia
abdominal pain in, 214t
acute, 1444-1449
clinical features of, 1446-1447
diagnosis of, 1447-1448, 1448f
differential diagnosis in, 1448
in mesenteric venous thrombosis, 1446, 1446b
in superior mesenteric artery emboli, 1445-1446, 1446b
in superior mesenteric artery thrombosis, 1446
management of, 1448
chronic, 1444-1445
nonocclusive, 1446, 1446b
Mesenteric tear, in seat belt injuries, 491
Mesenteric venous thrombosis, acute mesenteric ischemia in, 1446, 1446b
Mesoridazine, toxicity of, 2445, 2446t
Mesothelioma, pericardial, 1916
Meta-analysis, 3057-3058
Metabolic acidosis, 1926-1930, 1927f, 1931b. *See also* Ketoacidosis.
dialysis for, 1549
etiology of, 1927-1929, 1927b
high anion gap, 1927-1929, 1927b
delirium in, 1651
in cyanide poisoning, 2437
in ethylene glycol poisoning, 2399, 2400-2401
in methanol poisoning, 2396, 2397
seizure in, 1622
in abdominal trauma, 495
in acute renal failure, 1539, 2650
in diarrhea, 2624
in salicylate overdose, 2340
Metabolic acidosis *(Continued)*
management of, 1929-1930
physiologic compensation in, 1929
renal compensation in, 1923-1924
with normal anion gap, 1927b, 1929
Metabolic alkalosis, 1930-1931, 1931b
causes of, 1930, 1930b
from vomiting, 201
renal compensation in, 1924
saline-resistant, 1931
saline-responsive, 1930-1931
Metabolic changes, in pregnancy, 2724
Metabolic disorders
delirium in, 1648, 1649
in acute tumor lysis syndrome, 1912
in opioid overdose, 2454
in substituted phenol poisoning, 2464
myopathy in, 1708-1709, 1978
neuropathy in, 1692
seizure in, 1622
Metabolic encephalopathy, in cancer patient, 1920-1921
Metabolic optic neuropathy, 1060
Metacarpal arches, 578, 580f
Metacarpal base fracture, 599
Metacarpal bones, 577-578, 579f-580f
Metacarpal fracture, 595-600, 597f-599f
Metacarpal head fracture, 596-597, 597f
Metacarpal neck fracture, 597-598, 597f, 598f
Metacarpal shaft fracture, 598-599, 598f
Metacarpophalangeal joint, 578, 579f
dislocation of
finger, 602-603, 602f, 603f
thumb, 603-604
extensor tendon injuries at, 608
laceration of, with metacarpal head fracture, 596-597
stability testing of, 601
Metal, elemental, skin injuries from, 937
Metal detector
in esophageal foreign body, 872
in esophageal obstruction, 1383
Metal poisoning, 2418-2426
arsenic in, 2423-2424, 2424b
iron in, 2418-2421, 2419t, 2420f, 2420t
lead in, 2421-2423, 2422t
mercury in, 2424-2426, 2425b, 2425t
Metaphyseal fracture, 2699
Metaphyseal spurs, normal-variant, 2699
Metaphysis, 2175, 2175f
Metaplasia, Barrett's, 1389
Metaproterenol, for chronic obstructive pulmonary disease, 1105
Metaraminol, for junctional tachycardia, 1234
Metastatic cancer
epidural spinal cord compression in, 1919
hyperuricemia in, 1913
Metatarsal base fractures, 832-834, 833f
Metatarsal bones
fractures of, 831-836
stress fracture of, 837
Metatarsal head and neck fractures, 832
Metatarsal shaft fractures, 831-832
Metatarsalgia, 837
Metatarsophalangeal dislocations, 835
Metered-dose inhaler plus spacer/holding chamber
for asthma, 2538, 2539t, 2540
for chronic obstructive pulmonary disease, 1105
instructions for, 1094b
nebulizer vs., 1087-1088
Metformin, 1972-1973
alcohol interactions with, 2877
during pregnancy and lactation, 2790
lactic acidosis from, 1928-1929
Methadone, 2922t, 2925
for opioid withdrawal, 2455
respiratory effects of, 2453t
Methamphetamine, 2393, 2893-2896
Methanol poisoning, 2395-2398, 2887
antidotes to, 2329t
disposition in, 2402
management of, 2400-2402, 2401t
metabolic acidosis in, 1928
pharmacology and metabolism in, 2395, 2396f
vs. ethylene glycol poisoning, 2397-2398
Methantheline, anticholinergic toxicity of, 2345

Methazolamide, for increased intraocular pressure, 292
Methcathinone, 2393, 2893
Methemoglobinemia, 268, 269b, 269f, 273, 936, 2889, 2891. *See also* Cyanosis.
Methemoglobin forming agents, antidotes to, 2329t
Methicillin-nafcillin, for pneumonia, 2558t
Methicillin-resistant *Staphylococcus aureus*, 1130
Methimazole
 for hyperthyroidism in pregnancy, 2773
 for thyroid storm, 1988
Methohexital
 as induction agent, 15
 for procedural sedation and analgesia, 2940t-2941t, 2945-2946, 2949-2950, 2951t, 2953
Methotrexate, 2844
 for ectopic pregnancy, 2746
 for rheumatoid arthritis, 1791
Methoxamine, for junctional tachycardia, 1234
Methyl mercury poisoning, 2425, 2426
Methyldopa, 1321t, 2789
Methylene blue
 for methemoglobinemia, 273
 for nitrite abuse, 2890
Methylene chloride, toxicity of, 2887
Methylergonovine, after miscarriage, 2742
Methylparaben, allergy to, 847
Methylprednisolone
 for anaphylactic shock, 54
 for anaphylaxis, 2549
 for asthma, 1088, 2539t, 2541, 2543t
 for chronic obstructive pulmonary disease, 1106
 for Goodpasture syndrome, 1816
 for hypothermia, 2246
 for multiple sclerosis, 1673
 for optic neuritis, 1059-1060
 for rheumatologic disease, 2776
 for spinal cord injury, 309
 for spinal injuries, 438
 for systemic lupus erythematosus, 1809
 for temporal arteritis, 1060
Methylxanthines
 for asthma, 1090, 1090t
 for chronic obstructive pulmonary disease, 1105
 for postdural puncture headache, 1641
Methysergide, for migraine prophylaxis, 1634
Metoclopramide
 alcohol interactions with, 2875
 for gastroesophageal reflux, 1390
 for migraine, 2680
 for nausea and vomiting, 206
Metolazone, 1321t
Metoprolol, 1209, 1321t
 during pregnancy and lactation, 2788
 overdose of, 2373t
Metronidazole
 during pregnancy and lactation, 2758, 2785
 for amebic abscess, 1416
 for amebic dysentery, 235
 for bacterial vaginosis, 1567t, 1568
 for *Clostridium difficile* enterocolitis, 1475
 for *Giardia* gastroenteritis, 1479-1480
 for tetanus, 2011
 for trichomoniasis, 1567-1568, 1567t
Metropolitan Medical Response Systems, 3019
Mexican beaded lizard, 896, 902
Mexiletine, 1207
Mezlocillin, for cholangitis, 1422
Miconazole, during pregnancy and lactation, 2785
Microangiopathic hemolytic anemia, 1883
Microbiology
 in sepsis, 2210-2217
 in tuberculosis, 2154-2157, 2154f, 2157b, 2158t
Microcytic anemia, 1871-1873
Micrognathia, 2522
Microhematuria
 in bladder rupture, 521
 in kidney trauma, 528
 in pelvic fracture, 719
 in ureteral trauma, 531
Microreentry, 1204
Microscopic polyangiitis, 1813-1814
Microscopy, direct, in tuberculosis, 2154, 2154f
Microsomal ethanol-oxidizing system (MEOS), 2859
Microwave irradiation, 2319
 for rewarming in accidental hypothermia, 2250
Midazolam, 2484, 2484t
 as induction agent, 16
 for anxiety disorders, 1750
 for procedural sedation and analgesia, 2940t-2941t, 2944-2945
  in children, 2953
  with fentanyl, 2950, 2951t
 for seizure, 166, 166t, 1626, 1627t
 for status epilepticus, 2672t, 2673
 for tetanus, 2011
 in ventilated patient, 30
Midcarpal joint
 anatomy of, 622, 623f
 collapse of, 631-632, 632f, 633f
Middle ear
 barotrauma to, 2281-2282, 2282f, 2286-2287, 2287t, 2292
 infection of. *See* Otitis media.
Middle phalanx
 extensor tendon injuries at, 607
 fracture of, 594-595, 594f-596f
Midface fracture, 393-394, 394f
Midfoot
 anatomy of, 820, 820f
 cuboid fracture of, 828
 cuneiform fracture of, 828
 dislocation of cuneiform, cuboid, or navicular bones of, 828
 Lisfranc injuries in, 828-831, 829f, 830f
 navicular fracture of, 827-828
 pain in, 837
Midgut volvulus, malrotation with, 2606-2608, 2607f, 2608f
Midline lethal granuloma, oral manifestations of, 1035
Midpalmar space infection, 617-618, 617f
Midrin, for migraine, 2680
Midtarsal joint
 anatomy of, 820, 820f
 injuries to, 827
Migraine, 1631-1634
 basilar artery, 1632
 clinical features of, 1631-1633
 diagnosis of, 1633
 differential diagnosis in, 1633
 hemiplegic, 1632
 ophthalmoplegic, 1632
 pathophysiology of, 1631
 pediatric, 2678-2679, 2678b
 prophylactic therapy for, 1634
 seizure in, 1624
 seizures vs., 2668
 status migrainosus and, 1632-1633
 treatment of, 1633-1634, 1633t
 types of, 2678-2679
 with aura, 1631, 1632, 1632b, 2678, 2678b
 without aura, 1631, 1632b, 2678, 2678b
Miliaria rubra, 2259
Miliary tuberculosis, 2152, 2159-2160, 2160f
Military Assistance to Safety and Traffic (MAST) program, 2995
Military forces, disaster response responsibility of, 3019
Milk thistle, adverse effects of, 2476t
Milk-alkali syndrome, hypercalcemia in, 1945
Milker's node virus, 2040
Milrinone
 for acute pulmonary edema in hypotensive patient, 1274
 for cardiogenic shock, 54
 for heart failure, 2583t, 2584
Mineralocorticoids
 excess of, metabolic alkalosis in, 1930
 replacement of, for adrenal insufficiency, 1990
Minimal sedation, 2938, 2939b
Minimally conscious state, 156
Mini-mental state examination, 151, 152f, 1650, 1650f
Minor. *See also* Adolescent; Child.
 consent to treatment on behalf of, 3167-3168
 emancipated, 3168
 mature, 3168
 refusal of medical care for, by parent or guardian, 3171
Minor burn injury, 920
Minoxidil, 1321t
Minute ventilation
 carbon dioxide arterial pressure and, 1923
 during acclimatization to high altitude, 2297-2298
 in metabolic acidosis, 1080
Miosis
 in nerve agent exposure, 3030
 in opioid overdose, 2453
 traumatic, 1049
Mirtazapine, overdose of, 2362-2363
Miscarriage, 2740-2742
 clinical features of, 2740-2741
 diagnosis of, 2741, 2741b, 2741t
 differential considerations in, 2741
 ectopic pregnancy vs., 2745
 management of, 2741-2742
 pathophysiology of, 2740
 terminology in, 2740
Misoprostol
 after miscarriage, 2742
 for upper gastrointestinal disorders, 1399
Mist therapy, for viral croup, 2526
Mites
 in HIV/AIDS, 2085
 skin lesions in, 1854-1855, 1854f
Mithramycin, for hypercalcemic cancer patient, 1916
Mitochondrial function, in shock, 42, 43f
Mitral insufficiency, heart failure in, 1265
Mitral regurgitation, 1306
 heart failure in, 1265
 in pregnancy, 2763t, 2767
Mitral stenosis, 1305-1306
 in pregnancy, 2763t, 2767
Mitral valve prolapse, 1304-1305, 1747
Mixed cryoglobulinemia, 1815
Mixed venous oxygen saturation, in shock, 50
MOANS mnemonic, for evaluation of difficult bag/mask ventilation, 4, 4b
Mobitz type I (Wenckebach) second-degree atrioventricular block, 1218-1219, 1218t, 1219b, 1220f
Mobitz type II second-degree atrioventricular block, 1218t, 1219-1220, 1220f
Moderate burn injury, 920
Moderate sedation, 2938, 2939b
Molar pregnancy, 2741, 2746-2747
Molindone, 2446t
Molluscum contagiosum, 1861f, 2040, 2085
Monash method for snakebite management, 899
Mongolian spots, 974, 975f
Monitoring, 35-40
 blood gas, 36-39
  capnography/capnometry in, 37-39, 38f
  pulse oximetry in, 36-37
  transcutaneous and conjunctival, 36
 blood pressure, 35-36
 cardiac. *See also* Electrocardiography.
  during cardiopulmonary resuscitation, 79-82, 80f-82f, 80t
  in hypothermia, 2245
  in myocardial infarction, 1173-1174, 1173f
 core temperature
  in heatstroke, 2263
  in hypothermia, 2244
 during procedural sedation and analgesia, 2942-2943
 during ventilatory support, 29-30, 29t
 fetal
  electronic, 2800
  in pregnant trauma patient, 39, 319, 323-324, 324f
 home, for apparent life-threatening event or SIDS, 2720
 in asthma, 1085
 in cardiac arrest, 79-82, 80f-82f, 80t
 in heart failure, 1209, 1270t, 2773
 in multiple trauma, 304, 305
 in shock, 50
Monkey hand, 587, 588f
Monkeypox virus, 2040
Monoamine oxidase inhibitors
 classification of, 2363b
 for anxiety disorders, 1751, 1751t
 hypertension in patient taking, 1313, 1314b
 meperidine interactions with, 2923
 overdose of, 2363-2365, 2363b-2365b, 2364t

Monocytes, 1886t
Monomethylhydrazine, overdose of, 2329t
Mononeuropathy
  common peroneal, 1698-1699, 1698f
  diabetic, 1669-1670, 1971
  isolated, 1693-1699, 1694b
  lateral femoral cutaneous, 1698
  median, 1696-1697, 1697b, 1697f
  radial, 1693-1695, 1694f
  sciatic, 1697-1698, 1698f
  ulnar, 1695-1696, 1695f, 1696f
Mononeuropathy multiplex, 1699-1700, 1699b, 1971
Monosodium urate crystals, in synovial fluid, 1781-1782
Monospot tests, in pharyngitis, 1111
Monteggia fracture-dislocation, 551t, 642, 642f, 2697
Montelukast, for asthma, 1090
Mood disorders, 1734-1742. *See also* Bipolar disorder; Depression.
  caused by general medical condition, 1739, 1739b
  cerebral anatomy and, 1735
  clinical features of, 1736-1740, 1736b, 1737b, 1738b
  cyclothymic disorder and, 1739
  diagnosis of, 1740
  differential considerations in, 1740-1741
  epidemiology of, 1735
  genetics of, 1736
  hypothalamic-pituitary-adrenocortical system in, 1735-1736
  management of, 1741-1742, 1741b
  neurotransmitters in, 1735
  psychosocial theories of, 1736
  substance-induced, 1739-1740, 1740b
  suicide and, 1769
  with psychotic features, 1729
Mood stabilizers, for bipolar disorder, 1742
Moral rules, 3130, 3130b
Moraxella (Branhamella) catarrhalis, 1130
Morbilliform rash, drug-induced, 1844, 1844f
Moricizine hydrochloride, 1207
Morphine, 2921-2923, 2921t
  during pregnancy and lactation, 2784
  for acute coronary syndromes, 1184
  for acute pancreatitis, 1433
  for acute pulmonary edema, 1270t, 1271-1272
  for anxiety disorders, 1750
  for burn patient, 924
  for high-altitude pulmonary edema, 2304
  for hypoxic (tet) spells, 2580-2581
  for knee trauma, 776
  for pulmonary edema in chronic renal failure, 1546
  for sickle cell disease, 1880
  meperidine vs., 2920-2921, 2920t
  oral, 2925
  respiratory effects of, 2453t
Morrison's pouch, 498, 498f
Morton's neuroma, 837
Morulae, in ehrlichiosis, 2138
Motility disorders. *See also* Constipation; Diarrhea.
  esophageal, 1388, 1395-1396, 1397
  in opioid overdose, 2453
  small bowel, 1440, 1441b, 1443
Motive, medical liability and, 3161
Motor disturbances
  in cerebral palsy, 2904
  in ischemic stroke, 1609
  in multiple sclerosis, 1672
  in spinal cord disorders, 1678f, 1679
Motor examination
  in head trauma, 357
  in spinal injuries, 416, 417t
Motor function, developmental milestones in, 2495-2497, 2496t
Motor innervation of hand, 586-587, 588f, 589f
Motor neuron disease
  clinical characteristics of, 1680t, 1703t, 1704
  in amyotrophic lateral sclerosis, 1700
  upper vs. lower, 1704t
Motor strength, grading score for, 1704b
Motor tracts, 1676, 1676f
Motor vehicle crashes. *See also* Pedestrian collisions.
  aortic injury from, 476, 477
Motor vehicle crashes *(Continued)*
  biomechanical risk factors in, 946-947
  cardiac trauma from, 467
  death from, 300
  facial trauma from, 382, 383
  forensic aspects of, 963-966, 964b, 965f-966f, 966b
  hip dislocation from, 756
  in elderly person, 344-345
  in pregnancy, 318
  injury control in, 943, 943t, 944t, 946-947, 948
  mechanism of injury of, 303t
  myocardial contusion from, 467
  myocardial rupture from, 470
  spinal injuries from, 399
  sternal fracture from, 456
Motorcycle accidents
  death from, 300
  facial trauma from, 382
Mottling of skin, in pediatric assessment, 2499, 2499f
Mountain sickness, acute, 2296, 2299, 2299f, 2300-2303, 2301b
Mouth. *See also* Oral *entries.*
  anatomy of, 384
  laceration of, 391
Movement disorders
  alcohol-induced, 2870
  pediatric, ataxia as, 2681-2682, 2681b
  seizures vs., 2668
Moxifloxacin, for tuberculosis, 2164t, 2165
MPTP, parkinsonism caused by, 2452
Mucin clot test, in acute septic arthritis, 2705, 2706t
Mucocutaneous hyperpigmentation, in Addison's disease, 1997
Mucocutaneous lymph node syndrome. *See* Kawasaki disease.
Mucokinetic medications, for chronic obstructive pulmonary disease, 1106
Mucormycosis, 1123, 1124, 1126
Mucous clearance strategies, for chronic obstructive pulmonary disease, 1106
Muerto Canyon virus, 2055
Multicollinearity, 3055
Multiculturalism, 3107-3117. *See also* Cultural competence.
Multifocal atrial tachycardia, 1228, 1229f
Multi-infarct dementia, 1657
Multiple comparisons, and risk of type I error, 3053-3054
Multiple gestations
  incidence of, 2722
  labor and delivery in, 2816
Multiple myeloma
  hypercalcemia in, 1914
  hyperuricemia in, 1913
  hyperviscosity syndrome in, 1912
Multiple organ dysfunction syndrome (MODS)
  definition of, 2211
  in pancreatitis, 1427, 1429
  in sepsis, 2213-2214
  in solvent abuse, 2888
  trajectory of dying in, 3140-3141, 3140f
Multiple sclerosis, 1671-1674, 2909-2911
  anxiety in, 1747-1748
  ataxia in, 2682
  clinical features of, 1672
  diagnosis of, 1672-1673
  differential considerations in, 1673
  disposition in, 1674
  in pregnancy, 2763t, 2769-2770
  management of, 1673
  optic neuritis and, 1059
  pathophysiology of, 1671-1672
  seizure in, 1624
  spinal cord lesions in, 1681-1682
  vertigo in, 148t, 2684
Multiple trauma, 300-314
  clinical features in, 309-311, 310f
  diagnostic strategies in, 311-313, 313f
  disposition in, 311
  epidemiology of, 300
  etiology of, 302, 303t
  examination and reassessment in, 305
  in elderly person, 345
  management of, 302-309, 304b
  monitoring in, 305
  prehospital care in, 302-304
Multiple trauma *(Continued)*
  radiologic imaging in, 311-313, 313f
  stabilization in, 305-309
  team approach in, 304
  trauma system and, 300-302, 301f, 302b
Multiple victim incidents, prehospital end-of-life issues related to, 3145
Multisystem disease, in tuberculosis, 2159-2160, 2160f
Multivariate models, 3054-3055
Mumps, 1428, 2052
Mumps vaccine, 2035t
Munchausen's syndrome, 1761-1765
  by proxy, 1761, 1763, 1763t, 1765
  clinical features of, 1763
  diagnosis of, 1764
  differential considerations in, 1764, 1764b
  disposition in, 1765
  management of, 1765
Mupirocin, for impetigo, 1842
Murmur
  in aortic regurgitation, 1307
  in aortic rupture, 478
  in aortic stenosis, 1306
  in arteriovenous fistulas, 1347
  in chronic obstructive pulmonary disease, 1100
  in hypertrophic cardiomyopathy, 1295
  in infective endocarditis, 1301
  in mitral regurgitation, 1306
  in mitral stenosis, 1305
  in mitral valve prolapse, 1305
  in myocardial rupture, 471
  in tetralogy of Fallot, 2580
  in tricuspid stenosis and regurgitation, 1307
  innocent, 2572
  pediatric, 2571-2572, 2572b
Murphy's sign
  in cholecystitis, 1420
  in pancreatitis, 1429
Muscarinic acetylcholine receptors, 2345, 2346, 2347f
Muscimol, 2479
Muscle
  of forearm, 640t
  of hand, 578, 580-585, 581f-585f
  of hip and thigh, 737, 737t, 738f
  of knee, 770, 771f
  of lower leg, 797
  of shoulder, 672, 673f
  of upper arm, 648
Muscle contraction headache, in pregnancy, 2732
Muscle cramps, heat-induced, 2258, 2258b
Muscle fasciculations, in nerve agent exposure, 3030
Muscle relaxation, in reduction of glenohumeral joint dislocation, 688-689
Muscle spasm, in tetanus, 2009
Muscle weakness. *See* Weakness.
Muscles of mastication, 1026, 1027f
Muscular dystrophy, 2900t
Musculocutaneous nerve, 672
Musculoskeletal disorders
  in chronic renal failure, 1542-1543
  in developmentally disabled patient, 2901-2902
  pediatric, 2689-2711
    anatomy and physiology in, 2689
    apophyseal, 2709-2711, 2711f
    child abuse and, 2698-2701
    physeal, 2690, 2691f, 2691t, 2692, 2692f
    rhabdomyolysis as. *See* Rhabdomyolysis.
Musculoskeletal pain, during pregnancy, 2733
Musculoskeletal system
  aging and, 345
  examination of, in spinal cord injury, 310-311
  in pregnancy, 2727
Musculoskeletal trauma. *See* Orthopedic injuries.
Mushrooms
  anticholinergic, 2412-2413, 2412f
  cholinergic, 2413
  psilocybin, 2406-2408, 2407f
  toxicity of, 2477-2479, 2478t
Mustard exposure, 938-939, 3031
Mutilating injuries, to hand, 609
Muzzle contusion, 956, 956f
Myalgia
  during pregnancy, 2733
  in rhabdomyolysis, 1979

Myasthenia gravis, 1705-1707, 1706b
  diagnosis of, 1705-1706, 1706b
  exacerbation of, drug-induced, 1706, 1706b
  in pregnancy, 2764t, 2770-2771
  management of, 1706-1707
  oropharyngeal dysphagia in, 1397
  weakness in, 141
Mycobacterial infection
  fungal and nontuberculous, 2157
  in cancer patient with impaired cell-mediated immunity, 2840
  in organ transplant patient, 2849
Mycobacterium avium, 2076
Mycobacterium tuberculosis. *See also* Tuberculosis.
  in HIV/AIDS, 1136, 1140-1141, 2078-2079
  in pneumonia, 1130-1131
Mycobacterium tuberculosis direct test (MTDT), 2155
Mycophenolate, 2844
  for organ transplant patient, 2850, 2851f
Mycoplasma pneumoniae, 1130, 1132
  in children, 2558-2559, 2563t
  in myocarditis, 1292
  in pharyngitis, 1109, 1111, 1112, 1113
Mycotic aneurysm, 1356, 1357t
Mydriasis
  in psychedelic intoxication, 2408
  pharmacologic, 1061
  traumatic, 1049
Mydriatics, 1063b, 1064
  for red and painful eye, 292, 297t
Myelitis, 1710
  transverse, 1682
Myeloid leukemia, chronic, neutrophilia in, 1887-1888, 1887f
Myeloma
  hypogammaglobulinemia in, 2840-2841
  multiple
    hypercalcemia in, 1914
    hyperuricemia in, 1913
    hyperviscosity syndrome in, 1912
Myelopathy
  clinical characteristics of, 1680t, 1703t, 1704
  cystic, in spinal cord injury, 2909
  in HIV/AIDS, 1683
Myeloperoxidase, as cardiac marker, 1178
Myelophthisic anemia, 1876, 1876f
Mylohyoid muscle, 1027
Myocardial biopsy
  in dilated cardiomyopathy, 1294
  in myocarditis, 1290, 1290f
Myocardial cell action potential, 1200, 1201f, 1202f
Myocardial cell membrane, electrophysiology of, 1199-1201, 1200f-1202f
Myocardial concussion, 467
Myocardial contusions
  in children, 340
  observation in, 3068
Myocardial dysfunction, after resuscitation, 77
Myocardial fibrosis and scarring, heart failure from, 1263-1264
Myocardial hypertrophy, 1169-1170, 1172f. *See also* Hypertrophic cardiomyopathy.
Myocardial infarction. *See also* Acute coronary syndromes.
  anatomic location of, 1164-1166, 1164t, 1165f-1167f
  angina in, 1158, 1158t
  anterior, 1164, 1165f
  anxiety in, 1746
  atypical symptoms of, 1158-1159, 1159t
  cardiogenic shock in, 54, 1160
  chest pain centers and, 1181-1182
  chest pain in, 183, 186, 188, 189f, 190t-191t
  clinical features of, 1157-1161, 1158t, 1159t
  cocaine-related, 2001
  creatine kinase MB isoenzyme in, 1176f, 1176t, 1177-1178
  definition of, 1156
  Dressler syndrome after, 1189-1190, 1283
  early complications of, 1160-1161
  echocardiography in, 1179
  electrocardiography in, 1161-1174
    abnormalities in, 1161-1163, 1162f-1164f, 1162t
    additional lead, 1171-1173, 1172f, 1173f
    adjuncts in, 1171-1174
Myocardial infarction *(Continued)*
    anatomic location of infarct on, 1164-1166, 1164t, 1165f-1167f
    body surface mapping and, 1174
    fibrinolytic therapy eligibility and, 1190
    limitations of, 1174
    noninfarct ST segment elevation and, 1166-1170, 1167f-1172f
    NSTEMI and, 1170-1171
    QT dispersion and, 1174
    serial, 1173-1174, 1173f
  epidemiology of, 1155
  free wall rupture in, 1160
  graded exercise testing in, 1180-1181
  heart failure in, 1268
  historical perspective of, 1155
  in aortic dissection, 1326
  in diabetes mellitus, 1970
  in elderly person, 2828
  in Kawasaki disease, 2025, 2026, 2595
  in left bundle branch block, 1167, 1170f
  in pregnancy, 2766-2767
  inferior, 1164, 1165f, 1166, 1167f
  ischemic stroke after, 1608
  lateral, 1164, 1165f
  management of
    angiotensin-converting enzyme inhibitors in, 1185
    antiplatelet therapy in, 1185-1187
    antithrombotic therapy in, 1187-1188
    aspirin in, 1185
    beta blockers in, 1184-1185
    calcium channel blockers in, 1185
    chest pain centers and, 1181-1182
    delay in, reasons for, 1183
    direct thrombin inhibitors in, 1188
    fibrinolytic therapy in, 1189-1192, 1192b
    glycoprotein IIb/IIIa receptor inhibitors in, 1186, 1194
    heparins in, 1187-1188
    morphine in, 1184
    nitroglycerin in, 1184
    percutaneous coronary intervention in, 1186, 1192-1193, 1195
    physical examination in, 1159, 1159t
    prehospital care in, 1157
    reperfusion therapy in, 1189-1195
      choice of, 1193-1194
      combination, 1194-1195
      in cardiogenic shock, 1194
      process time points for, 1183, 1184f
      time to, 1182-1184, 1183f, 1184f
    thienopyridines in, 1186-1187
    time to treatment and, 1182-1184, 1183f, 1184f
    transfer of patient with, 1195
  missed diagnosis of, 1160
  myoglobin in, 1175f, 1176t, 1178
  nausea and vomiting in, 205t
  non-ST segment elevation, 1170-1171
  observation in, 3064, 3065
  outcome of, time to treatment and, 1182-1184, 1183f, 1184f
  pathophysiology of, 1156-1157
  pericarditis in, 1160, 1282-1283
  pneumothorax vs., 1146
  posterior, 1166, 1166f
  previous, fibrinolytic therapy eligibility and, 1191
  Q waves in, 1156, 1164
  radionucleotide scanning in, 1179-1180
  right ventricular, 1166, 1167f, 1172-1173
  ST segment abnormalities in
    monitoring of, 1173-1174, 1173f
    regional, 1164t
  ST segment depression in, 1162-1163, 1163f, 1171
  ST segment elevation, 1161-1162, 1162t, 1163f
  stroke in, 1161
  T wave in
    hyperacute, 1161, 1162f
    inverted, 1163-1164, 1164f, 1171
  time from symptom onset in, fibrinolytic therapy eligibility and, 1190-1191
  transmural, 1156
  troponins in, 1175-1177, 1175f, 1176t
  without chest pain, outcomes in, 1159
Myocardial ischemia
  acute
    observation in, 3064, 3065
Myocardial ischemia *(Continued)*
    risk stratification in, 3065
    time insensitive predictive instrument for, 3065
  chest pain in, 188t, 189f
  heart failure in, 1268
  hypertension in, 1316
  in hypomagnesemia, 1949
  in pathophysiology of acute coronary syndromes, 1156-1157
  orofacial pain in, 1034
Myocardial lavage, for rewarming in accidental hypothermia, 2250
Myocardial stunning, 77
Myocarditis, 1289-1293
  clinical features of, 1289
  cocaine-related, 1292-1293
  diagnostic strategies in, 1289-1290
  differential diagnosis in, 1290
  disposition in, 1290-1291
  doxorubicin-related, 1292
  epidemiology of, 1289
  etiology of, 1289
  heart failure in, 1264-1265, 1268
  in Chagas' disease, 1291
  in connective tissue disorders, 1297-1298
  in diphtheria, 1291
  in HIV/AIDS, 1292
  in infants and children, 2591-2592
  in Kawasaki disease, 1293, 2025, 2594
  in Lyme disease, 1291-1292
  in meningococcal disease, 2022
  in Rocky Mountain spotted fever, 2134
  in systemic lupus erythematosus, 1807
  in trichinosis, 1291
  management of, 1290
  pathophysiology of, 1289
  risk factors for, 186b
  sudden death in, 1298
Myoclonic seizure, 1621
Myoclonus
  alcoholic, 2870
  from etomidate, 2947-2948
Myofascial pain, temporomandibular, 1034-1035
Myofibrils, 1259
Myoglobin
  in myocardial infarction, 1175f, 1176t, 1178
  in renal pathology of rhabdomyolysis, 1977
  in sarcoplasm, 1976
  release of. *See* Rhabdomyolysis.
  urine, in rhabdomyolysis, 1980
Myoglobinuria
  in electrical and lightning injuries, 2276
  in heatstroke, 2264
Myonecrosis, 2196t, 2208-2209
Myonephropathic-metabolic syndrome, in arterial embolism, 1343
Myopathy
  alcohol-induced, 2870
  clinical characteristics of, 1680t, 1703t, 1704
  in hyperthyroidism, 1987
  inflammatory, 1708
  metabolic, 1708-1709, 1978
Myosin heavy chain, mutation of, in hypertrophic cardiomyopathy, 1294
Myositis, 2196t, 2208-2209
Myositis ossificans–heterotopic ossification, of femur and hip, 741-742, 743f-754f
Myringitis, bullous, 1066-1067
Myringotomy, for otitis media with effusion, 1069-1070
Myxedema, in hypothyroidism, 1863f
Myxedema coma, 1990, 1990b, 1991, 1991b, 1993-1994, 2239

NADH methemoglobin reductase deficiency, cyanosis in, 200
Nadolol, 1209, 1321t, 2373t, 2374
Naegleria infection, neurologic disorders in, 2107
Nafcillin, for staphylococcal scalded skin syndrome, 1845
Nägele's rule, 2727
Nail
  ingrown, 837
  paronychia and, 614-615, 615f
  structural framework of, 589

Nail bed
  avulsion of, 611
  laceration of, 594, 611
  trauma to, 610-611
Nail matrix, 589
Nalbuphine, 2924, 2924b
Nalmefene, for opioid overdose, 2455
Naloxone
  for alcohol intoxication, 2860
  for alcohol withdrawal syndrome, 2861
  for opioid overdose, 2328, 2455
  for opioid reversal, 2948-2949
  for overdosed/poisoned patient, 2326
  for Wernicke-Korsakoff syndrome, 2869
  in neonatal resuscitation, 123t, 124
Naproxen, for migraine, 2680
Narcissistic personality disorder, 2979b
Narcotic, 2451. *See also* Opioid(s).
Narrow-complex tachycardia, 1226-1235
  atrial fibrillation as, 1230-1233, 1231f, 1232b, 1232f
  atrial flutter as, 1229-1230, 1230f-1231f
  atrial tachycardia as, 1228-1229, 1228f, 1229f
  in infants and children, 2586-2587, 2588f
  junctional tachycardia as, 1233-1235, 1233f, 1234f
  P wave in, 1234f
  sinus tachycardia as, 1227-1228, 1227f
Nasal capnography, in asthma, 1085
Nasal congestion, in bronchiolitis, 2545
Nasal flaring, in pediatric assessment, 2498-2499, 2499f
Nasal pack, for epistaxis, 1074, 1075
Nasal polyp, 1082
Nasoethmoid complex fracture, 393-394
Nasogastric intubation
  esophageal perforation from, 483
  in abdominal trauma, 494
  in acute pancreatitis, 1433-1434
  in burn injury, 923
  in gastric volvulus, 1394
  in gastrointestinal bleeding, 223-224
  in hypothermia, 2244
  in neck trauma, 444
  in small bowel obstruction, 1444
Nasogastric suctioning, metabolic alkalosis from, 1930
Nasotracheal intubation, 12
  esophageal perforation from, 483
  in multiple trauma, 306
  in neck trauma, 444
National Clinicians' Postexposure Prophylaxis Hotline, 3083
National Disaster Medical System, 3018
National Guideline Clearing House, 3037, 3037t
National Heart Attack Alert Program, 1181
National Institute on Drug Abuse, drug testing guidelines of, 3080
National Institute on Elder Abuse, 1009
National Institutes of Health Expert Panel Report 2, on asthma diagnosis and management, 1083
Natriuretic peptides, in heart failure, 1263, 1269-1270
Natural killer cells, 2833
Naturalistic process, clinical decision making by, 127, 131t, 132
Nausea, 200-207
  ancillary studies in, 202-203
  chest pain associated with, 185, 186t
  definition of, 200
  differential considerations in, 201-202, 201t, 203, 204t-206t, 207f
  disposition in, 207, 209
  epidemiology of, 200
  history in, 202
  in abdominal aortic aneurysm rupture, 1333
  in abdominal trauma, 493
  in *Aeromonas hydrophila* gastroenteritis, 1467
  in appendicitis, 2619
  in *Bacillus anthracis* gastroenteritis, 1469
  in cholecystitis, 1420
  in cholelithiasis, 1418
  in chronic renal failure, 1542
  in ciguatera fish poisoning, 1473
  in esophagitis, 1387
  in gastritis, 1391
  in hemorrhagic *Escherichia coli* serotype O157:H7 gastroenteritis, 1467
Nausea *(Continued)*
  in infants and children, 203, 208t
  in opioid overdose, 2453
  in pancreatitis, 1429
  in *Plesiomonas shigelloides* gastroenteritis, 1468
  in pregnancy, 204t, 206, 2756
  in salmonellosis, 1463
  in *Vibrio* fish poisoning, 1472
  in *Vibrio parahaemolyticus* gastroenteritis, 1466
  in viral gastroenteritis, 1476
  management of, 203, 206, 207f, 208b, 208t
  palliative care for, 3153-3154
  pathophysiology of, 200-201, 201f
  physical examination in, 202, 202t
  rapid assessment and stabilization in, 201t, 202
Navicular
  accessory, 822, 822f, 837
  dislocation of, 828
  fracture of, 827-828
  stress fracture of, 837-838
Nebulizer, for asthma, 1087-1088
Neck. *See also* Head and neck.
  examination of, in dyspnea, 178t
  mass in, 1075-1076, 1075f, 1076b
  mobility of, difficult airway and, 4
  nuchal rigidity and
    causes of, 2663
    in bacterial meningitis, 2658, 2659
    in central nervous system infection, 1714
  zones of, 442, 442f, 443b
Neck stiffness
  causes of, 2663
  in bacterial meningitis, 2658, 2659
  in central nervous system infection, 1714
Neck swelling
  in aortic rupture, 478
  in *Bacillus anthracis* gastroenteritis, 1469
  in diphtheria, 2003
  in spinal cord injury, 2906
  in superior vena cava syndrome, 1910
Neck trauma, 441-451
  airway management in, 444-445
  anatomy in, 442-443, 442f, 443b
  clinical features of, 443, 443b
  diagnostic strategies in, 443
  disposition in, 446
  laryngotracheal injuries in, 447-448
  management of, 443-446
  near-hanging and strangulation in, 450-451
  nerve injuries in, 450
  pathophysiology of, 441-442, 442t
  pharyngoesophageal injuries in, 446-447
  thoracic duct, glandular, and retropharyngeal injuries in, 450
  tracheobronchial injury in, 466, 466f
  transcervical gunshot wounds in, 446
  vascular injuries in, 448-450
  venous air embolism in, 444, 450
  vertigo in, 144, 147t
Neck vein distention
  in neoplastic cardiac tamponade, 1917
  in superior vena cava syndrome, 1910
Necrobiosis lipoidica diabeticorum, 1972
Necrotizing abscess, 1515
Necrotizing anorectal infection, 1515
Necrotizing cellulitis, synergistic, 2209
Necrotizing enterocolitis, 2608-2609, 2609f
Necrotizing fasciitis, 2196t, 2207-2208
Necrotizing otitis externa, 1071
Necrotizing ulcerative oral diseases, 1033, 1033f
Needle, suturing, 853
Needle aspiration
  in osteomyelitis, 2182
  in peritonsillar abscess, 1118
Needle cricothyroidotomy
  for airway foreign body, 2530
  in pediatric resuscitation, 108
Needle cricothyrotomy, with transtracheal jet ventilation, 22, 22f
Needle decompression, for pneumothorax, 1147
Needle electromyography, 1689
Neer classification
  of proximal humerus fractures, 680-681, 681f
  of subacromial syndromes, 694, 694t, 695f
Neer's test, in rotator cuff tendinopathy, 1797
Negative predictive value, 3059t
Negative pressure rewarming, 2248
Negative reactions of physicians, 2975-2976
Negative symptoms in schizophrenia, 1726, 1728
Neglect
  child. *See* Child abuse.
  elder, 1010. *See also* Elderly person, abuse of.
Neisseria gonorrhoeae, 1518t, 1519, 1559t, 1565-1567, 1565f. *See also* Gonorrhea.
Neisseria meningitidis, 2021. *See also* Meningococcal disease.
Nematocysts, in marine animal envenomations, 909, 910
Nematode infections, parasites in, 2099t
Neologisms, in schizophrenia, 1727-1728
Neomycin, for hepatic encephalopathy, 1412
Neonatal abstinence syndrome, 2794
Neonatal resuscitation, 118-124
  chest compressions in, 123
  discontinuation of, 120
  disposition in, 124
  in anatomic abnormalities, 121
  in late decelerations of fetal heart rate, 2801
  in meconium aspiration, 120, 120f
  indications for, 119-120
  medications in, 123-124, 123t
  oxygen therapy, ventilation, and intubation in, 122-123
  positioning, suctioning, and stimulation in, 121-122
  preparation for, 121, 121b
  transition from fetal to extrauterine life and, 118-119, 119t
Neonate. *See also* Infant.
  acute bacterial meningitis in, 2657, 2658-2659
  air medical transport of, 2999
  Apgar score of, 122, 122t
  apnea in, 119
  assessment of, 2804
  circulation in, 2568-2569
  clavicle fracture in, 2693
  developmental milestones in, 2496, 2496t
  fever in, management of, 2512-2514, 2513b
  herpes simplex virus infection in, 1559
  hyperthyroidism in, 2773
  hypoglycemia in, 119
  hypomagnesemia in, 1948
  hypothermia in, 119, 2239
  hypoxia in, 119
  jaundice in, 2601-2603, 2602t, 2603b, 2603t, 2604f-2605f
  lupus erythematosus in, 1810
  necrotizing enterocolitis in, 2608-2609, 2609f
  osteomyelitis in, 2183-2184
  otitis media in, 1067
  pulmonic flow murmur of, 2572
  red and painful eye and, 292
  seizure in, 2667
  urinary tract infection in, 1583, 1583t
  vital signs in, 119t
  vomiting in, 203, 208t
Neoplasm. *See* Tumor.
Neoplastic cardiac tamponade, 1916-1918
Neoplastic constrictive pericarditis, 1917
Neoplastic pericardial tamponade, 1916-1918
Neostigmine, for myasthenia gravis, 1706
Nephritis, lupus, 1806-1807
Nephropathy
  diabetic, in pregnancy, 1972
  heroin, 2453
  HIV-associated, 2086
  pigment, 1536, 1536b
Nephrotic syndrome
  in children, 2648-2649
  proteinuria in, 1531, 1531b
Nephrotomography, bolus infusion intravenous pyelography with, in renal trauma, 528
Nephrotoxicity
  of acetaminophen, 2333
  of cyclosporine, 2850
  of ethylene glycol, 2398, 2399
Nephrotoxins, acute tubular necrosis from, 1536-1537, 1536b, 1538, 1539
Nerium oleander, 2474, 2474f
Nerve block
  for trigeminal neuralgia, 1666
  intercostal, for multiple rib fractures, 456
Nerve conduction studies, 1689
Nerve gases, 939, 2458b, 2461, 3030-3031, 3030b, 3031b

Nerve injury
in electrical and lightning injuries, 2271
in fracture, 559, 559t
in hand trauma, 614
in high-altitude cerebral edema, 2306
in hip trauma, 762-763
in neck trauma, 450
in pelvic fracture, 719-720
in supracondylar fracture, 2696-2697
Nerve supply
to distal humerus and elbow, 648-649, 648f
to face, 383-384
to femur and hip, 737-738
to foot, 821
to forearm, 640t
to hand, 586-587, 588f, 589f
to knee, 771
to lower leg, 797
to shoulder, 672
to wrist, 622, 625f
Nervous system. *See* Central nervous system; Neurologic *entries;* Peripheral nervous system.
Nesiritide, for acute pulmonary edema, 1270t, 1272
Networks, in medical information systems, 3104
Neurapraxia, 559
Neurocysticercosis, seizure in, 1623
Neuroendocrine tumor, pancreatic, 1437
Neurofibrillary tangles, in dementia, 1657
Neurofibromatosis, vertigo in, 2683
Neurogenic bladder, in spinal cord injury, 2908
Neurogenic hypotension, secondary to spinal shock, 437
Neurogenic obstruction of small bowel, 1440
Neurogenic pulmonary edema
after head trauma, 371
after seizure, 1625
Neurohormonal alterations, in heart failure, 1262-1263
Neuroimaging studies
in central nervous system infection, 1719-1720
in headache, 2679, 2680b
in HIV/AIDS, 2079-2080, 2080f
in minor head trauma, 364-365
in severe head trauma, 361-362, 362t
Neuroleptic agents. *See* Antipsychotic agents.
Neuroleptic malignant syndrome, 2257-2258, 2961-2962
clinical features of, 2447, 2447t
differential diagnosis in, 2448, 2448t
from antipsychotic agents, 1732-1733
management of, 2449
serotonin syndrome vs., 2359
Neurologic abnormalities
in acoustic neuroma, 1668-1669
in acute renal failure, 1540
in antidepressant overdose, 2354t, 2356
in bacterial meningitis, 2658
in carbon monoxide poisoning, 2439
in central nervous system infection, 1714
in cerebral venous thrombosis, 1670
in cervical vascular injury, 449
in chronic renal failure, 1542
in ciguatera fish poisoning, 1473
in electrical and lightning injuries, 2273-2274, 2274
in epidural abscess, 1684
in epidural hematoma, 1683
in ethylene glycol poisoning, 2399
in head trauma, 370-371
in headache, 172t
in heatstroke, 2260-2261, 2262
in hemodialysis patient, 1551-1552, 1552b
in HIV/AIDS, 1683
in hypothermia, 2241
in idiopathic spastic paraparesis, 1683
in intracerebral hemorrhage, 1611
in ischemic stroke, 1009-1010
in lithium toxicity, 2442
in MAOI toxicity, 2305
in mitral valve prolapse, 1305
in multiple sclerosis, 1672, 1601
in opioid overdose, 2452
in organophosphate poisoning, 2460
in osteogenesis imperfecta, 2700-2701
in serotonin toxicity of, 2360
in shigellosis, 1464
in spinal subarachnoid hemorrhage, 1682
Neurologic abnormalities *(Continued)*
in substituted phenol poisoning, 2464
in syringomyelia, 1682-1683
in systemic lupus erythematosus, 1807
in transverse myelitis, 1682
in vitamin B_{12} deficiency, 1874
mushrooms associated with, 2478-2479
Neurologic disorders, 1606-1723
airway foreign body aspiration and, 866
anxiety in, 1747-1748
cranial nerve, 1664-1670, 1665t
delirium in, 1645-1655
dementia in, 1655-1662
headache in, 1631-1643
in botulism, 1707-1708, 2014
in HIV/AIDS, 2079-2082, 2080f
in Lyme disease, 2123, 2128
in pregnancy, 2768-2771
in Rocky Mountain spotted fever, 2134
in spinal cord injury, 2909
pediatric, 2657-2686
peripheral, 1687-1701
seizure in, 1619-1629
spinal cord, 1675-1685
stroke in, 1606-1617
Neurologic emergencies, in cancer patient, 1918-1921
Neurologic examination
in back pain, 263
in chest pain, 187t
in comatose patient, 159-161, 159t
in dyspnea, 178t
in facial trauma, 388
in head trauma, 356-357, 357t
in multiple trauma, 309
in nausea and vomiting, 202, 202t
in seizure, 168
in spinal injuries, 415-417
in vertigo, 145
of distal upper extremity, 2694t
Neuroma
acoustic, 147t, 1668-1669
Morton's, 837
Neuromuscular blocking agents
competitive, for rapid sequence intubation, 14-15, 15t
for critically ill asthmatic patient, 1092-1093
for intubation, 13-15
for tetanus, 2011
in intubated, mechanically ventilated patient, 31
Neuromuscular disorders, 1702-1709
clinical characteristics of, 1680t, 1703-1704, 1703t
diagnosis of, 1704-1705
differential considerations in, 1703t, 1704
history in, 1703
in hyperkalemia, 1940
laboratory studies in, 1704-1705
oropharyngeal dysphagia in, 1396
physical examination in, 1703-1704
weakness and, 139, 139t, 140b, 1702-1709
Neuromuscular junction, 1703
Neuromuscular junction disease, 1705-1708
clinical characteristics of, 1680t, 1703t, 1704
in botulism, 1707-1708, 2014
in myasthenia gravis, 1705-1707, 1706b
in tick paralysis, 1708
Neuronal theory of headache, 2676
Neuronitis, vestibular, vertigo in, 147t
Neuronopathy
in amyotrophic lateral sclerosis, 1700
sensory, 1700, 1700b
Neuroophthalmologic visual loss, 1059-1061
Neuropathic pain, 1692
Neuropathy, 1687-1701. *See also* Mononeuropathy; Polyneuropathy.
alcoholic, 1692, 2869
anatomy in, 1000-1009, 1000f
ancillary studies in, 1700-1701, 1701b
asymmetric proximal and distal, 1092-1093, 1693b
autonomic
diabetic, 1971
in alcohol withdrawal syndrome, 2861
in tetanus, 2009
clinical features of, 1689-1700, 1703t, 1704
cranial, 1664-1670, 1665t
diabetic, 1669-1670
Neuropathy *(Continued)*
eye movement disorders in, 1062-1063
in ethylene glycol poisoning, 2399
in Lyme disease, 2123
in tetanus, 2009
diabetic, 1669-1670, 1691-1692, 1970-1971
in pregnancy, 1972
lower extremity ulcers in, 1351, 1972
epidemiology of, 1688
in alcoholism, 1692
in Guillain-Barré syndrome, 1690-1691
in hip trauma, 762-763
in HIV/AIDS, 1692, 2082
in Lyme disease, 2124
in plexopathies, 1692-1693, 1693b
median nerve, 639, 639f
metabolic, 1692
optic
compressive, 1060
glaucoma as, 1055-1056, 1056f
in ethylene glycol poisoning, 2399
in methanol poisoning, 2395-2396
ischemic, 1060
toxic and metabolic, 1060
traumatic, 1050-1051
pathophysiology of, 1689
patterns and prototypes of, 1690t
peripheral vascular injury and, 539
toxic, 1691b, 1692
Neuroprotective agents, for ischemic stroke, 1616
Neuropsychiatric symptoms, in cocaine overdose, 2388
Neurosis, hysterical, conversion type, 1755, 1755b
Neurotmesis, 559
Neurotoxin
botulinum, 2014
tetanospasmin, 2009
Neurotransmitters
in anxiety disorders, 1744-1745
in delirium, 1646-1647
in mood disorders, 1735
Neurovascular bundle, proximity wounds and, 540, 540f
Neutron exposure, 2319-2320, 2320f
Neutropenia, 1888-1889, 1889t
in cancer patient, 1907-1909, 1908b, 2834-2839, 2836t, 2838t
in children, 2516
Neutrophil(s), 2834
function of, 1886
in arthritis, 1777
in asthma, 1083
in bacterial meningitis, 2662
normal values for, 1886t
Neutrophilia, 1887-1888, 1887b, 1887f
Nevirapine, for HIV/AIDS, 2088
Newborn. *See* Neonate.
Nicardipine, 1321t
for hypertensive emergencies, 1319
for premature labor, 2807
overdose of, 2377t
Nicotiana tabacum, 2474
Nicotine
dermal exposure to, 2474
ingestion of, 2474
inhalation of. *See* Smoking.
Nicotinic acetylcholine receptors, 2345, 2347f
Nifedipine, 1321t
during pregnancy and lactation, 2788
for anal fissures, 1513
for aortic dissection, 1329
for chilblains, 2230
for dysphagia, 1398
for high-altitude pulmonary edema, 2304-2305
for premature labor, 2807
for thrombosed hemorrhoids, 1512
overdose of, 2376, 2377t
Nifurtimox, for Chagas' disease, 2112
Night terrors, 2008
Nightstick fracture, 551t
Nikolsky's sign, in pemphigus vulgaris, 1857
Nimodipine
for aneurysmal subarachnoid hemorrhage, 1607
overdose of, 2377t
9-1-1 universal emergency access number, 2988
Nisoldipine, 1321t
overdose of, 2377t

Nitrates
  abuse of, 936, 2889-2891, 2890b
  burn injury from, 936
  for chronic heart failure, 1276
  for urinary tract infection, 1575-1576
Nitric oxide
  in cerebral ischemia, 65-66
  in heart failure, 1263
  in sepsis, 2213
Nitrogen bubble formation, decompression sickness and, 2283-2284
Nitrogen narcosis, in scuba diving–related disorders, 2283, 2293
Nitroglycerin
  for acute coronary syndromes, 1184
  for acute pulmonary edema, 1270t, 1272
  for anal fissures, 1513
  for aortic dissection, 1329
  for chest pain, 184
  for hypertensive emergencies, 1318
  for pulmonary edema in chronic renal failure, 1546
  for pulmonary edema–related hypertension, 1316
Nitroprusside
  during pregnancy and lactation, 2765t, 2789
  for acute pulmonary edema, 1270t, 1272-1273
  for aortic dissection, 1328
  for heart failure, 2583t, 2584
  for hypertension
    in MAOI toxicity, 2365
    pulmonary edema–related, 1316
  for hypertensive emergencies, 1317-1318, 2653, 2765t
  for hypertensive encephalopathy, 1315
  for intracerebral hemorrhage, 1616
  for pulmonary edema in chronic renal failure, 1546
Nitrous oxide intoxication, solvent abuse vs., 2888
Nitrous oxide-oxygen mixtures, for procedural sedation and analgesia, 2929-2930, 2940t-2941t, 2948, 2950, 2951t
Nitrox I, 2279
Nits, in pediculosis, 1853, 1853f
Nizatidine, 1390t
NMDA receptor antagonists, after cerebral ischemia, 71
"No harm" contract, in suicide, 1773-1774
Nocardiosis
  in cancer patient with impaired cell-mediated immunity, 2840
  in organ transplant patient, 2848
Nociception, 2914-2916, 2915f, 2915t, 2916f, 2916t
Nociceptor, 2914, 2914b
Nocturnal enuresis, 2668
Nodule, 1839t, 1856-1857
  in milker's node virus, 2040
  in molluscum contagiosum, 2040
  in tuberculosis, 2151
  subcutaneous, in rheumatic fever, 1304
Noise stress, during air medical transport, 2995
Noninvasive positive pressure ventilation (NPPV), 28-29, 28f
  evolving therapies in, 33
  in asthma, 1091-1092
  in chronic obstructive pulmonary disease, 1104, 1104t
  initial settings and ongoing monitoring in, 29-30, 29t
  outcomes in, 32-33
  patient management in, 31
  patient selection for, 29
Nonmaleficence, 3129, 3129b
Nonnucleoside reverse transcriptase inhibitors, 2087t, 2088
  rifamycins and, drug interactions between, 2166
Nonparametric statistical tests, 3053
Nonpenetrating ballistic injury, in chest wall trauma, 458-459
Nonshivering thermogenesis, in burned infant, 923
Nonsteroidal antiinflammatory drugs, 2925-2926, 2927b, 2927f
  alcohol interactions with, 2876
  allergy to, 1828
  aspirin-exacerbated respiratory disease from, 1082
Nonsteroidal antiinflammatory drugs *(Continued)*
  during pregnancy and lactation, 2776, 2781, 2784
  for back pain, 267
  for colic syndromes, 2926
  for dental caries pain, 1031
  for gouty arthritis, 1786
  for migraine, 1633, 1633t, 2680
  for pericarditis, 1282
  for pseudogout, 1787
  for reactive arthritis, 1790
  for rheumatoid arthritis, 1791-1792
  for sprain, 566
  for strain, 567
  for subacromial syndromes, 696
  for systemic lupus erythematosus, 1808
  for tendinopathy, 568
  gastritis from, 1390
  guidelines for, 2928
  heart failure from, 1269
  in elderly person, 2826
  mechanisms of action of, 2927f
  ophthalmic, 1063b, 1064
  overdose of, 2342-2344
  peptic ulcer disease from, 1392, 1394
  pharmacokinetics of, 2342-2343
  physiology of, 2342
  renal insufficiency from, 1533
  routes of administration of, 2927
  safety of, 2926
  side effects of, 2926-2927
Nonunion, 564
Noradrenergic system, in mood disorders, 1735
Norepinephrine
  for acute pulmonary edema in hypotensive patient, 1273
  for cyclic antidepressant poisoning, 2356
  for sepsis, 2219t, 2220
  in anxiety disorders, 1744-1745
  in glucose regulation, 1957
  in heart failure, 1263
  in mood disorders, 1735
Norfloxacin
  for *Plesiomonas shigelloides* gastroenteritis, 1468
  for prostatitis, 1586
  for salmonellosis, 1463
  for shigellosis, 1461t, 1464
  for traveler's diarrhea, 1487
Normal-pressure hydrocephalus, dementia in, 1658, 1660
Normeperidine, 2923
Normochromic and normocytic anemia, 1875-1876, 1875t, 1876f
Norovirus gastroenteritis, 1475-1476
Northern Command (NorthCom), 3019
Northridge earthquake, 3016, 3017
Norwegian scabies, 1854, 1855
Nose. *See also* Nasal *entries.*
  anatomy of, 384
  choanal atresia of, 2522
  examination of, in facial trauma, 388
  foreign body in, 863-864
  fracture of, 391-392
  medial wall of, arterial supply to, 1073, 1073f
  soft tissue injuries to, 391
Nosebleed, 394, 863, 1072-1075, 1073f, 1074t
Notification
  death
    by phone, 3148
    empathy in, 3147-3149, 3148b
    training in, bioethical dilemnas in, 3135
  of foodborne diseases and conditions, 1463b
  to referring physician, computerized, 3102
Noxious stimulus, 2914b
Nuchal rigidity
  causes of, 2663
  in bacterial meningitis, 2658, 2659
  in central nervous system infection, 1714
Nuchal signs, as indication for lumbar puncture, 2659
Nuclear explosion injury, 2316-2317, 2317t
Nuclear reactor incidents, 2317
Nuclear studies. *See* Radionucleotide scanning.
Nuclear weapons, disaster preparedness for, 3017-3018, 3022
Nucleic acid amplification tests (NAATs)
  for chlamydia, 1565
Nucleic acid amplification tests (NAATs) *(Continued)*
  for gonorrhea, 1566
  for tuberculosis, 2154
Nucleoside analogue reverse transcriptase inhibitors, 1928, 2087-2088, 2087t
Nucleus pulposus
  anatomy of, 702, 702f
  herniation of, 702-703
Null hypothesis, 3051, 3051t
Number needed to treat, 3059t, 3060
Numbness, in frostbite, 2230
Nurse staffing, for observation, 3062
Nursemaid's elbow, 666, 666f, 2697-2698, 2697f
Nursery care, in emergency department, 2798, 2798b
Nursing home, institutional abuse in, 1009, 1015
Nutcracker esophagus, 1397
Nutcracker fracture, 828
Nutmeg, 2409-2410
Nutrition. *See also* Diet.
  in acute pancreatitis, 1433-1434
  in burn injury, 918
Nutritional deficiency
  dementia from, 1656
  hypothermia and, 2239
  in AIDS-related diarrhea, 1483
Nylon suture, 852t
Nystagmus, 1062
  in PCP intoxication, 2891
  vertigo and, 142-143, 144-145, 145t
Nystatin
  during pregnancy and lactation, 2785
  for oral thrush, 1841

Obese patient
  pulmonary embolism in, 1380-1381
  slipped capital femoral epiphysis in, 2708
Obidoxime, for organophosphate poisoning, 2461
Oblique fracture, 552, 552f
Oblique radiographs, of spinal injuries, 426-428, 426f, 427f, 428f
Observation medicine, 3062-3073
  approach in, 3062-3063
  in abdominal pain, 3063-3064, 3064b
  in asthma, 3069-3070, 3070b
  in atrial fibrillation, 3070-3071, 3070b
  in chest pain, 3064-3065, 3065b
  in congestive heart failure, 3071, 3071b
  in critical diagnostic syndromes, 3063-3069
  in deep vein thrombosis, 3065-3066
  in dehydration, 3071-3072, 3072b
  in emergency conditions, 3069-3073
  in head trauma, 3069
  in infection, 3072-3073, 3072b, 3073t
  in peripheral vascular injury, 544
  in syncope, 3066-3067, 3066b
  in trauma, 3067-3069
  in upper gastrointestinal bleeding, 3066
  principles of, 3062, 3063b
  staffing requirements for, 3062-3063
Observation unit, structure of, 3063
Observational study, longitudinal, 3047
Obsessive-compulsive disorder, 1746b, 1749
Obstetric trauma, 318-326, 320-321, 2733
  blunt, 318
  diagnostic strategies in, 320-321, 320t, 321t
  disposition in, 326
  fetal evaluation in, 323-324, 323f, 323t, 324f
  fetal injury in, 319
  fetomaternal hemorrhage and, 321
  management of, 321-326, 322f
  maternal resuscitation in, 322-323
  penetrating, 318-319
  perimortem cesarean section in, 325-326
  placental injury in, 319-320
  prehospital end-of-life issues related to, 3145
  primary survey in, 322-323
  secondary survey in, 323
  uterine injury in, 320
Obstipation, in large bowel obstruction, 1496
Obstructive acute renal failure, 1533-1534, 1533b, 1538
Obstructive biliary tract disorders, jaundice in, 243, 244f
Obstructive pancreatitis, 1435

Obstructive pulmonary disorders, chronic, 1097-1107. *See also* Chronic obstructive pulmonary disease.
Obtundation, 156, 2865
Obturator dislocation, 756, 757f
Obturator hernia, 1441
Obturator sign, in appendicitis, 1452, 2619
Occlusive injury in peripheral vascular trauma, 537-538, 538f
Occult blood tests, in gastrointestinal bleeding, 222
Occupational health issues in emergency department
  blood-borne pathogen exposure protocol and, 3081-3087, 3084t, 3085t, 3086b
  material safety data sheet and, 3081, 3082b
  tuberculosis prevention and, 2170-2171, 2170b
Occupational medicine, 3076-3081
  definition of, 3076
  drug and alcohol testing in, 3080-3081
  ethical issues in, 3077
  overview of, 3076-3077
  return-to-work issues in, 3078-3080
  workers' compensation and, 3077-3078
Octreotide
  for diarrhea, 236t
  for gastrointestinal bleeding, 225
Ocular bobbing, 161
Ocular dipping, 161
Ocular foreign body, 859-861, 860f, 861f
Ocular hypertension, 1055
Ocular migraine, 2679
Ocular tonometry, in red and painful eye, 286-287
Ocular trauma, 1044-1052
  acid and alkali burns in, 1046, 1046f
  blunt, 1044-1051
  complications of, 1052, 1052f
  in acid and alkali burns, 932
  in anhydrous ammonia exposure, 935
  in bipyridyl compound exposure, 2466
  in child abuse, 971
  in hydrofluoric acid exposure, 933
  in methanol poisoning, 2395-2396
  in mustard exposure, 3031
  of anterior chamber and iris, 1048-1049, 1048f, 1049f
  of cornea and conjunctiva, 1046-1048, 1047f-1048f
  of orbit and lid, 1044, 1045f, 1046, 1051-1052
  of posterior segment, 1050-1051, 1050f
  of sclera and lens, 1049-1050, 1050f
  penetrating, 290, 1051-1052, 1051f
  red and painful eye in, 283, 290, 292, 297
Oculocephalic testing
  in comatose patient, 161
  in head trauma, 357
Oculogyric crisis, antipsychotic-induced, 2446
Oculomotor nerve, 1665t
Oculovestibular testing
  in comatose patient, 161, 162f
  in head trauma, 357
Odds, 3059t
Odds ratio, 3059t
Odontalgia. *See also* Oral pain.
  atypical, 1034
  in scuba diving–related disorders, 2286
Odontoid fracture
  type II, 405, 406f-407f
  type III, 432f
  with anterior dislocation, 399, 401, 402f
Odontoid radiographs, of spinal injuries, 424, 424f-425f
Odors, in poisoning, 2327, 2327t
Odynophagia
  in achalasia, 1397
  in esophagitis, 1387
  in gastroesophageal reflux, 1388
  in neck masses, 1076
Ofloxacin
  for gonococcal dermatitis, 1843-1844
  for pelvic inflammatory disease, 1571t
  for prostatitis, 1586
Ogilvie's syndrome, 1105-1106
Ointment
  for burn wounds, 926
  ophthalmic, 1063
OKT3, for organ transplant patient, 2850-2851
Olanzapine
  for agitation in delirious patient, 1654
  for mood disorders, 1741
  for rapid tranquilization, 2962
  for thought disorders, 1730-1731
  toxicity of, 2446, 2446t, 2448
Oleander, 2474, 2474f
Olecranon
  anatomy of, 647, 647f
  fracture of, 663
Olecranon bursa, 649
Olecranon bursitis, 667, 1801-1803
Olfactory nerve, 1665t
Oligoanalgesia, 2917-2918
Olmesartan, 1322t
Omeprazole, 1390t
Onchocerca volvulus, 2100t, 2109, 2109f
Oncologic emergencies, 1907-1921
  acute tumor lysis syndrome in, 1911-1912, 1911b, 1912b
  central nervous system infections in, 1920
  cerebral herniation in, 1918
  encephalopathy in, 1920-1921
  epidural spinal cord compression in, 1919-1920
  fever in, 1907-1909, 1908b
  hypercalcemia in, 1914-1916, 1915b
  hyperuricemia in, 1913-1914
  hyperviscosity syndrome in, 1912-1913
  neoplastic cardiac tamponade in, 1916-1918
  seizures in, 1919
  superior vena cava syndrome in, 1909-1911, 1910f
Oncovirus, type C, 2056
Ondansetron
  during pregnancy and lactation, 2790
  for nausea and vomiting, 203
One-way analysis of variance (ANOVA), 3052-3053, 3052t
Onychia, candidal, 1841
Open fracture, 552, 558, 558b
  classification of, 749t
  of ankle, 813-814
  of hip, 748-749, 749t
  of pelvis, 719
  of skull, 373-374
  of tibial shaft, 800-801
Open-book pelvic fracture, 727, 728f, 733f
Open-chest cardiac massage, 89-90
Ophthalmia, sympathetic, 1052
Ophthalmic division of trigeminal nerve, 383-384
Ophthalmic drugs, 1063-1064, 1063b
Ophthalmologic conditions, 1044-1064
  acute visual loss and, 1056-1061, 1057f-1059f
  anatomy in, 1045f
  anisocoria and, 1061-1062
  corneal disease and, 1053-1054, 1054f
  epidemiology of, 1044
  extraocular movement disorders and, 1062-1063
  eyelid and ocular soft tissue disorders and, 1054-1055, 1055f
  glaucoma and, 1055-1056, 1056f
  in Graves disease, 1987
  in HIV/AIDS, 2085-2086, 2085-2087
  in Lyme disease, 2124
  in opioid overdose, 2453
  nystagmus and, 1062
  ocular trauma and, 1044-1052. *See also* Ocular trauma.
  ophthalmic drugs for, 1063-1064, 1063b
  optic disk abnormalities and, 1062
Ophthalmologic system, in pregnancy, 2727
Ophthalmologists, disposition requirements related to, 3164
Ophthalmoplegia, in diabetes mellitus, 1669-1670
Ophthalmoplegic migraine, 1632, 2679
Opioid(s), 2916-2920
  adjuvant analgesic agents with, 2921
  agonist-antagonist group of, 2924-2925, 2924b
  allergy to, 1828
  classification of, 2921t-2922t
  common therapeutic mistakes in, 2918-2921, 2919b
  during pregnancy, 2784, 2793-2794
  for abdominal pain, 217, 2925-2926
  for acute pancreatitis, 1433
  for appendicitis, 1450
Opioid(s) *(Continued)*
  for back pain, 264, 267
  for chronic pancreatitis, 1436
  for dental caries pain, 1031
  for migraine, 1633t, 1634
  for procedural sedation and analgesia, 2940t-2941t, 2944, 2952-2953
  for sickle cell disease, 1880
  for urolithiasis, 1592
  in children, 2935, 2952-2953
  in elderly person, 2826-2827
  in HIV/AIDS, side effects of, 2079t
  in rapid sequence intubation, 11b
  in ventilated patient, 31
  injection of
    medicolegal issues in, 3159
    skin lesions associated with, 1864-1865, 1865f, 2453-2454
  intramuscular, disadvantages of, 2919-2920, 2919b
  mechanism of action of, 2918, 2918t
  oral, 2925
  overdose of, 2327t, 2328, 2451-2456
    antidotes to, 2329t
    clinical features of, 2452-2454, 2453t
    diagnosis of, 2454
    differential diagnosis in, 2454
    disposition in, 2455
    management of, 2454-2455
    pathophysiology and pharmacology of, 2451-2452
  parenteral, 2921-2924
  patient given, informed consent in, 3169
  receptors for, 2451
  reversal agents for, 2948-2949
  withdrawal from, 2451-2456
    alcohol withdrawal syndrome vs., 2860
    clinical features of, 2454
    diagnosis of, 2454
    differential diagnosis in, 2454
    disposition in, 2455
    management of, 2455-2456
    pathophysiology and pharmacology of, 2452
Opioid receptors, 2918, 2918t
Opioid/sedative/ethanol syndrome, 2327t, 2328
Opisthorchis felineus, 2101t
Opium tincture, for diarrhea, 236t
Opponens digiti minimi, 580-581, 581f
Opponens pollicis, 580, 581f
Opportunistic infections
  after liver transplantation, 1417
  allograft rejection and, 2848-2849, 2849f
  in cancer patient, that mimic neoplasms, 2841
  respiratory, 1135-1136
Opsoclonus-myoclonus syndrome, ataxia in, 2681
Opsonin, 2834
Opsonization, 2833
Optic disk papilledema, 1062
Optic nerve, 1045f, 1665t
  blunt injury to, 1050-1051
Optic neuritis, 1059-1060
  in multiple sclerosis, 1672, 2910
Optic neuropathy
  compressive, 1060
  glaucoma as, 1055-1056, 1056f
  in ethylene glycol poisoning, 2399
  in methanol poisoning, 2395-2396
  ischemic, 1060
  toxic and metabolic, 1060
  traumatic, 1050-1051
Oral cavity
  examination of, 1029-1030, 1029f, 1030f
  pyogenic granuloma in, 1035
Oral contraceptives, hepatotoxicity of, 1414
Oral flora, 1128
Oral hemorrhage, 1036, 1042
Oral hypoglycemic agents, 1972-1973
  alcohol interactions with, 2077
  overdose of, hypoglycemia from, 1961
  rash from, 1972
Oral infection, extension of, into head and neck, 2229, 2230-2231, 2232f
Oral medicine
  acute necrotic ulcerative gingivitis and, 1032, 1033f
  alveolar bone fracture and, 1040
  anatomy in, 1026-1027, 1027f-1030f
  aphthous stomatitis and, 1036

Oral medicine *(Continued)*
atypical odontalgia and, 1034
blood dyscrasias and, 1036
dental caries and, 1028-1029, 1030-1032, 1030f, 1031f
drug-induced gingival hyperplasia and, 1036
examination of oral cavity in, 1029-1030, 1029f
nontraumatic dental emergencies and, 1027-1029, 1030f
oral hemorrhage and, 1042
oral manifestations of systemic disease and, 1035, 1035f
oral pain and, 1033-1034
paroxysmal pain of neuropathic origin and, 1034
pathophysiology of, 1027-1029
pericoronitis and, 1035
periodontal disease and, 1032-1033
postextraction pain and, 1034
soft tissue injuries and, 1040
subluxated and avulsed teeth and, 1037-1040, 1038f, 1039f
temporomandibular joint dislocation and, 1041-1042, 1041f
temporomandibular myofascial pain dysfunction syndrome and, 1034-1035
tooth fracture and, 1036-1037, 1036f
Oral mucosa
in Kawasaki disease, 2026
laceration of, 391, 1040
antibiotic prophylaxis for, 855
ulcers of, 1036
Oral pain
atypical, 1034
dental caries and, 1030-1031
in acute necrotic ulcerative gingivitis, 1033, 1033f
in cracked tooth and split root syndromes, 1033-1034
in maxillary sinusitis, 1034
in pericoronitis, 1035
in pulp exposure, 1037
in sinusitis, 1124
in temporomandibular myofascial pain dysfunction syndrome, 1034-1035
paroxysmal, of neuropathic origin, 1034
periapical abscess and, 1033
postextraction, 1034
root canal, 1033
Oral pharynx, visibility of, assessment of, 4, 5f
Oral rehydration therapy
for diarrhea, 234-235
for pediatric infectious diarrhea, 2629-2630, 2630t
for *Vibrio* fish poisoning, 1472
Oral thrush, 1840-1841
Oral ulcers, 1036
in Behçet's disease, 1814
in HIV/AIDS, 2083
OraQuick test, for HIV, 2074
Orbit
contusion of, 1044
examination of, in facial trauma, 387-388
foreign body in, 1051-1052
hemorrhage of, 1046
Orbital cellulitis, 293t, 2197-2198
Orbital emphysema, 393, 1044, 1045f
Orbital fracture, 393
Orbital hematoma, 393
Orbital septum, laceration through, 1051
Orbital tumor, red and painful eye in, 294t
Orbital wall fracture, traumatic, 1044, 1045f
Orbivirus, 2047
Orchitis, 1598
in children, 2639
in mumps, 2052
Order entry systems, computerized, 3043, 3043f, 3101, 3102f
Orelline/orellanine, in mushrooms, 2479
Organ damage, in sickle cell disease, 1881, 1881t
Organ radiosensitivity, 2321, 2321f
Organ system dysfunction
definition of, 2211
in pancreatitis, 1427, 1429
in sepsis, 2213-2214
in solvent abuse, 2888
trajectory of dying in, 3140-3141, 3140f
Organ transplant patient, 2846-2856
complications in, 2847-2851, 2850t, 2851f
disposition of, 2856
Organ transplant patient *(Continued)*
drug toxicity in, 2849-2851, 2850t, 2851f
heart, 2851-2854, 2852f, 2853f
immune defects in, 2846-2847
immunosuppressive therapy for, 2849-2851, 2850t
infectious complications in, 2847-2849, 2847b
kidney, 2855
liver, 2854-2855, 2854f
lung, 2855-2856
pancreas, 2856
rejection in, 2848-2849, 2849f
Organic brain syndrome, 1645-1662. *See also* Delirium; Dementia.
Organoaxial volvulus, 1394
Organogenesis, drug exposure during, 2781
Organophosphate poisoning, 2457-2461, 2458b, 2459b, 2459f
antidotes to, 2329t
as chemical weapon, 939, 3030-3031, 3030b, 3031b
O'Riain wrinkle test, in nerve injuries, 559
Ornithodoros tick, 2117
Oropharyngeal anthrax, 3026
Oropharyngeal disorders, in HIV/AIDS, 2083
Oropharyngeal dysphagia, 1396-1397
Oropharynx
examination of
in airway foreign body aspiration, 866
in facial trauma, 388
foreign body in, 870, 1384
inflammation or irritation of. *See* Pharyngitis.
Orphaned patient, as problem area in emergency care, 3124-3125
Orthodromic tachycardia, in Wolff-Parkinson-White syndrome, 1235, 1237
Orthomyxovirus, 2034t, 2054-2055
Orthopedic consultation, for ankle fractures, 812, 812b
Orthopedic infections, 2174-2194. *See also* Osteomyelitis; Septic arthritis.
Orthopedic injuries. *See also specific anatomic locations.*
ankle, 808-820
dislocations in, 564-566, 565f. *See also* Dislocation.
elbow and humerus, 647-668
femur and hip, 735-768
foot, 820-839
forearm, 639-644
fractures in, 552-564. *See also* Fracture.
hand, 589-618
in spinal cord–injured patient, 2909
injury prevention and control in, 940-950
knee, 770-796
low back pain and, 701-715
lower leg, 796-805
management principles in, 549-552, 550t-551t
pelvic, 717-734
shoulder, 670-699
soft tissue injuries in, 566-568. *See also* Soft tissue injuries.
subluxation in, 564-566. *See also* Subluxation.
treatment modalities for
casts in, 571-573, 573f
splinting and bandaging in, 568-571, 569f, 570f
thermal therapy in, 573-574
wrist, 622-639
Orthopedic repair, vascular repair vs., 544
Orthopedic surgeons, disposition requirements related to, 3164
Orthopnea, 176, 177
in heart failure, 1269
Orthoses, knee, in Osgood-Schlatter disease, 799
Orthostatic hypotension
from antipsychotic agents, 1732
in spinal cord injury, 2906
Orthostatic proteinuria, 1531, 2647
Orthotic supports, in sesamoid fractures, 835
Ortolani reduction maneuver in developmental hip dysplasia, 2701, 2702b
Orungo virus, 2047
Os acromiale, 680
Os peroneum, 822, 822f, 837
Os tibiale externum, 822, 822f, 837
Os trigonum, 822, 822f
Os trigonum syndrome, 836
Os vesalianum, 822, 822f
Osborn wave, in hypothermia, 2237, 2238f
Oseltamivir
for influenza, 2055
indications for, 2037-2038
Osgood-Schlatter disease, 798, 799, 2710
Osmol gap, elevated
differential diagnosis in, 2397
in ethylene glycol poisoning, 2400
in isopropyl alcohol poisoning, 2403
in methanol poisoning, 2397
Osmotic agents
for constipation, 241t, 242
for elevated intracranial pressure, in severe head trauma, 360
Osmotic diarrhea, 228, 2624
Osmotic equilibrium, 1933
Ossicles, accessory, of foot, 821-822, 822f
Ossification, heterotopic
after tibial femoral knee dislocation, 790
of femur and hip, 741-742, 743f-754f
Ossification centers
in elbow, 652, 652f, 653t, 2694, 2694f, 2694t
in hip, 763, 763f
Osteitis, alveolar, acute, 1034
Osteoarthritis, 1787
of hip, 739, 739f-741f
of knee, 796
Osteochondral fracture
of talar dome, 824-825, 825f
patellar dislocation and, 786
Osteochondritis dissecans, in knee trauma, 781-782
Osteochondroma, in femur, 742, 745f
Osteoclast inhibitors, for hypercalcemia, 1946
Osteocytes, 2175
Osteodystrophy, renal, 1542-1543
Osteogenesis imperfecta, 975, 2700-2701, 2700f, 2700t, 2901t
Osteoid osteoma, in femur, 742, 745f
Osteomyelitis, 558, 2174-2187
anatomy in, 2174-2175, 2175f
chronic, 2186
classification of, 2174
clinical features of, 2179-2186
complications of, 2186
cranial, after head trauma, 371
diagnostic imaging in, 2179-2182, 2179f-2183f
differential considerations in, 2186
disposition in, 2187
epidemiology of, 2174
etiology and microbiology of, 2177-2179, 2178t
hematogenous, 2175-2176, 2183, 2184f
history in, 2179
imaging in, 2179f-2182f
in children, 2183-2184, 2184f, 2516
in diabetic foot, 2185-2186
in hand, 618
in sickle cell anemia, 2186
in tuberculosis, 2159
laboratory studies in, 2179
management of, 2186-2187, 2189t
pathophysiology of, 2175-2176
pediatric limp and, 764-765
physical examination in, 2179
posttraumatic, 2185
skull-base, 1071
vertebral, 261, 265t, 2159, 2178, 2182, 2182f, 2184-2185
Osteonecrosis
after fracture, 562
after talar fracture, 824
in knee trauma, 782
in scuba diving–related disorders, 2286
of femoral head, 739-741, 741b, 742f
after femoral neck fracture, 740, 742f, 750-751
pediatric, 767
of proximal femoral epiphysis, 2706-2707, 2707f
Osteopenia of prematurity, 975
Osteoporosis, of femur, 739, 739f-741f
Ostiomeatal complex, 1123
Otalgia
differential diagnosis in, 1068
in mastoiditis, 1072
in neck masses, 1076
in otitis externa, 1070
in otitis media, 1067
referred, 1076

Otic encephalitis, in otitis media, 1068
Otitis externa, 1070-1071
  facial paralysis and, 1667
  necrotizing (malignant), 1071
Otitis media, 1066-1070
  acute, 1066, 1068-1069, 1069t, 1070t
  chronic suppurative, 1066, 1067
  facial paralysis and, 1667
  mastoiditis and, 1071
  recurrent, 1066
  screening for, 2509b
  with bronchiolitis, 2545
  with effusion, 1066, 1069-1070
Otolaryngologic conditions, 1066-1077
  epistaxis and, 1072-1075, 1073f, 1074t
  mastoiditis and, 1071-1072
  neck masses and, 1075-1076, 1075f, 1076b
  necrotizing otitis externa and, 1071
  otitis externa and, 1070-1071
  otitis media and, 1066-1070, 1069t, 1070t
  sialolithiasis and, 1075
  sudden hearing loss and, 1072, 1073b
Otolith, 142
Otomycosis, 1070-1071
Otorrhea
  in malignant otitis externa, 1071
  in otitis externa, 1070
  in otitis media, 1067
Ototoxic drugs, vertigo from, 2683
Ottawa Ankle Rules, 810-811, 3036, 3042
Ottawa Knee Rule, 774
Outcome data, collection of, 3050
Ovarian abscess, 248, 251t
Ovarian cyst, 251t
Ovarian torsion, 251t
Oven cleaner, ingestion of, 2381t
Overcrowding in emergency department, 3120-3121
Overdose. *See* Poisoning/overdose.
Overdose history, 2326, 2326b
Overflow proteinuria, 1531
Overuse injuries
  of foot, 836-838
  of knee, 793-796
  tendinopathy and bursitis in, 1794-1801
Overwhelming postsplenectomy infection (OPSI), 2018
Ovulation, cyclic, hormonal role in, 2723
Oxacillin, for pneumonia, 2558t
Oxalic acid, in ethylene glycol poisoning, 2398
Oxalosis, facial auditory nerve, in ethylene glycol poisoning, 2399
Oxazepam, 2484, 2484t
Oxidative stress, in chronic obstructive pulmonary disease, 1098
Oxime therapy, for organophosphate poisoning, 2461
Oxprenolol, overdose of, 2373t
Oxycodone, 2920, 2921t, 2925
  during pregnancy and lactation, 2784
  for migraine, 2680
  respiratory effects of, 2453t
Oxycontin, 2920
Oxygen
  desaturation of, in rapid sequence intubation, 10, 10f
  partial pressure of
    altitude and, 2297, 2307, 2307f
    cerebral blood flow and, 351-352, 351f
    conjunctival, 36
  saturation of
    during cardiopulmonary resuscitation, 82, 82f
    in asthma, 2537
    in shock, 50
  toxicity of, in scuba diving–related disorders, 2283
Oxygen therapy
  during procedural sedation and analgesia, 2942
  for acute mountain sickness, 2302-2303
  for acute pulmonary edema, 1271
  for asthma, 1086, 1091-1092, 2538
  for burns, 921
  for carbon monoxide poisoning, 2439-2440
  for cardiac arrest, 93
  for chronic obstructive pulmonary disease, 1103-1105, 1103t-1105t
  for cluster headache, 1635
Oxygen therapy *(Continued)*
  for cyanosis, 271, 273
  for high-altitude cerebral edema, 2306
  for high-altitude pulmonary edema, 2304
  for pulmonary edema, in chronic renal failure, 1546
  for scuba diving–related disorders, 2292
  for sepsis, 2218
  for sickle cell disease, 1880
  for toxic shock syndrome, 2030
  hyperbaric
    for carbon monoxide poisoning, 2439-2440
    for frostbite, 2233
    for high-altitude cerebral edema, 2306
    for high-altitude pulmonary edema, 2304, 2305f
    for myonecrosis, 2209
    for nitrite abuse, 2891
    for peripheral arteriovascular disease, 1350
    for scuba diving–related disorders, 2288-2292, 2288b, 2289f-2291f
    for simultaneous carbon monoxide and cyanide poisoning, 2440-2441
  in neonatal resuscitation, 122, 123, 123t
  in postresuscitation care, 86-87, 86f
Oxygenation
  altitude and, 2307, 2307f, 2994, 2995t
  before rapid sequence intubation, 10, 10f
  failure of, as indication for intubation, 2-3
  for sepsis, 2222
  in hypothermia, 2249, 2249t
  in pediatric resuscitation, 98-99
Oxygen-enriched air, 2279-2280
Oxygen-enriched Tri-Mix, 2280
Oxyhemoglobin dissociation curve
  altitude and, 2296, 2297f
  in cyanosis, 268, 269f
  shift of, during acclimatization to high altitude, 2298
Oxymetazoline, for sinusitis, 1125
Oxymorphone, respiratory effects of, 2453t
Oxytocin, during labor and delivery, 2805

P wave
  in complete atrioventricular block, 1221
  in multifocal atrial tachycardia, 1228, 1229f
  in narrow-complex tachycardia, 1234f
  in sinoatrial block, 1216
P′ wave
  in junctional tachycardia, 1233
  in premature atrial contractions, 1222-1223, 1222f, 1223f
  in premature junctional contractions, 1223
  in premature ventricular contractions, 1224
Pacemaker(s), 1246-1255
  components of, 1247-1248
  DDD, 1248t, 1249, 1249f, 1251, 1252f
  DDDR, 1248t
  defibrillation in patient with, 1255
  electrocardiography with, 1248-1250, 1249f, 1250f
  failure to capture by, 1252-1253, 1252f
  for atrial tachycardia, 1228
  for bradycardia, 1215
  for complete atrioventricular block, 1221
  for digitalis toxicity, 2371
  for Mobitz type II second-degree atrioventricular block, 1220
  for sinoatrial block, 1218
  for sinus node dysfunction, 1218
  for torsades de pointes, 1244
  inappropriate rate by, 1254
  inappropriate sensing by, 1253
  indications for, 1246-1247, 1247b
  infection from, 1250
  leads for, 1247-1248
    problems with, 1253
  malfunction of
    disposition in, 1255
    management of, 1254-1255
    types of, 1251-1254, 1251b, 1252f-1254f
  oversensing by, 1253-1254, 1254f
  terminology for, 1247, 1248t
  thrombophlebitis from, 1250
  undersensing by, 1253, 1253f
  ventricular, ICDs as, 1255
Pacemaker(s) *(Continued)*
  VVI, 1248t, 1249, 1249f, 1251
    with fusion beats, 1250, 1250f
  VVIR, 1248t
Pacemaker cells
  action potential of, 1200-1201, 1201f
  in atrioventricular node, 1203
  in sinoatrial node, 1201-1202
  infranodal, 1203
Pacemaker syndrome, 1250-1251
Pacing
  external noninvasive, in hypothermia, 2246
  for pediatric bradycardia, 111
  in adult resuscitation, 91
Packed red blood cells, 52, 58-59
Paget's disease of bone, hypercalcemia in, 1915, 1915f
Pain. *See also specific anatomic locations, e.g.,* Abdominal pain.
  acute vs. chronic, 2913-2914, 2914b
  anginal. *See* Angina.
  definition of, 2914b
  evaluation and documentation of, 2916-2917, 2917b, 2917t
  in abdominal aortic aneurysm, 1332-1333
  in acute arterial occlusion, 1345
  in aortic dissection, 1325
  in arthritis, 1778, 1778t
  in cholangitis, 1421
  in cholecystitis, 1420
  in cholelithiasis, 1418
  in chronic arterial insufficiency, 1345, 1346
  in compartment syndrome, 561
  in dislocation, 564
  in diverticular disease, 1493
  in frostbite, 2230
  in Osgood-Schlatter syndrome, 2710
  in peptic ulcer disease, 1392
  in peptic ulcer perforation, 1393
  in sickle cell disease, 1880
  in snakebite, 898
  in sprain, 566
  in strain, 567
  in tendinopathy, 568
  in thoracic outlet syndrome, 1359
  in toxic shock syndrome, 2200
  ischemic rest, in chronic arterial insufficiency, 1346
  management of. *See* Analgesia.
  palliative care for, 3153
  pathophysiology of, 2914-2916, 2915f, 2915t, 2916f, 2916t
  undertreatment of, 2917-2918
Pain behavior, 2916-2917
Pain conduction pathways, 2914-2916, 2915f, 2915t, 2916f, 2916t
Pain disorder, 1755
Pain scales, 2916, 2917b, 2917t
Pain threshold, 2915-2916
Painful arc syndrome
  in calcific tendinitis, 698
  in rotator cuff tear, 696
  shoulder, 693-696, 694t, 695f
Paint, in high-pressure injection injuries to hand, 612
Paint sniffer, 2430, 2430f
Paint thinner, in high-pressure injection injuries to hand, 612
Palivizumab, for respiratory syncytial virus prophylaxis, 2582, 2582b
Palliative care, 3143, 3151-3154
  establishing goals of, 3151-3153, 3152t
  in advanced dementia, 3154
  in chronic obstructive pulmonary disease, 3154
  in heart failure, 3154
  in renal failure, 3154
  medical treatment options in, 3153-3154, 3153b
  prehospital care and end of life issues related to, 3145
Pallor, in pediatric assessment, 2499
Palmar erythema, in pregnancy, 2724
Palmar lesions, in Kawasaki disease, 2594, 2595f
Palmar rash, in syphilis, 1561, 1561f
Palmar surface of hand, 576, 577f
Palmaris longus
  anatomy of, 582, 584f
  laceration of, 609

Palpation
in peripheral vascular injury, 541
of fetus, 2728
of knee, 772-773, 772f
of spine, 416
Palpitations
in mitral valve prolapse, 1305
in scombroid fish poisoning, 1472
Palsy. *See also* Paralysis.
Bell's, 1666-1667, 1668, 2123
bridegroom's, 1695
cerebral, 2903-2904
failure to thrive in, 2900
musculoskeletal disorders in, 2901-2902
fourth-nerve, eye movement disorders in, 1062-1063
median nerve, 587, 588f
radial nerve, 586, 588f
humeral shaft fracture and, 655
in radial mononeuropathy, 1695
Saturday night, 1694-1695
sixth-nerve, eye movement disorders in, 1063
third-nerve
anisocoria in, 1061
eye movement disorders in, 1062
ulnar nerve, 586, 588f
Pamidronate
for hypercalcemia, 1946
for hypercalcemic cancer patient, 1916
Pancarditis, in rheumatic fever, 1304
Pancreas
anatomy and physiology of, 1426, 1427f
carcinoma of, 1437-1438, 1817
transplantation of, 1973, 2856
tumor of, 1437
Pancreatic disorders, 1426-1438
Pancreatic enzymes, 1426
in abdominal trauma, 495
in acute pancreatitis, 1430-1431
replacement of, in chronic pancreatitis, 1436
Pancreatitis
acute, 1426-1434
abdominal pain in, 215t
clinical features of, 1429
complications of, 1429-1430, 1430f
diagnosis of, 1430-1433
differential diagnosis in, 1433, 1433b
imaging studies in, 1432-1433
laboratory tests in, 1430-1432, 1431t, 1432b
management of, 1433-1434
pathophysiology of, 1427
prognostic scoring systems for, 1431-1432, 1432b
alcoholic, 2868
chronic, 1434-1437
classification of, 1435
clinical features of, 1435
diagnosis of, 1435-1436, 1436f
management of, 1436-1437
drug-induced, 1428, 1429b
etiology of, 1427-1428, 1428b, 1429b
in child abuse, 971
in children, 2618, 2618t
nausea and vomiting in, 205t
panniculitis in, 1817
severe, definition of, 1432, 1432b
Pancuronium
for tetanus, 2011
in intubation, 14, 31
Panencephalitis, sclerosing, subacute, 2054
Panic attack, 1746b, 1748-1749, 2668
in primary psychiatric disorders, 1748-1749
management of, 1749-1751, 1750t
Panic buttons, in emergency department, 2966
Panic disorder
asthma and, 1082
primary, depression with, 1748-1749
suicide and, 1769
with agoraphobia, 1746b
Panic reactions
in marijuana intoxication, 2411
in psychedelic intoxication, 2408
in psychostimulant intoxication, 2410
Panniculitis, 1817
Panoramic radiography, 1030, 1030f
Panorex imaging of facial fracture, 388
Pantoprazole, 1390t
Papaverine, for acute mesenteric ischemia, 1449
Papaya, drug interactions with, 2478t
Papillae, interdental, edematous, in acute necrotic ulcerative gingivitis, 1033
Papillary dermis, 914
Papillary examination, in overdosed/poisoned patient, 2326
Papilledema
in cerebral venous thrombosis, 1670
of optic disk, 1062
Papilloma, laryngeal, 2045, 2525
Papillomavirus infection, 2034t, 2045
drugs for, 2037t
genital warts from, 1518t, 1519-1520
in condylomata acuminata, 1563-1564, 1564f
in HIV/AIDS, 2085
Papular purpura, 1839t
Papule
scaly, skin disorders with, 1841-1842
skin disorders with, 1839t, 1851-1856
Paracentesis, in ascites, 1410
Paradoxical central nervous system acidosis, from sodium bicarbonate, 1930
Paradoxical undressing, in hypothermia, 2241
Paragonimus westermani, 2101t, 2110-2111
Parainfluenza, 2051
in bronchiolitis, 2544
in pneumonia, 1130, 2555, 2557
Paraldehyde poisoning, metabolic acidosis in, 1928
Paralysis. *See also* Palsy.
facial nerve, 1666-1668
flaccid, in botulism, 2014
in acute arterial occlusion, 1345
in botulism, 1707
in rabies, 2065
induced, in intubated, mechanically ventilated patient, 31
periodic, 1708-1709
familial, 1709
hyperkalemia in, 1940
hypokalemia in, 1938
thyrotoxic, 1709, 1987
tick, 1708, 2141-2142
Todd's, 1625
vocal cord, 2524-2525
Paralysis with induction phase of rapid sequence intubation, 11
Paralytic PICE, 3012, 3012b
Paralytic poliomyelitis, 2056-2057
Paramedic, 2987, 2987t
Parametric statistical tests, 3053
Paramyxovirus, 2034t, 2051-2054
Paranoid personality disorder, 2979b
Parapharyngeal abscess, 1121-1123, 1122f
Parapharyngeal space, 1027, 1117
Paraphimosis, 2637, 2637f
Parapneumonic pleural effusion, 1148, 1149, 1152, 1153
Parapoxviruses, 2040
Paraquat poisoning, 2465-2466, 2465b
Parasitic infection, 2096-2104
abdominal pain in, 2113
anemia in, 2107
cardiovascular disease in, 2111-2112
challenges related to, 2096
diarrhea in, 228, 230b, 2112, 2112f, 2113f
drug therapy for, 2098-2099, 2098t, 2100t-2103t
fever in, 2099, 2103-2105
gastrointestinal disorders in, 2112-2114
in cancer patient with impaired cell-mediated immunity, 2840
in HIV/AIDS, 2114
neurologic disorders in, 2105-2107
peripheral edema in, 2107-2108
pruritus ani in, 2113-2114
pulmonary disorders in, 2110-2111
skin disorders in, 2108-2109
travel history and, 2097, 2099t
visual disturbances in, 2109-2110
Parasitic pathogens, in central nervous system infection, 1711t
Parasitosis, delusion of, in amphetamine abuse, 2894
Paraspinal cold abscess, in tuberculosis, 2159
Parasystole, 1225-1226, 1226b, 1226f
Parathyroid disease, hypertension in, 1313
Parathyroid hormone
in calcium homeostasis, 1941-1942
in phosphate homeostasis, 1950
Paravaccinia, 2040
Paregoric, respiratory effects of, 2453t
Parental advice
on simple febrile seizures, 2674b
on vomiting and diarrhea, 2628b
Parental consent, 3167-3168
Parental refusal of medical care, 3171
Paresthesia
in acute arterial occlusion, 1345
in ciguatera fish poisoning, 1473
in frostbite, 2234
in hypothyroidism, 1992
in thoracic outlet syndrome, 1359
Parity, 2722
Parkinsonian motor dysfunction
in antipsychotic overdose, 2447
in methanol poisoning, 2395
Parkinson's disease, anxiety in, 1747-1748
Parkland formula, for fluid resuscitation of burn patient, 922-923
Paromomycin, for AIDS-related diarrhea, 1484
Paronychia, 614-615, 615f, 1841
Parotid gland and duct, 385, 386f
Parotitis, infectious, 1428, 2052
Paroxysmal atrial tachycardia, 1228
Paroxysmal choreoathetosis, 2668
Paroxysmal nocturnal dyspnea, 176
Paroxysmal nocturnal hemoglobinuria, hemolytic anemia in, 1879
Paroxysmal pain of neuropathic origin, 1034
Paroxysmal supraventricular tachycardia, 1233-1235, 1233f, 1234f
Paroxysmal tachycardia, in Wolff-Parkinson-White syndrome, 1235
Paroxysmal vertigo, benign, 147t, 2683
Parsley, adverse effects of, 2476t
Partial thromboplastin time (PTT)
abnormal, differential diagnosis in, 1899-1900
in bleeding disorders, 1895
in pregnancy, 318
Partial-thickness burn, 918-919, 919f
Parvovirus B19 infection, 1850, 2046, 2046f
Pascal's law, 2280
Pasteurella multocida infection
in cat bites, 883-884, 888
in dog bites, 883
Patch, 1839t
Patchy skin disorders, 1838-1841
Patella
anatomy of, 770, 771f
dislocation of, 564, 565f, 785-786, 785b
fracture of, 784-785, 785f
lateral compression of, 794
Patella alta, 782, 783, 784f
Patella baja, 782
Patellar tendinitis, 794
Patellar tendinopathy, 1799
Patellar tendon
anatomy of, 770, 771f
injury to, 761, 782-784, 783f, 784f
Patellofemoral compartment, 770, 771f
Patellofemoral joint, 770, 771f
Patellofemoral pain syndrome, 786-787
Patent ductus arteriosus, 2568
Patent foramen ovale, decompression sickness and, 2284
Pathogen exposure, blood-borne, 3081-3087, 3084t, 3085t, 3086b
Pathologic apnea, 2714
Pathologic fracture, tibial shaft, 799-800
Pathologic lying, in Munchausen's syndrome, 1762
Patient
combative, 2956-2969
assault by, 2963
diagnostic studies in, 2964
differential considerations in, 2964-2965, 2965b
disposition of, 2969
epidemiology of, 2956-2957
functional vs. organic etiology of, 2963, 2964t
history taking and physical examination of, 2963-2964, 2964t
medical clearance of, 2965
medicolegal issues of, 2967-2969
pathophysiology of, 2957
physical restraints for, 2958-2961, 2960f
preparation of emergency department for, 2965-2967

Patient *(Continued)*
rapid tranquilization of, 2961-2963
risk assessment and, 2957-2958
verbal management techniques for, 2958
difficult, 2972-2982
as stressor for emergency physician, 3175
behavioral classification of, 2978-2981, 2978t
combative patient as, 2956-2969. *See also* Combative patient.
definition of, 2972-2973
emergency department factors in, 2973
impaired patient-physician relationship and, 2973, 2974f
management of, 2973-2981
crisis intervention in, 2976-2977, 2977b
dealing with negative reactions in, 2975-2976
general strategies in, 2973-2975, 2973b
personality disorder classification of, 2978, 2979b
physician factors in, 2973
Patient education
information technology for, 3098-3099
on back pain, 710-711
on wound management, 855-856, 856b
Patient information, security and confidentiality of, 3102-3103
Patient population in clinical trials
definition of, 3048
measurement of baseline characteristics of, 3049
recruitment and enrollment of, 3048-3049
Patient rights, 2967
Patient safety in emergency department, 3119-3126
problem areas and, 3124-3126, 3125t
sources of failure and, 3119-3123, 3120f, 3120t
Patient Self-Determination Act, 3144
Patient transfer
disposition requirements related to, 3165, 3165b
in acute coronary syndromes, 1195
in labor and delivery, 2797-2798
in myocardial infarction, 1195
interfacility and specialized, 2991-2992, 2991b, 2992b
to burn center, 927, 927b
Patient transport
by air, 2994-2999
administrative structure in, 2995
aviation physiology and, 2994-2995, 2995t
clinical concepts and patient care in, 2998-2999
criteria for, 2998b
efficacy and cost effectiveness of, 2999
flight crew in, 2996
future of, 2999
medical direction in, 2996
safety issues in, 2997, 2997b, 2997f, 2998b
types of missions in, 2995
interfacility and specialized, 2991-2992, 2991b, 2992b
Patient-controlled analgesia, 2920
Patient-physician relationship
and racial/ethnic disparities in health outcomes, 3109-3110
pathology of, difficult patient and, 2973, 2974f
Pattern injuries
in child abuse, 969, 969f
in intimate partner violence and abuse, 997
in motor vehicle crashes, 964-966, 965f
in pedestrian collisions, 965-966, 965f
in physical assault, 960-963, 961b, 961f-964f
Pattern recognition process, clinical decision making by, 126, 131t, 132
Pavlik harness, for developmental hip dysplasia, 2702
PCP (phencyclidine) intoxication, 2413, 2414-2415, 2414t, 2415t, 2416, 2882b, 2891-2893
during pregnancy, 2792
rhabdomyolysis in, 1979
Peak expiratory flow rate (PEFR)
in asthma, 1084, 1086t, 2535t, 2536, 2536f
in chronic obstructive pulmonary disease, 1101
Peak inspiratory pressure, 30
Pedestrian collisions
death from, 300
forensic aspects of, 965-966, 966b, 966f
in elderly person, 345
mechanism of injury of, 303t
Pediatric assessment triangle, 2497-2499
appearance in, 2497-2498, 2498t
circulation to skin in, 2498t, 2499, 2499f
interpretation of, 2500t
work of breathing in, 2498-2499, 2498f, 2498t, 2499f
Pediculosis, skin lesions in, 1853-1854, 1853f
Pelvic examination
in abdominal pain, 213, 215
in fever, 135
in genitourinary trauma, 515
in pelvic fracture, 718-719
in pelvic pain, 249, 250t
in vaginal bleeding, 256t
Pelvic fracture, 717-734
acetabular, 728-729, 728b, 731, 731f, 732f
anatomy in, 717-718, 718f
and blunt abdominal trauma, 509, 510f
classification of, 723, 723b
clinical features of, 718-720
diagnostic peritoneal lavage in, 722-723, 722f
epidemiology of, 717
general management of, 722f, 723
gynecologic injury in, 720
hemorrhage in, 718
evaluation of, 722-723, 722f
management of, 731-734, 731b, 733f
high-energy, 726-728, 727b, 733f
in bladder trauma, 520-521
in elderly person, 346
low-energy, 723-726, 724f
neurologic injury in, 719-720
open, 719
penetrating injuries in, 720
posterior urethral trauma and, 516, 516f
prehospital care in, 718
radiologic imaging in, 720-722, 721f
retrograde urethrogram and, 517-518
thoracic aortic injury in, 720
urologic injury in, 719
visceral and soft tissue injuries in, 719
Pelvic hematoma, 718
Pelvic inflammatory disease, 1569-1571
appendicitis vs., 1453, 1453t
clinical features of, 1570
differential diagnosis in, 1570-1571
ectopic pregnancy after, 2743
in pregnancy, 2759
pelvic pain in, 248, 251t
treatment of, 1571, 1571t
Pelvic ligaments, 717, 718f
Pelvic pain, 248-253. *See also* Abdominal pain.
diagnostic approach to, 248-250, 250t
differential diagnosis in, 249b, 250, 251t-252t
empiric management of, 250, 252-253, 252f, 253f
epidemiology of, 248
pathophysiology of, 248
Pelvic vessel embolization, for postpartum hemorrhage, 2819
Pelvirectal abscess, 2206
Pelvis, anatomy of, 717-718, 718f
Pemphigus vulgaris, skin lesions in, 1857, 1857f
Penbutolol sulfate, 1321t
Pendular shoulder exercises, 679f
Penetrating trauma
abdominal
diagnosis and management of, 502-507
epidemiology of, 489
history in, 493
in children, 342
observation in, 3067-3068
pathophysiology of, 490-491
physical examination in, 494
cardiac, 472-476
chest
observation in, 3068-3069
pneumothorax and, 482
esophageal, 483-484
facial, 386, 387f
head, 368-370
in pelvic fracture, 720
in pregnancy, 318-319
neck
in transcervical gunshot wounds, 446
mandatory vs. selective exploration of, 445-446
pathophysiology of, 441-442, 442t
Penetrating trauma *(Continued)*
pharyngoesophageal injuries in, 446-447
vascular injuries in, 448-450
ocular, 1051-1052, 1051f
peripheral vascular, 536, 537
renal, 528, 530
ureteral, 530
Penetration syndrome, in airway foreign body impaction, 865
Penicillamine
for lead poisoning, 2422
for mercury poisoning, 2426
for radioactive lead poisoning, 2324
Penicillin
allergy to, 1826
during pregnancy and lactation, 2775, 2784
for *Bacillus anthracis* gastroenteritis, 1469
for diphtheria, 2004
for diphtheria-related myocardial disease, 1291
for febrile, neutropenic cancer patient, 2838t
for Lyme disease, 1292, 1789
for mastoiditis, 1072
for orofacial infections, 1032
for pharyngitis, 1113
for pneumonia, 2558t
for scarlet fever, 1851
for streptococcal pharyngitis, 1304
for syphilis, 1856
for tetanus, 2011
in frostbite, 2232
prophylactic, in rheumatic fever, 2597
Penicillin G
for Lyme disease, 1789, 2127t, 2128
for meningococcal disease, 2023
for pneumococcal disease, 2019
for syphilis, 1559t, 1562
Penicillin V, for rheumatic fever, 1791
Penile disorders, in children, 2635-2638, 2637f-2638f
Penile entrapment and tourniquet injuries, 878, 2638
Penis
anatomy of, 532, 532f
physical examination of, 1573
trauma to, 532-534, 532f-534f
Pennyroyal, adverse effects of, 2476t
Pentachlorophenol, 2463, 2463b
Pentamidine
for pneumonia, in HIV-infected patient, 1139
in HIV/AIDS, side effects of, 2079t
Pentazocine, 2924, 2924b
Pentobarbital
for GHB withdrawal, 2490
for status epilepticus, 1627, 1627t, 2672t, 2673
Pentoxifylline, in frostbite, 2233
Penumbra, ischemic, 1607
Pepper sprays, capsaicin in, 2472
Peptic ulcer disease, 1391-1394
abdominal pain in, 210t
causes of, 1391-1392, 1391b
clinical features of, 1392
complications of, 1393
diagnosis of, 1393
in spinal cord injury, 2907
management of, 1393-1394, 1394t
nausea and vomiting in, 204t
PERC rule, 1372b, 1374
Perceptual disturbances, in delirium, 1649
Percutaneous coronary intervention, in myocardial infarction, 1192-1193
after fibrinolytic therapy, 1193
facilitated, 1195
guidelines on, 1193-1194
in cardiogenic shock, 1194
with glycoprotein IIb/IIIa receptor inhibitors, 1186, 1194
Percutaneous cricothyrotomy, 22-23, 23f
Percutaneous embolotherapy, for hemoptysis, 282
Percutaneous transluminal angioplasty, for acute mesenteric ischemia, 1449
Percutaneous transluminal peripheral angioplasty, for peripheral arteriovascular disease, 1349
Percutaneous transtracheal jet insufflation, in neck trauma, 445
Percutaneous transtracheal ventilation, in multiple trauma, 306
Perforating wounds to head, 369

Performance shaping factors, as source of failures in emergency department, 3120t, 3121-3123
Perfumes, caustic injuries from, 2381
Perianal abscess, 2206
Perianal itching, 1509
Periapical abscess, 1028, 1030f, 1031, 1032
Pericardial disease, 1280-1298. *See also* Pericardial effusion; Pericarditis.
acquired immunodeficiency syndrome and, 1287
cardiac tamponade in, 1285-1286, 1286f
connective tissue disorders and, 1284
epidemiology of, 1280
etiology of, 1280, 1281b
heart failure in, 1265
neoplastic, 1283-1284
pneumopericardium in, 1287-1288
pregnancy and, 1287
uremic, 1282
Pericardial effusion, 1284-1285, 1285f
in cardiac tamponade, 474, 474f
in chronic renal failure, 1542
in HIV/AIDS, 1287
in hypothyroidism, 1993
in myocardial contusion, 468
in pregnancy, 1287
malignant, 1283-1284
transudative vs. exudative, 1285
uremic, 1282
Pericardial friction rub, 1281, 2592
Pericardial knock, in constrictive pericarditis, 1288
Pericardial mesothelioma, 1916
Pericardial rupture, 471
Pericardial tamponade. *See* Cardiac tamponade.
Pericardial tumor, malignant, 1283-1284
Pericardiocentesis
in cardiac tamponade, 475, 1286
in hemodialysis patient, 1551
in myocardial rupture, 471
in neoplastic cardiac tamponade, 1917-1918
in pericardial effusion, 1285
Pericardiotomy
in myocardial rupture, 471
pericarditis after, 2581
Pericarditis
chest pain in, 183, 186b, 190t-191t
constrictive, 1288
heart failure in, 1265
neoplastic, 1917
restrictive cardiomyopathy vs., 1296
epidemiology of, 1280
etiology of, 1280, 1281b
iatrogenic, 1287
idiopathic, 1280-1282, 1281f
in acute renal failure, 1540
in amyloidosis, 1287
in chronic renal failure, 1542
in giant cell arteritis, 1284
in hemodialysis patient, 1551
in HIV/AIDS, 1287
in infants and children, 2592-2593, 2593f
in inflammatory bowel disease, 1287
in pregnancy, 1287
in rheumatoid arthritis, 1284
in Sjögren's syndrome, 1284
in systemic lupus erythematosus, 1284, 1807
infarct, 1160
miscellaneous infectious causes of, 1284
neoplastic, 1916
pathophysiology of, 1280
post-myocardial infarction, 1282-1283
post-pericardiotomy, 2581
posttraumatic, 1283
purulent, 1286-1287
radiation-induced, 1284, 1916-1917
risk factors for, 186b
ST segment elevation in, 1167, 1167f, 1168f
tuberculous, 1287, 2151
uremic, 1282
Pericardium, anatomy and physiology of, 1280
Pericoronitis, 1035
Perihepatitis, 1570
Perilunate dislocation, 630, 631f
Perilymphatic fistula, vertigo in, 2685
Perindopril, 1322t
Perineal laceration, 719
Periodic breathing
definition of, 2714
Periodic breathing *(Continued)*
in acute mountain sickness, 2301, 2302
in infants, 2495
Periodic paralysis, 1708-1709
familial, 1709
hyperkalemia in, 1940
hypokalemia in, 1938
thyrotoxic, 1709, 1987
Periodontal abscess, 1031, 1033
Periodontal disease, 1032-1033
in diabetes mellitus, 1035
in HIV/AIDS, 2083
Periodontal ligament, 1027, 1027f
Periodontal surgery, hemorrhage after, 1042
Periodontitis, 1032-1033
Periodontium, anatomy of, 1027, 1027f
Perionychium, 589
Perioral tremor, antipsychotic-induced, 2447
Periorbital cellulitis, 294t, 2197-2198
Periorbital edema
in hypothyroidism, 1992
in superior vena cava syndrome, 1910
Periosteum, in children, 2689
Periostitis, physiologic, 2699-2700
Peripatellar tendinitis, 794
Peripheral arterial aneurysm
infected, 1356-1357, 1357t
lower extremity, 1354
traumatic, 1357
upper extremity, 1354-1355
visceral, 1355-1356
Peripheral arteriovascular disease, 1342-1366
acute arterial occlusion in, 1345, 1345f, 1352-1354, 1353f
arterial anatomy and, 1342
arterial embolism in, 1343-1344, 1346, 1347t, 1352-1353
arterial thrombosis in, 1344, 1347, 1347t, 1353-1354
arteriosclerosis obliterans in, 1350-1351
arteriovenous fistula in, 538-539, 541, 1344, 1347, 1360
atheroembolism in, 1343-1344, 1353, 1353f
Buerger's disease in, 1351-1352
chronic arterial insufficiency in, 1345-1346, 1350-1352
clinical features of, 1344-1347
diagnosis of, 1348
drug abuse–related, 1360-1361
history in, 1344-1346, 1345f
inflammatory, 1344, 1347
management of, 1348-1350
pathophysiology of, 1342-1344
physical examination in, 1346-1347, 1347t
thoracic outlet syndrome in, 1358-1360, 1358f, 1359f
trauma in, 1344
vasospastic disorders in, 1344
Peripheral nerve disorders. *See* Mononeuropathy; Neuropathy; Polyneuropathy.
Peripheral nerve fibers, in pain transmission, 2914, 2915t
Peripheral nervous system
anatomy of, 1688-1689, 1688f
cyclic antidepressant effects on, 2353b
Peripheral vascular injury, 536-547
clinical features of, 539-541, 540f
diagnostic strategies in, 541-543
disposition in, 547
epidemiology of, 536-537
of lower extremity, 546-547
of upper extremity, 544-546
pathophysiology of, 537-539, 538f
treatment of, 543-544
Peripheral venous access
in adult resuscitation, 91
in pediatric resuscitation, 99
Perirectal abscess, 1513t, 1514, 2205-2206, 2206f
Perirenal hematoma, 498f
Peristaltic activity, decreased, causes of, 1440, 1441b
Peritalar dislocation, 825-826, 825f
Peritendinitis, calcifying, of femur and hip, 742
Peritoneal dialysis
chronic ambulatory, 1547
complications of, 1552-1554, 1553t
continuous cyclic, 1547
for acute renal failure, 2650
Peritoneal dialysis *(Continued)*
for chronic renal failure, 1547-1548
for rewarming in accidental hypothermia, 2249
Peritoneal irritation, in ectopic pregnancy, 2743
Peritoneal lavage
in abdominal trauma, 499-501, 500t
in multiple trauma, 312
in pregnant trauma patient, 321
Peritoneal signs
in abdominal stab wound, 503
in small bowel obstruction, 1442
Peritoneal violation, laparotomy and, 504, 506
Peritonitis
bacterial
in small bowel obstruction, 1441
spontaneous, 245-246, 1412-1413
eosinophilic, 1552
from corticosteroids, 2844
iatrogenic, 492
in peritoneal dialysis patient, 1552-1553, 1553t
in tuberculosis, 2161-2162
pelvic pain in, 250t
Peritonsillar abscess, 1117-1118, 1118f
Peritonsillar space, 1117
Peritonsillitis, 1117-1118, 1118f
Permethrin
for pediculosis, 1854
for *Phthirus pubis* infestation, 1569
for *Sarcoptes scabiei* infestation, 1569
for scabies, 1855
prophylactic, for tick-borne illness, 2142
Permissive hypercapnia
for chronic obstructive pulmonary disease, 1104
for critically ill asthmatic patient, 1092
Pernicious anemia, optic neuropathy from, 1060
Pernio, 2228, 2230
Peroneal arteries
anatomy of, 797
injury to, 547
Peroneal nerve, 797
anatomy of, 771, 797
injury to
in proximal tibial epiphyseal fracture, 781
in tibial femoral knee dislocation, 788
in tibial plateau fracture, 778
in tibial shaft fracture, 800
Peroneal retinaculum, 808, 809f
Peroneal tendon dislocation or tear, 818-819, 819f
Perphenazine, 2446t
Perseverations, speech, in schizophrenia, 1728
Persistent fetal circulation, 119
Personal integrity, 3129, 3129b
Personal protective equipment
for tuberculosis, 2170
in tactical emergency medical support, 3004
in terrorism incidents, 3013
Personality changes, in central nervous system infection, 1714
Personality disorders
classification of, 2978, 2979b
with brief psychotic episodes, 1729
Perthes' disease, 767
Perthes-Bankart lesion, in anterior glenohumeral joint dislocation, 690
Pertussis, 2004-2007, 2005f, 2006b, 2559-2560
Pes anserinus, 770, 771f
Pesticide poisoning, 2452-2469
bipyridyl compounds in, 2465-2466, 2465b
carbamate insecticides in, 2458b, 2461-2462
chlorinated hydrocarbon pesticides in, 2462-2463, 2462b
chlorophenoxy compounds in, 2464-2465, 2465b
DEET in, 2468-2469
glyphosate in, 2467-2468
hydrocarbons in, 2430
organophosphate insecticides in, 2457-2461, 2458b, 2459b, 2459f
pyrethrins and pyrethroids in, 2466-2467, 2467b
substituted phenols in, 2463-2464, 2463b
Petechiae
fever and, as indication for lumbar puncture, 2660
in infective endocarditis, 1301

Petechiae *(Continued)*
in meningococcal disease, 2022
pediatric fever and, 2507-2508
Petroleum asphalt burns, 926-927, 937
Petroleum distillates, toxicity of, 2428, 2429t
Peyote, 2409, 2409f
Peyronie's disease, 534
pH
in metabolic acidosis, 1929
in metabolic alkalosis, 1930
in mixed acid-base disorders, 1931
in respiratory acidosis, 1925
in respiratory alkalosis, 1926
of blood
changes in, compensatory responses to, 1923-1924
normal values for, 1923
Phagocytes, 2834
Phagocytosis, 2834
Phalangeal bones, 577-578, 579f-580f
Phalanx
extensor tendon injury at
distal, 605-607, 606f, 607f
proximal, 608
fracture of, 834
distal, 593-594, 593f
proximal, 594-595, 594f-596f
Phalen's sign, in carpal tunnel syndrome, 639, 639f, 1697
Pharmacokinetics
in children, 2935, 2952
in elderly person, 2826
Pharyngeal pain, in pharyngitis, 1109
Pharyngitis, 274-279, 1109-1114
ancillary studies in, 277-278, 277t
clinical features of, 1109-1111, 1110f
diagnosis of, 275-278, 276t, 277f, 277t, 1111-1112
differential diagnosis in, 278, 1112
disposition in, 1113-1114
epidemiology of, 274
etiology of, 1109
high-altitude, 2304
history in, 275-276
in children, screening for, 2509b
in epiglottitis, 2523
in lingual tonsillitis, 1114
in parapharyngeal abscess, 1122
management of, 278-279, 278f, 1112-1113
pathophysiology of, 274-275, 275t
physical examination in, 276-277, 276t
streptococcal, 274-275, 1109, 1110, 1111, 1112-1113, 1114
adult epiglottitis vs., 1115
in rheumatic fever, 1303, 1304
Pharyngoesophageal trauma, 446-447
Pharyngomaxillary space, 1121-1123, 1122f
Pharynx, foreign body in, 870-873
Phencyclidine intoxication, 2413, 2414-2415, 2414t, 2415t, 2416, 2882b, 2891-2893
during pregnancy, 2792
rhabdomyolysis in, 1979
Phenelzine, overdose of, 2365
Phenobarbital
during pregnancy and lactation, 2787
for alcohol-related status epilepticus, 2865
for bupropion-induced seizure, 2361
for cyclic antidepressant poisoning, 2356
for seizure, 166t, 167, 1627, 1627t, 1628t
in children, 2675, 2675t
for status epilepticus, 2672t, 2673
overdose of, 2482, 2483
side effects of, 1628t
Phenol and derivatives
burn injury from, 935-936
for wound cleansing, 848t
ingestion of, 2384
poisoning from, 936, 2463-2464, 2463b
Phenothiazine
adjuvant, with opioids, 2921
anticholinergic toxicity of, 2346b
cardiotoxicity of, 2445
during pregnancy and lactation, 2790
for nausea and vomiting, 203, 208b, 208t
Phenoxybenzamine
for hypertensive emergencies, 1319
in frostbite, 2233
Phentolamine
for cocaine overdose, 2390, 2391
for hypertension, 1319, 2693
Phentolamine *(Continued)*
in cocaine overdose, 2390
in MAOI toxicity, 2365
Phenylbutazone, overdose of, 2343
Phenylephrine
for sepsis, 2219t, 2220
for sinusitis, 1125
mydriasis from, 1061
Phenylephrinemethoxamine, for junctional tachycardia, 1234
Phenylpropanolamine, during pregnancy and lactation, 2790
Phenytoin, 1207
alcohol withdrawal syndrome and, 2865-2866
drugs affecting levels of, 1207b
during pregnancy and lactation, 2786
for alcohol-related status epilepticus, 2865
for digitalis toxicity, 2371
for seizure, 166, 166t, 1626-1627, 1627t, 1628t
in cancer patient, 1919
in children, 2675, 2675t
for status epilepticus, 2672t, 2673
gingival hyperplasia from, 1036
hyperglycemic hyperosmolar nonketotic coma from, 1969
prophylactic, in head trauma, 361, 370
side effects of, 1628t
Pheochromocytoma
anxiety in, 1747
hypertension in, 1313
Phimosis, in children, 2636
Phlebotomy, for polycythemia, 1885
Phlegmasia cerulea dolens, 1352, 1370
Phlegmonous gastritis, 1390, 1391
Phobia, 1746b, 1749
Phosgene, as chemical weapon, 939, 3032
Phosphate
for hypophosphatemia, 1952
imbalance of. *See* Hyperphosphatemia; Hypophosphatemia.
in diabetic ketoacidosis, 1966
normal physiology of, 1950-1951
Phosphodiesterase inhibitors
for beta blocker overdose, 2375
for calcium channel blocker overdose, 2378
for chronic heart failure, 1276
Phosphorus. *See* Phosphate.
Photographic documentation
in intimate partner violence and abuse, 1001, 1003
in sexual assault cases, 989, 989b
Photosensitivity, drug-induced, 1845, 1847t
Phototherapy, for kernicterus prophylaxis, 2603, 2605f
Phrenic nerve injury, 450
Phthirus pubis infestation, 1569
Physeal injuries, 2690, 2691f, 2691t, 2692, 2692f
Physical abuse
in pregnancy, 318
of child, 969-971, 969f, 970f, 970t, 972, 973, 974-975
of elder, 1009-1010
of intimate partner, 995-996, 997. *See also* Intimate partner violence and abuse.
Physical assault
by combative patient, 2963
forensic aspects of, 960-963, 961b, 961f-964f
victim identification in, 960
Physical fitness, as wellness strategy for emergency physicians, 3177-3178, 3177b
Physically disabled patient, 2904-2911
abuse of, 1015
hearing impairment in, 2904-2905
multiple sclerosis in, 2909-2911
pulmonary disorders in, 2907-2908
spinal cord injury in, 2905-2909
visual impairment in, 2905
Physician, emergency. *See* Emergency physician.
Physician staffing, for observation, 3062-3063
Physician-patient relationship
and racial/ethnic disparities in health outcomes, 3109-3110
pathology of, difficult patient and, 2973, 2974t
Physiologic jaundice of the newborn, 2601-2603, 2602t, 2603b, 2603t, 2604f-2605f
Physostigmine, for anticholinergic poisoning, 2350
Phytobezoar, 873
Phytolacca americana, 2474-2475, 2474f
Phytophotodermatitis, 974-975
Pick's disease, dementia in, 1657, 1659
Picornavirus, 2034t, 2056-2057
Picric acid, 935
Picture Archiving and Communications Systems and Imaging Systems, 3101
Piece of pie sign, in lunate dislocation, 630
Piedmont fracture, 551t
Pierre Robin syndrome, neonatal resuscitation in, 121
Pigment nephropathy, 1536, 1536b
Pigmentation changes
in Addison's disease, 1997
in pregnancy, 2723-2724, 2728
Pigmented gallstones, 1418, 2620
Pigmenturia, differential diagnosis in, 1981-1982, 1981b
Pill esophagitis, 1386, 1387
Pilocarpine, for closed-angle glaucoma, 1056
Pilon fractures, 814-815, 815f
Pilonidal abscess, 2206-2207
Pilonidal disease, 1515
Pimozide, 2446t
Pinch-off syndrome, 1362, 1363
Pindolol, 1321t, 2373t, 2374
Ping-pong fracture, in head-injured child, 368
Pinguecula, 296t, 1053-1054
"Pink puffer," 1099
Pinworm, 1479-1482
drug therapy for, 2100t
gastroenteritis in, 1479-1482
pruritus ani in, 2113-2114
Pipe-stem cirrhosis, in chronic schistosomiasis, 2112, 2113f
Pirbuterol, for asthma, 2538, 2539t
Pisiform
anatomy of, 622, 623f, 625
fracture of, 629
Pit viper envenomation, 896-897, 897f, 898, 900t
Pittsburgh Knee Rule, 774
Pituitary gland, in pregnancy, 2726
Pityriasis rosea, 1841
Pivot shift test, in knee trauma, 774
Placenta
abruption of, 319-320, 2747-2748, 2809-2810
circumvallate, 2810
delivery of, 2804-2805
drug transfer across, 2780-2781
examination of, 2805
retained, postpartum hemorrhage from, 2819
surgical removal of, 2819
Placenta accreta, increta, and percreta, 257-258, 257t, 2819
Placenta previa, 257, 257t, 2748, 2808-2809
Plague, 1131, 3027-3028, 3027f, 3028b
Plant poisoning, 2471-2479
anticholinergic agents in, 2345, 2346t
botanical identification in, 2471-2475, 2472f-2475f
epidemiology of, 2471
herbal medicines and, 2475-2477, 2476t
mushrooms in, 2477-2479, 2478t
unintentional childhood exposure in, 2471
Plantar fascial rupture, 836
Plantar fasciitis, 836
Plantaris strain and rupture, 804
Plaque, 1839t
dental bacterial, 1028
skin disorders with, 1838-1841
Plasma exchange
for Goodpasture syndrome, 1816
for hyperviscosity syndrome, 1913
for myasthenia gravis, 1707
for thrombotic thrombocytopenic purpura, 1898
Plasmids, antibiotic resistance and, 1575
Plasmodium falciparum, 2104. *See also* Malaria.
Plaster cast, 571-573
Plaster splint, 569
Plastic deformation of forearm, 644, 645f
Platelet(s)
adhesion defects of, 1898
aggregation defects of, 1899
in hemostasis, 1892, 1893b, 1893f
release defects of, 1898-1899
Platelet count
in bleeding disorders, 1895

Platelet count *(Continued)*
in gastrointestinal bleeding, 222
in pregnancy, 2725
Platelet disorders. *See also specific disorders, e.g.,* Thrombocytopenia.
differential diagnosis in, 1896-1899, 1896b
in alcoholism, 2874
in polycythemia, 1884
Platelet transfusions, 59, 1899
in acute radiation syndrome, 2324
in disseminated intravascular coagulation, 1904
in multiple trauma, 307
Platelet-activating factor, as anaphylaxis mediator, 1823, 1823b
Platysma muscle, 443
Plesiomonas shigelloides
dysenteric colitis in, 229t
gastroenteritis in, 1461t, 1462t, 1468
Plethysmography, in deep venous thrombosis, 1370
Pleural disease
pleural effusion and, 1148-1153
spontaneous pneumothorax and, 1143-1147
Pleural effusion, 1134, 1148-1153
clinical features of, 1150-1151, 1151f
exudative vs. transudative, 1149-1150, 1152, 1152b
in pneumonia, 2561, 2562
in superior vena cava syndrome, 1911
in systemic lupus erythematosus, 1808
in tuberculosis, 2152, 2152f, 2158-2159
loculated, 1148
malignant, 1149, 1153
management of, 1151-1153, 1152b
parapneumonic, 1148, 1149, 1152, 1153
pathophysiology of, 1148-1150, 1149b, 1149f
Pleural fluid analysis, 1152-1153, 1152b
Pleural fluid cell count, 1152
Pleural friction rub, 1150
Pleural irritation, in pneumonia, 2556
Pleuritic chest pain
in esophageal perforation, 484
in pneumothorax, 1145
Pleuritis, 1148, 1150
uremic, 1542
Plexopathy
brachial, 1692-1693, 1693b
in pelvic fracture, 720
lumbosacral, 1692-1693, 1693b
Plica syndrome, 794-795
Plicamycin, for hypercalcemia, 1946
Plummer-Vinson syndrome, esophageal web in, 1383
PMA (paramethylenedioxymethamphetamine), 2409
Pneumatic antishock garment, 2991
Pneumatocele, 1134
Pneumatosis intestinalis, in necrotizing enterocolitis, 2609, 2609f
Pneumococcal disease, 2016-2020, 2020b
after splenectomy, 2842-2843
drug-resistant, 1137-1138, 2019
in children, 2556, 2557, 2557f
meningitis in, 1711, 1714, 1715, 1720, 1721t, 1723, 2019
pediatric bacteremia in, 2505
Pneumococcal vaccine, 1129, 1723, 2017, 2019-2020, 2020b
Pneumocystis pneumonia (PCP), 1130, 2110
chest radiography in, 1136, 1136f
in cancer patient with impaired cell-mediated immunity, 2840
in HIV/AIDS, 1135-1136, 2077-2078, 1140
in organ transplant patient, 2848, 2849f
pneumothorax in, 1144
Pneumomediastinum
in asthma, 2536
in scuba diving–related disorders, 2286, 2293
spontaneous, 1146
subcutaneous emphysema and, 459
tracheobronchial injury and, 466, 466f
Pneumonia, 1128-1141
aspiration, 1136, 2560
atypical, 1131-1132
bacterial, 1129, 1130-1131
in children, 2555, 2556-2557, 2556f, 2557f, 2558t, 2563t
tuberculosis vs., 2157

Pneumonia *(Continued)*
chlamydial, 2559, 2559f, 2563t
clinical features of, 1131-1132
diagnostic strategies in, 1132-1135, 1133f, 1134f
differential diagnosis in, 1136
disposition in, 1140-1141, 1140t
dyspnea in, 179t
epidemiology of, 1128
etiologic agents in, 1129-1131
high-altitude pulmonary edema vs., 2304
host defenses and, 1128-1129
in alcoholism, 2870
in bronchopulmonary dysplasia, 2565, 2565f
in chronic obstructive pulmonary disease, 1102, 1106
in elderly person, 2828
in HIV-infected patient, 1135-1136, 1136f, 1138-1139, 1140-1141
in immunocompromised patient, 2560, 2841
in pertussis, 2006
in physically disabled patient, 2907
in pulmonary contusion, 461
isolation in, 1136, 1140-1141
management of, 1136-1139, 1138t, 1139t
mortality in, 1128, 1140, 1140t
mycoplasmal, 2558-2559, 2563t
observation in, 3072, 3072b, 3073t
pediatric, 2554-2564
complications of, 2562
diagnosis of, 2560-2561, 2561f
differential diagnosis in, 2561, 2562b
epidemiology of, 2555
management of, 2558t, 2562-2564
pathophysiology of, 2555
physical examination in, 2556
screening for, 2509b
signs and symptoms of, 2555-2556
Pneumocystis, 1130, 2110
chest radiography in, 1136, 1136f
in cancer patient with impaired cell-mediated immunity, 2840
in HIV/AIDS, 1135-1136, 2077-2078, 1140
in organ transplant patient, 2848, 2849f
pneumothorax in, 1144
tropical eosinophilic, 2110
viral, 1129, 1130, 1139, 2555, 2557-2560, 2563t
Pneumonia Severity Index, 3072, 3073t
Pneumonic plague, 3027
Pneumonitis, in systemic lupus erythematosus, 1808
Pneumopericardium, 1287-1288
Pneumoperitoneum
iatrogenic, 492
peptic ulcer perforation and, 1393
Pneumothorax, 1134, 1143-1147
catamenial, 1144
chest pain in, 183, 184, 186b, 187, 190t-191t
clinical features of, 1145-1146, 1145f, 1146f
communicating, 462, 462f, 464
dyspnea in, 179t
etiology of, 1143-1144, 1144b
in abdominal trauma, 497f
in asthma, 2536
in chronic obstructive pulmonary disease, 1102, 1143-1144, 1145
in scuba diving–related disorders, 2286, 2293
in tuberculosis, 2150, 2150f
management of, 1146-1148
occult, 463
open, 339
outcome of, 1148
pathophysiology of, 1144-1145, 1144f
risk factors for, 186b
simple, 461-462, 461f, 463-464, 464b
subcutaneous emphysema and, 459
tension, 339, 462, 462f, 463f, 464
tracheobronchial injury and, 466
traumatic, 338-339, 461-464, 461f-463f, 464b
Podofilox
for condylomata acuminata, 1564
for genital warts, 1520
Poikilocytosis, in myelophthisic anemia, 1876, 1876f
Poinsettia, 2474
Poison hemlock, 2472, 2473f
Poisoning/overdose, 2418-2426. *See also* Substance abuse.
acetaminophen, 2331-2337, 2332f

Poisoning/overdose *(Continued)*
antidotes to, 2329t
chronic exposure in, 2334b, 2335
clinical features of, 2332-2333
diagnosis of, 2333-2335, 2333b, 2334b
disposition in, 2337
in children, 2335
management of, 2333b, 2334b, 2335-2337
risk assessment using treatment nomogram in, 2333-2335, 2334f
anticholinergic, 2345-2350, 2346b, 2346t, 2347f
antidotes to, 2329t
clinical presentation in, 2347-2348, 2347t
diagnosis of, 2349
differential diagnosis in, 2348, 2348b
disposition in, 2350
management of, 2349-2350
antidepressant, 2352-2366
bupropion in, 2361, 2361t
cyclic antidepressants in, 2352-2357, 2353b, 2353f, 2354b, 2355f, 2357t
mirtazapine in, 2362-2363
monamine oxidase inhibitors in, 2363-2365, 2363b-2365b, 2364t
neurologic complications of, 2354t, 2356
selective serotonin reuptake inhibitors in, 2357-2360, 2358b, 2358t, 2359b, 2360t
trazadone in, 2361-2362
venlafaxine in, 2362, 2362t
antidotes to, 2329t
antipsychotic agent, 2445-2450, 2446t
arsenic, 2423-2424, 2424b
aspirin, 2339-2342, 2340f
clinical features of, 2341, 2341b
diagnosis of, 2341
disposition in, 2342
management of, 2341-2342, 2341b
cardiovascular drug, 2368-2379
beta blockers in, 2373-2376, 2373t, 2374b, 2375b
calcium channel blockers in, 2329t, 2376-2379, 2377b, 2377t, 2378b
digitalis in, 2368-2373
caustic, 2380-2385, 2381f, 2381t, 2382f
cocaine, 2386-2392
body packing/stuffing and, 2391-2392
clinical features of, 2386-2388, 2387b
diagnosis of, 2388-2389
differential diagnosis in, 2389, 2389b
disposition in, 2392, 2392t
management of, 2389-2391, 2389b, 2390b
dialysis for, 1549
digitalis, 2368-2373
acute vs. chronic, 2369, 2370t
antidotes to, 2329t
clinical features of, 2369, 2370b
diagnosis of, 2369-2370
differential diagnosis in, 2370
disposition in, 2372-2373
in children, 2372, 2372t
management of, 2370-2371, 2372b
pathophysiology of, 2368-2369, 2369b
ethanol. *See* Alcohol intoxication; Alcoholism.
general approach to, 2325-2331
consultation in, 2331
decontamination in, 2330
disposition in, 2330-2331
initial, 2326-2327
overdose history in, 2326, 2326b
physical examination in, 2326-2327, 2327t
toxic syndromes in, 2327-2328, 2327t
hallucinogen, 2406-2416
dissociative agents in, 2413-2426, 2414t, 2415t
entactogens in, 2408-2411, 2409f
marijuana and miscellaneous plants and fungi in, 2411-2413, 2412f
serotonin-like agents in, 2406-2408, 2407f
heavy metal, 2418-2426
arsenic in, 2423-2424, 2424b
iron in, 2418-2421, 2419t, 2420f, 2420t
lead in, 2421-2423, 2422t
mercury in, 2424-2426, 2425b, 2425t
hydrocarbon, 2428-2432, 2429t, 2430f, 2431f
inhaled toxin, 2432-2441, 2443t
carbon monoxide in, 2438-2441
cyanide and hydrogen sulfide in, 2436-2438, 2437f

Poisoning/overdose *(Continued)*
pulmonary irritants in, 2433t, 2434-2435, 2434f
simple asphyxiants in, 2432-2433
smoke in, 2435-2436
lithium, 2442-2444, 2443t
nonsteroidal antiinflammatory drug, 2342-2344
odors in, 2327, 2327t
opioid, 2327t, 2328, 2451-2456
antidotes to, 2329t
clinical features of, 2452-2454, 2453t
diagnosis of, 2454
differential diagnosis in, 2454
disposition in, 2455
management of, 2454-2455
pathophysiology and pharmacology of, 2451-2452
pesticide, 2452-2469
bipyridyl compounds in, 2465-2466, 2465b
carbamate insecticides in, 2458b, 2461-2462
chlorinated hydrocarbon pesticides in, 2462-2463, 2462b
chlorophenoxy compounds in, 2464-2465, 2465b
DEET in, 2468-2469
glyphosate in, 2467-2468
hydrocarbons in, 2430
organophosphate insecticides in, 2457-2461, 2458b, 2459b, 2459f
pyrethrins and pyrethroids in, 2466-2467, 2467b
substituted phenols in, 2463-2464, 2463b
plant, 2471-2479
anticholinergic agents in, 2345, 2346t
botanical identification in, 2471-2475, 2472f-2475f
epidemiology of, 2471
herbal medicines and, 2475-2477, 2476t
mushrooms in, 2477-2479, 2478t
unintentional childhood exposure in, 2471
sedative hypnotic, 2327t, 2328, 2481-2490
barbiturates in, 2481-2483, 2482b, 2482f
benzodiazepines in, 2483-2486, 2484t
buspirone in, 2486
chloral hydrate in, 2487
flunitrazepam in, 2486
γ-hydroxybutyrate in, 2488-2490, 2488b
OTC sleep aids in, 2487-2488, 2488t
zolpidem and zaleplon in, 2486-2487
suicide by, 1768
sympathomimetic, 2386-2393
toxic alcohol, 2395-2404
ethylene glycol in, 2398-2402, 2401t
isopropyl alcohol in, 2402-2404
methanol in, 2395-2398
Pokeweed, 2474-2475, 2474f
Police dogs, bites by, 882
Poliomyelitis, 1704
paralytic, 2056-2057
Poliovirus, 2035t, 2056-2057
Polle syndrome, 1761, 1763, 1765
Poloxamer, for sickle cell disease, 1880
Polyarteritis nodosa, 1813-1814
Polyarthritis, 1303-1304, 1784f, 1787-1792, 1790b, 2596
Polycythemia, 273, 1884-1885, 1884f, 1885b
Polycythemia vera, 1885, 1885b
Polydioxanone suture, 852t
Polydipsia, psychogenic, 1934
Polyethylene glycol therapy, for phenol burn, 935-936
Polymerase chain reaction testing
in bacterial meningitis, 2662
in central nervous system infection, 1719
in HIV, 2074
in trichomoniasis, 1567
in tuberculosis, 2155
Polymorphonuclear leukocytes. *See* Neutrophil(s).
Polymyalgia rheumatica, 1638
Polymyositis, 1396, 1708
Polyneuropathy
demyelinating, 1690-1691, 1690b
distal symmetrical sensorimotor, 1691-1692, 1691b
Polyomaviruses, 2034t, 2045-2046
Polyoxyethylene amine, in glyphosate poisoning, 2467-2468
Polyoxyethylene sorbitan, for tar removal, 927
Polyp, nasal, 1082
Polypropylene suture, 852t
Polysorbate, for tar removal, 927
Polytetrafluoroethylene (PTFE) vascular shunt, in arterial injury, 544
Polythiazide, 1321t
Pontine myelinolysis, central, in hyponatremia, 1935
Popliteal aneurysm, 1354
Popliteal artery, 540, 540f
anatomy of, 771
injury to, 546-547
in proximal tibial epiphyseal fracture, 781
in tibial femoral knee dislocation, 787, 788, 789
in tibial plateau fracture, 778
Popliteal cyst, 796, 797f
Popliteal disease, pain in, 1345
Popliteal fossa, 771
Popliteofibular ligament, 770-771, 771f
Popliteus tendinitis, 795
Porcelain gallbladder, 1423
Porphyrin, defective synthesis of, in sideroblastic anemia, 1873
Portuguese man-of-war, 909
Positional testing, in vertigo, 145, 145f
Positional vertigo, benign, 147t, 2683
Positioning, in neonatal resuscitation, 122
Positive airway pressure
bilevel, 28, 28f
in critically ill asthmatic patient, 1092
continuous, 27-28
in acute pulmonary edema, 1271, 1271f
in sleep apnea in chronic heart failure, 1277
in submersion victim, 2314
Positive end-expiratory pressure (PEEP), 27-28
Positive predictive value, 3059t
Positive-pressure insufflation technique, for nasal foreign body, 864
Positive-pressure ventilation
adverse effects of, 26b
basic approaches to, 26-27
modes of, 27-28
noninvasive, 28-29, 28f
evolving therapies in, 33
in asthma, 1091-1092
in chronic obstructive pulmonary disease, 1104, 1104t
initial settings and ongoing monitoring in, 29-30, 29t
outcomes in, 32-33
patient management in, 31
patient selection for, 29
Positive symptoms in schizophrenia, 1726, 1727-1728
Positron emission tomography
in minor head trauma, 365
in osteomyelitis, 2181
Postanal abscess, 1513t, 1514-1515
Postconcussive syndrome, 366
Postdural puncture headache, 1641
Posterior arch, 717, 718f
Posterior columns, 1676, 1676f
Posterior cruciate ligament injury, 790-791, 792
stability testing in, 773-774
tibial femoral knee dislocation and, 788
Posterior drawer test, in posterior cruciate ligament injury, 773-774
Posterior elbow dislocation, 664-665, 664f, 665f
Posterior fat pad, in elbow, 651, 651f
Posterior fossa, epidural hematoma in, 375, 376f
Posterior longitudinal ligament, 702
Posterior malleolus, fracture of, 813
Posterior neural arch fracture, of atlas, 410, 410f
Posterior sag sign, in posterior cruciate ligament injury, 774
Posterior segment, traumatic injury to, 1050-1051, 1050f
Posterior tibial artery
anatomy of, 797
injury to, 547
Posterior tibial nerve
compression of, heel pain in, 836-837
injury to
in tibial femoral knee dislocation, 788
tibial shaft fracture and, 800
Posteroinferior cerebellar artery syndrome, 420
Posterolateral corner, 770, 771f
Postexposure prophylaxis
for hepatitis, 1406, 1407t, 1408f
for hepatitis B, 1406, 3083-3084, 3084t
for hepatitis C, 3083, 3084
for HIV, 3083, 3084-3087, 3085t, 3086b
for rabies, 2066-2069, 2067t, 2068b
Postexposure testing, for HIV, 3087
Postmortem teaching, bioethical dilemnas in, 3136
Postnecrotic cirrhosis, 1410
Postoperative pancreatitis, 1428
Postpartum cardiomyopathy, 2821
Postpartum depression, 2821-2822
Postpartum endometriosis, 2821
Postpartum hemorrhage, 258t, 2818-2820
Postprandial hypoglycemia, 1961
Postresuscitation syndrome, 77
Poststreptococcal glomerulonephritis, 2647-2648
Poststreptococcal reactive arthritis, 1791
Post-test odds, 3059t
Post-test probability, 3059t
Posttraumatic corneal ulcer, 1052, 1052f
Posttraumatic headache, 1640
Posttraumatic osteomyelitis, 2185
Posttraumatic pericarditis, 1283
Posttraumatic pseudoaneurysm, 789-790, 1356-1357, 1357t
Posttraumatic reversible arterial spasm, 538
Posttraumatic seizure, 370, 373, 1623
prophylaxis against, 361, 361b
Posttraumatic stress disorder, 1746b
panic attack in, 1749
suicide and, 1769
Posttraumatic syrinx, 435, 436f, 2909
Postural strangulation, 450
Posturing, in head trauma, 357
Potassium
administration of
for diabetic ketoacidosis, 1966
for digitalis toxicity, 2370
for hypokalemia, 1939
for metabolic alkalosis, 1931
imbalance of. *See* Hyperkalemia; Hypokalemia.
in resting membrane potential, 1200, 1200f
normal physiology of, 1937
serum, in diabetic ketoacidosis, 1964, 1964t
serum pH and, 1924
skin injury from, 937
Potassium channel antagonists, after cerebral ischemia, 71
Potassium chloride
for alcoholic ketoacidosis, 2873
ingestion of, gastric injury from, 2381, 2381f, 2382f
Potassium hydroxide, ingestion of, 2380, 2381t
Potassium hydroxide (KOH) examination, in dermatophyte infections, 1838
Potassium iodide
for erythema nodosum, 1856-1857
for internal radioactive contamination, 2324
for radioactive iodine exposure, 3023, 3023t
for thyroid storm, 1989
Potassium loss, in salicylate overdose, 2340
Potassium phosphate, for hypophosphatemia, 1952
Potassium-sparing diuretics, 1321t
Potential injury-creating event (PICE) nomenclature, 3011-3012, 3011t, 3012b, 3012t
Pott's disease, 261, 265t, 2159, 2178, 2182, 2182f, 2184-2185
Pott's fracture, 551t
Povidone-iodine
for rabies postexposure prophylaxis, 2068
for skin disinfection, 847
for wound cleansing, 847-848, 848t
Powder burn, 953
Power of attorney, durable, 3133
Power of clinical trial, 3051t, 3052
Poxviruses, 2034t, 2039-2040, 2039f
PPD testing, 2156-2157, 2157b, 2158t
PR interval, 1202
in first-degree atrioventricular block, 1218
in infants and children, 2574, 2574t
in Wolff-Parkinson-White syndrome, 1235
PR segment, in pericarditis, 1281, 1282
Practice guidelines. *See* Guidelines for emergency medicine.

Practice patterns, computer-based analysis of, 3099
Practolol, overdose of, 2373t
Pralidoxime
for nerve agent exposure, 3030-3031, 3031t
for organophosphate poisoning, 2461
Prazosin, 1321t
Prechiasmal visual loss, 1059
Precordial thump, 90
Prednisolone
for asthma, 1088, 2539t, 2541, 2543t
for caustic ingestion, 2383
Prednisone
during pregnancy and lactation, 2776, 2789
for anaphylaxis, 2549
for asthma, 1088, 1089, 2539t, 2541, 2543t
for autoimmune hemolytic anemia, 1883
for Bell's palsy, 1667
for chronic obstructive pulmonary disease, 1106
for Churg-Strauss syndrome, 1816
for contact dermatitis, 1852
for erythema multiforme, 1853
for giant cell arteritis, 1638
for gouty arthritis, 1786
for Henoch-Schönlein purpura, 1815
for hypercalcemic cancer patient, 1916
for inflammatory bowel disease, 2616
for inflammatory myopathy, 1708
for kerion, 1839
for Lyme disease–related myocarditis, 1292
for mixed cryoglobulinemia, 1815
for nephrotic syndrome, 2648
for pemphigus vulgaris, 1857
for pericarditis, 1282
for *Pneumocystis* pneumonia in HIV/AIDS, 2078
for rheumatic fever, 1791
for rheumatoid arthritis, 1791
for systemic lupus erythematosus, 1809
for Takayasu's arteritis, 1813
for temporal, 1813
immunosuppressive effects of, 2843-2844
prophylactic, for cluster headache, 1635
Preeclampsia, 2749-2751, 2750b
Preexcitation, 1203, 1235-1237, 1236f, 1237f
Preexposure prophylaxis, for rabies, 2069, 2069t
Prefreeze phase of frostbite, 2229, 2229b
Pregnancy, 2722-2872
abdominal pain in, 2733, 2752-2756, 2753t
abruptio placentae in, 2747-2748, 2809-2810
acetaminophen overdose in, 2336-2337
acute complications of, 2739-2759
early, 2740-2747
late, 2747-2752
medical and surgical problems associated with, 2752-2759, 2753t
acute coronary syndromes in, 2763t, 2766-2767
acute fatty liver of, 1417, 2755-2756
air medical transport in, 2999
alcohol consumption during, 2877-2878
alkalemia in, 1926
altitude and, 2308-2309
amniotic fluid embolus in, 2751-2752
anatomic changes in, 317-318
anemia in, 2724, 2763t, 2767-2768
antituberculous agents during, 2168
appendicitis in, 1453, 2752-2754, 2754f
asthma in, 1091, 2761-2762, 2763t, 2765t
bacterial vaginosis in, 1568
bleeding diathesis in, 2753t
carbon monoxide poisoning in, 2440
cardiomyopathy in, 1297
carpal tunnel syndrome in, 1697
chest pain in, 2732-2733
cholelithiasis in, 1419, 2754-2755
cholestasis in, 1416-1417
intrahepatic, 2756
chorioamnionitis in, 2759
chronic medical illness during, 2761-2776, 2763t-2765t
decompression sickness in, 2285
definitions related to, 2722-2723
depression following, 1738
diabetes mellitus in, 1972, 2764t, 2771-2772
differential considerations in, 2731-2733
disease and injury prevention in, 2735-2737
domestic violence in, 997, 2734-2735, 2734t
Pregnancy *(Continued)*
drug therapy during, safety of, 2781-2790, 2782t-2783t
dyspnea in, 2725, 2753t
ectopic, 2742-2746
ancillary studies in, 2745
clinical features of, 2743
diagnosis of, 2743-2744
differential considerations in, 2745
hormonal assays in, 2744
management of, 2745-2746, 2746f
miscarriage vs., 2741
pelvic pain in, 251t
risk factors for, 2743, 2743b
ruptured, abdominal pain in, 214t
ultrasonography of, 2730, 2744, 2744b
vaginal bleeding in, 257, 257t
electrical injuries in, 2277
emergency equipment needs in, 2735
epidemiology of, 2722, 2723f
epilepsy in, 2763t, 2768-2769
genitourinary infections in, 2757-2759
gynecologic problems in, 2752, 2753t
headache in, 2732
heart failure in, 1268
hemorrhoids in, 1510
hepatitis in, 2775
heterotopic, 2743
history in, 2727
HIV/AIDS in, 2764t, 2774, 2810
hyperemesis gravidarum in, 2756
hypertension in, 1317, 2727, 2765t
chronic, 2762, 2763t, 2765t
gestational, 2749-2751, 2750b
pulmonary, 2762, 2766
hypomagnesemia in, 1948
jaundice in, 2726, 2753t
laboratory studies in, 2728-2730, 2729f
liver disorders in, 1416-1417, 2755-2756
Lyme disease in, 2128-2129
miscarriage in, 2740-2742, 2741b
ectopic pregnancy vs., 2745
molar, 257, 2741, 2746-2747
multiple sclerosis in, 2763t, 2769-2770
musculoskeletal pain in, 2733
myasthenia gravis in, 2764t, 2770-2771
nausea and vomiting in, 204t, 206, 2756
pancreatitis in, 1428
pelvic inflammatory disease in, 2759
pelvic pain in, 248, 249b, 250, 252
pericardial disease in, 1287
physical examination in, 2727-2728
physiologic changes in, 316-317, 317t, 2723-2727, 2724f-2726f, 2727t
placenta previa in, 2748, 2808-2809
prevention of, after sexual assault, 991, 991t
pulmonary embolism in, 1380
pyelonephritis in, 2754, 2757, 2758
radiologic studies in, 2730-2731, 2730f, 2731f
renal disorders in, 2771
rheumatic diseases in, 2775-2776
salicylate poisoning in, 2342
seizure in, 1624, 2753t, 2763t, 2768-2769
sexually transmitted diseases in, 2758-2759
spinal cord injury in, 2770
spurious, 2731-2732
substance abuse in, 2736, 2790-2794, 2791b, 2883
syphilis in, 1562, 2764t, 2775
systemic lupus erythematosus in, 1810, 2775-2776
thromboembolic disease in, 317, 2756-2757
thyroid disorders in, 2764t, 2772-2773
trauma in, 318-326, 2733
blunt, 318
diagnostic strategies in, 320-321, 320t, 321t
disposition in, 326
fetal evaluation in, 323-324, 323f, 323t, 324f
fetal injury in, 319
fetomaternal hemorrhage and, 321
management of, 321-326, 322f
maternal resuscitation in, 322-323
penetrating, 318-319
perimortem cesarean section in, 325-326
placental injury in, 319-320
prehospital end-of-life issues related to, 3145
primary survey in, 322-323
secondary survey in, 323
uterine injury in, 320
Pregnancy *(Continued)*
trichomoniasis in, 1568
tuberculosis in, 2764t, 2773-2774
ultrasonography in, third trimester, 2802, 2802b, 2802t
urinary tract infection in, 1578, 2757-2758
vaginal bleeding in, 2727
differential diagnosis in, 2753t
during second half, 2747-2748
epidemiology of, 254
first-trimester, 2740-2741, 2746f
pathophysiology of, 254
third-trimester, 2808-2810
treatment of, 257, 259
vaginitis in, 2758
valvular heart disease in, 2763t, 2767
vulvovaginal candidiasis in, 1568
Pregnancy test, 2728-2730, 2729f
in abdominal pain, 216
in appendicitis, 1454
in pelvic pain, 249
Pregnancy tumor, 1035
Prehospital care
airway management in, 2990
controversies in, 2990-2991
during air medical transport, 2998-2999
end-of-life issues in, 3144-3146
equipment in, 2988
in abdominal trauma, 502
in acute coronary syndromes, 1157
in alcohol withdrawal syndrome, 2861
in anaphylaxis, 1830
in aortic rupture, 481
in bleeding disorders, 1894
in cardiac tamponade, 475
in cardiovascular emergencies, 2990-2991
in central nervous system infection, 1721
in delirium, 1653
in eclampsia, 2750
in elder abuse, 1011
in elderly trauma patient, 348
in facial trauma, 389-390
in injury prevention and control, 948
in ischemic stroke, 1613-1614
in PCP intoxication, 2415
in pediatric asthma, 2537
in pediatric fever, 2511
in pelvic fracture, 718
in respiratory emergencies, 2990
in severe head trauma, 358
in snakebite, 899
in spinal injuries, 435
in splinting and bandaging of fractures, 568, 569f
in sudden infant death syndrome, 2717
in suicide, 1771
in thermal burns, 921
in trauma emergencies, 2991
medications in, 2987-2988, 2990-2991
protocols for, 2989
Prehospital directives, 3132-3133
Prehospital information systems, 3099, 3101, 3105
Prehospital response, in disaster preparedness, 3014-3015
Prehospital resuscitation, bioethical dilemmas in, 3132-3133
Prehypertension, 1310
Preload
in heart failure, 1259-1260, 1260f
normalization of, in sepsis, 2218
Premature atrial contractions, 1222-1223, 1222f, 1223f
Premature infant
sudden death in, 2714-2715
symptomatic, definition of, 2714
Premature junctional contractions, 1223-1224
Premature labor, 2805-2807, 2806b, 2807b
Premature rupture of membranes, 2807-2808, 2808t
Premature ventricular contractions, 1223t, 1224-1225, 1224f
causes of, 1224, 1224b
Lown classification of, 1225, 1225t
treatment of, 1225
Prematurity, apnea of, definition of, 2714
Preoxygenation, in rapid sequence intubation, 10, 10f
Prepatellar bursitis, 795-796, 1801-1803

Prerenal azotemia, 1527t, 1532-1533, 1533b, 1538
Preschool children
  developmental milestones in, 2496t, 2497
  fever in, management of, 2515
Prescriptions, medicolegal issues in, 3160
Preseptal cellulitis, 2197-2198
Pressure urticaria, 1848
Pressure-cycled ventilation, 27
Pressure-support ventilation (PSV), 27
Pressure-volume relationships
  and scuba diving–related disorders, 2281f
  in dysbarisms, 2280-2281, 2281f
Preterm labor, 2805-2807, 2806b, 2807b
Pretest odds, 3059t
Pretracheal layer, 442-443
Prevention and control of injury, 940-950
  acute trauma care and, 948
  advocacy of public policy for, 948, 950
  epidemiology and documentation in, 945-946
  in elderly person, 2829-2830
  in gang violence in emergency department, 1021-1022
  in pregnancy, 2735-2737
  in youth violence, 1020
  methods of prevention in, 944-945
  prehospital care in, 948
  principles of, 940, 941f, 943-945, 943t, 944t
  public health and, 943-944, 944t
  risk factor assessment in, 946-948
  scientific approach to, 940, 941b
Preventive services
  for elderly person, 2829-2830
  in tactical emergency medical support, 3004
  medicolegal issues in, 3159
Prevertebral space, 1027, 1117
Priapism
  in children, 2635-2636
  in sickle cell disease, 1880
Prickly heat, 2259
Primaquine, for malaria, 2104
Primary care physician, emergency physician and, differences between, 3131, 3131t
Primary survey
  in obstetric trauma, 322-323
  in pediatric trauma, 329-330, 329t, 331t-333t
Primate bite, 884, 888-889, 889b, 889t
Primidone, during pregnancy and lactation, 2787
Prinzmetal angina, 1156
Prion disease, 1657-1658, 1659, 2058
Prisoners
  consent and, 3168
  foreign body ingestion by, 873, 874f
Private patient, screening requirements for, 3157
Probability, 3051t, 3052
  a priori, 3055-3056
  post-test, 3059t
  pretest, 3059t
Probenecid
  during pregnancy and lactation, 2784
  for gouty arthritis, 1786
Problem patient. *See* Combative patient; Difficult patient.
Problem-solving, developmental milestones in, 2495-2497, 2496t
Procainamide, 1206
  during pregnancy and lactation, 2787
  for atrial fibrillation, 1232b, 1233
  for dysrhythmia, in infants and children, 2586b
  for pediatric resuscitation, 103t, 105
  for ventricular tachycardia, 1242
  for wide-complex tachycardia, 1240
  for Wolff-Parkinson-White syndrome, 1237
Procaine, 2931t
Procedural sedation and analgesia, 2938-2954
  agents for, 2940t-2941t
  barbiturates for, 2945-2946
  benzodiazepines for, 2944-2945
  consent prior to, 2940
  contraindications to, 2939
  discharge criteria and instructions after, 2943
  drug selection and administration in, 2949-2952, 2950t, 2951b
  etomidate for, 2940t-2941t, 2947-2948
  fasting prior to, 2939-2940
  in children, 2952-2954
  ketamine for, 2940t-2941t, 2946-2947
  monitoring of, 2942-2943
  nitrous oxide for, 2940t-2941t, 2948
Procedural sedation and analgesia *(Continued)*
  opioids for, 2944
  personnel providing, 2941-2942
  preprocedure patient assessment in, 2938-2940
  propofol for, 2940t-2941t, 2947
  recovery from, 2943
  reversal agents in, 2948-2949
  route of administration for, 2943-2944
  sedation continuum and, 2938, 2939f
  supplies and equipment for, 2942
  terminology in, 2938, 2939b
Process improvement in emergency department, 3119-3126
  problem areas and, 3124-3126, 3125t
  sources of failure and, 3119-3123, 3120f, 3120t
Prochlorperazine, 2446t
  for migraine, 1633t, 1634, 2680
  for nausea and vomiting, 203, 208b, 208t
  for vertigo, 146
Procidentia, 1521, 1521f
Proctalgia fugax, 1509, 1516 *See also* Anorectal pain
Proctitis
  Chlamydia trachomatis, 1519
  herpes, 1519
  radiation, 1520-1521
Proctocolitis, radiation, 1505-1506
Proctosigmoidoscopy, in gastrointestinal bleeding, 224
"Professional disclosure" standard, 3166
Professional relationships, as stressor for emergency physician, 3175
Professional values, 3129, 3129b
Progesterone, serum, in ectopic pregnancy, 2744
Progressive multifocal leukoencephalopathy, 2045-2046
  dementia in, 1658, 1659
  in HIV/AIDS, 2082
Prokinetic agents, for nausea and vomiting, 206, 208b
Prolactin, serum, in pregnancy, 2726
PROM (premature rupture of membranes), 2807-2808, 2808t
Promethazine, 2446t
  for migraine, 2680
  for vertigo, 146
Pronation, of hand, 577f
Pronator quadratus line, 626, 628f
Prone sleeping, in sudden infant death syndrome, 2715
Propafenone, 1208
Propantheline, anticholinergic toxicity of, 2345
Proparacaine, for red and painful eye, 291
Propofol
  for procedural sedation and analgesia, 2940t-2941t, 2947, 2950-2952, 2954
  for status epilepticus, 1627, 1627t, 2672t, 2673
  for tetanus, 2011
  in cyclic antidepressant poisoning, 2356
Proportional assist ventilation, 33
Propoxyphene, 2452, 2453, 2453t, 2920
Propranolol, 1209, 1321t
  alcohol interactions with, 2875
  for alcohol withdrawal syndrome, 2862
  for chloral hydrate poisoning, 2487
  for hypoxic (tet) spells, 2581
  for migraine prophylaxis, 1634
  for tetanus, 2011
  for thyroid storm, 1989
  overdose of, 2373t, 2374
  prophylactic, for migraine, 2680
Propylthiouracil
  for hyperthyroidism in pregnancy, 2773
  for thyroid storm, 1988
Prospective observational study, 3047
Prostacyclin
  as anaphylaxis mediator, 1823, 1823b
  in heart failure, 1262
Prostaglandin
  as anaphylaxis mediator, 1823, 1823b
  for upper gastrointestinal disorders, 1399
  in asthma, 1080f, 1081, 1081f
  in burn edema, 917
  in frostbite, 2229
  in heart failure, 1262
  in sepsis, 2213
Prostaglandin E1, for ductal-dependent congenital heart disease, 2576-2577, 2577b
Prostaglandin E2, in fever, 104
Prostaglandin synthetase inhibitors, for premature labor, 2807
Prostate, physical examination of, 1573
Prostatitis, 1585-1586
Prosthesis, joint, infection after, 2191
Prosthetic graft, for peripheral arteriovascular disease, 1350
Prosthetic valve
  complications of, 1307-1308
  endocarditis as complication of, 1300
Protease inhibitors
  for HIV/AIDS, 2087t, 2088
  rifamycins and, drug interactions between, 2166
Protease-antiprotease relationship, in chronic obstructive pulmonary disease, 1098
Protective body armor, nonpenetrating ballistic injury associated with, 458-459
Protective equipment
  for tuberculosis, 2170
  in tactical emergency medical support, 3004
  in terrorism incidents, 3013
Protein
  cerebrospinal fluid
    in bacterial meningitis, 2661
    in central nervous system infection, 1718
  urine, 1525
Protein buffers, 1923
Protein C, in sepsis, 2214
Protein kinases, in cerebral ischemia, 66
Proteinuria, 1530-1532
  clinical features of, 1531
  glomerular, 1531
  in children, 2646-2647
  in glomerulonephritis, 1534
  in nephrotic syndrome, 1531, 1531b
  in preeclampsia/eclampsia, 2749-2751, 2750b
  laboratory studies in, 1532
  orthostatic, 1531
  overflow, 1531
  tubular, 1531
Proteolytic enzymes, in sarcoplasm, 1976
Proteus infection, in urinary tract infection, 1583
Prothrombin time (PT)
  abnormal, 1899
  in bleeding disorders, 1895
  in factor VII deficiency, 1899
  in gastrointestinal bleeding, 222
  in hepatitis, 1404
  in pregnancy, 318
Protocols, decision making errors in using, 131t, 132
Proton pump inhibitors
  for gastroesophageal reflux, 1389-1390, 1390t
  for gastrointestinal bleeding, 224-225
  for upper gastrointestinal disorders, 1390t, 1399
Protozoal gastroenteritis, 1476-1482, 1477t
  Cryptosporidium, 1476-1478, 1477t
  Cyclospora cayetanensis, 1477t, 1478-1479
  Entamoebaa histolytica, 1477t, 1480-1481
  Enterobius vermicularis, 1479-1482
  Giardia, 1477t, 1479-1480
  Isospora belli, 1476-1478, 1477t
Protozoal infections
  drug therapy for, 2098t
  parasites in, 2099t
Proximal femoral epiphysis, avascular necrosis of, 2706-2707, 2707f
Proximal femoral fracture, 750-752, 750f-751f, 752b
Proximal fibula, fracture of, 801-802, 802f, 814f
Proximal humeral epiphysis, fracture of, 682-683, 683f
Proximal humerus
  anatomy of, 672, 673f
  fracture of, 680-682, 681f, 682f
Proximal interphalangeal joint, 578, 579f
  dislocation of, 601-602
  extensor tendon injuries at, 607-608, 607f
Proximal phalanx
  extensor tendon injuries at, 608
  fracture of, 594-595, 594f-596f
Proximal radioulnar joint, 639-640
Proximal radius, 647, 647f
Proximal tibia
  anatomy of, 770, 771f
  fracture of

Proximal tibia *(Continued)*
extra-articular, 797-799
intra-articular, 777-781
Proximal tibiofibular joint, dislocation of, 802-803
Proximity wounds, 540, 540f, 543
Pruritus
in anaphylaxis, 1829, 2548
in atopic dermatitis, 1842
in ciguatera fish poisoning, 1473
in decompression sickness, 2284
in HIV/AIDS, 2084-2085
in *Sarcoptes scabiei* infestation, 1569
internal malignancy associated with, 1864
Pruritus ani, 1509, 1517-1518, 1517b
causes of, 1517, 1517b
in *Enterobius vermicularis* gastroenteritis, 1481
in parasitic infection, 2113-2114
Pruritus gravidarum, 2726, 2756
Prussian blue, for cesium and thallium ingestion, 3023, 3023t
Pseudarthrosis, 564
Pseudoaneurysm, 538, 538f, 1348
after abdominal aortic aneurysm repair, 1340
infected, in drug abusers, 1361
posttraumatic, 789-790, 1356-1357, 1357t
repair of, 544
Pseudocholinesterase activity, conditions and drugs that reduce, 13, 13b
Pseudoclaudication, in spinal stenosis, 705
Pseudoclawing, 595
Pseudocoarctation syndrome, in aortic rupture, 478
Pseudocyanosis, 268
Pseudocyst, pancreatic, 1427, 1430, 1430f, 1435
Pseudodementia, 1656, 1659-1660, 1660t
Pseudodysrhythmias, 1215, 1215f
Pseudoephedrine
during pregnancy and lactation, 2790
prophylactic, for middle ear barotrauma, 2292
Pseudofracture, 558
Pseudogout, 1786-1787
Pseudohematuria, 1604
Pseudohyperkalemia, 1939
Pseudohyperphosphatemia, 1952
Pseudohyponatremia, 1933
Pseudohypoparathyroidism, hypocalcemia in, 1943
Pseudohypotension, in aortic dissection, 1326
Pseudologica fantastica, in Munchausen's syndrome, 1702
Pseudomembranous colitis, in *Clostridium difficile* infection, 2625
Pseudomonas aeruginosa
in bone or joint infections, 2178, 2178t
in cystic fibrosis, 2564
Pseudoneurologic symptoms, 1755, 1755b
Pseudoparkinsonism, from antipsychotic agents, 1732
Pseudoseizure, 1624-1625, 2668
Pseudosubluxation, cervical spine, 337, 337f, 421
Pseudotattooing, in long-range handgun wounds, 957, 957f
Pseudotumor cerebri
headache in, 2678
in pregnancy, 2732
Pseudotumor sign, in small bowel obstruction, 1443
Psilocybin, 2406-2408, 2407f, 2478-2479
Psittacosis, pneumonia in, 1131
Psoas sign, in appendicitis, 1452, 2619
Psoriatic arthropathy, 1790
Psychedelics, ingestion of, 2406-2408, 2407f
Psychiatric consultation, for somatoform disorders, 1758-1759
Psychiatric disorders
anxiety disorders as, 1744-1752
factitious disease and malingering as, 1761-1765
in developmentally disabled patient, 2903
in intimate partner violence and abuse, 997-998
in substance abuse, 2885
mood disorders as, 1734-1742
panic attack in, 1748-1749
seizures vs., 2668
sexual assault and, 979
somatoform disorders as, 1753-1759
suicide and, 1768, 1769
Psychiatric disorders *(Continued)*
thought disorders as, 1726-1733
violent behavior and, 2957
Psychiatric interview, 1730
Psychiatric presentations, hypothermia-induced, 2242
Psychiatric short-procedure unit, 1733
Psychic pain, in grief response, 3149
Psychoactive substances
ingestion of, 2406-2408, 2407f
syncope from, 195b
Psychogenic casualties, in terrorism incidents, 3013
Psychogenic polydipsia, 1934
Psychological abuse of elder, 1010
Psychological issues
after sexual assault, 991-992, 991b
in alcoholism, 2879-2880
in asthma, 1082
in elderly person, 2827
in HIV/AIDS, 2086-2087
Psychological symptoms, factitious disorder with, 1761-1762
Psychological techniques, in pain management, 2934
Psychomotor agitation. *See* Agitation.
Psychomotor epilepsy, 1621
Psychomotor processes, in clinical decision making, 130, 131t
Psychomotor retardation, in depression, 1737
Psychosis, 1726-1733
clinical features of, 1726-1728
delirium vs., 1652, 1652t
depression with, 1737
diagnosis of, 1728
disposition in, 1733
in anticholinergic poisoning, 2348
in HIV/AIDS, 2087
in psychostimulant intoxication, 2410
in systemic lupus erythematosus, 1807
Korsakoff's, 2869
LSD-induced, 2408
management of, 1730-1733, 1731b
organic vs. functional, 1727b, 1728-1729, 1728b, 1729t, 1771t
panic attack in, 1748
psychiatric diagnoses associated with, 1729
suicide and, 1769
Psychosocial considerations
in elderly person, 2827
in sudden infant death syndrome, 2717, 2717b
Psychosocial stress, somatoform disorders and, 1753
Psychosocial support, for bipolar disorder, 1742
Psychosocial theories of mood disorders, 1736
Psychostimulant intoxication, 2408-2409, 2410-2411
Psychotherapy
for anxiety disorders, 1751
for depression, 1741-1742
for somatoform disorders, 1758-1759
Psychotic disorder, brief, 1729
Psychotropics, for dysphagia, 1398
Psyllium, drug interactions with, 2478t
PTCA (percutaneous transluminal coronary angioplasty). *See* Percutaneous coronary intervention.
Pterygium, 296t, 1053-1054
Ptosis, in coral snakebite, 898
Pubic dislocation, reduction of, 759
Pubic ramus, fracture of, 724-725
Pubis, 717, 718f
Public health, injury prevention and control and, 943-944, 944t
Public health reporting, syndromic surveillance and, 3105
Public utility model, for EMS programs, 2985
Publication bias, 3050-3051, 3058
Puffy hand syndrome, in intravenous drug abusers, 1361
Pulled elbow, 666, 666f, 2697-2698, 2697f
Pulled muscle. *See* Strain.
Pulmonary. *See also* Lung; Respiration; Respiratory.
Pulmonary abscess, 1033, 1134, 1134f
Pulmonary agents, as chemical weapons, 3032
Pulmonary angiography, in pulmonary embolism, 1375-1377, 1377b
Pulmonary artery, congenital absence of, high-altitude pulmonary edema and, 2303
Pulmonary artery catheterization, in shock, 50
Pulmonary artery occlusive pressure (PAOP), in heart failure, 1260, 1260f
Pulmonary barotrauma, in scuba diving–related disorders, 2285-2286, 2293
Pulmonary compensation, in acid-base disorders, 1923
Pulmonary contusion, 340, 460-461, 460f
Pulmonary decompression sickness, 2284-2285, 2288, 2288t
Pulmonary disorders. *See also specific diseases, e.g.,* Asthma.
altitude and, 2307-2308, 2307f
anxiety in, 1747
aspirin-exacerbated, 1082
chronic
in children, 2565, 2565f
nonobstructive, 1102-1103
obstructive, 1097-1107. *See also* Chronic obstructive pulmonary disease.
heart failure in, 1265-1266
in airway foreign body aspiration, 866
in chronic renal failure, 1542
in Churg-Strauss syndrome, 1816
in developmentally disabled patient, 2903
in HIV/AIDS, 2076-2079, 2076t
in hydrocarbon poisoning, 2428
in hypothyroidism, 1992
in intracerebral hemorrhage, 1610
in opioid overdose, 2452-2453, 2453t
in pancreatitis, 1429
in parasitic infection, 2110-2111
in physically disabled patient, 2907-2908
in sepsis, 2214, 2214b
in substance abuse, 2885
in systemic lupus erythematosus, 1808
in thermal burns, 918
infectious. *See* Respiratory tract infection.
pleural, 1143-1153
Pulmonary edema
acute
in mitral regurgitation, 1306
pathophysiology of, 1261-1262
treatment of, 1270-1274, 1271f
with adequate perfusion, 1271-1273
with hypotension, 1273-1274
cardiogenic, 1261-1262
cardiomegaly with, 1174, 1175f
dialysis for, 1540
high-altitude, 2296, 2298-2299, 2299f, 2300f, 2303-2305, 2303b
hypertension in, 1316
in chronic renal failure, 1542, 1546, 1546b, 1546f
in cyclic antidepressant poisoning, 2354
in near-hanging and strangulation, 450-451
in peritoneal dialysis patient, 1554
in salicylate overdose, 2340, 2341
in scuba diving–related disorders, 2286
in spinal injuries, 438
neurogenic
after head trauma, 371
after seizure, 1625
noncardiogenic, 1261
in barbiturate overdose, 2482
in irritant gas exposure, 2434, 2435
in opioid overdose, 2453
in overdosed/poisoned patient, 2330
in sickle cell disease, 1880
in smoke inhalation, 2435
transfusion-related, 60
Pulmonary embolism, 1371-1381. *See also* Venous thrombosis.
anticoagulation in, 1377
chest pain in, 183, 186b, 190t-191t, 1372, 1380
clinical course in, unpredictability of, 1378-1380, 1379f
complications of, predictors of, 1377, 1378t
diagnosis of, 1372-1377, 1373f, 1375f, 1376t, 1377b
dyspnea in, 179t
heart failure in, 1269
high-altitude, 2304
in chronic obstructive pulmonary disease, 1102
in elderly person, 1368
in mitral stenosis, 1306
in obese patient, 1380-1381

Pulmonary embolism *(Continued)*
in pregnancy, 1380, 2733, 2756-2757
in spinal cord injury, 2906
management of, 1377-1381
massive, 1372f, 1378f
pathophysiology of, 1371-1372, 1371t, 1372b, 1372f
pleural effusion in, 1150-1151
pneumothorax vs., 1146
risk factors for, 186b, 1371, 1371t
rule-out criteria for, 1372b, 1374
thrombolytic therapy in, 1377-1378, 1378t, 1379
with lung infarction, 1373
Pulmonary function tests
in asthma, 1084-1085, 1086t, 2535t, 2536, 2536f
in chronic obstructive pulmonary disease, 1101
Pulmonary hemorrhage, in Goodpasture syndrome, 1816
Pulmonary hypersecretion, in organophosphate poisoning, 2459
Pulmonary hypertension
altitude and, 2308
from high altitude exposure, 2298-2299
in pregnancy, 2762, 2766
Pulmonary irritants, inhalation of, 2433t, 2434-2435, 2434f
Pulmonary laceration, 461
Pulmonary oxygen toxicity, in scuba diving–related disorders, 2283
Pulmonary system
aging and, 345
alcohol consumption and, 2866-2867
in hypothermia, 2239
in pregnancy, 2725
in transition from fetal to extrauterine life, 118-119, 119t, 2568
Pulmonary trauma, 459-466
hemothorax in, 464-465, 465b, 465f
in bipyridyl compound poisoning, 2466
in electrical and lightning injuries, 2274
in hydrocarbon poisoning, 2428
in scuba diving–related disorders, 2285-2286, 2293
in smoke inhalation, 2435
in submersion victim, 2312-2313
pneumothorax in, 461-464, 461f-463f, 464b
pulmonary contusion in, 460-461, 460f
pulmonary laceration in, 461
subcutaneous emphysema in, 459-460
tracheobronchial injury in, 466, 466f
Pulmonary tularemia, 2131
Pulmonary vascular bed, destruction of, in chronic obstructive pulmonary disease, 1097-1098
Pulmonary vascular occlusion, 1371-1372
Pulmonary vascular resistance, in thermal burns, 918
Pulmonic flow murmur of neonates, 2572
Pulp, 1026, 1027f
exposure of, fractures resulting in, 1037
Pulpitis, 1031
Pulpotomy, 1037
Pulse
absent
in electrical and lightning injuries, 2271
in pulmonary embolism, 1380
in tibial femoral knee dislocation, 788
during cardiopulmonary resuscitation, 79
in aortic regurgitation, 1307
in peripheral arteriovascular disease, 1346
in peripheral vascular injury, 539, 541
Pulse oximetry, 36-37
during procedural sedation and analgesia, 2942
in asthma, 1085, 2537
in bronchiolitis, 2545
in children, 2504
in chronic obstructive pulmonary disease, 1100
in comatose patient, 162
in confirmation of endotracheal tube placement, 7
in cyanosis, 270
in delirium, 1651
in peripheral vascular injury, 541
in pneumonia, 1134
in pulmonary embolism, 1377, 1378t
Pulseless disease, 1813
Pulseless electrical activity
capnography in, 82
in infants and children, 112, 2586t, 2590
treatment of, 84, 112
Pulseless ventricular tachycardia, treatment of, 84, 112-113, 112f
Pulsus alternans, in neoplastic cardiac tamponade, 1917
Pulsus paradoxus
in asthma, 1084, 2534, 2535t
in cardiac tamponade, 473
Punctate burns, 2273
Puncture wounds, antibiotic prophylaxis for, 855
Pupil
Adie's tonic, 1061
Horner's, 1061-1062
Pupillary abnormalities
in intracerebral hemorrhage, 1610-1611
in red and painful eye, 286
Pupillary block, in closed-angle glaucoma, 1056, 1056f
Pupillary examination, in head trauma, 357
Purkinje fibers, 1202
digitalis effects on, 2368
Purpura, 1839t
anaphylactoid, 2615, 2615f
causes of, 1864b
drug-induced, 1844-1845, 1845f, 1847t, 1864b
Henoch-Schönlein, 1815, 2615, 2615f, 2653-2654
in meningococcal disease, 2022
internal malignancy associated with, 1864
thrombocytopenic
autoimmune, 1897-1898
oral manifestations of, 1036
thrombotic, 1467, 1898
Purulent arthritis, gonococcal, 2191
Pustule, 1839t
Putaminal lesions, in methanol poisoning, 2396, 2397
Pyarthrosis, pediatric limp and, 764-765, 765f
Pyelography
intravenous
in renal trauma, 528
in ureteral trauma, 531, 531f
in urinary tract infection, 1578
in urolithiasis, 1589, 1592f
retrograde, in ureteral trauma, 531, 531f-532f
Pyelonephritis
acute, 1573
hypertension in, 1312
in children, 2642, 2643, 2644
in kidney transplant patient, 2855
in men, 1585
in pregnancy, 2757, 2758
appendicitis vs., 2754
in urinary tract infection, 1575, 1581t, 1582-1583
observation in, 3072-3073
urolithiasis vs., 1590
Pyloric stenosis
in infants and children, 2603-2606, 2605f, 2606t
malrotation with midgut volvulus vs., 2608
Pyogenic abscess, 1414-1415, 1415f
Pyogenic granuloma, 1035
Pyopneumopericardium, 1287-1288
Pyracantha, 2475
Pyrantel pamoate, for *Enterobius vermicularis* gastroenteritis, 1482
Pyrazinamide, for tuberculosis, 2162, 2163t, 2164t
Pyrazolone, overdose of, 2343
Pyrethrin and pyrethroid poisoning, 2466-2467, 2467b
Pyridostigmine, for myasthenia gravis, 1706
Pyridoxine
deficiency of, seizure in, 2667
for gyromitrin-containing mushroom poisoning, 2479
for sideroblastic anemia, 1873
for toxic alcohol poisoning, 2402
Pyrilamine, anticholinergic toxicity of, 2345
Pyrimethamine
for isosporiasis, 1478
for *Toxoplasma gondii* infection, 2082
in HIV/AIDS, side effects of, 2079t
Pyrogens, 134, 2258
Pyruvate kinase deficiency, in hemolytic anemia, 1878
Pyuria, in urinary tract infection, 1576

Q fever, 1131, 2137
Q waves, in myocardial infarction, 1156, 1164
QRS axis, in infants and children, 2574-2575, 2574t
QRS complex, 1202-1203
in atrial fibrillation, 1230, 1231f
in complete atrioventricular block, 1221
in infants and children, 2574, 2574t
in premature atrial contractions, 1222
in premature ventricular contractions, 1224
in Wolff-Parkinson-White syndrome, 1235
QRS prolongation
in cyclic antidepressant poisoning, 2352, 2354
in OTC sleep aid overdose, 2488
QT dispersion, in acute coronary syndromes, 1174
QT interval, 1203, 2574, 2574t
QT prolongation
antipsychotic-induced, 2447, 2449
classification and causes of, 1244b
seizures vs., 2668
submersion injuries and, 2312
sudden death in, 2598-2599
Quadriceps, overuse of, popliteus tendinitis and, 795
Quadriceps angle, in patellar dislocation, 785
Quadriceps tendon
anatomy of, 770, 771f
injury to, 761, 782-784, 783f, 784f
Quadriplegia
in cerebral herniation, 356
spastic, in cerebral palsy, 2904
Quality of life, end of life and, 3142
Quality/performance improvement, in emergency medical services, 2989
Quazepam, 2484t
Quetiapine
for thought disorders, 1731
toxicity of, 2446, 2446t
Quick Confusion Scale, 151, 153f
Quinapril hydrochloride, 1322t
Quincke's sign, in aortic regurgitation, 1307
Quinidine, 1206
during pregnancy and lactation, 2787
immune thrombocytopenia from, 1897
Quinine
for babesiosis, 2140
for malaria, 2104
thrombocytopenia from, 1897, 1898
Quinsy, 1117-1118, 1118f
Quinton-Mahurkar catheter, 1362f, 1364-1365

Rabeprazole, 1390t
Rabies, 2061-2069
clinical features of, 2065-2066
epidemiology of, 2061-2065, 2062f-2064f
pathophysiology of, 2065
postexposure prophylaxis for, 2066-2069, 2067t, 2068b
preexposure prophylaxis for, 2069, 2069t
vaccine for, 2035t, 2068, 2068b
Raccoon, rabies in, 2062, 2062f, 2063-2064, 2063f
Race, definition of, 3111
Racial/ethnic differences. *See also* Cultural competence.
demographics of, 3108, 3108t
discrimination based on, health consequences of, 3110
in atypical symptoms of myocardial infarction, 1159
in health beliefs, values, and life experiences, 3113-3114
in health care access and outcomes, 3108-3111, 3109t
in hepatitis A infection, 1402
in HIV/AIDS, 2072
in sudden infant death syndrome, 2715
in use of emergency department, 3115-3116, 3115b
Racism, 3110

Radial artery, 540f, 585-586, 587f, 588f, 622, 625f
injury to, 545-546
Radial bursa, flexor tendons and, 585, 586f
Radial collateral ligament, injury to, 604
Radial deviation, of hand, 577f
Radial head, 647
dislocation of, in Monteggia's fracture, 642, 642f
fracture of, 663, 663f, 664
subluxation of, 666, 666f, 2697-2698, 2697f
Radial keratotomy, altitude and, 2309
Radial length measurement, 625, 626f
Radial mononeuropathy, 1693-1695, 1694f
Radial neck, fracture of, 664
Radial nerve, 586, 588f, 589f, 622, 625f, 648, 648f
palsy of, 586, 588f
humeral shaft fracture and, 655
in radial mononeuropathy, 1695
Radial styloid, 625
Radial surface, of hand, 576, 577f
Radiation
external, 2320
heat transfer by, 2255
ionizing, 2318f, 2319
nonionizing, 2318-2319, 2318f
types of, and possible hazards, 2319-2320, 2320f
Radiation absorbed dose, 2321
Radiation accident protocol, 2322-2323
Radiation burns, ocular, 1046-1047
Radiation dose
indicators of, 2317t, 2321, 2321f
median lethal whole-body, 2322
Radiation Emergency Assistance Center/Training Site, 2324-2325
Radiation exposure, 2316-2325
as weapon of mass destruction, 3022-3023, 3023t
disaster preparedness for, 3017-3018
disposition in, 2324
epidemiology of, 2316-2318, 2317t
intrauterine, 320, 320t, 2731, 2731t
management of, 2322-2325, 2323f
pathophysiology of, 2318-2320, 2318f
prehospital care in, 2322-2323
resources for, 2324-2325
signs and symptoms of, 2321-2322, 2321f
types of, 2320-2321
Radiation therapy
acute tumor lysis syndrome from, 1911
esophagitis from, 1386, 1388
pericarditis after, 1284
proctocolitis from, 1505-1506
Radicular artery of Adamkiewicz, 1676
Radicular pain
in diskitis, 1684
in epidural abscess, 1684
in epidural hematoma, 1683
in intervertebral disk herniation, 264
in spinal cord tumor, 1685
pathophysiology of, 261
Radiculopathy
in Lyme disease, 2123
lumbar, 704
Radiocarpal joint, 622, 623f
Radiogardase, for cesium and thallium ingestion, 3023, 3023t
Radiography
abdominal
in abdominal aortic aneurysm, 1334, 1334f
in abdominal pain, 216, 216t
in abdominal trauma, 495-496, 496f, 497f
in constipation, 239
in iron overdose, 2420, 2420f
of calcified gallstones, 1418, 1418f
chest
in airway foreign body aspiration, 867, 867f-869f, 2551, 2551f
in anthrax exposure, 3025, 3025f
in aortic dissection, 1326-1327, 1326t
in aortic rupture, 478-479, 478f
in asthma, 1085, 2537, 2537f
in bronchiolitis, 2545
in cardiac tamponade, 474, 475f, 1285
in chest pain, 186, 188, 188t
in chronic obstructive pulmonary disease, 1100-1101
in confirmation of endotracheal tube placement, 7
Radiography *(Continued)*
in cyanosis, 271
in cystic fibrosis, 2564, 2565f
in esophageal obstruction, 1383
in esophageal perforation, 484-485, 485f
in fever, 137
in flail chest, 457-458
in heart failure, 1269
in hemoptysis, 281
in hemothorax, 465, 465f
in high-altitude pulmonary edema, 2299, 2300f, 2303
in HIV/AIDS, 2076t, 2077
in hydrocarbon poisoning, 2430, 2431f
in hypothyroidism, 1993
in mitral regurgitation, 1306
in mitral stenosis, 1305
in multiple trauma, 312
in neoplastic cardiac tamponade, 1917
in osteomyelitis, 2179-2180, 2179f, 2180f
in pacemaker malfunction, 1254-1255
in pediatric cardiovascular disorders, 2573-2574, 2573f, 2574f
in pediatric fever, 2510
in pericardial effusion, 1285
in pleural effusion, 1150, 1151f
in *Pneumocystis carinii* pneumonia, 1136, 1136f
in pneumonia, 1132-1134, 1133f, 1134f, 2561, 2561f
in pneumothorax, 462f, 463, 1145, 1145f, 1146f
in pulmonary embolism, 1373
in rib fracture, 454, 454b, 455f
in sepsis, 2217
in tetralogy of Fallot, 2580
in tuberculosis, 2152-2154, 2152f-2153f, 2159, 2159f
computed (digital), in fracture, 557
in acromioclavicular joint dislocation, 686, 687f
in acute mesenteric ischemia, 1447
in acute pancreatitis, 1432
in acute renal failure, 1538
in adult epiglottitis, 1115-1116, 1116f
in airway foreign body aspiration, 866-867, 867f-869f
in ankle trauma, 810-811, 810f, 811f
in anterior glenohumeral joint dislocation, 688, 688f
in appendicitis, 1454, 2619, 2620f
in arthritis, 1779-1780, 1780t
in back pain, 264, 707-708, 708b, 708f-709f
in calcaneal fracture, 826-827, 826f, 827f
in calcific tendinitis, 698
in cervical vascular injury, 449
in child abuse, 973, 2699
in chronic pancreatitis, 1435-1436, 1436f
in clavicle fracture, 2693, 2693f
in colonic ischemia, 1504
in diarrhea, 233
in distal tibiofibular syndesmotic ligament injury, 816
in diverticular disease, 1494
in elbow and humeral trauma, 641f, 650-652, 651f
in elderly trauma patient, 347
in esophageal foreign body, 868f, 869f, 871
in esophageal perforation, 1385
in facial fracture, 389
in fetal identification, 2730
in foot trauma, 821-822, 822f
in forearm trauma, 640-641, 640f
in fracture, 557-558
in frostbite, 2231
in hematuria, 1530
in hip dislocation, 757, 758f
in hypothermia, 2244
in inferior glenohumeral joint dislocation, 693, 694f
in inflammatory bowel disease, 1502, 1502f
in intercondylar eminence fracture, 780
in intussusception, 2611, 2611f
in knee extensor tendon injuries, 783, 784f
in knee ligament injuries, 791
in knee trauma, 774
in Legg-Calvé-Perthes disease, 2707, 2707f
in Lisfranc injuries, 829-830, 830f
in lower leg stress fractures, 803-804
Radiography *(Continued)*
in metatarsal base fractures, 832, 833f
in multiple trauma, 308-309, 312
in osteoarthritis of knee, 796
in osteochondral fracture of talar dome, 825, 825f
in patellar dislocation, 786
in patellar fracture, 784-785, 785f
in patellofemoral pain syndrome, 787
in pediatric cervical spine injury, 337, 337f
in pediatric pyarthrosis, 765, 765f
in pediatric trauma, 333
in pelvic fracture, 720-721, 721f
in peripheral vascular injury, 541
in posterior elbow dislocation, 665, 665f
in posterior shoulder dislocation, 691, 692f
in pregnant trauma patient, 320, 320t
in proximal tibial epiphyseal injuries, 781
in red and painful eye, 288
in renal disorders, 1528
in retropharyngeal abscess, 1120-1121, 1120f
in scaphoid fracture, 628
in septic arthritis, 2189
in sesamoid fractures, 835
in shoulder trauma, 674-676, 674f-676f
in sinusitis, 1124, 1124f
in slipped capital femoral epiphysis, 2708, 2708f
in small bowel obstruction, 1443, 1443f
in supracondylar fracture, 2694-2695, 2695f
in talar fracture, 823, 824f
in tendinopathy, 1800-1801
in tibial femoral knee dislocation, 788, 789f
in tibial plateau fracture, 778-779
in tibial shaft fracture, 800, 801f
in tibial tubercle fracture, 798
in upper airway obstruction, 2521, 2521f
in wrist trauma, 625-627, 626f-628f, 628t
of normal hip, 746, 747f
of teeth, 1030, 1030f
skull
in head-injured child, 336, 368
in minor head trauma, 364-365
in severe head trauma, 362, 362t
in skull fracture, 372
Radiohumeral bursa, 649
Radiology, misinterpretation errors in, 3125
Radionucleotide scanning, 2319
in acute coronary syndromes, 1179-1180
in appendicitis, 1454
in cholecystitis, 1420
in frostbite, 2231
in myocardial contusion, 469
in testicular torsion, 2640
in urinary tract infection, 1578
of bone. *See* Bone scan.
Radiosensitivity, organ and tissue, 2321, 2321f
Radioulnar joint
distal
anatomy of, 622, 623f, 639-640
dislocation of, 636-637, 642-643, 643f
proximal, 639-640
Radius, 639
distal. *See* Distal radius.
fracture of
in Galeazzi's fracture, 642-643, 643f
pediatric, 644, 644f
plastic deformation of, 644, 645f
proximal, 647, 647f
shaft fracture of, with ulnar shaft fracture, 641
Radon exposure, 2317-2318, 2318f
RAFFT score, for substance abuse in adolescents, 2884
Rales
in bronchiolitis, 2545
in high-altitude pulmonary edema, 2303
in tuberculosis, 2150
Ramipril, 1322t
Ramsay Hunt syndrome, 1071, 1667
Randomization, 3049
Range of motion
of elbow, 650
of foot, 821
of knee, 773
of shoulder, 674
Ranitidine, 1390t
during pregnancy and lactation, 2790
for anaphylaxis, 1831b, 1832, 2549

Ranke complex, in tuberculosis, 2152
Ranson's criteria for acute pancreatitis, 1431-1432, 1432b
Rape trauma syndrome, 991-992, 991b
Rapid diagnostic tests, for viral antigens, 1135
Rapid diagnostic treatment unit. *See* Observation medicine.
Rapid sequence intubation, 9-12, 10b
  in asthma, 16
  in elevated intracranial pressure, 17, 18t
  in head trauma, 358-359
  in neck trauma, 444
  in shock, 51
  indications for, 7-8
  paralysis with induction phase in, 11
  pediatric, 18, 107-108, 107b, 107t
  post-intubation management in, 11-12
  prehospital, 2990, 2991
  preoxygenation in, 10, 10f
  preparations for, 9-10
  pretreatment agents for, 10, 11b
  tube placement in, 11
  vs. blind nasotracheal intubation, 12
  with competitive neuromuscular blocking agent and etomidate, 14-15, 15t
Rapid streptococcal tests, 1111
Rapid tranquilization, 2914b
  for mood disorders, 1741
  for thought disorders, 1730-1731, 1731b
  of combative patient, 2961-2963
Rash. *See also* Skin lesions.
  drug-induced, 1844, 1847t
  glue sniffer's, 2430
  heat, 2259
  in bacterial meningitis, 2658, 2659
  in Colorado tick fever, 2141
  in dermatomyositis, 1708
  in disseminated gonococcal infection, 1566
  in ehrlichiosis, 2138
  in erythema infectiosum, 1850
  in gonococcal arthritis, 1788
  in halothane-induced hepatitis, 1414
  in Henoch-Schönlein purpura, 1815, 2615, 2615f, 2653
  in herpes zoster, 1859, 1860f
  in Kawasaki disease, 2026, 2594, 2595f
  in Lyme disease, 2122, 2122f
  in measles, 1849, 2053, 2053f
  in Rocky Mountain spotted fever, 1849, 2133-2134, 2133f, 2134f
  in roseola infantum, 1850
  in rubella, 1850
  in scarlet fever, 1851, 1851f
  in smallpox, 2039, 2039f, 3028-3029, 3028f, 3029f
  in syphilis, 1561, 1561f
  in systemic lupus erythematosus, 1806
  in toxic shock syndrome, 1847, 2029, 2200
  oral hypoglycemic agent–induced, 1972
Rat-bite fever, 884
Rattlesnake bite, 896, 2329t
Raynaud's disease, 1347, 1357
Raynaud's phenomenon, 273, 1357
Reactionary anxiety, 1746b
Reactive arthritis, 1789-1790, 1791, 2192
Reactive hypochondriasis, 1756
Reactive oxygen species, in cerebral necrosis, 66
Reanastomosis, end-to-end, in arterial injury, 544
"Reasonable person" standard, 3166
Reassurance, in somatoform disorders, 1757-1758
Rebleeding, in traumatic hyphema, 1048-1049
Rebreathers, in diving, 2280
Recommendations for emergency medicine. *See* Guidelines for emergency medicine.
Rectal biopsy, in AIDS-related diarrhea, 1484
Rectal bleeding, 1508
  in Meckel's diverticulum, 2613
  with defecation, 1508
Rectal examination, 1573
  in abdominal pain, 213, 215
  in abdominal trauma, 494
  in back pain, 263
  in constipation, 239
  in diarrhea, 233
  in gastrointestinal bleeding, 222
  in genitourinary trauma, 515
  in pelvic fracture, 719
  in sexual assault victim, 988
Rectal pain, 1509
  in anal fissures, 1512-1513
  in appendicitis, 1452
  in hemorrhoids, 1510
  in levator ani syndrome, 1516
Rectal sphincter tone, in head trauma, 357
Rectal tonography, in shock, 50-51
Rectum
  disorders of. *See* Anorectal disorders.
  foreign bodies in, 875-877, 876f, 1521-1522, 1522f
Recurrent laryngeal nerve, injury to, 450
Red and painful eye, 283-297
  ancillary studies in, 288
  diagnostic approach to, 283-288, 284b, 285b, 287f
  differential diagnosis in, 288-290, 288f-291f
  disposition in, 293t-297t, 297
  empiric management of, 290-292, 293t-297t
  epidemiology of, 283
  history in, 285
  in infants and children, 292
  physical examination in, 285-288, 285b
  traumatic, 283, 290, 292, 297
Red blood cell casts
  in glomerulonephritis, 1534
  in urinary sediment, 1526, 1526f
Red blood cell count
  decreased. *See* Anemia.
  in alcoholism, 2874
  in hypothermia, 2243
  in pregnancy, 318
  increased, 273, 1884-1885, 1884f, 1885b
  normal values for, 1868t
  peritoneal lavage, 500, 500t
Red blood cell indices, normal values for, 1871t
Red blood cell mass, in thermal burns, 918
Red macules, skin disorders with, 1844-1848
Redistributive hyponatremia, 1933
Red-red tears, meniscal, 792
Reduction
  of dislocation, 565-566
    ankle, 820
    anterior elbow, 666
    carpometacarpal joint, 603
    distal interphalangeal joint, 601
    glenohumeral joint, 688-690, 689f, 690f
    hip, 757-759, 758f-759f
    hip prosthesis, 760
    inferior glenohumeral joint, 693, 694f
    metacarpophalangeal joint, 602-603, 602f
    metatarsophalangeal joint, 835
    patellar, 786
    posterior elbow, 665
    posterior glenohumeral joint, 691-692
    proximal interphalangeal joint, 602
    proximal tibiofibular joint, 803
    sternoclavicular, 684-685, 685f
    subtalar, 826
    temporomandibular joint, 1041-1042, 1041f
    tibial femoral knee, 788-789
  of femoral head fracture-dislocation, 759-760, 760f
  of fracture
    ankle, 812
    Colles', 633, 634f
    displaced supracondylar, 657, 658f
    distal femur, 776-777
    humeral shaft, 654, 654f
    intercondylar, 659-660, 659f
    intercondylar eminence, 780
    metacarpal neck, 597-598, 598f
    metatarsal shaft, 831
    phalangeal, 834
    proximal humeral epiphysis, 683
    supracondylar, 2695, 2696f
    talar, 824
  of radial head subluxation, 666, 666f, 2697-2698
Red-white tears, meniscal, 792
Reentry mechanisms, for dysrhythmias, 1204-1205, 1204f
Refeeding syndrome, hypophosphatemia in, 1951
Referral
  in elder abuse, 1013-1014
  in intimate partner violence and abuse, 1004
  in substance abuse, 2886
Referred pain
  abdominal, 212
  to back, 703, 706
Reflex(es)
  brainstem, in comatose patient, 159t, 160-161
  cremasteric, 1594
    loss of, in testicular torsion, 1595
  deep tendon
    in head trauma, 357
    in spinal injuries, 417, 417t
    pseudomyotonic, in hypothyroidism, 1992
  diving, 2312
  doll's eye, 161, 2503
  in hypothermia, 2241
  in spinal cord disorders, 1679-1680
Reflex airway closure in physically disabled patient, 2907-2908
Reflex sympathetic dystrophy, 562-563
Reflex sympathetic response to laryngoscopy, 16-17
Reflex syncope, 2685
Reflux
  gastroesophageal. *See* Gastroesophageal reflux.
  vesicoureteral, in urinary tract infection, 1574
Refractory periods of action potential, 1200, 1202f
Refusal of medical care
  by Jehovah's Witnesses, 3171-3172
  federal rules governing, 3170-3171
  for minors, by parent or guardian, 3171
  informed, 3169-3170
  medicolegal issues in, 3169-3172
Regional anesthesia
  in wound care, 845-846
  intravenous, 2934
Regional health information network (RHIN), 3104
Regression models, 3055
Regurgitation
  in achalasia, 1397
  in gastroesophageal reflux, 1388
Rehydralyte, for pediatric infectious diarrhea, 2630, 2630t
Reimplantation
  in hand trauma, 613, 613b
  of avulsed tooth, 1038f, 1040
  penile, 533
Reiter syndrome, arthritis in, 1789-1790
Rejection
  in heart transplant patient, 2852-2853, 2853f
  in kidney transplant patient, 2855
  in liver transplant patient, 2854
  in lung transplant patient, 2855-2856
  opportunistic infections associated with, 2848-2849, 2849f
  phases of, 2849
Relapsing fever, 2129-2130
Relative afferent pupillary defect (RAPD), in red and painful eye, 286
Relative refractory period, 1200, 1202f
Relative risk, 3059t
Relaxation, as wellness strategy for emergency physicians, 3178
Relevance of study, 3059, 3059t
Reliability, 3059, 3059t
Religious values, 3129-3130, 3130b
Remifentanil, 2922t, 2923
Renal artery
  aneurysm of, urolithiasis vs., 1591
  fibromuscular dysplasia of, hypertension in, 1311-1312
  stenosis of, hypertension in, 1312
  trauma to, 529, 530
Renal blood flow, in hypothermia, 2239
Renal cell carcinoma, urolithiasis vs., 1590
Renal colic, 1586-1593, 1586b, 1589f-1592f, 1593b, 2645-2646. *See also* Urolithiasis.
Renal compensation
  in acid-base disorders, 1923-1924
  in metabolic acidosis, 1923-1924
  in metabolic alkalosis, 1924
Renal dialysis. *See* Dialysis.
Renal disorders
  diagnosis of, 1525-1528, 1527t, 1528b
  hypermagnesemia in, 1949
  hypomagnesemia in, 1947-1948
  in acetaminophen poisoning, 2333
  in acute tumor lysis syndrome, 1911
  in diabetes mellitus, 1970
  in ethylene glycol poisoning, 2398, 2399
  in heatstroke, 2262
  in HIV/AIDS, 2086

Volume 1 pp 1–1024 • Volume 2 pp 1025–2226 • Volume 3 pp 2227–3180

Renal disorders *(Continued)*
in hypertension, 1311-1312
in hyperuricemia, 1913
in infants and children, 2635-2655
in lithium toxicity, 2443
in pregnancy, 2771
in spinal cord injury, 2908
in submersion victim, 2313
in thermal burns, 918
in tuberculosis, 2159
Renal failure
acute, 1532-1540
clinical features of, 1532b, 1537
diagnosis of, 1537-1538
disposition in, 1540
in acute interstitial nephritis, 1534-1535, 1534b
in acute tubular necrosis, 1534b, 1535-1537, 1536b
in children, 2649-2651, 2649b
in glomerulonephritis, 1534, 1534b
in prerenal azotemia, 1532-1533, 1533b, 1538
in renal vascular disease, 1534b, 1535
in rhabdomyolysis, 1977, 1977f
intrinsic, 1534-1537, 1534b
management of, 1538-1540
organ system effects of, 1540
pigment-induced, 1536, 1536b
postrenal (obstructive), 1533-1534, 1533b, 1538
prevention of, 1538-1539
volume and metabolic complications of, 1539-1540
chronic, 1540-1554
causes of, 1541, 1541b, 1543, 1544b
clinical features of, 1542-1543, 1542f
definition of, 1541
diagnosis of, 1543-1544, 1543b, 1544b
dialysis for, 1547-1554
complications of, 1549-1554, 1550b, 1552b, 1553t
emergency, 1548-1549, 1548b
hyperkalemia in, 1545-1546, 1545t
hypertension in, 1316-1317
infection in, 1543, 1546-1547
kidney size in, normal or large, 1543, 1543b
management of, 1544-1554
pulmonary edema in, 1542, 1546, 1546b, 1546f
reversible factors and treatable causes of, 1543, 1544b
uremia in, 1541-1543, 1542f
hyperphosphatemia in, 1952
hypocalcemia in, 1943
immune defects in, 2842
in crush injury, 3007
in ethylene glycol poisoning, 2399, 2400
in HIV/AIDS, 2086
in hyperuricemia, 1913
in pregnancy, 2771
in salicylate overdose, 2340
in sepsis, 2214
in tetanus, 2009
infections in, 2842
metabolic acidosis in, 1929
palliative care in, 3154
pseudo-, in isopropyl alcohol poisoning, 2403-2404
renal function evaluation in, 1524-1528, 1526f, 1527t, 1528b, 1528f
seizure in, 1622
Renal function tests, 1524-1528, 1526f, 1527t, 1528b, 1528f
Renal infarction, urolithiasis vs., 1591
Renal ischemia, in acute tubular necrosis, 1536
Renal osteodystrophy, 1542-1543
Renal pedicle injuries, 530
Renal pelvis, 527, 527f
Renal trauma, 342, 526-530, 527f, 529f-530f
Renal tuberculosis, urolithiasis vs., 1590-1591
Renal tubular acidosis, hypokalemia in, 1937
Renal tumor, 2646
Renal vascular disease, 1534b, 1535
Renal vein
thrombosis of, urolithiasis vs., 1591
trauma to, 529-530
Renewal, as wellness strategy for emergency physicians, 3178
Renin-angiotensin-aldosterone system, 527
in heart failure, 1262
in hypertension, 1311, 1312f
in sodium homeostasis, 1933
Renovascular hypertension, 1311
in renal trauma, 526-527
Reovirus infection, 2034t, 2046-2047
Colorado tick fever in, 2140-2141
gastroenteritis, 1475-1476
Repaglinide, 1973
Reperfusion, cerebral, after cardiac arrest, 62-64
Reperfusion therapy
for acute mesenteric ischemia, 1449
in myocardial infarction, 1189-1195
choice of, 1193-1194
combination, 1194-1195
in cardiogenic shock, 1194
process time points for, 1183, 1184f
time to, 1182-1184, 1183f, 1184f
Repolarization, 1200
abnormalities of, in ventricular tachycardia, 1242
early, benign, ST segment elevation in, 1166-1167, 1167f, 1168f
Reporting requirements, 3172-3173
in child abuse, 976
in elder abuse, 1014-1015
in hepatitis, 1406
in intimate partner violence and abuse, 1004-1005
Reptile envenomation, 895-903, 897f, 897t, 900t
Rescue, search and, urban, 3005-3008, 3006b, 3008f
Rescue breathing, in pediatric resuscitation, 98
Research question, definition of, 3047-3048
Reserpine, 1321t
intra-arterial, for frostbite, 2233
Residents, in observation unit, 3063
Resistance, electrical injury and, 2268-2269, 2269b, 2269t
Resorcinol, 935
Resource limitations, as stressor for emergency physician, 3175
Respiration
accessory muscles of
in asthma, 1084
in chronic obstructive pulmonary disease, 1100
agonal, 97
Kussmaul's
in diabetic ketoacidosis, 1963
in metabolic acidosis, 1929
Respiratory acidosis, 1924-1926, 1925b, 1925f, 1931b
causes of, 1925b
clinical features of, 1924-1925
in chronic obstructive pulmonary disease, 1100
management of, 1925-1926
physiologic compensation in, 1925
Respiratory alkalosis, 1926, 1931b
causes of, 1926, 1926b
during acclimatization to high altitude, 2297-2298
hypophosphatemia in, 1951
in chronic obstructive pulmonary disease, 1100
in salicylate overdose, 2340
Respiratory arrest, 97
asthma-related, 2540
definition of, 79
in organophosphate poisoning, 2459
Respiratory depression
in barbiturate overdose, 2482
in benzodiazepine poisoning, 2484
with apnea, in GHB intoxication, 2489
Respiratory disease. *See* Pulmonary disorders.
Respiratory distress
acute, 1141, 1141b
in ethylene glycol poisoning, 2399
in pancreatitis, 1429
in sepsis, 2214, 2214b
mechanical ventilation in, 32
pulmonary contusion vs., 461
in anaphylaxis, 1829
in cystic fibrosis, 2564-2565, 2565f
in pediatric airway obstruction, 2519-2530, 2532-2552
Respiratory distress *(Continued)*
evaluation of, 2521, 2521f
in aeroesophageal foreign body, 2529-2530
in anaphylaxis, 2546-2550
in asthma, 2532-2544
in bronchiolitis, 2544-2546
in congenital lesions, 2522, 2524-2525, 2524f, 2527-2528, 2528f
in croup, 2525-2527, 2526f, 2527b
in epiglottitis, 2523-2524, 2524f
in foreign body aspiration, 2550-2551, 2551f
in laryngeal disease, 2524-2525, 2524f
in retropharyngeal abscess, 2522-2523, 2523f
in subglottic tracheal disease, 2525-2527
in supraglottic disease, 2522-2524
in tracheal disease, 2527-2529, 2529t
pathophysiology of, 2519, 2520f
stridor in, 2519-2520, 2521t
in pneumonia, 2554-2564
severe acute, 1130, 2034t, 2050-2051
Respiratory dyskinesia, antipsychotic-induced, 2447
Respiratory emergencies, prehospital care in, 2990
Respiratory failure
cardiac arrest in, 77
in acute respiratory distress syndrome, 1141
in botulism, 2015
in chronic obstructive pulmonary disease, 1100
in meningococcal disease, 2022
in myasthenia gravis, 1706
in pulmonary embolism, 1378-1379
in tetanus, 2009
Respiratory insufficiency
in botulism, 1707
in hypophosphatemia, 1952
Respiratory muscles
accessory
in asthma, 1084, 2534, 2535t
in chronic obstructive pulmonary disease, 1100
weakness of, 139
Respiratory rate
fever and, 135
in asthma, 1084
in infants and children, 2495, 2495t, 2571, 2571t
Respiratory stimulants, for chronic obstructive pulmonary disease, 1106
Respiratory syncytial virus infection, 2051-2052
congenital heart disease and, 2581-2582, 2582b
drugs for, 2037t
in bronchiolitis, 2544-2545
in pneumonia, 1130, 2555, 2557
Respiratory tract infection
high-altitude pulmonary edema and, 2299
host defenses against, 1128-1129
in diphtheria, 2001-2004, 2003b
in HIV/AIDS, 2076-2079, 2076t
in immunocompromised patient, 2841
in meningococcal disease, 2020-2024
lower
in bronchiolitis, 2544-2546
in pertussis, 2004-2007, 2005f, 2006b, 2559-2560
in pneumococcal disease, 2016-2020, 2020b
in pneumonia, 1128-1141, 2554-2564. *See also* Pneumonia.
upper, 1109-1126
in adult epiglottitis, 1114-1116, 1115f, 1116f
in deep space infections of head and neck, 1116-1117, 1116f
in laryngitis, 1114
in lingual tonsillitis, 1114, 1114f
in Ludwig's angina, 1118-1119
in parapharyngeal abscess, 1121-1123, 1122f
in peritonsiillitis, 1117-1118, 1118f
in pharyngitis, 1109-1114, 1110f
in retropharyngeal abscess, 1120-1121, 1120f, 1121f
in sinusitis, 1123-1126, 1124f, 1125f
pediatric screening for, 2509b
Restaurant syndromes, anaphylaxis vs., 2548-2549
Restless legs syndrome, in chronic renal failure, 1542
Restraint
in delirium, 1653-1654
in PCP intoxication, 2416

Restraint *(Continued)*
in suicide, 1772
physical
for combative patient, 2958-2961, 2960f
in alcohol withdrawal syndrome, 2861
in PCP intoxication, 2892
in thought disorders, 1730
Restrictions, return-to-work, 3079
Restrictive cardiomyopathy, 1296-1297
constrictive pericarditis vs., 1288
heart failure in, 1264
Resuscitation
adult, 75-94
airway and breathing management in, 87
algorithm for, 83f
cardiopulmonary resuscitation in, 88-90
defibrillation in, 90-91
epidemiology of cardiac arrest and, 76
etiology of cardiac arrest and, 77-78, 78t
history and physical examination in, 78-79, 79t
in asystole, 84-85
in pulseless electrical activity, 84
in ventricular fibrillation and pulseless ventricular tachycardia, 84
monitoring in, 79-82, 80f-82f, 80t
outcomes in, 93
pacing in, 91
pathophysiology of cardiac arrest and, 76-77
pharmacologic therapy in, 91-93
postresuscitation management of cardiac arrest and, 85-87, 88f
therapeutic modalities in, 87-93
brain, 62-73
clinical outcomes in, 72-73
experimental therapies in, 70-72
pathophysiology of cerebral ischemia and, 62-67, 63f-64f
standard strategies for, 67-70, 69t
family presence during, 3149
fluid. *See* Fluid resuscitation
honoring advance directive wishes to withhold, 3144-3145, 3152
hypotensive, in peripheral vascular injury, 543
in electrical and lightning injuries, 2275
in heatstroke, 2264-2265, 2265f
in hemorrhagic shock, 46, 52-53
myocardial dysfunction after, 77
neonatal, 118-124
chest compressions in, 123
discontinuation of, 120
disposition in, 124
in anatomic abnormalities, 121
in late decelerations of fetal heart rate, 2801
in meconium aspiration, 120, 120f
indications for, 119-120
medications in, 123-124, 123t
oxygen therapy, ventilation, and intubation in, 122-123
positioning, suctioning, and stimulation in, 121-122
preparation for, 121, 121b
transition from fetal to extrauterine life and, 118-119, 119t
of elderly trauma patient, 348
of implantable cardioverter-defibrillator patient, 1256-1257
of pregnant patient, 322-323
pediatric, 97-116
adenosine for, 101t, 104
advanced life support techniques in, 99, 99f
airway management in, 97-98, 105-109, 106f, 107b, 107t
amiodarone for, 101t, 104-105
antidiuretic hormone for, 100, 103t
atropine for, 99, 100, 101t-102t, 103-104
basic life support techniques in, 97-99
breathing management in, 98, 108-109
calcium for, 101t, 104
cardiac rhythm and etiology of arrest in, 109-113, 109t, 110f-112f, 110t
circulatory management in, 98-99, 109-113
defibrillation and cardioversion in, 113
epinephrine for, 111, 114
family presence during, 114-116, 3149
glucose for, 100, 101t, 103
lidocaine for, 102t, 105
magnesium for, 104
Resuscitation *(Continued)*
pharmacologic therapy in, 100-105, 101t-103t, 109-113
postresuscitation stabilization in, 113-114, 113f
procainamide for, 103t, 105
rapid sequence intubation in, 107-108, 107b, 107t
sodium bicarbonate for, 100, 101t
tape measurement system in, 114, 114f-115f
termination of, 116
research in, bioethical dilemmas in, 3136-3137
training in, bioethical dilemmas in, 3135
Resuscitative hypothermia, for comatose survivors of cardiac arrest, 68-70, 69t
Retching, definition of, 200
Reticular activating system, 156
Reticulocyte count
in normochromic and normocytic anemia, 1875
in sickle cell disease, 1881
Reticulocytes, 1868, 1868f
Reticuloendothelial system, 2832
Retina, 1045f
blunt injury to, 1050, 1050f
detachment of, 1050, 1050f, 1057-1058
tear of, 1050, 1057-1058
Retinal hemorrhage, 1050
high-altitude, 2306-2307, 2307f
in child abuse, 971
Retinitis, cytomegalovirus, in HIV/AIDS, 2086
Retinopathy
diabetic, 1970, 1972
fibrinolytic therapy eligibility and, 1191
Retrobulbar abscess, 288, 295t
Retrobulbar emphysema, 294t
Retrobulbar hematoma, 288, 295t
Retrobulbar hemorrhage, 1046
Retrograde cystography
computed tomography, in bladder trauma, 521, 525, 526f
conventional, in bladder trauma, 521, 521f-526f
Retrograde intubation, 20
Retrograde pyelography, 531, 531f-532f
Retrograde urethrogram, 517-519, 518f-520f
Retroperitoneal air, 497f
Retroperitoneal hematoma, pelvic fracture and, 500
Retropharyngeal abscess, 1120-1121, 1120f, 1121f
in children, 2522-2523, 2523f
Retropharyngeal injuries, in neck trauma, 450
Retropharyngeal space, 1027
soft tissues of, 424, 426f
Retrospective observational study, 3047
Retrosternal pain, in aortic rupture, 478
Retrovirus, 2034t, 2056
Return-to-work issues, in occupational medicine, 3078-3080
Reverse straight leg raise test, in lumbar radiculopathy, 704
Revised trauma score (RTS), 300
Rewarming
active, 2247-2251, 2247b
core, 2248-2251
external, 2248
airway, 2248-2249, 2249t
arteriovenous, continuous, 2250t, 2251
arteriovenous anastomoses, 2248
diathermic, 2250
external, 2247, 2248
extracorporeal blood, 2250-2251, 2250t
forced air, 2248
heated irrigation for, 2250
in accidental hypothermia, 2247-2251, 2247b, 2250b
in frostbite, 2231-2232, 2232b
negative pressure, 2248
peritoneal lavage, 2249
venovenous, 2250t, 2251
Reynolds' pentad in cholangitis, 1421
Rh (anti-D) immunoglobulin, in pregnancy, 2742, 2752
Rhabdomyolysis, 1975-1983
acute tubular necrosis in, 1536
anatomy and physiology in, 1976, 1977f
clinical features of, 1980
diagnosis of, 1980-1981, 1981f
differential considerations in, 1981-1982, 1981b
Rhabdomyolysis *(Continued)*
disposition in, 1983
etiology of, 1978-1980, 1978b
in amphetamine abuse, 2896
in electrical and lightning injuries, 2276
in hypokalemia, 1939
in hypophosphatemia, 1952
in hypothermia, 2243
in overdosed/poisoned patient, 2330
in PCP intoxication, 2892-2893
management of, 1982-1983, 1983f
pathophysiology of, 1976-1978, 1977b, 1977f
pigmenturia in, 1981-1982, 1981b
psychostimulant-induced, 2408
Rhabdovirus, 2034t, 2054
Rhegmatogenous retinal detachment, 1058
Rheumatic disease. *See also specific diseases, e.g.,* Arthritis.
historical perspective of, 1776-1777
in hypothyroidism, 1992
in pregnancy, 2775-2776
in systemic lupus erythematosus, 1806
orofacial pain in, 1034
sites and types of, 1777f
synovial fluid analysis in, 1781-1782, 1781t
Rheumatic fever, 1303-1304, 1304b
acute, 1790-1791, 1790b, 2596-2597, 2596f
after streptococcal pharyngitis, 1112, 1114
mitral stenosis after, 1305
Rheumatic heart disease, infective endocarditis in, 1300
Rheumatoid arthritis, 1791-1792
in pregnancy, 2776
myocarditis in, 1297
pericarditis in, 1284
skin lesions in, 1862t
Rheumatoid factor, in rheumatoid arthritis, 1791
Rhinitis
allergic, exercise-induced asthma and, 1082
in anaphylaxis, 1825t
in asthma, 1084
vs. sinusitis, 1125
Rhinitis medicamentosa, 1125
Rhinovirus, 2057
Rhizotomy, dorsal, for spasticity in cerebral palsy, 2904
Rhododendron, 2475
Rhomboid muscle, 672, 673f
Rib fracture, 454-456, 454b, 455f
anatomy in, 455f
aortic rupture and, 479
flail chest and, 457
in children, 2699
in chronic obstructive pulmonary disease, 1102
pneumothorax and, 461-462
pulmonary contusion and, 460
RICE therapy, for ankle sprain, 817
Rickets
fracture in, 2701
of prematurity, 975
Rickettsia rickettsii, 2132. *See also* Rocky Mountain spotted fever.
Rifabutin
for tuberculosis, 2163t
in HIV/AIDS, side effects of, 2079t
Rifamate, for tuberculosis, 2164
Rifampin
during pregnancy and lactation, 2785
for meningococcal meningitis, 1722-1723
for pharyngitis, 1113
for tuberculosis, 2162, 2163t
prophylactic, for meningococcal disease, 2024
Rifamycins, antiretroviral therapy and, drug interactions between, 2166
Rifater, for tuberculosis, 2164
Rifle wounds, centerfire, forensic evaluation of, 959, 959f, 960f
Rift Valley fever virus, 2055
Right bundle branch block, in pulmonary embolism, 1378, 1379f
Right subclavian artery, anomalous, dysphagia in, 1383
Right to refuse medical care, 3169-3172
Right ventricular collapse, in cardiac tamponade, 474, 474f
Right ventricular myocardial infarction, 1166, 1167f, 1172-1173

Rights
legal, 3128
patient, 2967
Right-sided aortic arch, 2574
Right-sided heart failure, 1266-1267
Rigidity
in appendicitis, 1452
nuchal
causes of, 2663
in bacterial meningitis, 2658, 2659
in central nervous system infection, 1714
Rigors, in pneumonia, 2556
Rimantadine, for influenza, 1139, 2035, 2037
Ring avulsion injuries, in hand trauma, 612-613, 613b
Risk assessment
combative patient and, 2957-2958
in acetaminophen overdose, 2333-2335, 2334f
in anaphylaxis, 1819-1820
in ectopic pregnancy, 2743, 2743b
in elder abuse, 1010-1011, 1010b
in endocarditis, 1302, 1303b
in injury prevention and control, 946-948
in intimate partner violence and abuse, 1000, 1002b, 1003b
in pulmonary embolism, 186b, 1371, 1371t
in sudden infant death syndrome, 2714-2716, 2715b
in tuberculosis, 2149-2150, 2149b, 2150b
Risk management, 3156-3173
consent to medical care and, 3166-3169
disposition requirements and, 3164-3165, 3165t
emergency medical condition and, 3156-3157
Emergency Medical Treatment and Active Labor Act and, 3156
medical screening examination and, 3160-3163
refusal of medical care and, 3169-3172
reporting requirements and, 3172-3173
screening requirements and, 3157-3158
stabilization requirements and, 3163-3164
testing requests and requirements and, 3158-3160
Risk stratification
in acute coronary ischemia, 3065
in gastrointestinal bleeding, 225-226, 225b, 226t
in minor head trauma, 363-364, 364b
in suicide, 1772-1773
Risperidone
for agitation, in delirious patient, 1654
for mood disorders, 1741
for thought disorders, 1730-1731
toxicity of, 2446, 2446t
Ritgen maneuver, modified, 2804
Ritodrine, for premature labor, 2806-2807, 2806b
Ritonavir, in HIV/AIDS, side effects of, 2079t
River blindness, 2109, 2109f
RNA viruses, 2034t, 2046-2058
Roberts v. Galen, 3164
Rochester method, for hip reduction, 759
Rocky Mountain spotted fever, 2132-2137
clinical features of, 2132-2134, 2133f, 2133t, 2134f
diagnosis of, 2134-2135, 2135b
differential considerations in, 2135
management of, 2136-2137, 2136t
skin lesions in, 1849-1850
Rocuronium
for tetanus, 2011
in rapid sequence intubation, 15, 15t, 16
Rodent bite, 884
Roentgen-equivalent-man (rem), 2321
Rofecoxib, 2927-2928
Rolandic epilepsy, benign, 2666
Rolando's fracture, 551t, 600
Rome II criteria for irritable bowel syndrome, 1491, 1491b
Root, 1026, 1027f
split, 1033-1034
Root canal pain, 1033
Rosary pea, 2471-2472, 2472f
Roseola infantum, 1850, 2044
Rotational injuries, cervical spine, 405-409, 408f-410f
Rotator cuff, 672, 673f
calcific tendinitis of, 698
hemorrhage into, in scapula fracture, 680
tears of, 696
Rotator cuff *(Continued)*
in anterior glenohumeral joint dislocation, 690
tendinitis of, 693-696, 694t, 695f
tendinopathy of, 1796-1797
Rotavirus, 2047
Rotavirus gastroenteritis, 1475-1476, 2624-2625
Roundup, 2467-2468
Roundworm, 2100t, 2113
Rovsing's sign, in appendicitis, 1452, 2619
R-plasminogen activator (r-PA), in myocardial infarction, 1189-1190
Rubber bullet, ballistic injury associated with, 458-459
Rubella, 2048-2049, 2049f
arthritis in, 1788
skin lesions in, 1850
Rubella vaccine, 2035t, 2048-2049
Rubeola, 2052-2053, 2053f
Kawasaki disease vs., 2594
screening for, 2509b
skin lesions in, 1849
Rubin syndrome, 1910
Rubin's maneuver, in shoulder dystocia, 2815, 2815f
Rue, adverse effects of, 2476t
Rule of 80, in neck masses, 1075
Rule of nines, in burn wound assessment, 919-920, 920f
Rule-using process, clinical decision making by, 126, 131t, 132
Rumination, definition of, 201
Rust remover, ingestion of, 2381t
Rust ring, in iron-containing corneal foreign body, 1047, 1048f

Saccharomyces boulardii, 1475
Sacral plexus, 718
Sacrum, 400f
fracture of, 725-726
SAD PERSONS scale, 1770, 1770t, 1772
Safety concerns, as stressor for emergency physician, 3175
Safety issues
in air medical transport, 2997, 2997b, 2997f, 2998b
in emergency department, 3119-3126
in intimate partner violence and abuse, 1004b
in suicide, 1772
Sager splint, 570, 570f
Sail sign
in infants and children, 2573, 2574f
in supracondylar fracture, 2695, 2695f
St. John's wort
adverse effects of, 2476t
drug interactions with, 2478t
St. Louis encephalitis, 2049-2050
Salicylates
during pregnancy and lactation, 2781
for rheumatic fever, 1791
for rheumatoid arthritis, 1791-1792
lactic acidosis from, 1929
metabolism of, 2339-2340, 2340f
overdose of, 2339-2342, 2340f
chronic exposure in, 2340
clinical features of, 2341, 2341b
diagnosis of, 2341
disposition in, 2342
management of, 2341-2342, 2341b
Salicylic acid, for prickly heat, 2259
Saline
for diabetic ketoacidosis, 1966
for diarrhea, 235
for elevated intracranial pressure, 360
for hypercalcemia, 1946
for hyperglycemic hyperosmolar nonketotic coma, 1969
for hypernatremia, 1936-1937
for hyponatremia, 1935
for hypovolemia, in adrenal insufficiency, 1998
for metabolic alkalosis, 1930-1931
for multiple trauma patient, 307
for rhabdomyolysis, 1982
for seizure in acute renal failure, 2650
for wound cleansing, 848
Saliva
microorganisms in, 1128
Saliva *(Continued)*
recovery of, in sexual assault examination, 985, 986b
Salivary glands, 385-386, 386f
stones of, 1075
Salmeterol
for asthma, 1088
for chronic asthma, 2542, 2543t
for chronic obstructive pulmonary disease, 1105
Salmonella infection
in cancer patient with impaired cell-mediated immunity, 2839-2840
in dysenteric colitis, 229t
in gastroenteritis, 1461-1463, 1461t, 1462t, 1482, 2625
Salpingitis, 248, 251t
Salt depletion heat exhaustion, 2259-2260
Salt solutions, for heat cramps, 2258
Salt tablets, heat illness and, 2256
Salter-Harris fracture classification system, 551t, 555-556, 557t, 2690, 2691f, 2691t, 2692, 2692f
Salvia, 2412
SAMPLE mnemonic, 2501, 2501b
Sample size, 3052
Sandifer's syndrome, 2610, 2668
Saphenous vein, thrombosis of, 1370
Saphenous vein graft, in arterial injury, 544
Saquinavir, in HIV/AIDS, side effects of, 2079t
Sarcoidosis
cardiac, 1297
hypercalcemia in, 1945
in chronic obstructive pulmonary disease, 1103
Sarcolemma
damage to, in rhabdomyolysis, 1976-1977, 1977f
ionic pumps in, 1976, 1977f
Sarcomeres, 1259
Sarcoplasmic reticulum, 1259
Sarcoptes scabiei, 1569
Sarin exposure, 2461
as chemical weapon, 939, 3030-3031, 3030b, 3031b
in children, 3021
Saturday night palsy, 1694-1695
"Save-a-Tooth" system, 1038-1039, 1039f
Saw palmetto, adverse effects of, 2476t
Scabies
in HIV/AIDS, 2085
skin lesions in, 1854-1855, 1854f
Scald burn, 913-928. *See also* Thermal burn.
Scalded skin syndrome, staphylococcal, 1845, 2199
Scalenus anticus syndrome, thoracic outlet syndrome in, 1359
Scales, 1838-1841, 1839t
Scalp
abrasion of, 372
anatomy and physiology of, 350
avulsion of, 372
laceration of, 371-372, 850
Scalp injury complexes, in children, 334
Scaly papules, skin disorders with, 1841-1842
Scaphoid fracture, 627-629, 628f
Scaphoid tubercle, 622, 623f, 625
Scaphoid view of wrist, 627, 627t
Scapholunate angle, 626, 627f
Scapholunate dissociation, 630, 631f
Scapholunate joint, 625
Scapholunate ligament, 622, 624f
Scapula
anatomy of, 672, 673f
fracture of, 679-680, 680f
manipulation of, in reduction of glenohumeral joint dislocation, 689-690, 690f
Scapular neck, fracture of, 680
Scapulothoracic dislocation, 693
Scarlet fever, 1110, 1851, 1851f
Schatzki's ring, 1383
Scheduling systems, computerized, 3104-3105
Schefflera, 2472
Schistosomiasis
chronic, 2112, 2112f, 2113f
drug therapy for, 2102t
fever in, 2105
neurologic disorders in, 2107
Schizoaffective disorder, 1729
Schizocytes, in hemolytic anemia, 1877, 1877f

Schizophrenia, 1726-1733
alcohol withdrawal syndrome vs., 2860
clinical features of, 1726-1728
criteria for, 1727, 1727b
diagnosis of, 1728
differential considerations in, 1727b, 1728-1729, 1728b, 1729t
disposition in, 1733
in alcoholism, 2875
management of, 1730-1733, 1731b
panic attack in, 1748
phases of, 1726-1727
suicide and, 1769
Schizophreniform disorder, 1729
School-age children
developmental milestones in, 2496t, 2497
fever in, management of, 2515-2516
Schools, violence in, 1017-1018
Schwannoma, 147t, 1668-1669
Sciatic mononeuropathy, 1697-1698, 1698f
Sciatic nerve, 738
Sciatic neuropathy, in hip trauma, 762-763
Sciatica, 702-703, 704-705, 711-712
Scintigraphy. *See* Radionucleotide scanning.
Sclera, 1045f
laceration of, 1051
penetration of, red and painful eye in, 296t
traumatic rupture of, 1049-1050, 1050f
whitening of, in alkali burn, 1046, 1046f
Scleral icterus, in hepatitis, 1404
Scleritis, 289-290, 290f, 295t
Scleroderma
myocarditis in, 1297-1298
oral manifestations of, 1035
Scleroderma renal crisis, 1535, 1543-1544
Sclerosing cholangitis, 1422
Sclerosing panencephalitis, subacute, 2054
Scoliosis, in cerebral palsy, 2901
Scombroid fish poisoning, 1470t, 1472-1473
Scopolamine
anticholinergic toxicity of, 2345, 2346
for nausea and vomiting, 206
mydriasis from, 1061
Scorpion bites, 907-908
Scorpion fish envenomation, 910
Scratch, rabies transmission from, 2065
Screening
for alcoholism, 2858
for elder abuse, 1011, 1011b
for gestational diabetes, 2772
for HIV, 2074-2075
for intimate partner violence and abuse, 998-999, 999b, 1000f, 1001f, 1002b
for pediatric upper respiratory tract infection, 2509b
for substance abuse in adolescents, 2884
for tuberculosis, 2169
requirements for, 3157-3158. *See also* Medical screening examination.
toxicologic. *See* Toxicologic screen.
Scrofula, 2158
Scrotal pain, in testicular torsion, 1595, 2640
Scrotal skin loss, 532
Scrotum
anatomy of, 1594, 1594f
carcinoma of, in children, 2642
dog bites to, 534-535
masses and swelling of, 1593-1598
anatomy and physiology in, 1594, 1594f
differential considerations in, 1594-1598
in children, 2638-2642, 2639f-2640f
physical examination of, 1573, 1594
Scuba diving–related disorders, 2279-2294
alternobaric vertigo in, 2286, 2287t
arterial gas embolism in, 2285-2286, 2288, 2288t
avascular osteonecrosis in, 2286
barodontalgia in, 2286
barosinusitis in, 2282
clinical features of, 2281-2286
contaminated air in, 2283
decompression sickness in, 2283-2285
diagnostic strategies in, 2286-2287, 2286b, 2287f, 2287t
differential considerations in, 2287-2288, 2288t
disposition in, 2293-2294, 2293t
external ear barotrauma in, 2282, 2292
facial barotrauma in, 2282, 2293
gastrointestinal barotrauma in, 2286
Scuba diving–related disorders *(Continued)*
inner ear barotrauma in, 2282, 2287-2288, 2287t, 2292
management of, 2288-2293
middle ear barotrauma in, 2281-2282, 2282f, 2286-2287, 2287t, 2292
nitrogen narcosis in, 2283, 2293
not requiring recompression therapy, 2292-2293, 2292b
oxygen toxicity in, 2283
pathophysiology of, 2280-2281, 2281f
pneumomediastinum in, 2286, 2293
pneumothorax in, 2286, 2293
pulmonary barotrauma in, 2285-2286, 2293
pulmonary edema in, 2286
recompression therapy for, 2288-2292, 2288b, 2289f-2291f
subcutaneous emphysema in, 2286
temporomandibular joint dysfunction in, 2283
Sea nettle, 909
Sea urchin, 909-910
Sea wasp, 909
Search and rescue, urban, 3005-3008, 3006b, 3008f
Seasonal affective disorder, 1738
Seat belt
injuries from, 341, 491-492, 947
use during pregnancy, 2735-2736
"Seatbelt sign," 491-492
Seatworm, 1479-1482
Sebaceous glands, 915
Seborrheic dermatitis, in HIV/AIDS, 2085
Seclusion, emergency, 2958-2961, 2960f
Second impact syndrome, 365-366
Second stage of labor, 2800-2804, 2802b, 2802t, 2803f
Secondary assessment of victim endpoint (SAVE) system, 3013
Secondary survey
in obstetric trauma, 323
in pediatric trauma, 330, 330b, 333, 333b
Second-degree burn, 918-919, 919f
SECONDS mnemonic, 1779-1780
Second-trimester fetal death, 2740
Secretory diarrhea, 228, 2624
Security
in emergency department, 2965-2966
of patient information, 3102-3103
Sedation, 2938-2954
agents for, 2940t-2941t
barbiturates for, 2945-2946
benzodiazepines for, 2944-2945
consent prior to, 2940
continuum of, 2938, 2939f
contraindications to, 2939
definitions of, 2914b, 2938, 2939b
discharge criteria and instructions after, 2943
drug selection and administration in, 2949-2952, 2950t, 2951b
etomidate for, 2940t-2941t, 2947-2948
fasting prior to, 2939-2940
for agitation in delirious patient, 1653-1654
for PCP intoxication, 2892
in children, 2952-2954
in cocaine overdose, 2389
in comatose survivors of cardiac arrest, 70
in PCP intoxication, 2416
in severe head trauma, 358
in ventilated patient, 30-31
ketamine for, 2940t-2941t, 2946-2947
monitoring of, 2942-2943
nitrous oxide for, 2940t-2941t, 2948
opioids for, 2944
personnel providing, 2941-2942
preprocedure patient assessment in, 2938-2940
propofol for, 2940t-2941t, 2947
rapid, 2944b
for mood disorders, 1741
for thought disorders, 1730-1731, 1731b
of combative patient, 2961-2963
recovery from, 2943
reversal agents in, 2948-2949
route of administration for, 2943-2944
supplies and equipment for, 2942
terminology in, 2938, 2939b
Sedative hypnotics
in elderly person, 2827
overdose of, 2481-2490
Sedative hypnotics *(Continued)*
barbiturates in, 2481-2483, 2482b, 2482f
benzodiazepines in, 2483-2486, 2484t
buspirone in, 2486
chloral hydrate in, 2487
flunitrazepam in, 2486
γ-hydroxybutyrate in, 2488-2490, 2488b
opioid/sedative/ethanol syndrome and, 2327t, 2328
OTC sleep aids in, 2487-2488, 2488t
zolpidem and zaleplon in, 2486-2487
Segmental ileus, 1440
Segond fracture, 777, 777f
Seidel's test, in corneal laceration, 287-288, 1051, 1051f
Seizure, 164-168, 1619-1629. *See also* Epilepsy.
absence, 1621
after cerebral ischemia, 70
alcohol-related, 2863-2866, 2863b, 2879
ataxia in, 2682
brain damage and, 2665
cerebrospinal fluid shunt–related, in developmentally disabled patient, 2899
classification of, 164, 165t, 1619-1620, 2665, 2666b
clinical features of, 1620-1625
confusion after, 154
diagnosis of, 165-168, 165t, 1625-1626
differential considerations in, 165-166, 165t, 1626
disposition in, 168
drug-induced, 1623, 2669-2670, 2670b
epidemiology of, 164
episodic disorders that mimic, 2668b
febrile, as indication for lumbar puncture, 2660
focal (partial), 164, 1620, 1621
from antipsychotic agents, 2448
generalized, 164, 1620, 1621
history in, 167
ictal events in, properties of, 167
imaging studies in, 168
in acute renal failure, 2650
in amphetamine abuse, 2896
in anticholinergic poisoning, 2349
in apparent life-threatening event, 2719
in arteriovenous malformations, 1624
in asthma, 2536
in beta blocker overdose, 2374
in bupropion overdose, 2361
in cancer patient, 1919
in central nervous system degenerative diseases, 1624
in central nervous system infection, 1721
in central nervous system tumor or vasculitis, 1624
in cerebral venous thrombosis, 1670
in chlorinated hydrocarbon poisoning, 2462, 2463
in cicutoxin poisoning, 2472
in cyclic antidepressant poisoning, 2354t, 2356
in developmentally disabled patient, 2898-2899
in eclampsia, 1627, 2749-2750, 2751
in HIV/AIDS, 2079
in infectious diseases, 1623
in mefenamic acid poisoning, 2343
in metabolic disorders, 1622
in migraine, 1624
in organophosphate poisoning, 2459
in pertussis, 2006
in pregnancy, 1624, 2753t, 2763t, 2768-2769
in severe head trauma, prophylaxis against, 361, 361b
in stroke, 1624
in systemic lupus erythematosus, 1007
laboratory tests in, 168
management of
immediate, 166-167, 166t, 168, 1626-1628, 1627t, 1628t
long-term, 1628-1629, 1629t
myoclonic, 1621
neonatal, 2667
pathophysiology of, 164-165, 1620
pediatric, 367, 2665-2676
after head trauma, 334
anticonvulsant therapy for, 2674-2676, 2675t
clinical features of, 2665-2667, 2666b
diagnosis of, 2670-2671

Seizure (Continued)
disposition in, 2674-2676, 2674b, 2675t
etiology of, 2667-2670, 2668b-2670b
febrile, 2507, 2666-2667, 2674, 2674b
management of, 2671-2673, 2671b, 2672t
pathophysiology of, 2665
precipitators of, identification and treatment of, 2673
secondary survey in, 2502
status epilepticus and, 2667, 2668b, 2672-2673, 2672t
physical examination in, 167-168
postictal states in, 1625
posttraumatic, 370, 373, 1623
prophylaxis against, 361, 361b
primary. *See* Epilepsy.
pseudoseizure and, 1624-1625, 2668
rapid assessment and stabilization in, 166-167, 166t
reactive, 1622-1624
recurrent
diagnosis of, 1625-1626
risk of, 2674
submersion injuries and, 2312
syncope vs., 194
temporal lobe, 1621
terminology in, 1620
tonic, 1621
toxin-induced, 1623
Selection bias, 3049
Selective serotonin reuptake inhibitors, 2328
for anxiety disorders, 1751, 1751t
for depression, 1741
for neuropathic pain, 1692
metabolism of, 2357
overdose of, 2357-2360, 2358b, 2358t, 2359b, 2360t
Selenium sulfide
for tinea capitis, 1839
for tinea versicolor, 1840
Self-destructive patient, 2978t, 2981
Self-neglect, by elder, 1009
Sellick's maneuver, in rapid sequence intubation, 11b
Semicircular canal, 142
Senescent forgetfulness, dementia vs., 1660
Sengstaken-Blakemore tube, in gastrointestinal bleeding, 225
Senile plaques, in dementia, 1657
Sensitivity analyses, 3058
Sensitization, to allergens, 1819
Sensorineural hearing loss, 1072
Sensorium, altered, in cholangitis, 1421
Sensory ataxia, 2682
Sensory dermatomes, 418f
Sensory disturbances
in carpal tunnel syndrome, 1697
in ischemic stroke, 1609
in multiple sclerosis, 1672
in spinal cord disorders, 1678f, 1679
in syringomyelia, 1683
Sensory examination
in lumbar radiculopathy, 704, 705f
in spinal injuries, 417, 417t, 418f
Sensory nerves, to hand, 587, 589f
Sensory neuronopathy, 1700, 1700b
Sensory tracts, ascending, 1676, 1676f, 2915, 2915f, 2916f
Sentinel loop, 1440
Sentinel pile, in anal fissures, 1512
Separation anxiety, 1746b
Sepsis, 2211-2222. *See also* Bacteremia.
as indication for lumbar puncture
in immunocompromised child, 2660
in young infant, 2659
clinical features of, 2214-2216
definitions in, 2211, 2212b
diagnosis of, 2216-2217
differential considerations in, 2217, 2218b
disposition in, 2222
epidemiology of, 2211-2212
in asplenic patient, 2842-2843
in cholangitis, 1421
in febrile cancer patient, 1907-1909, 1908b
in pneumococcal disease, 2017-2018
inflammatory mediators in, 2213
management of, 2217-2222, 2218f, 2219t, 2221t
mortality in, 2216, 2216t
pathophysiology of, 2212-2213
Sepsis (Continued)
pelvic pain and, 250
progression of disease in, 2211, 2212f
severe
definition of, 2211, 2212b
treatment of, 51, 51f
Septal branch of superior labial artery, 1073, 1073f
Septal defects, traumatic, 472
Septal myomectomy, for hypertrophic cardiomyopathy, 1296
Septic arthritis, 1782-1785, 2174
clinical features of, 1784-1785, 2188-2191
complications of, 2190
differential considerations in, 2191-2192
disposition in, 2193
etiology and microbiology of, 2177-2179, 2178t
gonococcal, 2190-2191
history and physical examination in, 2188
in atypical joints, 2191
in disseminated gonococcal infection, 1566
in hand, 618
in knee, 796
in tuberculosis, 2159
joint aspiration and joint fluid analysis in, 2188-2190, 2189f
management of, 1785, 2178t, 2192-2193
pathophysiology and epidemiology of, 1782-1784
pathophysiology of, 2177
pediatric, 2190, 2509b, 2704-2706, 2705t, 2706t
pediatric limp from, 764
with existing joint disease, 2191
Septic bursitis, 1801-1803
Septic olecranon bursitis, 667
Septic shock
adrenal insufficiency in, 1995-1996
causes of, 46-47
clinical features of, 2215
definition of, 49, 49b, 2211, 2212b
differential considerations in, 2218b
pediatric fever in, 2511
treatment of, 51, 51f, 52b, 53-54
Septic thrombosis, 1123, 1363
Septicemia
following hypothermia, 2247
postanginal, parapharyngeal abscess and, 1123
Septicemic plague, 3027
Sequestra, in osteomyelitis, 2175
Sequestration
abnormal, hemolytic anemia, 1884
splenic, 1896
Serologic tests
in babesiosis, 2140
in Colorado tick fever, 2141
in hepatitis, 1405t
in Lyme disease, 2125
in pneumonia, 1135
in Q fever, 2137
in Rocky Mountain spotted fever, 2135
in syphilis, 1561-1562
in tuberculosis, 2156
Serotonin
in mood disorders, 1735
suicide and, 1768
violent behavior and, 2957
Serotonin reuptake inhibitors
nonselective, 2328
selective, 2328
for anxiety disorders, 1751, 1751t
for depression, 1741
for neuropathic pain, 1692
metabolism of, 2357
overdose of, 2357-2360, 2358b, 2358t, 2359b, 2360t
Serotonin syndrome, 2328, 2358-2359
antidotes to, 2329t
clinical manifestations of, 2358b
diagnostic criteria for, 2358-2359, 2359b
differential diagnosis in, 2359
drugs associated with, 2359b
lithium-induced, 2442
opioid-induced, 2452
Serotonin-like agents, psychoactive, ingestion of, 2406-2408, 2407f
Serratus anterior muscle, 672, 673f
Sertraline, metabolism of, 2357
Serum sickness, 901, 1815-1816
Sesamoid fractures, 834-835
Severe acute respiratory distress syndrome (SARS), 1130, 2034t, 2050-2051
Sever's disease, 2710
Sexual abuse
of child, 969, 971, 972-973, 974, 975
of elder, 1010
of intimate partner, 997
Sexual assault, 977-992
debriefing after, 991-992, 991b
emergency department preparation for victim of, 978
epidemiology of, 977-978
examination protocol in, 980f-983f
male victim of, examination of, 992
medicolegal issues in, 3159-3160
obtaining history and consent in, 978-979, 978b, 979b, 979t, 984
of intimate partner, 997
perpetrators of
detection avoidance methods used by, 984
sexual dysfunction in, 984, 984b
suspected, examination of, 992
physical examination and evidence collection in, 984-989, 985b-987b, 987f, 987t, 988f, 988t
pregnancy prophylaxis and, 991, 991t
sexually transmitted disease and, 989-990, 989b, 989t
Sexual dysfunction
in depression, 1737
in multiple sclerosis, 1672
in perpetrators of sexual assault, 984, 984b
pelvic fracture and, 719, 720
Sexual intercourse, during pregnancy, 2736
Sexually transmitted disease, 1556-1571
after sexual assault, 989-990, 989b, 989t
anorectal involvement in, 1518-1520, 1518t
differential diagnosis in, 1557t
epididymitis and, 1595, 1596-1597, 1597t
in bacterial vaginosis, 1567t, 1568-1569
in Bartholin cyst and abscess, 1559-1560
in candidiasis, 1567t, 1568
in chancroid, 1557t, 1559t, 1562-1563, 1562f
in *Chlamydia trachomatis*, 1559t, 1564-1565
in condylomata acuminata, 1559t, 1563-1564, 1564
in granuloma inguinale, 1559t, 1563
in herpes simplex virus infection, 1557-1559, 1557t, 1558f, 1559t
in HIV/AIDS, 2087
in lymphogranuloma venereum, 1557t, 1559t, 1562
in nongonococcal urethritis, 1565
in pelvic inflammatory disease, 1569-1571
in pregnancy, 2758-2759
in syphilis, 1557t, 1559-1562, 1559t, 1560f, 1561f
in trichomoniasis, 1567-1568, 1567t
prophylaxis against, after sexual assault, 973-974, 974t, 989-990, 989t
treatment of, 1559t
with genital discharge, 1564-1571
with genital ulcers, 1557-1564, 1557t
Shaken-baby syndrome, 367, 970-971
Shear injuries, cervical spine, 405, 406f-407f
Sheep liver fluke, 2101t, 2113
Shenton's line, in hip dislocation, 757, 758f
Shepherd's purse, adverse effects of, 2476t
Shift work
performance and, 3122-3123, 3122t, 3123b
rational approaches to, 3123b
strategies for, 3176, 3177b
Shigella infection
in dysenteric colitis, 229t
in gastroenteritis, 1461t, 1462t, 1464-1465, 2625
in myocarditis, 1292
Shikani Optical Stylet, 21, 22f
Shin splints, 804-805
Shingles, 1054, 1859-1860, 1860f, 2042-2043
Shivering thermogenesis, 2236, 2247
Shock, 41-55
acid-base calculations in, 1924
anaphylaxis vs., 1830
burn, 918
cardiogenic
causes of, 47
definition of, 49, 49b
in myocardial infarction, 1160, 1194

Shock *(Continued)*
reperfusion therapy in, 1194
treatment of, 52b, 54, 113-114, 113f, 1273
classification of, 41-42, 42b
clinical features of, 47-49, 47b, 48f, 49b
compensated, in children, 2499
epidemiology of, 42
goal directed therapy for, 50-52, 51f
heart function in, 45
hemorrhagic
causes of, 44f, 45-46
definition of, 49, 49b
in subclavian artery injury, 545
treatment of, 52-53, 52b
hypovolemic
in cardiac tamponade, 473
in diabetic ketoacidosis, 1966
mechanical ventilation in, 32
in bacterial meningitis, 2663
in children, 2499, 2503
in meningococcal disease, 2022
in multiple trauma, 307-308
in pancreatitis, 1429
management of, 50-54, 51f, 52b
monitoring perfusion status in, 50
pathophysiology of, 42-47, 43f, 44f
septic. *See also* Sepsis.
adrenal insufficiency in, 1995-1996
causes of, 46-47
clinical features of, 2215
definition of, 49, 49b, 2211, 2212b
differential considerations in, 2218b
pediatric fever in, 2511
treatment of, 51, 51f, 52b, 53-54
spinal, 436-437, 1677
complete spinal cord lesion vs., 417
neurogenic hypotension secondary to, 437
toxic. *See* Toxic shock syndrome.
undifferentiated, classification of, 48f
ventilation in, 51-52
volume replacement in, 52
vs. hemodynamic changes in pregnancy, 316-317, 317t
Shored-exit wound, 958-959, 958f
Shotgun wounds. *See also* Firearm injuries
abdominal, 491, 507
peripheral vascular, 537
Shoulder
exercises for
in clavicle fracture, 677, 679f
in proximal humerus fractures, 682
frozen, 682, 698-699, 699t, 1797
immobilization of, 569, 677, 678f
pain in
in ectopic pregnancy, 2743
sources of, 672, 674
physical examination of, 674, 674t, 1778
tendinopathy of, 1796-1798
Shoulder dystocia, 2811, 2813-2815, 2814f, 2815f, 2816b
Shoulder girdle, 670, 671f
Shoulder trauma, 670-699
anatomy in, 670-672, 671f, 673f
clinical features of, 672, 674, 674t
dislocations in, 683-693
acromioclavicular, 685-687, 686f, 687f
glenohumeral, 687-693, 688f-694f
scapulothoracic, 693
sternoclavicular, 683-685, 684f-685f
fractures in, 676-683
clavicle, 676-679, 676f-679f
proximal humeral epiphysis, 682-683, 683f
proximal humerus, 680-682, 681f, 682f
scapula, 679-680, 680f
radiography in, 674-676, 674f-676f
soft tissue injuries in, 693-699
adhesive capsulitis, 698-699, 699t
biceps muscle lesions, 697-698, 697f
calcific tendinitis, 698
rotator cuff tears, 696
subacromial syndromes and impingement, 693-696, 694t, 695f
Shrug sign, in rotator cuff tendinopathy, 1797
Shudder attacks, 2668
Shunt
cerebrospinal fluid, in developmentally disabled patient, 2899
vascular, in arterial injury, 544
ventriculoperitoneal, pediatric fever in, 2517
Sialolithiasis, 1075
Siberian ginseng
adverse effects of, 2476t
drug interactions with, 2478t
Sick sinus syndrome, 1218
Sickle cell disease, 1879-1882
altitude and, 2308
clinical features of, 1000-1001, 1001f, 1001t
in pregnancy, 2763t, 2768
management of, 1001-1002
osteomyelitis in, 2186
pathophysiology of, 1879-1880
pediatric fever in, 2516-2517
urinary tract infection in, 1578
Sickle cell trait, 1880
Sickle cell–ß-thalassemia, 1882
Sideroblastic anemia, 1873, 2874
Sigmoid volvulus, 1497, 1498, 1498f, 1499
Sign language, 2905
Signet ring sign, in scapholunate dissociation, 630, 631f
Sign-overs, 3124
Silent perilobular fibrosis, 1435
Silk suture, 852t
Silver nitrate, for epistaxis, 1074
Simon's foci, in tuberculosis, 2152
Simple asphyxiants, inhalation of, 2432-2433
Simple obstruction of small bowel, 1440
Simple triage and rapid treatment (START) technique, 3012-3013, 3013f
Simulator technology, 3099, 3099f
Sin Nombre virus, 2055
Sinding-Larsen-Johansson disease, 794
Singh score for hip osteoporosis, 739, 740f-741f
Sinoatrial block, 1216-1218, 1217f
Sinoatrial node, 1201-1202, 1203f
digitalis effects on, 2368
Sinus, nasal, 384
Sinus bradycardia, 1215-1216, 1216f
from succinylcholine, 13
in hypothyroidism, 1992
Sinus dysrhythmias, 1216, 1216f
Sinus node dysfunction, 1218
Sinus tachycardia, 1227-1228, 1227f
in hyperthyroidism, 1987
in myocardial contusion, 468
in pediatric cardiac arrest, 109-110, 109t
Sinus thrombosis, lateral venous, in otitis media, 1068
Sinusitis, 1123-1126, 1124f, 1125f
allergic vs. infectious, 1123
clinical features of, 1124
complications of, 1125-1126
diagnostic strategies in, 1124, 1124f, 1125f
differential diagnosis in, 1125
management of, 1125
maxillary, oral pain in, 1034
Sirolimus, 2844
Sixth disease, 1850
Sixth-nerve palsy, eye movement disorders in, 1063
Sjögren's syndrome
myocarditis in, 1297
pericarditis in, 1284
Skeletal muscle
hyperactivity of, in organophosphate poisoning, 2459-2460
ionic pump function of, 1976, 1977f
Skeletal muscle relaxants, for analgesia, 2928-2929
Skeletal system. *See also* Bone; Musculoskeletal system; Orthopedic *entries.*
aging and, 345
in electrical and lightning injuries, 2273
Skeletal tuberculosis, 2159
Skew deviation, 160
Skier's thumb, 604
Skin
anatomy of, 912, 914-915
biomechanical properties of, 849
biopsy of, in Rocky Mountain spotted fever, 2135
changes in
in acute radiation syndrome, 2322
in pregnancy, 2723-2724, 2728
disinfection of, in wound care, 847
dry, in HIV/AIDS, 2084-2085
examination of
in dyspnea, 178t
in sexual assault victim, 985-986, 985b, 986b
Skin *(Continued)*
injury to. *See also* Chemical injuries; Thermal burn.
in acid and alkali burns, 931-933
in anhydrous ammonia exposure, 935
in bipyridyl compound exposure, 2466
in chlorinated hydrocarbon exposure, 2463
in elderly person, 347
in electrical and lightning injuries, 2272-2273, 2272f, 2273f
in frostbite, 2229
in hydrofluoric acid exposure, 933-934
in organophosphate exposure, 2460
in substituted phenol exposure, 2464
in tobacco workers, 2474
of hand, 576-577
of scalp, 350
resistance of, 2269b
Skin abscess, 2202-2204, 2203t
Skin disorders, 1838-1865
carbuncle as, 1843
in developmentally disabled patient, 2903
in HIV/AIDS, 2084-2085
in parasitic infections, 2108-2109
in spinal injuries, 438
in traumatic asphyxia, 459
with erythema, 1839t, 1844
with exanthems, 1848-1851
with nodular lesions, 1856-1857
with papular lesions, 1851-1856
with pustules, 1842-1844
with red macules, 1844-1848
with scales, plaques, and patches, 1838-1841
with scaly papules, 1841-1842
with vesicular lesions, 1857-1860
Skin lesions. *See also* Skin rash.
definitions of, 1839t
from opioid injection, 1864-1865, 1865f, 2453-2454
in anaphylaxis, 1829
in atopic dermatitis, 1841-1842
in *Candida* infection, 1840-1841
in chronic renal failure, 1542, 1542f
in Churg-Strauss syndrome, 1816
in contact dermatitis, 1851-1852, 1851f, 1852f
in cutaneous anthrax, 1860, 1861f, 3025, 3026f
in decompression sickness, 2284
in dermatomyositis, 1708, 1862t, 1863f
in diabetes mellitus, 1861f, 1862t, 1863f, 1971-1972
in diaper dermatitis, 1852
in diphtheria, 2003, 2004
in drug eruptions, 1844-1845, 1844f, 1845f, 1846t-1847t
in erythema infectiosum, 1850
in erythema multiforme, 1852-1853, 1853f
in erythema nodosum, 1816, 1856-1857, 1856f
in folliculitis, 1843
in fungal infection, 1838-1840, 1839f, 1840f
in gonococcal dermatitis, 1566, 1843-1844, 1843f
in herpes simplex virus infection, 1857-1858, 1858f
in herpes zoster, 1859-1860, 1860f
in hidradenitis suppurativa, 1843
in HIV/AIDS, 1861f, 1862t, 2085
in hypersensitivity vasculitis, 1815
in hyperthyroidism, 1862t, 1987
in hypothyroidism, 1862t, 1863f
in impetigo, 1842-1843, 2202
in inflammatory vascular disease, 1347
in Lyme disease, 2122, 2122f, 2124-2125
in measles, 1849
in meningococcal disease, 2022
in mustard exposure, 3031
in panniculitis, 1817
in pediculosis, 1853-1854, 1853f
in pemphigus vulgaris, 1857, 1857f
in pityriasis rosea, 1841
in rheumatoid arthritis, 1862t
in Rocky Mountain spotted fever, 1849-1850, 2133-2134, 2133f, 2134f
in roseola infantum, 1850
in rubella, 1850
in scabies, 1854-1855, 1854f
in scarlet fever, 1851, 1851t
in smallpox, 1860, 1860t, 1861f, 2039, 2039f
in staphylococcal scalded skin syndrome, 1845, 2199

Skin lesions (Continued)
in syphilis, 1855-1856, 1855f
in systemic lupus erythematosus, 1806, 1862t, 1863f
in toxic epidermal necrolysis, 1845-1846, 1846f
in toxic shock syndrome, 1846-1847
in ulcerative colitis, 1862t
in urticaria, 1847-1848, 1848f
in varicella, 1858-1859, 1859f
malignant diseases associated with, 1862-1864
nodular, 1856-1857
papular, 1851-1856
systemic diseases associated with, 1860, 1861f, 1862t, 1863f
vesicular, 1857-1860
Skin rash. *See also* Skin lesions.
drug-induced, 1844, 1847t
glue sniffer's, 2430
heat, 2259
in bacterial meningitis, 2658, 2659
in Colorado tick fever, 2141
in dermatomyositis, 1708
in disseminated gonococcal infection, 1566
in ehrlichiosis, 2138
in erythema infectiosum, 1850
in gonococcal arthritis, 1788
in halothane-induced hepatitis, 1414
in Henoch-Schönlein purpura, 1815, 2615, 2615f, 2653
in herpes zoster, 1859, 1860f
in Kawasaki disease, 2026, 2594, 2595f
in Lyme disease, 2122, 2122f
in measles, 1849, 2053, 2053f
in Rocky Mountain spotted fever, 1849, 2133-2134, 2133f, 2134f
in roseola infantum, 1850
in rubella, 1850
in scarlet fever, 1851, 1851f
in smallpox, 2039, 2039f, 3028-3029, 3028f, 3029f
in syphilis, 1561, 1561f
in systemic lupus erythematosus, 1806
in toxic shock syndrome, 1847, 2029, 2200
oral hypoglycemic agent–induced, 1972
Skin tension lines, 843, 843f, 844f
Skinfold asymmetry, in developmental hip dysplasia, 2701
Skull
anatomy of, 350
fetal, 2800f
radiography of
in minor head trauma, 364-365
in pediatric head trauma, 336, 368
in severe head trauma, 362, 362t
in skull fracture, 372
Skull fracture, 372-374
basilar, 373
clinical assessment and significance of, 372
depressed, 373
frontal, 393
in children, 334-335, 2699
linear, 372-373
open, 373-374
Skull-base osteomyelitis, 1071
Skullcap, adverse effects of, 2476t
Skunk, rabies in, 2062, 2062f, 2063, 2063f, 2064
Sleep aids, OTC, overdose of, 2487-2488, 2488t
Sleep apnea, hypertension in, 1313
Sleep deprivation, from shift work, performance and, 3123, 3123b
Sleep disturbance
in acute mountain sickness, 2301, 2302
in depression, 1737
seizures vs., 2668
Sleep talking, 2668
Sleeping, prone, sudden infant death syndrome and, 2715
Sleep-wake disturbances, in delirium, 1649
Sleepwalking, 2668
Sling and swathe, 569, 677, 678f
Sling immobilization
in clavicle fracture, 677, 678f
in scapula fracture, 680
Slipped capital femoral epiphysis, 765-767, 765f, 766f, 2707-2709, 2708f
Slit ventricle syndrome, in developmentally disabled patient, 2899
Slit-lamp examination
in corneal trauma, 1047, 1047f, 1051, 1051f
Slit-lamp examination (Continued)
in red and painful eye, 287, 287f
in traumatic hyphema, 1048, 1048f
of ocular foreign body, 860
Slow virus infections, 1657-1658, 1659, 2058
SLUDGE mnemonic, 2328, 2459, 2459b
Small intestine
biopsy of, in AIDS-related diarrhea, 1484
disorders of, 1440-1449
ischemia of, 1444-1449. *See also* Mesenteric ischemia.
motility disorders of, 1440, 1441b, 1443
obstruction of, 1440-1444, 1441b, 1443f
adynamic ileus in, 1440, 1441b, 1443
causes of, 1441-1442, 1441b, 1500b
clinical features of, 1442
complications of, 1442
diagnosis of, 1442-1443, 1443f
differential diagnosis in, 1443-1444
in malrotation with midgut volvulus, 2607, 2607f, 2608f
management of, 1444
mechanical vs. neurogenic, 1440
pseudoobstruction and, 1440
trauma to, 489, 490
volvulus of, 1441
Smallpox, 2034t, 2039-2040, 2039f, 3028-3029, 3028f, 3029f
skin lesions in, 1860, 1860t, 1861f
vaccine for, 2035t, 3029
Smith's fracture, 551t, 633-635, 635f
Smoke inhalation, 2435-2436
airway management and respiratory care in, 921-922
carbon monoxide with cyanide poisoning in, 2440-2441
prehospital care in, 921
Smoking
Buerger's disease and, 1351, 1352
chronic obstructive pulmonary disease and, 1098
Snakebite, 895-903, 897f, 897t, 900t, 1979
Sniffing position, in pediatric resuscitation, 105, 106f
Snowbird technique for reduction of anterior glenohumeral joint dislocation, 689
Snowblower injuries, 609
Soap, for rabies postexposure prophylaxis, 2068
Social phobia, 1746b, 1749
Social problems, in alcoholism, 2879-2880
Social relationships, promotion of, as wellness strategy for emergency physicians, 3177
Social/adaptive milestones, 2495-2497, 2496t
Societal factors, in suicide, 1767-1768
Societal values, 3129, 3129b
Soda lime dust particles, in scuba diving–related disorders, 2283
Sodium
dietary excess of, heart failure from, 1268
fractional excretion of, 1527-1528, 1527t, 1528b
imbalance of. *See* Hypernatremia; Hyponatremia.
normal physiology of, 1933
serum
in bacterial meningitis, 2662
in diabetic ketoacidosis, 1964, 1964t
skin injury from, 937
urine, 1527-1528, 1527t, 1528b, 1934
Sodium bicarbonate
for acute renal failure, 2650
for cardiac arrest, 93
for cyanide poisoning, 2437
for cyclic antidepressant poisoning, 2355, 2356
for diabetic ketoacidosis, 1966-1967
for hyperkalemia, 1941
in acute renal failure, 1539
in chronic renal failure, 1545, 1545t
for hyperuricemia, 1914
for metabolic acidosis, 1929-1930
for pediatric asystole, 111-112
for pediatric bradycardia, 111
for pediatric resuscitation, 100, 101t
for QRS prolongation in OTC sleep aid overdose, 2488
for rhabdomyolysis, 1982
for salicylate overdose, 2342
for sepsis, 2219t, 2220
Sodium bicarbonate (Continued)
for toxicant-induced metabolic acidosis, 2400-2401
for ventricular fibrillation and pulseless ventricular tachycardia, 84
for white phosphorus burn, 936
topical anesthetic with, 846
Sodium channel antagonists, after cerebral ischemia, 71
Sodium chloride
for hyponatremia, 1935
hypertonic, in cyclic antidepressant poisoning, 2356-2357
in hydrotherapy for acid and alkali burns, 933
Sodium hydroxide, ingestion of, 2380, 2381, 2381t
Sodium nitrite, for cyanide poisoning, 939, 2438
Sodium phosphate
for hypercalcemia, 1915
for hypophosphatemia, 1952
Sodium thiosulfate
for cyanide poisoning, 2438
for simultaneous carbon monoxide and cyanide poisoning, 2440
Sodium-calcium exchanger, 1199-1200, 1200f
Sodium-potassium pump, 1200, 1200f, 1976, 1977f
Soft tissue examination, in spinal cord injury, 311
Soft tissue infection, 2195-2209
clinical characteristics of, 2195-2196, 2196t
in abscess, 2202-2207. *See also* Abscess.
in cellulitis, 2196-2199, 2196t, 2197t
in impetigo, 2201-2202
in myonecrosis, 2196t, 2208-2209
in necrotizing fasciitis, 2196t, 2207-2208
in toxic shock syndrome, 2199-2201, 2200b, 2201b
superficial, antibiotics for, 2197, 2197t
Soft tissue injuries, 566-568. *See also specific types, e.g.,* Sprain.
foreign body in, 878-879
from dentoalveolar trauma, 1040
in ankle trauma, 815-820
in elbow and humeral trauma, 667-668
in elderly person, 347
in eye, 1054-1055, 1055f
in facial trauma, 390-392
in hand, 600
in hip trauma, 761-763
in lower leg trauma, 804-805
in pelvic fracture, 719
in shoulder, 693-699
in wrist trauma, 639, 639f
wound management in, 842-857
Solar urticaria, 1848
Solid-organ transplant patient. *See* Organ transplant patient.
Solvents, inhaled, 2428-2432, 2430f, 2886-2889, 2887t, 2888f, 2889b
Soman, 2461, 3030-3031, 3030b, 3031b
Somatic pain, 211-212
Somatization, 1753
Somatization disorder, 1754-1755, 1754b
Somatoform disorders, 1753-1759
clinical features of, 1753-1756, 1754b, 1755b
diagnosis of, 1756
differential considerations in, 1756-1757, 1757b
disposition in, 1759
management of, 1757-1759
panic attack in, 1748
undifferentiated, 1755
Somatoform pain disorder, 1755
Somatostatin analogues, for gastrointestinal bleeding, 225
Somogyi phenomenon, in hypoglycemia, 1960
Sore throat. *See* Pharyngitis.
Sotalol, 1210, 2373t
Space infections of head and neck, 1027, 1028-1029, 1030f, 1032, 1116-1117, 1116f
parapharyngeal, 1121-1123, 1122f
peritonsillar, 1117-1118, 1118f
retropharyngeal, 1120-1121, 1120f, 1121f
submandibular, 1028, 1032, 1118-1119
Space of Poirier, 622, 624f
Spasmodic croup, 2527
Spastic paraparesis, idiopathic, 1683

Spasticity
in cerebral palsy, 2904
in multiple sclerosis, 1673, 2910
Spathiphyllum, 2475
Specificity, 3059t
Spectinomycin, for gonococcal dermatitis, 1843
Specula, 2735
Speech
disorganized, in schizophrenia, 1727-1728
pressured, in mania, 1739
Speech disorders
in botulism, 2014
in neck masses, 1076
Speed's test, in bicipital tendinopathy, 1797
Sperm, recovery of, in sexual assault victim, 987-988, 988t
Spermatic cord, torsion of, in children, 2639-2640, 2640f
Sphenoid sinus, 1123
Sphenoid sinusitis, 1124, 1126
Sphenopalatine artery, 1073, 1073f
Spherocytosis, in hemolytic anemia, 1877, 1878f
Sphygmomanometer, in wound assessment, 845
Spider angioma, in hepatitis, 1404
Spider bites, 905-907, 2329t
Spider nevi, in pregnancy, 2724
Spill scalds, 915-916
Spilled teacup sign, in lunate dislocation, 630, 632f
Spinal abscess, 1684, 1712, 1715, 1716
Spinal accessory nerve, 1665t
Spinal arteries, 1676
Spinal carcinoma
back pain in, 261, 703, 706, 712-713
magnetic resonance imaging in, 712-713
radiography in, 708, 709f
Spinal column
anatomy of, 399, 400f-401f
injuries of. *See* Spinal injuries.
Spinal cord
infarction of, 1683
ligaments of, 401f
membranes of, inflammation of. *See* Meningitis.
pain transmission in, 2914-2915, 2915f, 2916f
tracts in, illustration of, 2916f
tumor of, 1685
vascular damage to, 413, 415f
Spinal cord compression, 1680-1681, 1681t, 1683-1685
epidural, in cancer patient, 1919-1920
with superior vena cava syndrome, 1910
Spinal cord disorders, 1675-1685
anatomy in, 1676, 1676f
classification of, 1677-1679, 1678f
clinical features of, 1679-1680
demyelinating
in multiple sclerosis, 1681-1682
in transverse myelitis, 1682
diagnosis of, 1680
differential considerations in, 1680-1681, 1681b
in diskitis, 1684-1685
in epidural abscess, 1684
in epidural hematoma, 1683-1684
in HIV/AIDS, 1683
in idiopathic spastic paraparesis, 1683
in subarachnoid hemorrhage, 1682
in syringomyelia, 1682-1683
management of, 1681
Spinal cord syndromes, 417-420, 419f, 420f, 1677-1679, 1678f
anterior, 419f, 420, 1678, 1678f
Brown-Séquard, 418, 419f, 420, 1677-1678, 1678f
cauda equina, 1678f, 1679
central, 417-418, 419f, 1677, 1678f
conus medullaris, 1678f, 1679
transverse, 417, 1677, 1678f
Spinal fracture
anatomy and physiology in, 399, 402f
back pain in, 706
computed tomography in, 429-430, 429f
disposition in, 439
extension, 410-411, 410f-411f
flexion, 399, 401-404, 402f-405f
minor, 439
rotational, 405-409, 408f-410f
Spinal fracture *(Continued)*
vertical compression, 411-413, 411f-414f
with cord impingement, back pain in, 265t
Spinal hemorrhage, magnetic resonance imaging in, 434, 434f
Spinal immobilization, 435, 436
Spinal infection, back pain in, 703, 706, 712
Spinal injuries, 398-439, 2905-2909
airway management in, 436
anatomy and physiology in, 399, 400f-402f
autonomic dysreflexia in, 2906
classification of, 399, 399t, 413
clinical features of, 415-420
complete (transverse), 417, 1677, 1678f
computed tomography in, 427, 429-431, 429b, 429f-432f
definitive treatment and prognosis in, 438-439
disposition in, 439
epidemiology of, 399
extension, 410-411, 410f-411f
flexion, 399, 401-404, 402f-405f
gastrointestinal disorders in, 438, 2907
genitourinary disorders in, 438
in children, 336-338, 337f
in decompression sickness, 2284
in elderly person, 346, 413, 415f
in electrical and lightning injuries, 2273-2274
in multiple trauma, 309
in pregnancy, 2770
incomplete, 417-420, 419f, 420f, 437-438, 1677-1679, 1678f
ligamentous, 434, 435f, 439
magnetic resonance imaging in, 431-435, 433f-436f
management of, 435-439, 437f
motor examination in, 416, 417t
neurologic disorders in, 2909
neurologic examination in, 415-417
orthopedic disorders in, 2909
orthostatic hypotension in, 2906
pathophysiology of, 399, 401-413
prehospital care in, 435
primary, 413, 415f
pulmonary edema in, 438
radiographic evaluation of, 420-427, 422f-428f
anteroposterior view in, 424, 426, 426f, 427f
cross-table lateral view in, 421, 424, 425f, 426f
flexion-extension views in, 428
indications for, 420-421
oblique views in, 426-428, 426f, 427f, 428f
odontoid view in, 424, 424f-425f
standard trauma series in, 421, 422f-424f
reflex examination in, 417, 417t
rotational, 405-409, 408f-410f
secondary, 413, 416f
sensory examination in, 417, 417t, 418f
shear, 405, 406f-407f
skin disorders in, 438
stabilization in, 435-436
thromboembolic disease in, 2906-2907
urinary tract disorders in, 2908-2909
vascular damage in, 413, 415f
vertical compression, 411-413, 411f-414f
without radiographic abnormality, 420
Spinal nerve, 1688f, 1689
Spinal shock, 436-437, 1677
complete spinal cord lesion vs., 417
neurogenic hypotension secondary to, 437
Spinal stenosis, back pain in, 705, 712
Spinal trigeminal tract, damage to, Dejeune onion skin pattern from, 420
Spinal tuberculosis, 261, 265t, 2159, 2178, 2182, 2182f, 2184-2185
Spinning sensation, 144
Spinoreticular tract, 2915, 2915f, 2916f
Spinothalamic tract, 2915, 2915f, 2916f
lateral, 1676, 1676f
Spiral fracture, 2690, 2691f
Spirochetemia, in Lyme disease, 2119
Spironolactone, 1321t
for chronic heart failure, 1276
Splash burns, 963, 2271
Spleen
infarction of, in sickle cell disease, 2308
trauma to, 341, 489, 490, 491
Splenectomy
immune defects in, 2842-2843
pneumococcal infection after, 2018
Splenic artery aneurysm, 1355
Splenic sequestration, 1880, 1896
Splenomegaly
in hepatitis, 1404
in tricuspid stenosis and regurgitation, 1307
Splint immobilization, 568-571, 569f, 570f
in ankle sprain, 817
in carpal tunnel syndrome, 639
in clavicle fracture, 677, 678f, 2603
in developmental hip dysplasia, 2702
in distal femur fracture, 776-777
in distal phalanx fracture, 593, 593f
in humeral shaft fracture, 654, 654f
in mallet finger, 606, 606f
in medial epicondylar fracture, 662
in metacarpal neck fracture, 597
in metacarpal or phalangeal fractures, 595, 595f, 596f
in pelvic fracture, 723
in sternoclavicular joint dislocation, 684
in tibial shaft fracture, 800
Split root syndromes, 1033-1034
Spondylitis
ankylosing, arthritis in, 1789
back pain in, 703, 706, 712
radiography in, 708, 709f
Spondyloarthropathies, seronegative, arthritis in, 1789-1790
Spondylolisthesis, degenerative
back pain in, 703, 705, 712
radiography in, 708, 708f
Spongiform encephalopathy, dementia in, 1657-1658, 1659
Spongiform leukoencephalopathy, from inhaled heroin, 2452
Spontaneous bacterial peritonitis, 245-246, 1412-1413
Sports injuries
concussion in, 365-366, 367
in facial trauma, 382
in foot trauma, 837-838
in hip trauma, 761-762
Spousal abuse. *See* Intimate partner violence and abuse.
Sprain, 566-567
ankle, 815-818, 817b, 817f
foot, 838
Spurious pregnancy, 2731-2732
Sputum, mucopurulent, in pneumonia, 1132
Sputum studies
in chronic obstructive pulmonary disease, 1101
in pneumonia, 1134-1135
in tuberculosis, 2154-2155, 2154f
Squeeze test, 816
ST segment
depression of
differential diagnosis in, 1163, 1163f
in myocardial infarction, 1162-1163, 1163f, 1171
reciprocal, 1162-1163, 1163f
elevation of
differential diagnosis in, 1161-1162, 1162t
electrocardiographic differential diagnosis of, 1166-1170, 1167f-1172f
in benign early repolarization, 1166-1167, 1167f, 1168f
in left bundle branch block, 1167, 1169, 1169f, 1170f
in left ventricular aneurysm, 1167, 1168f
in left ventricular hypertrophy, 1169-1170, 1172f
in pericarditis, 1167, 1167f, 1168f
in ventricular paced rhythms, 1169, 1171f
in myocardial infarction, 1164t, 1173-1174, 1173f
in pericarditis, 1281, 1282
ST segment elevation myocardial infarction (STEMI), 1101-1102, 1102t, 1103f
Stab wounds
abdominal
diagnostic studies in, 502
history in, 493
management of, 502-505, 503f, 503t
pathophysiology of, 490
physical examination in, 494
acute cardiac tamponade from, 473
in physical assault, 963, 963f
observation in, 3068-3069

Stab wounds *(Continued)*
  peripheral vascular, 537
  to neck, 442
Stabilization
  in abdominal pain, 213
  in anaphylaxis, 1830
  in back pain, 261-262, 263f
  in central nervous system infection, 1721
  in cervical spine injuries, 435-436
  in chest pain, 184-185, 184f
  in coma, 157-158
  in confusion, 150-151
  in diarrhea, 228, 232
  in dyspnea, 181f
  in fever, 135
  in gastrointestinal bleeding, 220-221
  in hemoptysis, 280
  in mood disorders, 1741
  in multiple trauma, 305-309
  in nausea and vomiting, 201t, 202
  in pediatric trauma, 329
  in seizure, 166-167, 166t
  in syncope, 196, 198, 199f
  in vaginal bleeding, 254-255
  in weakness, 138-139
  mechanical. *See* Fixation.
  medicolegal requirements for, 3163-3164
  of avulsed tooth, 1038f, 1040
  postresuscitation
    adult, 85-87, 88f
    pediatric, 113-114, 113f
Staffing requirements for observation, 3062-3063
Staining techniques, in sexual assault examination, 988-989, 988f
Stainless steel wire suture, 852t
Stanford classification of aortic dissection, 1325, 1325f
Staphylococcal infection
  in catheter-related infections, 1363
  in cellulitis, 2198-2199
  in dacryocystitis, 1055
  in food poisoning, 1469-1470, 1480t
  in gastroenteritis, 2626
  in impetigo, 1842, 2202
  in infective endocarditis, 1301
  scalded skin syndrome in, 1845, 2199
Staphylococcus aureus
  in bone or joint infections, 2177, 2178t
  in pneumonia, 1130, 2556-2557, 2556f
  in septic arthritis, 1784
  in toxic shock syndrome, 2027-2031, 2028b, 2029b, 2029t, 2199-2200, 2200b
  methicillin-resistant, 1130
Staphylococcus lugdenesis, 1301
Staphylococcus saprophyticus, 1574
Staples
  for scalp laceration repair, 850
  for wound closure, 853
"Star of Life," 2988, 2988f
Stasis, zone of, in burn injury, 917, 917f
Statins, rhabdomyolysis from, 1979
Statistical analysis
  bayesian, 3056
  in clinical trials, 3050
Statistical tests, 3052-3053, 3052t
Status asthmaticus, 1083, 1091, 2535-2536
  intubation and, 16, 17t
  mechanical ventilation in, 32
Status epilepticus, 167, 1621, 1622b
  alcohol-related, 2865
  complications of, 2668b
  convulsive vs. nonconvulsive, 2667
  in children, 2667, 2668b, 2672-2673, 2672t
  in pregnancy, 2769
  treatment of, 1627-1628, 1627t
Status migrainosus, 1632-1633
Steakhouse syndrome, 1383
Steal phenomenon, in arteriovenous fistula or graft, 1366
Steatorrhea, in viral gastroenteritis, 1476
Steatosis, in alcoholic liver disorders, 1409
Stellate tear, in handgun contact wound, 955-956, 955f
"STEMI alert" system, 1193
Stener fracture, 551t
Stenosing tenosynovitis, in hand, 618
Stensen's duct, 385, 386f
Stephania tetrandra, 2476
Sternal fracture, 456-457
Sternbach's diagnostic criteria for serotonin syndrome, 2359b
Sternoclavicular arthritis, 2191
Sternoclavicular joint
  anatomy of, 670, 671f
  dislocation, 683-685, 684f-685f
Sternoclavicular ligaments, 670, 671f
Steroids. *See* Corticosteroids.
Stevens-Johnson syndrome, 1853, 1853f
Still's murmur, 2572
Stimson technique
  for anterior glenohumeral joint dislocation reduction, 689, 689f
  for hip reduction, 758, 758f
Stimulation, in neonatal resuscitation, 122
Stinging hydroids, 909
Stingray, 910
Stings
  hymenoptera, 903-905
    allergy to, 1827, 2547
    rhabdomyolysis from, 1979
  venomous, marine animals in, 909-910, 911
Stokes sign
  in neoplastic cardiac tamponade, 1917
  in superior vena cava syndrome, 1910
Stomach. *See also* Gastric *entries.*
  foreign body in, 873-875, 875f, 1384-1385
  inflammation of. *See* Gastroenteritis.
  perforation of, in peptic ulcer disease, 1393
  secretory cells of, 1391
Stomatitis
  aphthous, 1036
  vesicular, 2054
Stomatocytosis, in alcoholism, 2874
Stomatognathic system, anatomy of, 1026-1027, 1027f-1030f
Stonefish envenomation, 910
Stool culture
  in *Aeromonas hydrophila* gastroenteritis, 1468
  in AIDS-related diarrhea, 1483
  in *Bacillus anthracis* gastroenteritis, 1469
  in *Campylobacter* gastroenteritis, 1460
  in *Clostridium difficile* enterocolitis, 1475
  in coccidial gastroenteritis, 1478
  in diarrhea, 233
  in *Giardia* gastroenteritis, 1479
  in hemorrhagic *Escherichia coli* serotype O157:H7 gastroenteritis, 1467
  in infectious diarrhea, 2626-2627
  in intestinal amebiasis, 1480
  in pediatric fever, 2510
  in *Plesiomonas shigelloides* gastroenteritis, 1468
  in salmonellosis, 1463
  in shigellosis, 1464
  in *Vibrio* fish poisoning, 1472
  in *Vibrio parahaemolyticus* gastroenteritis, 1466
  in *Yersinia enterocolitica* gastroenteritis, 1465
Stool examination
  in diarrhea, 233
  in gastrointestinal bleeding, 222
Stool softener, for constipation, 241t, 242
Stools
  black tarry, 221
  bloody, 221
    in hemolytic uremic syndrome, 2654
    in hemorrhagic *Escherichia coli* serotype O157:H7 gastroenteritis, 1466
    in inflammatory bowel disease, 2616
    in intussusception, 2610
    in *Plesiomonas shigelloides* gastroenteritis, 1468
Straddle fracture, pelvic, 725, 726f
Straddle injuries, 975
Straight leg raise
  in back pain, 264
  in lumbar radiculopathy, 704
Strain, 567
  gastrocnemius, 804
  in hip trauma, 761-762
  plantaris, 804
Strangulation, 450-451
  penile, 532, 533f
Strangulation obstruction of small bowel, 1440
Stratified randomization, 3049
Stratum corneum, 842, 914
Stratum germinativum, 842
Street gangs, violence by, 1017-1018, 1020-1022
Streptococcal infection
  in cellulitis, 2198
  in impetigo, 1842, 2202
  in infective endocarditis, 1301
  in rheumatic fever, 1303
  in toxic shock syndrome, 2028, 2028b, 2029, 2029t, 2200-2201, 2201b
Streptococcal pharyngitis, 274-275, 1109, 1110, 1111, 1112-1113, 1114
  adult epiglottitis vs., 1115
  in rheumatic fever, 1303, 1304
Streptococcus bovis, 1301
Streptococcus pneumoniae, 1129, 1132, 2016-2020, 2020b. *See also* Pneumococcal disease.
Streptokinase
  in myocardial infarction, 1189
  in pulmonary embolism, 1378t
Streptomycin
  for tuberculosis, 2163t, 2164
  for tularemia, 2131
Stress disorder
  acute, 1746b
  posttraumatic. *See* Posttraumatic stress disorder.
Stress echocardiography, in acute coronary syndromes, 1179
Stress fracture, 553
  femoral neck, 755-756
  foot, 837-838
  lower leg, 803-804
  pelvic, 725
  tibial shaft, 800
Stress management, disaster, 3018
Stress polycythemia, 1884-1885
Stress radiographs, in fracture, 557
Stress response
  in anxiety disorders, 1744
  in hemorrhagic shock, 46
  in mood disorders, 1735
  in shock, 43, 44f
Stress test
  ankle, 816-817
  collateral ligament, 774
  elevated arm, 1359
Stress ulcer, in burn injured patient, 924
Stressors, in emergency medicine, 3174-3175
Striae gravidarum, 2723, 2728
Stricture
  esophageal, from caustic ingestion, 2383
  in gastroesophageal reflux, 1389
Stridor
  anaphylaxis vs., 1829
  biphasic, 2520
  causes of, 2521t
  in airway foreign body aspiration, 865, 866
  in anaphylaxis, 2549
  in bacterial tracheitis, 2528
  in epiglottitis, 2523
  in laryngomalacia, 2524
  in laryngotracheal stenosis, 2525
  in neck masses, 1076
  in pediatric upper airway obstruction, 2519-2520, 2521t
  in retropharyngeal abscess, 2522
  in subglottic hemangioma, 2525
  in viral croup, 2525
  in vocal cord paralysis, 2524
String of beads sign, in small bowel obstruction, 1443
Stroke, 1606-1617. *See also* Intracerebral hemorrhage; Subarachnoid hemorrhage.
  acute drug therapy for, 1615-1616, 1615t
  alcohol consumption and, 2869-2870
  anatomy and physiology in, 1607
  antihypertensive drug therapy for, 1614, 1614t, 1616
  anxiety in, 1748
  cardioembolic, 1608
  clinical features of, 1609-1611, 1610t, 1611f
  diagnosis of, 1612-1613, 1612f
  differential diagnosis in, 1611-1612
  disposition in, 1616-1617
  epidemiology of, 1607-1609, 1607t, 1608b
  fibrinolytic therapy for, 1615, 1615t
  in central retinal artery occlusion, 1057
  in myocardial infarction, 1161
  in systemic lupus erythematosus, 1807

Stroke *(Continued)*
management of, 1613-1616, 1613t, 1614t, 1615b
oropharyngeal dysphagia in, 1396-1397
pathophysiology of, 1606-1607
previous, fibrinolytic therapy eligibility and, 1191
seizure in, 1624
thrombotic, 1607-1608
time goals in, 1613t
vs. high-altitude cerebral edema, 2306
Stroke in evolution, 1609
Stroke syndromes, hypertension in, 1315-1316
Stroke volume
in heart failure, 1260, 1260f, 1262
in infants and children, decreased, causes of, 2569, 2569b
Strongyloides stercoralis, 2102t
dysenteric colitis in, 230t
gastroenteritis in, 1477t
in cancer patient with impaired cell-mediated immunity, 2840
in organ transplant patient, 2849
neurologic disorders in, 2107
skin disorders in, 2109
Struvite kidney stones, 1587
Strychnine poisoning, tetanus vs., 2010
Student's *t* test, 3052, 3052t, 3053
Stun gun, injuries from, 2274
Stupor, 156, 2482
Subacromial bursitis, 1803
Subacromial dislocation, 691
Subacromial syndromes, 693-696, 694t, 695f
Subacute sclerosing panencephalitis, 2054
Subarachnoid hemorrhage, 1635-1637, 1636t, 1637f
diagnosis of, 1636-1637, 1637f
dysrhythmia after, 371
headache in, 174t, 1637, 2677
Hunt and Hess scale for, 1636, 1636t
in pregnancy, 2732
risk factors for, 171b
spinal, 1682
traumatic, 377
treatment of, 1637
Subcalcaneal heel pain, 836-837
Subclavian artery
aneurysm of, 1354
compression of, thoracic outlet syndrome from, 1358
injury to, 544-545
Subclavian steal syndrome, 147t
Subclavian vein
compression of, thoracic outlet syndrome from, 1358
injury to, 544-545
thrombosis of, 1363
Subclavian-axillary artery aneurysm, 1354
Subclavicular dislocation, 697, 698f
Subconjunctival hemorrhage, 285, 296t, 1048, 1048f
Subcoracoid dislocation, 697, 698f
Subcutaneous drug abuse, skin lesions associated with, 1864-1865, 1865f
Subcutaneous emphysema
chest wall trauma and, 459-460
in esophageal perforation, 484
in scuba diving–related disorders, 2286
tracheobronchial injury and, 466, 466f
Subcutaneous nodules
in acute rheumatic fever, 2596
in rheumatic fever, 1304
Subcutaneous tissue, 915
Subdiaphragmatic thrusts, for airway foreign body, 2530
Subdural empyema, in otitis media, 1068
Subdural hematoma, 375-377, 376f
headache in, 2678
in children, 335
Subdural hygroma, 377
Subfascial web space infection, 617, 617f, 618
Subglenoid dislocation, 691, 697, 698f
Subglottic hemangioma, 2525
Subglottic stenosis, 2525
Subglottic tracheal disease, 2525-2527
Sublingual capnography, 39
Sublingual glands, 385-386
Subluxation, 564-566
biceps tendon, 698
cervical spine, 401, 404, 404f-405f, 427, 428f
Subluxation *(Continued)*
glenohumeral joint, 690, 691f
lens, 1049
radial head, 666, 666f, 2697-2698, 2697f
tooth, 1037, 1038f
Subluxation provocation test, in knee trauma, 774
Submandibular gland, stones of, 1075
Submandibular space, 1117
Submersion injuries, 2311-2315
Subperiosteal abscess
in mastoiditis, 1072
in osteomyelitis, 2175
Subscapular nerve, 672
Subscapularis muscle, 672, 673f
Subspinous dislocation, 691
Substance abuse, 2882-2896. *See also* Poisoning/overdose.
alcohol. *See* Alcohol intoxication; Alcoholism.
amphetamines and amphetamine-like drugs in, 2893-2896, 2894t, 2895b
ancillary studies in, 2885-2886
anxiety from, 1746b
by emergency physicians, 3176
by sexual assault victim, 979
cocaine in, 2386-2392
complications of, 2885
differential diagnosis in, 2885
epidemiology of, 2882-2883, 2884f
GHB in, 2489
hallucinogens in, 2406-2416
history in, 2883-2884
in intimate partner violence and abuse, 998
in pregnancy, 2736, 2790-2794, 2791b, 2883
ketamine in, 2893
management of, 2886
marijuana in, 2411-2412
mood disorders from, 1739-1740, 1740b, 1740f
opioids in, 2327t, 2328, 2451-2456
phencyclidine in, 2413, 2414-2415, 2414t, 2415t, 2416, 2882b, 2891-2893
physical examination in, 2884-2885
plant and mushroom poisoning associated with, 2471, 2477
psychosis from, 1727b, 1728-1729
referral in, 2886
reporting requirements for, 3173
solvents/hydrocarbons in, 2428-2432, 2430f, 2886-2889, 2887t, 2888f, 2889b
suicide and, 1769
youth violence and, 1018
Substance dependence, alcohol, 2858
Substituted judgment, 3134
Substituted phenol poisoning, 2463-2464, 2463b
Subtalar joint
anatomy of, 808, 809f, 820, 820f
dislocation of, 825-826, 825f
Subtrochanteric fracture, 753-755, 754f
Subungual hematoma, nail bed trauma and, 594, 610-611
Succimer
for arsenic poisoning, 2424
for lead poisoning, 2422
for mercury poisoning, 2426
Succinylcholine
for emergency intubation, 13-14, 17, 18
for scleral rupture, 1050
for tetanus, 2011
hyperkalemia from, 14, 14t, 1940
refrigeration of, 14
Sucking chest wound, 462
Sucralfate
for gastroesophageal reflux, 1390
for upper gastrointestinal disorders, 1399
Sudden asphyxic asthma, 1084
Sudden death
epidemiology of, 77
in heart failure, 1259
in hydrocarbon poisoning, 2429
in hypertrophic cardiomyopathy, 1295, 1296
in mitral valve prolapse, 1305
in myocardial disease, 1298
of infant. *See* Sudden infant death syndrome.
of young athletes, 2597-2599, 2597b
trajectory of dying in, 3140, 3140f
Sudden infant death syndrome, 2713-2717
apparent life-threatening event and, 2718
caffeine/theophylline and, 2719-2720
Sudden infant death syndrome *(Continued)*
definition of, 2714
diagnosis of, 2716
epidemiology of, 2713-2714
etiology and pathophysiology of, 2716, 2716f
future directions in, 2720
home monitoring for, 2720
management of, 2716-2717
prehospital care in, 2717
prehospital end-of-life issues related to, 3145-3146
psychosocial considerations in, 2717, 2717b
risk factors for, 2714-2716, 2715b
SUDS (single-use diagnostic system) assay for HIV, 2074
Sufentanil, 2922t, 2923
Sugar-tong splint, in humeral shaft fracture, 654, 654f
Suicide, 1766-1774
by hanging and strangulation, 450
clinical features of, 1769-1771
definitions in, 1767
depression and, 1737, 1768, 1769
diagnostic strategies in, 1771
disposition in, 1773-1774, 1773b
documentation in, 1774
epidemiology of, 1767, 1767b
etiology and pathophysiology of, 1767-1769
history in, 1770-1771, 1770t
hospitalization indications in, 1773
in adolescence, 1769
in elderly person, 1767, 1769-1770
in terminal illness, 1770
management of, 1771-1773
methods used in, 1768-1769
physical examination in, 1771, 1771t
prehospital care end-of-life issues related to, 3145
prevention of, 1774
psychiatric disorders and, 1768, 1769
risk determination in, 1772-1773
risk factors for, 1767, 1767b
safety precautions in, 1772
substance abuse and, 1769
Sulfadiazine, for *Toxoplasma gondii* infection, 2082
Sulfasalazine
for Behçet's disease, 1815
for inflammatory bowel disease, 1502
for rheumatoid arthritis, 1791
Sulfhemoglobin toxicity, cyanosis in, 272-273
Sulfites, allergy to, 1827
Sulfonamides, during pregnancy and lactation, 2784
Sulfonylurea drugs, 1972
antidotes to, 2329t
during pregnancy and lactation, 2790
Sulfur mustard exposure, 938-939, 3031
Sulindac, for premature labor, 2807
Sumatriptan
for cluster headache, 1635
for migraine, 1633t, 1634, 2680
Sundown syndrome, 2827
Sunflower oil, for tar removal, 927
Super glue, ocular trauma from, 1046
Superficial fascia
anatomy of, 842
neck, 442
Superficial femoral vein, 1368
Superficial partial-thickness burn, 918, 919f
Superficial peroneal nerve, 797
Superficial punctate keratitis, 1054
Superfund Amendments and Reauthorization Act of 1986, 930
Superinfection
in pertussis, [illegible]
in tuberculosis, 2151, 2151f
Superior gluteal artery, 717-718
Superior mesenteric artery, 1445
acute mesenteric ischemia and, 1445-1446, 1446b
aneurysm of, 1355-1356
in spinal cord injury, 2907
Superior orbital fracture, 393
Superior peroneal retinaculum, injury to, 818-819, 819f
Superior vena cava syndrome
in cancer patient, 1909-1911, 1910f
pacemaker lead–induced, 1250

Supination, of hand, 577f
Supine hypotensive syndrome, in pregnancy, 316, 2725
Suppositories, for constipation, 241t, 242
Suppurative gastritis, 1390, 1391
Supracondylar fracture, 2693-2697, 2694f-2696f, 2694t
extension, 655-658, 656f-658f
flexion, 657f, 658-659
Supracondylar process, 648, 648f
Supradiaphragmatic volvulus, 1394
Supraglottic airway disease, 2522-2524
Supralevator abscess, 1513t, 1514
Suprapatellar bursitis, 795-796
Suprascapular nerve, 672
Supraspinatus muscle, 672, 673f
Supraventricular tachycardia, 1226
in infants and children, 2585-2589, 2586t, 2587f, 2587t, 2588f
in pediatric cardiac arrest, 109-110, 109t
paroxysmal, 1233-1235, 1233f, 1234f
with abnormal conduction, vs. ventricular tachycardia, 1237-1239, 1238t, 1239f, 1240f
Sural nerve, 797
Surface tension of hydrocarbons, 2428
Surgery, recent, fibrinolytic therapy eligibility and, 1191-1192
Surgical mask, for tuberculosis exposure prophylaxis, 2170
Surrogate decision-makers, 3134-3135
Surrogate lists, 3134-3135
Sutural diastasis, 373
Suture
corner stitch, 851
half-buried horizontal mattress, 851
horizontal mattress, 850
in laceration of extensor mechanism over distal interphalangeal joint, 607, 607f
interrupted, 849-850
intradermal (buried), 850
removal of, 856
running, 849
simple, 850
subcutaneous, for reducing wound tension, 849
vertical mattress, 850
Suturing
materials for, 851-853, 852t
of animal bites, 886-887, 887t
techniques in, 849-851
Swallowing
disturbances of. *See* Dysphagia.
physiology of, 1395
Swallowing study, in dysphagia, 1397
Swan neck deformity, 607, 607f
SWAT units, tactical emergency medical support in, 3000-3005
Sweat glands, 915
Sweating
heat loss through, 2255
in anticholinergic poisoning, 2348
Swimmer's itch, 2109
Swimming pool cleaner, ingestion of, 2381t
Sympathectomy
for frostbite, 2233
for peripheral arteriovascular disease, 1350
Sympathetic blockage, for complex regional pain syndrome, 563
Sympathetic nervous system, hyperactivity of, in organophosphate poisoning, 2459
Sympathetic response, to laryngoscopy, 16-17
Sympathomimetic syndrome, in overdosed/poisoned patient, 2327-2328, 2327t
Sympathomimetics. *See also specific agents, e.g.,* Cocaine.
overdose of, 2386-2393
Synchronized intermittent mechanical ventilation (SIMV), 27
Syncope, 193-198
anaphylaxis vs., 1830
ancillary studies in, 195-196, 196t
chest pain associated with, 185, 186t
diagnostic approach to, 193-196, 194b, 195b, 195t, 196t
differential diagnosis in, 194b, 196, 196t, 197t, 198f
disposition in, 198
drug-induced, 195, 195b
Syncope *(Continued)*
empiric management of, 196, 198, 199f
epidemiology of, 193
heat, 2259
in abdominal aortic aneurysm rupture, 1333
in aortic dissection, 1325
in aortic stenosis, 1306
in children, 2685-2686
in hypertrophic cardiomyopathy, 1295
observation in, 3066-3067, 3066b
pathophysiology of, 193
physical examination in, 195, 195t
reflex, 2685
seizure vs., 165-166, 1626, 2667-2668
Syndesmotic ligaments, anatomy of, 808, 809f
Syndrome of inappropriate antidiuretic hormone (SIADH), 1934, 1934b
Syndromic surveillance, public health reporting and, 3105
Synergistic necrotizing cellulitis, 2209
Synovial fluid analysis
in acute septic arthritis, 2705, 2706t
in rheumatic diseases, 1781-1782, 1781t
in septic arthritis, 1785
Synovial joint, 1777, 1777f
Synovial membrane, glenohumeral, 672, 673f
Synovial spaces, in hand, 585, 586f
Synovitis
toxic, pediatric limp from, 764
transient, in children, 2703-2704
Syphilis, 1518t, 1519, 1557t, 1559-1562, 1559t, 1560f, 1561f
congenital, 2701, 2775
fracture in, 2701
in HIV/AIDS, 2087
in pregnancy, 2764t, 2775
skin lesions in, 1855-1856, 1855f
vertigo in, 2683
Syphilitic pharyngitis, 1111, 1112, 1113
Syringomyelia, spinal cord lesions in, 1682-1683
Syrinx, posttraumatic, 435, 436f, 2909
Systemic disease
diarrhea in, 231b
in tuberculosis, 2149
oral manifestations of, 1035, 1035f
skin lesions associated with, 1860, 1861f, 1862t, 1863f
Systemic infection
delirium in, 1649
in animal bite, 885
in pregnancy, 2773-2775
Systemic inflammatory response, in burn injury, 917-918
Systemic inflammatory response syndrome (SIRS), 49, 49b, 2211, 2212b
Systemic lupus erythematosus, 1805-1812
clinical features of, 1806-1808, 1806b
diagnosis of, 1808
disposition in, 1811-1812
epidemiology of, 1805
immune thrombocytopenia in, 1896-1897
in pregnancy, 1810, 2775-2776
management of, 1808-1810
myocarditis in, 1297
oral manifestations of, 1035, 1035f
panniculitis in, 1817
pathophysiology of, 1806
pericarditis in, 1284
skin lesions in, 1862t, 1863f
Systemic mastocytosis, 1835
Systemic vascular resistance, in heart failure, 1262
Systolic dysfunction, in heart failure, 1267

T cells
development of, 1820, 1820f
in asthma, 1080, 1080f, 2533
in cell-mediated immunity, 2833
monoclonal antibody to, for organ transplant patient, 2850-2851
types of, 1820, 2833
t test, 3052, 3052t, 3053
T wave, 1203
hyperacute, in myocardial infarction, 1161, 1162f
in premature ventricular contractions, 1224-1225
T wave *(Continued)*
inverted
differential diagnosis in, 1164
in acute coronary syndromes, 1163-1164, 1164f
in pericarditis, 1282
in Wellen's syndrome, 1163
pseudonormalization of, 1164
Tabun, 939, 2461, 3030-3031, 3030b, 3031b
TAC, topical, 846, 2933
Tachycardia
atrial, 1228-1229, 1228f, 1229f
in asthma, 1084
in cardiac tamponade, 473
in high-altitude pulmonary edema, 2303
in pericarditis, 2592
in pulmonary embolism, 1372
in tension pneumothorax, 462
in Wolff-Parkinson-White syndrome, 1235, 1237
junctional, 1233-1235, 1233f, 1234f
narrow-complex, 1226-1235
atrial fibrillation as, 1230-1233, 1231f, 1232b, 1232f
atrial flutter as, 1229-1230, 1230f-1231f
atrial tachycardia as, 1228-1229, 1228f, 1229f
in infants and children, 2586-2587, 2588f
junctional tachycardia as, 1233-1235, 1233f, 1234f
P wave in, 1234f
sinus tachycardia as, 1227-1228, 1227f
pediatric, 109-110, 109t
pseudotachycardia and, 1226
sinus, 1227-1228, 1227f
in hyperthyroidism, 1987
in myocardial contusion, 468
in pediatric cardiac arrest, 109-110, 109t
supraventricular. *See* Supraventricular tachycardia.
ventricular, 1240-1243, 1241f-1243f
wide-complex, 1237-1244
adenosine-induced, 2588, 2589f
differential diagnosis in, 1237-1239, 1238t, 1239f, 1240f
in cocaine overdose, 2390
in infants and children, 2586, 2587f
torsades de pointes as, 1243-1244, 1243f, 1244b
treatment of, 1239-1240
ventricular tachycardia as, 1240-1243, 1241-1243f
Tachycardia-bradycardia syndrome, 1231
Tachydysrhythmia
in heatstroke, 2264
in infants and children, 2585-2590
Tachypnea, 175
in asthma, 1084
in high-altitude pulmonary edema, 2303
in pediatric assessment, 2499
in pneumonia, 2556
Tacrine, for dementia, 1661
Tacrolimus, 2844
for organ transplant patient, 2851
toxicity of, 1417
Tactical emergency medical support, 3000-3005
equipment in, 3003-3004
forensic science and, 3004
goals of, 3001, 3001b
hazardous materials and, 3004
history of, 3001
liability in, 3004-3005
medical threat assessment in, 3004
phases in, 3002-3003, 3002b
preventive medicine in, 3004
remote patient assessment in, 3004
tactical team structure, training, and integration in, 3001-3003
training in, 3002, 3002f, 3003
Taenia saginata, 2102t, 2105
Taenia solium, 2102t, 2105, 2109
Takayasu's arteritis, 1813
Talar dome, osteochondral fracture of, 824-825, 825f
Talar neck fracture, 823, 823f
Talar tilt test, 817
Talocalcaneal joint
anatomy of, 808, 809f, 820, 820f
dislocation of, 825-826, 825f
Talocrural joint, 808, 809f

Talonavicular dislocation, 825-826, 825f
Talus
  anatomy of, 808, 809f, 810f
  dislocation of, 820, 826
  fracture of, 822-824, 823f, 824f
Tamarind, drug interactions with, 2478t
Tanapox viruses, 2040
Tangential wounds, to head, 369
Tap water irrigation, for wound cleansing, 848
Tape, wound closure, 853
Tape measurement system, in pediatric
    resuscitation, 114, 114f-115f
Tapeworm infection
  anemia in, 2107
  drug therapy for, 2102t
Tar burns, 926-927, 937
Tarasoff v Regents of California, 2967-2968
Tardieu's spots, in near-hanging and
    strangulation, 451
Tardive dyskinesia, antipsychotic-induced, 1732,
    2445, 2447
Tarsal tunnel syndrome, 836-837
Tarsometatarsal joint
  anatomy of, 820, 820f
  fractures and dislocations of, 551t, 828-831,
    829f, 830f
Taser gun injuries, 2274
Taste alterations, in scombroid fish poisoning,
    1472
Tattooing
  in facial trauma, 390
  in intermediate-range handgun wounds, 956-
    957, 956f
Taxus, 2475, 2475f
Teardrop fracture, 551t
  extension, 410-411
  flexion, 401, 403f
Teardrop sign, in orbital wall fracture, 1044,
    1045f
Tears, artificial, 1063b, 1064
Technetium 99m labeled bone scan, in
    osteomyelitis, 2180-2181, 2180f, 2181f
Teeth. *See* Tooth (teeth).
Telemedicine, 3105-3106
Telmisartan, 1322t
Temazepam, 2484, 2484t
  for sleep disturbances in demented patient,
    1662
Temperature
  altered perceptions of, in ciguatera fish
    poisoning, 1473
  body. *See* Body temperature.
  duration of exposure to, burn injury and, 915-
    916, 916f
  of material, burn injury and, 915, 915t
Temporal arteritis, 1813
  headache in, 174t
  risk factors for, 171b
  visual loss in, 1060
Temporal lobe epilepsy, 148t, 1621
Temporomandibular joint
  anatomy of, 1026, 1027f
  dislocation of, 396, 1041-1042, 1041f
  in scuba diving–related disorders, 2283
  trauma to, 395-396
Temporomandibular myofascial pain dysfunction
    syndrome, 1034-1035
Tendinitis/tendinopathy, 567-568, 1794-1801
  Achilles, 1799-1800
  bicipital, 1797
  calcific, 568, 698, 1797-1798
  common sites for, 1796f
  diagnosis of, 1800-1801
  disposition in, 1801
  history in, 1795
  management of, 1801
  of ankle, 818-820, 819f, 1799-1800
  of elbow, 1798-1799
  of foot, 838
  of hand, 604-609, 605f-607f
  of hip, 761-762
  of knee, 791, 795, 1799
  of shoulder, 1796-1798
  of wrist, 1799
  patellar, 1799
  physical examination in, 1795-1796
  rotator cuff, 1796-1797
Tenecteplase, with enoxaparin, in myocardial
    infarction, 1194-1195
Tenesmus
  in inflammatory bowel disease, 1501
  in intestinal amebiasis, 1480
  in radiation proctocolitis, 1505
Tennis elbow. *See* Epicondylitis.
Tenosynovitis
  bicipital, 697, 697f
  De Quervain's, 1799
  flexor, 616-617
  in gonococcal arthritis, 1788, 2191
  stenosing, in hand, 618
Tensilon test, in myasthenia gravis, 1705
Tension headache, 1635, 2679
Tension pneumomediastinum, 459
Tension pneumopericardium, 1288
Tension pneumothorax, 339, 462, 462f, 463f,
    464
Tenting, in dehydrated infant, 2629
Teratogen, 2779-2780, 2780b
Terazosin, 1321t
Terbinafine, for tinea capitis, 1839
Terbutaline
  for asthma, 1088, 2539t, 2541
  for premature labor, 2806-2807, 2806b
Teres minor muscle, 672, 673f
Terminal illness
  suicide in, 1770
  trajectory of dying in, 3140, 3140f
Terrorism
  role of informatics in, 3105
  weapons used in, 3021-3032. *See also*
    Weapons of mass destruction.
Terry Thomas sign, in scapholunate dissociation,
    630
Testicular appendage, torsion of, 1597, 2641
Testing requests and requirements, medicolegal
    issues in, 3158-3160
Testis
  anatomy of, 1594, 1594f
  cancer of, 1597
    in children, 2642
    superior vena cava syndrome in, 1909
  physical examination of, 1573, 1594
  torsion of, 1594-1595, 2639-2640, 2640f
  trauma to, 534-535, 535f
  tumor of, 1597
Tetanospasmin neurotoxin, 2009
Tetanus, 2007-2012, 2008f, 2010b, 2012t, 2013t
  cephalic, 2009, 2010
  neonatal, 2009
  prophylaxis against
    in burn injury, 925-926
    in human bites, 891, 891t
    in wound management, 856-857, 857b, 2012,
      2013t
Tetany, hyperventilation, heat cramps vs., 2258
Tetracaine, 846, 2931, 2931t, 2933
Tetracycline
  during pregnancy and lactation, 2784
  for ehrlichiosis, 2138
  for epididymitis, 1597t, 2639
  for Lyme disease–related myocarditis, 1292
  for periodontal abscess, 1033
  for reactive arthritis, 1790
  for relapsing fever, 2129-2130
  for Rocky Mountain spotted fever, 1850
  for syphilis, 1856
Tetrahydrocannabinol (THC), 2411
Tetralogy of Fallot, 2573, 2574f, 2579-2581,
    2579f, 2580f, 2581b
Text teletype writer (TTY), 2905
Thalassemia, 1872-1873, 1872f
Thallium ingestion, radiogardase for, 3023,
    3023t
Thenar mass or eminence, 576, 577f
Thenar muscles, 580, 581f
Thenar space infection, 617, 618
Theophylline
  during pregnancy and lactation, 2780
  for asthma, 1090, 1090t, 2542, 2543t
  for postdural puncture headache, 1641
  serum, in asthma, 1095
  sudden infant death syndrome and, 2719-2720
Thermal burn, 913-928
  airway management and respiratory care in
    921-923
  anatomy of skin and, 914-915
  burn shock and, 918
  burn wound assessment in, 919-920, 920f
Thermal burn *(Continued)*
  burn wound care in, 924-927, 925f
  catheterization of patient in, 923
  depth of burn injury in, 918-919, 919f
  disposition in, 927, 927b
  epidemiology of, 913-914, 914f
  fluid resuscitation in, 921, 922-923
  gastrointestinal disorders in, 924
  in child abuse, 969-970, 970f, 970t
  in lightning injury, 2273
  in physical assault, 963, 964f
  metabolic response to therapy in, 919
  ocular, 1046
  pain management in, 924
  patient categorization in, 920
  pediatric considerations in, 923
  physiologic changes in, 917-918
  prehospital care in, 921
  thermodynamics of burn injury in, 915-917,
    915t, 916f, 917t
  transportation of patient in, 923-924
  white phosphorus in, 936
  zones of tissue injury in, 917, 917f
Thermal therapy, for fracture, 573-574
Thermogenesis
  decreased, hypothermia and, 2239-2240, 2240b
  increased, heat illness and, 2257
  nonshivering, in burned infant, 923
  physiology of, 2254-2255
  shivering, 2236, 2247
Thermometry
  in heatstroke, 2263
  pediatric, 2508
Thermoregulation
  hypothalamus in, 134
  impaired, hypothermia and, 2240-2241, 2240b
  mechanisms of, 2255-2256
  physiology of
    in cold exposure, 2228, 2236-2237, 2237f
    in heat exposure, 2254-2256
Thermosensors, 2255
Thiamine
  deficiency of
    in alcoholic hepatitis, 1409
    optic neuropathy from, 1060
  for alcohol intoxication, 2860
  for alcohol withdrawal syndrome, 2861, 2863
  for benzodiazepine overdose, 2326
  for toxic alcohol poisoning, 2402
  for Wernicke-Korsakoff syndrome, 2869
Thiazide diuretics
  during pregnancy and lactation, 2788
  hypercalcemia from, 1945
Thiazolidinediones, 1973
Thienopyridines, in acute coronary syndromes,
    1186-1187
Thigh
  compartments of, 737, 737t, 738f
  pain in, atraumatic, 756b
Thioamides, for thyroid storm, 1989
Thiopental
  as induction agent, 15-16
  for procedural sedation and analgesia, in
    children, 2953
Thioridazine, toxicity of, 2445, 2446t
Thiothixene, 2446t
Third stage of labor, 2804-2805
Third trimester
  complications in, 2805-2810
  fetal ultrasonography in, 2802, 2802b, 2802t
Third-degree atrioventricular block, 1220-1221,
    1221f
Third-degree burn, 919, 919f
Third nerve palsy
  anisocoria in, 1061
  eye movement disorders in, 1062
Thompson test, in Achilles tendon rupture, 818
Thoracentesis, in pleural effusion, 1151-1152
Thoracic aorta
  aneurysm of
    chronic, 482
    superior vena cava syndrome in, 1909
  injury to, in pelvic fracture, 720
  rupture of, 476-482, 477f-479f, 481b
Thoracic duct, injury to, in neck trauma, 450
Thoracic endometriosis syndrome, 1144
Thoracic examination, in multiple trauma, 309
Thoracic lavage, for rewarming in accidental
    hypothermia, 2250

Volume 1 pp 1–1024 • Volume 2 pp 1025–2226 • Volume 3 pp 2227–3180

Thoracic outlet syndrome, 1358-1360, 1358f, 1359f, 1693
Thoracic pump model of chest compression, 77, 98
Thoracic spine
anatomy of, 400f
fracture-dislocation of, 410f
vertebral osteomyelitis in, 2184
vertical body fracture of, 426
Thoracic trauma, 453-486
cardiovascular injuries in, 467-482
chest wall injury in, 454-459
epidemiology of, 453
esophageal perforation in, 482-485, 482b, 484b, 485f
in elderly person, 346
pulmonary injuries in, 459-466
Thoracic vertebrae, 399, 400f
Thoracoabdominal gunshot wounds, 506
Thoracoabdominal stab wounds, 505
Thoracoscopy, in hemothorax, 465
Thoracostomy
abdominal trauma after, 492
in children, 339
in hemothorax, 465
in pleural effusion, 1151-1152
in pneumothorax, 463, 464, 464b, 1147-1148
in tension pneumothorax, 464
Thoracotomy
in abdominal trauma, 502
in cardiac tamponade, 475-476, 476t
in children, 339
in hemothorax, 465, 465b
in multiple trauma, 308
in myocardial rupture, 471
in tracheobronchial injury, 466
Thought disorders, 1726-1733
clinical features of, 1726-1728
diagnosis of, 1728
differential considerations in, 1727b, 1728-1729, 1728b, 1729t
disposition in, 1733
management of, 1730-1733, 1731b
Threat assessment, in tactical emergency medical support, 3004
Three Mile Island nuclear reactor incident, 2317
3-3-2 rule, in direct laryngoscopy, 4, 5f
Thrill, in arteriovenous fistula, 539
Throat culture, in pharyngitis, 1111, 1112
Thrombasthenia, 1899
Thrombectomy
for arterial thrombosis, 1354
for peripheral arteriovascular disease, 1349
Thrombin, in bleeding disorders, 1895
Thrombin-sensitive factors, 1892, 1893f
Thromboangiitis obliterans, 1351-1352
Thrombocytopathy, differential diagnosis in, 1896b, 1898-1899
Thrombocytopenia
cold-induced, 2244
differential diagnosis in, 1896-1898, 1896b
dilutional, 1898
heparin-induced, 1897
idiopathic, 1897-1898
immune, 1896-1897
in alcoholism, 2874
in systemic lupus erythematosus, 1808
nonimmune, 1898
thrombotic, 1467, 1898
Thrombocytopenic purpura
autoimmune, 1897-1898
oral manifestations of, 1036
thrombotic, 1467, 1898
Thrombocytosis, differential diagnosis in, 1896b, 1899
Thromboembolism
in nephrotic syndrome, 1531
in pregnancy, 317, 2756-2757
in prosthetic valve patient, 1308
in spinal cord injury, 2906-2907
pathophysiology of, 1343-1344
Thrombolytic therapy
during pregnancy and lactation, 2766, 2786
for acute arterial embolism, 1352-1353
for acute mesenteric ischemia, 1449
for cerebral venous thrombosis, 1671
for pacemaker-induced thrombophlebitis, 1250
for pulmonary embolism, 1377-1378, 1378t, 1379
for stroke, 1613t, 1615, 1615b
Thrombophlebitis, pacemaker-induced, 1250
Thrombosis
arterial, 1344, 1347, 1347t, 1353-1354
embolism vs., 1347t
in acute coronary syndromes, 1157
in infective endocarditis, 1301
in nephrotic syndrome, 2648
in peripheral vascular injury, 537-538, 538f, 544
lateral venous sinus, 1068
of arteriovenous fistula or graft, 1365
of hemorrhoids, 1510, 1511-1512, 1511f, 1512f
of saphenous vein, 1370
pathophysiology of, 1368
septic, 1123, 1363
venous, 1368-1371. *See also* Pulmonary embolism.
anatomy in, 1368-1369
cerebral, 1670-1671
clinical presentation in, 1369
complications of, 1370-1371
diagnosis of, 1369-1370, 1369t
differential diagnosis in, 1369b
in pregnancy, 2733, 2756-2757
in spinal cord injury, 2906-2907
isolated calf, 1370
mesenteric, 1446, 1446b
observation in, 3065-3066
of upper extremity, 1370
pretest probability of, 1369, 1369t
proximal vs. distal, 1369
septic, 1363
treatment of, 1370
Thrombotic ischemic stroke, 1607-1608
Thrombotic thrombocytopenic purpura, 1467, 1898
Thrombovasculitis, cerebral, in Rocky Mountain spotted fever, 2134
Thromboxane
as anaphylaxis mediator, 1823, 1823b
in frostbite, 2229
in sepsis, 2213
inhibitors of, in frostbite, 2232
Thrush, oral, 1840-1841
Thumb
dislocation of
carpometacarpal joint, 604
interphalangeal joint, 564, 565f, 603
metacarpal fractures of, 599-600, 599f
extra-articular, 599
intra-articular, 599-600, 599f
Rolando's, 600
motions of, 578f
radial collateral ligament injuries of, 604
radiography of, 590-591
ulnar collateral ligament injuries of, 604
Thumb spica cast, in scaphoid fracture, 628, 628f
"Thumbprint sign," in epiglottitis, 2523, 2524f
Thurston Holland's fragment, 551t, 555
Thymectomy, for myasthenia gravis, 1706-1707
Thyroid disorders, 1985-1994
hypertension in, 1313
in pregnancy, 2764t, 2772-2773
Thyroid function tests
in hyperthyroidism, 1987-1988
in hypothyroidism, 1992-1993
Thyroid gland
in mood disorders, 1736
in pregnancy, 2726
Thyroid hormone
abnormal levels of. *See* Hyperthyroidism; Hypothyroidism.
hypercalcemia from, 1945
replacement of
for hypothyroidism, 1993-1994
in pregnancy, 2773
Thyroid storm, 1985-1986, 1986b, 1987
management of, 1988-1989, 1989t
vs. heat stroke, 2263
Thyroiditis, 1986, 2773
Thyroid-stimulating hormone
in hyperthyroidism, 1988
in hypothyroidism, 1992-1993
Thyrotoxic crisis, 1985
Thyrotoxicosis, 1985-1989
clinical features of, 1986-1987, 1987b
diagnosis of, 1987-1988
differential considerations in, 1988, 1988t
Thyrotoxicosis *(Continued)*
etiology of, 1985-1986, 1986b
management of, 1988, 1989, 1989t
Thyroxine
in comatose patient, 163
in hypothermia, 2246-2247
Tibia
anatomy of, 797
fracture of
epiphyseal, 780-781
proximal
extra-articular, 797-799
intra-articular, 777-781
shaft, 799-801, 801f
stress, 803-804
subcondylar, 797-798
tibial plateau, 777-779, 777f-778f
tibial spine, 779-780, 780f
tibial tubercle, 798-799, 798f
proximal, anatomy of, 770, 771f
Tibial arteries, 797
anatomy of, 771, 797
injury to, 547
Tibial condyles
anatomy of, 770, 771f
fracture of, 777-779, 777f-778f
Tibial femoral knee dislocation, 787-790, 789f
Tibial nerve, 771, 797
Tibial plateau fracture, 347, 553, 555f
Tibial tubercle apophysitis, 799
Tibialis anterior tendon rupture, 820
Tibialis posterior tendon rupture, 819-820
Tibiofemoral compartments, 770, 771f
Tibiofemoral joint, 770, 771f
Tibiofibular joint
anatomy of, 797
fracture at, 799-801, 801f
proximal, dislocation of, 802-803
Tibiofibular syndesmotic ligaments, distal, injury to, 816, 817
Tibiotalar joint, fracture at, 813, 813f
Tic douloureux, 1664, 1666
headache in, 1642
pain in, 1034
Ticarcillin, for mastoiditis, 1072
Tick-borne illness, 2116-2142
babesiosis as, 2138-2140, 2139f
Colorado tick fever as, 2140-2141
ehrlichiosis as, 2137-2138
identification of ticks in, 2116-2117, 2119f
Lyme disease as, 2118-2129. *See also* Lyme disease.
physiology of, 2117-2118, 2118f
prophylaxis against, 2142
Q fever as, 2137
relapsing fever as, 2129-2130
Rocky Mountain spotted fever as, 2132-2137. *See also* Rocky Mountain spotted fever.
tick paralysis as, 1708, 2141-2142
tick removal procedure in, 2142, 2142b
toxin-induced, 908
tularemia as, 2130-2132
types of, 2117t
Ticlopidine
in acute coronary syndromes, 1186-1187
thrombocytopenia from, 1898
Tics, 2668
Tile's classification of pelvic fractures, 723, 723b
Tillaux fracture, 551t
Tilt table testing, for syncope, 3067
Timolol, 1321t
for closed-angle glaucoma, 1056
for increased intraocular pressure, 292
overdose of, 2373t
Timolol maleate, for central retinal artery occlusion, 1057
Tinea capitis, 1838-1839
Tinea corporis, 1839-1840, 1839f
Tinea pedis, 1840
Tinea unguium, 1840
Tinea versicolor, 1840, 1840f
Tinel's sign
in carpal tunnel syndrome, 639, 1697
in thoracic outlet syndrome, 1359
Tinnitus
in acoustic neuroma, 1668
vertigo and, 144
Tiotropium, for chronic obstructive pulmonary disease, 1105

Tirofiban, in myocardial infarction, 1186
Tissue
  conductivity of, burn injury and, 916-917
  injury to
    in bone or joint infections, 2176
    zones of, in burn injury, 917, 917f
  ischemia of, in compartment syndrome, 560-561, 560b, 561b, 561f
  radiosensitivity of, 2321, 2321f
  resistance of, 2269b
Tissue adhesives, for wound closure, 853-854
Tissue factor, in hemostasis, 1892, 1893f
Tissue plasminogen activator (t-PA)
  during pregnancy and lactation, 2786
  for ischemic stroke, 1615, 1615b
  in myocardial infarction, 1189
    vs. percutaneous coronary intervention, 1192-1193
  in pulmonary embolism, 1377-1378, 1378t
  mutant forms of, 1189-1190
TMP-SMX. *See* Trimethoprim-sulfamethoxazole.
Tobacco
  dermal exposure to, 2474
  ingestion of, 2474
  inhalation of. *See* Smoking.
Tobramycin, for febrile, neutropenic cancer patient, 2838t
Tocainide, 1207
Tocolysis
  for placenta previa, 2809
  for premature labor, 2806-2807, 2806b, 2807b
  for PROM, 2808
Toddlers
  developmental milestones in, 2496t, 2497
  fever in
    management of, 2514-2515, 2515f
    pathophysiology of, 2505
  temperature determination in, 2508
Toddler's fracture, 2698, 2698f
Todd's paralysis, 1625
Toe
  decompression of, in burn injury, 925
  fracture of, 834
  interphalangeal dislocation of, 835-836
  metatarsophalangeal dislocation of, 835
  pain in, 837
Toenail, ingrown, 837
Togavirus, 2047-2049
Toilet bowl cleaner, ingestion of, 2381t
Tokaimura, Japan, radiation incident in, 2317
Toluene abuse, 2886-2889
Toluidine blue dye staining technique, in genital trauma, 988-989, 988f
Tomography
  computed. *See* Computed tomography.
  positron emission
    in minor head trauma, 365
    in osteomyelitis, 2181
Tongue
  adult vs. child, 2519, 2520f
  laceration of, 391, 1040
Tonic seizure, 1621
Tonka bean, adverse effects of, 2476t
Tonography, in shock, 50-51
Tonometry, ocular, in red and painful eye, 286-287
Tonsillar herniation, 1918
Tonsillectomy, for peritonsillar abscess, 1118
Tonsillitis
  lingual, 1114, 1114f
  recurrent or chronic, treatment of, 1113
Tonsillopharyngitis. *See* Pharyngitis.
Tooth (teeth), 384. *See also* Dental *entries.*
  anatomy of, 1026, 1027f-1029f
  aspiration of, 395, 866
  avulsed, 389-390, 395, 1037-1040, 1038f, 1039f
  cracked, 1033-1034
  extraction of
    hemorrhage after, 1042
    pain after, 1034
  fracture of, 1036-1037, 1036f
  radiography of, 1030, 1030f
  reimplantation of, 395
  subluxated, 1037-1040, 1038f, 1039f
Tooth sign, in quadriceps rupture, 700
Topical anesthesia, 2933-2934
  allergy to, 846-847
  in wound care, 846
Topiramate
  for seizure, 2675t
  side effects of, 1628t
Torsades de pointes, 1243-1244, 1243f, 1244b
  antipsychotic-induced, 2447, 2449
  in infants and children, 2589-2590
Torsemide, 1321t
Torso examination, in genitourinary trauma, 515
Torus fracture, 554, 556f, 637, 637f, 2690, 2690f
Tossy and Allman classification of acromioclavicular joint dislocations, 685-686, 686f
Total body surface area assessment, in burn injury, 919-920, 920f
Total hip arthroplasty, 749-750, 750f
Toulene
  abuse of, 2429
  inhalation of, metabolic acidosis from, 1928
Tourniquet injury, of penis, 2638
Toxic alcohol poisoning, 2395-2404
  ethylene glycol in, 2398-2402, 2401t
  isopropyl alcohol in, 2402-2404
  methanol in, 2395-2398
Toxic appearance, as indication for lumbar puncture, 2659
Toxic conjunctivitis, 297t
Toxic disaster preparedness, 3017
Toxic encephalopathy, in cancer patient, 1920-1921
Toxic epidermal necrolysis
  drug-induced, 1846t
  skin lesions in, 1845-1846, 1846f
Toxic goiter
  diffuse, 1985-1986, 1987
  in pregnancy, 2764t, 2772-2773
  multinodular, 1986
  uninodular, 1986
Toxic megacolon, 1501, 1502f, 2613, 2616
Toxic optic neuropathy, 1060
Toxic shock syndrome, 2027-2031, 2028b, 2029b, 2029t, 2199-2201, 2200b, 2201b
  pediatric fever in, 2511, 2511b
  skin lesions in, 1846-1847
  streptococcal, 2028, 2028b, 2029, 2029t, 2200-2201, 2201b
Toxic syndromes, 1651, 2327-2328, 2327t, 2964t
Toxicologic screen, 2328-2330, 2328b
  drugs, chemicals, and groups not detected by, 2328b
  for cocaine, 2388
  in abdominal trauma, 495
  in anticholinergic poisoning, 2349
  in comatose patient, 162
  in delirium, 1651
  in hypothermia, 2244
  in substance abuse, 2885-2886
Toxicology. *See* Poisoning/overdose.
Toxicology laboratory, 2328-2330, 2328b
Toxin(s)
  aplastic anemia from, 1875, 1875t
  botulinum, 2013, 2014
  chronic renal failure from, 1544
  cyanosis from, 269t
  delirium from, 1648
  diarrhea from, 231b
  in bacterial gastroenteritis, 1469-1475, 1480t
  in diphtheria, 2002
  in pertussis, 2005
  in snake venoms, 897-898, 897t
  in toxic shock syndrome, 2029
  inhaled, 2432-2441, 2443t
    carbon monoxide in, 2438-2441
    cyanide and hydrogen sulfide in, 2436-2438, 2437f
    pulmonary irritants in, 2433t, 2434 2435, 2434f
    simple asphyxiants in, 2432-2433
    smoke in, 2435-2436
  neuropathy from, 1601b, 1603
  pediatric fever from, 2510-2511
  rhabdomyolysis from, 1979
  seizure from, 1623
  tetanospasmin, 2009
  uremic, 1541
Toxocariasis, 2107t, 2109, 2110
Toxoplasma gondii infection
  in cancer patient with impaired cell-mediated immunity, 2840
  in HIV/AIDS, 2081-2082, 2082f
Toxoplasma gondii infection *(Continued)*
  in organ transplant patient, 2848-2849
  myocarditis in, 1292
  visual disturbances in, 2110
Tracheal disease
  subglottic, 2525-2527
  upper airway obstruction in, 2527-2529, 2529t
Tracheal foreign body, 867, 868f
Tracheal stenosis, 2527
Tracheal tuberculosis, 2151
Tracheitis
  bacterial, 2528-2529, 2529t
  in children, screening for, 2509b
Tracheobronchial injury, 466, 466f
Tracheomalacia, 2527
Tracheostomy
  in neck trauma, 445
  in physically disabled patient, 2907
Tracking systems, computerized, 3101
Traction, in femoral and hip fractures, 746, 748
Traction retinal detachment, 1058
Traction-countertraction reduction method
  for anterior glenohumeral joint dislocation, 689, 689f
  for hip fracture, 759
  for inferior glenohumeral joint dislocation, 693, 694f
  for tibial femoral knee dislocation, 789
Tramadol, 1692, 2925
Trandolapril, 1322t
Tranquilization. *See also* Sedation.
  rapid, 2914b
    for mood disorders, 1741
    for thought disorders, 1730-1731, 1731b
    of combative patient, 2961-2963
Transabdominal ultrasonography, in pregnancy, 2730, 2730f
Transcondylar fracture, 659, 659f
Transcutaneous blood gas monitoring, 36
Transcutaneous electrical nerve stimulation, 2934
Transection, in peripheral vascular injury, 537
Transesophageal echocardiography
  in aortic dissection, 1327, 1327t
  in aortic rupture, 480, 480f
  in multiple trauma, 313
Transfer. *See* Patient transfer.
Transferrin, in iron overdose, 2419
Transfusional hemosiderosis, 61
Transfusional therapy, 56-61
  adjuncts in, 58
  clinical features in, 58
  decision making in, 58-59
  hepatitis C infection risk in, 1403
  hypocalcemia after, 1943
  in autoimmune hemolytic anemia, 1883
  in gastrointestinal bleeding, 222
  in hemolytic uremic syndrome, 2655
  in kernicterus prophylaxis, 2603, 2604f
  in multiple trauma, 307-308
  in pelvic fracture, 723, 728, 731
  in peripheral vascular injury, 543
  in placenta previa or abruptio placentae, 2748
  in sickle cell disease, 1880
  in thalassemia, 1872-1873
  massive, 57-58
  outcomes in, 59-61
  pathophysiologic principles in, 57-58, 58t
  refusal of, 3171-3172
  therapeutic modalities in, 59
  thrombocytopenia after, 1897
  viral infection transmission and, 57t, 61
Transfusion-associated graft-versus-host-disease, 60
Transient ischemic attack (TIA)
  antihypertensive drug therapy for, 1614, 1614t
  anxiety in, 1747
  disposition in, 1617
  epidemiology of, 1607, 1607t, 1608
  previous, fibrinolytic therapy eligibility and, 1191
Transitional circulation, 118-119, 119t, 2568
Transitions in patient care, as problem area in emergency care, 3124
Transplantation, 2846-2856, 3151
  bone marrow
    for aplastic anemia, 1875-1876
    for sickle cell disease, 1881
  complications in, 2847-2851, 2850t, 2851f
  disposition of, 2856

Transplantation *(Continued)*
drug toxicity in, 2849-2851, 2850t, 2851f
heart, 2851-2854, 2852f, 2853f
immune defects in, 2846-2847
immunosuppressive therapy for, 2849-2851, 2850t
infectious complications in, 2847-2849, 2847b
kidney, 2855
liver, 2854-2855, 2854f
lung, 2855-2856
pancreas, 2856
rejection in, 2848-2849, 2849f
Transport
by air, 2994-2999
administrative structure in, 2995
aviation physiology and, 2994-2995, 2995t
clinical concepts and patient care in, 2998-2999
criteria for, 2998b
efficacy and cost effectiveness of, 2999
flight crew in, 2996
future of, 2999
medical direction in, 2996
safety issues in, 2997, 2997b, 2997f, 2998b
types of missions in, 2995
interfacility and specialized, 2991-2992, 2991b, 2992b
Transtentorial herniation, after head trauma, 355-356, 355f
Transthoracic echocardiography, in aortic dissection, 1327
Transtracheal jet ventilation, needle cricothyrotomy with, 22, 22f
Transvaginal ultrasonography, in pregnancy, 2730, 2731f
Transverse fracture, 2690, 2691f
Transverse myelitis, 265t, 1682
Transverse spinal cord syndromes, 417, 1677, 1678f
Trapezium
anatomy of, 622, 623f
fracture of, 630
Trapezoid
anatomy of, 622, 623f
fracture of, 630
Trapezoid ligament, 670-671, 671f
Trauma. *See also specific anatomic locations.*
abdominal, 489-512
air medical transport in, 2998
alcohol consumption and, 2878
ankle, 000-020
birth, postpartum hemorrhage from, 2818
blunt. *See* Blunt trauma.
cardiac, 467-482
chest wall, 454-459
dental, 1036-1042
elbow and humerus, 647-668
esophageal, 446-447
facial, 382-396
femur, 735-768
foot, 820-839
forearm, 639-644
from animal bites, 882-892
from chemical injuries, 929-939
from electrical and lightning injuries, 2267-2277
from motor vehicle crashes. *See* Motor vehicle crashes; Pedestrian collisions.
from thermal burns, 913-928
from venomous animal bites and stings, 894-911
genitourinary, 514-535
hand, 592-618
head, 349-379
hip, 735-768
hypothermia and, 2241
in elderly person, 344-348, 2829
background of, 344
clinical features of, 347
diagnostic strategies in, 347
disposition in, 348
epidemiology of, 344-345
management of, 348
pathophysiology of, 345
specific disorders and injuries related to, 345-347
in pregnancy, 318-326, 2733
blunt, 318
diagnostic strategies in, 320-321, 320t, 321t

Trauma *(Continued)*
disposition in, 326
fetal evaluation in, 323-324, 323f, 323t, 324f
fetal injury in, 319
fetomaternal hemorrhage and, 321
management of, 321-326, 322f
maternal resuscitation in, 322-323
penetrating, 318-319
perimortem cesarean section in, 325-326
placental injury in, 319-320
prehospital end-of-life issues related to, 3145
primary survey in, 322-323
secondary survey in, 323
uterine injury in, 320
injury prevention and control in, 940-950. *See also* Injury prevention and control.
knee, 770-796
lower leg, 796-805
multiple, 300-314
clinical features in, 309-311, 310f
diagnostic strategies in, 311-313, 313f
disposition in, 311
epidemiology of, 300
etiology of, 302, 303t
examination and reassessment in, 305
in elderly person, 345
management of, 302-309, 304b
monitoring in, 305
prehospital care in, 302-304
radiologic imaging in, 311-313, 313f
stabilization in, 305-309
team approach in, 304
trauma system and, 300-302, 301f, 302b
neck, 441-451
observation in, 3067-3069
ocular, 1044-1052
pediatric, 328-342
abdominal, 340-342
blunt, 492, 510
epidemiology of, 489-490
history in, 493
cardiothoracic, 338-340
cervical spine, 336-338, 337f
child abuse and, 349, 367, 383, 490
clinical features of, 329-330
disposition in, 342
epidemiology of, 328
facial, 382, 383
general management principles in, 331-333, 332b, 332t, 333t
head, 333-336, 334b, 335b, 366-368, 369b
hip, 763-767, 763f, 765f-767f
primary survey in, 329-330, 329t, 331t-333t
renal, 528
secondary survey in, 330, 330b, 333, 333b, 2501, 2501b, 2502b
surgical indications in, 332b
pelvic, 717-734
penetrating. *See* Penetrating trauma.
peripheral vascular, 536-547
prehospital care in, 2991
pressure-induced. *See* Barotrauma.
pulmonary, 459-466. *See also* Pulmonary trauma.
recent, fibrinolytic therapy eligibility and, 1191-1192
renal, 526-530, 527f, 529f-530f
rhabdomyolysis in, 1978
scoring systems for, 300, 301f, 302b
shoulder, 670-699
single vs. multisystem, 502, 509
soft tissue, 566-568. *See also* Soft tissue injuries.
spinal, 398-439, 2905-2909
testicular, 534-535, 535f
thoracic, 453-486
urinary tract, 514-535
vascular. *See* Vascular injury.
wound management in, 842-857. *See also* Wound management.
wrist, 622-639
Trauma captain, 304
Trauma care system, 948
Trauma series, in child abuse, 973
Trauma system, 300-302, 301f, 302b
Traumatic aneurysm, 1357
Traumatic anxiety, 1746b
Traumatic asphyxia, in chest wall trauma, 459
Traumatic axonal injury, in child abuse, 971

Traumatic brain injury, 349-350. *See also* Head trauma.
basilar skull fracture and, 357, 358b
disseminated intravascular coagulation after, 371
in children, 366-367
indirect, 352
primary, 352
secondary, 352-353, 353f
subarachnoid hemorrhage in, 377
Travel restrictions, during pregnancy, 2736
Traveler's diarrhea, 1484-1487, 1486t, 1487b
Trazadone, overdose of, 2361-2362
Treatment
consent for. *See* Consent.
in clinical trials, 3050
minor category of, medicolegal issues in, 3159
withholding and withdrawing, bioethical dilemmas in, 3132
Treatment effect, 3051, 3051t
Trematode infections
drug therapy for, 2098t
parasites in, 2099t
Trematodicides, 2098t
Tremor
alcoholic, 2870
in multiple sclerosis, 1673
perioral, antipsychotic-induced, 2447
Trench foot, 2228, 2230-2231
Trench mouth, 1033
Treponemal tests, for syphilis, 1562
Triage
bioethical dilemmas in, 3136
disaster, 3012-3014, 3013f
catastrophic casualty, 3013-3014
routine multiple-casualty, 3012-3013, 3013f
special categories in, 3014
failures in emergency care and, 3124
in electrical and lightning injuries, 2275
in multiple trauma, 303-304
in pediatric assessment, 2500, 2500t
in radiation exposure, 2324, 3023
marker of death in, 2251
of private patient, 3157
scoring systems for, 300, 301f, 302b
Triamcinolone, for asthma, 1089
Triamterene, 1321t
Triangular fibrocartilage complex, 640
Triazolam, 2484, 2484t
Tribec virus, 2047
Trichinella spiralis, 2106
Trichinosis, 1291, 2103t
Trichloroacetic acid, for condylomata acuminata, 1564
Trichlorophenoxyacetic acid, 2465b
Trichobezoar, 873
Trichomoniasis, 1557t, 1567-1568, 1567t, 2103t, 2758
Trichuriasis, 2107
Tricuspid stenosis and regurgitation, 1307
Tricyclic antidepressants
anticholinergic toxicity of, 2346b
antidotes to, 2329t
for anxiety disorders, 1751, 1751t
for neuropathic pain, 1692
metabolism of, 2352
overdose of, 2352-2357, 2353b, 2353f, 2354b, 2355f, 2357t
Trifluoperazine, 2446t
Trifluridine, 2038
Trigeminal nerve, 383-384, 1665t
Trigeminal neuralgia, 1664, 1666
headache in, 1642
pain in, 1034
Trigeminovascular theory of headache, 2676
Trigeminy, 1222
Trigger finger, 585, 618
Trihexyphenidyl
anticholinergic toxicity of, 2345
for spasticity in cerebral palsy, 2904
Trimalleolar fractures, 813
Trimethadione, during pregnancy and lactation, 2787
Trimethoprim
for epididymitis, 2639
for *Pneumocystis* pneumonia in HIV/AIDS, 2077
Trimethoprim-sulfamethoxazole
for *Aeromonas hydrophila* gastroenteritis, 1461t, 1468

Trimethoprim-sulfamethoxazole *(Continued)*
for AIDS-related diarrhea, 1484
for *Cyclospora cayetanensis* gastroenteritis, 1479
for epididymitis, 1597t
for *Escherichia coli* food poisoning, 1474
for granuloma inguinale, 1559t, 1563
for isosporiasis, 1478
for otitis media, 1069
for pertussis, 2006
for *Plesiomonas shigelloides* gastroenteritis, 1468
for *Pneumocystis* pneumonia in HIV/AIDS, 2077
for pneumonia, 2558t
in HIV-infected patient, 1138-1139
for prostatitis, 1586
for *Toxoplasma gondii* infection, 2082
for urinary tract infection, 1581t, 1582, 1583
for *Vibrio* fish poisoning, 1472
hyperkalemia from, 1940
in HIV/AIDS, side effects of, 2078, 2079t
prophylactic, in cat bites, 888
Tri-Mix diving, 2280
Tripod fracture, midface, 393, 394f
Tripod position
in epiglottitis, 2523
in pediatric assessment, 2498, 2498f
Triptans, for migraine, 1633t, 1634
Triquetral fracture, 629
Triquetrum
anatomy of, 622, 623f, 625
dislocation of, 630
Triradiate cartilage, 729
Trismus
in dental infection, 1032
in peritonsillitis, 1117
in temporomandibular joint dislocation, 1041
in tetanus, 2009
Trisomy 21, 2900t, 2901
Trochanteric bursal calcification, 742, 744f
Trochanteric bursitis, 1803
Trochlea
anatomy of, 647, 647f
fracture of, 662
Trochlear nerve, 1665t
Troponin(s), cardiac-specific, in myocardial infarction, 1175-1177, 1175f, 1176t
Troponin-I
cardiac specificity of, 1177
in chest pain, 188
in myocardial contusion, 469
in pulmonary embolism, predictive value of, 1377, 1378t
Troponin-T
in chest pain, 188
in myocardial contusion, 469
in renal failure, 1177
mutation of, in hypertrophic cardiomyopathy, 1294-1295
Trousseau's sign, in hypocalcemia, 1943
Truncal mononeuropathy, diabetic, 1971
Trust, failure of, and racial/ethnic disparities in health outcomes, 3110
Truth-telling, as value, 3129
Trypanosomiasis
African, neurologic disorders in, 2106
American, 2103t
fever in, 2105
myocarditis in, 1291, 2111-2112
myocarditis in, 1291
Tryptamines, 2406-2408, 2407f
Tryptase, in anaphylaxis, 2548
Tube thoracostomy
abdominal trauma after, 492
in children, 339
in hemothorax, 465
in pleural effusion, 1151-1152
in pneumothorax, 463, 464, 464b, 1147-1148
Tuberculin skin test, 2156-2157, 2157b, 2158t
Tuberculoma, 2152, 2161, 2161f
Tuberculosis, 2145-2171
chest radiography in, 2152-2154, 2152f-2153f, 2159, 2159f
clinical features of, 2148-2150, 2149t
complications of, 2150-2151, 2150f
diagnosis of, 2151-2157, 2152f-2154f
differential considerations in, 2157
disposition in, 2169
Tuberculosis *(Continued)*
drug-resistant, 2166-2167, 2167b, 2167t
epidemiology of, 2146
etiology of, 2147
extrapulmonary, 2158-2162, 2160f, 2161f, 2167-2168
history in, 2145-2146
in alcoholism, 2870
in bone or joint infections, 2178
in chronic obstructive pulmonary disease, 1103
in HIV/AIDS, 1136, 1140-1141, 2078-2079, 2149, 2153-2154, 2166
in pregnancy, 2764t, 2773-2774
isolation precautions for, 2147, 2169-2170
laboratory tests in, 2151-2152
latent
testing for, 2158t
treatment of, 2168-2169, 2168t
management of, 2162-2169. *See also* Antituberculous agents.
meningitis in, 2160-2161
complications of, 1715
in HIV/AIDS, 2082
management of, 1722, 2161
signs and symptoms of, 1714
spinal, 2161
microbiology in, 2154-2157, 2154f, 2157b, 2158t
miliary, 2152, 2159-2160, 2160f
occupational exposure protocol for, 2170-2171, 2170b
oral manifestations of, 1035
pathogenesis of, 2147-2148
patient history in, 2149, 2149t
pericarditis in, 1287
pharyngitis in, 1111, 1112, 1113
physical examination in, 2150
postprimary, 2148-2149, 2152-2154, 2153f
primary, 2152, 2152f
pulmonary, 2149-2157, 2149t
renal, urolithiasis vs., 1590-1591
risk factors for, 2149-2150, 2149b, 2150b
spinal, 261, 265t, 2159, 2178, 2182, 2182f, 2184-2185
surgical management of, 2168
transmission of, 2147
in emergency department, prevention of, 2169-2171, 2170b
Tuberculostearic acid test, in tuberculosis, 2155
Tuberosity fracture
in glenohumeral joint dislocation, 698
ischial, 724, 724f
navicular, 828
Tubular necrosis, acute, 1534b, 1535-1537, 1536b
in rhabdomyolysis, 1977, 1977f
urinary findings in, 1527t
Tubular proteinuria, 1531
Tuft fracture, of distal phalanx, 593-594, 593f
Tularemia, 1131, 2130-2132
Tumor
atheroembolism from, 1344
bone, osteomyelitis vs., 2186
brain
ataxia in, 2681
cerebral herniation in, 1918
headache in, 1637-1638, 2678
in pregnancy, 2732
central nervous system, seizure in, 1624
facial nerve, paralysis from, 1667
femur or hip, 742, 745f
malignant. *See* Cancer.
orbital, red and painful eye in, 294t
ovarian, 251t
pancreatic, 1437
pericardial, 1283-1284
pregnancy, 1035
renal, in children, 2646
spinal cord, 1685
testicular, 1597
vertebral body, spinal cord compression in, 1919
Tumor lysis syndrome, acute, 1911-1912, 1911b, 1912b
Tumor necrosis factor, in sepsis, 2213
Tunica adventitia, 1342
Tunica albuginea, 533, 533f
Tunica intima, 1342
Tunica media, 1342
Turf toe, 837
Turner's syndrome, 2901t
Turtle sign, in shoulder dystocia, 2814
Twin gestations
incidence of, 2722
labor and delivery in, 2816
Two-dimensional echocardiography, in acute coronary syndromes, 1179
Two-point discrimination test
for hand, 587
in nerve injuries, 559
Tympanic membrane
in otitis media, 1067
perforation of, in otitis media, 1067
rupture of, in middle ear barotrauma, 2282
Tympanic membrane thermometer, 2508
Tympanocentesis, in otitis media, 1068
Tympanostomy tubes, for otitis media with effusion, 1070
Type I error
definition of, 3051t, 3052
risk of, multiple comparisons and, 3053-3054
Type II error, 3051t, 3052
Typhoidal tularemia, 2131
Tyramine, hypertension and, 1313, 1314b

Uhthoff's phenomenon, in multiple sclerosis, 1672
Ulcer
atherosclerotic aortic, 1325
corneal, 289, 289f, 294t, 1052, 1052f, 1054
decubitus
in developmentally disabled patient, 2903
in physically disabled patient, 2907
in spinal injuries, 438
foot, in diabetes mellitus, 1351, 1971
genital, 1557-1564
in Bartholin cyst and abscess, 1559-1560
in chancroid, 1557t, 1559t, 1562-1563, 1562f
in condylomata acuminata, 1559t, 1563-1564, 1564
in granuloma inguinale, 1559t, 1563
in herpes simplex virus infection, 1557-1559, 1557t, 1558f, 1559t, 1858
in lymphogranuloma venereum, 1557t, 1559t, 1562
in syphilis, 1557t, 1559-1562, 1559t, 1560f, 1561f
oral, 1036
in Behçet's disease, 1814
in HIV/AIDS, 2083
peptic, 1391-1394, 1391b, 1394b
stress, in burn-injured patient, 924
vascular, in diabetes mellitus, 1863f
Ulcerative colitis, 1500-1503, 1502b, 1502f, 1503b
in children, 2615-2616
skin lesions in, 1862t
Ulcerative gingivitis, acute necrotic, 1033, 1033f
Ulceroglandular tularemia, 2131
Ulna, 639
Ulnar artery
anatomy of, 540f, 585-586, 587f, 588f, 622, 625f
aneurysm of, 1355
injury to, 546
Ulnar bursa, flexor tendons and, 585, 586f
Ulnar collateral ligament
anatomy of, 647, 648f
injury to, 604
Ulnar deviation, of hand, 577f
Ulnar injuries
fracture in
Monteggia's, 642, 642f
pediatric, 644, 644f
shaft, 641-642
styloid, 643
plastic deformation in, 644, 646f
radioulnar joint disruption in, 636-637
Ulnar nerve
in elbow, 648-649, 648f
in hand, 586, 588f, 589f
in wrist, 622, 625f
mononeuropathy of, 1605-1606, 1605f, 1606f
palsy of, 586, 588f
Ulnar slant, of distal radius, 625, 626f
Ulnar styloid, 625
Ulnar surface, of hand, 576, 577f

Ulnar tunnel, 586
Ultrafiltration, for chronic heart failure, 1277
Ultrasonography
B-mode, 542
color flow Doppler, 542, 774
Doppler, 542
in peripheral arteriovascular disease, 1346, 1348
in peripheral vascular injury, 541
in testicular torsion, 1595, 2640
in testicular trauma, 534, 535f
duplex, 449, 542
fetal, in third trimester, 2802, 2802b, 2802t
in abdominal aortic aneurysm, 1334-1335, 1335f
in abdominal pain, 216, 216t
in abdominal trauma, 498-499, 498f
in acute pancreatitis, 1432-1433
in acute renal failure, 1538
in aortic rupture, 480
in appendicitis, 1454, 1456
in arthritis, 1780
in cardiac tamponade, 473-474, 474f
in cervical vascular injury, 449
in cholangitis, 1422f
in cholecystitis, 1419f, 1420
in cholelithiasis, 1419, 1419f
in chronic pancreatitis, 1436
in deep venous thrombosis, 1369
in diverticular disease, 1494
in ectopic pregnancy, 2745
in gastrointestinal foreign body, 874
in hematuria, 1530
in jaundice, 244
in knee trauma, 774
in multiple trauma, 312-313, 313f
in ocular foreign body, 860
in pelvic pain, 250
in peripheral arteriovascular disease, 1348
in peripheral vascular injury, 542
in placenta previa, 2748
in pneumothorax, 463
in pregnancy, 2730, 2730f, 2731f
in pregnant trauma patient, 320
in renal disorders, 1528
in renal tumor, 2646
in septic arthritis, 2188, 2189f, 2190
in soft tissue foreign body, 878-879
in tendinopathy, 1801
in urinary tract infection, 1578
in urolithiasis, 1589, 1590f, 1591f
in vaginal bleeding, 256-257, 256t
Ultraviolet keratitis, 1046-1047
Umbilical cord
clamping and cutting of, 2804
entanglement of, 2817-2818
prolapse of, 2817, 2817t
Umbilical cord soufflé, 2728
Umbilical vein cannulation, in neonatal resuscitation, 123
Umbrella tree, 2472
Uncal herniation, 355, 1918
Unconscious sedation, 2914b
Undermining, for reducing wound tension, 849
Undressing, paradoxical, in hypothermia, 2241
Union, in fracture healing, 564
United States, changing demographics in, 3108, 3108t
Univariate models, 3055
Universal donor blood, 57, 58
Universal precautions, noncompliance with, 3081-3082
Universalizability Test, in ethical case analysis, 3132
Unna's boot, for ankle immobilization, 571
Unstable angina
definition of, 1156
in differential diagnosis of chest pain, 190t-191t
management of
antiplatelet therapy in, 1185-1187
beta blockers in, 1184-1185
heparins in, 1187-1188
morphine in, 1184
missed diagnosis of, 1160
ST segment depression in, 1163f
Upper airway obstruction, pediatric, 2519-2530
evaluation of, 2521, 2521f
in congenital lesions, 2522, 2524-2525, 2524f, 2527-2528, 2528f
Upper airway obstruction, pediatric *(Continued)*
in croup, 2525-2527, 2526f, 2527b
in epiglottitis, 2523-2524, 2524f
in foreign body aspiration, 2529-2530
in laryngeal disease, 2524-2525, 2524f
in retropharyngeal abscess, 2522-2523, 2523f
in subglottic tracheal disease, 2525-2527
in supraglottic disease, 2522-2524
in tracheal disease, 2527-2529, 2529t
pathophysiology of, 2519, 2520f
stridor in, 2519-2520, 2521t
Upper extremity
aneurysm of, 1354-1355
deep venous thrombosis of, 1370
distal, neurologic examination of, 2694t
escharotomy of, 924-925, 925f
fracture of, in elderly person, 346
immobilization of, 569, 569f
isolated mononeuropathy of, 1693-1697, 1694b
vascular injury of, 544-546
Upper gastrointestinal bleeding, 220-227
diagnostic approach to, 220-223, 221b
differential diagnosis in, 220, 221b, 223
disposition in, 225-227, 225b, 226t
management of, 223-225, 223f
observation in, 3066
Upper respiratory tract infection, 1109-1126
in adult epiglottitis, 1114-1116, 1115f, 1116f
in deep space infections of head and neck, 1116-1117, 1116f
in laryngitis, 1114
in lingual tonsillitis, 1114, 1114f
in Ludwig's angina, 1118-1119
in parapharyngeal abscess, 1121-1123, 1122f
in peritonsiillitis, 1117-1118, 1118f
in pharyngitis, 1109-1114, 1110f
in retropharyngeal abscess, 1120-1121, 1120f, 1121f
in sinusitis, 1123-1126, 1124f, 1125f
pediatric screening for, 2509b
Upper sulcus, examination of, in red and painful eye, 286
Upper urinary tract trauma
renal injuries in, 526-530, 527f, 529f-530f
ureteral injuries in, 530-531, 531f-532f
Upward transtentorial herniation, after head trauma, 356
Uranium, radon exposure from, 2317-2318, 2318f
Urate oxidase, for hyperuricemia, 1914
Urban search and rescue, 3005-3008, 3006b, 3008f, 3019
crush injury and crush syndrome in, 3007-3008
medical team operations in, 3006, 3006b
specific disorders in, 3006-3008, 3008f
team structure and components in, 3005-3006
Uremia. *See also* Azotemia.
clinical manifestations of, 1541-1543, 1542f
metabolic acidosis in, 1928
pericarditis in, 1282
Uremic frost, 1542, 1542f
Ureter
anatomy of, 527, 527f
obstruction of, in urolithiasis, 1587, 1588f
trauma to, 530-531, 531f-532f
Ureteral stones, 1586-1593, 1586b, 1589f-1592f, 1593b. *See also* Urolithiasis.
abdominal pain in, 210t
pelvic pain in, 252t
Urethra
obstruction of, 1538
prolapse of, 975
trauma to, 515-519, 516f-520f, 719
Urethral catheterization
for urinary retention, 1599
in children, 2643
Urethritis, 1573
gonococcal, 1565, 1565f
in urinary tract infection, 1575, 1579-1580, 1579t
nongonococcal, 1565
Urethrogram, retrograde, in urethral trauma, 517-519, 518f-520f
Urgent care centers, screening requirements related to, 3158
Uric acid crystals, in gouty arthritis, 1785
Uric acid kidney stones, 1587
Uric acid therapy, for gouty arthritis, 1786
Urinalysis, 1525-1527, 1526f, 1527t
in abdominal pain, 215, 216t
in acute renal failure, 2649
in appendicitis, 1454
in bacterial meningitis, 2662
in comatose patient, 162
in diarrhea, 233
in epididymitis, 2639
in fever, 137
in hematuria, 1530, 1602-1603, 2644
in pediatric urinary tract infections, 2643, 2643t
in proteinuria, 1532
in renal stones, 2645
in rhabdomyolysis, 1980
in urinary tract infection, 1575-1576
in urolithiasis, 1588
Urinary alkalinization. *See* Sodium bicarbonate.
Urinary catheterization
in children, 2643
in genitourinary trauma, 515, 517, 518f
in hypothermia, 2244-2245
in urinary retention, 1599-1600
Urinary disorders, 1524-1604. *See also specific disorders, e.g.,* Renal failure.
Urinary fluorescence, in ethylene glycol poisoning, 2400
Urinary outlet obstruction
acute renal failure in, 1533-1534, 1533b, 1538
in phimosis, 2636
Urinary retention, 1598-1601, 1598b, 1599b, 1600f
clinical features of, 1599, 1599b
drug-induced, 1599, 1599b
in cauda equina syndrome, 706
in spinal cord injury, 2908-2909
management of, 1599-1601, 1600f
Urinary sediment, microscopic examination of, 1525-1527, 1526f
Urinary tract. *See also* Genitourinary *entries.*
foreign body in, 877-878
in pregnancy, 2725-2726
Urinary tract infection, 1573-1586
bacteriology in, 1574-1575
complicated, 1573
definition of, 1573
diagnosis of, 1575-1578, 1577b
differential considerations in, 1579-1581, 1579t, 1580f
epidemiology of, 1573-1574
in chronic renal failure, 1547
in diabetes mellitus, 1578
in elderly person, 2828
in men, 1573, 1574, 1585-1586
in patient with indwelling catheters, 1578-1579
in pregnancy, 1578, 2757-2758
in sickle cell disease, 1578
in spinal cord injury, 2909
in women, 1573, 1574
lower, 1576, 1581-1582, 1581t
pathophysiology of, 1574
pediatric, 1573, 1583-1585, 2510, 2642-2644, 2643b, 2643t
clinical features of, 1583, 1583t
diagnosis of, 1583-1584, 1584f
treatment of, 1584-1585
pelvic pain in, 251t
signs and symptoms of, 1575
terminology related to, 1573
uncomplicated, 1573
upper, 1581t, 1582-1583
Urinary tract trauma, 514-535
bladder injuries in, 519-526, 521f-526f
clinical features of, 515
Foley catheter placement in, 515, 517, 518f
in pelvic fracture, 719
penile injuries in, 532-534, 532f-534f
renal injuries in, 526-530, 527f, 529f-530f
testicular injuries in, 534-535, 535f
ureteral injuries in, 530-531, 531f-532f
urethral injuries in, 515-519, 516f-520f
Urine collection methods, 1575
in children, 1584, 2642-2643
Urine culture
in epididymitis, 2639
in pediatric fever, 2509-2510
in urinary tract infection, 1576-1577, 1577b
Urine dipstick tests, in urinary tract infection, 1575-1576

Urine microscopy, in urinary tract infection, 1576
Urine output, 1525
Urine protein/creatinine ratio, in proteinuria, 2647
Urine test
  for PCP, 2415
  in nausea and vomiting, 203
Urokinase
  for occluded catheters, 1060b
  in frostbite, 2233
  in pulmonary embolism, 1378t
Urolithiasis, 1586-1593
  clinical features of, 1588
  diagnosis of, 1588-1590
  differential considerations in, 1590-1591, 1593b
  epidemiology of, 1586-1587, 1586b
  imaging of, 1589-1590, 1589f-1592f
  laboratory tests in, 1588-1589
  management of, 1591-1593, 1593b
  pathophysiology of, 1587, 1588f
  risk factors for, 1586b, 1587
  types of, 1587
Urologic disorders, 1524-1604. *See also specific disorders, e.g.,* Renal failure.
Urologic examination, 1572-1573, 1573f
Uropathogens, in urinary tract infection, 1574-1575
Urticaria, 1834, 1834f, 1835
  causes of, 1865t
  drug-induced, 1844-1845, 1844f, 1846t-1847t
  in anaphylaxis, 1825t, 2547
  internal malignancy associated with, 1864
  skin lesions in, 1847-1848, 1848f
  transfusion-related, 60
Urticaria pigmentosa, 1835
Uterine activity, measurement of, 2800
Uterine atony
  postpartum hemorrhage from, 2818
  vaginal bleeding in, 258
Uterine contractions, in maternal trauma, 320
Uterine curettage, after miscarriage, 2742
Uterine exploration, and placental removal, for postpartum hemorrhage, 2819
Uterine inversion, 2820
Uterine packing, for postpartum hemorrhage, 2819
Uterine rupture, 2820
  in maternal trauma, 320
  vaginal bleeding in, 257, 257t
Uterine size, gestational age and, 323, 323f, 2728
Uterine soufflé, 2728
Uterus, in pregnancy, 317, 2723
Uveitis, anterior, 287, 287f, 289, 295t
Uvular deviation, in peritonsillitis, 1117, 1118f

Vaccine. *See also* Immunization.
  anthrax, 3026
  BCG, 2170-2171, 2170b
  diphtheria, 2002, 2004, 2012, 2012t
  Haemophilus influenzae, 1723
  hepatitis A, 2035t
  hepatitis B, 1406, 2035t
  influenza, 2055
  influenza A and B, 2035t
  Japanese encephalitis virus, 1723
  Lyme disease, 2126-2127
  measles, 2035t, 2053
  meningococcal, 1723, 2024
  mumps, 2035t
  pertussis, 2005, 2007
  pneumococcal, 1129, 1723, 2017, 2019-2020, 2020b
  polio, 2035t, 2056-2057
  rabies, 2035t, 2068, 2068b
  rubella, 2035t, 2048-2049
  smallpox, 2035t, 3029
  tetanus, 856-857, 857t, 2008, 2011-2012, 2012t, 2013t
  varicella, 1859, 2035t, 2043
  yellow fever, 2035t
Vaccine Information Statement (VIS), 925-926
Vaccinia virus, 2040
Vacuum device, for anorectal foreign body removal, 876, 876f
Vagal maneuvers, for supraventricular tachycardia, 2588
Vagal nerve stimulation, for seizures in developmentally disabled patient, 2899
Vagina
  foreign body in, 877-878
  in pregnancy, 2723
  tear of, postpartum hemorrhage from, 2818-2819
Vaginal birth after cesarean section, 2820
Vaginal bleeding, 254-259
  ancillary studies in, 256-257, 256t
  diagnostic approach to, 254-257, 255t, 256t
  differential diagnosis in, 255t, 257, 257t-258t
  disposition in, 259
  empiric management of, 257, 259, 259f, 260f
  epidemiology of, 254
  history in, 255-256
  in ectopic pregnancy, 2743
  in pelvic fracture, 720
  in pregnancy, 2727
    differential diagnosis in, 2753t
    during second half, 2747-2748
    epidemiology of, 254
    first-trimester, 2740-2741, 2746f
    pathophysiology of, 254
    third-trimester, 2808-2810
    treatment of, 257, 259
  pathophysiology of, 254
  pelvic pain associated with, 249
  physical examination in, 256, 256t
  rapid assessment and stabilization in, 254-255
Vaginal breech delivery, 2813, 2813b
Vaginal examination
  in genitourinary trauma, 515
  in pelvic fracture, 719
  in sexual assault victim, 987-988, 987b
Vaginitis
  atrophic, 1569
  chemical, 1569
  dysuria in, 1580
  in pregnancy, 2758
Vaginosis, bacterial, 1567t, 1568-1569, 2758
Vagus nerve, 1065t
Valacyclovir
  for genital herpes, 1557t, 1559, 1858
  for herpes simplex esophagitis, 1387
  for herpes simplex virus infection, 2042
  indications for, 2038
  prophylactic, in monkey bites, 888, 889t
Valerian, adverse effects of, 2476t
Valgus displacement of fracture, 552, 553f
Validity of study, 3059, 3059t
Valproic acid
  during pregnancy and lactation, 2786-2787
  for bipolar disorder, 1742
  for seizure, 1627, 1627t, 1628t, 2675, 2675t
  for status epilepticus, 2672t, 2673
  overdose of, antidotes to, 2329t
  side effects of, 1628t
Valsalva maneuver, for dysrhythmias, 1214
Valsartan, 1322t
Values
  religious, 3129-3130, 3130b
  societal and bioethical, 3129, 3129b
Valve replacement
  for aortic regurgitation, 1307
  for aortic stenosis, 1306-1307
Valvular heart disease, 1304-1308. *See also specific types, e.g.,* Aortic stenosis.
  heart failure in, 1265, 1268
  in children, 2517
  in pregnancy, 2763t, 2767
Valvular injuries, traumatic, 472
Vancomycin
  for *Clostridium difficile* enterocolitis, 1475
  for febrile, neutropenic cancer patient, 2838, 2838t
  for febrile cancer patient, 1000
  for pediatric fever, 2514
  for peritonitis in dialysis patient, 1552, 1553t
  for pneumococcal disease, 2019
Vapor-permeable dressings, in wound management, 855
Varicella, 2042-2043, 2042f
  in children, screening for, 2509b
  skin lesions in, 1858-1859, 1859f
  smallpox vs., 1860, 1860t, 1861f, 3029
Varicella vaccine, 1860, 2035t, 2043
Varicella-zoster virus, 2042-2043, 2042f. *See also* Herpes zoster.
  drugs for, 2037t
Varicella-zoster virus *(Continued)*
  in cancer patient with impaired cell-mediated immunity, 2840
  in HIV/AIDS, 2085
  in organ transplant patient, 2848
  in pneumonia, 1130
Varicocele, 2641
Variola virus, 3028
Varus displacement of fracture, 552, 553f
Vasa previa, 257, 257t, 2810
Vascular access
  during cardiopulmonary resuscitation, 91-92
  in adult resuscitation, 91-92
  in hemodialysis, problems related to, 1364-1366, 1549-1550
  in multiple trauma, 307
  in neonatal resuscitation, 123
  in pediatric resuscitation, 99, 99f
  in procedural sedation and analgesia, 2942
  in shock, 50
Vascular dementia, 1656, 1657, 1659
Vascular disorders
  abdominal aortic aneurysm in, 1330-1340
  aortic dissection in, 1324-1329
  cyanosis in, 273
  differential diagnosis in, 1896, 1896b
  hypertension in, 1310-1322
  peripheral, 1342-1366. *See also* Peripheral arteriovascular disease.
  pulmonary embolism and venous thrombosis in, 1368-1381
Vascular endothelial cells, in hemostasis, 1892, 1893f
Vascular injury
  hard vs. soft findings of, 539
  high-risk, 540, 540f
  in electrical and lightning injuries, 2271, 2273
  in foot trauma, 838
  in hand trauma, 613-614
  in hip trauma, 762
  in spinal injuries, 413, 415f
  in tibial femoral knee dislocation, 787, 788, 789
  major, 544
  minor, 544
  peripheral, 536-547
    clinical features of, 539-541, 540f
    diagnostic strategies in, 541-543
    disposition in, 547
    epidemiology of, 536-537
    of lower extremity, 546-547
    of upper extremity, 544-546
    pathophysiology of, 537-539, 538f
    treatment of, 543-544
  to neck, 448-450
Vascular ring, 2527-2528, 2528f
Vascular shunt, in arterial injury, 544
Vascular steal, in arteriovenous fistula or graft, 1366
Vascular supply. *See* Blood supply.
Vascular theory of headache, 2676
Vascular ulcer, in diabetes mellitus, 1863f
Vasculitis, 1812-1817
  central nervous system, seizure in, 1624
  classification of, 1812b
  drug-induced, 1844-1845, 1846t
  granulomatous, 1814
  hypersensitivity, 1815-1817
  in Kawasaki disease, 2025
  in systemic lupus erythematosus, 1807, 1808
  large vessel, 1813
  medium vessel, 1813-1815
  mononeuropathy multiplex in, 1699
  pathophysiology of, 1344, 1812-1813
  small vessel, 1815-1817
Vasoconstriction, cold induced, [illegible]
Vasodilation
  heat loss through, 2255
  in sepsis, 2213
Vasodilators, 1321t
Vasogenic cerebral edema
  after head trauma, 354
  in high-altitude cerebral edema, 2299-2300, 2306, 2306f
Vaso-occlusive crisis, in sickle cell disease, 1880
Vasopressin. *See* Antidiuretic hormone.
Vasopressors
  for anaphylaxis, 1833
  for cardiac arrest, 92

Vasopressors *(Continued)*
for sepsis, 2219-2220, 2219t
for septic shock, 53
for toxic shock syndrome, 2030
for ventricular fibrillation and pulseless ventricular tachycardia, 84
Vasospasm
cerebral, in traumatic subarachnoid hemorrhage, 377
coronary, in acute coronary syndromes, 1157
Vasospastic disorders, 1344, 1347, 1357
Vater's ampulla carcinoma, 1423
Vault fracture of skull, 373
VDRL (Venereal Disease Research Laboratory) test, in syphilis, 1856
Vecuronium
for tetanus, 2011
in intubated, mechanically ventilated patient, 31
in rapid sequence intubation, 14-15, 15t
Vegetation, in infective endocarditis, 1301, 1302
Vegetative state, 156
Vegetative symptoms, in depression, 1737
Vein graft, for peripheral arteriovascular disease, 1350
Velpeau bandage, 569
Vena caval interruption, in pulmonary embolism, 1377
Venereal Disease Research Laboratory test, in syphilis, 1856
Venlafaxine, overdose of, 2362, 2362t
Venography
in cerebral venous thrombosis, 1670
in deep venous thrombosis, 1369
in pulmonary embolism, 1377
in thoracic outlet syndrome, 1360
Venomous animal injuries, 894-911
arthropods in, 903-908
epidemiology of, 894-895, 895t
hymenoptera in, 903-905
allergy to, 1827, 2547
rhabdomyolysis from, 1979
marine animals in, 908-911
scorpions in, 907-908
snakes and other reptiles in, 895-903, 897f, 897t, 900t
spiders in, 905-907
venom delivery in, 895
Venous access
in adult resuscitation, 91-92
in pediatric resuscitation, 99
Venous admixture, in pulmonary embolism, 1372
Venous air embolism, in neck trauma, 444, 450
Venous catheterization, postresuscitation, 87
Venous hypertension
from arteriovenous fistula or graft, 1366
in superior vena cava syndrome, 1910
Venous injuries, 544
Venous insufficiency, chronic, lower extremity ulcers in, 1351
Venous pressure, in pregnancy, 2725, 2726f
Venous system
of femur and hip, 737, 737t
of hand, 586
of pubis, 718
Venous thrombosis, 1368-1371. *See also* Pulmonary embolism.
anatomy in, 1368-1369
cerebral, 1670-1671
clinical presentation in, 1369
complications of, 1370-1371
diagnosis of, 1369-1370, 1369t
differential diagnosis in, 1369b
in pregnancy, 2733, 2756-2757
in spinal cord injury, 2906-2907
mesenteric, 1446, 1446b
observation in, 3065-3066
of upper extremity, 1370
pretest probability of, 1369, 1369t
proximal vs. distal, 1369
septic, catheter-related, 1363
treatment of, 1370
Venovenous rewarming, 2250t, 2251
VENTIDC mnemonic, in central nervous system oxygen toxicity, 2283
Ventilation
assisted. *See* Ventilatory support.
differential lung, in pulmonary contusion, 461
Ventilation *(Continued)*
failure of, as indication for intubation, 2-3
mechanical. *See* Mechanical ventilation.
minute
carbon dioxide arterial pressure and, 1923
during acclimatization to high altitude, 2297-2298
in metabolic acidosis, 1929
transtracheal jet, needle cricothyrotomy with, 22, 22f
Ventilation-perfusion inequality, in pulmonary embolism, 1372
Ventilation-perfusion scan, in pulmonary embolism, 1375, 1376t
Ventilatory support, 26-33. *See also* Airway management; Intubation
after brain resuscitation, 68
basic approaches to, 26-27
evolving therapies in, 33
in acute respiratory distress syndrome, 1141
in adult resuscitation, 87
in asthma, 1092-1093
in chronic obstructive pulmonary disease, 1103-1105, 1103t-1105t
in flail chest, 458
in multiple trauma, 306
in neonatal resuscitation, 122-123
in pediatric resuscitation, 108-109
in pediatric trauma, 329-330, 332t
in pregnant trauma patient, 322
in shock, 51-52
initial settings and ongoing monitoring in, 29-30, 29t
invasive, 27-28. *See also* Mechanical ventilation.
noninvasive, 28-29, 28f
evolving therapies in, 33
in asthma, 1091-1092
in chronic obstructive pulmonary disease, 1104, 1104t
initial settings and ongoing monitoring in, 29-30, 29t
outcomes in, 32-33
patient management in, 31
patient selection for, 29
outcomes in, 32-33
patient management in, 30-31
special clinical circumstances in, 31-32
Ventricle
penetrating injury to, 472
rupture of, 470-472
Ventricular assist device, for chronic heart failure, 1277
Ventricular bigemy, 1222, 1222f
Ventricular contractility abnormalities, in dilated cardiomyopathy, 1294
Ventricular dysrhythmias
in beta blocker overdose, 2375
in chlorinated hydrocarbon poisoning, 2463
in myocardial contusion, 469
Ventricular fibrillation
in hypothermia, 2238, 2246
in infants and children, 112-113, 112f, 2586t, 2590
treatment of, 84, 112-113, 112f
Ventricular paced rhythms, ST segment elevation in, 1169, 1171f
Ventricular pacemaker, ICDs as, 1255
Ventricular parasystole, 1226, 1226b, 1226f
Ventricular septal defect, in infants and children, 2577
Ventricular tachycardia, 1240-1243, 1241f-1243f
bidirectional (alternating), 1241, 1243f
electrocardiography in, 1238-1239, 1241f-1243f
in infants and children, 2586t, 2589-2590
monomorphic, 1240-1241, 1242f
polymorphic, 1241, 1243-1244, 1243f
pulseless, in infants and children, 2586t, 2590
sustained vs. nonsustained, 1240
vs. supraventricular tachycardia with abnormal conduction, 1237-1239, 1238t, 1239f, 1240f
Ventriculoperitoneal shunt, pediatric fever in, 2517
Verapamil, 1210-1211, 1321t
during pregnancy and lactation, 2788
for atrial flutter, 1229
for dysphagia, 1398
for hypertrophic cardiomyopathy, 1295
Verapamil *(Continued)*
overdose of, 2376, 2377t
side effects of, 1210-1211
Verbal management techniques, for combative patient, 2958
Vertebrae, 399, 400f
Vertebral artery
dissection of
ataxia in, 2681
headache in, 1638-1639
injury to, 448
occlusion of, spinal cord syndromes from, 420, 420f
stroke involving, 1607, 1609-1610
Vertebral body
compression fracture of, 553, 555f
tumor of, spinal cord compression in, 1919
Vertebral column. *See* Spinal column.
Vertebral osteomyelitis, 261, 265t, 2159, 2178, 2182, 2182f, 2184-2185
Vertebrobasilar arterial injuries, 448
Vertebrobasilar insufficiency, 146, 147t
Vertebrobasilar migraine, 148t
Vertical body burst fracture, 411-412, 411f-413f, 426, 427f
Vertical compression injuries of spinal cord, 411-413, 411f-414f
Vertical mattress suture, 850
Vertical shear pelvic fracture, 727, 730f
Vertigo, 142-149
alternobaric, in scuba diving–related disorders, 2286, 2287t
benign paroxysmal positional, 147t, 2683
causes of, 143b
diagnostic approach to, 143-146, 143b, 143t, 145b, 145t, 148f
differential diagnosis in, 143, 143b, 143t, 146, 147t-148t
disposition in, 146, 149
hearing loss and, 144, 2684b, 2684f
management of, 146, 149f
pathophysiology of, 142-143
pediatric, 2682-2685, 2683b, 2684b, 2684f
Very important persons (VIPs), 2978t, 2980
Vesical calculus, 1593
Vesicants, as chemical weapons, 938-939, 3031
Vesicoureteral reflux, 1574
Vesicular lesions, 1839t, 1857-1860
Vesicular stomatitis, 2054
Vestibular apparatus, 142
cold water testing of, in comatose patient, 161, 162f
Vestibular neuronitis, 147t, 2683
Vestibular system, 142-143
Vestibule, 384
Vestibule cardiopulmonary resuscitation, 89
Vestibulocochlear nerve, 1665t
Veterans Affairs, 3018-3019
Vibration stress, during air medical transport, 2995
Vibrio fish poisoning, 1470t, 1471-1472
Vibrio gastroenteritis, 2626
Vibrio parahaemolyticus
dysenteric colitis in, 229t
gastroenteritis in, 1461t, 1462t, 1465-1466
Vicryl suture, 852t
Victim identification, in physical assault, 960
Vidarabine, 2038
Video and rigid fiberoptic laryngoscopy, 21, 22f
Videoesophagram, in dysphagia, 1397
Vigabatrin, for infantile spasms, 2666
Villous adenoma, 1938
Vincent's angina, 1033, 1111-1112, 1113
Violation producing factors, as source of failures in emergency department, 3121, 3121t
Violence. *See also* Abuse; Combative patient.
differential considerations in, 2964-2965, 2965b
functional vs. organic etiology of, 2963, 2964t
in PCP intoxication, 2414, 2415-2416, 2891, 2892
intimate partner. *See* Intimate partner violence and abuse.
barriers to diagnosis of, 998
clinical features of, 996-998
definitions of, 995, 995t
disposition in, 1004-1005, 1005b
documentation of, 1000-1001, 1003-1004
during pregnancy, 997, 2734-2735, 2734t
epidemiology of, 995-996

Violence *(Continued)*
improving emergency department response to victims of, 1005-1006
legal considerations in, 1004-1005
referral in, 1004
risk assessment in, 1000, 1002b, 1003b
risk factors for injury related to, 996
screening for, 998-999, 999b, 1000f, 1001f, 1002b
use of emergency department in, 996
validation of patient's experience in, 999-1000
media, 1018
pathogenesis of, 2957
reporting requirements for, 3172
sexual. *See* Sexual abuse; Sexual assault.
suicide and, 1768
youth, 1017-1022
drug abuse and, 1018
firearms and, 1018-1019
in schools, 1017-1018
prevention strategies for, 1019-1020, 1021-1022
street gangs and, 1017-1018, 1020-1022
Viral detecting testing, for HIV, 2074
Viral infection, 2033-2058
antiviral chemotherapy for, 2035-2039, 2036t-2037t
classification of, 2033, 2034t
DNA, 2034t, 2039-2046
exanthems in, 1849
immunization for, 2033-2034, 2035t
in acute gastroenteritis, 1475-1476, 2624-2625
in arthritis, 1788
in cancer patient with impaired cell-mediated immunity, 2840
in conjunctivitis, 297t
in COPD exacerbation, 1099
in croup, 2525-2527, 2526f, 2527b, 2529t
in diarrhea, 228, 230b
in encephalitis. *See* Encephalitis, viral.
in esophagitis, 1386, 1387
in febrile cancer patient, 1908
in hepatitis, 1402-1406, 1403f, 1403t, 1405t, 1407t, 1408f
in HIV/AIDS. *See* HIV/AIDS.
in laryngotracheobronchitis, 2525-2527, 2526f, 2527b
in meningitis. *See* Meningitis, viral.
in otitis media, 1066
in pancreatitis, 1428
in pharyngitis, 274, 275t, 1109
in pneumonia, 1129, 1130, 1139, 2555, 2557-2560, 2563t
in sinusitis, 1123
pediatric hyperpyrexia in, 2506
risk of, blood transfusions and, 57t, 61
RNA, 2034t, 2046-2058
unclassified, 2058
urticaria in, 1848
Viral vaccines, 2033, 2035t
Visceral aneurysm, 1355-1356
Visceral bias, 3122
Visceral injuries, in pelvic fracture, 719
Visceral larva migrans, 2103t, 2109, 2110
Visceral pain, 209, 211
Viscosity, of hydrocarbons, 2428
Viscus, perforated, abdominal pain in, 215t
Visual acuity assessment, in red and painful eye, 285-286
Visual agnosia, in ischemic stroke, 1609
Visual Analogue Pain Scale, 2917b
Visual disturbance
in botulism, 2014
in ethylene glycol poisoning, 2399
in hyperviscosity syndrome, 1912
in methanol poisoning, 2396
in parasitic infection, 2109-2110
Visual field testing, in red and painful eye, 286
Visual loss. *See also* Blindness.
acute, 1056-1061, 1057f-1059f
chiasmal, 1060
functional, 1060-1061
in central retinal artery occlusion, 1057, 1057f
in central retinal vein occlusion, 1057, 1057f
in macular disorders, 1059, 1059f
in methanol poisoning, 2395, 2396
in multiple sclerosis, 2910
in posterior vitreous detachment, 1058
Visual loss *(Continued)*
in retinal breaks and detachments, 1057-1058
in vitreous hemorrhage, 1058-1059
neuroophthalmologic, 1059-1061
postchiasmal, 1060
prechiasmal, 1059
Visually impaired patient, 2905
Vital signs
in abdominal pain, 213
in asthma, 2534, 2535t
in back pain, 262-263
in chest pain, 187t
in comatose patient, 159, 159t
in cyanosis, 269
in dyspnea, 178t
in gastrointestinal bleeding, 222
in headache, 172t
in infants and children, 2495, 2495t, 2571, 2571t
in nausea and vomiting, 202, 202t
in newborn, 119t
in overdosed/poisoned patient, 2326
in pancreatitis, 1429
in pelvic pain, 250t
in pregnancy, 2727-2728
in seizure, 167
in syncope, 195t
in vaginal bleeding, 256t
in vertigo, 144
monitoring of
during procedural sedation and analgesia, 2943
in multiple trauma, 304
toxic syndromes and, 2964t
Vitamin A intoxication, hypercalcemia from, 1945
Vitamin B deficiency, causes of, 1874b
Vitamin B12 deficiency, megaloblastic anemia from, 1873-1875, 1874f, 1874t, 1875t
Vitamin C, for complex regional pain syndrome, 563
Vitamin D
deficiency of, hypocalcemia in, 1942
in calcium homeostasis, 1941-1942
in phosphate homeostasis, 1950
Vitamin E
for dementia, 1661
for Peyronie's disease, 534
Vitamin K, for cholestasis, 1416-1417
Vitamin K–sensitive factors, 1892, 1893f, 1894
Vitamin supplementation, during pregnancy, 2736
Vitrectomy, 1050
Vitreous
hemorrhage of, 1050, 1058-1059
posterior detachment of, 1058
Vocal cord paralysis, 2524-2525
Volar compartment of forearm, 640, 640t
Volar extrinsic ligaments of wrist, 622, 624f
Volar intercalated segment instability (VISI), 631-632, 633f
Volar surface, of hand, 576, 577f
Volar tilt, of distal radius, 626, 626f
Volatility, of hydrocarbons, 2428
Voltage, electrical injury and, 2269, 2270
Volume
depletion of. *See* Hypovolemia.
excess of. *See* Hypervolemia.
repletion of. *See* Fluid resuscitation.
Volume-cycled ventilation, 27
Volvulus
cecal, 1497-1498, 1499, 1499f
colonic, 1497-1499, 1498f, 1499b, 1499f
gastric, 1394-1395
midgut, malrotation with, 2606-2608, 2607f, 2608f
sigmoid, 1497, 1498, 1498f, 1499
small bowel, 1441
Vomiting, 200-207
after pediatric head trauma, 334
ancillary studies in, 202-203
chest pain associated with, 185, 186t
definition of, 200
differential considerations in, 201-202, 201t, 203, 204t-206t, 207f
disposition in, 207, 209
epidemiology of, 200
history in, 202
hypokalemia from, 1938
in abdominal aortic aneurysm rupture, 1333
in abdominal trauma, 493
Vomiting *(Continued)*
in *Aeromonas hydrophila* gastroenteritis, 1467
in appendicitis, 2619
in asthma, 2536
in *Bacillus anthracis* gastroenteritis, 1469
in *Bacillus cereus* food poisoning, 1471
in bacterial meningitis, 2659
in cholecystitis, 1420
in cholelithiasis, 1418
in chronic renal failure, 1542
in ciguatera fish poisoning, 1473
in *Escherichia coli* food poisoning, 1474
in esophagitis, 1387
in gastric volvulus, 1394
in gastritis, 1391
in gastroesophageal reflux, 2610
in hemorrhagic *Escherichia coli* serotype O157:H7 gastroenteritis, 1467
in hypertrophic pyloric stenosis, 2604-2605
in infants and children, 203, 206, 208t, 2605, 2606t, 2627t, 2628b
in intracerebral hemorrhage, 1610
in intussusception, 2610
in large bowel obstruction, 1496
in malrotation with midgut volvulus, 2606
in necrotizing enterocolitis, 2608
in opioid overdose, 2453
in pancreatitis, 1429
in *Plesiomonas shigelloides* gastroenteritis, 1468
in pneumonia, 2556
in pregnancy, 204t, 206, 2756
in salmonellosis, 1463
in small bowel obstruction, 1442
in staphylococcal food poisoning, 1470
in urolithiasis, 1588
in *Vibrio* fish poisoning, 1472
in *Vibrio parahaemolyticus* gastroenteritis, 1466
in viral gastroenteritis, 1476
management of, 203, 206, 207f, 208b, 208t
metabolic alkalosis from, 1930
of blood, 221
palliative care for, 3153-3154
parental instruction sheet for, 2628b
pathophysiology of, 200-201, 201f
physical examination in, 202, 202t
rapid assessment and stabilization in, 201t, 202
sequelae of, 201-202
Vomiting center, 200, 201f
Vomitus, content of, 202
Von Willebrand's disease, 1898, 1902-1903
Vulvar tears, postpartum hemorrhage from, 2818-2819
Vulvovaginal candidiasis, 1567t, 1568
Vulvovaginitis, 1567-1569, 1567t
VX, 2461, 3030-3031, 3030b, 3031b
V-Y wound closure, 851

Waiting times in emergency department, violent behavior and, 2966
Waldenstrom's macroglobulinemia, hyperviscosity syndrome in, 1912
Waldvogel classification of osteomyelitis, 2174
Wall motion abnormalities, 1179
Wallenberg's syndrome, 147t
War, role of informatics in, 3105
Warfarin
during pregnancy and lactation, 2785-2786
for acute mesenteric ischemia, 1449
for deep venous thrombosis, 1370
Warm ischemia, in peripheral vascular injury, 537
Warm-reacting antibodies, in autoimmune hemolytic anemia, 1883
Warts
genital, 1518t, 1519-1520, 1563-1564, 1564f, 2045
laryngeal, 2045
WASH regimen
for anal fissures, 1513
for hemorrhoids, 1511, 1511b
Wasp stings. *See* Hymenoptera stings.
Water balance, regulation of, 1933
Water brash, in gastroesophageal reflux, 1388
Water deficit, calculation of, 1937

Water depletion heat exhaustion, 2259
Water hemlock, 2472, 2472f
Water moccasins, 896
Water retention, in pregnancy, 2724
"Water-bottle" appearance of heart, 474, 475f
Water-hammer pulse, 1307
Waterhouse-Friderichsen syndrome, 2022
Water-soluble contrast enema
  in diverticular disease, 1494
  in large bowel obstruction, 1496-1497
Weakness, 138-141. *See also* Palsy; Paralysis.
  acute, emergent, causes of, 1689b
  definitive management of, 141
  diagnostic approach to, 138-139, 139f, 139t, 140b, 140t
  differential diagnosis in, 138, 139t, 140, 140b
  disposition in, 141
  empiric management of, 140-141, 141b
  epidemiology of, 138
  in botulism, 2014
  in rhabdomyolysis, 1979
  in toluene abuse, 2888
  neuromuscular disorders and, 139, 139t, 140b, 1702-1709
  neuropathies and, 1687-1701
  pathophysiology of, 138
  shoulder, 674
Weapon searches, in emergency department, 2966
Weapons of mass destruction, 3021-3032
  anthrax and, 3021, 3024-3026, 3025f, 3026b, 3026f
  biologic, 3023-3029, 3024b
  chemical, 937-939, 938t, 3029-3032, 3030b, 3031b
  disaster preparedness for, 3017-3018
  likely candidates for use in, 3022b
  nuclear, 2316, 3022
  plague and, 3027-3028, 3027f, 3028b
  planning and response to events involving, resources and contact for, 3022b
  radiologic, 3022-3023, 3023t
  smallpox and, 3028-3029, 3028f, 3029f
  threat of, features of, 3022b
Web Bulb Globe Thermometer index, 2257
Wedge fracture, of cervical spine, 401, 402f
Wegener's granulomatosis, 1035, 1814
Weight gain
  during pregnancy, 2724, 2736
  in hypothyroidism, 1991
Weight loss
  in hyperthyroidism, 1986
  in inflammatory bowel disease, 1501
  in intestinal amebiasis, 1480
  in pancreatic carcinoma, 1437
  products for, misidentification of plant used in, 2476
Wellens criteria, 1237, 1238t
Wellen's syndrome, 1163
Wellness strategies for emergency physician, 3176-3178, 3176b, 3177b
Wenckebach phenomenon
  in atrioventricular block, 1218-1219, 1218t, 1219b, 1220f
  in other conduction disorders, 1219
Wernicke-Korsakoff syndrome, 2869
Wernicke's aphasia, 1609
West Nile virus, 2049-2050
West syndrome, 2665-2666
Western blot assay
  for HIV, 2073-2074
  for Lyme disease, 2125
Western medicine, role expectations in, 3115-3116
Wharton's ducts, 385-386
Wharton's jelly, 2805
Wheal, 1839t
Wheezing
  in airway foreign body aspiration, 865, 866
  in asthma, 1081, 1083, 1084, 2532-2533, 2537
  in bronchiolitis, 2545
  in pediatric assessment, 2498
  in pneumonia, 2556
Whiplash, 2684-2685
Whipworm infestation, 2107
Whirlpool hydrotherapy, for frostbite, 2234
White blood cell casts, in urinary sediment, 1526, 1526f
White blood cell count
  agents and conditions that elevate, 1889b
White blood cell count *(Continued)*
  decreased, 52, 1888-1889, 1889f
  in abdominal trauma, 495
  in alcoholism, 2874
  in asthma, 1085
  in back pain, 707
  in bacterial meningitis, 2661-2662, 2661t
  in diarrhea, 233
  in hypothermia, 2243
  in osteomyelitis, 2179
  in pediatric bacteremia, 2506
  in pediatric fever, 2508-2509, 2513
  in pertussis, 2006
  in pneumonia, 1134, 2560-2561
  in pregnancy, 318
  in septic arthritis, 2189, 2705
  in transient synovitis, 2703
  increased. *See* Leukocytosis.
  normal values for, 1886t
  peritoneal lavage, 501
  rationale for selection of, 1889
White blood cell differential count
  normal values for, 1886t
  rationale for selection of, 1889
White blood cell disorders, 1886-1889. *See also specific disorder, e.g.,* Eosinophilia.
  abnormal values in, 1887
  in alcoholic hepatitis, 1409
  normal values and influences in, 1886-1887, 1886t
  physiology and pathophysiology of, 1886
White phosphorus, thermal burn from, 936
White-white tears, meniscal, 792
Whole blood
  anaphylactic-type reactions to, 1827
  transfusion of, 58
Whole-body irradiation, acute radiation syndrome after, 2317t, 2321-2322, 2321f
Whole-bowel irrigation
  in beta blocker overdose, 2374
  in cocaine body packing/stuffing, 2391
  in iron overdose, 2420
  in lithium toxicity, 2444
  in opioid overdose, 2455
  in overdosed/poisoned patient, 2330
Whooping cough, 2004-2007, 2005f, 2006b, 2559-2560
Wide-complex tachycardia, 1237-1244
  adenosine-induced, 2588, 2589f
  differential diagnosis in, 1237-1239, 1238t, 1239f, 1240f
  in cocaine overdose, 2390
  in infants and children, 2586, 2587f
  torsades de pointes as, 1243-1244, 1243f, 1244b
  treatment of, 1239-1240
  ventricular tachycardia as, 1240-1243, 1241-1243f
Wilcoxon rank sum test, 3052, 3052t, 3053
Wilcoxon signed rank test, 3053
Wild animal bite, 885
Will, living, 3133
Winterbottom's sign, in African trypanosomiasis, 2106
Wire suture, 852t
Withdrawal
  anxiety in, 1748
  from alcohol, 2860-2863
    clinical features of, 2860-2861
    differential considerations in, 2860
    disposition in, 2879
    hypertension in, 1314
    management of, 2861-2863
    pathophysiology of, 2860
    seizure in, 1623, 2863
  from barbiturates, 2482
  from benzodiazepines, 2486, 2486b
  from GHB, 2490
  from opioids, 2451-2456
    clinical features of, 2454
    diagnosis of, 2454
    differential diagnosis in, 2454
    disposition in, 2455
    management of, 2455-2456
    pathophysiology and pharmacology of, 2452
    seizure in, 2670
Withholding and withdrawing treatment, bioethical dilemmas in, 3132
Wolff-Parkinson-White syndrome, 1235-1237, 1235b, 1236f, 1237f, 2589
Wood distillates, toxicity of, 2429t
Woodruff, adverse effects of, 2476t
Wood's corkscrew maneuver, for shoulder dystocia, 2815
Wood's lamp, in sexual assault examination, 985, 985b
Word catheter, for Bartholin abscess, 1560
Word salad, in schizophrenia, 1728
Workers' compensation, 3077-3078
Work-related injuries/illness. *See* Occupational medicine.
Wormwood, adverse effects of, 2476t
Wound
  assessment of, in thermal burns, 919-920, 920f
  cleansing of, 847-848, 848t
  closure of, 849-854
    decision making in, 849
    in animal bites, 886-887, 887t
    materials in, 851-854, 852t
    suture technique in, 849-851
    wound tension considerations in, 849
  contraction of, skin tension lines and, 843, 843f, 844f
  debridement of, 847
  healing of, phases in, 842-843
  infection of
    in animal bites, 883-884, 885-886, 885t
    risk factors for, 844-845, 844b
  irrigation of, 848
  microscopic examination of, in forensic emergency medicine, 960
  radioactive contamination of, 2321
  tetanus-prone, 2008
Wound ballistics, handgun, 954-955
Wound botulism, 2013, 2014, 2015
Wound management, 842-857
  anesthesia in, 845-847
  antibiotic prophylaxis in, 854-855
  biomechanical properties of skin and, 843
  burn, 924-927, 925f
  clinical features and diagnostic strategies in, 843-845
  disposition in, 855-857, 856b, 857b
  drains, dressings, and immobilization in, 855
  foreign body assessment in, 845, 878
  history taking in, 843
  in animal bites, 886-889, 886b, 887t
  in electrical and lightning injuries, 2276
  in facial trauma, 390-391
  in fingertip amputation, 610
  in human bites, 891-892, 891t
  in rabies, 2068, 2068b
  in radiation exposure, 2323
  in snakebite, 902
  physical examination in, 845
  skin preparation in, 847
  tetanus prophylaxis in, 856-857, 857b, 2012, 2013t
Wrist
  anatomy of, 622, 623f-625f
  as link mechanism, 632f
  examination of, in arthritis, 1778
  tendinopathy of, 1799
Wrist flexion test, 639, 639f
Wrist splint, 569, 569f
Wrist trauma, 622-639
  carpal injuries in, 627-632, 628f, 630f-633f
  clinical features of, 622, 625
  distal radius and ulna injuries in, 632-639, 634f-638f
  radiography in, 625-627, 626f-628f, 628t
  soft tissue injuries in, 639, 639f
Wristdrop, 586, 588f
  humeral shaft fracture and, 655
  in radial mononeuropathy, 1695

Xanthochromia, in subarachnoid hemorrhage, 1636-1637, 1718
Xanthoma diabeticorum, 1972
Xerosis, in HIV/AIDS, 2084-2085

Yarrow, adverse effects of, 2476t
Yellow fever, 2035t, 2049-2050
Yellow jacket stings. *See* Hymenoptera stings.
Yellow-bellied sea snake envenomation, 901

Yergason's test
in bicipital tendinopathy, 1797
in bicipital tenosynovitis, 697, 697f
Yersinia enterocolitica
in dysenteric colitis, 229t
in gastroenteritis, 1461t, 1462t, 1465, 2625
Yew trees, 2475, 2475f
Yohimbine
adverse effects of, 2476t
drug interactions with, 2478t
Youth violence, 1017-1022

Zafirlukast
for asthma, 1090
for chronic asthma, 2542, 2543t
Zalcitabine, in HIV/AIDS, side effects of, 2079t
Zaleplon, overdose of, 2486-2487
Zanamivir
for influenza, 2055
indications for, 2037-2038
Zebra fish envenomation, 910
Zidovudine
for HIV/AIDS, 2087-2088
side effects of, 2079t
Zieve's syndrome, 2874
Zileuton, for chronic asthma, 2542, 2543t
Zinc supplement therapy, in infectious diarrhea, 2628
Ziprasidone
for agitation in delirious patient, 1654
Ziprasidone *(Continued)*
for mood disorders, 1741
for psychosis in demented patient, 1662
for rapid tranquilization, 2962
for thought disorders, 1731
toxicity of, 2446, 2446t
Zolendronate, for hypercalcemic cancer patient, 1016
Zollinger-Ellison syndrome, peptic ulcer disease in, 1391
Zolmitriptan, for migraine, 2680
Zolpidem
for insomnia in acute mountain sickness, 2302
overdose of, 2486
Zoonotic infection, in pneumonia, 1131
Zygomatic fracture, 394